Begin Thinking LIKE A NURSE using your PEARSON RESOURCES

Simplify your study time by using the resources included with this textbook at **http://www.nursing.pearsonhighered.com**

Further enhance your Clinical Reasoning with the additional resources below.
For more information and purchasing options visit **www.mypearsonstore.com**.

Break Through
to improving results

MyNursingApp™

Clinical references across the nursing curriculum available!

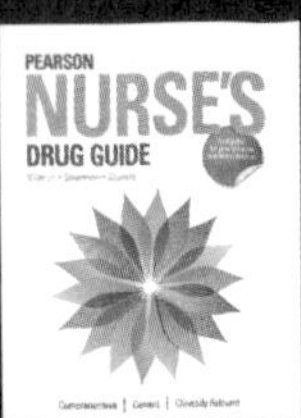

Pearson's Nurse's Drug Guide

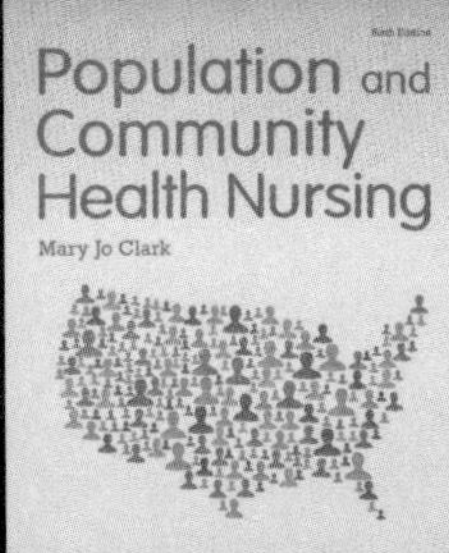

Thinking Like a Nurse in Clinical

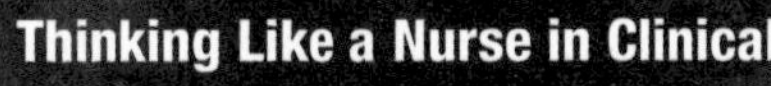

Real Nursing Skills 2.0 for the RN offers students the complete foundation for competency in performing clinical nursing skills.

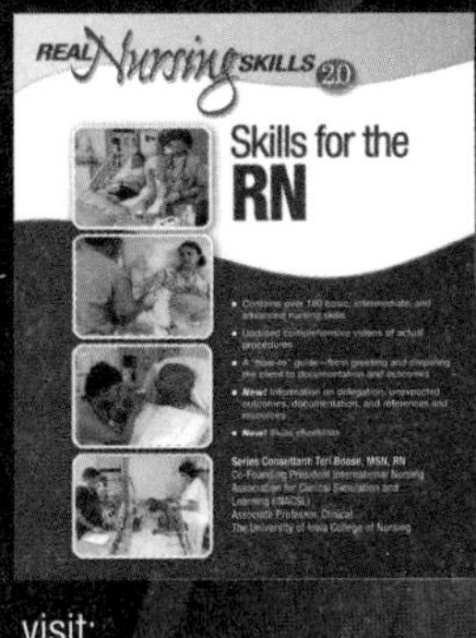

visit:
www.realnursingskills.com

Thinking Like a Nurse for NCLEX Success

MaryAnn Hogan, MSN, RN provides clear, concentrated, and current review of "need to know" information for effective classroom and NCLEX-RN® preparation.

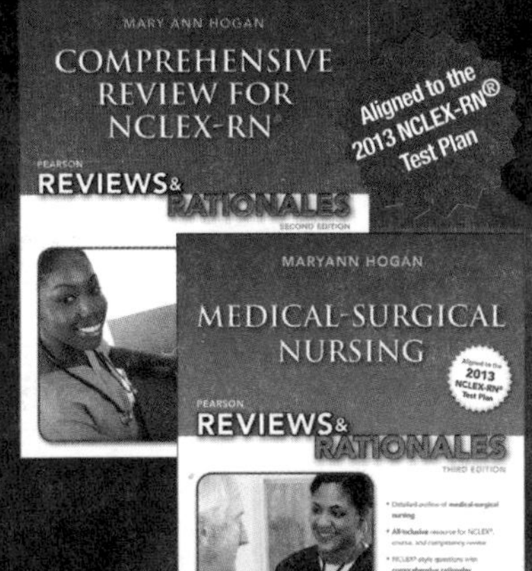

ALWAYS LEARNING

PEARSON

Publisher: Julie Alexander
Product Manager/Executive Editor: Pamela Fuller
Development Editor: Elisabeth Garofalo
Program Manager: Erin Rafferty
Editorial Assistant: Erin Sullivan
Director of Marketing: David Gesell
Senior Product Marketing Manager: Phoenix Harvey
Field Marketing Manager: Debi Doyle
Marketing Specialist: Michael Sirinides
Director, Product Management Services: Etain O'Dea
Project Management Team Lead: Cynthia Zonneveld
Project Managers: Maria Reyes, Jonathan Cheung
Manufacturing Manager: Maura Zaldivar-Garcia
Art Director: Maria Guglielmo
Cover and Interior Design: Wanda Espana
Cover Art: Getty Images by Iconeer
Full-Service Project Management: Revathi Viswanathan
Composition: Lumina Datamatics, Inc.
Printer/Binder: RR Donnelley / Willard
Cover Printer: Phoenix Color/Hagerstown

Library of Congress Cataloging-in-Publication Data
Clark, Mary Jo Dummer, author.
[Community health nursing]
Population and Community Health Nursing / Mary Jo Clark. — Sixth edition.
p. ; cm.
Preceded by: Community health nursing / Mary Jo Clark. 5th edition. 2008.
Includes bibliographical references and index.
ISBN 978-0-13-385959-1
ISBN 0-13-385959-2
I. Title.
[DNLM: 1. Community Health Nursing. 2. Nursing Process. WY 106]
RT98
610.73'43—dc23

2014024175

10 9 8 7 6 5 4 3 2 1

PEARSON

ISBN-10: 0-13-385959-2
ISBN-13: 978-0-13-385959-1

POPULATION AND COMMUNITY HEALTH NURSING

SIXTH EDITION

Mary Jo Clark

PEARSON

Boston Columbus Indianapolis New York San Francisco Hoboken Amsterdam
Cape Town Dubai London Madrid Milan Munich Paris Montreal Toronto
Delhi Mexico City São Paulo Sydney Hong Kong Seoul Singapore Taipei T

About the Author

Mary Jo Clark, PhD, RN, PHN, has been practicing and teaching population health nursing for 50 years. After completing her BSN degree at the University of San Francisco, she received her introduction to global population health nursing as a U.S. Peace Corps Volunteer in Vita, India, a rural town with a population of about 3,000. Returning to the United States, Dr. Clark employed her cross-cultural expertise as a Public Health Nurse in the Los Angeles County Department of Health Services. In 1973, she became a pediatric nurse practitioner, and later began teaching population health nursing at East Tennessee State University. She completed a master's degree as a community health clinical nurse specialist at Texas Women's University and a PhD in nursing at the University of Texas at Austin. Moving with her army nurse husband to Augusta, Georgia, she taught graduate and undergraduate population health at the Medical College of Georgia. For the past 29 years, Dr. Clark has taught at baccalaureate, master's, and doctoral levels at the University of San Diego, Hahn School of Nursing and Health Science. In addition to her full-time teaching and writing, Dr. Clark has maintained an active population health nursing practice. She is well known in the population health nursing field and has provided consultation and made presentations across the country and overseas. Her many and varied experiences in population health nursing in the United States and abroad form the core of the material presented in this book.

Dedication

This book is lovingly dedicated to Phil the elder, Phil the younger, and Heather, who are the wind beneath my wings, and to my fellow population health nurses and faculty across the country and around the globe. Little by little we are improving the health status of the world's population.

Thank You!

Reviewers

Our heartfelt thanks go to our colleagues from schools of nursing across the country and others who have given time generously to help create this exciting new edition of our text. These individuals helped us plan and shape our book and resources by reviewing chapters, art, design and more. *Population and Community Health Nursing* has reaped the benefit of your collective knowledge and experience as nurses and teachers, and we have improved the materials due to your efforts, suggestions, objections, endorsements and inspiration. Among those who gave their time to help us are the following:

Dr. Sue Bhati, PhD,FNP-BC,NP-C,MSN,RN
Northern Virginia Community College
Springfield, Virginia

Terese Blakeslee, MSN, RN, Ed
University of Wisconsin
Oshkosh, Wisconsin

Anne Watson Bongiorno, Ph.D., APHN-BC, CNE
SUNY Plattsburgh
Plattsburgh, New York

Angeline Bushy, PhD, RN, FAAN, PHC
University of Central Florida
Daytona Beach, Florida

Kim Clevenger, EdDc, MSN, RN, BC
Morehead State University
Morehead, Kentucky

Angela Cox, RN, MS
Ball State University—School of Nursing
Muncie, Indiana

Mary P. Curtis, RN, PhD, ANP-BC, PHCNS-BC
Barnes-Jewish College, Goldfarb School of Nursing
St. Louis, Missouri

Pamela Davis, MSN, RN, ANP, CPHQ
Northern Kentucky University
Highland Heights, Kentucky

Julia K. Donegan, MS, APHN-BC, RN
The Ohio State University—College of Nursing
Columbus, Ohio

Charlene Douglas, PhD, MPH, RN
George Mason University
Fairfax, Georgia

Janice Edelstein, RN, EdD
University of Wisconsin
Oshkosh, Wisconsin

Susan England, PhD, RN
Texas State University
Round Rock, Texas

Melissa Garno, EdD, RN
Georgia Southern University—School of Nursing
Statesboro, Georgia

Camille Groom, RN,MS
Miami-Dade College School of Nursing
Miami, Florida

Lisa Rae Dummer, Transgender Law Center
San Francisco, California

Tammy Haley, PhD, CRNP
University of Pittsburgh at Bradford
Bradford, Pennsylvania

Linda James, MSc, RN
Sam Houston State University
Huntsville, Texas

Nancy Jones, MSN, RN
Kent State University
Kent, Ohio

Toshua Kennedy, MSN/MPH, BSN, ADN
The University of South Carolina Upstate
Greenville, South Carolina

Nancy Laplante, PhD, RN
Neumann University
Aston, Pennsylvania

Sherry Lovan, PhD, RN
Western Kentucky University
Bowling Green, Kentucky

Paula McNiel, DNP, RN, APHN-BC
University of Wisconsin Oshkosh—College of Nursing
Oshkosh, Wisconsin

Richard Ralls, RN, BSN
Florida International University
Miami, Florida

Kate Shade, PhD, RN
Samuel Merritt University
Oakland, California

Ashley Shroyer, MSN, RN, CNE
Fairmont State University
Fairmont, West Virginia

Virginia Teel, DHSc, RN
Georgia Southern University
Statesboro, Georgia

Anne Watson Bongiorno, Ph.D., APHN-BC, CNE
SUNY Plattsburgh
Plattsburgh, New York

Kim White, PhD, MS, CNS-BC
Southern Illinois University Edwardsville—School of Nursing
Edwardsville, Illinois

Preface

This book represents the lessons learned and the progress made in more than 100 years of population health nursing in the United States. The year 1993 marked the 100th anniversary of the founding of the Henry Street Settlement, the acknowledged beginning of modern American population health nursing. Since then, the work of population health nurses and others has led to better health for individuals, families, and population groups. In this book, I have tried to distill the wisdom of early pioneers and present-day practitioners to guide and direct future generations toward nursing excellence.

Locally, nationally, and globally, society is in greater need of population health nursing services than at any time since our beginning. Although expected longevity has increased significantly in the last century, quality of life has not kept pace for a large portion of the world's population. Previously controlled communicable diseases are resurfacing, and new diseases are emerging to threaten the public's health. Malnutrition is a fact of life for many people. Chronic physical and emotional diseases are taking their toll on the lives of large numbers of people. Substance abuse and violence are rampant, and more and more frequently, environmental conditions do not support health. All of these are problems that population health nurses can and do help to solve.

Population health nurses must have the depth and breadth of knowledge that allows them to work independently and in conjunction with clients and others to improve the health of the world's populations. In part, this improvement occurs through care provided to individuals and families, but it must also occur on a larger scale through care provided to communities and population groups. *Population and Community Health Nursing*, Sixth Edition, provides population health nurses with the knowledge needed to intervene at these levels. This knowledge is theoretically and scientifically sound, yet practical and applicable to society's changing demands.

Nursing Excellence Through Advocacy

Like prior editions, this edition focuses on the central facet of population health nursing—advocating for the health of the public. The theoretical concept of advocacy is introduced in Chapter 1 and is based on qualitative research by the author that examines the process of advocacy as it is performed by population health nurses. Practical application of the concept occurs in each of the subsequent chapters.

Advocacy Then and Advocacy Now

The *Advocacy Then* and *Advocacy Now* vignettes that open each chapter showcase the efforts of population health nurses, other health professionals, and members of the lay public to advocate for the health of populations. Some of the *Advocacy Now* vignettes were contributed by population health nurses and are gratefully acknowledged. Other vignettes celebrate the past and present contributions of population health nurses and others to promoting health and addressing health needs in the United States and the world. We offer our appreciation to these contributors for their heartfelt descriptions of nursing in the population and for their generosity in permitting us to tell their stories. The *Advocacy Now* vignette that opens Chapter 2 describes the work of Susie Walking Bear Yellowtail, the first Native American registered nurse and an exemplary population health nurse advocate. The other stories, past and present, are equally inspiring for the population health nurses of today and those in the ages to come.

Population and Community Health Nursing, Sixth Edition, provides students with a strong, balanced foundation for population health nursing practice. The book is designed to help students first achieve excellence in the classroom through the many features and exercises that accompany the narrative. The additional tools and supplemental information will help students succeed at applying those concepts in clinical settings with families, communities, and population groups, with the ultimate goal of preparing nurse generalists who will exhibit nursing excellence in any setting.

The underlying intent of this book is to convey to nursing students at the beginning of the 21st century the excitement and challenge of providing nursing care to populations. As we begin a new era of population health nursing, I believe that well-educated population health nurses can provide a focal point for resolution of the global health problems presented throughout the book. Early population health nurses changed the face of society; we can be a strong force in molding the society of the future by striving for nursing excellence through advocacy.

Organization

This textbook is designed to present general principles of population health nursing and to assist students to apply those principles in practice. It is organized in five units. The first three units address general concepts and strategies of population health nursing practice, and the last two examine the application of those concepts to specific populations, settings, and population health problems.

UNIT I sets the stage for practice by describing population health nursing and the context in which it occurs. Readers are introduced to population health nursing as an area of specialized practice and to its emphasis on advocacy for the health of individuals, families, and population groups. The attributes and features that make population health nursing unique, standards for practice, and typical roles and functions of population health nurses are addressed. Then, the concept of populations as recipients of nursing care and the historical and theoretical underpinnings and development of population health nursing are presented followed by a discussion of epidemiology as a core content area for population health care.

A unique feature of this book is the consistent use of the Population Health Nursing model to structure the discussion of principles of practice. The model is introduced in Chapter 1. *Further Information* about other theoretical models that may be useful in population health nursing practice is provided in ancillary materials found at www.nursing.pearsonhighered.com. Other relevant models dealing with epidemiology, family nursing, health promotion, and so on, are included in specific chapters.

The population health nursing (PHN) model is used as the organizing framework for most of the chapters in the book, providing students with a systematic approach to determining factors that influence health and relevant strategies designed to promote health, prevent illness and injury, resolve existing health problems, and restore health in individuals, families, communities, and populations. The consistent use of the PHN model permits students to readily identify commonalities and differences among processes, populations, settings, and health problems.

UNIT II examines influences on population health and addresses environmental, cultural, economic, healthcare delivery system, and global influences on population health. Knowledge of the influence of these factors on population health leads to the application of specific strategies to improve population health addressed in **UNIT III**. Strategies addressed include political, empowerment, health promotion and health education, case management, and home visiting approaches to population health nursing as a specialized area of practice. Other aspects of population health nursing practice (e.g., community engagement, referral, delegation, social marketing, group dynamics, and leadership) are integrated into these and other chapters as appropriate.

UNIT IV addresses health care provided to special population groups. In each chapter, students are assisted to apply principles of care to individuals and families, as well as to these populations as aggregates. For example, Chapter 16 emphasizes population health nursing care for children and adolescents as population groups, as well as strategies for improving the health of individual children and adolescents. Similar approaches are taken to other population groups in the unit: families, communities, men, women, the elderly, the GLBT population, and people experiencing poverty and homelessness.

UNIT IV also addresses population health nursing in specialized settings such as the school, work, correctional, and disaster settings. For example, Chapter 22 examines the role of the population health nurse in school settings, whereas Chapter 23 addresses employee health in the work setting. In each chapter in the unit, students are guided in the use of the nursing process and application of the PHN model in the special practice setting. Consideration is given to factors influencing determinants of health in each setting, and population health nursing interventions related to health promotion, illness and injury prevention, resolution of existing health problems, and health restoration are discussed.

UNIT V focuses on population health nursing practice related to the control of common population health problems such as communicable diseases, chronic physical and mental health conditions, substance abuse, and societal violence. Again, students are assisted to apply the nursing process and the PHN model to identify factors contributing to problems in each of these areas and in designing nursing interventions at each of the four levels of health care. Consideration is given to the care of individuals and families with these problems as well as to resolving common health problems at the population level.

How to use this book to foster success in POPULATION HEALTH advocacy

The various features in the sixth edition of *Population and Community Health Nursing* provide tools to help you succeed in the classroom and in practice. They offer opportunities to apply the principles presented in the book in real and virtual practice settings, promoting your ability to be an advocate for health at multiple levels.

Learning Outcomes

Learning outcomes at the beginning of each chapter help you to focus on the outcomes expected of you in relation to your knowledge and application of principles of population health nursing. They highlight the important content for each chapter and assist you in applying the PHN model to specific circumstances and settings.

Key Terms

The list of key terms at the beginning of each chapter alerts you to significant concepts to be addressed in the chapter, concepts with which an effective population health nurse needs to be familiar. At the point of definition within the chapter, each term is set in boldface type.

Healthy People 2020: Objectives for Population Health

These boxes present relevant objectives from *Healthy People 2020* to familiarize you with these important population health goals. You also learn about the current status of objectives here and sources of further information on the objectives on the Nursing Portal for students at www.nursing.pearsonhighered.com.

Focused Assessments

These boxes present a series of questions that assist you in conducting health assessments focused on a particular client, specific population groups, or particular aspects of care. They are framed in the context of determinants of health included in the PHN model and help you to tailor your nursing assessment to the specific needs of the client population, setting, or health problem addressed in the chapter.

Global Perspectives

This feature presents an international view of population health nursing practice, examining issues that affect health throughout the world. The feature also addresses differences in population health nursing as practiced outside the United States and highlights global solutions to health problems facing mankind.

Evidence-Based Practice

These boxes discuss the evidence base (and sometimes the lack of evidence) that underlies specific aspects of population health nursing practice. They also pose questions that stimulate thinking about the development or critical review of the evidence base for practice.

Client Education

These boxes identify important content for educating clients and the public regarding particular health issues and topics, equipping you for successful clinical encounters as you begin your career.

Highlights

A feature intended to aid your review of content from the chapter; these bulleted summaries of main points or special foci appear periodically in the text.

Case Studies

Each chapter concludes with a case study designed to assist you to apply the principles addressed in the chapter to the real world of population health nursing practice. Many of the case studies foster application of the PHN model in clinical practice with individual, families, and/or population groups. Each case study is followed by questions designed to promote critical thinking in practice.

References

References contained in each chapter present an up-to-date picture of principles and concepts related to the topic presented. References provide a balanced view of population health nursing, exploring a variety of issues from several perspectives, and provide a wide range of supplemental materials, including research reports, for the interested reader.

Additional Student Resources

A variety of supplemental information and assessment tools are provided on the Nursing Portal for students at www.nursing.pearsonhighered.com. The site includes the following features:

- **Testing Your Understanding:** This feature assists you in evaluating your comprehension of concepts and principles presented in each chapter and assessing your achievement of the chapter learning outcomes. Questions are open-ended to facilitate thought and discussion.
- **Clinical Reasoning Questions:** Additional short answer questions are provided to assist readers in applying content from the chapters and to promote clinical reasoning. These questions maintain a balance between application of practice concepts to individuals/families and population groups.
- **Exam Review Questions:** Multiple-choice review questions are provided for each chapter to assist readers in evaluating their comprehension of chapter content.
- **Assessment Guidelines:** The Nursing Portal for students also contains a wide variety of assessment tools and guidelines to assess the health needs of individuals, families, and population groups in a variety of settings. Formerly included in a separate companion text, these tools and guidelines are made available to assist you with the practical aspects of assessing the health needs of various populations as well as individual clients and their families. Most of the guidelines are organized around the elements of the PHN model, making it even easier to apply the model to a variety of client populations, settings, and population health issues. Tools range from comprehensive assessment and intervention guides for care of specific population groups (e.g., children and adolescents, prisoners) or in specific settings (e.g., schools) to more specialized assessments (e.g., fall risk assessment in the elderly or client suitability for case management services). The tools and guidelines can be downloaded for immediate use in practice.
- **Cultural Considerations:** Relevant cultural considerations are provided for each chapter of the book to assist you in developing expertise in caring for a wide variety of culturally and ethnically diverse populations.
- **Further Information:** For some chapters, the Nursing Portal for students contains additional information related to chapter topics that may be of interest to readers. As noted earlier, additional information about other theoretical models for population health nursing is provided in this feature. Similarly, detailed cultural information tables are provided for a wide variety of cultural groups, including ethnic groups, healthcare professionals, and the dominant U.S. culture.
- **Resource Exchange:** This section of the Nursing Portal for students provides resources for further information on a variety of topics addressed in the book.

Instructor Resources

- **Test Bank:** An electronic test generator with questions for each chapter is available for instructors to download from the Instructor Resource Center via the Nursing Portal.
- **Instructor's Resource Manual:** This guide, available in the Instructor Resource Center, provides a wealth of helpful information for planning learning opportunities for students. Included are learning objectives that provide instructors with student goals for each chapter. Suggested classroom activities promote student participation in learning and help bring community health nursing practice to life.
- **Lecture Note PowerPoints**: PowerPoint slides for each chapter are available to instructors in the Instructor Resource Center to help convey key points to students in class and facilitate discussion.

Contents

UNIT

1

Population Health Nursing: An Overview

Chapters

1 — Population Health and Nursing

2 — Population Health Nursing: Yesterday, Today, and Tomorrow

3 — Epidemiology and Population Health Nursing

CHAPTER

1 Population Health and Nursing

Learning Outcomes

After reading this chapter, you should be able to:

1. Define population health and population health nursing.
2. Describe the *Healthy People 2020* national objectives for population health.
3. Describe advocacy as a critical function of population health nurses.
4. Summarize the standards for population health nursing practice.
5. Identify the eight domains of competency for population health nursing.
6. Describe the components of the population health nursing (PHN) model.
7. Describe a systematic process for implementing evidence-based population health nursing practice.

Key Terms

advocacy
aggregates
assessment
assurance
case finding
case manager
clinical practice guidelines
coalition building
collaboration
community
community mobilization
coordination
counseling
education
evidence-based practice
geopolitical community
health determinants
health promotion
liaison
neighborhood
policy advocate
policy development
population health
population health management
population health nursing
populations
prevention
primary prevention
referral
resolution
restoration
role model
secondary prevention
social capital
social marketing
surveillance
tertiary prevention

Advocacy Then

Florence Nightingale and Population Health

Florence Nightingale, considered the founder of modern nursing practice, was also a consummate advocate for population health. In her work in the Crimean War, she was a strong advocate for both the use of statistics to provide a population level of health and of environmental sanitation to improve the conditions of the ill and injured (Lewis, 2010). Ms. Nightingale used her influential media contacts with *The Times* of London to force the British government to support women's involvement in care of the sick and injured soldiers (Simkin, n.d.). Throughout her career, she continued to advocate for social conditions that promoted health and was influential in creating the system of district nursing that was the British version of public health nursing. She also was instrumental in workhouse reform in England (Workhouse, n.d.) and in the establishment of the Indian Sanitary Department to deal with environmental sanitation in India (Bloy, 2010). In a letter to a friend, Nightingale wrote of the need for nursing advocacy, stating "One's feelings waste themselves in words; they ought all to be distilled into actions . . . which bring results" (cited in Hallett, 2010, p. 50).

Advocacy Now

A Picture Is Worth a Thousand Words

Residents of a small community and staff members of local health and social service agencies in a small southern California community were involved in an assessment of community health status and health needs. One of the concerns voiced most often by community members were discriminatory practices by absentee landlords in which tenants, many of whom were newly arrived immigrants, were evicted if they complained about needed repairs and safety hazards. Because many of them had arrived in the United States from countries with repressive regimes, the residents were reluctant to present their concerns to the local housing authority. The local public health nurse, who was well respected in the community and knowledgeable about many housing code violations, took pictures of violations in the homes of many of her clients. Her pictures depicted stoves situated immediately next to walls without adequate ventilation, stairs in poor repair, stairs without handrails, and bars on windows that prevented escape in the event of fire. Armed with her pictures, the Community Collaborative held a town forum to which they invited members of the local housing authority. The pictures graphically reinforced the concerns voiced by community members at the meeting. As a result, the housing authority acted on a number of code violations, which encouraged community members to report other safety issues. In addition, the efforts of the Collaborative resulted in the creation of a city-funded position of housing ombudsman to assist residents in dealing with a variety of housing issues.

Emphasis on the health of populations as a focus for care arose out of growing evidence that individual-oriented health care has only limited effects on improving the health of the general public. A population health focus may occur at a variety of levels, and populations may encompass smaller or larger groups of people.

Defining Populations as a Focus for Care

Populations are groups of people, who may or may not interact with each other, but who have common health concerns and needs. According to the second edition of the American Nurses Association (ANA) *Public Health Nursing: Scope and*

Standards of Practice, a population, in the population health nursing context, refers to the residents of a specific geographic area, but the population health nurse's focus may include specific targeted groups of people with some trait or attribute in common (e.g., a minority group, employees, the elderly) or who "may be at risk for, experience, a disproportionate burden of poor health outcomes" (ANA, 2013, p. 3). Three other commonly used, similar, but different terms for these smaller subgroups are *neighborhood, community*, and *aggregate.*

A **neighborhood** is a smaller, frequently more homogeneous group than a community that involves an interface with others living nearby and some level of identification with those others. Neighborhoods are self-defined, and although they may be constrained by natural or man-made factors, they often do not have specifically demarcated boundaries. For example, a major highway may limit interactions between residents on either side, thus creating separate neighborhoods. Or a neighborhood may be defined by a common language or cultural heritage. Thus, non-Hispanic residents of a "Hispanic neighborhood" are not usually considered, nor do they consider themselves, part of the neighborhood.

A community may be composed of several neighborhoods. Some people define communities in terms of specific geographic locations or settings, but most definitions of community go beyond locale as a primary defining characteristic. In addition to location, other potential defining aspects of communities include a social system or social institutions designed to carry out specific functions; identity, commitment, or emotional connection; common norms and values; common history or interests; common symbols; social interaction; and intentional action to meet common needs. A community is described as an "interactional whole" different from the people who comprise it (ANA, 2013, p.65). For our purposes, then, a **community** is defined as a group of people who share common interests, who interact with each other, and who function collectively within a defined social structure to address common concerns. By this definition, geopolitical entities, such as the city of San Diego, a school of nursing, and a religious congregation can be considered communities. A **geopolitical community** is one characterized by geographic and jurisdictional boundaries, such as a city.

Aggregates are subpopulations within the larger population who possess some common characteristics, often related to high risk for specific health problems. School-aged children, persons with human immunodeficiency virus (HIV) infection, and the elderly are all examples of aggregates.

Population health nurses may work with any or all of these population groups—aggregates, neighborhoods, and communities—in their efforts to enhance the health status of the general public or overall population. Population health addresses the health needs of entire groups, and those health needs are affected by factors influencing individuals, families, neighborhoods and communities, as well as the society at large. Issel and Bekemeier (2010) used the *population-patient* to reflect this focus on providing care at the population level.

Defining Population Health

The health of a population goes beyond the health status of the individuals or subgroups that comprise it, but involves the collective health of the group. Several authors have noted the lack of a precise definition of population health, but note that definitions range from health outcomes affecting total populations defined by geography (e.g., a county or state) to "accountability for health outcomes in populations defined by health care delivery systems such as health plans or Accountable Care Organizations" (Stoto, 2013, p. 2). This latter perspective requires health care systems to address "upstream" factors such as health promotion and illness and injury prevention as well management of disease. Both of these perspectives embody a "population health perspective" characterized by conceptualization of the population as a unit separate from its members, incorporation of upstream factors in measures of population health, and the goal of reducing disparities within the population. Other characteristics of a population health perspective include consideration of a broad array of determinants or factors that influence health and recognition that responsibility for population health is shared by many segments of society that must work collaboratively to achieve health, because none of them can do so alone (Stoto, 2013).

Thirty years ago, the World Health Organization conceptualized population health as both a measure of the health status of a given population and "a resource for everyday life, not the object of living. Health is a positive concept, emphasizing social and personal resources as well as physical capacities." (World Health Organization, 1984, p. 1).

The Public Health Agency of Canada (2012) combined these perspectives to describe population health as "the health of a population as measured by health status indicators and as influenced by social, economic and physical environments, personal health practices, individual capacity, and coping skills, human biology, early childhood development, and health services" (para 2). The Institute of Medicine (IOM) adopted Kindig and Stoddart's (2003) definition of population health as "the health outcomes of a group of individuals, including the distribution of such outcomes within the group" (p. 380) as the working definition of population health for its *Roundtable on Population Health Improvement* (IOM, 2013). The Institute also noted the distinction between population health as the health status of residents in a geopolitical area versus the clinical health outcomes of a subpopulation served by a given health care system. Notice was also given to Jacobsen and Teutsch's (2012) recommendation that the term "total population health" be used to denote the health status of people within a geopolitical jurisdiction, but the Institute anticipated further refinement of the definition of population health in the work of the Roundtable (2013). The outcome of that work is yet to be realized.

In the interim, for purposes of this book, **population health,** as an outcome of care, can be defined as the attainment of the greatest possible biologic, psychological, and social well-being of the total population as an entity and of its individual members. Population health can also be viewed as a capability or resource that allows members of the population to pursue goals, develop skills, and grow. A population health approach to care focuses on improving the health of the population and decreasing inequities in health status among subgroups within the population. Key elements of a population health approach include the following:

- A focus on the health of the overall population
- Attention to determinants of health and their interactions
- Decision making based on scientific evidence of health status, health determinants, and the effectiveness of interventions
- "Upstream" investment in strategies that maintain and promote health and address root causes of health and illness
- Application of multiple strategies
- Collaboration across sectors and levels of society
- Mechanisms for public participation in health improvement
- Demonstrated accountability for health outcomes (Public Health Agency of Canada, 2013)

Population Health Practice

In the United States, the terms "public health" and "population health" are often used interchangeably, but have the same focus on the health of the overall population. Elements of public or population health practice include core functions and essential services.

Core Public Health Functions

In 1988, the Institute of Medicine (IOM) released a report entitled "The Future of Public Health," which identified three core functions related to public or population health. These core functions of assessment, policy development, and assurance form the foundation for population health practice and population health nursing activities (ANA, 2013). These functions were reinforced in a 2002 revision of the report. The revised report also recommended adoption of a population health approach similar to that described above to address multiple determinants of health (IOM, 2002).

In their assessment function, public health agencies are expected to identify the health needs of the population. The National Public Health Performance Standards Program (n.d.) defined **assessment** as "the systematic collection and analysis of data in order to provide a basis for decision-making" (p. 3).

The **policy development** function of public health practice involves advocacy and political action to develop local, state, and national policies conducive to population health. Policy development has been described as the process of making informed decisions about issues related to the public's health (National Public Health Performance Standards Program, n.d.). The third core function, **assurance**, reflects the responsibility of the public health care system to see that needed services are available to the population through other entities, regulatory processes, or direct provision of care (National Public Health Performance Standards Program, n.d.).

Essential Public Health Services

In 1994, the core public health functions were operationalized in 10 essential public health services delineated by the Public Health Functions Steering Committee (American Public Health Association, 2014). These services and their relationship to the core functions are presented in Table 1-1●.

The statement of the essential functions of public health agencies led in 2001 to the development of core competencies for public health professionals performing these functions. Revised in 2010, the core competencies reflect eight domains of public health practice: analytic assessment skills, knowledge of basic public health sciences (e.g., epidemiology), cultural competence, communication skills, capacity for community-level practice, financial planning and management skills, leadership and systems thinking capabilities, and policy development and program planning skills (Council on Linkages Between Academia and Public Health Practice, 2010). Based on feedback

TABLE 1-1 Core Public Health Functions and Related Essential Services

Core Function	Essential Services
Assessment	• Monitor health status to identify health problems • Diagnose and investigate health problems and hazards in the community • Evaluate the effectiveness, accessibility, and quality of personal and population-based health services
Policy Development	• Develop policies and plans that support individual and community health efforts • Enforce laws and regulations that protect health and ensure safety • Inform, educate, and empower people with respect to health issues
Assurance	• Link people to needed personal health services and assure the provision of health care when otherwise unavailable • Assure a competent public and personal health care workforce • Inform, educate, and empower people about health issues • Mobilize community partnerships to identify and solve health problems • Conduct research into innovative solutions for health problems

from the community of public professionals, the competencies are currently undergoing another revision. The revised competencies will continue to include the same eight domains and three tiers of practice (entry level practice, program management/supervisory practice, and senior management/executive level practice). The revised competencies are expected to be completed by June 2014 (Public Health Foundation, n.d., 2014a, 2014b). The development of these general competencies led, in turn, to the development of specific competencies for population health nursing practice, which are discussed later in this chapter.

Objectives for Population Health

The goals and desired outcomes for population health in the United States have been operationalized in several sets of national objectives. The *Healthy People* initiative began in 1979 with the publication of the *Healthy People: Surgeon General's Report on Health Promotion and Disease Prevention* (Office of Disease Prevention and Health Promotion [ODPHP], n.d.a). A subsequent set of more detailed national objectives was established in 1980 in the publication *Promoting Health/ Preventing Disease: Objectives for the Nation* (U.S. Department of Health and Human Services [USDHHS], 1980). Later sets of objectives were published in 1990 and 2000. See the materials provided on the student resources site for a discussion of the changes in the objectives over time.

In 2007, work commenced on a two-phase process for developing the *Healthy People 2020* objectives. Phase I involved the development of the framework and format to be used in the revision and culminated in a report from the Secretary's Advisory Committee on National Health Promotion and Disease Prevention Objectives for 2020 in October of 2008 (Advisory Committee, 2008). The committee recommended an interactive, searchable, web-based format for the document rather than the prior print format. The framework consists of a vision, mission statement, overarching goals, four foundation health measures, and a graphic model. The vision is one of a "society in which all people live long, healthy lives" (ODPHP, n.d.b), and the mission statement is as follows:

Healthy People 2020 strives to:

- Identify nationwide health improvement priorities
- Increase public awareness and understanding of the determinants of health, disease, and disability and the opportunities for progress
- Provide measurable objectives and goals that are applicable at the national, state, and local levels
- Engage multiple sectors to take actions to strengthen policies and improve practices that are driven by the best available evidence and knowledge
- Identify critical research, evaluation, and data collection needs (ODPHP, n.d.b)

The primary emphasis for *Healthy People 2020* is on achieving health equity and eliminating disparities among segments of the population by addressing the determinants that influence health. Actual delivery of health care services is a secondary emphasis (ODPHP, n.d.a; USDHHS, n.d.). **Health determinants** as defined in *Healthy People 2020* are "the range of personal, social, economic, and environmental factors that influence health status" (USDHHS, 2012a, para 3). Determinants of health addressed by *Healthy People 2020* include policy making, social factors, health services, individual behavior, and biology and genetics (USDHHS, 2012a).

The overarching goals for the *Healthy People 2020* are to:

- Attain high-quality, longer lives free of preventable disease, disability, injury, and premature death.
- Achieve health equity, eliminate disparities, and improve the health of all groups.
- Create social and physical environments that promote good health for all.
- Promote quality of life, healthy development, and healthy behaviors across all life stages (ODPHP, n.d.b).

The final element of the framework was the development of a graphic model for *Healthy People 2020*. The model is depicted in Figure 1-1●. Within the model, actions, consisting of policies, programs, and interventions, influence determinants of health to achieve the overarching goals. The feedback cycle indicated by the two-way arrow in the model relies on assessment, monitoring, evaluation, and dissemination of best practices to inform action (ODPHP, n.d.b).

Healthy People 2020, released in December 2010, incorporates nearly 600 objectives across the 42 topical areas depicted in Table 1-2●. Objectives were developed by experts from lead federal agencies and then reviewed for comment by multiple constituencies including the Federal Interagency Workgroup as well as the general and professional population. Some objectives focus on specific health conditions, whereas others address broader issues such as health disparities, access to care, dissemination of health-related information, strengthening of public health services, and addressing social determinants of health (USDHHS, n.d.). Figure 1-2● depicts the stakeholders who influenced the development of the 2020 objectives.

Generally, objectives are of two kinds: measurable and developmental. Measurable objectives include the current national baseline status of a health issue derived from existing reliable data sources, as well as the target for achievement by 2020. Developmental objectives do not have available baseline data and are targeted for the development of national data collection systems and processes. Objectives for some of the topical areas are still in development, but each topical area will include an overview of the topic, a list of related objectives to be achieved by 2020, and information on interventions and resources. The interventions and resources information will include clinical recommendations for evidence-based interventions and links to relevant consumer health information (USDHHS, n.d.).

Monitoring progress toward achieving the objectives will be the primary responsibility of a designated lead federal

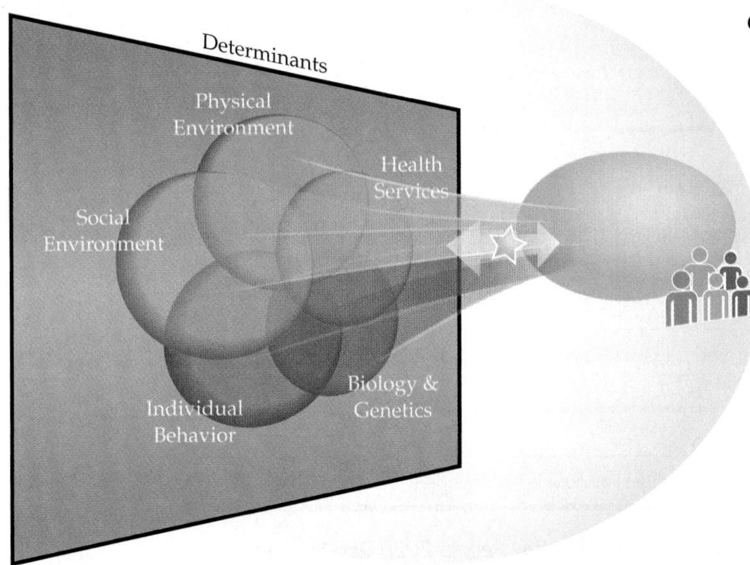

FIGURE 1-1 Model for *Healthy People 2020*

Source: Office of Disease Prevention and Health Promotion. (n.d.a). *Healthy People 2020: A resource for promoting health and preventing disease throughout the nation.* Retrieved from http://www.healthypeople.gov/2020/consortium/HealthyPeoplePresentation_2_24_11.ppt

agency for each topical area. Overall progress will be assessed in terms of four foundation health measures: general health status, health-related quality of life and well-being, determinants of health, and disparities. Specific measures included within each of the general measures are summarized in Table 1-3●. In addition, a revised set of leading health indicators, first established for *Healthy People 2010*, have been established as a focus for assessing goal attainment (USDHHS, 2012b, 2012c). The health indicators consist of 26 objectives addressing 12 topical areas that have been selected as high-priority health issues. The 26 indicator objectives are included in Table 1-4●.

You can access data related to the health indicators through the Healthy People 2020 website. For further information

TABLE 1-2 *Healthy People 2020* Topical Areas

• Access to health services • Adolescent health* • Arthritis, osteoporosis, and chronic back conditions • Blood disorders and blood safety* • Cancer • Chronic kidney disease • Dementias, including Alzheimer's disease* • Diabetes • Disability and health • Early and middle childhood* • Educational and community-based programs • Environmental health • Family planning • Food safety • Genomics*	• Global health* • Health communication and health information technology* • Health care–associated infections* • Health-related quality of life and well-being* • Hearing and other sensory or communication disorders • Heart disease and stroke • HIV • Immunization and infectious diseases • Injury and violence prevention • Lesbian, gay, bisexual, and transgender health • Maternal, infant, and child health	• Medical product safety • Mental health and mental disorders • Nutrition and weight status • Occupational safety and health • Older adults* • Oral health • Physical activity • Preparedness* • Public health infrastructure • Respiratory diseases • Sexually transmitted diseases • Sleep health* • Social determinants of health* • Substance abuse • Tobacco use • Vision

* Indicates new focus area for 2020, not included in prior sets of objectives.

Based on: U.S. Department of Health and Human Services. (2014). *About Healthy People.* Retrieved from http://www.healthypeople.gov/2020/about/default.aspx

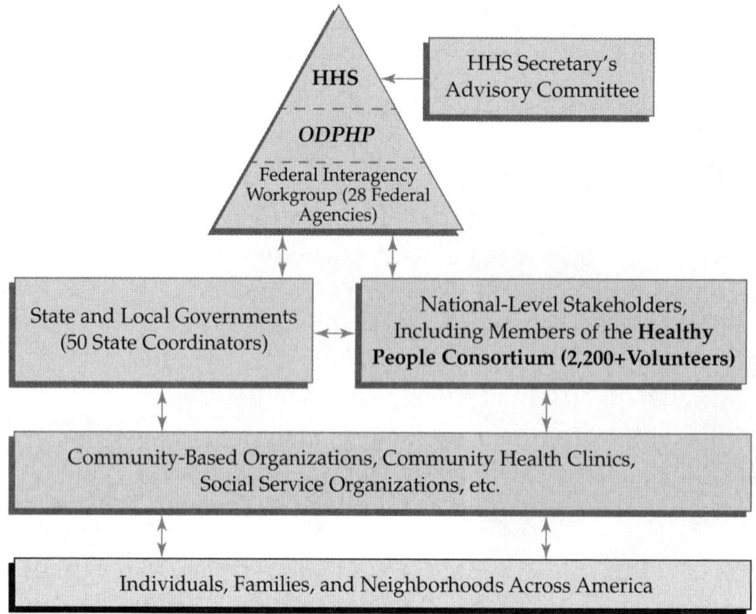

FIGURE 1-2 Stakeholders in the *Healthy People 2020* Development Process

Source: Office of Disease Prevention and Health Promotion. (n.d.a). *Healthy People 2020: A resource for promoting health and preventing disease throughout the nation.* Retrieved from http://www.healthypeople.gov/2020/consortium/HealthyPeoplePresentation_2_24_11.ppt

about the *Healthy People 2020* objectives, see the *External Resources* section of the student resources site.

Population health care is designed to improve the overall health status of the public through modification of factors that influence health either positively or negatively. National health objectives, as exemplified in *Healthy People 2020* and its precursors, guide the design of care delivery systems and serve as a means for evaluating the effectiveness of population health care.

TABLE 1-3 Foundation Health Measures for *Healthy People 2020* and Related Specific Measures

Foundation Measure	Specific Measures
General health status	• Life expectancy • Healthy life expectancy • Years of potential life lost • Physically and mentally unhealthy days • Self-assessed health status • Limitation of activity • Chronic disease prevalence
Health-related quality of life and well-being	• Physical, mental, and social health-related quality of life • Well-being/satisfaction • Participation in common activities
Determinants of health	• A range of personal, social, and environmental factors including biology, genetics, individual behavior, access to health services, and environment
Disparities	Differences in health status based on: • Race/ethnicity • Gender • Physical and mental ability • Geography

Based on: U.S. Department of Health and Human Services. (2014). *About Healthy People.* Retrieved from http://www.healthypeople.gov/2020/about/default.aspx

TABLE 1-4 Leading Health Indicators for *Healthy People 2020*

Topical Area	Leading Health Indicator Objectives	Target
Access to health services	**AHS 1.1** Increase the proportion of persons with medical insurance.	100%
	AHS 3 Increase the proportion of persons with a usual primary care provider.	83.9%
Clinical preventive services	**C-16** Increase the proportion of adults who receive a colorectal cancer screening based on the most recent guidelines.	70.5%
	HDS-12 Increase the proportion of adults with hypertension whose blood pressure is under control.	61.2%
	D-5.1 Reduce the proportion of the diabetic population with an A1c value greater than 9%.	14.6%
	IID-8 Increase the proportion of children aged 19 to 35 months who receive the recommended doses of DTaP, polio, MMR, Hib, hepatitis B, varicella, and PCV vaccines.	80%
Environmental quality	**EH-1** Reduce the number of days the Air Quality Index (AQI) exceeds 100.	10 days
	TU-11.1 Reduce tobacco use by adults.	12%
Injury and violence	**IVP-1.1** Reduce fatal injuries.	53.3/100,000 pop
	IVP-29 Reduce homicides.	5.5/100,000 pop
Maternal, infant, and child health	**MICH-1.3** Reduce infant deaths (within 1 year).	6/1,000 live births
	MICH-9.1 Reduce preterm births.	11.4%
Mental health	**MHMD-1** Reduce the suicide rate.	10.2/100,000
	MHMD-4.1 Reduce the proportion of adolescents who experience major depressive episodes.	7.4%
Nutrition, physical activity, and obesity	**PA-2.4** Increase the proportion of adults who meet the objectives for aerobic physical activity and for muscle-strengthening activity.	20.1%
	NWS-9 Reduce the proportion of adults who are obese.	30.6%
	NWS-10.4 Reduce the proportion of children and adolescents aged 2 to 19 years who are obese.	14.6%
	NWS-15.1 Increase the contribution of total vegetables to the diets of the population aged 2 years and older.	1.1 cup equivalents per 1,000 calories
Oral health	**OH-7** Increase the proportion of children, adolescents, and adults who used the oral health care system in the past 12 months.	49%
Reproductive and sexual health	**FP-7.1** Increase the proportion of sexually active females aged 15 to 44 years who received reproductive health services in the past 12 months.	86.7%
	HIV-13 Increase the proportion of persons living with HIV who know their serostatus.	90%
Social determinants	**AH-5.1** Increase the proportion of students who graduate with a regular diploma 4 years after starting 9th grade.	82.4%
Substance abuse	**SA-13.1** Reduce the proportion of adolescents reporting use of alcohol or any illicit drugs during the past 30 days.	16.5%
	SA-14.3 Reduce the proportion of persons engaging in binge drinking during the past 30 days—Adults aged 18 years and older.	24.3%
Tobacco	**TU-1.1** Reduce cigarette smoking by adults.	12%
	TU-2.2 Reduce cigarette smoking by adolescents.	16%

Based on: U.S. Department of Health and Human Services. (2013). *2020 LHI topics.* Retrieved from http://www.healthypeople.gov/2020/LHI/2020indicators.aspx

Nursing and Population Health: Labeling the Specialty

As noted in the description of historical advocacy by Florence Nightingale at the beginning of this chapter, nursing has long had a focus on the health of population groups. The specialty area that has had this primary focus has been variously known as public health nursing, community health nursing, population-based nursing, community-based nursing, community-focused nursing, community-driven nursing, and community-focused health care. Each of these terms, however, has slightly different connotations and may give rise to misconceptions.

The original term for the specialty, *public health nursing*, was coined by its U.S. founder Lillian Wald (Fee & Bu, 2010). At the time, Wald used the term to describe a nursing focus on the myriad ills of populations, particularly poor immigrants. These first nurses in the specialty were not associated with any official government agency, but functioned independently, often relying on charitable donations to fund their services. Subsequently, however, the term was most often used to describe nurses working for official local, state, or national public health departments or agencies. Current critics of the term *public health nursing* note that it implies the clientele of these official public health agencies, who are often the underserved sick poor, as the primary recipients of care. In fact, however, the specialty addresses the needs of whole populations, including those who are well and affluent as well as those who are poor and sick.

Community health nursing, as a name for the specialty, also has the potential for inappropriate connotations. The term *community health nursing* was coined by the American Nurses Association (ANA) as a general term for all nurses who worked outside of institutional settings such as hospitals. Work outside of an institutional setting, however, may not be focused on the health of the population. These nurses might be more appropriately described as engaged in "community-based" nursing (Levin, Swider, Breakwell, Cowell, & Reising, 2013). "Community-focused" care involves "consideration of health across a whole population; working with communities and other agencies to plan interventions based on local need, valid evidence, and national health priorities" (Poulton, 2009, p. 74).

"Community-driven" care focuses on the needs of the community as a whole and emphasizes community participation in determining those needs. This terminology, however, has the potential for limiting the focus of practice to those health needs identified by members of the community or population group. Although community involvement in the identification and resolution of health needs and issues is important, it is also true that part of community health nursing practice is raising community consciousness levels to the point where community members recognize the existence of health needs they may have previously ignored. Similarly, "community-oriented" care can be somewhat limiting, focusing program development on small aggregates while potentially ignoring health issues that affect larger population groups.

The Public Health Nursing Section of the American Public Health Association (APHA) has traditionally labeled the specialty as "public health nursing." According to the section, public health nursing incorporates nursing, public health, and social science concepts to foster the health of population groups (APHA, Public Health Nursing Section, 2013).

The American Nurses Association (1986) used the term *community health nurse*, in the introduction to *Standards of Community Health Nursing Practice*. The 1999 definition by the Quad Council of Public Health Nursing Organizations (Quad Council) reinstated the term *public health nursing*, and the current *Public Health Nursing: Scope and Standards of Practice* defined the specialty as nursing practice "focused on population health through continuous surveillance and assessment of the multiple determinants of health with the intent to promote health and wellness; prevent disease, disability, and premature death; and improve neighborhood quality of life" (ANA, 2013).

Despite the disagreement regarding labels and definitions, there is basic agreement that the defining characteristic of the specialty is population-focused nursing care directed toward the overall health of communities or population groups. For this reason, in this book, we will use the term *population health nursing* to describe the specialty. **Population health nursing** is a synthesis of nursing knowledge and practice and the science and practice of public health to affect determinants that influence the health of population groups.

Population Health Nursing as Advocacy

Improving the overall health of populations requires advocacy, usually at multiple levels. As noted in one article related to population health practice, action to modify determinants of health at the societal level is not for the faint of heart. Public health proponents, including population health nurses, must be actively involved in advocacy within and outside the health care delivery system to create conditions that promote health and prevent illness and injury as well as provide access to care for existing conditions (Baum, Bégin, Houweling, & Taylor, 2009).

Defining Advocacy

Dictionary definitions of advocacy involve adoption of a cause or pleading in favor of a cause (Advocacy, n.d.a, n.d.b). Wikipedia distinguishes *health* advocacy as a specific form of advocacy and notes that health advocacy "encompasses direct service to the individual or family as well as activities that promote health and access to health care in communities and the larger public. Advocates support and promote the rights of the patient in the health care arena, help build capacity to improve community health and enhance policy initiatives focused on available, safe and quality care" (Health Advocacy, 2014).

In nursing, advocacy was originally defined by the American Nurses Association in its 1976 *Code for Nurses with Interpretive Statements* as protecting clients from "incompetent, unethical, or illegal practice of any person" (p. 8). The *Public Health Nursing Scope and Standards of Practice* (ANA, 2013) defined advocacy as "the act of pleading or arguing in favor of a cause, idea, or policy on someone else's behalf, with a focus on developing the community, system, individual, or family's capacity to plead their own cause or act on their own behalf" (p. 65). Nursing authors have noted that social advocacy is a legal and moral imperative, particularly for population health nurses who need to return to their commitment to caring for the most vulnerable. **Advocacy** can be defined from a population health nursing perspective, as action taken on behalf of, or in concert with individuals, families, or populations to create or support an environment that promotes health.

Advocacy by Population Health Nurses

Advocacy in the acute care setting has been described as focusing on informing and educating patients, protecting patients, and promoting access to care (Young, 2009). These latter activities, however, primarily support the interests and welfare of individual clients. For population health nurses, on the other hand, advocacy for the health of populations, as well as individuals and families, has historically been a large part of their practice. As we will see in Chapter 2∞, community or public health nursing was synonymous with political activism and population advocacy for early nurse leaders such as Florence Nightingale, Clara Barton, Lillian Wald, Lavinia Dock, and Margaret Sanger. Florence Nightingale was a consumate advocate for human rights and population health, although she never used the term advocacy (Selanders & Crane, 2012). Margaret Sanger, an early advocate of contraceptive rights for women, highlighted the need for continuing advocacy by population health nurses: "Though many disputed barricades have been leaped, you can never sit back smugly content, believing that victory is forever yours; there is always the threat of its being snatched from you" (quoted in Drevdahl, Kneipp, Canales, & Dorcy, 2001, p. 28).

Advocacy for social justice is an essential aspect of the core mission of population health nursing, yet the last century has witnessed a decline in the social activist efforts of these nurses. In part, this decline has been attributed to a shift in control of population health nursing practice. In the early days of public health nursing, the practice of population health nurses was outside the control of the medical profession. After World War II, medicine began to dominate public health, and population health nurses were less autonomous (Drevdahl et al., 2001). Another contributing factor, as we will see later, was the shift from a focus on health promotion and illness prevention to provision of direct care to individuals and families (Barnum, 2011). Recently, however, population health nurses have begun to reclaim their population advocacy function, while still maintaining advocacy activities for individual clients and families.

The Advocacy Process

How does one engage in advocacy, particularly at the population level? There is a great deal in the literature about the need for advocacy and its importance as an element of nursing practice. There is very little discussion, however, of how advocacy occurs. Two qualitative research studies provide some information on the process involved in advocacy. One study examined advocacy events in general and the other focused primarily on advocacy in a population health nursing context (Clark, 2001, 2008).

In the studies, advocacy arose out of a precipitating situation that resulted in vulnerability. Vulnerability may be experienced by clients at any level—individual, family, community, or population. Carel (2009) noted that at the individual level, vulnerability stems from a loss of ability to do something for oneself that one is accustomed to doing without assistance from others. This may be the result of actual physical inability or because one is prohibited from doing something by the rules of the setting (e.g., getting up without assistance). At the population level, vulnerability may stem from a variety of physical and social conditions that prohibit group members from taking action for themselves. Situations that contribute to vulnerability may relate to health status (e.g., mentally retarded individuals or persons with HIV/AIDS), behavior (e.g., substance abuse), culture, social status (e.g., unemployment or poverty), environment, or other social factors that lessen people's abilities to promote and protect their health. Vulnerability is reflected in a loss of control over factors that impinge on health and that result in some kind of unmet need. Vulnerability prevents the person or group affected from acting on their own behalf and requires the efforts of an outside agent (the population health nurse) to act for or support action by the vulnerable person or group.

The advocacy situations described in the studies involved three essential categories of participants: a recipient of the advocacy, an advocate, and an "adversary." The recipient of advocacy was the vulnerable individual, family, or population group who could not act for themselves for a variety of reasons (e.g., fear, lack of knowledge, poverty). The advocate was the person or persons who acted for or enabled action by the recipient. Not all of the advocates in the situations reviewed were nurses. Family, friends, and other health care providers also functioned as advocates in some situations.

Adversaries were persons, institutions, or societal systems that impeded action to address unmet needs. Individual clients may need advocacy with family members or health care professionals to meet their needs. For example, a nurse may have to intervene with overly protective parents who are not allowing a handicapped child to achieve his or her full potential. Similarly, advocacy may be needed with a physician who ignores a client's request for information about treatment options for breast cancer. A health department that charges fees for immunizations may be a health system adversary prohibiting access to preventive care for indigent segments of the population. Similarly, legislation prohibiting access to care for undocumented immigrants is a societal adversary impeding health promotion for this population.

An additional participant, an "intermediary," was also present in many advocacy situations. Intermediaries were of two types: adversarial or supportive. Adversarial intermediaries interpreted and supported the adversary's position. For example, a nurse case manager may merely inform clients that their health insurance does not support a specific intervention rather than searching for a way to provide the desired intervention or discover an acceptable alternative. Unfortunately, adversarial intermediaries were often other nurses (Clark, 2001). Supportive intermediaries, on the other hand, supported the efforts of the advocate to meet client needs. A legislator interested in changing eviction practices to protect vulnerable groups, such as non-English-speaking residents, would be an example of a supportive intermediary.

The research identified three major factors influencing participants in an advocacy situation: knowledge, conviction, and emotion. *Knowledge* influenced all of the participants. For example, knowledge of current eviction regulations (or lack thereof) may lead unscrupulous landlords to evict tenants for complaints about unsafe housing conditions; conversely, lack of knowledge of appropriate channels to report housing violations may make tenants more vulnerable to coercion. Knowledge also influences the actions of the advocate when he or she knows what is allowable under the law.

Conviction was a factor that primarily influenced the advocates in the study situations. Advocates frequently voiced their conviction that their action was warranted. Often this conviction was upheld in the face of knowledge about possible consequences and even in the event of negative consequences for the advocate. Advocates repeatedly spoke of knowing they were doing "the right thing."

Emotion also played a role in advocacy situations. Emotions such as fear and anxiety may contribute to the vulnerability of the advocacy recipient. For example, fear of eviction may prevent tenants from filing complaints about unsafe housing conditions. The effect of both conviction and emotion can be seen in recent debates regarding gay marriage and granting spousal rights (e.g., to insurance coverage) to members of same-sex marriages.

In each advocacy situation, effective advocacy required action on the part of the advocate. The type of action taken depended on the situation as well as on the personality of the advocate. Some actions were collaborative, with the advocate attempting to work cooperatively with the adversary to meet clients' needs. Other actions were more adversarial in nature. Types of actions taken by advocates included adjusting (e.g., changing a therapeutic regimen or adjusting clinic hours to accommodate clients' schedules), connecting or "hooking up" clients with outside resources, supporting clients' decisions, helping (e.g., helping a sexually active adolescent to obtain contraceptives), and assuring (e.g., promoting access to care, assuring informed consent). Other approaches to advocacy included educating the advocacy recipient or adversary, confronting the adversary, requesting a change, showing (e.g., providing legislators with photographs of housing violations to promote effective legislation), explaining (e.g., explaining the effects of unprotected intercourse to sexually active adolescents), and enlisting the help of others (e.g., forming coalitions to promote legislation to enhance access to care for underserved segments of the population).

The last element of the advocacy process was its consequences. Advocacy had consequences for multiple participants in the advocacy situations. Generally the consequences were positive ones, but that was not always the case. Advocacy always entails an element of risk and may never be completely politically safe. Some authors see exposure to client vulnerabilities and the stress involved in addressing them as contributing to vulnerability of the part of the nurse advocate (Carel, 2009).

Population Health Nursing Functions in the Advocacy Role

As an advocate, the population health nurse engages in a number of activities or functions. The first function is determining the need for advocacy and factors that prevent clients from acting on their own behalf. A second function involves determining the point at which advocacy will be most effective. For example, should the nurse raise concerns of safety violations in rental housing with the landlord, with the housing authority, or with the media? Answers to such questions might be derived from knowledge of what has been tried previously and the effects of prior action. Related questions involve how the case should be presented. Should one, for example, ask for a meeting with interested parties, or stage a demonstration?

Collecting facts related to the problem is another advocacy-related function. An advocate is considerably less effective when he or she does not have all the facts about a situation. A population health nurse advocate should get a detailed chronological account of events related to the problem for which advocacy is needed. The nurse should also try to validate or verify the information obtained to support the claim that a problem exists and action is needed.

The fourth task in advocacy is presenting the case to the appropriate decision makers. This function requires tact and interpersonal skill. Threatening or confrontational behavior should be avoided whenever possible, as both can set up an adversarial relationship rather than a collaborative one, which may be detrimental to the cause. When other avenues fail, threats may have to be employed, but nurse and client population must be committed to acting on them. For example, if the nurse threatens to report a landlord for safety code violations

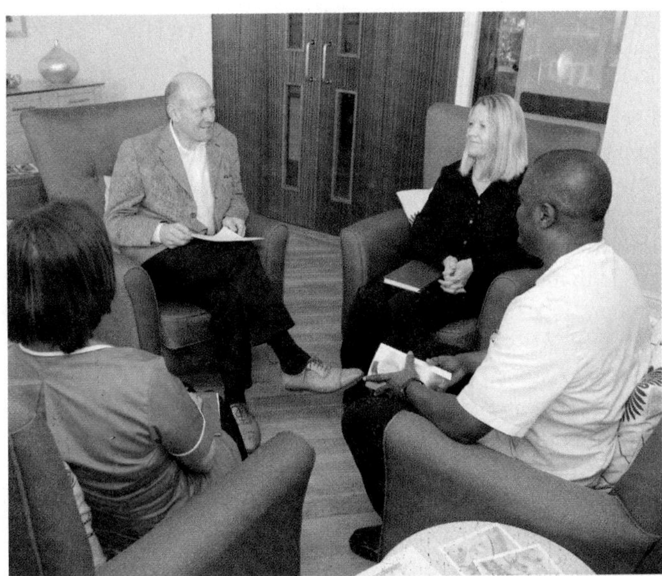

Population health nurses collaborate with people from widely varied segments of the population. *(MindStudio/Pearson Education. Inc)*

unless action is taken to remove hazards, he or she should actually be prepared to make the report.

The final function of the nurse as an advocate is to prepare clients to speak for themselves. The activities and functions of advocacy should not be carried out by the nurse alone, but should be a collaborative effort between nurse and client population. In this way, clients learn how to develop and present a forceful argument for their own needs and may, in the future, be able to act without nursing intervention.

Population health nurses must speak for those who cannot speak for themselves and articulate their needs to those in power. Nurses must also assist members of the population to learn how to speak for themselves rather than remain dependent on the nurse. Advocacy is a twofold obligation to take the part of others and, in time, to prepare them to stand alone.

A final comment is necessary with respect to advocacy. Because advocacy promotes clients' right to self-determination, population health nurses must be prepared to support clients' decisions even when they run counter to health interests. For instance, the nurse may need to accept a community's decision not to act on an issue that the nurse believes to be important in favor of focusing on other issues of greater community concern.

Population Health Nursing Standards and Competencies

One of the hallmarks of a profession is the establishment of standards of practice. Nursing, like other health-related professions, has set up standards for nursing practice and nursing service. The standards for nursing practice are further delineated in standards established for each of several specialty areas in nursing. Among these, and of particular interest to population health nurses, is the American Nurses Association's *Public Health Nursing: Scope and Standards of Practice* (2013) which addresses 16 standards for population-focused nursing care.

The standards of care for population health nursing practice have been developed within the framework of the nursing process and the core functions of public health. They relate to the areas of assessment, population diagnosis and priority setting, outcomes identification, planning, implementation, and evaluation. Additional standards address expected levels of professional performance and deal with ethics, education, evidence-based practice and research, quality of practice, communication, leadership, collaboration, professional practice evaluation, resource utilization, environmental health, and advocacy. The first standard addresses assessment. Under this standard, the population health nurse collects data needed to assess the health status of the population and to identify factors contributing to health and illness in the population. Under Standard 2, the nurse analyzes health assessment data to derive population health diagnoses which are then prioritized to promote effective action. Standard 3 addresses determination of expected outcomes of population-based care for the diagnoses and priorities identified. Standard 4 focuses on planning to address population health diagnoses; planning is based on best practices derived from available evidence (ANA, 2013).

Under Standard 5, the population health nurse implements the plan of care, partnering with others as appropriate. Competencies related to this standard include the abilities to coordinate efforts, promote health and prevent illness, and engage in health teaching. Skill in consultation, prescriptive authority, and identification, interpretation, and implementation of health-related laws, regulations, and policies are also addressed in this standard. Standard 6 focuses on evaluating the health status of the population and the effectiveness of population-based interventions (ANA, 2013).

Standards 7 through 17 address standards of professional performance in the public health nursing role. Under Standard 7, the population health nurse promotes ethical practice, whereas under Standard 8, he or she attains knowledge and maintains competency in nursing and public health practice. Standard 9 addresses the nurse's responsibility to integrate evidence and research into practice. Standard 10 requires the nurse to promote the quality of practice in the specialty (ANA, 2013).

The focus of Standard 11 is on effective communication with a variety of audiences including the public, policy makers, and interprofessional colleagues, whereas Standard 12 addresses the requirements for leadership in the practice setting and the profession. Standard 13 focuses on the nurse's ability to collaborate with others in addressing the health needs of the population, and Standard 14 addresses the nurse's ability to evaluate his or her own practice in light of professional standards and guidelines, laws, rules, and regulations (ANA, 2013).

Standard 15 focuses on the population health nurse's responsibility to use resources wisely and to consider factors related to safety, effectiveness, and cost in planning systems of care. Standard 16 addresses the expectation that the population health nurse will promote environments that are conducive to health and will support environmental justice for all segments of the population. Finally, under Standard 17, the population health nurse functions as an advocate to protect the health, safety, and rights of members of the population (ANA, 2013).

As noted earlier, the Council on Linkages between Academia and Public Health Practice (COL) (2010) has developed a set of competencies reflecting the skills, knowledge, and attitudes required for effective public or population health practice. In 2003, the Quad Council developed a set of related competencies for public/population health nursing at two levels of practice, the staff nurse/generalist and the manager/specialist/consultant. The Quad Council initially examined the applicability of the COL competencies specifically to public health nursing practice and developed performance expectations related to each competency for two levels of practice, generalist and specialist. The generalist competencies were intended to reflect baccalaureate-level educational preparation, and the specialist competencies reflected master's-level preparation (Swider, Krothe, Reyes, & Cravetz, 2013).

The nursing competencies incorporate expectations for care of individuals and families within an overall context of population-focused practice, a unique feature compared to the COL competencies that deal only with population-focused practice (Quad Council of Public Health Nursing Organizations, 2011). The competencies address eight domains of practice: (a) analytic and assessment skills, (b) policy development and program planning, (c) communication, (d) cultural competence, (e) community dimensions of practice, (f) public health science, (g) financial planning and management, and (h) leadership and systems thinking. The competencies were intended to reflect the practice of experienced population health nurses at both generalist and specialist levels, not novices, and expectations ranged from awareness through knowledge to proficiency on any given item. In 2011, the Quad Council undertook a revision of the competencies to address three tiers of practice. Tier 1 competencies are skills to be possessed by public health nurses who engaged in day-to-day care in official state and local public health agencies. Tier 2 competencies address the practice of program managers or supervisors. Tier 3 competencies are intended for public health nurses in senior management and leadership positions with responsibility for major programs and strategy development (Quad Council of Public Health Nursing Organizations, 2011). Any particular population health nursing position may incorporate components from some or all domains. For further information about the competencies, see the *External Resources* section of the student resources site.

Population Health Nursing Education

Because of the autonomy and breadth of knowledge required in population health nursing at the generalist level, the minimum level of educational preparation should be a baccalaureate degree. Even in the early days of district nursing in England, Florence Lee, a former student of Nightingale's, proposed that district nurses be educated beyond the basic nursing preparation. In the United States, the first postgraduate course in public health nursing was offered by the Instructive District Nursing Association of Boston in 1906 (Howse, 2009).

As noted above, specialist level population health nursing competencies were predicated on master's level educational preparation, and many nurses in the specialty were prepared in master's programs as community health clinical nurse specialists. More recently, however, the nursing professional has established the Doctor of Nursing Practice (DNP) degree. Based on the *Essentials for Doctoral Education for Advanced Nursing Practice* (American Association of Colleges of Nursing [AACN], 2006), the guiding document for DNP programs, the DNP may have one of two foci, advanced practice directed toward individuals (e.g., nurse practitioners, nurse midwives, etc.) or population or aggregate-focused practice. AACN data for 2009 indicated that 14% of the existing DNP programs had a population or public health option. A survey of leaders in community/public health settings indicated that the competencies included in the *Essentials* document would be appropriate for population health nursing, but that their organizations did not have positions designated for DNPs (Swider et al., 2009). It remains to be seen whether or not DNP level education will be required for specialist level population health nursing in the future.

The current shortage of nurses prepared for population health nursing practice has led many public health agencies to hire nurses prepared at the Associate Degree level despite the fact that Associate Degree program curricula do not include content on population-level nursing. Issel and Bekemeier (2010) cautioned that employment of unprepared nurses may jeopardize the safety of whole populations and advance the concept of population-patient safety comparable to safety concerns in acute care settings.

A Population Health Nursing Model

Effective nursing practice is facilitated when nurses use a systematic approach to clients, their health status, and the nursing interventions needed to promote, maintain, or restore health. Conceptual or theoretical models provide such an approach. A conceptual model is usually "a diagram that defines theoretical entities, objects, or conditions of a system and the relationships between them" (Conceptual model, n.d.). In nursing, conceptual models describe the relationships between health care needs and nursing interventions to meet those needs. Conceptual models can assist population health nurses to evaluate health status and to plan, implement, and evaluate effective nursing care to improve the health of populations. The model directs attention to relevant aspects of a client situation and to interventions that are apt to be most effective in that situation. The Population Health Nursing (PHN) model used in this text has been developed specifically for use in population health nursing and consists of three components: determinants of population health, population health nursing interventions, and levels of health care. The model is depicted in Figure 1-3●.

Determinants of Population Health

Determinants of health are factors that determine whether people are healthy or unhealthy. The World Health Organization (WHO, 2014) has categorized determinants of health as reflecting social and economic environments, the physical environment, and personal characteristics and behaviors. The Canadian government has identified a number of determinants of health to include biology and genetics, physical environment, early childhood development, education, employment and working conditions, culture, gender, housing, the social environment, personal health practices, income and social status, social support networks, and the health care system (Senate Subcommittee on Population and Health, 2009). As indicated in Figure 1-1, *Healthy People 2020* has conceptualized determinants of health as arising from human biology and genetics, individual behavior, social and physical environments, and health service systems.

Emphasis on broad determinants of health and illness marks a change from individually focused explanations of disease to a focus on social and environmental contributions to health and illness. A focus on broad determinants of health acknowledges that individual behaviors are shaped by interaction with the environment (WHO, 2014) and that contextual variables found in the environment probably interact in complex ways with individual variables to determine health and illness. In the PHN model, the determinants that influence health have been grouped into six categories of determinants: biological, psychological, environmental, sociocultural, behavioral, and health system determinants. Factors in each of the six categories influence the health of individuals as well as the overall health status of a population.

BIOLOGICAL DETERMINANTS. Biological determinants of health are factors related to human biology that influence health and illness. These factors may be related to age and developmental level, genetic inheritance, and physiologic function. Age can affect one's susceptibility to illness or the potential for exposure to other risk factors. Genetic inheritance encompasses gender and racial/ethnic characteristics as well as

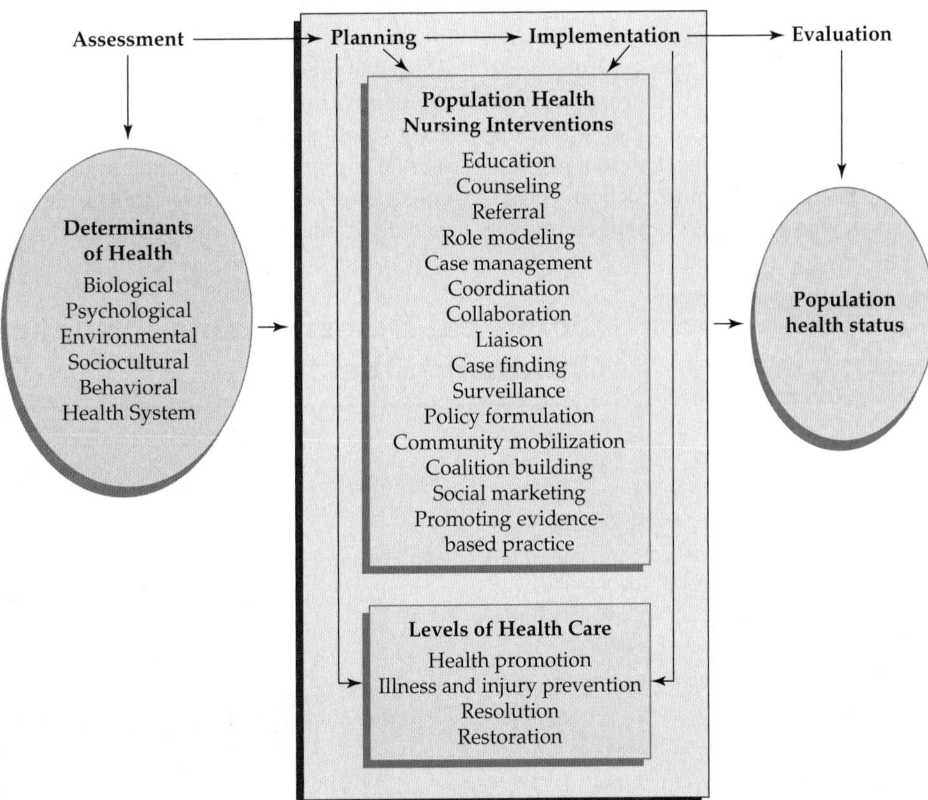

FIGURE 1-3 Elements of the Population Health Nursing Model

the specific gene pattern transferred by one's parents. Certain health problems (e.g., hemophilia and sickle cell disease) are more frequently associated with some gender or racial/ethnic groups than with others. The presence of certain genetically transmitted traits also increases one's risk of developing some health problems, such as heart disease and some forms of cancer. Concern for genetic influences on health is evident in the increased focus on genetics and genomics in baccalaureate nursing education (AACN, 2008).

Factors related to physiologic function include one's basic state of health as it affects the probability of developing other health problems. Considerations in this area would include the presence or absence of other disease states. For example, obesity is a physiologic factor that contributes to a variety of health problems, including heart disease, diabetes, and stroke. Immunity, discussed in more detail in Chapter 26∞, is another aspect of physiologic function that affects susceptibility to disease.

When assessing populations, rather than individuals, the age, gender, and racial/ethnic composition of the groups would be determined. Other information related to biological determinants include the prevalence of genetic traits for specific health conditions, the prevalence of specific physiologic conditions in the population (e.g., pregnancy, diabetes), and population levels of immunity. The *Focused Assessment* below includes questions that address biological determinants related to the population-level problem of increased incidence and prevalence of childhood obesity.

PSYCHOLOGICAL DETERMINANTS. Psychological determinants of health include both internal and external psychological environments. Depression and low self-esteem are two factors in one's internal psychological environment that contribute to a variety of health problems, including suicide, substance abuse, family violence, and obesity. External psychological factors can also influence the development of health problems. For example, a person who has a great deal of emotional support in a crisis is less likely to attempt suicide than a person who faces a crisis without such support. Stress is another factor in the external psychological environment that is associated with a variety of health problems. The ability to cope with stress, on the other hand, is a factor in one's internal psychological environment.

Psychological determinants at the population level would include the incidence and prevalence of psychiatric disorders, the amount of stress experienced by members of the population, and the coping abilities of the population as a whole. For example, some populations or communities are better able to cope with increased numbers of homeless individuals or with increasing unemployment than others. Questions to guide assessment of psychological determinants contributing to childhood obesity in the population are presented in the *Focused Assessment* on the next page.

ENVIRONMENTAL DETERMINANTS. Although psychological determinants address aspects of one's psychological environment, the environmental dimension encompasses the health effects of factors in the physical environment. The physical environment consists of weather, geographic locale, soil composition, terrain, temperature and humidity, and hazards posed by poor housing and unsafe working conditions. Additional elements of the physical environment that affect health include light and heat, exposure to pathogens and allergens, radiation, pollution, and noise. Similarly, elements of the built environment, such as areas to congregate or obtain exercise, have been shown to affect both physical and psychological health in general.

The health effects of environmental factors will be addressed in greater detail in Chapter 4∞. Using the PHN model, the population health nurse would assess the overall population, as well as individual clients, for the presence of environmental conditions detrimental to health. For example, poorly constructed highways may contribute to high rates of motor vehicle accidents for the population. At the individual level,

FOCUSED ASSESSMENT Biological Determinants Influencing Childhood Obesity

Age and developmental level

- What age groups within the child and adolescent population are most affected by overweight and obesity?
- Are there infant feeding practices common in the population that contribute to obesity?
- To what extent are infants breastfed in the population?
- To what extent do parents supervise the eating habits of children of different ages?

Genetics

- Is there a genetic predisposition to obesity in the population?
- Are there gender or ethnic group differences in the prevalence of overweight and obesity in the child population?

Physiologic function

- What physical conditions or disabilities are present in the population that might contribute to lack of physical activity and obesity? What is the incidence and prevalence of such conditions?
- What physiologic effects has obesity had on the child population? For example, what are the incidence and prevalence of type 2 diabetes or hypertension among children in the population?

FOCUSED ASSESSMENT Psychological Determinants Influencing Childhood Obesity

External psychological environment

- Is food used by members of the population as a reward for children's good behavior?
- Is food seen as a symbol of love and affection in the population?
- What attitudes do members of the population hold toward childhood overweight and obesity?
- What value do members of the population place on physical activity by children?

Internal psychological environment

- What is the effect of overweight and obesity on the self-image and psychological health of children affected?

poor lighting, stairs, and other hazards may increase the potential for falls in an elderly client. The *Focused Assessment* below includes questions that address environmental determinants related to the population-level problem of childhood obesity.

SOCIOCULTURAL DETERMINANTS. Sociocultural determinants of health include those factors within the social environment that influence health, either positively or negatively. Elements of the social structure such as employment, economics, politics, ethics, and legal influences all fall within this dimension of health. The sociocultural dimension also includes societal norms and culturally accepted modes of behavior.

Another important sociocultural determinant is prevailing attitudes toward specific health problems. For example, the fear and stigma attached to HIV infection may seriously hamper efforts to control the spread of disease. Substance abuse, mental illness, family violence, and adolescent pregnancy are other examples of health problems in which social attitudes contribute to the problem or hinder the solution.

Societal action with respect to health behaviors also falls within this category. For example, legislation requiring immunization of preschool children may significantly decrease rates of illness in the population. Legislative action can have both positive and negative effects on population health. For example, increases in cigarette taxes in New York City led to decreased levels of smoking, but also increased black market sales and decreased tax revenues targeted for smoking cessation programs (Shelley, Cantrell, Moon-Howard, Ramjohn, & VanDevanter, 2007).

Social capital is another sociocultural determinant of health that has been receiving increased attention in public health arenas. **Social capital** is the extent of one's access to and participation in relationships that can provide one with the necessities for life. Social capital is comprised of two components: social relationships that permit claims to available resources and the actual resources received. Social capital, at the population level, is akin to the concept of social support networks available to individuals and families. As an example, the existence of and access to educational opportunities afforded a population group is one element of social capital that can affect health status in a number of ways.

Sociocultural determinants can also influence health in other ways. Media portrayals of a variety of healthy and unhealthy behaviors are an example of the influence of social mores on health and illness. Occupation is another sociocultural determinant that may influence health. Conversely, unemployment may have adverse effects on physical and emotional health. Several sociocultural determinants will be addressed further in the chapters related to culture, economics, and politics (Chapters 5, 6, and 9∞, respectively).

FOCUSED ASSESSMENT Environmental Determinants Influencing Childhood Obesity

- What are the opportunities and environment for physical activity among children? For example, do traffic patterns or personal safety issues prohibit physical activity?
- Are there parks, sports fields, and other environmental features that promote physical activity?
- What is the extent of access to healthy foods in the environment?
- What is the extent of fast food establishments in the environment? How often are they frequented by members of the population?

FOCUSED ASSESSMENT Sociocultural Determinants Influencing Childhood Obesity

- What is the socioeconomic level of members of the population? How does socioeconomic status influence the ability to obtain and consume healthy or unhealthy foods?
- What are the cultural influences on food preferences and modes of preparation? Do they contribute to the development of overweight and obesity among children?
- What are the typical attitudes of members of the population to food, nutrition, and physical activity? Is physical activity among children valued, or are other activities (e.g., school work) given higher priority?
- What is the educational level of the population? Are they aware of factors contributing to obesity? Do they understand the long-term consequences of obesity for physical, emotional, and social health?
- What policies in the social environment contribute to or prevent obesity? For example, do local schools have "no junk food on campus" policies, or is the sale of sodas, fast food, and candy perceived as a way to generate funds for school activities?
- What are school policies related to physical activity among children? Are regular physical education activities that involve vigorous physical activity incorporated into school curricula at all levels?
- Are there sports teams available to promote physical activity among children? Do all children have access to them, or are some barred from participation due to expense?
- What is the level of funding provided by policy makers for programs related to nutrition and physical activity? Does funding for these programs receive priority within the community?
- What is the employment status of parents in the population? Do many parents work making it more difficult to find time to prepare healthful meals?
- To what extent do children prepare their own meals in parents' absence?

Population health nurses using the PHN model would assess the effects of sociocultural determinants on the health of the public. For example, the nurse might examine the unemployment rate in the population and the consequent effects on access to health care services. Sample assessment questions related to childhood obesity are presented in the focused assessment above.

BEHAVIORAL DETERMINANTS. Behavioral determinants involve personal behaviors that either promote or impair health. Behavioral factors are often those most amenable to change in efforts to prevent disease and promote health and, so, are of particular importance in population health nursing practice. Health-related behaviors include dietary patterns, recreation and exercise, substance use and abuse, sexual activity, and use of protective measures.

Dietary habits can either enhance or undermine health, and both leanness and obesity can predispose one to other health problems. Exercise patterns also influence health status, as do smoking, drinking, and drug use. Recreational activities are another behavioral factor that may pose health risks, but may also improve both physical and emotional health. Sexual activity poses risks related to pregnancy and sexually transmitted diseases. Failure to use protective measures such as contraceptives or barrier devices during intercourse can also increase one's chances of health problems. Similarly, not wearing seat belts or motorcycle helmets increases the potential for serious injury. Population health nurses can assess the extent of these and other health-related behaviors in individuals and in population groups and use this information to design appropriate interventions. Examples of assessment questions that might be used to assess the population health problem of childhood obesity are presented in the focused assessment on the next page.

HEALTH SYSTEM DETERMINANTS. The final category of health determinants included in the PHN model is related to the health care system. The way in which health care services are organized and their availability, accessibility, affordability, appropriateness, adequacy, acceptability, and use influence the health of individual clients and population groups. Availability refers to the type and number of health services present in a community, and accessibility reflects the ability of clients to make use of those services. Affordability, the ability to pay for services, also influences health outcomes. Service appropriateness refers to a health care system's ability to provide those services needed and desired by its clientele. The adequacy of health services refers to the quality and amount of service provided relative to need, and acceptability reflects the level of congruence between services provided and the expectations, values, and beliefs of the target population. Acceptability of services is also related to the level of trust that people have in health care providers and may differ significantly from one population group to another (Abel & Elfird, 2013). Finally, the extent to which members of the population actually make use of available health care services will influence health status.

Health system factors can influence health status either positively or negatively. For example, immunization services that are available and easily accessible to all community members promote control of communicable diseases such as measles, polio, and tetanus. Conversely, the failure of health professionals to take advantage of opportunities to immunize people contributes to increased incidence of these diseases.

FOCUSED ASSESSMENT Behavioral Determinants Influencing Childhood Obesity

- What is the typical daily calorie consumption among children in the population? What is the source of these calories?
- What is the average daily consumption of fruits and vegetables among children in the population?
- How many empty calories are consumed by children on a daily or weekly basis (e.g., sodas, unhealthy snacks, sweets)?
- What are the food preferences of children in the population?
- To what extent do families consume extensive fast food? How often do families eat meals prepared at home?
- Do children eat breakfast every day?
- Do children take lunches to school, or do they purchase lunch or eat in the cafeteria at school? How healthful are school meal menus?
- What is the extent of physical activity among children in the population?
- What types of physical activity are preferred? Do these types of physical activity require specialized training or equipment that might make them unaffordable for lower income children?
- To what extent do children walk or bicycle to school?
- What kinds of after-school activities do children engage in?
- How many hours per week are spent in vigorous physical activity by children?
- How many hours per week are spent in sedentary activities like watching television or playing video games?
- What household chores do children engage in? Do these chores promote physical activity (e.g., vacuuming the house)?

As we will see in Chapter 6∞, some health care system contributions to health problems stem from the economics of health care delivery. The high cost of health services limits the ability of many individuals to take advantage of them. Continuity of care may also affect health outcomes for individuals and population groups. In other instances, inappropriate actions on the part of health care providers may actually contribute to health problems. For example, inappropriate use of antibiotics has contributed to the development of antibiotic-resistant strains of gonorrhea and syphilis. Other health system activities may also contribute to disease. For example, blood transfusion has been associated with transmission of diseases such as HIV and hepatitis B and C. The focused assessment below provides questions addressing health system determinants related to childhood obesity in the population.

Elements of the determinants of health component of the PHN model are summarized below. Health determinants related to specific kinds of community health problems will also be addressed in relevant chapters of this book.

The population health nurse collects and organizes data regarding determinants of health. Factors in each of the six categories may apply to clients at multiple levels, including individuals, families, groups, communities, and populations. From the data, the population health nurse derives community health diagnoses that guide the planning of nursing interventions. Table 1-5● summarizes the contribution of various determinants of health to the problem of high incidence and prevalence of obesity in a university population.

FOCUSED ASSESSMENT Health System Determinants Influencing Childhood Obesity

- To what extent do health care providers focus on healthy weight, nutrition, and physical activity? Does this focus extend to children with physical conditions that necessitate physical activities specifically tailored to their abilities?
- What percentage of children in the population has access to a regular health care provider who can promote healthy eating and physical activity?
- What population-based programs are available in the community to promote good nutrition and physical fitness? For example, are there educational programs available for new parents that emphasize healthy diet? Are there educational programs for parents and children of other ages?
- What health care programs are available for weight management for overweight or obese children? What is the level of accessibility of these programs to all children in need of services?
- What is the level of funding available for programs to promote healthy eating and physical activity among children or to provide weight management services when needed?
- To what extent are programs to promote healthy diets and physical activity among children culturally sensitive and appropriate to various segments of the population?

Highlights

Determinants of Health

Biological Determinants

- Age and developmental level
- Genetics
- Physiologic function

Psychological Determinants

- Internal psychological environment
- External psychological environment

Environmental Determinants

- Physical environment
- Environmental hazards

Sociocultural Determinants

- Social structure
- Societal norms
- Societal attitudes
- Social action

Behavioral Determinants

- Dietary practices
- Recreation and exercise
- Substance use and abuse
- Sexual activity
- Use of protective measures

Health System Determinants

- Availability
- Accessibility
- Affordability
- Appropriateness
- Adequacy
- Acceptability
- Use

Population Health Nursing Interventions

The second component of the PHN model reflects interventions taken by population health nurses to address health problems within a population. Several categories of population health nursing intervention have been identified and are summarized below. Each type of intervention will be discussed briefly and examples of particular interventions will be included throughout this book.

Education is the process of facilitating learning that leads to positive health behavior. In the educator role, the population health nurse provides clients and others with information and insights that allow them to make informed decisions on health matters. Population health nurses often provide educational services to individuals, families, and groups, and they are frequently involved in the development of population-based health education programs. Population health nurses, for example, educate individuals and their families about adequate nutrition. At the same time, they may educate the general public regarding the harmful effects, say, of a high-cholesterol, low-fiber diet. Similarly, population health nurses may educate legislators and other policy makers regarding societal factors that impede population health. Educational interventions are discussed in greater detail in Chapter 11∞.

Although many people do not distinguish between counseling and education, they *are* different. **Counseling** is the process of helping a client to choose viable solutions to health problems. In educating, one is presenting facts and developing attitudes and skills. In counseling, one is *not* telling people what to do but helping them to employ the problem-solving process and decide on the most appropriate course of action. In the role of counselor, population health nurses explain the problem-solving process and guide clients/populations through each step. In this way, the nurse is not only helping the individual, family, or population to solve the immediate problem but also assisting in the development of problem-solving abilities.

Counseling involves several steps on the part of the community health nurse. The first step is helping to clarify the problem to be solved. The nurse and client/population together examine the factors that contribute to a problem and those

TABLE 1-5 Determinants of Health and Their Influence on the Problem of Obesity in a University Population

Model Concept	Application
Biological determinants	Age composition of the population; prevalence of obesity in the population
Psychological determinants	Stress of college life; extent of use of food as stress reliever; extent of exposure to stressful circumstances; prevalence of eating disorders on campus
Environmental determinants	Weather conducive to outdoor exercise; facilities available for obese members of the population (e.g., size of classroom chairs)
Sociocultural determinants	Use of eating and drinking as social activities; population attitudes toward obesity; extent of peer support for healthy lifestyles; availability of education for healthy lifestyles
Behavioral determinants	Dietary practices in campus population; availability of healthy foods in campus dining facilities; availability of recreational activities and equipment; extent of participation in physical activity among campus population; sedentary nature of university life
Health system determinants	Health center staff attention to weight problems among campus community members; availability of weight/diet counseling programs; availability of stress-reduction/counseling programs

that may enhance or impede problem resolution. The second step involves identifying alternative solutions to the problem. If, for example, a large proportion of pregnant women in the population do not receive prenatal care, one could suggest an educational campaign, outreach efforts by lay health promoters, financial subsidies for care by available providers, or the use of nurse midwives.

Assisting the client or population group to develop criteria for an acceptable solution to the problem is the third step in counseling. For example, an acceptable solution to the problem of poor nutrition among family members would need to fit the family's budget and might need to conform to cultural dietary preferences. A program to address nutritional needs at the population level would need to address the same constraints.

Next, the population health nurse would assist the client to evaluate each of the alternative solutions in terms of criteria established for an acceptable solution. The most appropriate alternative is one that best meets the acceptability criteria. This alternative is then implemented. Evaluation is the fifth step of the problem-solving process. If the alternative selected solves the problem, fine! If not, the process begins again.

Referral is one of the key functions of population health nurses. **Referral** is the process of directing clients to resources required to meet their needs. These resources may be other agencies that can provide necessary services or sources of information, equipment, or supplies that the client needs and the population health nurse cannot supply. A distinction must be made between the functions of referral and consultation. In a referral, the client is directed toward another source of services. In *consultation*, on the other hand, the nurse may seek assistance or information needed to help the client from another source, but the client does not receive services directly from the consultant. Population health nurses also provide consultation to other professionals and to policy-making bodies. The referral process is discussed in more detail in Chapter 12∞.

A **role model** is someone who consciously or unconsciously demonstrates behavior to others who will perform a similar role. Population health nurses serve as role models for a variety of people with whom they come in contact. Through their own behavior, nurses influence the behavior of others. For instance, the population health nurse's ability to engage in systematic planning may promote similar skills in community planning groups.

Although case management is a new concept for many nurses, it has long been an integral component of population health nursing. A **case manager** is a health professional who coordinates and directs the selection and use of health care services to meet client needs, maximize resource utilization, and minimize the expense of care. The aims of case management include identifying high-risk clients or those with the potential for high-cost service needs, making appropriate choices among available services and providers, controlling costs, and coordinating care to achieve optimal client outcomes. The process of case management will be addressed in more detail in Chapter 12∞.

Highlights

Population Health Nursing Interventions

Education: Providing clients/populations with information to make informed health-related decisions

Counseling: Assisting clients/populations to choose viable solutions to health problems

Referral: Directing clients to resources needed to meet their needs

Role modeling: Demonstrating desired behaviors to promote learning and change

Case management: Coordinating and selecting health care services to meet identified client needs

Coordination/care management: Organizing and integrating health care delivery services to best meet population health care needs

Collaboration: Engaging in joint decision making with clients/populations, other health care providers, and non-health sectors of society to resolve client/population health problems

Liaison: Facilitating relationships between clients/populations and other health care providers or policy makers

Case Finding/screening: Identifying individual cases of health problems or the incidence and prevalence of conditions in the population

Surveillance: Monitoring occurrence and trends in specific health problems within the population

Policy formulation: Promoting and assisting in the development of social and health care policies that support the health of the population

Community mobilization: Assisting populations to identify goals and implement strategies to improve health and promote conditions that support health

Coalition building: Assisting in the creation of alliances of individuals or groups to achieve health-related goals

Social marketing: Using commercial marketing strategies to change public attitudes or behaviors

Promoting evidence-based practice: Critically examining scientific evidence to identify and effectively implement strategies that improve population health

Population health nurses frequently care for clients who are receiving services from a variety of sources. Because of their awareness of the needs of the client as a whole being, population health nurses are in an ideal position to serve as coordinators of care. **Coordination** is the process of organizing and integrating services to best meet client needs in the most efficient manner possible. Unlike the case manager, the coordinator does not plan the care to be carried out by other health care professionals, but organizes that care to meet clients' needs as effectively as possible. At the population level, coordination may be referred to as **population health management**, or the "coordination of care across a population to improve clinical and financial outcomes" (Population Health Management, 2010, p. 1).

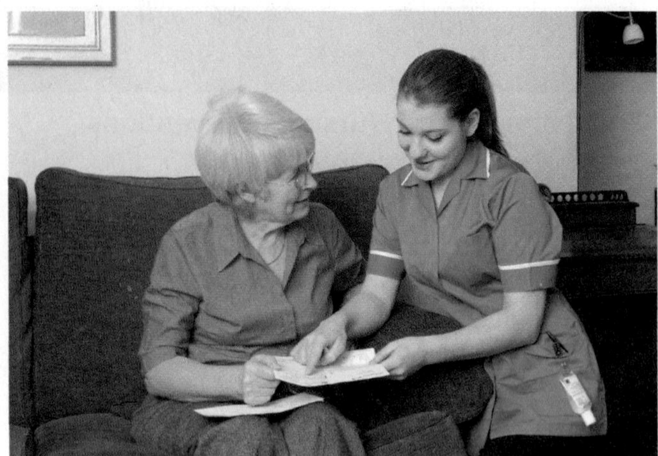

Population health nurses provide health education to individuals, families, communities, and population groups. *(Jules Selmes/Pearson Education. Inc)*

Collaboration involves joint decision making regarding action to be taken to resolve health problems. Collaboration is frequently confused with the nurse's coordination role. Coordination is essentially a management function and involves making sure that efforts to provide services are consistent and occur without gaps or overlaps. Collaboration, on the other hand, entails joint decision making. Both collaboration and coordination, of course, necessitate working with members of the population and other professionals (and nonprofessionals) to address population health problems.

Collaboration is not a matter of each health care provider or agency designing and providing a program in his or her area of expertise with a certain amount of coordination between efforts. Rather, it is a joint effort on the part of health care providers, members of the population, and representatives from other sectors of society to set mutual goals and to arrive at a mutually acceptable plan to achieve them. A **liaison** is a person who provides a connection, relationship, or intercommunication. The population health nurse working with clients dealing with multiple health and social agencies may serve as that connection or liaison. In referral, the nurse may function as the initial point of contact between client and agency. The liaison's role might involve continued communication between client and other providers via the nurse. Sometimes this communication includes the additional function of interpretation and reinforcement of provider recommendations to the client or advocacy for the client with the provider agency. At the population level, the population health nurse may serve as a liaison between community residents and policy makers.

Case finding has been described as basic to population health nursing. **Case finding** involves identifying individual cases or occurrences of specific diseases or other health-related conditions requiring services. As we will see in Chapter 26∞, case finding is an important strategy in preventing the spread of communicable diseases in large population groups. Case finding may involve screening or conducting tests to identify the presence of a particular disease or condition. Population health nurses may screen individual clients or assist in planning and implementing population-based screening efforts.

Case finding is closely related to the public health nursing intervention of **surveillance**, which is defined as "the systematic collection, analysis, interpretation, and dissemination of data to assist in the planning, implementation, and evaluation of public health interventions and programs" (ANA, 2013, p. 68). For example, identifying more instances of child abuse may be an indication of a community health problem.

As noted earlier in this chapter, policy development is one of the core functions of public health practice, and population health nurses have a definite role as policy advocates in the execution of this function. A **policy advocate** is a person or group of people who work for and argue on behalf of policy formation or changes in policy that influence population health. Policy advocacy may occur at institutional, community, state, national, or international levels. Population health nurses may assist in determining the need for policy formation or change, developing policy goals, analyzing factors influencing the policy situation, identifying key decision makers involved in policy formation, assisting in the formulation of proposed policies, communicating the proposed policy to the general public and to policy makers, and monitoring the progress of policy formation. These functions will be discussed in more detail in Chapter 9∞.

Community mobilization is assisting populations to identify areas of concern and to develop and implement strategies to address them. Community mobilization promotes the participation of members of population groups in the control of their own lives and gives them the power to enact changes in circumstances that affect their health. Community mobilization will be discussed in more detail in Chapter 10∞.

As we will see in Chapter 9∞, coalition building is a strategy often used in political activism. **Coalition building** is the process of creating temporary or permanent alliances of individuals or groups to achieve a specific purpose. Coalitions have the advantage of fostering community-wide problem solving and collaborative policy and program development bringing to bear the assets and resources and perspectives of multiple segments of the population. Population health nurses may initiate coalition building activities among members of the population and between both health-related and other sectors of society to influence the determinants of health.

Social marketing is another population health nursing intervention. The most frequently quoted definition of **social marketing** in the literature is that provided by Andreasen (1995): "the application of commercial marketing technologies to the analysis, planning, execution, and evaluation of programs designed to influence the voluntary behavior of target audiences to improve their personal welfare or that of their society" (p. 7). Social marketing is consumer focused in that it is tailored to the needs and characteristics of a specific target population and is designed to address societal problems at the population level.

Population health nurses involved in social marketing may assist in identifying a needed change in societal behavior, analyzing behavioral motivations and perceived benefits and barriers to action, identifying particular target markets for interventions and determining the unique features of those markets, developing and testing strategies to promote the desired change, implementing those strategies, and evaluating their effectiveness. Concepts and principles of social marketing and related community health nursing functions are discussed in more detail in Chapter 11∞.

Promoting evidence-based practice is an overarching intervention by population health nurses that involves translating research findings into practice and may inform all of the other interventions described above. **Evidence-based practice** is a

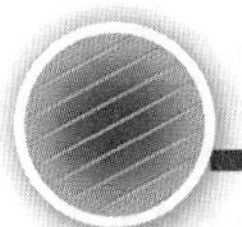

Evidence-Based Practice

Understanding the Process

Effective population health nursing should be based on scientific evidence combined with clinical expertise and client preferences. Use of a systematic process to critically evaluate available evidence can promote evidence-based practice. A number of models for evidence-based practice are found in the literature (Mitchell, Fisher, Hastings, Silverman, & Wallen, 2010), but they generally incorporate similar steps for integrating evidence as a basis for practice.

The first step in evidence-based practice is to identify a clinical question or problem that needs resolution. Clinical questions may be framed in the PICO format in which **P** stands for the population of interest, **I** reflects a potential intervention, **C** is a comparison intervention or group, and **O** is the desired outcome to be achieved. Some authors add a **T** to the acronym to make it PICOT, with the **T** reflecting the time period in which the outcome is expected to be measured (Melnyk, Fineout-Overholt, Stillwell, & Williamson, 2010).

The second step in promoting evidence-based practice in a practice setting is finding the relevant evidence. Evidence frequently includes published research, both quantitative and qualitative (Owens, 2009), but may also include non-research-based evidence from within or outside the setting. Such evidence might include quality improvement data, case studies, or expert opinion (Bednarski, 2010). In addition to bringing to light individual research studies, a literature review may produce meta-analyses of several related studies or previously developed clinical practice guidelines related to the topic of interest. **Clinical practice guidelines** (CPGs) are "general practice recommendations to aid clinical decision making for specific clinical situations" (American Professional Wound Care Association, 2010, p. 161) that are usually based on a critical review of research findings, expert opinion, and client preferences.

Once various forms of evidence have been identified, the body of evidence must be critically evaluated in terms of its level, quality, and strength. The level of evidence refers to the hierarchy of research methodologies used to develop evidence, with randomized controlled strategies having greater credibility than other methods, such as observational studies, cross-sectional studies, qualitative studies, case reports, and expert opinion or consensus (Stillwell, Fineout-Overholt, Melnyk, & Williamson, 2010). The quality of the evidence refers to the way in which the study was conducted, the validity of the research design and methods for addressing the research question, the clinical relevance of the findings, and the potential applicability of the findings to one's own practice population (the generalizability of the findings). Finally, the strength of the evidence reflects the extent to which different credible studies support the effectiveness of the intervention being considered (Shapiro, 2010). This process of appraisal frequently involves grading each study or other piece of evidence using a critical appraisal guide, or criteria appropriate to the type of study being reviewed (Fineout-Overholt, Melnyk, Stillwell, & Williamson, 2010). Existing clinical practice guidelines should also be critically evaluated using a systematic approach such as that provided by the AGREE instrument (AGREE Next Steps Consortium, 2013; Zadvinskis & Grudell, 2010).

The fourth step in implementing evidence-based practice is to integrate the research evidence with clinical expertise and patient preferences and values (Melnyk et al., 2010). Client situations differ, so the applicability of research findings to a particular client or population must also be evaluated. When there is sufficient evidence for the effectiveness of the proposed intervention, it is implemented on a trial basis and the outcomes of the trial evaluated. Finally, the outcomes of implementation should be disseminated to add to the evidence base for practice in other similar settings. Throughout the remainder of this book, we will examine the evidence for specific interventions as well as address some additional considerations related to evidence-based population health nursing practice.

Evidence-based practice is not a new concept. We opened this chapter with a discussion of the advocacy activities of Florence Nightingale, who was one of the forerunners of evidence-based nursing practice. Nightingale used her notes and observations on mortality in the Crimean War to improve hygiene and sanitation in treating the ill and injured (Pasley, 2010).

strategy for improving patient outcomes by integrating "the best evidence from studies and patient care data with clinician expertise and patient preferences and values" (Melnyk, Fineout-Overholt, Stillwell, & Williamson, 2009, p. 49). In promoting evidence-based practice, population health nurses will be actively involved in searching and critically analyzing related research literature and identifying practice interventions that have significant research support and are appropriate to the population to be served.

The population health nursing interventions presented here are similar to those included in the interventions wheel model developed by Public Health Nursing Section of the Minnesota Department of Health in 2001 (Wisconsin Department of Health Services, 2014). The 17 interventions included in the model were derived from research on actual practice by public health nurses.

Levels of Health Care

The population health nursing interventions described above and those included in the interventions wheel may be employed to address health concerns at one of four levels of care: health promotion, illness and injury prevention, resolution, and restoration. The *American Journal of Health Promotion* (O'Donnell, 2009) has adopted the definition of **health promotion** as "the art and science of helping people discover the synergies between their core passions and optimal health, enhancing their motivation to strive for optimal health, and supporting them in changing their lifestyle to move toward a state of optimal health" (p. 1). Health promotion, then entails activities designed to foster a healthy lifestyle and develop a state of good health in the population. For example, the population health nurse might engage in a number of interventions, such as education and advocacy for access to healthy foods, designed to foster good nutrition as a health promoting strategy.

Prevention, also referred to as health protection, involves strategies aimed at preventing the occurrence of specific health problems. For example, immunization is a preventive measure for certain communicable diseases. Illness and injury prevention may also involve reducing or eliminating risk factors as a means of preventing the occurrence of health problems. Legislation to require helmet use for bicycle riders is an example of risk factor modification to prevent injury.

The aim of the **resolution** level of health care is elimination of an existing health problem. At this level, a health problem has already occurred and population health nursing interventions are directed toward its solution and preventing further serious consequences. Resolution activities may include screening and early diagnosis as well as treatment for existing health problems. Treatment for a sexually transmitted disease is an example of resolution. Removing a child from an abusive home situation and providing respite for caregivers who are overwhelmed are other resolution strategies. **Restoration**, or rehabilitation, involves activities designed to assist the client's or population's return to a prior state of good health and functional ability. For many health problems restoration is not needed (e.g., after a minor cold) or is not possible (e.g., with a terminal diagnosis). At the population level, resolving immediate problems related to an earthquake, such as rescuing victims and restoring power, are examples of resolution. Rebuilding damaged buildings and highways would constitute restoration.

As depicted in Table 1-6●, the levels of care are similar to the public health concept of levels of prevention, which includes primary prevention, secondary prevention, and tertiary prevention. Health promotion and illness and injury prevention are elements of **primary prevention**, which is the intervention aimed at preventing health problems from occurring. **Secondary prevention** focuses on the early identification and treatment of existing health problems and occurs after the health problem has arisen. **Tertiary prevention** is an activity aimed at returning the client (individual or population) to the highest level of function and preventing further deterioration in health (Gerstman, 2013). Because of the confusion engendered by different uses of the term "prevention," however, we will use the terms of health promotion, illness and injury prevention, resolution, and restoration for the levels of health care throughout this book.

Appropriate population health nursing interventions would be used at each level of health care to prevent population health problems or deal with identified problems. Table 1-7● presents interventions at each level of health care related to the problem of increased prevalence of obesity in the population. The elements of the PHN model are used within the context of the nursing process as depicted in Figure 1-3.

TABLE 1-6 Levels of Health Care and Levels of Prevention

Level of Health Care	Level of Prevention
Health promotion	Primary prevention: Focus on preventing occurrence of health problems
Prevention	Primary prevention: Focus on preventing occurrence of health problems
Resolution	Secondary prevention: Focus on identification and treatment of existing health problems
Restoration	Tertiary prevention: Focus on restoring health status and preventing further deterioration

TABLE 1-7 Levels of Health Care and Population Health Nursing Interventions for Obesity

Levels of Health Care	Selected Population Health Nursing Interventions
Health promotion	• Promoting regular exercise in the population • Developing environments that foster physical activity
Prevention	• Educating the public on good nutrition • Referring needy families to nutrition support programs • Promoting access to healthy foods • Limiting access to unhealthy food choices
Resolution	• Assuring access to weight-reduction programs in the community
Restoration	• Providing services to deal with long-term consequences of obesity

In the assessment stage of the nursing process, the population health nurse assesses the impact of the six categories of determinants on the health of the population (or individual client/family) and derives nursing diagnoses related to population health. Nursing diagnoses may be positive or negative. Positive diagnoses are areas in which the population is functioning effectively. Negative diagnoses are areas in which intervention is required to address identified health problems. In the planning and implementation stages of the nursing process, the nurse develops and carries out, often in collaboration with members of the population and others, interventions designed to support population health or to address identified problems. The population health nursing uses evaluation findings to assess the effectiveness of interventions and to inform subsequent interventions.

Other models have been developed or modified for use in population health nursing. Information about some of these models is provided on the student resources site.

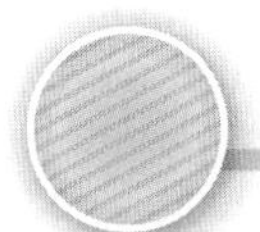

Global Perspectives

Population Health Models

The population health nursing (PHN) model described in this chapter forms the theoretical foundation for the rest of the book. The PHN model is one approach to population health nursing. Other models that can be used to direct population health nursing activity are discussed in the *Further Information* section of the student resources. The point has been raised, however, that models developed for practice in the United States may not always be appropriate and applicable to population health nursing practice in other countries. Another concern in adopting U.S. practice models in other countries is the abstract language that is sometimes used in describing such models and the educational level and facility with English exhibited by nurses in other countries. Of the theoretical models presented in the text and on the website, which ones do you think would be most applicable in other countries? Why?

CHAPTER RECAP

As we have seen in this chapter, population health is the health status of an entire population and is more than the cumulative health of its individual members. Population health practice is guided by three core public health functions of assessment, policy development, and assurance, and by 10 essential public health services. *Healthy People 2020* provides national objectives for the improvement of population health.

Population health nursing is nursing care directed toward the improvement of the health of the overall population. It is guided by a set of standards and competencies expected of population health nurses. Population health nurses use the PHN model, in the context of the nursing process, to direct their practice. Elements of the model include the determinants of health, factors that influence the health of the population, and population health nursing interventions that are employed at four levels of health care, health promotion, illness and injury prevention, resolution, and restoration. Throughout this book, we will use the PHN model to address a variety of population health problems and conditions.

CASE STUDY Transportation Services for Older Clients

Vista Hills is a small, low-income community within a major metropolitan area. In home visits to several older clients, the population health nurse assigned to the area discovers that they have not been able to keep medical appointments or get prescriptions filled due to lack of available transportation. There is a bus that traverses the area, but it only has stops on major thoroughfares, and most older residents have difficulty walking from their homes to the bus stops. In the past, the community had access to a Dial-a-Ride service that provided door-to-door transportation for elderly residents for 50 cents a ride (one-way). This service was discontinued several years ago because of escalating costs.

The city in which the community is located has some funds for transportation services for elderly clients, but they have not been allocated to this community because older residents comprise only 11% of the overall population. Some residents use taxi services to meet their transportation needs, but find this very expensive given their limited incomes.

1. What are some of the determinants of health operating in this situation?
2. What population health nursing interventions might be needed to address this community health problem? Why are these interventions appropriate to this situation?
3. Give examples of some specific activities the population health nurse might carry out in relation to each intervention.

REFERENCES

Abel, W. M., & Elfird, J. T. (2013, December 5). The association between trust in health care providers and medication adherence among Black women with hypertension. *Frontiers in Public Health, 1*, 66. doi: 10.3389/fpubh.2013.00066

Advisory Committee on National Health Promotion and Disease Prevention Objectives for 2020. (2008). *Phase I report: Recommendations for the framework and format of Healthy People 2020*. Washington, DC: U.S. Department of Health and Human Services.

Advocacy. (n.d.a). *Dictionary.com unabridged*. Retrieved from Dictionary.com website: http://dictionary.reference.com/browse/advocacy

Advocacy. (n.d.b). Retrieved from http://en.wikipedia.org/wiki/Advocacy

The AGREE Next Steps Consortium. (2013). *Appraisal of guidelines for research and evaluation II*. Retrieved from http://www.agreetrust.org/wp-content/uploads/2013/10/AGREE-II-Users-Manual-and-23-item-Instrument_2009_UPDATE_2013.pdf

American Association of Colleges of Nursing. (2006). *Essentials for doctoral education for advanced nursing practice*. Washington, DC: Author.

American Association of Colleges of Nursing. (2008). *The essentials of baccalaureate education for professional nursing practice*. Washington, DC: Author.

American Nurses Association. (1976). *Code for nurses with interpretive statements*. Kansas City, MO: Author.

American Nurses Association. (1986). *Standards of community health nursing practice*. Kansas City, MO: Author.

American Nurses Association. (2013). *Public health nursing: Scope and standards of practice* (2nd ed.). Silver Spring, MD: Author.

American Professional Wound Care Association. (2010). SELECT: Evaluation and implementation of clinical practice guidelines: A guidance document from the American Professional Wound Care Association. *Advances in Skin & Wound Care, 23*, 161–168.

American Public Health Association. (2014). *10 essential public health services*. Retrieved from http://www.apha.org/programs/standards/performance-standardsprogram/resexxentialservices.htm

American Public Health Association, Public Health Nursing Section. (2013). *The definition of public health nursing*. Retrieved from http://www.apha.org/NR/rdonlyres/284CE437-6AF3-4B23-88BA-52F2A0E329E6/0/PHNdefinitionNov2013_final125142.pdf

Andreasen, A. R. (1995). *Marketing social change: Changing behavior to promote health, social development, and the environment*. San Francisco, CA: Jossey-Bass.

Barnum, N. C. (2011). Public health nursing: An autonomous career for World War II nurse veterans. *Public Health Nursing, 28*, 379–386. doi: 10.1111/j.1525-1446.2011.00949.x

Baum, F. E., Bégin, M., Houweling, T. A. J., & Taylor, S. (2009). Changes not for the fainthearted: Reorienting health care systems toward health equity through action on the social determinants of health. *American Journal of Public Health, 99*, 1967–1974.

Bednarski, D. (2010). Integrating evidence-based practice. *Nephrology Nursing Journal, 37*, 113–114.

Bloy, M. (2010). *Florence Nightingale (1820–1910)*. Retrieved from http://www.victorianweb.org/history/crimea/florrie.html

Carel, H. (2009). A reply to "Towards and understanding of nursing as a response to human vulnerability" by Derek Sellman: vulnerability and illness. *Nursing Philosophy, 10*, 214–219. doi: 10.1111/j.1466-769X.2009.00401.x

Clark, M. J. (2001). *Voicing their voice: The structure of advocacy*. Unpublished raw data.

Clark, M. J. (2008). *Advocacy in community health nursing*. Unpublished raw data.

Conceptual model. (n.d.). *Dictionary.com's 21st century Lexicon*. Retrieved from Dictionary.com website: http://dictionary.reference.com/browse/conceptual model

Council on Linkages Between Academia and Public Health Practice. (2010). *Core Competencies for Public Health Professionals: Revisions adopted: May 2010*. Retrieved from http://www.phf.org/resourcestools/Documents/Core_Competencies_for_Public_Health_Professionals_2010May.pdf

Drevdahl, D., Kneipp, S. M., Canales, M. K., & Dorcy, K. S. (2001). Reinvesting in social justice: A capital idea for public health nursing? *Advances in Nursing Science, 24*(2), 19–31.

Environmental Health Services. (2011). *Core functions of public health and how they relate to the 10 essential services*. Retrieved from http://www.cdc.gov/nceh/ehs/ephli/core_ess.htm

Fee, E., & Bu, L. (2010). The origins of public health nursing: The Henry Street visiting nurse service. *American Journal of Public Health*, 100, 1206–1207.

Fineout-Overholt, E., Melnyk, B. M., Stillwell, S. B., & Williamson, K. M. (2010). Critical appraisal of the evidence: Part I. *American Journal of Nursing, 110*(7), 47–52.

Gerstman, B. B. (2013). *Epidemiology kept simple: An introduction to traditional and modern epidemiology* (3rd ed.). Hoboken, NJ: Wiley Blackwell.

Hallett, C. E. (2010). *Celebrating nurses: A visual history*. Hauppauge, NY: Barron's.

Health Advocacy. (2014). *Wikipedia, the free encyclopedia*. Retrieved from http://en.wikipedia.org/wiki/Health_advocacy

Howse, C. (2009). "The reflection of England's light": The Instructive District Nursing Association of Boston, 1884–1914. *Nursing History Review, 17*, 47–79. doi: 10.1891/1062-8061.17.47

Institute of Medicine. (1988). *The future of public health*. Washington, DC: National Academies Press.

Institute of Medicine, Committee on Assuring the Health of the Public in the 21st Century. (2002). *The future of the public's health in the 21st century*. Washington, DC: National Academies Press.

Institute of Medicine. (2013). *Working definition of population health*. Retrieved from http://iom.edu/~/media/Files/Activity%20Files/PublicHealth/PopulationHealthImprovementRT/Pop%20Health%20RT%20Population%20Health%20Working%20Definition.pdf

Issel, L. M., & Bekemeier, B. (2010). Safe practice of population-focused nursing care: Development of a public health nursing concept. *Nursing Outlook, 58*, 226–232. doi:10.1016/j.outlook.2010.06.001

Jacobsen, D. M., & Teutsch, S. (2012). *An environmental scan of integrated approaches for defining and measuring total population health by the clinical care system, the government public health system, and stakeholder organizations*. Washington, DC: The National Academies Press.

Kindig, D., & Stoddart, G. (2003). What is population health? *American Journal of Public Health, 93*, 380–383.

Levin, P. F., Swider, S. M., Breakwell, S., Cowell, J. M., & Reising, V. (2013). Embracing a competency-based curriculum for community-based nursing roles. *Public Health Nursing, 30*, 557–565. doi: 10.1111/phn.12042

Lewis, J. J. (2010). *Florence Nightingale*. Retrieved from http://womenshistory.about.com/od/nightingale/p/nightingale.htm?p=1

Melnyk, B. M., Fineout-Overholt, E., Stillwell, S. B., & Williamson, K. M. (2009). Igniting a spirit of inquiry: An essential foundation for evidence-based practice. *American Journal of Nursing, 109*(11), 49–52.

Melnyk, B. M., Fineout-Overholt, E., Stillwell, S. B., & Williamson, K. M. (2010). The seven steps of evidence-based practice. *American Journal of Nursing, 110*(1), 51–53.

Mitchell, S.A., Fisher, C. A., Hastings, C. E., Silverman, L. B., & Wallen, G. R. (2010). A thematic analysis of theoretical models for translational science in nursing: Mapping the field. *Nursing Outlook, 58*, 287–300. doi:10.1016/j.outlook.2010.07.001

National Public Health Performance Standards Program. (n.d.). *Acronyms, glossary, and reference terms*. Retrieved from http://www.cdc.gov/od/ocphp/nphpsp/PDF/glossary.pdf

O'Donnell, M. P. (2009). Definition of health promotion 2.0: Embracing passion, enhancing motivation, recognizing dynamic balance, and creating opportunities. *American Journal of Health Promotion, 24*, iv. Retrieved from http://www.healthpromotionjournal.com

Office of Disease Prevention and Health Promotion. (n.d.a). *Framework: The vision, mission and goals of Healthy People 2020*. Retrieved from http://www.healthypeople.gov/2020/consortium/HP2020Framework.pdf

Office of Disease Prevention and Health Promotion. (n.d.b). *Healthy people 2020: A resource for promoting health and preventing disease throughout the nation*. Retrieved from http://www.healthypeople.gov/2020/consortium/HealthyPeoplePresentation_2_24_11.ppt

Pasley, J. (2010, Fall). What would Florence think? *Vanderbilt Nurse*, pp. 8–13.

Population health management. (2010). *Thefreedictionary.com*. Retrieved from http://medical-dictionary.thefreedictionary.com/population+health+management

Poulton, B. (2009). Barriers and facilitators to the achievement of community-focused public health nursing practice: A UK perspective. *Journal of Nursing Management*, 17, 74–83. 10.1111/j.1365-2834.2008.00949.x

Public Health Agency of Canada. (2012). *What is the population health approach?* Retrieved from http://www/phac-aspc.gc.ca/ph-sp/approach-approche/index-eng.php

Public Health Agency of Canada. (2013). *What is the population health approach? Key elements of a population health approach*. Retrieved from http://www.phac-aspc.gc.ca/ph-sp/approach-approche/appr-eng.php#key_elements

Public Health Foundation. (n.d.). *Core Competencies for Public Health Professionals: Tiers*. Retrieved from http://www.phf.org/programs/corecompetencies/Pages/COL_CorePublicHealthCompetencies_Guidance_Definitions.aspx

Public Health Foundation. (2014a). *About the Core Competencies for Public Health Professionals*. Retrieved from http://www.phf.org/programs/corecompetencies/Pages/About_the_Core_Competencies_for_Public_Health_Professionals.aspx

Public Health Foundation. (2014b). *Behind the scenes of the Core Competencies for Public Health Professionals revisions*. Retrieved from http://www.phf.org/phfpulse/Pages/Amos_Behind_the_Scenes_of_the_Core_Competencies_Revisions.aspx?utm_source=Council+on+Linkages+Update+-+March+2014&utm_campaign=Council+on+Linkages+Update+-+March+2014&utm_medium=email

Quad Council of Public Health Nursing Organizations. (2011). *Quad Council Competencies for Public Health Nurses*. Retrieved from http://www.achne.org/files/Quad%20Council/QuadCouncilCompetenciesforPublicHealthNurses.pdf

Selanders, L. C., & Crane, P. C. (2012) The Voice of Florence Nightingale on Advocacy. *OJIN: The Online Journal of Issues in Nursing, 17*(1), Manuscript 1. doi: 10.3912/OJIN.Vol17No01Man01

Senate Subcommittee on Population and Health. (2009). *A healthy, productive Canada: A determinant of health approach*. Ottawa, ON: Author.

Shapiro, S. E. (2010). Grading evidence for practice. *Advanced Emergency Nursing Journal, 32*, 59–67.

Shelley, D., Cantrell, M. J., Moon-Howard, J., Ramjohn, D. Q., & VanDevanter, N. (2007). The $5 man: The underground economic response to a large cigarette tax increase in New York City. *American Journal of Public Health, 97*, 1483–1488.

Simkin, J. (n.d.). *Florence Nightingale*. Retrieved from http://www.spartacus.schoolnet.co.uk/REnightingale.htm

Stillwell, S. B., Fineout-Overholt, E., Melnyk, B. M., & Williamson, K. M. (2010). Searching for the evidence. *American Journal of Nursing, 110*(5), 41–47.

Stoto, M. A. (2013). *Population health in the Affordable Care Act era*. Retrieved from http://www.academyhealth.org/files/AH2013pophealth.pdf

Swider, S. M., Krothe, J., Reyes, D., & Cravetz, M. (2013). The Quad Council practice competencies for public health nursing.*Public Health Nursing, 30*, 519–536. doi: 10.1111/phn.12090

Swider, S. M., Levin, P., Cowell, J., Breakwell, S., Holland, P., & Wallinder, J. (2009). Community/public health nursing practice leaders' views of the Doctorate of Nursing Practice. *Public Health Nursing, 26*, 405–411.

University of Oxford. (n.d.). PICO: Formulate an answerable question. Retrieved from http://learntech.physiol.ox.ac.uk/cochrane_tutorial/cochlibd0e84.php

U.S. Department of Health and Human Services. (1980). *Promoting health/preventing disease: Objectives for the nation*. Washington, DC: Government Printing Office.

U.S. Department of Health and Human Services. (2012a). *Healthy people 2020 leading health indicator topics*. Retrieved from http://healthypeople.gov/2020/LHI/2020indicators.aspx

U.S. Department of Health and Human Services. (2012b). *Leading health indicators*. Retrieved from http://healthypeople.gov/2020/LHI/default.aspx

U.S. Department of Health and Human Services. (2012c). *Leading health indicators*. Retrieved from http://healthypeople.gov/2020/LHI/default.aspx

U.S. Department of Health and Human Services. (2013). *2020 LHI topics*. Retrieved from http://www.healthypeople.gov/2020/LHI/2020indicators.aspx

U.S. Department of Health and Human Services. (2014). *About healthy people*. Retrieved from http://www.healthypeople.gov/2020/about/default.aspx

Wisconsin Department of Health Services. (2014). *Public health nursing: The public health intervention wheel*. Retrieved from http://www.dhs.wisconsin.gov/phnc/InterventionWheel/

Workhouse. (n.d.). *The Metropolitan Asylums Board*. Retrieved from http://www.workhouses.org.uk/MAB/

World Health Organization. (1984). *Health promotion: A discussion document on the concept and principles*. Copenhagen, Denmark: WHO Regional Office for Europe.

World Health Organization. (2014). *The determinants of health*. Retrieved from http://www.who.int/hia/evidence/doh/en/print.html

Young, S. (2009). Professional relationships and power dynamics between urban community-based nurses and social work case managers. *Professional Case Management, 14*, 312–320.

Zadvinskis, I. M., & Grudell, B. A. (2010). Clinical practice guideline appraisal using the AGREE instrument. *Clinical Nurse Specialist, 24*, 204–214.

CHAPTER

2 Population Health Nursing: Yesterday, Today, and Tomorrow

Learning Outcomes

After reading this chapter, you should be able to:

1. Describe the contributions of historical figures who influenced the development of population health nursing.
2. Discuss the contributions of population health nurses to social and health care reform.
3. List significant historical events in the development of population health nursing in the United States.
4. Describe evidence for a shift in public health policy toward a greater emphasis on health promotion.
5. Describe events that are shaping current and future population health nursing practice.

Key Terms

diagnosis-related groups (DRGs)

missionary nurses

Nursing Interventions Classification (NIC)

Nursing Outcomes Classification (NOC)

variolation

visiting nurse associations

Advocacy Then

The Henry Street Settlement

Known as the founder of American public health nursing and the originator of the term, Lillian Wald was a staunch advocate of population health nursing. A daughter of a well-to-do Jewish family, she chose nursing as a career and worked for a short time in New York City's Juvenile Asylum. Appalled by the lack of quality care, Wald entered medical school, but left after an exposure to the disease and squalor experienced by immigrant populations in New York City (van Betten & Moriarty, 2004). One day, when called to visit a woman who had been attending a home nursing class she was teaching, Wald encountered the poverty and deprivation in which the family and others around them lived. Wald wrote of her experience, "to me personally it was a call to live near such conditions; to use what power an individual may possess as a citizen to help them." (quoted in Keeling, 2007, p. 6). As a result, she began her lifelong crusade to improve the health of this population by founding the Henry Street Settlement with colleague Mary Brewster in 1893. She believed that by living among their clients, she and other nurses could teach them routine health measures as well as care for their illnesses and refer them to other sources of care. In addition to her work at Henry Street, Wald was active in a number of other reform initiatives related to the health of children, workers, and women and world peace (Hallett, 2010; Judd, 2010). Her peace-related activities included marching in a parade to protest World War I and led to the loss of donor funds for Henry Street (Jewish Women's Archive, 2010).

Advocacy Now

Susie Walking Bear Yellowtail

Born in 1903 on the Montana Crow Indian reservation, Susie Walking Bear Yellowtail was an orphan at the age of 12. In 1923, she became the first Native American registered nurse after graduating from the Boston City Hospital School of Nursing. Returning to the Montana Crow Agency, Ms. Yellowtail worked at the Bureau of Indian Affairs Hospital and later worked for the U.S. Public Health Service.

Experiences of Native American women sterilized without their consent and children dying on their mothers' backs while being carried 20 to 30 miles to a hospital led Ms. Yellowtail to a career of advocacy for Native American health care (*Susie Walking Bear Yellowtail*, RN, 2004). Her advocacy activities encompassed 30 years of midwifery services in the Little Horn Valley and travel to many North American Indian reservations to evaluate health and health care. Through her membership on tribal councils and state health advisory boards, she became well known to health policy makers. She was appointed to the former U.S. Department of Health, Education, and Welfare's Council on Indian Health, the President's Special Council on Aging, and the President's Council on Indian Education and Nutrition, on which she served as an ambassador between her people and the federal government. She and her husband, Tom Yellowtail, also promoted understanding of American Indian culture in Europe and the Middle East as part of a U.S. cultural delegation in 1950 (American Society of Registered Nurses, 2007a; Scozzari, 2009). Throughout her life, she maintained her own cultural heritage, wearing Native American dress and engaging in the artistry of traditional Native American beadwork.

Ms. Yellowtail was also active in promoting the profession of nursing and was the founder of the Native American Nurses Association, which honored her as the "Grandmother of American Indian Nurses" (*Susie Walking Bear Yellowtail*, 2010). Through her advocacy activities at tribal and federal levels, she was able to win funding for nursing education of Native American women.

In 1962, Ms. Yellowtail received the president's Award for Outstanding Nursing Health Care, and six years after her death her picture was included in the Outstanding Montanans Gallery at the Montana State Capitol. Ms. Yellowtail has been included among the 100 most influential Montanans of the 20th century and on July 1, 2002, became the first American Indian nurse admitted to the American Nurses Association Hall of Fame (ANA, n.d.; First American Indian Nurse, n.d.).

The history of population health nursing provides important insights into the events and factors that have shaped our practice. Knowledge of where we have been and how we got where we are today gives us a sense of the present and future directions that population health nursing should take to achieve its goal—improved health for all people. Historical events that gave rise to a concern for the health of population groups influenced the development of both public health science and population health nursing.

Historical Roots

The roots of modern public health and population health nursing practice go far back in history. For 5,000 years different cultural groups have developed a variety of approaches to dealing with common community health problems. Historical records provide evidence of concern for health and prevention of disease in several ancient civilizations. Ancient Mesopotamia, the possible birthplace of humanity, and the Harappan civilization along the Indus River in what is now India employed sewage systems to prevent the spread of disease (Carr, n.d.). Similarly, primitive tribes engaged in public health measures by not burying human wastes where they would contaminate water supplies (Association of State and Territorial Directors of Nursing, 2000). The Egyptians, Romans, and Aztecs were all known to emphasize the importance of clean water supplies. Healing in these ancient civilizations was thought to be the province of supernatural beings, and healers often functioned as priests of healing gods (Hallett, 2010).

The ancient Greeks spent a good deal of time theorizing about health and disease causation. Empedocles of Acragas, who lived from 493 to 433 CE, originated the theory of imbalance among four "humors" as the cause of disease. These four humors (blood, yellow bile, phlegm, and black bile) corresponded to the four elements believed to compose the world (fire, air, water, and earth) as well as to specific temperaments exhibited by individuals (sanguine, choleric, phlegmatic, or melancholic) (Kalisch & Kalisch, 2004). The humoral theory, however, was borrowed and expanded upon a theory of balance between three components of the human body, spirit, phlegm, and bile, derived from 6th century Indian medicine (Reeves, n.d.).

Hippocrates, an eminent Greek physician, rejected the prior concept of disease, as caused by supernatural intervention, in favor of natural causation (Kalisch & Kalisch, 2004). He accepted the theory of the four humors, but believed they were influenced by environmental factors that shaped the physiologic response of people living in specific areas (Watts, 2003).

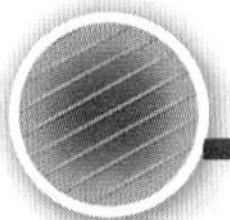

Evidence-Based Practice

A Nursing Historiography

Connolly (2004) presented a history of nursing historiography (the study of nursing history) and noted that research in nursing history, as in other fields of historical inquiry, has evolved in the last several decades. She pointed out that early nursing histories were "only weakly linked to the broader social, economic, and cultural contexts in which events unfolded" (p. 10) and tended to focus on the development of institutions in which nurses worked and the "great women" of nursing. These histories lauded nursing's accomplishments and recounted the profession's "purity, discipline, and faith [but] contained little about the less glorious aspects of the past" (p. 10).

Historians of this genre engaged in "political history," examining how public officials, legislation, and formal mechanisms of local, state, and federal government affected nursing. According to Connolly, history from this perspective assumed a coherence and unanimity in nursing that may not have truly existed. She maintained that early nursing political history, like much of history in general, was written from an elitist point of view and neglected the perspectives of other, less visible groups within and outside nursing.

During the 1960s and 1970s, historical research in general and nursing history in particular began to focus on those unheard voices, and a "social history" perspective was born. Connolly defined social history as "that which focuses on the experience, behavior, and agency of those at society's margins, rather than on its elite" (p. 5). Social historians examined nursing in the context of social factors influencing it (e.g., gender socialization, race relations, etc.).

Connolly recommended melding the two perspectives and examining political influences on nursing and nursing's influence on policy making in the context of social factors that influence both. For example, the Nurse Reinvestment Act could be examined in the light of the social factors that led to the shortage as well as the political history of legislative efforts to resolve past nursing shortages. Both perspectives can provide information that can direct policy development in ways that capitalize on past successes and avoid past mistakes.

1. How might you combine political and social history to examine some of the issues that affect population health nursing today? (As an example, you might examine the nursing shortage in terms of the lack of ethnic diversity in the profession and how current legislation does or does not address this issue.)
2. What other issues can you think of that could be addressed from a combined political/social historical perspective?

There is some controversy regarding which of the writings on health and medicine ascribed to Hippocrates were actually composed by him. There is evidence, however, that he did write the famous treatise entitled *On Airs, Waters, and Places* as well as two books about epidemics in which he expounded on his theory of environmental contributions to disease (Udwadia, 2001).

The humoral theory, along with other selected elements of Hippocratic thinking, was adopted by the famous physician teacher, Galen. Galen's teachings were perpetuated in medical education until well into the Middle Ages, to the point that medical students would discard as anatomic abnormalities dissection evidence that did not support Galen's teachings. Despite his many other contributions, Galen has been credited by some authors with retarding the development of medical science for several hundred years through his erroneous description of blood flow in the body (Reeves, n.d.).

Nursing of the sick at this period in history was primarily the function of the women of the family (Kalisch & Kalisch, 2004). In the case of large and wealthy households, the matron of the family cared for the health needs of both family members and servants or slaves. The care provided, however, was primarily palliative and was only slightly related to today's concept of nursing.

The Influence of Christianity

Christianity, with its ethic of service to others, did a great deal to foster health care for particularly vulnerable populations such as lepers and the poor. Gradually that focus expanded to provision of care to other members of the population (e.g., in the many hospitals and other health-related institutions sponsored by Christian religious groups).

The Early Christian Church

The advent of Christianity brought an emphasis on personal responsibility for the corporal and spiritual welfare of others. Care of the sick was seen as one means of fulfilling this responsibility, and early Christians employed their time and monetary wealth ministering to the sick. Such efforts were intended to provide comfort and material goods to the sick and suffering and bore little resemblance to modern nursing. Such services, although lacking an emphasis on prevention and health promotion or cure, did serve to bring about an awareness of illness within the population.

With the growth of Christianity and charitable giving by Christians, the wealth of the early Christian Church began to accumulate. A large portion of this wealth was used for organized care of the sick and needy through almshouses, asylums, and hospitals rather than through personal visitation to the sick. Hospitals or hospices of this time were not designed exclusively for care of the sick but ministered to all in need, including the sick, the poor, and travelers or pilgrims. The first hospital exclusively for the care of the sick was the Nosocomia, or "house for the sick," established by the Roman matron Fabia in the 4th century (Udwadia, 2001).

The Middle Ages

The mystical tradition of Christianity during the Middle Ages (500–1500 A.D.) led to a decline in population and personal health status. Castigation and neglect of the body to purify the soul resulted in a number of health problems. Many of the health-promotive activities of antiquity were abandoned in favor of fasting and the wearing of sackcloth and ashes. Care of the sick was often undertaken by wise women, women healers who used herbal remedies and extended the usual caring duties of family members (Hallett, 2010).

The need for healthy warriors to fight in the Crusades sparked a slight renewal of interest in health. The Crusades also led to the development of the first hospitals, built in the Holy Land to care for Christian pilgrims and later for wounded Crusaders. The first of these was the Hospital of St. John in Jerusalem. Following the capture of Jerusalem in 1099 by the Christian forces, many Crusader knights were impressed with the care provided at the hospitals and sought to participate in the care of the sick. Their interest eventually led to the establishment of the Knights Hospitalers of St. John of Jerusalem, the first of the religious military orders that were to dominate the provision of nursing care for some time. The establishment of the Hospitalers was followed by the creation of the Knights Templar in 1118 and the Knights of the Teutonic Order in 1190. Interestingly, there were some women involved in the care of the sick under the auspices of female chapters of military orders, such as the Hospitaler Dames of the Order of St. John of Jerusalem (Hallett, 2010).

Following the Crusades, other religious orders were formed to look after the sick. Groups of monks and nuns established hospitals to care for the ill. Initially, these hospitals provided care primarily for members of religious orders and their lay employees. For example, the Benedictine rule required each monastery to have a hospital for the care of ill brothers. Later, religious orders expanded the focus of their services to the sick poor. Care was often provided by secular orders, called "tertiaries," groups of people who did not want to join a religious order, but wished to provide service to others. Village wise women and healers unaffiliated with the church, however, were often subject to witch hunts and hideous deaths (Hallett, 2010).

In many instances, particular orders would focus on the care of specific groups or illnesses. For instance, the Antonites cared for persons with skin conditions, whereas Lazarites emphasized care of those with leprosy (Kalisch & Kalisch, 2004). Thus, the concept of specialization among health care providers is not as recent as one might believe.

Changes in social structure in the Middle Ages led to the development of cities, which increased the potential for the spread of disease. War and the attendant starvation and poor sanitation in cities have been described as the two most significant contributions to disease at this time. During the 14th century, recurring epidemics of plague killed nearly one fourth of the population of Europe. Periodic epidemics led to the establishment of some public health regulations, such as those related to burials and quarantine. Quarantine was first initiated in the city of Ragusa in 1347, then in Venice and Marseilles (Udwadia, 2001). It is interesting to note that the concept of quarantine was developed in Europe by town magistrates, not health care professionals. Similarly, an Egyptian Pasha instituted quarantine regulations in defiance of the recommendations of his French medical advisor (Watts, 2003).

Other Religious Influences

Other religious groups contributed to the health of populations as well. In ancient times, the Jews developed a significant body of health regulations, incorporated into the Book of Leviticus (Association of State and Territorial Directors of Nursing, 2000). Similarly, Jewish physicians are credited with preserving scientific medicine through the Dark Ages by translating Greek and Arabic texts into Latin and promulgating Greco-Arabic medical knowledge in Europe. Similarly, Islamic medicine was a basis for the revival of the medical profession, embodied in the formation of the medical school at Salerno, Italy (Kalisch & Kalisch, 2004). Similarly, Ayurveda, based on traditional Indian philosophies, originated many of the alternative therapies gaining popularity today (Udwadia, 2001).

During the 6th century, nursing was established in Islam by Rufaidah bint Sa'ad. Rufaidah was taught her skills by her physician father and functioned as both nurse and community advocate, seeing to the needs of soldiers wounded in battle as well as the poor and the handicapped. In addition, she taught her nursing skills to other women (Kasule, 2004).

The European Renaissance

From 1500 to 1700, the European Renaissance gave rise to the beginnings of scientific thought. Also evident were the development of a social conscience and early recognition of social responsibility for the health and welfare of the population (Udwadia, 2001). England enacted the first Poor Law in 1601, making families financially responsible for the care of their aged and disabled members and creating publicly funded almshouses for those with no families. This development reflected the concept of "pauper stigma," under which the poor were believed to be responsible for their own condition due to lack of effort. The Belle Vue "pest-house," established in 1794 in Manhattan, was the first public institution developed for the sick in the United States, but charity hospitals were established as early as 1851 (Jonas, Goldsteen, & Goldsteen, 2007). Another development in this period was the collection of vital statistics as a basis for public health policy decisions. Collection of vital statistics was pioneered by Johann Peter Sussmilch in the 1700s and systematized nationally in Sweden in 1748 and in Britain in 1801 (Udwadia, 2001).

For most of the population, nursing was performed by family members. In 1610, however, Saint Francis DeSales and Madame de Chantal established a Parisian voluntary organization of well-to-do women to care for the sick in their homes. Care of the sick was institutionalized by some orders in the vows of consecration. For example, the Sisters of Charity, established in Paris in 1633 by Saint Vincent de Paul and Mademoiselle Louise De Marillac, and the Sisters of Bon Secours, established in 1822, took a fourth vow to care for the sick in addition to the traditional vows of poverty, chastity, and obedience (Hallett, 2010; Kalisch & Kalisch, 2004).

During the Protestant reformation, the monastic orders and the hospitals they provided were dismantled in Protestant countries. Health care in nations that retained their Roman Catholic heritage continued to be provided by religious orders and independent healers, particularly women in rural areas, continued to be persecuted (Hallett, 2010).

A New World

The discovery and colonization of the American continents led to different health issues and solutions to them. Communicable disease and poor health habits, for instance, traveled across the oceans in both directions. Native Americans were devastated by such diseases as measles and smallpox brought by European settlers (Hogan, Harchelroad, & McGovern, 2005). Europeans, on the other hand, took tobacco back with them.

The Colonial Period

While new avenues of scientific thought were being opened in Europe, some of the ideas generated were being translated into a new way of life on a new continent. Some groups of colonists included members of religious orders who provided care for the sick and injured. For example, Jeanne Mance and the Grey nuns nursed those wounded in battles between French soldiers and the Iroquois, and Dutch deaconesses were among the early settlers in New Amsterdam. Early hospitals, however, were frequently linked to poor houses and care was often provided by the untrained paupers residing in them (Hallett, 2010).

In the early colonial period in America, the health status of the colonists was good compared with that of their European counterparts, and longevity approached today's figures. The relative good health of the population was primarily due to low population density and, interestingly, poor transportation. Communities remained relatively isolated, and the spread of communicable diseases, the major health problem of the era, was curtailed by lack of movement between population groups.

Because doctors were few, health care was primarily a function of the family. Nursing care in the United States was most often provided by the women of the family, with assistance from neighbors where this was possible. The Sisters of Charity also provided services to the sick in the United States, starting in 1809 under the direction of Mother Elizabeth Seton (Kalisch & Kalisch, 2004). In Canada, public health practice was carried out by Christian religious orders as early as the 17th century.

Early Public Health Efforts

The growth of population centers led to concern for sanitation and vital statistics, the foci of early public health efforts in the colonies. In 1639, both Massachusetts and Plymouth colonies mandated the reporting of all births and deaths, instituting the official reporting of vital statistics in what would later become the United States. Environmental health and sanitation were also of concern in the early colonies. Concern for the spread of communicable diseases was manifested in the establishment of "pesthouses" for people with contagious conditions (Kalisch & Kalisch, 2004) as well as isolation and quarantine measures.

For the most part, health was seen as a personal responsibility with little governmental involvement. Temporary boards of health were established in response to specific health problems, usually epidemics of communicable disease, and were disbanded after the crisis had passed.

Recognition of the need for a consistent and organized approach to health problems was growing, however, and in 1797, the state of Massachusetts granted local jurisdictions legal authority to establish health services and regulations. The following year, Congress passed the Act for Relief of Sick and Disabled Seamen to create hospitals for the care of members of the merchant marine. The group of hospitals created under this Act was renamed the Marine Hospital Service in 1871. Responsibility for quarantine was shifted to the Marine Hospital Service in 1878 as one of the first efforts to deal with health problems at a national, rather than state or local, level (Jonas et al., 2007).

Nursing during this period remained a function of the family. Although the care given was primarily palliative, the women of the house might also engage in some health-promotive practices, such as regular purging with castor oil. Treatment tended to consist of home remedies, and the literature of the era is replete with housewives' recipes for the treatment of a variety of ailments.

In 1813, the Ladies' Benevolent Society of Charleston, South Carolina, was established. This was the first organized approach to home nursing of the sick in the United States. This organization was initiated in response to a yellow fever epidemic and was completely nondenominational and nondiscriminatory in an era characterized by widespread racial discrimination. Care was provided to the sick in their homes by upper-class women. Because these women had no background in nursing, care focused on relieving suffering and providing material aid (Buhler-Wilkerson, 2001). With the exception of a 20-year period during and after the Civil War, the Ladies' Benevolent Society provided services until the 1950s.

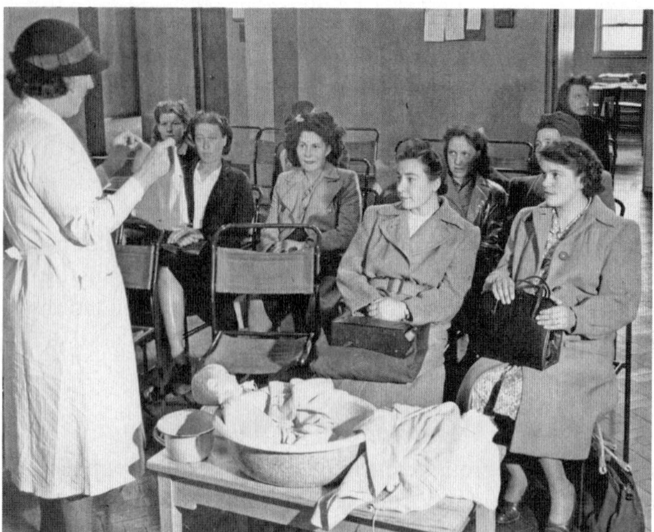

Population health nurses often demonstrated appropriate hygiene practices as well as teaching about them. *(Popperfoto/Getty Images)*

A similar service was instituted in 1819 in Philadelphia's Jewish community by the Hebrew Female Benevolent Society of Philadelphia. This service was organized by Rebecca Gratz, a Jewish society woman who engaged in nursing activities within her own family and later initiated a number of community service activities directed toward poor Jewish women and children (Ashton, 2009).

Another early attempt at home care nursing also saw upper-class women visiting the homes of indigent women during childbirth. The Lying-in Charity for Attending Indigent Women in Their Home was established in 1828 by Dr. Joseph Warrington to assist poor women during and after delivery. Dr. Warrington also established the Philadelphia Nurse Society to train women in obstetric nursing, who then provided services to this population (Obstetrics, n.d.).

The Industrial Revolution

The Industrial Revolution profoundly influenced health in both Europe and the United States. Movement, on both continents, from agricultural to industrial economies led to the development of large industrial centers and the need for a large workforce to labor under unhealthy conditions in mines, mills, and factories. By 1850, half of England's population lived in urban areas (Watts, 2003). The demand for manufactured goods and the necessity to get goods to market prompted advancements in transportation, which increased mobility and the potential for spreading communicable diseases. In the United States, rural–urban migration and the presence of large contingents of poor immigrants led initially to the conversion of single-family dwellings in less affluent areas of town and then to the development of crowded tenement

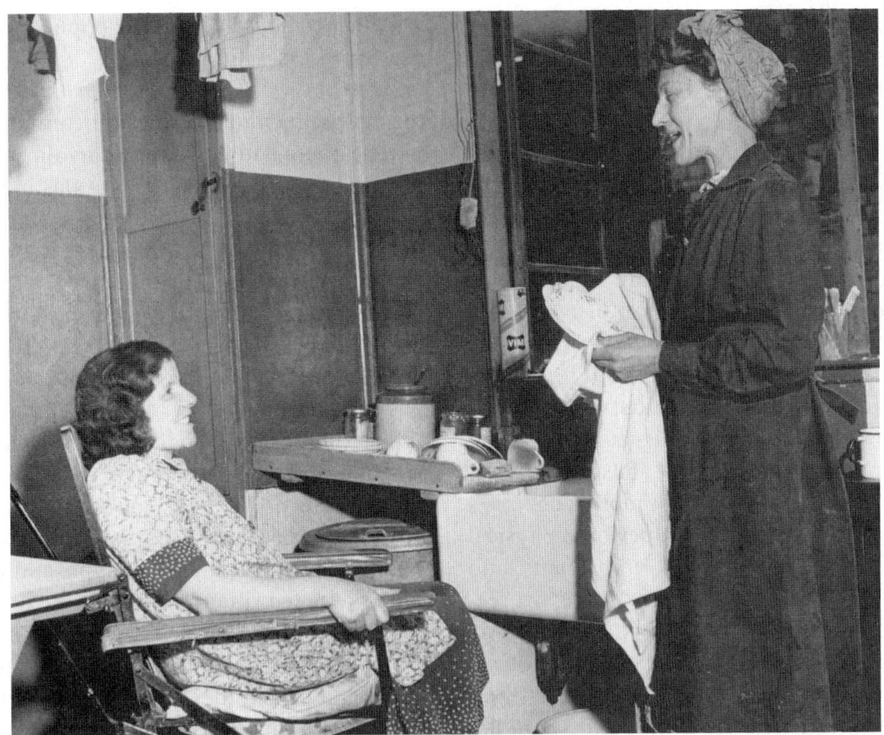

Many families who received population health nursing services lived in a single room.
(Popperfoto/Getty Images)

houses (Fee, Brown, Lazarus, & Theerman, 2002). From 1820 to 1910, 30 million immigrants came to the United States, representing almost half of the populations of urban slums in major U.S. cities. By the mid-1890s, for example, two thirds of the population of New York City lived in 90,000 tenement houses (Kalisch & Kalisch, 2004).

The poor were overworked and underpaid. Poor nutrition contributed to increased incidence of a variety of diseases, particularly tuberculosis. Recognition of tuberculosis as a growing problem among the poor led to the creation of the first tuberculosis hospital in England in 1840 (Zilm & Warbinek, 1995). The use of children in the workforce, coupled with low wages, inadequate food, and hazardous living and working conditions, led to many preventable illnesses and deaths among the children of the poor. In the 1870 census, more than 750,000 working children were recorded. This number does not include children of farm families who often worked alongside their parents. In 1930, the Fair Labor Standards Act abolished child labor (excluding farm labor) in the United States, but this practice remains rampant in other parts of the world (Helfand, Lazarus, & Theerman, 2001).

The 19th century saw a beginning recognition of the effects of these social and economic conditions on health, and the concept of social responsibility for public health began to take root. The growth of this concept was fostered by the publication in the mid-1800s of several landmark reports. The first of these publications was C. Turner Thackrah's treatise on occupational health, *The Effects of Arts, Trades, and Professions . . . on Health and Longevity*. In this document, Thackrah described the effects of working conditions on health.

In 1842, Edwin Chadwick's *Inquiry into the Sanitary Conditions of the Labouring Population of Great Britain* provided additional fuel for efforts to change the working and social conditions that contributed to disease. Chadwick's committee recommended extensive changes to sanitation practices, particularly removal of sewage and other noxious toxins (Del Col, 2002). Chadwick's report led to sanitary engineering solutions, and annual local government spending for sanitary improvements increased from £5 million in 1856–1871 to £30 million by 1910 (Watts, 2003). Chadwick's report heralded a shift in the view of public health from one of social reform to one of sanitary engineering.

While Thackrah and Chadwick addressed the effects of working conditions on health and instigated reforms to prevent disease, Henry W. Rumsey focused on health promotion. Rumsey's *Essays on State Medicine* emphasized health promotion and illness prevention as social obligations of government. Some nations acted on this concept by establishing national health care systems. For example, Germany instituted a state-funded medical insurance program for working men and civil servants as early as 1869. Similar attempts were initiated in Britain in the 1860s, but the National Health Insurance

Act was not passed until 1911 (Sigerist, 2003; Watts, 2003). In the United States, national health insurance was an element of Theodore Roosevelt's election platform in 1912 (Jonas et al., 2007).

Documents similar to those of Rumsey, Chadwick, and Thackrah were also published in the United States. The Massachusetts Sanitary Commission was established in response to concern over the effects of crowded living conditions, poverty, and poor sanitation on health. In 1850, Lemuel Shattuck drafted the commission's findings (Koslow, 2002). The *Report of the Massachusetts Sanitary Commission* included recommendations for establishing state and local health departments, systematic collection of vital statistics, and sanitation inspections, and for instituting programs for school health and control of mental illness, alcohol abuse, and tuberculosis. Other recommendations included public education regarding sanitation, control of nuisances, periodic physical examinations, supervision of the health of immigrants, and construction of model tenements. In addition, the report recommended improved education for nurses and the inclusion of content on preventive medicine and sanitation in medical school curricula.

The publication of the *Report of the Massachusetts Sanitary Commission* marks the beginning of public health practice as we know it today (Koslow, 2002). Recommendations of the report form the basis for much of the present work of official state and local public health agencies. The eventual effect of the commission's report was the establishment of state boards of health. The first state board was established in Louisiana in the early 1800s (Louisiana Department of Environmental Quality, n.d.), but was not developed along the lines recommended in the report. In 1869, nearly 90 years after the advent of the first temporary boards of health and 19 years after the publication of Shattuck's report, Massachusetts established the first working board of health (Commonwealth of Massachusetts, 1870), followed by California in 1870 (Timeline, California Board of Health, n.d.).

Collection of vital statistics at the national level was another activity undertaken in the latter half of the 19th century. The first national mortality statistics, for example, were published by the U.S. federal government in 1850 (Epidemiology Program Office, 1999).

During this period, great strides were made in the fledgling science of epidemiology. In 1854, without knowledge of the nature of the causative organism, John Snow determined the source of a London epidemic of cholera to be something in the water of the Broad Street pump (Centers for Disease Control and Prevention [CDC], 2004; Robinson, 2009). Jacob Henle was the first to postulate microorganisms as a cause of disease rather than miasmas (harmful vapors) or humors (Paneth, n.d.). It was not, however, until 1876 that Louis Pasteur and Robert Koch, working independently, identified specific bacteria (Watts, 2003). These and other epidemiologic findings allowed more scientific measures to be applied to the control of communicable disease and contributed greatly to the armamentarium used by later population health nurses in preventing disease.

Another significant advance in public health practice was the development of vaccines for communicable diseases. Early practitioners had developed **variolation**, a process in which material from smallpox lesions was inoculated into the skin, nose, or veins of a healthy person to induce immunity. The first recorded instance of variolation involved the activities of a Buddhist nun at the beginning of the second millennium. In 1713, the Greek physician Timoni submitted a report on variolation to the Royal Society, but his conclusions were ignored until Lady Mary Montagu, wife of the British Ambassador to Turkey, wrote about her use of the practice for her children and recommended it to the British royal family (Riedel, 2005). Variolation was widely practiced in the Orient and was used by some European physicians but was not widely accepted. Edward Jenner later used material from cowpox lesions to vaccinate people against smallpox, and this process was more widely adopted (Brannon, 2004).

In 1888, Emil Von Behring used immune serum to provide protection against diphtheria. Tetanus toxoid was introduced in 1914, and vaccines for other communicable diseases followed (Immunization Action Coalition, n.d.). Some of the significant events in the development of public health prior to the 20th century are summarized in Table 2-1●.

Organized advocacy for the health of the population by public health professionals began in 1872 with the establishment of the American Public Health Association (APHA). APHA consists of members of more than 50 public health disciplines and is the oldest and largest association of public health professionals in the world (APHA, 2010a). Throughout its history, APHA has focused on the development of standards and policies that promote population health. APHA is organized

TABLE 2-1 Significant Public Health Events Prior to the 20th Century

Date	Event
1347	Quarantine first instituted in Ragusa, Italy.
1797	Jurisdiction to establish local boards of health first granted in Massachusetts.
1798	Marine Hospital Service, forerunner of the U.S. Public Health Service, created.
1854	Contaminated water demonstrated to be the cause of cholera by John Snow.
1869	State-funded medical insurance instituted for German workers. First modern state board of health established in Massachusetts.
1872	American Public Health Association established.
1876	Specific bacteria first isolated by Koch and Pasteur.
1888	Immune serum first used to prevent diphtheria.

in 27 discipline-based sections and 8 special interest groups that cut across disciplines (APHA, 2010c). The APHA section of greatest interest to population health nurses is the Public Health Nursing Section, developed to provide leadership in population health nursing practice, policy development, and research (APHA, 2010b).

Nursing in War

Throughout history, war has necessitated the care of sick and injured combatants. Nursing, as a profession has been actively involved in these efforts from the time of the crusader orders dedicated to the care of the sick. Florence Nightingale first gained prominence for her work with the British Army in the Crimean war, but other nurses were actively involved in that conflict as well. For example, several groups of Roman Catholic nuns and Protestant nursing sisters were part of Nightingale's contingent.

Jamaican-born self-proclaimed "nurse-doctress" Mary Seacole also volunteered to join Nightingale in her efforts. Her offer was repeatedly rejected, however, perhaps because of her Creole background. Seacole learned her nursing skills in apprenticeship with her mother, a boarding house mistress, and many of her treatments involved herbal remedies (Hallett, 2010). Using her own funds, she traveled to the Crimea and established the British Hotel in Balaclava, where she cared for injured officers. Seacole also ventured onto the battlefields to provide care to injured soldiers on both sides of the conflict. She also provided care during cholera and yellow fever epidemics in Jamaica and Panama and later cared for employees of a mining camp run by a relative (Lewis, 2010a). In recognition of her contributions, Seacole has been designated the greatest Black Briton (Anionwu, 2006).

In the United States, nurses were actively involved from the beginning of American Independence. In fact, George Washington called for the employment of women to care for the colonial army at a salary of $2 per month. Most of their work entailed washing and cooking for the troops, but these women and camp followers were also involved in the care of the ill and injured (Sitzman, 2010). Nurses were involved in official and unofficial capacities during both the Spanish American and American Civil wars. For example, Anna Maxwell, known as the "American Florence Nightingale," organized the nurses who cared for soldiers wounded in the Spanish American war at Camp Thomas, Georgia. Maxwell and 160 nurses cared for more than 1,000 men affected by typhoid, malaria, and measles, with only 67 deaths. Maxwell also organized nurses for Red Cross units during World War I and supported military rank for nurses in the Army Nurse Corps (Hanink, 2010a).

During the American Civil War, more than 2,000 nurses were engaged in the care of the sick and wounded on both sides. Care was initially provided for the northern army by Roman Catholic nursing orders, but their numbers proved insufficient to meet the need. Perhaps the two most famous of the Civil War nurses were Dorothea Dix and Clara Barton, both of whom gained nursing experience within their families. Dorothea Dix was a social reformer who did much to improve the conditions of people with mental illness in institutions throughout the nation (Bumb, n.d.). During the war, she was engaged by the federal government to establish a volunteer nursing service and served as superintendent of female nurses for the army (Hallett, 2010). Many of the volunteer nurses, such as Walt Whitman and Louisa May Alcott, had no formal nursing education, but had cared for sick family members. Whitman entered the war to care for his purportedly injured brother and stayed to care for other sick and injured soldiers, supporting himself as a paymaster's clerk in the interim (Hallett, 2010).

Clara Barton entered the war as a private citizen to gather needed food and medical supplies (American Red Cross, 2014). Known as the "Angel of the Battlefield," Barton and one other nurse cared for 3,000 injured after the Battle of Bull Run. Barton later served as the first woman to run a U.S. government office, the Office of Correspondence with the Friends of the Missing Men of the United States Army, in her rôle locating missing Civil War soldiers (Behling, n.d.). Barton was also instrumental in the establishment of the Red Cross of the United States of America (Hallett, 2010). Harriet Tubman was a former slave who also functioned as a nurse during the Civil War (Lewis, n.d.b). She is probably best known for her activities with the underground railroad in bringing approximately 300 former slaves to freedom in the north (Lewis, n.d.a). In addition, Tubman organized a spy network for the north and personally led troops during the Combahee River expedition to disrupt southern supply lines (Lewis, n.d.b). Following the war, Tubman was active in women's suffrage activities and in advocacy and service to aged and poor African Americans (Lewis, n.d.c; Ripley & Hembree, 1992). Sojourner Truth was another African American who served during the Civil War and then for the Freedman's Relief Association during reconstruction (Aetna, 2003).

District Nursing in England

The "three great revolutions" of the late 18th and early 19th centuries—the intellectual revolution, the French and American political revolutions, and the Industrial Revolution—set the stage for the development of population health nursing. In England, the same spirit that motivated industrial and prison reform led to concern for the health of large urban populations and the development of nursing practices to address these concerns.

In addition to being the acknowledged founder of modern hospital nursing, Florence Nightingale was instrumental in the development of population health or district nursing. Nightingale received her training in nursing at the school for deaconesses established by Theodor Fliedner. Fliedner's second wife, Caroline Bertheau, conceived the idea of extending the nursing services offered in the hospital to the sick in their homes. This concept influenced Nightingale, who endorsed the idea of health promotion as well as home care for illness (Hallett, 2010).

In 1840, Elizabeth Frye, a Quaker woman, founded the Institution of Nursing Sisters in London to train lower-class women to provide care to the sick poor. Their training consisted of 3 months of work in London hospitals. Frye was also actively involved in attempts by reformers to improve conditions in British prisons (Hallett, 2010).

William Rathbone, another Quaker philanthropist, instituted professional home care for the sick poor in Liverpool in 1859 after seeing the effectiveness of a trained nurse in caring for his dying wife. Although in the early days of the experiment, the nurse hired was often tempted to leave, the initiative was considered a success and spread to other cities in England (Kalisch & Kalisch, 2004). Unable to recruit sufficient trained nurses on his own, Rathbone turned to Florence Nightingale for assistance. Nightingale was instrumental in developing the concept of visiting nursing and viewed public health nursing as including specific nursing care for the sick poor as well as attention to environmental and sanitation issues. The nursing services provided were organized in terms of local districts—hence the term *district nursing* (Buhler-Wilkerson, 2001). Similar services were also provided by the Ladies Sanitary Association in Manchester and Salford. In 1928, certification by the Royal Sanitary Institute was made mandatory for health visitors (Hallett, 2010).

The need to standardize population health nursing services was recognized early in the development of district nursing. A committee chaired by Rathbone undertook to conduct a study of district nursing services coordinated by Florence Lee, a nurse trained in one of the Nightingale schools. Lee's report, published in 1875, noted that many visiting nurses were not adequately trained, that their practice included responsibilities beyond hospital nursing, and that they required additional training. In addition, Lee recommended the employment of educated women for district nursing services. The report led to the formation in 1876 of the Metropolitan and National Nursing Association for Providing Trained Nurses for the Sick Poor (Hallett, 2010). Prior to the employment of professional nurses to visit the sick poor, home visiting often provided the opportunity for proselytizing and attempts to convert the client to a specific religious persuasion or to redeem them from moral decrepitude.

Visiting Nurses in America and the World

In the United States, proselytizing was also part of the role of women who visited the sick poor in their homes, providing for their material needs. These women were often ill prepared to meet illness care needs, however; so wealthy women in several large cities hired trained nurses to visit the sick. For example, the Women's Branch of the New York City Mission first employed trained nurses to provide home visiting services in 1877 (Kalisch & Kalisch, 2004). The role of these and many other **missionary nurses** was to provide nursing care and religious instruction for the sick poor. Often, visiting of the sick was motivated by beliefs that poverty was a result of moral deficiency and that the poor needed exposure to the "elevating experience of their moral betters" (Buhler-Wilkerson, 2001, p. 18).

In 1839, the Nurse Society of Philadelphia received referrals from physicians to care for women after delivery. Their services were later expanded to care for medical and surgical patients (Hallett, 2010). In the next few years, **visiting nurse associations**, agencies that provided nursing care to people in their homes, were established in Buffalo (1885) (Visiting Nursing Association of Western New York, 2010), and in Boston and Philadelphia (1886) (Visiting Nurse Association of Boston, 2010; Visiting Nurse Association of Greater Philadelphia, 2010). The Philadelphia agency was the first to institute a nurse's uniform, a fee for services, and a community nursing supervisor. The Boston Instructive District Nursing Association emphasized the population health nurse's educative function as well as the role in the care of the sick (Kalisch & Kalisch, 2004), signaling the beginning of the health promotion emphasis that now characterizes population health nursing. By 1890, there were 21 visiting nursing organizations in the United States (Kalisch & Kalisch, 2004), and 22 years later, when the National Organization for Public Health Nursing (NOPHN) was founded, there were 3,000 visiting nurses in the United States (Winslow, 1993).

Similar events were taking place in Canada, with the establishment of the Victorian Order of Nurses (VON) in 1897. VON nurses were required to have basic nursing preparation and additional education in community work. In 1898, the VON sent four district nurses to the Klondyke region, who were faced with a typhoid epidemic on their arrival. In addition, Canadian Red Cross outposts provided public health and midwifery services in remote parts of the frontier (Hallett, 2010).

In Australia, the Bush Nursing Associations were initiated in 1910 by philanthropic women to provide trained nurses for local communities who would pay their salaries (Hallett, 2010). Plunket Society nurses offered visiting nurse services for mothers and their children in New Zealand, starting in 1907. The society was established by volunteer groups of women with some government support and minimal medical supervision (Bryder, 2002). On a global level, the International Council of Nurses was founded in 1899, with the help of Mrs. Bedford Fenwick, to address international nursing issues (Hallett, 2010).

Nursing and the Settlement Houses

The settlement movement was based on the belief espoused by Arnold Toynbee that educated persons could promote learning, morality, and civic responsibility in the poor by living among them and sharing certain aspects of their poverty. Reformers, acting on this belief, "settled" in homes in the London slums with the idea that their poor neighbors would learn through watching their behavior (Lewis, 2010b).

In the United States, the settlement idea was adapted by nurses such as Lillian Wald, who believed that the most effective way to bring health care to the poor immigrant population was for nurses to live and work among them. Accordingly, Wald and her associate Mary Brewster established the forerunner of the Henry Street Settlement from their Jefferson Street tenement apartment in New York City in 1893 (Kalisch & Kalisch, 2004). The actual Henry Street establishment was purchased in 1895. The house on Henry Street differed from many other settlement houses of the era in its incorporation of visiting nurse services. In addition, visiting nurse services in the United States differed from those in England in their acceptance of the germ theory and its use as a foundation for many of their interventions.

The Henry Street Settlement is usually considered the first American public health agency because of its incorporation of modern concepts of population health nursing. At Henry Street, Wald redefined the basic principles of home care. She believed that access to the services of a nurse should be determined by the client and not based on a decision by a physician (Keeling, 2007). In spite of the focus on health promotion at the Henry Street Settlement, Wald contended that the primary function of the visiting nurse was care of the sick in their homes, with health education as a secondary focus. She also felt that care of the poor should be equivalent to that available to the rich and that services provided should respect the client's individual dignity and independence (Buhler-Wilkerson, 2001). The latter principle led her to establish a 3-month probationary period for nurses employed at Henry Street to orient the nurses to the culture of the immigrant populations they served (Kalisch & Kalisch, 2004). Although the nurses were expected to view other cultures with tolerance, they often experienced culture shock that subsided as they were exposed to a variety of different cultures (Keeling, 2007).

The nurses of the Henry Street Settlement did more than visit the sick in their homes. Lillian Wald coined the term *public health nurse* to reflect the focus on service to the whole community to improve both individual and societal conditions affecting health (Fee & Bu, 2010). Health promotion and disease prevention were heavily emphasized, as was political activism. In Wald's words, "The call of the nurse is not only for bedside care of the sick, but to help in seeking out the deep-lying basic causes of illness and misery. That in the future, there may be less sickness to nurse and cure" (quoted in Buhler-Wilkerson, 2001, p. 98). Wald herself was a prime example of the political activist, supporting many changes in social conditions that would benefit the health of the public (Jewish Women's Archive, 2010). In fact, the Henry Street Settlement served as the site for the opening reception of the 1909 National Negro Conference, one of the few places that would host an interracial gathering. This conference led to the establishment of the National Association for the Advancement of Colored People (NAACP) (Buhler-Wilkerson, 2001).

Other early population health nurses like Margaret Sanger, Clara Barton, and Dorothea Dix were also actively involved in promoting social change. Margaret Sanger's contributions to contraceptive services for women are addressed in more detail in Chapter 18∞. Care at Henry Street was often provided under standing orders that allowed the nurses to avoid charges of practicing medicine without a license. Charges were further defused by pointing out that services were usually provided to those who could not afford a doctor and were not in competition with local physicians. The nurses "used both physician-prescribed medications and middle-class household remedies as they attended lower-class patients and their families. In essence, they practiced somewhere between pharmacists and physicians, between domestic care and professional care" (Keeling, 2007, p. 11).

The nurses of Henry Street, like other population health nursing pioneers, were able to accomplish more in the way of social activism than their hospital counterparts because their practice was essentially free of external control (Buhler-Wilkerson, 2001). In fact, the Henry Street nurses have been described as "virtually independent practitioners in sick and preventive care, health, education, and school nursing" in an era when other nurses were experiencing medical domination (Roberts & Group, 1995, p. 82).

Other nursing settlement houses patterned on the Henry Street model were established. One particularly inspiring example was the Nurse's Settlement established in 1900 in Richmond, Virginia, by nurses working at the Old Dominion Hospital. These nurses had been exposed to the needs of Richmond's poor during student experiences and were concerned about clients discharged too soon from the hospital. Services were provided by the eight founding nurses during their after-work hours (Instructive Visiting Nurse Association, 2008). The settlement they founded differed from the Henry Street Settlement in that it did not have any wealthy patrons to provide support and was initiated with the limited resources of the graduates themselves and on money raised from renting out rooms in the house as well as donations from local churches and women's groups. Like Henry Street, the Richmond settlement focused on health promotion and education as well as care of the sick (Green, 2005).

Expanding the Focus on Prevention

The effectiveness of population health nurses in preventing sickness and death among the poor was recognized and became the basis for visiting nurse services offered by the Metropolitan Life Insurance Company. This program was begun at the instigation of Lillian Wald. Wald convinced the Metropolitan board that providing nursing services to its policyholders would improve the public image of an industry tarnished by economic scandal. The compelling argument, though, was evidence that community health nursing reduced mortality and would limit the death benefits paid by the company. Services were begun on an experimental basis in 1909 at a cost to the company of 50 cents per visit. The 3-month experiment was such a success that the program was extended nationwide in 1911 (Buhler-Wilkerson, 2001) and continued to provide services until 1953. In 1923 alone, the nurses made more than 37,000 visits, and by 1926, more than 300,000 visits were made each year (Keeling, 2007). This association with the business world was an education for population health nurses, who had no conception of marketing or the economic bases for programs. The program was finally discontinued because of nursing's failure to grasp economic realities and the realization of diminishing returns by the insurance company.

The emphasis of population health nursing on health promotion began with health education in the home during visits to the poor in large cities. Gradually, however, the concepts of health promotion and illness prevention were expanded to other population groups to include services to mothers and young children, school-age youngsters, employees, and the rural population.

Concern for the health of mothers and children was growing, and the nurses of the Henry Street Settlement and other similar programs spent a large portion of their time in health promotion for this group of clients. Because they recognized that services to individual families would not overcome the effects of poverty, they worked actively to improve social conditions affecting health. Through the efforts of Lillian Wald and other social activists, the first White House Conference on Children was held in 1909. As a result of the conference, the U.S. Children's Bureau was established in 1912 to address the issue of child labor. Its efforts were later expanded to encompass a variety of initiatives related to child health (Judd, 2010).

School nursing, another arena for health promotion, actually began in London in 1893 (Wolfe & Selekman, 2002) and was introduced in the United States by Lillian Wald in 1902. The initial impetus for school health nursing was the high level of school absenteeism due to illness. In New York City in 1902, 15 to 20 children per school were being sent home daily. In response, Wald assigned Lina Rogers Struthers from the Henry Street Settlement to a pilot project in school nursing. Because of the overwhelming success of the project (a 90% decline in school exclusions in the first year), the New York Board of Health absorbed the program and hired additional nurses to continue the work (Hanink, 2010b; Kalisch & Kalisch, 2004). The program resulted in school exclusion only for those children who were not able to be treated in "dressing rooms" at the schools, where the nurses provided treatments under protocols or "cards of instruction" developed by

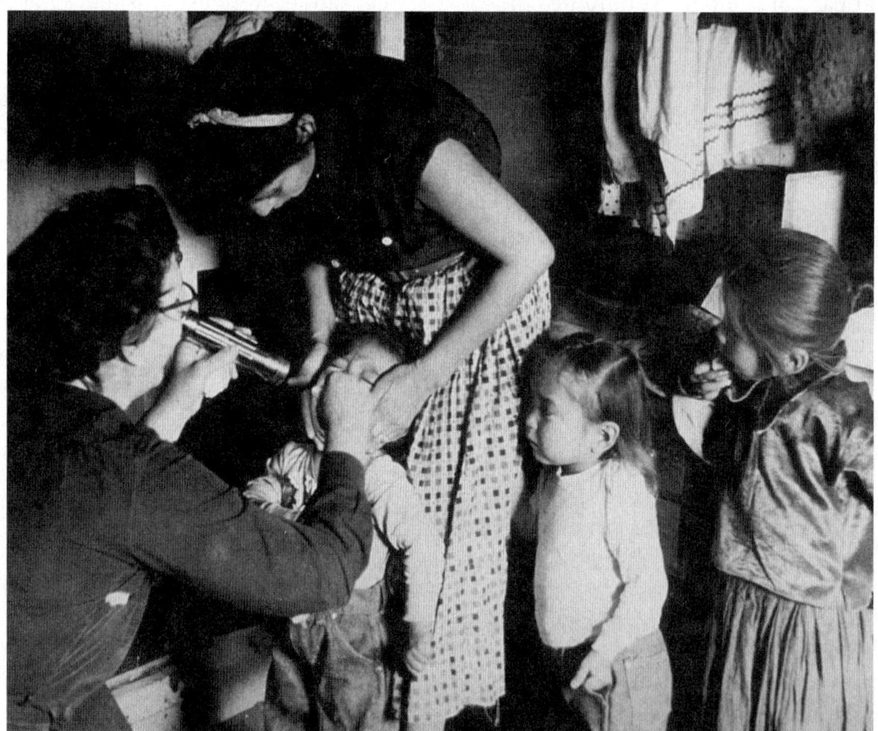

In addition to school inspections, population health nurses made home visits to children excluded from school for communicable diseases. *(National Library of Medicine.)*

the New York City Department of Health. After school hours, the nurses made home visits to the families of the children (Keeling, 2007).

The concept of school nursing spread to other parts of the country and to Canada. In 1904, Los Angeles became the first of many municipalities to employ nurses in schools (Spotsylvania County Public Schools, 2009). In 1907, Canada initiated medical inspections of schoolchildren in Ontario. Later Lina Rogers moved from New York City to Toronto to supervise the school inspection efforts (Rutty & Sullivan, 2010).

Early school nursing focused on preventing the spread of communicable diseases and treating ailments related to compulsory school life. More recently, however, the focus has shifted to preventive and promotive activities, including case finding, integrating health concepts into school curricula, and maintaining a healthful school environment, as well as caring for sick children.

The first rural nursing service was established in 1896 in Westchester County, New York, by Ellen Morris Wood and was followed in 1906 by the initiation of a nursing service for both the poor and the well-to-do of Salisbury, Connecticut. Despite her usual sphere of activity in the city, Lillian Wald was also involved in the growth of rural population health nursing. She convinced the American Red Cross, founded in 1881, to direct its peacetime attention to expanding community health services in rural America. In 1912, the Red Cross established the Rural Nursing Service (later the Town and Country Nursing Service) to extend population health nursing services to rural areas (Kalisch & Kalisch, 2004). In Canada, rural nursing services were provided to large immigrant populations by such organizations as the Victorian Order of Nurses for Canada and the Canadian Red Cross Society (Hallett, 2010).

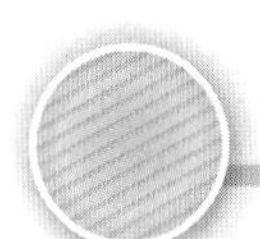

Global Perspectives

Developing the Role of the Population Health Nurse

Cho and Kashka (2004) described the contributions of Korean nurse leader Mo Im Kim in the development of a population health nurse practitioner role to meet the needs of rural communities in Korea. Kim's vision of the skills needed for population health nursing included political acumen, program management, and community leadership. The authors' description of Kim's activities in the development and support of the rural population health nurse practitioner role provides an excellent example of advocacy for the specialty itself.

Explore how population health nursing practice has developed in another country. What events led to the development of the role? What factors have influenced how the population health nursing role is conceptualized in that country?

Another pioneer in the provision of health services in rural settings was Mary Breckenridge. In 1928, Breckenridge initiated the Frontier Nursing Service (FNS) in the remote areas of rural Appalachia (American Society of Registered Nurses, 2007b). The FNS provided midwifery services by nurses who traveled on horseback and served families in isolated rural Appalachia. An assessment of its outcomes in the first 1,000 cases indicated no maternal mortality and fewer stillbirths and infant deaths than in the general population (Kalisch & Kalisch, 2004). Although midwifery was the primary focus of the FNS, the nurses provided a variety of other services from health education to pulling teeth (Hallett, 2010).

Other largely rural populations experiencing significant health problems were the Native American population on federal reservations and the African Americans in the South. Population health nursing services on the reservations arose out of a 1922 study of health conditions by the American Red Cross commissioned by the Bureau of Indian Affairs (Ruffing-Rahal, 1995). Nurses in this setting often found themselves breaking official rules in order to provide effectively for the needs of their clients (Abel, 1996). To meet the needs of Black women in the South, some states co-opted local Black midwives to work closely with public health nurses. As on the reservations, the rules imposed frequently violated accepted cultural health practices. For example, the nurses "forbade midwives to use any folk medicine or herbal remedies in their childbirth work" (Smith, 1994, p. 31). In spite of the cultural insensitivity displayed, the partnership between public health nurses and midwives helped to create a modern public health system in the rural South. In Arkansas, for example, Mamie Odessa Hale Garland was made a midwife consultant and developed a training and supervision program for untrained lay midwives, resulting in dramatic declines in maternal and infant mortality. Later, her work led to the establishment of maternal–child clinics in several counties throughout the state (Bell, 2010).

Occupational health nursing provided another avenue for health promotion by population health nurses. This specialty area began in 1895 when Vermont's Governor Proctor employed nurses to see to the health needs of villages where employees of his Vermont Marble Company lived. These first employment-based services focused on care of the sick rather than prevention and care of occupation-related conditions (Kalisch & Kalisch, 2004). In 1897, the Employees' Benefit Association of John Wanamaker's department store in New York City hired nurses to visit employees' homes. These nurses soon expanded their role to include first aid and prevention of illness and injury in the work setting.

Dying clients constitute another more recent population for which population health nursing services are required. The hospice movement, initiated in London in 1967 by Cecily Saunders, was established in the United States by Florence Wald in 1974 (Hallett, 2010). Wald founded the Connecticut Hospice to provide interdisciplinary services to dying clients, both in their homes and in hospital settings. From this beginning, there are now more than 2,500 independent hospice centers in the United States (American Society of Registered Nurses, 2007c). More recently, care has been expanded to palliation of long-term symptoms such as chronic pain, for both terminal and nonterminal clients, and in 2007 the Worldwide Palliative Care Alliance was formed to address end-of-life issues at the global level (National Hospice and Palliative Care Organization, 2010).

Standardizing Practice

The need to standardize population health nursing practice was recognized in both the United States and England. Early American attempts to standardize visiting nursing services included publications related to public health nursing and the development of a national logo by the Cleveland Visiting Nurse Association (VNA). This logo, or seal, was made available to any visiting nurse organization that met established standards. Both the Chicago (1906) and Cleveland (1909) VNAs published newsletters titled *Visiting Nurse Quarterly* to aid attempts to standardize care (Brainerd, 1985). Another attempt to standardize practice was the development of a list of standing orders for public health nurses by the Chicago Visiting Nurse Association in 1912 (Kalisch & Kalisch, 2004).

In 1911, a joint committee of the American Nurses Association (ANA) and the Society for Superintendents of Training Schools for Nurses met to consider the need for standardization. The result was a second meeting, held in 1912. Letters inviting representation were sent to 1,092 organizations employing visiting nurses at that time. These organizations included VNAs, city and state boards of health and education, private clubs and societies, tuberculosis leagues, hospitals and dispensaries, businesses, settlements and day nurseries, churches, and charitable organizations. A total of 69 agencies responded with their intent to send a representative to the meeting. The result of this second meeting was the formation of the National Organization for Public Health Nursing (NOPHN) (Brainerd, 1985). The objective of this organization was to provide for stimulation and standardization of public health nursing. This was the first professional body in the United States to include lay membership. Similar activity was undertaken in Canada, leading to the creation in 1920 of the public health section of the Canadian Association of Trained Nurses (Duncan, Liepart, & Mill, 1999).

The NOPHN was influential in maintaining population health nursing services at home during World War I and in the organization of the Division of Public Health Nursing within the U.S. Public Health Service in 1944. The NOPHN also provided advisory services regarding postgraduate education for public health nursing in colleges and universities. The NOPHN was incorporated into the National League for Nursing (NLN) in the restructuring of professional nursing organizations in the 1950s (Kalisch & Kalisch, 2004).

In 1986, the American Nurses Association developed the *Standards of Community Health Nursing Practice*. As we saw in Chapter 1∞, the standards are based on the use of the nursing process in population health nursing practice. In 1999, the standards were revised by the Quad Council of Public Health Nursing Organizations as the *Scope and Standards of Public Health Nursing Practice* and have subsequently undergone additional revisions (ANA, 2013).

Attempts were also made over the years to standardize the functions and competencies of population health nurses. These culminated in the Quad Council's 2003 adoption of the public health nursing competencies discussed in Chapter 1∞ (Quad Council, 2003, 2004, 2011), but began as early as 1931, when the Field Studies Committee of NOPHN developed functions and related objectives for generalized and specialized practice (King & Erickson, 2006). These objectives were revised in 1936 and 1944 and again in 1949 in a document entitled *Public Health Nursing Responsibilities in a Community Health Program* (Abrams, 2004). Although the Quad Council accepted the Council on Linkages competencies for public health practice as the basis for the public health nursing competencies, they were modified to reflect the dual focus of population health nursing on the care of individuals and families as well as populations (King & Erickson, 2006).

Educating Population Health Nurses

As Steven Jonas, noted public health author, has observed, whenever a new area of nursing practice is established, it is inevitably followed by the development of practice standards and related curricula (Jonas et al., 2007). Public health nursing was no exception, and during the 1920s, nursing education was under study. The Goldmark Report, *Nursing and Nursing Education in the United States*, published in 1923, dealt with nursing education in general and pointed out the need for advanced preparation for population health nursing. The report recommended that nursing education take place in institutions of higher learning (Kalisch & Kalisch, 2004). As a result, the Yale University School of Nursing and the Frances Payne Bolton School of Nursing at Western Reserve University opened in 1923. Canada's first baccalaureate program in nursing (also the first in the British Empire) was established in 1918 at the University of British Columbia (Canadian Museum of Civilization, 2004). The curricula of both U.S. and Canadian programs included population health nursing content.

Prior to the education of nurses in university settings, special postgraduate courses in public health nursing had been established by various agencies. The first of these in the United States was undertaken by the Instructive District Nursing Association of Boston in 1906 (Buhler-Wilkerson, 2001). In 1910, Teachers' College of Columbia University offered the first course in public health nursing in an institution of higher learning (Brainerd, 1985), and in 1927 the NLN curriculum document, *A Curriculum for Schools of Nursing*, emphasized the need for specific training for public health nursing (Kalisch & Kalisch, 2004).

In addition to witnessing the movement of population health nursing education to institutions of higher learning, the 1920s saw a shift in the employment of population health nurses. Before this time, most population health nursing services were provided by voluntary agencies such as the Red Cross and similar organizations. Although some local jurisdictions, such as Los Angeles, employed public health nurses in communicable disease control, no state recognized the role of this nursing specialty in an official health or education agency until 1907, when Alabama became the first state to approve public health nurse employment by government agencies. By 1924, a survey by NOPHN found that half of all nurses employed in public health nursing worked for official government agencies and approximately 41% of all U.S. counties had access to public health nursing services (Kalisch & Kalisch, 2004). This same movement of public health nurses from charitable organizations to governmental agencies also occurred in Canada (McKay, 2009).

The Brown Report of 1948, *Nursing for the Future*, reemphasized the need for nurses to be educated in institutions of higher learning to prepare them to meet population health needs (Kalisch & Kalisch, 2004). A similar, but earlier, report in Canada, *Survey of Nursing Education in Canada* (Weir, 1932), also known as the Weir Report, had recommended advanced educational preparation for population health nurses, particularly those practicing in rural areas. In 1964, the American Nurses Association (ANA) formally defined the public health nurse as a graduate of a baccalaureate program in nursing. In 1995, the Pew Health Professions Commission report, *Critical Challenges: Revitalizing the Health Professions*, reinforced baccalaureate education as the entry level for population-based practice. Today, in some states, such as California, only graduates from baccalaureate programs in nursing can be certified as public health nurses. Moreover, there are now master's and doctoral programs with a population health nursing focus, including recently developed Doctor of Nursing Practice Programs with an aggregate focus (American Association of Colleges of Nursing [AACN], 2006). Table 2-2● presents a summary of significant events in the development of population health nursing practice.

TABLE 2-2 Historical Events in the Development of Population Health Nursing

Date	Event
1813	Ladies' Benevolent Society of Charleston, South Carolina, organized as first home nursing service in the United States.
1819	Visiting nursing services organized through the Hebrew Female Benevolent Society of Philadelphia.
1832	Lying-in Charity for Attending Indigent Women in Their Homes established.
1840	Institute of Nursing in London founded by Elizabeth Frye to provide care in homes and prisons.
1859	District nursing initiated in Liverpool, England, by William Rathbone.
1876	Metropolitan and National Nursing Association for Providing Trained Nurses for the Sick Poor founded in England.
1877	Women's Branch of the New York City Mission is first to employ trained nurses for home visiting.
1880	Health promotion and education focus initiated by the Boston Instructive District Nursing Association.
1881	American Red Cross founded by Clara Barton.
1885–86	Visiting nurse associations established in Buffalo, Boston, and Philadelphia.
1893	First school nurse employed in London. Henry Street Settlement founded by Lillian Wald.
1896	First rural nursing service established (Westchester County, New York).
1897	Victorian Order of Nurses (VON) founded to pioneer community health nursing in Canada.
1899	International Council of Nurses established.
1900	Nurse's Settlement house founded in Richmond, Virginia.
1902	First school nursing program in the United States established by Henry Street Settlement.
1903	Henry Street Settlement school nursing program absorbed by New York City Department of Health.
1904	First school nurse is employed by a municipality (Los Angeles, California).
1906	The *Visiting Nurse Quarterly* first published (Chicago). First postgraduate course in public health nursing established by Instructive District Nursing Association of Boston.
1907	Public health nurse employment by government agencies first approved by Alabama.
1909	Metropolitan Life Insurance Company offers visiting nurse services to policyholders. Red Cross Nursing Service established.
1910	First postgraduate course in community health nursing in an institution of higher learning is established at Columbia University.

(Continued)

TABLE 2-2 (Continued)

Date	Event
1911	Metropolitan Life Insurance visiting nurse services expanded nationwide.
1912	National Organization for Public Health Nursing (NOPHN) established. Red Cross Town and Country Nursing Service established. Standing orders for public health nursing activities adopted by Chicago Visiting Nurse Association.
1918	University of Alberta offered first Canadian course in public health nursing.
1919	Alberta District Nursing Service established to meet the needs of frontier families.
1920	Public health section of the Canadian National Association of Trained Nurses established.
1921	Maternity and Infancy (Sheppard–Towner) Act passed.
1923	Goldmark Report recommended education for nurses in institutions of higher learning and additional preparation for population health nursing.
1928	Frontier Nursing Service initiated by Mary Breckenridge.
1929	NOPHN established criteria and procedures for grading courses in public health nursing, initiating the accreditation process.
1931	Functions of public health nurses and related objectives first developed by the Field Studies Committee of NOPHN.
1932	Weir Report on nursing education in Canada recognized need for advanced education for public health nurses and recommended an increase in the public health nurse workforce.
1933–1935	Nurses employed during the Depression in the Federal Emergency Relief Administration (FERA), Civil Works Administration (CWA), and Works Progress Administration (WPA).
1934	First public health nurse employed by USPHS.
1936	Public health nursing functions and objectives revised.
1944	Division of Public Health Nursing established in USPHS. Public health nursing functions and objectives revised.
1948	Brown Report reemphasized the need to educate nurses in institutions of higher learning and to include population health nursing content in curricula.
1949	Public health nursing functions and objectives revised in *Public Health Nursing Responsibilities in a Community Health Program.*
1952	NOPHN absorbed into National League for Nursing (NLN).
1964	*Public health nurse* defined by American Nurses Association as a graduate of a baccalaureate program in nursing.
1973	Provision of home health services mandated for health maintenance organizations.
1974	First U.S. hospice established by Florence Wald
1986	*Standards of Community Health Nursing Practice* published by the American Nurses Association.
1988	Institute of Medicine report published, recommending restructuring of public health.
1993	National Center for Nursing Research established.
1995	Pew Health Professions Commission reinforced baccalaureate as entry level for population health nursing practice.
1999	Population health nursing standards revised by Quad Council of Public Health Nursing Organizations as *Scope and Standards of Public Health Nursing.*
2003	Public health nursing competencies established by the Quad Council of Public Health Nursing Organizations.
2006	*Essentials for doctoral education for advanced nursing practice* published by the American Association of Colleges of Nursing including an aggregate/populations focus.
2007	*Public Health Nursing: Scope and Standards of Practice* revised. Worldwide Palliative Care Alliance established.
2013	*Public Health Nursing: Scope and Standards of Practice* (2nd ed.) published.

Federal Involvement in Health Care

For most of its history, the federal government has left health matters to the states. It was not until 1879 that the United States established a National Board of Health in response to a yellow fever epidemic. This board continued to function until 1883, when it was dissolved. In 1912, the need for a permanent national agency responsible for the country's health was recognized, and the U.S. Public Health Service (USPHS) was created out of the reorganization of the Marine Hospital Service (Timeline, U.S. Public Health Service, n.d.). In that same year, federal legislation created the office of the Surgeon General and mandated federal involvement in health promotion. It was not until 1953, however, that the need for advisement on health matters at the cabinet level was recognized with the creation of the Department of Health, Education, and Welfare. This department was reorganized in 1980 to create the present Department of Health and Human Services (DHHS).

Since the beginning of the 20th century, the federal government has become progressively more involved in health care delivery. Unfortunately, this involvement has been rather haphazard, dependent on the interests and concerns of different administrations. In the early years of the 20th century, the health needs of specific segments of the population began to be recognized, resulting in federal programs designed to enhance the health of mothers and children, the poor, those with sexually transmitted diseases, the mentally ill, and others. For example, in 1921, Congress passed the Sheppard–Towner Act to help state and local agencies meet the health needs of mothers and children. In addition to providing funds for maternity centers, prenatal care, and child health clinics, the legislation provided monies to enhance visiting nurse services (Kalisch & Kalisch, 2004). These funds allowed local agencies—for example, the San Diego County Health Department—to hire additional public health nurses, known as "Sheppard–Towner nurses" (Interview with Harney M. Cordua, son of Dr. Olive Cordua, San Diego County Medical Officer). In 1930, recognition of the need for federal support of health care research to address the health needs of mothers and children and other special groups led to the development of the National Institutes of Health.

As a result of the Great Depression of the 1930s, the federal government became even more active in health and social welfare programs. Jobs were created to employ thousands of the unemployed. Nurses were employed under Regulation 7 of the Federal Emergency Relief Act (1933), the Civil Works Administration (1933–34), and the Works Progress Administration (1935) to meet the health needs of the population (Kalisch & Kalisch, 2004). The first public health nurse was employed by the USPHS in 1934.

Recognition of the economic plight of the elderly led to passage of the Social Security Act in 1935, 60 years after the efforts of Lavinia Dock and others to provide health care to the elderly poor. This act established the Old-Age and Survivors Insurance (OASI, better known as Social Security) to improve the financial status of the elderly. Interestingly, the Act also provided funds for the education of public health professionals, including public health nurses (Kalisch & Kalisch, 2004).

World War II also influenced health care delivery. Wage and price freezes and a dearth of skilled labor led industries to offer health insurance benefits in an attempt to compete for competent workers. During the war, some 15 million U.S. service members were exposed to quality health care, some for the first time in their lives. Afterward, these veterans began to demand the same quality of care for themselves and their families in the civilian sector. This increased demand for care led to new arrangements for financing health care and the subsequent burgeoning of the health insurance industry. The growth in health insurance was further influenced by the 1954 inclusion of premiums as legitimate tax deductions. This development led to the use of insurance benefits as a tax-deductible substitute for higher wages in business and industry. Because such benefits were tax exempt for employees, they were readily accepted in lieu of salary increases by unions and other bargaining agents. Blue Cross hospitalization insurance was initiated at this time under the leadership of the American Hospital Association (Kalisch & Kalisch, 2004).

Increased demands for services also led to a lack of adequate facilities, especially in nonurban areas. In 1946, pressured by USPHS officials, Congress responded with passage of the Hill–Burton Act to finance hospital construction in underserved areas (Kalisch & Kalsich, 2004). Hospital construction and insurance coverage for care provided in the hospital further strengthened the national emphasis on curative rather than preventive care and widened the gap between bedside nursing and health promotion and prevention. In fact, a 1928 Bureau of Indian Affairs (BIA) circular directed BIA public health field nurses to promote the use of hospitals over home care (Abel, 1996). Hospitals became a major focus for health and illness care. Ironically, during this same period, the first hospital-based home care program was established at Montefiore Hospital in New York (Fondiller, n.d.), setting a precedent for the burgeoning home care industry of today. The present emphasis on cost containment has led to a shift away from institutional care and more toward home and community-based care. This development has also resulted in a growing need for population health nurses to provide home health services.

The Latter Half of the 20th Century

In 1966, the Social Security Act was amended to create the Medicare program to address the health care needs of older Americans. Medicaid, a program that funds health care for the indigent, was instituted in 1967. These two programs contributed to increased demands for health care services and resulted in rapid increases in the cost of health care. In 1965, when they were introduced as part of Lyndon Johnson's "Great Society" program, Medicare and Medicaid were seen by some as initial steps toward universal health care coverage in the United States, a vision that has yet to be fulfilled (Jonas et al., 2007).

Acknowledging the growing demand for health care and recognizing the differing abilities of certain areas of the country to meet those needs, the U.S. federal government responded with the Comprehensive Health Planning Act of 1966 and the National Health Planning and Resources Development Act of 1974. Both pieces of legislation were attempts to organize the planning of health care delivery to meet differing needs throughout the country. Unfortunately, both efforts failed. One positive effect of the 1974 Act was recognition of the contribution of nurse practitioners to the health status of the public, 9 years after the establishment of the first nurse practitioner program in 1965 (Jenkins & Sullivan-Marx, 1994).

The Child Health Act of 1967 and the Health Maintenance Organization Act of 1973 also recommended the use of nurses in extended roles. The 1971 publication of a report entitled *Extending the Scope of Nursing Practice* provided additional support for the use of nurses in expanded capacities (Kalisch & Kalisch, 2004). Subsequent legislation has led to the increased use of nurse practitioners in a variety of settings. Over the last few years, there has been increased use of population health nurses with advanced educational preparation as nurse practitioners providing primary care to selected populations. Many of these nurses are employed in nurse-managed community health centers that continue the vision of Wald and Breckenridge of providing care to people where they are. Established in the 1970s with funding from the Office of Economic Opportunity during Lyndon Baine Johnson's presidency, the number of nurse-managed centers had increased to 150 within a decade (Malka, 2007).

While the United States was attempting to decentralize health care policy making through health planning legislation, efforts were being made elsewhere to focus attention on risk factors for population health problems. The Lalonde Report, *New Perspectives for the Health of Canadians*, was published in Canada in 1974, identifying the importance of biological, environmental, and lifestyle risks as determinants of health and recommending greater attention to the elimination of risks in each of these areas. The Lalonde Report marked the initial shift away from a treatment paradigm to a health promotion focus at the national level in Canada (Stachenko, Legowski, & Geneau, 2009). As a result of the Lalonde Report, the Health Promotion Directorate was formed in Canada in 1978 (Glouberman & Millar, 2003).

In 1978, at an international conference on primary health care, the Declaration of Alma-Ata was developed, calling for access to primary health care for all. The resulting slogan for this campaign was "Health for all by the year 2000," a goal which has not yet been achieved (Watts, 2003). In 1984, the *Beyond Health Care* conference in Toronto established two key health promotion concepts: healthy public policy and healthy cities. These developments were followed by the adoption of health-for-all strategies in many nations, including the Canadian Epp report, *Achieving Health for All: A Framework for the Health of Canadians*, in 1986 (Glouberman & Millar, 2003).

The comparable movement in the United States is the focus on the achievement of the national health objectives discussed in Chapter 1∞. The need for systematic data collection relative to the achievement of the objectives was recognized in the introduction of the Behavioral Risk Factor Surveillance System (BRFSS). The system involves periodic surveys of the U.S. public to determine trends in specific health behaviors and health indicators (National Center for Chronic Disease Prevention and Health Promotion, 2008).

The health-for-all concept was further developed in the World Health Organization's *Global Strategies for Health for All by the Year 2000*, published in 1981, and the *Ottawa Charter for Health Promotion*, developed at the First International Conference on Health Promotion in 1986. Both focused on social, economic, and political reform and empowerment as strategies for improving the health of the world's populations (Glouberman & Millar, 2003). The importance of health promotion at the global level was reinforced in the *Jakarta Declaration on Health Promotion into the 21st Century* (World Health Organization [WHO], 2010).

Reform efforts in the United States in the late 20th century focused more on health care financing and the organization of services than on changes in social conditions affecting health. The Tax Equity and Fiscal Responsibility Act (TEFRA) of 1982 had a profound effect on health care and community health nursing. This Act, passed in an effort to reduce Medicare expenditures, led to the development of **diagnosis-related groups (DRGs)** as a mechanism for prospective payment for services provided under Medicare (Kalisch & Kalisch, 2004). Basically, prospective payment means that health care institutions are paid a flat fee set in advance under Medicare. The fee is based on the client's diagnosis. The effect of this legislation has been earlier discharge of sicker clients and greater demand for home health and population health nursing services. Diagnosis-related groups and their effects have changed the role of population health nurses, who may need to return to the earlier role of care of the sick in their homes in addition to their roles in promoting health and preventing illness in populations.

Public health practice, including population health nursing, is being restructured in light of the 1988 Institute of Medicine report, *The Future of Public Health*. This report identified the three core functions of public health as assessment, policy formation, and assurance discussed in Chapter 1∞. Similarly, the September 11, 2001, terrorist attacks on New York and the Pentagon and the development of new and reemerging communicable diseases, such as autoimmune deficiency syndrome (AIDS), later labeled acquired immunodeficiency syndrome, and, more recently, severe acute respiratory syndrome (SARS), Ebola virus, and hantavirus, have highlighted inadequacies in the public health infrastructure here and internationally (CDC, 2002; Watts, 2003). These events are beginning to result in increased funding for public health efforts, including those related to terrorism.

Another event that could have a significant impact on population health nursing is the development of the **Nursing Interventions Classification (NIC)** system to categorize nursing services and facilitate their direct reimbursement (McCloskey, Butcher, & Bulechek, 2007). The NIC system should lend itself to direct reimbursement for nursing services under managed care, the new focus of the U.S. federal government. The **Nursing Outcomes Classification (NOC)** system is a parallel development that will allow nurses to document the effectiveness of intervention (Moorhead, Johnson, Maas, & Swanson, 2007).

Another significant accomplishment was the international eradication of smallpox. The World Health Organization initiated its campaign to eradicate smallpox in 1966, and the last reported naturally occurring case in the world occurred in 1977. In 2002, the world marked the 25th anniversary of its freedom from this previously devastating disease (CDC, 2002). Significant events in American public health in the 20th and 21st centuries are presented in Table 2-3●. Table 2-4● summarizes recent international events related to global public health.

The Present and Beyond

The eradication of smallpox highlighted the effectiveness of international cooperation in health matters, which we will discuss in more detail in Chapter 5∞. Unfortunately, this accomplishment has had a negative consequence. The last case of smallpox in the United States occurred in 1949, prompting

TABLE 2-3 Significant 20th- and 21st-Century Events in American Public Health

Date	Event
1906	Pure Food and Drug Act passed.
1912	Children's Bureau established to foster child health. Marine Hospital Service changed to U.S. Public Health Service.
1915	Tetanus antitoxin introduced.
1929	Blue Cross insurance instituted. Penicillin discovered by Alexander Fleming (discovery not acted on until World War II).
1930	National Institutes of Health established to conduct health-related research. Food and Drug Administration established. National Fair Labor Standards Act passed.
1935	Social Security Act established Old-Age and Survivors Insurance (OASI).
1938	Garfield/Kaiser Prepaid Group Practice established (forerunner of managed care).
1946	Hospital Survey and Construction (Hill–Burton) Act passed. Communicable Disease Center (CDC) established.
1953	U.S. Department of Health, Education, and Welfare (USDHEW) established.
1954	Health insurance premiums first allowed as tax deductions.
1955	Salk polio vaccine widely used.
1957	Nationalized Canadian health care system established.
1964	U.S. Surgeon General's report on smoking published.
1966	Comprehensive Health Planning and Public Health Services Act passed. Medicare program instituted to fund health care for the elderly.
1967	Medicaid program initiated to fund health care for the medically indigent.
1970	Occupational Safety and Health Administration established. Environmental Protection Agency established.
1974	National Health Planning and Resources Development Act passed. Lalonde Report, *New Perspectives for the Health of Canadians*, published.
1978	Canadian Health Promotion Directorate formed.
1979	*Healthy People: Surgeon General's Report on Health Promotion and Disease Prevention* published.
1980	USDHEW reorganized to form U.S. Department of Health and Human Services (USDHHS). *Promoting Health/Preventing Disease: Objectives for the Nation* published, creating the first set of national health objectives for the United States.
1981	Autoimmune deficiency syndrome (AIDS) identified (later labeled acquired immunodeficiency syndrome).
1982	Tax Equity and Fiscal Responsibility Act (TEFRA) passed.
1983	Prospective payment system based on diagnosis-related groups (DRGs) initiated.
1984	Behavioral Risk Factor Surveillance System (BRFSS) initiated.
1986	*Achieving Health for All: A Framework for the Health of Canadians* published.
1988	Institute of Medicine report, *The Future of Public Health*, published.
1989	*U.S. Public Health Services Task Force: Guide to Clinical Preventive Services* published, recommending standardized evidence-based screening and prevention strategies for specific populations.
1990	*Healthy People 2000: National Objectives for Health Promotion and Illness Prevention* published.
1993	Health Plan Employer Data and Information Set (HEDIS) created.
1996	*Report on the Health of Canadians* identified environmental challenges to health.
2000	*Healthy People 2010* published. Public Health Improvement Act passed to assist state and local agencies in enhancing public health services.
2010	*Healthy People 2020* published. Affordable Care Act passed.

TABLE 2-4 International Events Influencing Public Health

Date	Event
1902	Pan-American Health Organization (PAHO) founded.
1919	Health Organization of the League of Nations established.
1948	World Health Organization (WHO) established.
1977	Smallpox eradicated worldwide.
1979	Call for access to primary care for all established in Declaration of Alma-Ata.
1981	Need for primary health care emphasized by World Health Organization report, *Global Strategies for Health for All by the Year 2000.*
1986	Prerequisites to and strategies for achieving health for all identified in *The Ottawa Charter for Health Promotion.*
1988	WHO goal for poliomyelitis eradication set.
1992	WHO goal for integration of hepatitis B vaccination into childhood immunization programs set.
1993	Global emergency declared by WHO in response to worldwide incidence of tuberculosis.
1994	Goal of measles elimination established by WHO Region of the Americas.
1998	Concepts of global health promotion reinforced in *Jakarta Declaration on Health Promotion into the 21st Century.*
2000	World Health Report 2000, *Health Systems: Improving Performance*, published.
2001	United Nations General Assembly Special Session on HIV/AIDS held.
2002	European Region of WHO declared polio-free. WHO goal of reducing worldwide measles mortality by 50% established.

discontinuation of smallpox vaccination in 1971 (Immunization Action Coalition, n.d.). This development has led to a generation of Americans who are vulnerable to the use of smallpox as a mechanism of bioterrorism and has prompted plans for preventive immunization of persons at greatest risk and mass immunization campaigns in the event of an attack.

Other advances of previous eras may also be undone in the current political climate. For example, in 2001, the U.S. Congress repealed the ergonomic standards put forth by the Occupational Safety and Health Administration under pressure from businesspeople who feared the cost of implementing measures to prevent repetitive motion injuries and other related conditions (Fee & Brown, 2001). Similarly, activities taken to prevent terrorist initiatives may undermine individual freedoms, and the focus on terrorism may serve to detract attention from other critical issues in public health, such as disparities in health status and societal conditions that affect the health of all. The wars in Iraq and Afghanistan also drew away resources that could have been used to improve the overall health of the population. Population health nurses will need to reemerge as social activists to maintain a balance among these concerns that fosters the health of populations, both nationally and internationally.

Growing evidence indicates a shift to greater emphasis on health promotion and illness prevention in national and international health policy. The U.S. national health objectives published first in 1980 and again in 1990, 2000, and 2010, and discussed in Chapter 1∞, are one sign of this shift. A second bit of evidence is the 1988 creation of the Center for Nursing Research (now the National Institute for Nursing Research) within the National Institutes of Health. One reason given in Senate testimony favoring the center was the health promotion and illness prevention focus in much of nursing research. Another somewhat encouraging sign is the passage of the Public Health Improvement Act of 2000, which provides funds for the development of public health activities at state and local levels (CDC, 2001).

In addition, one of the focus areas for *Healthy People 2010* and continued in the current *Healthy People 2020* was the development of the public health infrastructure. The public health infrastructure includes the organizational structure of official government health agencies, the public health workforce, and the information systems employed in public health practice (Advisory Committee on National Health Promotion and Disease Prevention Objectives for 2020, 2008). The most recent development is the March 23, 2010, signing of the Affordable Care Act by President Barack Obama. The primary provisions of the bill include the provision of affordable health care through new consumer protections against denial of coverage due to pre-existing conditions and removal of lifetime limitations on coverage; support for the Medicare program, particularly for drug costs; provision of insurance assistance for small business owners through tax credits; and inclusion of preventive services in coverage (Internal Revenue Service, 2010; U.S. Department of Health and Human Services, 2010). This legislation will be discussed in more detail in Chapter 7∞.

Recently the Global Public Health Achievements Team (2011) within the Centers for Disease Control and Prevention highlighted 10 of the most significant worldwide public health accomplishments of the first decade of the 21st century. These accomplishments are summarized in Table 2-5•.

TABLE 2-5 Worldwide Public Health Achievements, 2001–2010

Focus Area	Achievements
Child mortality	• Decrease of 2 million deaths in children under 5 years of age from 77 deaths to 62 deaths per 1,000 live births
Vaccine-preventable diseases	• 2.5 million deaths prevented each year in children under 5 years of age • 78% decline in measles mortality • Decrease in the number of countries with endemic poliomyelitis from 20 to 4 • Fewer than 1,500 cases of poliomyelitis in 2010 • Global coverage with a third dose of DTP vaccine increased from 74% to 82% • Global coverage with hepatitis B vaccine increased to 70% • Global coverage with Hib vaccine increased to 38% and 130,000 pneumonia and meningitis deaths prevented
Safe water and sanitation	• Increase in the proportion of the world's population with access to improved drinking water sources from 83% to 87% • Increase in the proportion of the world's population with access to improved sanitation from 58% to 61%
Malaria prevention and control	• Increased annual funding for prevention in endemic countries from $100 million to $1.8 billion • Reduction in annual number of cases to 225 million • 21% decrease in malaria deaths
HIV/AIDS prevention and control	• Annual number of new infections dropped from 3.1 million to 2.6 million • Annual AIDS-related deaths decreased to 1.8 million • Antiretroviral therapy (ART) provided to 5.25 million persons in low- and middle-income countries
Tuberculosis control	• 20% increase in case detection and treatment success rates • Declining incidence and prevalence in every region worldwide
Control of neglected tropical diseases	• Annual number of dracunculiasis cases reduced to 1,797 with probable global eradication by 2012 • Elimination of new cases of onchocercal blindness in all 13 regions of the Americas, with transmission completely interrupted in 8 regions • 9.5 million cases of filariasis prevented and 32 million disability-adjusted life years averted
Tobacco control	• WHO Framework Convention on Tobacco Control adopted by 168 countries • 50% of the world's population protected from second-hand smoke in health care and educational facilities (but only 5% in all public places) • Population covered by comprehensive smoke-free laws increased from 3.1% to 5.4% from 2007 to 2008
Global road safety	• 36% reduction in annual traffic-related fatalities in Europe • 2009 adoption of UN General Assembly resolution initiating 2011–2020 Decade of Action for Road Safety
Preparedness and response to global health threats	• Adoption of the 2005 International Health Regulations • Increased global laboratory and epidemiologic capacity • Development of 21 new field epidemiology training programs • Most rapid and effective response to a global pandemic ever in relation to the H1N1 influenza epidemic in 2009, with vaccine development within 20 weeks of virus detection and deployed in 86 countries

Based on: Global Public Health Achievements Team. (2011). Ten great public health achievements—Worldwide, 2001–2010. *Morbidity and Mortality Weekly Report, 60,* 814–818.

CHAPTER RECAP

In this chapter, we have seen how population health nursing grew to its present state. The future direction of population health nursing will be determined by the population health nurses of today and tomorrow. The times we live in are not dissimilar to those encountered by Lillian Wald and other population health nursing pioneers. Lack of access to care and environmental conditions that are not conducive to health impede the ability of the world's citizens to live healthy and productive lives. It may be time to return to the dual nature of the initial public health nursing role: personal care in conjunction with population-based health promotion and illness prevention.

CASE STUDY Continuing the Focus on the Population's Health

Population health nursing in the United States arose in response to identified health needs among European immigrants.

1. What recently arrived immigrant populations live in the area where you live?
2. In what ways are these new immigrants similar to and different from those arriving in the United States at the end of the 19th century?
3. How do their health needs compare to those encountered by the nurses on Henry Street?
4. What population health nursing interventions might be needed to improve their health status?

REFERENCES

Abel, E. K. (1996). "We are left so much alone to work out our own problems": Nurses on American Indian reservations during the 1930s. *Nursing History Review, 4*, 43–64.

Abrams, S. E. (2004). From function to competency in public health nursing, 1931 to 2003. *Public Health Nursing, 21*, 507–510.

Advisory Committee on National Health Promotion and Disease Prevention Objectives for 2020. (2008). *Phase I report: Recommendations for the framework and format of Healthy People 2020.* Washington, DC: U.S. Department of Health and Human Services.

Aetna. (2003). *African American history calendar: History.* Retrieved from http://www.aetna.com/diversity/aahcalendar/2003/history.html

American Association of Colleges of Nursing. (2006). *Essentials for doctoral education for advanced nursing practice.* Washington, DC: Author.

American Nurses Association. (n.d.). *Susie walking bear yellowtail (1903–2002).* 2002 Inductee. Retrieved from http://www.nursingworld.org/FunctionalMenuCategories/AboutANA/Honoring-Nurses/HallofFame/20002004Inductees/SusieWalkingBearYellowtail.aspx

American Nurses Association. (2013). *Public health nursing: Scope and standards of practice (2nd ed.).* Silver Spring, MD: Author.

American Public Health Association. (2010a). *About APHA.* Retrieved December 14, 2005, from http://www.apha.org/about

American Public Health Association. (2010b). *APHA sections and special interest groups.* Retrieved December 14, 2005, from http://www.apha.org/sections/sectdesc.htm

American Public Health Association. (2010c). *Sections, SPIGs and caucuses.* Retrieved December 14, 2005, from http://www.apha.org/sections

American Red Cross. (2014). *Founder Clara Barton.* Retrieved from http://www.redcross.org/about-us/history/clara-barton

American Society of Registered Nurses. (2007a). *Big heart.* Retrieved from http://www.asrn.org/newsletter_article.php?journal=&issue_id=37&article_id=205

American Society of Registered Nurses. (2007b). *Mary Breckenridge.* Retrieved from http://www.asrn.org/newsletter_article.php?journal=&issue_id=37&article_id=206

American Society of Registered Nurses. (2007c). *Meet Florence Wald.* Retrieved from http://www.asrn.org/newsletter_article.php?journal=&issue_id=37&article_id=224

Anionwu, E. (2006). *About Mary Seacole.* Retrieved from http://www.maryseacole.com/maryseacole/pages/aboutmary.html

Ashton, D. (2009). *Rebecca Gratz. Jewish women: A comprehensive historical encyclopedia.* Retrieved from http://jwa.org/encyclopedia/article/gratz-rebecca

Association of State and Territorial Directors of Nursing. (2000). *Public health nursing: A partner for healthy populations.* Washington, DC: American Nurses Publishing.

Behling, S. (n.d.). *Note on Clara Barton.* Retrieved September 12, 2004, from http://www.rootsweb.com/~nwa/barton.html

Bell, P. L. (2010). Mamie Odessa Hale Garland (1911–1968?). The Encyclopedia of Arkansas History & Culture. Retrieved from http://www.encyclopediaofarkansas.net/encyclopedia/entry-detail.aspx?entryID=1662

Brainerd, A. M. (1985). *The evolution of public health nursing.* New York: Garland. Reprinted from Brainerd, 1922 Brainerd, A. M. (1922). *The evolution of public health nursing.* Philadelphia: Saunders.

Brannon, H. (2004). *The history of smallpox: The rise and fall of a disease.* Retrieved from http://dermatology.about.com/cs/smallpox/a/smallpoxhx.htm

Bryder, L. (2002). *The Plunket nurses as a New Zealand icon.* Retrieved from http://www.nursing.manchester.ac.uk/ukchnm/publications/seminarpapers/plunketnurse.pdf

Buhler-Wilkerson, K. (2001). *No place like home: A history of nursing and home care in the United States.* Baltimore: Johns Hopkins University.

Bumb, J. (n.d.). *Dorothea Dix.* Retrieved from http://www.webster.edu/~woolflm/dorotheadix.html

Canadian Museum of Civilization. (2004). *A brief history of nursing in Canada from the establishment of new France to the present.* Retrieved from http://www.civilization.ca/cmc/exhibitions/tresors/nursing/nchis01e.shtml

Carr, T. J. (n.d.). *The Harappan civilization.* Retrieved from http://www.archaeologyonline.net/artifacts/harappa-mohenjodaro.html

Centers for Disease Control and Prevention. (2001). *The Public Health Improvement Act: Priority Capacities, Section 319 (A).* Retrieved from http://www.publichealthgrandrounds.unc.edu/performance/pshandout_phimprovement.htm

Centers for Disease Control and Prevention. (2002). 25th anniversary of last case of naturally occurring smallpox. *Morbidity and Mortality Weekly Report, 51*, 952.

Centers for Disease Control and Prevention. (2004). 150th anniversary of John Snow and the Pump Handle. *Morbidity and Mortality Weekly Report, 53*, 783.

Cho, H. S. M., & Kashka, M. S. (2004). The evolution of the community health nurse practitioner in Korea. *Public Health Nursing, 21*, 287–294.

Commonwealth of Massachusetts. (1870). *First annual report of the State Board of Health of Massachusetts*. Boston, MA: Wright & Potter. Retrieved from http://www.archive.org/details/annualreportofst1869mass

Connolly, C. A. (2004). Beyond social history: New approaches to understanding the state of and the state in nursing history. *Nursing History Review, 12,* 5–24.

Del Col, L. (2002). *Chadwick's report on sanitary conditions*. Retrieved from http://www.victorianweb.org/history/chadwick2.html

Duncan, S. M., Leipart, B. D., & Mill, J. E. (1999). "Nurses as health evangelists"? The evolution of public health nursing in Canada, 1918–1939. *Advances in Nursing Science, 22*(1), 40–51.

Epidemiology Program Office, Centers for Disease Control and Prevention. (1999). Changes in the public health system. *Morbidity and Mortality Weekly Report, 48,* 1141–1147.

Fee, E., & Brown, T. (2001). Editor's note. *American Journal of Public Health, 91,* 1381.

Fee, E., Brown, T. M., Lazarus, J., & Theerman, P. (2002). Baxter Street then. *American Journal of Public Health, 92,* 753.

Fee, E., & Bu, L. (2010). The origins of public health nursing: The Henry Street visiting nurse service. *American Journal of Public Health, 100,* 1206–1207.

First American Indian nurse named to nursing hall of fame. (n.d.). Retrieved from http://www.minoritynurse.com/vital-sign/first-American-Indian-nurse-named-nursing-hall-fame

Fondiller, S. H. (n.d.). *The promise and the reality: Our history from 1944 to 1993*. Retrieved from http://www.vnsny.org/mh_about_history_more.html

Global Public Health Achievements Team. (2011). Ten great public health achievements—Worldwide, 2001–2010. *Morbidity and Mortality Weekly Report, 60,* 814–818.

Glouberman, S., & Millar, J. (2003). Evolution of the determinants of health, health policy, and health information systems in Canada. *American Journal of Public Health, 93,* 388–392.

Green, E. C. (2005). Gendering the city, gendering the welfare state. *Virginia Magazine of History and Biography, 113,* 277–308.

Hallett, C. E. (2010). *Celebrating nurses: A visual history*. Hauppauge, NY: Barron's.

Hanink, E. (2010a). *Anna Maxell, the American Florence Nightingale*. Retrieved from http://www.workingnurse.com.articles/anna-maxwell-the-American-florence-nightingale

Hanink, E. (2010b). *Lina Rogers, the first school nurse*. Retrieved from http://www.workingnurse.com.articles/Lina-Rogers-the-First-School-Nurse

Helfand, W. H., Lazarus, J., & Theerman, P. (2001). Night shift in a glass factory. *American Journal of Public Health, 91,* 1370.

Hogan, C. J., Harchelroad, F., & McGovern, T. W. (2005). *Smallpox*. Retrieved from http://www.emedicinehealth.com/smallpox/article_em.htm

Immunization Action Coalition. (n.d.). *Historic dates and events related to vaccines and immunization*. Retrieved from http://immunize.org/timeline

Instructive Visiting Nurse Association. (2008). *IVNA home health care*. Retrieved from http://www.ivna.org/history.html

Internal Revenue Service. (2010). *Small business health care tax credit for small employers*. Retrieved from http://www.irs.gov/newsroom/article/0,id=223666,00.html

Interview with Harney M. Cordua, son of Dr. Olive Cordua, San Diego County Medical Officer. San Diego: San Diego Historical Society.

Jenkins, M. L., & Sullivan-Marx, E. M. (1994). Nurse practitioners and community health nurses: Clinical partnerships and future visions. *Nursing Clinics of North America, 29,* 459–470.

Jewish Women's Archive. (2010). *Lillian Wald, 1867–1940*. Retrieved from http://jwa.org/historymakers/wald

Jonas, S., Goldsteen, R., & Goldsteen, K. (2007). *An introduction to the U.S. health care system* (6th ed.). New York: Springer.

Judd, D. (2010). Nursing in the United States from 1900 to the early 1920s: A new century brings novel ideas and social concerns. In D. Judd, K. Sitzman, & G. M. Davis (Eds.), *A history of American nursing: Trends and eras* (pp. 60–93). Boston, MA: Jones and Bartlett.

Kalisch, P. A., & Kalisch, B. J. (2004). *American nursing: A history*. Philadelphia: Lippincott Williams & Wilkins.

Kasule, O. H. (2004). *History of medicine (Tarikh al tibb)*. Retrieved from http://omarkasule-03.tripod.com/id782.html

Keeling, A. W. (2007). *Nursing and the privilege of prescription, 1893–2000*. Columbus, OH: Ohio State University Press.

King, M. G., & Erickson, G. P. (2006). Development of public health nursing competencies: An oral history. *Public Health Nursing, 23,* 196–201.

Koslow, J. (2002). Lemuel Shattuck. In L. Breslow & G. Cengage (Eds.), *Encyclopedia of public health*. Retrieved from http://www.enotes.com/public-health-encyclopedia/shattuck-lemuel

Lewis, J. J. (n.d.a). *Harriet Tubman—From slavery to freedom: Civil war service: Nurse, scout, spy*. Retrieved from http://womenshistory.about.com/od/harriettubman/a/tubman_civilwar.htm

Lewis, J. J. (n.d.b). *Harriet Tubman—From slavery to freedom: Later years of activism and reform*. Retrieved from http://womenshistory.about.com/od/harriettubman/a/tubman_later.htm

Lewis, J. J. (n.d.c). *Harriet Tubman—From slavery to freedom: Underground railroad conductor, abolitionist, women's rights*. Retrieved from http://womenshistory.about.com/od/harriettubman/a/tubman_moses.htm

Lewis, J. J. (2010a). *Mary Seacole: British black nurse*. Retrieved from http://womenshistory.about.com/od/nursesandnursing/a/mary_seacole_2.htm?p=1

Lewis, J. J. (2010b). *Settlement houses: Basics about the settlement house movement*. Retrieved from http://womenshistory.about.com/od/settlementhouses/a/settlements.htm?p=1

Louisiana Department of Environmental Quality. (n.d.). *History of the department*. Retrieved from http://www.deq.louisiana.gov/portal/ABOUT/HistoryoftheDepartment.aspx

Malka, S. G. (2007). Daring to care: American nursing and second-wave feminism. Urbana, IL: University of Illinois Press.

McCloskey, J. C., Butcher, H. K., & Bulechek, G. M. (Eds.). (2007). *Nursing interventions classification* (5th ed.). St. Louis, C: Mosby.

McKay, M. (2009). *Public health nursing in early 20th century Canada*. Retrieved from http://www.thefreelibrary.com/Public+health+nursing+in+early+20th+century+Canada%2FLes+services...-a0209404149

Moorhead, S., Johnson, M., Maas, M., & Swanson, E. (2007). *Nursing outcomes classification (NOC)*. St. Louis, MO: Mosby.

National Center for Chronic Disease Prevention and Health Promotion. (2008). *BRFSS history*. Retrieved from http://www.cdc.gov/brfss/history.htm

National Hospice and Palliative Care Organization. (2010). *History of hospice*. Retrieved from http://www.nhpco.org/i4a/pages/index.cfm?pageid=3285

Obstetrics: A brief history of obstetrical care at Pennsylvania Hospital. (n.d.). Retrieved from http://www.uphs.upenn.edu/paharc/timeline/

Paneth, N. (n.d.). *Jacob Henle*. Retrieved from http://www.enotes.com/public-health-encyclopedia/henle-jacob

Pew Health Professions Commission. (1995). *Critical challenges: Revitalizing the health professions for the twenty-first century*. San Francisco: UCSF Center for the Health Professions.

Quad Council of Public Health Nursing Organizations. (2003). *Quad Council PHN competencies*. Retrieved from http://www.uncc.edu/achne/quadcouncil/final_phn_competencies.doc

Quad Council of Public Health Nursing Organizations. (2004). Public health nursing competencies. *Public Health Nursing, 21,* 443–452.

Quad Council of Public Health Nursing Organizations. (2011). *Quad Council competencies for public health nurses.* Retrieved from http://www.achne.org/files/Quad%20Council/QuadCouncilCompetenciesforPublicHealthNurses.pdf

Reeves, C. (n.d.). *History of medicine.* Retrieved from http://www.historyworld.net/wrldhis/plaintexthistories.asp?historyid=aa52

Riedel, S. (2005). Edward Jenner and the history of smallpox and vaccination. *Baylor University Medical Center Proceedings, 18*(1), 21–25.

Ripley, C. P., & Hembree, M. F. (Eds.). (1992). *The black abolitionist papers: Vol. V, the United States, 1859–1865.* Chapel Hill, NC: University of North Carolina Press.

Roberts, J. I., & Group, T. M. (1995). *Feminism and nursing: An historical perspective on power, status, and political activism in the nursing profession.* Westport, CT: Praeger.

Robinson, B. (2009). *Victorian medicine—From fluke to theory.* Retrieved from http://www.bbc.co.uk/history/British/victorians/victorian_medicine_01.shtml

Ruffing-Rahal, M. A. (1995). The Navajo experience of Elizabeth Foster, public health nurse. *Nursing History Review, 3,* 173–188.

Rutty, C., & Sullivan, S. C. (2010). *This is public health: A Canadian history.* Retrieved from http://cpha100.ca/sites/default/files/History-book-print_ALL_e.pdf

Scozzari, T. E. (2009). *The journey of America's first native nurse.* Retrieved from http://yellowstonevalleywoman.com/view_article?id=202

Sigerist, H. E. (2003). Medical care for all the people. *American Journal of Public Health, 93,* 57–59. (Reprinted from "Medical care for all people," by H. E. Sigerist, 1944, *Canadian Journal of Public Health, 35,* 253–267.)

Sitzman, K. (2010). Nursing in the American colonies from the 1600s to the 1700s: The influence of past ideas, traditions, and trends. In D. Judd, K. Sitzman, & G. M. Davis (Eds.), *A history of American nursing: Trends and eras* (pp. 8–21). Boston, MA: Jones and Bartlett.

Smith, S. L. (1994). White nurses, black midwives, and public health in Mississippi, 1920–1950. *Nursing History Review, 2,* 29–49.

Spotsylvania County Public Schools. (2009). *Celebrating 100 years of school nursing.* Retrieved from http://www.spotsylvania.k12.va.us/Page/546

Stachenko, S., Legowski, B., & Geneau, R. (2009). Improving Canada's response to public health challenges: The creation of a new public health agency. In R. Beaglehole & R. Bonita (Eds.), *Global public health: A new era* (2nd ed., pp. 123–137). Oxford: Oxford University Press.

Susie Walking Bear Yellowtail. (2010). Retrieved from http://www.nurses.info/personalities_susie_yellowtail.htm

Susie Walking Bear Yellowtail, RN (1903–1981). (2004). Retrieved from http://nsweb.nursingspectrum.com/NursesWeek/SusieWalkingBearYellowtail.htm

Timeline, California Board of Health. (n.d.). *California Board of Health.* Retrieved from http://www.google.com/search?q=California+board+of+health+history&hl=en&rls=com.microsoft:en-US&tbs=tl:1&tbo=u&ei=7-BqTLv2O4v0tgPborwb&sa=X&oi=timeline_result&ct=title&resnum=11&ved=0CD8Q5wIwCg

Timeline, U.S. Public Health Service. (n.d.). *U.S. Public Health Service.* Retrieved from http://www.google.com/search?q=US+public+health+service+history&hl=en&rls=com.microsoft:en-US&tbs=tl:1&tbo=u&ei=qONqTOHpOJHCsAPk5OBH&sa=X&oi=timeline_result&ct=title&resnum=11&ved=0CEgQ5wIwCg

Udwadia, F. E. (2001). *Man and medicine: A history.* Cary, NC: Oxford University Press.

U.S. Department of Health and Human Services. (2010). *About the law.* Retrieved from http://www.healthcare.gov/law/about

Van Betten, P., & Moriarty, M. (2004). *Nursing illuminations: A book of days.* St. Louis, MO: Mosby.

Visiting Nurse Association of Boston. (2010). *About the VNA of Boston.* Retrieved from http://www.bostonvna.org/site/c.frLJKYPJLuF/b.3890097/k.64F6/About_the_VNA_of_Boston.htm

Visiting Nurse Association of Greater Philadelphia. (2010). *Mission and history of the VNA.* Retrieved from http://www.vnaphilly.org/visiting-nurse-mission-history.aspx

Visiting Nursing Association of Western New York. (2010). *The first in 1885… the largest today.* Retrieved from http://www.vna-wny.org/

Watts, S. (2003). *Disease and medicine in world history.* New York: Routledge.

Weir, G. M. (1932). *Survey of nursing education in Canada.* Toronto: University of Toronto Press.

Winslow, C. E. A. (1993). Nursing and the community. *Public Health Nursing, 10,* 58–63. (Reprinted from *The Public Health Nurse,* April 1938).

Wolfe, L. C., & Selekman, J. (2002). School nurses: What it was and what it is. *Pediatric Nursing, 28,* 403–407.

World Health Organization. (2010). *Jakarta declaration on leading health promotion into the 21st century.* Retrieved from http://www.who.int/healthpromotion/conferences/previous/jakarta/declaration/en/index1.html

Zilm, G., & Warbinek, E. (1995). Early tuberculosis nursing in British Columbia. *Canadian Journal of Nursing Research, 27*(3), 65–81.

CHAPTER

3 Epidemiology and Population Health Nursing

Learning Outcomes

After reading this chapter, you should be able to:

1. Describe at least two theories of disease causation.
2. Identify at least three criteria for determining causality in a relationship between two events.
3. Define risk, relative risk, and absolute risk.
4. Distinguish between morbidity and mortality rates.
5. Identify the six steps of the epidemiologic process.
6. Apply three epidemiologic models.

Key Terms

absolute risk
agent
antigenicity
attack rate
case fatality rate
causality
epidemiology
exposure potential
host
incidence
infectivity
mode of transmission
morbidity
mortality
pathogenicity
populations at risk
portal of entry
portal of exit
prevalence
relative risk
relative risk ratio
resistance
risk
survival rate
survival time
susceptibility
target group
toxigenicity
virulence

Advocacy Then

The Father of Epidemiology

John Snow, a physician and anesthesiologist known as the father of epidemiology, used epidemiologic statistical mapping methods to determine the source of a cholera epidemic (Centers for Disease Control and Prevention [CDC], 2004; Robinson, 2009). Prior to the outbreak, Snow had sought to convince medical colleagues that several diseases thought to be spread by air were, in fact, spread through contaminated drinking water. In 1854, an epidemic of cholera began in the Soho district. On one day, 56 new cases occurred, with 143 cases and 70 deaths by the next day. Snow plotted each case on a map of the area and found that all of the early cases were in the vicinity of one particular municipal pump (see Figure 3-1●). His early investigations indicated that workers at a nearby brewery and a workhouse were not affected, as one might have expected them to be, and additional cases were found in the outlying villages of Hampstead and Islington (The puzzle, 2002).

Conducting house-to-house interviews, Snow discovered that the workhouse had its own well and the workers drank only beer, being leery of public water. In addition, the woman affected by the disease in Hampstead had her water delivered each day from the Broad Street pump and had shared the water with her visiting niece from Islington (The puzzle, 2002). Based on this knowledge of disease incidence, he deduced that the source of the infection was the water from the Broad Street pump. Snow was able to persuade local government officials to remove the handle of the pump, preventing access to the contaminated water (Ludwig, 2000). This action led to a decrease in the number of new cases of cholera and the end of the epidemic. Later examination of the pump indicated that a nearby sewer pipe was allowing seepage into the well (The puzzle, 2002). Snow published his theories on the transmission of cholera in a book entitled *On the Mode of Communication in Cholera* before there was evidence of bacteria as a source of infection (Snow, 1855). A 2003 poll of readers of the journal *Hospital Doctor* selected Snow as the "greatest doctor" in history (*John Snow*, n.d.).

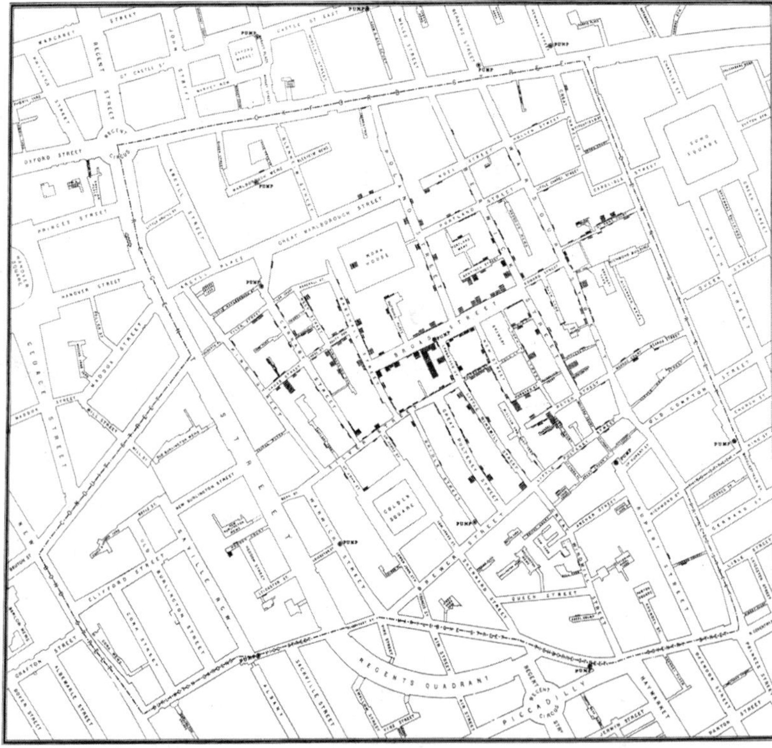

FIGURE 3-1 John Snow's Map of Cholera Cases in London, 1854

Advocacy Now

Uncovering an *Escherichia coli* Outbreak

A population health nurse employed by a local county health department made several home visits to families in her district. Throughout the day, she heard reports of family members in several households experiencing diarrhea. The families involved did not tend to interact much, and had not attended any common functions in the neighborhood. Operating on a hunch that the increase in diarrhea incidence was more than coincidental, the nurse made visits to several families in the area who were not part of her normal case load, explaining to them that she was checking on reports of diarrhea in the neighborhood and asking if any family members in those households had been having gastrointestinal problems. In this way, she uncovered several more cases of diarrhea and initiated an epidemiologic investigation. As part of the investigation, she went house to house for several blocks locating additional people who were affected and collecting stool specimens from those with diarrhea.

The majority of the stool specimens tested positive for *E. coli*. When the source of the infection was identified, it proved to be the city water system. One of the water mains providing water to that particular neighborhood had developed a leak. Recent heavy rains in the area had caused contaminated water to seep into the water supply. Ordinarily such a leak would have been addressed by the chlorination process, but further investigation indicated that one of the chlorinators in the city water system was malfunctioning. In addition to identifying people in the neighborhood affected by the problem, the population health nurse referred them for treatment. Fortunately, there were no long-term consequences for those affected.

Population health nurses deal with conditions affecting whole populations as well as subgroups within populations; therefore, they need to be conversant with the basic principles of epidemiology. The term *epidemiology* derives from three Greek words: *epi* meaning among, *demos* or people, and *logos* meaning discourse or study (*Epidemiology – Definition*, n.d.). Literally, then, epidemiology is a study of what occurs among the people. A more formal definition of **epidemiology** is the science that deals with the study of the causes, distribution, and control of disease in populations (*epidemiology*, n.d.).

Epidemiology involves examination of the distribution of health and illness within a population, factors that determine the population's health status, and use of the knowledge generated to control the development of health problems (Friis & Sellers, 2014). Epidemiologic perspectives on the factors that contribute to disease and illness have changed remarkably over time, and some authors describe four eras of epidemiologic thought. The first was the sanitary era, with interventions based on the ancient theory of miasmas discussed in Chapter 2∞. The second era was that of communicable diseases, in which interventions were based on the germ theory. Emphasis in the third or chronic disease era was on multiple layers of personal risk factors contributing to chronic diseases. The focus of the fourth era, at the beginning of the 21st century, remains to be seen, but the era may turn out to be what some have termed an "ecosocial" perspective (Krieger, 2011), emphasizing the multiple interactions among biological, environmental, and social factors that lead to health or illness in population groups. An alternative direction for epidemiology in this fourth era might be molecular epidemiology, which focuses on the contribution of genetic–environmental interactions to the development, distribution, and prevention of disease (Cabaret, Morand, & Beaudeau, 2012).

Basic Epidemiologic Concepts

Three basic concepts underlie epidemiologic perspectives on health and illness. These concepts are causality, risk, and rates of occurrence.

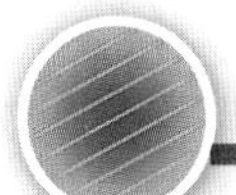

Evidence-Based Practice

Incorporating Epidemiologic Findings

Epidemiologic findings are part of the evidence base used by population health nurses to identify health problems in the population and the factors that contribute to them. Knowing the epidemiology of a specific problem in a specific population permits the population health nurse, in collaboration with others, to design interventions tailored to the needs and circumstances of a particular population, making interventions more likely to achieve the desired outcomes.

Causality

To control health problems, epidemiologists and population health nurses must have some idea of their causes. The concept of **causality** is based on the idea that one event is the result of another event. The main purpose of epidemiology is to identify causal links between contributing factors and resulting states of health and illness.

THEORIES OF CAUSATION. Theories about the cause of disease and ill health have evolved over time. The first recognized attempt to attribute a cause to illness occurred during the "religious era," which extended from roughly 2000 CE through the age of the early Egyptian and Greek physicians to around 600 CE. During this period, disease was thought to be caused directly or indirectly by divine intervention, possibly as punishment for sins or as a trial of faith.

Subsequent to the religious era, disease was often attributed to various physical forces, such as miasmas, or mists. A rudimentary theory of disease was put forth by Hippocrates in the famous treatise, *On Airs, Waters, and Places*, written about 400 CE. The primary belief at that time was that disease was caused by harmful substances in the environment (Friis & Sellers, 2014).

The bacteriologic era commenced in the late 1870s with the discovery of specific organisms as etiologic (causative) agents for specific diseases. As we saw above, early hypotheses were derived by John Snow during the 1854 London cholera epidemic. Subsequently, actual bacteria were isolated and found to be the source of this and other infectious diseases. These discoveries gave rise to theories of a single cause for any specific disease. Single-cause theories were further supported by the identification of specific agents as causative elements in the development of other health problems. For example, lack of vitamin C was found to result in scurvy. The discovery of specific agents responsible for particular diseases did not, however, explain why some people exposed to an agent developed the disease, while others did not. The result of this explanatory failure was the movement into the current era of multiple causation or the ecosocial perspective described above.

The era of multiple causation is characterized by the recognition that multiple factors interact in the development of health or illness in a given person or population and that there is seldom one single cause. Recent advances in epidemiology and biomolecular technology are moving toward an era of multiple causation that encompasses the gene–environment interactions discussed earlier.

Epidemiology examines the interaction among factors at the population level with an eye toward controlling particular health problems. Prevention or control of any disease within population groups depends on knowledge of these factors and determination of the point at which intervention will be most feasible and most effective. The historical development of theories of disease causation is summarized in the *Highlights* box on the left.

Highlights

Historical Development of Theories of Causation

- Religious era (2000–600 CE)

  Disease is thought to be caused by divine intervention, possibly as punishment for sins or as a test of faith.
- Environmental era (circa 400 CE)

  Disease is believed to be caused by harmful miasmas, or mists, or other substances in the environment.
- Bacteriologic era (1870–1900)

  Disease is thought to be caused by specific bacteriologic or nutritive agents.
- Era of multiple causation/Ecosocial perspective (1900 to present)

  Occurrence of disease and other health problems is a result of the interaction of multiple individual risk factors and population exposure patterns.
- Molecular epidemiology perspective (future)

  Occurrence of health-related conditions results from a complex interaction of genetic and environmental factors.

CRITERIA FOR CAUSALITY. With the advent of single-cause/single-effect theories of disease causation during the bacteriologic era, the scientific community began to look for specific causes for all health problems. Now, however, the concept of causality has become more complicated in view of the recognized interplay among several factors in the development of a particular health problem. A factor may be considered causative if the health condition is more likely to occur in its presence and less likely to occur in its absence. Even when these conditions are met, however, a specific factor may not necessarily cause a particular condition. Several criteria can be used in determining causality (Friis & Sellers, 2014). These criteria include the consistency of the relationship, strength of the association, specificity, the temporal relationship between the supposed cause and effect, and coherence.

Consistency. The first criterion for establishing a causal relationship is the consistency of the association between the supposed causal factor and its presumed effect. The condition in question must occur when the factor is present, not when it is absent. For example, people cannot develop measles without being exposed to the measles virus. In addition, the association must always occur in the same direction. Exposure cannot result in disease in one case, and disease result in exposure to the virus in another.

Strength of association. The second criterion for establishing causality is the strength of the association. The greater the correlation between the occurrence of the factor and the condition, the greater the possibility that the relationship is one of cause and effect. For example, not every susceptible person who is exposed to the measles virus develops the disease, but most of them do. The association between exposure and disease, in this instance, is quite strong and supports the idea that the measles virus caused measles. The strength of the association may reflect a *dose-response gradient* in which the greater the exposure to the presumed cause, the greater the likelihood of developing the problem (Gordis, 2014). For example, the fact that people who smoke two packs of cigarettes a day are more likely to develop lung cancer than those who smoke one pack is strong evidence for a causal relationship between smoking and lung cancer.

Specificity. Specificity is the third criterion for causality. Specificity is present when the factor in question results in one specific condition. For example, exposure to measles virus results only in measles, not mumps or varicella (chicken pox). Specificity is the weakest of the criteria with respect to causation in noninfectious conditions. For example, smoking is known to be related to lung cancer, but is also related to stomach and bladder cancer and heart disease.

Temporal relationship. The fourth criterion for establishing causality is the time (or temporal) relationship between the factor and the resulting condition. The factor thought to be causative should occur before the condition occurs. For example, one has to be exposed to the measles virus before, not after, one gets the disease.

Coherence. Coherence with the established body of scientific knowledge is the last criterion for determining causality. The idea that one condition causes another must be logical and should be congruent with other known facts. For example, it is known that alcohol consumption increases the time required for voluntary muscles to react to stimuli. Therefore, it is reasonable to consider alcohol consumption as a causative factor in many accidents because this interpretation is consistent with the idea of a slowed response to changing driving conditions.

The only criterion absolutely required for attributing causation is the presence of a correct temporal relationship. For example, Snow's hypothesis that the water from the Broad Street pump was the cause of the cholera epidemic was certainly not congruent with the prevalent belief that such diseases were caused by the presence of *effluvia* or noxious substances in the air. The greater the number of criteria met, however, the more credible the idea that the factor in question causes the condition of interest. The criteria for determining causality are summarized in the *Highlights* box at the right.

Highlights

Criteria for Determining Causality

- **Consistency:** The association between the supposed cause and its effect is consistent and always occurs in the same direction.
- **Strength of Association:** The greater the correlation between supposed cause and effect, the greater the possibility the relationship is a causal one.
- **Specificity:** The supposed cause always creates the same effect.
- **Temporal relationship:** The supposed cause always occurs before the effect.
- **Coherence:** The supposition that one event causes another is coherent with other existing knowledge.

Risk

In addition to establishing the causes of health-related conditions, epidemiologists are interested in estimating the likelihood that a particular condition will occur. **Risk** is the probability that a given individual will develop a specific condition. Risk may be absolute or relative. **Absolute risk** is the probability that anyone in a given population will develop a particular condition. **Relative risk** is the probability that someone in a group of people with a particular characteristic will develop the condition when compared to people without that characteristic (*Absolute risk and relative risk*, 2011). For example, the absolute risk of breast cancer is about one in every eight U.S. women, but the relative risk of developing breast cancer is much higher for women with a family history of breast cancer than for those without a family history. One's risk of developing a particular condition is affected by a variety of physical, emotional, environmental, lifestyle, and other factors. When epidemiologists speak of **populations at risk**, they are referring to groups of people who have the greatest potential to develop a particular health problem because of the presence or absence of certain contributing factors. "Risk factor epidemiology" may underplay the role of social structure and social relationships in people's response to risk factors. Risk factor epidemiology also tends to assume that people are free to choose their responses, which may or may not be the case.

The basis for risk may lie in one's personal susceptibility to a condition or the potential for exposure to causative factors. **Susceptibility** is the ability to be affected by factors contributing to a particular health condition. For example, very young unimmunized children are susceptible to, and constitute the greatest population at risk for, pertussis (whooping cough). In this case, the basis for increased risk lies in the increased susceptibility of this group. Children who have been immunized against pertussis are less likely to develop the disease and therefore are not part of the population at risk. Another example of risk based on susceptibility is found in the population of sexually active women of childbearing age who are at risk for pregnancy. Men, children, and older women are not susceptible to pregnancy and, therefore, are not considered part of the population at risk.

Exposure potential is another factor in one's risk of developing a particular health problem. **Exposure potential** is the likelihood of encountering or being exposed to factors that contribute to a condition. For example, those most at risk for sexually transmitted diseases are adolescents and young adults. In this instance, the basis of risk is not increased susceptibility, as is the case in pertussis, but an increased potential for exposure due to more frequent and less selective sexual activity than may occur among older adults. Another population at risk through increased chance of exposure includes individuals whose occupations bring them in contact with toxic substances.

Members of a population at risk have a greater probability of developing a specific health problem than those who are not affected by factors known to contribute to its occurrence. This difference in the probability of developing a given condition between those exposed to causative factors and those who are not is known as the **relative risk ratio** (*Relative risk*, 2014). This ratio is derived by comparing the frequency of occurrence of the condition in a group exposed to known risk factors with its occurrence among individuals who have not been exposed. For example, if 50% of smokers develop heart disease versus only 5% of nonsmokers, smokers have a relative risk ratio of 10:1, or have a 10 times greater risk of heart disease than their nonsmoking counterparts.

The relative risk ratio is useful in identifying areas in which preventive interventions will have the greatest impact on the occurrence of the condition. When the relative risk is greater than 1:1, there is a positive association between the factors and the condition, suggesting that eliminating the factor may prevent the condition from occurring. A negative association, in which the relative risk ratio is less than 1:1 (e.g., 1:5), suggests that enhancing the factor or causing it to be present may prevent the condition. For example, smoking has a positive relationship with heart disease and regular exercise has a negative relationship, so both preventing smoking and promoting exercise should decrease the incidence of heart disease in the population.

The population at risk becomes the target group for any intervention designed to prevent or control the problem in question. The **target group** includes those individuals who would benefit from an intervention program and at whom the program is aimed. The target group for an immunization campaign against pertussis, for example, would include unimmunized children under the age of 10 as well as college students whose immunity is waning.

Highlights

Basic Formula for Calculating Statistical Rates

$$\text{Rate} = \frac{\text{Number of events over a time period}}{\text{Population at risk at that time}} \times \begin{array}{c}1{,}000\\ \text{(or 100,000)}\end{array}$$

For example, in a community with a population of 10,000 females aged 13 to 18 years, there were 200 teenage pregnancies in 2010. What is the rate of teenage pregnancy?

$$\text{Rate of teenage pregnancy} = \frac{\text{200 pregnancies in females 13–18 during 2010}}{\text{10,000 females aged 13–18 in the population at midyear}} \times 1{,}000 = \text{20 pregnancies per 1,000 females}$$

Rates of Occurrence

The rate of occurrence of a health-related condition is also of concern to population health nurses. *Rates of occurrence* are statistical measures that indicate the extent of health problems in a group. A rate is simply the number of a particular event (e.g., cases of illness) divided by the size of the population at risk for the event in a given time period (e.g., annually, per quarter) (CDC, 2011). Rates of occurrence allow comparisons between groups of different sizes with respect to the extent of a particular condition. For example, a community with a population of 1,000 may report 50 cases of syphilis this year, whereas another community of 100,000 persons may report 5,000 cases. On the surface, it would seem that the second community has a greater problem with syphilis than the first; however, both communities have experienced 50 cases per 1,000 population. In other words, both have a problem with syphilis of comparable magnitude.

Computing the statistical rates of interest in population health nursing involves dividing the *number of instances of an event* during a specified period by the *population at risk* for that event and *multiplying by 1,000* (or 100,000 if the numbers of the event are so small that the result of the calculation using a multiplier of 1,000 would be less than 1). The basic formula for calculating statistical rates of interest to community health nurses is presented at left.

Both mortality and morbidity rates are of concern in population health nursing. **Mortality** is the ratio of the number of deaths in various categories to the number of people in a given population, whereas **morbidity** is the ratio of the number of cases of a disease or condition to the number of people in the population. Mortality rates describe deaths; morbidity rates describe cases of health conditions that may or may not result in death. For example, the number of people in a particular group who die as a result of cardiovascular disease is reflected in the mortality rate; however, the number of people experiencing cardiovascular disease is indicated by the morbidity rate.

MORTALITY RATES. Mortality rates of interest in population health nursing include the overall or "crude" death rate, cause-specific death rates, infant and neonatal mortality, fetal and perinatal mortality, and the maternal death rate. Each rate is calculated from the number of events during a specified time period (e.g., a year) and the average population at risk during that same time. Formulas for calculating some specific rates of interest are presented on the next page.

Rates are reported in terms of the multiplier used to calculate them. For example, overall cancer deaths usually occur in fairly large numbers, so a cause-specific death rate for all cancers would be calculated using 1,000 as the multiplier. The resulting death rate is reported as the number of deaths per 1,000 population. For example, if City A, with a population of 50,000, had 100 cancer-related deaths in 2010, the cause-specific death

Highlights

Formulas for Calculating Selected Mortality Rates

$$\text{Crude death rate} = \frac{\text{Total number of deaths during year}}{\text{Total population at midyear}} \times 1{,}000$$

$$\text{Cause-specific annual death rate} = \frac{\text{Number of deaths from specific cause during year}}{\text{Total population at midyear}} \times 1{,}000$$

$$\text{Annual infant mortality rate} = \frac{\text{Number of deaths during year (birth to 1 year of age)}}{\text{Number of live births during year}} \times 1{,}000$$

$$\text{Annual neonatal mortality rate} = \frac{\text{Number of deaths during year (birth to 28 days of age)}}{\text{Number of live births during year}} \times 1{,}000$$

$$\text{Annual fetal death rate} = \frac{\text{Number of fetal deaths during year (20 to 28 weeks' gestation)}}{\text{Number of live births plus fetal deaths during year}} \times 1{,}000$$

$$\text{Annual perinatal death rate} = \frac{\text{Number of perinatal deaths during year (20 weeks' gestation to 1 week of age)}}{\text{Number of live births plus fetal deaths during year}} \times 1{,}000$$

$$\text{Annual maternal death rate} = \frac{\text{Number of maternal deaths during year}}{\text{Number of live births during year}} \times 100{,}000$$

rate for cancer for that year would be reported as 2 deaths per 1,000 population. Deaths from pancreatic cancer, on the other hand, occur relatively infrequently, so 100,000 would be the multiplier used to calculate the pancreatic cancer death rate for 2010. If there were six deaths from pancreatic cancer in City B in 2010, and City B had a total population of 500,000 people at midyear, the annual pancreatic cancer mortality rate would be reported as 1.2 deaths per 100,000 population.

Age-adjusted mortality rates can be calculated to account for differences in age distribution between groups. This allows the population health nurse to make more accurate comparisons of mortality between groups with varying age distributions. For example, City A might have a considerably higher crude death rate for influenza than City B. If, however, City A also has a larger proportion of elderly people in the population, more influenza deaths would be expected, because older people are more vulnerable to this condition. Age-adjusted mortality rates, on the other hand, allow the population health nurse to compare the effects of influenza on Cities A and B as if they had similar proportions of elderly residents. If City A's death rate remains higher when adjusted for age, the nurse would look for other factors in the community to explain this difference.

A case fatality rate is another form of mortality rate. The **case fatality rate** is the percentage of persons who develop a health problem and who die as a result of it. For example, at present many people infected with Ebola virus die because of the lack of an effective treatment and the case fatality rate for Ebola virus infection is close to 100%. In the early days of the AIDS epidemic, case fatality rates were also extremely high. Now, with more effective treatment, many people with AIDS can live for significantly longer periods.

A related concept is **survival time**, or the average length of time from diagnosis to death. For example, given current health care technology, the survival time for children with Down syndrome is much longer today than at the turn of the century. Caution should be used, however, when interpreting trends in both survival rate and survival time. Diagnostic technology has permitted earlier diagnosis of many conditions, increasing the time from diagnosis to death, but not appreciably lengthening one's life (Gordis, 2014).

MORBIDITY RATES. Morbidity rates reflect the number of persons within the population who experience a particular condition. Like mortality rates, morbidity rates can be calculated for specific subsets of the population; for example, extent of diabetes or heart disease occurring among people in specific age groups or from different ethnic backgrounds. Morbidity is further described in terms of the incidence and prevalence of a condition. **Incidence** reflects the number of *new* cases of a particular condition identified during a specified period of time. **Prevalence** is the *total number* of people affected by a particular condition at a specified point in time.

To illustrate the concepts of incidence and prevalence, consider a town with a population of 30,000 in which 15 new cases of hypertension were diagnosed in June. This is an indication of the incidence of hypertension. People who were diagnosed as hypertensive prior to June and who continue to live in the town still have hypertension. These additional cases of hypertension, however, are not reflected in the hypertension incidence rate for June, but are included in the prevalence, the total number of people in the community affected by hypertension. The formulas on the next page are used to calculate annual incidence and prevalence rates. Again, the results of the calculations are reported in terms of the multiplier used (e.g., per 1,000 population or per 100,000 population).

The converse of the case fatality rate discussed earlier under mortality rates is the survival rate. The **survival rate** is the proportion of people with a life-threatening condition who remain alive for a specific period of time (usually 5 years) (National Cancer Institute, n.d.). For example, the 5-year survival rate for women with breast cancer is relatively high compared to the survival rate for those with pancreatic cancer.

Highlights

Formulas for Calculating Annual Incidence and Prevalence Rates

$$\text{Annual incidence rate} = \frac{\text{Number of new cases of a condition last year}}{\text{Total population at risk at midyear}} \times 1{,}000$$

$$\text{Annual prevalence rate} = \frac{\text{Total number of cases of a condition last year}}{\text{Total population at risk at midyear}} \times 1{,}000$$

Other rates that may be of interest to population health nurses include marriage and divorce rates, unintended pregnancy rates, employment rates, utilization rates for health services and facilities, and rates for alcohol and drug use and abuse. Population health nurses use morbidity and mortality data and information about other rates in assessing the health status of the population. Population morbidity or mortality rates that are generally higher than state or national rates indicate health problems that require intervention at the population level. For example, the nurse may note that local morbidity rates for vaccine preventable illnesses such as measles and rubella are twice those of the rest of the state. These differences indicate that a significant portion of the population is not immunized. The nurse then uses these data to begin an investigation of factors involved in the problem and to plan a solution. Is it a matter of inaccessibility of immunization services, lack of education on the need for immunization, or poor surveillance of immunization levels in the schools? The solution to the problem must be geared to the cause. Statistical data merely serve to indicate the presence of a problem; they do not delineate its specific nature.

Low morbidity and mortality rates do not indicate the absence of health problems in the population because biostatistics are only one indicator of population health status. Many health problems are not reported statistically, and their presence in the population is not reflected in morbidity and mortality rates. The nutritional status of the population is one area not addressed by biostatistics such as morbidity and mortality rates. Other indicators that the population health nurse employs in assessing the population's health status are discussed in Chapter 15∞. A software program for creating epidemiologic questionnaires to capture some of these forms of data is available from the Centers for Disease Control and Prevention. Source information for the program is included in the student resources site.

The Epidemiologic Process

Epidemiologists use a systematic process, similar to the nursing process, to study states of health and illness in an effort to control disease and promote health. The steps of the *epidemiologic process* are:

- Defining the condition
- Determining the natural history of the condition
- Identifying strategic points of control
- Developing control strategies
- Implementing control strategies
- Evaluating the effects of control strategies

Determining the natural history of the condition is analogous to the assessment and diagnosis phases of the nursing process. Identifying strategic points of control and designing control programs reflect the planning aspects of the nursing process, and the implementation and evaluation steps are equivalent to similar steps in the nursing process.

Defining the Condition

The first step in the epidemiologic process is defining the health condition requiring intervention. As we will see in Chapter 11∞, the epidemiologic process can be applied to health as well as illness. In either case, it is necessary to define specifically the state or condition for which intervention is required. Taking a health promotion focus, one needs to define what is meant by health. With respect to a specific disease or health problem, one must clearly define what is and what is not an instance of the problem. For example, to study the factors contributing to child abuse one must be able to differentiate abuse from accidental harm to a child. Similarly, one must be able to differentiate cases of measles from other similar diseases in order to study and control the disease.

Determining the Natural History of the Condition

The natural history of a disease or condition is a description of the events that precede its development and occur during its course, as well as its typical outcomes. Determining a condition's natural history involves identifying factors that contribute to its development, typical signs and symptoms of the condition, its effects on the human system, and its typical outcomes and factors that may affect those outcomes. For example, crowded living conditions, lack of immunization, and exposure to influenza virus are some of the factors involved in the development of influenza. The typical course of influenza includes a short incubation period and rapid onset of respiratory and/or gastrointestinal symptoms. Most cases of influenza resolve after several days, but the eventual outcome depends on such factors as the individual's overall health, age, nutritional status, and personal habits such as smoking. All of these bits of information are part of the natural history of influenza.

The description of the natural history of a particular condition also incorporates information on the frequency of occurrence, severity of outcomes, and its geographic distribution. Information is obtained on time relationships and trends related to the condition. Time relationships refer to the occurrence of the condition at specific times or during particular seasons. For example, influenza occurs primarily in the winter, and the incidence of suicide rises around holidays. Similarly, a first incident of spousal abuse is often associated with the victim being pregnant. Trends refer to patterns of occurrence for the condition. Incidence of vaccine preventable diseases, for example, declined considerably when vaccines became available, but several of these diseases have shown a trend of increasing incidence, particularly among certain population groups.

The natural history of a condition is often divided into four stages: susceptibility, preclinical, clinical, and resolution (CDC, 2011). In the *susceptibility stage*, factors contributing to development of the condition are present and the person is at-risk for its development. When exposure to causative factors has occurred, but no symptoms have appeared, the condition is in the *preclinical stage*. The *clinical stage* begins with the onset of signs and symptoms characteristic of the disease or condition. In the *resolution stage*, the condition culminates in a return to health, death, or continuation in a chronic state. These stages are depicted in Figure 3-2●. We can use the example of arthritis to clarify the stages of the natural history. In the preexposure stage, factors contributing to arthritis (e.g., overweight, history of prior joint injury, etc.) are present, but the disease has not manifested yet. In the preclinical stage, changes have begun to occur in joint tissue, but no symptoms are present. In the clinical stage, the person begins to experience pain, joint swelling, and other symptoms typical of arthritis. Because arthritis is a lifelong condition, the resolution stage does not involve a return to a prearthritic state, but involves continuation as a chronic condition that will require continuing care.

Determining the factors involved in the natural history of a condition is usually undertaken from the perspective of a particular epidemiologic model. Three such models are presented later in this chapter. The PHN model discussed in Chapter 1∞ is based on one of these epidemiologic models.

Identifying Strategic Points of Control

Knowledge of the natural history of a disease or condition allows epidemiologists and population health nurses to identify strategic points at which the development or course of the condition might be controlled. One might, for example, design interventions to eliminate or modify the factors contributing to the condition to prevent it from occurring. Similarly, knowledge of factors affecting the course of a condition might lead to interventions designed to minimize its effects.

Strategic points of control might occur at any of the levels of health care. For example, health promotion and illness or injury prevention strategies might be employed in the preexposure and preclinical stages of the condition. As an example, good nutrition and immunization are health promotion and prevention strategies that might prevent a child from developing varicella (chickenpox). Resolution strategies might be used during the clinical stage when symptoms of the condition have

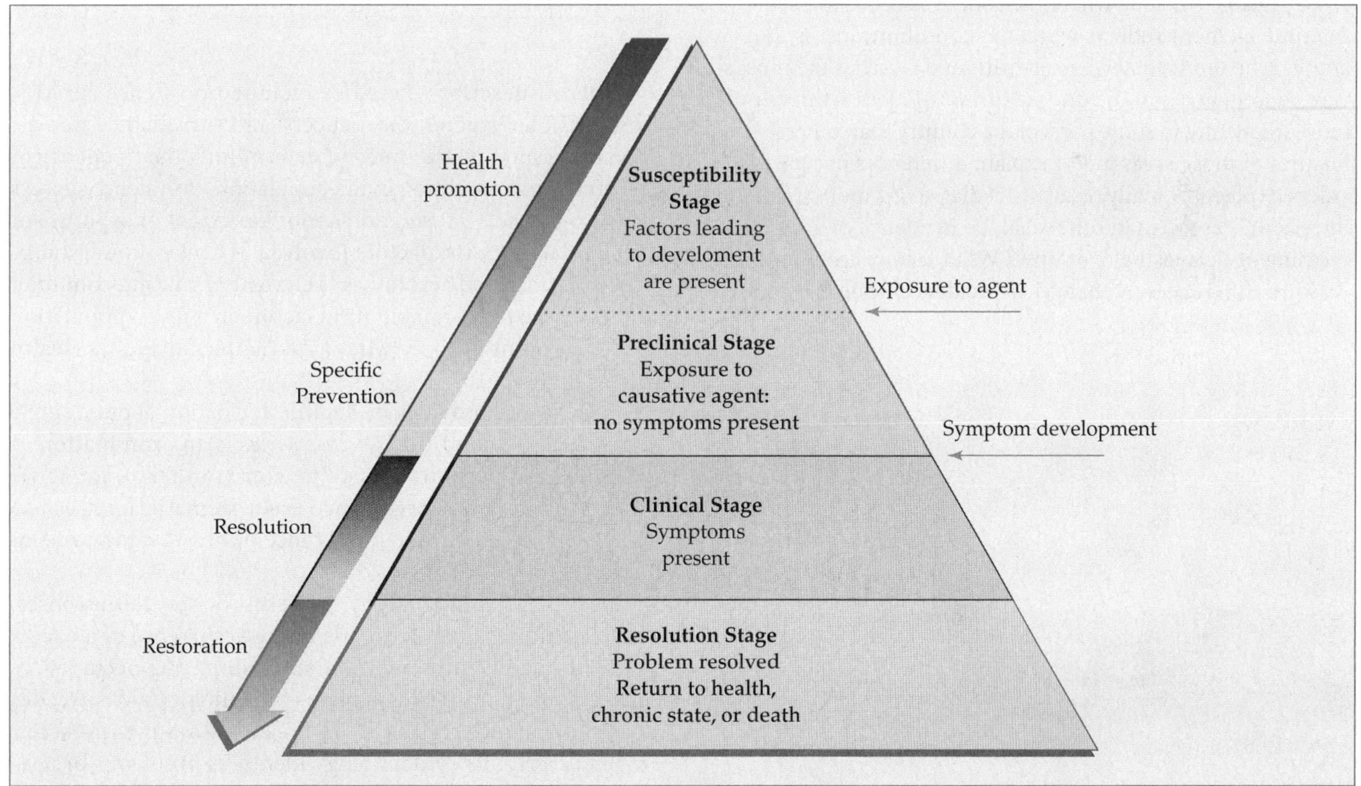

FIGURE 3-2 Stages in the Natural History of a Condition and Their Relationship to the Levels of Health Care

occurred. If long-term complications arise from the condition, other strategies might be needed to restore normal function or prepare for a peaceful death.

Designing, Implementing, and Evaluating Control Strategies

Once strategic points of control have been identified, health care interventions or programs can be designed to prevent or minimize the effects of the condition on the health of the population. These interventions or programs are then implemented and evaluated in terms of their effects on the occurrence and outcomes of the particular condition.

Epidemiologic Investigation

The basic requirement for using the epidemiologic process to control health and illness is information on contributing factors as well as on effective control strategies. Information about any given condition is usually obtained over time from multiple epidemiologic investigations. Epidemiologic studies are of three general types: descriptive, analytic, and experimental.

Descriptive Epidemiology

Descriptive epidemiology is the study of the distribution of a given health state in a specified population in terms of person, place, and time (CDC, 2011). The person element reflects the characteristics of people who develop the condition, such as age, gender, race and ethnicity, economic status, and so on. Place variables include where the condition tends to occur, and the time element reflects when the condition occurs. For example, who tends to develop arthritis and who has the most severe consequences of the disease (person)? Does arthritis occur more frequently in some parts of the country than others? What features of those areas might explain differences in arthritis incidence (place)? Finally, is arthritis diagnosed more frequently in certain seasons than others? Is the incidence of arthritis increasing or decreasing over time? What factors account for the seasonal differences or changes in incidence (time)

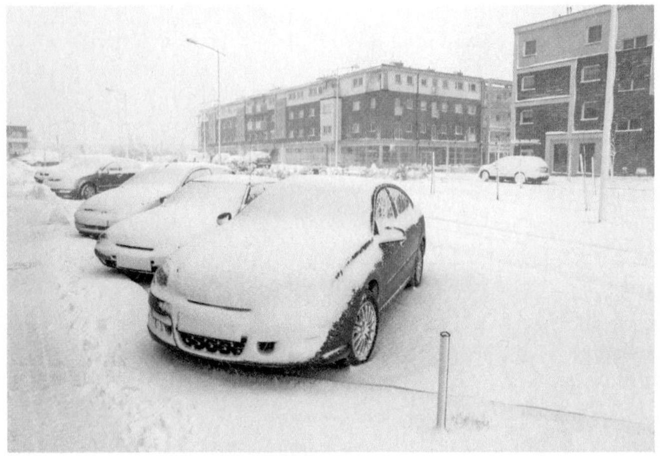

Some diseases occur primarily in winter. *(Patryk Kosmider/Fotolia)*

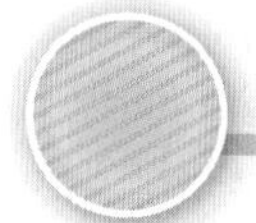

Global Perspectives

Epidemiologic Investigation

Questions related to person, place, and time address three of the key features of an epidemiologic investigation. The person component of epidemiology addresses who is affected by the condition? Are certain age groups more likely to develop the condition than others? Does the condition occur more frequently in members of certain ethnic groups or those of a particular socioeconomic level?

The time component reflects when the condition occurs. Is incidence higher at certain times of the year? Does the condition tend to occur after certain other events or does it occur before other events. What else is happening about the time the condition is noted?

Place reflects the locales where the condition tends to occur. Does it occur in areas with certain weather patterns? Is it confined to certain geographic areas or particular neighborhoods? The place component was a key feature of Snow's identification of the Broad Street pump as the source of the London cholera epidemic. Place may also affect the way in which a particular condition develops. How might the epidemiology of a particular condition, such as HIV/AIDs, differ in a place like the United States versus a rural African village? What are the features of place that influence the development of HIV infection and AIDS disease in these two parts of the world?

Types of descriptive studies include prevalence surveys, cross-sectional studies, case reports, and surveillance studies. Prevalence surveys are aimed at determining the frequency of occurrence of a condition in the population. Prevalence surveys may also provide information about the extent of exposure of the population to risk factors involved in a given condition. A cross-sectional study examines the extent of a health condition and exposure to its contributing factors in a given population at a given point in time (Michigan Center for Public Health Preparedness, 2010).

A *case report* provides in-depth information about a single instance of the condition. A *case series* is an examination of several case reports to determine common features. As we saw in Chapter 1∞, surveillance is a systematic approach to monitoring trends in the occurrence of health conditions of interest.

Descriptive epidemiology is useful for several purposes. These include evaluating trends in the occurrence of a condition within a given population and comparing occurrences between populations. Descriptive epidemiology also provides a basis for planning health services and allocating resources. Finally descriptive epidemiology identifies problems for analytic epidemiologic investigations. Descriptive studies may provide causal hypotheses that can be tested in other types of

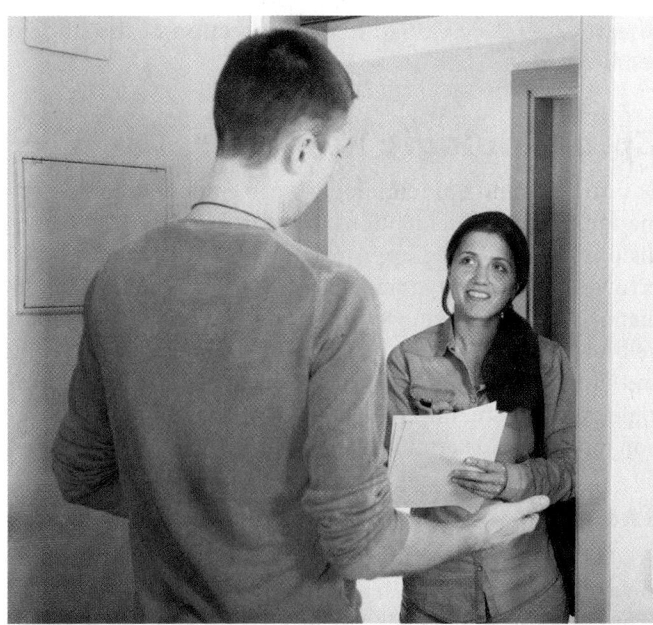

Door-to-door surveys are one way of obtaining epidemiologic data. *(JackF/Fotolia)*

epidemiologic studies, but do not themselves provide evidence of causation (Friis & Sellers, 2014).

Analytic Epidemiology

Analytic epidemiology is the study of factors contributing to health states. Its purposes are to (a) suggest mechanisms of causation, (b) generate etiologic (causal) hypotheses, and (c) test those hypotheses. Analytic epidemiology can be divided into three categories of investigations: ecological studies, case–control studies, and cohort studies (Friis & Sellers, 2014). Ecological studies compare rates of disease occurrence among several population groups, usually 10 or more. For example, one might compare the rates of HIV infection among heterosexuals and sexual minority group members of different races/ethnicities. Ecological studies are useful when the extent of exposure of specific individuals to factors contributing to a problem is unknown, but information about the general level of exposure in the population is available. Ecological studies can be used to assess relationships between exposure rates and disease rates in different populations. They also provide information on trends in exposures as compared to trends in disease occurrence. For example, frequency of sexual activity among persons of different age groups would suggest differential probabilities of being exposed to HIV infection.

Case–control studies involve comparisons between people with a specific condition and those without it. Differences in characteristics of members of these two groups may suggest causative or preventive factors related to the health condition of interest. For example, we might compare people who develop bladder cancer with those who do not with respect to their smoking behavior. Cohort studies, also called prospective or longitudinal studies, follow over time people exposed to a supposed causative factor, but without the condition, to determine the proportion of people who actually develop the condition of interest. For example, we might follow a group of smokers over time to determine how many of them develop bladder cancer, or examine the levels of certain chemicals in the body to determine links to mental illness.

Experimental Epidemiology

Experimental epidemiology is a subset of analytic epidemiology in which exposure to certain variables is manipulated by the researcher to determine the results (Friis & Sellers, 2014). Experimental studies are used to test the effectiveness of interventions. Application of an intervention by the researcher is called a *trial. Clinical trials* apply interventions to individuals; *community trials* test interventions with population groups (Friis & Sellers, 2014). Trials can involve removal of a risk factor for a condition or addition of some other factor and can be either prophylactic or therapeutic in nature, depending on the timing of the intervention.

In prophylactic trials, the intervention is designed to prevent the occurrence of a condition. Interventions designed to promote health are also tested in prophylactic trials. Therapeutic trials, on the other hand, investigate the effects of treatments at the resolution and restoration levels of health care. In these studies, the researcher exposes a group of people to an intervention designed to resolve an existing health problem. The intervention may be either positive or negative. Positive interventions add a factor to the situation being studied (e.g., a new form of education to prevent smoking among teens). Negative interventions reduce or eliminate causative factors (e.g., preventing access to tobacco products among teens). In another example, a population health nurse might explore the effects of teaching parenting techniques (a positive intervention) or reducing environmental stressors (a negative intervention) on the incidence of child abuse by already abusive parents. The

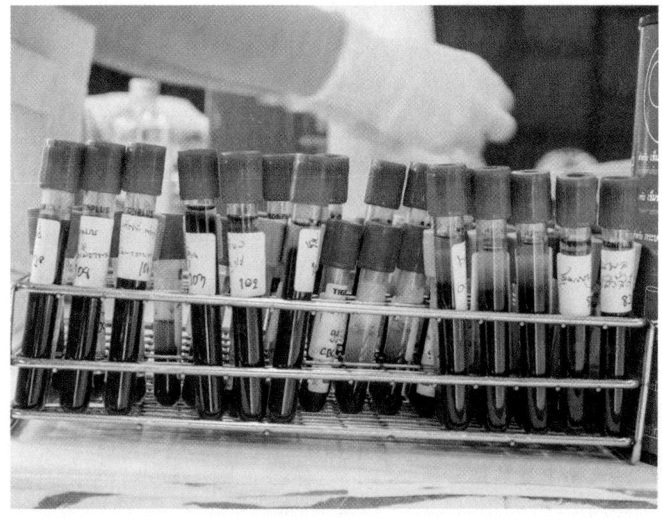

Tests of biomarkers may help to identify populations at risk for specific diseases. *(Panupong1982/Fotolia)*

relationships among the types of epidemiologic investigations presented here are depicted in Figure 3-3●. The selection of a particular investigative approach depends on the study to be conducted and the extent of prior research on the topic. For example, descriptive studies are appropriate in studying conditions about which little is known. For example, a descriptive study might be conducted among male-to-female transgender individuals regarding their access to and use of mammography screening services. In other areas where there is already evidence of possible relationships between variables, analytic or experimental studies might be more appropriate. Choice of an analytic or experimental approach depends primarily on whether the situation permits the researcher to manipulate the variables of interest. In some instances, manipulation of variables is not possible; in others, manipulation of the variables involved would be unethical. For example, if a particular vaccine has been shown to be effective in preventing a specific disease, it would not be ethical to give some people the vaccine and others a placebo to see what the rate of infection in the two groups is.

Population health nurses may be actively involved in epidemiologic investigations. For information about agencies and organizations that support epidemiology and epidemiologic research, see the *External Resources* section of the student resources site.

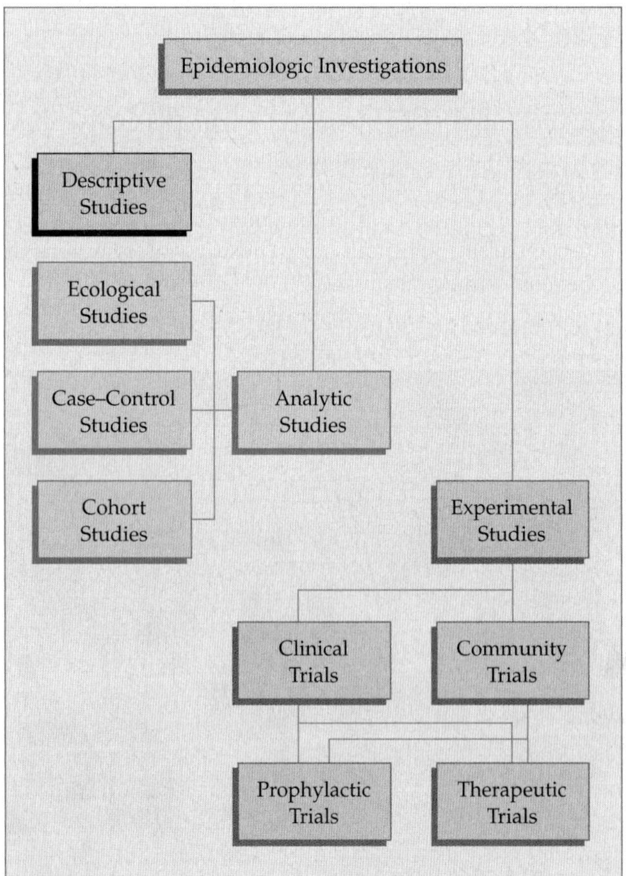

FIGURE 3-3 Approaches to Epidemiologic Investigation

Epidemiologic Models

Both nurses and epidemiologists use epidemiologic information to direct interventions to control health-related conditions. Determining appropriate control strategies often involves collecting large amounts of data about multiple factors that may be contributing to the condition. For this reason, it is helpful to have a model or framework to direct the collection and interpretation of these data. We explore three epidemiologic models here: the epidemiologic triad, the web of causation model, and determinants-of-health models.

The Epidemiologic Triad Model

Traditionally, epidemiologic investigation has been guided by the epidemiologic triad. In this model, data are collected with respect to a triad of elements: host, agent, and environment (Friis & Sellers, 2014). The interrelationship of these elements results in a state of relative health or illness. The relationships among host, agent, and environment and specific considerations under each are depicted in Figure 3-4●.

HOST. The **host** is the client system affected by the particular condition under investigation. Population health nursing is concerned with the health of human beings, so, for our purposes, the host is a human being. A variety of factors can influence the host's exposure, susceptibility, and response to an agent. Host-related factors include intrinsic factors (e.g., age, race, and sex), physical and psychological factors, nutritional status, genetics, and the presence or absence of disease states or immunity, among others (Friis & Sellers, 2014).

AGENT. The **agent** is the primary cause of a health-related condition. After specific microorganisms were found to cause specific diseases, the concept of agents of disease originated in the context of communicable diseases. Although the causes of some health problems may be so complex that no single agent can be identified, the concept of agent remains useful for exploring many health problems.

Agents can be classified into six types: physical agents, chemical agents, nutritive elements, infectious agents, genetic agents, and psychological agents. Physical agents include heat, trauma, and radiation. Chemical agents include various substances to which people may develop untoward reactions. Some plants such as poison ivy and ragweed can be considered chemical agents because they cause a chemical reaction resulting in an allergic response. An absence or an excess of a variety of nutritive elements is known to result in disease, as do the presence of and exposure to a number of infectious agents that cause communicable diseases. Genetic agents arise from genetic transmission from parent to child. Finally, psychological agents such as stress can produce a variety of stress-related

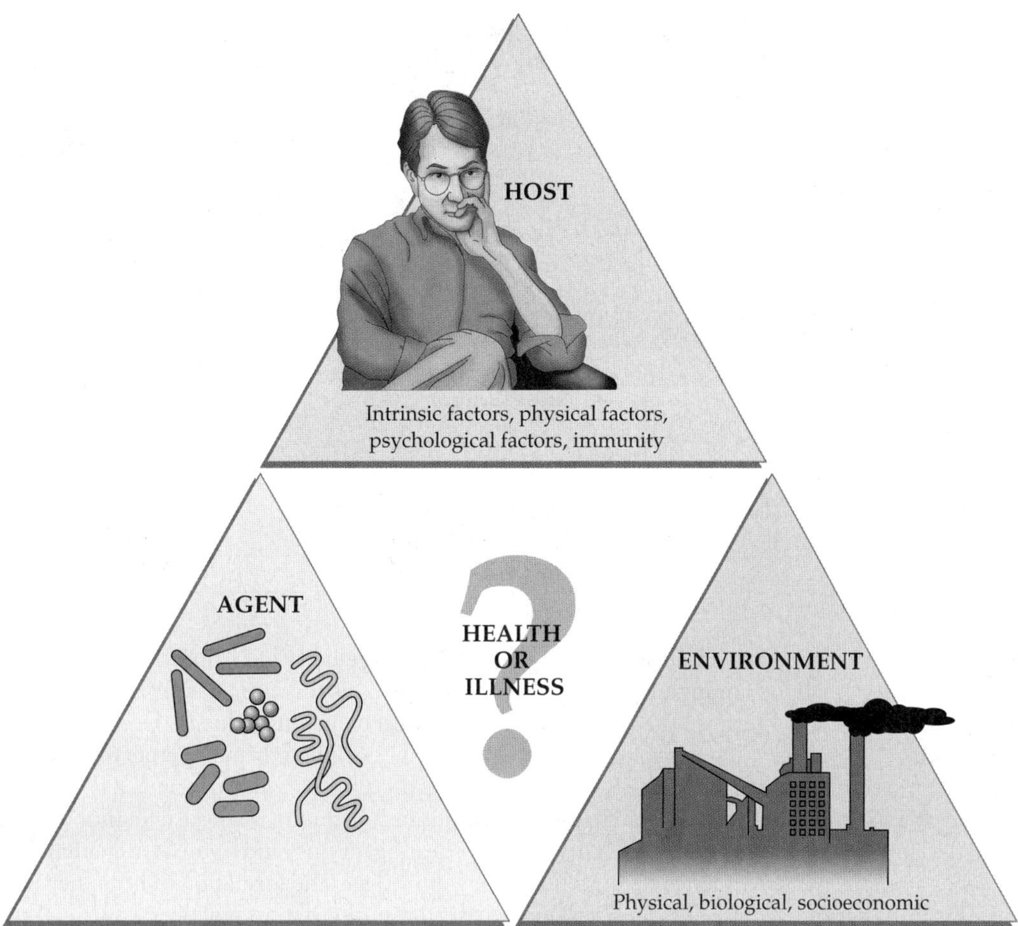

FIGURE 3-4 Elements of the Epidemiologic Triad Model

conditions. The types of agents and examples of health conditions to which they contribute are listed in Table 3-1●.

An agent's characteristics influence whether a given individual develops a particular health-related condition. These characteristics vary somewhat depending on the type of agent involved.

Characteristics of infectious agents. Characteristics that influence the effects of infectious agents include the extent of exposure to the agent and the agent's infectivity, pathogenicity, and virulence. Additional characteristics of infectious agents include toxigenicity, resistance, and antigenicity (Friis & Seller, 2014). The *extent of exposure* to a disease-causing microorganism, or the *infective dose*, affects the outcome of the exposure. For example, a person exposed to a few *Mycobacterium tuberculosis* organisms is unlikely to develop tuberculosis (TB). The greater the number of disease organisms inhaled, however, the greater the likelihood of developing TB.

Infectivity is the ability of an infectious agent to enter, survive and reproduce within, and cause disease in an individual host (*Infectivity*, 2014). Infectivity is determined, in part, by the organism's portals of entry and exit. The **portal of entry** is the means by which the agent invades the host; the **portal of exit** is the avenue by which the agent leaves the host. The portals of entry and exit also influence the **mode of transmission**, or the means by which an infectious agent is transmitted from a source (an infected person, animal, or other source) to a susceptible host. Modes of transmission are discussed in more detail in Chapter 26∞. Measles virus, for example, has a higher infectivity than does tetanus bacillus. The measles virus enters the body quite easily through the respiratory system, whereas tetanus gains entry through a break in the skin, usually a deep puncture wound. Similarly, variola virus, the causative agent for smallpox, is usually inhaled and can be transmitted by means of an aerosol cloud, making it a possible weapon of biological terrorism.

Pathogenicity is the ability of an agent to cause disease when a susceptible person is exposed or the proportion of people who develop clinical disease when infected by the agent (CDC, 2011). In terms of infectious agents, measles virus causes disease in most of the susceptible exposed individuals. *M. tuberculosis*, on the other hand, produces disease in only a small portion of the individuals exposed.

Another concept closely related to pathogenicity is that of **attack rate**, which is the proportion of those exposed to an agent who develop the disease. As is the case with pathogenicity,

TABLE 3-1 Agents and Selected Health Problems to Which They Contribute

Type of Agent	Example	Problems
Physical	Heat	Burns, heat stroke
	Trauma	Fractures, concussion, sprains, contusions
	Radiation	Genetic changes
Chemical	Medications	Accidental poisoning, suicide
	Chlorine	Poisoning, asphyxiation (in gas form)
	Poison ivy	Rash and pruritus
Nutritive	Vitamin C	Scurvy (in absence of vitamin C)
	Iron	Anemia (in absence of iron)
	Vitamin A	Poisoning (in excess)
Infectious	Measles virus	Measles, measles encephalitis
	HIV	AIDS
	Varicella virus	Chickenpox
	Influenza virus	Influenza
Genetic	Genetic predisposition to disease	Sickle cell disease
	Genetic abnormality	Down syndrome, Turner's syndrome
Psychological	Stress	Ulcerative colitis, heart disease, suicide, asthma, alcoholism, drug abuse, violence

measles has a high attack rate, whereas tuberculosis has a low attack rate. The attack rate for smallpox among unvaccinated individuals is greater than 37% of those exposed (*Smallpox of poxviruses infection*, n.d.).

Virulence is the term used to describe the severity of the health problem caused by an agent or the proportion of people with the disease who develop serious illness or die (CDC, 2011). Rubeola or measles has a relatively low virulence because uncomplicated measles is not a serious disease. Tetanus, on the other hand, is extremely virulent because it results in fatality unless treatment is instituted. The virus that causes AIDS is another infectious agent with a very high virulence. Virulence is frequently confused with pathogenicity, but the two terms refer to different agent characteristics. For example, cold viruses that cause disease in exposed individuals are highly pathogenic, but have a low virulence because the diseases caused are relatively minor. Virulence is closely related to case fatality rates discussed earlier in this chapter.

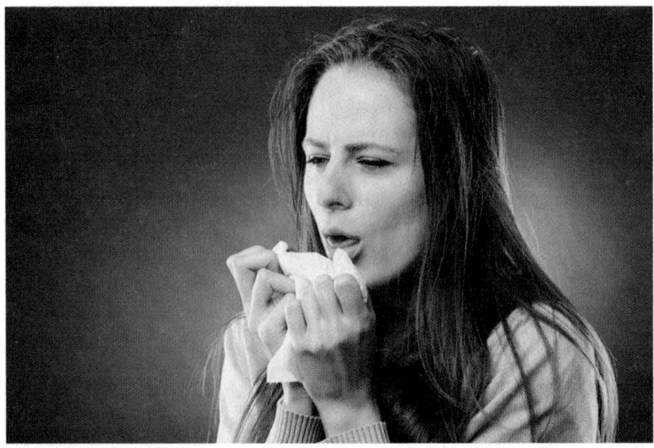

Many diseases are spread by respiratory transmission. *(Xalanx/Fotolia)*

The **toxigenicity** of an infectious agent refers to its ability to produce toxins that are harmful to the human body. The primary effect of tetanus is due to the effects of the toxin produced by tetanus bacilli on the human nervous system. **Resistance** refers to the ability of an infectious agent to survive in adverse conditions, including exposure to antibiotics, but also including heating, drying, and so on. **Antigenicity** is the ability of the agent to trigger the formation of immune antibodies and is the basis for immunization practices.

Characteristics of noninfectious agents. Noninfectious agents share some of the characteristics of infectious agents. For example, the extent of exposure to an agent affects its ability to cause health problems. Ingesting moderate amounts of alcohol or aspirin does not cause problems, and may, in fact, be beneficial. Excessive consumption of either substance, however, can cause difficulties. The amount of stress, a psychological agent, to which one is exposed can also affect the development of stress-related health problems.

The concept of infectivity can also be applied to other types of agents, although the term was developed in relation to infectious agents. For example, asbestos, which can be inhaled, has a higher "infectivity" than an overdose of aspirin, which must be ingested. Stress, as an agent of health problems, also has a high infectivity because it is an everyday factor impinging on people. All of us are "infected" by stress.

Stress can also be viewed in terms of its ability to cause disease. Although everyone experiences some degree of stress, not all people develop stress-related illnesses. Stress, therefore, has a relatively low pathogenicity. Noninfectious agents may vary in terms of their virulence as well. Stress may produce a mild stomach upset in some individuals and drive others to suicide. In the first instance, stress has a low virulence, and in the second, a high virulence.

ENVIRONMENT. The third element of the epidemiologic triad includes factors in the physical, biological, and socioeconomic environments that contribute to health-related conditions (Friis & Sellers, 2014). The physical environment consists of such factors as weather, terrain, and buildings. A variety of physical environment factors can influence health. For example, air pollution contributes to respiratory disease as well as other physiologic and psychological effects in human beings. Similarly, elements of community design such as walking trails have been shown to affect exercise behavior and health status (Parra et al., 2010).

The biological environment, in the triad model, consists of all living organisms other than humans. Components of the biological environment include plants and animals as well as microorganisms, all of which can influence health.

The socioeconomic environment includes factors related to social interaction that may contribute to health or disease. For example, cultural factors, which are part of the social environment, can influence health behaviors. In a similar fashion, social norms may influence health and illness. For example, societal views of alcoholism and drug abuse as character weaknesses have hampered efforts to control these problems. Growing societal acceptance of marijuana use is another example of the effects of culture on health. Conversely, in a health conscious culture, behaviors such as smoking are considered unacceptable.

Factors in each of these three environments were addressed in more detail in the discussion of the PHN model in Chapter 1∞. Because of the triad model's failure to address multiple causative factors completely, it has not been as useful for chronic diseases or other health problems (e.g., societal violence) as it has for communicable diseases.

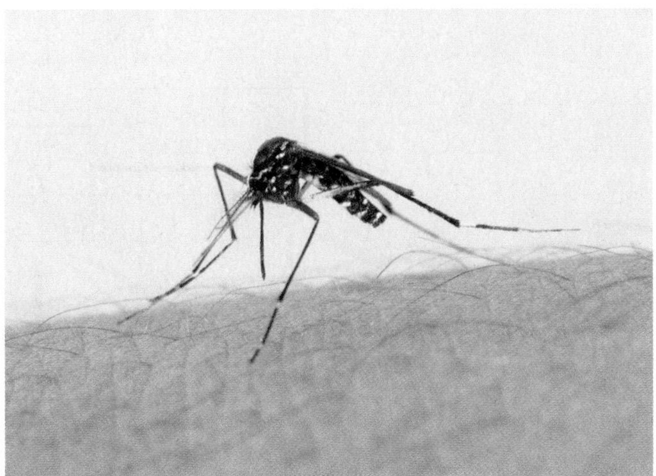

Insect vectors in the biological environment are responsible for the spread of a variety of diseases. *(Panupong/Fotolia)*

The Web of Causation Model

The "web of causation" is a second model for exploring the influence of multiple factors on the development of a specific health condition. In this model, factors are explored in terms of their interplay, and both direct and indirect causes of the problem are identified. The web of causation approach allows the epidemiologist to map the interrelationships among factors contributing to the development (or prevention) of a particular health condition. This approach also assists in determining areas where efforts at control will be most effective.

Some of the factors in a web of causation for the problem of adolescent tobacco use are depicted in Figure 3-5•. It is obvious from the complexity of Figure 3-5 that multiple factors contribute to adolescent tobacco use. The interplay of these factors determines whether or not the problem occurs. The most direct causes are those linked directly to tobacco use—purchase of tobacco products and the decision to use them. Numerous other factors, however, contribute to the adolescent's decision to engage in the use of tobacco. These include perceptions of tobacco use as grown-up or "cool," peer pressure, and easy access to tobacco products. Perceptions of tobacco use are influenced by media messages and adult role models as well as by peer perceptions. Easy access to tobacco products is influenced by poor enforcement of laws regarding the sale of tobacco products to minors, which is in turn influenced by public acceptance of tobacco use. Other contributing factors and their interrelationships are also depicted in Figure 3-5.

Determinants-of-Health Models

Because of the complexity of causal associations in many health problems, the triad and web of causation models have largely been replaced by models that focus on a variety of determinants of health. As we saw in Chapter 1∞, determinants of health are categories of factors that influence health and illness. Emphasis on broad determinants of health and illness marks a change from individually focused explanations of disease to a focus on social and environmental contributions to health and illness. A focus on broad determinants of health acknowledges that individual behaviors are shaped by interaction with the environment and that contextual variables found in the environment probably interact in complex ways with individual variables to determine health and illness.

McKeown has been credited with coining the term *determinants of health*, which was incorporated into The Lalonde Report discussed in Chapter 2∞. The Lalonde Report incorporated the concept of four general determinants (human biology, health system, environment, and lifestyle) into the health field concept (The Social Determinants of Health, 2008).

Over the years, the number and categories of determinants have varied among models. For example, Evans and Stoddart (2003) developed the Producing Health, Consuming Health Care (PHCHC) model in 1990, which included determinant categories such as social environment, physical environment, genetic endowment, individual biological and behavioral response, health and function, disease, health care, well-being,

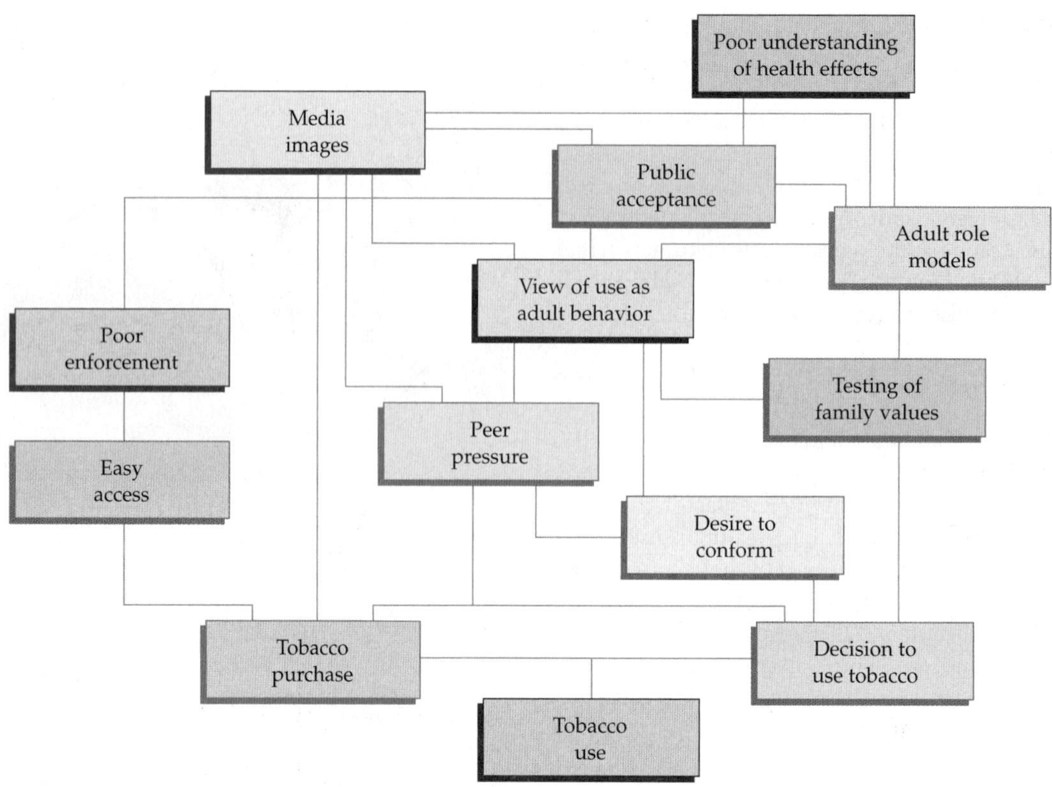

FIGURE 3-5 The Web of Causation for Adolescent Tobacco Use, Indicating the Interplay Between Multiple Direct and Indirect Causes

and prosperity. The Mandala model developed by Hancock and Perkins and embodied in the Ottawa Charter included only seven categories of determinants. The Population Health Promotion model included nine categories (Evans & Stoddart, 2003) and other conceptualizations include as few as six categories. Some of the models focus primarily on social determinants of health and illness, whereas others address biophysical, psychological, and environmental determinants as well.

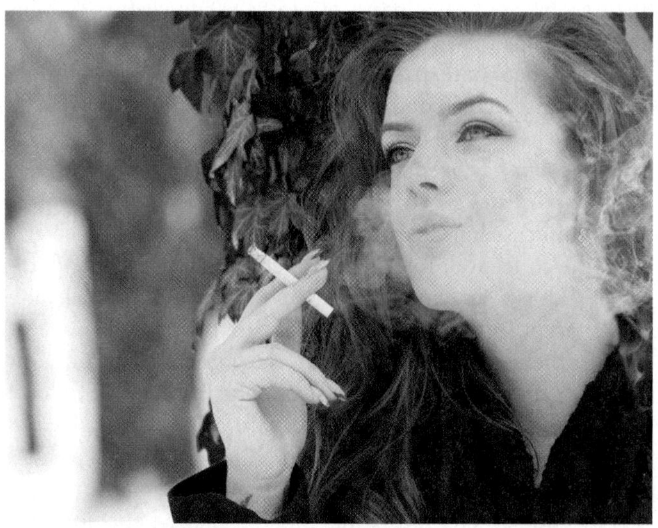

Behavioral determinants, such as smoking, are contributing factors in the development of many diseases. *(Nickolae/Fotolia)*

Determinants-of-health models examine the interplay of factors at each level (individual, family and social network, community, and general societal conditions) and their contribution to the development of health-related problems. The broad array of factors contributing to a problem, as suggested by determinants-of-health models, underscores the fact that resolution of population health problems lies outside the realm of individual effort or medical science and involves action in multiple societal sectors. For example, addressing the issue of handicapping conditions involves not only providing the needed medical care for the condition, but may also require making changes in the built environment to promote access, as well as making changes in work environments to permit handicapped individuals to make productive contributions to society. Figure 3-6● depicts a composite determinants-of-health model that reflects elements included in many of the models found in the literature.

Population health nurses use epidemiologic models to understand the multiple influences on the health of the population. These models highlight the factors contributing to, or in some cases preventing, the occurrence of population health problems and suggest strategic points and interventions that may help in controlling them.

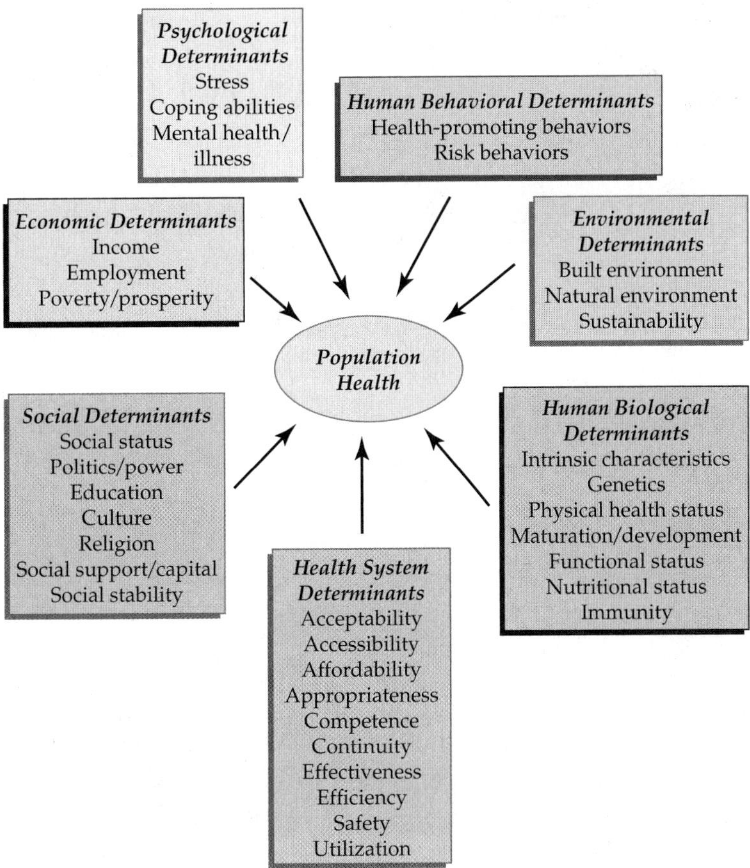

FIGURE 3-6 A Composite Determinants-of-Health Model

CHAPTER RECAP

Epidemiology is concerned with the development of an understanding of factors that influence the health of population groups. Originally developed for use in examining communicable diseases, epidemiologic principles and processes can be used to study any health-related issue.

Population health nurses use epidemiologic strategies to assess the health of the population and identify factors affecting health status. Epidemiologic findings may also help to identify points at which intervention may help to prevent or minimize the consequences of population health problems.

CASE STUDY Absences from Work

As the population health nurse responsible for five census tracts in a small city, you are making a Monday home visit to a young mother with a newborn infant who lives in your area. In asking about the health of other family members, you discover that the woman's husband has been experiencing vomiting and diarrhea for the last day and a half. She says her husband thinks it is something "going around at work" because several people in his office called in sick yesterday and today with similar symptoms. She and the baby have been fine.

The company the client's husband works for is outside of your census tracts, but he happens to mention that he went to the company picnic on Saturday. His wife didn't go because the baby was too young and she was feeling pretty tired after being up for several night-time feedings. When you talk to the husband, you discover that several of the other people who called in sick also attended the picnic, but he is not sure about the others as this is a large company with about 200 employees and he doesn't know exactly who attended the picnic and who did not.

1. What is your first step in determining whether or not an epidemiologic investigation is warranted?
2. How would you go about initiating such an investigation in the jurisdiction where you are doing your population health nursing clinical rotation?
3. What is the usual role of population health nurses in epidemiologic investigations in that jurisdiction?

REFERENCES

Absolute risk and relative risk. (2011). Retrieved from http://www.patient.co.uk/health/Risks-of-Disease-Absolute-and-Relative.htm

Cabaret, J., Morand, S., & Beaudeau, F. (2012). Introduction. In S. Morand, F. Beaudeau, & J. Cabaret (Eds.), *New frontiers of molecular epidemiology in infectious diseases* (pp. 1–8). New York: Springer.

Centers for Disease Control and Prevention. (2004). 150th anniversary of John Snow and the pump handle. *Morbidity and Mortality Weekly Report, 53*, 783.

Centers for Disease Control and Prevention. (2011). *Principles of epidemiology in public health practice* (3rd ed.). Retrieved from http://www.cdc.gov/osels/scientific_edu/SS1978/index.html

Epidemiology. (n.d.). Retrieved from http://www.answers.com/topic/epidemiology

Epidemiology—Definition. (n.d.). Retrieved from http://www.wordiq.com/definition/Epidemiology

Evans, R. G., & Stoddart, G. L. (2003). Consuming research, producing policy? *American Journal of Public Health, 93*, 371–379.

Friis, R. H., & Sellers, T. A. (2014). *Epidemiology for public health practice* (5th ed.). Sudbury, MA: Jones & Bartlett.

Gordis, L. (2014). *Epidemiology: With student consult online access*. Philadelphia, PA: Saunders Elsevier.

Infectivity. (2014). Retrieved from http://medical-dictionary.thefreedictionary.com/infectivity

John Snow. (n.d.). Retrieved from http://www.ph.ucla.edu/epi/snow.html

Krieger, N. (2011). Ecosocial theory of disease distribution: Embodying societal and ecologic context. In N. Krieger (Ed.), *Epidemiology and people's health: Theory and content* (pp. 202–235). Oxford, UK: Oxford University Press.

Ludwig, J. (2000, June 13). UCLA epidemiologist creates a web site about a pioneer in the field. *Chronicle of Higher Education*. Retrieved from http://www.ph.ucla.edu/epi/snow/chronicle_article.html

Michigan Center for Public Health Preparedness. (2010). *Cross sectional study/prevalence study*. Retrieved from http://practice.sph.umich.edu/micphp/epicentral/cross_sectional.php

National Cancer Institute. (n.d.). *NCI dictionary of cancer terms*. Retrieved from http://www.cancer.gov/dictionary?cdrid=44301

Parra, D. C., McKenzie, T. L., Ribeiro, I. C., Hino, A. A. F., Dreisinger, M., Coniglio, K., ..., Simoes, E. J. (2010). Assessing physical activity in public parks in Brazil using systematic observation. *American Journal of Public Health, 100*, 1420–1426. doi:10-2105/AJPH.2009.181230

Relative risk. (2014). Retrieved from http://medical-dictionary.thefreedictionary.com/Risk+ratio

Robinson, B. (2009). *Victorian medicine—From fluke to theory*. Retrieved from http://www.bbc.co.uk/history/british/victorians/victorian_medicine_01.shtml

Smallpox of poxviruses infection. (n.d.). Retrieved from http://virology-online.com/viruses/Poxviruses2.htm

Snow, J. (1855). *On the mode of communication of cholera*. London: John Churchill. Retrieved from http://www.ph.ucla.edu/epi/snow/snowbook.html

The puzzle was a maddening one. (2002, Fall). *The Handle: The Magazine of the University of Alabama School of Public Health*, pp. 4–5.

The social determinants of health. (2008). *Health Affairs, 27*, 320. doi:10.1377/hlthaff.27.2.320

UNIT

2

Influences on Population Health

Chapters

4 — Environmental Influences on Population Health

5 — Cultural Influences on Population Health

6 — Economic Influences on Population Health

7 — Health System Influences on Population Health

8 — Global Influences on Population Health

CHAPTER

4 Environmental Influences on Population Health

Learning Outcomes

After reading this chapter, you should be able to:

1. Analyze the interrelationships among environmental factors, human behavior, and human health.
2. Discuss elements of the natural, built, and social environments that affect population health.
3. Analyze the role of the population health nurse with respect to environmental health issues at the individual/family and population levels.
4. Analyze the role of the population health nurse in prevention measures for environmental issues that affect population health.
5. Identify measures to resolve environmental health problems in individuals and populations and the role of the population health nurse in their implementation.
6. Discuss health restoration measures related to environmental health problems in individuals and populations and the role of the population health nurse related to each.

Key Terms

built environment
ecological footprint
environmental health
hazardous waste
mixed-use development
natural environment
smart growth
sustainable development
urban sprawl
zoonoses

Advocacy Then

Walt Whitman

As we saw in Chapter 2∞, Walt Whitman, in addition to being a renowned writer, was a nurse during the American Civil War. What is even less well known is his advocacy of public health issues, such as personal hygiene and clean water. Whitman used his position as editor of the *Brooklyn Daily Eagle* to advocate for health promotion and conditions to promote health. In one essay, Whitman spoke of the "great sanitative power of the bath, as a general aid to health among the laboring classes" (quoted in Rezick & Fee, 2011, p. 1051) and recommended "immersion in water as often as once every other day" (p. 1050). In another essay, he expounded on the need for clean water and noted that "rum and bad milk [other public health issues of the day] are not as nasty as city pump-water, which is the most stinking and villainous liquid known upon land or sea" (p. 1052). He pointed out the potential for contamination of water through filtration of sewage and decomposing matter into the water system. In his paper, he actively supported the development of the Brooklyn waterworks and later described its completion as "a feather in my wings" (p. 1053).

Advocacy Now

Game Day Challenge

In 2010, 77 colleges and universities participated in the Environmental Protection Agency's "Game Day Challenge" to reduce the amount of waste generated during football games. Schools competed in recycling, composting, reusing, or donating waste generated during one home football game. As a result of the competition, more than 500,000 pounds of materials were diverted from landfills, contributing greatly to environmental sustainability (Schools divert trash, 2011).

Concerns for environmental effects on human health were documented nearly 2,500 years ago when Hippocrates wrote his famous treatise, *On Airs, Waters, and Places*. Although Hippocrates and his contemporaries mistakenly believed illness resulted from *miasmas*, or unhealthy vapors, in specific locales, their conception of environmental effects on health was correct. Nursing, as a profession, has also had an abiding concern for the effects of environment on health. Florence Nightingale's campaign for cleanliness in the surroundings of wounded British soldiers in the Crimean War is a legendary example of this concern. What are less well known are her support for reforestation (McDonald, 2004) and a paper she presented in 1887 to the International Congress of Hygiene and Demography castigating the British government for the unsanitary conditions found in India. This last activity is particularly interesting since Miss Nightingale did not believe that diseases such as cholera, often seen in India, were contagious and perceived quarantine measures as "evil" (Watts, 2003).

Other early population health nurses were equally concerned about the contribution of the environment to human disease. Lillian Wald and her compatriots were concerned about both physical and social environmental effects on health, and much of their work was directed toward changing social conditions that contributed to disease and illness. Population health nurses remain concerned with the effects of environmental factors on health and regularly engage in interventions related to environmental concerns that affect individuals, families, and population groups. To engage in effective action at all levels, population health nurses must have an understanding of environmental influences on health.

Environment and Health

According to the World Health Organization (2011), **environmental health** involves action that

> addresses all the physical, chemical, and biological factors external to a person, and all the related factors impacting behaviors. It encompasses the assessment and control of those environmental factors that can potentially affect health. It is targeted towards preventing disease and creating health-supportive environments. (para. 1)

According to WHO data, approximately 24% of the global burden of disease and 23% of mortality worldwide are related to environmental conditions (Prüss-Üstün & Corvalán, 2006). In recent years, greater attention has been given to the health risks posed by environmental conditions. This attention is evident in the number of national health objectives that focus on environmental health issues.

The *Healthy People 2020* objectives for environmental health encompass 24 objectives, several of which have a number of subobjectives. The objectives address six major environmental themes, including outdoor air quality, surface and groundwater quality, toxic substances and hazardous wastes, homes and communities, infrastructure and surveillance for environmental hazards, and global environmental health. The objectives are presented on pages 75–77, and progress on their achievement can be tracked on the *Healthy People* website.

Many environmental forces influence human health. Microorganisms such as bacteria, viruses, and fungi cause communicable diseases, and animals contribute to the spread of these diseases. Plants may contribute to accidental poisoning or to allergic reactions. Industry, vehicles, and buildings add to air and water pollution and excess noise. Climate and terrain contribute to natural disasters, which are discussed in Chapter 25∞. In addition, climate and terrain may promote air and water pollution, which have long-term effects on health. Community design and the incorporation of walking and biking areas influence opportunities for healthy physical activity, and the quality of interpersonal interactions within the population influence people's willingness to take advantage of these opportunities. All of these facets of the environment give rise to environmental hazards that affect human health. Some of the environmental components that produce health hazards are presented in Figure 4-1●.

Human health requires a viable environment that incorporates the local ecosystem, including the air, water, and soil, and the availability of safe and adequate food. In addition, a viable environment requires **sustainable development**, which has been defined as economic development that complies with "maintaining the function and integrity of the ecosystems that support human societies and the things that they value" (Michael & Beaglehole, 2009, p. 4).

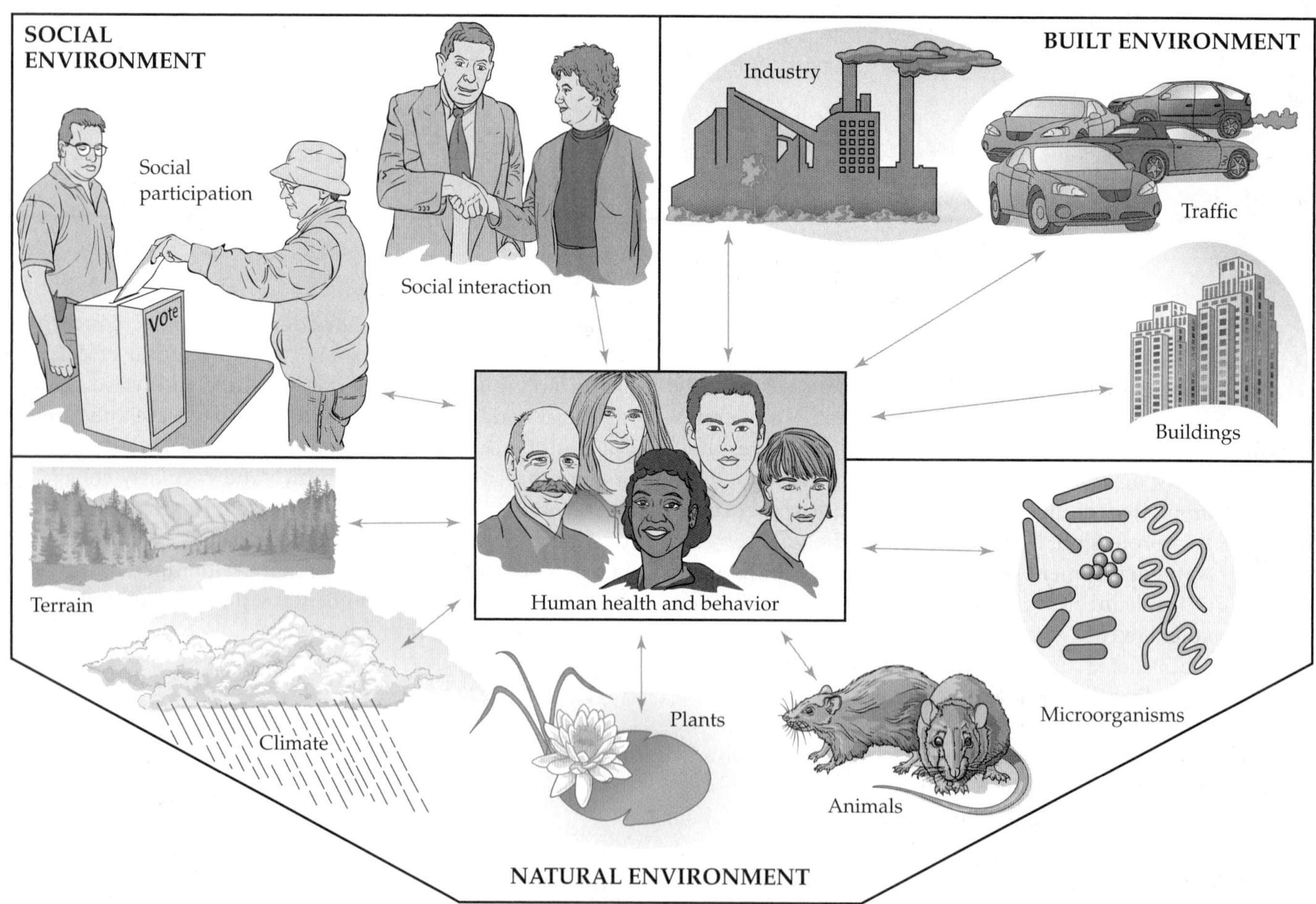

FIGURE 4-1 Selected Environmental Components Influencing Health

Healthy People 2020

Objectives for Environmental Health

OBJECTIVE	BASELINE (YEAR)	TARGET	CURRENT DATA (YEAR)	DATA SOURCE
EH-1: Reduce the number of days the Air Quality Index (AQI) exceeds 100	11 (2008)	10	NDA	Air Quality System, EPA
EH-2: Increase the use of alternative modes of transportation for work	(2008)			American Community Survey, U.S. Bureau of the Census
• Bicycling	0.5%	0.6%	NDA	
• Walking	2.8%	3.1%	NDA	
• Transit	5%	5.5%	NDA	
• Telecommute	4.1%	5.3%	NDA	
EH-3: Reduce air toxic emissions to decrease the risk of adverse effects caused by airborne toxics	(2005)			National Emissions Inventory (NEI), EPA, Office of Air and Radiation (OAR), Office of Air Quality Planning and Standards (OAQPS)
• Mobile sources	1.8 mil tons	1 mil tons	NDA	
• Area sources	1.3 mil tons	1.7 mil tons	NDA	
• Major sources	0.8 mil tons	0.7 mil tons	NDA	
EH-4: Increase the proportion of persons served by community water systems who receive a supply of drinking water that meets the regulations of the Safe Drinking Water Act	(2008) 92%	91%	NDA	Potable Water Surveillance System, Safe Drinking Water Information System, EPA, OW, OGWDW
EH-5: Reduce waterborne disease outbreaks arising from water intended for drinking among persons served by community water systems	7 per year (1999–2008)	2 per year	NDA	Waterborne Disease Outbreak Surveillance System (WBDOSS) Morbidity and Mortality Weekly Report, CDC, NCID, State Health Departments
EH-6: Reduce per capita domestic water withdrawals with respect to use and conservation	99 gallons (2005)	89.1 gallons	NDA	U.S. Department of the Interior, U.S. Geological Survey, USGS National Water-use Information Program
EH-7: Increase the number of days that beaches are open and safe for swimming	95% of beach days (2008)	96% of beach days	NDA	BEACH program, EPA, Office of Water
EH-8: Reduce blood lead levels in children	(2005–2008)			National Health and Nutrition Examination Survey (NHANES), CDC, NCHS
• Elevated blood lead levels	0.9%	0%	NDA	
• Mean blood lead levels	1.5 μg/dL	1.4 μg/dL	NDA	
EH-9: Minimize the risks to human health and the environment posed by hazardous sites	(2010) 1, 279 sites	1,151 sites	NDA	Comprehensive Environmental Response and Cleanup Liability Information System (CERCLIS), EPA, OSWER, OSRTI
EH-10: Reduce pesticide exposures that result in visits to a health care facility	15,965 (2008)	10,377	NDA	Nation Poison Data System, American Association of Poison Control Centers

Continued on next page

Healthy People 2020 (Continued)

OBJECTIVE	BASELINE (YEAR)	TARGET	CURRENT DATA (YEAR)	DATA SOURCE
EH-11: Reduce the amount of toxic pollutants released into the environment	3.9 billion pounds (2008)	3.5 billion pounds	NDA	U.S. National toxics Release Inventory (TRI), EPA
EH-12: Increase recycling of municipal solid waste	33.2% (2008)	36.5%	NDA	Characterization of Municipal Solid Waste, EPA, OSW
EH-13: Reduce indoor allergen levels				American Healthy Homes Survey, HUD
• Cockroach	0.51 units/g settled dust	0.46 units/g	NDA	
• Mouse	0.16 mcg/g (2006)	0.14 mcg/g		
EH-14: Increase the number of homes with operating radon mitigation system for persons in homes at risk for radon exposure	10.2% (2007)	30%	NDA	EPA report by Radon Vent Fan Manufacturers, EPA, Indoor Environments Division
EH-15: Increase the percentage of new single-family homes constructed with radon-reducing features, especially in high-radon-potential areas	28.6% (2007)	100%	NDA	Annual Builder and Consumer Practices Surveys, National Association of Home Builders Research Center, reported to EPA, Indoor Environments Division
EH-16: Increase the proportion of the nation's elementary, middle, and high school students that have official school policies and engage in practices that promote a healthy and safe physical school environment	(2006)			School Health Policies and Programs Study, CDC
• Indoor air quality management program	51.4%	56.5%	NDA	
• Plan for addressing mold problems	67%	74%	NDA	
• Plan for hazardous materials	85.9%	94.5%	NDA	
• Reduction of pesticide exposures	57.9%	63.7%	NDA	
• Drinking water inspection for				
• Lead	55.7%	61.3%	NDA	
• Bacteria	58.8%	64.7%	NDA	
• Coliforms	55.2%	60.7%	NDA	
EH-17: Increase the proportion of persons living in pre-1978 housing that has been tested for the presence of lead-based paint or related hazards	Developmental	Developmental	NDA	Potential data source: National Health Interview Survey
EH-18: Reduce the number of U.S. homes that are found to have lead-based paint or related hazards	(2005–2006)			American Healthy Homes Survey, HUD, Office of Health Homes and Lead Hazard Control
• Lead-based paint	37 mil homes	3.7 mil fewer homes	NDA	
• Paint-lead hazards	15.3 mil homes	1.5 mil fewer homes	NDA	
• Dust-lead hazards	13.7 mil homes	1.4 mil fewer homes	NDA	
• Soil-lead hazards	3.8 mil homes	380,000 fewer homes	NDA	
EH-19: Reduce the proportion of occupied housing units with moderate or severe physical problems	5.2% of units (2007)	4.2% of units	NDA	American Housing Survey, U.S. Department of Commerce, Bureau of the Census

Healthy People 2020 (Continued)

OBJECTIVE	BASELINE (YEAR)	TARGET	CURRENT DATA (YEAR)	DATA SOURCE
EH-20: Reduce exposure to selected environmental chemicals in the population as measured by blood and urine concentrations	(2003–2004 unless otherwise indicated)			National Report on Human Exposure to Environmental Chemicals, CDC, NCEH, NHANES, CDC, NCHS
• Arsenic	50.4 µg/g of creatinine	35.28 µg/g of creatinine	NDA	
• Cadmium	1.6 µg/L	1.12 µg/L	NDA	
• Lead	4.2 µg/dL	2.94 µg/L	NDA	
• Mercury (children 1–5 years)	1.8 µg/L	1.26 µg/L	NDA	
• Mercury (women 16–49 years)	4.6 µg/L (2001–2002)	3.22 µg/L	NDA	
• Chlordane	37.7 ng/g of lipid	26.39 ng/g of lipid	NDA	
• DDT	1,860 ng/g of lipid	1,302 ng/g of lipid	NDA	
• Beta-hexachlorocyclohexane	56.5 ng/g of lipid	39.55 ng/g of lipid	NDA	
• Paranitrophenol	2.89 µg/g of creatinine	2.02 µg/g of creatinine	NDA	
• 3,4,6-Trichloro-2-pyridinol	9.22 µg/g of creatinine (2001–2002)	6.45 µg/g of creatinine	NDA	
• 3-Phenobenzoic acid	3.1 µg/g of creatinine (2001–2002)	2.32 µg/g of creatinine	NDA	
• PCB 153	97.1 ng/g of lipid (2001–2002)	67.97 ng/g of lipid	NDA	
• PCB 126	68.7 ng/g of lipid	48.09 µg/g of creatinine	NDA	
• 1,2,3,6,7,8-Hexachlorodibenzo-*p*-dioxin	68.5 ng/g of lipid	47.95 ng/g of lipid	NDA	
• Bisphenol A	11.2 µg/g of creatinine	7.84 µg/g of creatinine	NDA	
• Perchlorate	12.0 µg/g of creatinine	8.4 µg/g of creatinine	NDA	
• Mono-*n*-butyl phthalate	91.6 µg/g of creatinine	64.12 µg/g of creatinine	NDA	
• BDE 47	163 ng/g of lipid	114.1 ng/g of lipid	NDA	
EH-21: Improve quality, awareness, and use of existing information systems for environmental health	16 states	51 states and the District of Columbia	NDA	National Environmental Health Tracking Network, CDC, NCEH
EH-22: Increase the number of states, territories, tribes, and the District of Columbia that monitor diseases or conditions caused by exposure to environmental hazards		Total coverage in 56 states, territories, and District of Columbia for all subobjectives	NDA	Council of State and Territorial Epidemiologists, State Reportable Conditions Data Inventory
• Lead poisoning	29 states, DC			
• Pesticide poisoning	28 states			
• Mercury poisoning	24 states			
• Arsenic poisoning	22 states			
• Cadmium poisoning	21 states			
• Acute chemical poisoning	17 states			
• Carbon monoxide poisoning	20 states			
EH-23: Reduce the number of new schools sited within 500 feet of an interstate or Federal or State highway	18.9%	18.9% or less	NDA	GRASP/ATSDR geocoded data from Homeland Security Information Program
EH-24: Reduce the global burden of disease due to poor water quality, sanitation, and insufficient hygiene	2.2 mil deaths	2 mil deaths	NDA	Global Burden of Disease Project, WHO

NDA: No data available on objective status from Healthy People 2020 site.

Based on: U.S. Department of Health and Human Services. (2014). *Environmental health.* Retrieved from http://www.healthypeople.gov/2020/topicsobjectives2020/overview.aspx?topicId=12

Components of the Human Environment

The environmental context that influences human health incorporates a number of components. These include the natural and constructed, or built, environments, as well as the social and psychological environments. In this chapter, we will deal with aspects of the natural, built, and social environments. Other elements of the social environment and the psychological environment are addressed in other chapters throughout this book.

The Natural Environment

The **natural environment** consists of those features of the environment that exist in a natural state, unmodified in any significant way by human beings. Elements of the natural environment include plants, animals, and biological agents; weather and climate, terrain (e.g., mountains, rivers, oceans), and natural resources (air, wood, water, fuel). Some of the concerns related to the natural environment include air and water pollution, global climate change and its consequences, radiation and temperature extremes, biological hazards, and the depletion of natural resources. As we will see, many of these concerns are interrelated and are connected to the features of the social and built environments.

PLANTS, ANIMALS, AND BIOLOGICAL AGENTS. A variety of living organisms found in the environment affect human health. These include plants, animals, and a myriad of biological agents such as bacteria, viruses, and so on. Some of these living organisms are beneficial to human beings and others contribute to a variety of health problems. For example, plants serve as food sources for humans as well as for animals that, in turn, provide food for people. On the other hand, many plants are poisonous if ingested or cause different types of allergies through pollens (e.g., hay fever-type allergies) or toxins (e.g., poison oak or poison ivy).

Animals also have both beneficial and negative effects on human health. We have already noted animals as a food source for omnivorous human beings. Animals, particularly as pets, serve as a source of companionship and promote psychological health for many people. Similarly, many animals help control other nuisance organisms. For example, birds and fish eat a variety of insects that may cause human disease or destroy food crops.

Animals are also a source of exposure to a variety of pathogens. Both wild and domestic animals may contribute to human illness. **Zoonoses**, or diseases transmitted from animals to people, are occurring with greater frequency than in the past because of greater potential for human–animal interaction. The U.S. Agency for International Development (USAID) has developed a tracking system for animal-to-human disease transmission throughout the world. This PREDICT system permits identification of animal-to-human disease outbreaks that promote early intervention and prevent further spread of disease (USAID, 2011). For further information about the system, see the *External Resources* section of the student resources site.

As a result of growth of human populations and encroachment on the habitats of wild animals, there is greater potential for interaction between humans and wild animals (UC Davis Veterinary Medicine, n.d.). This interaction can lead to disease transmission and injury. For example, a variety of diseases, such as Lyme disease, human granulocytic anaplasmosis, and babesiosis, are transmitted by ticks found on wild animals (Joseph et al., 2011). Ticks may also be transferred to domestic animals and then infect people.

Humans encounter animals in several other settings in addition to their wild habitats. The National Association of State Public Health Veterinarians (2011) has noted that many venues promote human–animal interactions including, zoos, petting zoos, pet stores, circuses, farms, state fairs, and in educational settings. Each of these settings promotes interaction and may result in health problems such as enteric diseases, injuries, rabies exposure, and other bacterial, viral, fungal, and parasitic infections. For example, tuberculosis has been transmitted from elephants to human handlers in a Tennessee elephant refuge. In addition, the disease was transmitted to several nonhandlers in nearby offices due to aerosolized bacteria that entered the facility's ventilation system when barns were pressure washed or swept (Murphree, Warkentin, Dunn, Schaffner, & Jones, 2011).

The National Association of State Public Health Veterinarians (2011) has developed a set of guidelines for settings in which human–animal interactions occur to limit the transmission of diseases from animals to humans. Use of these guidelines is particularly important in the protection of young children, pregnant women, and persons who are immunocompromised.

Pets also serve as a source of disease for humans. An estimated 60% of U.S. households have pets, including approximately 60 million dogs and 75 million cats. As much as 33%

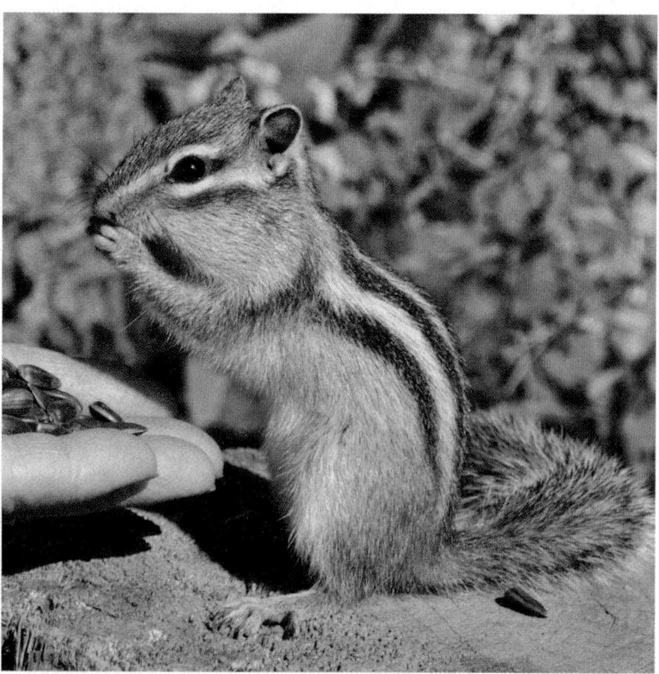

Increased interaction between wild animals and human beings increases the potential for transmission of diseases such as plague. *(© 46boris48/Fotolia)*

of dogs and 60% of cats sleep in or on their owners' bed increasing the potential for disease transmission. In addition, kissing or being licked by a pet may transmit disease. Examples of diseases transmitted by pets include plague (from fleas), chagas disease, cat-scratch disease, pasteurella infection, staphylococcus (including methicillin-resistant infection), rabies, and parasitic infections. Bites are also a source of potential injury particularly when overly possessive dogs are kept in their owners' bedrooms (Chomel & Sun, 2011).

More and more people are also keeping more exotic pets, which increases the potential for more unusual disease occurrences. For example, pet African dwarf frogs have been associated with cases of *salmonella* infection (National Center for Emerging and Zoonotic Infections, 2011). Similarly, pet kinkajous pose a risk of human infestation with raccoon roundworms, which may result in serious neurological disease (Division of Parasitic Diseases and Malaria, 2011). Foreign travel may also increase the risk of exposure to zoonotic diseases. For example, nearly a fourth of U.S.-reported cases of rabies were acquired outside of the country, and travelers visiting areas where zoonoses are common should use precautions in interacting with animals (National Center for Emerging and Zoonotic Infections, 2010).

In addition to being spread by animals, biological agents of disease are transmitted from human to human through social interaction as a part of the social environment, which will be discussed later in this chapter. Biological agents are also transmitted by food and water. Waterborne illnesses will be discussed in more detail in the section on water pollution. Although foodborne disease incidence reached the *Healthy People 2010* target for reduction to less than 1 case per 100,000 population (Division of Foodborne, Waterborne, and Environmental Diseases, 2011b), the Centers for Disease Control and Prevention (CDC, 2011a) estimates that 48 million people are affected by foodborne illness in the United States each year. Of these people, 128,000 are hospitalized and 3,000 die. Many of these illnesses result from 31 pathogens known to cause foodborne illnesses, many of which are tracked by public health surveillance systems. Eight pathogens account for an estimated 91% of foodborne illnesses. Noroviruses, for example, cause approximately 58% of the foodborne disease cases in the United States, and nontyphoidal *Salmonella* infections cause an estimated 28% of the related deaths. Other offending agents include *Clostridium perfringens, Campylobacter, Staphylococcus aureus, Toxoplasma gondii, E. coli,* and *Listeria monocytogenes* (CDC, 2011a).

Foodborne disease outbreaks occur as a result of contamination of food with pathogens and other disease-causing agents (e.g., mercury in fish). Contamination may occur when food is being produced, during processing, or prior to consumption. For example, contamination of oysters and other shellfish occurs when shellfish grow in contaminated waters. Similarly, use of human waste as fertilizer or irrigation with untreated waste water for foods crops imported from Mexico and other countries contaminates fresh foods such as strawberries, tomatoes, sprouts, and other fruits and vegetables. Contamination may also occur during food processing or as a result of failure to properly refrigerate foods. For example, cases of botulism have been associated with commercially produced potato soups that were improperly refrigerated (Division of Foodborne, Waterborne, and Environmental Diseases, 2011a). Finally, contamination may occur during preparation in the home, as when fresh foods are prepared on a cutting board that has been used in the preparation of contaminated meats, such as chicken.

WEATHER AND CLIMATE. As we will see in Chapter 25∞, the natural environment contributes to a variety of human health hazards in the form of disasters related to high winds, precipitation, earthquakes, and so on. Weather and climate also have positive effects on human health. For example, a moderate level of precipitation (both rain and snow) is required for crop growth and adequate water supplies for human consumption.

Weather has multiple effects on human health. For example, in 2010, weather-related events resulted in 490 deaths, 2,369 injuries, and nearly $9.9 million in damages (National Weather Service [NWS], 2011c). More than a quarter (28%) of weather-related deaths were due to exposure to excessive heat, and the number of deaths was three times higher than in 2009 (NWS, 2011b, 2011d). From 2000 to 2010, an average of 115 heat-related deaths occurred each year in the United States (NWS, 2011d). Conversely, hypothermia, primarily due to cold weather, accounted for an average of 25 deaths per year during the same period (NWS, 2011a). About half of both cold- and heat-related deaths occurred among elderly persons (NWS, 2011a, 2011b). In addition, poor weather conditions contribute to a significant portion of motor vehicle accidents. Other health-related effects of weather events are summarized in Table 4-1•.

Although there have always been deaths due to hypo- and hyperthermia and motor vehicle accidents caused by weather conditions, the potential for illness and injury due to temperature extremes and adverse weather conditions has increased recently as a result of global climate changes. Population health nurses can educate individuals, families, and communities to prevent weather-related mortality. For example, education tips for preventing heat-related deaths are provided on page 80. Guidelines for governmental response to heat waves have also been developed by the WHO European Region (Mathies, Bickler, Marin, & Hales, 2008). For further information about the guidelines, see the *External Resources* section of the student resources site.

Global climate change has been described as the "biggest global health threat of the 21st century" (Bell, 2011, p. 804). Climate change is a natural phenomenon, but is occurring much more rapidly than it normally would due to human activities. Mean global temperatures increased by 0.6° to 0.9° Celsius from 1906 to 2005, and the rate of temperature increase has more than doubled in the last half century (National Aeronautics and Space Administration, Earth Observatory, n.d.). A team of U.S. and WHO scientists has estimated that more than 150,000 excess deaths and 5 million illnesses occur yearly due to climate change (West, 2014).

Climate change has both direct and indirect health effects. Direct effects relate primarily to severe weather events discussed above and their impact on human health. Indirect effects arise out of changes in plant allergens and their effect on

TABLE 4-1 Health Effects and Populations Affected by Selected Weather Events

Weather Event	Health Effects	Populations Most Affected
Heat waves	Heat stress	Extremes of age, athletes, people with respiratory disease
Extreme weather events (rain, hurricane, tornado, flooding)	Injuries, drowning	Coastal, low-lying land dwellers, low SES
Drought, floods, increased mean temperature	Vector-, food-, and waterborne diseases	Multiple populations at risk
Sea level rise	Injuries, drowning, water and soil salinization, ecosystem and economic disruption	Coastal areas, low SES
Drought, ecosystem migration	Food and water shortages, malnutrition	Low ES, elderly, children
Extreme weather events, drought	Mass population movement, international conflict	General population
Increases in ground-level ozone, airborne allergens, and other pollutants	Respiratory disease exacerbations (COPD, asthma, allergic rhinitis, bronchitis)	Elderly, children, those with respiratory disease
Climate change generally, extreme events	Mental health	Young, displaced, agricultural sector, low SES

Data from: Centers for Disease Control and Prevention. (2009). *CDC policy on climate change and public health.* Retrieved from http://www.cdc.gov/climatechange/pubs/Climate_Change_Policy.pdf

asthma prevalence and severity, increases in insect populations and consequent insect-borne diseases, mental health issues, and increasing health disparities between segments of populations. A number of disease vectors, such as mosquitos, sandflies, ticks, tsetse flies, and black flies, have become more numerous or moved to other areas as a result of climate change (West, 2014). Many diseases have also been found to be climate sensitive (Bell, 2011), and climate change is contributing to the emergence of new diseases and reemergence of several tropical diseases (Yumul, Cruz, Servando, & Dimalanta, 2011). Indirect effects may also include social disruption related to population dislocation and civil conflict over scarce food and water resources created by climate changes.

Global efforts have been initiated to address the reduction in CO_2 emissions, one of the most significant of greenhouse gases contributing to global warming, within the context of the Kyoto Protocol, which went into effect in February 2005. The Kyoto Protocol amends the United Nations Framework Convention on Climate Change to control emissions of CO_2 and five other greenhouse gases. Unfortunately, the protocol remains unsupported by the United States, which contributes a significant proportion of the world's CO_2 emissions. In December 2009, the U.S. Environmental Protection Agency (EPA) promulgated an administrative report that included both "endangerment" and "cause" findings. The endangerment findings noted that current and projected concentrations of six greenhouse gases, including CO_2, threaten the public health and the welfare of current and future generations. The cause findings specifically implicated motor vehicle engines as contributing to greenhouse gas pollution leading to public endangerment (EPA, 2011e). In spite of these findings, however, the greenhouse gas emission regulations implemented by the EPA in January 2011 are being challenged by entities such as the American Petroleum Institute and other producers (Isakower, 2011). Several challenges to the endangerment finding have been made in Congress and in the court system. Unfortunately, the 1996 Congressional Review Act allows congress to veto agency regulations (OMB Watch, 2010). For this reason, it is important for population health nurses to stay abreast of environmental legislation and motivate the public to speak out against actions that imperil the environment.

CLIENT EDUCATION

Preventing Heat-Related Deaths

During heat waves:

- Check on infants, young children, elderly, disabled, mentally ill, or homebound persons frequently.
- Evaluate persons at risk for heat-related death frequently for heat-related hazards and illnesses, and take appropriate preventive action.
- Never leave anyone unattended in a closed vehicle.
- Drink plenty of fluids. Refrain from alcohol consumption.
- Stay indoors or seek air-conditioned environments.
- Take cool showers or baths.
- Wear lightweight, light-colored, loose-fitting clothing.

If exposure to heat cannot be avoided:

- Reduce, eliminate, or reschedule strenuous activities.
- Limit activity to morning and evening hours.
- Reduce exercise or replace fluids and electrolytes during exercise.
- Drink water or nonalcoholic fluids frequently.
- Wear a wide-brimmed hat and sunglasses and use broad spectrum (UVA/UVB protection) sunscreen of SPF 15 or higher.
- Avoid direct sunlight and rest in shady areas.

Data from: Centers for Disease Control and Prevention. (n.d.). *Tips for preventing heat-related illness.* Retrieved from http://www.bt.cdc.gov/disasters/extremeheat/heattips.asp

POLLUTION. Pollution is another area of environmental concern that has significant health effects for populations. Considerations to be addressed in this chapter include water and air pollution, and radiation.

Water pollution. The safety and adequacy of the world's water supply is of serious concern. Approximately 97.5% of the world's water is either salt water or is contaminated. Seventy percent of what remains is frozen in the polar ice caps, which leaves only approximately 0.01% of the earth's water for human consumption. The World Bank estimates that 100 to 200 gallons of water are needed per person per day to meet basic personal needs, excluding water needs for agricultural and industry, yet about 1 billion people lack access to safe water throughout the world. It is anticipated that this number will increase as populations grow (Levy & Sidel, 2011).

As water shortages become more acute, it is likely that waste water will be used increasingly to irrigate food crops. Although waste water has been used for irrigation for more than 3,000 years in China and for centuries in Vietnam, its use poses the risk of disease transmission through contamination of food crops with bacteria-laden water. Because of increasing interdependence among nations for food products and greater movement of produce worldwide, the potential for global spread of disease is vastly enhanced compared to preglobalization eras, and there is a need for both local and international regulation of water safety and food production.

In the United States, threats to the safety of water supplies arise from an aging water infrastructure, chemical and pathogenic contamination, the impact of climate change on water availability, and the development of new ways to obtain and use water (CDC, 2011b). Some of the health effects of water pollution include diarrheal diseases, malaria, trachomatis infection, intestinal helminths, Japanese encephalitis, heavy metal poisoning, and hepatitis A. The most current U.S. Geological Survey (USGS) data on water sources in the United States indicate that about 80% of water is derived from surface water and only 20% from ground water sources (USGS, 2014). Both water sources can become contaminated, with some contamination resulting naturally, and significant pollution arising from pollutants derived from land use, such as use of fertilizers, agricultural runoff, and industrial pollutants.

Groundwater resources are covered by drinking water regulations promulgated by the EPA. Well water, on the other hand, is not covered. The EPA has developed both primary and secondary drinking water regulations. Primary drinking water regulations are legally enforceable standards for public water systems that specify acceptable limits of seven categories of contaminants. These categories include seven microorganisms (including turbidity or the amount of suspended solids in water), four disinfection by-products, three disinfectants, 16 inorganic chemicals, 53 organic chemicals, and four radionuclides. Secondary drinking water regulations are unenforceable guidelines for water contaminants that cause cosmetic effects (e.g., discoloration of teeth and skin), aesthetic effects (e.g., odor, color, or taste), corrosivity, and so on (EPA, 2011d).

There is some fear that diminishing water availability will result in increasing conflict throughout the world. For example, there have been predictions of conflict between India and Pakistan over use of the waters of the Indus River (Pappas, 2011). Similarly, conflicts, although not armed, occur among states drawing water from the Colorado River for irrigation as well as for human consumption. In addition, there is a need to assist jurisdictions with water management strategies that conserve water and prevent flooding as climate change occurs.

Several public health roles have been identified for protection of water supplies throughout the world, and population health

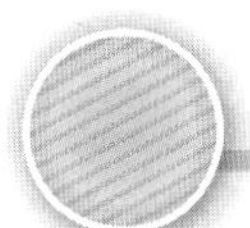

Global Perspectives

Water Quality and Health

According to the World Health Organization (WHO) and UNICEF (2014) , 11% or 748 million of the world's people continued to lack access to improved drinking water sources and 2.5 billion people were without improved sanitation facilities in 2012. An estimated 173 million people rely on untreated surface water sources open to myriad contaminants. Improved drinking water sources are those that protect water supplies against outside contamination, particular fecal contamination. Improved sanitation facilities are those that prevent contact with human excreta.

Globally, the Millenium Development Goal (MDG) of halve the proportion of the world's population without access to improved drinking water sources was met in 2010; however, specific areas have failed to do so and are not on track to meet the goal by the 2015 target. Lack of safe drinking water and sanitation, for example, are more common in rural areas where residents encompass 90% of those without improved water sources or improved sanitary facilities. Similarly, in sub-Saharan Africa, 40% of people are without access to improved drinking water sources and sanitary facilities and this number is increase due to population growth. Open defecation, defined as defecation in open space areas, such as fields, forests, bushes or open bodies of water, continues to be practiced by 1 billion people or 17% of the world's population who have no access to sanitary facilities of any kind. Open defecation is most common in India where more than 597 million people engage in this practice. Open defecation, is actually increasing in sub-Saharan Africa, again, due to a sanitation infrastructure that has not kept up with population growth (WHO & UNICEF, 2014).

Lack of access to safe water supplies and sanitation has a variety of health-related effects. Contaminated water transmits enteric pathogens and other harmful substances resulting in diarrheal disease and other health problems. In addition, the need to collect water from infested sources contributes to diseases caused by contact rather than ingestion (e.g., guinea worm infestation). Limited water resources also limit peoples' abilities to engage in appropriate hygiene, particularly handwashing, which would limit the transmission of communicable diseases. In some places, women and girls face the added threat of violence as well as lost time and productivity through the need to travel significant distances to acquire water. The need to defecate or urinate in open fields also places them at risk for assault (WHO & UNICEF, 2014).

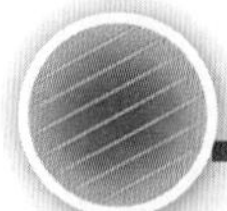

Evidence-Based Practice

Access to Safe Drinking Water

Worldwide, 768 million people lacked access to improved drinking water sources in 2011 (WHO & UNICEF, 2013). Even if the Millennium Development Goal of halving the number of people without access to safe water by 2015 is achieved, an estimated 600 million people will still lack access to safe water systems. Unsafe water contributes to more than 5 billion waterborne disease fatalities and more than 2 million deaths from diarrhea in young children each year (Natural Resources Defense Council, n.d.). Research suggests that in developing countries, significant water contamination occurs between water sources and home use and that use of household water treatment and safe storage (HWTS) strategies in individual homes can minimize the health effects of waterborne diseases.

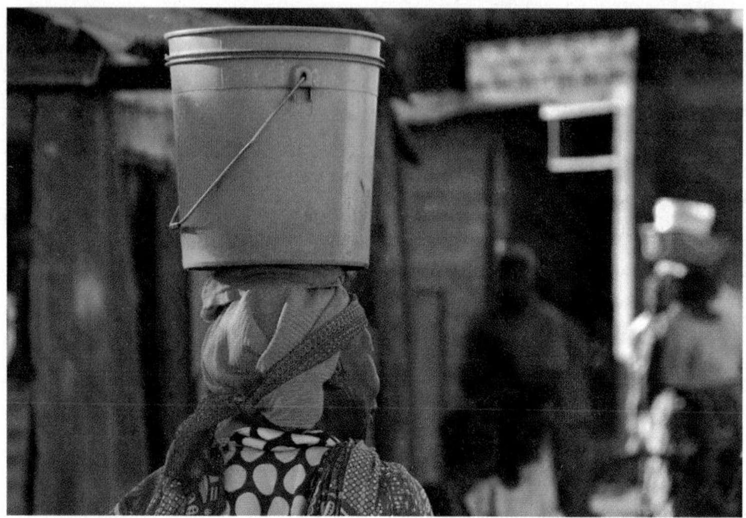

Much of the world's population does not have access to potable water sources. *(africa/Fotolia)*

The U.S. Centers for Disease Control has developed an evidence-based strategy for HWTS that includes three aspects: (a) use of an easily accessible, inexpensive chlorine solution in water for home use, (b) storage in safe containers, and (c) education on hygiene and water use practices. The CDC Safe Water System (SWS) has been implemented in more than 30 countries since 1998 and has provided thousands of people with safe drinking water (Division of Foodborne, Waterborne, and Environmental Diseases, n.d.).

Based on the results of multiple projects to promote SWS use in households in numerous countries, a number of lessons have been learned that can inform other similar projects. These lessons are summarized in Table 4-2●.

---

nurses can be actively involved in these roles. They include raising awareness of the need for clean water access among the public and policy makers, documenting water conflicts and their effects on human health, and promoting water conservation and efforts to prevent water contamination. Additional roles include promoting nonviolent conflict resolution strategies, promoting proactive cooperation on water issues, and working toward achievement of Millennium Development Goal 7 to reduce the proportion of people without access to safe water and basic sanitation (Levy & Sidel, 2011). This goal reflects the last of the *Healthy People 2020* environmental health objectives presented earlier in this chapter.

Air pollution. Hazardous air quality is another issue of concern at both national and global levels. Air pollution arises from the discharge of gaseous and particulate emissions into the air. Four general categories of air pollution sources are recognized: biogenic sources, mobile sources, point sources, and area sources (EPA, 2011a). Biogenic sources are natural sources of pollutants, such as volcanic eruptions or wild fires that create numerous gaseous pollutants and particulate matter. Plant pollens and dust are other biogenic sources of pollutants. Mobile sources include most forms of transportation as well as lawn mowers and other devices that move and pollute the air (EPA, 2010b, 2011a). Point sources are stationary sources that arise from a single point, such as a factory smoke stack or a storage tank. Area sources are a collection of stationary sources in a specific locale, for example, a residential area in which many homes use coal- or oil-based heating systems (EPA, 2010b).

Six major pollutants, also called criteria pollutants, affect air quality in the United States and their emissions are

TABLE 4-2 Lessons Learned about Safe Water System Campaigns

Category	Lessons Learned
Project design	Target populations in need who have sufficient resources to purchase the products needed and existing distribution systems Develop long-term funding strategies by creating a locally viable market for the products that is self-sustaining Incorporate a range of technical expertise in planning including consultants and locally knowledgeable staff
Production of safe water product	Enable local production of product (bottle, cap, chlorine solution, label) in standardized packaging, considering technical and production capabilities and internal and external quality control mechanisms Provide ongoing product quality monitoring to maintain safety and effectiveness Produce products with an extended shelf life (at least 12 months) Standardize correct chlorine dosage Standardize plastic water containers to assure correct chlorine dose Use packaging appropriate for rural transport and distribution
Regulatory environment	Involve all relevant government agencies from the beginning Respond immediately to government concerns Educate program staff to answer technical questions about the product
Marketing and communication	Focus on rural communities with unsafe water for program launch rather than high-profile political figures in prominent areas Address specific safe water program behavioral constructs by providing an understanding of diarrheal disease severity, transmission, and effectiveness of SWS strategies and handwashing Use a positive and aspirational branded marketing campaign with focus on positive aspect of use (versus disease severity) Use campaign messages complementary to related campaigns Consider timing of launch efforts (e.g., just before seasonal disease peaks) Choose communication channels appropriate to the context (e.g., media in urban areas and personal communication in rural areas) Use targeted technical information to address concerns about chlorine use Provide for sustained funding Develop marketing templates that can be adapted to local needs (verbal, pictorial, or combination designs)
Sales and distribution	Combine commercial sector and project push for distribution of the product Capitalize on NGO networks to promote the project, particularly in rural areas Encourage commercial sector participation by use of a socially marketed product
Creating partnerships	Develop partnerships at all levels (e.g., government, nongovernment, local, international, etc.) Promote donor advocacy and support for the project through integration into other project contracts Coordinate with NGOs to reach rural and high-risk populations Use trusted spokespersons and product champions
Product costs, pricing, and cost recovery	Recover product costs through sales (usually no need for subsidies, but other costs usually covered by external donors)
Integrating safe water into HIV/AIDS programming to meet the needs of the most at risk populations for waterborne diseases	Partner with local NGOs that serve the HIV/AIDs population Use interest in reaching the HIV/AIDs population to stimulate a national safe water campaign

Data from: U.S. Agency for International Development. (2007). *Best practices in social marketing safe water treatment solution for household water treatment: Lessons learned from Population Services International Field Programs.* Washington, DC: Author. Retrieved from http://pdf.usaid.gov/pdf_docs/PNADI479.pdf

monitored by the EPA. These include carbon monoxide, lead, nitrogen dioxide, volatile organic compounds, particulate matter, and sulfur dioxide. In 2009, for example, 70 million tons of carbon monoxide were discharged into U.S. air. Similar discharges for other pollutants were as follows: lead—2000 tons, nitrogen oxides—14 million tons, volatile organic compounds—13 million tons, particulate matter—2 million tons, and sulfur dioxide—9 million tons (EPA, 2011b). Ozone is another major pollutant. Ozone is not typically discharged directly into the air from a pollution source, but results from chemical interactions of nitrous oxide and hydrocarbons produced by burning or evaporation of volatile substances (American Lung Association, 2011). Ozone production is exacerbated by heat. From 1980 to 2009, emissions of six of the criteria pollutants decreased by 57%, but carbon dioxide emissions increased by 28%. Despite decreases, more than 80 million people in the United States lived in areas where air quality concentrations were above the National Ambient Air Quality Standards for at least part of the year in 2009 (EPA, 2011b). In addition, half of the population lived in areas with dangerous levels of ozone or particulate matter in 2010 (American Lung Association, 2011).

Each of these pollutants has a variety of health consequences. The most obvious are, of course, respiratory effects including lung cancer and exacerbation of asthma and other respiratory diseases. Air pollution has also been associated with cardiovascular disease, and there is some evidence that exposure

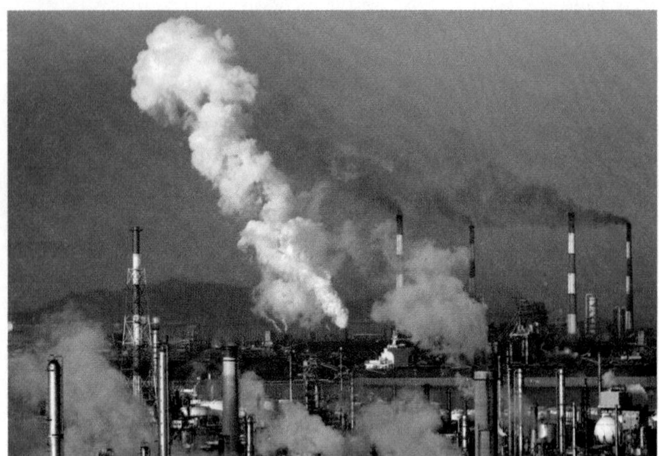

Uncontrolled industrial processes may contribute to a variety of environmental health concerns. *(Akiyoko/Shutterstock)*

to particulate matter may contribute to insulin resistance in persons with diabetes (American Lung Association, 2011). Population health nurses can educate the public to prevent air pollution as well as assist them in avoiding the worst effects of pollution. Specific strategies are addressed later in this chapter, but population health nurses can also alert people regarding warning mechanisms for unsafe air conditions. Client education information regarding air quality and health implications is included below.

In addition to exposure to pollutants in the outside or ambient air, many people are also exposed to indoor air pollution, the primary source of which is environmental tobacco smoke. Exposure to environmental tobacco smoke contributes to an estimated 50,000 deaths each year in adult nonsmokers due to lung cancer and heart disease. Environmental tobacco smoke exposure has also been implicated in sudden infant death syndrome (SIDS) and contributes to nasal and eye irritation. Approximately 35% of U.S. children (21 million children) are exposed to tobacco smoke in the home, and 49% of nonsmoking children with in-home exposure to tobacco smoke have detectable cotinine blood levels indicating increased risk for long-term consequences (Cramer, Roberts, & Stevens, 2011).

Radiation. Radiation also affects the natural environment, often in conjunction with features of the built and social environments. Human health is affected by two types of radiation, ionizing and nonionizing radiation. Ionizing radiation is created through decay of unstable isotopes of certain elements. The term ionizing indicates that the energy created is sufficient to break molecular bonds resulting in charged or "ionized" atoms. Ionizing radiation is of two types; radioactive particles and high-frequency electromagnetic radiation (e.g., X-rays). Human exposure to ionizing radiation occurs both naturally (e.g., radon in the ground in some areas) and by artificial means, such as medical use, radioactive discharges from nuclear plants, and so on. Human effects of ionizing radiation include somatic effects, such as cancer, genetic effects, and teratogenic effects on infants exposed *in utero* (Environmental Protection Agency, 2012).

An estimated 21,000 lung cancer deaths each year are related to radon exposure. Lung cancer incidence is increased by the interaction of radon exposure in the natural environment and smoking behavior. Although the *Healthy People 2020* objectives address radon testing and remediation for homes in areas with high radon levels, it is estimated that declines in

CLIENT EDUCATION Air Quality and Health Implications

Code	Air Quality	Health Implications
Green	Good	Continue routine activity
Yellow	Moderate	Limited outdoor exertion for highly sensitive people
Orange (advisory)	Unhealthy for sensitive groups	Limited outdoor exertion for active children, adults, and people with respiratory conditions
Red (alert)	Unhealthy	Avoid outdoor exertion by active children, adults, and people with respiratory conditions; limited outdoor exertion by all others
Purple (health alert)	Very unhealthy	Avoid outdoor exertion by active children, adults, and people with respiratory conditions; limited outdoor exertion by all others

Data from: AIRNow. (2010). *Air Quality Index (AQI) – A guide to air quality and your health.* Retrieved from http://www.airnow.gov/index.cfm?action=aqibasics.aqi

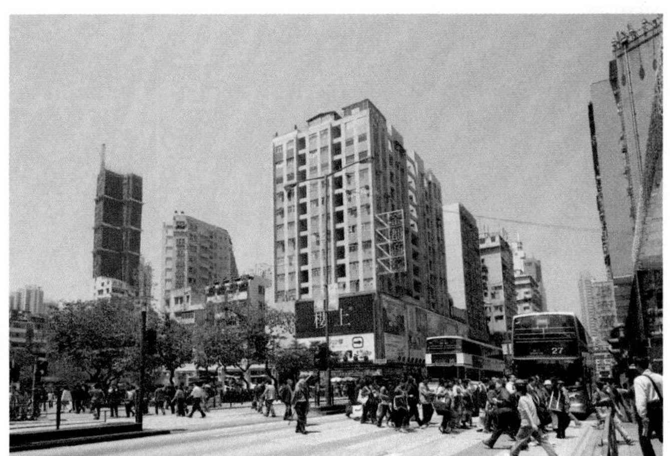

Both natural and built environments affect human health. *(Joey Chan/ Pearson Education, Inc)*

smoking behaviors will have a greater effect on radon-related lung cancer than home remediation (Mendez, Alshanqeety, Warner, Lantz, & Courant, 2011).

Nonionizing radiation is produced by sources such as power lines, mobile telephones, and so on. There are known effects of exposure to high levels of nonionizing radiation resulting from the sudden heating of body tissue. The Occupational Safety and Health Administration (OSHA) has developed standards for exposures to sources of nonionizing radiation such as electromagnetic radio waves, due to the potential for adverse health effects of chronic exposure (OSHA, 2013).

ENVIRONMENTAL SUSTAINABILITY. The last consideration with respect to the natural environment to be discussed here is the concept of environmental sustainability. Sustainability is often viewed as continued growth of the economy and may be conceptualized from both public and business perspectives. From a public perspective, environmental sustainability can be defined as "the satisfaction of basic economic, social, and security needs now and in the future without undermining the natural resource base and environmental quality on which life depends" (EPA, 2011h). A business perspective views the goal of sustainability as increasing value while decreasing use of materials and minimizing negative environmental impacts. A synergistic perspective entails "recognition of the need to support a growing economy while reducing the social and economic costs of economic growth" (EPA, 2011h).

Population health nurses can assist members of the population to recognize environmental sustainability issues and to promote a sustainable environment. This may be done through conservation initiatives and through development of more effective and less environmentally damaging industrial, personal, and transportation-related activities. Strategies that may be used by population health nurses to achieve these ends are presented later in this chapter.

The Built Environment

The U.S. Department of Health and Human Services, (USDHHS, 2012) defined the **built environment** as "human-made (versus natural) resources and infrastructure designed to support human activity" (p. 64). Elements of the built environment include homes, schools, workplaces, roads, and features such as transportation systems, highways, electrical transmission and waste management systems, and parks and recreation areas. Public health experts have broadened the concept of the built environment to incorporate land use planning and environmental policy, which will be considered in the discussion of the social environment.

The built environment has both direct and indirect effects on health. Direct effects derive from exposure to hazardous conditions arising from the built environment. Examples of direct health effects include lead poisoning arising from ingestion or inhalation of lead from older structures painted with lead-based paints or respiratory disease due to air pollution. The focused assessment on page 86 provides tips for assessing the potential for lead exposure.

Indirect effects are the result of the effects of the built environment on the natural environment (e.g., contamination of air and water) or on human health-related behaviors. As we saw earlier, much of the contamination of the natural environment arises from features of the built environment. For example, air pollution is a result of motor vehicle use in the built environment, and pollution tends to be worse in areas near major highways and other heavily traveled areas.

Home safety is another area of concern related to the built environment. In 2009, for example, more than 5% of U.S. housing units were considered inadequate, with deficiencies in plumbing, heating, electricity, hallways, or upkeep. An additional 21% of housing units were considered unhealthy due to potential for exposure to toxins, rodents, water leaks, peeling paint, and lack of functional smoke detectors (Raymond, Wheeler, & Brown, 2011). Home conditions can also influence a variety of chronic illnesses for better or worse. For example, homes specifically constructed to minimize the presence of asthma triggers have been associated with an increase in asthma-free days and a decrease in urgent care visits for people affected by asthma (Takaro, Krieger, Song, Sharify, & Beaudet, 2011).

Rural environments have traditionally been considered natural and more healthful than urban environments. However, the built environment also influences rural areas. For example, "factory farms" or concentrated animal feeding operations (CAFOs) cause significant air and water pollution, but are exempt from enforcement of provisions of the Clean Air Act pending further study. Particulate emissions, for example, have been found to be three times higher than permitted levels at some factory farms, and thousands of pounds of ammonia may be produced on the worst days. In addition, hydrogen sulfides have been found to exceed acceptable levels for other industries and are often worse than in many cities (Environmental Integrity Project, 2011).

The built environment also influences human health-related behavior. For example, the proximity of tobacco outlets in residential areas has been associated with success or failure of tobacco cessation initiatives (Reitzel et al., 2011), and a preponderance of small grocery stores in urban neighborhoods has been related to higher BMIs and greater prevalence of obesity. Similarly, moving from a rural to an urban area has been shown to result in lower BMIs, possibly due to greater availability of healthy food choices (Gibson, 2011).

The presence of parks and recreation areas in the built environment influences health-related physical activity levels in the population, and parks with supervised activity classes have been shown to promote physical activity more than parks without such programs (Parra et al., 2010). Unfortunately, many such programs are being eliminated as a result of city, county, and state budget cuts. A number of studies have demonstrated the link between access to physical activity venues in the built environment and engagement in physical activity. For example, James and colleagues (2013) found that elements of the built environment were associated with physical activity levels and body mass index (BMI) (James et al., 2013). Similarly, greater density of fast-food restaurants in a community is associated with increased BMI, particularly for low-income residents (Reitzel et al., 2014). The presence of parks also influences physical activity, and public parks have been suggested as avenues of escape from stress for victims of natural disasters (Rung, Broyles, Mowen, Gustat, & Sothern, 2011).

Urban sprawl is another feature of the built environment that has drawn considerable attention in recent years. **Urban sprawl** has been defined as "a pattern of uncontrolled development around the periphery of a city," (Resnick, 2010, p. 1853) and is characterized by low population density, loss of open spaces,

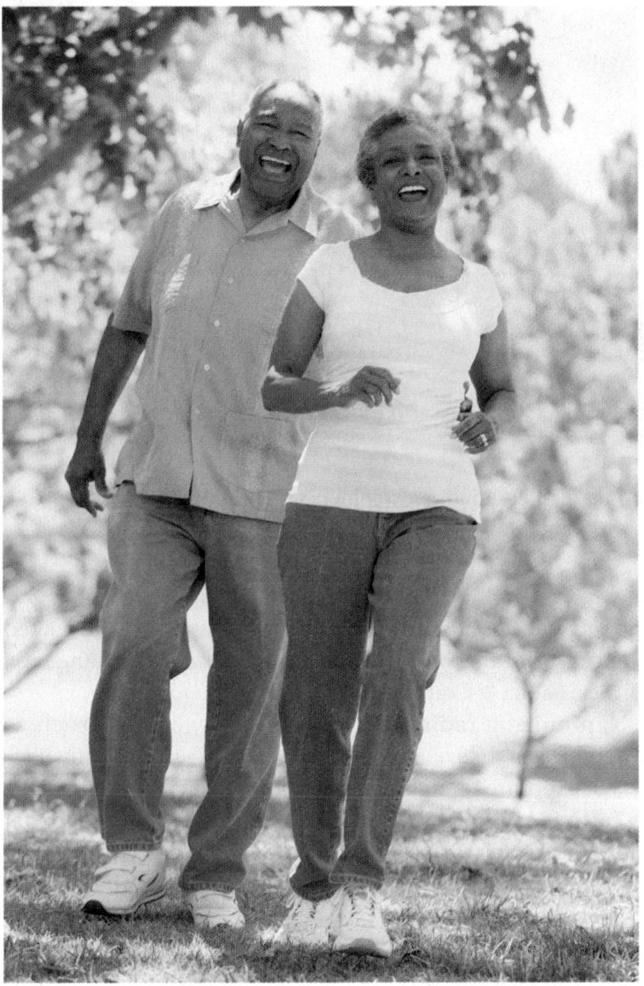

Aspects of the built environment strongly influence health-related behaviors such as physical activity. *(Monkey Business Images/Shutterstock)*

FOCUSED ASSESSMENT Lead Exposure Risk

- Do you live in or regularly visit a house or building built before 1978 with chipped or peeling paint or current or recent renovation?
- Have you ever lived outside of the United States?
- Is anyone you know (family member, neighbor's child, child's playmate) being treated for lead poisoning?
- Do any jobs or hobbies of family members involve exposure to lead?
- Do you live near an active lead smelter or battery recycling plant or other industry that may release lead into the environment?
- Do you live near a heavily traveled road or highway?
- Do you or family members use products from other countries that may contain lead (pottery, medicines, spices, food, candy)?
- Do you serve food in leaded crystal, pottery, or pewter dishes?
- Do you or members of your family chew on nonfood items (e.g., dirt, paint chips)?

An affirmative answer to any of these questions suggests the need for blood lead testing.

Adapted from: New York State Department of Health. (2009). *Lead exposure risk assessment questionnaire for children.* Retrieved from http://www.health.state.ny.us/environmental/lead/exposure/childhood/risk_assessment.htm; Texas Department of State Health Services. (2011). *Risk assessment for lead exposure: Parent questionnaire.* Retrieved from http://www.dshs.state.tx.us/lead/pdf_files/pb_110_parent_questionnaire.pdf

automobile dependence due to low connectivity between destinations, air and water pollution, and limited opportunities to walk or bicycle to work or school. Other characteristic features of urban sprawl include poor land use mix, limited activity centers and downtown areas, "leapfrogging" development, and employment dispersion.

Urban sprawl can be counteracted by **smart growth**, which has been defined as a "policy framework that promotes an urban development pattern characterized by high population density, walkable and bikeable neighborhoods, preserved green spaces, mixed use development (i.e., development projects that include both residential and commercial uses), available mass transit, and limited road construction" (Resnick, 2010, p. 1853).

Smart growth has been resisted by some entities for a variety of reasons. These include possible decreases in property values, diminished affordability of housing, restrictions on property owners on their use of their land, and the potential to increase, rather than decrease, urban sprawl as new planned communities are built. In addition, smart growth may disrupt existing communities and displace low-income minority residents from center city areas (Resnick, 2010).

Mixed-use development refers to the extent to which urban development creates areas that combine residential and commercial endeavors. Poor land use mix has a long historical tradition in the United States, mandating segregated land use for residential and commercial purposes. Leapfrogging development is the practice of developing distant parcels of land while skipping over those closer to developed areas. Both types of arrangements result in the necessity for people to commute to work or shopping areas and increase motor vehicle traffic while decreasing opportunities for physical activity through walking and bicycling. Urban sprawl wastes available land and converts valuable agricultural land to other uses as well as increasing energy use and contributing to pollution.

All of the characteristic features of urban sprawl lead to increased resource use. The extent of resource use is conceptualized in terms of humanity's **ecological footprint**, which has been defined as the amount of environmental resources in terms of productive land or water required by a population to support a current lifestyle (World Wildlife Federation, n.d.). An ecological footprint is usually measured in hectares per person (one hectare is 10,000 square meters or 2.47 acres). Worldwide, the current ecological footprint is 2.7 hectares per capita, but only 2.1 hectares can be regenerated each year, suggesting that we are outpacing our resources. The ecological footprint of industrialized nations is even greater. Earlier in this chapter, we referred to the need for sustainable development. In this context, a sustainable or ecological community is one with an acceptable ecological footprint. For further information on determining your own ecological footprint, see the *External Resources* section of the student resources site.

The Social Environment

Throughout this book, we discuss the effects of several elements of the social environment on the health of populations. For example, Chapter 5∞ discusses the cultural aspects of the social environment, and Chapter 6∞ addresses the economic aspect. In this chapter, we will focus on four aspects of the social environment as they affect health: social capital, social policy, energy consumption, and waste management.

SOCIAL CAPITAL. A basic definition of social capital was presented in Chapter 1∞. The World Bank (2011) conceptualized social capital as "the institutions, relationships, and norms that shape the quality and quantity of a society's social interactions" (para 1). Social capital is derived from relationships that make resources available to members of a group and depends on the overall level of resources available to the group. These relationships may involve both horizontal and vertical associations and are facilitated by an enabling social and political environment. Horizontal relationships are social networks of people that increase their productivity by facilitating cooperation and coordination. Interactions with your classmates that facilitate assimilation of educational concepts (e.g., study groups) are examples of horizontal relationships. Vertical relationships may also provide social capital. For example, the expertise of your nursing faculty may also facilitate your learning. The culture of a nursing program that promotes open interaction between faculty and students is an example of an enabling environment.

The social capital available to a population or to a segment of the population has been shown to be related to population health status, independent of the economic status of the individual or family. For example, higher economic-level neighborhoods have been associated with lower obesity risk for adults. Similarly, a study in Brazil indicated that people in the richest residential areas had a healthy life expectancy more than twice as high as that of slum dwellers (Szwarcwald, de Mota, Damacena, & Pereira, 2011).

Resources, in the context of social capital, include those available to individual members of the group as well as to the group as a whole. Because of the relationships among group members, resources available to one member become available to others. The extent of social capital in a community or population group depends on the resources available to the group as well as the relationships that permit access to those resources.

Communities with high levels of social capital have also been characterized by cohesion and collective efficacy. The extent of social capital in a community or population group may also be affected negatively by community or neighborhood characteristics. These negative effects also have health-related implications. For example, overall neighborhood poverty has been associated with higher cardiovascular disease risk for women, and neighborhood crime rates and segregation have been linked to cancer risk in both men and women (Freedman, Grafova, & Rogowski, 2011).

Some authors, however, note the potential for disadvantages to social capital. These disadvantages lie in the group norms and in the relationship of the group to the outside world. Group norms can, in some instances, promote "antisocial capital"—that is, social capital put to inappropriate uses. Examples given include social norms and behaviors related to drug rings, nepotism, cronyism, and crime. Neighborhood crime rates have been linked to health-related behaviors such as physical activity, particularly among youth (Moore et al., 2010).

Another area for consideration is the differential effect of social capital on some subgroups within the population. For example, young people in the community may not have access to some elements of community social capital. As another example, homeless individuals are denied access to community social capital when they are prohibited from using public facilities such as parks. With respect to interactions with the larger society, some authors have warned that an emphasis on building social capital within groups and communities may be used as an excuse not to redistribute economic resources to address structural inequalities in access to resources.

SOCIAL POLICY. Social policy also has multiple effects on the environment and on human health and health-related behaviors. Policies may relate directly to environmental conditions or to behaviors that affect the environment. For example, smoke-free policies for multiunit housing may prevent tobacco smoke exposure. Approximately 40 million Americans live in multiunit housing in which smoke is easily transmitted among units. Landlords have resisted initiation of smoke-free policies for a variety of reasons. Chief among these is an expectation that smoke-free policies will lead to higher vacancy and turnover rates. In actual fact, however, in units with smoke-free policies, vacancy rates increased by only 11% compared to an expected 54%, and turnover rates were less than 4% compared to an anticipated 50%. Other reasons for not instituting smoke-free policies in rental properties include difficulties in enforcement, anticipated tenant objections, and loss of rental market share (Cramer et al., 2011).

Policies related to smoking in the workplace are also an issue with respect to environmental health. The National Center for Chronic Disease Prevention and Health Promotion (2011) reported an increase from zero to 26 in the number of states that prohibit smoking in the workplace, bars, and restaurants from 2000 to 2010, and nearly half of U.S. residents live in smoke-free jurisdictions. Unfortunately, more than 88 million nonsmokers over 3 years of age continue to be exposed to second-hand smoke. The *Healthy People 2020* objective is to increase the prevalence of smoke-free workplace, bar, and restaurant laws to all states. In addition to decreasing exposure of nonsmokers to second-hand smoke, such laws assist smokers in cessation efforts, change social norms regarding smoking, and decrease hospitalizations related to heart disease and asthma.

At the national level, the EPA has promulgated a wide variety of social policies with regulatory enforcement to reduce environmental health risks. Two prominent examples are the Clear Air Act of 1970 and the Clean Water Act of 1972. The EPA (2011c) estimates that the Clean Air Act will prevent more than 230,000 premature deaths in 2020 through its enforcement of emission standards related to industry and transportation. Several amendments have been made in the legislation since its enactment, the most recent being regulations regarding the emission of greenhouse gases discussed earlier. The precursor to the Clean Water Act was passed in 1948 as the Federal Water Pollution Control Act, but was substantially reorganized in 1972 and labeled the Clean Water Act in 1977. This act regulates wastewater and sets standards for contaminants in surface water (EPA, 2011f). The EPA also develops policy in a variety of other areas of environmental concern, including waste management, radon exposure, acid rain, lead and other heavy metal exposures, climate change, pesticide exposures, and so on.

The EPA (2010a) has developed a set of five strategic goals for 2011 to 2025. These goals and related objectives are presented in Table 4-3●. Similar environmental-policy-making bodies may also operate at local and state levels. At the international level, WHO provides a focus for global health initiatives and policy development.

Other types of social policies also affect human health. For example, minimum wage policies have been shown to affect access to health. States with higher minimum wage laws also tend to have a lower risk of unmet health needs among low-skilled workers. Such findings refute contentions that minimum wage laws might actually decrease access to care due to lowered numbers of workers hired, fewer hours worked to eliminate the need to provide health insurance benefits, or reductions in available benefits (McCarrier, Zimmerman, Ralston, & Martin, 2011). Many other social policies also affect health, from enactment of seat belt legislation to food labeling laws. Political influences on health and the role of population health nurses in policy formation are discussed in more detail in Chapter 9∞.

ENERGY CONSUMPTION. Energy consumption is another aspect of the social environment to be considered. Energy consumption, which plays a large part of the human ecological footprint discussed earlier, arises out of social mores and standards of living. Total energy use in the United States during 2012 was 95 quadrillion British thermal units (Btus), nearly three times the energy use in 1950. Less than 10% of 2012 energy consumption resulted from residential and commercial use, 20.5% from industrial use, and nearly 27% from transportation (U.S. Energy Information Administration [EIA], 2013a). Results of the Residential Energy Consumption Survey indicate that per-household residential energy use in the United States decreased from 1980 to 2009, but that each household still used an average of 90 Btus per year. In 2013, less than 10% of energy consumption came from renewable energy sources (EIA, 2014).

In large part, reductions in home energy consumption are related to use of more energy-efficient appliances and heating

TABLE 4-3 EPA Strategic Goals and Related Objectives

Strategic Goal	Related Objectives
Goal 1: Taking action on climate change and improving air quality	Address climate change by reducing greenhouse gas emissions and assisting the public to deal with effects of climate change. Improve air quality by reducing the extent of toxic pollutants. Restore ozone layer, protecting the public from ultraviolet radiation. Reduce unnecessary radiation exposure, minimizing exposure and dealing with exposures that occur.
Goal 2: Protecting America's water	Reduce human exposure to contaminants in drinking water, shellfish, fish, and recreational water. Protect and restore watersheds and aquatic ecosystems.
Goal 3: Cleaning up communities and advancing sustainable development	Promote sustainable and livable communities by promoting smart growth, land reclamation, and emergency preparedness. Preserve land by decreasing waste generation, recycling, and effective waste management. Restore land by cleaning up and restoring contaminated land and responding to toxic releases. Strengthen health and environmental protection on Indian lands.
Goal 4: Ensuring the safety of chemicals and preventing pollution	Ensure chemical safety and reduce chemical exposures. Promote pollution prevention.
Goal 5: Enforcing environmental laws	Implement environmental law with vigorous enforcement and use of sanctions.

Data from: Environmental Protection Agency. (2010a). *FY 2011–2011 EPA strategic plan: Achieving our vision.* Washington, DC: Author.

and cooling systems as well as housing units with more energy-conserving features. For example, in 2009, 58% of homes surveyed had multipane windows and 80% of new homes built after 2000 had energy-efficient windows. Similarly, 39% of households used an Energy Star refrigerator and 36% had an Energy Star clothes washer. On the other hand, more homes (40%) use DVRs rather than VCRs and DVD players. DVRs consume more energy than VCRs or DVD players. In addition, 75% of homes now have computers and 35% have two or more computers. Another 50 million homes have three or more televisions, adding to the level of home energy consumption (EIA, 2011).

Manufacturing or industrial energy consumption declined by nearly 17% from 2002 to 2010, but still accounted for 14 quadrillion Btu in 2010 (EIA, 2013b). All forms of energy consumption are contributing to rapid depletion of natural resources, and there is a serious need to develop alternative forms of energy production.

Some alternative energy sources, however, pose environmental health hazards themselves. For example, depletion of oil resources has motivated the development of new methods of natural gas extraction, which make natural gas a more cost-effective alternative fuel than in the past. The extraction process, called "fracking," uses chemicals that leak into groundwater supplies and are known to cause damage to lungs, liver, kidneys, blood, and the brain (Finkel & Law, 2011). As was seen in the aftermath of the tsunami and flooding of nuclear reactors in Japan, use of nuclear power has other potential health-related risks. Similarly, conversion of food products, such as corn, to fuel alternatives minimizes their availability as food supplies for humans and domestic animals. Wind and solar power may be more healthful as well as renewable energy sources, but their long-term health effects are not yet known. Population health nurses need to stay current on the research on the health effects of various energy sources and educate the public and policy makers to make informed decisions. In addition, nurses can be instrumental in promoting energy conservation.

WASTE MANAGEMENT. The final aspect of the social environment to be addressed is the issue of waste management. Categories of waste to be considered include solid waste, hazardous waste, chemical waste, heavy metals, and biological waste. Solid waste consists of paper products, glass, metal, plastics, rubber and leather, textiles, wood, and other wastes, which include food scraps, yard trimmings, and other organic wastes. According to the U.S. Census Bureau (2011a), U.S. residents generated nearly 250 million tons of solid waste in 2008, an increase of 65% over 1980. Approximately one third of the solid waste generated in 2008 was recovered by recycling, composting, or burning as an energy source. Another 135 million tons were discarded to landfills and other sites.

Hazardous waste is defined as "waste that is dangerous or potentially harmful to our health or the environment. Hazardous wastes can be liquids, solids, gases, or sludges. They can be discarded commercial products, like cleaning fluids or pesticides, or the by-products of manufacturing processes" (EPA, 2011i). Hazardous wastes are of concern in terms of their disposal and in terms of transportation from one place to another. In 2007, the United States generated more than 32 million tons of hazardous waste, 655,000 tons of which were transported posing risk for major exposures due to accidents in transit (U.S. Census Bureau, 2011c).

PLEASE TAKE
YOUR RUBBISH HOME
THIS IS A NATIONAL
NATURE RESERVE AND
HOME TO MANY PEOPLE,
ANIMALS AND PLANTS

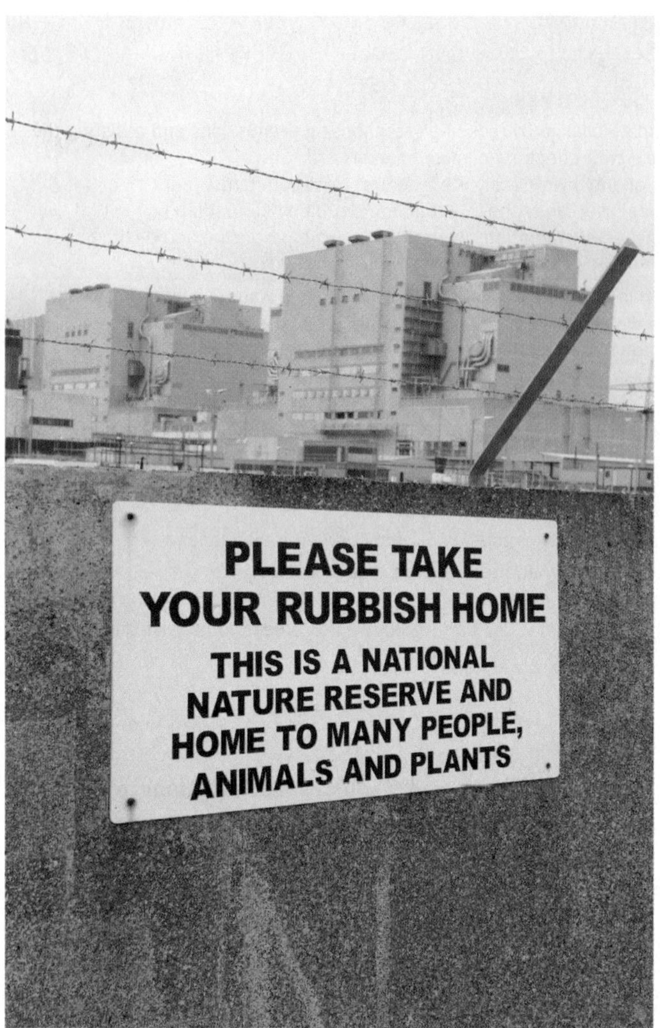

Pollution affects everyone's health. *(Jules Selmes/Pearson Education, Inc.).*

Hazardous wastes are primarily generated by human activities, and may be biological, chemical, or metal. Biological hazardous wastes occur when harmful bacteria and other biological agents are discharged into water supplies or contaminate foods. Chemical hazardous wastes are generated by a variety of industrial processes and frequently contaminate water supplies. Use of personal products such as cleansing agents in the home may also lead to generation of hazardous waste. Metal contamination of water supplies or land may also occur as a result of industrial processes or home use of products that contain heavy metals such as lead, arsenic, and so on. For example, in 2009, the prevalence of elevated blood lead levels (BLLs) in U.S. adults was 6.3 per 100,000 employed persons. Control strategies have resulted in a decreased prevalence of lead poisoning in adults, however. For example, the prevalence of elevated blood lead levels declined by more than 50% from 1994 to 2009 (Division of Surveillance, Hazard Evaluation, and Field Studies, 2011).

Toxic chemical waste releases actually decreased by 15% from 2003 to 2008, but total industrial releases in 2008 still totaled more than 3,861 million pounds. The greatest releases occurred from metal mining, followed by electric utilities (U.S. Census Bureau, 2011b). Agriculture also produces chemical wastes related to pesticides and fertilizers that contaminate water supplies through runoff. As we noted earlier, ammonia production at factory farms is also of concern.

In the past, many toxic hazardous wastes were stored or dumped in a variety of places that permitted their release into air and water. During the 1970s, the health implications of these hazardous waste sites were recognized prompting the development of the *Superfund* program; *Superfund* is the EPA program initiated to clean up these hazardous waste sites. It was established under the Comprehensive Environmental Response, Compensation, and Liability Act of 1980 and permits EPA cleanup of sites placed on the National Priorities List, to compel parties responsible for hazardous waste dumping to engage in cleanup or compensate EPA for cleanup activities. Since the passage of the legislation, tens of thousands of sites throughout the nation have been cleaned up (EPA, 2011g). For further information on remaining Superfund sites, see the *External Resources* section of the student resources site.

Biological wastes are created by humans, animals, and insects, as well as by decomposing plant matter. Biological wastes become hazardous to human health when they contain pathogens that contaminate water and food supplies. In developed countries, most human biological wastes are controlled through sewage treatment systems. In other parts of the world, however, sanitation is rudimentary and the consequent risk of exposure to fecal pathogens is high. Animal and insect droppings are also sources of many communicable diseases. For example, the presence of mouse droppings in the environment increases the risk of hantavirus exposure. Similarly, flies, cockroaches, and other insects contaminate food and water supplies. Population health nurses can help to educate populations for control of biological wastes and prevention of food and water contamination by biological agents.

Interactions Among Environmental Components

Although we have discussed the natural, built, and social environments as if their effects on health are independent of one another, they are actually intimately related. For example, industrial and human wastes deposited into the ocean from the built environment have polluted waters and altered the marine food chain. Overfishing of coastal waters has, in turn, led to an increasing dependence on farmed fish, which may have higher levels of contaminants than wild fish, thereby increasing the potential for human health effects. Similarly, ozone levels that contribute to air pollution peak during traffic rush hours (part of the built environment) and with increasing temperatures during the day (the natural environment). Surprisingly, ozone levels may be worse in less densely populated areas due to increased vehicle use as a result of urban sprawl.

Elements of the natural environment also interact with human development, human behavioral factors, and elements of the social environment to contribute to health problems. For instance, the effects of severe heat waves are associated with increased age, decreased socioeconomic status, poor housing quality, and lack of air conditioning, as well as with the use of alcohol and some medications. Another example of the interactions between built and natural environments lies in the aging water systems in most U.S. cities, leading to breakdowns and contamination of natural water supplies.

We noted before the effects of the built environment on human health-related behaviors such as walking. Community design also affects the natural environment. Urban development, for example, increases the amount of impervious surfaces that do not absorb rain water, leading to greater storm water volume and runoff, which have the potential to contaminate water sources or increase flood risk in residential areas. The built environment also affects levels of social capital through its effects on opportunities for people to congregate and interact with each other. For example, communities with walkable, mixed-use neighborhoods tend to exhibit higher levels of social capital than automobile-dependent ones.

Social environmental changes such as the move to smaller, nuclear families requires more housing, uses more natural resources, and creates a larger ecological footprint. These effects, as well as those of global climate change in the natural environment, are anticipated to result in major social upheavals such as water wars and environmental refugees (Pappas, 2011).

Population Health Nursing and Environmental Influences on Health

Because of their consistent presence in the community, population health nurses are some of those most likely to become aware of environmental health problems, yet they are often unprepared to recognize and deal with them. Protection of the environment is one of the essential functions of public health, and the participation of population health nurses in this function is critical. Population health nursing activity related to environmental health issues occurs at individual/family client and population levels.

Standards and competencies for occupational and environmental health nursing practice have been developed and are discussed in Chapter 23∞. In addition, a number of national initiatives support the role of nursing with respect to environmental health issues. The first of these initiatives was an offshoot of the Agency for Toxic Substances and Disease Registry (ATSDR). ATSDR, part of the *Superfund* legislation passed in 1980, was created to prevent or minimize public exposure to hazardous substances. In 1994, ATSDR established the Environmental Health Nursing Initiative to promote research, collaboration, and educational opportunities related to environmental health. The ATSDR initiative was designed to promote a more active role for the nursing profession in addressing environmental health with a goal of making environmental health "an integral component of nursing practice, education, and research" (ATSDR, n.d.). To that end, the initiative has developed a series of education resources and training programs and roundtable discussions around nursing involvement in environmental health.

In 1995, the Institute of Medicine report, *Nursing, Health, and the Environment* (Pope, Snyder, & Mood, 1995), promulgated four general competencies for nursing with respect to environmental health. The first of these competencies addressed knowledge related to mechanisms for environmental exposure, prevention and control strategies, and the need for evidence-based approaches to dealing with environmental issues. The second competency dealt with the ability to take an environmental exposure history and make appropriate referrals for health care services as well as informing the public regarding environmental hazards. The third competency underscored the need for advocacy to support environmental justice in resolving environmental health problems, and the fourth reflected knowledge and use of legislative and regulatory processes to address environmental conditions that jeopardize health.

In 2010, the Alliance of Nurses for Healthy Environments joined the American Nurses Association (ANA) to incorporate a standard related to environmental health in ANA's revised *Nursing: Scope and Standards of Practice*. The standard addresses competencies for both the basic registered nurse and graduate-prepared nurses (Gilden, 2010). For further information on the competencies, see the *External Resources* section of the student resources site.

Population health nurses can use the population health nursing model to address environmental health problems. Use of the model focuses on assessment, intervention planning, and evaluation of environmental interventions.

Assessing Environmental Health Influences

The first step in ameliorating environmental health problems is an assessment of the factors contributing to them and their effects on human health. In addition to identifying environmental factors in the community that may affect health, population health nurses assess the population for factors that may increase the risk or severity of the health effects of environmental conditions. Factors in each of the determinants of health categories may be addressed.

BIOLOGICAL DETERMINANTS. Biological determinants such as age, genetics, and existing health problems may increase a population's risk of environmentally caused health problems. For example, children's higher metabolic rate increases the rate of absorption of toxins, and very young children are closer to the floor, where air pollutants, in particular, accumulate. In addition, the rapid rate of growth and cell differentiation in children fosters genetic alteration and carcinogenesis. Older adults, because of changes in their cardiovascular, renal, pulmonary, and immune systems, are less able to detoxify environmental toxins and, consequently, have a higher risk of adverse health effects. The population health nurse would determine the age composition of the population as it affects risk for and presence of health problems related to environmental factors.

Existing genetic and physiologic conditions may also increase the potential for health effects of environmental factors. For example, levels of environmental toxins that might not harm an adult may be harmful to the fetus in a pregnant woman. A higher prevalence of chronic respiratory conditions, such as asthma, increases the adverse health effects of plant pollens and air pollution.

Population health nurses also assess population groups and individual clients for evidence of environmentally caused disease. Air pollution, for example, affects the respiratory system primarily, but may also produce cardiovascular, central nervous system, or hematopoietic effects. Air pollution also irritates the eyes and mucous membranes of the respiratory system. Water pollution can affect the gastrointestinal system, skin, liver, and reproductive, hematopoietic, lymphatic, cardiovascular, and genitourinary systems. Pesticides can adversely affect the central nervous system and produce kidney damage, a variety of cancers, and chromosomal changes. Radiation can cause skin cancer, visual impairment, cataracts, and genetic mutations, as well as lung and other cancers. Lead poisoning damages the central nervous system as well as the gastrointestinal system and can impair growth and development. Other metals and hazardous chemicals may cause cancers or central nervous system, gastrointestinal, and metabolic damage. High levels of noise not only compromise human hearing but can also contribute to gastrointestinal, dermatologic, central nervous system, cardiovascular, and psychological problems. Finally, built environments that hinder physical activity contribute to obesity, osteoporosis, and depression. Some of the effects of these environmental hazards are presented in Figure 4-2●.

PSYCHOLOGICAL DETERMINANTS. Psychological determinants within the population may influence behaviors that contribute to environmental risk or affect the consequences of environmental conditions for members of the population. For example, stress may increase smoking behavior, leading to greater levels of smoke exposure for both smokers and nonsmokers. Conversely, environmental conditions may affect the mental health of the population. For example, persistent rain may lead people to stay indoors and lead to a higher incidence of depression. Certainly, environmentally caused disasters have significant psychological effects on the population.

ENVIRONMENTAL DETERMINANTS. Population health nurses would also assess the environmental conditions that may affect the health of the population. What is the extent of air and water pollution? To what extent do weather conditions affect health? What features of the built environment contribute to health or ill health?

SOCIOCULTURAL DETERMINANTS. Sociocultural determinants such as occupation, income, and educational levels; cultural beliefs, behaviors, and attitudes; and social and environmental policies influence environmental conditions that affect health. Occupational settings give rise to multiple opportunities for exposure to environmental hazards, and population health nurses should assess the potential for exposure to hazardous environmental conditions created by local occupations and industries. A related issue is the extent of recreational pursuits that entail exposure to toxins. Other social factors, such as socioeconomic status, may influence exposure to environmental hazards. For example, children living in housing of lower economic value are at higher risk for lead poisoning or injury resulting from home safety deficiencies. Similarly, social capital available to the population may affect their ability to address environmental risk factors. Educational levels influence the population's knowledge of environmental issues and their awareness of strategies to prevent environmentally caused health problems or recognition when those problems exist.

Cultural attitudes toward the environment may also influence concern for environmental issues and the population health nurse would assess public awareness of environmental concerns and willingness to take relevant actions to prevent or ameliorate problems. The population health nurse would also examine policies related to environmental issues and the extent to which they promote or impede environmental health. Closely aligned with policies is the existence of special interest groups that may resist social policies that promote and protect environmental health. For example, economic costs have been used to argue against implementation of clean air regulations in some industries. What groups within the population support or resist policies aimed at promoting environmental health and what is the basis for their support or resistance?

BEHAVIORAL DETERMINANTS. Certain personal behaviors prevalent in the population may interact with elements of the physical environment to cause or exacerbate health problems. Smoking, for example, increases lead absorption levels for both smokers and their children. Similarly, reliance on biomass fuels for cooking and heating creates indoor air pollution. Recreational activities are also affected by environmental factors. For example, after-school sports and after-work physical activity at times of peak ozone levels increase the potential for respiratory health effects. Similarly, swimming and other water-related recreational activities increase the potential for exposure to microorganisms and chemical agents when water is contaminated.

Population health nurses would also assess the extent of behaviors within the population that prevent environmental pollution and environmental health effects. What is the attitude to and extent of recycling in the population? To what extent do members of the population limit energy consumption or conserve water? What protective measures do members of the population take to prevent environmental exposures (e.g., use sunscreen, wear hats, fence swimming pools)?

HEALTH SYSTEM DETERMINANTS. Finally, factors related to the health care delivery system may contribute to or exacerbate environmental health problems. For example, screening for lead levels in high-risk children and adults does not always occur when indicated. Health care providers in general have little knowledge of the manifestations or treatment of many environmentally caused diseases. The focused assessment on page 94 provides tips to assist you in your assessment of environmental health issues.

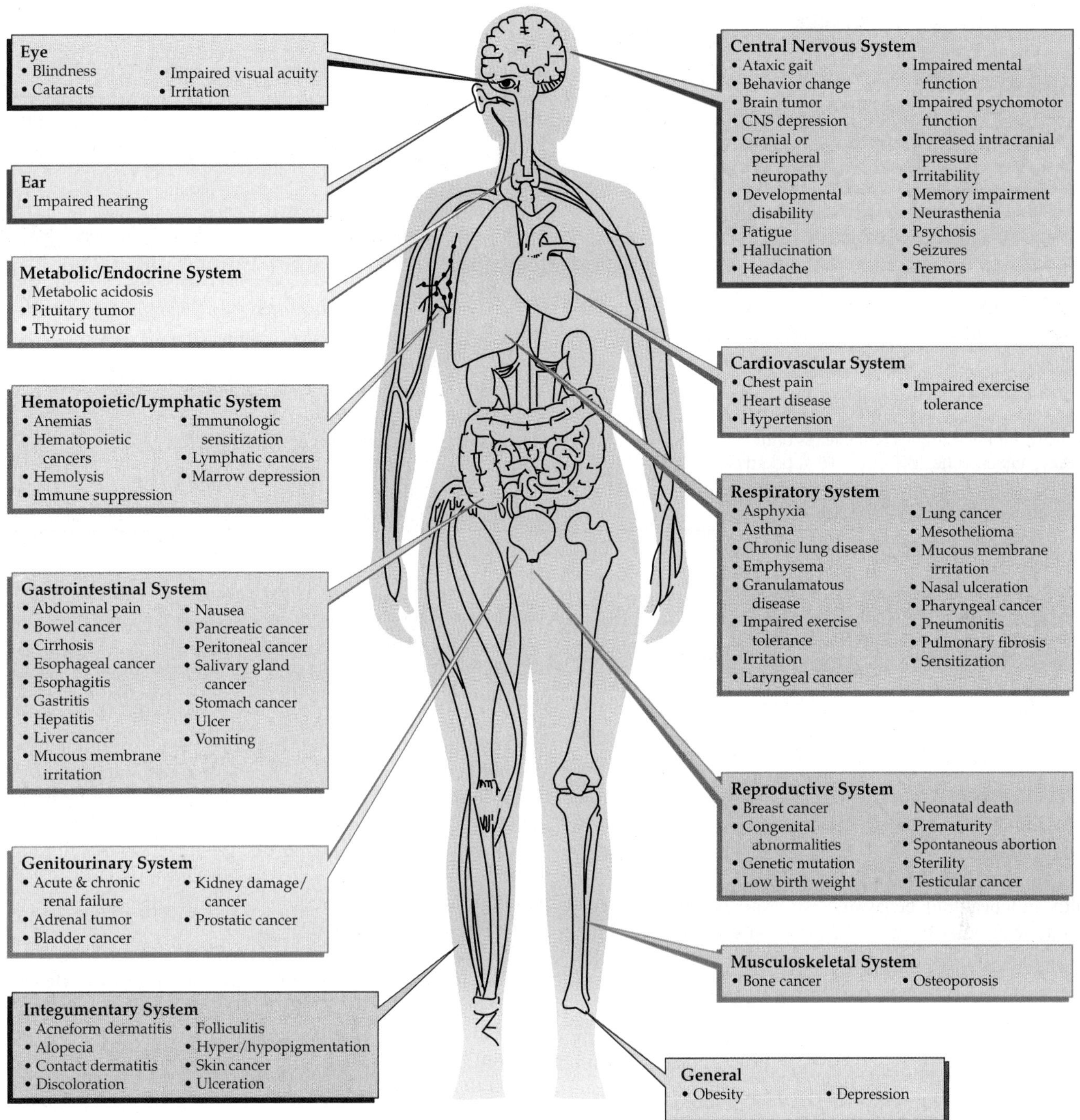

FIGURE 4-2 Human Health Effects of Environmental Conditions

Some environmental assessment data can be obtained primarily by observation in the home or community. For example, elements of the built environment such as traffic safety hazards or recreational opportunities are easily observed. Data related to environmental health effects may be available from local health departments or environmental protection agencies or from state agencies. Information on human behaviors that contribute to environmental health problems (e.g., smoking) is best obtained by asking family members or in community surveys. Information on environmental policy can be obtained from local government, environmental protection agencies, and local businesses and industries. Other elements of environmental assessment are addressed in relevant chapters in this book (e.g., community assessment in Chapter 15∞ and school and occupational settings in Chapters 22∞ and 23∞, respectively), as well as in assessment tools included on the student resources site.

FOCUSED ASSESSMENT Assessing Environmental Influences on Population Health

- What natural, built, and social environmental conditions have the potential to influence the health of the population? How do these conditions affect health? What is the extent of their influence on health at the present time?
- What segments of the population are most likely to be adversely affected by environmental conditions? Why?
- What factors contribute to the presence and influence of environmental conditions within the population?
- To what extent do environmental conditions arise from or are influenced by individual behavior (e.g., smoking, recycling, water conservation)?
- What are the attitudes of members of the population to environmental health issues? What priority is given to resolution of environmental health issues?
- What barriers exist to improving environmental conditions?
- What is the potential for eliminating hazardous environmental conditions? What is the potential for limiting human exposure if hazardous environmental conditions cannot be eliminated?
- What actions will be required to address environmental health concerns within the population?
- Does the health care system contribute to environmental health hazards? If so, how?
- Is the health care system adequate to address environmentally caused diseases in the population?
- Are health care providers adequately prepared to recognize and treat environmentally caused diseases in individual clients?

Planning to Address Environmental Health Issues

Population health nurses assess for environmental hazards present in the community, the factors contributing to them, and the health effects that result. They then use this information to plan interventions, in conjunction with others in the population, to address environmental health problems affecting the population. These interventions can address promotion, prevention, resolution, and restoration.

PROMOTION. With respect to promotion, population health nurses can advocate for environments that promote health and healthful behaviors. For example, they can collaborate with other segments of the population to foster built environments that promote physical activity. Similarly, they can advocate for environments in which access is provided to healthful and nutritious foods at reasonable prices.

PREVENTION. A significant portion of population health nurses' efforts, with respect to environmental health, will relate to prevention efforts. Prevention strategies may focus on prevention of environmental degradation or prevention of human exposure to adverse environmental conditions. These activities may include education of the public regarding prevention as well as advocacy for environmental policies that protect the environment or minimize human exposures. For example, the population health nurse can educate members of the public for energy conservation while advocating for the development of new energy resources and industrial processes that can minimize energy consumption and decrease emission of greenhouse gases, reducing the effects of global warming. Nurses can initiate recycling campaigns within the community or in health care facilities. They can also educate the public regarding vector control measures that do not jeopardize human health (e.g., care in use of rodenticides or pesticides).

Prevention within the built environment would include the development of well-designed communities that minimize urban sprawl, limit resource use, promote mixed land use and the development of social capital, and foster healthy behaviors such as walking and bicycling. In addition, the contributions of the built environment to degradation of the natural environment could be minimized by investing in more effective water systems that make use of newer technological approaches that are more effective and more environmentally friendly. For example, use of waterless toilets, recycling, and rainwater harvesting can conserve water and make it available for human needs (Natural Resources Defense Council, 2012). Population health nurses can advocate for water treatment systems that do not damage the natural environment and yet provide safe water for human consumption. In addition, they can educate the population with respect to water conservation, use of drought tolerant landscaping, and other measures to conserve water. They can also educate clients on inexpensive water treatment measures when more technologically advanced systems are not available (e.g., in underdeveloped countries or on a camping trip).

Developing countries that will not be able to initiate water treatment systems in the near future can encourage point-of-use water treatment systems that incorporate use of dilute solutions of sodium hypochlorite (laundry bleach), solar disinfection by means of ultraviolet light projected through clear plastic bottles or bags, and safe water storage in narrow-mouth containers that require pouring or the use of a spigot to prevent recontamination of the water by dipping. Use of such systems will require access to the needed supplies and public motivation to offset the added costs in terms of time and money.

Public education and social support will be required for all of these initiatives, and many of them will require political advocacy as well. For example, there is a need for additional lead poisoning prevention legislation, funding for programs, and public education to foster identification of risk groups and intervention to reduce exposure risks. Similarly, developers and community development agencies will need to be convinced of the need for smart growth and for provision of affordable mass transit located near schools, homes, and workplaces in those communities already affected by urban sprawl. Population health nurses can be actively involved in all of these activities. For example, they may organize local residents to work with developers to plan mixed-use communities and community designs that promote fitness and exercise. Such strategies can be employed in the design of new communities, but are also appropriate to the redevelopment of older existing communities. Additional prevention activities by population health nurses directed at promoting environmental health for individuals/families and for populations are presented in Table 4-4●.

RESOLUTION. Resolution-related activities also reflect care of individuals and families as well as population groups. Population health nursing interventions with individuals and their families would be geared to identifying and resolving existing health problems caused by environmental conditions. For example, population health nurses might be involved in screening for elevated lead levels or for hearing loss. They might also make referrals for testing of water supplies for clients who are concerned about potential contamination. When possible environmentally caused health conditions are identified, population health nurses might make referrals for medical diagnosis and treatment as needed. They might also make referrals for assistance with eliminating environmental hazards. For example, the nurse might be aware of lead-based paint in dwellings in some parts of town. He or she can screen young children in the area for elevated blood lead levels (BLLs) and make referrals for treatment for children with positive test results. The nurse might also make a referral for assistance in removing lead-based paint from the homes of affected children. Finally, the nurse might monitor children's responses to therapy and the potential for continued exposure to lead.

At the population level, population health nurses might promote targeted screening programs to identify the prevalence of risk factors in the community. Population health nurses can also encourage policy makers to adopt targeted screening practices for appropriate populations in the community.

TABLE 4-4 Prevention Measures for Populations, Individuals, and Families Related to Selected Environmental Concerns

Environmental Concern	Population	Individual/Family
Radiation	Educate the public on the hazards of radon exposure and preventive measures.	Educate the public on the hazards of radon exposure and preventive measures.
	Engage in political activity to promote building standards that safeguard occupants in areas with high levels of natural radiation.	Encourage spending most of one's time in higher levels of the home.
	Educate public about the hazards of overuse of diagnostic X-rays.	Discourage overuse of diagnostic X-rays.
	Engage in political activity to promote and enforce safety standards for nuclear reactors. Educate the public about the hazards of exposure to ultraviolet radiation.	Encourage adequate cleaning of door seals on microwave ovens and maintenance of safe distance while microwave is in operation. Discourage sunbathing. Encourage use of sunscreen and protective clothing when outdoors.
	Promote availability of smoking cessation services.	Discourage smoking in home; refer for smoking cessation assistance.
Lead and heavy metals	Encourage communities to remove lead-based paint from older homes. Advocate for funds for lead remediation of older homes.	Encourage families to remove lead-based paint from older homes.
		Encourage covering surfaces on which paint is peeling.
		Encourage families to wash small children's hands as well as toys to remove lead-contaminated dust.
		Encourage close supervision of small children.
	Encourage policy makers to set and enforce standards for solid waste sites to prevent metal contamination in waters.	Encourage calcium intake to limit lead absorption. Encourage families to use cold water to drink and cook with and to allow the tap to run for a few minutes.

(Continued)

TABLE 4-4 (*Continued*)

Environmental Concern	Population	Individual/Family
Noise	Promote noise abatement ordinances.	Encourage families to limit noise in the home.
	Encourage use of ear protection in high-noise areas.	
Infectious agents	Educate the public on the need for immunizations.	Promote routine immunization for all ages.
	Encourage policy makers to provide low-cost immunization services.	
		Encourage good hygiene, particularly handwashing.
	Promote enforcement of regulations for food processing and food handlers.	Encourage washing fruits and vegetables before eating.
		Encourage adequate cooking and refrigeration of food.
	Advocate for adequate sanitation, waste disposal, and water treatment.	Encourage susceptible individuals to boil water for cooking and drinking in areas with unsafe water.
Insects and animals	Advocate for development and enforcement of pet immunization and leash laws.	Encourage immunization of family pets. Discourage exotic pets and educate owners regarding hazards and prevention.
	Advocate for ordinances controlling insect-breeding areas.	Refer for assistance in eliminating insects, rats, and other pets from the home.
		Encourage use of insect repellant and protective clothing when outdoors.
Plants	Promote elimination of poisonous plants from recreation areas.	Eliminate poisonous houseplants.
	Educate the public about poisonous plants.	Eliminate poisonous plants from yards.
		Eliminate other hazardous plants (e.g., poison ivy, plant allergens) from home environment.
		Encourage close supervision of small children.
Poisons	Educate the public on hazards of household chemicals and medications.	Educate families on proper use, storage, and disposal of household chemicals and medications.
		Encourage close supervision of children.
	Advocate for legislation to limit use of hazardous chemicals in home and industry.	Encourage proper disposal of hazardous wastes.
	Advocate for effective hazardous waste disposal services.	
Air pollution	Promote legislation to prevent air pollution.	Encourage limiting physical activity on days with high air pollutant levels.
	Promote incentives for carpooling.	Encourage carpooling.
	Advocate for legislation to develop and enforce safety standards for home-heating devices.	Discourage use of space heaters in poorly ventilated areas.
	Promote building standards that ensure adequate ventilation.	Encourage frequent cleaning or replacement of heater and air-conditioning filters.
		Encourage opening doors and windows to permit air exchange.
	Advocate replacement of hazard-producing industrial processes.	Encourage replacement of asbestos insulation as needed.
	Advocate legislation mandating CO monitors in residential units.	Encourage installation of CO monitors in home.
		Educate for use of hazardous household products with adequate ventilation.
Water pollution	Promote development and enforcement of legislation to prevent water pollution.	Encourage use of bottled water by high-risk persons in areas with heavily polluted water.
	Promote replacement of hazard-producing industrial processes.	Encourage use of fewer polluting products.
	Promote filtration of water sources for new pathogens, etc.	Educate about water purifying techniques as needed.
Energy consumption	Advocate for policies that conserve resources, promote smart growth, and limit urban sprawl.	Educate regarding interventions to conserve electricity, water, natural gas, etc.
	Advocate for recycling programs.	Promote recycling.

Political activity by population health nurses might also be needed to influence health policy makers to provide adequate access to diagnostic and treatment facilities for people with health problems caused by environmental conditions. Or a nurse might campaign for stricter standards for pollutant emissions in air and water. Table 4-5● provides additional examples of resolution measures that might be taken to improve environmental health in families and population groups.

RESTORATION. Population health nurses may need to work with individuals or families to prevent recurrence or complications of environmentally caused health problems. For example, a nurse might assist a family to find housing where exposure to lead is not a problem. Or the nurse might provide parents with referrals for assistance in coping with the mental effects of long-standing lead poisoning in their children. Another restoration measure might involve suggestions for decreasing noise levels in the home to prevent further impairment of hearing.

Restoration activities might also be needed to deal with environmental problems at the aggregate or group level. An example might be political activity to mandate standards that prevent the recurrence of a leak at a nuclear power plant or to pass a bond issue to renovate a water treatment plant and prevent recontamination of drinking water with sewage. Advocacy for funds to remove lead hazards from older homes or legislation mandating lead removal in rental units are other possible population health nursing interventions related to restoration. Advocacy for continued funding of *Superfund* clean-up activities is another

TABLE 4-5 Resolution Measures for Individuals, Families, and Populations Related to Selected Environmental Concerns

Environmental Concern	Population	Individual/Family
Radiation	Monitor incidence of health problems caused by radiation. Promote access to diagnostic and treatment facilities. Monitor longevity to determine effects of treatment in groups of people affected.	Look for signs of health problems that may be caused by radiation among clients and members of their families. Refer for diagnosis and treatment as needed. Monitor effectiveness of treatment.
Lead and heavy metals	Promote access to screening services. Promote compliance with Medicaid lead-screening guidelines for children. Promote adequate reimbursement for lead-screening services. Monitor incidence of heavy metal poisoning. Promote access to diagnostic and treatment facilities. Monitor prevalence of complications due to heavy metal poisoning.	Screen for elevated blood levels of heavy metals in persons at risk. Observe for signs of heavy metal poisoning. Refer for diagnosis and treatment as needed. Monitor effects of treatment.
Noise	Promote access to hearing-screening services. Promote access to diagnostic and treatment services.	Screen for hearing loss in persons at risk. Refer for diagnosis and treatment as needed. Monitor effects of treatment.
Infectious agents	Promote access to screening services for infectious diseases. Monitor incidence of communicable diseases.	Screen for selected communicable diseases in high-risk persons. Observe for signs of communicable diseases.
Insects and animals	Promote access to treatment for animal bites. Monitor the incidence of diseases caused by insects or animals. Promote access to diagnostic and treatment services for diseases caused by insect or animal bites.	Educate families about first aid for insect and animal bites. Observe for signs and symptoms of diseases caused by insects or animals. Refer for medical assistance as needed.
Plants	Educate the public about poison control activities. Promote community support of poison control centers.	Inform families of poison control center activities. Refer families for poison control center services as needed. Refer for treatment of allergies and other conditions caused by plants.
Poisons	Educate the public about first aid for poisoning. Monitor the incidence of accidental poisoning. Promote access to poison control services.	Educate families about first aid for poisoning. Observe for signs and symptoms of poisoning. Refer families for poison control services as needed.
Air pollution	Advocate development and enforcement of legislation to reduce pollutant emissions. Promote access to diagnostic and treatment services.	Observe for signs and symptoms of diseases caused by air pollution. Refer for diagnosis and treatment as needed.
Water pollution	Promote legislation to control water pollution. Promote access to diagnostic and treatment services for water-related diseases.	Observe for signs and symptoms of water-related diseases. Refer for diagnosis and treatment of water-related diseases.

TABLE 4-6 Restoration Measures for Populations, Individuals, and Families Related to Environmentally Caused Health Conditions

Population	Individual/Family
Monitor effects of environmental changes on incidence of environmentally caused conditions.	Monitor for long-term effects of environmentally caused conditions.
Promote access to services for members of the population affected by environmentally caused conditions.	Promote adjustment to the long-term effects of environmentally caused conditions.
	Refer families to personal or environmental health services to deal with consequences of adverse environmental conditions.
Advocate environmental policies to prevent recurrence of environmental health problems.	Promote changes in environmental conditions or minimize subsequent exposure to prevent recurrence of environmentally caused disease.

population-level restoration intervention. Table 4-6• presents several restoration interventions related to environmental health in the care of individuals/families and populations.

Evaluating Environmental Health Measures

Population health nurses are also involved in evaluating the effectiveness of environmental control measures. Evaluation would focus on the effectiveness of promotion, prevention, resolution, and restoration measures related to individuals, families, and population groups. For example, the nurse might monitor blood lead levels of children in housing with lead-based paint to determine whether preventive measures have prevented initial elevation. For those children who already have elevated blood lead levels, evaluation would focus on the effects of chelating agents in reducing blood levels and the prevention of symptoms of lead poisoning. Evaluation of restoration measures would be aimed at the effectiveness of abatement procedures in preventing blood lead levels from rising again after treatment. Similar approaches to evaluation of promotion, prevention, resolution, and restoration interventions could be used for each of the environmental health problems addressed in this chapter. Evaluation at the aggregate level would focus on the extent to which national objectives for environmental health have been achieved as well as on the effectiveness of specific promotion, prevention, resolution, and restoration interventions.

CHAPTER RECAP

Population health nurses are in a prime position to identify environmental influences on health and to initiate measures to foster health promoting environments. They assess factors related to each of the six categories of determinants of health arising from natural, built, and social environments and collaborate with others to plan and implement environmental strategies related to health promotion, illness and injury prevention, problem resolution, and health restoration. They are also involved in the evaluation of the effectiveness of interventions in modifying environmental factors that influence population health.

CASE STUDY Environmental Advocate

Janice Wu, a community health nurse, is visiting a new client in a nursing home in an inner-city area in Los Angeles. As she enters the nursing home, she notices that several of the residents are doing calisthenics in the yard. Some of the residents are sitting on the sidelines and appear quite short of breath. When Janice checks to make sure they are all right, they tell her that they usually have a hard time breathing when they exercise on smoggy days like today. The residents say that they usually try to continue their exercises because it is one of the few activities that get them out of the building. They also enjoy the social aspects of the exercise sessions. Many of them state that they have always been active and want to maintain their strength and mobility as long as possible. They express fears of being bedridden and unable to care for themselves.

After Janice is sure that all of the residents will be all right, she goes on to see her client. When she enters the building, she notices that it is quite hot inside, even though all the windows and doors are open. Although it is only 10 A.M., it promises to be one of L.A.'s scorching summer days. After seeing her client, Janice talks to the director about the heat in the building. The director tells her that the building is always hot and that the air conditioning has never worked properly. The last time the service people came to fix the air-conditioning unit, they said it could not be repaired and would have to be replaced. The nursing home is run by a large national corporation, and the director says she has been told they will have to wait until the next budget year (October) before money will be available for a new air conditioner. Fortunately, the heating system is separate, so there will be heat when the colder weather starts. The director says that staff members have been particularly careful about maintaining hydration in the residents during the hot weather, but many of the residents seem fatigued and listless with the heat.

1. What hazards are present in the natural, built, and social environments in this situation? What health effects, if any, are these hazards causing?
2. What levels of intervention are warranted in this situation? What might Janice do to intervene?

REFERENCES

Agency for Toxic Substances and Diseases Registry. (n.d.). *The ATSDR environmental health nursing initiative.* Retrieved from http://www.atsdr.cdc.gov/EHN/

AIRNow. (2010). *Air Quality Index (AQI)—A guide to air quality and your health.* Retrieved from http://www.airnow.gov/index.cfm?action=aqibasics.aqi

American Lung Association. (2011). *State of the air 2011.* Retrieved from http://www.stateoftheair.org/2011/assets/SOTA2011.pdf

Bell, E. (2011). Readying health services for climate change: A policy framework for regional development. *American Journal of Public Health, 101,* 804–813. doi:10.2105/AJPH.2010.202820

Centers for Disease Control and Prevention. (n.d.). *Tips for preventing heat-related illness.* Retrieved from http://www.bt.cdc.gov/disasters/extremeheat/heattips.asp

Centers for Disease Control and Prevention. (2009). *CDC policy on climate change and public health.* Retrieved from http://www.cdc.gov/climatechange/pubs/Climate_Change_Policy.pdf

Centers for Disease Control and Prevention. (2011a). *CDC 2011 estimates: Findings.* Retrieved from http://www.cdc.gov/foodborneburden/2011-foodborne-estimates.html

Centers for Disease Control and Prevention. (2011b). Drinking water week 2011. *Morbidity and Mortality Weekly Report, 60,* 517.

Chomel, B. B., & Sun, B. (2011). Zoonoses in the bedroom. *Emerging Infectious Diseases, 17,* 167–171. doi:10.3201/eid1702101070

Cramer, M. E., Roberts, S., & Stevens, E. (2011). Landlord attitudes and behaviors regarding smoke-free policies: Implications for voluntary policy change. *Public Health Nursing, 28,* 3–12. doi:10.1111/j.1525-1446.2010.00904.x

Division of Foodborne, Waterborne, and Environmental Diseases. (n.d.). *CDC and the safe water system.* Retrieved from http://www.cdc.gov/safewater/PDF/SWS-Overview-factsheet508c.pdf

Division of Foodborne, Waterborne, and Environmental Diseases. (2011a). Botulism caused by consumption of commercially produced potato soups stored improperly—Ohio and Georgia, 2011. *Morbidity and Mortality Weekly Report, 60,* 890.

Division of Foodborne, Waterborne, and Environmental Diseases. (2011b). Vital signs: Incidence and trends of infection with pathogens transmitted commonly through food—Foodborne Diseases Active Surveillance Network, 10 U.S. sites, 1996–2010. *Morbidity and Mortality Weekly Report, 60,* 749–755.

Division of Parasitic Diseases and Malaria, (2011). Raccoon roundworms in pet kinkajous—Three states, 1999 and 2010. *Morbidity and Mortality Weekly Report, 60,* 302–305.

Division of Surveillance, Hazard Evaluation, and Field Studies. (2011). Adult blood lead epidemiology and surveillance—United States, 2008–2009. *Morbidity and Mortality Weekly Report, 60,* 841–845.

Environmental Integrity Project. (2011). *Hazardous pollution from factory farms: An analysis of EPA's National Air Emissions Monitoring study.* Retrieved from http://www.environmentalintegrity.org/documents/HazardousPollutionfromFactoryFarms.pdf

Environmental Protection Agency. (2010a). *FY 2011-2011 EPA strategic plan: Achieving our vision.* Washington, DC: Author.

Environmental Protection Agency. (2010b). *Sources of pollutants in the ambient air.* Retrieved from http://www.epa.gov/apti/course422/ap3.html

Environmental Protection Agency. (2011a). *Air pollution emissions overview.* Retrieved from http://www.epa.gov/airquality/emissns.html

Environmental Protection Agency. (2011b). *Air quality trends.* Retrieved from http://www.epa.gov/airtrends/aqtrends.html

Environmental Protection Agency. (2011c). *Clean Air Act.* Retrieved from http://www.epa.gov/air/caa/

Environmental Protection Agency. (2011d). *Drinking water contaminants.* Retrieved from http://water.epa.gov/drink/contaminants/index.cfm

Environmental Protection Agency. (2011e). *Endangerment and cause or contribute findings for greenhouse gases under Section 202(a) of the Clean Air Act.* Retrieved from http://www.epa.gov/climatechange/endangerment.html

Environmental Protection Agency. (2011f). *Summary of the Clean Water Act.* Retrieved from http://www.epa.gov/regulations/laws/cwa.html

Environmental Protection Agency. (2011g). *Superfund—Basic information.* Retrieved from http://www.epa.gov/superfund/about.htm

Environmental Protection Agency. (2011h). *Sustainability: Basic information.* Retrieved from http://www.epa.gov/sustainability/basicinfo.htm#sustainability

Environmental Protection Agency. (2011i). *Wastes—Hazardous waste.* Retrieved from http://www.epa.gov/osw/hazard/

Environmental Protection Agency. (2012). *Radiation protection: Health effects.* Retrieved from http://www.epa.gov/rpdweb00/understand/health_effects.html

Finkel, M. L., & Law, A. (2011). The rush to drill for natural gas: A public health cautionary tale. *American Journal of Public Health, 101,* 784–785. doi:10.2105/AJPH.2010.300089

Freedman, V. A., Grafova, I. B., & Rogowski, J. (2011). Neighborhoods and chronic disease onset in later life. *American Journal of Public Health, 101*, 79–86. doi:10.2105/AJPH.2009.178640

Gibson, D. M. (2011). The neighborhood food environment and adult weight status: Estimates from longitudinal data. *American Journal of Public Health, 101*, 71–78. doi:10.2105/AJPH.2009.187567

Gilden, R. (2010). *Environmental health scope and standards of practice*. Retrieved from http://envirn.org/pg/groups/3755/environmental-health-scope-and-standards-of-practice/

Global Health Council, (2009). *Improving global health with clean water and sanitation*. Retrieved from http://www.globalhealth.org/images/pdf/publications/200903_fact_sheet_clean_water.pdf

Isakower, I. (2011). *The impact of GHG regulations*. Retrieved from http://blog.energytomorrow.org/2011/02/the-impact-of-ghg-regulations.html?gclid=CMmfzuj2kKoCFSE_gwodJT2Xzg

James, P. J., Troped, P. J., Hart, J. E., Joshu, C. E., Colditz, G. A., Brownson, R. C., . . . Laden, F. (2013). Urban sprawl, physical activity, and body mass index: Nurses' Health Study and Nurses' Health Study II. *American Journal of Public Health, 103*, 369-375. doi: 10.2105/AJPH.2011.300449

Joseph, J. T., Roy, S. S., Shams, N., Visitainer, P., Nadelman, R. B., Hosur, S., ..., Wormser, G. P. (2011). Babesiosis in Lower Hudson Valley, New York, USA. *Emerging Infectious Diseases, 17*, 843–847.

Kovats, S. (2006). Climate change: Vector-borne diseases. In P. Wilkinson (Ed.), *Environmental epidemiology* (pp. 160–172). New York: McGraw-Hill Education.

Levy, B., S., & Sidel, V. W. (2011). Water rights and water fights: Preventing and resolving conflicts before they boil over. *American Journal of Public Health, 101*, 778–779. doi:10.2105/AJPH.2010.194670

Mathies, F., Bickler, G., Marin, N. C., & Hales, S. (Eds.). (2008). *Heat health action plans: Guidance*. Retrieved from http://www.euro.who.int/__data/assets/pdf_file/0006/95919/E91347.pdf

McCarrier, K. P., Zimmerman, F. J., Ralston, J. D., & Martin, D. P. (2011). Associations between minimum wage policy and access to health care: Evidence from the Behavioral Risk Factor Surveillance System, 1996–2007. *American Journal of Public Health, 101*, 359–367. doi:10.2105/AJPH.2006.108928

McDonald, L. (Ed.). (2004). *Florence Nightingale public health care*. Waterloo, ON: Wildfrid Laurier University Press.

Mendez, D., Alshanqeety, O., Warner, K. E., Lantz, P. M., & Courant, P. N. (2011). The impact of declining smoking on radon-related lung cancer in the United States. *American Journal of Public Health, 101*, 310–314. doi:10.2105/AJPH.2009.1892250

Michael, A., & Beaglehole, R. (2009). The global context for public health. In R. Beaglehole & R. Bonita (Eds.), *Global public health: A new era* (2nd ed., pp. 1–22). Oxford, UK: Oxford University Press.

Moore, J. B., Jilcott, S. B., Shores, K. A., Evenson, K. R., Brownson, R. C., & Novick, L. F. (2010). A qualitative examination of perceived barriers and facilitators of physical activity for urban and rural youth. *Health Education Research, 25*, 355–367. doi:10.1093/her/cyq004

Murphree, R., Warkentin, J. V., Dunn, J. R., Schaffner, W., & Jones, T. F. (2011). Elephant-to-human transmission of tuberculosis, 2009. *Emerging Infectious Diseases, 17*, 366–370. doi:10.3201/eid1703101668

National Aeronautics and Space Administration, Earth Observatory. (n.d.). *Global warming*. Retrieved from http://earthobservatory.nasa.gov/Features/GlobalWarming/page2.php

National Association of State Public Health Veterinarians. (2011). Compendium of measures to prevent disease associated with animals in public health settings, 2011. *Morbidity and Mortality Weekly Report, 60*(RR-4), 1–23.

National Center for Chronic Disease Prevention and Health Promotion. (2011). State smoke-free laws for worksites, restaurants, and bars—United States, 2000–2010. *Morbidity and Mortality Weekly Report, 60*, 472–475.

National Center for Emerging and Zoonotic Infections, (2010). Human rabies—Virginia, 2009. *Morbidity and Mortality Weekly Report, 59*, 1236–1238.

National Center for Emerging and Zoonotic Infections, (2011). Update on human *Salmonella typhimurium* infections associated with aquatic frogs—United States, 2009–2011. *Morbidity and Mortality Weekly Report, 60*, 628.

National Weather Service. (2011a). *2010 cold-related fatalities*. Retrieved from http://www.weather.gov/om/hazstats/cold10.pdf

National Weather Service. (2011b). *2010 heat-related fatalities*. Retrieved from http://www.weather.gov/om/hazstats/heat10.pdf

National Weather Service. (2011c). *Summary of natural hazard statistics for 2010 in the United States*. Retrieved from http://www.weather.gov/om/hazstats/sum10.pdf

National Weather Service. (2011d). *Weather fatalities*. Retrieved from http://www.weather.gov/om/hazstats.shtml

Natural Resources Defense Council. (n.d.). *Bringing safe water to the world*. Retrieved from http://www.nrdc.org/international/safewater.asp

Natural Resources Defense Council. (2012). *Water facts*. Retrieved from http://www.nrdc.org/water/sanitation/files/sani.pdf

New York State Department of Health. (2009). *Lead exposure risk assessment questionnaire for children*. Retrieved from http://www.health.state.ny.us/environmental/lead/exposure/childhood/risk_assessment.htm

Occupational Safety and Health Administration. (2013). *Non-ionizing radiation*. Retrieved from https://www.osha.gov/pls/oshaweb/owadisp.show_document?p_table=STANDARDS&p_id=9745

OMB Watch. (2010). *As Senate defeats challenges to climate finding, EPA faces additional trials*. Retrieved from http://www.ombwatch.org/node/11070

Pappas, G. (2011). Pakistan and water: New pressures on global security and human health. *American Journal of Public Health, 101*, 786–788. doi:10.2105/AJPH.2010.300009

Parra, D. C., McKenzie, T. L., Ribeiro, I. C., Hino, A. A. F., Dreisinger, M., Coniglio, K., ..., Simoes, E. J. (2010). Assessing physical activity in public parks in Brazil using systematic observation. *American Journal of Public Health, 100*, 1420–1426. doi:10-2105/AJPH.2009.181230

Pope, A. M., Snyder, M. A., & Mood, L. H. (Eds.). (1995). *Nursing, health, and environment: Strengthening the relationship to improve the public's health*. Washington, DC: National Academy Press.

Prüss-Üstün, A., & Corvalán, C. (2006). *Preventing disease through healthy environments: Toward an estimate of the environmental burden of disease*. Geneva, Switzerland: World Health Organization.

Raymond, J., Wheeler, W., & Brown, M. J. (2011, January 14). Inadequate and unhealthy housing, 2007 and 2009. *Morbidity and Mortality Weekly Report, 60*(Suppl.), 21–27.

Reitzel, L. R., Cromley, E. K., Li, Y., Cao, Y., Dela Mater, R., Mazas, C. A., ..., Wetter, D. W. (2011). The effect of tobacco outlet density and proximity on smoking cessation. *American Journal of Public Health, 101*, 315–320. doi:10.2105/AJPH.2010.191676

Reitzel, L. R., Regan, S. D., Nguyen, N., Cromley, E. K., Strong, L. L., Wetter, D. W., & McNeill, L. H. (2014). Density and proximity of fast food restaurants and body mass index among African Americans. *American Journal of Public Health, 104*, 110–116. doi: 10.2105/AJPH.2012.301140

Resnick, D. B. (2010). Urban sprawl, smart growth, and deliberative democracy. *American Journal of Public Health, 100*, 1852–1856. doi:10.2105/AJPH.2009.182501

Rezick, J. S., & Fee, E. (2011). Voices from the past. *American Journal of Public Health, 101,* 1050–1053. doi:10.2105/AJPH.2010.300022

Rung, A. L., Broyles, S. T., Mowen, A. J., Gustat, J., & Sothern, M. S. (2011). Escaping to and being active in neighborhood parks: Park use in a post disaster setting. *Disasters, 35,* 383–403. doi:10.1111/j.0361-3666.2010.01217.x

Schools divert trash at football games. (2011, April). *The Nation's Health, 17.*

Szwarcwald, C. L., de Mota, J. C., Damacena, G. N., & Pereira, T. G. S. (2011). Health inequalities in Rio de Janeiro, Brazil: Lower health life expectancy in socioeconomically disadvantaged areas. *American Journal of Public Health, 101,* 517–523. doi:10.2105/AJPH.2010.195453

Takaro, T. K., Krieger, J., Song, L., Sharify, D., & Beaudet, N. (2011). The breathe-easy home: The impact of asthma-friendly home construction on clinical outcomes and trigger exposure. *American Journal of Public Health, 101,* 55–62. doi:10.2105/AJPH.2010.300008

Texas Department of State Health Services. (2011). *Risk assessment for lead exposure: Parent questionnaire.* Retrieved from http://www.dshs.state.tx.us/lead/pdf_files/pb_110_parent_questionnaire.pdf

UC Davis Veterinary Medicine. (n.d.). *PREDICT: Building a global early warning system for emerging diseases that move between animals and people.* Retrieved from http://www.vetmed.ucdavis.edu/ohi/predict/index.cfm

U.S. Agency for International Development. (2007). *Best practices in social marketing safe water treatment solution for household water treatment: Lessons learned from Population Services International Field Programs.* Washington, DC: Author. Retrieved from http://pdf.usaid.gov/pdf_docs/PNADI479.pdf

U.S. Agency for International Development. (2011). *Predict.* Retrieved from http://www.healthmap.org/predict/

U.S. Census Bureau. (2011a). *Statistical abstract of the United States—Table 373. Municipal solid waste generation, materials recovery, combustion with energy recovery, and discards: 1980–2008* (p. 229). Retrieved from http://www.census.gov/compendia/statab/2011/tables/11s0373.pdf

U.S. Census Bureau. (2011b). *Statistical abstract of the United States—Table 377. Toxic chemical releases and transfers by media: 2003 to 2008* (p. 231). Retrieved from http://www.census.gov/compendia/statab/2011/tables/11s0377.pdf

U.S. Census Bureau. (2011c). *Statistical abstract of the United States—Table 381. Hazardous waste generated, shipped, and received by state and other areas* (p. 233). Retrieved from http://www.census.gov/compendia/statab/2011/tables/11s0381.pdf

U.S. Department of Health and Human Services. (2012). *2012 Environmental justice strategy and implementation plan.* Retrieved from http://www.hhs.gov/environmentaljustice/strategy.pdf

U.S. Department of Health and Human Services, (2014). Environmental health. Retrieved from http://www.healthypeople.gov/2020/topicsobjectives2020/overview.aspx?topicId=12

U.S. Energy Information Administration, (2011). *What's new in our home energy use?* Retrieved from http://www.eia.gov/consumption/residential/reports/2009overview.cfm

U.S. Energy Information Administration, (2012). *Residential Energy Consumption Survey data show decreased household energy consumption per household.* Retrieved from http://www.eia.gov/todayinenergy/detail.cfm?id=6570#

U.S. Energy Information Administration. (2013a). *Energy in brief: What are the major sources and users of energy in the United States?* Retrieved from http://www.eia.gov/energy_in_brief/article/major_energy_sources_and_users.cfm

U.S. Energy Information Administration. (2013b). *Manufacturing Energy Consumption Survey (MCES).* Retrieved from http://www.eia.gov/consumption/manufacturing/reports/2010/decrease_use.cfm?src=‹Consumption-f2

U.S. Energy Information Administration. (2014). *Primary energy consumption by source.* Retrieved from http://www.eia.gov/totalenergy/data/monthly/pdf/sec1_7.pdf

U.S. Geological Survey, (2014). *Source and use of water in the United States, 2005.* Retrieved from http://water.usgs.gov/edu/wateruse-diagrams.html

Watts, S. (2003). *Disease and medicine in world history.* New York: Routledge.

West, L. (2014).*Global warming leads to 150,000 deaths every year.* Retrieved from http://environment.about.com/od/globalwarmingandhealth/a/gw_deaths.htm

World Bank. (2011). What is social capital? Retrieved from http://web.worldbank.org/WBSITE/EXTERNAL/TOPICS/EXTSOCIALDEVELOPMENT/EXTTSOCIALCAPITAL/0,,contentMDK:20185164~menuPK:418217~pagePK:148956~piPK:216618~theSitePK:401015,00.html

World Health Organization. (2011). Environmental health. Retrieved from http://www.who.int/topics/environmental_health/en/

World Health Organization & United Nations Children's Fund. (2014). *Progress on drinking water and sanitation, 2014 update.* Retrieved from http://apps.who.int/iris/bitstream/10665/112727/1/9789241507240_eng.pdf

World Wildlife Federation. (n.d.). *Ecological footprint.* Retrieved from http://wwf.panda.org/about_our_earth/teacher_resources/webfieldtrips/ecological_balance/eco_footprint/

Yumul, G. P. Jr., Cruz, N. A., Servando, N. T., & Dimalanta, C. B. (2011). Extreme weather events and related disasters of the Philippines, 2004–08: A sign of what climate change will mean? *Disasters, 35,* 262–282. doi:10.1111/j.0361-3666.2010.01216.x

CHAPTER

5 Cultural Influences on Population Health

Learning Outcomes

After reading this chapter, you should be able to:

1. Differentiate among culture, race, nationality, and ethnicity.
2. Discuss direct and indirect influences of culture on health and health care.
3. Describe cultural competence.
4. Identify barriers to cultural competence.
5. Conduct a cultural assessment of an individual, family, group, or health system.
6. Design, implement, and evaluate culturally competent care and health care delivery systems.

Key Terms

ableism

acculturation

assimilation

complementary and alternative medicine

cultural competency

culturally congruent care

cultural imposition

culture

culture-bound syndromes

discrimination

ethnicity

fatalism

health culture

health literacy

individual religiosity

integrative medicine

linguistic competence

nationality

organizational culture

pluralism

prejudice

race

racism

social religiosity

stereotyping

worldview

xenophobia

Advocacy Then

Helper Woman

Like many nurses of her generation, Elinor Delight Gregg went against the expectations of her family to pursue a career in nursing. As the youngest daughter, Elinor was expected to stay at home to care for aging parents, and at one point actually interrupted her career to care for her increasingly debilitated father. Elinor's early career encompassed positions in a variety of different fields, including industrial nursing, as Assistant Superintendent of Nurses at Cleveland City Hospital, as Superintendent of Infant's Hospital in Boston, and as a Red Cross Nurse in Europe during World War I (Pflaum, 1996). After the war, she completed postgraduate work in public health nursing at Simmons College (van Betten & Moriarty, 2004).

In 1922, Elinor accepted a position as a Red Cross Nurse on loan to the Bureau of Indian Affairs and was assigned to the Pine Ridge and Rosebud Reservations in South Dakota. In an era when the focus in the Bureau was on assimilation into the mainstream society, Elinor displayed a level of cultural sensitivity that led to her adoption as a member of the Sioux with the name "Helper Woman." Throughout her 2-year tenure on the reservation, she focused on trying to improve the living conditions of the residents as well as their access to health care. In one report, she wrote:

> "This report sounds as if my mind were more occupied with social problems than with nursing activities. After all, what is done effectively in nursing lines depends so much on the proper adjustment to the existing social structures that the thorough knowledge of the social structure should come first" (quoted in Pflaum, 1996, p. 100).

In addition to providing direct care in a clinic in her home, she traveled the reservation noting the needs of the population and agitating among supervisors in Washington, DC, for appropriate medical and nursing personnel. As a result of her work on the reservation, Elinor was made Supervisor of Public Health Nursing for the Bureau of Indian Affairs and spent the remainder of her career traveling to reservations across the country assessing needs and recruiting qualified nurses to address those needs. During her tenure in the Bureau, the size of the health workforce increased by 600%. Even in retirement, Elinor continued her advocacy for the needs of ethnic populations through volunteer work at a free clinic serving the Hispanic population in Santa Fe, New Mexico (Pflaum, 1996).

Advocacy Now

Meeting the Needs of an Ethnic Population

Hollywood, California, is often equated with wealthy movie stars, but there is a growing ethnic population in the area as well. In fact, one local area is officially known as Koreatown, with 23% of its population of Korean descent. Members of this community, like other ethnic groups, often experience culture shock when encountering scientific health care systems. Problems encountered are as widely varied as language barriers, lack of ethnic food choices in hospital menus, and the inability to have family members present. Recognizing the effects of these issues on the health of the population, Hollywood Presbyterian Medical Center created a Korean Care Center (KCC) which later became the Asian Pavilion dedicated to meeting the needs of clients from multiple Asian countries. The KCC employs bilingual nurses who speak Korean and provides culturally appropriate food choices as well as access to Korean television and newspapers. In addition, the center provides an environment in which family can engage in their traditional roles in the care of ill members. In fact, nursing staff are asked to identify a family member as a patient care partner during the client's hospital stay (Magda, 2010).

Efforts to modify health care services to meet the needs of ethnically diverse clients do not have to be as extensive as those initiated by Hollywood Presbyterian Medical Center. What actions might be taken in health care systems with which you are familiar to better meet the needs of these populations?

Why study culture? The most obvious answer, of course, is to enable us to provide effective care for the increasingly diverse populations that we serve. There are, however, other reasons as well. Each of us is the product of a cultural background that influences, often unconsciously, our thoughts, beliefs, values, attitudes, and behaviors. When we are unaware of the influences of culture on our own behaviors, we are less able to recognize how our attitudes and behaviors influence others. The more we know about culture in general, and our own culture in particular, the better able we are to modify our interactions with others to provide effective care. In addition, as nurses, we are immersed in a biomedical culture; the influences of which are again often unrecognized. Awareness of the influences of the biomedical culture on our practice can assist us to modify elements of that culture that impede effective health care. Finally, as nurses, we generally work with health care institutions and organizations that have their own distinct cultures. If we are to work effectively within these organizations, we must conform to the cultural expectations others have of us. Similarly, recognition of organizational culture and its influence on practice can help us modify health care systems to better meet the needs of clients from diverse cultural backgrounds.

The principles of cultural assessment and cultural competence can be applied in client care situations as well as professional interactions within nursing and between nursing and other disciplines. Throughout this chapter, we will examine cultural principles as they relate to traditional ethnic cultures, the dominant U.S. culture, biomedical culture, and organizational culture.

Basic Concepts Related to Culture and Health

Culture is often equated with ethnicity, nationality, or race. As we saw above, however, groups other than ethnic minorities or national populations are influenced by culture. Similarly, culture may cut across racial or ethnic groups. For example, both White nurses and nurses of color are imbued with the culture of nursing, which cuts across racial boundaries. Similarly, Arab Muslims and African American Muslims subscribe to similar aspects of culture derived from their adherence to Islam, but display other cultural beliefs and behaviors unique to their ethnic heritage. As an example of the interaction of race and ethnicity, the population categories included in the most recent census subdivided racial categories of Black and White into subcategories of Black/Hispanic, Black/non-Hispanic, White/Hispanic, and White/non-Hispanic, combining features of race and ethnicity to create more informative categories.

Culture has been described as "a system of symbols and meanings that members of a group use to make sense of their world" (Green, 2010, p. 28). In other words, culture is the way that people think about their world and interact with it. For our purposes, **culture** is defined as the ways of thinking and acting developed by a group of people that permit them to interact effectively with their environment and to address concerns common to the human condition. A group's **worldview**, which shapes culture, is their way of looking at their universe and their relationship to that universe.

Ethnicity, on the other hand, is defined as "belonging to a common group with shared heritage, often linked by race, nationality and language" (Edmonton Seniors Coordinating Council, n.d.). An ethnic group usually has a relatively homogeneous social culture. Ethnicity is self-defined and may be influenced by one's personal, social, and political experiences. Ethnicity is also a fluid concept and may change over time or with the situation. For example, I generally perceive myself as American, but in some contexts, I would describe myself in terms of my largely German heritage. **Nationality** usually refers to one's country of birth, but may also refer to a country adopted for permanent residence. Again, nationality may cut across ethnic and racial designations. For example, citizens of the United States consider themselves Americans (nationality), but include members of all three racial groups (White, Black, and Asian) as well as multiple ethnicities (e.g., German Americans, Irish Americans, African Americans).

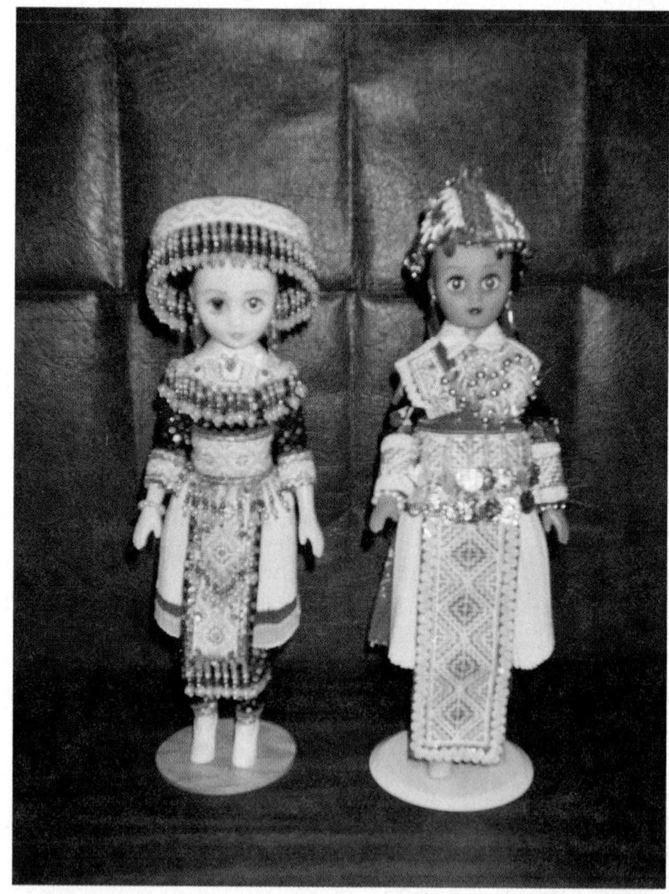

Hmong residents in the United States maintain their cultural heritage with traditional New Year's costumes and celebrations.
(Photo by Mary Jo Clark)

Race is an artificial categorization of people based on genetic inheritance and such physical characteristics as skin color, blood type, hair color and texture, and eye color or shape. Much of the demographic and other information used for planning health care delivery services (e.g., census data, morbidity, and mortality data) is categorized on the basis of race. The five categories currently used by the Office of Management and Budget (OMB) for national data purposes are Black or African American, White, Asian, American Indian or Alaska Native, and Native Hawaiian or Other Pacific Islander. The OMB also collects ethnicity data related to Hispanic or non-Hispanic origin. In a 2009 report, however, the Institute of Medicine (IOM) recommended the expansion of data categories to include the OMB racial and ethnic designations along with "granular ethnicity" data and information about preferred language and English proficiency in the population. Granular ethnicity refers to more in-depth exploration of ethnicity as, for example, Puerto Rican or Cuban, rather than merely Hispanic (Ulmer, McFadden, & Nerenz, 2009).

Societal or ethnic culture is most often learned within the family, but is also transmitted in one's day-to-day interactions with other members of the group. Biomedical and professional cultures, on the other hand, are learned in the context of specific educational preparation and through interactions with others in professional practice. Similarly, the organizational culture of the workplace is transmitted through both formal and informal mechanisms in the workplace (e.g., through formal orientation programs and through everyday interactions with supervisors and coworkers).

Culture is not static and is undergoing constant change even if that change is very slow. The culture of a specific group is influenced by interactions within and outside the group and is constantly being renegotiated and redefined in different contexts. For example, migration from one's country of origin to another country usually results in profound changes in culture as a result of interactions between members of the cultural group and those of the dominant culture. The aspects of culture that influence the behavior of members include values, beliefs, and customs or behaviors. The interrelationship of these factors has been conceptualized as a pyramid. Values serve as the broad foundation or base of the pyramid and are the component of culture that is the least amenable to change. Beliefs rest on the foundation of values and are somewhat more open to change. Finally, customs or behaviors flow from beliefs and form the apex of the pyramid. Customs and behaviors with a cultural basis are much more easily modified than either beliefs or values (Hulme, 2010).

Even though culture affects virtually every aspect of life, its influence is largely unconscious. The influence of culture is rarely consciously noted, unless one purposefully undertakes a study of one's own culturally determined behavior. This is why nurses need to become aware of their own cultural beliefs, biases, and behaviors in order to understand their influence on interactions with clients and with members of other health care disciplines.

Some authors have noted that culture is an individual concept as well as a group phenomenon. In addition, culture is a facet of organizations. The culture of any particular group is unique. Although several cultures may exhibit certain commonalities, no two cultures, like no two individuals, are exactly alike. The beliefs and behaviors that constitute a particular culture arise from the unique constraints faced by a given group of people in dealing with problems common to humanity. These unique situational constraints are the source of cultural variation among groups of people. For example, the arid nature of the southwestern United States has led to water conservation practices among residents of the region that would not be seen in other parts of the country. Similarly, although the cultures of nursing and medicine have some commonalities, they also have many distinct differences. Likewise, the organizational culture of one health care institution may differ markedly from that of another institution even though both exist for the same basic purpose.

Even within a cultural group, there is considerable variation among group members. Each individual exhibits a unique blending of various cultures to which he or she belongs. Some authors note that culture is "taken up selectively" by individuals within a group, with adherence to some aspects of the typical culture and nonadherence to others. Intracultural variability exists within cultural groups because culture is not the only factor that influences behavior and because people engage in interactions with others outside the cultural group and respond differently to circumstances based on those interactions. Not only do members of a particular group vary with respect to adherence to the behavioral aspects of culture, but they may also not be homogenous even with respect to genetic traits. African Americans, for example, represent a gene pool of more than 100 different genetic strains, making for a great deal of variation within the group (Campinha-Bacote, 2009).

Variability also occurs within professional cultures. A particular nurse, for example, may not always believe or act in ways typical of nursing's culture. Similarly, not all members of an ethnic population exhibit the beliefs and behaviors typical of the group. Adherence to the values and behaviors of a particular culture is influenced by the extent of one's acculturation. **Acculturation** is a process by which people react to contact with another culture, adopting some features of the new culture, while retaining elements of their own culture, to develop a new composite culture (Acculturation, n.d.). Acculturation involves the acquisition of at least some of the beliefs, values, and behaviors of another culture (Hulme, 2010). Acculturation usually occurs because such adaptation is required for survival in a new environment. For members of ethnic groups, acculturation is usually considered in terms of their acquisition of beliefs, values, and behaviors typical of the dominant societal culture, and members of a given cultural group may exhibit various levels of adherence to the beliefs, values, and behaviors of that group. Some people, for example, maintain a traditional cultural stance, adhering strongly to the culture of their family of origin. Others are bicultural, and are equally at home in traditional and dominant cultures.

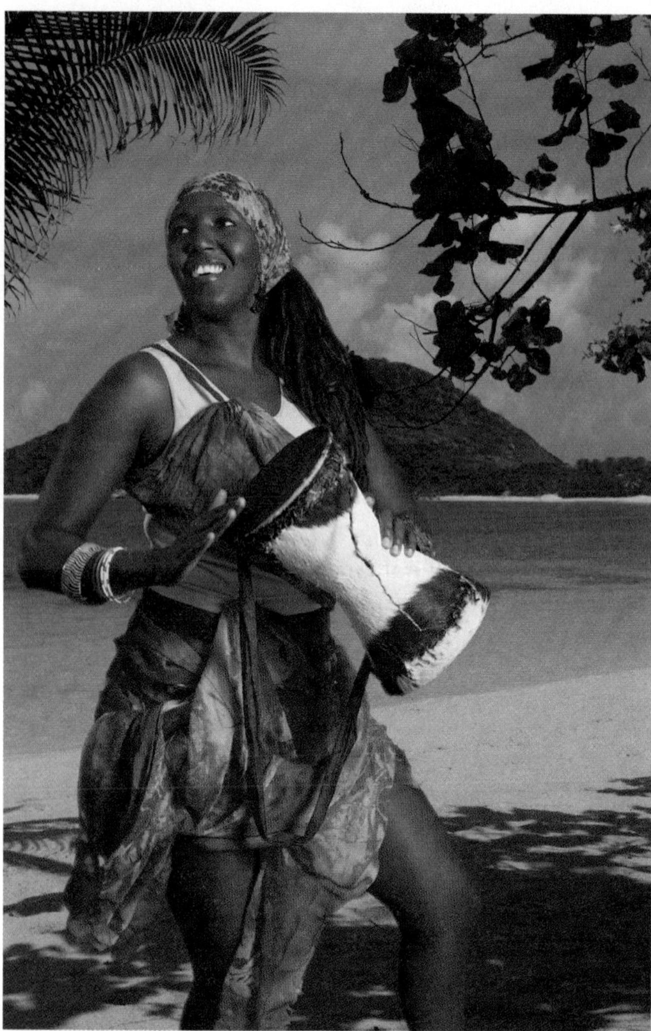

Traditional music enables some cultural groups to maintain their heritage. *(Abbitt/Fotolia)*

Acculturation is not only seen in movement from ethnic cultural traditions to those of the dominant culture, but is also reflected in the degree to which gay and lesbian individuals subscribe to the mores of those subcultural groups. Finally, some people may be marginal in their cultural affiliations, with little interaction with either a culture of origin or the dominant culture. Many homeless individuals may be considered culturally marginalized.

Acculturation also takes place in other venues. Your nursing education, for example, is designed to promote your acculturation to the nursing profession and its unique culture. In the same way, you are becoming acculturated to the overall biomedical culture. You will also need to become acculturated to a certain extent to the health care institution or agency that employs you, if you are to be successful there. In all of these examples, acculturation may have both positive and negative effects. **Assimilation** is a process similar to acculturation, but goes even further. Assimilation involves complete acceptance of the values, beliefs, customs, behaviors, and so on of another cultural group (Hulme, 2010). In other contexts, assimilation may be conceived of as "going native."

Additional concepts that relate to cultural considerations include pluralism, stereotyping, cultural imposition, discrimination, and cultural competence. **Pluralism** involves the presence of multiple distinct entities or groups within a society. These distinct groups may be the result of differences in culture, ethnicity, nationality, religion, or other characteristics (Hulme, 2010). **Stereotyping** is defined as an "exaggerated over-generalization" about a group of people based on limited knowledge (Campinha-Bacote, 2009). Stereotyping often results from a tendency to react to people on the basis of what one thinks is typical of a group with which they are associated. One is tempted to apply what one knows about a given culture to all of the members of the culture in spite of the intracultural variation discussed earlier. Knowledge of some facets of a culture may be used as a starting point for intercultural interactions, but should not be acted upon until its accuracy has been validated with the individual client.

Cultural imposition is an expectation that others will conform to the dictates of one's own culture. Expecting hospitalized clients to bathe at times convenient to hospital routine is an example of imposing health care culture on clients whose own behaviors may be quite different. **Discrimination** involves being treated differently than others based on some perceived trait or characteristic or membership in a particular group. At the health care organizational level, discrimination may take the form of "institutional racism," which has been described as "collective failure of an organization to provide an appropriate and professional service to people because of their color, culture, or ethnic origin" (as quoted in Hulme, 2010, p. 275). We will explore some of the health-related effects of discrimination later in this chapter.

Cultural competence, on the other hand, is a positive response to the cultural diversity encountered in today's health care system. **Cultural competency** has been defined as

> A developmental process in which individuals or institutions achieve increasing levels of awareness, knowledge, and skills along a cultural competence continuum. Cultural competence involves valuing diversity, conducting self-assessments, avoiding stereotyping, managing the dynamics of differences, acquiring and institutionalizing cultural knowledge, and adapting to diversity and cultural contexts in communities. (Office of Minority Health [OMH], 2013a, p. 139)

Characteristics of cultural competence and strategies for promoting culturally congruent health care encounters will be addressed in more detail later in this chapter.

Culture and Health

Culture, whether it is that of an ethnic group, the dominant society, a professional discipline, or health professionals as a group, has both positive and negative health consequences. For example, the dominant U.S. culture values cure of disease, often through the use of expensive technology. This cultural value results in extensive expenditures for costly high-technology therapies and little attention to health promotion and illness prevention needs. At the same time, the dominant culture values an attractive physical appearance, which may lead people to engage in more exercise activities than they would if uninfluenced by this value.

Ethnic/Societal Culture and Health

Ethnic minority cultures and the dominant societal culture have both direct and indirect effects on health. Direct effects stem from specific culturally prescribed practices related to diet and food or to health and illness. For example, all cultures have prescribed practices intended to promote health and prevent illness or to restore health when illness occurs. Similarly, all cultures have particular dietary practices that influence nutritional status and, thereby, the health status of their members. For example, the typical diets of many ethnic minority groups are basically healthful, but some dietary practices (e.g., the preponderance of fried food in the southern United States) have negative health effects. Similarly, the prevalence of fast food and "super sizing" in the dominant culture contributes to obesity and other adverse health effects.

Ethnic and societal cultures also affect health indirectly. Some of these indirect effects result from cultural definitions of health and illness, acceptability of health care programs and providers, and cultural influences on compliance with suggested health or illness regimens. Cultural definitions of health and illness determine what kinds of health problems are considered worthy of attention and what conditions are likely to be disregarded. If, for example, certain behaviors that are perceived as evidence of mental illness by health professionals are considered normal in the client's culture, then the client is unlikely to take any action to deal with those behaviors. Similarly, minor illnesses may be ignored if health is defined in terms of one's ability to work or to perform other social roles. In general, people are likely to disregard any type of condition that is not defined as illness in their own culture. This cultural propensity can lead to serious health consequences.

Cultural factors may also determine the acceptability of both health programs and health providers. For example, cultures that eschew scientific medicine in favor of healing based on faith in God may view immunization programs as inimical to their beliefs. In other cultures, health care providers may be considered lower-class persons not to be associated with, effectively preventing people from taking advantage of many health opportunities.

Cultural factors often determine whether clients will comply with recommendations when they do seek professional help. Culture gives rise to certain expectations regarding treatment. If health care providers' recommendations are too far removed from these expectations, the provider loses credibility, and the client is unlikely to comply with those recommendations. For example, in the dominant U.S. culture, clients have come to expect health care providers to address most health problems with prescription medications. When no prescription is provided, even though the health problem doesn't really require medication, clients may be dissatisfied with care and fail to follow through on other more appropriate recommendations, such as dietary changes, weight loss, and so on.

Biomedical Culture and Health

Health culture has been defined as "a system that attempts to explain and treat sickness and to maintain health. Health cultures are a component of the larger culture or tradition of a people and may be a popular or folk system or a technical or scientific one" (Health culture, n.d.). As this definition implies, health cultures exist within ethnic cultures as well as within the biomedical health care system, although many health care providers do not realize that their actions are often dictated by a biomedical culture.

Biomedical culture is characterized by several prominent features, including mind–body dualism, conceptualizations of disease versus illness, and a focus on cure over care (Crowley-Matoka, Saha, Dobscha, & Burgess, 2009). Mind–body dualism refers to the generalized belief in the biomedical system that the mind and body are separate entities, with the physical body taking priority over issues related to the mind. In addition, biomedical culture tends to focus on disease, the visible manifestations of ill health noted in anatomical and physiological changes. An illness focus, on the other hand, emphasizes the social context of ill health and its effects on clients' lives in addition to physical signs and symptoms. Finally, biomedical culture revolves around strategies for the cure of physical diseases rather than on the care of the individual who is experiencing it. These characteristic features differ markedly from the conceptualizations of ethnic health cultures and may contribute to difficulties in intercultural interactions.

Like ethnic and dominant societal cultures, the overall biomedical culture and the cultures of professional health disciplines and organizations may have both positive and negative influences on the health of population groups. The emphasis on the provider as an authority and the client as subordinate that pervades the biomedical culture may lead clients to forgo health care in an effort to control their own lives and health or to fail to accept responsibility for health actions on their own behalf. Unfortunately, health professionals often fail to recognize the influence of the biomedical culture and the dominant societal culture on their practice, and may see biomedicine as having been "purged" of cultural influences by its reliance on objective scientific evidence.

Authors in the health professions and other disciplines give a variety of examples of the cultural rituals and artifacts embedded in the biomedical culture. For example, the use of the hospital gown in biomedically oriented hospitals is a ritual that conveys the dependence of the client on the institution and their loss of autonomy with respect to even their own apparel. Similar rituals include meals served at specific times whether clients are hungry or not and the need to schedule an appointment to receive services in most biomedical organizations. These cultural rituals within the biomedical and health professional communities are primarily based on dominant cultural values of efficiency and time consciousness.

The biomedical culture in the United States has also been characterized by vacillation between risk taking and risk avoidance. There is a tendency to want to try new things, such as experimental therapies, mixed with distrust of new ideas. Negative health effects can result from either perspective. For example, clients may be pressured to agree to new treatments with undetermined efficacy. Conversely, providers may resist implementation of evidence-based practice guidelines.

Culture may also have adverse effects on the health professions themselves. For example, some nurse authors have cited the lack of cultural sensitivity in the NCLEX-RN exam as a contributing factor in the dearth of nurses representative of ethnic minority groups and in the exacerbation of the nursing shortage. In addition, the cost of preparing for and taking the examination itself may disadvantage minority nurses. This may be particularly true for nurses prepared in other countries whose programs may not include some of the content tested on the examination. Even within the United States, nurses educated in Puerto Rico are successful on Puerto Rican advanced practice certification examinations, but have difficulty with national certification examinations due to language and cultural differences.

Ethnic Diversity in the United States

As we noted earlier, one of the primary reasons for becoming knowledgeable about culture and its effects on health lies in the ethnic and cultural diversity of the clients that we serve. Beyond the period of early colonization of North America by settlers primarily from England, the United States has always been ethnically and culturally diverse. Even in the early colonial periods, there were cultural differences in the groups that settled here. For example, many of the first settlers were members of specific religious groups seeking religious freedom that brought their own cultures with them. Later immigrant groups came from other Western European countries, particularly Ireland and Germany, and from other parts of the world as well. Although possessed of their own distinct cultures, these groups had more in common than many later immigrant groups.

Today, the United States is more ethnically and culturally diverse than ever before. For example, the Latino/Hispanic population, constituted 12.5% of the total U.S. population in 2002, but had increased to 15.7% of the population by 2009, and is expected to comprise 17.7% of the population by 2015. In 2009, African Americans constituted 12.9% of the population, and Asians comprised another 4.5% of the population. In addition, there were 3.1 million Americans of American Indian or Alaskan Native descent and more than 578,000 native Hawaiians and Pacific Islanders compared to more than 244 million White Americans. Each of these groups is expected to increase at a greater rate than the White population between 2010 and 2015 (U.S. Census Bureau, 2013f, 2013g). Much of the change in population composition in the United States is a result of natural increase through birth, but a significant portion of it results from international migration (U.S. Census Bureau, 2013a). In 2010, for example, slightly over 12% of the U.S. population was foreign born (U.S. Census Bureau, 2013c).

Even these figures do not give a full picture of the extent of diversity in the population because of the different ethnicities represented within each of these large groups. For example, in 2009, 20% of the U.S. population spoke a language other than English at home, ranging from 35.4 million Spanish speakers to speakers of various European languages and multiple Asian languages, to those who speak Arabic or a variety of Native American languages. There is great variation even within groups that speak the same language. For example, Arabic speakers may include people from Egypt, Iraq, Jordan, Lebanon, Morocco, Palestine, and Syria among others (U.S. Census Bureau, 2013d). Similarly, the Hispanic population includes people from Spain, Mexico, Puerto Rico, and a variety of Central and South American countries, each with its own unique culture and different health problems and service needs.

Even among the Anglo population of the United States, there are distinct cultural groups. For example, dietary patterns among Southern Whites may differ significantly from those of Caucasian groups in other areas of the country (e.g., Midwestern German Americans or Italian Americans in the northeast). Diversity also exists within cultural groups with respect to other population characteristics. For example, as an aggregate group, Asian Americans had higher mean family incomes than their White, Black, or American Indian/Native Alaskan counterparts in 2009, and lower rates of poverty than all groups except White Americans (U.S. Census Bureau, 2013e). On the other hand, there are considerable differences in income among different Asian subgroups. This is particularly true for foreign-born ethnic populations among whom 10.5% of households had annual family incomes below $15,000 in 2010 compared to only 7% of native-born residents (U.S. Census Bureau, 2013c). European immigrants are less likely than their Asian or Latin American counterparts to have low family incomes (U.S. Census Bureau, 2013b).

The United States is not the only country to experience cultural diversity, yet diversity may be even less well recognized in other nations than in the United States. For example, a group of Japanese nursing students visiting the United States to study social and health care cultures were amazed to note the cultural diversity present there. When they were asked about cultural diversity in their own country, they indicated that there was no diversity. They were unable to recognize the cultural diversity posed by the Ainu, the original population of Japan, and the large resident Korean population as well as the wide variety of foreign visitors to Japan.

Assessing Cultural Influences on Health and Health Care

As noted earlier, population health nurses must incorporate cultural concepts into the care of individuals and their families as well as the development and implementation of health care programs for population groups. In addition, nurses must be able to function effectively within the biomedical, professional, and organizational cultures in which they work and modify those cultures to improve population health care. To accomplish these tasks, nurses must have knowledge of the cultural groups with which they interact. Such knowledge is derived from a cultural assessment, including assessment of the group to determine typical beliefs, values, and behaviors, and assessment of individual members of the group in terms of their adherence to those beliefs, values, and behaviors.

Principles of Cultural Assessment

Four basic principles should guide the study of a culture. First, view the culture in the context in which it developed. As noted earlier, cultural practices arise out of a need to meet common human problems in a particular human setting. That setting must be considered in exploring culture.

Second, examine the underlying premise of culturally determined behavior. What was the intended purpose for the behavior when it originated? Does the behavior still fulfill this purpose? When one knows the underlying reason for behaviors that seem strange, the behaviors may not seem quite so strange after all. Third, the nurse examines the meaning of behavior in the cultural context. The meaning of certain behaviors from the perspective of the nurse may be very different from the behavior's meaning to others. Using the previous example of the hospital gown, its original purposes were to minimize spread of microorganisms via clothing brought in from the outside, promote ease of access to clients for therapeutic procedures, and prevent ruin of clients' personal clothing by blood and other substances. With the advent of washing machines, however, the first and third purposes are really no longer relevant in many situations. In fact, given the rate of nosocomial infection in hospitals, wearing one's personal clothing might actually be safer than wearing a hospital gown. Similarly, when faced with the potential meaning attached to the practice from a client perspective of dependence and loss of autonomy, is the advantage of the hospital gown to providers outweighed by its disadvantages in the provider–client relationship? Using another example, the dominant U.S. cultural values of independence and self-sufficiency make sense in the light of the historical development of the United States, but do they still serve their underlying purpose in the context of an increasingly interdependent global society?

Finally, there is the need to recognize intracultural variation. Not every member of any given cultural group displays all of the beliefs and behaviors typical of that culture. As we saw earlier, subgroups within a cultural group may exhibit different behavior patterns. Or individuals may be more or less adherent to the beliefs, values, attitudes, and behaviors typically expected by members of the culture. Not all Mexican Americans, for example, will demonstrate a belief in the "evil eye." Similarly, not all perinatal providers believe that an enema is a necessary part of preparation for birth. Another term used to denote the degree of adherence or nonadherence to elements of a culture is *heritage consistency*, or the degree to which one conforms to one's cultural heritage. Although this concept was obviously developed in relation to ethnic cultural heritages, it is equally applicable to the "tribal culture" of nursing or biomedicine. Principles of cultural assessment are summarized above.

> **Highlights**
>
> **Principles of Cultural Assessment**
>
> - View all cultures in the context in which they developed.
> - Examine underlying premises for culturally determined beliefs and behaviors.
> - Interpret the meaning and purpose of behavior in the context of the specific culture.
> - Recognize the potential for intracultural variation.

Obtaining Cultural Information

How does one become knowledgeable about a culture? Perhaps the best way to begin is to recognize the influences of culture on one's own life and behavior. Personal insights regarding culture will enable the nurse to recognize and accept cultural beliefs and behaviors that may differ from his or her own. Once familiar with his or her own cultural heritage, the nurse can begin to read literature related to other cultures of interest. In reading, the community health nurse should examine the qualifications of the authors writing. Was the book or article written by a member of the culture? Is it based on empirical data derived from research, on personal experience with a particular culture, or on stereotypes? Information about a culture from the perspective of nonmembers of the culture can also be instructive. For example, some of the sociological and social anthropological research on professional cultures can assist us to see the elements of culture that are embedded in biomedicine or in nursing practice that we might not have identified when viewing them from inside the culture.

A second means of acquainting oneself with a culture is to interview colleagues who are members of that culture. Explore with them their concepts of health and illness and attitudes and practices affecting health. Discover how these concepts may differ from those held by previous generations or other members of their family. Health care professionals, by virtue of their knowledge of health matters, are likely to have achieved a greater degree of acculturation and conformity with the dominant U.S. culture with respect to health practices than nonprofessionals from the same group. These individuals, however, usually remain a valid source of information regarding cultural health beliefs and practices. Such strategies are also effective in understanding the "culture" of other groups, such as members of the gay, lesbian, bisexual, and transgender (GLBT) populations (see Chapter 20∞).

You can also use this strategy of interviewing members of a culture when newly employed or considering employment in a particular health care organization. Talk about the organizational culture with people who are already members of the organization. How are clients viewed? How are employees viewed? How are employees expected to interact with each other? With clients? If the organizational culture seems to be too alien to your own personal culture, you may not want to work there. Clients' perspectives on the biomedical culture can also be enlightening. How do they perceive some of the attitudes and behaviors typical of the culture? Do these perceptions enhance or impede effective health care delivery?

Another effective way to become familiar with a particular culture is to spend time living within it. For example, prospective nursing students may be encouraged to engage in volunteer work or to shadow practicing nurses to explore the culture of nursing as a career option. Similarly, one might spend time living within an ethnic cultural group. This approach, however, is not always feasible. Alternatives include home visits to families within the group to observe daily living in the cultural context and questioning clients and families regarding health-related beliefs and practices. Another possible approach is observing activities and interactions at health facilities and community or religious functions.

When assessing another culture directly, whether it is an ethnic cultural group or the organizational culture of a health care institution, the population health nurse should follow a few general guidelines. First, look and listen before asking questions or taking action. Observation aids in asking pertinent and timely questions and forestalls actions that may be inappropriate. Second, explore how the group feels about being studied. Explain that your reasons for studying the culture are practical and do not arise out of idle curiosity. Third, discover any special protocols. Should one speak to a local leader or agency supervisor before beginning to observe a group? Is there a council or leadership group who should grant permission for participation in group activities? Fourth, foster human relations, putting them before the need to obtain information. Information will not assist the nurse to provide care or function effectively in a work setting if he or she alienates members of the group. Social amenities are important in many cultures and should be attended to before the "business" of information gathering begins in earnest. In fact, information about social amenities is part of the data needed by the nurse.

Many people, in exploring another culture, look for differences from their own culture. The nurse, however, should also look for cultural similarities to use as a foundation in aiding clients to accept and use health care services. Cultural differences should be accepted as normal.

Locate group leaders and respected residents, those considered wise, "ordinary" group members, and clients who can converse knowledgeably about the culture. Critics of traditional aspects of the culture may also be interviewed to provide a balanced picture.

Participate as well as observe. The nurse must assess each cultural situation as it occurs to determine whether participation or observation is the more appropriate activity. Participation conveys an openness to cultural differences and a willingness to engage in culturally prescribed activities rather than ridicule them. Some activities, however, are closed to outsiders, and the population health nurse's participation would not be welcomed.

When exploring another culture, the nurse should also consider the feelings of group members about questions asked. The nurse should ascertain what types of questions are acceptable or offensive in a particular culture. For example, U.S. Peace Corps volunteers in India found it difficult to adjust to frequent questions about their salary or how much their clothes cost. Such questions were perfectly acceptable in Indian society, but considered impolite or "nosy" in the United States. Similarly, there may be certain questions that can safely be asked within the biomedical culture. For example, some physicians may respond readily to questions about a particular element of their practice or the plan of care for a client, whereas others would perceive questions as threatening to their authority. The same may be true in the employment setting, where certain questions are acceptable and others are not.

A little forethought as to the phrasing and timing of questions can prevent serious mistakes. Ask questions positively without implying value judgments. For example, "I notice you put garlic on a string around the baby's neck; can you tell me what it's used for?" is far more acceptable than "Why in the world do you hang garlic around the baby's neck?" Nurses might ask the same questions themselves and gauge their own emotional reaction to the questions. A nurse can also try out questions on colleagues who are members of the culture being explored. Suggested modes of cultural exploration are summarized below.

Highlights

Modes of Cultural Exploration

- Become conversant with your own culture and its influences on your life.
- Review the existing literature on beliefs, values, and behaviors of specific cultural groups.
- Interview colleagues who are members of the cultural group in question.
- Immerse yourself in the culture to be studied.
- Observe members of specific cultural groups.
- Interview members of cultural groups, particularly group leaders.
- Interview other persons who are conversant with the culture.

Cultural Assessment Data

General areas to be considered in a cultural assessment based on the population health nursing model include factors related to biological, psychological, physical, environmental, sociocultural, behavioral, and health system determinants.

Biological Determinants

Biological considerations in cultural assessment include those related to maturation and aging, genetics, and physiologic function. Each of these areas will be explored with respect to ethnic cultures and the dominant U.S. culture. Where appropriate, aspects of biomedical and professional cultures and organizational culture are also discussed.

MATURATION AND AGING. Cultural groups may display different attitudes toward age. For example, the dominant U.S. culture is oriented toward youth, and youth is valued over age. A significant proportion of the gross domestic product is expended each year on trying to look, feel, and act young. In many traditional ethnic cultures, on the other hand, older persons tend to be highly respected and influential within the family and the social group.

Biomedical and organizational cultures may also display differential attitudes toward age. For example, many health care providers believe that because older clients are nearing the end of their lives health promotion interventions will have little effect and are unwarranted. Research, however, indicates that health promotion activities with the elderly can have profound, positive effects on health status and self-care capacity. As we will see in Chapter 19∞, ageism and stereotypes of the elderly significantly affect the type of health care services provided to older clients. Similarly, age may be viewed differently in different organizational cultures. How are older employees treated in the organization? Is their expertise valued, or are they expected to move aside in favor of younger employees?

In addition to the attitudes of the cultural group toward aging and people of different age groups, the population health nurse would want to consider the age composition of the cultural group because this information will help identify potential age-related health concerns. For example, if a large percentage of the cultural group is young children, different types of services will be required. Similarly, if a large portion of the workforce in the organization is close to retirement age, consideration needs to be given to finding replacements. This is currently a problem for health care professions in general and nursing in particular.

GENETIC INHERITANCE. Considerations related to genetics would be more relevant in the assessment of ethnic cultural groups than for biomedical or organization cultures. Generally, ethnic groups differ with respect to several genetically determined physical characteristics, such as body build and structure, skin color, enzymatic variations, and susceptibility to disease (Spector, 2012).

Physical differences based on genetic inheritance in some ethnic groups have implications for nursing, and nurses need to be conversant with these physiologic variations. For example, different ethnic groups may experience enzymatic variations such as the lactose intolerance of many Asian and Native American groups. Similarly, "normal" skin color varies widely between groups based on the amount of melanin typically found in the skin. Campinha-Bacote (2009) described the need to assess skin from a "melanocentric" perspective, based on the amount of pigment in the skin, rather than a Eurocentric perspective based on what is considered normal for light-complected people of European ancestry. She suggested several basic considerations in assessing skin, including: (a) establishing a baseline color by asking or comparing with family members, (b) observing the skin in direct sunlight rather than artificial light, (c) observing areas with the least pigmentation, (d) palpating, rather than observing, for evidence of rashes, and (e) comparing the skin in corresponding areas when possible.

Genetic inheritance may also play a part in the types of health problems commonly seen in members of some ethnic groups. For example, African Americans and people of Kurdish and Sephardic Jewish descent experience higher rates of glucose-6-phosphate dehydrogenase (G-6-PD) deficiency, an enzyme deficiency that causes red blood cell hemolysis, than members of other groups (Dugdale & Mason, 2010). Similarly, data from the 2009 National Patient Information Reporting System (NPIRS) indicate that diabetes prevalence was 77% higher in non-Hispanic Blacks, 66% higher in Hispanics, and 18% higher in Asian Americans than among non-Hispanic White adults (Centers for Disease Control and Prevention [CDC], 2011). Knowledge of the prevalence of these diseases in certain population groups can promote accurate diagnosis and treatment. Ethnic groups may also vary in their capacity to metabolize drugs, resulting in the need to adjust dosages to accommodate these differences (Purnell, 2012). There may also be differences among groups with respect to their susceptibility to adverse health effects of environmental hazards.

PHYSIOLOGIC FUNCTION. Considerations related to physiologic function are the third aspect of biological determinants of health addressed in a cultural assessment. Areas to be considered include health problems prevalent in a particular group (beyond those with a genetic component discussed above) and attitudes to body parts and functions. Population health nurses should be familiar with the kinds of health problems experienced by a particular ethnic cultural group. This permits the development of health delivery programs to meet specific needs in the population. At the same time, such knowledge may lead to stereotyping and inappropriate individual diagnosis and treatment within the biomedical culture. Uncertainty about a clinical diagnosis on the part of a professional provider may lead him or her to rely on probability to make a diagnosis. Knowing that a certain ethnic group has a high prevalence of a specific condition may lead to a diagnosis of that condition, when the symptoms are actually the result of some other disease.

ATTITUDES TOWARD BODY PARTS AND PHYSIOLOGIC FUNCTIONS. There may be considerable difference in the attitudes toward body parts and physiologic functions among ethnic cultural groups and between these groups and the dominant U.S. culture. For example, Muslims are extremely modest and may be reluctant to bare their bodies to health care providers, particularly a provider of the opposite gender (Wehbe-Alamah, 2008). In India, it is common for women to bare their midriff, but in village society in many parts of the country, baring the shoulders is considered indecent. Similarly, the head is considered sacred in many Asian cultures (Purnell, 2012), and touching the head of another may be considered threatening or insulting.

Clothing and exposure of different body parts is an area of culture that may change drastically over time. It was not so very long ago when women wore floor-length skirts, and to show even as much as an ankle was considered "fast" behavior in the dominant U.S. culture. Today, short skirts or shorts and bare legs and midriffs are common among youth in the United States and other parts of the world, but may be shocking to older people, even within the dominant culture. Among many Muslim groups, modest women are expected to be completely covered, including their hair and face, but the style of dress varies among Muslim groups (Wehbe-Alamah, 2008).

Different ethnic cultural groups also have different attitudes toward specific physiologic functions. In many cultures, menstruating women are considered unclean and are expected to remove themselves from the flow of daily life. In the previous century in the United States, menstruation was sometimes viewed as a time of weakness and vulnerability in the dominant culture, and women were expected to rest and not engage in strenuous activity during their menstrual periods. Today, most menstruating women continue their normal life activities. Breast-feeding, urination, defecation, and sexual activity are other bodily functions that are viewed differently by different cultural groups.

Many members of the dominant U.S. societal culture are embarrassed to see women breast-feeding in public, yet this is a commonly accepted practice in many ethnic cultural groups. Similarly, urinating, defecating, and spitting in public are practices that are generally frowned upon in "polite" U.S. society, but may be common, or even necessary, in places without private sanitation facilities. Groups may also differ with respect to the position assumed for defecation or cleansing themselves afterward. For example, most American homes are equipped with sit-down flush toilets. Even in some areas in rural America that still use "outhouses," a seating area is provided. In other countries, such as Japan and India, even some modern toilets are designed for squatting rather than sitting. Similarly, most people in the United States would use toilet paper to cleanse themselves after urinating or defecating. This practice, however, is considered very unsanitary by those in other cultures (e.g., rural India) who wash themselves with water using the left hand. The left hand is then considered contaminated and is not used for clean activities such as eating. Similarly, many Muslims eat only with the right hand and will not accept something offered with the left hand (Wehbe-Alamah, 2008).

Different groups also differ with respect to the types of touch that are permissible in public and who may touch whom. In the dominant U.S. culture, kissing and holding hands is permissible between men and women, but may be less so in certain settings and situations (e.g., in church). In other cultural groups, such intimate behaviors are not condoned between members of opposite genders, but may be acceptable between members of the same gender without connoting a same-sex sexual orientation.

FOCUSED ASSESSMENT Biological Determinants in Cultural Assessment

Maturation and Aging

- What is the age composition of the cultural group?
- What attitudes toward age and aging are prevalent in the culture? How do these attitudes affect health and health care?
- At what age are members of the culture considered adults?
- Are there cultural rituals associated with coming of age?

Genetics

- What is the gender composition of the cultural group? Are there differences in the cultural value given to one gender over the other?
- Does gender play a role in the acceptability of health care providers?
- Do members of the cultural group display genetically determined physical features or physiologic differences?
- Do group members display differences in normal physiologic values (e.g., hematocrit, height)?
- What genetically determined illnesses, if any, are prevalent in the cultural group?

Physiologic Function

- What physical health problems are common within the cultural group?
- What are the cultural attitudes to body parts and physiologic functions? How do these attitudes affect health and health care delivery?

In the biomedical culture, providers usually think nothing of baring whatever body part needs to be examined or treated. Often, there is scant concern for clients' modesty and the embarrassment that results. Although nurses are taught to respect clients' privacy and to protect their modesty during procedures, often the pace of the work setting leads nurses to forget these "amenities." Similarly biomedical culture often undertakes invasive procedures (e.g., shaving the head for surgery) that may have very negative connotations in other cultures. Tips for a focused assessment of biological factors in cultural assessment are included on page 112.

Psychological Determinants

Areas to be considered in assessing psychological determinants of health related to culture include the extent of and typical sources of stress experienced by members of the group, the importance of group versus individual goals, attitudes toward change, and attitudes toward mental health and mental illness. An additional area for exploration is that of culture-bound syndromes. The importance of culture in relation to mental health is highlighted by findings that treatment programs specifically designed for certain ethnic groups have better outcomes than generalized mental health programs.

EXTENT AND SOURCES OF STRESS. The extent of stress experienced by the cultural group affects the health status of its members. As we will see later, stressful interactions with the dominant culture in the form of prejudice and discrimination affect health both directly and indirectly. Members of ethnic cultural groups may also experience stress related to intergenerational conflict as some generations become more acculturated to the dominant culture while others attempt to retain traditional cultural orientations. Similarly, some members of the gay, lesbian, bisexual, and transgender cultures may experience rejection or estrangement from family because of their sexual identity or orientation. Membership in the biomedical culture can itself be a source of stress given the life-and-death decisions that are sometimes required of members of this cultural group. Similarly, members of professional cultures may experience stress and frustration in situations in which they are unable to achieve desired outcomes for their clients. This stress may be exacerbated by the relative loss of control of one's own practice that has accompanied the move to manage systems of health care.

INDIVIDUAL VERSUS GROUP GOALS. Cultural groups differ with respect to the priority given to individual goals versus those of the larger group, and may be characterized as either collectivist or individualist societies. Collectivist societies emphasize the good of the group, harmonious relationships, traditional values, and group loyalty. Individualist societies are characterized by the primacy of individual needs over those of the larger group. In individualist societies, people expect to be able to make and act on their own decisions independent of influence or coercion by others. Although these perspectives might also be considered part of the sociocultural determinants of health, they are included under psychological determinants because of their potential for adverse effects on the psychological health of members of a cultural group when there is conflict between individual and group goals.

The dominant U.S. culture is highly individualistic. Many traditional ethnic cultures, on the other hand, have a collectivist perspective. For example, in many Asian and Latino cultural groups, family goals take precedence over the personal goals of members. Many Native American tribal cultures are community oriented, and illness may be perceived as resulting from estrangement from the community. For these reasons, family and community members are important participants in health and illness care in many Latino and Native American groups, as well as among Muslims (Center for Health and Healing, n.d.; Green, 2010; Wehbe-Alama, 2008).

Medicine as a culture has some elements of collectivism. For example, the previous taboo against advertising medical services and the reluctance to criticize the medical practice of others might be seen as attempts to protect the professional group. Certainly, much political activity undertaken by medical groups has collectivist underpinnings in promoting the welfare of the medical profession. Nursing, on the other hand, although also a collectivist culture, has worked more often for the benefit of the collective society than for the profession itself. A move away from individualism in medicine can also be seen in the dwindling number of independent practitioners and the expansion of group practice and managed care.

ATTITUDES TOWARD CHANGE. Group attitudes toward change also influence the psychological environment and health care for members of cultural groups. The dominant U.S. culture is positively oriented toward change, which is frequently labeled "progress." Biomedical culture tends to vacillate between the desire for change and the tendency to stick to traditional forms of care. In the biomedical culture, change is often linked to technological advances, and more particularly, to public knowledge of and demand for care based on those advances. One of the interesting areas of change in biomedical culture that is occurring primarily in response to public demand is the incorporation of what were once considered traditional "folk" health practices, now termed complementary and alternative medicine (CAM). We will discuss CAM in more detail later in this chapter.

The culture of nursing is also characterized by a certain degree of ambiguity with respect to attitudes toward change. On the one hand, nursing is attempting to move toward evidence-based practice. On the other, many nurses are unwilling to give up practices that have not demonstrated therapeutic effectiveness or that are no longer practical in the current health care system because they learned to provide care that way. Nursing education has been criticized for its willingness to "jump on every bandwagon that comes by," but cannot agree on a single mechanism for entry into the profession. Changes in nursing education often lack a sound basis in student and societal needs and evidence of the effectiveness of specific educational activities.

Ethnic cultural groups vary with respect to their eagerness to engage in change, but many tend to hold to traditional ways of doing things. Attitudes toward change also differ within cultural groups (and within professional groups, as well), based on the level of acculturation to the dominant culture.

Closely allied to group attitudes toward change are culturally based attitudes of resignation and acceptance. In many areas of the world, notably underdeveloped countries but also among the poor of the developed world, people have little access to the means to change the circumstances of their lives. Over many years or generations, people in such groups may become resigned and develop fatalistic attitudes. Widespread resignation within a cultural group can hinder health promotion and disease prevention initiatives, and may even affect willingness to seek care for existing health problems. For example, cancer fatalism has been associated with unwillingness to participate in screening activities in general (Baron-Epel, Friedman, & Lernau, 2009) and breast cancer screening in particular (Clark & Natipagon-Shah, 2008). **Fatalism** is defined as the belief that one's fate is fixed and that personal efforts can do little to affect that fate (Fatalism, n.d.). Population health nurses working with members of other cultural groups should determine the effects that fatalistic beliefs have on health behaviors.

PREVALENCE AND PERCEPTIONS OF MENTAL HEALTH AND ILLNESS. Cultural groups also differ in their definitions of what constitutes mental health and mental illness and their attitudes toward mental illness. For example, in some groups, symptoms that would be construed as mental illness in the biomedical culture are considered normal behavior or a fact of life. In addition, cultural groups often differ with respect to the extent of mental illness present in the population.

In many cultural groups, including segments of the dominant U.S. culture, mental illness carries an unpalatable stigma, leading members of the group to avoid seeking care. Mental illness may also be seen as a stigma for the family as well as for the individual involved. Chinese Americans, for example, may experience strong stigma attached to mental illness (Yeung et al., 2010). Asian Indian families have been known to hide family members with mental illness in the home to avoid social stigma against the family. Some American families may abandon mentally ill/disabled family members in public institutions. Among Islamic cultures, mental illness may be perceived as punishment or a test of one's faith (Ciftci, Jones, & Corrigan, 2013). In the dominant U.S. culture, those with a history of mental illness or substance abuse may encounter difficulty with employment or election to public office, among other social effects. Among some cultural groups, mental illness may be perceived as possession by an evil spirit or failure to honor good spirits, warranting religious intervention rather than psychotherapy. Psychological distress may be concealed or expressed psychosomatically due to perceptions of stigma attached to mental illness. Other cultural groups are more tolerant of mental health problems.

In the dominant U.S. culture, and even in the biomedical and professional cultures, mental illness also continues to carry a stigma, although much progress has been made in this area. The degree of stigma varies with the type of condition and is less severe for problems like depression than for chronic mental health problems, such as schizophrenia, in which bizarre behavior may be displayed.

Some ethnic cultural groups may recognize a variety of emotional conditions that are not documented in the *Diagnostic and Statistical Manual* (DSM-5), which serves as the compendium of mental illness in the biomedical culture. These conditions are often referred to as *culture-bound syndromes*. The general diagnosis of culture-bound syndrome has, however, been added to later versions of the DSM-IV and defined as recurrent patterns of behavior or symptoms that lie outside the biomedical system.

Culture-bound syndromes are conditions involving behavioral, affective, and cognitive symptoms that manifest within a specific culture and represent behaviors different from those expected in the culture (Singh Balhara, 2011). Although unique to a given culture, similar conditions may occur, with some variations, in other cultural groups. For example, *dhat*, is an Asian Indian culture-bound syndrome that involves weakness, loss of vitality, sexual dysfunction, and loss of virility attributed to loss of bodily fluid through urine, nocturia, or masturbation. Other variants of *dhat* are found in China, Europe, Russia, and the Americas (Singh Balhara, 2011). *Amok* is another example of culture-bound syndromes found in Malaysia. *Amok* involves a period of brooding followed by a sudden violent outburst. *Nerviosismo* is a culture-bound syndrome noted in Latin America and the Caribbean. It is characterized by somatization, anxiety, dizziness, emotional lability, and difficulties with sleeping and concentrating, and is believed to be brought on by stress (Hulme, 2010).

Care should be taken in attributing symptoms of emotional distress or unusual behavior to culture-bound syndromes without exploring other possible causes. Several authors note that culture-bound syndromes can only be understood in the context of the cultures in which they occur and that therapy often depends on the "deep grammar" or underlying circumstances resulting in disease (Yang, Tranulis, & Freudenreich, 2009). Assuming that symptoms experienced by a client from another culture represent a culture-bound syndrome may prevent accurate diagnosis of underlying mental health problems (Green, 2010). Rather, it may be more appropriate to accept the client's explanation of the underlying issues and combine conventional and traditional therapies in addressing their cause.

Culture-bound syndromes are not unique to ethnic cultural groups, but may also be seen in the dominant U.S. and biomedical cultures. For example, *anorexia nervosa* is a recognized illness in Western cultures, particularly in the United States, that is not seen in many other cultural groups and has been described as a culture-bound syndrome (Isaac, 2013). Its incidence in U.S. women may reflect the cultural pressure to be thin (National Alliance on Mental Illness, 2013). Similarly, seasonal affective disorder, a form of depression recognized by the biomedical culture and believed to be caused by diminished light in winter, is seen in some Western cultures (e.g., in the United States), but not in others.

Population health nurses should also assess the prevalence of specific mental illness diagnoses in the population as well as the extent of use of mental health services. For example, it has been estimated that 17% of Asian Americans may experience psychiatric illness at some point in their lives, but that their use of formal mental health system services is low. Often, informal support systems are sought instead (Spencer, Chen, Gee, Fabian, & Takeuchi, 2010). Other authors have suggested that Asian Americans do seek health providers' assistance with mental health issues but are often undiagnosed due to failure of providers to recognize symptoms reported as evidence of mental health problems (Yeung, et al., 2010).

As we have seen, psychological determinants related to culture may have profound effects on the health of population groups. Tips for a focused assessment of psychological determinants in cultural assessment are provided below.

Environmental Determinants

Cultural groups differ in their perceptions of relationships between people and their environment. The dominant U.S. culture seeks mastery over the environment. Many traditional ethnic cultures, on the other hand, seek harmonious relationships with the external physical environment. For example, traditional African American cultural groups have often perceived a need for cooperation with a powerful natural environment in order to promote survival. Similarly, some cultural groups also view seasonal changes as directly affecting human health and behavior. Again, seasonal affective disorder is an example recognized in the biomedical culture.

Other aspects of relationships to the external environment include perceptions of space and time. With respect to time, some cultural groups, such as the dominant culture in the United States and African American culture, are future oriented, whereas others are past or present oriented. Many Asian cultures, for example, attach great importance to the past and are considered past oriented. Native American and Latino groups, on the other hand, tend to be oriented to the present moment (Spector, 2012). Both past- and present-oriented cultural groups may have difficulty in long-range planning for future events or may not be attuned to preventive health care.

Other perceptions related to time may also be of importance in planning nursing care for individual clients or for population groups. Care of a Muslim client, for example, may need to be planned to prevent interference with specified times for prayer (Wehbe-Alamah, 2008). At the group level, effective health programs targeted to Jewish clients or Seventh-day Adventists would not be scheduled on Saturday. Similarly, many cultural groups have fluid concepts of time that make appointment-based health care delivery, a biomedical cultural norm, less effective.

Cultural groups also have differing attitudes to space. Most population health nurses in the United States subscribe to European American notions of acceptable personal space in certain situations. Preferred distance between people in European American culture can be described as follows:

- Public distance: greater than 12 feet
- Social distance: 4 to 12 feet
- Personal distance: 1.5 to 4 feet
- Intimate distance: within 1.5 feet (Spector, 2012)

European Americans are frequently uncomfortable when their perceived personal space is invaded by another person. Among other cultural groups, however, there is considerable variation in what is perceived as one's personal space, leading to the potential for discomfort and conflict.

One final consideration with respect to the physical environment relates particularly to immigrant and refugee groups.

FOCUSED ASSESSMENT Psychological Determinants in Cultural Assessment

- Does the culture have an individualist or collectivist perspective?
- How do members of the cultural group prioritize individual, family, and group welfare and goals?
- What is the extent of stress experienced by members of the cultural group? What are the usual sources of stress? How do group members typically cope with stress?
- Is there intergenerational conflict within the cultural group that contributes to stress?
- How do members of the cultural group perceive change? How do they adapt to change?
- Do members of the cultural group exhibit attitudes of resignation and fatalism? If so, what effect does this have on the use of health care services?
- What attitudes toward mental health and illness are held by members of the cultural group? Is there stigma attached to mental illness for the individual? For the family?
- Does the group recognize any culture-bound syndromes? If so, what are they? What are their characteristic features?

FOCUSED ASSESSMENT Environmental Determinants in Cultural Assessment

- How do members of the cultural group perceive their relationship to the environment?
- How do members of the cultural group perceive personal space?
- What is the orientation of the cultural group to time?
- What changes in their physical environment have members of the cultural group experienced? What influence do these changes have on the health status of the group?

The change in their physical environment may lead to a variety of health problems not encountered in their homelands. For example, the heavy traffic patterns in most U.S. cities have contributed to traffic fatalities among Hmong children whose parents are not accustomed to having to teach traffic safety. Similarly, exposure to a variety of household cleaning products common in U.S. households has led to a number of accidental poisonings among refugees. In addition, research has indicated that refugee children may experience elevated blood lead levels several months after coming to the United States due to the need to find housing in older run-down areas with a high degree of lead contamination. Tips for assessing elements of the physical environmental dimension of culture as they affect health are presented above.

Sociocultural Determinants

Cultural elements related to the sociocultural determinants of health can have profound effects on health and health-related behaviors. Each cultural group has norms that govern the interaction of its members. Considerations to be addressed in assessment include cultural values, relationships with the supernatural, interpersonal roles and relationships, relationships with health care providers and the larger society, socioeconomic status, and life experiences such as those related to sexuality and reproduction, coming of age, marriage, immigration, and death.

VALUES. As we noted earlier, the values held by a cultural group are some of the elements most resistant to change. Cultural groups may differ significantly on the value attached to certain conditions and differences in strongly held values between group members and the dominant culture may give rise to difficulties. Data from the World Values Survey of 79 nations from 2005 to 2008 indicated that cultural values differ along two main dimensions. The first is the traditional/secular-rational dimension, which denotes differences between cultures in which religion is very important and those that have a more secular view of the world in which religion is less important. Other related values tend to vary along traditional/secular lines. For example, groups with more traditional values tend to emphasize deference to authority and traditional family values. Groups with a secular-rational values orientation tend to value self-determination and rationality (Inglehart & Welzel, n.d., 2010).

The second major dimension on which values vary among cultural groups is the survival/self-expression dimension. In this dimension, according to the theory posed by Inglehart and Welzel (2010), societies that have major concerns with basic survival tend to emphasize values that support survival, such as order, economic security, and conformity. On the other hand, in societies in which survival is more or less taken for granted, higher value is placed on self-expression, subjective well-being, and quality of life. These values are accompanied by modifications in other areas of life such as more permissive parenting, fostering of tolerance for diversity, and so on (Inglehart & Welzel, n.d., 2010).

For example, the dominant culture, including the biomedical culture, strongly values being on time. Appointments are made for specific times and clients are expected to arrive at that time or earlier. This value, however, frequently does not seem to apply to providers themselves, who may keep clients waiting to be seen for significant periods of time. Examples of other values that may differ among cultural groups or between members of these groups and the dominant culture are those related to autonomy and self-sufficiency, work ethic, dignity of life, importance of family, and the need for education or health-related activities.

The population health nurse explores with members of the culture the areas of strongly held values. Often this is done through observation since people may be unable to adequately articulate values in conversation.

RELATIONSHIPS WITH THE SUPERNATURAL. Human psychological health is often intertwined with spiritual health, particularly among many ethnic cultural groups. Even in the dominant societal culture, spiritual interventions, such as prayer, are commonly invoked in health promotion and restoration. Attitudes and behaviors with respect to the supernatural world are often exhibited in the form of religious affiliation and magical practices.

Religiosity, the belief or participation in religious observances, is conceptualized as having two aspects: social

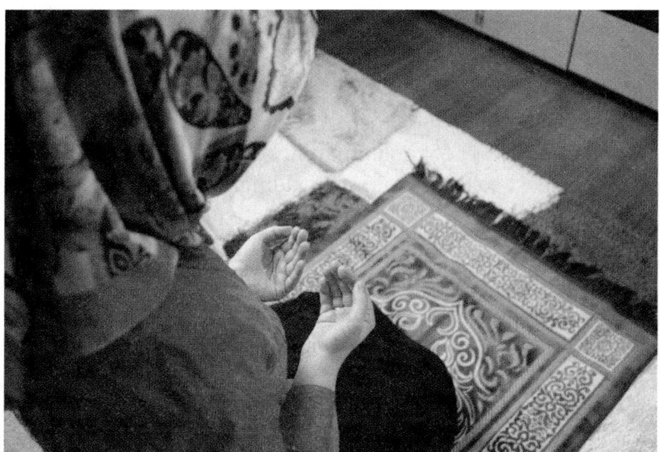

Religion is an important aspect of a group's culture. *(Eray/Fotolia)*

religiosity and individual religiosity. **Social religiosity** reflects the extent to which members of the population affiliate with religious organizations and spend time in religion-oriented activities. **Individual religiosity** addresses individual beliefs in a God and the importance of God and religious observance in one's life (Okulicz-Kozaryn, 2010). These two aspects of religiosity may also be referred to as extrinsic and intrinsic religiosity (Abdel-Khalek, 2009).

The influences of religion and spiritual beliefs may be seen in five areas. First, specific religious beliefs or practices may influence health, either positively or negatively (Rabinowitz, Mausbach, Atkinson, & Gallagher-Thompson, 2009). Second, religious groups may be involved in the provision of health care. In addition, participation in organized religious activities may contribute to a sense of belonging (Okulicz-Kozaryn, 2010). Religious beliefs may also act as a source of personal support in times of adversity, and religiosity has been associated with better life satisfaction and mental health (Abdel-Khalek, 2009; Okulicz-Kozaryn, 2010). Finally, the type and quality of interactions between religious leaders and the health care system can profoundly influence the acceptability and use of health care services.

Biomedical culture tends to separate health care and religion or spirituality as distinct and unrelated fields, despite evidence that religious practices may enhance well-being. There is growing recognition, however, that spirituality may play a significant role in clients' well-being. In fact, the National Cancer Institute (2012) has recommended spiritual assessment of clients with cancer. This assessment has been adapted in the *Focused Assessment* below to assess religious and spiritual influences on population groups.

Religious belief and magic are closely intertwined in some cultures. In other cultures, magic is conceived as antithetical to religion and as an act against God (Greenwood, 2009). Magical effects may be conceptualized as resulting from sympathetic magic or analogical thinking. Sympathetic magic may be based on two perspectives: homeopathic magic or contagious. In homeopathic magic, effects occur based on associations of similarity in which a desired effect can be achieved by imitation (Greenwood, 2009). In rural Appalachia, for example, scissors may be placed beneath the mattress of a woman in labor to "cut" or reduce her pain. The basic concept is that "like causes like." In contagious magic, effects result from contact. For example, an object in contact with a person is believed to absorb the attributes of that person. For example, a pair of a laboring woman's husband's pants might be placed on the bedpost to impart his strength to her.

In analogical thinking, reasoning is based on similarities perceived between one thing and another in the view of the person making the analogy (Greenwood, 2009). Analogical thinking is the basis for some religious rituals. For example, baptism with water is symbolic of being cleansed of one's sins, the analogy

FOCUSED ASSESSMENT Population Spiritual Assessment

- What religious denominations are represented in the population?
- What beliefs or philosophies are prevalent in the population?
- How important are spiritual practices or rituals within the population?
- To what extent do members of the population view religion or spirituality as a source of support?
- To what extent does religion or spirituality contribute to a feeling of belonging among members of the population?
- To what extent do members of the population engage in prayer or meditation as a source of comfort or help?
- To what extent are adverse events (e.g., serious illness, natural disaster) likely to result in a loss of faith in the population?
- What conflicts, if any, exist between religious beliefs and health care practices?
- To what extent do religious beliefs and spirituality contribute to healthy behaviors?
- What views of death and afterlife are held by members of the population? How do these views affect their participation in health-related behaviors?

Adapted from: National Cancer Institute. (2012). *Spiritual assessment.* Retrieved from http://www.cancer.gov/cancertopics/pdq/supportivecare/spirituality/Patient/page3

being that as water washes dirt from the physical body, it also washes sins from the soul. Greenwood (2009), an anthropologist who has studied magic extensively, adds a third view of magic as "magical consciousness," which is seen as expanded awareness of the world and participation through multiple connectedness between persons, between persons and other features of the physical world (e.g., animals), and between the living and the dead.

Belief in magic as a means of causing or curing disease is common in many traditional ethnic cultures, including African American, Italian, Native American, and Latino groups (Spector, 2012). Magic may even be perceived as the origin of scientifically diagnosed illnesses. For example, when health care providers were unable to provide Thai clients and their families with an explanation for the development of schizophrenia, many family members attributed the disease to supernatural powers or black magic (Sanseeha, Chontawan, Sethabouppha, Disayavanish, & Turale, 2009).

Belief in and practices related to magical thinking are not only found among members of ethnic cultural groups. In the dominant culture, as well, many of us engage in "magical rituals" that comfort us or give us confidence in tricky situations, like wearing your "lucky poker shirt." Population health nurses would assess the place of magic in the belief system of a given population and the relationship of those beliefs to health and health-related behaviors.

FAMILY AND COMMUNITY RELATIONSHIPS. Culturally defined roles and relationships are learned first within the family, and may differ by family type, age, and gender. The predominant family form in U.S. societal culture remains the two-parent nuclear household, with loose relationships with kin in both parents' families of origin. As we will see in Chapter 14∞, however, this family form is being supplanted by a variety of other family forms, including single-parent families, nuclear dyads, extended families, and cohabiting couples. In many ethnic cultural groups, the extended family remains the predominant family type, but in many countries this is changing as younger family members move away from the family of origin in search of employment opportunities.

Roles within the family are frequently defined by age, gender, and family position. In the traditional U.S. culture of the past, men were considered the family providers and women were responsible for care of the home and family, except in families that were dependent on women's income to replace or supplement that of male family members. Gender role expectations in the dominant culture, however, have experienced a number of changes with women more often employed outside the home and men taking on more traditionally female tasks with respect to homemaking and child rearing.

In many traditional ethnic cultures, on the other hand, gender roles are more specifically defined. Men are often considered the head of the family and the primary decision maker on major family issues. In other ethnic cultural groups (e.g., some Native American tribes), women are the primary decision makers. Women's traditional role is often defined in terms of childbearing and care of the home and family. Gender roles may also entail strict separation of men from women except within the immediate family. In same-sex families, family roles may be shared by both partners or may be divided in ways that best meet the needs of the family.

Age may also play a role in family decision making. For example, in most cultural groups, including the dominant U.S. culture, parents often make decisions related to their children. In the dominant culture, however, adolescents are often given more decision latitude regarding their own behavior than their counterparts in other cultural groups. Middle adults in the dominant culture may also find themselves in the position of making decisions for older parents. In some ethnic cultural groups, on the other hand, decision making is the province of family elders.

Children in many ethnic cultural groups are expected to respect and obey their parents without question. Children in the dominant U.S. culture, however, are generally given more latitude to question parents' decisions or the rationale for those decisions. As we saw earlier, the dominant culture is youth oriented, and the elderly are not as well respected as may be the case in many ethnic cultural groups.

Family relationships may also be affected by illness or disability among family members. In some cultures, ill or disabled family members may be hidden to escape social stigma for the family. In others, they may be overprotected and prohibited from developing to their full potential.

Relationships with extended family members also have many cultural aspects. As noted earlier, extended families in some cultural groups have often lived together in joint households or in close proximity to other family members. Members of the GLBT population, on the other hand, may experience strained relationships with their families of origin and strive to create their own "families" with other individuals like themselves. Transgendered women, in particular, may create a "sisterhood" to replace or augment family ties.

Age and gender also influence roles within the biomedical and health professional cultures. Traditionally, as a largely female profession, nurses were expected to be subservient to physicians, and only recently have nurses begun to be respected as equally expert providers of care. An interesting twist to this hierarchy is seen in the military health care culture, where respect and authority are based on rank, not professional discipline. The influence of age in the biomedical and professional cultures is less forthright. Older professionals have greater experience than their younger counterparts, but in many instances, this advantage is offset by better education among younger practitioners.

COMMUNICATION AND LANGUAGE. Communication plays a significant role in interpersonal interactions within and between cultures. In assessing cultures, population health nurses attend to all types of communication, including oral and written communication, the language spoken, forms of nonverbal communication and acceptable behavior, speed of speech and intonation, slang, and culturally inappropriate words, phrases, and topics.

The language spoken by members of ethnic cultural groups and group members' facility with the language of the dominant culture, will affect intercultural interactions, particularly as they influence health. Differences in dialects within cultural groups may also impede communication. In the United States, 21% of the population over 5 years of age, speak a language other than English at home. Although many of these people also speak English, 8.5% of them speak English less than "very well" (U.S. Census Bureau, American Fact Finder, 2012). Non-English speakers are more likely than English speakers to have incomes below poverty level and less than a high school education. The Office of Minority Health (OMH, 2013a) defined **linguistic competency** as the ability to communicate effectively and convey information in ways that are easily understood by persons with limited English proficiency, low literacy or health literacy levels, or communication disabilities.

Patient and provider concordance with respect to language is important in providing culturally competent care. Language differences make for miscommunication and may compromise care and client outcomes resulting in increased disparities, inequities, dissatisfaction, and inefficiency in health care delivery systems (Tang, Lanza, Rodriguez, & Chang, 2011). Ideally, health care providers should be able to speak a client's native tongue, but this is not always possible or practical. In such cases, interpreters or other linguistic services may be needed to assist with communication.

Linguistic services generally consist of four components: oral services, interpretation services, written services, and translation services. Interpretation services are used in the context of oral communication. Interpretation is not a word-for-word rendering of what is said, but involves conveying meaning for meaning. Translation, on the other hand, is the rendering of the written word in another language (Partnership for the Public's Health, n.d.). Interpretation services are not always available in many health care settings due to their cost, yet research has shown that clients who receive interpretation services made more visits to providers, received more preventive services, and were given more prescriptions than those who needed, but did not receive, interpretation services. It is hypothesized that ultimate health care costs may be decreased enough, due to prevention and earlier intervention, to warrant the added cost of interpretation services.

Approaches to interpretation in health care settings range from the ideal of bilingual and bicultural providers to using family members as interpreters. Unfortunately, the lack of qualified bicultural providers and the cultural diversity encountered in many health care settings often prohibits this solution to problems of interpretation. Even when providers speak the same language as the client, there may be difficulties related to dialect or socioeconomic status that make communication difficult. Health care agencies may also employ other bilingual staff who serve as interpreters. This approach is most effective, but also most costly, when staff are used exclusively for interpretation rather than being pulled away from other responsibilities to provide interpretation services. Another option is the use of outside interpreters or telephonic interpretation. These approaches usually need to be arranged in advance and so are not particularly useful in emergency situations. In addition, these services tend to be expensive, and the interpreter may not be conversant with medical terminology. Telephonic interpretation also has the disadvantage of the loss of communication through body language. Family members should be a last resort in meeting interpretation needs. Use of family members to interpret runs the risk of violating client confidentiality and creates the potential for family conflict or other adverse effects. Tips for assessing the need for interpretation services with a particular client are provided below.

Interpretation and translation are usually considered in terms of communication between providers and members of ethnic cultural groups. It is wise to keep in mind, however, that both interpretation and translation may be required to render biomedical terminology intelligible to clients and other members of the lay public. The Program for International Assessment of Adult Competencies (PIAAC) assesses health literacy (ability to read and understand information), numeracy (ability to calculate), and problem-solving skills in the United States and 22 other countries. The 2012 PIAAC data indicated that 16 countries had literacy levels higher than those in the United States,

FOCUSED ASSESSMENT Assessing Interpretation Needs

- What language does the client speak at home?
- How long has the client been speaking the language of the dominant culture?
- What is the client's level of literacy in the language of origin? In the language of the dominant culture?
- What types of things does the client read in each language?
- When does the client prefer an interpreter?
- Can the client rephrase instructions to staff in the language of the dominant culture?

Data from: McLaurin, J. A. (2002). *Assimilation, acculturation, and alternative medicines.* MCN Streamline: The Migrant Health News Source, 8(6), 1–3.

and only 7 countries had lower scores. Since the assessment is only given in English, these scores vastly underrepresent literacy levels among non-English-speakers. The U.S. scores were not significantly different from those derived from the National Assessment of Adult Literacy (ALL) in 2003–2008 (National Center for Education Statistics, 2012). **Health literacy** has been defined by the World Health Organization (WHO, 2009) as cognitive and social skills that motivate and enable people to obtain, understand, and use health-related information to promote their health.

Two *Healthy People 2020* objectives related to health communication and information technology deal specifically with health literacy and communication with health care providers. These objectives are summarized below. The first objective, with its subobjectives, is developmental in nature, so there are no existing baseline data or established targets

Healthy People 2020

Selected Objectives Related to Cultural Competence

OBJECTIVE	BASELINE (YEAR)	TARGET	CURRENT DATA (YEAR)	DATA SOURCE
HC/HIT-1 Improve the health literacy of the population				
1.1 Increase the proportion of persons who report that their health care provider always gave them easy-to-understand instructions about what to do to take care of their illness or health	Developmental	Developmental	NDA	Medical Expenditure Survey, AHRQ
1.2 Increase the proportion of persons who report that their health care provider always asked them to describe how they will follow the instructions	Developmental	Developmental	NDA	Medical Expenditure Survey, AHRQ
1.3 Increase the proportion of persons who report that their health care providers' office always offered help in filling out a form	Developmental	Developmental	NDA	Medical Expenditure Survey, AHRQ
HC/HIT 2 Increase the proportion of persons who report that their health care providers have satisfactory communication skills				
2.1 Increase the proportion of persons who report that their health care provider always listened carefully to them	59% (2007)	65%	61.9% (2010)	Medical Expenditure Survey, AHRQ
2.2 Increase the proportion of persons who report that their health care provider always explained things so they could understand them	60% (2007)	66%	60.6% (2010)	Medical Expenditure Survey, AHRQ
2.3 Increase the proportion of persons who report that their health care provider always showed respect for what they had to say	62% (2007)	68.2%	64.9% (2010)	Medical Expenditure Survey, AHRQ
2.4 Increase the proportion of persons who report that their health care provider always spent enough time with them.	49% (2007)	54%	51.4% (2010)	Medical Expenditure Survey, AHRQ

NDA = No data available.
U.S. Department of Health and Human Services. (2013). *Health communication and health information technology.* Retrieved from http://www.healthypeople.gov/2020/topicsobjectives2020/overview.aspx?topicid=18

for accomplishment. As data collection systems are developed, baseline data will be collected and appropriate targets determined.

There may also be difficulties in communication within the biomedical culture itself due to the different languages employed by many health care disciplines. For example, how well do members of other disciplines understand the language of nursing diagnosis? Similarly, health care professionals recruited internationally to address shortages in the United States may face a variety of communication difficulties with clients and other providers. These health care providers need to learn the language of the profession as employed in the United States as well as the conventions of interprofessional communication, which may differ significantly from those of their countries of origin. Language proficiency tests are not specific to the nursing profession and may not adequately assess English proficiency in a professional context. Communication difficulties are often exacerbated on the telephone and in reading and writing charts. Some of the problems that may occur include basic grammar, use of lay vocabulary and that of other professionals, pronunciation difficulties, lack of understanding of different levels of interaction (formal, informal), and failure to recognize the variability of cultural norms among clients seen.

In addition to the words used, *paralanguage* variations may be important in communication between cultures. *Paralanguage* includes the tone of voice, volume, and inflection typically used in verbal communication (Purnell, 2012). For example, some cultural groups may use loud volume for urgent messages and repeat messages for emphasis. Others routinely use a louder voice and more rapid speech in ordinary conversation than is common in some cultural groups. In the dominant U.S. culture, a loud voice may convey an emergency but may also be interpreted as anger.

Inflections also signal meaning in conversation. For example, in English, a question is indicated with an upswing in tone at the end of the sentence. In other languages, such as Marathi, an Asian Indian language, questions may be indicated by appending a word to the end of the sentence or by means of an interrogative word at the beginning of the sentence (similar to English).

Nonverbal communication also varies among cultural groups. For example, nurses often rely on nonverbal cues to identify clients in pain; however, when the cues differ between the nurse's and the client's culture, effective pain relief may be compromised. Gestures are another element of nonverbal communication that may differ among cultural groups. For example, when you want someone to come closer to you in the dominant U.S. culture, you might crook your finger. In India, on the other hand, you would use a sweeping motion of the fingers toward you with the hand held prone. In yet other cultures, beckoning in any form is considered rude.

Another aspect of communication to be considered in a cultural assessment is the level of prescribed reticence within the group—the extent to which people are expected or willing to share private information. In the dominant U.S. culture, it is not uncommon for people to tell much of their life story during a chance encounter in the grocery store. Yet, there are certain things that one does not ask or tell. For example, it would be considered rude to ask a chance acquaintance how much money they make or whether they are sexually active. Yet, these kinds of questions are routinely asked by health care professionals and may insult even members of the dominant culture if the reason for them is not carefully explained. Among many other cultural groups, there may be even greater reluctance to provide personal or family information, particularly when it relates to emotions.

RELATIONSHIPS WITH THE LARGER SOCIETY. The relationship between members of different cultural groups and the dominant society may also have significant effects on health status. Many people in the dominant U.S. culture display **xenophobia**, an irrational fear of strangers (Spector, 2012), particularly those who are significantly different from oneself in appearance or behavior. When this fear centers on those of different sexual orientations, it is termed *homophobia*. Xenophobia, homophobia, and other negative reactions to persons of a cultural group may lead to racism, prejudice, and discrimination. **Racism** is the belief that people can be classified on the basis of biophysical traits into groups that differ in terms of mental, physical, and ethical capabilities, with some groups being intrinsically superior or inferior to other groups. **Prejudice** is the holding of negative attitudes or feelings toward members of another group. It is an internal perspective, and may or may not be acted upon. Discrimination, as we saw earlier, is a behavioral demonstration of racism or prejudice involving differential treatment of an individual or group based on unfavorable attitudes toward the group. When discrimination is directed toward persons with a handicapping condition or disability, it is termed **ableism**.

Discrimination has been shown to have negative effects on health through both direct and indirect mechanisms. Discrimination by health care providers leads to inappropriate and ineffective care. Discrimination may be seen in response to members of ethnic cultural groups, but also in response to other individuals as well. For example, GLBT individuals report significant discrimination against them by members of the dominant U.S. society, as well as among health care providers. As noted earlier, the elderly and disabled populations may also face discrimination from the general public or from health care providers who believe certain health services (e.g., health promotion and illness prevention) are not warranted. Discrimination may have indirect effects in terms of willingness to seek health care services or via the stress caused by exposure to culture-related discrimination or harassment.

Responses to negative experiences with the larger society can also have adverse effects on health. A large body of research has linked various forms of discrimination and even perceptions of discrimination to the health status of multiple groups characterized by differences from the mainstream population (Juang & Alvarez, 2010; Pascoe & Smart, 2009). Perceived discrimination against members of racial and ethnic minority groups by health care providers has also been reported (Sorkin, Ngo-Metzger, & De Alba, 2010).

Members of the biomedical culture also experience different relationships with the larger societal culture. In most ethnic cultures and in the dominant U.S. culture, health care providers are held in high esteem by the society in which they function. In the dominant U.S. culture, this can be seen in the incomes of physicians and in the trust placed in nurses. Nursing has not always been as highly valued as a profession, however. In the early days of the history of modern nursing, for example, nursing was seen as an occupation of lower-class women that most families would not want to see their daughters enter. This was also true on the Indian subcontinent as few as 40 years ago and may still be true in some parts of the world. Even in cultures in which nursing is esteemed, the profession may not be valued as highly as medicine. Although the status of nursing is changing within the biomedical culture, nursing has not usually been as highly valued as medicine and some other health professional disciplines. In fact, nursing is still viewed in some settings and by some members of other professional disciplines as a handmaiden group.

SOCIOECONOMIC STATUS. The socioeconomic status of a cultural group also influences its health status. Generally speaking, most members of the biomedical culture are of relatively high socioeconomic status. Even within this group, however, there is considerable variation, with physicians and dentists more often included in the upper to upper middle class and nursing and other health care disciplines considered to be middle- to lower-middle-class occupations. Members of many ethnic minority groups in the United States, on the other hand, tend to have relatively low socioeconomic status, but even that status varies among groups. For example, some Asian cultural groups enjoy relatively high educational and income levels, while others, particularly more recent immigrants and refugees, include large numbers of the poor or poorly educated. In general, members of the GLBT population tend to be fairly highly educated, but may have lower incomes than their "straight" counterparts due to the need to accept positions in organizations that are accepting of their sexual orientation or identity.

Income, education, and the resulting lower socioeconomic status are some of the major contributing factors in health disparities noted in the United States. Health disparities are particularly prevalent among immigrant and refugee populations, who tend to have lower education and economic levels than the general population. Chapter 6∞ presents a general discussion of poverty and health insurance and their influence on health disparities. Specific health disparities and their underlying causes are discussed in relevant chapters throughout this book. Population health nurses assess the typical socioeconomic status of the cultural groups with whom they interact. They also examine the effects of these factors on the health status of the population.

LIFE EVENTS. Cultural groups may differ significantly in the ways they address life experiences common to human existence. Although all cultural groups deal with these common life experiences, cultural beliefs and behaviors related to them can vary considerably. Life experiences that will be addressed here include experiences related to sexuality and reproduction, coming of age, marriage, and death.

Sexuality and reproduction. Different cultures have differing perspectives on and attitudes toward human sexuality and sexual activity. Some groups (e.g., fundamentalist Muslims and Christians) perceive sexual activity as inherently sinful and to be tolerated only within the bounds of marriage. Other groups are more tolerant of sexual activity outside of marriage, but may differ in terms of their application of this norm to men and women. For example, among some populations extramarital sexual activity is accepted for men but not women. "Good" women are not sexually experienced or knowledgeable and may not be willing to discuss sexual issues with their partners for fear of being thought a prostitute. These cultural attitudes place these women at risk for sexually transmitted diseases and cervical cancer since sexual beliefs have been found to influence willingness to obtain pap smears.

Attitudes toward homosexuality are another area that should be explored by the population health nurse engaged in a cultural assessment of a group of people. Homosexuality may be defined and perceived differently in some cultures than in the dominant U.S. culture. For example, Muslims and traditional Christians and Jews generally consider homosexuality sinful. In some Asian cultures, homosexuality can be viewed as expressing disdain for societal norms that include expectations for marriage and children and brings shame to the family of the homosexual individual. China and Iran are particularly repressive of homosexual behavior, and such attitudes may accompany recent immigrants (Purnell, 2012). The dominant U.S. culture is generally homophobic and members of the GLBT populations experience considerable discrimination as we will see in Chapter 20∞.

Cultural groups also vary with respect to attitudes and behaviors related to contraception. In societies where childbearing is an expectation, contraception is not approved and abortion is not permitted. Nonetheless, even in these cultures, there may be a variety of methods employed to induce abortion, some of which can be extremely dangerous. For example, poisoning with pennyroyal, a common abortifacient that is highly toxic, occurs periodically in the United States and elsewhere (Natural Medicines Comprehensive Database, 2012).

Many ethnic cultural groups also engage in a variety of behaviors designed to prevent conception, some of which are based on traditional explanatory models for conception. For example, some African Americans believe that one is more apt to get pregnant if one has intercourse during menses and is "safe" at mid-cycle or that it is impossible to become pregnant until one has had a menstrual period following delivery of a baby. This latter belief may also be seen among some Italians (Purnell, 2012) and members of other cultural groups. Members of cultural groups may also engage in a variety of behaviors to promote conception. Selected cultural beliefs and behaviors related to menstruation, conception, and contraception are included in tables presented in the *Further Information* section of the student resources for this book.

All cultural groups have prescribed and proscribed behaviors to be performed when pregnancy does occur, as well as during labor and delivery. Some authors have noted the relatively positive birth outcomes among immigrant women, particularly Latinas, compared to other low-income women, suggesting that healthful behaviors and social support arising out of cultural beliefs about pregnancy should be emulated by other groups.

Birth rituals occur in some form in all cultures. Birthing systems usually prescribe a specific locale for the birth event to take place, as well as specific practices to be employed. Generally speaking, the technocratic society of the United States and other developed nations advocates birth in a specialized locale, usually a delivery room within a hospital setting. Some authors have noted that this locale is designed to make the birth easy for the birth attendants rather than the mother. The second locale specified for births is the woman's local sphere. In many ethnic cultural groups, this is the home. Home births are a growing phenomenon in some segments of the dominant U.S. culture, as is the use of birthing centers. For members of other groups, birth should take place outside of the home because it is an unclean event and would contaminate the home.

Cultural groups also forbid some practices during pregnancy and engage in a number of others to promote a positive pregnancy outcome. For example, some ethnic cultural groups perceive pregnancy as a hot condition and, thus, refuse prenatal vitamins, a hot medication. In some cultures, part of the role of the traditional midwife or an older family member is to instruct the pregnant woman on the cultural taboos to be observed.

Biomedical culture is not exempt from birthing rituals, many of which have little scientific basis or evidence of effectiveness. For example, the practice of performing an episiotomy to keep the perineum from tearing has no scientific evidence of its efficacy and may be a function of the dominant U.S. cultural value for trying to speed up a natural process. Similarly, the routine practices of fetal monitoring and giving an enema prior to delivery have not demonstrated any difference in pregnancy outcomes. Advances in reproductive technology have made it possible for members of the GLBT population to have children and biomedical cultural birthing practices may need to be modified to accommodate same-sex parents or surrogate parents. Selected cultural beliefs and behaviors related to the perinatal period are presented in the *Further Information* section of the student resources.

Coming of age. Some ethnic cultural groups have specific ceremonies that mark the movement of children into adulthood. For Jewish children, for example, the bar mitzvah for boys and the bat mitzvah for girls mark their entry into adult life. Similarly, in the southern United States, some groups still hold debutante parties as a rite of passage for young girls. Initiation of dating may be seen as a coming-of-age ritual in some segments of the dominant U.S. culture. In rural India, this change is typically signaled by a change in female clothing from a short dress or skirt and blouse to the traditional sari.

Female genital mutilation (FGM) is an extreme coming-of-age ritual for young girls in some cultural and religious groups in which portions of the female genitalia (clitoris and possibly the labia) are excised to promote chastity. Some authors suggest that immigrant women may be at greater risk for FGM in resettlement areas than in their country of origin due to attempts by the group to maintain their cultural identity. Although FGM is illegal in the United States and other countries, it does still occur. Population health nurses should be alert to the possible practice of FGM in client populations with whom they work because of the serious physical and psychological health effects, including infection and difficulties with fertility, pregnancy, and delivery.

Marriage. Some of the issues that may affect health include the typical age at marriage, who is considered an appropriate marriage partner, how marriages are contrived, and the roles and rights of the partners in marriage. In cultural groups where marriage takes place soon after a woman's first menstrual period, the potential for complications of pregnancy increase. Conversely, in the dominant U.S. society, marriage is occurring at later ages, and women may be nearing the end of their childbearing years when a first pregnancy occurs, which may also increase the risk of adverse maternal and infant outcomes.

Who is considered an appropriate spouse within the cultural group is also a consideration. In some societies, excessive consanguinity may result in a high prevalence of genetically determined diseases. In others, marriage to an "outsider" is not considered acceptable and may cause significant stress for the couple and their children. Finally, the nurse should consider the attitude of the cultural groups to same-sex couples. In the dominant U.S. culture, for instance, this is a current issue that is being hotly debated and cultural attitudes and family reactions to same-sex couples have been shown to create increased stress on the marriage and for the participants.

In the dominant U.S. culture, most marriages are "love matches," but in other parts of the world and in some ethnic groups within the United States, marriages may still be arranged by parents. Such marriages do not necessarily create negative health effects unless one party or the other resents being forced to marry, which may lead to individual as well as family stress. Pressure to marry may also occur in some groups when a girl becomes pregnant out of wedlock, although such pressure is less likely to occur today with the increasing number of single-parent families. Cultural attitudes toward divorce may also lead to stigma for couples who become divorced. Although this is not usually a problem in the dominant U.S. culture today, it may create family conflict in cultural groups that have a more traditional concept of the permanence of marriage.

Finally, the population health nurse would assess the roles and responsibilities expected of marital partners within the cultural group. Is the wife expected to be subservient to her husband? Is she allowed to own property in her own right? What are either partner's rights in the event of abuse? Answers to all of these questions have implications for the physical and emotional health of the couple as well as other family members.

Death and dying. All cultural groups have beliefs and practices related to death and dying that may vary considerably from those of other groups. Culture influences attitudes toward death and dying in a number of ways. One area of influence is the need for comfort experienced by the dying client. In those cultures in which death is seen as a normal part of life, there may be less need to comfort the dying and his or her family; conversely, in cultures in which death is feared, comfort may be needed and appreciated. Members of the biomedical culture, because of their focus on cure and promoting longevity, tend not to deal well with the concept of death and may need assistance in dealing with the death of a client or a loved one. They may also need to be encouraged to accede to clients' requests to die with dignity and without heroic lifesaving measures. For the GLBT population, the right of the significant other to be present during hospitalization, particularly when death is imminent is an area that may require advocacy on the part of population health nurses.

The population health nurse should assess whether those he or she is dealing with have a cultural belief in an afterlife. Some non-Western religions, including Hinduism, believe in reincarnation until the soul has achieved perfection and passes to Nirvana. Do religious beliefs regarding death and afterlife offer a source of comfort to clients and families, or do they engender fear and anxiety?

Culture also influences the selection and perception of health care providers when death is imminent. People from some cultures, including a growing body of mainstream Americans, believe that death should occur at home and are therefore unlikely to seek medical care for a dying client for fear that he or she will be removed from the home and placed in a hospital to die. For many people, going to the hospital means that death is inevitable.

Care of the body following death and funeral and burial practices are also influenced by culture, as are expectations regarding grief and mourning and practices to be observed during this period. Mourning is a cultural expression of grief following death, and mourning practices may vary from group to group.

Finally, culture influences communication regarding death, particularly with respect to children and their knowledge of and participation in the rites that accompany a death. Some groups are quite open in their communication about death; children may help with the care of the dying family member and participate in funeral and grieving practices. Despite this participation, members of many cultural groups may resist telling the client or others regarding imminent death (Purnell, 2012).

Similarly, some cultural groups may resist the discussion or use of advance directives for fear that such a discussion implies a belief that death is near and may cause the ill client to lose hope. For these groups, discussion of death is avoided. Use of advance directives may also be resisted in some cultures because of a perceived lack of need for them. For example, among African Americans, the family usually makes end-of-life decisions (Purnell, 2012).

Other questions relate to who should attend the dying client. The eldest son of a Chinese patient is often expected to be present with his dying parent, whereas in some Native American tribes, the maternal aunt is the more important figure. Some members of other tribes believe that the spirit cannot leave the body until family members are present.

Nurses should be familiar with the death rites of specific cultural groups so they can assist the family through their time of grief. Should the nurse wash and prepare the body, or is a family member responsible for this? Should personal belongings be left with the body or given to the family? The nurse should learn the answers to such questions when working with clients from other cultures. Death rites and the presence of family members may violate institutional policies in some health care settings, and nurses may need to function as advocates for culturally congruent care in these instances.

Members of many Native American tribes see the body as a "seed to be planted" and believe that the body must be disposed of in its entirety. Thus, family members may request amputated limbs to be kept until death and disposal of the body. They may also resist having an autopsy performed. Autopsy may also be resisted by members of some other cultural groups. In a similar vein, members of some cultural groups may request the return of hair or nail clippings from hospitalized clients to prevent their use by witches. Disposal of the body can vary among cultures and may include burning, burial, or exposure to the elements.

Mourning can be very emotional in some cultural groups and very subdued in others and may last for varying periods of time. For instance, following 4 days of mourning, the Cheyenne and Quechan cease grieving, as do members of some other tribes. In some tribes, the name of the deceased is never spoken again, and memory of the deceased is actively suppressed. Among Hmong clans, mourning may last until the following New Year celebration (which usually occurs in late December).

Clothing may assume special meanings in relationship to death. The clothing of a deceased person is believed, in some cultural groups, to contain evil spirits. Family members of hospitalized clients should be encouraged to take clothing home until the client is discharged. If the client should die, the family may be reluctant to accept the deceased's personal effects. In the dominant U.S. culture, family members are usually responsible for going through and disposing of the deceased person's belongings, although who takes responsibility and how items are allocated vary considerably from family to family.

Clothing is also used to symbolize mourning, and mourning garments are worn for varying lengths of time in different cultures. The color of mourning can also vary. For example, black is the color of mourning for many cultures, including the dominant U.S. culture, but among the Hmong and Vietnamese, white signifies mourning and black is worn for weddings and other celebrations.

Non-Anglo cultural groups often celebrate death in a way that is foreign to many members of the dominant U.S. culture. The dominant culture, and particularly the biomedical culture, is more likely to try to defy death. In traditional African American culture, death is perceived as a passage from one realm of

FOCUSED ASSESSMENT Sociocultural Determinants in Cultural Assessment

Values

- What are the strongly held values of the group?
- In what ways do values affect health and illness within the group?
- What is the value given to health in the cultural group? What priority is given to health over other group values?

Relationships with the Supernatural

- What are the perceptions of members of the cultural group with respect to supernatural forces?
- What roles, if any, do supernatural forces have in health and illness?
- What are the religious affiliations of members of the cultural group? What are the major tenets of the religion(s)?
- What influence does religious affiliation or spirituality have, if any, on health care beliefs and practices?
- Do religious leaders have a role with respect to health and illness within the cultural group? If so, what is that role?
- Do magical influences play a part in health and illness within the cultural group?

Family and Community Relationships

- What are the gender roles expected within the cultural group?
- What roles are expected of family members in various positions (e.g., parent, child, elder)?
- What is the typical family structure within the cultural group? Has this structure changed with recent life events? If so, what are the health effects of change in family structure?
- Who is responsible for decisions within the family? Within the larger cultural group?
- What behaviors are expected in interactions with others within the cultural group? Outside the group?
- What is the primary language of the cultural group? What is the level of fluency with the language of the dominant culture among members of the group?
- What other forms of communication are employed by members of the cultural group?
- What is the level of prescribed reticence expected of members of the cultural group?

Relationships with the Larger Society

- What is the quality of interaction between the larger society and members of the cultural group?
- What is the attitude of members of the dominant culture toward the cultural group? What is the attitude of members of the cultural group toward the dominant culture?
- To what extent are members of the cultural group subjected to or perceive prejudice, discrimination, hostility, or harassment?

Socioeconomic Status

- What is the attitude of members of the cultural group toward material wealth and possessions?
- What is the education level typical of members of the cultural group? What is the group's attitude toward education?
- What is the socioeconomic status typical of members of the cultural group? What effect does socioeconomic status have on health and access to health care services?

Life Events

- What attitudes and beliefs do members of the cultural group hold toward sexuality?
- What are the attitudes of group members toward differences in sexual orientation and gender identity?
- What attitudes and practices related to conception and contraception are displayed by members of the cultural group?
- What are the attitudes, beliefs, and practices of the cultural group related to pregnancy, birth, and the postpartum period?
- Are there specific coming-of-age rituals within the cultural group? What are the health effects of these rituals and practices, if any?
- How is marriage perceived within the cultural group? At what age does marriage usually occur?
- Who is considered an appropriate spouse for a member of the cultural group? How are marriages contracted?
- What are the expected roles and responsibilities of couples? How are they expected to interact with other family members?
- What are the attitudes, beliefs, and practices of the group with respect to death?
- Is there a cultural belief in an afterlife? If so, what effect does this belief have on attitudes toward death and dying?
- What cultural practices are typical of the group in its care of dying members, mourning, and funeral rites?

life to another. Funerals are generally occasions for celebration despite the grief of family members left behind. As is true in the larger society, funerals and wakes are seen as a psychosocial mechanism that facilitates grieving. Funerals for many Latinos are evidence of their deep religious belief in an afterlife. Among the Hmong, funerals are very elaborate functions that may last for several days. As we have seen, beliefs and behaviors regarding death and dying vary among different cultures. Selected cultural behaviors related to death and dying and presented in the *Further Information* section of the student resources for this book. Tips for a focused assessment of sociocultural determinants in cultural assessment, including the consideration of life events, are provided on page 125.

Behavioral Determinants

Culturally determined lifestyle patterns and related behaviors may also influence the health status of members of a cultural group. Aspects of the behavioral dimension to be addressed in a cultural assessment include dietary practices, other consumption patterns, and other health-related behaviors.

DIETARY PRACTICES. Apparel and dietary practices are some of the more obvious differences among ethnic cultural groups, with dietary practices having significant implications for health and illness. Some dietary practices have a religious basis. For example, for both Jews and Muslims, pork is eschewed on religious grounds, and both groups follow strict butchering practices. Other religiously motivated dietary practices among Muslims relate to *halal*, permitted food and actions, and *haram*, prohibited food and actions (Katme, 2009). Muslims also fast during the month of Ramadan, eating and drinking nothing between sunrise and sunset. Among Orthodox Jews who keep kosher, separate utensils are used for preparing meat and dairy products, and these foods are not eaten together. In addition, only mammals with cloven hooves and fish with fins and scales are eaten (Keeping kosher: Jewish dietary laws, n.d.). Jains, a religious group found primarily on the Indian subcontinent, are strict vegetarians because of their beliefs in the sanctity of all life. For Jains and other cultural groups, including the dominant U.S. culture, food is a way of establishing community, particularly in a new place. Food may have religious connotations aside from specifically prescribed and proscribed foods. For instance, bread and wine are the staples of the Christian communion rite.

Among other ethnic cultural groups, food preferences and dietary practices are more a function of foods available than of religious beliefs and practices. For example, poverty and climate gave rise to the staple items of Southern Black diets. Immigration and acculturation to the dominant culture may have a negative effect on the healthier aspects of some traditional diets. Ethnic cultural groups are not the only ones to experience changes in dietary patterns. For example, the move from home-cooked meals to fast foods in the dominant U.S. and other cultures contributes to the increasing prevalence of obesity. Patterns of food consumption have also changed, with

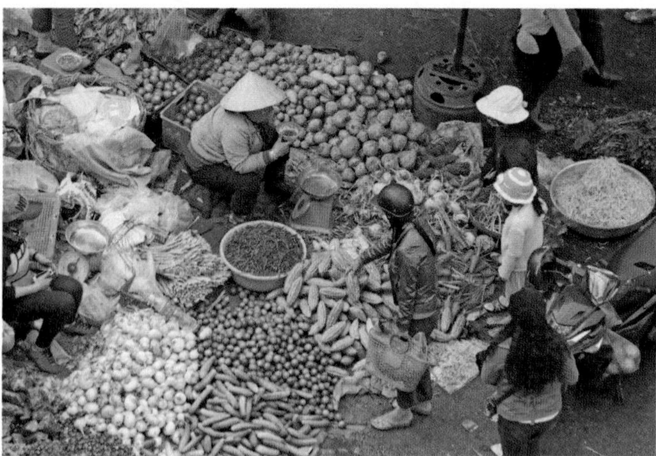

Ethnic markets support cultural food preferences. *(xuanhuongho/Fotolia)*

fewer meals eaten as a family group and more special family occasions celebrated with dinner in a restaurant than a celebratory home-cooked meal. Generally speaking, the health impact of these and other similar changes in dietary patterns is a negative one.

In addition to considering the food preferences and meal patterns of a particular cultural group, the nurse may also want to assess the meaning of food (and specific food items) within the culture. Other considerations relate to what constitutes food for a cultural group (e.g., snails or hamburger, tomatoes or dandelion greens), who does the cooking and how, and the uses of food for specific health purposes. For example, corn is used for religious ceremonies in some Native American groups, and turkey is the traditional Thanksgiving meat in the dominant U.S. culture. With respect to cooking practices, some groups (e.g., some Asian cultures) use stir-fry methods that preserve vitamins; others (e.g., residents of the southern United States) eat a lot of fried foods that increase fat intake. Still other groups may boil vegetables until vitamins are lost. Finally, some foods (e.g., the classic chicken soup or Jell-O in the dominant U.S. culture), are used to promote or restore health.

OTHER CONSUMPTION PATTERNS AND HEALTH-RELATED BEHAVIORS. Other consumption patterns are also addressed in an assessment of behavioral determinants within a cultural group. Areas that the population health nurse might explore are the extent of tobacco use, alcohol consumption, attitudes toward and use of prescription and nonprescription medications, caffeine consumption, and so on. Additional considerations include use of safety precautions, leisure-time pursuits, and exercise.

Smoking and other forms of tobacco use are prevalent in many cultural groups, including the dominant U.S. culture. Other stimulants may also be used; for example, betel leaves are frequently chewed in some parts of India. Cultural groups also vary with respect to physical activity. For instance, large segments of the dominant U.S. culture and many ethnic cultural groups do not engage in the recommended level of physical activity. Cultural fatalism may influence safety behaviors such as seat belt or helmet use.

Use of and attitudes toward alcohol are other areas in which cultural groups may vary. For example, French and Italian groups usually include wine with most meals, yet experience low prevalence of alcohol abuse. In other groups, however, where drinking alcohol is seen to be a sign of adulthood or manliness, alcohol abuse is more prevalent. Ease of access to controlled substances is an area of concern in the biomedical culture. Cultures also vary in their perceptions of alcohol and other substance abuse, with some cultures perceiving it as a disease (biomedical culture) and others as a character weakness (e.g., some fundamentalist religious groups).

Another area for assessment with respect to behavioral factors influencing the health of cultural groups is the use of health-related and safety practices. Among many immigrants, for example, the use of child car seats is limited due to the number of children in the family and the cost of car seats. Members of the biomedical culture may also vary in the degree to which they engage in safety practices such as the use of gloves during routine procedures such as immunization.

Culturally determined behaviors and attitudes toward health-related behaviors can have a profound effect on a group's health status. Tips for a focused assessment of behavioral considerations in cultural assessment are provided below.

Health System Determinants

Factors related to health systems also affect the health of population groups. In assessing cultural groups, one would address health system factors related to perceptions of health and illness and disease causation, the design of health systems, health care providers, and health care practices.

PERCEPTIONS OF HEALTH AND ILLNESS AND DISEASE CAUSATION. Cultural groups may differ significantly in their perceptions of what constitutes health and illness and beliefs about what causes disease. To protect or restore health, one must be able to identify health and illness and devise interventions that address their causes. Based on their perceptions of health and disease, cultural groups develop explanatory models that address causation, symptomatology, pathological processes, the course of the disease, and appropriate treatment. For many Asians and some Latinos, health is a balance between hot and cold forces, and intervention is directed toward restoring that balance. Other groups view health as the ability to stay active and to participate in desired activities and functions.

For some groups, disease may have natural or supernatural causes. In keeping with common cultural beliefs in *karma*, fate, or God's will, disease may be perceived as punishment for one's own wrongdoing or that of one's ancestors. A variety of beliefs about disease causation are also seen in the dominant U.S. culture, where illness may be thought to occur as a result of exposure to cold, wrong living (e.g., drinking, sexual activity), pathogens, poor diet, and so on. In the past, in the biomedical culture, disease was perceived to have a discrete external causative agent (e.g., a microorganism, exposure to environmental carcinogens). More recently, greater attention is being given to mind–body interactions in psychoneuroimmunology and to concepts of multiple causation.

Cultural groups may also develop complex disease taxonomies or types and categories of diseases encountered in the population. The International Classification of Disease (ICD-10) is the biomedical culture's comparable classification system. Cultural conceptions of disease causation and treatment are discussed in more detail below.

HEALTH CARE SYSTEMS. Health care is provided in several domains and each may be used to a different degree by members of different cultural groups or by individuals within those groups. These three domains include the professional, popular, and folk or alternative care domains. The professional domain involves care by biomedical providers. The popular domain consists of health care engaged in by individuals themselves or family members. This domain has been expanded considerably by the availability of health-related information on the Internet. The folk domain involves care by specialized members of the cultural group, usually after a period of apprenticeship. Each domain is characterized by explanatory models of health and illness, social roles for the players involved, and appropriate settings in which health care occurs (Gupta, 2010).

FOCUSED ASSESSMENT — Behavioral Determinants in Cultural Assessment

- What dietary practices are typical of members of the cultural group? What are the preferred foods? How are they typically prepared? Are any foods proscribed?
- Do certain foods or dietary practices (e.g., fasting) have religious significance for members of the cultural group?
- What is the effect of acculturation on dietary practices?
- What are the other consumption patterns of the cultural group (e.g., tobacco and alcohol use, caffeine consumption)?
- To what extent do members of the cultural group engage in health and safety behaviors?

Use of health systems in any of the three domains is the result of health-seeking behavior, which is a dynamic process of self-evaluation of symptoms, possible self-treatment, and seeking and acting on professional advice. Health-seeking behavior is greatly influenced by culture, and conventional providers need to consider each of these areas in interacting with clients from any cultural group. Areas for consideration include the meaning of the experience as viewed through a client's cultural lens, use of popular and alternative therapies, the meaning of health advice within the context of the culture, and the resulting effects on behavior (Gupta, 2010).

Considerations related to health care systems address the perceptions of members of the cultural group with respect to health care and the design and philosophical underpinnings of the health care system. Health systems may differ in their focus and their perspectives on individual responsibility for health and illness (Purnell, 2012). The biomedical culture and many health professional cultures focus heavily on curative practices. The dominant U.S. culture emphasizes restoration of health rather than health promotion and illness prevention, as seen in the level of funding provided for these various activities. The U.S. health system is generally focused on disease entities. Only recently has there been somewhat greater attention paid to health promotion and illness prevention in the biomedical culture. Health and illness tend to be seen as individual or family responsibilities, with less attention to societal factors influencing health. Illness is often seen as the result of personal behaviors over which the client has considerable control. As we saw in Chapter 1∞, it is only relatively recently that attention has been given to the effects of social determinants of health.

Many ethnic cultural health systems, on the other hand, place significant emphasis on health promotion and illness prevention. Health is viewed holistically, and in some cultural groups, health and illness may have significant implications for the group or community in terms of both cause and resolution. Naturopathy, for example, is a health system that places special emphasis on illness prevention, and therapeutic interventions in this system often focus on promoting healthy lifestyles and facilitating the body's natural ability to heal (American Association of Naturopathic Medicine, 2011).

Recent biomedical literature abounds with references to CAM. The National Center for Complementary and Alternative Medicine (NCCAM, 2012c) defined **complementary and alternative medicine** as "a group of diverse medical and health care systems, practices, and products that are not generally considered part of conventional medicine" (p. 2). Complementary medicine involves the use of CAM in conjunction with conventional medicine; alternative medicine systems use CAM in place of conventional therapy (NCCAM, 2012a). The term integrative medicine may also be used, denoting the integration of these nonconventional practices into mainstream health promotion and treatment (NCCAM, 2013b).

NCCAM has identified several broad categories of CAM to include natural products, mind–body medicine, manipulative and body-based practices, and other CAM practices (NCCAM, 2012b). Natural products include herbal remedies, vitamins, minerals, and other natural products, such as probiotics, live microorganisms that are similar to those found normally in the gastrointestinal tract. Mind–body medicine encompasses therapies that emphasize interconnections between the mind and the body and use of the mind to affect physical health. Some examples of mind–body practices include meditation, yoga, acupuncture, hypnotherapy, progressive relaxation, and tai chi. Manipulative and body-based practices include chiropractic and other practices that may involve rubbing, pressing, or manipulating the spinal column, muscles, or soft tissue. Other CAM practices involve such interventions as movement therapy, healing practices of traditional healers, manipulation of energy fields, (e.g., qigong or healing touch), and whole medicine systems. Whole medicine systems are complete theoretical systems outside of conventional medicine, such as homeopathy, Chinese medicine, and Ayurveda (NCCAM, 2012a). Shamanism is another alternative health

Tea and toast are a common popular remedy in mainstream U.S. culture. *(Jannyjus/Fotolia)*

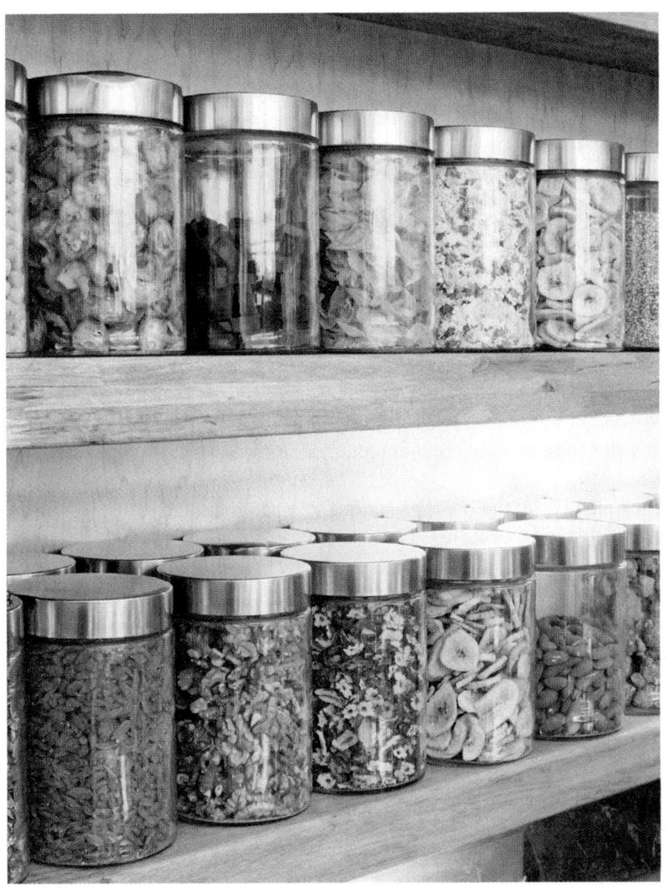

Herbal remedies are common in many cultures. *(Photobee/Fotolia)*

system employed in some ethnic cultural groups. Each of these health care systems, including the biomedical or allopathic system, includes basic theoretical and philosophical concepts, perceptions of disease causation, and specific diagnostic and therapeutic practices. Table 5-1● describes salient features of some of these health care systems. For more information about categories of CAM, see the *Further Information* section of the student resources site.

A number of concerns have been raised regarding the increasing use of CAM in the United States, particularly regarding herbal preparations. These concerns deal with issues of regulation, standardization, quality, safety, and efficacy. Because herbals are considered dietary supplements by the U.S. Food and Drug Administration (FDA), they must carry labels indicating that they are not intended for use to prevent or treat illness. Unfortunately, herbals are often used by the public for these purposes without FDA evaluation of their safety or efficacy. In addition, there is no standardization regarding the strength of active ingredients or their biological activity, which often vary from batch to batch due to differences in plants and growing conditions. Quality is an issue in that preparations do not always contain what they are supposed to, possibly due to incorrect plant identification, contamination and adulteration, inability to disintegrate completely in the body, or misleading product information. Safety is another area of concern. Herbals are considered "natural substances," so people may not be aware of their potential side effects, allergic reactions, or adverse events (NCCAM, 2012b). In addition, the safety of many herbals for children and pregnant women has not been determined. Finally, although many herbals are the basis for many pharmaceuticals, there is limited information about the efficacy of many other herbs. One other area of concern is the potential for interaction with prescription medications and the fact that many clients who use CAM do not disclose that use to biomedical providers (NCCAM, 2012b). Reasons given for nondisclosure include failure of the provider to ask, lack of importance, lack of understanding by providers, and fear that providers would disapprove of or discourage CAM use (IOM, 2005).

Complementary and alternative therapies may be used for health promotion, illness prevention, or curative purposes. An array of cultural approaches to health promotion, prevention, and treatment is included in the *Further Information* section of the student resources site. Many of the health promotion preventive strategies could also be used to prevent recurring health problems.

HEALTH CARE PRACTICES AND PRACTITIONERS. Each of the health care systems described in Table 5-1 makes use of a cadre of providers who function in accord with the precepts of that system. There are also a few independent providers who do not subscribe to a particular system of care as the basis for their activities. Health care providers within cultural health systems vary with respect to how they enter their profession, the type of training they receive, their degree of specialization and focus of care, the health promotion and curative practices they employ, and the way in which they are viewed by members of the culture.

Health practitioners may come to their calling in several ways, including inheritance, family position, birth portents, revelation, apprenticeship, self-study, and formal education. Healing skills are sometimes believed to be passed down in families from generation to generation. One's position within the family may also indicate special abilities, for instance, a seventh or ninth child or a child born after twins. Unusual occurrences during pregnancy or at birth, such as being born with a "caul," or amniotic membrane over the face, may also herald healing skills. Other practitioners may be called in a dream or vision or after recovering from a life-threatening illness themselves. Others show an aptitude for healing and may be apprenticed to an experienced healer. A few practitioners learn their calling on their own because of personal interest. In the biomedical culture, professional health care providers receive specific training in their discipline, most often in a recognized institution for postsecondary education. Even within the biomedical culture, however, there are variations in educational preparation for practice in a specific discipline (e.g., diploma, associate degree, and bachelor's degree preparation for entry into the nursing profession versus post-baccalaureate education for physicians and dentists).

TABLE 5-1 Selected Health Care Systems

System	Description
Ayurveda	**Source:** India **Basic Concepts:** All matter is composed of five elements: ether, air, fire, water, and earth. Human beings are composed of body (*dhatus*—body tissues, *malas*—waste products, and *doshas*—physiologic elements) and soul (*atma*—soul or spirit, and *nana*—mood, cognition). *Doshas* are the embodiment of the five elements in the body: *Vata dosha:* composed of ether and air; controls functions of the central and sympathetic nervous systems; regulates feelings and emotions; prevalent after age 55 years *Pitta dosha:* composed of fire and water; controls heat production and metabolism, vision, skin texture; influences intellect and cheerfulness, anger, hate, and jealousy; prevalent from puberty to middle age *Kapha dosha:* composed of water and earth; influences strength, cell reproduction, memory, emotional bonding, greed, and envy; prevalent in childhood Individuals differ in the preponderance of each element in the body, giving rise to seven different "constitutions" that influence physical and behavioral aspects of the individual. **Cause of Disease:** Disease is caused by imbalance among elements of mind and body or ineffective functioning of one or more elements. **Diagnosis:** Diagnostic processes include observation, touch, questioning, assessment of pulses; examination of urine, stool, tongue, bodily sounds, eyes, skin, and total appearance; and assessment of digestive capacity, personal habits, and individual resilience. **Treatment:** Treatment entails four types of therapies: *Shodan:* cleansing by means of five *panchakarma:* intestinal cleansing, cleansing of the stomach and duodenum, medicinal enemas, medicinal nasal oils, and, occasionally, bloodletting *Shaman:* palliation through burning toxic wastes, fasting, yoga, lying in the sun, breathing exercises, and meditation *Rasayan:* rejuvenation through herbal remedies and dietary supplements *Satwajaya:* stress reduction, mental nurturing, and spiritual healing
Biomedicine (Allopathy)	**Source:** Cartesian worldview of mind–body separation **Basic Concepts:** The body functions mechanically, based on complex physical and chemical interactions and independent of the influence of the mind. **Cause of Disease:** Disease causation is perceived from a mechanistic perspective, that is, changes in structure or function of the human "machine" in response to specific factors (e.g., microorganisms, fat intake, genetics) result in disease. **Diagnosis:** Diagnosis tends to rely on symptom presentation, invasive tests, and technological processes. **Treatment:** Treatment focuses on repair or replacement of bodily processes by means of pharmaceutical, immunological, and surgical interventions.
Chinese Medicine	**Source:** Originated in China, but has spread throughout much of Asia **Basic Concepts:** The human body is composed of several vital substances: Qi (pronounced "chee") is the body's vital energy force, responsible for effective physiologic function. It forms the basis for the other bodily substances. Blood moistens and nourishes the body. Jing (essence) is a specific hereditary energy force contained in the kidney that determines constitution and regulates growth, development, and reproduction. Body fluids such as saliva, mucus, sweat, urine, and excretory fluids may be deficient or stagnant. Shen encompasses the mental, emotional, and spiritual aspects of the individual. Qi flows through a network of 12 principal meridians or channels within the body and can be adjusted through acupuncture. All life is composed of male and female aspects of yang and yin. Yin is related to the water element and has properties of moistness, coolness, and substance. Yang is related to fire and has properties of warmth, dryness, and lack of substance. **Cause of Disease:** Disease is caused by an imbalance between forces of yin and yang and among the five elements of wood, fire, earth, metal, and water. Yin/yang imbalance may be related to deficiency, stagnation, counterflow, or sinking Qi. **Diagnosis:** Diagnosis relies on two primary mechanisms: examination of the depth and quality of pulses in multiple locations, and examination of the color, shape, coating, and moistness of the tongue, which indicates the nature of imbalance between yin and yang.

TABLE 5-1 (*Continued*)

System	Description
	Treatment: Traditional treatments in Chinese medicine include: Acupuncture: insertion of slender needles at specific points on the meridians to influence the flow of Qi within the body Qigong: meditative movements and breathing exercises to improve the flow of Qi Herbal preparations
Chiropractic	**Source:** Roots in ancient Chinese and Greek writings; promoted in the United States with the establishment of a chiropractic professional organization by Daniel David Palmer in 1895 and the Palmer School of Chiropractic in 1897 **Basic Concepts:** Natural and conservative methods are best used to promote and restore health. The human body has a vast capacity to heal itself. Adjustment and manipulation of musculoskeletal articulations, particularly in the area of the spine, and adjacent tissues can be used to treat functional disorders. **Cause of Disease:** Disease is caused by misalignment of body parts. **Diagnosis:** Based on perceptions of misalignment, may include specific measures of alignment through physical examination or X-ray. **Treatment:** Treatment focuses on manipulation of body parts.
Homeopathy	**Source:** Developed by a German allopathic physician, Samuel Hahnemann, who was disenchanted with 19th-century biomedicine **Basic Concepts:** One's vital force can promote self-healing. Stimulation of vital force promotes the body's healing response. Based on the law of similars—"like cures like"—and the law of infinitesimals—disease can be cured by use of very dilute doses of substances that are similar to the disease and would produce symptoms similar to those of the disease in a healthy person. Small doses of substances cure; larger doses damage the body's ability to heal itself. The smaller the dose, the more effective in healing. Hering's laws of cure: Healing occurs from head to foot. Healing occurs from internal to external. Healing progresses from more-vital to less-vital organs. Symptoms disappear in the reverse order of their appearance. **Cause of Disease:** Disease is caused by an imbalance or disruption in vital energy. **Diagnosis:** Diagnosis occurs by means of case taking or an interview to determine the client's problem and all symptoms experienced, and involves categorizations of the client's constitutional type. **Treatment:** Treatment is individualized and holistic, considering lifestyle as well as emotional state and other factors. Treatment involves prescription of remedies that are akin to the symptoms experienced, based on the *Materia Medica*, a compendium of remedies and their uses. Remedies may be derived from plant, mineral, or animal sources and are regulated by the FDA.
Native American Healing	**Source:** North American tribes **Basic Concepts:** Health is a reflection of harmony between the individual and nature, supernatural beings, and other people. Body and spirit are one entity. Health and disease have both physical and spiritual aspects. **Cause of Disease:** Disease results from disharmony and may be caused by: Internal factors, such as negative thinking or disturbance in life energy External factors, such as: pathogenic forces (e.g., microorganisms, sorcery, or supernatural beings) environmental poisons (e.g., pollution, alcohol abuse, poor diet) traumatic physical, emotional, or spiritual events breach of taboo and inharmonious relationships with nature, other people, or spiritual beings **Diagnosis:** Diagnostic approaches vary from group to group and may include hand trembling, crystal gazing, dream interpretation, divination, questioning, and observation. **Treatment:** Treatment also varies among groups, but may include prayer, music and chanting, purification rituals and ceremonies, herbs, massage, counseling, and fasting. Family and community are frequently intimately involved in healing practices.

(*Continued*)

TABLE 5-1 (Continued)

System	Description
Naturopathy	**Source:** Initiated in the United States by Benjamin Lust, a proponent of hydrotherapy **Basic Concepts:** The body has the ability to heal itself. Natural substances have healing properties. Treatment should encompass the whole person. Prevention and health promotion are important to health. **Cause of Disease:** Disease results from alterations in the mechanisms by which the body heals itself. **Diagnosis:** Diagnosis is made by history and physical examination. **Treatment:** Treatments include a variety of therapies such as nutrition, botanicals, fasting, heat, cold, exercise, counseling, and lifestyle modification.
Shamanism	**Source:** Siberia and Central and Southeast Asia. Variations also found among indigenous people worldwide. **Basic Concepts:** Shamanism focuses on harmony with nature, healing of self and community, daily spiritual practice, connection with sacred places. Health and illness result from the imbalance between the person and natural forces. **Cause of Disease:** Disease results from an imbalance between the individual and the spiritual world. **Diagnosis:** Diagnosis occurs by means of communication with the spirits responsible. **Treatment:** Ceremonies to honor natural spirits and promote harmony and balance
Traditional African Healing	**Source:** African tribal, Native American, and White colonial practices **Basic Concepts:** Human beings are composed of body and spirit (which includes mind). The balance between hot and cold in the body is important for health. **Cause of Disease:** Disease may be caused by natural and supernatural causes or an imbalance between hot and cold. **Treatment:** Treatment varies with the identified cause of disease and may employ spiritual or magic practices, herbs and diet therapy, massage, and dermabrasive practices such as cupping, pinching, rubbing, and burning.

Data from: American Chiropractic Association (2014a, 2014b); Mhame, Busia, & Kasilo, 2010; National Center for Complementary and Alternative Medicine (2012a, 2012b, 2012c, 2012d, 2013a, 2013b, 2013c, 2013e). (See References in this chapter for full citations.)

There is also wide variation in the types of people who provide health care in different cultural groups, from the family member or friend with expertise in dealing with illness to the specialist practitioner. Many people first seek advice on health from knowledgeable family members or friends before seeking more professional assistance. In the dominant U.S. culture, as well, people may rely on the wisdom and expertise of family members and friends for the care of minor illnesses or in making the decision to seek the assistance of a professional health care provider.

Professional assistance may be sought from a variety of different practitioners, depending on one's cultural background. There is also a growing tendency among the general public to seek health care from providers in non-biomedical health systems. Many clients with back pain or headache, for example, are seeking pain relief through acupuncture and the use of chiropractic services. The National Health Interview Survey indicated that 38% of U.S. adults and 12% of children used some form of CAM (NCCAM, 2008). In 2007, national out-of-pocket expenditures for CAM were almost $34 billion. This figure represents only 1.5% of total health care expenditures, but more than 11% of out-of-pocket spending (NCCAM, 2013d). Some health insurance plans are beginning to cover some CAM practices such as chiropractic and acupuncture; however,

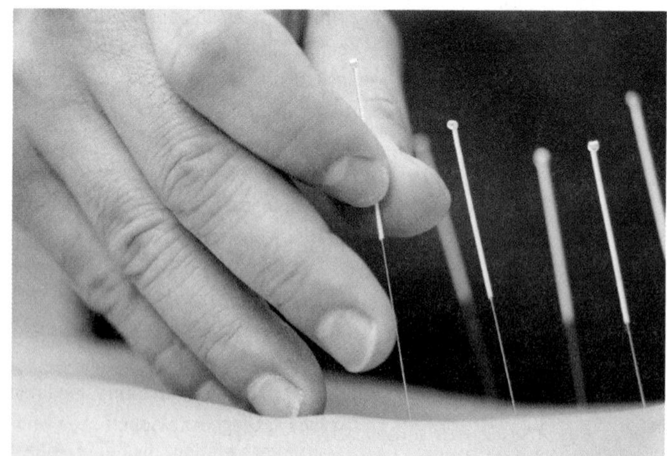

Members of many cultural groups seek the services of traditional practitioners. *(Max Tactic/Fotolia)*

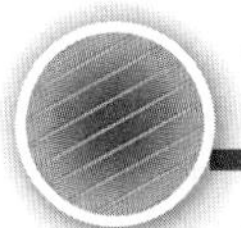

Evidence-Based Practice

CAM for HIV Symptom Relief

The advent of highly active antiretroviral therapy (HAART) has resulted in the transformation of HIV/AIDS from an acute and frequently fatal communicable disease to a chronic disease with multiple symptoms and undesirable treatment effects. HAART can often result in total viral suppression with rigid adherence to the treatment regimen. Adherence, however, is compromised by the experience of unpalatable side effects. Many people experiencing the chronic effects of both the disease and side effects of therapy have turned to a variety of complementary and alternative methods of symptom control. For example, in one study, 38% of HIV infected persons used a CAM provider and 89% used a variety of micronutrients. In another study, nearly half of the patients seen in an HIV/AIDS treatment program reported using some form of CAM. For these reasons, it is important that the evidence base for CAM use in conjunction with HAART be examined.

A systematic review of 40 studies conducted from 2000 to 2009 examined the effectiveness of four categories of CAM and specific interventions related to each. The four categories of therapy included whole medicine systems (homeopathy, naturopathy, Ayurvedic medicine, and traditional Chinese medicine), body–mind medicine (e.g., support groups, cognitive behavioral therapy, meditation, prayer, etc.), biologically based practices (e.g., herbs, dietary supplements, and specific foods), and energy therapies (e.g., therapeutic touch, qigong, reiki). Two prior systematic reviews in 2002 and 2005 had found limited evidence to support CAM use, with some suggestion that stress management strategies might eventually be found to improve quality of life.

After the present review, Hoogbruin (2011) concluded that there is insufficient evidence that any particular complementary or alternative therapy was effective in managing HIV disease. Many CAM therapies interact with HAART or may lead to noncompliance with therapy in the belief that the disease is adequately controlled using CAM. For these reasons, population health nurses should educate the population of HIV-infected persons regarding the overall lack of evidence of effectiveness of CAM in addressing HIV symptoms and HAART side effects. Clients in this population should be cautioned to discuss intended use of CAM with their conventional health care provider. Population health nurses should cultivate an awareness of the effectiveness of CAM for other health conditions in order to assist clients to make informed decisions about CAM use.

---

there are frequent restrictions on the type and extent of CAM covered, and deductibles and copayments may be higher than for conventional care (NCCAM, 2013d). Increases in insurance coverage for CAM are a function of consumer demand and the growing body of research indicating the effectiveness of some forms of CAM for a variety of health problems.

Some cultural groups include a wide array of health providers, many of whom are highly specialized. Zuni (Native American) healers, for example, are divided into several highly secret medicine societies, each of which specializes in the treatment of specific conditions. Specialization is also an emphasis in biomedicine, and there is a variety of specialty areas of practice in medicine and in nursing. Population health nursing is one example of specialization in nursing. Among the Navajo, healers may be divided into medicine men or women and diagnosticians. The function of the diagnostician is to determine the cause of illness through divination, whereas the medicine man or woman treats it (Spector, 2012). Singers are considered the most specialized practitioners among the Navajo and cure by means of specific songs and ceremonies (Purnell, 2012). Asian practitioners are often divided into the categories recognized in Chinese medicine, including acupuncturists and herbalists. Herbalists are also found among African American, Latino, and Appalachian cultural groups.

Religious healers, faith healers, or spiritualists are found among many cultural groups, including Asians, Latinos, African Americans, and Appalachians. Religion as a source of healing is common, and prayer and other religious rituals may accompany more scientific forms of healing for many. The charismatic healing tradition of the Roman Catholic Church is another example of the use of religious practices in healing. Other cultural groups embrace the practice of psychic healers thought to possess healing energy that can be transmitted to others, usually by some form of touch. Belief in this transfer of energy underlies the practice of therapeutic touch as a nursing intervention.

Practitioners of healing magic may also be found in a number of ethnic cultural groups. For example, *espiritistas* in the Latino alternative health tradition of spiritualism specialize in the treatment of illness caused by witchcraft (Purnell, 2012). Spiritual healers may also be seen among African American cultural groups, and the voodoo priest or priestess found among some African American groups is another example of magic used in healing (Spector, 2012).

Another group of health practitioners found in many cultures specializes in massage and is exemplified by the *sabador* in some Latino cultures. Massage and manipulation of body parts are also employed in chiropractic practice. Finally, many cultural groups include midwives as recognized health practitioners. In fact, midwifery as a specialized practice is a growing phenomenon in nursing that is gaining in popularity throughout the United States.

In assessing health system determinants for any cultural group, the population health nurse explores several areas related to health care providers. Among these are the types of practitioners recognized by the group, the health-related services provided, and the methods employed. Who and where are the practitioners? Is there a recognized hierarchy among practitioners? Who uses what type of provider, and what is the prevailing attitude of community members toward different types of providers?

INTERACTIONS WITHIN AND AMONG HEALTH CARE SYSTEMS. Another component of cultural assessment is the exploration of relationships and interactions between and among health care systems. Do members of an ethnic cultural group use the services of both biomedical and traditional health systems? If so, what is the effect of this dual usage? Another area for consideration lies in the attitudes of providers in one system toward providers in other systems. To what extent do providers in different systems interact with each other? What is the character of that interaction? For example, is it collaborative or adversarial?

Providers in one system may fail to see the value of practices of another system. This attitude is not restricted to biomedical practitioners. For example, a few biomedical and alternative providers believe that having a disease such as measles provides more effective immunity than immunization. Similarly, biomedical providers may perceive spiritual or magico-religious health practices employed in some traditional health systems as evidence of superstition.

Varying degrees of interaction occur between and among health care systems. In this discussion, we will focus primarily on interactions between the biomedical system and other systems of health care. Some of the failure of interactions among systems is the result of repression of traditional systems of health care. For example, the practice of lay midwives attending births was actively discouraged by the medical community in the United States, and many practiced their calling outside the law. On the other hand, interaction between systems may be encouraged. For example, CAM has been integrated into the national health systems of several countries. Referrals between health systems may be somewhat uneven, however, rather than equally reciprocal. In general, CAM practitioners may be more likely to make referrals to the biomedical system than vice versa.

Lack of interaction between and among health care systems may lead to a variety of problems for their users. As we saw earlier, for example, failure to tell providers of one system that one is using the services of another may contribute to health problems such as drug–drug interactions. Many CAM users believe that biomedical physicians are prejudiced against herbals and other traditional practices or that they know little about them. In some instances, reliance on traditional health care practices may lead to delay in seeking care and more severe illness when biomedical care is sought.

People in ethnic cultural groups may encounter a variety of barriers to obtaining care in the biomedical system, resulting in a preference for seeking care in traditional systems. Racial and cultural biases and inappropriate services, philosophical differences, language barriers, and a lack of knowledge of available biomedical services are some of the reasons given for not seeking care in the biomedical system. In addition, some members of ethnic cultural groups report "language discrimination," being treated unfairly because of their language or accent. As we will see in Chapter 20∞, members of the GLBT culture may experience discrimination from biomedical health care providers.

Some authors have noted that Eastern and Western systems of mental health care differ greatly due to their different philosophical traditions and conceptualizations of mental illness. Differences in interpersonal boundaries and language issues also complicate the use of conventional mental health services by members of some cultural groups. In addition, nonlinear thinking patterns typical of some cultural groups may be interpreted by Western practitioners as confusion or resistance to treatment, and culturally unfamiliar behaviors may be viewed as pathological. Similarly, key concepts (e.g., death, rape, suicide) may have significantly different meanings in different cultural contexts, resulting in different emotional responses. All of these factors may lead to inappropriate diagnoses and treatment approaches in the Western mental health tradition.

Another health system determinant involves expectations of interactions between clients and health care providers. In many ethnic cultural groups, as well as in the dominant U.S. and biomedical cultures, the provider is seen as dominant and the client as subordinate. In some respects, this expectation is changing as many members of the dominant U.S. culture gain

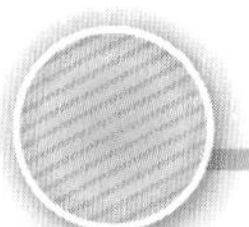

Global Perspectives

Decline of Traditional Medicine Use in China

Although traditional Chinese medicine is gaining greater acceptance and use in the United States, its use in China is declining. Some of the reasons for its decline are an increased emphasis on profit, decentralization, and movement to a fee-for-service and private insurance system for health care. In addition, there are a growing number of for-profit Western hospitals in China and greater emphasis on Western medicine in the education of younger providers. Another reason for the decline is the increasingly busy lifestyle of modern Chinese, who no longer have the time for frequent provider visits or preparation of herbal teas and other remedies. These pressures to move to a Westernized approach to health care are viewed by some as a threat to the cultural significance of traditional Chinese medicine, a reduction in the availability of low-cost services, and loss of a valuable source of care for major segments of the population (Burke, Wong, & Clayson, 2003). How might the principles of integrative health care discussed in this chapter help to prevent this loss?

FOCUSED ASSESSMENT Health System Determinants in Cultural Assessment

Perceptions of Health and Illness and Disease Causation

- How do members of the cultural group define health and illness? What do they perceive as the cause(s) of disease?
- How does the cultural group classify disease?

Health Practices

- What practices do members of the cultural group typically employ to promote health and prevent illness?
- What home remedies, if any, do members of cultural groups employ to treat health problems? For what problems are they used? How are they used?
- What over-the-counter remedies are used by the cultural group? For what and how are they used?
- What provider-prescribed medications and treatments are used by the cultural group? By whom are they prescribed? If therapies are prescribed by multiple providers, are all providers aware of this?
- What are the client's/cultural group's preferences with respect to the type of treatment modalities prescribed (e.g., massage, medications in liquid or tablet form)?
- What measures are used by the cultural group to deal with the consequences of long-term health problems (e.g., pain relief, mobility limitation)?
- Are any of the health practices or therapies employed by the cultural group potentially harmful?

Health Care Providers and Systems

- From whom do members of the cultural group seek advice on health promotion and illness prevention?
- From whom do members of the cultural group first seek assistance with health care problems?
- For what types of health issues is assistance sought by members of the cultural group?
- Do members of the cultural group seek assistance from different types of providers for different problems? If so, whom do they seek for what kinds of problems? What is the rationale for the types of providers selected?
- Who are the recognized providers of health care within the cultural group? What types of care do they provide? What is the extent of their use by members of the group?
- Do members of the cultural group voice a preference for providers with certain characteristics (e.g., nurse practitioners over physicians, providers of a specific gender, herbalists over biomedical providers)? If so, on what beliefs and attitudes are these preferences based?
- Are there barriers to the use of specific types of health care providers? If so, what are they?
- If members of the cultural group use multiple providers, are the providers aware of this? If not, why?

knowledge of health-related matters from the Internet and are exposed to marketing initiatives by health-related vendors such as pharmaceutical companies.

Members of some groups expect providers to spend time in casual conversation or even to share meals before addressing intimate health issues. In the biomedical culture, however, the focus is on obtaining health-related information rather than on observing social amenities. Similarly, health care providers are taught to withhold personal information, which may make it difficult for clients from other cultural groups to develop a trusting relationship. Differences in relationships between provider and client may lead members of some cultural groups to prefer traditional healers to professional providers. Some of the reasons for this preference may be perceptions of low risk in the interaction, an emphasis on high-touch interpersonal relationships, and a perception that traditional healers stimulate one's innate healing mechanisms rather than using chemicals and other approaches that may seem unnatural to the client (Jackson, 2010). Tips for a focused assessment of health system determinants of health in cultural groups are presented above.

As we have seen, cultural assessment includes exploration of factors in each of the six categories of determinants of health. A comprehensive tool for cultural assessment based on the determinants of health can be found on the student resources site.

Planning Culturally Congruent Care and Delivery Systems

Providers in all health systems should engage in culturally congruent care. Doing so requires that individual providers and health delivery systems emphasize cultural congruence with the populations served. The need for culturally appropriate care and care systems lies in the increasing diversity of populations throughout the world, the increasing provision of care in the home setting where cultural factors are more influential, and the increasing disparities in health status among many ethnic cultural minorities (OMH, 2013a). Benefits of culturally competent care include more appropriate and accurate diagnoses of health problems and better compliance with treatment recommendations, reduced delay in care seeking and use of services, enhanced client/provider communication, and greater compatibility of biomedical and traditional health care systems.

Cultural Competence

A number of terms are used to describe nursing and health care that take into account elements of clients' culture. These include cultural congruence, ethnic nursing care, culture care, and culturally congruent care. The term that will be used in this book is cultural competence or culturally and linguistically appropriate care. **Culturally congruent care** has been defined as "actions and decisions that fit with people's lifeways to support satisfying health care and promote well-being or dignified death" (McFarland, Mixer, Wehbe-Alamah, & Burk, 2012, p. 263). Campinha-Bacote's (2009) definition of cultural competence was presented earlier in this chapter. Another widely accepted definition of cultural competence is that advanced by the Office of Minority Health (2013b, para. 1), "a set of congruent behaviors, attitudes, and policies that come together in a system, agency, or among professionals that enables effective work in cross-cultural situations." Basically, culturally appropriate care is care that meets, or is congruent with, the expectations of the recipient whatever their cultural orientation.

Culturally appropriate care incorporates several components. These include cultural diversity, cultural awareness, cultural sensitivity, and cultural competence. Cultural diversity reflects the cultural differences that exist between health care professionals and a given population or cultural group (e.g., differences between "straight" health care providers and members of the GLBT population or between "able" providers and disabled clients). Cultural awareness encompasses providers' recognition of the influence of culture on health and health-related behaviors. Cultural sensitivity involves assuming a learner role with respect to the cultures of the populations served, and being willing to recognize cultural factors that influence our interactions with others. Cultural competence, on the other hand, is the ability to interact effectively with people from all backgrounds (Edmonton Seniors Council, n.d.).

Several models of cultural competence have been developed that delineate the critical elements of the concept. Two of these are Leininger's (2006) theory of culture care diversity and universality and Campinha-Bacote's (2009) process of cultural competence in health care services model. Leininger's theory addresses the similarities (universalities) and differences (diversities) among cultures and incorporates three modes of nursing activity, preservation and maintenance, accommodation/negotiation, and restructuring/repatterning (McFarland et al., 2012). In the preservation and maintenance mode, the population health nurse assists members of the cultural group to maintain and promote healthful beliefs and practices, often by incorporating them in the plan of care. In the accommodation/negotiation mode, the nurse assists the cultural group to adapt care delivery services or negotiate for culturally congruent care. When cultural beliefs and practices may be harmful to health, the nurse assists group members to restructure or repattern lifeways to more healthful ones. Restructuring and repatterning may also lead to changes in health professional behaviors or health care systems (Hulme, 2010).

A significant amount of repatterning has already occurred among many biomedical providers, resulting in a willingness to employ CAM in their practices. Similarly, repatterning has taken place in the insurance world, leading to coverage for some complementary and alternative therapies. As more such therapies are integrated into the biomedical system, it is anticipated that the system itself may be repatterned in ways that will change the overall delivery of care to a more humanistic, less mechanistic perspective.

Repatterning may also be warranted for members of ethnic cultural groups to be able to function effectively within the dominant culture. For example, there may be a need to explain host country laws regarding child care and neglect to immigrants whose cultural practice is to have older siblings care for younger children. The presence of lead and other toxic substances in some traditional remedies is another area in which repatterning may be required. For example, lead in Cambodian protective amulets has been linked to lead poisoning in young children (Healthy Homes and Lead Poisoning Prevention Bureau, 2011).

Clients from ethnic cultural groups, particularly immigrants, may need nursing assistance in dealing with intergenerational conflicts arising from different levels of acculturation among family members. For example, traditional food preparation may create difficulty, conflict, and guilt for younger women who do not have time to prepare traditional cultural dishes due to changes in their roles with the necessity to work outside the home to support their families. Culturally competent population health nurses could engage in interventions that could assist families experiencing these and other stresses of relocation.

Leininger's theory gives rise to the Sunrise model in which culture is situated within the group's worldview and social and cultural dimensions of life. The model also includes guidance for cultural assessment addressing elements of technological factors; religious and philosophical factors; kinship and social factors; cultural values, beliefs, and lifeways; political and legal factors; economic factors; and educational factors as they influence the health of the cultural group (McFarland et al., 2012).

Campinha-Bacote's model of the process of cultural competence in the delivery of health care services encompasses components of cultural desire, cultural awareness, cultural knowledge, cultural skill, and cultural encounters. The cultural desire component reflects the population health nurse's motivation to provide culturally congruent care. Cultural desire includes the concept of cultural humility, which involves "seeing the greatness in others and coming into the realization of the dignity and worth of others" (Campinha-Bacote, 2009, p. 49). Cultural awareness involves exploration of one's own biases, stereotypes, prejudices, and assumptions about those who differ from oneself. The element of cultural knowledge includes seeking information about the health-related beliefs and practices of the cultural group, incidence and prevalence of specific conditions within the group, and knowledge of treatment efficacy (e.g., rates of drug metabolism, responses to treatment). Cultural skill is the ability to collect data in a culturally sensitive way and to perform a culturally based physical assessment attending to differences in normal and abnormal findings. Finally, the process involves deliberately seeking opportunities for interactions with members of another cultural group in order to learn (Campinha-Bacote, 2009).

CHARACTERISTICS OF CULTURAL COMPETENCE. Provision of culturally congruent care requires the development of cultural competence on the part of individual health care providers and health care organizations. Individual cultural competence encompasses several characteristics. First among these is an awareness of one's own culturally determined perspectives without letting them influence one's interactions with others. Cultural competence is also characterized by knowledge and understanding of another culture and by acceptance of and respect for other cultures. The culturally competent health care provider does not assume that other cultures are similar to his or her own and is nonjudgmental in examining the beliefs, values, attitudes, and practices of other cultural groups. In addition, the competent provider displays an openness to and comfort with encounters with persons from other cultural heritages. Finally, cultural competence is characterized by a conscious process of adaptation of care to the cultural context (Purnell, 2012).

At the health system level, culturally and linguistically appropriate health care programs also display certain characteristic traits. These include a broad definition of culture beyond considerations of race, language, ethnicity, and recognition of value in clients' cultural heritage. Culturally competent systems are also characterized by a recognition of the complexities involved in language interpretation and an awareness of the need to consider linguistic variation within cultural groups (including professional cultures), cultural variation within language groups (e.g., among the multiple cultural groups that speak Spanish), and variation in literacy levels among members of a particular cultural group. Culturally competent systems of care facilitate learning between providers and communities and involve communities in defining and addressing their health care needs. They also foster interagency collaboration and take steps to institutionalize cultural competency within the system. Characteristics of cultural competence at the individual provider and health system levels are summarized in Table 5-2●. These characteristics are exemplified in adherence to the "National Standards for Culturally and Linguistically Appropriate Services (CLAS) in Health and Health Care" developed by the OMH (2013a). These standards are discussed in more detail below.

CHALLENGES IN DEVELOPING CULTURAL COMPETENCE. A number of challenges have been identified that may impede the development of cultural competence in individual providers or in health care systems. The first challenge is the recognition of clinical differences among cultural groups. Providers may be "culturally blind" and fail to recognize the differences among cultures (including biomedical culture) and the influence of culture on health and health care. Communication among cultural groups may also be a challenge in developing cultural competence, even among those that share a common language. The challenge in that case arises from differences in the way words are used, their particular meanings, and the interpretation of paralanguage and nonverbal aspects of communication. A third challenge is developing a sense of ethics and recognizing when it is appropriate to incorporate elements of culture in the plan of care and when those elements of culture may be harmful and should be eliminated or modified. Developing trust between members of a cultural group and those of the biomedical culture may be another challenge in developing cultural competence. As we will see in Chapter 20∞, many members of the gay, lesbian, bisexual, and transgender cultures have reason to distrust health care providers. Distrust of biomedical providers is also a relatively common occurrence among members of some other cultural groups.

Cultural competence may also be impeded by stereotypes held by providers. Development of culture-specific knowledge has both benefits and disadvantages. On the plus side, knowledge of other cultures leads to recognition of cultural differences, opens the mind to alternative viewpoints, and serves as a starting point for cultural assessment of individual clients or subgroups within the population. However, such knowledge may give providers a false sense of security in working with members of other cultures and may lead to stereotyping as discussed earlier. Stereotyping is a useful cognitive strategy for organizing information about the complex world in which we live, and is not necessarily associated with negative attitudes

TABLE 5-2 Individual and System-Level Characteristics of Cultural Competence

Individual Characteristics	System Characteristics
• Awareness of personal perspectives • Knowledge and understanding of other cultures • Not assuming similarity to one's own culture • Nonjudgmental view of other cultures • Openness to and comfort with cultural encounters • Conscious adaptation of care to the cultural context	• Broad definition of culture • Value attributed to cultural beliefs • Recognition of complexity in language interpretation • Facilitation of learning between providers and cultural communities • Involvement of cultural communities in defining and addressing health needs • Interagency collaboration • Institutionalization of cultural competence

toward members of other cultural groups. It is when providers fail to assess individuals or segments of a population group to see how closely they conform to beliefs and behaviors typical of the cultural group that stereotyping interferes with culturally competent care.

Other barriers to the provision of culturally competent care include viewing cultures as "them," not "me," without recognizing the influence of culture on one's own life; confusing race, culture, and ethnicity; and misdiagnosing ethnic-specific medical concerns due to lack of knowledge or communication difficulties. Cultural mismatches may also impede culturally competent care. Ideally, both an ethnic match and a language match exist between the provider and the client. An ethnic match occurs when both the client and the provider have the same ethnic identity. Given the dearth of biomedical providers from many ethnic cultural minority groups, ethnic matches are often difficult to obtain. In a language match, the client's native language is one in which the provider is fluent. Ethnic and language matches seem to be particularly important in the area of mental health.

DESIGNING CULTURALLY AND LINGUISTICALLY APPROPRIATE HEALTH CARE DELIVERY SYSTEMS. Organizations, like individuals and other groups, have their own distinct culture. **Organizational culture** is the shared assumptions, beliefs, and values that result in shared behavioral norms and expectations for members of the organization. The organizational cultures of health care agencies and systems may make it more or less difficult for providers to engage in culturally congruent care.

In addition to providing culturally and linguistically appropriate care for individual clients, families, and population groups, population health nurses can contribute to the development of culturally appropriate health care delivery systems. In 2000, the Office of Minority Health developed the National Standards for Culturally and Linguistically Appropriate Services, better known as the CLAS standards, to guide health care organizations in providing culturally competent care. Those standards were revised and enhanced in 2013 (OMH, 2013a), and are summarized in Table 5-3●.

TABLE 5-3 National Standards for Culturally and Linguistically Appropriate Services (CLAS)

Focus	Related Standards
Principal Standard	• Provide effective, equitable, understandable, and respectful quality care and services that are responsive to diverse cultural health beliefs and practices, preferred languages, health literacy, and other communication needs.
Governance, leadership, workforce	• Advance and sustain organizational leadership that promotes CLAS and health equity through policy, practices, and allocated resources. • Recruit, promote, and support a culturally and linguistically diverse governance, leadership, and workforce that are responsive to the population in the service area. • Educate and train governance, leadership, and workforce in culturally and linguistically appropriate policies and practices on an ongoing basis.
Communication and language assistance	• Offer language assistance to individuals who have limited English proficiency and/or other communication needs, at no cost to them, to facilitate timely access to all health care and services. • Inform all individuals of the availability of language assistance services clearly and in their preferred language, verbally and in writing. • Ensure the competence of individuals providing language assistance, recognizing that the use of untrained individuals and/or minors as interpreters should be avoided. • Provide easy to understand print and multimedia materials and signage in the languages commonly used by the populations in the service area.
Engagement, continuous improvement, and accountability	• Establish culturally and linguistically appropriate goals, policies, and management accountability, and infuse them throughout the organization's planning and operations. • Conduct ongoing assessments of the organization's CLAS-related activities and integrate CLAS-related measures into measurement and quality improvement activities. • Collect and maintain accurate and reliable demographic data to monitor and evaluate the impact of CLAS on health equity and outcomes and to inform service delivery. • Conduct regular assessments of community health assets and needs and use the results to plan and implement services that respond to the cultural and linguistic diversity of populations in the service area. • Partner with the community to design, implement, and evaluate policies, practices, and services to ensure cultural and linguistic appropriateness. • Create conflict and grievance resolution processes that are culturally and linguistically appropriate to identify, prevent, and resolve conflicts or complaints. • Communicate the organization's progress in implementing and sustaining CLAS to all stakeholders, constituents, and the general public.

Source: Office of Minority Health. (2013a). *National standards for culturally and linguistically appropriate services (CLAS) in health and health care: A blueprint for advancing and sustaining CLAS policy and practice.* Retrieved from https://www.thinkculturalhealth.hhs.gov/pdfs/EnhancedCLASStandardsBlueprint.pdf

Movement toward cultural proficiency and provision of culturally and linguistically appropriate care requires that a health system provide care with an understanding of and respect for culture and its influences on health and that the care provided incorporates community participation in its planning and delivery. In addition, it requires staff who respect the cultures of others and who reflect and respond to the values and demographics of the population served. Finally, movement toward cultural proficiency and competent care requires policies that assure a consistent response to cultural differences in the population served and continual improvement and accountability (OMH, 2013a). For further information about the CLAS standards, see the *External Resources* section of the student resources site.

The incorporation of CAM into biomedical practice through "integrative medicine" is another means providing culturally and linguistically appropriate health care services. **Integrative medicine** is defined by the American Association of Integrative Medicine (AAIM, 2011) as "health care that views the patient as the most important member of the medical team and applies all safe and effective therapies without subservience to any one school of medical thought." The intent of integrative medicine is to deal with symptoms of illness as well as causes, whether those causes are mental, physical, or spiritual or a combination of these, through the best possible application of conventional and traditional therapies.

The World Health Organization's (WHO) *Traditional Medicines Strategy 2002–2005* identified four areas for action to promote the integration of CAM into biomedicine. Although these strategies were developed several years ago, they continue to be relevant to population health nursing practice. The action areas identified included strategies to address needs related to policy; safety, efficacy, and quality; access; and rational use (WHO, 2002). Table 5-4● highlights each strategy and the related actions needed for effective integration of CAM into biomedical practice.

A 2005 report by the "Institute of Medicine, 2005" suggested a systematic process for evaluating the appropriateness of incorporating CAM into biomedical health systems. The process should begin with a determination of the persons responsible for gathering information about various forms of CAM and for making incorporation decisions. Both the informal and formal mandates affecting the system should be examined, as should the system's mission and values and their congruence with various forms of CAM. In addition, an assessment of the internal and external environments as they affect incorporation of CAM in the institution should also be conducted. For example, are qualified practitioners of desired CAM available to the system? What forms of CAM are covered by insurance plans among the system's clientele? All of this information can lead to an informed decision on whether or not to incorporate CAM in the setting.

Education regarding appropriate and inappropriate use of CAM is another way in which population health nurses may assist with repatterning for members of ethnic cultural groups as well as members of the dominant culture. WHO (2004) identified several considerations in educating the public regarding safe and effective use of CAM that are still appropriate for population health nursing care. Categories of education

TABLE 5-4 WHO-Defined Areas for Action in Integrating CAM in Biomedical Practice

Area for Action	Expected Outcomes
Policy	Increased government support for and policies related to CAM Integration of relevant CAM into national health care systems Preservation of indigenous knowledge of CAM
Safety, efficacy, quality	Increased knowledge of CAM through exchange of accurate information Review of research on use of CAM Selective support for clinical research on CAM Regulation of herbal medicines Safety monitoring of herbals, other CAM products, and practices Development of guidelines for evaluating the safety, efficacy, and quality of CAM Development of criteria for evidence-based data related to CAM
Access	Development of criteria and indicators to measure cost-effectiveness of and access to CAM Official recognition of CAM providers Increased provision of CAM through national health systems Increased number of national organizations of CAM providers Development of guidelines for good agricultural practice related to medicinal plants
Rational use	Training in CAM therapies for allopathic providers Training in basic primary care practice for CAM practitioners Provision of reliable consumer information on proper use of CAM Improved communication between CAM providers and conventional health care professionals

Source: World Health Organization. (2002). *WHO traditional medicine strategy: 2002–2005.* Retrieved from http://apps.who.int/medicinedocs/en/d/Js2297e/8.1.html#Js2297e.8.1

needed include general considerations, such as the need to be informed consumers and for both CAM and biomedical providers to be conversant with CAM; knowledge of how to find reliable information; information about specific therapies; information regarding providers; and information about the costs of and insurance coverage for CAM. Specific areas of public education related to CAM are delineated in the client education box at right.

Population health nurses can be involved in the development of culturally and linguistically appropriate health care services in a number of ways. If they are employed in a particular organization that needs to adopt more culturally appropriate approaches to health care, they can assess current practices and the barriers to culturally and linguistically appropriate care that they represent. They can also be involved in the development of policies and procedures that promote cultural competence in the organization. In addition, population health nurses can help the agency conduct an assessment of the cultural groups served and assist in the development of agency–community partnerships to better meet the needs of the population. If the nurse is not an employee of an agency that needs to improve the cultural congruence of its services, he or she can bring to the attention of agency administrators the concerns of members of local cultural groups regarding the services provided. Community assessment and policy development may also be areas of involvement for nonemployee population health nurses. The process used in the development of culturally and linguistically appropriate health care systems is essentially the same process used to develop any kind of health care program discussed in Chapter 15∞.

CLIENT EDUCATION

Safe Use of Complementary and Alternative Medicine

General Considerations

- Use of CAM by informed consumers, knowledgeable about appropriate uses and safety considerations
- Extent of provider knowledge regarding CAM including knowledge of CAM use by particular clients

Finding and Identifying Reliable Information Regarding CAM

- Credibility and objectivity of information sources
- Purpose of the information source (e.g., if product sales are the primary purpose, information may be slanted)
- Relevance and accuracy of information presented
- Frequency with which information is updated

Information Regarding Specific Therapies

- Claims and evidence supporting them
- Product quality information regarding active ingredients, recognition of quality standards, storage information, expiration date, quality control of raw materials
- Precautions for use
- Adverse events/potential toxicity
- Interactions and contraindications
- Information regarding dose, time, frequency, duration, method of administration, preparation instructions
- Safety for use with children, pregnant women, the elderly

Information Regarding CAM Practitioners

- Qualifications for practice, education, and experience related to the therapy
- Certification, if relevant
- Surveillance and monitoring

Cost/Insurance Coverage

- Typical costs of CAM
- What forms of CAM are covered under insurance

Source: World Health Organization. (2004). *Guidelines on developing consumer information on proper use of traditional, complementary and alternative medicine.* Geneva, Switzerland: Author.

Evaluating Cultural Competence

Evaluation of care provided to clients from another cultural group should focus on both the outcomes of care and the delivery processes employed. In terms of outcomes, nurses should examine indicators of health status for individual clients and for subcultural groups. For example, has the nurse been able to improve the client's nutritional status without changing his or her cultural dietary pattern? Has the frequency of successful pregnancy outcomes been increased for members of a given cultural group? Have inappropriate biomedical practices been modified to promote better care?

Health care delivery systems should also be examined in terms of their cultural congruence. The assessment profile discussed earlier provides direction for assessing the cultural congruence of care provided by health care delivery systems. At the population level, the extent to which disparities in health among culturally diverse populations have been decreased is another way of evaluating the cultural congruence of the national health care system. A particular health system could look also at the extent of disparities among its clientele as one measure of its cultural competence.

CHAPTER RECAP

Many groups display unique cultural beliefs, values, and behavior, including the dominant U.S. and biomedical cultures as well as other groups such as ethnic cultural groups and members of the GLBT and disabled populations. Culture influences health in a variety of ways, both direct and indirect. Culture affects definitions of health and illness within a population group and influences how health and illness are viewed, as well as the value of health to members of the population. Culture also influences how population groups seek to promote health and prevent and deal with health problems.

Cultural assessment can be directed by the six categories of determinants of health included in the population health nursing model. Culturally congruent care may include preserving elements of a cultural heritage, negotiation and accommodation of clients' cultures or that of the biomedical community, or repatterning to eliminate cultural practices that are harmful to health. Culturally congruent health care occurs at the individual client/family level and in the design of health care systems to provide care that is congruent with the values and expectations of the client population.

CASE STUDY Culture and Care

Apple Valley is a rural agricultural community approximately 100 miles from the U.S.–Mexico border. Because of the mild climate, there are crops to be tended and harvested much of the year, and many Latino migrant workers are involved in this work. Although there is work for a significant portion of the year, many of the laborers have extended families still in Mexico. They frequently work for several months, then return to Mexico to share their earnings and visit family members. When they return to the United States, they often come as nuclear family groups, and both parents work in the fields. Children may or may not attend school while in Apple Valley.

There are high infant and maternal mortality rates among this group as the women do not usually receive care during their pregnancies. In part, this is because of the high cost of care, but it also results from lack of facility with English and inability to take time from work to receive care. Although most of the workers are legal immigrants, they are not eligible for financial assistance or care at the local health department prenatal clinic. Complicated deliveries often occur in the local hospital, however, and contribute to the burden of "uncompensated care" since the migrant families are usually unable to pay the hospital bills. According to some of the workers, there is a Latino woman living year round in Apple Valley who serves as a midwife for some of the women.

1. What cultural factors are operating in this situation? What other circumstances, not necessarily cultural in origin, complicate the situation?
2. What interventions by the population health nurse could help reduce the infant and maternal mortality rates?
3. Who else should be involved in efforts to resolve the problem? Why?
4. How could the population health nurse motivate involvement by other segments of the population?

REFERENCES

Abdel-Khalek, A. M. (2009). Religiosity, subjective well-being, and depression in Saudi children and adolescents. *Religion, & Culture, 12*, 803–815. doi:10.1080/13674670903006755

Acculturation. (n.d.). In *Dictionary of cross-cultural terminology/intercultural terminology*. Retrieved from http://www.dot-connect.com/Dictionary_of_Cross-Cultural_terminology_Inter_cultural_terminology.html

American Association of Integrative Medicine. (2011). *About integrative medicine*. Retrieved from http://www.aaimedicine.com/about/

American Association of Naturopathic Medicine. (2011). *What is naturopathic medicine?* Retrieved from http://www.naturopathic.org/content.asp?contentid=59

American Chiropractic Association. (2014a). *History of chiropractic care*. Retrieved from http://www.acatoday.org/level3_css.cfm?T1ID=13&T2ID=61&T3ID=149

American Chiropractic Association. (2014b). *What is chiropractic?* Retrieved from http://www.acatoday.org/level2_css.cfm?T1ID=13&T2ID=61

Baron-Epel, O., Friedman, N., & Lernau, O. (2009). Fatalism and mammography in a multicultural population. *Oncology Nursing Forum, 36*, 353–361.

Burke, A., Wong, Y., & Clayson, Z. (2003). Traditional medicine in China today: Implications for indigenous health systems in a modern world. *American Journal of Public Health, 93*, 1082–1083.

Campinha-Bacote, J. (2009). A culturally competent model of care for African Americans. *Urologic Nursing, 29*(1), 49–54.

Center for Health and Healing. (n.d.). *Native American medicine*. Retrieved from http://www.healthandhealingny.org/tradition_healing/native.html

Centers for Disease Control and Prevention. (2011). *National diabetes fact sheet: National estimates and general information on diabetes and prediabetes in the United States, 2011*. Retrieved from http://www.cdc.gov/diabetes/pubs/estimates11.htm#4

Ciftci, A., Jones, N., & Corrigan, P. W. (2013). Mental health stigma in the Muslim community. *Journal of Muslim Mental Health, 7*, 17–32. permalink: http://hdl.handle.net/2027/spo.10381607.0007.102

Clark, M. J., & Natipagon-Shah, B. (2008). Thai American women's perceptions regarding mammography participation. *Public Health Nursing, 25*, 212–220.

Crowley-Matoka, M., Saha, S., Dobscha, S. K., & Burgess, D. J. (2009). Problems of quality and equity in pain management: Exploring the role of biomedical culture. *Pain Management, 10*, 1312–1324.

Dance of the Deer Foundation Center for Shamanic Studies. (2014). *What is shamanism?*. Retrieved from http://www.shamanism.com/what-is-shamanism/

Dugdale, D. C., & Mason, J. R. (2010). *Glucose-6-phosphate dehydrogenase deficiency*. Retrieved from http://www.nlm.nih.gov/medlineplus/ency/article/000528.htm

Edmonton Seniors Coordinating Council. (n.d.). *Glossary of cross cultural terms*. Retrieved from http://www.seniorscouncil.net/uploads/files/Issues/Mobilizing_Action_Report/Glossary%20of%20Cross%20Cultural%20Terms.pdf

Fatalism. (n.d.). *In Merriam-Webster's online dictionary* (11th ed.). Retrieved from www.merriam-webster.com/dictionary/fatalism

Green, B. L. (2010). Culture is treatment: Considering pedagogy in the care of aboriginal people. *Journal of Psychosocial Nursing, 48*(7), 27–34. doi:10.3928/02793695-20100504-04

Greenwood, S. (2009). *The anthropology of magic*. New York, NY: Berg.

Gupta, V. B. (2010). Impact of culture on healthcare seeking behavior of Asian Indians. *Journal of Cultural Diversity, 17*, 13–19.

Health culture. (n.d.). *Free online dictionary*. Retrieved from http://medical-dictionary.thefreedictionary.com/health+culture

Healthy Homes and Lead Poisoning Prevention Bureau. (2011). Lead poisoning of a child associated with use of a Cambodian amulet—New York City, 2009. *Morbidity and Mortality Weekly Report, 60*, 69–71.

Hoogbruin, A. (2011). Complementary and alternative therapy (CAT) use and highly active retroviral therapy (HAART): Current evidence in the literature, 2000–2009. *Journal of Clinical Nursing, 20*, 925–939.

Hulme, P. A. (2010). Cultural considerations in evidence-based practice. *Journal of Transcultural Nursing, 21*, 271–280.

Inglehart, R., & Welzel, C. (n.d.). *The WVS cultural map of the world*. Retrieved from http://www.worldvaluessurvey.org/wvs/articles/folder_published/article_base_54

Inglehart, R., & Welzel, C. (2010). Changing mass priorities: The link between modernization and democracy. *Perspectives on Politics, 8*, 551–567. doi:10.1017/S1537592710001258

Institute of Medicine. (2005). *Complementary and alternative medicine in the United States*. Washington, DC: Author.

Isaac, D. (2013). Culture-bound syndromes in mental health: A discussion paper. *Journal of Psychiatric and Mental Health Nursing, 20*, 355–361. doi: 10.1111/jpm.12016

Jackson, C. (2010, May–June). Evidence-based practice: Pushback from a holistic perspective. *Holistic Nursing Practice*, pp. 120–124.

Juang, L. P., & Alvarez, A. A. (2010). Discrimination and adjustment among Chinese American adolescents: Family conflict and family cohesion as vulnerability and protective factors. *American Journal of Public Health, 100*, 2403–2408. doi:10.2105/AJPH.2009.185959

Katme, A. M. (2009). *Foodandfaith fact files – Islam*. Retrieved from permalink: http://www.faithandfood.com/Islam.php

Keeping kosher: Jewish dietary laws. (n.d.). Retrieved from http://www.religionfacts.com/judaism/practices/kosher.htm

Leininger, M. M. (2006). Culture care diversity and universality theory and evolution of the ethnonursing method. In M. M. Leininger & M. R. McFarland (Eds.), *Culture care diversity and universality: A worldwide theory of nursing* (2nd ed., pp. 1–41). Sudbury, MA: Jones and Bartlett.

Magda, R. (2010). Lifting the language barrier. *Advance for Nurses, 7*(8), 8–9.

McFarland, M. R., Mixer S. J., Webhe-Alamah, H., & Burk, R. (2012). Ethnonursing: A qualitative research method for studying culturally competent care across disciplines. *International Journal of Qualitative Methods, 11*, 259–279.

McLaurin, J. A. (2002). Assimilation, acculturation, and alternative medicines. *MCN Streamline: The Migrant Health News Source, 8*(6), 1–3.

Mhame, P. P., Busia, K., & Kasilo, M. J. (2010). *Clinical practices of African traditional medicine*. Retrieved from https://www.aho.afro.who.int/en/ahm/issue/13/reports/clinical-practices-african-traditional-medicine

National Alliance on Mental Illness. (2013). *What is anorexia nervosa?* Retrieved from http://www.nami.org/Template.cfm?Section=By_Illness&template=/ContentManagement/ContentDisplay.cfm&ContentID=7409

National Cancer Institute. (2012). *Spiritual assessment*. Retrieved from http://www.cancer.gov/cancertopics/pdq/supportivecare/spirituality/Patient/page3

National Center for Complementary and Alternative Medicine. (2008). *The use of complementary and alternative medicine in the United States*. Retrieved from http://nccam.nih.gov/news/camstats/2007/camsurvey_fs1.htm

National Center for Complementary and Alternative Medicine. (2012a). *Acupuncture: An introduction*. Retrieved from http://nccam.nih.gov/health/acupuncture/introduction.htm

National Center for Complementary and Alternative Medicine. (2012b). *CAM basics: What is complementary and alternative medicine?* Retrieved from http://nccam.nih.gov/sites/nccam.nih.gov/files/D347_05-25-2012.pdf

National Center for Complementary and Alternative Medicine. (2012c). *Naturopathy: An introduction*. Retrieved from http://nccam.nih.gov/health/naturopathy/naturopathyintro.htm

National Center for Complementary and Alternative Medicine. (2012d). *Terms related to complementary and alternative medicine*. Retrieved from http://nccam.nih.gov/health/providers/camterms.htm

National Center for Complementary and Alternative Medicine. (2013a). *Ayurvedic medicine: An introduction*. Retrieved from http://nccam.nih.gov/health/ayurveda/introduction.htm

National Center for Complementary and Alternative Medicine. (2013b). *Complementary, alternative, or integrative health: What's in a name?*. Retrieved from http://nccam.nih.gov/health/whatiscam

National Center for Complementary and Alternative Medicine. (2013c). *Homeopathy: An introduction*. Retrieved from http://nccam.nih.gov/health/homeopathy

National Center for Complementary and Alternative Medicine. (2013d). *Paying for complementary health approaches*. Retrieved from http://nccam.nih.gov/health/financial/

National Center for Complementary and Alternative Medicine. (2013e). *Traditional Chinese medicine: An introduction*. Retrieved from http://nccam.nih.gov/health/whatiscam/chinesemed.htm

National Center for Education Statistics. (2012). *PIAAC 2012 results.* Retrieved from http://nces.ed.gov/surveys/piaac/results/summary.aspx

Natural Medicines Comprehensive Database. (2012). *Pennyroyal.* Retrieved from http://www.nlm.nih.gov/medlineplus/druginfo/natural/480.html

Office of Minority Health. (2013a). *National standards for culturally and linguistically appropriate services (CLAS) in health and health care: A blueprint for advancing and sustaining CLAS policy and practice.* Retrieved from https://www.thinkculturalhealth.hhs.gov/pdfs/EnhancedCLASStandardsBlueprint.pdf

Office of Minority Health. (2013b). *What is cultural competency?* Retrieved from http://minorityhealth.hhs.gov/templates/browse.aspx?lvl=2&lvlid=11

Okulicz-Kozaryn, A. (2010). Religiosity and life satisfaction across nations. *Mental Health, Religion, & Culture, 13,* 155–169. doi:10.1080/13674670903273801

Partnership for the Public's Health. (n.d.). *Tips and tools: Working effectively across languages.* Oakland, CA: Author.

Pascoe, E. A., & Smart, R. L. (2009). Perceived discrimination and health: A meta-analytic review. *Psychological Bulletin, 135,* 531–554. doi: 10.1037/a0016059

Pflaum, J. S. (1996). *Helper woman: A biography of Elinor Delight Gregg* (Unpublished doctoral dissertation). University of San Diego, San Diego, CA.

Purnell, L. D. (2012). *Transcultural health care: A culturally competent approach* (4th ed.). Philadelphia, PA: F. A. Davis.

Rabinowitz, Y. G., Mausbach, B. T., Atkinson, P. J., & Gallagher-Thompson, D. (2009). The relationship between religiosity and health behaviors in female care givers of older adults with dementia. *Aging & Mental Health, 13,* 788–798. doi:10.1080/13607860903046446

Sanseeha, L., Chontawan, R., Sethabouppha, H., Disayavanish, C., & Turale, S. (2009). Illness perspectives of Thais diagnosed with schizophrenia. *Nursing and Health Sciences, 11,* 306–311. doi:10.1111/j.1442-2018.2009.00474.x

Singh Balhara, Y. P. (2011). Culture-bound syndrome: Has it found its right niche? *Indian Journal of Psychological Medicine, 33,* 210–215. doi: 10.4103/0253-7176.92055

Sorkin, D. H., Ngo-Metzger, Q., & De Alba, I. (2010). Racial and ethnic discrimination in health care: Impact on perceived quality of care. *Journal of General Internal Medicine, 25,* 390–396. doi: 10.1007/s11606-010-1257-5

Spector, R. E. (2012). *Cultural diversity in health and illness* (8th ed.). Upper Saddle River, NJ: Prentice Hall.

Spencer, M., S., Chen, J., Gee, G. C., Fabian, C. G., & Takeuchi, D. T. (2010). Discrimination and mental health—Related services use in a national study of Asian Americans. *American Journal of Public Health, 100,* 2397–2402. doi:10.2105/AJPH.2009.176321

Tang, G., Lanza, O., Rodriguez, F. M., & Chang, A. (2011). The Kaiser Permante Clinician Cultural and Linguistic Assessment Initiative: Research and development in patient-provider language concordance. *American Journal of Public Health, 101,* 205–208. doi:10.2105/AJPH.2009.177055

Ulmer, C., McFadden, B., & Nerenz, D. R. (Eds.). (2009). *Race, ethnicity, and language data: Standardization for healthcare quality improvement.* Retrieved from http://www.nap.edu/catalog/12696.html

U.S. Census Bureau. (2013a). *Statistical abstract of the United State 2012s: Components of population change.* Retrieved from https://www.census.gov/compendia/statab/2012/tables/12s0005.pdf

U.S. Census Bureau. (2013b). *Statistical abstract of the United States, 2012: Foreign-born population—selected characteristic by region of origin: 2010.* Retrieved from https://www.census.gov/compendia/statab/2012/tables/12s0041.pdf

U.S. Census Bureau. (2013c). *Statistical abstract of the United States, 2012: Native and foreign-born population by selected characteristics: 2010.* Retrieved from https://www.census.gov/compendia/statab/2012/tables/12s0040.pdf

U.S. Census Bureau. (2013d). *2011 Statistical abstract of the United States, 2012: Languages spoken at home.* Retrieved from https://www.census.gov/compendia/statab/2012/tables/12s0053.pdf

U.S. Census Bureau. (2013e). *Statistical abstract of the United States, 2012: Population: Elderly, Selected characteristics of racial groups and Hispanic or Latino population, 2009.* Retrieved from https://www.census.gov/compendia/statab/2012/tables/12s0036.pdf

U.S. Census Bureau. (2013f). *Statistical Abstract of the United States, 2012: Resident population by sex, race, and Hispanic origin status: 2000 to 2009.* Retrieved from https://www.census.gov/compendia/statab/2012/tables/12s0006.pdf

U.S. Census Bureau. (2013g). Statistical Abstract of the United States, 2012: Resident population projections by race, and Hispanic origin status, and age: 2010 and 2015. Retrieved from https://www.census.gov/compendia/statab/2012/tables/12s0012.pdf

U.S. Census Bureau, American Fact Finder. (2012). *Languages spoken at home?* Retrieved from http://factfinder2.census.gov/faces/tableservices/jsf/pages/productview.xhtml?pid=ACS_12_1YR_S1601&prodType=table

U.S. Department of Health and Human Services. (2013). *Health communication and health information technology.* Retrieved from http://www.healthypeople.gov/2020/topicsobjectives2020/overview.aspx?topicid=18

van Betten, P. T., & Moriarty, M. (2004). *Nursing illuminations: A book of days.* St Louis, MO: Mosby.

Wehbe-Alamah, H. (2008). Bridging generic and professional care practices for Muslim patients through use of Leininger's culture care model. *Contemporary Nurse, 28,* 83–97.

World Health Organization. (2002). *WHO traditional medicine strategy: 2002-2005.* Retrieved from http://apps.who.int/medicinedocs/en/d/Js2297e/8.1.html#Js2297e.8.1

World Health Organization. (2004). *Guidelines on developing consumer information on proper use of traditional, complementary and alternative medicine.* Geneva, Switzerland: Author.

World Health Organization. (2009). *Health Promotion Track 2: Health literacy and health behavior.* 7th global conference on health promotion. Retrieved from http://www.who.int/healthpromotion/conferences/7gchp/track2/en/index.html

Yang, H., Tranulis, C., & Freudenreich, O. (2009). Keeping culture-bound syndromes in cultural context: The case of koro. *International Journal of Culture and Mental Health, 2,* 86–91. doi:10.1080/03637750902792964

Yeung, A., Shyu, I., Fisher, L., Wu, S., Yang, H., & Fava, M. (2010). Culturally sensitive collaborative treatment for depressed Chinese Americans in primary care. *American Journal of Public Health, 100,* 2397–2402. doi:10.2105/AJPH.2009.184911

CHAPTER

6 Economic Influences on Population Health

Learning Outcomes

After reading this chapter, you should be able to:

1. Analyze the interrelationships among economic conditions, health care services, and health status.
2. Discuss factors contributing to escalating health care costs.
3. Discuss the effects of economic factors on the provision of public health services.
4. Analyze the effects of selected health care reimbursement mechanisms.
5. Distinguish among selected approaches to financing health care services.

Key Terms

assignment
block grant
capitation
charity care
consumer price index (CPI)
copayment
cost shifting
deductible
devolution
economics
health disparity
limiting charge
managed care organization (MCO)
medigap plans
pay-for-performance reimbursement
per capita expenditures
per diem payment
premiums
prospective reimbursement
reimbursement
Resource-Based Relative Value Scale (RBRVS)
retrospective reimbursement
uncompensated care

Advocacy Then

Establishing a "Shoestring" Clinic

Economic issues related to access to health care are a continuing problem in American Society and were part of the impetus for such developments as the Henry Street Settlement. In much of the nation, these issues have continued to undermine the health of the population, and various strategies have been undertaken to address them.

Upper East Tennessee is on the edge of the Appalachian region and shares a number of features of that region, including lack of access to health care for a significant portion of the population. Awareness of this need prompted population health nursing students and faculty to create a weekly "clinic" to meet the health care needs of low-income residents of a federal housing project. The clinic was first held in a recreation room at the housing project, but this proved untenable because the landlord was not willing to permit regular use of the room. The clinic was moved to rooms provided by a nearby church, and members of the congregation became part of its clientele. Clinic services included health histories and physical examinations, blood pressure monitoring, health education, and referral for needed health care services.

During the academic year, the clinic was staffed 1 day a week by population health nursing faculty and students. Faculty members continued to staff the clinic during breaks and over the summer to assure continuity of services. Students were involved in planning the services and developing a record system, forms, and referral contacts in the larger community. In addition to the weekly clinic, students and faculty made home visits to clients needing additional follow-up. Local physicians were contacted to inform them of the availability of the clinic for low-income clients who needed monitoring or health education. Several physicians took advantage of the services to request follow-up for their clients regarding issues of medication compliance or health education.

Although the clinic was initiated in the 1980s, long before the days of Health Insurance Portability and Accountability Act (HIPAA), strict measures were taken to promote client confidentiality. Client records (and equipment) were not left at the clinic site, but were locked in the trunk of one faculty member's car and transported to the site each week. Over the course of several years, several hundred clients were seen and multiple referrals were initiated to obtain low cost services for clients in need of them.

Advocacy Now

Promoting a Living Wage

A community needs assessment conducted by a collaborative of community agencies and residents and coordinated by a population health nurse indicated that low salaries were a significant influence on the health status of the community. After additional data gathering, the members of the collaborative initiated a campaign to promote a living wage for as large a segment of the population as possible. As a result of their efforts, a living wage ordinance was passed by the city. The ordinance required payment of a living wage, approximately three times the minimum wage level in the state, to all city employees. In addition, all businesses that contracted with the city were required to guarantee the same living wage to their employees before submitting bids for contract services. Although the ordinance did not cover the entire population, it provided an adequate income for a large proportion of the city's residents.

Economics can be defined as the way in which a society distributes its resources to address human wants and needs. Scarcity results when there are insufficient resources to satisfy the wants and desires of the population, and economics determines how those scarce resources will be distributed among the population. Currently, the federal government and the states are experiencing an economic crisis that affects the health of the population as well as the health care services that are provided. This crisis is the result of several factors, including recent tax cuts, poor economic performance, and increased expenditures in areas such as defense and national security. In 2010, for example, federal spending related to national defense was more than twice the funds spent on all nondefense activities (U.S. Census Bureau, 2013). These factors are unlikely to change in the near future for a number of reasons. Congress is unlikely to reduce federal spending and likely to extend tax cuts under pressure from many constituencies. These factors will maintain expenditures while reducing the revenues that could fund them. Although tax cuts and low interest rates will stimulate the economy in the short run, they are likely to cause a long-term imbalance, leading to increasing deficits, lower rates of national savings, higher interest rates, and a slowed economy as well as reductions in government-supported services. All of these factors will lead to a greater scarcity of health resources and more severe effects on the health of the population.

When we consider the economic context of health, we often think of the effects of poverty on health status or the increasing cost of health care. However, there are many different aspects to the economic context in which population health nursing takes place. The two major considerations in this area are the interrelationships between economics and health and the financing of health care services. Each of these aspects will be discussed here.

Economics and Health—The Interrelationships

Three fundamental economic principles must be considered in examining the effects of economic conditions on health and health care services. The first principle is that resources are always more limited than what is needed for desired levels of consumption. Second, resources have alternative uses. Third, different people will have differing ideas as to what those uses should be. Based on these principles, the basic question related to health care economics is how limited resources should be used. What types of health services should consume the resources available?

The interrelationships among economic factors and health status are many and varied. In this chapter, we will discuss three specific relationships: (a) the relationship between health and societal productivity and stability, (b) health care spending and rising costs, and (c) the effects of socioeconomic factors on health status.

Societal Productivity and Stability

As we noted earlier, we often think of the effects of economic factors on health status. What we tend to forget, however, is that health also affects a nation's economic welfare. A healthy population is more productive than an unhealthy one and is better able to learn and to use education effectively to increase society's overall productivity. When people are unable to work due to health deficiencies, society loses their productive capability. In addition, the productive capacity of other family members may also be lost. For example, diseases leading to disability result in lost productivity for those affected and for family members who must leave work to care for them.

Poverty and ill health lead to lower income and slowed economic growth as well as social instability and conflict. Conversely, nations with strong economies are better able to afford health care and other determinants of health.

Health care programs may also have a more direct effect on the economy than that seen in increased capacity for production. For example, state Medicaid programs generate revenue for states beyond the costs of the programs. This revenue comes from a number of sources, including federal block grants that would otherwise not come to the states, new business, and new jobs. A **block grant** is a lump sum made available to the states by the federal government to be used as each state sees fit within certain broadly defined parameters. Similarly, health care services in general generate revenues that support the overall economy.

Health Care Spending

The amount of money spent on health care services in the United States has been increasing at an alarming rate for the last several years. For example, national personal health care expenditures increased from $27.3 billion in 1960 to nearly $2.5 trillion in 2009 (U.S. Census Bureau, 2013). Health spending is expected to continue to grow by an average rate of 6.2% per year from 2015 through 2022 (Centers for Medicare and Medicaid Services [CMS], 2014b).

Overall, health care spending has risen from 5% of the gross domestic product (GDP) in 1960 to 17.2% in 2012 (CMS, 2014d), and is expected to rise to 19.9% of the GDP by 2022. U.S. per capita expenditures for health care in 2012 were $8,195 (CMS, 2014c). **Per capita expenditures** reflect the average amount spent on health care per person per year. Health care expenditures have increased consistently from 1 year to the next. From 1990 to 2009, per capita health care expenditures more than doubled (U.S. Census Bureau, 2013). Figure 6-1● presents a breakdown of different types of health care expenditures as well as the sources of funding for health care, which will be discussed in more detail later.

Factors that have contributed to increasing health care spending include an aging population, greater use of technology, an emphasis on costly specialty care, costs of care for the uninsured, and the labor-intensive nature of health care delivery (Sultz & Young, 2010). An aging population contributes

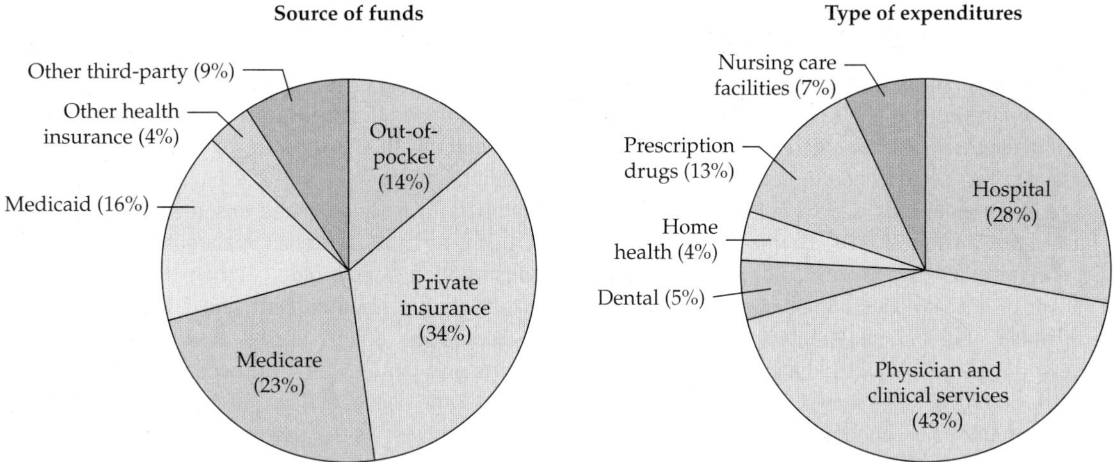

FIGURE 6-1 Distribution of Health Care Funding Sources and National Expenditures, 2012

Source: Centers for Medicare and Medicaid Services. (2013c). *Medicare and Medicaid research review/ 2013 statistical supplement.* Retrieved from http://www.cms.gov/Research-Statistics-Data-and-Systems/Statistics-Trends-and-Reports/MedicareMedicaidStatSupp/Downloads/2013_Section1.pdf

to greater demand for and use of services, particularly as the prevalence of chronic diseases with high costs for disease management increases in older age groups. The size of the older population relative to other age groups in the United States has increased consistently over the last several decades. In 1990, for example, people over the age of 65 years comprised only 29.6% of the U.S. population; by 2010 the proportion of the population over 65 years of age had increased to 38.6% of the population (U.S. Census Bureau, 2013). People over age 65 consume a large portion of the health care services provided each year.

Greater use of technology, particularly in response to fears of malpractice, and greater use of specialty care have also contributed to an increase in health care spending. Nearly two thirds of U.S. physicians are specialists, who tend to command higher reimbursement than generalists and employ more expensive technology. In addition, specialists have been associated with more inappropriate use of costly therapies. Greater use of technology also creates a demand for a better prepared health care workforce at all levels, thereby increasing the costs of its use (Sultz & Young, 2010).

Health care spending differs for different elements of the health care system. For example, as indicated in Figure 6-1, an estimated 28% of health care dollars was spent on hospital care, 43% on physician and clinical services (physicians, nurse practitioners, and others), 5% on dental care, 7% on nursing home care, 4% on home health care, and 13% on prescription drug costs (CMS, 2013c). Health care delivery is a labor-intensive segment of the economy, requiring 24-hour-a-day and 7-day-a-week coverage in some settings.

Costs of uncompensated care for the uninsured and increasing prescription drug prices are two other factors implicated in rising health care costs. **Uncompensated care** is that proportion of care for which the provider receives no reimbursement and includes both charity care and bad debt (American Hospital Association [AHA], 2014). A large segment of the population is uninsured or underinsured, resulting in large amounts of uncompensated care provided by health care institutions and providers. Approximately three fourths of uncompensated care is provided by federal, state, and local government agencies (Clemans-Cope, Garrett, & Buettgens, 2010).

Before the enactment of the Patient Protection and Affordable Care Act, uncompensated care amounted to about $61 billion per year, but this is expected to drop to $25 billion as the provisions of the Act are implemented (Clemans-Cope et al., 2010). AHA data indicate that uncompensated hospital care in the United States amounted to $45.9 billion in 2012 or 6.1% of U.S. hospitals' total expenses (AHA, 2014).

Uncompensated care leads to a phenomenon known as **cost shifting**, the passing on of the cost of uncompensated care to those who do pay for care, either those who pay out-of-pocket or those covered by health insurance. Cost shifting leads in turn to higher insurance premiums and higher overall costs for health care.

U.S. drug prices have risen considerably more than the consumer price index. **The consumer price index (CPI)** is "a measure of the average change over time in the prices paid by urban consumers for a market basket of consumer goods and services" (U.S. Bureau of Labor Statistics, 2013a, para. 1). In 2009, U.S. prescription drug costs amounted to $249.9 billion, and prescription drug spending increased by nearly 9% from 2008 to 2009 alone (U.S. Census Bureau, 2013). In 2011,

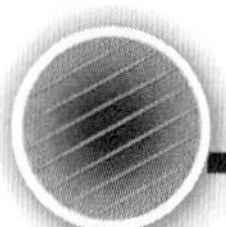

Evidence-Based Practice

Health and Neighborhood Socioeconomic Status

Numerous recent research studies have demonstrated links between the socioeconomic status of one's neighborhood and a variety of adverse health events. These associations have been found independent of one's own socioeconomic status in the United States as well as other countries such as Japan (Murakami, Sasaki, Takahashi, & Uenishi, 2010), Germany (Dittmann & Goebel, 2010), and Israel (Gerber, Myers, Goldbourt, Benyamini, & Drory, 2011). For example, neighborhood socioeconomic status has been linked to psychosocial functioning and frailty in older adults (Everson-Rose et al., 2011; Lang et al., 2009) and overall health status among persons with diabetes (Gary-Webb et al., 2011). Neighborhood socioeconomic status has also been linked to rates of fatal coronary heart disease (Foraker et al., 2011) and hospitalizations for injuries (Zarzaur, Croce, Fabian, Fischer, & Magnotti, 2010).

In addition, neighborhood socioeconomic levels have been associated with health-related behaviors. For example, youth from lower socioeconomic status neighborhoods were found to be less involved in physical activity than those from more affluent neighborhoods (Boone-Heinonen et al., 2011). Similar findings were noted with respect to physical activity following myocardial infarction (Gerber et al., 2011). Neighborhood socioeconomic status has even been linked to screen-time in preschool children (Carson, Spense, Cutumisu, & Cargill, 2010), fruit and vegetable consumption among older women (Nicklett et al., 2010), and overall life satisfaction (Dittmann & Goebel, 2010).

Population health nurses may be able to help individual clients and families deal with economic issues, but they cannot address the issue of low neighborhood socioeconomic status by themselves. As we saw in the *Advocacy Now* feature at the beginning of this chapter, however, they can advocate for a living wage, more effective economic assistance programs, and better overall economic status for members of the population in conjunction with other groups and organizations. What might you do to promote improvements in socioeconomic status for low-income neighborhoods in your community?

---

the average retail price for each drug prescribed for people over 65 years of age was $28 (Kaiser Family Foundation, 2011).

Many authors have suggested allowing U.S. citizens to purchase less expensive prescription drugs from international markets or discounted drugs from U.S. manufacturers. The Veterans Administration (VA) and other federal agencies, for example, have very successfully negotiated for drug discounts with U.S. pharmaceutical companies.

A large proportion of Americans are without any assistance in paying for prescription medications. With increasing costs, many employers are reducing or eliminating prescription coverage from health care plans or requiring higher copayments by beneficiaries. As a result, many people fail to take medications as directed due to the costs. Those most seriously affected by rising prescription drug costs have been the elderly who live on fixed incomes that do not increase with rising inflation rates. Some effort has been made to improve prescription drug access for Medicare beneficiaries through the Medicare Prescription Drug, Improvement, and Modernization Act of 2003. This legislation initiated Medicare Prescription Drug Coverage to assist older Americans with drug costs. This program will be discussed in more detail in the section related to the Medicare program.

Socioeconomic Factors and Health Status

Socioeconomic status affects health directly, in terms of access to health care, as well as indirectly, through factors such as social and educational opportunities, knowledge of health promotion and prevention measures, and shaping health behaviors. Despite the relatively high standard of living in the United States, the point has been made that "there are considerable pockets of the population for whom access to care and the effects on health status are much more similar to those of poorer and less successful Third World countries than they are to the rest of the industrial world" (Vladek, 2003, p. 16). This statement was supported by the findings of *Crossing the Quality Chasm*, an Institute of Medicine report published in 2001, and continues to be supported by current data.

Socioeconomic factors have a variety of effects on the health status of the population. Two major factors that will be discussed here are poverty and lack of health insurance. Questions for assessing the economic status of a population are provided in the *Focused Assessment* on page 149. A more in-depth assessment tool is available on the student resources site.

POVERTY. Poverty affects one's ability to gain access to the necessities of life that support health and wellness, including food, shelter, and access to health care services. Poverty is measured in terms of one's income relative to the current federal or state income guidelines. The poverty level is defined in terms of both household income and size. In 2013, for example, the poverty level for a family of five was an annual income less than $25,570 in all states except Alaska and Hawaii, which had slightly higher income levels defining poverty (CMS, 2012a).

In 2011, 46.2 million people in the United States were living in poverty. This figure represents 15% of the U.S. population. The median household income declined by 8.1% between 2007 and 2011, with steeper declines for Blacks and non-Hispanic Whites (DeNavas-Walt, Proctor, Smith, 2012). In large part, these declines are due to the overall economic downturn

FOCUSED ASSESSMENT Assessing the Economic Status of a Population

- What is the average income of the group?
- What proportion of the group has incomes at or below poverty level?
- What subpopulations are included in the low-income group?
- What proportion of low-income families receives some form of public assistance? Are all those eligible for assistance receiving it? If not, why not?
- What is the level of unemployment in the population? For those who are employed, what are the typical salaries?
- What proportion of the population receives employment-based health insurance benefits? Why do others not receive benefits (e.g., part-time employment, cannot afford premiums, etc.)?
- How are most health care services for the population funded?
- What revenue sources fund public health services for the population? Are these revenues adequate to provide needed services?

beginning in 2007. Poverty rates differ considerably among racial and ethnic groups with the highest rates among U.S. Blacks (25.8% in 2009) followed by Hispanics (25.3%), and Whites and Asians (12.2% and 12.5%, respectively) (U.S. Census Bureau, 2013). Children constitute a significant proportion of those living in poverty, and in 2011, 21.9% of U.S. children under 18 years of age were living in poverty (DeNavas-Walt et al., 2012).

Poverty contributes to a variety of disparities related to health among segments of the population. A **health disparity** is defined by *Healthy People 2020* as:

> a particular type of health difference that is closely linked with social or economic disadvantage. Health disparities adversely affect groups of people who have systematically experienced greater social or economic obstacles to health based on their racial or ethnic group, religion, socioeconomic status, gender, mental health, cognitive, sensory, or physical disability, sexual orientation or gender identity, geographic location, or other characteristics historically linked to discrimination or exclusion. (U.S. Department of Health and Human Services [USDHHS], 2010, para.6)

Disparities occur with respect to morbidity and mortality as well as access to preventive health services. Poverty leads to malnutrition, poor housing, lack of health care, and lack of adequate child care, all of which have negative health implications. In addition, poverty is associated with low literacy levels, which limit earning power and access to health care.

LACK OF HEALTH INSURANCE. The second major way in which economic factors affect health is through diminished access to needed health care services. Diminished access occurs as a result of the mixed effects of poverty and lack of health care insurance. In fact, 38% of the uninsured are people with incomes below poverty level. During 2011, 48 million non-elderly people in the United States were uninsured. This is a decrease of 1.3 million from 2010 (Kaiser Commission on Medicaid and the Uninsured, 2012a). Lack of insurance is not confined to those living in actual poverty. In 2009, for example, 32% of people with incomes 200% to 300% above the federal poverty level were uninsured, and more than one fifth of those 300% to 400% above poverty were without health insurance. People who remain uninsured for a year or more are seven times more likely to forgo needed health care due to costs, and even being without coverage for 1 to 3 months results in a fourfold likelihood of forgoing or delaying care (Fox & Richards, 2010). The likelihood of going without needed care is twice as high for uninsured persons with disabilities as it is for those without a disability (National Center for Health Statistics [NCHS], 2010). Data from 2002 to 2004 suggested that 21% of the 92 million adults with chronic conditions were uninsured for at least 1 month, and 23% of those with both chronic conditions and disabilities were uninsured at some point. Lack of insurance among these groups led to greater problems accessing needed care, fewer ambulatory care visits, less prescription drug use, and higher out-of-pocket expenses than for their insured counterparts (Gulley, Rasch, & Chan, 2011).

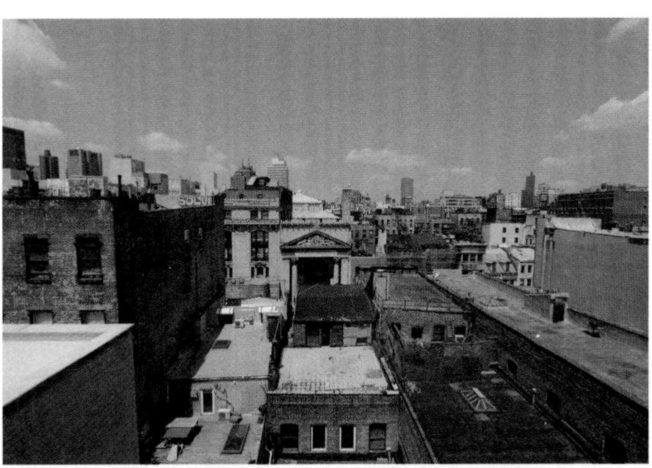

Research has shown that low-income neighborhoods affect the health of even those of moderate income who live in them.

Lack of health insurance is most common among young to middle-aged adults. More than 83% of those uninsured for the entire year in 2009 were 18 to 64 years of age, compared to 14.8% of children under age 18 and only 1.3% of persons over 65 years of age (U.S. Census Bureau, 2013). In large part, these coverage differences are due to the availability of Medicare for the elderly and the Medicaid and Children's Health Insurance Programs (CHIP) for children. Each of these programs will be discussed in more detail later in this chapter.

Differences in health insurance coverage are also noted by race and ethnicity, with members of ethnic minority groups less likely to be covered. For example, in 2009, only 16% of the White U.S. population was uninsured compared to 32% of Hispanic, 21% of Black, and 17% of Asian residents (U.S. Census Bureau, 2013).

There are a number of reasons for lack of health insurance in such a large portion of the population. Slightly more than half (55.8%) of people under 65 years of age who had health insurance in 2009 received it as an employment-based benefit (DeNavas-Walt et al., 2012). Those without insurance may be unemployed or work in jobs that do not provide insurance coverage. Others may lose coverage due to job loss; loss of eligibility for Medicaid or State Children's Health Insurance Programs (SCHIP); or loss of coverage through a spouse due to death, separation, or divorce (Kaiser Commission on Medicaid and the Uninsured, 2012a, 2012b). Even those eligible for employment-based health insurance may not be covered due to inability to pay the beneficiary portion of premiums or competing priorities for limited incomes. For example, the average family cost for employment-related health insurance was $15,745 in 2012, comprising about 28% of total premium costs, beyond the ability of many families to afford. From 2002 to 2012, the overall cost of premiums increased by 97% and workers' share of premiums increased by the same amount while wages increased by only 33% on average. In the 2009 National Health Interview Survey, 48% of those who were uninsured indicated that it was because of cost. Another 28% reported they had lost or changed jobs and so lost coverage, and 12% said their employers did not provide health insurance benefits or they were refused coverage by an insurance company (NCHS, 2011).

Lack of health insurance is associated with a variety of health effects. For example, the uninsured are less likely than those with insurance to receive cancer screening and other preventive services and are often less healthy in general than their insured counterparts. They are also less likely to comply with medication regimens for chronic diseases due to costs and may experience greater mortality.

Having health insurance is associated with better health status, a regular source of care, and more appropriate use of health care services. In addition, people with insurance are more likely to receive health-promotive and illness-preventive services (Kaiser Commission on Medicaid and the Uninsured, 2012a). For example, in 2012, uninsured adults were five times more likely than insured adults not to have a regular source of care. Similarly, the uninsured were more than six times more likely to go without needed care due to cost and nearly five times more likely not to get a prescription filled than those with insurance (Kaiser Commission on Medicaid and the Uninsured, 2012a).

According to a critical Institute of Medicine report (IOM, 2003), lack of health insurance has implications for society as well as for the individuals involved. For example, lack of insurance leads to premature death and loss of social productivity. In addition, the uncompensated care related to high numbers of uninsured individuals in the population may lead to health system closure and loss of providers, resulting in decreased community health care capacity. Because health problems have been allowed to escalate due to the inability to afford care, the ultimate societal costs for treatment are much higher than they would be if treatment was initiated earlier.

Lack of health insurance and its implications for access to needed health care services was recognized in the development of the national health objectives. Access to health care services is the first topical area addressed in *Healthy People 2020*. According to the U.S. Department of Health and Human Services (USDHHS, 2013b), lack of access to health care leads to both personal and societal consequences that include unmet health needs, delay in receiving needed care, inability to obtain preventive services, and increased hospitalizations that might have been prevented. *Healthy People 2020* objectives related to access to care are presented on page 151. Many of the objectives are developmental in nature, indicating that there is no baseline data for the current status of a particular objective. During the course of implementation of the objectives, baseline data will be obtained and appropriate targets set for achievement by 2020.

Health Care Reimbursement Systems

When people receive health care, those who provide care need to be paid for their services. Payment for health services or reimbursement, involves two aspects, the way in which payments are made and the source of the funds for payment. In this section, we will discuss the approaches to paying for services, or reimbursement systems. **Reimbursement** is compensation, usually through a public or commercial insurance plan, for health services provided. Payment approaches to be addressed include retrospective and prospective reimbursement, capitation, and a new approach termed pay-for-performance.

Retrospective Reimbursement

Retrospective reimbursement is payment for services rendered based on the cost of those services; cost is determined after the fact. Forms of retrospective reimbursement include fee-for-service payment and discounted fee-for-service payment as well as per diem payment. In a fee-for-service system, providers are paid for each service rendered after that service has been provided. Fee-for-service payment is based on the unit of service, such as a single visit to a provider or a single

Healthy People 2020

Objectives for Access to Health Services

OBJECTIVE	BASELINE (YEAR)	TARGET	CURRENT DATA (YEAR)	DATA SOURCE
AHS-1.1: Increase the proportion of persons with health insurance	83.2% (2008)	100%	82.8% (2011)	National Health Interview Survey (NHIS), CDC, NCHS
AHS-1.3: Increase the proportion of persons with prescription drug coverage	Developmental	Developmental	NDA	National Health Interview Survey (NHIS), CDC/NCHS
AHS-2: Increase the proportion of insured persons with coverage for clinical preventive services	Developmental	Developmental	NDA	Children's Health Insurance Program (CHIP), CMS, AGing Integrated Database (AGID), AoA, CMS claims data, Medicare Current Beneficiary Survey (MCBS), CMS
AHS-3: Increase the proportion of people with a usual primary care provider	76.3% (2007)	83.9%	76.8% (2010)	Medical Expenditure Panel Survey (MEPS), AHRQ
AHS-4: Increase the number of practicing primary care providers	Developmental	Developmental	NDA	
AHS-5.1: Increase the proportion of persons of all ages who have a specific source of ongoing care	86.4% (2008)	95%	86.8% (2011)	National Health Interview Survey (NHIS), CDC, NCHS
AHS-6.2: Reduce the proportion of individuals who are unable to obtain or delay in obtaining necessary medical care	7% (2007)	4.2%	4.6% (2010)	Medical Expenditure Panel Survey (MEPS), AHRQ
AHS-6.3: Reduce the proportion of people who are unable to obtain or delay in obtaining necessary dental care	5.5% (2007)	5%	5.8% (2010)	Medical Expenditure Panel Survey (MEPS), AHRQ
AHS-6.4: Reduce the proportion of people who are unable to obtain or delay in obtaining necessary prescription medicines	3.1% (2007)	2.8%	3.3% (2010)	Medical Expenditure Panel Survey (MEPS), AHRQ
AHS-7: Increase the proportion of persons who receive appropriate evidence-based clinical preventive services	Developmental	Developmental	NDA	Medical Expenditure Panel Survey (MEPS), AHRQ
AHS-8: Increase the proportion of persons who have access to rapidly responding prehospital emergency medical services	Developmental	Developmental	NDA	National EMS Information System (NEMSIS)
AHS-9: Reduce the proportion of hospital emergency department visits in which the wait time to see an emergency department clinician exceeds the recommended time	Developmental	Developmental	NDA	National Hospital Ambulatory Medical Care Survey (NHAMCS), CDC, NCHS

NDA= No data available

Source: U.S. Department of Health and Human Services. (2013a). *Access to health services: Objectives.* Retrieved from http://www.healthypeople.gov/2020/topicsobjectives2020/objectiveslist.aspx?topicId=1

procedure. Discounted fee-for-service mechanisms are used when third parties (e.g., an insurance company or health care plan) negotiates with providers who agree to charge less than their usual fee in return for being designated a "preferred provider" to whom patients are routinely referred.

Per diem payment is a reimbursement arrangement in which a health care facility is paid retrospectively, at a flat rate per day, for the number of days a client was hospitalized or received care. Per diem reimbursement is usually used for institutional providers such as hospitals, skilled nursing facilities, and long-term-care facilities.

Retrospective reimbursement has the disadvantage of encouraging health care providers to give services that may not be necessary, merely because they are reimbursable. A provider who can be reimbursed for each office visit may be tempted to see a client three times when two visits would suffice. Or tests and treatments may be given that are not strictly necessary. For example, a surgeon might suggest a hysterectomy to a woman when other, less expensive measures would be equally effective.

Prospective Reimbursement

In 1983, prompted by rising costs, the federal government instituted prospective reimbursement for services provided under Medicare. **Prospective reimbursement** is payment at a predetermined, fixed rate for a specific health care program or set of services (CMS, 2013f). Prospective payment rates are based on the extent of resources typically used in providing a given type of service. Prospective payment minimizes the impetus for providers to render unneeded services because they are paid on a per incident basis rather than on the basis of the number of services provided. Because prospective payment is based on the average amount of service required for a particular condition, health care providers actually lose money if they provide unneeded services.

Forms of prospective payment include diagnosis-related groups (DRGs), the Resource-Based Relative Value Scale (RBRVS), and capitation. Both DRG and RBRVS systems are based on payment for each episode of illness.

Prospective payment for services provided under the Medicare program is based on clients' diagnoses, with set fees for care of clients who fall into specific diagnosis-related groups. As we saw in Chapter 2∞, DRGs are categories of client diagnoses for which typical costs of care have been calculated, based on the cost of specific services required. In the DRG system, health care organizations, such as hospitals and skilled nursing facilities, are paid a set fee based on a client's diagnosis and the typical costs of care for someone with that diagnosis.

A similar prospective payment system, the **Resource-Based Relative Value Scale (RBRVS)**, was initiated in 1992 for physician services provided to Medicare clients. In this system, the typical costs of a given health service have been calculated based on the prevailing cost for that service in a particular locale. Physicians providing a given service are paid a flat fee based on the estimated cost of the service. Costs are based on the coding categories of the *Current Procedural Terminology Manual* (CPT) developed by the American Medical Association (AMA) and used for Medicare billing purposes. The Healthcare Common Procedure Coding System (HCPCS), also based on the AMA's CPT codes, is used in the National Correct Coding Initiative for providers billing Medicaid (CMS, 2014a). Variations of the RBRVS are also used by commercial insurance organizations to reimburse health care providers.

Capitation

Capitation is a particular type of prospective reimbursement in which the provider or health care system is paid a set predetermined fee for a defined set of health services for each client enrolled in a particular health plan (Goldsteen & Goldsteen, 2012). In a capitated system, a third-party payer, such as an insurance company or health plan, pays providers on the basis of the number of persons enrolled in the plan who select the particular provider. Capitation has the advantages of certainty for the payer in terms of the cost of services and for the provider in a guaranteed patient population. However, the provider must provide all needed services under a fixed budget and may lose money if clients' service needs exceed the amount of payment. Capitation is a prominent feature of many managed care plans, which will be discussed in the section on commercial insurance.

Pay-for-Performance

Pay-for-performance reimbursement is a relatively new approach to paying for health care services in which providers and health care institutions receive bonus payments for achieving specific quality outcomes. For example, providers whose immunization rates reach certain targets may be given additional income by insurance providers. Pay-for-performance may occur in the form of additional payments for meeting global threshold targets for an entire client population or using a piece-rate performance reimbursement approach in which the provider is rewarded for each client that meets designated benchmarks. This system has the advantage of rewarding high performing providers and organizations, but may not promote improvement in low performers. In addition, it may encourage providers and health care delivery systems to avoid high-risk clients for whom it is more difficult to achieve the targeted outcomes. Pay-for-performance has been shown, however, to improve immunization rates in systems in which it has been implemented (Chien, Li, & Rosenthal, 2010).

A reverse approach to pay-for-performance has been initiated by Medicare with its "never events." In 2002, the National Quality Forum (NQF) developed a list of serious reportable events (SREs) that are serious errors and events that include both "errors caused by care management (rather than the underlying disease) and errors that occur from failure to follow standard care or institutional practices and policies" (NQF, 2006, p. 1).The list includes 28 events in six categories: surgical events, product or devices events, patient protection events, care management events, environmental events, and criminal events. These SREs or "hospital-acquired conditions" (HACs) are basically preventable with quality care and should "never occur." Based on the concept of SREs, Medicare developed a list of hospital-acquired conditions incorporating multiple diagnostic codes, for which health care institutions will not be reimbursed for care (although care to address adverse patient effects must be provided). An initial list of eight non-reimbursable conditions was instituted in 2008, but has since been expanded (CMS, 2012b; Healy & Cromwell, 2012). The Affordable Care Act required that similar provisions for non-reimbursement of these events be incorporated into the Medicaid reimbursement system (Medicaid.gov, n.d.c). These events have significant financial implications in that health care organizations are not reimbursed for care provided for these preventable conditions. Institution of non-reimbursement for such events, however, has led to a decline in the rates of several HACs including falls and trauma, catheter-associated urinary tract infections, and deep vein thrombosis/pulmonary embolism (Healy & Cromwell, 2012).

Health Care Funding Sources

The second aspect of payment for health care services involves the source of funds for payment. Sources of health care funding include personal payment, commercial insurance, government-funded programs, and charity.

Personal Payment

Perhaps the easiest to understand and least often used approach to financing health care is personal payment. In a personal payment system, when you see a provider for care, you pay him or her directly out of your pocket. Personal payment tends to be used by the very wealthy, by the uninsured (if they can afford any payment at all), or for certain specific goods and services that are not covered under an insurance plan. For example, if you do not have vision coverage in your health insurance plan, you would personally pay for your eye examination, new glasses, and so on. The entire risk for the costs of health care rests on the recipient of care.

Personal payment for health care services and products comprises one part of out-of-pocket expenses incurred by people who receive health care services. Insurance premiums, deductibles, and copayments are the other components of out-of-pocket funding. **Premiums** are the periodic, usually monthly, amounts paid for health insurance benefits. A **deductible** is the amount of money that you must pay out-of-pocket before an insurance plan begins to pay for any care. A **copayment** or coinsurance payment is a fixed amount or percentage of costs that a client pays for each visit or service provided (Goldstein & Goldstein, 2012). Copayment is over and above the amount that is covered by one's health insurance. In 2012, out-of-pocket payments accounted for 14% of U.S. health care expenditures, compared to nearly 34% from private insurance and 45% from public sources (CMS, 2013c). Out-of-pocket expenses can be fairly significant, with more than 8% of people with health care expenses paying more than $2,000 out-of-pocket in 2006 (NCHS, 2013).

Personal payment is also the funding approach used in flat-rate medical clinics that are becoming more common in the United States. Flat-rate clinics charge clients a fixed or flat rate, typically on a monthly (e.g., $100 a month) or per-visit basis (e.g., a flat rate of $30 for each visit) for routine health care. Many of the recipients of care at flat-rate clinics have health insurance coverage for hospitalization, but use the clinics to address routine illness needs (McDonald, 2012). In flat-rate clinics, the risk for the cost of care is borne by the clinic.

Commercial Insurance

Commercial insurance may involve either traditional fee-for-service retrospective reimbursement or a managed care approach to health care services. In traditional indemnity insurance plans, the client or his or her employer pays for insurance coverage. When services are provided, the insurance plan "indemnifies" the client, compensating him or her for the expenses incurred in obtaining services. Sometimes the client pays for services and is reimbursed for the payment; more often, however, insurance companies pay providers directly. Payment is made retrospectively after services are provided and is based on whatever fee the provider charges.

Managed care has no single definition but refers to a set of principles that govern provider–payer–recipient relationships or "a system of health care delivery that influences or controls utilization of services and costs of services by providing both the financing of care and the health services for covered individuals" (Goldsteen & Goldsteen, 2012, p. 290). In managed care, the payer and provider functions of health care are combined in the same organization. This is in contrast to more traditional indemnity insurance, in which the insurance company pays for care but does not actually provide the care given. A **managed care organization (MCO)** is a system of health care delivery that attempts to control costs while being accountable for the health outcomes of a group of enrolled individuals (Goldsteen & Goldsteen, 2012). MCOs are characterized by integration of funding and delivery systems and a comprehensive array of services. In 2010, 99% of the U.S. population who received health insurance through an employer were enrolled in some form of managed care plan (Claxton et al., 2010), and managed care plans covered more than 135 million people (Managed Care On-line, 2011).

Despite a wide and growing variety, managed care plans usually have two elements in common. First, they generally require some form of authorization for services, particularly specialty services, and second, they usually include some restriction on choice of providers. The types and forms of MCOs create a veritable alphabet soup and include open- and closed-panel health maintenance organizations (HMOs), preferred provider organizations (PPOs), point of service (POS) plans, and others. Managed care organizations are usually characterized by a specific enrolled population, a designated set of covered services (usually including a variety of health-promotive and illness-preventive services), and a fixed subscription or enrollment premium that covers all designated services. Table 6-1● summarizes key features of some of the more common forms of MCOs.

Commercial insurance may be purchased individually by private individuals or through employment-based group health plans. Both forms of commercial insurance will be discussed briefly.

INDIVIDUAL INSURANCE. Individual health insurance is purchased by an individual directly from an insurance company. It tends to be expensive because the individual does not have the bargaining power of a large entity such as a corporation that can guarantee the insurance company a number of subscribers. Individual policies also tend to have limited coverage, again because of the expense. Some people may not be eligible for such policies because of existing health conditions that make them a poor economic risk for the insurance company. Under the Consolidated Omnibus Reconciliation Act (COBRA), individuals who have been insured under an employment-based group plan may continue individual coverage at the group premium rate for 18 months after termination of employment. This legal provision is available whether or not there is a preexisting medical condition, but the individual is responsible for the entire cost of the premium, which makes it unaffordable for many people following a job loss (U.S. Department of Labor, n.d.).

EMPLOYMENT-BASED GROUP HEALTH PLANS. By far the greatest number of people with commercial insurance obtains it by way of employment. Because of the number of people they insure, employers are able to obtain insurance for whole groups of employees at discounted rates not available to individual purchasers. Employment-based insurance is popular because it is purchased with pretax dollars. Employee health benefits are a pretax deduction for the employer and are not

TABLE 6-1 Key Features of Common Forms of Managed Care Organizations

Type of MCO	Key Features
All MCOs	Provide comprehensive health care to an enrolled group for a specified fee (premium). Emphasize health promotion and illness prevention as means of minimizing costs. Attempt to minimize costs by providing care in the least expensive environment with the least expensive provider.
Health maintenance organization (HMO)	Depends on subtype (see below). Members are generally restricted to services from providers within the plan. Services provided outside the plan are not covered and the member is liable for the full cost of outside services. Primary care providers (PCPs) function as "gatekeepers" preventing members from seeking specialty care without authorization.
Open-panel HMO	HMO contracts with groups of providers who may see clients from other MCOs as well as fee-for-service clients. • Direct contract—HMO contracts directly with independent physicians for service for its members • Individual Practice Association (IPA)—HMO contracts with groups of physicians
Closed-panel HMO	Providers see only members of the particular HMO, usually in facilities provided by the HMO. • Group model—HMO contracts with a group of providers and hospitals separately to provide services exclusively for HMO members (also known as an exclusive provider organization, EPO) • Staff model—HMO employs providers on a salaried basis
Network model HMO	HMO contracts with several large multispecialty groups of providers that operate independently of each other.
Mixed model HMO	Same HMO incorporates two or more of the above types of arrangements. So a given HMO might have separate closed-panel and open-panel segments that usually operate independently of each other.
Individual Practice Association (IPA)	Group of independent providers (usually physicians) forms an association to contract with managed care organizations to provide services to MCO enrollees.
Preferred provider organizations (PPOs)	MCO includes a group of independent "preferred providers" (hospitals, physicians, and other providers) that provide services at a discounted rate to MCO members. If members choose to obtain services outside the plan, they are covered at a reduced rate, and the member must pay the difference (usually 20% of costs).
Point of service (POS) plans	Plan members choose a participating PCP who serves as a gatekeeper for specialty care. Specialty care requires a referral, but the member may choose to see a specialist outside the plan and pay a higher deductible, copayment, or both. Differentials may be as high as 20% to 40% of the cost of services.
Integrated delivery systems (IDSs)	Coordinated network of health care organizations that provide a continuum of services to a defined population. Characterized by a defined population, a defined set of services, clinical and administrative integration of services and information systems, a capitated payment system, and pooled revenues from several sources. Emphasizes centralized planning and management and a shared mission and vision. Includes hospital beds and at least one long-term-care service. May include contracts with several HMOs for the provision of services.
Other weird arrangements (OWAs)	Because of the proliferation and combination of features of many different models of MCOs, there are other types of plans that defy description. These models are collectively referred to as OWAs.

currently considered taxable income for employees. In 2011, 56% of the U.S. population under 65 years of age obtained health insurance through an employer (NCHS, 2013), and 67% of the total U.S. population were enrolled in some sort of group health insurance plan (U.S. Census Bureau, 2013).

As we saw earlier, however, significant segments of the population are not eligible for employment-based health insurance. In 2013, only 72% of civilian workers in the United States had access to employment-based health benefits, and only 56% actually participated in benefits plans. Participation rates were even lower for low-income workers, with only 42% of those with wages in the lowest 25% participating (U.S. Bureau of Labor Statistics, 2013b). Access to health insurance benefits is somewhat dependent on the size of the employer's workforce with 86% of companies with more than 100 employees providing access to health benefits compared to only 57% of those with fewer than 100 workers (U.S. Bureau of Labor Statistics, 2013b). Retirees may also lack access to continued employer-sponsored health insurance benefits. In 2010, for example, less than 18% of workers were employed by companies that provided health benefits to early retirees who were not yet eligible for Medicare. Those organizations that do offer retiree health insurance coverage are changing to less expensive benefits packages, increasing premiums, or reducing eligibility (Fronstin & Adams, 2012).

In addition, the cost of group health plan premiums, while not as expensive as individual insurance coverage, has continued to escalate, with annual increases in insurance premiums consistently outstripping wage increases and overall inflation rates. From 2003 to 2013, the average annual health insurance premium increased by 80%, and the contribution required of the average employee increased by 89% (Kaiser Family Foundation and Health Research & Educational Trust, 2013). In 2013, the average monthly premium for employment-based family insurance was $901 for all U.S. civilian workers, with approximately 31% of the cost of premiums contributed by the employee (U.S. Bureau of Labor Statistics, 2013b).

Employers are faced with one of several unpalatable options due to rising premium costs: (a) pay the increased premiums, thereby reducing their profit margins, (b) reduce the level of benefits covered, (c) pass a larger share of health insurance costs on to employees (e.g., a greater percentage of premiums and larger deductibles and copayments), or (d) discontinue coverage altogether (Kaiser Family Foundation and Health Research & Educational Trust, 2013). For example, in 2009, a single-person employment-based insurance policy required an average deductible of $917, and the average deductible for family coverage was $1,761. Similarly, nearly 73% of employer-sponsored health plans required a copayment for each doctor visit, with an overall average copayment of $21.53. In addition, covered employees were required to pay 18.6% of the cost of care as a coinsurance payment (Davis, 2011).

Increases in the cost of health insurance have led to a proliferation of types of employment-based coverage in an effort to reduce costs to employers, including defined benefits plans, defined contribution plans, fixed contribution plans, and consumer-driven plans. In defined benefits plans, employers select a predetermined set of benefits that are covered by the plan. Differing sets of benefits may be available under different plans or from different companies. For example, benefits may or may not cover reproductive services such as contraception. Similarly, dental insurance plans may or may not cover any amount for orthodontics. Employees of large companies may have a choice among several different defined benefits plans.

In a defined contribution plan, the employer provides a set amount of money to each employee, which the employee can use to purchase whatever type of insurance plan is desired. Defined contribution plans have more advantages for employers than employees. Employers' health insurance costs remain constant, but employees may find that the amount provided does not go far to cover the costs of a desirable health insurance plan. In a fixed contribution plan, the employer chooses a specific benefits package and provides a fixed amount toward the premiums for that package, with the expectation that the employee will pay the difference in the cost of the plan.

A fourth approach is a consumer-driven plan, in which the employer usually provides a defined catastrophic coverage for serious illness or injury as well as a flexible health care spending account. The employee can then use the amount in the health spending account to pay directly for any other health care expenses incurred. Health spending accounts are similar to the health savings accounts allowed by the Internal Revenue Service. A health savings account is money contributed by the employee through payroll deduction prior to taxes that is available for certain health care expenses not covered by insurance plans. The health spending account included in a consumer-driven health plan differs in that the contribution is made by the employer rather than the employee. In many such plans, monies left in a health spending account can be carried over in subsequent years; in others, whatever money is not spent in a given year is forfeited.

Consumer-driven plans have the advantage of covering catastrophic events, the most expensive area of health care, with flexibility for addressing other health care needs. They have the disadvantage of controlling only the small portion of health care expenditures outside of catastrophic coverage. In addition, there is concern that ill-informed consumers may make poor health choices that later lead to the need for more costly services. Attempts to prevent this from occurring include the incorporation of online access to health-related information and nurse counseling and coaching. There is also the possibility that if many people who receive employment-based health care coverage opt for consumer-driven plans, it will reduce the number of people with traditional commercial insurance, driving prices beyond the capacity of many to afford.

The options available to most employees whose employers provide health insurance benefits include some form of managed care plan. Most employers who provide access to health insurance (84%) offer only one option, with larger employers more likely to offer more than one plan option. Among all U.S. civilian firms, 24% offered access to HMOs, 53% to PPOs, and 25% to POSs. Only 2% offered employees the option of conventional fee-for-service insurance. A growing percentage of businesses (15% in 2010) offered eligible employees the choice of high- deductible health plans with a savings option (HDHP/SOs). These plans are similar to consumer-driven plans discussed earlier and are characterized by a high annual deductible amount (averaging $1,700 to $2,000) to be paid by the employee before the insurance plan provides any coverage coupled with a Health Savings Account or Health Reimbursement Arrangement. In the health savings account, the employee makes nontaxable contributions to the account to be used for health-related expenses. In a health reimbursement arrangement, the contribution is made by the employer (Claxton et al., 2010). HDHP/SOs generally have lower premium costs than other group plans (Kaiser Family Foundation and Health Research & Educational Trust, 2013). Figure 6-2 • depicts the process of health care funding through employment-based managed care participation.

Self-funded insurance is another option selected by some businesses to minimize insurance costs. Self-funded insurance and self-insurance are more radical approaches taken by some large employers and unions. In a self-funded insurance plan, an employer collects pooled premiums from its employees and uses funds that would have paid insurance company premiums to pay for the costs of care provided to employees and their dependents. Self-insured programs are similar, but the employing organization hires a third party (often a commercial insurance company) to administer the program and process claims. Some physician networks assist companies in developing self-funded insurance plans and may negotiate to provide services under the plan. Plans may also include PPO and POS managed care options (PhysiciansCare Health Plans, n.d.b). Self-funded insurance is one component of the "other third-party" source of health care funding depicted in Figure 6-1.

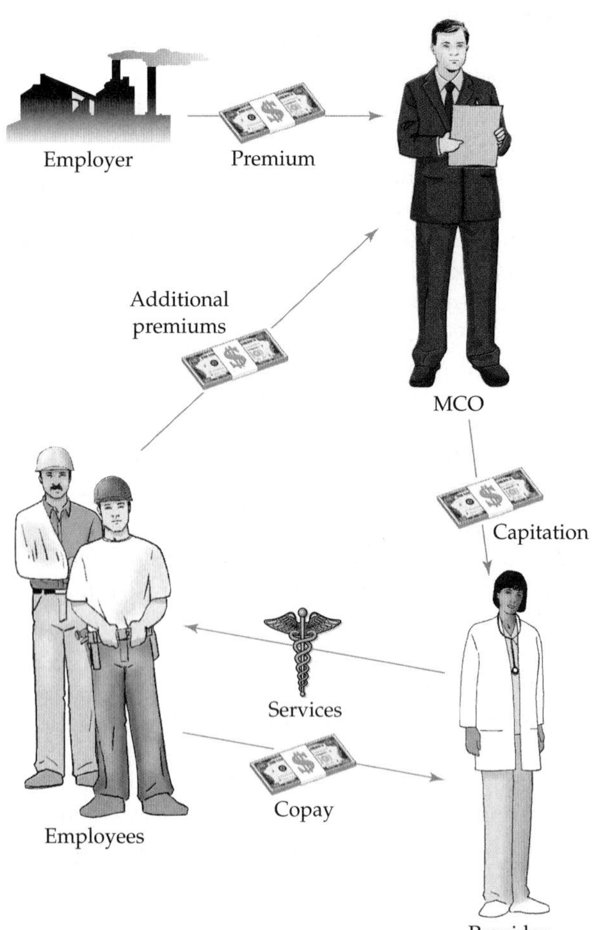

FIGURE 6-2 Health Care Funding Through Employment-based Managed Care Plan Enrollment

Self-funded plans have a number of advantages for employers allowed under the Employee Retirement Income Security Act (ERISA). They avoid the third party that increases premium costs. In addition, costs are based on the level of pooled risk of the company's employees, not all participants in an insurance program. Since employees of many companies are relatively young and healthy, this decreases costs. Self-funding avoids the premium tax collected by state governments as a percentage of commercial insurance premiums, and self-funded programs are exempt from state insurance regulations. Although they are regulated by the U.S. Department of Labor, they do not have to meet the minimum benefits requirements of commercial plans and can provide a health benefits package tailored to the needs of the company's employees (PhysiciansCare Health Plans, n.d.a).

In self-funded plans, the risk for excessive health care costs is borne by the employer or union. However, these organizations often get around this disadvantage by purchasing corporate insurance protecting them against catastrophic losses (PhysiciansCare Health Plans, n.d.b).

HEALTH INSURANCE EXCHANGES. Under the Patient Protection and Affordable Care Act [HP 3590], enacted in 2010, each state is required to establish some form of health insurance exchange by 2014. The exchanges are designed to permit individuals and small businesses to shop for affordable health insurance coverage. States have some options in the development of the exchanges. The state may create its own exchange or separate exchanges for individuals and small businesses or let the federal government administer a state exchange. States may also choose to cooperate with other states to create regional exchanges (Alliance for Health Reform, 2010a).

State insurance exchanges will offer a variety of plans providing federally designated tiers of coverage. These tiers are as follows:

- Bronze tier: Covers 60% of costs for all services included in the plan (exclusive of premiums)
- Silver tier: Covers 70% of costs for all services included in the plan
- Gold tier: Covers 80% of costs for all services included in the plan
- Platinum tier: Covers 90% of costs for all services included in the plan (Healthcare.gov, n.d.a).

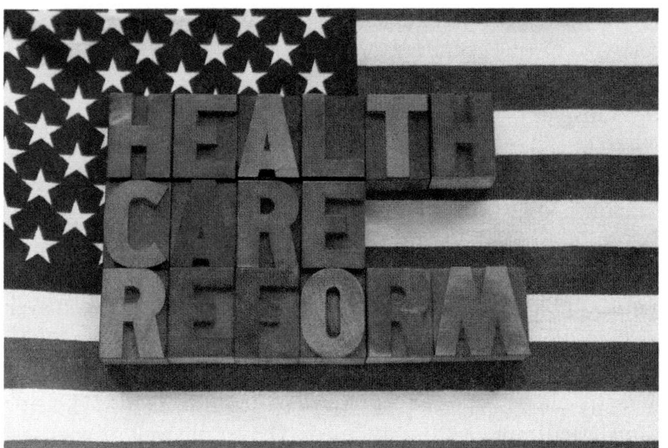

Health care reform. *(Nebari/Fotolia)*

The exchanges will have the advantage of buying power due to the number of people involved, so coverage will be less expensive than is currently the case for individuals and companies with small numbers of employees. State exchanges may be administered by state government agencies or by nonprofit groups (Alliance for Health Reform, 2010b) and will be available only to citizens and legal residents of the United States. They will not be available to anyone who is incarcerated, so it will not assist state and local law enforcement agencies to reduce the costs of health care to prisoners (Kaiser Family Foundation, 2013). They may, however, be available to persons awaiting trial. Whether or not coverage will terminate if conviction occurs or will merely be suspended is yet to be determined. The requirements to be met by state insurance exchanges are highlighted at right. Data from one of the largest existing state risk pools cover too few of the uninsured to resolve the overall problem of access to care, and concerns exist over how those enrolled will be integrated into the reformed health care system. As of September 2010, 27 states and the District of Columbia had chosen to administer their own risk pools, and the other 23 states had opted for a federally administered plan (Blewett, Spencer, & Burke, 2011).

Government-Funded Care

Federal, state, and local governments are another significant source of health care funding in the United States. In government-funded health programs, the risk for the costs of care is borne by the government, and ultimately by taxpayers. In 2012, 43% of the insured population in the United States was covered by government health insurance (U.S. Census Bureau, 2013), and government funding sources paid for 45% of personal health care expenditures in the United States. (CMS, 2014d). These funds primarily fall into the Medicare and Medicaid sources of funding depicted in Figure 6-1. The remainder of federal government programs (e.g., Department of Veterans Affairs, Department of Defense, and so on) fall into the "other third-party" category in the figure.

Federal, state, and local governments have a variety of programs that finance health care. The two major federal government programs are Medicare and Medicaid. Medicare is designed to provide care for the elderly and certain individuals who are disabled. The Medicaid program is jointly financed by federal and state funds and was developed to address the health care needs of the poor. Other federal health care programs include the Department of Veterans Affairs, military programs including Department of Defense facilities and the TRICARE program, the Federal Employee Health Benefits Program (FEHBP), the Indian Health Service, and the National Health Service Corps.

The Department of Veterans Affairs and the Indian Health Service provide services for selected population groups, military

Highlights

Requirements for State Insurance Exchanges

- Provide easy web-based access to information on plan options, benefits, and costs in a standard format.
- Operate a toll-free hotline to provide information to consumers.
- Assist in screening and enrolling eligible persons in existing public insurance programs.
- Use a standardized enrollment form for all plans and programs.
- Use consumer navigators to help consumers or employers make health insurance decisions.
- Inform consumers of satisfaction and quality ratings of insurance plans available through the exchange.
- Offer plans that:
  - Cover the basic federal benefits package and any additional benefits mandated by the state.
  - Include caps on out-of-pocket spending for plan enrollees.
  - Offer only designated tiers of coverage and offer at least one silver and one gold level plan.
  - Have an adequate number of health care providers in the plan.
  - Meet specified marketing standards.
  - Meet relevant quality, quality improvement, and accreditation standards.
  - Meet transparency standards, including disclosure of claims denials.
  - Make prior justification for premium increases.
- Solicit consumer and public input.
- Publish financial information and be audited by the Department of Health and Human Services.
- Be self-financing through premiums and other state resources by January 2015.

Data from: Families USA. (2010). *Implementing health insurance exchanges: A guide to state activities and choices.* Retrieved from http://familiesusa.org/sites/default/files/product_documents/Guide-to-Exchanges.pdf

veterans and Native Americans, respectively. Both Department of Defense and TRICARE programs provide services to active-duty members of the military, retirees, and their dependents. Department of Defense facilities are managed and staffed by the military. TRICARE, on the other hand, is a program by which members of the military, retirees, and their dependents receive care in the civilian sector with funding provided by the federal government. TRICARE is also available to members of the National Guard and Reserves and their families. TRICARE functions much like traditional commercial health insurance or managed care plans and provides several options including dental and pharmacy coverage options. A similar type of program, FEHBP, serves employees of federal agencies outside of the military. In this program, the federal government functions primarily as an employer purchasing employment-based health insurance for employees, just as in the private sector (U.S. Office of Personnel Management, n.d.). The National Health Service Corps is designed to provide health care services in underserved areas of the country. Like Medicaid, the SCHIP is funded by the federal government but administered by the states. The SCHIP program was initiated to provide care for poor children who did not meet eligibility requirements for Medicaid (Medicaid.gov, n.d.a). Medicare, Medicaid, and SCHIP are discussed in more detail below. Local jurisdictions, such as counties, often have programs that fund health services for indigent persons who are not eligible for Medicaid.

MEDICARE. Medicare is part of the social insurance program arising from provisions of the Social Security Act. Under Medicare, people over 65 years of age who are eligible for Social Security benefits receive partial coverage of health services. Certain other individuals, such as the disabled and those with end-stage renal disease who require renal dialysis or transplant, are eligible for Medicare coverage before age 65 (CMS, 2013d; Social Security Administration, 2010). In 2011, Medicare provided coverage for approximately 48.6 million people, including 39 million over 65 years of age and 8.3 million non-elderly people with permanent disabilities. Federal expenditures for Medicare in 2011 amounted to nearly $514.3 million and the federal allocation for 2012 was over $545 million (CMS, 2011).

At its inception in 1965, Medicare was intended to protect the elderly against expensive hospitalizations. The optional Medicare Part B was added to cover physician expenses. Medicare Part C, previously called Medicare + Choice and now Medicare Advantage, was instituted in 1997 to provide beneficiaries with a choice of options among traditional fee-for-service practices and managed care plans (Social Security Administration, 2010). Medicare Part D, Medicare Prescription Drug Coverage, was initiated under the Medicare Prescription Drug, Improvement, and Modernization Act of 2003 and was fully implemented in 2006. Each of the components of Medicare will be discussed briefly. Elements of each component are summarized in Table 6-2●.

Medicare Part A covers medically necessary hospitalization, care in a skilled nursing facility (SNF), some home health care, hospice services, and blood administered in an inpatient setting. Part A coverage is available to all participants in the Social Security program and is provided without additional premiums to those who are eligible for Social Security or railroad retirement

TABLE 6-2 Components of Medicare

Medicare Component	Services	Premiums (2014)	Deductible (2014)	Copayment
Part A	• Hospitalization • Skilled nursing facility • Home health • Hospice • Blood (given in an inpatient setting)	• None for 99% of Medicare beneficiaries • $426/month for those who are otherwise ineligible	$1,216/benefit period	Hospitalization • None for first 60 days • $304/day for days 61–90 • $608/day for days 91+
Part B	• Physician services • Outpatient services • Some home health care • Durable medical equipment • Screening/preventive services	$104.90/month (2014)	$147/year for approved services	• 20% of cost for most services
Medicare Advantage Plans	• Replaces Medicare A & B for enrollees • May include additional services	Based on plan	Based on plan	Based on plan
Medicare Part D	Prescription drug services	Based on plan	Maximum/year determined by CMS	• 25% of drug costs from $250 to $2,850 • 47.5% of the cost of brand name drugs and a variable amount for generic drugs (2014)

benefits, a dependent parent of an eligible dead child, those meeting disability eligibility criteria, and spouses of those who paid Medicare taxes through their employment, and those with kidney failure (Social Security Administration, 2010). Funding for Medicare Part A is derived from nonvoluntary Social Security payroll taxes on one's income with a matching payment from the employer. Elderly people who do not meet the eligibility criteria may enroll in Medicare Part A with payment of a monthly premium, and state assistance with premiums is available for low-income elderly (CMS, 2013d, 2013e; Cubanski et al., 2010).

Part A benefits begin after the beneficiary has incurred the specified annual deductible amount ($1,216 in 2014) (CMS, 2013b). Benefits are paid within a *benefit period.* A benefit period begins with admission to a hospital or SNF and ends when no further hospital or SNF care has been received for 60 consecutive days. One may have several benefit periods within a given year and must pay the deductible for each benefit period. Within each benefit period, Medicare pays all covered costs for the first 60 days. For hospitalizations longer than 60 days, the beneficiary pays a copayment for each additional day ($304 a day for days 61 to 90 and $608 a day after 90 days in 2014) (CMS, 2013b).

Medicare Part B covers medically necessary provider services, outpatient care, some home health care, and other services that are not covered under Part A (CMS, 2012c). Part B also covers a variety of preventive services including colorectal, breast, cervical, and prostate cancer screening; osteoporosis screening; immunizations; and so on.

Part B coverage is optional and entails payment of an additional premium similar to that paid for private health insurance, but much less costly. Due to recent changes in regulations, premiums are now somewhat higher for recipients with higher incomes than for the general population (Social Security Administration, 2010). By law, the Medicare Part B premium must be sufficient to cover 25% of the program's costs, so the premium increases each year as health care costs increase. For 2014, the monthly premium was $104.90; the same as for 2013 (CMS, 2013b). Part B premiums may be slightly higher for Medicare beneficiaries who did not enroll in Part B when they first became eligible. Beneficiaries with incomes less than 135% of the federal poverty level may receive assistance with their Part B premiums, and for some Medicare enrollees, the Medicaid program pays their Medicare Part B premiums.

Like Part A, there is a deductible amount that must be paid before Part B coverage begins ($147 in 2014), but unlike Part A, the Part B deductible is paid only once a year. In addition to the monthly premiums and annual deductible, beneficiaries pay a copayment for Medicare-approved services or supplies. Provisions of the Affordable Care Act eliminate cost-sharing (deductible and copayment) requirements for preventive services under Medicare.

If health service providers accept Medicare assignment, beneficiaries do not have any additional costs for Medicare-approved services. **Assignment** is an agreement whereby the Medicare beneficiary agrees to allow the service provider to bill Medicare directly for services or goods (e.g., a walker or ventilator) provided. In return, the provider agrees to accept the Medicare reimbursement amount as full payment. If providers do not accept assignment, the greatest amount that the beneficiary can be charged for a Medicare-approved service or product is 15% above the Medicare-approved amount for that service or product. This is called the **limiting charge.**

As noted earlier, Medicare Part C, or Medicare Advantage, was intended to permit Medicare enrollees to exercise the same options with respect to their health care as others in the U.S. population and to take the place of **medigap plans** or supplemental insurance to cover costs for services not provided under Medicare. Specifically, the program allowed beneficiaries to apply their Medicare funding to enrollment in a Medicare-approved managed care plan. Medicare Advantage Plans may include health maintenance organizations, preferred provider organizations(PPOs), and Medicare private fee-for-service plans, depending on what is available in a given locale (Medicare.gov, n.d.b). In 2010, 24.6% of Medicare Part A and 20.4% of Part B disbursements were made to managed care organizations (CMS, 2011).

Medicare HMOs and PPOs are similar to those discussed in the section on employment-based group health plans. Medicare special needs plans provide coverage to select groups of people, such as nursing home residents, those who are eligible for both Medicare and Medicaid, and those with certain chronic or disabling conditions. Medicare private fee-for-service plans allow recipients to choose any provider that accepts the plan, and the plan determines what the recipients' share of the cost will be. Some Medicare Advantage Plans also include prescription drug coverage and services not included under the Original Medicare Plan (Parts A & B). Like Medicare Part B, there is usually an additional premium for a Medicare Advantage plan that is paid by the enrollee.

In 2006, the major provisions of the Medicare Prescription Drug, Improvement, and Modernization Act of 2003 were implemented as Medicare Part D, Medicare Prescription Drug Plans. This drug subsidization program is available to all Part A, B, and C recipients and requires beneficiaries to enroll in one of many Medicare Prescription Plans offered by private insurance companies. Although described as a "voluntary" plan, Medicare beneficiaries who choose not to enroll in a prescription plan will be required to pay increased premiums of 1% for every month that they delay coverage, unless their drug coverage during that time was as good as Part D coverage (Social Security Administration, 2010). For some Medicare recipients, prescription drug coverage may be provided under Medicare Advantage plans rather than specific Part D plans (Medicare.gov, n.d.a). Prescription drug coverage plans vary in terms of costs, drugs covered, and pharmacies participating. Medicare beneficiaries with incomes below 135% of poverty level can get assistance with Part D premiums, and those between 135% and 150% of poverty level can receive partial assistance (CMS, 2013a). In 2010, more than 28 million Medicare beneficiaries were enrolled in Part D prescription plans (CMS, 2011).

Plan beneficiaries pay a deductible amount prior to coverage. The deductible varies from plan to plan, but cannot exceed the amount specified by CMS for a given year. After the deductible is paid, the beneficiary pays a copayment (typically 25% of the cost) for each prescription until costs reach a specified amount ($2,850 in 2014). Once total drug costs have reached that amount, the beneficiary pays 47.5% of brand name drug costs and a specified amount for generic drugs that will decrease to 25% by 2010 until total drug expenditures for the year reach another set amount, at which point the beneficiary resumes paying a small copayment for each prescription. Drug costs in the specified window are referred to as the "doughnut hole," or gap in prescription drug care coverage under Medicare (Medicare.gov, n.d.a). The Affordable Care Act provided a $250 rebate for Medicare beneficiaries in the doughnut hole during 2010 and will eventually close the coverage gap completely (Alliance for Health Reform, 2010b).

Although the Medicare program has provided significant assistance to the elderly population with respect to hospitalization and, to a lesser extent, provider services, it does not provide adequate coverage in a number of areas. For example, mental health services are only partially covered, and long-term custodial health care is not addressed at all by the program. As we saw earlier, prescription drug coverage may be inadequate even with Medicare Part D. Medicare has begun to provide for some preventive services such as influenza and pneumonia immunization and mammography, but these are generally considered insufficient to meet the health promotion needs of the elderly population.

MEDICAID. The Medicaid program was established in 1965 to provide health care services to a large segment of the population who could not otherwise afford care. Its original purpose was to integrate the indigent into mainstream health care services. Medicaid and the Children's Health Insurance Program (CHIP) provide services for more than 60 million people in the United States, including 31 million children, 11 million non-elderly low-income parents, caretakers, pregnant women, and other adults, and 8.8 million people with disabilities. Medicaid also funds care for 4.6 million low-income seniors who need assistance with Part B Medicare premiums and prescription drug coverage and 3.7 million people with disabilities who also receive Medicare assistance (Medicaid.gov, n.d.b, 2014). Based on the most recent CMS *Data Compendium*, federal Medicaid expenditures for 2010 were $383.4 million, with a 2012 allocation of more than $997 million (CMS, 2011). Despite the availability of Medicaid coverage, however, many children remain uninsured. Given the economic downturn since 2007, however, the number of uninsured U.S. children would have been far higher without the Medicaid program (Kaiser Commission on Medicaid and the Uninsured, 2012a).

Medicaid is a means-tested program, which means that eligibility for services is based on one's income (Goldsteen & Goldsteen, 2012). Under the program, the federal government provides block grants to the states that are combined with matching state funds. Matching rates depend on the per capita income of the state, with lower-income states receiving more federal money for every state dollar expended.

The Medicaid program is administered by the states, but state programs must provide a minimum set of federally defined benefits. Beyond that, states are free to determine the level of service provided as well as eligibility requirements for the program, and both benefits and requirements may differ drastically from state to state. States may choose to expand eligibility for Medicaid to cover people with incomes too high to meet regular eligibility requirements, but with extensive medical expenses. Eligibility expansions may also encompass other groups of people such as institutionalized low-income persons, low-income women diagnosed with breast or cervical cancer through Centers for Disease Control and Prevention (CDC) screening programs, and others (Medicaid.gov, 2014).

In the past, Medicaid covered most prescription drug costs for enrollees. Now prescription drug costs for "dual eligibles," persons eligible for both Medicare and Medicaid, will be covered under a Medicare Prescription Drug Plan. Medicaid will cover the costs of Medicare Prescription Drug Plan premiums, but it is anticipated that the change will increase copayments for prescription drugs from those previously paid under the Medicaid program.

Because both Medicare and Medicaid are programs that arise out of federal legislation, they are often confusing. Table 6-3 • provides characteristic features that may help differentiate the two programs.

STATE CHILDREN'S HEALTH INSURANCE PROGRAM (SCHIP). The State Children's Health Insurance Program was authorized by Congress in 1997 to address the health insurance needs of low-income children and pregnant women who do not meet the income eligibility requirements for Medicaid. The enacting legislation gave states the option of either expanding existing Medicaid programs or creating separate SCHIP

TABLE 6-3 Differentiating Features of Medicare and Medicaid

Feature	Medicare	Medicaid
Funding source	Social Security contributions	General tax revenues (federal and state)
Program administration	Federal	State
Beneficiaries	Elderly and disabled persons	Medically indigent
Benefits	Standardized for each component Hospitalization, primary care (under Part B only), prescription drugs, selected preventive services, no dental services	Vary from state to state Primary care, preventive services, prescription drug coverage, hospitalization, may include dental services

programs to include uninsured children who were eligible for Medicaid but unenrolled, or with family incomes too high for Medicaid eligibility but too low to afford commercial insurance coverage (Medicaid.gov, 2014). Most SCHIP programs provide services to children in families with incomes at or below 200% of the federal poverty level, but eligibility thresholds may be higher or lower in some states. The SCHIP program gave the states extraordinary latitude in determining how to deal with the problem of uninsured children and is an example of a phenomenon called **devolution**, or the transfer of responsibility for an area from federal to state governments or other jurisdictions (Devolution, 2011).

In 2010, 7.7 million children were enrolled under a SCHIP (CHIP Statistical Enrollment Data System, 2011). Under the provisions of the 2009 reauthorization bill, coverage was expanded to 11 million to provide coverage for nearly half of the uninsured children in the United States (Alliance for Health Reform, 2010c). Total federal funding for 2010 for the CHIP program was $11.4 billion and the 2012 federal funding allocation was $13.4 billion (CMS, 2011).

Like Medicaid, SCHIP is state administered but funded jointly by federal and state governments. The federal government pays an average of 72% of the costs of SCHIP in a given state. SCHIP, in conjunction with Medicaid, was responsible for decreasing the number of uninsured children by 2.7 million in spite of increasing child poverty and family loss of employment-based insurance. Both SCHIP and Medicaid have been shown to be effective in meeting the care needs of those insured. In addition, expansion of both SCHIP and Medicaid programs have been credited with decreases in child mortality as a result of external causes (e.g., accidental injury) (Howell, Decker, Hogan, Yemane, & Foster, 2010). For further information about Medicare, Medicaid, and SCHIP, see the *External Resources* section of the student resources site.

Charity Care

Charity care is the "other private" source of health care funding depicted in Figure 6-1. **Charity care** is defined as care that is provided free of charge to individuals who meet established financial criteria and that was never expected to generate revenue. There is no reliable estimate of the amount of charity care provided in the United States, because the costs for charity care are accounted for in different ways in health care organizations' accounting systems. IRS data indicated that the percentage of charity care by U.S. hospitals in 2009 ranged from 7.3% for small hospitals to 9.8% for large hospitals (Dunn & Becker, 2013).

Private charitable giving for all purposes (not just health) amounted to $298.4 billion in 2010. Approximately 8.3% of charitable contributions are made to health care organizations; another 32% is given to religious organizations, and approximately 12% is contributed to human services agencies, both of which provide some health-related services. In addition, nearly 27% of the U.S. population provided voluntary services, amounting to 15.2 billion hours in 2011 (Blackwood, Roeger, & Pettijohn, 2012). Charitable giving tends to decrease during hard economic times and frequently does not keep pace with inflation and the cost of providing charity care. In addition, many nonprofit organizations are faced with growing demands for assistance during economic downturns stretching their resources even further.

Charity care may be provided by individual health care organizations or funded by a wide variety of voluntary organizations and philanthropic foundations. For example, the Gates Foundation has funded a massive international immunization campaign. Other organizations and foundations fund similar health care programs as well as providing services or funding services for individual needy clients and families. The National Center for Charitable Statistics (n.d.) lists three types of nonprofit organizations that may provide health-related services: 501c3 organizations that include health care and community service agencies, 501c3 private foundations that most often provide funding grants to other nonprofit agencies, and other tax-exempt groups, such as unions, veterans groups, and social and recreational clubs. Voluntary health organizations will be discussed in more detail in Chapter 7∞.

Both the Better Business Bureau (BBB, 2003) Wise Giving Alliance and the Federal Trade Commission (FTC) (2012) provide tips on selecting reputable charities to which one might wish to give donations. In addition, the BBB has promulgated standards for charity accountability against which a potential donor can judge a charity's worthiness. The Alliance also publishes reports about major charity organizations that are available to the general public on its website.

Health Insurance and Reform

In March of 2010, President Barack Obama signed the Patient Protection and Affordable Care Act instituting a variety of reforms to health insurance and programs to improve the health of the U.S. population. Some of the effects of the law have been presented earlier, but we will discuss others here. General categories of provisions within the law address mandatory coverage, employer requirements, expansion of public programs, premium and cost-sharing subsidies, tax changes, and the health insurance exchanges discussed earlier. Other areas addressed in the bill include creation of an essential benefits package, changes to private insurance, the role of the states in implementing the law, cost containment, quality improvement, prevention and wellness services, long-term care, and other investments (Kaiser Family Foundation, 2013).

Under the law, individual U.S. citizens and legal residents will be required to have health insurance coverage that meets minimum requirements or pay a tax penalty, which may be a flat fee or a percentage of family income. Similarly, employers with 50 or more employees will be required to provide health insurance coverage for their employees or pay a fee of $2,000 per full-time employee. Some individuals and employers may be eligible for subsidies or tax credits to offset the costs of insurance premiums. In addition, some individuals may qualify

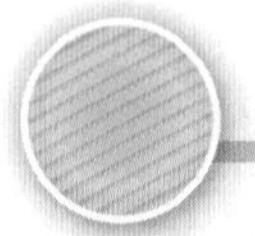

Global Perspectives

Health Care Funding in Other Countries

Select three other countries and explore how health care services are funded in those countries. How does health care funding differ from that in the United States? What are the advantages and disadvantages of these other approaches to funding health care delivery? What effects do they have on population health status? What effects, if any, do they have on the role of the population health nurse?

for cost-sharing subsidies to assist with deductibles and copayments. Employers may also receive reimbursement for health claims of retirees not yet eligible for Medicare to offset the costs of allowing retirees to participate in employment-based group plans (Kaiser Family Foundation, 2013).

The law also provides for expansion of Medicaid eligibility to all non-Medicare eligible individuals with incomes up to 133% of the federal poverty level and maintains state requirements for SCHIP programs. After 2015, states will receive an increase in their federal CHIP matching rates (Kaiser Family Foundation, 2013).

Some changes in tax provisions include removal of unprescribed over-the-counter drugs from eligible expenses that can be reimbursed from health savings accounts and limiting contributions to flexible spending accounts to $2,500 per year (adjusted for cost of living increases). The law also changes the threshold for including unreimbursed health expenses as itemized deductions in computing income taxes, imposes new annual fees for pharmaceutical manufacturers, and initiates annual fees for the insurance sector (with lower fees for nonprofit insurers). The law also provides for the creation of an essential health insurance benefits package that provides a comprehensive set of services, covers 60% of the cost of services, and limits cost-sharing requirements. The Act, however, specifically prohibits the inclusion of abortion services in the essential benefits package (Kaiser Family Foundation, 2013).

Some of the most far-reaching provisions of the Affordable Care Act involve changes to private insurance. These include increasing the age for dependent children's coverage to 26 years, prohibiting lifetime limits on coverage and withdrawal of coverage except in the case of client fraud, and requiring justification of premium increases. Additional provisions require all new plans to conform to one of the tiers of coverage discussed earlier, limit deductibles and waiting times for coverage and provide for the creation of an Internet website to assist individuals to explore insurance options, and the development of standards for providing benefits information (Kaiser Family Foundation, 2013). The legislation also prohibits denial of coverage due to the presence of a preexisting condition and requires that 85% of insurance premiums from large employers and 80% from small employers be spent on health care services rather than administrative costs (U.S. Department of Health and Human Services [USDHHS], n.d.a).

Cost-containment provisions in the law include adoption of a single set of rules for eligibility verification and filing claims as well as a variety of cost-containment strategies for Medicare and Medicaid. Research funding is included for quality improvement pilot projects. Another system improvement strategy is an increase in Medicaid payments to providers to conform to Medicare rates (Kaiser Family Foundation, 2013).

This far-reaching piece of legislation might go some way to providing coverage to the millions of uninsured residents of the United States and would also result in needed insurance reform. Unfortunately, however, provisions of the law are already being challenged. Recently, a federal judge ruled the mandate for individual health insurance coverage to be unconstitutional because it exceeds the federal government's authority to regulate interstate commerce. In doing so, however, the judge refrained from issuing an injunction to stop implementation of the mandate pending appeal of his ruling (Lowes, 2010). In addition, powerful lobbies and members of the Republican party have already vowed to move toward repeal of the law. Population health nurses and other concerned citizens need to be actively involved in efforts to sway legislators to prevent this from happening. Thus far, most legal challenges to the law have not been successful.

One of the arguments against the legislation is the cost of its implementation. According to the Congressional Budget Office (CBO, 2010b), as much as $50 billion may be involved in implementation. Much of this funding is not included in the law itself, but would require additional congressional appropriations for functions added to existing federal agencies and grants and other program funding required under the legislation. There would also be costs associated with Internal Revenue Service activities in verifying premium and cost-sharing credits included in income tax deductions and the increased eligibility under Medicare, Medicaid, and CHIP programs. On the other hand, it is also estimated that the direct spending and revenue effects at the federal level would result in a reduction of federal deficits of $118 billion from 2010 to 2019. During that time, federal financial commitment for health care would be expected to increase by about $210, but this increase would be offset by provisions of the law that would generate revenue and decrease the costs of providing health care through greater efficiency. Costs for state and local governments related to health care funding are expected to increase substantially, but overall the implementation of the law would reduce the number of uninsured non-elderly people in the United States by more than half (CBO, 2010a).

Health Care Reform and Population Health

The Patient Protection and Affordable Care Act also includes a variety of provisions that will influence the health of the overall population beyond the effects of providing access to care through health insurance. Significant attention is given in the law to coverage of preventive health services and elimination of cost-sharing requirements for health promotion and illness prevention services (Kaiser Family Foundation, 2013). Some of the specific preventive services for adults, women, and children addressed in the law include screenings (e.g., for abdominal aortic aneurysm, alcohol misuse, blood pressure, depression, and mammography, among others), immunizations for adults and children, tobacco counseling and cessation assistance, and other counseling services (e.g., diet, sexually transmitted infection prevention) (USDHHS, n.d.b). Specific provisions include restriction of federal coverage to preventive services with significant levels of evidence of their effectiveness, removal of barriers to preventive services under Medicare and Medicaid (particularly for adults), initiation of annual wellness visits and personalized prevention plans for Medicare beneficiaries, and incentives to states to initiate activities among Medicaid recipients to change lifestyle behaviors to prevent chronic illness (Trust for America's Health, n.d.).

HR 3590 also created the National Prevention, Health Promotion and Public Health Council to coordinate federal efforts related to prevention, wellness and health promotion, and public and integrative health systems. The council is also charged with creating a national strategy with goals and objectives to improve health through federally supported prevention and promotion programs. In addition, the legislation established a Prevention and Public Health Fund to support prevention and public health initiatives, including research, screening, and intervention activities (Trust for America's Health, n.d.).

HR 3590 also directs the Secretary of Health and Human Services to support planning and implementation of a public–private partnership and media campaign to promote public awareness and education related to health promotion and prevention. Other provisions support school-based health centers and community transformation grants for community initiatives to prevent chronic disease and sequellae, address health disparities, and develop a stronger evidence base for preventive activities; and grants to develop and evaluate promotion and prevention programs for Medicare beneficiaries (Trust for America's Health, n.d.). Population health nurses can acquaint communities with the opportunities for funding of health promotion and prevention programs and assist them in writing grant proposals and implementing and evaluating such programs.

CHAPTER RECAP

Economic conditions have both direct and indirect effects on the population's health. Direct effects stem from funding allocated to health care services. Indirect effects reflect the ability of members of the population to obtain the resources needed for good health (e.g., appropriate housing, good nutrition) as well as their ability to afford health care services.

The cost of providing health care services in the United States has increased dramatically in the last few decades without an appreciable increase in the population's health status. Some of the factors involved in this increase include an aging population, greater use of technology, emphasis on costly specialty care, costs of care for the uninsured, and the labor-intensive nature of health care delivery. Failure to engage in health promotion and illness prevention activities has also increased the costs of health care when problems occur.

Funding for health care services in the United States derives from several sources. These include personal payment, commercial health insurance, government services and government-funded insurance programs, and charity care. Approaches to reimbursement for health care services include retrospective payment, prospective payment, and pay-for-performance. Population health nurses need to be conversant with health services funding mechanisms to assist clients to obtain needed services. They can also campaign for allocation of sufficient funding for health care, particularly to cover the uninsured elements of the population, and develop and test cost-effective interventions to meet population health needs.

CASE STUDY Financing Care for the Underserved

You have been appointed to the mayor's task force on health care in the midsize community in which you work as a population health nurse. The assessment of population health and economic status conducted by the task force indicates that most of the population's health care needs are adequately met at all levels of health care. The exception to this, however, is the population of the migrant farm camp at the edge of town.

This group consists primarily of male Mexican workers who have entered the United States on legal work visas. Very few of the workers have brought their families with them. Most of this population receives no health care except for treatment in the emergency room of the community hospital. Usually, this care is provided for work-related injuries or serious illness. Members of this group receive no health promotion or preventive care and do not seek care for minor illnesses because of their inability to pay.

Because most of these people are in the United States legally, they would be eligible for county medical assistance (CMA); however, very few have applied for this program because of language barriers, lack of transportation to the social services office, and inability to afford to take the time off work to submit an application. Even if they did receive assistance, they would be unlikely to find a regular health care provider who has a contract with the county to provide services under CMA reimbursement. Only one community clinic and one independent nurse practitioner, in addition to the community hospital, have county contracts. Local physicians receive adequate income from private paying clients and those with private health insurance. Because of the extended time between provision of services and receipt of reimbursement, these physicians no longer accept county assistance clients.

The rest of the population is well off when compared with average state and national incomes. With the exception of the migrant workers, most residents are employed by three large industries and receive salaries that are quite adequate to meet the cost of living. Because of the industry present in the community, the local tax base is more than adequate. The community does not budget any public funds for health care as the majority of the population is adequately served by private providers. There is no local health department, but the county offers public health services in a town 50 miles away.

1. What factors are influencing the health status of the migrant group?
2. How would you finance health care for this population group?
3. Would fee-for-service care or managed care arrangements be more appropriate for providing care to the migrant population? Why?

REFERENCES

Alliance for Health Reform. (2010a). *Designing a marketplace that works: Steps to affordable coverage.* Retrieved November 10, 2010, from http://www.allhealth.org/briefing_detail.asp?bi=197

Alliance for Health Reform. (2010b). *The future of children's health coverage.* Retrieved November 10, 2010, from http://www.allhealth.org/publications/Child_health_insurance/The_Future_of_Childrens_Health_Coverage_98.pdf

Alliance for Health Reform. (2010c). *Implementing health reform: Federal rules and state roles.* Retrieved November 10, 2010, from http://www.allhealth.org/publications/State_health_issues/Implementing_Health_Reform_-_Federal_Rules_and_State_Roles_100.pdf

American Hospital Association. (2014). *Uncompensated hospital care cost fact sheet.* Retrieved from http://www.aha.org/content/14/14uncompensatedcare.pdf

Better Business Bureau. (2003). *Standards for charity accountability.* Retrieved November 10, 2010, from http://www.bbb.org/us/Charity-Standards

Blackwood, A., Roeger, K. L., & Pettijohn, S. L. (2012) *The nonprofit sector in brief.* Retrieved from http://www.urban.org/UploadedPDF/412674-The-Nonprofit-Sector-in-Brief.pdf

Blewett, L. A., Spencer, D., & Burke, C. E. (2011). State high-risk pools: An update on the Minnesota Comprehensive Health Association. *American Journal of Public Health, 101,* 231–237. doi:10.2105/AJPH.2009.185975

Boone-Heinonen, J., Diex Roux, A. V., Kiefe, C. I., Lewis, C. E., Guilkey, D. K., & Gordon-Larsen, P. (2011). Neighborhood socioeconomic status predictors of physical activity through young to middle adulthood: The CARDIA study. *Social Science & Medicine, 72,* 641–649. doi:10.1016/josocscimed.2010.12.013

Carson, V., Spence, J. C., Cutumisu, N., & Cargill, L. (2010). Association between neighborhood socioeconomic status and screen time among pre-school children: A cross-sectional study. *BMJ Public Health, 10.* Retrieved from http://www.biomedcentral.com/1471-2458/10/367.

Centers for Medicare and Medicaid Services. (2011). *Data compendium.* Retrieved from http://www.cms.gov/Research-Statistics-Data-and-Systems/Statistics-Trends-and-Reports/DataCompendium/2011_Data_Compendium.html

Centers for Medicare and Medicaid Services. (2012a). *2013 poverty guidelines.* Retrieved from http://www.medicaid.gov/Medicaid-CHIP-Program-Information/By-Topics/Eligibility/Downloads/2013-Federal-Poverty-level-charts.pdf

Centers for Medicare and Medicaid Services. (2012b). *Hospital-acquired conditions (HACs) in acute inpatient prospective payment system (IPPS) hospitals.* Retrieved from http://www.cms.gov/Medicare/Medicare-Fee-for-Service-Payment/HospitalAcqCond/Downloads/HACFactsheet.pdf

Centers for Medicare and Medicaid Services. (2012c). *Medicare part B.* Retrieved from http://www.cms.gov/Medicare/Medicare-General-Information/MedicareGenInfo/Part-B.html

Centers for Medicare and Medicaid Services. (2013a). *Bridging the coverage gap.* Retrieved from http://www.cms.gov/Medicare/Prescription-Drug-Coverage/PrescriptionDrugCovGenIn/bridgingthegap.html

Centers for Medicare and Medicaid Services. (2013b). *CMS announces major savings for Medicare beneficiaries.* Retrieved from http://www.cms.gov/Newsroom/MediaReleaseDatabase/Press-Releases/2013-Press-Releases-Items/2013-10-28.html

Centers for Medicare and Medicaid Services. (2013c). *Medicare and Medicaid research review/ 2013 statistical supplement.* Retrieved from http://www.cms.gov/Research-Statistics-Data-and-Systems/Statistics-Trends-and-Reports/MedicareMedicaidStatSupp/Downloads/2013_Section1.pdf

Centers for Medicare and Medicaid Services. (2013d). *Medicare part A*. Retrieved from http://www.cms.gov/Medicare/Medicare-General-Information/MedicareGenInfo/Part-A.html

Centers for Medicare and Medicaid Services. (2013e). *Medicare Program - General Information*. Retrieved from http://www.cms.gov/Medicare/Medicare-General-Information/MedicareGenInfo/index.html?redirect=/MedicareGenInfo

Centers for Medicare & Medicaid Services. (2013f). *Prospective payment systems—General information*. Retrieved from http://www.cms.gov/Medicare/Medicare-Fee-for-Service-Payment/ProspMedicareFeeSvcPmtGen/index.html?redirect=/ProspMedicareFeeSvcPmtGen

Centers for Medicare and Medicaid Services. (2014a). *National Correct Coding Initiative edits*. Retrieved from http://www.cms.gov/Medicare/Coding/NationalCorrectCodInitEd/index.html

Centers for Medicare and Medicaid Services. (2014b). *National health expenditure projections 2012–2022*. Retrieved from http://www.cms.gov/Research-Statistics-Data-and-Systems/Statistics-Trends-and-Reports/NationalHealthExpendData/Downloads/Proj2012.pdf

Centers for Medicare and Medicaid Services. (2014c). *National health expenditures 2012 highlights*. Retrieved from https://www.cms.gov/Research-Statistics-Data-and-Systems/Statistics-Trends-and-Reports/NationalHealthExpendData/Downloads/highlights.pdf

Chien, A. T., Li, Z., & Rosenthal, M. B. (2010). Improving timely childhood immunizations through pay for performance in medicaid-managed care. *Health Services Research, 45*, 1934–1945. doi:10.1111/j.1475-6773.2010.01168.x

CHIP Statistical Enrollment Data System. (2011). *CHIP ever enrolled in year*. Retrieved from http://www.medicaid.gov/Medicaid-CHIP-Program-Information/By-Topics/Childrens-Health-Insurance-Program-CHIP/Downloads/CHIPEverEnrolledYearGraph.pdf

Claxton, G., DiJulio, B., Finder, B., Lundy, J., McHugh, M., Osel-Anto, A., …, Gabel, J. (2010). *Employee health benefits: 2010 annual survey*. Retrieved January 5, 2011, from http://ehbs.kff.org/pdf/2010/8085.pdf

Clemans-Cope, L., Garrett, B., & Buettgens, M. (2010). *Health care spending under reform: Less uncompensated care and lower costs to small employers*. Retrieved November 15, 2010, from http://www.urban.org/uploadedpdf/412016_health_care_spending.pdf

Congressional Budget Office. (2010a). *HR 3590, patient protection and Affordable Care Act: Cost estimate for the bill as passed on December 24, 2009*. Retrieved from http://www.cbo.gov/ftpdocs/113xx/doc11307/Reid_Letter_HR3590.pdf

Congressional Budget Office. (2010b). *Potential effects of the patient protection and Affordable Care Act on discretionary spending*. Retrieved from http://www.cbo.gov/ftpdocs/113xx/doc11307/Specified_Authorizations_HR3590.pdf

Cubanski, J., Huang, J., Damico, A., Jacobson, G., & Neuman, T. (2010). *Medicare chartbook* (4th ed.). Menlo Park, CA: Henry J. Kaiser Family Foundation.

Davis, K. E. (2011). *Co-pays, deductibles, and coinsurance percentages for employer-sponsored health insurance in the private sector, by industry classification, 2009*. Retrieved from http://meps.ahrq.gov/mepsweb/data_files/publications/st323/stat323.pdf

DeNavas-Walt, C., Proctor, B. D., & Smith, J. C. (2012). *Income, poverty, and health insurance coverage in the United States: 2011*. Retrieved November 15, 2010, from http://www.census.gov/prod/2012pubs/p60-243.pdf

Devolution. (2011). *Encyclopædia Britannica*. Retrieved from http://www.britannica.com/EBchecked/topic/155042/devolution

Dittmann, J., & Goebel, J. (2010). Your house, your car, your education: The socioeconomic situation of the neighborhood and its impact on life satisfaction in Germany. *Social Indicators Research, 96*, 497–513. doi:10.1007/s11205-009-9489-7

Dunn, L., & Becker, S. (2013). *50 things to know about the hospital industry*. Retrieved from http://www.beckershospitalreview.com/hospital-management-administration/50-things-to-know-about-the-hospital-industry.html

Everson-Rose, S. A., Sharupski, K. A., Barnes, L. L., Beck, T., Evans, D. A., & Mendes de Leon, C. F. (2011). Neighborhood socioeconomic conditions are associated with psychosocial functioning in older people. *Health & Place, 17*, 793–800. doi:10.1016/j.healthplace.2011.02.007

Families USA. (2010). *Implementing health insurance exchanges: A guide to state activities and choices*. Retrieved from http://familiesusa.org/sites/default/files/product_documents/Guide-to-Exchanges.pdf

Federal Trade Commission. (2012). *Before giving to charity*. Retrieved from http://www.consumer.ftc.gov/articles/0074-giving-charity

Foraker, R. E., Rose, K. M., Kucharska-Newton, A. M., Ni, H., Suchindran, C. M., & Whitsel, E. A. (2011). Variation in rates of fatal coronary heart disease by neighborhood socioeconomic status: The atherosclerosis risk in communities surveillance. *Annals of Epidemiology, 21*, 580–588.

Fox, J. B., & Richards, C. L. (2010). Vital signs: Health insurance coverage and health care utilization—United States, 2006–2009 and January–March 2010. *Morbidity and Mortality Weekly Report, 59*, 1448–1454.

Fronstin, P., & Adams, N. (2012). *Employment-based retiree health benefits: Trends in access and coverage, 1997–2010*. Retrieved from http://www.ebri.org/pdf/briefspdf/EBRI_IB_10-2012_No377_RetHlth.pdf

Gary-Webb, T. L., Baptiste-Roberts, K., Pham, L., Wesche-Thobaben, J., Patricio, J., Pi-Sunyer, F. X., …, Look AHEAD Research Group. (2011). Neighborhood socioeconomic status, depression, and health status in the Look AHEAD (Action for Health in Diabetes) study. *BMJ Public Health, 11*, 349. Retrieved from http://www.biomedcentral.com/1471-2458/11/349

Gerber, Y., Myers, V., Goldbourt, U., Benyamini, Y., & Drory, Y. (2011). Neighborhood socioeconomic status and leisure time physical activity after myocardial infarction: A longitudinal study. *American Journal of Preventive Medicine, 3*, 266–273. doi:10.1016/j.amepre.2011.05.016

Goldsteen, R. L., & Goldsteen, K. (2012). *Introduction to the U.S. health care system* (7th ed.). New York, NY: Springer.

Gulley, S. P., Rasch, E. K., & Chan, L. (2011). Ongoing coverage for ongoing care: Access, utilization, and out-of-pocket spending among uninsured working-aged adults with chronic health needs. *American Journal of Public Health, 101*, 368–375. doi:10.2105/AJPH.2010.191569

Healthcare.gov. (n.d.a). *Health plan categories*. Retrieved from https://www.healthcare.gov/glossary/health-plan-categories/

Healy D., & Cromwell, J. (2012). *Hospital-acquired conditions - Present on admission: Examination of spillover events and unintended consequences*. Retrieved from https://www.cms.gov/Medicare/Medicare-Fee-for-Service-Payment/HospitalAcqCond/Downloads/HAC-SpilloverEffects.pdf

Howell, E., Decker, S., Hogan, S., Yemane, A., & Foster, J. (2010). Declining child mortality and continuing racial disparities in the era of Medicaid and SCHIP insurance coverage expansions.*American Journal of Public Health, 100*, 2500–2506.`doi:10.2105/AJPH.2009.184622

Institute of Medicine. (2001). *Crossing the quality chasm*. Washington, DC: National Academies Press.

Institute of Medicine. (2003). *Hidden costs, value lost: Uninsurance in America*. Washington, DC: National Academies Press.

Kaiser Commission on Medicaid and the Uninsured. (2012a). *Five facts about the uninsured*. Retrieved November 15, 2010, from http://kaiserfamilyfoundation.files.wordpress.com/2013/01/7806-05.pdf

Kaiser Commission on Medicaid and the Uninsured. (2012b). *The uninsured and the difference health insurance makes*. from http://www.kff.org/uninsured/upload/1420-12.pdf

Kaiser Family Foundation. (2011). *Retail prescription drugs filled at pharmacies (annual per capita by age)*. Retrieved from http://kff.org/other/state-indicator/retail-rx-drugs-by-age/

Kaiser Family Foundation. (2013). *Summary of new health reform law*. Retrieved from http://kaiserfamilyfoundation.files.wordpress.com/2011/04/8061-021.pdf

Kaiser Family Foundation and Health Research & Educational Trust. (2013). *Employer health benefits: 2013 summary of findings*. Retrieved from http://kaiserfamilyfoundation.files.wordpress.com/2013/08/8466-employer-health-benefits-2013_summary-of-findings2.pdf

Lang, I., Hubbard, R. E., Andrew, M. K., Llewellyn, D. J., Melzer, D., & Rockwood, K. (2009). Neighborhood deprivation, individual socioeconomic status, and frailty in older adults. *Journal of the American Geriatrics Society, 57*, 1776–1780. doi:10.1111/j.1532-5415.2009.02480.x

Lowes, R. (2010). *Individual mandate in health care reform law ruled unconstitutional by federal judge*. Retrieved from www.medscape.com/viewarticle/734110?src=nl_newsalert

Managed Care On-line. (2011). *Managed care fact sheets: National statistics*. Retrieved January 5, 2011, from http://www.mcareol.com/factshts/factnati.htm

McDonald, R. (2012). *For uninsured in Ore.: A flat rate for health care*. Retrieved from http://www.npr.org/2012/06/11/154738940/for-uninsured-in-ore-a-flat-fee-for-health-care

Medicaid.gov. (n.d.a). *Children's Health Insurance Program*. Retrieved from http://www.medicaid.gov/CHIP/CHIP-Program-Information.html

Medicaid.gov. (n.d.b). *Medicaid by population*. Retrieved from http://www.medicaid.gov/Medicaid-CHIP-Program-Information/By-Population/By-Population.html

Medicaid.gov. (n.d.c). *Provider preventable conditions*. Retrieved from http://www.medicaid.gov/Medicaid-CHIP-Program-Information/By-Topics/Financing-and-Reimbursement/Provider-Preventable-Conditions.html

Medicaid.gov. (2014). *Eligibility*. Retrieved from http://www.medicaid.gov/Medicaid-CHIP-Program-Information/By-Topics/Eligibility/Eligibility.html

Medicare.gov. (n.d.a). *Costs for Medicare drug coverage*. Retrieved from https://www.medicare.gov/part-d/costs/part-d-costs.html

Medicare.gov. (n.d.b). *Medicare Advantage plans*. Retrieved from https://www.healthcare.gov/glossary/health-plan-categories/

Medicare.gov. (n.d.c). *Medicare special needs plans*. Retrieved from http://www.medicare.gov/sign-up-change-plans/medicare-health-plans/medicare-advantage-plans/special-needs-plans.html

Murakami, K., Sasaki, S., Takahashi, Y., & Uenishi, K. (2010). Neighborhood socioeconomic status in relation to dietary intake and insulin resistance syndrome in female Japanese dietetic students. *Nutrition, 26*, 508–414. doi:10.1016/j.nut.2009.08.025

National Center for Charitable Statistics. (20n.d.). *Key data concepts*. Retrieved November 15, 2010, from http://nccs.urban.org/database/concepts.cfm

National Center for Health Statistics. (2010). Delayed or forgone medical care because of cost concerns among adults aged 18–64 years, Y disability and health insurance coverage status—National Health Interview Survey, United States, 2009. *Morbidity and Mortality Weekly Report, 59*, 1456.

National Center for Health Statistics. (2011). Reasons for no health insurance coverage among uninsured persons aged <65 years—National Health Interview Survey (NHIS), United States, 2009. *Morbidity and Mortality Weekly Report, 60*, 19.

National Center for Health Statistics. (2013). *Health, United States, 2013: With Special Feature on Emergency Care*. Retrieved from www.cdc.gov/nchs/data/hus/hus12.pdf

National Quality Forum. (2006). *Serious reportable events (SREs): Transparency, accountability critical to reducing medical errors and harm*. Retrieved from http://www.qualityforum.org/projects/sre2006.aspx

Nicklett, E. J., Szanton, S., Sun, K., Ferrucci, L., Fried, L. P., Guralnik, J. M., & Semba, R. D. (2010). Neighborhood socioeconomic status is associated with serum carotenoid concentrations in older, community-dwelling women. *Journal of Nutrition, 141*, 284–289. doi:10.3945/jn.110.129684

Office of the Assistant Secretary of Defense. (n.d.). *TRICARE overview*. Retrieved from http://ra.defense.gov/benefits/tricare/overview.html

Physicians Care Health Plans. (n.d.a). *Advantages of self-funding*. Retrieved January 6, 2011, from http://www.physicianscare.com/content/public/default.aspx?d=327

Physicians Care Health Plans. (n.d.b). *Is self-funding or fully insured right for your company?* Retrieved January 6, 2011, from http://www.physicianscare.com/content/public/default.aspx?d=330

Social Security Administration. (2010). *Medicare*. Retrieved August 7, 2010, from http://www.socialsecurity.gov/pubs/10043.html

Sultz, H. A., & Young, K. M. (2010). *Health care USA: Understanding its organization and delivery* (7th ed.). Sudbury, MA: Jones and Bartlett.

Trust for America's Health. (n.d). *Patient protection and affordable care act (HR 3590): Selected prevention, public health & workforce provisions*. Retrieved from http://healthyamericans.org/assets/files/Summary.pdf

U.S. Bureau of Labor Statistics. (2013a). *Consumer price index: Frequently asked questions (FAQs)*. Retrieved from http://www.bls.gov/cpi/cpifaq.htm#Question_1

U.S. Bureau of Labor Statistics. (2013b). *National Compensation Survey: Employee benefits in the United States, March 2013*. Retrieved from http://www.bls.gov/ncs/ebs/benefits/

U.S. Census Bureau. (2013). *Statistical abstract of the United States, 2012*. Retrieved from http://www.census.gov/compendia/statab/

U.S. Department of Health and Human Services. (n.d.a). *About the law*. Retrieved from http://www.hhs.gov/healthcare/rights/index.html

U.S. Department of Health and Human Services. (n.d.b). *Prevention and wellness*. Retrieved from http://www.hhs.gov/healthcare/prevention/index.html

U.S. Department of Health and Human Services. (2010). *Disparities*. Retrieved from http://www.healthypeople.gov/2020/about/DisparitiesAbout.aspx

U.S. Department of Health and Human Services. (2013a). *Access to health services: Objectives*. Retrieved from http://www.healthypeople.gov/2020/topicsobjectives2020/objectiveslist.aspx?opicId=1

U.S. Department of Health and Human Services. (2013b). *Access to health services: Overview*. Retrieved from http://www.healthypeople.gov/2020/topicsobjectives2020/overview.aspx?opicid=1

U.S. Department of Labor. (n.d.). *Health plans and benefits: Continuation of health coverage – COBRA*. Retrieved from http://www.dol.gov/dol/topic/health-plans/cobra.htm

U.S. Office of Personnel Management. (n.d.). *Federal Employees Health Benefits Program*. Retrieved from http://www.opm.gov/healthcare-insurance/healthcare/

Vladek, B. (2003). Universal health insurance in the United States: Reflections on the past, the present, and the future. *American Journal of Public Health, 93*, 16–19.

Zarzaur, B. L., Croce, M. A., Fabian, T. C., Fischer, P., & Magnotti, L. J. (2010). Population-based analysis of neighborhood socioeconomic status and injury admission rates and in-hospital mortality. *Journal of the American College of Surgeons, 211*, 216–223. doi:10.1016/j.jamcollsurg.2010.03.036

CHAPTER

7 Health System Influences on Population Health

Learning Outcomes

After reading this chapter, you should be able to:

1. Describe the components of the U.S. health care system.
2. Describe the organizational structure of the U.S. health care delivery system.
3. Compare and contrast official and voluntary health agencies.
4. Describe at least five functions performed by voluntary health agencies.
5. Discuss the involvement of local, state, and national governments in health care in the United States.
6. Compare selected features of national health care systems.

Key Terms

complementary/alternative health care subsystem
health care system
local public health system
official health agencies
pass-through funds
personal health care sector
popular health care subsystem
population health care sector
public health practice
public health system
scientific health care subsystem
state public health system
voluntary health agencies

Advocacy Then

Lemuel Shattuck and Public Health Organization

Although not a health professional, Lemuel Shattuck was known as a public health advocate. Following his career as an educator and merchant at age 46, he devoted the remainder of his life to improving public health. Shattuck was convinced of the need for the accurate collections of vital statistics as a means of monitoring the health of the public and was instrumental in the passage of the Massachusetts Registration Act (Koslow, 2011). In addition, Shattuck recommended a decennial federal census (*Lemuel Shattuck Biography (1739–1859*), 2011).

Shattuck conducted a census of the city of Boston in 1845 and was shocked by the mortality figures collected, particularly with respect to maternal and infant mortality (*Lemuel Shattuck (1793–1789): Prophet of American Public Health,* 1959). As a member of the Massachusetts legislature, he instigated the appointment of a state commission chaired by himself to investigate the sanitary conditions of the state. The commission's report, published in 1850, made broad recommendations for measures to improve the public's health. The members of the committee drafted sweeping legislation that addressed such issues as creation of state and local boards of health, sanitary laws, health promotion and illness prevention, immunization, sanitation and nuisance control, school health, food and medication safety, and communicable disease control. At the end of the report, the commission provided a series of reasons for approving the recommended plan of action as follows:

- Because it is a practical measure
- Because it is a useful measure
- Because it is an economical measure
- Because it is a philanthropic and charitable measure
- Because it is a moral measure
- Because the progress of the age demands it
- Because it involves an important duty (Shattuck, 1850)

Although the commission's legislative proposal was not passed, the vision for the organization of public health care services outlined in the report served as the foundation for the later development of boards of health in Massachusetts and throughout the country (London School of Hygiene and Tropical Medicine, 2010).

Advocacy Now

Nursing and Health System Reform

On February 22, 2010, a letter was sent to President Barack Obama and leaders in the U.S. Senate and House of Representatives presenting the nursing profession's perspectives on the proposed health care reform legislation, which eventually became the Patient Protection and Affordable Care Act. The letter was drafted by a coalition of 47 national nursing organizations called the Nursing Community and addressed multiple provisions of the proposed bill. Specifically, the letter supported provisions to expand the nursing workforce, nurse-managed health clinics, and primary care, prevention, health promotion, and emergency services. In addition, support was voiced for provisions to improve patient outcomes and reduce hospitalizations while reducing the costs of care, improving care coordination, increasing nursing home visitation programs, and incorporating best practices and evidence-based care into health care delivery systems, as well as provisions related to reimbursement for advanced practice nursing services.

The letter also addressed provisions of the bill requiring modification. These included inclusion of nurse midwives and nurse anesthetists in pay-for-performance plans along with nurse practitioners and clinical nurse specialists, equal representation from health disciplines on the National

Health Care Workforce Commission, and inclusion of nurse-sensitive quality and performance indicators in evaluation research.

Throughout the letter, the writers highlighted facts and figures that supported their positions. Given nursing's often-divisive approach to change, the ability to develop a common voice with respect to health care reform legislation was a major accomplishment and one that advocated for both the status of the profession and the needs of the American public.

Population health nursing occurs in the context of a health care delivery system that creates constraints and provides opportunities for practice. For example, the lack of emphasis on health promotion in the health care delivery system increases the need for health promotion efforts by population health nurses but simultaneously limits funds available for health promotion activities. In order to function effectively within the system and to achieve improvements in the public's health, population health nurses must understand how the health care delivery system is organized, how it works, and how it influences population health nursing practice and the public's health status.

Exploring the organization of health care delivery systems can help us to understand how these systems developed, how they work, and how and why they sometimes fail to work. Moreover, we can identify factors that positively or negatively influence population health nursing practice. Finally, we can identify areas where change is needed in the health care delivery system to best fulfill our goal as population health nurses, namely, the promotion of the public's health. We will look first at the U.S. health care system and then make some comparisons with the systems of other developed and developing nations.

The U.S. Health Care System

Sometimes referred to as a "nonsystem," the health care delivery system in the United States is a mixture of multiple sources of care at multiple levels. Each source and level is affected by a variety of external forces.

Forces Influencing the Health Care System

Health system observers have identified several forces that influence the organization and effectiveness of the U.S. health care system. Some of these factors include changing population demographics, growing numbers of uninsured residents, increasing demands for accountability, technological advances and innovation, professional labor issues, economic globalization, changes in delivery systems, and information management issues (Sultz & Young, 2014). The population in the United States, as in every other nation, is growing older, and older people tend to be the greatest users of health care services due to the prevalence of chronic disease in this population. In addition, the U.S. population is changing in terms of the ethnic groups represented; necessitating changes in health care delivery systems to accommodate clients from multiple cultures.

At the same time, there is a growing number of uninsured and underinsured individuals in the population, particularly among members of ethnic and cultural minority groups. In Chapters 6∞ and 21∞, we have and will examine some of the factors leading to this growth, but the very existence of a large population of uninsured individuals results in unmet needs in the health care system as it currently exists. From 1994 to 2007, the number of uninsured people in the United States increased from 15.8% of the non-elderly population to 17.1%, and an estimated 45 million people had no health insurance coverage in 2008 (Cover the Uninsured, 2009). The Affordable Care Act passed in 2010 was designed to provide insurance coverage for non-elderly persons with incomes below 133% of the federal poverty level (Kaiser Family Foundation, 2010); the legislation appears to have had a positive effect on the number of uninsured. For example, the percentage of people without health insurance had declined to 15.4% by 2012 (U.S. Census Bureau, 2013). Projections indicate that by 2019 the Act will result in decreases in the rate of uninsured persons to less than 14% in all but one state, with a large number of states' rates reduced below 8% (Commonwealth Fund, 2011).

Lack of health insurance is equivalent to lack of access to health care services for many people. In addition to the loss of health of individuals, lack of access to care poses significant costs to society. These costs lie in the loss of productive citizens through early death and disability as well as higher health care costs due to increasingly serious diseases that could have been treated at lower cost early in their course. Access to health care through affordable health insurance is perhaps the most important focus for advocacy to promote population health in the United States.

Another influence on health care systems is increasing public demand for accountability for both the quality of care provided and the use of resources to provide that care. Initiatives to assure standards of quality and limit the escalating costs of health care services have profoundly affected how health care is delivered. These and other economic influences on the health care system are addressed in more detail in Chapter 6∞. Technological advances significantly influence the cost of health care and greatly affect health care delivery systems. Furthermore, the widespread availability of high-tech information sources, such as the Internet, allows the U.S. public to be better informed of technological advances in care and encourages them to demand costly, high-tech services.

The primary professional labor issue facing health care delivery systems is the shortage of health care personnel, particularly nurses. With many other occupational choices available to potential recruits, health care systems have had to make many changes to attract young people to health care occupations and to specific practice locales (e.g., rural or inner-city areas). A second issue related to the professional workforce is the increasing need for advanced education for effective practice. The cost of educating providers and the need to provide the technology required to support the level of practice for which they are educated further increase the cost of health care services. In addition, health care systems are facing a need to change the ways they do business in order to attract providers (e.g., more flexible schedules, opportunities for job sharing, etc.).

Chapter 8∞ will address the effects of globalization on health and health care delivery. As we will see, the effects of globalization on health and health care delivery are both positive and negative. Changes in the organization of health care delivery systems also affect the operation and overall effectiveness of the U.S. health care system. For example, mergers of several institutions into large, for-profit organizations and competition among systems have a definite impact on health care delivery. Finally, changes in information management systems have led to changes in the completeness, accuracy, and transferability of information within and among health care organizations (Sultz & Young, 2014). For the most part this influence has been positive, leading to faster access to client care information, but it also raises issues of privacy and confidentiality.

All of these forces, as well as others that will be addressed elsewhere in this book (e.g., political activity and threats of terrorism), have contributed to the U.S. health care system as it presently exists and as it continues to evolve. Exploration of the health care system within the context of these forces can help us develop strategies to guide that evolution to greater effectiveness.

Components of the U.S. Health Care System

The World Health Organization (WHO, 2014) has defined a **health care system** as the network of personnel, agencies and organizations, and resources designed to promote, maintain, and restore the health of the population. No two health systems are alike, but many national health care systems share a number of commonalities. The major exception to this perception of commonality is the United States, which is the only developed nation in the world without a comprehensive approach to funding or providing health care services (Goldsteen & Goldsteen, 2012). Health care delivery in the United States has been described as an "unsystematic system" (Budrys, 2012) because of its multicentric and uncoordinated nature. Despite the relative accuracy of this description, we can still examine U.S. health care delivery in terms of the structure depicted in Figure 7-1●.

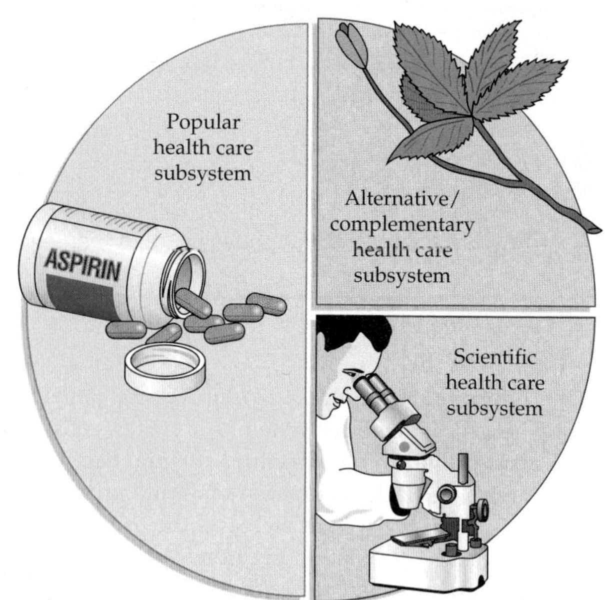

FIGURE 7-1 Organizational Structure of the U.S. Health Care Delivery System

The organizational structure for health care delivery in the United States consists of three major elements or subsystems, depicted in Figure 7-1. These subsystems include the popular health care subsystem, the complementary or alternative health care subsystem, and the scientific health care subsystem.

THE POPULAR HEALTH CARE SUBSYSTEM. Most health-related care is provided within the popular health care subsystem. The **popular health care subsystem** is the component of the health care system in which care is provided by oneself, family members, or friends, in short by people who are not considered health care providers. It is estimated that 70% to 90% of illness care is provided within this system. The popular subsystem includes health care that each of us provides for ourselves and our families. When you have a headache, for example, you may take an over-the-counter analgesic. If you are constipated, you may either increase the bulk, fiber, and fluid in your diet or take a laxative. If your child has a mild fever, you might give him or her an antipyretic. All of these self-care or family care practices constitute popular subsystem health care.

Although health care in this subsystem is provided by oneself or by family members, population health nurses have an educational role in the popular subsystem. As we shall see in Chapter 9∞, one of the purposes of health education is to prepare clients to make informed self-care decisions. For example, a population health nurse might caution a client against overuse of laxatives and suggest dietary approaches to dealing with constipation, or the nurse may inform parents about the hazards of giving aspirin to children and recommend a nonaspirin substitute.

THE COMPLEMENTARY/ALTERNATIVE HEALTH CARE SUBSYSTEM. When self-care fails or seems inappropriate, people often turn to other sources of health care. Some of these sources might be folk health practitioners. The **complementary/alternative health care subsystem** consists of providers and practices outside the scientific health care subsystem that are specifically focused on promotion of health and prevention of and care for illness. The terms *complementary* and *alternative* are often used interchangeably when discussing this subsystem, but actually differ in terms of their relationship to the scientific subsystem. Complementary health care practices are those that are used in conjunction with scientific care to *complement* and enhance its effects. Alternative practices, on the other hand, are used in place of, or as *alternatives* to, scientific interventions. Any given health practice may be considered complementary or alternative depending on its use in relation to scientific subsystem practices.

Practitioners in this subsystem are individuals who are believed to have special health-related knowledge or training beyond that of the average member of the society. Examples of alternative/complementary health care providers are the *curanderas* found among Latinos in the northeastern and southwestern regions of the United States and the herbalists found in these and other areas. The role of the population health nurse in the complementary/alternative health care subsystem is to assess the influence of this subsystem on health and to incorporate traditional health practices into the plan of care as appropriate. On occasion, the nurse may also need to caution clients against specific alternative practices that may be harmful to health (e.g., the use of traditional remedies that contain lead or other contaminants) or educate clients regarding the interactions between alternative and scientific therapies. The complementary/alternative health care subsystem was discussed in Chapter 5∞.

THE SCIENTIFIC HEALTH CARE SUBSYSTEM. The professional or **scientific health care subsystem** is the system of care based on scientific research–derived evidence. Health care provided in the scientific subsystem is based on knowledge derived from the biological, physical, and behavioral sciences and includes the services of nurses, physicians, pharmacists, social workers, and other health care professionals.

The scientific health care subsystem consists of two sectors that differ primarily in their focus of care. These sectors are the personal health care sector and the public, or population, health care sector.

The personal health care sector. The **personal health care sector** is the segment of the scientific health care subsystem that provides health-related services to individual clients. The primary emphasis in this sector is cure of disease and restoration of health, although individuals may also receive some health-promotive and illness-preventive services.

There are five major components to this sector of the health care system: health care institutions, personnel, health commodities firms, education/research institutions, and financing systems (Goldsteen & Goldsteen, 2012). The institutional component consists of health provider office settings, clinics, hospitals, nursing homes, and other places where care is dispensed to individual clients. The personnel component is composed of the professionals who provide services. Health commodities firms include industries that manufacture or supply the materials and equipment required to implement health care services. Some examples of commodities firms include pharmaceutical companies and manufacturers of durable medical equipment or health-related computer software.

Both educational and research institutions are components of the personal health sector in that they educate health professionals to provide individual client care services and conduct research related to therapeutic interventions and delivery systems. The final component of the sector comprises the systems that finance care, which include insurers, philanthropic institutions, and government agencies.

Any given element of the sector may embody several of these components. For example, a university hospital may provide services, educate providers, and conduct research. As we saw in Chapter 6∞, some health care organizations, such as managed care organizations (MCOs), also incorporate the financing element.

The personal health care sector may be further divided into for-profit and not-for-profit segments. In the for-profit segment, health care services are provided with the intention of deriving monetary gain. Within this segment are the "proprietary" service providers, such as physicians and health care institutions designed to create revenue, and corporations that provide health care to employees (and occasionally their families) in order to limit the drain of health insurance costs on company revenue (Goldsteen & Goldsteen, 2012). Population health nurses' primary relationship with the personal health care sector is linking clients to sources of health care and advocating for the availability of personal health care services needed by members of the population. A few population health nurses, who also function in advanced practice nursing roles (e.g., nurse practitioner, clinical nurse specialist, etc.) may also provide direct services in the personal health care sector.

The population health care sector. The **population health care sector** consists of both public and private organizations whose focus is the health of the total population. This sector is also referred to as the **public health system**, which has been defined as "All public, private, and voluntary entities that contribute to the delivery of essential public health services within a jurisdiction. These systems are a network of entities with differing roles, relationships, and interactions that contribute to the health and well-being of the community or state" (National Public Health Performance Standards Program [NPHPSP], n.d., p. 32).

Public health practice is defined as "the art and science of preventing disease, promoting population health and extending life through organized local and global efforts" (McMichael & Beaglehole, 2009, p. 2). General goals for public health practice include improving population health, reducing health inequalities within the population, and developing environments that support health (McMichael & Beaglehole, 2009).

In a classic report on "The Future of the Public's Health in the 21st Century," the Institute of Medicine (IOM) (2003) identified six areas of action and change that must be undertaken to assure effective population health in the United States:

- Adopting a population health approach that considers the multiple determinants of health;
- Strengthening the governmental and public health infrastructure, which forms the backbone of the public health system;
- Building a new generation of intersectoral partnerships that also draw on the perspectives and resources of diverse communities and actively engage them in health action;
- Developing systems of accountability to assure the quality and availability of public health services;
- Making evidence the foundation of decision making and the measure of success; and
- Enhancing and facilitating communication within the public health system (e.g., among all levels of the governmental public health infrastructure and between public health professionals and community members). (p. 4)

One segment of the IOM that focuses specifically on population health is the Board on Population Health and Public Health Practice. This 16-member board focuses on issues affecting the public's health from general public health principles to addressing specific population health issues. Recent activities of the board have ranged from examination of issues related to specific communicable diseases, to integration of public health and primary care activities, to action related to chronic disease, health literacy, and tobacco cessation (IOM, 2011).

A particularly salient recent activity of the board has been the constitution of a committee to develop public health strategies to improve health. The committee examined population health strategies in the context of the provisions of the Affordable Care Act (ACA) discussed in Chapter 6∞ and in more detail later in this chapter. A report by the committee noted that ACA contains a number of provisions that support population health, including an emphasis on health promotion and illness prevention and the requirement for hospitals receiving federal funding to conduct periodic community needs assessments and to develop plans to address identified needs. The committee noted, however, that in order to achieve the "Triple Aim" identified by the Institute for Healthcare Improvement (2014) (improved population health, enhanced patient experience of care, and reduced or controlled costs), the health care system needs to "move from a culture of sickness to a culture of care and then to a culture of health" (Alper, 2013, p. 17). There is a need to create a market for health, rather than a market for disease or care, by creating a payment system that rewards improvements in health, rather than treatment of disease. Strategies identified to enhance population health included:

- Public health collaboration with multiple stakeholders in addressing health
- Use of financial incentives to align provider and hospital interests with a health focus
- Creation of information systems to assess and monitor population health, including development of metrics to measure progress
- Integration of a health focus into all areas of care
- Developing an agreed-upon vision, culture, and goals
- Community engagement in priority setting and action
- Effective training for health professionals to integrate and advocate for a health focus in care
- Development of certification and licensing that supports new population health roles
- Creation of learning and improving environments (Alper, 2013)

Population health nurses will be actively involved in initiating and implementing all of these strategies.

Care provided in the population health care sector has traditionally centered on promoting health and preventing disease, although some curative care does occur in this sector. Emphasis is on designing health care programs that meet the needs of population groups.

Official public health agencies. **Official health agencies** are agencies of local, state, and national governments that are responsible for the health of the people in their jurisdictions. Official agencies are supported by tax revenues and other public funding. They are accountable to the citizens of their jurisdiction, usually through an elected or appointed governing body. Many of the activities conducted by official agencies are mandated by law. For example, local health departments are required by state law to report cases of certain diseases. We will discuss specific functions of official agencies at local, state, and national levels in more detail later in this chapter. Generally speaking, however, official public health agencies are responsible for providing the ten essential public health services discussed in Chapter 1∞.

Voluntary health agencies. **Voluntary health agencies** are nonprofit organizations that provide adjuncts to services provided by government agencies. These may include institutional and personal services that address the needs of special groups, education for public health, or prevention, screening, health maintenance, rehabilitation, or terminal care services (Sultz & Young, 2014). Voluntary agencies may focus on a specific disease entity, an organ system, or a population group. Voluntary agencies are funded primarily by donations. They are accountable to their supporters, and their activities are determined by supporter interests rather than legal mandate. Their primary emphasis is on research, education, and policy development, although they may provide some direct health care services.

Voluntary agencies can be categorized on the basis of their source of funding. The first category consists of agencies supported by citizen contributions, such as the American Cancer Society. The first agency of this type in the United States was the Antituberculosis Society founded in Philadelphia in 1892. The focus of this type of agency frequently changes as health needs change. For example, the Antituberculosis Society is known today as the American Lung Association, indicating its broader focus on a variety of respiratory conditions. The second category consists of foundations established by private philanthropic contributions. An example of this type of voluntary organization would be the Kellogg Foundation, which provides funding for health care research. Today, more than 3,000 philanthropic foundations support health efforts. The third category of voluntary agency is funded by member dues. The American Public Health Association and the American Nurses Association are examples of this type of agency.

Integrating agencies, such as the United Way, coordinate the fund-raising activities of several voluntary agencies. A fifth type of voluntary agency includes religious organizations that derive their funds from contributions by members of a congregation. These groups often focus on local needs and are particularly effective because of their ability to draw on volunteers. The final category of voluntary health agency is the commercial organization that engages in health care activities. For example, the American Dairy Association provides literature and visual aids for nutrition education. Similarly, health insurance companies often disseminate literature on health promotion and illness prevention.

Voluntary agencies often explore areas that are poorly addressed by the other components of the health care system. For example, research that culminated in the development of a vaccine for polio was the early focus of the March of Dimes. Now, polio immunization is largely a function of official agencies. Education of the public and health professionals regarding health-related issues is another major focus of voluntary agencies. For example, the American Cancer Society has spearheaded educational campaigns on the hazards of smoking. Voluntary agencies may also supplement services provided by official health agencies. For instance, some voluntary agencies provide transportation to clinics, respite care, special equipment, and other ancillary services.

Advocacy for the public's health is a major role for voluntary agencies. For example, a voluntary agency may campaign against reduction of health care services due to budget cuts. In this role, voluntary agencies often promote legislation related to health. In one community, for example, a collaborative organization of residents and service providers was successful in promoting legislation to prevent tenants from being evicted without cause and to extend required eviction notice from 30 to 60 days. Voluntary agencies may also assist official agencies in determining health care needs in the population and in planning programs to address those needs. They also support and conduct research related to interventions to address population health problems.

Levels of care in the population health sector. Health care delivery in the United States takes place at local, state, and national levels. Each level has certain responsibilities with respect to the health of the population. Both official and voluntary agencies exist at each level, but official agencies are the focus of this discussion. Public health agencies at each of the three levels—local, state, and national—perform the essential public health services, but the degree to which they are emphasized varies from level to level.

Although official health agencies at all three levels address public health needs, state governments hold primary responsibility for preserving and protecting the health of the public. The power to protect the safety and welfare of the public is reserved to the states by the United States Constitution. In fact, any power not specifically delegated to the federal government by the Constitution remains within the purview of state governments. In the same way that the states, through the Constitution, have delegated certain responsibilities to the federal government, they may also delegate some health-related functions and responsibilities to agencies at the local level (Goldsteen & Goldsteen, 2012).

The Local Level. A **local public health system** is defined as "the collection of public, private and voluntary entities, as well as individuals and informal associations, that contribute to the public's health within a jurisdiction" (NPHPSP, n.d., p. 24). The official agency at the local level is usually the *local health department.* Some local public health agencies are large health systems serving the populations of major jurisdictions such as New York City or Los Angeles County. Many, however, serve smaller populations and do not have the resources to perform all of the essential public health services. The local health department's authority is derived, in part, from responsibilities delegated by the state. For example, the state delegates to the local level the responsibility for collecting statistics on births and deaths. Because this responsibility has been legally delegated, the local health department has the authority to ensure that a death certificate is filed for every death that occurs. The local agency also derives authority from local health ordinances. For instance, local government might pass an ordinance requiring all residential rental units to have functioning smoke detectors. Enforcement of this ordinance might then become the responsibility of the local health department.

Funding at the local level comes from both local taxes and state and federal subsidies. A portion of local public health agency funding comes from the state, including federal **pass-through funds**, money granted to the states by the federal government that is allocated to local government agencies. Other operating funds derive from local revenues, including local taxes. A small percentage of funding comes directly from federal monies (excluding Medicaid and Medicare funds). In recent years, local health departments have attempted to augment revenue sources by providing personal care services reimbursable under Medicare and Medicaid. Another small percentage of local health department funding is derived from client fees, private health insurance, regulatory fees, and so on.

Figure 7-2● depicts the typical organizational structure of a local health department. The staff and programs included will vary from place to place. In some areas, the district health officer might also fulfill the role of administrative officer. Small counties or districts may not be able to afford the full-time services of some types of personnel, and the services of nutritionists, social workers, dentists, and other personnel might be shared by several counties or provided at the state level. Nurses and clerical staff would be found in almost any local

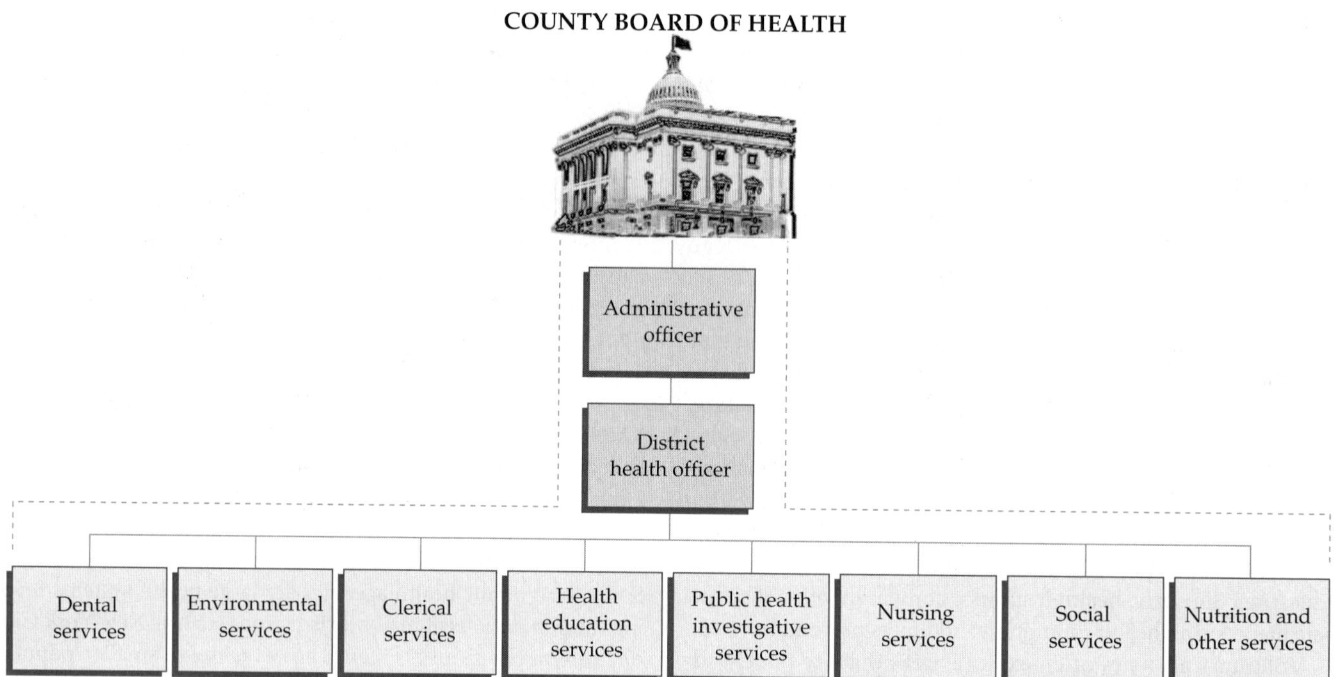

FIGURE 7-2 Typical Organizational Structure of a Local Health Department

health department. Other personnel who may be available include environmental specialists, physical therapists, psychologists, laboratory and X-ray technicians, and pharmacists.

Because delegation of specific responsibilities to local jurisdictions is the function of the state, the responsibilities assumed vary from state to state. Local responsibilities may also vary within regions of a particular state, depending on the local jurisdiction's capabilities and resources. Within the context of the core public health functions, local health agencies assess and monitor local health needs and resources, develop policies that foster local involvement in decision making and equitable allocation of resources, and assure availability of high-quality services to meet local health needs. The assurance function also includes educating the community on how to access available services. Typical responsibilities performed by local health agencies include collection of vital statistics, communicable disease control, disease screening and surveillance, immunization, and health education. Other responsibilities include chronic disease control, sanitation, school health and maternal–child health programs, and population health nursing services. Local public health services may or may not include mental health services and primary care services for the indigent. Specific services provided by local public health agencies will depend, in large part, on the needs of local populations.

The state level. A **state public health system** is "the state public health agency working in partnership with other state government agencies, private enterprises, and voluntary organizations that operate statewide to provide services essential to the health of the public" (NPHPSP, n.d., p. 37). The official agency at the state level has traditionally been a state department of health. As noted above, the state, not the federal government or the local jurisdiction, has primary authority in matters relating to health. The state retains the ultimate responsibility for the health of the public and possesses essential power to make laws and regulations regarding health.

The state health department derives funding from state tax revenues and may also receive monies from the federal government. A general organizational schema for a state department of health is depicted in Figure 7-3●. The various divisions coordinate services at the state level and provide assistance to the local level.

Because of their primary responsibility for the health of the population, state public health agencies have more mandated functions related to health than the federal government. General areas of responsibility for state health agencies include, for example, regulation and quality assurance for health care providers and facilities, health care planning, regulation of insurance companies, and workplace and environmental protection (Goldsteen & Goldsteen, 2012). Some state health departments also provide direct services to selected population, and as we saw in Chapter 6∞, state health agencies fund a significant portion of care provided under the Medicaid program.

The national level. Because the Constitution makes no reference to any responsibilities of the federal government regarding health, the federal government has no direct authority to regulate health-related matters. The authority of the federal government with respect to health is derived indirectly from two other constitutional powers (Goldsteen & Goldsteen, 2012). The first of these is the *power to regulate foreign and interstate commerce.* For example, because most cosmetics are transported across state lines, the federal Food and Drug Administration has the authority to establish standards of purity for the manufacture of cosmetics.

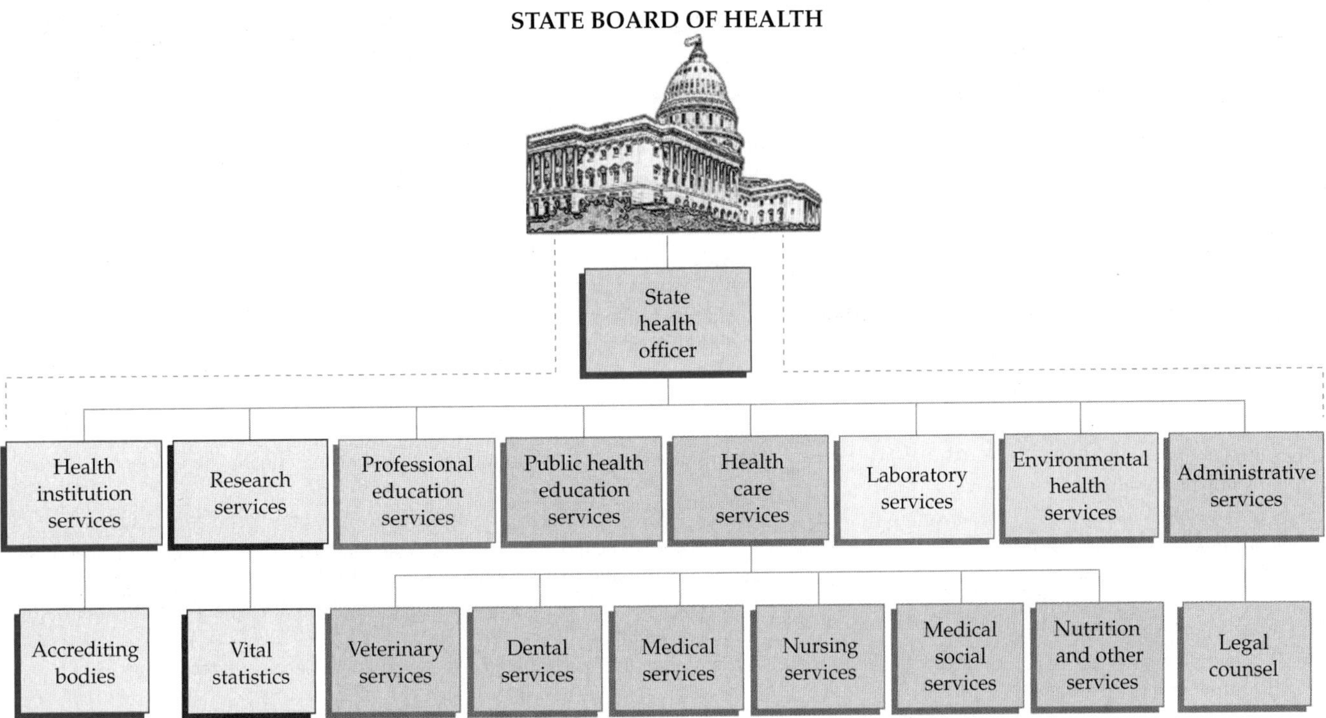

FIGURE 7-3 Typical Organizational Structure of a State Health Department

The second constitutional source of authority over health matters is the *power to levy taxes and spend to promote the general welfare*. For example, it can be argued that such programs as Medicaid and Medicare promote the general welfare and are therefore within the authority of the federal government.

The official health agency at the national level is the United States Department of Health and Human Services (USDHHS or HHS), created in 1980 with the division of the former Department of Health, Education, and Welfare into two separate departments. The head of the agency is the Secretary of Health and Human Services, who fills a cabinet post and acts in an advisory capacity to the president in matters of health. The Office of the Secretary incorporates staff divisions, operating divisions, and ten regional offices. The staff divisions oversee the overall operations of the department, provide guidance, and see that funding allocations are used appropriately and that legal requirements are met. The 11 operating divisions of HHS include eight agencies within the U.S. Public Health Service and three human service agencies. The regional offices oversee program implementation in specific regions throughout the country (USDHHS, n.d.a). Within HHS, the Office of the Assistant Secretary for Health (ASH) oversees a variety of public health-related agencies, including 12 core public health offices (USDHHS, n.d.b, n.d.c, 2011). These agencies are summarized in Table 7-1•. ASH also oversees the provision of services by the U.S. Public Health Services Commissioned Corps, an agency that provides health care personnel to meet the needs of specific underserved populations (USDHHS, 2013a).

Operating divisions within HHS are depicted in Figure 7-4• and include the Administration for Children and Families,

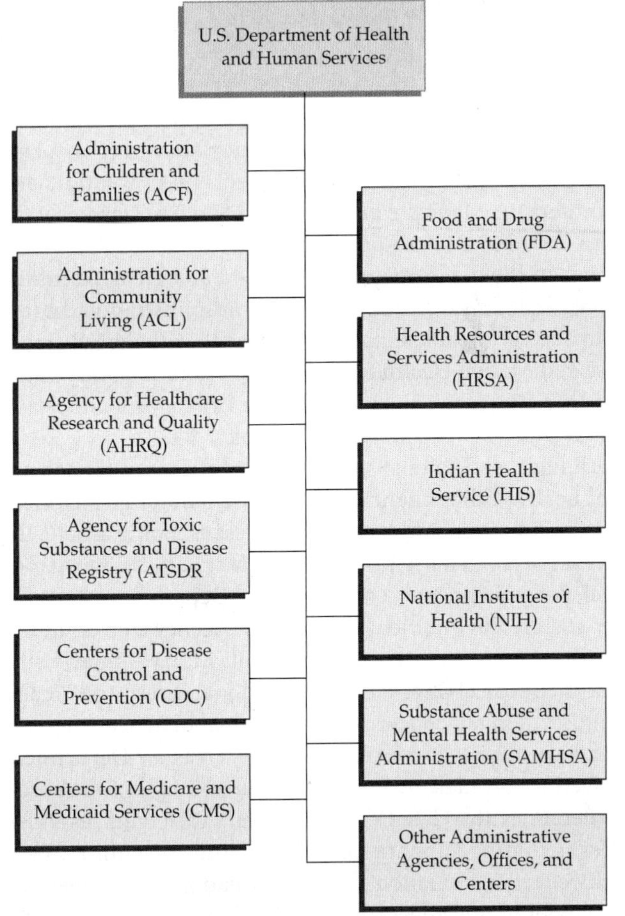

FIGURE 7-4 Operating Divisions of the U.S. Department of Health and Human Services

TABLE 7-1 Agencies Under the Assistant Secretary of Health

Agency	Function
National Vaccine Program Office (NVPO) http://www.hhs.gov/nvpo	Provides information on childhood, adolescent, and adult immunizations and ensures collaboration among federal agencies dealing with immunization activities
Office of Adolescent Health http://www.hhs.gov/ash/oah/	Coordinates adolescent health promotion and disease prevention programs across HHS
Office of Disease Prevention and Health Promotion (ODPHP) http://odphp.osophs.dhhs.gov	Provides leadership, coordination, and policy development related to public health and prevention activities. Leads the *Healthy People* initiative
Office of HIV/AIDS and Infectious Disease Policy (OHAIDP) http://www.hhs.gov/ash/ohaidp/	Coordinates, integrates, and directs HHS policies, programs and activities related to HIV/AIDS, viral hepatitis, and other infectious diseases, and blood safety and availability
Office for Human Research Protections (OHRP) http://www.hhs.gov/ohrp	Provides leadership and oversight in the protection of human subjects in HHS-supported research
Office of Minority Health (OMH) http://minorityhealth.hhs.gov/	Addresses health status and quality of life for U.S. minority populations
Office of Population Affairs (OPA) http://www.hhs.gov/opa/	Advises HHS officials regarding reproductive and other population issues
Office of Research Integrity (ORI) http://ori.hhs.gov/	Promotes integrity in intramural and extramural Public Health Service research and addresses allegations of research misconduct
Office on Women's Health (OWH) http://www.womenshealth.gov/owh/	Advances a comprehensive women's health agenda throughout HHS to improve the health of women
Presidential Commission for the Study of Bioethical Issues (PCSBI) http://www.bioethics.gov/	Advises on ethical issues related to biomedical science and technology
President's Council on Fitness, Sports, and Nutrition (PCFSN) http://www.fitness.gov/	Advises on issues related to fitness, sports, and nutrition

Data from: U.S. Department of Health and Human Services. (n.d.b). *Office of the Assistant Secretary of Health.* Retrieved from http://www.hhs.gov/ash/

Administration for Community Living, Agency for Healthcare Research and Quality, Agency for Toxic Substances and Disease Registry, Centers for Disease Control and Prevention, and the Centers for Medicare and Medicaid Services (formerly the Health Care Financing Administration). Other health-related agencies in the department are the Food and Drug Administration, Health Resources and Services Administration, Indian Health Service, National Institutes of Health, and the Substance Abuse and Mental Health Services Administration (USDHHS, 2013b). These agencies, along with their primary functions and Internet addresses, are presented in Table 7-2●.

Although HHS is the agency primarily responsible for national health, other agencies within the federal government are also involved in addressing health issues. For example, the Department of Defense provides health care for military personnel, dependents, and retirees, and the Department of the Interior and the Environmental Protection Agency address health concerns related to environmental pollution. Similarly, the Department of Labor and the Occupational Safety and Health Administration are concerned with occupational health as well as other employment concerns, and the Treasury Department is actively involved in efforts to control drugs subject to abuse.

Federal health-related agencies have a variety of responsibilities including support for research and dissemination of health-related information, developing national objectives and priorities for health, and assurance related to actions and services in the interests of national public health. In addition, the federal government provides assistance to state agencies in the form of technical assistance and funding to support state health initiatives. One of the major ways in which the federal government enacts its knowledge development and dissemination function is through the activities of the National Institutes of Health (NIH). NIH consists of the Office of the Director, 20 research institutes, 6 centers, and the National Library of Medicine. The institutes and many of the centers fund and conduct research related to specific health problems, conditions, and susceptible populations (National Institutes of Health, 2014). Figure 7-5● depicts the institutes and centers that comprise NIH.

U.S. Health System Reform

Due to the complexity and multicentric nature of the U.S. health care system, the system is frequently deficient in meeting the third core function of public health, assuring availability and provision of needed care, and in achieving desired health-related outcomes. As we saw earlier, significant portions of the U.S. public are uninsured and have limited access to care. In the 2011 National Interview Survey, 19.9 million people or 6.5% of the U.S. population did not receive needed medical care due to cost, and another 27.3 million delayed obtaining care (Adams, Kirzinger, & Martinez, 2012). In international comparisons, the United States lags behind many other developed nations with respect to health care outcomes. Some of these comparisons will be discussed in more detail later in this chapter.

TABLE 7-2 Operating Divisions Within the Department of Health and Human Services

Agency	Function
Administration for Children and Families (ACF) http://www.acf.hhs.gov	Promotes the economic and social well-being of families, children, individuals, and communities
Administration for Community Living (ACL) http://www.acl.gov	Combines the former Administration on Aging, Administration of Developmental Disabilities, and Office on Disabilities to promote access to community support and resources to meet the needs of the elderly and people with disabilities
Agency for Healthcare Research and Quality (AHRQ) http://www.ahrq.gov	Supports research to improve the quality of health care, decrease costs, promote safety, and broaden access to services for all Americans
Agency for Toxic Substances and Disease Registry (ATSDR) http://www.atsdr.cdc.gov	Prevents harmful exposures and disease related to toxic environmental substances
Centers for Disease Control and Prevention (CDC) http://www.cdc.gov	Promotes health and quality of life by preventing and controlling disease and other preventable conditions
Centers for Medicare and Medicaid Services (CMS) http://www.cms.hhs.gov	Oversees the federal health care programs under Medicare, Medicaid, the Children's Health Insurance Program (CHIP), and the Health Insurance Marketplace
Food and Drug Administration (FDA) http://www.fda.gov	Protects the public health by assuring the safety, efficacy, and security of human and veterinary drugs, biological products, medical devices, national food supply, cosmetics, and products that emit radiation
Health Resources and Services Administration (HRSA) http://www.hrsa.gov	Improves access to quality health care for the uninsured, isolated, or medically vulnerable
Indian Health Service (IHS) http://www.ihs.gov	Provides comprehensive health services to American Indians and Alaska Natives to the highest level
National Institutes of Health (NIH) http://www.nih.gov	Supports and conducts biomedical and behavioral research and promotes dissemination of medical knowledge
Substance Abuse and Mental Health Services Administration (SAMHSA) http://www.samhsa.gov	Provides leadership for the prevention and treatment of mental and addictive disorders

Data from: U.S. Department of Health and Human Services. (2013b). *Operating divisions.* Retrieved from http://www.usphs.gov/aboutus/

The relative lack of effectiveness of the U.S. health care system mandates significant reform, and reform efforts have a long, and generally unsuccessful, history. Reform proposals have been put forward since 1912 when Teddy Roosevelt's Progressive Party promoted the concept of social insurance, to include health insurance coverage. Efforts to promote compulsory health insurance at a national level were promulgated as early as 1915 by the American Association for Labor Legislation. During the Depression, Franklin Delano Roosevelt created a Commission on Economic Security to address medical care and health insurance as well as other economic issues. As a result, the Social Security Act was passed, but health insurance initiatives failed (Kaiser Family Foundation, 2011b).

During the 1940s, renewed calls for compulsory national health insurance were defeated due to fears of socialism and reluctance to grant a significant role to the federal government in health care matters. Similar initiatives continued to fail in the 1950s, but in 1965 the Medicare and Medicaid programs were initiated with federal legislation, and the neighborhood health centers program was established to provide care in poor and medically underserved communities. For the next 35 years, numerous plans for a national health insurance system were put forth and rejected, often in the name of cost containment.

Pay-for-performance, a system of rewards for meeting preestablished outcomes related to quality and efficiency, is one approach that has been taken in the attempt to control health care costs while improving outcomes. Some health care funders have instituted financial incentives to reward providers and systems that meet or exceed designated outcomes. Performance measures tend to be of four types: process measures, outcome measures, patient experience measures, and structure measures. Process measures address the extent to which demonstrated best-practice activities have been incorporated into care (e.g., annual eye exams for people with diabetes). Outcome measures reflect the effects of care on the client's health status (e.g., the extent of hypertension control achieved). Patient experience measures assess client's perceptions of the quality of care and satisfaction with that care. Finally, structure measures address how health care delivery is structured, for example, whether or not electronic health records are in place (*Pay for Performance*, 2012). The Human Resources and Services Administration (HRSA) has suggested adherence to evidence-based guidelines for care as a measure of provider or system performance rather than patient outcomes, which are less influenced by external factors (e.g., patient compliance with medication) (HRSA, n.d.).

Other agencies have taken the opposite approach and sanctioned providers and systems that do not meet established benchmarks. For example, as we saw in Chapter 6∞, the Centers for Medicare and Medicaid Services (CMS) has developed a set of adverse events, termed "never events," for which it will not reimburse hospitals for care. Positive reimbursement for performance is exemplified in the CMS Value-based Purchasing program expanded by the Affordable Care Act. This program

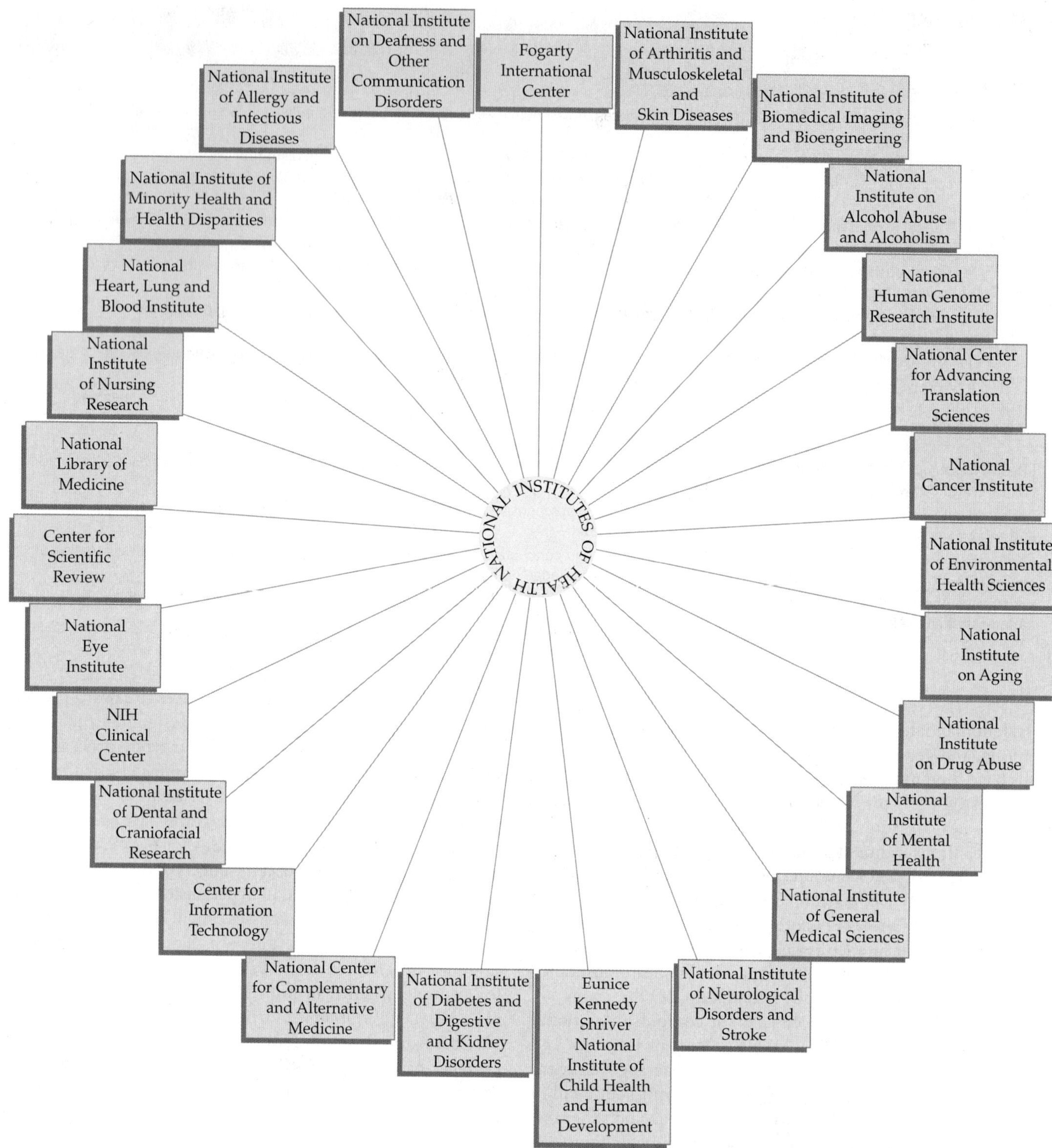

FIGURE 7-5 Institutes and Centers of the National Institutes of Health

links incentive payments to hospitals' ability to perform on a designated set of quality measures. Until recently, CMS also provided incentive payments to physicians who voluntarily reported specific quality data. In 2015, however, the incentives will cease and physicians who fail to report quality data will receive reduced Medicare payments. Pay-for-performance initiatives have been shown to have some effect on both the costs and quality of care, but have been criticized for the potential for unintended negative effects (*Pay for Performance*, 2012). Pay-for-performance was explored in more detail in Chapter 6∞.

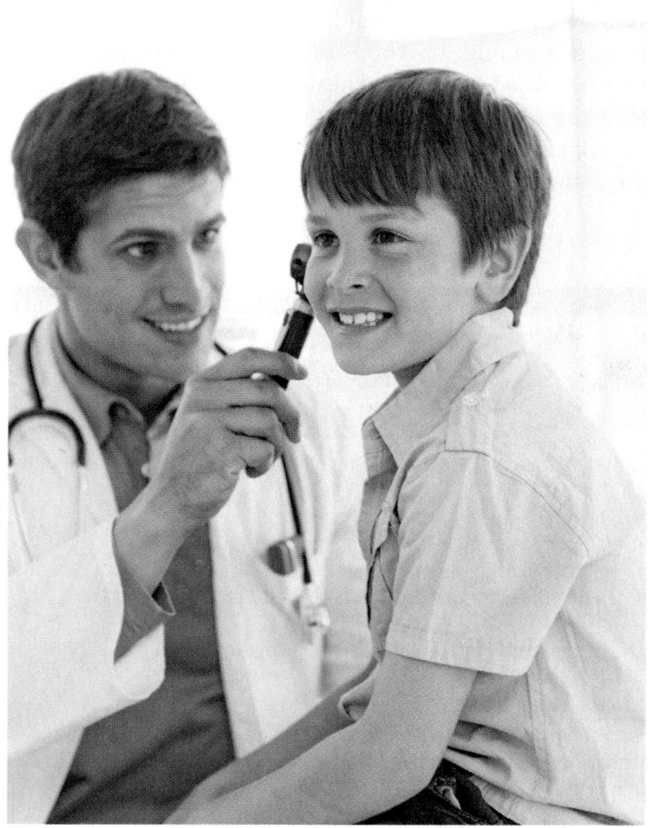

Assuring availability of health services is one of the core functions of public health. *(Wavebreakmedia/Shutterstock)*

In March of 2010, President Barack Obama signed the Patient Protection and Affordable Health Care Act in an effort to improve health care access and system function in the United States (Kaiser Family Foundation, 2011b). Provisions of the act are designed for incremental implementation through 2019. The provisions are far reaching and include a number of different initiatives. Major categories of initiatives include requirements for all U.S. citizens to have some form of health insurance coverage; employer requirements for coverage of employees; expansion of public insurance programs under Medicare, Medicaid, and the Children's Health Insurance Program (CHIP); provision of premium and cost-sharing subsidies to individuals and families with incomes between 133% and 400% of the federal poverty level and to small businesses; taxation of individuals without insurance coverage and of pharmaceutical, health insurance, and medical device companies; creation of state-based health insurance exchanges to assist in the purchase of coverage by individuals and small businesses; and creation of an "essential benefits" package. Additional provisions of the bill prohibit insurance companies from placing lifetime limits on coverage and denying coverage for preexisting conditions. The act also expands the role of state government in providing insurance coverage, promotes cost-containment initiatives, supports research on improving system quality and performance, promotes prevention and wellness initiatives and long-term care coverage, and supports health care workforce development, community- and school-based health centers, trauma care, and disaster preparedness (Kaiser Family Foundation, 2011a). For further information about the provisions of ACA, see the *External Resources* section of the student resources site.

Other National Health Care Systems

As we noted above, The U.S. health care system compares unfavorably with several other national health systems, in large part because of the lack of universal coverage of all its citizens. The United States is the only developed nation that does not have some form of universal health care coverage.

Public Health Functions: An International Perspective

In Chapter 1∞, we examined the core functions and essential public health services developed for the U.S. health care system. Similar descriptions have been developed elsewhere in the world. For example, the Pan American Health Organization (PAHO, 2011) developed a list of essential public health functions and defined them as "the fundamental set of actions that should be performed in order to achieve public health's central objective: improving the health of populations" (para. 1). PAHO also developed a methodology to evaluate public health capacity within a given country (PAHO, 2011). The essential functions and related public health activities are presented in Table 7-3●.

Features of Selected National Health Systems

Nations throughout the world have developed unique organizational structures for delivering health care services to their peoples. Although no two health systems are alike, they tend to have certain commonalities. For example, all health systems are designed to address three major considerations: how care

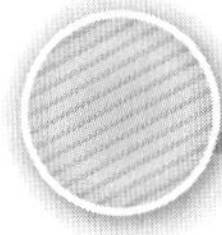

Global Perspectives

Barriers to Obtaining U.S. Health Care

People come to the United States from all over the world for many different purposes. Some intend only a short stay; others plan to relocate here permanently. What are some of the barriers within the U.S. health care system to obtaining care for those from other parts of the world? How might these barriers be eliminated or modified to improve their access to necessary care?

will be organized and delivered, how services will be funded, and the mechanisms to be used for reimbursing providers. In addition, national health systems have to address a number of policy dilemmas. These include balancing the need for regional or national coordination with the requirement to meet local health needs, distributing available resources equitably, balancing professional practice autonomy with accountability for population health outcomes, promoting the use of evidence-based best practices and guidelines, and addressing health disparities among subgroups in the population. Additional dilemmas faced by national health systems include assuring access to care in the face of cost constraints, balancing curative technology with allocations for prevention and promotion, maintaining a qualified health care workforce, ensuring

TABLE 7-3 Essential Public Health Functions of National Health Systems, Pan American Health Organization

Function	Related Activities
Monitoring, evaluation, and analysis of health status	• Evaluating health status, trends, and determinants, and identifying inequalities in risks, threats, and access to health services. • Identifying population health needs, health risks, and demand for services. • Managing important statistics and the situation of high-risk and/or specific groups. • Producing information to evaluate health services performance. • Identifying resources from outside the health sector that can improve health promotion and the quality of life. • Developing technology and methods to manage, interpret, and communicate information to public health's decision makers, external actors, suppliers, and citizens. • Defining and developing agencies to evaluate the quality of the collected data.
Surveillance, research, and control of risks and threats to public health	• Developing capacity for research and surveillance of epidemic outbreaks and communicable and non-communicable diseases models, behavioral factors, accidents, and exposure to toxic substances or environmental agents detrimental to health. • Developing a public health structure to support epidemiological research. • Supporting public health laboratory capacity to perform rapid analyses and process large volumes of tests to identify and control new health threats. • Implementing programs for epidemiological surveillance and infectious disease control. • Creating capacity to connect with international networks to better tackle the health problems of greatest concern. • Strengthening the ability to conduct surveillance at a local level and produce rapid responses to control health problems or risks.
Health promotion	• Promoting changes in lifestyle and environmental conditions that promote development of a health culture. • Strengthening intersectoral partnerships to make health promotion actions more effective. • Assessing the impact of public policies on health. • Developing educational actions and social communication that promote healthy conditions, lifestyles, behaviors, and environments. • Reorienting health services to develop models of care that support health promotion.
Social participation in health	• Empowering citizens to change their own lifestyles and take an active role in developing healthy behaviors and environments. • Facilitating organized community participation in decisions and actions related to programs of prevention, diagnosis, treatment, and rehabilitation.
Development of policy and institutional capacity for planning and management in public health	• Defining measurable public health objectives at all levels, consistent with a framework of values that promote equality. • Developing, monitoring, and evaluating political decisions concerning public health, through a participatory process consistent with the political and economic context of the decisions. • Creating institutional capacity to manage public health systems, including strategic planning to solve the population's health problems. • Developing decision-making capacity based on evidence that incorporates planning, evaluation, leadership, effective communication, organizational development, and resource management. • Developing public health capacity for international cooperation.
Strengthening of institutional capacity for regulation and enforcement in public health	• Creating institutional capacity to develop regulatory frameworks necessary to monitor and protect the population's health. • Developing the capacity to create new laws and regulations to improve population health and promote the development of healthy environments. • Protecting citizens in their relationship with the health system. • Ensuring compliance with the standards in a timely, correct, congruent, and complete manner.

TABLE 7-3 (*Continued*)

Function	Related Activities
Evaluation and promotion of equitable access to necessary health services	• Promoting equitable access to necessary health services for all citizens. • Developing actions to overcome access barriers to public health interventions and link vulnerable groups to health services. • Monitoring and evaluating access to necessary public and private health services, adopting a multisectoral, multitechnical and multicultural approach in conjunction with various agencies and institutions to resolve the injustices and inequalities in the utilization of services. • Fostering close collaboration with governmental and non-governmental organizations to promote equitable access to necessary health services.
Human resources training and development in public health	• Determining human resource profiles needed to provide public health services. • Educating, training, and evaluating public health personnel to identify public health services needs, effectively face pressing public health issues, and adequately evaluate action. • Defining accreditation requirements for general health professionals and fostering continuous quality improvement programs for public health services. • Constructing active partnerships with professional development programs that expose participants to relevant experiences in public health, as well as continuing human resources education for management and leadership development in the area of public health. • Developing capacities for interdisciplinary and multicultural work in public health. • Providing ethical training for public health personnel, with special attention to the values of solidarity, equality, and respect for human dignity.
Quality assurance in personal and population-based health services	• Promoting the implementation and improvement of evaluation systems. • Promoting the development of standards for quality assurance and improvement systems, as well as monitoring providers for compliance with these standards. • Defining, explaining, and guaranteeing service user's rights. • Developing an evaluation system for health technologies that can assist in health system decision making and that contributes to improving the quality of the health system as a whole. • Using scientific methods to evaluate health interventions of various degrees of complexity. • Implementing systems to evaluate user satisfaction and using these assessments to improve the quality of health services.
Research	• Conducting rigorous research to increase the knowledge that supports decision-making at various levels. • Developing and implementing innovative public health solutions, and measuring and evaluating their impact. • Establishing partnerships with research centers and academic institutions, both within and outside the health sector, to conduct studies to support the NHA's decision-making process.
Reduction of the impact of emergencies and disasters on health	• Developing policy and planning and implementing measures to prevent, mitigate, reduce, and prepare for the impact of disasters on public health. • Developing integrated approaches to the threats and the etiology of each possible emergency or disaster within the country. • Promoting health system-wide participation and broad intersectoral/interinstitutional collaboration in reducing the impact of emergencies and disasters. • Managing intersectoral and international cooperation in solving health problems caused by emergencies and disasters.

Data from: Pan American Health Organization. (2011). *Esssential public health functions.* Retrieved from http://www.paho.org/HQ/index.php?option=com_content&view=category&id=3175&layout=blog&Itemid=3617&lang=en

community participation in policy making, and reaching hard-to-serve populations (Fried & Gaydos, 2012). Unique features of selected health care systems in other countries indicate the many approaches that can be taken to address the considerations and dilemmas presented above. In 2012, the Commonwealth fund published a report providing profiles of several national health care systems (Thompson, Osborn, Squires, & Jun, 2012). Key features of those health systems are summarized below.

The United Kingdom has a National Health Service (NHS) under which the majority of health services is provided through a government-run system that is operated slightly differently in each of four administrative units (England, Scotland, Wales, and Northern Ireland), with separate administrative structures for the Isle of Man and the Channel Islands. Funding is derived from national taxes and care is free to all residents with the exception of some prescription, optical, and dental charges. In 2013, the NHS in England underwent a major reorganization. Health care is under the direction of the Secretary of State for Health and is funded through Parliamentary allocations to the Department of Health. Funding is derived from taxation (NHS Choices, 2013a).

NHS England is an independent body from the government designed to improve health outcomes in the population. The former Primary Care Trusts that administered the majority of the health care budget were abolished and replaced with Clinical Commissioning Groups (CCGs). All general practice physicians are employed by a particular CCG, which also includes other health professionals, including nurses. The CCGs are responsible for providing hospital, rehabilitative, and urgent/emergent care, as well as most community health services and mental health and learning disability services. CCGs can also incorporate outside entities that meet established standards (NHS Choices, 2013b). Health and Wellbeing Boards are being established at local levels to coordinate public health services and reduce health disparities (Harrison, 2012). The Health and Wellbeing Boards will also provide avenues for consumer input into strategic decisions and coordinate health and social services (NHS Choices, 2013b).

Until recently, the emphasis at the NHS has been on personal health care. However, the reorganization included the creation of a new entity, Public Health England (PHE), which is charged with coordinating a national public health service and delivering some services, creating an evidence base to support local public health services, supporting healthy choices by members of the public, and providing leadership to the public health delivery system. PHE is also responsible for supporting public health workforce development (NHS Choices, 2013b).

Canada's "Medicare" system is a single-payer system in which services are provided by a variety of public and private providers, but are co-funded by the federal and provincial or territorial governments. Health care service delivery is primarily the responsibility of provincial and territorial systems under federal standards for hospital, diagnostic, and physician services (Allin, 2012). Coverage is universal for medically necessary physician and hospital services, and in-patient prescription drugs; essential services are free (Health Canada, 2014). Services are funded by a combination of federal and provincial or territorial funds derived through personal and corporate income taxes. Some provinces provide supplementary benefits to certain groups of people (e.g., the elderly and low-income residents). People who do not qualify for supplementary benefits may obtain them through out-of-pocket payment, employment-based group insurance, or individual private insurance coverage. Federal monies are allocated to the provincial and territorial governments, who then pay for services provided (Health Canada, 2012). Two thirds of residents are covered under private insurance as well for services not covered under the national system (Allin, 2012). The basic service package for hospital, physician, and prescription drug coverage is mandated by the federal government, but provinces may cover additional services as well (Canadian Health Care, n.d.).

Like the United Kingdom, the Canadian system has been focused on personal health care service delivery with less attention to public health. In 2004, in response to the severe acute respiratory syndrome (SARS) outbreak of the previous year, Canada created the new Public Health Agency of Canada (PHAC). The designated functions of PHAC include population health assessment, surveillance, health promotion and disease and injury prevention, health protection, and public health emergency preparedness and response. These changes have led to an increased focus on health promotion and initiatives to address social determinants of health and illness (Stachenko, Legowski, & Geneau, 2009).

In Australia, the health care system is financed and regulated by the federal government, with oversight and autonomous administration of health services by states and territories. Coverage is universal, funded by taxes, patient fees, and other private sources. The national Medicare system covers both physician and hospital services as well as prescription medications, mental health care, and some dental care and allied health services if referred by a physician. Care is provided in a mix of public and private facilities, although most physicians are in private practice or combine a salary for seeing public patients with fee-for-service income from private clients. Approximately half of Australians also have private health insurance to assist with services not covered under the national plan. Private insurance coverage may involve "lifetime health coverage" for a fixed premium based on one's age at the time of enrollment. Recent foci in health care planning include targeted health issues, such as workforce planning, primary care, preventive care, hospital reform, and disability services funding (Healy, 2012). In the past, health promotion, in general, has received less emphasis, and there was little systematic attention to social determinants of health (Davis, Lin, & Gauld, 2009).

The New Zealand health care system is tax funded and provides universal coverage for physician and hospital care, medications, and a broad range of other health and disability services. About one third of the population also has private insurance coverage to cover cost-sharing expenses and for other services. Services are provided under District Health Boards and public hospitals. System reforms resulted in a network of self-employed provider groups that provide primary care services to the majority of the population on either a fee-for-service or capitated (prepaid per enrollee) basis. Specialists tend to work in both public and private hospitals and in their own private practices. There has been a growing emphasis on social determinants of health in New Zealand (Gauld, 2012).

As of 2009, health insurance coverage is mandatory for all German citizens and permanent residents. Health care services in Germany are provided within a system of non-governmental "sickness funds." Employer (or pension fund) and employee contributions are collected in a national fund that is then distributed to local sickness funds based on risk-adjusted capitation formulas. The sickness funds provide a universal benefit package with a wide array of preventive and curative services determined by the federal government. Some residents may opt out of the system in favor of substitutive private insurance, and private insurance may also be used for additional services. Providers are paid primarily on a fee-for-service basis negotiated between sickness funds and regional medical provider associations. Hospitals may be either private or public, but their physicians are usually salaried and are not permitted to see outside patients. Evidence-based disease management programs are in place for several chronic conditions, and sickness funds contract with providers for their implementation (Blümel, 2012).

Comparing Health System Outcomes

Each year, the Organization for Economic Cooperation and Development collects data on more than 1,200 health system performance measures for 34 industrialized countries. The Commonwealth Fund uses that data to rate the performance of the U.S. health care system (Squires, 2011). In 2012, the Commonwealth Fund examined U.S. health care system performance in five general areas: health care spending and coverage, health care supply and utilization, health promotion and disease prevention services, quality of care and patient safety, and the price of care. Highlights of the analysis in each of these areas are presented below.

HEALTH CARE SPENDING AND COVERAGE. In 2012, the United States ranked first in terms of average per capita spending on health care in comparison with 12 other countries. U.S. per capita spending was $8,233, more than 50% higher than the next highest ranked country, Norway, at $5,388 and 2.7 times higher than New Zealand with the lowest per capita expenditures ($3,022). In addition, the United States expends more of its gross domestic product (17.6%) on health care than any other country, again nearly 50% higher than Denmark, with next highest ranking (12%). Despite this level of expenditure, as we will see, health care outcomes in the United States lag far behind those of other countries in most areas addressed (Squires, 2013).

In comparisons of out-of-pocket spending for health care, the United States ranks second only to Switzerland ($970 and $1,325, respectively). Similarly, U.S. spending on pharmaceuticals was the highest among 14 nations at $983 per person, and was more than 30% higher than in Canada and 3.4 times higher than pharmaceutical expenditures in New Zealand.

HEALTH CARE SUPPLY AND UTILIZATION. U.S. residents make extensive use of costly health care services. For example, rates of coronary bypass surgery are higher in the United States (79 per 100,000 population) than in any country than Germany (116 per 100,000). These figures are most likely a function of a lack of preventive care in these systems. Similarly, the availability of magnetic resonance imaging units in the United States (31.6 per million population) is surpassed only by Japan (Squires, 2013).

As a measure of access to care, the United States ranked third lowest in terms of the average number of physician visits per person at 3.9, compared to highest ranking Japan at 13.1 visits per capita (Squires, 2013). In addition, the United States ranked next to last in terms of the number of practicing physicians per 1,000 people at 2.4, compared to first ranked Norway at 4.1. The number of hospital beds in the United States is only slightly higher at 2.6 beds per 1,000 population, lower than seven other countries and less than a third of the number of available beds in Japan (Squires, 2013).

HEALTH PROMOTION AND DISEASE PREVENTION. Only on two indicators in this area did the United States perform fairly well. With respect to cervical cancer screening rates, the United States ranked higher than another country with 85% of women screened in 2010. Similarly, the U.S. rate for adult smokers was second lowest, surpassed only by Sweden. On other measures, U.S. health system performance is less than stellar. For example, the United States ranked in the middle of the countries assessed with respect to influenza immunization among adults 65 years of age and older, and ranked highest in terms of obesity among adults, 29% higher than New Zealand, the second ranked country (Squires, 2013).

QUALITY AND SAFETY. As a measure of health care quality, the United States lagged behind 15 other nations with the highest rate of mortality preventable by adequate health

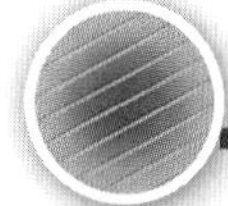

Evidence-Based Practice

The Medical Home

One approach to the delivery of both preventive and curative services is the patient-centered medical home (PCMH) model. The Agency for Healthcare Research and Quality (AHRQ, n.d.a) has defined PCMH as a model of organization for primary care that encompasses the following functions and attributes: patient centeredness, comprehensive care, coordinated care, superb access to care, and a systems-based approach to quality and safety. The Patient-Centered Primary Care Collaborative reported on a review of evidence related to the outcomes of implementing patient-centered medical home interventions in the United States. The review indicated improved quality of care and reduced hospitalization and emergency department use leading to reduced costs of care. The review explored cost and quality outcomes for integrated delivery system models, private payer initiatives, Medicaid-sponsored initiatives, and other PCMH programs (Grumbach & Grundy, 2010). In addition, AHRQ has collected multiple reports of studies of outcomes related to the PCMH model (AHRQ, n.d.b). For further information related to study findings, see the *External Resources* section of the student resources site.

care. Similarly, the United States had the second highest rate of lower extremity amputations due to diabetes, at 32.9 per 100,000 population, second only to Germany at 33.7 per 100,000. With respect to in-hospital mortality due to myocardial infarction, the U.S. rate was at the mid-point of the comparison nations, nearly twice the rate of best performing Denmark, but less than half of the rate for Japan. Conversely, the United States had the highest rate of any country for five-year breast cancer survival (Squires, 2013).

Measures of patient safety reported in the Commonwealth Fund analysis included the rate of foreign bodies left in a patient's body during a procedure and the rate of postoperative sepsis. With respect to foreign bodies, the United States had the fourth best rate at 4.9 instances per 100,000 hospital discharges, but still nearly three times higher on this indicator than best performing Denmark. The U.S. rate for postoperative sepsis was the third highest among the comparison countries at 1,077 per 100,000 hospital discharges, more than three times that of Switzerland (Squires, 2013).

PRICES. Health care in the United States is much more costly than in any of the comparison health systems in the Commonwealth Fund analysis. For example, U.S. prices for the 30 most commonly prescribed drugs are 23% higher than Canadian prices and three times higher than those in New Zealand. Similarly, U.S. prices for diagnostic imaging such as MRI and CT scans are higher than any of the comparison countries, and average hospital pending per discharge was 30% higher than the next highest country. In part these high costs are a function of physician incomes and reimbursement rates. For instance, physician fees from public payment sources for hip replacement amounted to $1,634 in the United States, compared to $652 in Canada. Fees charged to private payers were more than twice as much. Similarly, the average income for an orthopedic surgeon in the United States was $442,450, nearly three times the income of a French orthopedic surgeon. Similar differences in incomes are noted for primary care physicians with U.S. incomes twice those of Australian primary care physicians (Squires, 2013).

Another performance measure comparing the U.S. health care delivery system to other national systems is infant mortality, in which the United States ranked last among eight nations. Similarly, sicker adults in the United States are more likely to report difficulty in getting care after hours without going to an emergency department than residents of most other comparison countries. The United States also performed worst in terms of people who reported being unable to access care due to costs in 2010. In addition, the percentage of U.S. primary care physicians using electronic medical records in 2009 was below that for all the comparison countries except Canada (Commonwealth Fund, 2011).

Generally speaking, deficits in the U.S. health care system have been identified with respect to the quality of care provided, access to care, efficiency, equity, and indicators of healthy life. Quality issues include safety, care coordination, and the effectiveness of chronic disease management. Areas of concern with respect to access include inability to afford care due to costs and the extent of out-of-pocket expenditures by Americans for health care. Efficiency reflects the extent of the GDP allocated to health care expenditures, and equity is related to disparities in access to care as well as to disparities in health status across population groups in the United States. Major indicators of healthy life on which the United States performs abysmally include infant mortality, preventable mortality, and healthy life expectancy after age 60. U.S. health care system performance in all of these areas is considerably less than desired. Many of these areas are designed to be addressed by the *Healthy People 2020* initiatives discussed throughout this book. The provisions of the Affordable Care Act are also intended to address issues of access, equity, quality, and efficiency. The success of these endeavors, however, remains to be seen.

CHAPTER RECAP

Health care delivery in the United States occurs in multiple settings at multiple levels. The primary divisions of the U.S. health care system are the popular, complementary or alternative, and scientific health care subsystems. Care in the popular subsystem is provided by individuals to themselves or family members. Complementary or alternative care is provided by recognized ethnic healers or providers, while care in the scientific subsystem is based on research evidence.

The scientific health care subsystem includes the personal health care sector, which focuses on care to individuals, and the public health care sector, which emphasizes the health of population groups. Within the public health care sector, care is provided by both official and voluntary organizations. Official health agencies are the offices within local, state, or federal governments that are responsible for health issues and concerns. Voluntary agencies supplement the efforts of official health agencies.

Due to major concerns with quality, efficiency, and cost, there have been numerous attempts to reform the U.S. health care system, the most recent being the enactment of the Patient Protection and Affordable Health Care Act in 2010. Pay-for-performance is another strategy that has been employed to improve the quality of care provided and the efficiency of the system.

The United States is the only developed nation without some form of national health care system that provides universal coverage for its citizens. The health systems of other nations vary across a number of parameters, but are fairly consistently ranked more highly than the U.S. system on a number of outcomes.

CASE STUDY The Ideal Health Care System

Design a health care delivery system that would meet the health needs of the U.S. public. Diagram the organizational structure of the system, making sure that your system addresses the core functions and essential services of public health as well as the goals of medical care. Address the following questions:

1. What features (if any) would you incorporate from other national health care delivery systems?
2. How would you fund your system? How would health care providers be reimbursed? Why?
3. Would you offer comprehensive health care services? What would be included in the basic health services package? Would this basic coverage be available to all residents? Why or why not?
4. How would your system address the four levels of health care (health promotion, prevention, resolution, and restoration)? Would one level receive priority over the others? Why or why not?
5. What political, economic, and social changes would need to occur before your proposed system could be implemented in the United States?

REFERENCES

Adams, P. F. Kirzinger, W. K., & Martinez, M. E. (2012). Summary health statistics for the U.S. population: National Health Interview Survey, 2011. Retrieved from http://www.cdc.gov/nchs/data/series/sr_10/sr10_255.pdf

Agency for Healthcare Research and Quality. (n.d.a). *Defining the PCMH.* Retrieved from http://pcmh.ahrq.gov/page/defining-pcmh

Agency for Healthcare Research and Quality. (n.d.b). *Evidence and evaluation.* Retrieved from http://pcmh.ahrq.gov/page/evidence-and-evaluation

Allin, S. (2012). The Canadian health care system, 2012. In S. Thompson, R. Osborn, D. Squires, & M. Jun (Eds.). *International profiles of health care systems, 2012: Australia, Canada, Denmark, England, France, Germany, Iceland, Italy, the Netherlands, New Zealand, Norway, Sweden, Switzerland, and the United States* (pp. 19–25). Retrieved from http://www.commonwealthfund.org/~/media/Files/Publications/Fund%20Report/2012/Nov/1645_Squires_intl_profiles_hlt_care_systems_2012.pdf

Alper, J. (Rapporteur), Round Table on Population Health Improvement, Board on Population Health and Public Health Practice. (2013). *Population health implications of the Affordable Care Act.* Retrieved from http://www.nap.edu/download.php?record_id=18546

Blümel, M. (2012). The German health care system, 2012. In S. Thompson, R. Osborn, D. Squires, & M. Jun (Eds.). *International profiles of health care systems, 2012: Australia, Canada, Denmark, England, France, Germany, Iceland, Italy, the Netherlands, New Zealand, Norway, Sweden, Switzerland, and the United States* (pp. 46–52). Retrieved from http://www.commonwealthfund.org/~/media/Files/Publications/Fund%20Report/2012/Nov/1645_Squires_intl_profiles_hlt_care_systems_2012.pdf

Budrys, G. (2012). *Our unsystematic health system* (3rd ed.). Lanham, MD: Rowman & Littlefield.

Canadian Health Care. (n.d.). Retrieved from http://www.candian-healthcare.org

Commonwealth Fund. (2011). *Why not the best? Results from the national scorecard on U.S. health system performance, 2011.* Retrieved from http://www.commonwealthfund.org/~/media/Files/Publications/Fund%20Report/2011/Oct/1500_WNTB_Natl_Scorecard_2011_web_v2.pdf

Cover the Uninsured. (2009). *Overview.* Retrieved from http://covertheuninsured.org/content/overview

Davis, P., Lin, V., & Gauld, R. (2009). Public health in Australia and New Zealand. In R. Beaglehole & R. Bonita (Eds.), *Global public health: A new era* (2nd ed., pp. 225–247). Oxford, UK: Oxford University Press.

Fried, B. J., & Gaydos, L. M. (2012). Preface. In B. J. Fried & L. M. Gaydos (Eds.), *World health systems: Challenges and perspectives* (2nd ed., pp. ix–xii). Chicago: Health Administration Press.

Gauld, R. (2012). The New Zealand health care system, 2012. In S. Thompson, R. Osborn, D. Squires, & M. Jun (Eds.). *International profiles of health care systems, 2012: Australia, Canada, Denmark, England, France, Germany, Iceland, Italy, the Netherlands, New Zealand, Norway, Sweden, Switzerland, and the United States* (pp. 79–85). Retrieved from http://www.commonwealthfund.org/~/media/Files/Publications/Fund%20Report/2012/Nov/1645_Squires_intl_profiles_hlt_care_systems_2012.pdf

Goldsteen, R., & Goldsteen, K. (2012). *An introduction to the U.S. health care system* (7th ed.). New York, NY: Springer.

Grumbach, K., & Grundy, P. (2010). *Outcomes of implementing patient-centered medical home interventions: A review of the evidence from prospective evaluation studies in the United States.* http://www.pcpcc.net/files/evidence_outcomes_in_pcmh.pdf.

Harrison, A. (2012). The English health care system, 2012. In S. Thompson, R. Osborn, D. Squires, & M. Jun (Eds.). *International profiles of health care systems, 2012: Australia, Canada, Denmark, England, France, Germany, Iceland, Italy, the Netherlands, New Zealand, Norway, Sweden, Switzerland, and the United States* (pp. 32–38). Retrieved from http://www.commonwealthfund.org/~/media/Files/Publications/Fund%20Report/2012/Nov/1645_Squires_intl_profiles_hlt_care_systems_2012.pdf

Health Canada. (2012). *Canada's health care system.* Retrieved from http://www.hc-sc.gc.ca/hcs-sss/pubs/system-regime/2011-hcs-sss/index-eng.php

Health Canada. (2014). *Health care system.* Retrieved from http://www.hc-sc.gc.ca/hcs-sss/index-eng.php

Health Resources and Services Administration. (n.d.). *What is pay-for-performance?* Retrieved from http://www.hrsa.gov/healthit/toolbox/HealthITAdoptiontoolbox/QualityImprovement/whatispay4perf.html

Healy, J. (2012). The Australian health care system, 2012. In S. Thompson, R. Osborn, D. Squires, & M. Jun (Eds.). *International profiles of health care systems, 2012: Australia, Canada, Denmark, England, France, Germany, Iceland, Italy, the Netherlands, New Zealand, Norway, Sweden, Switzerland, and the United States* (pp. 11–18). Retrieved from http://www.commonwealthfund.org/~/media/Files/Publications/Fund%20Report/2012/Nov/1645_Squires_intl_profiles_hlt_care_systems_2012.pdf

Institute for Healthcare Improvement. (2014). *Triple Aim for populations: Overview. Retrieved from* http://www.ihi.org/Topics/TripleAim/Pages/Overview.aspx

Institute of Medicine. (2011). *Board on population health and public health practice.* Retrieved from http://www.iom.edu/About-IOM/Leadership-Staff/Boards/Board-on-Population-Health-and-Public-Health-Practice.aspx

Institute of Medicine, Committee on Assuring the Health of the Public in the 21st Century. (2003). *The future of the public's health in the 21st century.* Washington, DC: National Academies Press.

Kaiser Family Foundation. (2010). *Uninsured and untreated: A look at uninsured adults who received no medical care for two years.* Retrieved from http://www.kff.org/uninsured/8083.cfm

Kaiser Family Foundation. (2011a). *Summary of the Affordable Care Act.* Retrieved from http://kaiserfamilyfoundation.files.wordpress.com/2011/04/8061-021.pdf

Kaiser Family Foundation. (2011b). *Timeline: History of health reform in the U.S.* Retrieved from http://kaiserfamilyfoundation.files.wordpress.com/2011/03/5-02-13-history-of-health-reform.pdf

Koslow, J. (2011). *Encyclopedia of public health: Lemuel Shattuck.* Retrieved from http://www.enotes.com/public-health-encyclopedia/shattuck-lemuel/print.

Lemuel Shattuck Biography (1793–1859). (2011). Retrieved from http://www.faqs.org/health/bios/27/Lemuel-Shattuck.html

Lemuel Shattuck. (1793–1859): Prophet of American public health. (1959). *American Journal of Public Health, 49,* 676–677.

London School of Hygiene and Tropical Medicine. (2010). *Behind the frieze—Lemuel Shattuck (1793-1859).* Retrieved from http://www.lshtm.ac.uk/library/archives/history/frieze/shattuck.html

McMichael, A., & Beaglehole, R. (2009). The global context for public health. In R. Beaglehole & R. Bonita (Eds.), *Global public health: A new era* (2nd ed., pp. 1–22). Oxford, UK: Oxford University Press.

NHS Choices. (2013a). *The NHS in England: About the National Health Service (NHS).* http://www.nhs.uk/NHSEngland/thenhs/about/Pages/overview.aspx

NHS Choices. (2013b). *The NHS in England: The NHS structure explained.* Retrieved from http://www.nhs.uk/NHSEngland/thenhs/about/Pages/nhsstructure.aspx

National Institutes of Health. (2014). *Institutes, centers, and offices.* Retrieved from http://www.nih.gov/icd

National Public Health Performance Standards Program. (n.d.). *Acronyms, glossary, and reference terms.* Retrieved from http://www.cdc.gov/od/ocphp/nphpsp/PDF/glossary.pdf

Pan American Health Organization. (2011). *Essential public health functions. Retrieved from* http://www.paho.org/HQ/index.php?option=com_content&view=category&id=3175&layout=blog&Itemid=3617&lang=en.

Pay for performance. (2012). Retrieved from https://www.healthaffairs.org/healthpolicybriefs/brief.php?brief_id=78

Shattuck, L. (1850). *Report of a general plan for the promotion of public and person health: Devised, prepared and recommended by the commissioners appointed under a resolve of the Legislature of Massachusetts relating to a sanitary survey of the state.* Boston, MA: Dutton and Wentworth State Printers. Retrieved from http://biotech.law.lsu.edu/cphl/history/books/sr/index.htm

Squires, D. (2011). *The U.S. health system in perspective: A comparison of twelve industrialized nations.* Retrieved from http://www.commonwealthfund.org/~/media/Files/Publications/Issue%20Brief/2011/Jul/1532_Squires_US_hlt_sys_comparison_12_nations_intl_brief_v2.pdf

Squires, D. (2013). *Multinational comparisons of health systems data, 2012.* Retrieved from http://www.commonwealthfund.org/~/media/Files/Publications/In%20the%20Literature/2012/Nov/PDF_2012_OECD_chartpack.pdf

Stachenko, S., Legowski, B., & Geneau, R. (2009). Improving Canada's response to public health challenges: The creation of a new public health agency. In R. Beaglehole & R. Bonita (Eds.), *Global public health: A new era* (2nd ed., pp. 123–137). Oxford, UK: Oxford University Press.

Sultz, H. A., & Young, K. M. (2014). *Health care USA: Understanding its organization and delivery* (8th ed.). Burlington, MA: Jones and Bartlett.

Thompson, S., Osborn, R., Squires, D., & Jun, M. (Eds.). (2012). *International profiles of health care systems, 2012: Australia, Canada, Denmark, England, France, Germany, Iceland, Italy, the Netherlands, New Zealand, Norway, Sweden, Switzerland, and the United States.* Retrieved from http://www.commonwealthfund.org/~/media/Files/Publications/Fund%20Report/2012/Nov/1645_Squires_intl_profiles_hlt_care_systems_2012.pdf

U.S. Census Bureau. (2013). *Income, poverty, and health insurance coverage: 2012.* Retrieved from http://www.census.gov/hhes/www/hlthins/data/incpovhlth/2012/index.html

U.S. Department of Health and Human Services. (n.d.a). *HHS family of agencies.* Retrieved from http://www.hhs.gov/about/foa/index.html

U.S. Department of Health and Human Services. (n.d.b). *Office of the Assistant Secretary of Health.* Retrieved from http://www.hhs.gov/ash/

U.S. Department of Health and Human Services. (n.d.c). *Public health offices.* Retrieved from http://www.hhs.gov/ash/public_health/indexph.html

U.S. Department of Health and Human Services. (2011). *Office of Disease Prevention and Health Promotion.* Retrieved from http://www.aids.gov/federal-resources/federal-agencies/hhs/office-of-the-assistant-secretary-for-health/office-of-disease-prevention-and-health-promotion/

U.S. Department of Health and Human Services. (2013a). *About the U.S. Public Health Service Commissioned Corps.* Retrieved from http://www.usphs.gov/aboutus/

U.S. Department of Health and Human Services. (2013b). *Operating divisions.* Retrieved from http://www.usphs.gov/aboutus/

World Health Organization. (2014). *Health systems: About health systems.* Retrieved from http://www.who.int/healthsystems/topics/en/

CHAPTER

8 Global Influences on Population Health

Learning Outcomes

After reading this chapter, you should be able to:

1. Discuss the dimensions of globalization.
2. Describe factors contributing to the globalization of population health issues.
3. Distinguish between international and global health.
4. Discuss U.S. involvement in global health initiatives.
5. Describe recent global health initiatives.
6. Discuss the concept of global health governance and its effects on population health.
7. Describe health care organization at global and international levels.
8. Discuss selected global issues related to population health status and determinants of health.
9. Describe nursing involvement in global health.

Key Terms

bilateral agencies
burden of disease
civil society
civil society organizations (CSOs)
Declaration of Alma-Ata
disability-adjusted life year (DALY)
elimination
eradication
ethical poverty line
food insecurity
Global Alliance for Leadership in Nursing Education and Science (GANES)
global governance
global health
global health governance
globalization
gross domestic product (GDP)
health diplomacy
health governance
healthy life expectancy (HALE)
International Council of Nurses (ICN)
international health
millennium development goals (MDGs)
multilateral agencies
non-governmental organizations (NGOs)
Pan American Health Organization (PAHO)
policy
policy communities
primary health care (PHC)
sector-wide approaches (SWAPs)
Sigma Theta Tau International
World Health Organization (WHO)

Advocacy Then

ICN: Global Advocacy for Nurses

ICN, the International Council of Nurses, arose out of concerns for women's rights, health care reform, and the development of professional nursing practice. In 1899, three international nursing leaders, Ethel Gordon Fenwick (England), Lavinia Dock (USA), and Agnes Karll (Germany) established the first international organization for women and health care providers. Initiated as a federation of national nursing organizations, such as the American Nurses Association, ICN was often funded by the personal funds of participants (ICN, 2013c). Throughout its more than 100-year history, ICN has advocated for nurses around the world. Two examples of its activities are particularly salient.

At the start of World War II, the German Nurses Association, one of the founding members of ICN, was disbanded by National Socialist (Nazi) Party. Similar action was taken against the Italian National Nurses Association (ICN, 2013c). As a result of the war, more than 3,000 nurses were displaced, often without proof of their nursing credentials. In 1950, ICN took over from the International Refugee Organization, the task of verifying the credentials of these nurses and assisting them in obtaining the documents needed to practice their profession in their new countries of residence (Center for the Study of the History of Nursing, School of Nursing, University of Pennsylvania, n.d.).

More recently, in 1973, ICN challenged one of its older members, the South African Nurses Association, to integrate the organization. As ICN was preparing for a vote on expulsion of the South African Nurses Association, the association abruptly withdrew its membership. Today, a fully integrated South African association is once again an active member of ICN.

Advocacy Now

Holy Innocents Children's Hospital—A Nurse-Initiated Venture in Uganda

In August 2006, Fr. Bonaventure from Mbarara, Uganda, visited the University of San Diego and its School of Nursing to see if we could help him and the Archbishop realize a dream. That dream was to build a hospital to help save the 17,000 children under the age of 5 who died in their community in Uganda every year. As a nurse and a pediatric nurse practitioner, how does one say "no" to such a plea?

With the support of the university, six MSN students and I traveled to Mbarara, Uganda to conduct a needs assessment, identifying existing services, needs, in-country resources, the consequences of and barriers to intervening, and the lay and professional communities' perspectives. After traversing 600 square miles, conducting over two dozen focus groups with diverse lay and professional groups, we identified a place to build a hospital, developed plans for the hospital, and presented a proposal to the Archbishop and his community. The proposal was taken back to the San Rafael Catholic Church in Rancho Bernardo, California and parishioners who were interested in helping the Archbishop realize his dream.

The report we developed was used as the foundation for an NGO to finance the building of the first children's hospital. The organization's tax-deductible, 503-status, was acquired in May 2007, its website was developed (www.holyinnocentsuganda.org), and fund-raising began. By March 2008, enough money had been raised to break ground for the hospital in Uganda. A 60-bed hospital, outpatient department, and administrative wing were informally opened on July 4, 2009. By the time of the official opening on July 4, 2010, over 16,000 patients had been treated at Holy Innocents Children's Hospital.

Because the Uganda health care system uses the British model of care, all health professionals are educated accordingly. To be responsive to this health care orientation, Dr. Hunter contacted her nursing experts in Northern Ireland for input into the development of the hospital and its early leadership. As of January 2011, both the Medical Director and the Hospital Administrator are Ugandans.

From April 2007 to July 4, 2010 I made seven trips to Mbarara with over 100 nursing, chemistry, and business students and faculty from USD and health professionals from Children's Hospital, Oakland. Our purpose has been to conduct environmental, developmental, and business needs assessments, provide nurse and physician and lay community educator training, and initiate partnerships with the Mbarara University of Science and Technology Medical School and Business School and other entities in the community.

Nursing has advocated for the most vulnerable in Uganda, the age group birth–12 years, by helping to build the only children's hospital in Uganda. As of January 2011, over 25,000 children have been treated in both the inpatient and outpatient departments. Our patients are critically ill and in the United States would be categorized as pediatric intensive care unit (PICU) patients, yet there is no PICU due to financial constraints. A neonatal intensive care unit of sorts has been created that serves the needs of the critically ill neonates in this resource-poor environment. Nursing and medicine have now joined forces to help meet the hospital's mission—the sister relationship with Children's Hospital, Oakland will help solidify the standards of care necessary to provide pediatric care, and the ongoing affiliations with the schools of nursing committed to this project will help ensure the more global well-being of the children, their families, and the community.

The mission of the hospital is to provide health care services to improve the health of the children and their families and to promote opportunities for their future. This nursing initiative was developed around the framework of global health diplomacy, whereby partnerships between multiple disciplines, including medicine, nursing, environmental science, agriculture, politics, and business have been created to advocate for change, build local capacity, address factors that contribute to poor health, and promote stability in this community.

Anita Hunter, Phd, RN, PNP, FAAN

We live in a small world that can be circumnavigated in a matter of hours, increasing the potential for the spread of disease, ideas, and technological advances. Today you are a nursing student in one country; six months or a year from now you may be working or vacationing in another. Or you may be caring for a client from a distant part of the world. Health problems cross national boundaries, and their solutions will need to cross boundaries as well. For all these reasons, population health nurses need to be well versed in the global context in which health problems arise and health care is delivered.

Globalization

The interaction of health and other issues in multiple parts of the world arises from increasing globalization. Although there is no universally accepted definition of **globalization**, a useful definition from the World Health Organization (WHO), is a "process of growing interdependence that represents a fundamental change from a world of individual and independent states to a world of state interdependence" (WHO, 2014c, para.4). The results of globalization are reflected in a similar definition as a "process of increasing interconnectedness between societies such that events in one part of the world increasingly have effects on peoples and societies far away" (Fidler, 2001/2009, p. 125).

Dimensions of Globalization

Globalization has spatial, temporal, cognitive, and social dimensions. The spatial dimension reflects international trade, global political initiatives, communication, and increased cultural exchange. Similarly, movement back and forth across national borders is common and increasingly easy. The temporal dimension addresses changes in our experiences of time and the increased speed of transactions, political change, and resource depletion. For example, I can be in San Diego this morning and

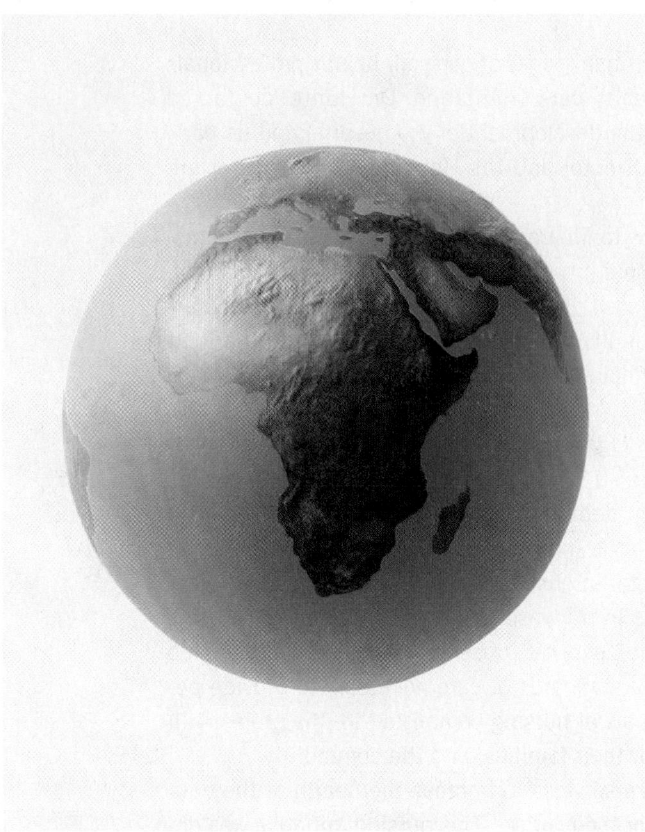

Many health concerns transcend national boundaries and require international cooperation. *(Steve Gorton/Dorling Kindersley)*

in Taiwan by late evening. Interchanges among people in different parts of the world may need to account for time changes. The cognitive dimension of globalization reflects thoughts about ourselves and our world. Positive effects of globalization in this dimension include expansion of democratic principles and support for human rights. Additionally, in order to work effectively to address worldwide problems, we need to begin to think of ourselves more as global citizens than as citizens of a specific nation. The social dimension of globalization is reflected in its effects on people in terms of its impact on culture, employment, working conditions, income, security, family life, and other aspects of social interaction, as well as redistribution of power from states to international bodies (WHO, 2014c).

Economic interconnectedness has been described as a core component of globalization that is fueled by technology and has a variety of societal effects. For example, a global economy is viewed by some as an impetus to increased productivity and standards of living based on economies of scale. Conversely, globalization of the economy may lead to destruction in jobs due to increased competition from low-wage countries. Other concerns related to globalization include loss of national sovereignty and self-determination and inequitable distribution of its benefits (WHO, 2014c).

Although international interchanges have occurred since ancient times, in the past they tended to take place between one nation and another, frequently between sovereign and independent national governments. Today's "new" globalization, on the other hand, is characterized by new entities that have a certain amount of authority over national governments (e.g., the World Trade Organization [WTO]). In addition, globalization is influenced by multinational business corporations with tremendous power to influence world events, global networks of non-governmental organizations (NGOs), new rules of governance such as international agreements, new modes of communication, and global movement among people.

Health Effects of Globalization

Globalization has a number of effects on the health of the world's populations, some of which are positive and some negative. Positive effects include broader dissemination of health care technology that permits prevention and cure of illness. The existence of multinational corporations may also lead to improvements in labor standards and wages in developing nations. Similarly, globalization may also have the effect of globalizing concern for human rights.

Negative effects include the increased potential for the spread of communicable diseases with increasing international travel (Association of State and Territorial Health Officials, 2013). Changes in culture and lifestyle have led to dietary changes, increased sedentary behaviors, and increased tobacco and alcohol use that contribute to the growing worldwide incidence of noncommunicable conditions. Growing reliance on motor vehicle transportation, combined with industrialization, and population growth has also led to global climate change, which in turn affects weather patterns, potential for natural disaster, and crop production.

Globalization also affects social determinants of health. For example, although the number of people in extreme poverty (persons living on incomes less than $1 a day) has decreased, globalization has increased disparities between the rich and the poor, with the poor being disproportionately affected by the negative consequences of globalization (Ezeani, 2012). Per capita income has increased substantially for some nations, but not as rapidly in others. For example, China, once one of the poorest nations in the world, now has a per capita income higher than 50% of the rest of the world (Ross, 2013). The gap between poor and middle-income countries has increased; Sub-Saharan Africa remains the poorest region in the world, with a 29% increase in per capita income from 2000 to 2010 compared to a 63% increase in middle-income countries (Stadtfeld, 2012).

Another negative effect of globalization has been the decreasing ability of national governments to address health issues because multiple factors affecting health lie outside the authority of the government health sector. These effects of globalization will be addressed in more detail in our discussion of specific global health issues later in this chapter. Some of the positive and negative effects of globalization are summarized in Table 8-1●.

TABLE 8-1 Positive and Negative Effects of Globalization

Positive Effects	Negative Effects
Promotion of economic growth	Increasing inequities between and within groups
Greater employment or entry into the workforce for some segments of the population	Job loss for some segments of the population
Positive environmental effects (e.g., safer water supplies)	Negative environmental effects (e.g., environmental degradation and increased resource consumption)
Greater financial prosperity and health for some	Creation of unhealthful working conditions
Rapid dissemination of health innovations and information	Marketing of unhealthful products (e.g., tobacco)
Development of global standards related to health (e.g., food safety standards)	Lack of access to available health innovations (e.g., antiretrovirals)
Changes in views of population health from a nation-specific perspective to a subgroup perspective across national boundaries	A shift away from the focus on social justice to an emphasis on market economies and efficiency
Positive effects of *geoculture* development (e.g., increasing autonomy for women)	Ease of spread of communicable diseases
	Ease of illicit trade in harmful substances
	Difficulty of keeping up with new developments and potential for information overload
	Increased time needed for decision making to incorporate input from diverse groups
	Negative effects of *geoculture* development (e.g., dissemination of poor health habits)

International and Global Health Perspectives

At this point, we need to make a distinction between international health activities and global health. **International health** involves health matters that affect two or more countries. **Global health**, on the other hand, involves multinational efforts to address health problems that cross national borders, and has been defined as "collaborative transnational research and action for promoting health of all" (Beaglehole & Bonita, 2010, p. 5142). Global health is also concerned with factors that affect the capacity of individual nation-states to deal with the determinants of health and illness. Global health issues are beyond the capability of one nation to resolve and require multinational cooperation.

Trends in Global Health Collaboration

Early international collaborative efforts related to health consisted primarily of attempts to control the international spread of epidemics. In 1903, these efforts led to the adoption of the International Sanitary Regulations, better known as International Health Regulations.

In 1946, the United Nations (UN) established the World Health Organization (WHO) to address global health issues. Over the years, WHO has adopted a number of international conventions, or agreements, related to health issues. These conventions are not legally binding and member nations can refuse to accept an entire convention or opt out of certain provisions of a convention. WHO activities were predicated on three primary strategies, each of which has been less than successful: global surveillance, transnational control measures, and multilateral funding. Global surveillance initiatives were designed to promote early identification of communicable disease outbreaks. Until recently, they have been largely unsuccessful because developing nations either did not have the public health infrastructure needed to conduct surveillance activities or were afraid to report outbreaks for fear of economic consequences associated with decreased trade or tourism. Transnational control measures have been unsupported by developed countries, which were able to care for their sick and were less concerned about the spread of disease, and developing countries that feared initiation of "excessive measures" that might, again, restrict trade. Finally, the concept of multilateral funding was largely unsuccessful because the developed nations that provided most of the funding did not trust recipient countries to use them wisely. Two WHO initiatives that have been successful are the worldwide elimination of smallpox and eradication of polio from significant portions of the globe.

From the 1990s onward, there has been greater multilateral cooperation on health issues due to the emergence of new diseases with increased potential for worldwide spread. In 2005, the International Health Regulations were revised, and WHO has taken a more active role in prescribing effective intervention for disease outbreaks that have been implemented by most of the international community (WHO, 2014c). There has also been a marked expansion of multilateral health aid, particularly from non-governmental organizations. In addition, some international agreements have been modified to address their health consequences. For instance, under the TRIPS agreement on Trade Related Aspects of Intellectual Property Rights, World Trade Organization (WTO) members are required to protect intellectual property rights, but that protection can be abrogated to address public health issues. As an example, member countries can issue compulsory licenses mandating in-country production of a necessary drug and avoid the high cost of importation from the country in which it was developed (WTO, 2014).

One particular WHO initiative that has changed over the years is the concept of primary health care and the goal of "health for all by 2000." The "health for all" concept arose out of the 1977 World Health Assembly. The central goal of the "health for all" movement was the provision of basic health care to all peoples of the world by the year 2000. Its three main objectives were promotion of healthy lifestyles, prevention of preventable conditions, and therapy for existing conditions. The strategy to achieve health for all centered on the concept of primary health care as described in the **Declaration of Alma-Ata**, a report generated by the International Conference on Primary Health Care held in Alma-Ata in 1978.

Primary health care (PHC) is an approach to providing health care resources that focuses on provision of essential health care using socially acceptable and affordable methods and technology, accessibility, public participation in policy development, and intersectoral collaboration. In 1978, the Declaration of Alma-Ata proposed a set of core activities to be included in primary health care and tailored to the needs of a particular population. These activities included:

- Education to prevent and control major health problems in the area
- Promotion of nutrition and a safe and sufficient food supply
- Provision of safe water and basic sanitation
- Provision of maternal and child health care, including family planning services
- Immunization
- Prevention and control of endemic diseases
- Adequate treatment of common illnesses and injuries
- Provision of essential medications (Hixon & Maskarinec, 2008).

Basic values of PHC include equity, universal access to care, people-centeredness, and communities that provide conditions conducive to health. Unfortunately, these values have been largely subverted by the effects of hospitalcentrism, commercialism, and fragmentation within health care systems. *Hospitalcentrism* refers to health care systems built around hospitals and specialty care rather than primary care. Commercialism has been defined by WHO (2008) as unregulated sale of health care services for purposes of profit. Under the values of PHC, health care services should not be a source of profit for individuals, businesses, or governments. Fragmentation of health care systems reflects a focus on "priority" programs, projects, and issues, rather than a comprehensive approach to health.

To address these issues, WHO has suggested four areas for reform in PHC initiatives. These include universal coverage reforms, service delivery reforms, public policy reforms, and leadership reforms. Universal coverage reforms include strategies to move toward access to health care services for all members of all populations, regardless of income or insurance status. Three approaches have been suggested to achieve universal access: (a) reducing cost sharing by recipients of care, (b) expanding the services covered by health care service plans, and (c) expanding the populations covered to include all residents (WHO, 2008).

Service delivery reform suggestions reflect the need for health care services to be socially relevant and to respond to the needs of the population. Such reforms would lead to people-centered care characterized by a focus on health needs of the population, enduring relationships between providers and clients, comprehensive and continuous care, and responsibility for the health of the total population as well as for determinants that affect health status and partnerships with recipients of care (WHO, 2008).

Public policy reform is needed to integrate public health initiatives with primary care services. There is also a need to develop policies across all sectors that support health and strengthen national and transnational health initiatives (WHO, 2008). Such policy development will require what has been referred to as sector-wide approaches. **Sector-wide approaches (SWAPs)** are approaches to the resolution of health-related problems through attention to conditions in the broader social and economic sectors that affect health (WHO, 2014b). An example of a sector-wide approach might be efforts to provide access to safe, drinkable water in a developing nation. Assistance might be sought from an NGO to build a water purification system, but local government initiatives will be required to support system maintenance. There may also be a need for cooperation from local agricultural businesses to prevent water contamination with agricultural runoff. At the same time, legislation might be needed that prohibits the dumping of human wastes within a prescribed distance of a water supply. For the safe water system to be developed and continue to function, activities will be required in several aspects of the health, social, and economic sectors.

Leadership reforms are needed to replace authoritarian or laissez-faire governmental approaches to health issues with participatory approaches (WHO, 2008). The aims of PHC will not be achieved without input from those affected in the planning and development of health care services. Other changes in the PHC approach suggested by WHO include an expanded focus on all members of the population rather than subpopulations such as mothers and children, promotion of healthier lifestyles and attention to social determinants of health, use of a primary health care team, comprehensive health care services rather than narrow foci on "priority" issues, adequate

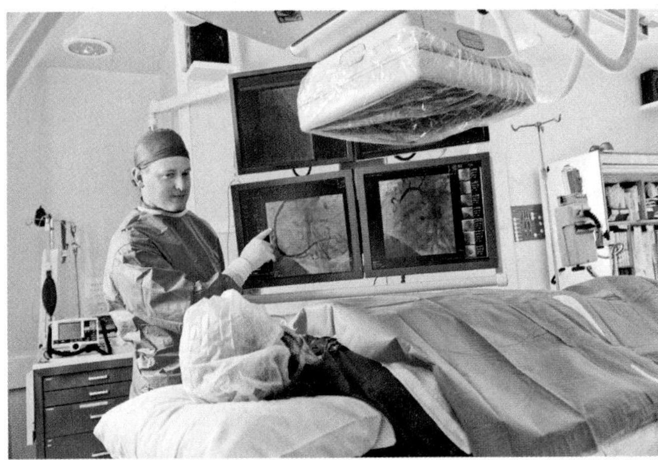

Many national health care systems incorporate advanced medical technology. *(EPSTOCK/Fotolia)*

funding for comprehensive PHC, and care coordination across levels of preventive and curative services (WHO, 2008).

U.S. Involvement and Global Health

The United States has long been actively involved in global health initiatives, but that involvement has been changing. In the past, much of U.S. involvement has occurred through federal government activities, but more recently there has been increased activity by U.S.-based non-governmental organizations and multinational corporations. In 2009, the Institute of Medicine (IOM) made five recommendations for U.S. action within the global health enterprise. These recommendations included the following:

- Expanding existing governmental and non-governmental interventions to achieve greater gains, with particular foci on supporting the achievement of the Millennium Development Goals (MDGs) (discussed below), preparation for emerging communicable and noncommunicable health challenges, and promoting health infrastructure and workforce development in developing nations.
- Generating and sharing knowledge to solve global health problems.
- Investing in global capacity building in line with local priorities. One suggested strategy is the creation of a global health service corps in which U.S. health care providers would serve in other nations much as they do in medically underserved areas of the United States.
- Increasing the U.S. commitment to funding global health initiatives by meeting existing commitments and increasing aid spending, moving from a treatment to a health promotion and illness prevention focus, and funding global health research.
- Setting an example for respectful partnerships by addressing the needs and concerns of partner nations and highlighting health as an integral component of foreign policy (IOM, 2009).

A 2010 report by the Kaiser Family Foundation noted that the United States was a party to only 36 of 50 recent international agreements. The study found the U.S. government to be most likely to participate in agreements related to control of specific diseases, trade and intellectual property, and security and international preparedness. The United States is not a party to several agreements related to environmental issues (e.g., the Kyoto Protocol to the United Nations Framework Convention on Climate Change and the WHO Framework Convention on Tobacco Control) and protection of some specific vulnerable populations such as the Convention on the Rights of Children and the Convention on the Elimination of All Forms of Discrimination Against Women. Greater U.S. involvement in such international efforts may be heralded by the Obama Administration's proactive stance on international partnerships for health and development (Kates & Katz, 2010).

For the first time, the *Healthy People 2020* objectives include a focus on global health. To a large extent, the objectives related to this focus area emphasize protection of the United States from global threats to health. Some of the objectives, however, are aimed at developing global health competencies that will benefit the rest of the world as well. The global *Healthy People 2020* objectives, with baseline data and target figures as well as related data sources for monitoring their achievement, are presented on the next page.

Global Health Initiatives

A number of global health initiatives have been recently undertaken, two of which will be addressed here. Other initiatives will be discussed in the context of global health issues to which they relate. The two initiatives to be presented here are the millennium development goals and the contributions of the G7/G8 nations to global health efforts.

MILLENNIUM DEVELOPMENT GOALS. In 2000, the UN General Assembly developed its **millennium development goals (MDGs)**, a set of goals for international development that address issues of health status and social determinants of health. Three of the goals, reducing child mortality, promoting maternal health, and combating HIV/AIDS, malaria, and other diseases address health directly. The other goals address determinants of health. Each goal encompasses one or more targets to be achieved by the international community. Specific indicators for achievement of each target have also been identified (United Nations, 2012). Table 8-2• summarizes the millennium development goals and specific targets. Like the U.S. *Healthy People 2020* objectives, the MDGs provide consensus on the most important goals to be accomplished in the coming years as well as a comprehensive agenda for international development to achieve and sustain those goals. Information on progress in attaining the MDGs is published annually by the United Nations (UN, 2013). For information on annual progress in meeting the goals, see the *External Resources* section of the student resources site.

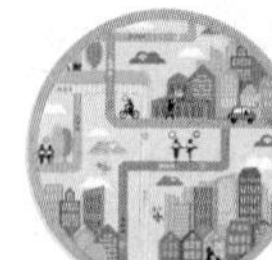

Healthy People 2020

Objectives for Global Health

OBJECTIVE	BASELINE (YEAR)	TARGET	CURRENT DATA (YEAR)	DATA SOURCE
GH-1: Reduce the number of new cases of malaria reported in the United States	1,298 cases (2008)	999 cases	1,691 (2010)	National Notifiable Disease Surveillance System (NNDSS), CDC/ PHSIPO, National Malaria Surveillance System (NMSS), CDC/CGH
GH-2: Decrease the tuberculosis (TB) case rate for foreign-born persons living in the United States	20.3 cases per 100,000 population (2008)	14 cases per 100,000 population	17.2 cases per 100,000 population (2011)	National Tuberculosis Indicators Project (NTIP), CDC
GH-3: Increase the number of Global Disease Detection (GDD) Regional Centers worldwide to detect and contain emerging health threats	7 centers (2009)	18 centers	8 centers (2012)	GDD Monitoring and Evaluation Database, CDC
GH-4: Increase the number of public health professionals trained by the Global Disease Detection (GDD) programs worldwide	37,221 health professionals (2009)	300,000 health professionals	73,905 (2012)	GDD Monitoring and Evaluation Database, CDC
GH-5: Increase diagnostic testing capacity in host countries and regionally through the Global Disease Detection (GDD) Regional Centers	156 tests established or improved (2009)	1000 tests	232 tests (2012)	GDD Monitoring and Evaluation Database, CDC

Data from: U.S. Department of Health and Human Services. (2013). *Global health.* Retrieved from http://www.healthypeople.gov/2020/topicsobjectives2020/overview.aspx?topicid=16

G7/G8 CONTRIBUTIONS TO GLOBAL HEALTH INITIATIVES. The United States is one of a group of six national governments formed in 1975 in response to a global oil crisis. Because of their monetary contributions to global initiatives, these organizations, which numbered eight until Russia became plagued with internal issues and now number seven, have greater voting strength in a number of world decision-making bodies such as World Bank, International Monetary Fund (IMF), and World Trade Organization. The seven countries that currently make up the group labeled G7 include Canada, France, Germany, Italy, Japan, the United Kingdom, and the United States. These seven nations account for nearly 40% of the world's total gross domestic product, with China and India accounting for another 20% (Quandl, 2014). The **gross domestic product (GDP)** is the total monetary value of all goods and services produced by a nation in a given period.

The G7 nations have committed themselves to contributing to the achievement of the millennium development goals. Unfortunately, that commitment has not been met, and only one country has lived up to its commitment to date.

A contribution of 0.1% of the GDP of all affluent countries would raise an estimated $35 trillion, roughly $35 per person for the one million people throughout the world who need assistance. In addition, low-income countries would be expected to dedicate 15% of their national budgets to address internal health issues (MacDonald, 2009). It is estimated, however, that achievement of the MDGs would require $40 to $70 billion more than is currently being contributed in annual aid and a goal of increasing aid contributions to 0.7% of affluent countries' GDP has been advanced. There is a need for considerably greater support of global health initiatives by the G7 nations and other relatively affluent countries before the MDGs can be realized.

Global Health Governance

Another perspective on global health that is undergoing relatively rapid change is the concept of global governance. **Health governance** is defined as "the actions and means adopted by a society to organize itself in the promotion and protection of the health of its population (Dodgson et al., 2002/2009,

TABLE 8-2 Millennium Development Goals (MDGs) and Selected Targets

Goal	Selected Targets
1. Eradicate extreme poverty and hunger	• Halve the proportion of people living on less than $1 per day • Halve the proportion of people suffering from hunger
2. Achieve universal primary education	• Ensure that all boys and girls are able to complete a full course of primary education
3. Promote gender equality and empower women	• Eliminate gender disparity in primary and secondary education by 2005 and at all levels by 2018
4. Reduce child mortality	• Reduce by two thirds the mortality rate among children under 5 years of age
8. Improve maternal health	• Reduce by 75% the maternal mortality ratio
6. Combat HIV/AIDS, malaria, and other diseases	• Halt and begin to reverse the spread of HIV/AIDS • Halt and begin to reverse the incidence of malaria and other major diseases
7. Ensure environmental sustainability	• Integrate principles of sustainable development into national policies and programs and reverse the loss of environmental resources (e.g., reduce energy use and carbon dioxide emissions) • Halve the proportion of people without sustainable access to safe drinking water and basic sanitation • Achieve significant improvement in lives of at least 100 million slum dwellers (e.g., adequate sanitation and secure housing tenure)
8. Develop a global partnership for development	• Develop an open, rule-based, predictable, non-discriminatory trading and financial system • Address the special needs of the least developed and land-locked and island countries • Deal with developing countries' debt • Make available the benefits of new technologies, especially information and communication

Data from: United Nations. (2012). *The Millennium Development Goals report 2012.* Retrieved from http://mdgs.un.org/unsd/mdg/Resources/Static/Products/Progress2012/English2012.pdf

p. 440). **Global governance** is defined by the World Health Organization as "an international process of consensus-forming which generates guidelines and agreements that affect national governments and international corporations" (WHO, 2014b, para. 2). **Global health governance** is the application of international laws, norms, and expectations to the management of health issues that cross international boundaries (WHO, 2014b). Global health governance requires the ability to influence health determinants outside the control of national governments due to the cross-border nature of many health issues and their contributing factors. International cooperation related to health risks began in the mid-19th century (Fidler, 2001/2009), and the International Sanitary Regulations discussed above constituted an early attempt at global health governance. These regulations were revised by the World Health Assembly as the International Health Regulations (IHRs) in 2005 and became binding international law as of June 2007. The purpose of the regulations is to prevent the spread of public health emergencies, particularly communicable diseases, without undue disruption of trade and travel. The regulations required WHO member states to develop national surveillance and response systems by 2012, specifying mechanisms for identification, reporting, and management of international health emergencies (WHO, 2014e).

International agreements such as the IHRs are the product of **health diplomacy**, which is the art of negotiating and reaching agreement with respect to competing health needs and goals. Most global governance does not involve the development of binding international law, but, instead, takes the form of accepted conventions or agreements that may exist between specific nations or a global collective of countries. Such international and global agreements have implications for national policy and vice versa (WHO, 2014b). For example, the waivers possible under the TRIPS Agreement discussed earlier have implications for intellectual property rights as recognized by U.S. law.

Some authors have noted that the world is in the process of transitioning from a system of international relations between specific countries to a "system of global politics" (Bartsch, Hein, & Kohlmorgen, 2007, p. 19). Such a system often involves direct action between non-governmental factors functioning independently rather than through national governments as negotiators. In addition, a global political system is characterized by multilevel modes of governance and regulation that involve power sharing among different groups or actors, including partnerships between public and private sectors, and a lack of central authority for enforcement of agreements. Only rarely does this system result in international law.

Several types of power play a role in global governance, and different actors involved in negotiation may exhibit different forms of power. Particular forms of power that may be involved include discursive power, decision-making power, legal power, and resource-based power. Discursive power reflects the ability to shape discourse regarding an issue or to set an agenda for negotiation. Decision-making power involves the ability to participate in decision making and formal norm setting. As noted earlier, the relative financial contribution of the G7 nations to global initiatives gives them a more decision-making power than is held by other countries involved in those institutions. Legal power is based on legal structures and laws and rarely is brought to bear in global health governance. Finally, resource-based power is power derived from the ability of a negotiator to provide both material and immaterial resources needed to achieve goals. Material resources might include money or personnel, while immaterial resources might involve knowledge and information resources (Bartsch et al., 2007).

Essential elements of global health governance include deterritorialization of thinking and the elimination of national boundaries in addressing health issues and their solutions. Global health governance also requires definition of health determinants from a multisectoral perspective, not from a biomedical outlook. For example, access to clean drinking water is a health issue that lies beyond the health care sector. In addition, global health governance necessitates the involvement of a variety of actors and interests, including governmental and non-governmental players, public and private sectors, and so on (Dodgson et al., 2002/2009).

Several challenges must be overcome in order for global health governance to be achieved. First, there is a need for consensus on the moral and ethical principles that should undergird global health governance. Decision makers need to agree on what are considered basic human rights related to health and health care and work toward support of those rights. Second, there is a need to define leadership and authority (Dodgson et al., 2002/2009). As noted earlier, the International Sanitary Regulations were largely ignored, in part due to a lack of sanctions for failure to follow them, in addition to other factors. What sanctions might be applied to the United States, for example, if it fails to uphold agreed upon provisions of the Framework Convention on Tobacco Control or agreements on human trafficking?

The third, and perhaps most significant, challenge to achieving global health governance is the need for resources needed to support global health cooperation. Funding is needed to organize and carry out agreed upon health-related initiatives. For example, the campaign to eradicate smallpox was a labor-intensive and costly endeavor, fortunately funded by a combination of WHO funds and money from donor countries. Overcoming national sovereignty concerns is another area that impedes global health governance. Nation-states are understandably reluctant to cede power to control health issues to international groups. There is also a need to agree on enforcement of agreements at the global level. Finally, there is a need to involve wider participation in global health governance, not just national governments, the traditional negotiators in international interactions (Dodgson et al., 2002/2009). In the end, developing global health governance structures will depend on achieving a balance between increased interdependence and desires to pool resources to address common problems and fears of loss of autonomy for individual nations (Kickbush, 2000/2009).

Some authors envision an expanded role for WHO in the development of a system of global health governance. Potential functions might include ensuring a reliable information base related to health issues, safeguarding global security through global response protocols and creation of a rapid response network to deal with emerging threats to health, supporting the competence of developing nations in addressing health issues, and acting as a global health broker in the creation of cooperative regulations and negotiation of health-related conflicts. In addition, WHO might function as an oversight body monitoring health-related networks and partnerships and could create a UN spokesperson on human rights and health to draw the attention of the international community to health issues (Kickbush, 2000/2009).

At present, however, three gaps exist that interfere with the development of global health policy and governance. The first of these is a jurisdictional gap. No organization or body has jurisdiction to enforce global health regulations or agreements. The second is a participation gap in that there is minimal representation of developing nations or citizens in policy development. Finally, there is an incentive gap. Many countries do not see the benefits to development and enforcement of global health-related policy and fear loss of autonomy related to internal affairs as they influence global health issues (Kickbush, 2000/2009).

Development of a true system of global health governance will require the accomplishment of several tasks to fill these gaps. The first of these is convincing the nations of the world that global health policy serves their needs and is of benefit to them. The second requirement is to widen the support base for global health, particularly in terms of funding sources. Finally, global health governance will require a shift to a moral argument for accountability for the health of the entire world and a focus on populations across national boundaries (e.g., the poor, children, the elderly, etc.) (Kickbush, 2000/2009).

Health Care Organization at Global and International Levels

There are a variety of agencies that undertake global or international health efforts. These agencies can be loosely grouped as bilateral agencies, multilateral agencies, and civil society organizations. Bilateral and multilateral agencies tend to be associations of member nations represented by official government health-related agencies. **Multilateral agencies** are those that involve several countries in joint activities related to health, whereas **bilateral agencies** are health-related agencies that generally involve only two countries in any single project.

Bilateral Agencies

A number of bilateral organizations with health emphases exist throughout the world. Virtually all developed countries provide some form of health-related aid to underdeveloped countries, with the contribution of some countries far in excess of that provided by the United States. This section will focus on the bilateral organizations involving the United States. One of the federal agencies concerned with international health is the United States Agency for International Development (USAID), which administers all federally financed projects for foreign development, including those that are health related. This agency is housed in the U.S. Department of State, and its twofold purpose is to promote U.S. foreign policy through expansion of democracy and free markets and to improve life in the developing world. To these ends, the agency supports economic growth, agriculture, and trade; global health; and democracy, conflict prevention, and humanitarian aid (USAID, 2014).

The U.S. Department of Health and Human Services includes several agencies with international foci. One is the Office of Global Affairs (OGA) which "promotes the health and well-being of Americans and of the world's population by advancing global strategies and partnerships in the coordination of global health policy" (OGA, n.d., para. 1). The second is the Center for Global Health within the Centers for Disease Control and Prevention (CDC). This center is involved in both bilateral and multilateral health activities sending health experts to specific countries in need of assistance and providing representation in multilateral organizations such as WHO, the World Bank, and the International Red Cross. CDC is involved in a number of global health initiatives related to control of specific diseases such as HIV/AIDS, malaria, influenza, measles, and polio, as well as programs related to environmental health, reproductive health, road safety, violence prevention, and food safety, to name a few areas of focus (Center for Global Health, n.d.). For further information on global health initiatives undertaken by CDC, see the *External Resources* section of the student resources site.

Within the National Institutes of Health (NIH), the Fogarty International Center (n.d.) focuses on international health research. Other branches of the NIH (e.g., the Geographic Medicine Branch of the Institute of Allergy and Infectious Diseases) are involved in activities that are international in focus. Many of the programs of the Peace Corps, the federal international volunteer program, have a health focus.

Some federal agencies that function primarily at the national level also have some international aspects to their roles. For example, the U.S. Food and Drug Administration (2014) houses the Office of International Programs, which focuses on bilateral as well as multilateral regulatory initiatives related to safe food and drug supplies throughout the world. In addition, federally chartered institutions such as the Institute of Medicine and the National Science Foundation are also concerned with problems of international health as well as with domestic problems.

Bilateral or binational initiatives are particularly needed along the U.S.–Mexico border. There are 15 million people in 44 U.S. countries and 90 Mexican municipalities who live along the border, and this number is expected to rise to 23 million by 2030 (McDonald, Mojarro, Sutton, & Ventura, 2013). The United States–Mexico Border Health Commission (n.d.) was established to address health needs in the border populations. Particular areas of emphasis include obesity and diabetes, strategic planning, research, data collection, and academic alliances.

Multilateral Agencies

The **World Health Organization (WHO)** is "the directing and coordinating authority on international health within the United Nations' system" (WHO, 2014a, para. 1), and is the primary multilateral agency dealing with global health issues. WHO was established in 1948 and is responsible for providing leadership in global health initiatives, supporting health-related research and setting a global research agenda, monitoring global health trends, and providing technical assistance in the control of health problems that threaten the global community (WHO, 2014a). WHO is funded through "dues" and donations by member nations and focuses on health promotion and disease prevention, cure of illness, health systems and health resources development, and health-related international research. The World Health Assembly is the governing body for WHO and sets global health policy (WHO, 2014a). For further information about WHO, see the *External Resources* section of the student resources site.

The **Pan American Health Organization (PAHO)** is the multilateral agency that deals with health-related concerns in the Americas and provides an avenue for collective efforts to promote the health status of people in all nations in the Western Hemisphere. PAHO is the oldest of the global health organizations and celebrated its 100th anniversary in 2002. PAHO originated in 1902 as the International Sanitary Bureau. Its original focus was the development of uniform sanitary regulations and laws in North and South America. In 1958, the organization expanded its focus to address broader health issues and changed its name to the Pan American Health Organization (PAHO, 2011, 2013).

One of PAHO's significant achievements is the development of the Regional Core Health Data Initiative, which monitors achievement of health goals in PAHO member states (PAHO, 2014b). To date, the data generated have been used to create health profiles for 47 jurisdictions, including the United States and Puerto Rico (PAHO, 2014c). Data collected provide direction for programs to enhance health status in the region of the Americas. For further information about PAHO and current indicator status for member nations, see the *External Resources* section of the student resources site.

Other multilateral agencies include the health components of the North Atlantic Treaty Organization (NATO) and the Southeast Asia Treaty Organization (SEATO). The United Nations International Children's Emergency Fund (UNICEF) and the United Nations Educational, Scientific, and Cultural Organization (UNESCO) are two other agencies within the UN that provide assistance with matters of global health. The Food and Agricultural Organization (FAO) is a multilateral agency designed to enhance the world's food supply. Finally, the World Bank provides both funding and technical assistance in dealing with health problems around the world.

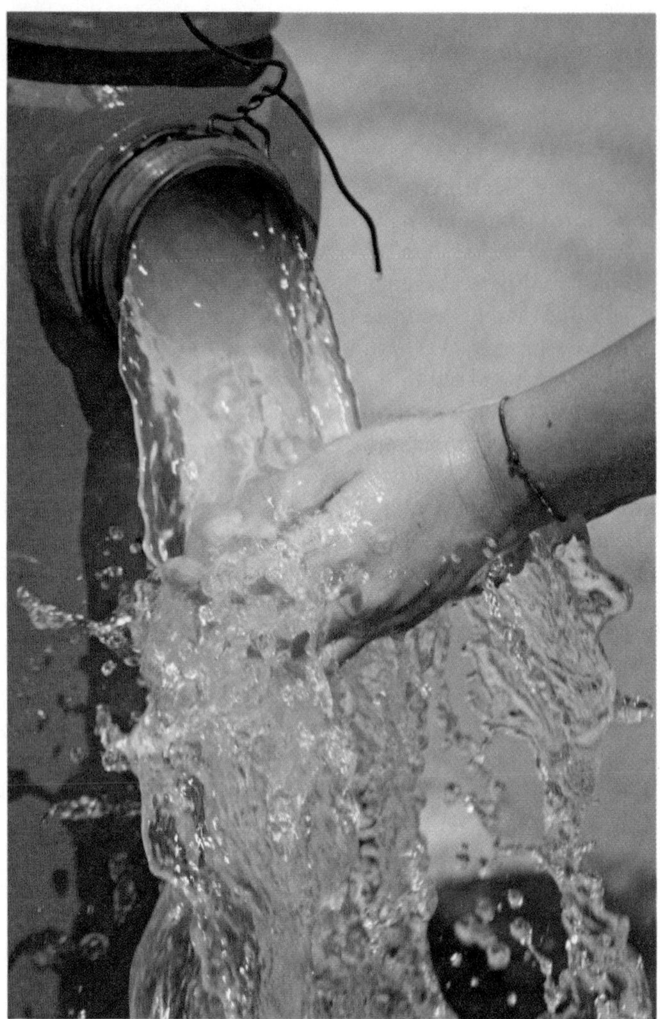

Hand washing is one of the most effective means of preventing communicable diseases. *(fotocociredef73/Fotolia)*

Civil Society Organizations

Civil society is one of three aspects of society, with the other two aspects being government and the economy. The definition of **civil society** adopted by the World Bank is as follows: "the wide array of non-governmental and not-for-profit organizations that have a presence in public life, expressing the interests and values of their members or others, based on ethical, cultural, political, scientific, religious or philanthropic considerations" (World Bank, 2013, para. 5). Civil society, then, determines the culturally acceptable directions for political and economic decisions. **Civil society organizations (CSOs)** are "community groups, non-governmental organizations (NGOs), labor unions, indigenous groups, charitable organizations, faith-based organizations, professional associations, and foundations" that represent the voice of the people in societal decision making (World Bank, 2013, para. 5). CSOs occur at local and national, as well as international, levels of society.

CSOs are characterized by their nonprofit nature, their organizational and financial independence from government, and, like voluntary agencies, their reliance on voluntary membership and contributions. CSOs carry out a variety of functions with respect to global health governance. These functions include raising awareness of health problems caused by economic or political factors, agenda setting, developing usable knowledge, monitoring problem status and policy implementation, rule making, and norm development. Additional functions include policy verification through scrutiny of policy initiatives and their implementation, capacity building in terms of technology transfer and organizational skill development, and financing (Lee, 2010).

There are several types of CSOs that are somewhat similar to the types of voluntary agencies discussed in Chapter 7∞. One distinct type of CSO that has no parallel among voluntary agencies is a social movement. Social movements are informal networks and groups who work for societal change, sometimes independently of each other. Social movements are usually issue-focused and frequently work through campaigns to educate the public and influence policy makers. Other types of CSOs include non-governmental organizations, social membership organizations (e.g., unions or professional organizations), national and ethnic organizations and movements, and foundations. Faith-based organizations are related to CSOs, but arise from religious groups to provide certain social and advocacy services while conducting related missionary activities.

Non-governmental organizations (NGOs) are nonprofit, voluntary, citizens' agencies outside of the official government-sponsored agencies that work toward the public good. NGOs differ from social movements in that they have a professional and sustainable organizational structure. They are characterized by their function of advocacy for the interests of others and the translation of private resources into public goods. Their foci are self-determined and are generally limited to one or more specific and related issues (e.g., women's rights, tobacco control, prevention of human trafficking, etc.) (NGO Global Network, n.d.). A great deal of humanitarian aid is contributed by NGOs, with much of it being disaster-related. Humanitarianism is based on a strongly held belief that all human life has value wherever it is found, in affluent countries or developing nations. Humanitarianism embodies both beneficence/charity and duty/justice perspectives (Walzer, 2011).

Social membership organizations focus on the interests of their members. Examples of social membership organizations include unions and professional organizations, both of which may engage in health-related initiatives to improve the public good as well as efforts to promote the interests of their membership. The final type of CSO is foundations. Foundations may be nonprofit organizations established by for-profit entities for the purpose of promoting the public good. For example, the Bill & Melinda Gates Foundation (n.d.), which is supported by profits from Bill Gates' technological enterprises, as well as some other donations, has undertaken significant efforts related to global development as well as global health issues such as communicable disease control and immunization, family planning, and nutrition. The Susan G. Komen Foundation (2014), on the other hand, was established in memory of Susan Komen, who battled breast cancer and campaigned for support of women with breast cancer. The foundation is a grassroots network of cancer survivors and advocates supported by donations from a variety of individual, organizational, and corporate sources.

Global Health Issues

There are a number of issues that affect the health status of the world's population. Although it is beyond the scope of this chapter to address them all, we will explore selected health issues in two major areas: issues related to population health status and those related to determinants of health.

Health Status Issues

General categories of global issues related to the health status of the world's population to be addressed here include life expectancy, maternal and child health, communicable diseases, and noncommunicable conditions.

LIFE EXPECTANCY AND MORTALITY. In spite of overall gains in life expectancy over the last several decades, there is a significant disparity in life expectancy between high- and low-to-moderate-income countries. For example, in 2011 overall life expectancy at birth ranged from 47 years in Sierra Leone to 83 years in Japan and Switzerland. From 1990 to 2011, life expectancy for both sexes actually decreased by 11 years in Zimbabwe (WHO, 2013c). U.S. life expectancy in 2011 was 79 years. Differences in **healthy life expectancy (HALE)**, or the number of years of life one can expect to attain in a state of relatively good health, were equally pronounced.

Differences in mortality rates are also substantial. Among adults between 15 and 60 years of age, the 2011 worldwide mortality was 190 deaths per 1,000 population. For low-income nations, however, the mortality rate was more than two times higher than the mortality experience of high-income countries for men and more than six times higher for women (WHO, 2013c).

WOMEN'S AND CHILDREN'S HEALTH. Most child caretakers throughout the world are women; therefore, the health of women and that of children is intimately connected. Women's health is a major area of concern in global health care. Maternal mortality continues to be high in many parts of the world. In 2010, maternal mortality ranged from 2 (Estonia) to 1,100 maternal deaths per 100,000 births (Chad) (WHO, 2013c). Many other women suffer complications of pregnancy and childbirth that lead to injury and disability.

Because of the biological effects of reproduction, women are more vulnerable to related health problems, but reproductive biology is only one of the reasons for poor health status among the women of the world. Gender inequities that contribute to discrimination and poverty are experienced by women throughout the world. For example, women are more vulnerable to the effects of poverty than men, primarily because they are less likely to be employed outside the home. Even when employed for pay, women may earn as much as 40% less than men, and women are often employed in low-paying, high-risk jobs. In many countries, women retain responsibility for the care of homes and children while shouldering the additional burden of out-of-home labor. Increased participation in the labor force has the advantage of increased material and social support, but also leads to increased workload and greater potential for occupational exposures. Even women working in the home experience greater environmental risks due to increased use of carbon-based cooking fuels (WHO, 2009b).

Traditional gender roles may also place women at higher risk for HIV infection due to the inability to negotiate condom use or other elements of sexual activity. In 2004, HIV/AIDS was the leading cause of death worldwide among women aged 20 to 59 years, contributing to 835,000 deaths or 13.3% of all mortality in this age group. Other causes of mortality in middle adult women included heart disease and stroke (12.5%), tuberculosis (5%), breast cancer (3.5%), suicide (3.2%), lower respiratory infection (3%), and road traffic accidents (2.7%). Among women over 60 years of age, the greatest causes of mortality included heart disease and stroke (39.7%), chronic obstructive pulmonary disease (8.2%), cancers (5.4%), lower respiratory infection (5.3%), diabetes mellitus (3.3%), and Alzheimer's and other dementias (2%) (WHO, 2009b).

Violence against women is another area of growing international concern. A WHO study found that as much as 71% of women in some countries had been subjected to intimate partner violence at some point in their lives (as much as 54% in the prior year). In addition, 40% to 70% of murders of women in countries such as Australia, Canada, Israel, South Africa, and the United States are perpetrated by their male partners (WHO, 2009b). Laws in many countries do not recognize intimate partner violence (IPV) as a crime. Even when they do, they may not include IPV that occurs outside of marriage (e.g., dating violence). IPV will be discussed in more detail in Chapter 30∞.

International trafficking in human beings, which affects primarily women and young girls and boys, is another source of societal violence. An estimated 600,000 to 800,000 individuals are trafficked across international borders each year, and thousands more are enslaved in their own countries. More than 12 million people are believed to be enslaved in forced labor and sexual servitude throughout the world. Much of the human trafficking is for the purpose of sexual exploitation, but trafficking also involves involuntary servitude. In the 2000 Trafficking Victims Protection Act, severe forms of trafficking in persons were defined as:

(a) sex trafficking in which a commercial sex act is induced by force, fraud, or coercion, or in which the person induced to perform such act has not attained 18 years of age; or

(b) the recruitment, harboring, transportation, provision, or obtaining of a person for labor or services, through the use of force, fraud or coercion for the purpose of subjection to involuntary servitude, peonage, debt bondage, or slavery. (U.S. Department of State, 2013, p. 8)

Approximately 12.3 million persons, mostly women and children, have been forced to provide labor or become prostitutes throughout the world, and nearly 2 in every 1,000 people in the world, including 1.2 million children a year, may be victims of trafficking (National Human Trafficking Resources Center, 2010). Unfortunately, far too many cases are unreported. For example, in 2012, more than 46,000 trafficking victims were identified worldwide, yet only 7,705 cases were prosecuted and only 4,746 perpetrators were convicted (U.S. Department of State, 2013). Trafficking of persons will be discussed in more detail in Chapter 30∞.

Because of income differentials, new health-related products and effective treatments may not be available to women. Women have also become a new global market for harmful products such as tobacco and products that undermine healthful behaviors, such as prepared formulas used in place of breast-feeding.

Many of the efforts related to global health have been prompted by the plight of the world's children. In spite of millions of dollars of international assistance, however, in 2012 children under 5 years of age in low-income countries had a mortality rate of 96 per 1,000 live births compared to only 6 per 1,000 for high-income nations (WHO, 2013c). Even in developed countries, children living in poverty have worse outcomes than their wealthier counterparts. Causes of inequalities in child health include financial barriers to health care and other necessities and lack of access to quality care.

In 2010, 7.6 million children under the age of 5 died. Three conditions accounted for 45% of these deaths: pneumonia, diarrheal diseases, and prematurity (WHO, 2013c). Maternal or child malnutrition was a significant contributing factor in many of these deaths.

Vaccine preventable diseases play a significant role in childhood mortality. Considerable progress has been made in providing routine immunizations for the children of the world. In 2011, however, 16% of the world's children under one year of age remained unimmunized for measles, 17% for diphtheria, tetanus, and pertussis (DTP), 25% for hepatitis B, and 43% for Hib (WHO, 2013c). The worldwide immunization rate for pneumococcal diseases was only 19% in 2012, and only 11% of young children had been immunized against rotoviruses. In 2012, an estimated 22.6 million children, half of them in three countries (India, Indonesia, and Nigeria) had not received routine immunization services (WHO, 2014d).

Diarrheal diseases are the leading cause of morbidity and mortality in children under 5 years of age. Diarrheal death rates have decreased somewhat due to the use of oral rehydration therapy, but this strategy has not been employed as widely as needed. Diarrheal diseases are not likely to be well controlled, however, until improvements in water quality and sanitation are achieved worldwide. Each day 1,400 children die of diarrheal diseases caused by contamination of drinking water, inadequate sanitation, and poor hygiene (United Nations Children's Fund [UNICEF], 2014).

Like their mothers, many children are subjected to unsafe and unhealthy working conditions and violence. An estimated 150 million children 5 to 14 years of age are engaged in child labor worldwide, and 500 million to 1.5 billion children have been affected in some way by violence (UNICEF, 2009).

In 2004, members of the WHO-World Bank Child Health and Poverty Working Group suggested that a simple set of six preventive activities and two therapeutic activities could significantly decrease the extent of disease burden among children. Basic preventive activities include prenatal care, breast-feeding, birth spacing, hygiene, immunization, and insect control. Recommended therapeutic interventions include effective home management of illness and prompt medical attention when needed. Unfortunately, much work needs to be done to implement these activities worldwide.

COMMUNICABLE DISEASES. Considerable progress has been made with respect to control of some communicable diseases throughout the world. For example, global eradication of smallpox was certified in 1979. Ironically, the last case of naturally occurring smallpox occurred in a smallpox vaccinator who received ineffective vaccine in Somalia in 1977 (WHO, 2014h). **Eradication** is the reduction of the worldwide incidence of a disease to zero through specific efforts to control its spread. **Elimination** is the same phenomenon on a smaller scale; that is, reduction of the incidence of the disease in question to zero in a specific area of the world. Development of effective vaccines is not sufficient for successful disease eradication. There is also a need for systematic worldwide campaigns to deliver immunization services to susceptible individuals (Centers for Disease Control and Prevention [CDC], 2013).

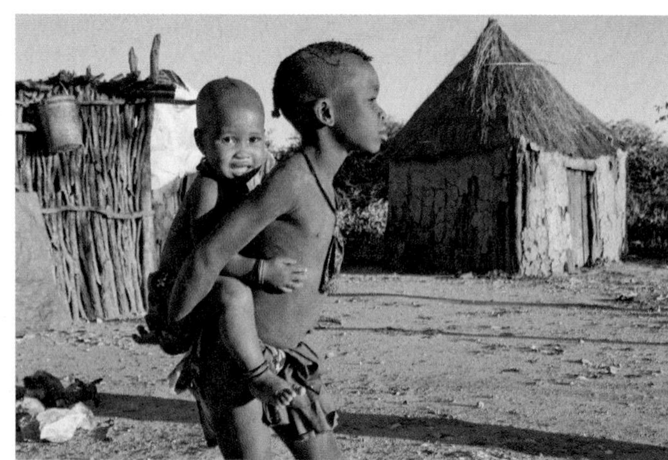

Health care workers often travel to remote villages to provide immunization services. *(Erichon/Fotolia)*

At present there are two perspectives regarding eradication efforts. From one perspective, eradication is an appropriate goal if it can be achieved. Feasibility is based on four primary premises:

- Eradication is biologically feasible (e.g., an effective vaccine or other strategy exists).
- Financial resources are sufficient to mount a worldwide campaign.
- Sufficient political will and commitment exist to implement the campaign.
- Social benefits go beyond the mere eradication of disease (e.g., improved economic productivity due to better health).

The second perspective is that eradication provides an avenue for later use of biologic agents as bioterrorist strategies and that global eradication campaigns divert resources away from other broader health and social problems. In 2003, CDC recommended smallpox vaccination for a small group of providers designated as first responders and caregivers for persons infected with smallpox in each U.S. hospital. Vaccination of people who will be handling or administering smallpox vaccine in an emergency situation has been recommended since 2009 (CDC, 2009).

Diseases currently targeted for worldwide eradication include dracunculiasis (guinea worm disease), poliomyelitis, filariasis, mumps, rubella, and pork tapeworm. Several of these efforts will be discussed here. In 1986, the World Health Assembly adopted a resolution to eradicate dracunculiasis, a disease spread by ingestion of contaminated water that causes skin lesions on the lower extremities through which worms up to a meter long exit the host. These lesions often become secondarily infected, causing considerable disease burden. There is no cure for the disease, but it can be prevented by filtering drinking water or treating it with a larvicide and encouraging infected persons to stay out of bodies of water when worms are emerging. At the time of the resolution, there were 3.5 million infected persons in 20 countries where the disease was endemic. By 2009, only 17 countries, all in Africa, continued to report cases of endemic dracunculiasis, and the number of cases reported worldwide had decreased to 3,185 (Division of Foodborne, Waterborne, and Environmental Diseases, 2010).

A similar initiative was undertaken in 1988 to eradicate poliomyelitis. The WHO strategy for polio eradication consisted of three aspects: (a) interruption of worldwide transmission of the disease, (b) global certification of eradication, and (c) preparation for the cessation of routine use of oral polio vaccine (Global Immunization Division, 2004). In 2013, the strategy expanded to address four aspects: (a) stopping all wild polio virus (WPV) transmission and circulating vaccine-derived polio virus (cVDPV) outbreaks, (b) hastening interruption of all polio virus transmission and strengthening immunization systems, (c) certifying all world regions as polio free and safely containing polio virus stocks, and (d) ensuring the permanence of a polio-free world (WHO, 2013c). From 1988 to 2013, the number of reported cases decreased by more than 99%, from 350,000 to 206 (WHO, 2014f). As of 2012, 84% of the world's children under 1 year of age had received three doses of oral polio vaccine. In 2014, the number of countries with endemic polio had decreased to three—Pakistan, Afghanistan, and Nigeria (WHO, 2014f). Similarly, the worldwide incidence of rubella declined 82% from 2000 to 2009 due, in large part, to increasing immunization levels (Strebel, Dabbaugh, Gacic-Dobo, Reef, & Cochi, 2010). The last case of endemic transmission of rubella in the Americas occurred in 2009, and experts are currently in the process of verifying its elimination from the region (PAHO, 2012).

Reduction of measles mortality is another global initiative related to communicable disease control The number of cases of measles has declined globally, but more than 354,000 still occurred in 2011, and nearly 54% of those cases occurred in the African Region (WHO, 2013e).

In 1994, the WHO Region of the Americas agreed on the goal of eliminating endemic measles by 2000, and the Pan American Health Organization set a goal of 95% vaccination coverage with two doses of measles vaccine among children in the Americas. From 2001 to 2014, more than 1.1 million children have been immunized, and 13.8 million deaths were averted worldwide between 2000 and 2012 due to measles immunization (Global Health, 2014). No cases of endemic measles have been reported in the Americas since 2002 (PAHO, 2014a). The potential for importation of new cases and possible epidemics remains high unless current immunization rates are maintained.

Despite these impressive successes, communicable diseases remain a significant problem affecting global health status. Changing patterns of communicable disease are creating increasing global concern. These changes include the emergence of new diseases, many of which are zoonotic viral diseases (those acquired from animals), such as H1N1 and avian influenza, Ebola virus, and others. A second change that impairs control strategies is the increasing development of antibiotic resistance in a number of disease-causing agents (Michael & Beaglehole, 2009).

Lower respiratory infection, diarrheal disease, HIV/AIDS, tuberculosis, neonatal infection, and malaria were among the top 10 causes of death in low-income countries. Vaccine preventable diseases remain a problem despite concerted efforts to increase immunization levels. In 1974, WHO began its Expanded Program on Immunization. At that time, less than 5% of the world's children under 1 year of age were effectively immunized with available agents. Current estimates suggest, however, that more than 23 million infants still do not receive routine immunizations (Department of Immunization, Vaccines, and Biologicals, World Health Organization, 2010), and vaccine preventable diseases continue to be a worldwide concern.

Other diseases that contribute significantly to the global disease burden include HIV/AIDS, tuberculosis (TB), and malaria. In 2007, HIV/AIDS was responsible for 30 deaths per 100,000 population with 174 deaths per 100,000 in the African region. It is estimated that one child under 15 years of age dies and another is infected with HIV virus each day throughout the world (MacDonald, 2009). As many as 700,000 infants may be infected with HIV virus by their mothers, approximately 40% through contaminated breast milk. International guidelines recommend discontinuing breast-feeding in the face of disease if other safe feeding methods are available, but this is often not the case.

HIV/AIDS has a variety of consequences other than morbidity and mortality. HIV infection and AIDS impairs people's ability to earn enough money to feed their families and diminishes the productive workforce in many high-incidence countries. For example, by 2015, an estimated 20% of the agricultural workforce in Africa will have died from AIDS. Societal and family repercussions from the HIV/AIDS epidemic will be felt for generations in many parts of the world (MacDonald, 2009).

During the 20th century, the incidence of tuberculosis declined in most of the developed world. At the same time, it increased in the rest of the world to the point where the World Health Organization has declared an international emergency. Worldwide tuberculosis killed 1.3 million people in 2010, and 8.6 million others developed the disease. Twenty-two high-burden countries account for 80% of tuberculosis cases worldwide, but 11 of them are on target to reach 2015 goals for reduced incidence. More than 75% of tuberculosis occurs in developing areas of the world; 29% in the Asian region alone. Not all cases of TB occur in poorer nations, however. In 2012, more than 360,000 cases occurred in Europe and another 280,000 in the region of the Americas. A significant portion of the tuberculosis in developed nations occurs in foreign-born individuals who migrate. Treatment of tuberculosis is complicated by the growing incidence of HIV co-infection, with approximately 1.1 million co-infections occurring in 2012 (WHO, 2013b).

Malaria is another significant cause of death; 219 million cases led to 660,000 deaths in 2010. The burden of malaria is significantly higher in some areas than others. An estimated 80% of cases in 2010, for example, occurred in 17 countries, and 80% of deaths occurred in only 14 countries (WHO, 2013e).

Despite higher standards of living and better medical care, the effects of malaria are felt in wealthy countries as well. Because of the limited incidence of malaria, residents in nonendemic areas such as the United States lack the protective immunity acquired from living in malaria-prone areas. In addition, providers are often unfamiliar with the diagnosis and treatment for the disease, leading to misdiagnosis or ineffective therapy. Malaria was virtually eliminated in the United States in the 1950s, but is now reemerging as a condition of concern due to international travel, transport of mosquitoes via trade, and land use changes that have produced new mosquito breeding grounds. Approximately 1,500 cases of malaria occur each year in the United States (CDC, 2012b).

Malaria interacts with malnutrition and common respiratory diseases to increase death rates, particularly among children. In fact, an estimated 32% of malaria deaths in girls under 5 years of age are attributable to malnutrition (WHO, 2009b). Malaria also increases the risk of maternal and fetal deaths and low birth weight in infants (CDC, 2012b). Elimination of malaria-causing mosquitoes or protection of the population from their bites is an effective preventive strategy for malaria, yet from 2000 to 2008 only 17% of those at risk for malaria in Africa and 5% in the Mediterranean region slept under insecticide-treated nets (WHO, 2010).

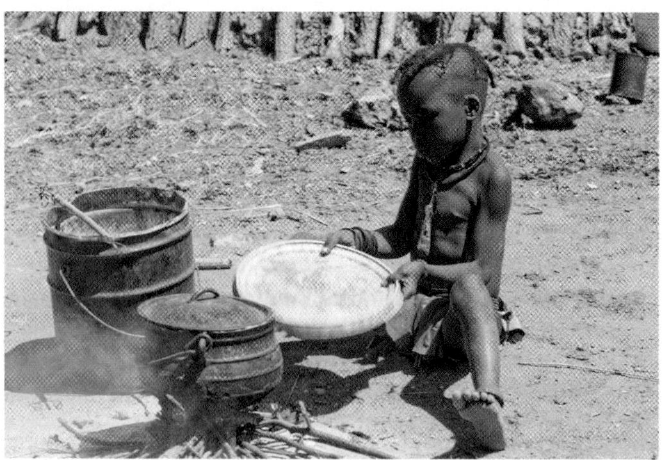

Malnutrition is a serious world health concern. *(Erichon/Fotolia)*

Other communicable diseases continue to contribute to worldwide mortality. For example, emerging diseases, such as Ebola virus and Hantavirus infections, have no known cure and result in significant mortality throughout the world. There is also increasing global concern for biological agents that might be used in bioterrorist attacks. Bioterrorism is discussed in more detail in Chapter 25∞. CDC has identified three foci for global security related to infectious diseases: preventing the likelihood of outbreaks, detecting threats early, and responding rapidly. Prevention includes immunization, preventing the spread of disease, and preventing the development of antimicrobial-resistant organisms, as well as promoting food safety. Detection involves linking global surveillance networks, developing rapid specimen testing capacities, and training a biosurveillance workforce. Elements of response include developing an interconnected global response network and improving worldwide access to medical and nonmedical countermeasures during health emergencies (CDC, 2014).

NONCOMMUNICABLE CONDITIONS. Noncommunicable conditions are fast approaching communicable diseases as the primary causes of death throughout the world. In 2011, six of the top ten causes of death worldwide were related to noncommunicable diseases. These causes of mortality included, in rank order, coronary heart diease; stroke; chronic obstructive pulmonary disease (COPD); cancers of the trachea, bornchus, and lungs; and diabetes mellitus (WHO, 2013d). This shift is predicted to continue until the vast majority of worldwide deaths will be related to noncommunicable conditions. In 2012, coronary heart disease and stroke

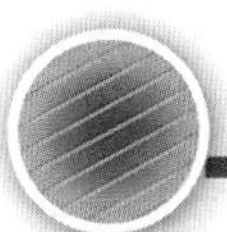

Evidence-Based Practice

Malaria

Malaria is one of the health problems affecting a significant portion of the world's population. CDC (2012b, 2012d) recommends the use of evidence-based malaria control strategies. Commonly used approaches include first line treatment of infected individuals, intermittent preventive therapy (IPT—giving full doses of medication at prescribed intervals) or chemoprophylaxis (use of medications to prevent a condition from occurring), and routine use of insecticide-treated mosquito nets (ITNs).

First line treatment effectiveness is influenced by the extent of drug resistance in the population and by the funding available for treatment with more or less expensive drugs. The report details the relative effectiveness and potential harmful effects of several individual drugs and drug combinations in the treatment of malaria in children. Evidence from systematic reviews of several, randomized controlled trials has indicated that sulfadoxine-pyrimethamine is an effective approach to both IPT and chemoprophylaxis, but that use of chloroquine, the most common prophylactic agent, is generally ineffective due to widespread drug resistance of the causative parasite. In other systematic reviews, ITNs were found to be effective in preventing malaria in children, but were less so in protecting pregnant women. In addition, the evidence indicated that relatively few persons at risk had access to or used ITNs.

1. How might population health nurses be involved in the selection of appropriate drugs for malaria treatment?
2. How could they advocate for access to both curative and preventive drug treatment for underserved populations?
3. How could population health nurses in high-risk areas for malaria promote the use of ITNs?
4. How might this information on evidence-based control strategies for malaria be of relevance to population health nurses in the United States?

together accounted for more than 29% of global mortality (WHO, 2013d).

Another measure of the effects of noncommunicable diseases on world health is the disability-adjusted life year. A **disability-adjusted life year (DALY)** is 1 year of "healthy" life lost as a result of disease (WHO, 2009a) and reflects the burden of disease due to noncommunicable conditions that are often not fatal. Globally, the **burden of disease** can be considered the gap between current global health status and the ideal of achieving a healthy, disease- and disability-free old age for all the world's populations (WHO, 2009a).

Despite the growing burden of noncommunicable conditions, there is little recognition of its effects in global health efforts, which continue to focus heavily on control of communicable diseases. Factors that contribute to the increase in noncommunicable conditions include an aging global population, changes in dietary habits, increased tobacco use, and decreased physical activity (Beaglehole & Yach, 2003/2009). Increases in motorized transportation and subsequent accidents are other contributing factors. In 2011, for example, road injuries accounted for 1.3 million deaths worldwide (WHO, 2013d).

Much of the global burden of noncommunicable disease can be attributed to tobacco use. Globalization affects national economies, frequently making more income available for purchase of "luxury" goods such as tobacco. In addition, global access to technology permits widespread tobacco advertising and targeting of marketing messages to world markets (Beaglehole & Yach, 2003/2009). These factors will require global efforts to control tobacco marketing and consumption. Unfortunately, these efforts are often undermined by the tobacco industry and by nations, such as the United States, that benefit from global exportation of tobacco products.

Similar global effects are noted with respect to dietary consumption, with limitations placed on importation of fresh products from other countries and changes from high fruit and vegetable diets to increasing consumption of fast food and high carbohydrate diets (Beaglehole & Yach, 2003/2009).

Many noncommunicable health conditions are not fatal, but significantly decrease people's quality of life due to disability. Like causes of death, causes of disability differ markedly among high-, middle-, and low-income countries. For example, depression and hearing loss are the leading causes of disability in persons from birth to 59 years of age in high-income countries. Hearing loss is also the most significant cause of disability in middle-income countries, but vision problems are the most common contributor to disability in low-income countries. Worldwide, the most common causes of disability in order of frequency are hearing loss, refractive vision problems, depression, cataracts, unintentional injury, osteoarthritis, alcohol dependence and abuse, infertility related to unsafe abortion and sepsis, macular degeneration, and chronic obstructive pulmonary disease, all of which caused a significant burden of disease (Mathers & Bonita, 2009).

Social Determinants of Health

A number of social factors play a significant role in global health. Among these are poverty, food and water resources, tobacco and alcohol control, motor vehicle traffic, climate change, and immigration, each of which is briefly discussed below. Disaster, another social determinant of health, which has increasingly dire global ramifications, is discussed in Chapter 25∞.

POVERTY. Poverty affects health in a number of ways, from reduced access to health care to inability to afford necessary food, housing, and other requisites for health. The World Bank has defined extreme poverty as an income less than $1.25 per day. By 2010, the millennium development goal of halving the number of people in poverty had been achieved. Even so, 21% of people in the developing world still live in extreme poverty, and 2.4 billion people live on less than $2 per day (World Bank, 2014). It has been suggested that these figures probably underestimate the extent of the world poverty because they do not reflect the income level required for an acceptable standard of living. When one considers the concept of an **ethical poverty line**, the level of income below which life expectancy is shortened; it is more likely that most of the world's population falls into this income category (McCoy, 2011).

FOOD AND WATER. Globalization has had a number of effects on food and water supplies. Increasing transportation of food products has had the advantage of opening markets to produce grown in other parts of the world, thus increasing revenues from exportation. At the same time, the advent of global food processors has often undermined local agricultural economies and put small growers out of business. In addition, there is the increased potential for contamination of foodstuffs due to lack of safe production standards.

Beyond the concern for contamination of food is the problem of insufficient food. According to the United Nations Food and Agricultural Organization, 854 million people throughout the world, 60% of whom are women, do not have enough food to eat, and the number of chronically hungry people increases by about 4 million persons per year. It is estimated that a child dies of starvation approximately every 5 seconds, and 350 to 400 million of the world's children are undernourished, 70% of them in just ten countries. Although overall poverty in the world declined by 20% in the 1990s, the number of hungry people increased by 18 million in the same time frame (MacDonald, 2009). The term currently used to describe chronic hunger is **food insecurity**, which is defined as a persistent lack of nutritionally adequate and safe food in one's diet resulting from a "nonsustainable food system that interferes with optimal self-reliance and social justice" (Kregg-Byers & Schlenk, 2010).

Growing hunger is a result of two phenomena: increases in the world's population and the increasing cost of food. World population estimates are expected to increase by 50% to 9 billion people by 2050. Even by 2030, it is estimated that we will need 50% more food than current requirements, yet food production is decreasing rather than increasing in many areas. Climate change has led to drought and poor crop yields in many parts of the world. At the same time, the increased use of biofuels and diversion of food crops to biofuel production has decreased the availability and increased the price of food-based oils necessary for human consumption. For example, the cost of palm oil, a significant source of calories in the developing world, increased 70% in 2007 alone. Maldistribution of food availability is also a factor with the richest 20% of the world's population consuming 16 times as many calories as the poorest 20% (MacDonald, 2009).

Changes in food consumption patterns and specific nutrient deficiencies are also of concern. For example, meat consumption is increasing in many developing countries. Meat is an inefficient source of calories because raising meat sources consumes significant amounts of grain crops which could provide better sources of food calories if eaten by humans than animals (MacDonald, 2009). Trade liberalization has also led to increased availability of high-calorie, low-nutrient foods such as fast food and processed foods that are contributing to obesity and other chronic health problems. Severe nutrient deficiencies are also noted in many areas of the world. An estimated 684,000 deaths per year could be prevented, for example, with diets adequate in vitamin A and zinc, and 180 million children under 4 years of age are iron deficient (MacDonald, 2009).

Availability of fresh drinking water is another area of global concern. Long perceived as a public good, water resources are being increasingly privatized in both developed and developing parts of the world. When water resources are publicly owned, guarantee of wholesome supplies with effective sanitation at reasonable costs is easier to achieve than when water is considered a profitable commodity. Privatization of water resources often leads to increased costs to consumers. For example, privatization in Bolivia let to a 35% increase in consumer costs, approximately 20% of some family incomes (MacDonald, 2009).

Although some progress has been made in providing safe drinking water and effective sanitation throughout the world, significant portions of the world's population still do not have clean water supplies. In 2011, safe drinking water was available to only 89% of the world's population. This figure meets the 11% target of the millennium development goals, but 768 million people remain without access to improved water sources (WHO & UNICEF, 2013).

Similar findings are noted for access to effective sanitation facilities. Sanitation coverage was at 64% in 2011 and is not expected to meet the MDG goal of 75% by 2015. Approximately 2.5 million people do not have access to sanitation facilities, and 15% continue to practice open defecation, increasing the risk of infectious diseases (WHO & UNICEF, 2013).

Lack of water for hygiene and efforts required to obtain water have a variety of other effects as well. For example, numerous deaths occur each year from diarrheal and respiratory illnesses that could be prevented with adequate hand washing. In addition, time spent by family members in fetching water from distant sources decreases time for education or employment. Women, in particular, may experience sexual assault while traveling long distances to obtain water or defecating in open areas. These dangers may lead to attempts to withhold bodily functions resulting in constipation and urinary tract infections. Water is also needed for effective treatment of HIV/AIDS and tuberculosis, and standing water provides breeding grounds for mosquitoes that spread malaria and other diseases.

Some jurisdictions are implementing the safe water management systems developed by CDC to promote access to clean water. Such programs incorporate several components, including: (a) household water treatment with chlorine disinfectant powder, solar irradiation, or ceramic or slow sand filtration, (b) safe water storage in vessels that prevent contamination, and (c) behavior change to promote hygiene and safe food and water handling practices. These low-cost programs have been found to be effective in improving water quality and decreasing the incidence of disease (CDC, 2012a).

TOBACCO AND ALCOHOL CONTROL. One in ten adult deaths, or a total of 4 million deaths each year, is attributable to tobacco use, and this figure is expected to rise to one in six deaths by 2030. Over the years, the burden of tobacco-related disease has shifted from high-income to low-income countries. By 2030, for example, an estimated 70% of tobacco-related deaths will occur in low-income nations (Collin, Lee, & Bissell, 2002/2009).

Much of this shift is the result of the globalization of the tobacco trade with increased access to international markets due to trade liberalizations, greater telecommunication marketing, economies of scale resulting from production by large multinational corporations, and the ability of transnational companies to undermine local anti-tobacco regulations (Collin et al., 2002/2009).

The WHO Framework Convention on Tobacco Control was initiated as a binding treaty designed to foster tobacco control legislation by signatory nations (Collin et al., 2002/2009). Unfortunately, the United States, a significant producer of tobacco products, has refused to sign the treaty, thereby undermining its effectiveness. The tobacco industry at large has undertaken a variety of measures to weaken the provisions of the convention. These include initiating ineffective youth smoking education and prevention activities to gain public good will, promoting government endorsement of such activities to draw attention away from effective control programs, and detracting from serious consideration of control measures by focusing attention on "more important" public health issues such as communicable diseases and terrorism (Collin et al., 2002/2009).

Unlike many other global public health issues, tobacco control, and control of other harmful substances such as illegal drugs, will require more than public education. Such activities are often undermined by the efforts of special interest groups such as the tobacco industry and the manufacturers and suppliers of illicit drugs. International regulatory efforts controlling advertising, sale, and use of such substances will be required. Such efforts, even within a single jurisdiction, may have cross-border effects. For example, California tobacco control policies related to no-smoking legislation, taxes, advertising limitations, community involvement, media campaigns, and smoking cessation assistance in border areas have decreased tobacco use in neighboring Tijuana, but not farther south in Mexico (Martinez-Donate et al., 2008).

MOTOR VEHICLE TRAFFIC. Globalization, in general, depends on mobility, which is fostered by use of motorized transportation, including cars and air planes. The automotive industry was one of the first to become globalized, with cars being mass produced and mass consumed. Unfortunately, the increase in automobile availability is often not accompanied by road infrastructure development, resulting in increased traffic congestion and environmental deterioration.

Although car ownership is beneficial at the individual level, its population effects are less advantageous. As noted earlier, increasing use of motor vehicles for transportation decreases physical activity among the population, contributing to obesity and other related noncommunicable conditions. Increased consumption of fuel oil to transport people and goods, has also led to a growing energy crisis, and as we saw earlier, has resulted in the diversion of food crops to the creation of biofuels. Greater use of motor vehicles also contributes to air pollution, noise, and environmental degradation.

In addition, the incidence of motor vehicle accidents has increased tremendously, resulting in significant trauma-related morbidity and mortality. More than 1.2 million deaths occur each year, and traffic fatalities are expected to become the fifth leading cause of death by 2030 (WHO, 2013a).

In response to this growing problem, the United Nations has initiated road safety collaboration. Recommendations for dealing with the problem of motor vehicle accidents have been grouped into four safety areas: safer transport and land use policies, safer roads, safer vehicles, and safer people. Safer transport and land use policies address the need for reduction of motor vehicle traffic and use of safer modes of transportation, including mass transportation systems. Such policies should also focus on restrictions in motor size and power, driving age restrictions, and the use of graduated licenses, so that new drivers receive adequate supervision. The recommendations also call for safer roads that incorporate safety features in their designs. Such features might include sidewalks for pedestrian protection, bicycle lanes, and speed reduction and traffic calming strategies such as speed bumps and traffic lights (WHO, 2013a).

Recommended features of safer vehicles include automatic day-time headlight use, safety testing for vehicles, and safety standards and requirements (e.g., seat belts, air bags). Finally, measures to develop "safer people" include restrictions and sanctions for driving under the influence of drugs or alcohol, no speeding, and use of protective helmets for motorcycle and scooter riders (WHO, 2013a).

CLIMATE CHANGE. Global climate changes have had a significant impact on population health throughout the world. The effects of climate change on health are both direct and indirect. Direct effects include the impact of increased heat, flooding, and drought that lead to changes in the distribution of vector- and waterborne diseases. The effect of climate change on food production was addressed earlier. Indirect effects are a result of the social upheaval that occurs with food scarcity, leading to violence and conflict, and changes in refugee and migration streams. These and other effects of climate change were addressed in Chapter 4∞.

IMMIGRATION. Population movement is a salient feature of globalization. Transient movement related to business, industry, and tourism may have beneficial effects on national and global economies. Other forms of immigration, however, arise from and create social problems that cause people to migrate from one place to another. It is estimated that there were approximately 232 million legal and illegal immigrants throughout the world in 2013, and the growth in the immigrant population has been about 1.6% per year since 2010. Half of the world's immigrant population lives in ten countries, with the United States having the largest number of immigrants. Nearly half of the immigrant population is composed of women (United Nations Population Division, 2013).

Migration may be forced or voluntary. People engage in voluntary migration when they choose to move from one place to another, often in search of better employment opportunities, better climate, or other factors. Forced migration arises out of conflict, persecution, natural or environmental disasters (such as famine or chemical or nuclear accidents), or the results of "development projects" as when people are displaced by dams that cause flooding in their original location. In 2013, there were an estimated 15.7 million refugees worldwide (United Nations Population Division, 2013). Unfortunately, developing countries, that are themselves poor, house 90% of the world's refugee population (66%% of them in Asia and nearly 19% in Africa (United Nations Population Division, 2013).

Migration sometimes occurs from developing to developed nations. For example, in 2012, more than 1 million people entered the United States as legal permanent residents and another 58,000 were admitted as refugees. In addition, more than 165.5 million non-immigrants arrived in the United States for limited periods of time, primarily on business, for study, or as tourists. Finally, more than 643,000 persons were apprehended entering illegally (Office of Immigration Statistics, 2013). An unknown number of undocumented immigrants also cross U.S. borders each year, contributing to the economy but also to the risk for health problems.

People engaged in both voluntary and forced migration may experience better opportunities, but they may also be subjected to exploitation and abuse because of their vulnerability and lack of familiarity with the laws and customs of their new homelands. Although they may be healthier than those who remain in their countries of origin, immigrants tend to be at greater risk for health problems than the native-born populations of their new homes. Immigrants tend to use health care services less than their native-born counterparts, particularly mental health services, and may have less access to care or be unaware of eligibility for services. In some immigrant populations, the incidence of mental health problems has increased with subsequent generations in the United States, possibly as a result of discrimination, social stress, and downward social mobility. They are also frequently less likely to engage in health promotion and illness prevention behaviors, although their preferred diets are often healthier at entry.

Mental health problems created by hardships during immigration may be compounded by social isolation and discrimination experienced in the host country (Park, Cho, Park, Bernstein, & Shin, 2013). Discrimination may lead to socioeconomic disadvantage and greater exposure to environmental hazards, pollution, and stress, and perceptions of discrimination have been associated with increased incidence of chronic diseases such as heart disease and respiratory illness. Perceived discrimination is also related to depression (Sirin, Ryce, Gupta, & Rogers-Sirin, 2013). In their new countries, immigrants may experience poverty and poor living and working conditions. In fact, immigrants may be at greater risk for workplace fatalities than the general population because of employment in the most dangerous jobs.

Poorer health status among refugee populations may also put the general population of the host country at risk. For example, legal requirements for vaccination do not apply to U.S. refugees, but they must be immunized prior to applying for permanent residence. Whether immigrants should be immunized before or after their arrival has long been debated, but the potential costs of both vaccination and care for those who become infected suggest that pre-arrival immunization would be of greater benefit to society. Failure to immunize immigrant populations may have other serious and costly consequences. For example, debilitated refugees may be subject to a variety of communicable diseases that may spread to the larger population. For all of these reasons, population health nurses should be involved in the delivery of services and development of policy related to immigrant health.

Population Health Nursing and Global Health

Why should a nurse working in a particular country, such as the United States, be concerned about globalization and global health issues? The most obvious answer to this question, of course, is to be able to understand the effects of global health issues on the health status of the local population, but there are other reasons as well. Some of these include delivery of health services to an international clientele, policy development, and involvement in global health issues through international nursing organizations.

Service Delivery

Nurses in most countries will encounter clients from a variety of other nations. These clients may need assistance in navigating the health system differences between their countries of origin and their current countries of residence. Knowledge of these other health systems will allow nurses to better educate clients with respect to similarities and differences between health systems and how to navigate the system in their country of residence. Similarly, knowledge of the health problems prevalent in their countries of origin can assist population health nurses in assessing the health status of individuals from other parts of the world.

At some point population health nurses may also work or travel in other countries, and knowledge of health systems and prevalent health problems can help them to better protect their own health or meet the health needs of their host countries. Finally, population health nurses may find themselves working with nurses from other countries, either at home or in international arenas, and knowledge of their health care systems will permit more effective collaboration in addressing the health care needs of all of the world's populations.

Framing Global Policy Issues

Health policy issues are those that rise to the consciousness of policy makers. **Policy** is a set of principles determining the direction for action and allocation of resources to achieve an identified prioritized goal. Many serious health problems, however, never rise to the level of policy issues. What, then, distinguishes these problems from identified policy issues?

Some authors have noted that attracting and sustaining attention from the global community to specific issues depends upon how they are framed. The point has been made that policy issues are not always related to the severity or impact of the problem, but to "institutions that create, negotiate, promote, and sustain" portrayals of the issues that keep attention centered upon them (Shiffman, 2009, p. 610). Institutions, in this context, are not specific organizations or agencies, but are the "rules, norms, and strategies adopted by individuals within or across organizations" (quoted in Shiffman, 2009, p. 610). Attention to specific issues may be mediated by social interpretations or understandings of the issue.

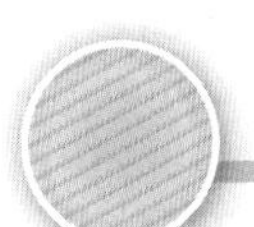

Global Perspectives

The Population Health Nursing Role

The role of population health nurses differs from one part of the world to another. Select another country in which you are interested and explore the role of population health nurses in that country. How does the role differ from that of population health nurses in your own area? What factors contribute to those differences? How easy or difficult would it be for a population health nurse educated in the United States to engage in population health nursing in that country? What factors would influence a U.S. nurse's ability to function in the expected population health role?

Many issues are backed by powerful institutions that may be preexisting or be created specifically to draw attention to issues (Shiffman, 2009). For example, we will see in Chapter 9∞ that the tobacco industry is a powerful institution that tries to frame the issue of tobacco use in ways that will not lead to restriction of sales. Other institutions are purposefully created to address a particular issue; for instance, time-limited political action groups arise to support or oppose specific ballot initiatives and then disappear after the election.

Institutions mobilize resources, initiate programs, and support research related to the problem of interest, but may also create portrayals of the problem that sustain the interest of the public or influential policy makers (Shiffman, 2009). For example, if the public is concerned about national security, framing an immunization issue around the concept of the potential for terrorist-engendered epidemics may promote public support and federal funding for vaccine development and immunization services.

Policy issues are framed by members of **policy communities**, which are defined as "networks of individuals (including researchers, advocates, policy makers and technical officials) and organizations (including governments, non-governmental organizations, United Nations agencies, foundations, and donor agencies) that share a concern for a particular issue" (Shiffman, 2009, p. 608). Issues that are successful in gaining the sustained attention of global policy makers "may be ones in which policy community members have discovered frames—ways of positioning an issue—that resonate with global and national political elites, and then established institutions that can sustain these frames" (Shiffman, 2009, p. 608).

Population health nurses can help to frame global health problems in ways that attract the attention of the public and policy makers. In general, there are five ways of framing health issues to focus attention on them. The first approach is to frame health problems as security issues that may contribute to risk of infection or political and economic instability. What, for example, would be the nutritional and economic effects of worldwide contamination of food with chemical toxins?

Health problems can also be framed as development issues or as desired outcomes of global economic development. For example, provision of clean water supplies easily accessible may free women from onerous household chores to join a labor force severely depleted by illness, in addition to preventing the spread of waterborne diseases. Thus, a health-related intervention can promote economic development as well as population health status.

A third approach to framing health issues is as global public goods. This approach lauds the collective benefit of intervention over individual gain, and promotes the good as something open to all that does not lessen its availability to others. Health-related issues can also be framed as "commodities" or tradable goods. For example, research to find newer and more effective medications for a variety of conditions have been supported as an avenue to increased profit. This approach to framing an issue may actually have negative health effects by limiting access to the resulting medications to those who can pay for them.

Finally, health issues may be framed in terms of a human right leading eventually to international rights agreements. Unfortunately, such agreements are difficult to enforce and require equal access to care and provision of access to basic survival needs. In actual fact, a combination of all of the above approaches (except the commodity approach) may be what is needed to frame health-related problems in such a way that they attain and sustain global attention and efforts to resolve them. There is a need for combined discussion of moral, legal, and economic parameters in the framing of global health issues, and population health nurses can help to support all of these levels of discussion.

International Nursing Organizations

Population health nurses are supported in their international activities by several agencies and organizations. WHO recognizes the importance of nursing (and midwifery) services to the accomplishment of global health objectives and so maintains a Nursing and Midwifery Office to assist with nursing development throughout the world. The division has outlined several strategic directions for its efforts including:

- Developing action plans to incorporate nursing and midwifery as an integral part of national health plans
- Forging strong interdisciplinary health teams to resolve priority health issues
- Improving nursing and midwifery education
- Collaborating with nursing and midwifery professions to strengthen regulatory processes
- Strengthening datasets on nursing and midwifery as an integral part of workforce information systems
- Utilizing the expertise of nursing and midwifery researchers
- Actively engaging nurses and midwives in health care planning, implementation, and evaluation and policy formation
- Implementing strategies to enhance interprofessional education and collaborative practice
- Including nurses and midwives in the development of strategies for recruitment and retention and improved working conditions
- Implementing the WHO *Global Code of Practice on the International Recruitment of Health Personnel* (WHO, n.d.).

Another avenue for international involvement by community health nurses is the **International Council of Nurses (ICN)**. ICN is a federation of national nurses' associations, including the American Nurses Association, representing nurses in more than 130 countries. Established in 1899, ICN was the first international organization for health professionals (ICN, 2013a). The organization was established to address three primary goals:

- To promote worldwide nursing exchange
- To advance the nursing profession
- To influence global health policy

In its efforts to achieve these three goals, ICN works to standardize professional nursing practice worldwide and to improve the socioeconomic welfare of nurses. ICN's mission is to "represent nursing worldwide, advancing the profession and influencing health policy" (ICN, 2013b). One of the major ways in which ICN works to achieve this mission is through the creation of nursing networks that serve as avenues for the exchange of nursing knowledge and expertise in specific areas. Current ICN initiatives focus on professional nursing practice, nursing regulation, and the socioeconomic welfare of nurses. Specific practice foci include the International Classification for Nursing Practice (ICNP), advanced nursing practice, entrepreneurship, women's health, primary health care, family health, safe water, and HIV/AIDS, tuberculosis, and malaria (ICN 2013b). For further information about ICN and its activities, see the *External Resources* section of the student resources site.

Sigma Theta Tau International is another international nursing organization. Established in 1922 by six U.S. nursing students, Sigma Theta Tau's goal is to provide leadership and support scholarship related to nursing practice, education, and research to improve the health of the world's population. The organization was the first funder of nursing research in the United States and currently supports a variety of nursing education and research initiatives. In 1985, the organization was incorporated as Sigma Theta Tau International, Inc. to better connect the worldwide network of scholars who promote health worldwide. Membership currently embraces nurses in 86 countries throughout the world (Sigma Theta Tau International, n.d.).

One final international nursing organization to be discussed here is the **Global Alliance for Leadership in Nursing Education and Science (GANES)**. GANES is an organization of national associations of nursing deans and schools of nursing established to support health care policy makers and nurse educators throughout the world. Its mandate is to "work in partnership with global and national organizations to raise awareness of the key role of nurse education in the improvement of global health and quality of care" (GANES, n.d.b). The founding members of GANES include the national nursing education organizations of the United Kingdom, Canada, the United States, and Australia and New Zealand. GANES activities include promoting sharing among nurse educators around the world, providing information and advice to global policy makers related to nursing education issues, and supporting development of a sound evidence base for nursing practice and education (GANES, n.d.a). For additional information about Sigma Theta Tau and GANES, see the *External Resources* section of the student resources site.

Population health nurses may also be actively involved in a wide variety of international nursing and multidisciplinary organizations that address special focus areas such as violence against women, menopause, child health, HIV/AIDS, family health, and so on. As we have seen, a wide variety of health problems cross national boundaries, and global approaches must be taken to resolve them.

CHAPTER RECAP

Globalization is affecting population health as well as other issues throughout the world. Globalization occurs within four dimensions, the spatial, temporal, cognitive, and social dimensions. Globalization has both positive and negative effects on population health. Positive health effects derive from dissemination of new knowledge and effective interventions, development of international standards, and increasing concern for global social justice. Negative effects include the rapid spread of disease, dietary and activity changes, increased substance abuse, traffic accidents, and global warming.

Global health differs from international health in its broader scope. Where international health issues usually lie between two countries, global health issues cross multiple international boundaries and affect large segments of the globe. Several global and international health organizations work to address global health issues including WHO and PAHO.

A number of current issues affect the health of the world's population. These include life expectancy, communicable and chronic diseases, poverty, safe food and water resources, tobacco and alcohol control, motor vehicle accidents, violence, climate change, immigration, and disaster response. Many of these issues center on the *Global Millennium Development Goals*, which are similar to the *Healthy People 2020* objectives in the United States. Population health nurses can be involved in the resolution of these issues through direct service delivery, policy formation, and participation in international professional nursing organizations such as ICN, Sigma Theta Tau, and GANES, and other organizations designed to address global health issues.

CASE STUDY **Cooperation for Polio Elimination**

Peace Corps volunteers (PCVs) in one small village in India in the 1960s initiated an immunization program for DTP and polio immunizations in the local Primary Health Center and its five substations in outlying villages. The volunteers got funding for an initial supply of vaccines from the International Rotary Club. Vaccines were purchased in Bombay, a trip of 250 miles from the health center, and transported on ice to the village. This trip needed to be made every 6 weeks because of the limited shelf-life of the oral polio vaccine.

Since the health center only possessed two syringes, the PCVs acquired used disposable syringes and needles from Peace Corps headquarters in Bombay. This equipment was of the type that could be resterilized by boiling and several hundred syringes were used each year to update immunizations for volunteers in the region. A very small fee was charged for each immunization. This revenue was used to pay for subsequent vaccine purchases and the program was essentially self-funding.

The PCVs gave the immunizations themselves, both in the health center itself and on specific immunization days in the subcenters. Immunizations were also begun in the local school. Unfortunately, after the first dose of DTP in the school setting, many of the children developed mild inflammation and soreness at the injection sites. Their parents complained to the physician director of the health center who stopped further immunization in the school setting. One member of the health center staff, whose daughter had been nursed by the volunteers through a life-threatening episode of typhoid, became a local proponent for immunization in the village. Many of her friends and family came to the health center requesting immunizations. Unfortunately, she was of lower-class status and did not have influence with upper-class residents.

Just before the volunteers were scheduled to leave India, they took one of the host-country staff to Bombay and showed him where to purchase the vaccines. They left a supply of syringes and needles that could be used by the staff of the health center to continue the program. The program was sustained for a year or so after the volunteers left, but then dwindled away.

1. What might the Peace Corps volunteers have done differently to create a sustainable immunization program in this village?
2. How might the program have been expanded to encompass other villages in the region?

REFERENCES

Association of State and Territorial Health Officials. (2013). *Global infectious disease*. Retrieved from http://www.astho.org/programs/infectious-disease/refugee-health/global-infectious-disease---impact-on-state-and-territorial-health/

Bartsch, S., Hein, W., & Kohlmorgen, L. (2007). Interfaces: A concept for the analysis of global health governance. In W. Hein, S. Bartsch, & L. Kohlmorgen (Eds.), *Global health governance and the fight against HIV/AIDS* (pp. 18–37). New York, NY: Palgrave Macmillan.

Beaglehole, R., & Bonita, R. (2010). What is global health? *Global Health Action, 3*, 5242. doi: 10.3402/gha.v3i0.5142

Beaglehole, R., & Yach, D. (2003/2009). Globalisation and the prevention and control of non-communicable disease: The neglected chronic diseases of adults. *The Lancet, 362*, 903–908. Reprinted in J. J. Kirton (Ed.), *Global health* (pp. 137–142). Farnham, Surrey, UK: Ashgate.

Bill & Melinda Gates Foundation. (n.d.). *Global health program*. Retrieved from http://www.gatesfoundation.org/global-health/Pages/overview.aspx

Center for the Study of the History of Nursing, School of Nursing, University of Pennsylvania. (n.d.). *International Council of Nurses Records, 1946–1970* (MC # 112). Retrieved from http://www.nursing.upenn.edu/history/Documents/ICN_MC112_Brief_Description.pdf

Centers for Disease Control and Prevention. (2009). *Questions and answers about smallpox vaccine*. Retrieved from http://emergency.cdc.gov/agent/smallpox/faq/characteristics.asp

Centers for Disease Control and Prevention. (2012a). *CDC and the safe water system*. Retrieved from http://www.cdc.gov/safewater/PDF/SWS-Overview-factsheet508c.pdf

Centers for Disease Control and Prevention. (2012b). *Malaria: Frequently asked questions*. Retrieved from http://www.cdc.gov/malaria/about/faqs.html

Centers for Disease Control and Prevention. (2013). *Preferred usage*. Retrieved from http://wwwnc.cdc.gov/eid/pages/preferred-usage.htm

Centers for Disease Control and Prevention. (2014). *Medicare and Medicaid research review/ 2013 statistical supplement*. Retrieved from http://www.cdc.gov/globalhealth/security/ghsagenda.htm

Collin, J., Lee, K., & Bissell, K. (2002/2009). The Framework Convention on Tobacco Control: The politics of global health governance. *Third World Quarterly, 23*, 265–282. Reprinted in J. J. Kirton (Ed.), *Global health* (pp. 137–142). Farnham, Surrey, UK: Ashgate.

Center for Global Health. (n.d.). *Global health: Who we are*. Retrieved from http://www.cdc.gov/globalhealth/index.html

Department of Immunization, Vaccines, and Biologicals, World Health Organization. (2010). Global routine vaccine coverage, 2009. *Morbidity and Mortality Weekly Report, 59*, 1367–1371.

Division of Foodborne, Waterborne, and Environmental Diseases. (2010). Progress toward global eradication of dracunculiasis, January 2009–June 2010. *Morbidity and Mortality Weekly Report, 59*, 1239–1242.

Dodgson, R., Lee, K., & Drager, N. (2002/2009). *Global Health Governance, a Conceptual Review, Discussion Paper No. 1, Centre on Global Change and Health, London School of Hygiene and Tropical Medicine, Department of Health and Development, World Health Organization*, 5–17. Reprinted in J. J. Kirton (Ed.), *Global health* (pp. 137–142). Farnham, Surrey, UK: Ashgate.

Ezeani, K. O. (2012). *Globalization, poverty, and inequality*. Retrieved from http://www.academia.edu/1829893/Globalisation_Poverty_and_Inequality

Fidler, D. P. (2001/2009). The globalization of public health: The first 100 years of international health diplomacy. *Bulletin of the World Health Organization, 79*, 842–849. Reprinted in J. J. Kirton (Ed.), *Global health* (pp. 125–132). Farnham, Surrey, UK: Ashgate.

Global Alliance for Leadership in Nursing Education and Science. (n.d.a). *GANES: Global Alliance for Leadership in Nursing Education and Science.*, from http://www.ganes.info/documents/GANESBrochure310.pdf

Global Alliance for Leadership in Nursing Education and Science. (n.d.b). *Mission*. Retrieved from http://www.ganes.info/About.php

Global Health. (2014). *Measles & rubella: Eliminating measles, rubella & congenital rubella syndrome (CRS) worldwide*. Retrieved from http://www.cdc.gov/globalhealth/measles/

Global Immunization Division, National Immunization Program. (2004). Global polio eradication initiative strategic plan, 2004. *Morbidity and Mortality Weekly Report, 53*, 107–108.

Hixon, A. L., & Maskarinec, G. G. (2008). The Declaration of Alma Ata on its 30th anniversary: Relevance for family medicine today. *Family Medicine, 40*, 585–588. No doi:

Institute of Medicine. (2009). *The U.S. commitment to global health: Recommendations for the public and private sectors*. Washington, DC: The National Academies Press.

International Council of Nurses. (2013a). *About ICN*. Retrieved from http://www.icn.ch/about-icn/about-icn

International Council of Nurses. (2013b). *The ICN story—1899–1999*. Retrieved from http://www.icn.ch/about-icn/the-icn-story-1899-1999

International Council of Nurses. (2013c). *Our mission*. Retrieved from http://www.icn.ch/about-icn/icns-mission

Fogarty International Center. (n.d.). *About the Fogarty International Center*. Retrieved from http://www.fic.nih.gov/About/Pages/default.aspx

Kates, J., & Katz, R. (2010). *U.S. global health policy: U.S. participation in international health treaties, commitments, partnerships, and other agreements*. Retrieved from http://www.kff.org/globalhealth/8099.cfm

Kickbush, I. (2000/2009). The development of international health policies—Accountability intact? *Social Science & Medicine, 51*, 979–989. Reprinted in J. J. Kirton (Ed.), *Global health* (pp. 396–405). Farnham, Surrey, UK: Ashgate.

Kregg-Byers, C. M., & Schlenk, E. A. (2010). Implications of food insecurity on global health policy and nursing practice. *Journal of Nursing Scholarship, 42*, 278–285.

Lee, K. (2010). Civil society organizations and the functions of global health governance. *Global Health Governance, III (2)*. Retrieved from http://blogs.shu.edu/ghg/files/2011/11/Lee_Civil-Society-Organizations-and-the-Functions-of-Global-Health-Governance_Spring-2010.pdf

MacDonald, T. H. (2009). *Removing the barriers to global health equity*. Abingdon, UK: Radcliffe.

Martinez-Donate, A. P., Hovell, M. F., Hofstetter, C. R., Gonzalez-Perez, G. J., Kotay, A., & Adams, M. A. (2008). Crossing borders: The impact of the California tobacco control program on both sides of the US–Mexico border. *American Journal of Public Health, 98*, 258–267.

Mathers, C., & Bonita, R. (2009). Current global health status. In R. Beaglehole & R. Bonita (Eds.), *Global public health: A new era* (2nd ed., pp. 23–61). Oxford, UK: Oxford University Press.

McCoy, D. (2011). *Humanitarianism – Moving beyond medical rescue to poverty reduction, sustainable development and justice?* Retrieved from http://www.phmovement.org/en/node/6254

McDonald, J. A., Mojarro, O., Sutton, P. D., & Ventura, S. J. (2013). A binational overview of reproductive health outcomes among US Hispanic and Mexican women in the border region. *Preventing Chronic Disease, 10*, 130019. doi: http://dx.doi.org/10.5888/pcd10.130019

Michael, A., & Beaglehole, R. (2009). The global context for public health. In R. Beaglehole & R. Bonita (Eds.), *Global public health: A new era* (2nd ed., pp. 1–22). Oxford, UK: Oxford University Press.

National Human Trafficking Resources Center. (2010). Human trafficking statistics: Polaris report. Retrieved from http://www.handsacrosstheworldmn.org/resources/Human+Trafficking+Statistics.pdf

NGO Global Network. (n.d.). *Definition of NGOs*. Retrieved from www.ngo.org/ngoinfo/define.html

Office of Global Affairs. (n.d.). *Who we are*. Retrieved from http://www.globalhealth.gov/about-us/

Office of Immigration Statistics. (2013). *2012 yearbook of immigration statistics*. Retrieved from https://www.dhs.gov/sites/default/files/publications/ois_yb_2012.pdf

Pan American Health Organization. (2011). *Values, vision and mission of the Pan American Sanitary Bureau*. Retrieved from http://new.paho.org/hq/index.php?option=com_content&task=view&id=95&Itemid=163

Pan American Health Organization. (2012). *Experts start verifying measles, rubella elimination from the Americas*. Retrieved from http://www.paho.org/hq/index.php?option=com_content&view=article&id=4558%3Aexperts-start-verifying-measles-rubella-elimination-americas&catid=1637%3Afgl-03-measles-featured-items&Itemid=1711&lang=en

Pan American Health Organization. (2013). *About PAHO*. Retrieved from http://new.paho.org/hq/index.php?option=com_content&task=view&id=91&Itemid=220

Pan American Health Organization. (2014a). *No endemic transmission of measles in the Americas since 2002*. Retrieved from http://www.paho.org/hq./index.php?option=com_content&view=article&id=9318%3Ano-endemic-transmission-of-measles-in-the-americas-since-2002&catid=1443%3Anews-front-page-items&Itemid=358&lang=fr

Pan American Health Organization. (2014b). *Regional Core Health Data Initiative*. Retrieved from http://www.paho.org/HQ/index.php?option=com_content&view=article&id=2151&Itemid=1876&lang=en

Pan American Health Organization. (2014c). *Regional Core Health Data Initiative: Profiles by country*. Retrieved from

Park, S. Y., Cho, S., Park, Y., Bernstein, K. S., & Shin, J. (2013). Factors associated with mental health service utilization among Korean American immigrants. *Community Mental Health Journal, 49*, 765-773. doi: 10.1007/s10597-013-9604-8

Quandl. (2014). *GDP as share of world GDP at PPP by country*. Retrieved from http://www.quandl.com/economics/gdp-as-share-of-world-gdp-at-ppp-by-country

Ram, P. K., Kelsey, E., Ratsoatioana, M. R. R., Rakotomalala, O., & Dunstan, C. (2007). Bringing safe water to remote populations: An evaluation of a portable point-of-use intervention in rural Madagascar. *American Journal of Public Health, 97*, 398–400.

Ross, J. (2013). *Only 30% of the world now has a higher GDP per capita than China*. Retrieved from http://ablog.typepad.com/keytrendsinglobalisation/2013/05/only-30-of-the-world-now-has-a-higher-gdp-per-capita-than-china.html

Shiffman, J. (2009). A social explanation for the rise and fall of global health issues. *Bulletin of the World Health Organization, 87*, 608–613. doi:10.2471/BLT.08.06749

Sigma Theta Tau International. (n.d.). *Organizational fact sheet*. Retrieved from http://www.nursingsociety.org/aboutus/mission/Pages/factsheet.aspx

Sirin, S. R., Ryce, P., Gupta, T, & Rogers-Sirin, L. (2013). The role of acculturative stress on mental health symptoms for immigrant adolescents: A longitudinal investigation. *Developmental Psychology, 49*, 736-748. doi: 10.1037/a0028398

Stadtfeld, R. (translator). (2012). *The evolution of the per capital income levels in the world*. Retrieved from http://www.inequalitywatch.eu/spip.php?article102

Strebel, P., Dabbaugh, A., Gacic-Dobo, M., Reef, S. E., & Cochi, S. (2010). Progress toward control of rubella and prevention of congenital rubella syndrome—Worldwide, 2009. *Morbidity and Mortality Weekly Report, 59*, 1307–1310.

Susan G. Komen Foundation. (2014). *About us*. Retrieved from http://ww5.komen.org/AboutUs/AboutUs.html

United Nations. (2012). The *Millennium Development Goals report 2012*. Retrieved from http://mdgs.un.org/unsd/mdg/Resources/Static/Products/Progress2012/English2012.pdf

United Nations. (2013). *Millennium development goals and beyond 2015*. Retrieved from http://www.un.org/millenniumgoals/reports.shtml

United Nations Children's Fund. (2009). *The state of the world's children, Special edition: Executive summary*. Retrieved from http://www.unicef.org/rightsite/sowc/pdfs/SOWC_SpecEd_CRC_ExecutiveSummary_EN_091009.pdf

United Nations Children's Fund. (2014). *The state of the world's children 2014 in numbers: Every child counts: Revealing disparities, advancing children's rights*. Retrieved from http://www.unicef.org/sowc2014/numbers/documents/english/SOWC2014_In%20Numbers_28%20Jan.pdf

United Nations Population Division. (n.d.). *International migration*. Retrieved from http://esa.un.org/unmigration/wallchart2013.htm

United States-Mexico Border Health Commission. (n.d.). *Overview*. Retrieved from http://www.borderhealth.org/about_us.php

U.S. Agency for International Development. (2014). *Who we are*. Retrieved from http://www.usaid.gov/who-we-are

U.S. Department of Health and Human Services. (2013). *Global health*. Retrieved from http://www.healthypeople.gov/2020/topicsobjectives2020/overview.aspx?topicid=16

U.S. Department of State. (2013). *Trafficking in persons report* June 2013. Retrieved from http://www.state.gov/documents/organization/210737.pdf

U.S. Food and Drug Administration. (2014). *International programs*. Retrieved from http://www.fda.gov/internationalprograms/default.htm

Wagstaff, A., Bustreo, F., Bryce, J., Cleason, M.; The WHO-World Bank Child Health and Poverty Working Group. (2004). Child health: Reaching the poor. *American Journal of Public Health, 94*, 726–736.

Walzer, M. (2011). On humanitarianism: Is helping others charity, or duty, or both? *Foreign Affairs, 90*(4). Retrieved from http://www.foreignaffairs.com/articles/67931/michael-walzer/on-humanitarianism

World Bank. (2013). Defining civil society. Retrieved from http://web.worldbank.org/WBSITE/EXTERNAL/TOPICS/CSO/0,,contentMDK:20101499~menuPK:244752~pagePK:220503~piPK:220476~theSitePK:228717,00.html

World Bank. (2014). *Poverty overview*. Retrieved from http://www.worldbank.org/en/topic/poverty/overview

World Health Organization. (n.d.). *Nursing and midwifery at WHO*. Retrieved from http://www.who.int/hrh/nursing_midwifery/en/

World Health Organization. (2008). *Primary health care: Now more than ever*. Retrieved from http://www/who.int/2008/whr08_en.pdf

World Health Organization. (2009a). *Global health risks: Mortality and burden of disease attributable to selected major risks*. Retrieved from http://www.who.int/healthinfo/global_burden_disease/GlobalHealthRisks_report_full.pdf

World Health Organization. (2009b). *Women and health: Today's evidence, tomorrow's agenda*. Retrieved from http://whqlibdoc.who.int/publications/2009/9789241563857_eng.pdf

World Health Organization. (2010). *World health statistics 2010.* Retrieved from http://www.who.int/whosis/whostat/EN_WHS10_Full.pdf

World Health Organization. (2013a). *Global status report on road safety 2013: Supporting a decade of action.* Retrieved from http://www.who.int/violence_injury_prevention/road_safety_status/2013/report/en/index.html

World Health Organization. (2013b). *Global tuberculosis report 2013.* Retrieved from http://apps.who.int/iris/bitstream/10665/91355/1/9789241564656_eng.pdf?ua=1

World Health Organization. (2013c). *Polio eradication & end game strategic plan, 2013-2018.* Retrieved from http://www.polioeradication.org/Portals/0/Document/Resources/StrategyWork/PEESP_ES_EN_A4.pdf

World Health Organization. (2013d). *The top 10 causes of death.* Retrieved from http://www.who.int/mediacentre/factsheets/fs310/en/

World Health Organization. (2013e). *World health statistics 2013.* Retrieved from http://www.who.int/gho/publications/world_health_statistics/2013/en/

World Health Organization. (2014a). *About WHO.* Retrieved from http://www.who.int/about/en/

World Health Organization. (2014b). *Global health governance.* Retrieved from http://www.who.int/trade/glossary/story038/en/

World Health Organization. (2014c). *Globalization.* Retrieved from http://www.who.int/trade/glossary/story043/en/

World Health Organization. (2014d). *Immunization coverage.* Retrieved from http://www.who.int/mediacentre/factsheets/fs378/en/

World Health Organization. (2014e). *International Health Regulations.* Retrieved from http://www.who.int/topics/international_health_regulations/en/

World Health Organization. (2014f). *Poliomyelitis.* Retrieved from http://www.who.int/mediacentre/factsheets/fs114/en/

World Health Organization. (2014g). Sector-wide approaches (SWAPs). Retrieved from http://www.who.int/trade/glossary/story081/en/

World Health Organization. (2014h). *Smallpox.* Retrieved from http://www.who.int/mediacentre/factsheets/smallpox/en/

World Health Organization. (2014i). *World Health Assembly.* Retrieved from http://www.who.int/mediacentre/events/governance/wha/en/

World Health Organization & UNICEF. (2013). *Progress on drinking water and sanitation, 2013 update.* Retrieved from http://www.wssinfo.org/fileadmin/user_upload/resources/JMPreport2013.pdf

World Trade Organization. (2014). *Intellectual property: Protection and enforcement.* Retrieved from http://www.wto.org/english/thewto_e/whatis_e/tif_e/agrm7_e.htm

UNIT

3

Population Health Nursing Strategies

Chapters

CHAPTER

9 Political Strategies

Learning Outcomes

After reading this chapter, you should be able to:

1. Analyze potential population health nursing roles in policy development.
2. Discuss four avenues for public policy development.
3. Describe at least four aspects of the policy development process.
4. Apply criteria for health policy evaluation.

Key Terms

allocative policies
bill
campaigning
coalitions
community organizing
electioneering
executive orders
governance
health impact assessment (HIA)
health policy
interest group
judicial decisions
laws
legislative proposals
lobbying
networking
pocket veto
policy agenda
political advocacy
politics
procedural policies
public policies
redistributive policies
regulation
regulatory policies
sin taxes
stakeholders
substantive policies

Advocacy Then

Creating the Children's Bureau

An early history of the U.S. Children's Bureau credits the development of this federal agency to "a hardy band of practical dreamers who, beginning about 1903, studied the past and present circumstances of children in order to chart a course for the future" (Oettinger, 1962, p. 1). Chief among those practical dreamers were Lillian Wald and Florence Kelley. It was actually Lillian Wald who conceived of the idea of a federal agency to address the needs of the nation's children over tea with her friend and colleague Florence Kelly, a social worker who lived and worked at the settlement.

Two letters received simultaneously addressed the needs of children, one asking for help and one offering to help in any way to reduce the numbers of children dying. They sparked a comment by Ms. Wald, "I wish there were some agency that would tell us what can be done about these problems" (Oettinger, 1962, p. 2). An article in the newspaper that same day described the activities of the Secretary of Agriculture related to weevil infestations in southern cotton crops, which led to the idea of a federal agency to address the needs of children. As expressed by Ms. Wald, "If the government can have a department to take such an interest in what is happening to the Nation's cotton crop, why can't it have a bureau to look after the Nation's crop of children?" (Bradbury & Eliot, 1956, p. 1). Even before that time, Florence Kelley had proposed a "Commission for Children" during a series of lectures at major universities and colleges.

Dr. Edward Devine, a member of Florence Kelley's diverse personal network informed President Theodore Roosevelt of the idea, and Ms. Wald was invited to the White House to discuss it with him. The next 9 years saw the introduction of 11 bills in the U.S. house or senate, nationwide campaigning by Ms. Wald, Mrs. Kelley, and other individuals and organizations including the National Child Labor Committee in which Florence Kelley was actively involved (Bradbury & Eliot, 1956, p. 2). During this period, Mrs. Kelley published several books, including *Some Ethical Gains Through Legislation*, in which she presented evidence of the need for federal intervention to support the health and welfare of children (Bradbury & Eliot, 1956). In 1912, their efforts culminated in the passage of the enabling legislation and its signature by then President William Howard Taft (Social Security Administration, n.d.). Both Lillian Wald and Florence Kelley were also involved in numerous other political advocacy activities related to women's and children's health, the laboring poor, rural nursing services, and women's suffrage (*Florence Kelley,* 2011; Jewish Women's Archive, 2010; Lewis, 2011).

Advocacy Now

The Campaign for APRN Consensus

In 2008, an alliance of professional nursing organizations, educational organizations, certifying bodies, and the National Council of State Boards of Nursing (NCSBN) collaborated to draft the "Consensus Model for APRN Regulation: Licensure, Accreditation, Certification, and Education," more popularly known as the "Consensus Model." The model is designed to provide for nationwide standardization in the education, licensure, and practice of advanced practice registered nurses (APRNs) in the roles of nurse practitioner, clinical nurse specialist, nurse anesthetist, and nurse midwife. The intent of the model is to assure safety and quality in the services provided by advanced practice nurses across the nation as well as to promote public access to APRN care and facilitate mobility among APRNs (American Association of Colleges of Nursing [AACN], 2008).

Among the model's several provisions is a mandate for independent practice by APRNs without physician oversight. Because nursing practice is regulated at the state level, however, implementation of the model will require modification of state nurse practice acts on a state-by-state basis. To that end, professional organizations have mobilized their members to educate state and territorial legislators about the model and the need for changes in nurse practice acts. The National Council of State Boards of Nursing has created a toolkit to facilitate legislative advocacy in pursuit of model implementation. The toolkit is designed to assist nurses in promoting relevant legislation in their own states and contains resources for nurse advocates (NCSBN, 2011) as well as a handbook that can be shared with legislators (NCSBN, n.d.). For further information about the toolkit, see the resources provided in the *External Resources* section of the student resources site.

As of April, 2014, the NCSBN reported that eight states had fully implemented the consensus model (NCSBN, 2014). What is being done in your state to implement the model? What can you do to promote the legislative changes needed to implement the model in your state?

Policy decisions affect every aspect of our lives, including our access to health care and the way in which health care is provided. Policy arises from a demand for action, or inaction, in relation to a particular issue. Unfortunately, policy development often excludes those most knowledgeable about the area of concern. Population health nurses need an awareness of the political context in which their practice occurs and must possess the skills and abilities to influence health policy development to achieve their goal of improving the health of the public. The need for policy development skills is one of the key nursing competencies recognized in the recent Institute of Medicine report, "The Future of Nursing: Leading Change, Advancing Health" (IOM, 2011b). Skills required to influence policy formation include social astuteness, interpersonal influence, networking ability, and sincerity (Chaffee, Mason, & Leavitt, 2012). *Social astuteness* involves the ability to understand oneself and others in the context of social situations. *Interpersonal influence* requires the ability to adapt to situations and to be a pleasant and productive person to work with. *Networking* involves the capacity to develop and bring into play diverse connections with others and to take advantage of opportunities as they present. Finally, *sincerity* demands personal integrity, authenticity, and honesty. To develop these skills, health policy content needs to be integrated into all levels of nursing education and nursing students need to develop the habit of examining the policy implications of everything they study in nursing (IOM, 2011b).

Policy and Politics

Policy is established by organizations and political units in both public and private sectors and reflects the values, beliefs, and attitudes of policy makers.

Policy was defined in Chapter 8∞ as a set of principles determining direction for action and allocation of resources to achieve identified goals.

As noted earlier, policy development takes place in both public and private sectors. **Public policies** are the ways in which public officials deal with public problems or government directives intended to influence the actions of others in areas that affect the public good (Chaffee et al., 2012), whereas private policies are enacted to deal with problems in private-sector organizations. Public policies include laws or statutes, regulations, executive orders, court rulings, and state development plans. Public policy is derived from **governance**, which is defined as the ways in which needs are articulated, power is exercised, and resources are used to meet those needs (Slokum-Bradley & Bradley, 2010). Public policies arise from several interdependent sectors beyond those directly related to health, including housing, national security, education, welfare services, and so on.

Public or private policy is created through the policy development process. Policy development was defined in Chapter 1∞. **Politics**, on the other hand, is the mechanisms by which scarce resources are allocated among members of the population (Chaffee, 2012), or the way in which conflicts arising from multiple sets of values or interests are addressed.

Relationships Between Public Policy and Health

As noted above, policy in a variety of arenas can influence the health status of the population. **Health policy** involves courses of action designed to achieve health-related goals (World Health Organization [WHO], 2014, para. 1), has a direct impact on health in the population. The overall goal of health policy is to promote the highest possible level of health in the population at a reasonable cost.

Many policies arising out of other social sectors have health implications that frequently go unrecognized until major problems arise. Awareness of this interaction between other social and economic policy initiatives and health consequences has prompted a call for health impact assessments for all major policy proposals, in much the same way that major building or development proposals trigger environmental impact assessments (EIAs) (Centers for Disease Control and Prevention [CDC], 2014). A recent Institute of Medicine report (IOM, 2011a) recommended that state and federal governments adopt a "health in all policies" approach, which would involve consideration of the potential positive and negative health effects of all policies through health impact assessments. A **health impact assessment (HIA)**, or health impact analysis is "a systematic process that uses an array of data sources and analytic methods, and considers input from stakeholders to determine the potential effects of a proposed policy, plan, program, or project on the health of a population and the distribution of those effects within the population" (National Research Council, 2011, p. 5). The intent of HIA is to assist policy makers in evaluating the potential health effects of a plan, policy, or program before it is implemented to minimize the potential for adverse health outcomes (CDC, 2014). Elements of HIA include the following:

- Screening and identification of projects and policies for which an HIA would be appropriate
- Identifying which specific potential health impacts should be examined
- Assessing the risks and benefits of the policy or project for those who will be affected
- Developing recommendations for changes to proposals to promote positive health effects and mitigate negative ones
- Reporting the results of the assessment to policy makers
- Evaluating the effects of the HIA on the policy decision (CDC, 2014).

Potential health effects of policies in other social sectors include the following examples. A study of the plan for community development in a San Francisco community was deemed to have potentially negative effects related to traffic congestion, creation of hazardous design features that might increase the incidence of injuries, and result in decreased emergency access, all of which have health implications. In addition, there were expectations of increases in noise and air pollutants during construction (San Francisco Planning Department, 2010).

A health impact assessment conducted in Columbia, Missouri, examined the probable health consequences of expanding the public transit system. Four specific health outcomes were addressed: (a) physical activity; (b) exposure to the outdoors; (c) access to health care, employment, education, and healthy food; and (d) creation of a livable, sustainable community. The assessment found that expansion of public transit would have favorable effects in all four areas (HIA Partner Team, 2012).

The focus of a health impact assessment in Saint Paul, Minnesota (Malekafzali & Bergstrom, 2011) was a proposal to construct a light rail transit line through the city's central corridor. Residents of the corridor comprised 60,000 of the lowest-income, most diverse people in the city. In addition to evaluating the potential health effects of the proposal, the HIA was intended to empower residents to make decisions that affected their health. The assessment addressed the probable effects of the proposal on 50 indicators directly and indirectly related to health (e.g., healthy and affordable housing, economic growth). The assessment identified several negative effects of the proposal, including displacement of local small businesses in the corridor, loss of jobs for residents with low educational attainment, increased gentrification and higher housing costs in the area that would displace many current low-income residents, and increased potential for unsafe pedestrian infrastructure in the area that could limit physical activity. Recommendations arising from the assessment included a city commitment to the creation of sustainable low-income housing, promoting commercial parking, and employment assistance.

A final example of a health impact assessment of economic policy revolves around the potential health effects of approving casino construction and gambling in an urban area. Some of the positive health consequences anticipated included increased employment, income, and health insurance coverage for casino employees, and increased state tax revenues that could be used for health-related initiatives. Negative consequences included sleep deprivation and increased second-hand smoke exposure for patrons and employees, increased traffic resulting in diminished air quality and driving under the influence of intoxicants, thus contributing to both motor vehicle crashes and pedestrian injuries, and increases in the transient population and gambling addictions possibly leading to increased crime. Finally, there were anticipated costs related to accident and addiction treatment, greater public safety costs (e.g., police presence), and a need for expansion of health care services to address the needs of tourists (Purtle, 2010). As we can see from these examples, numerous economic and social policies have health-related implications that need to be considered in policy development. We will consider health impact assessment in greater detail later in this chapter when we discuss the assessment of a policy situation in the context of the determinants of health in the population health nursing model.

Types of Policies

As noted earlier, health policies may be either public or private, depending on their source and focus. Policies may also be categorized as substantive or procedural. **Substantive policies** are those that dictate action to be taken. For example, a policy (in this case legislation) mandating helmet use by bicycle riders is a substantive policy, as is a policy funding health care services for the indigent. **Procedural policies** are those that determine how the action will occur. In the case of the helmet law, procedural policies would determine how the law would be implemented. In the health services funding policy, procedural policies would address who is eligible for services, how services are to be obtained, how providers will be reimbursed for services, and so on.

Policies can also be categorized as allocative or regulatory (Chaffee et al., 2012). **Allocative policies** distribute goods and services among members of the population. The Medicaid and

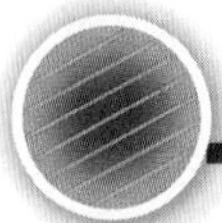

Evidence-Based Practice

Policy Development

Like all health care practice, health-related policy formation should be based on the evidence of effective interventions that is derived from sound research and consideration of the situational factors related to specific target populations. Nurses and other researchers need to make sure that policy makers are apprised of research findings that have a bearing on health-related policy development (Young, 2009). Some authors suggest an eight-step RAPID Outcome Mapping Approach (ROMA) to direct involvement of researchers in policy development. The eight steps of the approach are as follows:

1. Develop a clear policy objective to define the expected outcome of policy development.
2. Map the policy context in terms of factors influencing the policy process.
3. Identify key stakeholders in the policy area.
4. Identify desired behavior changes in stakeholders to promote support of the policy initiative.
5. Develop a strategy to promote those changes.
6. Analyze the internal capacity to make change.
7. Establish an action plan for the policy change.
8. Develop a monitoring and learning system to track progress in policy implementation (Young, 2009).

For population-based policy initiatives, the evidence base for effective intervention may come from a variety of sources. One useful source of evidence for population-based intervention strategies is the *Guide to Community Preventive Services* developed by the Community Preventive Services Task Force. The task force is an independent decision-making body, similar to the U.S. Preventive Services Task Force for individual-level interventions, convened by the U.S. Department of Health and Human Services. The task force evaluates the evidence base for population level interventions to address major public health problems and makes recommendations on the use of specific interventions, based on their effectiveness, economic efficiency, and feasibility. These recommendations can form the basis for evidence-based public health policy formation. Topics addressed in the Guide as of 2014 included adolescent health; alcohol; asthma; birth defects; cancer; diabetes; health communication; HIV/AIDS, STIs, and pregnancy; mental health; motor vehicle accidents; nutrition; obesity; oral health; physical activity; social environment; tobacco; vaccines; violence; and the worksite (Community Preventive Services Task Force, 2014). Specific guidelines will be addressed in relevant chapters later in this book.

Medicare programs are examples of allocative policies that determine who may receive care reimbursed by these funding sources. Similarly, Congressional funding decisions that promote specific research agendas over others (e.g., development of a vaccine for avian influenza) provide direction for allocation of federal research funds. When policies take goods and services away from some members of the population and give them to others, they are considered **redistributive policies**. For example, taxing the income of some citizens to fund services for others is a redistributive policy. **Regulatory policies** restrict or constrain behavior in some way. For example, nurse practice acts are regulatory policies that restrict the practice of nursing to people who meet identified criteria for licensure. Some policies are self-regulatory, as in the case of professional codes of ethics or standards for accreditation of schools of nursing.

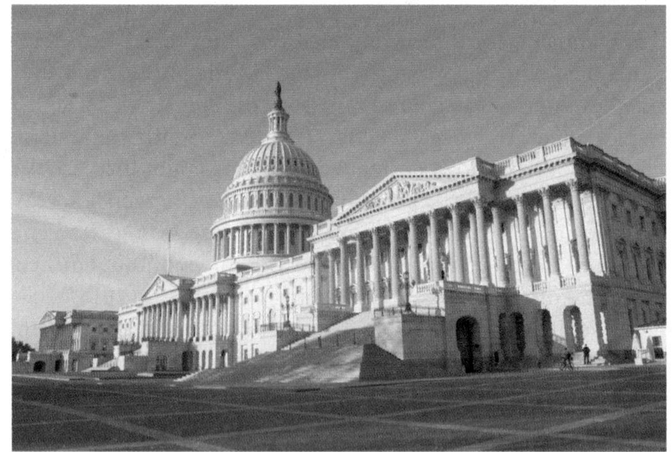

Federal legislation is only one way in which the political context influences health and health care services. *(Multitel/Shutterstock)*

Avenues for Public Policy Development

Health policy formation may take one of four major forms in the public sector: legislation and health programs created by legislation, rules and regulations for implementing legislation, administrative decisions, and judicial decisions. Development of state health plans is another avenue for health-related policy formation at the state level that may incorporate several of these approaches.

Legislation

Laws, or statutes, are public policy decisions generated by the legislative branch of government at the federal, state, or local level. Laws are created in a social system to express the collective values, interests, and beliefs of the society that generates them. Law is a mechanism for enforcing social norms within a given society. As a society develops, so do its beliefs, values, and interests. Some laws enacted in earlier periods of a society's evolution eventually become obsolete. Sometimes laws are created or revised to address new problems that surface as society changes. Modifications or changes in laws are legislative attempts to correct discrepancies that may have arisen between past and current social practices. Although this description of the function of legislation is highly simplified, the point is that laws reflect societal needs and values and are subject to revision. The 2011 IOM report, "For the Public's Health: Revitalizing Law and Policy to Meet New Challenges," noted that much of state and federal law related to public health is outdated (IOM, 2011a). The authors of the report recommended modernizing public health law to assure that "appropriate powers are in place to enable public health agencies to address contemporary challenges to population health" (p. S-3). Other recommendations made in the report include the following:

- States should enact legislation and allocate funds to assure that public health agencies have the capability of providing the essential public health services discussed in Chapter 1∞.
- States should mandate accreditation of state and local health departments to assure quality provision of services.
- The federal government should set minimum requirements for public health policy.
- Public health agencies should have access to legal counsel to prevent preemption of state and local prerogatives by higher levels of government.
- The federal government should facilitate local and state enforcement of federal and state health and safety standards, and governmental levels should share resources whenever possible.
- State and local governments should create health councils that assure stakeholder input into policy development and that conduct health impact assessments prior to and after implementation of all major legislation, regulations, and policies.
- The Department of Health and Human Services should create a group of experts to develop methods to assess evidence of the health effects of public policies and develop evidentiary standards to support translation of research findings into policy and practice (IOM, 2011a).

Figure 9-1• depicts the typical progress of a bill through the legislative process. The process is similar at federal and state levels, and the discussion here addresses both. The names of specific legislative bodies and committees will vary from one jurisdiction to another, however. A similar but more circumscribed process is used in the development of ordinances and policies by local government bodies (e.g., city council or county board of supervisors). Local communities may vary somewhat in the extent of and avenues for public input into policy decisions. The asterisks in Figure 9-1• indicate points in the state or federal process at which population health nurses might influence legislation.

Legislative proposals are statements of beliefs or interests that have been brought to the attention of a legislator. These interests may come to the legislator's attention through his or her constituents, personal experiences, or involvement on a legislative subcommittee dealing with specific issues. Population health nurses and nursing and other health-related organizations can influence the legislative process at this point by making lawmakers aware of the need to develop policy or to modify existing policies (Ridenour & Santa Anna, 2012). After due consideration, constituents' beliefs or interests are drafted in a **bill**, which is a formally worded statement of a desired legislative policy. There are two kinds of legislation: authorization and appropriation. *Authorization legislation* establishes laws or programs; *appropriation legislation*, on the other hand, provides funding for the implementation of laws and programs for the next fiscal year (American Association of Colleges of Nursing [AACN], 2010).

Once a bill has been drafted, the sponsoring legislator submits it for identification, meaning that the bill will carry the legislator's name as sponsor. It is not unusual for a proposed bill to have multiple sponsors. Many state and national nursing and other health-related organizations (e.g., AACN, the American Nurses Association [ANA] or the American Public Health Association [APHA]) maintain a legislative focus that allows them to keep members informed of pending legislation with health implications. They also typically provide their members with information on how to access drafts of legislation for review and how to contact legislators and specific committees. Membership in such organizations is an important avenue for keeping up-to-date on legislative initiatives that may affect the health of the population. For further information about the toolkits, see the resources provided in the *External Resources* section of the student resources site.

The bill is assigned a number, listed by the clerk of the appropriate legislative body, and sent to a general committee for review. The committee may revise the language of the bill or amend it. In the normal course of events, the bill would then be sent on to the House or Senate floor for its "first reading." After its first reading, the bill might be referred to the appropriate committee for hearings. Some bills are sent to multiple committees. Several congressional committees included in Table 9-1• deal with most health-related legislation at the federal level. Most of the committees presented in the table deal with authorization legislation. The House and Senate Appropriations Committees are responsible for allocating the funds for the various federal programs, and the Budget Committees develop broad budgetary directions for the legislature, respectively (Hendrickson, Ceccarelli, & Cohen, 2012). In addition to the committees listed in Table 9-1, members of the House of Representatives and Senate serve on several joint committees, the two most relevant of which are the Joint Economic Committee and the Joint Committee on Taxation (U.S. Senate, n.d.). A similar committee structure exists at the state level.

Once bills are referred to a committee, it is not unusual for them to be sent to a subcommittee, which does the most thorough review of the proposed legislation. Functions of subcommittees include hearings, markup, and reporting. Subcommittees may hold public hearings on the issue addressed by the bill.

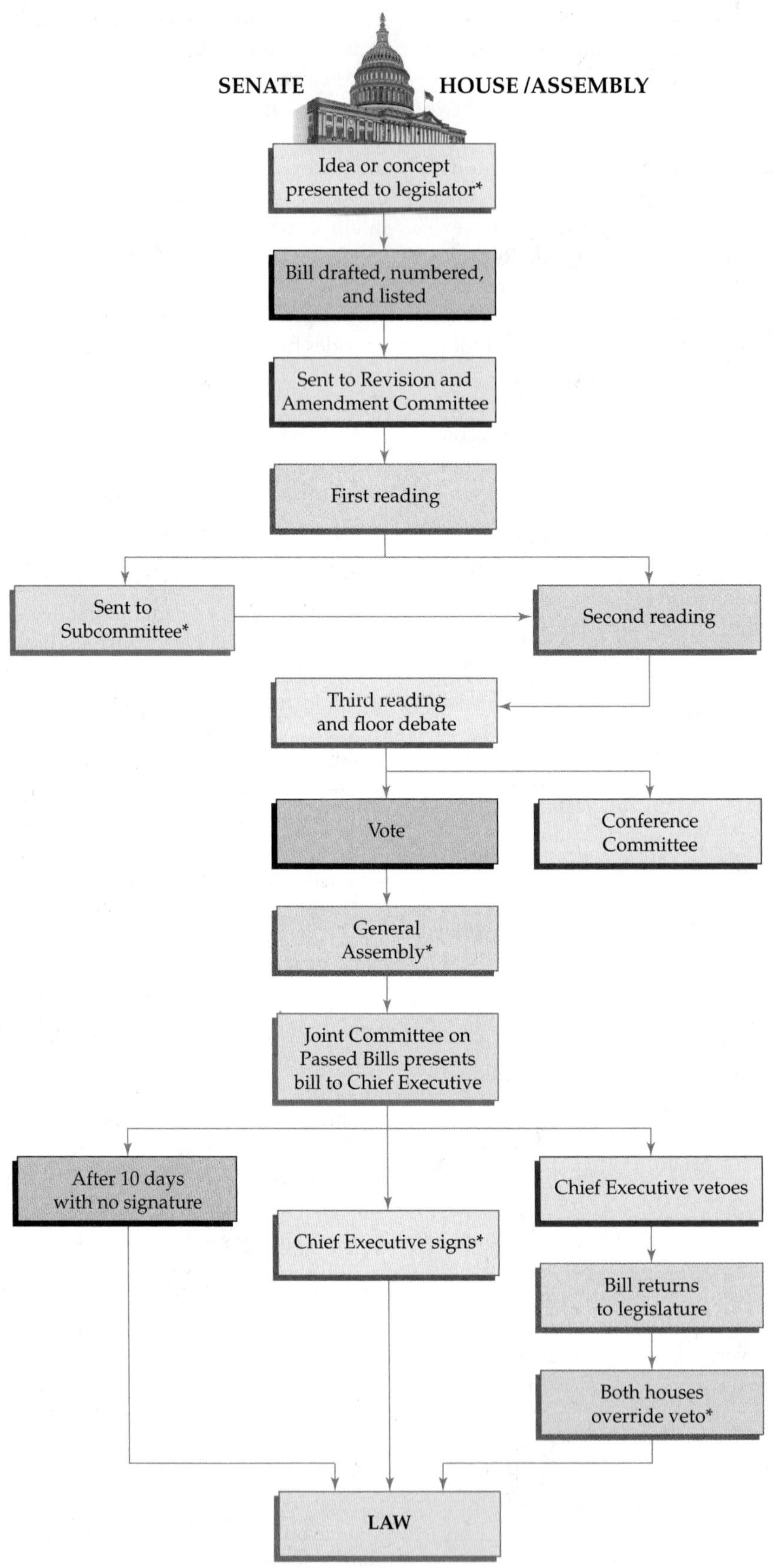

FIGURE 9-1 A Typical Legislative Process

*Points at which population health nurses can best influence the process.

TABLE 9-1 Congressional Committees with Health-Related Responsibilities

Senate Committees	Health-Related Responsibility	House of Representatives Committees	Health-Related Responsibility
Agriculture, Nutrition, and Forestry	• Food stamp program • Human nutrition • School nutrition programs	Agriculture	• Human nutrition and home economics • WIC and Food Stamps • Rural development • Bioterrorism • Animal diseases • Inspection of animal products
Appropriations	Allocation of funds	Appropriations	Allocation of funds of funds
Armed Services	• National defense issues • Military benefits	Armed Services	• Common defense • National security • Military benefits • Military research • Counter-drug programs
Banking, Housing, and Urban Affairs	• Nursing home construction • Public and private housing • Urban development and mass transit		
Budget	Annual budget planning	Budget	Budget resolutions and process
Commerce, Science, and Transportation	• Science, engineering, and technology research, development, and policy • Highway safety	Education and Workforce	• Child labor • Early childhood education • Child abuse and adoption • School food programs • Higher education and workforce training • Education and labor • Worker's compensation
Energy and Natural Resources	• Emergency preparedness • Nuclear waste • Energy development	Energy and Commerce	• Biomedical research • Health and health facilities • Public health and quarantine • Consumer protection and product safety • Motor vehicle safety
Environment and Public Works	• Air pollution and environmental policy • Solid waste disposal and recycling		
Finance	• Social Security Act health programs • Health programs financed by special tax or trust funds • National social security	Financial Services	• Public and assisted housing
Foreign Relations	• Foreign assistance • International treaties and foreign policy	Foreign Affairs	• Foreign assistance • HIV/AIDS in foreign countries • International law enforcement (including drug control)
Health, Education, Labor, and Pensions	• USDHHS • Education • Labor and employment law • Retirement plans and railroad pensions		
Homeland Security and Governmental Affairs	• Census and statistics • Government agency performance • Effects of legislation • National security • Civil Service	Homeland Security	• National security • Science and technology preparedness • Transportation security
Judiciary	• Immigration and naturalization • Civil liberties • Federal penitentiaries	Judiciary	• Federal penitentiaries
		Natural Resources	• Water and power • Indian Affairs

TABLE 9-1 (*Continued*)

Senate Committees	Health-Related Responsibility	House of Representatives Committees	Health-Related Responsibility
		Science, space and Technology	• Environmental and energy research • National Science Foundation
		Transportation and Infrastructure	• Clean water and waste water management • Flood damage reduction • Disaster preparedness and response
Veteran's Affairs	Veteran's hospitals, services	Veteran's Affairs	Veteran's hospitals, services
Indian Affairs	Indian health and special services	Ways and Means	• Customs • Tax exempt foundations • National Social Security • Social Security Act health programs and those funded by specific taxes • Health services payment • Health insurance tax credit and deductions
Special Committee on Aging	Advise on issues related to aging		

Sources: U.S. House of Representatives. (n.d.). *House committees.* Retrieved from http://www.house.gov/committees/; U.S. Senate. (n.d.). *Committees.* Retrieved from http://www.senate.gov/pagelayout/committees/d_three_sections_with_teasers/committees_home.htm

"Markup" refers to modifications made in the proposal. Finally, the subcommittee makes a report regarding the intent of the bill, any amendments made in the committee, ramifications in terms of changes to current laws, the costs of implementation, and any dissenting views on the bill (Ridenour & Santa Anna, 2012). Population health nurses can influence the legislative process during subcommittee review by contacting lawmakers and making their views known on legislation pending before them. Such contacts may be made by individual nurses or by lobbyists employed by nursing and other health-related interest groups. Lobbying is discussed in more detail later in the chapter.

Committee members considering a particular piece of legislation can either review and modify a bill or decide not to report the bill out of committee, thus effectively killing it. Legislation can also bypass assignment to a standing committee and be assigned to a specially created ad hoc committee or advance directly to a second reading on the floor of the particular legislative chamber. The bill may then proceed to a third reading, be referred back to committee, or be sent to another committee for review and revision before advancing to the third and final reading. Following the third reading, the proposed legislation is placed on the calendar for floor debate and, finally, voted on. At this point in the legislative process, population health nurses can contact their own representatives and try to persuade them to support nursing's position on a particular bill.

If the legislation is passed in the chamber of Congress or the state legislature where it originated, it is sent to the other chamber for approval. In many cases, when a bill has advanced to this point, it is passed by the second chamber without further modification. The bill can, however, be sent to another committee for review and modification. Once a bill has passed the second chamber, it is returned to the house or chamber where it originated for final approval. At the state level, a bill must be signed by the leaders of both houses of the legislature as well as the secretary of state before it is forwarded for the governor's signature. After the bill is signed by the governor, it is renumbered according to the appropriate lawbook code number and filed with the secretary of state, and becomes law. A similar process occurs at the federal level after a bill is signed by the president.

In most states and in Congress, if the two chambers of the legislature cannot agree on a similar version of a given bill, a special committee composed of members of both chambers is formed. The purpose of this *joint conference committee* is to develop a compromise bill. It is highly unusual for a joint committee recommendation not to be passed. If, however, the committee cannot reach agreement, the bill dies. Once the compromise bill has passed both houses of the legislature, it is sent to the executive branch of the government (governor or president) for final approval.

The chief executive (governor or president) can either sign the bill or hamper its progress by not signing it or vetoing it. If the chief executive does not sign the bill, it automatically becomes law after 10 days, unless the legislative session ends in the interim. In that case, the bill dies (Ridenour & Santa Anna, 2012). Holding a bill unsigned until the end of the legislative session is called a **pocket veto**. Lobbying may also be used at this point to influence the chief executive's disposition of a particular bill. If the executive vetoes a bill, it is returned to the legislature. The legislature is then required to meet a constitutionally prescribed majority vote (usually a two thirds majority) to override the veto and enact the bill into law. Any bill that does not complete the legislative process during the legislative session in which it is introduced is dead, and it must be reintroduced in a subsequent session if it is ever to become law.

Regulation

Policy decisions enacted as legislation are usually implemented by regulatory agencies charged with implementing specific types of legislation. For example, federal policies related to environmental issues are implemented by the Environmental Protection Agency (EPA); state health-related policies are usually implemented by a state board of health or a comparable agency.

These agencies develop regulations that determine how legislation will be implemented. A **regulation** is a rule or order having the force of law that deals with procedures to be followed in implementing a piece of legislation (Alliance for Health Reform, 2010). Regulations are intended to promote individual accountability for actions and to protect the public health and welfare. Regulations specify how policies are realized in actual behavior.

Regulatory agencies exert a great deal of control over health-related activities by both professionals and the general public. State agencies such as boards of nursing, for example, regulate who may practice nursing and how nursing licensure is granted. These same agencies might also be responsible for determining which health care providers can write prescriptions for medication in those states where such practices are authorized for personnel other than physicians.

When a piece of legislation authorizing an activity such as prescription writing is passed, the legislature usually designates an existing agency or creates a new agency to implement the legislation. This agency develops the regulations that govern implementation of the law. In the case of prescription-writing privileges, the regulatory agency would determine who can write prescriptions and what additional qualifications might be required of those persons. For example, in California, nurses who are certified by the state as nurse practitioners may write prescriptions, but only if they have completed an approved course in pharmacology. Other regulations specify who is eligible for certification as a nurse practitioner in the state.

Another example of regulations that implement legislation is the procedures for handling hazardous substances in the workplace, which were developed by the Occupational Safety and Health Administration (OSHA). The enabling legislation mandated protection of employees from exposure to hazardous substances, but regulations developed by OSHA specify how certain substances should be handled. For example, certain types of ventilatory equipment are required in manufacturing processes using hazardous aerosols to minimize the risk of exposure to employees.

Regulations instituted by various agencies may dramatically influence the actual impact of a law. For example, when prescription writing by nurse practitioners was first instituted in Tennessee, one proposal was to restrict the privilege to nurse practitioners prepared at the master's level. As this requirement would have excluded many nurse practitioners in rural counties where physicians were scarce, it would have undermined the intent of the enabling legislation—to provide greater access to health care for underserved populations.

Population health nurses can have input into regulations that affect their professional practice as well as into the legislation that shapes public health policy. When a regulatory agency is in the process of formulating regulations, the public is informed that the process is being initiated. Generally, the agency formulates some preliminary regulations that are published for public review and comment. At the federal level, proposed regulations are published in the *Federal Register* as a *Notice of Proposed Rulemaking (NPRM)*; similar registers exist in each state. Interested parties are then allowed to comment on the proposed regulations and suggest changes (Alliance for Health Reform, 2010).

When regulations deal with particularly sensitive areas, the regulatory body involved may hold public hearings to solicit input from interested parties. Population health nurses may either comment on proposed regulations in written communications to the regulatory agency or provide testimony at public hearings (Ridenour & Santa Anna, 2012). Nursing input should be provided early in the development process. It should also be supported by data and identify how nursing's position on proposed regulations supports the intent of the legislation. The regulatory agency may use the input to refine the regulations, but is not required to do so. Regulations are published in the appropriate state or federal publication and promulgated among individuals affected by them. Once regulations are published and go into effect, they have the force of law.

Administrative and Judicial Decisions

Health policy development can also occur by means of administrative or judicial decisions. Administrative decisions are those made by an individual or agency that affect the implementation of health care policies or programs. For example, a state board of nursing or other similar agency would develop the processes by which one becomes licensed in that state. One specific type of administrative decision is an executive order. **Executive orders** are legally binding orders that an executive officer (president or governor) gives governmental agencies and individuals on how they are to implement legislation. Executive orders do not have to be approved by the legislative branch and are occasionally used to contradict or add to the intent of legislation through interpretation. The legislature can override an executive order with more explicit legislation. Former President Clinton, used executive orders to achieve a number of health policy changes that were not originally included in legislation, such as instituting programs to promote Medicaid enrollment for eligible children. **Judicial decisions** are decisions within the court system regarding how laws are to be interpreted. As an example, a federal court ruled that the individual mandate for health insurance coverage included in the Patient Protection and Affordable Care Act violated constitutional provisions of freedom of choice and exceeded Congressional authority to regulate interstate commerce, but overturned a prior ruling that the entire Act was unconstitutional (Lowes, 2011). Subsequently, in response to further legislative challenges, the U.S. Supreme Court modified the individual mandate as a tax on most people who do not have health insurance coverage as of 2014 (National Federation of Small Business, 2012).

State Health Plans

Another avenue for health policy development that may involve legislation as well as regulation is the development of state health plans. State health plans are comprehensive policy statements that provide direction for efforts to improve the health of the state's population. They are analogous to the *Healthy People* documents, but at a state, rather than federal level. State health plans may vary in their depth and scope. The Wisconsin plan, for example, includes specific objectives in 23 focus areas to be achieved over the course of the next decade. The plan also encompasses a set of ten "pillar" objectives critical to the overall plan's success (Wisconsin Department of Health Services, 2010). These pillar objectives are presented in the *Highlights* box below.

State health plans for Vermont and California, on the other hand, are more circumscribed and deal primarily with the creation of state health care systems in a move to single-payer systems. Vermont's plan created a board to develop a payment system that incorporates the concept of the medical home and to design a health budgeting system for the state. Additional mandates include development of a single-payer plan to provide a minimum package of health care benefits established by the board, but yet to be approved by the legislature and to address the costs, revenue, and savings anticipated from the proposed reforms (State of Vermont, 2011).

California's plan, approved by the state Senate in 2010, also addresses the creation of a single-payer health plan and creates a California Health System that pools all state and federal money currently spent on health care with a to-be-determined payroll tax to provide health insurance coverage for basic health services for all state residents. Residents will have the option of purchasing additional private insurance coverage for uncovered services (*California Senate OKs single-payer health plan,* 2010).

Highlights

Pillar Objectives of the Wisconsin State Health Plan

- Develop and enforce policies and procedures for tracking health determinants for populations experiencing health disparities.
- Fund initiatives to eliminate health disparities to a level equal to the Midwest state average.
- Develop and implement policies to improve social cohesion and support by reducing racism and discrimination; creating healthy home, workplace, and community environments; and promoting diversity and social connectedness.
- Develop and implement programs that reduce poverty.
- Develop and implement educational policies that support healthy outcomes.
- Improve the system of primary care, behavioral screening and intervention, mental health services, oral health, alcohol and drug use treatment, chronic disease management, and reproductive and sexual health and enable secure and appropriate information exchange to support effective health decision making.
- Improve the health and resilience of youth and families through a variety of educational and health care services and interventions.
- Implement community designs that promote physical activity, healthy diets, and social interaction, while reducing air and water pollution and heat retention.
- Create the capacity to conduct health impact assessments related to proposed policies and to compare and disseminate information on the effectiveness of alternative population health policies and practice.
- Increase per capita public health funding at least to average levels in surrounding states.

Data from: Wisconsin Department of Health Services. (2010). *Healthiest Wisconsin 2020: Everyone living better, longer.* Retrieved from http://www.dhs.wisconsin.gov/hw2020/report2020.htm

Nursing and Policy Development

Florence Nightingale and other early population health nurses were adept at using the political process to promote the health of the population. We saw at the beginning of this chapter that Lillian Wald engaged in political activism to spur creation of the Children's Bureau. She and other early nursing leaders were alert to the political culture of the times, using that knowledge to gain important changes in societal conditions. For example, Clara Barton and Florence Nightingale minimized their active support for women's suffrage issues in order to address what they considered more critical social issues. Others, such as Margaret Sanger and Lavinia Dock, were more confrontational in their political activism, but all achieved significant social changes. These early leaders in population health nursing realized that the political process was a means of achieving their goal of improved health for all and that, because of its focus on the health of population groups population health nursing is, by definition, political in nature.

In addition to the political activities to improve the public's health and the plight of the poor, early nursing political activity focused on nursing education and its standardization and the creation of professional nursing organizations. Subsequently, however, many nurses became uncomfortable with the idea of political involvement, with the possible exception of exercising the right to vote. Politics had an unfavorable aura that was seen as incompatible with nursing's altruistic philosophy. With the advent of the women's movement in the 1960s, nurses once again began to recognize the need to influence health care policy decisions (Lewenson, 2012).

Among several reasons for nursing involvement in policy development is the level of power that nurses have in the health care arena. That power arises from several sources, the first of which is the sheer number of nurses in the country. When nurses speak with a united voice on policy issues, policy makers listen. Nurses also possess expert power by virtue of their health care expertise and legitimate power conferred by licensure as health care providers. In addition, nurses can exercise the referent power inherent in the respect and trust accorded to them by the general public. Finally, like other citizens, nurses can exercise reward power by voting for policy makers who support nursing's stance on health-related policy issues. In order to exercise their power, nurses need to understand the legislative and policy processes, know and become known to key players in policy formation, and communicate with policy makers. A *Political Astuteness Inventory* is included in the *Assessment Guidelines* section of the student resources for this book. The inventory can be used to assess the political activity and savvy of nurses.

Spheres of Nursing Influence in Policy Development

Political writers in nursing have identified four spheres in which nurses influence policy development (Chaffee et al., 2012). The first sphere of influence is the community sphere, in which nurses influence health-related policy through community activism. In this sphere, the nurse may become involved in civic organizations, planning boards, or other agencies and groups that develop policy that affects health directly or indirectly. The second sphere is in the workplace, where policies influence both health care delivery (e.g., policies related to fees for basic preventive services such as immunizations) and health determinants (e.g., policies banning smoking in the workplace). The third sphere is the governmental policy arena, in which nurses advocate for public policies that support health. Note that public policies often "bleed" into the private sector. For example, recent Medicare policies regarding reimbursement for "never events" (preventable adverse health outcomes) influence care for all clients in an institution, not just those whose care is paid for by Medicare. The final sphere of nursing influence in policy making is within professional organizations. Policy making in this sphere influences the regulation and education of the profession itself and provides impetus for public policy formation in the government sphere.

Principles of Policy Development

Effective policy making is based on several core principles. These principles include the following:

- Effective policy making is designed to achieve clearly defined future-oriented outcomes.
- The policy-making process considers a wide array of factors influencing the policy situation.
- The policy-making process is flexible and innovative, seeking creative solutions to identified problems.
- Effective policy making is evidence-based, and the best available evidence is accessible to key stakeholders.
- The policy-making process is inclusive, and considers the needs of all those directly or indirectly affected by the policy.
- Effective policy making takes a holistic view, examining the potential effects on multiple segments of society.
- Effective policy making takes account of lessons learned from previous policy initiatives.
- Effective policy making considers how policy will be communicated to the public and other stakeholders.
- Effective policy making incorporates processes for evaluating the effects of the policy.
- Existing policies are reviewed for their adequacy in addressing the problems they were designed to address (Office of the First Minister and Deputy First Minister, n.d.).

The Policy Development Process

Population health nurses can influence health-related policies at all levels. To do so, however, they must be conversant with the political process and its use. The ability of population health nurses to influence policy development is affected by their skill in assessing the policy situation, agenda setting, planning and implementing health care policy, and evaluating the effects of health policy development and the resulting health policies.

The policy development process is a series of steps analogous to the nursing process and begins with identification of a problem that can be resolved through policy formation. This entails an assessment of the nature of the problem, who is affected, and the factors contributing to the problem. The second step in the process is getting the policy issue on the agenda of policy makers, followed by development of a policy option designed to address the problem and based on scientific data and consideration of other relevant factors, such as public opinion, economic factors, and so on. Implementation of the policy usually requires involvement of interest groups and stakeholders. **Stakeholders** are persons interested in or affected by a specific issue, policy, or program. Following implementation of the policy, perhaps on a trial basis, its outcomes, costs, benefits, risks, and progress toward problem resolution are evaluated and modified as needed (Berkowitz, 2012). We will discuss each of these steps in policy development in more detail in the application of the population health nursing model to the policy context later in this chapter. Elements of the policy development process are summarized in the *Highlights* box below.

Highlights

The Policy Development Process

- Problem identification and assessment
- Agenda setting
- Formulation of proposed policy to address the problem
- Involvement of interest groups and stakeholders
- Policy implementation
- Evaluation of effects, benefits, costs, risks, and progress toward problem resolution
- Policy modification, as needed

Population Health Nursing Roles and Policy Development

Population health nurses may engage in one or more of four roles in their efforts to influence policy development in areas that affect health. These roles include those of citizen, activist, politician, and researcher. In their role as citizens, nurses engage in traditional political activities such as staying informed; voting; speaking out on local issues; participating in public forums; becoming acquainted with local, state, and federal officials; and participating in politically active nursing organizations. In the activist role, nurses contact public officials, register others to vote, contribute to and work for political campaigns, and engage in other activities to educate and influence policy makers. In their role as politicians, some nurses become policy makers themselves through elected or appointed office. In the researcher role, population health nurses may conduct research to create the foundation of evidence on which effective health policy should be based. Beyond conducting the actual research studies, however, nurse researchers need to make a concerted effort to acquaint policy makers with research findings and assist them to incorporate research evidence, with other considerations (e.g., economic implications, societal values, and so on), into policy decisions (Young, 2009). The IOM (2011b) "Future of Nursing" report notes in particular, that doctorally prepared nurses need to link their research to policy formation and develop skills in policy development as part of their doctoral education. Nursing activities in each of the four roles for policy involvement are summarized in Table 9-2●. Actions related to the citizen, activist, and politician roles will be discussed in more detail in the section on strategies for implementing policy.

Applying the Population Health Nursing Model to Policy Development

The elements of the population health nursing model can assist population health nurses to assess the context surrounding a policy issue and in formulating, implementing, and evaluating health-related policy. In the remainder of this chapter, we will explore the application of the model to policy development in general and then examine the Affordable Care Act as a critical example of health policy affecting the population's health.

ASSESSING THE POLICY SITUATION. Assessment of a policy situation involves two basic aspects: assessing the need for policy formulation and assessing factors that are influencing the policy situation and resolution of the underlying problem. Some health-related problems or issues cannot be resolved through policy formation, and population health nurses need to be able to identify those problems that are amenable to resolution through policy. For example, the incidence of traumatic brain injury in motorcycle riders might be reduced

TABLE 9-2 Population Health Nursing Roles and Activities in Policy Development

Role	Related Nursing Activities
Citizen	• Voting • Staying informed • Speaking out on policy issues • Participating in public forums • Becoming acquainted with elected officials • Joining politically active professional nursing organizations
Activist	• Contacting public officials • Registering members of the public to vote • Contributing to political campaigns • Working for political campaigns • Lobbying decision makers with relevant data • Forming or joining relevant coalitions • Writing letters to the editor • Inviting legislators to the workplace • Organizing media events to publicize issues • Providing testimony on health-related issues • Locating and soliciting grant funding
Politician	• Running for public office • Seeking appointment to a regulatory body • Seeking appointment to a governing board of a public or private entity • Using nursing experience as a frontline policy maker
Researcher	• Identifying health policy issues through research • Ensuring the inclusiveness of viewpoints in policy formation • Assuring the quality, integrity, and objectivity of data on which policy decisions are based • Recognizing and communicating uncertainty and risk (e.g., acknowledging when research evidence is equivocal) • Assuring transparency and openness regarding the bases for policy decisions • Reviewing policy decisions to assure that they reflect up-to-date knowledge

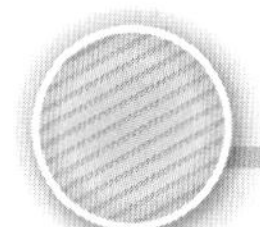

Global Perspectives

Developing a National Population Health Nurse Practitioner Program in Korea

Cho and Kashka (2004) described the political efforts of Mo Im Kim to establish a national population health nurse practitioner program in Korea. The intent of the program was to combine the skills of population health nurses with those of nurse practitioners to meet the health care needs of rural Koreans. Dr. Kim began by instituting a 6-month population health nurse practitioner program at Yon Sei University. The program addressed health policy formation, implementation and evaluation of community health programs, program management, and community development strategies as well as skills in physical assessment, prevention and detection of disease, and disease management. Dr. Kim and her associates made use of a number of political opportunities, including a government coup, to promote the concept of the CHNP to meet population health needs. Some of her strategies included capitalizing on the reform goals of the new regime, informing officials of the work of the CHNPs and inviting them to nursing seminars where firsthand stories of practice were shared, lobbying legislators and government officials, and publishing a collection of CHNP cases. Dr. Kim herself also held a congressional office. Dr. Kim used research data regarding the public popularity of the CHNP program to sway legislators and defuse resistance from vested interests such as physicians and obtained external assistance from the Asian Foundation and WHO. She also engaged in specific initiatives to educate government officials, such as arranging for the chair of the Congressional Health Policy Committee to visit the United States and observe population health nursing roles.

1. How might Dr. Kim's political strategies be adapted for use in another country or culture?
2. Would Dr. Kim's strategies be likely to be successful in the United States? Why or why not?

by legislation mandating helmet use or development of motorcycle lanes on major highways. Other issues, such as food or housing costs, are not as amenable to policy intervention. Determining a need for policy, even when policy might help resolve a problem, is also dependent on the extent and severity of a problem. Policy makers will not be interested in problems or issues that affect only a limited number of people or that have minimal consequences. For example, legislatures would be unlikely to legislate mandatory school absence for cases of the common cold, but do mandate school absence for serious conditions that are highly communicable, such as measles or chickenpox.

The second aspect of assessing the policy situation involves examination of the factors that affect the policy issue and its resolution (Leavitt, Mason, & Whelan, 2012). Such an assessment can occur in the context of the determinants of health component of the population health nursing model as described below.

Biological determinants. An assessment of biophysical factors influencing a policy situation would include a determination of who is affected by the health problem. For example, what age groups are most often affected by accidental injuries? What age-related factors contribute to the problem? For example, diminished strength, mobility, and sensory acuity are factors that lead to injury in the elderly. Are there gender differences in injury incidence? Does the existence of other health conditions, such as epilepsy or arthritis, contribute to injury? In this example, it is unlikely that factors related to genetic inheritance will affect injury incidence, but would be an influencing factor in problems related to diabetes mellitus or cardiovascular disease.

Psychological determinants. The population health nurse exploring factors that contribute to a particular health problem would also examine the contribution of psychological determinants. Do depression or anger contribute to accidental injury? Risk taking and perceptions of invulnerability common among adolescents are certainly contributors to accidental injury in this age group.

Environmental determinants. A variety of environmental elements are widely known to contribute to accidental injuries, from safety hazards in the home to driving conditions. The population health nurse would examine the effect of specific environmental conditions on injury incidence in the population affected by a proposed policy. Data in this area and that related to other categories of determinants might come from published research, epidemiologic studies, or personal observations by the nurse and other health care providers and interested parties.

Sociocultural determinants. A variety of sociocultural determinants influence policy situations. These may include the economic effects of the problem or issue or economic considerations in its resolution. For example, policy makers may favor a particular policy option that is less costly than other approaches to problem resolution. Educational, cultural, and legal factors may also influence policy development. For instance, educational levels among the population to be affected by the proposed policy may help or hinder its implementation or be part of the problem the policy is designed to address. Similarly, a proposed policy that conflicts with existing legislation may pose difficulties. Two other important sociocultural determinants that influence policy development are the values and ethical considerations operating in the situation and the influence of persons or groups with vested interests in the issue.

Values and ethical considerations. Conflicts among values are often noted in policy situations. For example, legislation designed to promote motorcycle or bicycle helmet use is often resisted on grounds that such mandates violate the strongly held U.S. value for individual liberty. For example, the slogan on the helmet issues page of an online bikers' rights organization is "let those who ride decide" (Bikersrights.com, 2013). At the same time, the values of protecting the health of individual riders and protecting both individuals and society from catastrophic economic burdens are also at play. In this instance, policy makers have to make a determination of which values should receive higher priority. Similarly, federal child labor laws prohibiting child labor under a certain age do not apply to children of any age working on their family-owned farms, presumably on the basis of the value that children should help with chores at home and that parents, not government, should control their behavior (OSHA, n.d.).

Another example of the influence of values and ethics in policy development lies in the issue of "sin taxes." **Sin taxes** are taxes levied on products that are deemed harmful to health, such as tobacco and alcohol (Green, 2010). The argument for sin taxes is that people who engage in unhealthful behavior (e.g., smoking) are choosing to jeopardize their health, and they, rather than society, should be responsible for the consequences. In initiating sin taxes, governments are usually responding to two values: improvement of the public's health by deterring unhealthy behavior and generation of revenue that can be used to offset the societal costs of such behaviors. For example, a $0.50 per pack tax on cigarettes in California has resulted in more than $4 billion in revenue designated for child health and education programs. Similarly, a 3% tax on beer sales in Arkansas generates more than $14 million per year used for preschool programming. The public perspective on sin taxes is usually split between approval of the revenues generated and complaints of discrimination by those who pay the additional taxes, and powerful lobbies are active on both sides. Again the conflicting values are societal good and individual autonomy and responsibility (Green, 2010).

Vested interests. An **interest group** is a group of people and/or organizations that have a common interest in the outcome of a specific policy initiative (Warner, 2012). Using our injury example, motorcycle groups that campaign against helmet laws are one example of interest groups and their influence on health care policy. On the other hand, emergency health care providers might be an interest group that would support helmet laws.

Tobacco industry organizations are possibly the classic example of interest groups that actively campaign against initiatives designed to prevent smoking and protect individual and public health. The tobacco industry has consistently campaigned against legislation designed to prohibit smoking. For example, industry claims of up to 20% decline in revenue and loss of patronage for bars that initiate smoking bans were used to argue against smoke-free bars. Research indicates, however, that there has been no decrease in alcohol sales revenue in such establishments following institution of smoking bans (Loomis, Shafer, & van Hasselt, 2013).

Similarly, the RJ Reynolds company capitalized on the exclusion of cigars from restrictions on cigarette advertising, but creating cigarettes marketed as "little cigars" with lower tax rates. Flavored little cigars are specifically targeted for a youth market. In 2012, 16.7% of high school boys smoked cigars, and a third of them smoked little cigars (CDC, 2013). In addition, tobacco manufacturers are now employing "front organizations" to present messages that do not appear to support the industry's self-interest but support their policy positions. A front group is a an organization that portrays itself as representing one agenda (e.g., responsible alcohol use) when it actually serves the interests of another group (e.g., alcohol distillers) that remains in the background (*Front groups, 2013*). Front groups frequently claim to represent the voice of the people. A "citizens for free choice" group might be such a front organization.

A recent U.S. Supreme Court ruling permits corporations to make unlimited contributions to election advocacy campaigns, permitting them to influence voters in favor of candidates that support their policy positions (Wiist, 2011). Due to the relative funding available to large corporations and public health interest groups, such contributions can undermine public health policy advocacy. Population health nurses working in the policy arena need to identify special interest groups and work to form coalitions with those that support nursing's policy positions and to counteract the efforts of those working against those positions.

Behavioral determinants. Behavioral determinants may also influence policy situations. Behavioral determinants, such as consumption behaviors, for example, may contribute to the problem to be addressed by a proposed policy. For instance, increased alcohol and drug use is a significant contributor to accidental injuries of all types, and policies may be advanced to attempt to control or minimize use as a means of reducing the incidence of injuries. Similarly, dietary behaviors and sedentary lifestyles contribute to the problems of obesity and consequent chronic disease. In this instance, policies to promote physical activity opportunities in communities may help to address obesity risk and other consequences. Health-related behaviors may also be the focus of policy formation. For example, economic policy and health insurance coverage may influence access to and use of screening services such as mammography.

Health system determinants. Finally, factors related to the health care system may influence both the need for and direction of policy formation. For example, the nursing shortage, in part the result of lack of qualified faculty to educate nurses led to the development of educational funding programs for nursing faculty. Similarly, the dearth of primary care physicians has contributed to expansion of the scope of practice of APRNs, in particular, nurse practitioners. Such shortages have also influenced changes in some nurse practice acts to permit APRNs to function without physician oversight and were part of the impetus for the development of the APRN Regulatory Model discussed earlier in this chapter. Other health system determinants, such as reimbursement mechanisms, availability of certain types of care, and access to care issues, also create a need for policy development or revision and influence the direction of policy initiatives.

AGENDA SETTING. The next step in policy development is setting the policy agenda. A **policy agenda** is the list of priority issues that become the focus for action by policy makers. Agenda setting is a process of getting a particular problem or policy issue incorporated in the agenda of issues to be addressed by policy makers (The Policy Circle, n.d.).

Priority among specific policy goals is promoted when there is widespread perception that the current status of a problem or issue is unacceptable, there is a high degree of cohesion among groups supporting the policy issue, and national political leaders champion the issue. Other conditions that bring issues to the forefront of a policy agenda include the use of credible evidence to educate policy makers, development of clear and feasible policy alternatives that are likely to address the issue, and the use of national events to promote public awareness of the issue. When a particular issue is given priority on the policy agenda, policy makers exhibit concern for the issue, government enacts policies to address it, and funding is allocated to support the policies enacted.

For a particular issue to become a focus for action, policy makers often need to be made aware of the issue through issue analysis. Population health nurses may engage in issue analysis resulting in a formal policy issue paper. The elements of a policy analysis are included in Table 9-3•. Some of the elements of policy analysis have been addressed in the discussion of the determinants of health affecting the policy situation presented above. Tips for assessing a policy situation are included in the *Focused Assessment* on the next page.

Effective policy analysis requires collection, interpretation, and use of data, which may be of two types: primary data and secondary data. *Primary data* is information that the nurse or affiliated groups collect. *Secondary data* is information from existing data sources. In an issue such as teenage pregnancy, adolescent pregnancy statistics collected by the local health department would be secondary data, whereas findings of a survey on why teens are sexually active collected by a teen pregnancy coalition would be primary data. Data have a variety of uses beyond validating a problem. For example, data can be used to convince others of the need for action, as a basis for developing policy goals and objectives, and to mark progress toward problem resolution.

PLANNING HEALTH CARE POLICY. Planning health care policy involves a number of activities in which population health nurses can be involved. These activities include developing and evaluating alternative policy solutions for identified problems, delineating the policy, and planning strategies to garner support for the selected alternative.

Evaluating policy alternatives. There may be multiple policy alternatives to resolving a particular health problem, and policy makers must evaluate potential alternatives in terms of what is feasible given the constraints operating in the situation (Leavitt et al., 2012). The first step in evaluating alternatives is determining the criteria that will be used for evaluation. Some of the criteria that may be used include the relative cost of one alternative over another, the ease of implementing a particular alternative, the acceptability of the policy to those who will be affected, and so on. One particular area that should always be considered is the

TABLE 9-3 Elements of an Issue Analysis

Element	Explanation
Problem identification and analysis	Description of the problem or issue, including information regarding causes and effects Description of factors affecting the problem (could be organized in terms of the determinants of health); a description of past history of attempts at problem resolution
Background	Description of the history of the issue and prior attempts at problem resolution
Political setting	Identification of the entities with jurisdiction over the problem
Stakeholders	Description of parties with an interest in the outcome of the issue (e.g., those affected by the problem, implementers of possible solutions, special interest groups, specific policy makers with an interest in the area)
Values assessment	Identification of underlying values shaping stakeholders' perspectives
Power analysis	Determination of power bases of stakeholders (both supporters and resisters of problem resolution)
Resources	Identification of the resources (financial and human) needed to address the issue
Alternatives	Potential solutions to the problem
Evaluation criteria	Development of criteria for judging the appropriateness of alternative solutions in light of desired outcomes; typical criteria might include cost, equity, quality, feasibility, and resource needs
Alternative analysis and scoring	Analysis of the extent to which any given alternative meets established criteria for evaluation; may employ a scoring mechanism that ranks each alternative based on weighted criteria
Policy recommendation	Recommendation to select one or more alternatives based on the analysis

Data from: Leavitt, J. K., Mason, D. J., & Whelan, M.E. (2012). Political analysis and strategies. In D. J. Mason, J. K. Leavitt, & M. W. Chaffee (Eds.), *Policy and politics in nursing and health care* (6th ed., pp. 65–76). St. Louis, MO: Saunders.

FOCUSED ASSESSMENT Assessing the Policy Situation

Effective participation in policy formation requires the ability to assess the policy situation and determine factors that are operating in the situation. Here are some considerations that should guide policy assessment.

- What is the health problem or issue to be addressed? Why has the need for policy development or change arisen? What are the data related to the problem or issue?
  - What biophysical, psychological, environmental, sociocultural, behavioral, and health system factors are contributing to the problem to be addressed by the proposed policy?
  - What biophysical, psychological, environmental, sociocultural, behavioral, and health system factors will influence the policy direction?
- What is the appropriate policy arena? Where does jurisdiction lie?
- What is the goal or desired outcome of policy development?
- What are the potential alternative strategies for the problem? What are the advantages and disadvantages of each alternative? Which alternative(s) is most likely to achieve the goal or desired outcome?
- Are there strongly held values that will be supported or threatened by the proposed policy?
- Who will be affected by the policy? Who will support the policy? Who might oppose it? Why? What influence does the opposition wield? What is the power base of supporters of the proposed policy?
- Who should be involved in policy development? Implementation?
- Does the proposed policy adequately address the issue?
- Does the policy safeguard individual rights as much as possible?
- Are proposed implementation strategies fair and equitable?
- How easy or difficult will it be to implement the proposed policy?
- What will be the cost of policy implementation? What resources will be needed? How will these resources be obtained?

political feasibility of the policy alternative. Political feasibility reflects the anticipated ease or difficulty of getting the proposed policy accepted by policy makers. Three sets of factors influence the political feasibility of a particular policy issue: issue-related factors, process factors, and institutional factors.

Issue-related factors include the comprehensiveness, complexity, and costliness of the proposed policy. Comprehensive policies that lead to massive change and those that are complex in their implementation are more difficult to achieve than those that result in modest or incremental change and are simple to implement. Similarly, less costly alternatives usually receive greater support from policy makers than more costly ones. For example, moving to a national health system in the United States would be a sweeping change in the health care delivery system and would be extremely complex in its implementation. Incremental policies that cover smaller subpopulations (e.g., Medicare for the elderly) have historically been easier to enact.

Process factors relate to the situational context rather than the policy itself. Examples of process factors include the importance of the issue to the general public and to policy makers and the timing of the proposal in relation to other issues and factors, such as an election year or major focus on other events and issues (e.g., national security). Institutional factors reflect the political context and include such things as a landslide political victory or control of both houses of government by a single party.

Delineating the policy. Once policy alternatives have been evaluated, an appropriate alternative or group of alternatives is selected and the policy itself is developed in detail. The program or plan should be made as clear and simple as possible. One of the reasons for the failure of the Health Security Act, proposed by former President Clinton, was its complexity and the inability of the general public, as well as legislators, to understand it. Many of these issues were more successfully addressed in the Patient Protection and Affordable Care Act, which is discussed in more detail later in this chapter.

An important consideration in outlining the details of the selected policy option is the identification of needed resources and their potential availability. What will be required to implement the planned policy? Is there a need for specially trained personnel? For equipment? Where will these resources be obtained, and how will they be financed? Where will funding for policy implementation be derived?

POLICY IMPLEMENTATION STRATEGIES. When the proposed policy has been outlined, strategies are developed to promote its adoption by policy makers. These may include developing a message, forming coalitions, mobilizing grassroots constituencies, and developing a specific action plan. The action plan should include long- and short-term goals, activity timeframes and areas of responsibility, strategies for developing community support, and identified target audiences and agents of change.

The message or issue should be framed in terms that are meaningful to stakeholders and target audiences (Leavitt, Mason, & Whelan, 2012). Different messages may be needed depending on the target. For example, messages designed for the general public might be different from those designed to enlist support from health professional organizations. Other specific strategies to promote adoption of a proposed policy by policy makers are discussed below.

Population health nurses alone cannot assure the development and implementation of effective health care policies. Although they may be actively involved in policy development, achieving policy approval and implementation usually requires broad-based support in many segments of society. Nurse policy makers can use a variety of strategies to create support for desired policy options. These include keeping informed of policy issues, communicating with policy makers, networking, coalition building, reciprocal action, creating media support, community organizing, lobbying, and providing testimony.

Staying informed and communicating with policy makers. Unlike the rest of the strategies for creating support for policy adoption, staying informed and communicating with policy makers are ongoing strategies that are not confined to a specific issue or policy. Population health nurses need to stay current on issues and problems related to health at local, state, national, and international levels. This can be accomplished through involvement in nursing and other health-related organizations and by keeping up with literature in public and professional domains (e.g., local news media and journal literature). For population health nurses, APHA is the single most effective advocacy group for public health policy in the United States and is also influential in international policy development. National and state nursing organizations (e.g., ANA and its state affiliates and nursing specialty organizations) also advocate for some health issues, but do not address population health issues with the breadth of APHA. As we saw in Chapter 8∞, the International Council of Nurses, composed of national nursing organizations, exerts a great deal of influence on international health policy, as do other international organizations.

To be seen as credible resources regarding specific issues, population health nurses need to become acquainted with policy makers at multiple levels. To do so, they should engage in regular contact with legislators and other policy makers, promote their visibility as issue experts, and provide clear, consistent messages. Population health nurses should develop strategies and tactics for becoming known to policy makers. *Strategies* are general approaches to be taken; *tactics* are the implementation details of a particular strategy. Population health nurses may communicate with legislators through letters supporting a particular position or by presenting data related to issues of interest to legislators or nurses. For example, a population health nurse may routinely send new information regarding a particular topic to legislators who are supporting (or not supporting) a related piece of legislation. Similarly, nurses may make periodic visits to legislators who represent their state or district. On the local level, nurses may invite policy makers or members of their staffs to important community meetings or extend an invitation to participate in regular meetings of community-based organizations.

When attempting to influence policy makers, the APHA (2011) recommends meeting them where they are and acknowledging the constraints under which they operate. Whenever possible, nurses and others working for health policy changes should link health policy to major issues of interest to legislators and other policy makers. In addition, they should present issues clearly, in terms that policy makers can understand, and address economic considerations as appropriate.

When communication relates to a particular issue, nurses or allied groups should create a clear public image and articulate key messages that are consistent and targeted to the intended audiences. Audiences may include the general public as well as legislators and other policy makers. Communication necessitates identifying the most appropriate means of reaching specific audiences. For example, members of an ethnic cultural group may be approached by means of ethnic radio and television stations or newspapers, whereas e-mail messages and telephone calls may be more appropriate for communicating with policy makers.

Networking, coalition building, and reciprocal action. Another group of related strategies for creating support for health policy initiatives includes networking, coalition building, and reciprocal action. **Networking** is a process of coming to know and becoming known to others with similar interests. Population health nurses can engage in networking by joining groups dedicated to addressing specific health-related issues or becoming involved in organizations that have a broader health focus. These groups or organizations may be local, regional, national, or international in their focus. At the local level, for example, a population health nurse might become a member of a community collaborative that addresses all kinds of community issues, including those that affect health. Or the nurse may become involved in the state nurses association or APHA. Nurses can also network by attending conferences related to specific areas of interest or by contacting authors who write about these areas.

Coalitions are alliances of individuals or groups who unite to address a common interest. Coalitions have several advantages in promoting adoption of a desired policy alternative including the ability to pool resources and to achieve more extensive results than individuals or single agencies operating alone. Membership in coalitions may also lead to involvement in broader issues or similar issues at broader levels. Coalitions can make efficient use of resources and prevent duplication of effort. In addition, coalitions promote communication, cooperation, and idea generation and build a broader, more stable constituency than a single organization might have. Finally, all of these characteristics of coalitions build to a final advantage, greater political clout than independent action (Rice Bowers-Lanier, 2012). It is critically important that coalitions include partnerships with groups of community residents as well as other groups and organizations working in the community.

In addition to their many advantages in supporting adoption of specific policy proposals, coalitions do have a few disadvantages. There is a need for staff time to carry out the work of the coalition that may draw staff of member agencies away from their usual responsibilities. There is also work needed to maintain the interactions of the coalition as well as to address the policy issue. For example, efforts must be undertaken to communicate among members. Another disadvantage is the increased time needed for group decisions and the potential for a weakened stance on an issue necessitated by the need to compromise to gain agreement among members. Finally, credit for the success of coalition endeavors must be shared among all members, which may make it more difficult for individual agencies to showcase their achievements to funders and other interested parties. Additional challenges posed by coalitions include getting the right participants, areas of distrust among members, and the need to protect one's own "turf" or agenda. One final difficulty is the potential for conflict among members posed by different perspectives on directions that should be taken to address policy issues or the strategies that should be employed to promote them (Rice Bowers-Lanier, 2012).

Usually a few salient issues must be addressed for effective coalition formation. Three of these issues are coalition leadership, structure, and funding. Generally, two types of leadership are required for effective coalitions—motivational leadership and organizational leadership—and it is unusual for one person to embody both. The motivational leader has a bold vision and can motivate others to pursue that vision. The organizational leader deals with the day-to-day operation of the coalition. Issues related to coalition structure deal with governance and decision making. How should decisions be made, and by whom? Finally, there is the issue of funding. Some coalitions acquire operating funds from dues paid by members, but many have to seek outside funding through grants and other sources. The need to actively seek funds adds to the work of the coalition (Rice Bowers-Lanier, 2012).

Coalition formation occurs in a series of steps, the first of which is determining whether or not a coalition is an appropriate approach to a given policy issue. If so, the next task is determining who should be invited to participate. Once participation has been solicited, the group must develop consensus on the goals to be achieved and the strategies used to achieve them. The coalition then engages in activities designed to achieve the designated goals and evaluates goal accomplishment. Throughout this process, the coalition must engage in activities that maintain its forward momentum.

Networking and coalition building may necessitate reciprocal action. This usually involves providing support for the issues and projects of interest to other members of the network or coalition in return for their support on issues of interest to nursing. For example, nurses may agree to support bond issues to expand police and fire services in return for the support of these groups in issues related to housing code violations.

Creating media support. Much of the information regarding policy issues received by the general public is transmitted by the media. To create public support for a policy initiative, population health nurses must carefully select and orchestrate media coverage.

Nurses need to help assure that policy debate is framed in the interests of the public's health while accounting for contextual factors that influence the policy situation. For example, a policy should not be perceived to unduly advantage one segment of the population to the disadvantage of others. Policy makers should seek out media that are favorable to the particular issue, and media messages should be targeted to specific audiences to create support for a given policy initiative. The burgeoning social media movement is an excellent way to educate the public about health-related issues (Daniels, Glickstein, & Mason, 2012). Media messages should be designed not only to inform the public, but also to encourage them to mobilize to support the initiative. Public support is only effective when it is visible to policy makers through organized efforts such as contacting legislators, and so on.

Community organizing. Another way population health nurses create support for policy directions is community organizing. **Community organizing** is the process of mobilizing community resources in support of planned change within the community. It is a systematic process of assessment, analysis, and planning, conducted within the context of the political process. Aspects of community organizing include locality development, social planning, and social action. Locality development involves promoting the ability of community members to help themselves. Training community members for leadership roles and promoting their ability to interact with policy makers would be examples of locality development. Social planning involves collecting problem-related data, goal setting, and planning policies that address community problems that later inform social action. Social action involves efforts to increase the power and resources available to members of the community to enable them to address problems and create change (Work Group for Community Development and Change, 2013). Population health nurses can be actively involved and provide a leadership role in data collection activities.

Lobbying and advocacy. Lobbying and advocacy are additional means for promoting adoption of a particular policy alternative. In the political context, these terms have different legal definitions. **Lobbying** refers to attempts to influence policy makers to take a particular action with respect to a specific piece of legislation. Lobbyists may be volunteers, but are often paid representatives of organizations, agencies, or businesses. **Political advocacy**, on the other hand, involves communicating with policy makers regarding an issue without requesting specific action. The U.S. federal government makes important distinctions between lobbying and advocacy. If a person spends more than 20% of his or her time in lobbying efforts, he or she must register as a lobbyist with Congress, report on the focus of lobbying efforts, and report funding contributions above a certain fixed limit. Advocacy activities, on the other hand, are not regulated and are often performed by ordinary citizens (Whelan & Woody, 2012).

Government agencies may or may not be permitted to engage in lobbying activities, but lobbying may be restricted to specific individuals within the organization. The federal Hatch Act specifically prohibits government employees of agencies receiving federal monetary support from engaging in any partisan political activity (Malone & Chaffee, 2012).

Presenting testimony. Policy makers sometimes hold public hearings or meetings to gather background information on an issue before attempting to draft legislative proposals or regulations. On occasion, such meetings are held by legislative subcommittees to explore the potential impact of a proposed piece of legislation. Writing and presenting testimony in a public hearing is another way population health nurses can influence policy makers.

Testimony presented by population health nurses should specifically address the issue in question and be brief, factual, and well documented. Legislative representatives are not usually health care providers, so testimony should avoid medical jargon and be clearly understandable. A copy of the testimony should be given to the legislative representatives and staff either immediately preceding or at the time of the hearing. Documentation of sources of data permits later verification by legislators or their staff members. Population health nurses should also be conversant with the format for hearings and the rules governing presentation of testimony. In addition, it is helpful to identify potential questions that might be asked by policy makers in order to be prepared to answer as fully as possible. If the answer to a question is not known, offer to get the relevant information (Whelan & Woody, 2012). On no account, however, should data be invented.

Population health nurses can also influence policy development and implementation through more traditional political activities. These activities influence the selection of policy makers and issues to be addressed and include voting, campaigning, obtaining political appointments, and holding office.

Voting. Voting is perhaps the easiest means of influencing health care policy formation at governmental levels. Nurses can themselves vote and motivate others to vote to support policy directions that enhance public health. One vote alone may not seem important, but it may be a key factor in determining the outcome on an important issue. Because lawmakers in the United States are elected, they are susceptible to the power their constituents hold through the ballot box. Thus, voting is a vital component of the political process in which all nurses can participate.

In addition to voting, nurses can educate others regarding the need to vote. Legislative networks among nurses are intended to keep members informed of health-related issues and the need for support or lack of support for certain policy directions. Nurses can also educate the general public on legislative issues that come up for public vote. Finally, nurses can participate in voter registration programs that motivate the general public to exercise their constitutional right to influence policy formation.

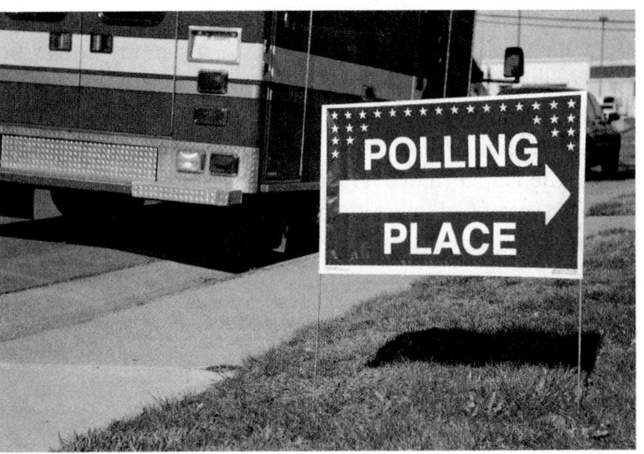

Voting is a common way to affect change. *(Karin Hildebrand Lau/ Shutterstock)*

Campaigning. Campaigning is a process designed to influence the public to vote in a particular way on an issue or a candidate. An issue or candidate is presented in a favorable light with the intent of influencing voters. Campaigning can be implemented via media presentations, in group meetings or rallies, or in face-to-face contacts with the public.

Campaigning for an issue involves presenting information related to the issue that persuades people to support nursing's position. Campaigning for a specific candidate can help ensure the election of policy makers who support nursing's position on important issues. Campaigning is an opportunity for nurses to become personally known to a candidate and other campaign workers. It is also an opportunity to become known as a reliable source of information about health and health care issues. Campaigning for a candidate also creates a debt on the part of an elected official that may result in future support for a position promoted by population health nurses.

Much of the work of political action committees (PACs) is designed to support the candidacy of specific individuals. The American Nurses Association Political Action Committee (ANA-PAC) was created in response to nursing's perceived lack of influence in the formulation of health care policy (ANA, 2014). The purpose of ANA-PAC is to promote constructive national health care legislation through the political "electioneering" process. **Electioneering** is the active process of endorsing candidates who have demonstrated support for nursing's political agenda and contributing time and money to their campaigns. ANA-PAC and similar political action committees supported by nurses seek to enhance the political influence of nurses by supporting the election of candidates who back the profession and its position on significant health-related issues.

There are some constraints on campaign involvement for certain groups of nurses. For example, nurses employed by government agencies (whether part-time or full-time, permanently or temporarily) are prohibited by the Hatch Act (also known as the Act to Prevent Pernicious Political Activities) from soliciting campaign contributions (even anonymously by telephone) or engaging in campaign activities while on duty, in uniform, or using an agency vehicle. They are also prohibited from running for office in a partisan election. The provisions of the Hatch Act cover all federal employees, employees of the District of Columbia, employees of state or local agencies funded by the federal government, and Commissioned Officers in the U.S. Public Health Service (Malone & Chaffee, 2012).

Holding political appointments and elected offices. A final means of creating support for policy directions promoted by population health nurses is to become a policy maker oneself. This may involve being appointed to a specific position or running for elective office. In either case, the population health nurse must first become politically active in some of the other ways described in this chapter to be sufficiently well known to be elected or appointed to a policy-making position (Hall-Long, 2012; Leavitt & Chaffee, 2012).

One may also work in the background in policy making by becoming a legislative staff person or a lobbyist for an organized group. Again, such positions require familiarity with the political process and well-developed interpersonal relationships with legislators and other policy makers. Strategies to influence policy development and implementation are summarized in Table 9-4●.

EVALUATING HEALTH POLICY DEVELOPMENT. Population health nurses should be involved in evaluating the policy development process as well as polices developed. In evaluating the process itself, the nurse would consider the extent to which all stakeholders, including those affected by a given policy, have been involved in policy development. In addition, the nurse would assess the adequacy of strategic management of the policy development process, gaining insights into what worked and what did not for application in future policy development efforts.

Population health nurses should also evaluate the adequacy of health policies developed. Criteria for evaluating health policies include their adequacy in meeting the health needs of the public, safeguards for the rights of individuals, equitable allocation of resources, their capacity for implementation, and the effects of the policy on the target population.

Health policies must be developed that effectively address the health needs of the affected population and identification of needs must derive from population-based data. For example, a local government policy allowing homeless persons to sleep in city-owned buildings addresses only one small part of the problem of homelessness. In this case, a more comprehensive policy that addresses both short-term and long-term solutions to the problems of homelessness is needed.

Safeguarding individual rights is another criterion for sound health care policy development. As an example, a policy that would require homeless individuals to surrender personal belongings to meet communal needs when admitted to a shelter would violate their property rights. There are circumstances, however, in which the good of society supersedes individual rights. For example, homeless persons may be prohibited from smoking in a shelter to prevent exposing others to smoke or to prevent a fire. Whenever possible, health policies should be written so that they do not violate the rights of individuals affected by them.

Health care policies should also promote equitable distribution of health care resources. This means that policies should not discriminate against certain subgroups within the population. For example, open housing policies in homeless shelters

TABLE 9-4 Strategies for Promoting Policy Adoption

Strategy	Description of Strategy
Staying informed	Keeping current on health-related issues at local, state, national, and international levels
Communicating with policy makers	Becoming known to policy makers Establishing credibility as a source of information
Networking	Becoming aware of and known to groups and individuals with similar policy-related interests
Coalition building	Creating a temporary alliance among individuals or groups to work toward common goals
Reciprocal action	Supporting the policy efforts of others in return for support of issues of interest to nursing
Creating media support	Selecting appropriate media and designing targeted media messages for specific audiences
Community organizing	Mobilizing community resources in favor of planned change or a proposed policy
Lobbying	Engaging in personal communications with policy makers in an attempt to elicit a specific action with respect to a specific policy
Presenting testimony	Providing information on an issue to policy makers at a public hearing
Voting	Exercising one's personal right to vote
	Encouraging others to vote
	Participating in voter registration drives
Campaigning	Providing endorsements or monetary support for specific policy proposals or candidates with the intent of influencing voters' responses
Holding a political appointment or elected office	Assuming a position as a policy maker by virtue of election or appointment to a specific office

may inadvertently discriminate against women and children who may be subjected to force to make them give way to adult men who desire shelter. Sex-segregated shelters that ensure access for both males and females provide for a more equitable allocation of resources.

For a specific health policy to be effective in promoting health or preventing illness, it must be capable of being implemented or enforced. For example, a local government might adopt a policy encouraging houses of worship to provide overnight shelter for homeless individuals. But unless the houses of worship are willing to cooperate, the policy cannot be implemented.

Population health nurses planning to influence health care policy formation should assess proposed policies or modifications of existing policies in light of these five criteria. Policies that do not meet the criteria should be redesigned, if possible, before they are presented to policy makers. If a proposed policy continues not to meet one or more criteria, its supporters should be prepared to justify the need for the policy. For example, nurses should be prepared to convince policy makers that a smoking ban in shelters for the homeless is warranted despite the violation of the individual's personal freedom of choice.

Population health nurses may also be actively involved in assessing the effects of health care policies on meeting the needs of the particular target group. Population health nurses could assist in collecting data related to the outcomes of programs put into operation. For example, data might be gathered on the incidence of health problems among the homeless to evaluate the effects of policies designed to foster health promotion, illness prevention, or treatment services in this population. In addition, information could be collected regarding the number of persons who continue to be homeless despite assistance from established programs.

The Patient Protection and Affordable Care Act—PL 111–148

The most sweeping piece of U.S. health-related legislation in several years culminated in the signing of the Patient Protection and Affordable Care Act in March 2010. In spite of political and legal challenges, broad segments of American society are currently engaged in implementing its provisions. A general overview of these provisions was provided in Chapter 7∞. For further information about the Affordable Care Act, see the resources provided in the *External Resources* section of the student resources site. Here we will briefly review some of the aspects of the development of this significant piece of legislation.

Efforts to provide health insurance coverage for the American people began as far back as 1912 when Theodore Roosevelt's Progressive Party included social insurance, including health insurance, in the election platform. As recently as 1993, the Clinton Administration developed a proposal for health care reform, the Health Security Act, which failed in Congress (Kaiser Family Foundation, 2011). What then was different in 2010 that permitted the passage of the Affordable Care Act (ACA)?

One factor influencing the success of the legislative initiative was the long-standing complaints from business and industry about the rising cost of health insurance premiums for employees. At the same time, there were concerns about increasing federal costs for Medicare and Medicaid programs. In addition, a greater percentage of the American people—nearly 50 million—were without health insurance coverage than ever before. These factors led to the impetus for major legislation to reform the health care delivery system (APHA, 2012b; Sparer, 2011).

Any possible legislation, however, faced three major obstacles: significant self-interest on the part of many organizations, disagreement about the appropriate role of the federal government in health care, and the need to circumvent a Senate filibuster designed to kill the legislation. Factors operating in favor of the legislative proposal included a mandate in the 53% of the popular vote that elected President Barack Obama, coupled with a Democratic majority in the U.S. Senate. In addition, the Obama administration designated health care reform a governmental priority and linked it to recovery from a serious economic recession. Rather than develop a proposal from the executive branch that was forwarded to Congress for action, Obama charged the Senate with developing a workable plan for reform and emphasized willingness to compromise, limiting the opposition from interest groups (Sparer, 2011).

In addition, the Obama administration highlighted the need to base reform on the current system rather than creating an entirely new system of care, again defusing some opposition from vested interests. Changes are incremental rather than overwhelming in nature, and some provisions left out of the initial bill were reincorporated in the reconciliation process between House and Senate versions of the legislation (Kaiser Family Foundation, 2011).

Several elements of the Affordable Care Act have far reaching implications for population health status. These include a significant reduction in the number of uninsured, an emphasis on health promotion and prevention, and provisions for improving chronic disease management, as well as elimination of discriminatory insurance practices (APHA, 2012a; Centers for Medicare and Medicaid Services [CMS], 2013b). In addition, the law is expected to result in considerable savings over the long term. In fact, CMS has reported $8.3 million in savings on prescription drug costs as of 2013. In addition, sufficient savings have been realized to hold Medicare Part B premiums at the prior year's level and to reduce both Part A and Part B deductibles (CMS, 2013a).

One of the most salient aspects of ACA for population health practice is the creation of the National Prevention, Health Promotion, and Public Health Council. This federal agency is charged with developing a National Prevention Strategy that incorporates evidence-based health promotion practices. In 2011, the "National Prevention Strategy: America's Plan for Better Health and Wellness" was released. The strategy delineates four strategic directions: (a) promoting healthy and safe communities, (b) enhancing clinical and community prevention services, (c) eliminating health disparities, and

(d) empowering people. The strategy also addresses seven targeted priority issues including (a) tobacco-free living, (b) drug abuse and excessive alcohol use, (c) healthy eating, (d) active living, (e) injury and violence-free living, (f) reproductive and sexual health, and (g) mental and emotional well-being (National Prevention, Health Promotion, and Public Health Council, 2013). ACA also includes a number of other provisions that focus on health promotion and prevention including insurance coverage for preventive services, requirements for community health needs assessments, and funding for health promotion and prevention initiatives (APHA, 2012a).

CHAPTER RECAP

Effective population health nurses use the political process to attain their primary objective, enhancing the health of the populations with which they work. Political activity by population health nurses may occur at the institutional or societal level and often involves efforts to influence legislation related to health issues. The political process begins with identification of health issues or problems that can be resolved through policy formation. Agenda setting and delineation of the actual policy are followed by development of strategies designed to get the desired policy adopted and implemented. These strategies may include staying informed on policy issues, communicating with policy makers, networking, coalition building, reciprocal action, creating media support, and community organizing. Additional strategies include lobbying, presenting testimony, voting, campaigning, and holding political appointments or elected offices. Policy development ends with an evaluation of the policy development process as well as the effectiveness of the policy in addressing the identified health issue. The Patient Protection and Affordable Care Act is a prime example of the use of the political process to enhance the health of the population.

CASE STUDY Influencing Housing Policy

In focus groups conducted to determine local health needs, residents of a low-income, culturally diverse neighborhood repeatedly voiced concerns about intimidation of tenants by landlords. Because of housing shortages, many tenants were (justifiably) worried that reporting inadequacies to landlords would result in evictions. With limited low-income housing available, people were not willing to take the risk of making complaints about needed repairs or noisy neighbors.

Cultural differences, the tenants' lack of facility with English, and the fact that most owners of rental units were absentee landlords complicated the situation. More than half of the residents in the community were members of ethnic cultural groups, including many relatively recent refugees from Southeast Asia and the Middle East. Long-time area residents were primarily older persons on fixed incomes who also could not afford to antagonize landlords.

There was a fledgling landlord/tenant association in the neighborhood, but few of the absentee landlords were active participants. There was also a neighborhood collaborative that had successfully mounted some initiatives to improve conditions for residents, including decreasing drug dealing in selected areas of the neighborhood and putting up antitobacco billboards. The collaborative had developed relatively close relationships with city council members and county supervisors in the wider community, although recently several political positions had been filled by newly elected officials. One or two long-time residents were particularly influential with local politicians. The nearby university law school provided landlord/tenant mediation services to individuals in the community. Other agencies and associations active in the neighborhood included local schools, the community center, Boys and Girls Club, the community health center, the local health department office, the university school of nursing, a Lao-Hmong Association, the Vietnamese Federation, and several programs geared toward children and the elderly.

1. What steps might the local population health nurses take to address the problem of intimidation by landlords?
2. What community groups might be appropriate coalition partners in resolving this problem? Why?
3. What approaches might be taken in terms of policy development to deal with intimidation?
4. Are there particular government agencies that should become involved? If so, what are they and how would you promote their involvement?
5. How might local residents become actively involved in resolving the issue?
6. What cultural considerations have relevance for this situation and its resolution?

REFERENCES

Alliance for Health Reform. (2010). *Implementing health reform: Federal rules and state roles.* Retrieved from http://www.allhealth.org/publications/State_health_issues/Implementing_Health_Reform_-_Federal_Rules_and_State_Roles_100.pdf

American Association of Colleges of Nursing. (2008). *Consensus model for APRN regulation: Licensure, accreditation, certification, and education.* Retrieved from http://www.aacn.nche.edu/education-resources/APRNReport.pdf

American Association of Colleges of Nursing. (2010). *From patient advocacy to political activism: AACN's guide to understanding healthcare policy and politics.* Washington, DC: Author.

American Nurses Association. (2014). *ANA-PAC: What is ANA-PAC?* Retrieved from http://www.nursingworld.org/MainMenuCategories/ANAPolitical-Power/ANAPAC.aspx

American Public Health Association. (2011). *Transportation and health toolkit.* Retrieved from http://www.apha.org/advocacy/priorities/issues/transportation/Toolkit.htm

American Public Health Association. (2012a). *Affordable Care Act overview: Selected provisions.* Retrieved from http://www.apha.org/NR/rdonlyres/26831F24-882A-4FF7-A0A9-6F49DFBF6D3F/0/ACAOverview_Aug2012.pdf

American Public Health Association. (2012b). *Why do we need the Affordable Care Act?.* Retrieved from http://www.apha.org/NR/rdonlyres/19BEA341-A7C3-4920-B2BC-65BDC846B803/0/WhyWeNeedtheACA_Aug2012.pdf

Berkowitz, B. (2012). The policy process. In D. J. Mason, J. K. Leavitt, & M. W. Chaffee (Eds.), *Policy & politics in nursing and health care* (6th ed., pp. 49–58). St. Louis, MO: Elsevier Saunders.

Bikersrights.com. (2013). Helmet issues: Use your head. Retrieved from http://www.bikersrights.com/helmets.html

Bradbury, D. E., & Eliot, M. M. (1956). *Four decades of action for children: A short history of the Children's Bureau.* Retrieved from http://www.ssa.gov/history/pdf/child1.pdf

California Senate OKs single-payer health plan. (2010, January 29). Retrieved from http://articles.sfgate.com/2010-01-29/bay-area/17840931_1_health-care-single-payer-state-plan

Centers for Disease Control and Prevention. (2013). *Emerging tobacco products gaining popularity among youth.* Retrieved from http://www.cdc.gov/media/releases/2013/p1114-emerging-tobacco-products.html

Centers for Disease Control and Prevention. (2014). *Health impact assessment.* Retrieved from http://www.cdc.gov/healthyplaces/hia.htm

Centers for Medicare and Medicaid Services. (2013a). *CMS announces major savings for Medicare beneficiaries.* Retrieved from http://www.cms.gov/Newsroom/MediaReleaseDatabase/Press-Releases/2013-Press-Releases-Items/2013-10-28.html

Centers for Medicare and Medicaid Services. (2013b). *CMS strategy: The road forward 2013–2017.* Retrieved from http://www.cms.gov/About-CMS/Agency-Information/CMS-Strategy/Downloads/CMS-Strategy.pdf

Chaffee, M. W. (2012). Science, policy, and politics. In D. J. Mason, J. K. Leavitt, & M. W. Chaffee (Eds.), *Policy & politics in nursing and health care* (6th ed., pp. 307–317). St. Louis, MO: Elsevier Saunders.

Chaffee, M. W., Mason, D. J., & Leavitt, J. K. (2012). A framework for action in policy and politics. In D. J. Mason, J. K. Leavitt, & M. W. Chaffee (Eds.), *Policy & politics in nursing and health care* (6th ed., pp. 1–11). St. Louis, MO: Elsevier Saunders.

Cho, H. S. M., & Kashka, M. S. (2004). The evolution of the community health nurse practitioner in Korea. *Public Health Nursing, 21,* 287–294.

Community Preventive Services Task Force. (2014). *What is the community guide?* Retrieved from http://www.thecommunityguide.org/index.html

Daniels, J., Glickstein, B., & Mason, D. J. (2012). Using the power of media to influence health policy and politics. In D. J. Mason, J. K. Leavitt, & M. W. Chaffee (Eds.), *Policy & politics in nursing and health care* (6th ed., pp. 88–104). St. Louis, MO: Elsevier Saunders.

Florence Kelley. (2011). Retrieved from http://www.nndb.com/people/460/000204845/

Front groups. (2013). Retrieved from http://www.sourcewatch.org/index.php/Front_groups

Green, R. (2010). The ethics of sin taxes. *Public Health Nursing, 28,* 68–77. doi:10.1111/j.1525-1446.2010.00907.x

Hall-Long, B. (2012). Taking action: Nurse, educator, and legislator: My journey to the Delaware General Assembly. In D. J. Mason, J. K. Leavitt, & M. W. Chaffee (Eds.), *Policy & politics in nursing and health care* (6th ed., pp. 579–582). St. Louis, MO: Elsevier Saunders.

Hendrickson, K. C., Ceccarelli, C., & Cohen, S. S. (2012). How government works: What you need to know to influence the process. In D. J. Mason, J. K. Leavitt, & M. W. Chaffee (Eds.), *Policy & politics in nursing and health care* (6th ed., pp. 480–493). St. Louis, MO: Elsevier Saunders.

HIA Partner Team. (2012). *Expanding public transit in Columbia, Missouri: A health impact assessment.* Retrieved from http://www.healthimpactproject.org/resources/document/Columbia-MO-Transit-HIA-Executive-Summary-FINAL-1.pdf

Institute of Medicine. (2011a). *For the public's health: Revitalizing law and policy to meet new challenges.* Washington, DC: National Academies Press.

Institute of Medicine. (2011b). *The future of nursing: Leading change, advancing health.* Washington, DC: National Academies Press.

Jewish Women's Archive. (2010). *Lillian Wald, 1867–1940.* Retrieved from http://jwa.org/historymakers/wald

Kaiser Family Foundation. (2011). *Timeline: History of health reform efforts in the U.S.* Retrieved from http://kff.org/health-reform/timeline/history-of-health-reform-efforts-in-the-united-states/

Leavitt, J. K., & Chaffee, M. W. (2012). Political appointments. In D. J. Mason, J. K. Leavitt, & M. W. Chaffee (Eds.), *Policy & politics in nursing and health care* (6th ed., pp. 533–539). St. Louis, MO: Elsevier Saunders.

Leavitt, J. K., Mason, D. J., & Whelan, E.-M. (2012). Political analysis and strategies. In D. J. Mason, J. K. Leavitt, & M. W. Chaffee (Eds.), *Policy and politics in nursing and health care* (6th ed., pp. 65–76). St. Louis, MO: Saunders.

Leavitt, J. K., Mason, D. J., & Whelan, E.-M. (2012). Political analysis and strategies. In D. J. Mason, J. K. Leavitt, & M. W. Chaffee (Eds.), *Policy & politics in nursing and health care* (6th ed., pp. 65–76). St. Louis, MO: Elsevier Saunders.

Lewenson, S. B. (2012). A historical perspective on policy, politics, and nursing. In D. J. Mason, J. K. Leavitt, & M. W. Chaffee (Eds.), *Policy and politics in nursing and health care* (6th ed., pp. 12–18). St. Louis, MO: Elsevier Saunders.

Lewis, J. J. (2011). *Florence Kelley.* Retrieved from http://womenshistory.about.com/od/workgeneral/p/florence_kelley.htm?p=1

Loomis, B. R., Shafer, P. R., & van Hasselt, M. (2013). The economic impact of smoke-free laws on restaurants and bars in 9 states. *Preventing Chronic Disease,10,* 120327. doi: http://dx.doi.org/10.5888/pcd10.120327. Retrieved from http://www.cdc.gov/pcd/issues/2013/12_0327.htm

Lowes, R. (2011). *US Appeals court in Atlanta strikes down individual mandate.* Retrieved from http://www.medscape.com/viewarticle/747987?sssdmh=dm1.709979&src=nl_newsalert

Malekafzali, S., & Bergstrom, D. (2011). *Healthy corridor for all: A community health impact assessment of transit-oriented development policy in Saint Paul, Minnesota.*Retrieved from http://www.healthimpactproject.org/news/project/body/Healthy-Corridor-summary-FINAL.pdf

Malone, T. A., & Chaffee, M. W. (2012). Political activity: Different rules for government-employed nurses. In D. J. Mason, J. K. Leavitt, & M. W. Chaffee (Eds.), *Policy & politics in nursing and health care* (6th ed., pp. 590–593). St. Louis, MO: Elsevier Saunders.

National Council of State Boards of Nursing. (n.d.). *Campaign for APRN consensus: Model for uniform national advanced practice registered nurse (APRN) regulation: A handbook for legislators.* Chicago, IL: Author. Retrieved from https://www.ncsbn.org/2010_APRN_HandbookforLegislators_web.pdf

National Council of State Boards of Nursing. (2011). *APRN consensus model toolkit.* Retrieved from https://www.ncsbn.org/2276.htm

National Council of State Boards of Nursing. (2014). *APRNs in the U.S.* Retrieved from https://www.ncsbn.org/2567.htm

National Federation of Small Business. (2012). *PPACA: The individual mandate tax.* Retrieved from http://www.nfib.com/cribsheets/individual-mandate/

National Prevention, Health Promotion, and Public Health Council. (2013). *2013annual status report.* Retrieved from http://www.surgeongeneral.gov/initiatives/prevention/2013-npc-status-report.pdf

National Research Council. (2011). Improving Health in the United States: The role of health impact assessment. Retrieved from http://www.nap.edu/catalog.php?record_id=13229

Occupational Safety and Health Administration. (n.d.). *Youth in agriculture.* Retrieved from https://www.osha.gov/SLTC/youth/agriculture/other.html

Oettinger, K. B. (1962). *It's your Children's Bureau.* Retrieved from http://www.ssa.gov/history/childb2.html

Office of the First Minister and Deputy First Minister. (n.d.). *A practical guide to policy making in Northern Ireland.* Retrieved from http://www.ofmdfmni.gov.uk/practical-guide-policy-making.pdf

Policy. (2011). *In Merriam-Webster's online dictionary.* Retrieved from http://www.merriam-webster.com/dictionary/policy

The Policy Circle. (n.d.). *The process: Policy development.* Retrieved from http://www.policyproject.com/policycircle/content.cfm?a0=4

Purtle, J. (2010). *Gambling on the health of the public: A rapid health impact assessment for an urban casino.* Retrieved from http://www.healthimpactproject.org/resources/document/sugarhouse-casino.pdf

Rice Bowers-Lanier, R. (2012). Coalitions: A powerful political strategy. In D. J. Mason, J. K. Leavitt, & M. W. Chaffee (Eds.), *Policy & politics in nursing and health care* (6th ed., pp. 626–632). St. Louis, MO: Elsevier Saunders.

Ridenour, N., & Santa Anna, Y. (2012). An overview of legislation and regulation. In D. J. Mason, J. K. Leavitt, & M. W. Chaffee (Eds.), *Policy & politics in nursing and health care* (6th ed., pp. 494–505). St. Louis, MO: Elsevier Saunders.

San Francisco Planning Department. (2010). *Initial study: Glen Park community plan.* Retrieved from http://www.hiaguide.org/sites/default/files/SF.pdf

Slokum-Bradley, N., & Bradley, A. (2010). Is the EU's governance "good"? An assessment of EU governance in its partnership with ACP states. *Third World Quarterly, 31*(1), 31–49. doi:10.1080/01436590903557314

Social Security Administration. (n.d.). *History: The Children's Bureau.* Retrieved from http://www.ssa.gov/history/childb1.html

Sparer, M. (2011). U.S. health care reform and the future of dentistry. *American Journal of Public Health, 101,* 1841–1844. doi:10.2105/AJPH.2011.300358

State of Vermont. (2011). *Brief summary of Act 48: Vermont health reform law of 2011I.* Retrieved from http://hcr.vermont.gov/sites/hcr/files/ACT%2048%20one%20page%20summary%20June%2014.doc

U.S. House of Representatives. (n.d.). *House committees.* Retrieved from http://www.house.gov/committees/

U.S. Senate. (n.d.). *Committees.* Retrieved from http://www.senate.gov/pagelayout/committees/d_three_sections_with_teasers/committees_home.htm

Warner, J. R. (2012). Interest groups in health care policy and politics. In D. J. Mason, J. K. Leavitt, & M. W. Chaffee (Eds.), *Policy & politics in nursing and health care* (6th ed., pp. 594–601). St. Louis, MO: Elsevier Saunders.

Whelan, E.-M., & Woody, M. P. (2012). Lobbying policy makers: Individual and collective strategies. In D. J. Mason, J. K. Leavitt, & M. W. Chaffee (Eds.), *Policy & politics in nursing and health care* (6th ed., pp. 519–526). St. Louis, MO: Elsevier Saunders.

Wiist, W. H. (2011). Citizens *United*, public health, and democracy: The Supreme Court ruling, its implications, and proposed action. *American Journal of Public Health, 101,* 1172–1179. doi:10: 2105/AJPH.2010.300043

Wisconsin Department of Health Services. (2010). *Healthiest Wisconsin 2020: Everyone living better, longer.* Retrieved from http://www.dhs.wisconsin.gov/hw2020/report2020.htm

Work Group for Community Development and Change. (2013). *Community tool box: Section 8: Some lessons learned on community organization and change.* Retrieved from http://ctb.ku.edu/en//tablecontents/sub_section_tools_1386.htm

World Health Organization. (2014). *Health policy.* Retrieved from http://www.who.int/topics/health_policy/en/

Young, J. (2009, September). Helping researchers become policy entrepreneurs. *Overseas Development Institute Briefing Paper, 53.* Retrieved from http://www.odi.org.uk/resources/download/1127.pdf

CHAPTER

10 Community Empowerment Strategies

Learning Outcomes

After reading this chapter, you should be able to:

1. Discuss the relationship of community empowerment to other similar concepts.
2. Identify levels of community empowerment.
3. Apply selected models for community empowerment.
4. Describe the process of community empowerment.
5. Apply criteria to evaluate community empowerment.
6. Analyze the role of population health nurses in community empowerment.

Key Terms

community building
community capacity
community competence
community development
empowerment
participatory evaluation
powerlessness

Advocacy Then

Harriet Tubman

Harriet Tubman epitomized the concept of a nurse empowering others. Born into slavery, Harriet Tubman suffered lasting consequences of a blow delivered by an overseer when, as a young girl, she thwarted his efforts to capture a runaway slave (Sahlman, 2011). After escaping to the North herself, she made multiple trips back to the South to lead an estimated 300 slaves, including members of her own family, to freedom, earning the title "the Moses of her people" (Maschi, n.d.; New York History Net, n.d.). These activities required her to employ a number of creative strategies including traveling in disguise and using hymns to spread the word that she would be in the area to guide willing slaves to freedom (Driggs, 1980). She collaborated with members of the underground railroad, and became an accomplished speaker at antislavery and women's rights meetings, gaining the support of such well-known figures as suffragette Susan B. Anthony, Secretary of State William H. Seward, and authors Ralph Waldo Emerson and Louisa May Alcott (Lewis, n.d.).

During the Civil War, Tubman worked as a nurse and teacher, meeting the needs of escaped slaves fighting with the U.S. Army and the Gullah people of the South Carolina Sea Islands, left behind by their White owners (Lewis, n.d.). In addition, she organized a network of scouts and coordinated the Union attack on Southern supply lines on the Combahee River (Conrad, n.d.). In addition to disrupting supply lines, the expedition freed several hundred slaves from plantations along the river (Conrad, n.d.). During her scouting missions, she continued to try to persuade slaves to leave their masters and join the Union Army. After the war, Tubman, herself illiterate, worked to establish schools for freed slaves in South Carolina and later to establish a home for indigent elderly former slaves.

Advocacy Now

Self-Empowerment of Indian Women

Self-employed women in the state of Gujarat, India, found themselves living in poverty with no employment security and no coverage under the national social security system. More than 1 million of these women organized a self-help trade union, the Self-Employed Women's Association (SEWA) to improve their living and working conditions. Starting their own bank, the women provided access to credit and kept the proceeds of their labor without being exploited by lenders charging high interest rates. In addition, vegetable producers and sellers started their own shops and eliminated exploitation by middlemen. Other initiatives undertaken by the group include child care and collective health insurance coverage. In 2008, SEWA campaigned for legislation for social security coverage for informal self-employed workers, including insurance, pension, and maternity benefits. In response, the Indian government established a commission to develop related laws and policies for informal workers (World Health Organization, 2008, 2009).

Throughout this book, we emphasize the advocacy role of the population health nurse. Population health nurses act on behalf of individuals, families, and population groups that, for whatever reason, cannot act for themselves. The ultimate outcome of advocacy by population health nurses, however, is the ability of the client to act independently. Community empowerment, as discussed in this chapter, is designed to accomplish that outcome, to enable communities to identify community health problems, and take steps to resolve them independently of or in concert with health care professionals and others. Just as successful nursing education programs prepare graduates to function effectively on their own in the practice milieu, so too does effective population health nursing, as community empowerment, prepare communities to deal with their own health problems and issues.

Although some authors trace the beginnings of community organization and empowerment to the settlement house activities of the late 1800s (Minkler & Wallerstein, 2012), the nurses of the Henry Street Settlement did not engage in community organization or empowerment activities as we know them today. Those nurses certainly functioned as advocates for the health and social welfare needs of the immigrant populations they served, but they did not work to enable those populations to act on their own behalf. On the contrary, they tried to work within the existing power structure to benefit these populations, rather than attempting to redistribute power in their favor. Today, however, community development and particularly community empowerment are key strategies to address health disparities throughout the world (Tsey et al., 2010). In fact, community empowerment, as exemplified in community participation in health care decisions, is one of the five principles of primary health care promoted by the World Health Organization (WHO) (Aston, Meagher-Stewart, Edwards, & Young, 2009). Community development may improve health directly by addressing specific health issues or indirectly through empowering communities to take action to address health issues.

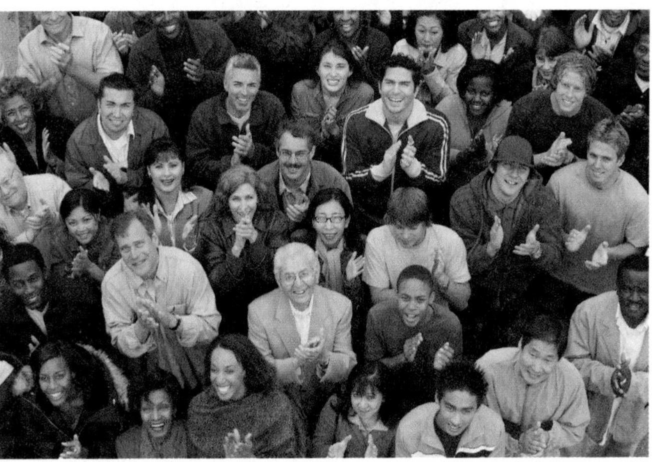

Community empowerment requires participation by diverse segments of the community. *(Bikeriderlondon/Shutterstock)*

Empowerment and Related Concepts

Community empowerment, the topic of this chapter, is closely related to a number of similar concepts. **Empowerment** is "a social action process that promotes participation of people and communities toward goals of increased individual and community control, improved quality of life and social justice" (World Health Organization [WHO], 2009, Empowerment focuses on assisting the community to develop its own capacity to resolve problems rather than relying on outside assistance (Burkett, 2013). At a very basic level, empowerment involves transferring power from official bodies, authorities, or experts to members of the community. In some instances, this may involve community ownership of resources as well as capitalization on existing community assets (Cooke, 2013).

Powerlessness is the antithesis of empowerment. **Powerlessness** is the belief that one's actions cannot determine the achievement of outcomes sought and is widely considered a significant contributor to health and social inequities throughout the world. As noted by some authors, "If powerlessness is the underlying factor among all adverse social conditions . . ., then empowerment takes precedence over other theoretical frameworks used to eliminate health disparities" (Wiggins et al., 2009, p. 12).

Community empowerment arises from activities related to community development, community organizing, community mobilization, and community building. Empowerment, in turn, leads to increased community capacity and competence. The relationships among these concepts are depicted in Figure 10-1•. Some authors have noted that community development as a concept has been co-opted by governments and other organizations in top-down efforts to further their own agendas rather than empowering communities to control power and resources themselves (Craig & Mayo, 2013). **Community development** has been linked to capacity building and has been defined as "a set of practices and methods that focus on harnessing the innate abilities and potential that exist in all human communities to become active agents in their own development and to organize themselves to address key issues and concerns that they share" (International Association for Community Development, 2014, para 2). Community development involves building people's skills and their ability to resolve common problems (Improvement and Development Agency, 2012).

The concept of community organization was presented in Chapter 9∞ and reflects the process of mobilizing resources to resolve community-identified problems. Community mobilization, a similar term, was defined as a community health

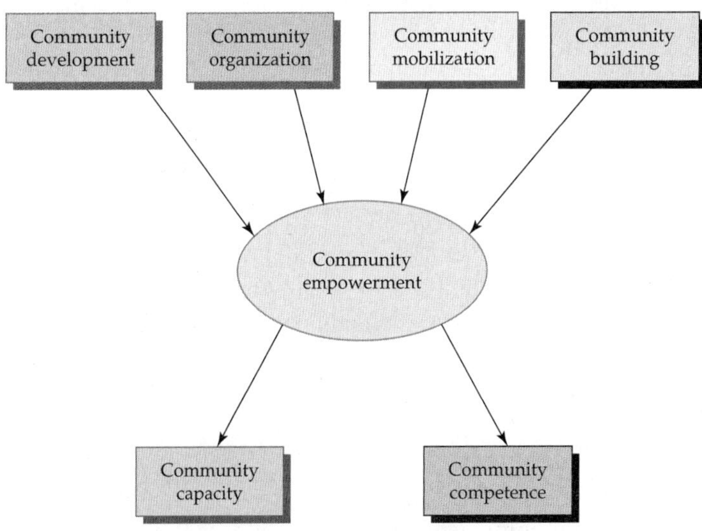

FIGURE 10-1 Community Empowerment and Related Concepts

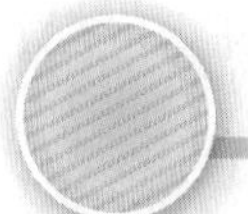

Global Perspectives

International Capacity Building

International capacity building has been described as the efforts of people in one country to help those in another to achieve their objectives. Examine the news media to identify examples of international capacity building or empowerment related to health issues. Who is providing the assistance? Who is receiving it? Based on the examples you have found, does capacity building always flow from the "haves" to the "have nots"? In what ways could underdeveloped nations contribute to international capacity building? As one example, what could the United States learn from countries with low neonatal death rates that could decrease U.S. neonatal mortality?

nursing role in Chapter 1∞, and involves assisting populations to identify areas of concern and to develop and implement strategies to address them. Both of these processes tend to be more problem specific than community empowerment, which is designed to develop overall community abilities to deal with a variety of problems. Community building is another similar, but more general, process that leads to community empowerment. **Community building** is defined as "continuous, self-renewing efforts that are led by residents, focused on collective action, aimed at relationship building and problem solving and build a stronger community" (Neighbor Works® America, 2014, para. 2). Community building efforts frequently lead to increases in community social capital as described in Chapter 1∞.

Other terms often associated with empowerment include public participation and community engagement. *Public participation* involves providing information and soliciting input from community members in decision-making processes, but with no real power over the final decision. *Engagement* involves community members in collaborative decision-making processes, but again does not result in ultimate power lying in the hands of the community (Bailey, 2010). These terms do not reflect true empowerment, and so are not included in the diagram in Figure 10-1.

Community empowerment results in increased community competence and capacity, as depicted in Figure 10-1. **Community competence** is defined as a community's ability to engage in problem identification and resolution. **Community capacity** is the abilities and resources of the community that enable it to carry out tasks and functions to achieve identified goals.

Levels of Empowerment

Empowerment may occur at several levels, including individual community members, organizations within the community, and the community at large. Individual empowerment is a process of increasing one's power to take action to improve one's own life. Empowered individuals gain new skills and power to influence others and to affect the outcomes of decision making (Bailey, 2010). For example, an individual community member may develop the knowledge and skills to bring housing code violations in their rental unit to the attention of the housing authority. Organizational empowerment involves increasing the power of community organizations to control decisions related to the health and welfare of the community. Using the former example, members of a Community Collaborative may develop the skills to present findings about widespread housing-code violations to the local housing authority. In this process, the balance of power may change among organizations involved in partnerships (Bailey, 2010). For example, in a university-community partnership, the university may initially exercise a great deal of power, particularly with respect to allocation of grant funding received. As the community develops greater competence and capacity, more of this power is transferred to the hands of community members, who are enabled to write independent funding grants.

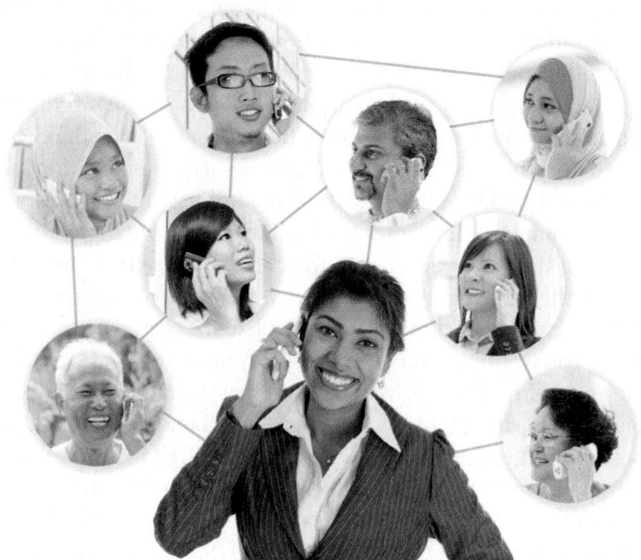

Effective group work requires communication and collaboration.
(Wong Sze Fei/Fotolia)

Population health nurses may be involved in individual, organizational, and community empowerment. For example, a nurse may assist an abused woman to obtain job training and to request a restraining order against her abuser, empowering her to leave the abusive situation. Organizational empowerment might involve advocacy for beneficiaries of a particular health program to have more control in the management of the program. At the community level, a population health nurse might assist residents of a low-income neighborhood to collect information on gang-related criminal activity and present a petition to the City Council requesting a greater police presence in the neighborhood.

Community empowerment may also occur at horizontal and vertical levels (de Wit & Berner, 2009). *Horizontal empowerment* is internal to the community and is reflected in the community's ability to solve problems by mobilizing its own resources. For example, a population health nurse might help neighborhood residents to form a neighborhood watch group to help control gang activity. *Vertical empowerment* involves efforts to change power structures outside the community and to leverage outside power and resources to address community concerns and may involve organizing marginalized groups to make demands on the larger society. Vertical empowerment is reflected in community members petitioning the City Council for better police coverage. Some authors point out that developing horizontal empowerment structures may be difficult in low-income populations who may not have the time, energy, or resources needed for grassroots organizing initiatives. They also note that vertical empowerment for these populations may have the unintended effect of increasing community dependence on outside assistance and decreasing community control in decision making and action.

Finally, community empowerment may be conceived as occurring along a continuum from personal empowerment to the development of small mutual support groups, to the development of community organizations, to the creation of coalitions and partnerships, to community-based social and political action related to community concerns. At the level of personal empowerment, a population health nurse might help a homeless man with a substance abuse problem find work and enroll in a recovery program. At the next level, the nurse might assist a group of homeless individuals to form a support group that permits them to share knowledge of resources. Helping to create an organization composed of homeless individuals and families and members of the social services community to address the health care needs of the homeless population would be an example of the third level of empowerment. Finally, at the fourth and fifth levels, the population health nurse might assist the community organization to link with legal advocates and others to promote legislation to protect the civil rights of homeless individuals.

Models for Community Empowerment

Community empowerment can be conceptualized in a number of ways, and various models for viewing community empowerment have been put forth. Bailey (2010) developed the concept of decision-making spaces occurring at three levels: closed, invited, and claimed or created spaces. In closed spaces, decisions are made behind closed doors without input from community members. In invited spaces, community members may be invited by authorities to provide input and work collaboratively to resolve community-identified problems. These spaces reflect the community participation and engagement approaches described earlier. At the third level, community members claim, create, or demand opportunities for input or to make decisions for themselves.

Laverack (2007) used the concept of a ladder with three sets of rungs to depict the process of community empowerment in health promotion program development that can be applied to empowerment of populations in general. The foot of the ladder rests on a foundation of community readiness to work with outside agents to resolve community problems. Ascending the ladder moves the community or population from participation in decision making to taking action for themselves. The first rung addresses community involvement and includes community participation in the identification of existing community needs and providing input for programs to address those needs. The next set of rungs encompasses the creation of community competence and includes fostering community engagement, community organizing, community development, and building community capacity. Community engagement, in Laverack's model, involves collaborative identification of solutions to problems and creation of partnerships to mobilize resources, influence systems, and change relationships. Community organization involves the development of structures within the community designed to achieve shared goals. Again, development of a Crime Watch program might be an example of community organization. In community development, outside assistance is received to improve the lives of members of the community or population. Often, this assistance occurs in the form of distribution of resources and opportunities. For example, a skills training program might be initiated to educate women in the community for employment opportunities. The final rung related to community competence involves building community capacity and includes the identification or development of community assets needed to resolve community-identified problems.

The third set of rungs on the ladder moving toward community or population action addresses community control. The first rung at this level incorporates community action, which involves community ownership of specific issues and their resolution. The final rung is that of community empowerment, in which members of the community or larger population group have achieved control over decisions and resources that affect their lives and engage in social and political action to exercise that control (Laverack, 2007).

Another model for approaching community empowerment is the Asset-based Community Development, or ABCD, model (Leech & Potts, 2010). This model builds on existing community strengths or assets and provides an inherent challenge to power hierarchies by putting the community in charge. An asset-based orientation also addresses frequent assumptions by community members that government agencies have and control the resources needed to address identified community problems. Such assumptions fail to recognize the existence of agency deficits that impede problem resolution and lead to dismissal of available community resources that might be brought to bear in the solution of community problems.

Steps in the ABCD model include recognition and identification of community strengths and building on those strengths and existing social capital to address problems (Leech & Potts, 2010). Identification of strengths might occur through the process of asset mapping in which the resources, skills, and capacities of individual community members are determined. For example, some members of the community might possess child care skills that could assist in the development of needed child care services for employed women. Community organizations may also possess resources and capabilities that can be used to solve community problems. For example, unused space in a church might be converted into a teen center with activities to discourage gang membership or drug and alcohol use.

Asset-based community development has several additional advantages beyond identifying assets that might be employed to resolve community problems. Working from a strengths orientation can increase collective beliefs in community competency and increase community perceptions of self-efficacy. In addition, just the process of asset mapping may increase public discussion and awareness of community issues and promote cooperation among members of the population. Finally, an asset-based approach portrays community members, community organizations, and government agencies as cooperative elements of the same community that represent mutual assets and avoids perceptions of the community as a "special needy population dependent on . . . an outside supplier of resources" (Leech & Potts, 2010, p. 82).

The natural helper model employs a particular type of community asset to address specific types of health-related problems. This model focuses on the use of natural helpers within the community to promote community empowerment. *Natural helpers* are "individuals who are naturally sought out for advice, assistance, and emotional support by community members." These natural helpers "possess the knowledge and tools that help foster health within their community" (Scott, 2009, p. 285). Several other types of informal helpers may exist as assets in a community. Among these are family, friends, and neighbors, role-related helpers, people with similar problems, and volunteers. The role of friends, family, and neighbors as informal helpers is well understood. Role-related helpers are people who, because of their role in the community, can provide help in certain circumstances. For example, educated shopkeepers could assist clients to make healthy food choices or could be sources of information and referral in other health-related areas. People who have similar kinds of problems can form self-help and support groups and share group resources, knowledge, and skills. Volunteers are people who are willing to contribute their time and energy to specific initiatives or program efforts. Natural and informal helpers are not the same as community health workers (CHWs), who are members of a community with some training hired by community agencies to work directly with their fellow residents. We will discuss the use of community members as health workers later in this chapter.

Population Health Nursing and Community Empowerment

The process of community empowerment is very similar to the nursing process. In this chapter, we will address some of the aspects of that process, focusing on the population health nurse's role in community empowerment and assessment, planning, implementation strategies, and evaluation of empowerment initiatives.

The Population Health Nurse's Role in Fostering Empowerment

Population health nurses and other health care professionals who desire to foster empowerment among individuals, organizations, communities, and population groups first need to foster perceptions of themselves as partners with community members and as an asset possessed by the community or population. This requires health professionals to recognize and shift power relationships with community members to move away from "professionally dominated decision making" to decision making by group members (Aston et al., 2009, p. 25). Leech and Potts (2010) were quite explicit in noting that failure by population health nurses and other professionals to self-identify as community assets supports a power hierarchy, in which the professional is seen as an expert and an employee of an institution or agency rather than as an active and equal member of the community.

Laverack (2005) described three primary roles of population health nurses and others in fostering empowerment. The first role involves becoming a more effective communicator who engages in listening, assists others to talk, gives advice, and obtains feedback. Some of the tasks involved in this role include providing information, increasing community members' understanding of the underlying causes of their lack of power, and combining media channels to foster communication. Such media channels might include one-on-one discussions with community members, use of printed materials, and use of population-specific and mass media.

The second major role of the empowering health care professional is increasing the critical self-awareness of members of the community. This may involve mapping positions of power, ranking complex issues, and developing decision-making skills. Mapping positions of power includes developing an understanding of how community members can build a power base from their existing positions of strength, identifying areas under their control, and identifying strategies for increasing their power (Laverack, 2005). For example, labor unions learned early on that they had the ability to influence business and industry through their power to stop production. This knowledge gives them power even when they choose not to exercise it through a strike. Just the possibility of a strike confers power and influence.

Fostering an empowering provider–client relationship is the third major role of the empowering health care professional. Such relationships can be fostered with individual clients as well as between professionals and communities or population groups. Activities involved in fostering empowering relationships include clearly defining and communicating the role of the professional to the client, promoting individual and group clients to political leaders, fostering support for community leaders and community organizations, serving as a liaison in the creation of new partnerships with other organizations and the private sector, facilitating change through skills training of community members, and facilitating the involvement of marginalized groups within the community or population (Laverack, 2005).

Empowering professionals may also engage in three other activities designed to empower communities. These include direction, facilitation, and collaboration, each of which occurs in a particular time period (Laverack, 2007). Initially, the health care professional may provide community members with direction in what needs to be done and how it may be accomplished. As the community or population becomes more competent, the population health nurse may shift into a facilitative role, asking questions and assisting community members to determine what they want to do and how they want to do it. Finally, the empowering professional may engage in collaboration with community members to bring about social and political changes, gradually relinquishing control of activities to community agents.

Assessing Community Strengths and Needs

Community assessment, in the context of community empowerment, has two general purposes. The first is to provide information for change—facts about the current situation, contributing factors, and assets that may be brought to bear to facilitate change. The second purpose is to provide information for empowerment. As the old adage states, "knowledge is power," and communities need knowledge in order to assess the situation and take action (Hancock & Minkler, 2012). The same elements of community assessment data can contribute to the achievement of both purposes. Community assessment may also result in several other indirect effects for community empowerment, including the creation of social cohesion among community members, encouragement of self-help within the community, persuasion for change, and identification and development of local leadership.

The actual assessment of the community can be framed in terms of the determinants of health from the population health nursing model, examining factors in each of the six categories of determinants that reflect community assets or contribute to community needs. The specifics of such an assessment are addressed in detail in Chapter 15∞. Some of the areas that might be examined in a community empowerment assessment include 16 elements of community strength and six dimensions of culture (Bartle, 2013). These elements of strength and dimensions of culture are described in Table 10-1•.

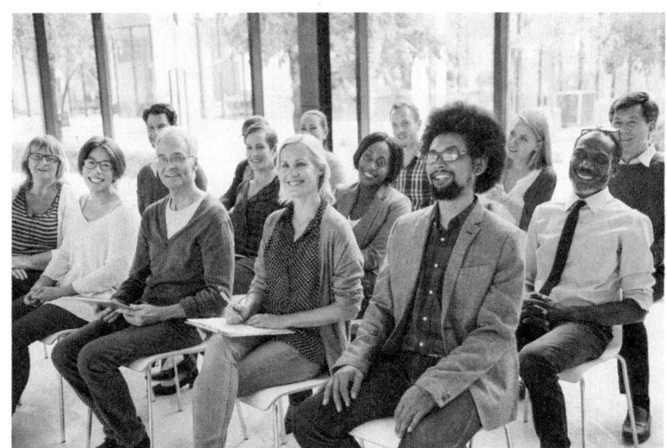

Town hall meetings can foster community empowerment.
(Rawpixel/Shutterstock)

Population health nurses can help members of the community to conduct an assessment as a first step in community empowerment. For example, the nurse can assist community members to identify relevant categories and sources of data needed and to develop effective data collection strategies. In addition, the nurse can help community members analyze assessment data and identify factors that impede and facilitate community empowerment. Clark et al. (2003) provided an example of a population health nurse facilitating resident involvement in a community assessment. In this process, the population health nurse assisted community members to conduct focus groups among multiple segments of the community to identify community needs and assets. The findings of the assessment were shared with the wider community and became the impetus for a variety of community-initiated efforts to improve living conditions in the community.

Planning and Implementing Empowerment Strategies

Community empowerment is most effective when it employs a planned and systematic process based on fundamental principles. In this portion of the chapter, we will discuss the principles of effective community empowerment, goals of community empowerment, issue selection, the process of group development as a foundation for community empowerment, and strategies that can be employed by population health nurses to facilitate community empowerment.

TABLE 10-1 Elements of Strength and Dimensions of Culture in Community Empowerment Assessment

Element of Strength	Description
Altruism	The extent to which community members are willing to sacrifice personal goals to achieve group goals
Common values	The extent to which values are shared among group members
Communal services	The extent of group members' access to needed services and facilities
Communication	The degree of willingness and ability to communicate effectively
Confidence	The degree of shared confidence in the group's ability to solve problems
Context • Political • Administrative • Approach	The existence of an environment that supports empowerment • Attitudes and values of political leaders • Attitudes and values of adminstrative agents • An approach in which needs are provided weakens groups, whereas an approach that enables people to provide for their own needs strengthens the group
Information	Access to and abilities to process and analyze information; level of knowledge; and the degree of wisdom among key individuals
Intervention focus	Extent of focus on increasing or decreasing dependency and levels of internal sustainability without external assistance
Leadership	The power of community leaders to influence and move the community in desired directions
Networking	The extent of existing links to useful resources
Organization	Perceptions of group members of their role in supporting the activities of the whole
Political power	The extent of participation and influence in decision making
Skills	The extent of abilities to get things done, including technical and management skills of group members
Trust	The degree of trust among group members
Unity	The degree of shared sense of belonging among group members
Wealth	The extent of community control over actual and potential resources, as well as their production and distribution
Dimension of Culture	**Description**
Technological dimension	Ideas and behaviors that allow community members to invent, use, and teach others about tools, including elements such as language, material resources, and community infrastructure (e.g., roads, sewers, etc.). Changes in this dimension result in changes in each of the other five dimensions
Economic dimension	• Ideas and behaviors that give value to cash • Ways and means of producing and allocating goods and services • Distribution of wealth, how and by whom
Political dimension	Ways of allocating power and influence • Types of leaders in community • Extent of member participation and ways of promoting participation in decision making • Mechanisms and changes in the distribution of power and influence
Institutional dimension	Ways in which people interact and are expected to interact
Values dimension	The community structure of ideas about good/bad, beautiful/ugly, and right/wrong
Worldview dimension	The population's world view, ideas about the nature of the universe and their place in it, cause and effect, and conceptions of time, matter, and behavior

Data from: Bartle, P. (2008). The human factor and community empowerment. *Review of Human Factor Studies Special Edition, 14*(1), 99–122; Bartle, P. (2013). *Community Empowerment Collective Society.* Retrieved from http://cec.vcn.bc.ca/cmp/collect.htm

PRINCIPLES OF COMMUNITY EMPOWERMENT. Effective community empowerment is based on several general principles that are summarized in the box on the next page.

DOMAINS OF COMMUNITY EMPOWERMENT. Four key domains or goals of empowerment have been identified. These domains include the following:

- Community activation: Promoting community members' participation in community problem solving.
- Competence development: Developing community members' expertise in problem solving.
- Program management skill development: Fostering program management and team-building skills among community members; promoting skill in planning, implementation, and evaluation methods; and promoting use of evidence-based solutions and strategies.
- Creation of a supportive environment: Developing lobbying and political advocacy skills and linking community groups to resources (Kasmel & Tanggaard, 2011).

ISSUE SELECTION. It may be helpful, and more meaningful for community members, to initiate community empowerment activities in the context of a specific health problem or issue. Hopefully, community empowerment engendered in the context of this particular issue will carry over to promote community action with respect to other issues. There may be any number of issues that can be used to foster community empowerment, but there are some criteria that might lead members of a community to select one issue over others.

The issue should be one that can be clearly articulated and explained by community members to give them confidence in presenting their case to policy makers. The issue should also be one that will serve to unite community members and foster their participation in its resolution. In addition, the issue should promote the visibility and credibility of the community or representative groups as entities who should be involved in decision making. Other criteria include the degree of consistency of the issue with the long-range goals of the community and have the potential to promote growth and capacity building in the community. To this end, the issue should provide opportunities for leadership development among community members. Other considerations include the effect of work related to the issue of community or organizational resources and assets and the potential of the issue for creating either new allies or enemies for the community. In addition, the issue should focus on an area for direct action and have significant potential for a positive outcome. The criteria for selection of an issue to promote community empowerment are reflected in the *Focused Assessment* presented below.

GROUP DEVELOPMENT. Engaging in community empowerment activities may necessitate the formation of effective groups or organizations within the community to spearhead empowerment initiatives. Group development occurs in a series of stages: orientation, accommodation, negotiation, operation, and dissolution, sometimes also labeled as forming, norming, storming, performing, and termination or ending (Stein, n.d.). These stages parallel the components of the nursing process, as indicated in Table 10-2●. Specific tasks must be accomplished during each stage of group development for the group to function effectively.

Highlights

Principles of Community Empowerment

- Holders of power must want the community to be more self-reliant and must be willing to cede power to community members.
- A trained facilitator is needed to guide the community in its efforts to be more self-reliant.
- Assistance should be offered in the form of a collaborative partnership rather than charity and should be designed to promote increased self-reliance and capacity in the community.
- Empowerment starts where community members are and does not try to force change on the community.
- Struggle and adversity strengthen social organizations and communities when they are overcome through community activity.
- Hands-on participation in decision making and problem resolution increases problem-solving capabilities. Decisions need to be made by community members, not for them by others, however well-intentioned.
- The community should supply a substantial portion of the resources needed for problem resolution or project implemenation to promote long-term sustainability.
- Community empowerment activities should be designed from the beginning to achieve the ultimate goal of community control of and responsibility for decision making and actions taken.

Data from: Bartle, P. (2013). *Community empowerment collective society.* Retrieved from http://cec.vcn.bc.ca/cmp/collect.htm

FOCUSED ASSESSMENT Selecting an Issue for Community Empowerment

- Is the issue simply and easily explained by community members?
- Will the issue unite community members and involve them in problem resolution?
- Does the issue provide greater visibility and credibility for the community or for the organizing group within the community?
- Is the issue consistent with the long-range goals of the community or organization?
- Does the issue have potential for promoting growth of the group?
- Will the issue provide educational or training experiences for community leaders?
- How will the issue affect community or organizational resources?
- Does the issue have potential for creating new community allies? New enemies?
- Does the issue focus on direct action?
- Will the issue result in victory?

Data from: Minkler, M., & Wallerstein, N. (2012). Improving health through community organization and community building. In M. Minkler (Ed.), *Community organizing and community building for health and welfare* (3rd ed., pp. 37–58). New Brunswick, NJ: Rutgers University Press; Staples, L. (2012). Selecting and cutting the issue. In M. Minkler (Ed.), *Community organizing and community building for health and welfare* (3rd ed., pp. 187–214). New Brunswick, NJ: Rutgers University Press.

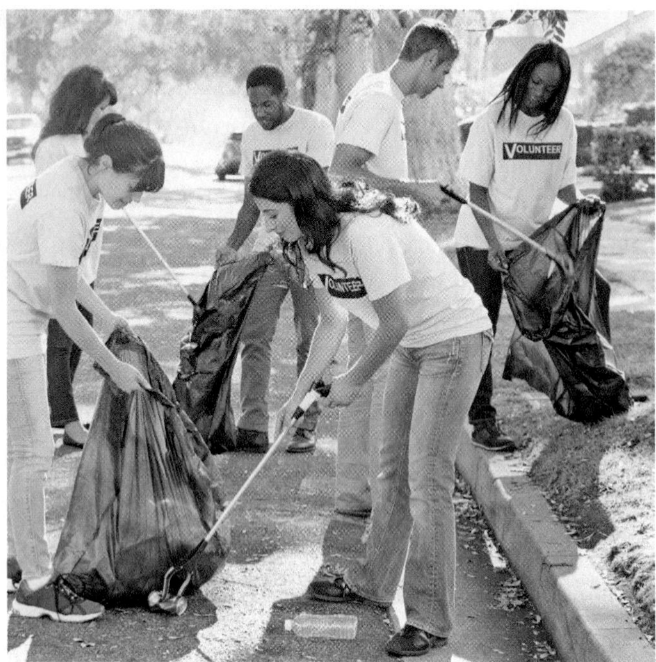

Empowered communities are able to deal with local problems.
(Monkey Business Images/Shutterstock)

Orientation. The orientation stage of group development, sometimes referred to as the "forming stage," is when group members come to know each other and assess their ability to function as a group. Tasks of this stage include selection of group members, training them for group participation, and identification of group goals and purposes. Also during this stage, the group assesses community empowerment needs and community assets.

Accommodation. The accommodation (or "norming") stage of group development focuses on the development of group dynamics, the ways in which the group will carry out its group-related functions. This does not relate to activities the group will undertake to resolve any identified community issues, but to the ways in which the group itself will operate. Tasks in this stage include developing an atmosphere conducive to group collaboration and establishing modes of group decision making, conflict resolution, and communication.

Group action requires group decisions, and decisions must be made after careful consideration by group members. To facilitate decision making, group members should agree on the method by which decisions will be made. Because most people are not familiar with group processes or the deliberate need to select a decision-making strategy, the population health nurse may need to guide the group in this task. Decisions can be made in one of six ways: by default, by the leader, by a subgroup, by majority vote, by consensus, or by unanimous consent. For the purposes of community empowerment, majority vote, consensus, and unanimous consent are the most appropriate methods of group decision making.

Establishing modes of group conflict resolution is the second task in the accommodation stage of group development. Breakdowns in the decision-making process are one source of conflict within the group. Other potential sources of conflict are unclear expectations, poor communication, differing values or attitudes, and competition for scarce resources. Lack of clear jurisdiction among group members and conflicts of interest may also be sources of conflict within the group. Additional sources of conflict are interdependence when needs are not met and the existence of prior unresolved conflict between members or subgroups.

Conflict is a normal component of group effort and is to be expected. In fact, many group behavior theorists include a conflict or "storming" stage in describing the development of groups over time. If the group has developed mechanisms for conflict resolution before conflicts arise, conflict can often be a positive rather than divisive experience for the group.

TABLE 10-2 Tasks of Group Development by Stage and Related Nursing Process Component

Nursing Process Component	Stage of Group Development	Group Development Tasks
Assessment and diagnosis	Orientation (forming)	1. Selection of group members 2. Training for group participation 3. Identification of goals and purposes
Planning	Accommodation (norming)	1. Establishment of modes of decision making 2. Development of mechanisms for conflict resolution 3. Development of communication network 4. Development of climate conducive to group collaboration
	Negotiation (norming)	1. Negotiation of member roles 2. Development of methods of task assignment
Implementation	Operation (performing)	1. Assignment of specific tasks to accomplish group goals 2. Performance of actions to accomplish goals
Evaluation	Dissolution (leaving)	1. Planning of evaluative mechanisms 2. Assignment of member roles and tasks in evaluation 3. Data collection 4. Analysis of evaluative findings 5. Possible group dissolution

Recognition of conflict as a normal phenomenon is essential if the group is to plan ahead for conflict resolution. Again, many groups do not anticipate conflict, and when conflict occurs they are unprepared to deal with it. Strategies for resolving conflict constructively involve creating a climate conducive to discussion, identifying and eliminating sources of conflict, capitalizing on areas of agreement, and rationally considering alternative solutions to conflict. The population health nurse can explore these approaches to conflict resolution with members of the group and assist members to select the most appropriate approach.

Creating a climate in which disagreement is acceptable can minimize or resolve conflict. Conflict resolution requires that all parties be fully able to express their perspectives through open communication. Open communication cannot take place when there is pressure to conform and there is the lack of acceptance of different opinions. Lack of communication hampers conflict resolution as well as contributing to conflict. As a group leader, the population health nurse may need to encourage group members to express thoughts and opinions that may not be congruent with those of other members. Through the use of interpersonal skills, the nurse can ensure that communications within the group are not accusatory, but deal with issues rather than personalities.

Recognizing the existence of conflict and identifying its sources and possible solutions are strategies for constructive use of conflict. A conflict that is ignored in the hope that it will resolve itself is likely to become worse. The population health nurse can encourage other group members to acknowledge that a conflict exists and help them explore the reasons for conflict. Again, the nurse should be alert to covert signs of conflict and bring them to the attention of the rest of the group. For example, a nurse working with a group trying to determine budget allocations among health care programs within the county may notice that representatives of programs for the elderly are maintaining a stony silence during the discussion. The nurse may comment on the fact that they have not participated in the discussion and ask why. In the ensuing discussion, it may be learned that these group members feel that too much money is being allocated to maternal–child health programs and that the elderly are being shortchanged. Once this conflict has been exposed, the group can begin work to resolve it.

Another strategy for resolving conflict involves identifying small areas of trust and agreement between group members that can be expanded. For example, although two group members may disagree on the "appropriate" approach to a problem, they can capitalize on their shared concern for clients' welfare. Finally, rational consideration of alternative solutions to a particular conflict using the group's decision-making and problem-solving processes can result in conflict becoming a valuable learning experience in group problem solving. The population health nurse can assist the group to explore a variety of alternative solutions to a conflict and to select an approach that is agreeable to all members.

Developing group communication strategies is another task in planning group operation. The importance of an effective communication network cannot be overemphasized. The group must develop a common language that facilitates communication, and members should refrain from using jargon familiar only to members of their own discipline. When it is necessary to use terminology unfamiliar to others, efforts should be made to translate it into the common language. The nurse in this situation can either play the part of the translator or ask other members for clarification. For example, some members of a group may use acronyms unfamiliar to others, such as CMS. The nurse should then explain to the group that this stands for the Centers for Medicare and Medicaid Services. If the nurse does not recognize the acronym, he or she can ask for an explanation of its meaning.

The group should also agree on the forms that communication will take. For example, communications may be verbal, written, or a combination of both, depending on the situation. Perhaps the group will decide that communication with sponsoring institutions should take the form of formal written memoranda, whereas communications between group members should be more informal verbal messages.

Consideration should also be given to the fact that communication takes place outside of regular group sessions. The content of these informal encounters between group members should not undermine group function or provide a forum for airing grievances or denigrating other members. The population health nurse who encounters unproductive communication outside of group meetings can bring relevant issues to the attention of the entire group, so open discussion can take place and conflict can be avoided or resolved.

Establishing a climate in which group members feel respected and in which differences are accepted contributes to an effective communication network. This means that all group members should be encouraged to participate and should receive positive reinforcement for their contribution whether or not others agree with it. In the beginning of the group's operation, the nurse group leader may need to ask reluctant group members for their ideas and opinions. As their participation is received positively, they will begin to volunteer remarks.

Negotiation. Tasks of the negotiation stage of group development include role negotiation and methods of task assignment. Professional roles often overlap, and role negotiation is crucial to effective group function. In addition, social change professionals working in a community empowerment context need to be careful not to usurp roles that should be performed by community members. The goal of community organizing and empowerment is to develop leadership within the community, not to provide that leadership. When two or more group members possess similar skills, the group must decide who will be responsible for exercising those skills. These decisions may be made as a general rule of thumb, so that one member always has responsibility for certain activities, or may change with the needs of the situation.

One particular group role that must be negotiated is the role of the leader. This position incorporates functions related to group administration, liaison with outside groups, teaching, and coordination of group effort. Additional group leadership roles may include providing information for group decision making, clarifying issues, refocusing the group's attention, and playing "devil's advocate" to promote exploration of alternative ideas. The leadership role may be assigned to one member, may shift with the situation, or may reside with the group as a whole. In the last instance, no one member acts as the leader and leadership functions are performed by the group as a unit. Ideally, as community empowerment progresses, group leadership is assumed by members of the community rather than by helping professionals.

Operation and dissolution. The operation stage of group development is analogous to the implementation stage of the nursing process. It is during this stage that the group assigns and performs specific roles and tasks to achieve group-designated goals and objectives.

The dissolution stage of group development focuses on evaluation of the group's accomplishments and decisions regarding the continuation or dissolution of the group. Depending on the focus of group empowerment initiatives, the group may shift its focus to address other community issues after achieving its original purpose. Or it may dissolve to reform with other participants to address additional issues. Tasks of the dissolution stage of group development include planning evaluative mechanisms related to both the process and outcomes of community empowerment, assignment of member roles in evaluation, data collection and analysis, and dissemination of findings. Evaluation of community empowerment activities will be discussed in more detail later in this chapter.

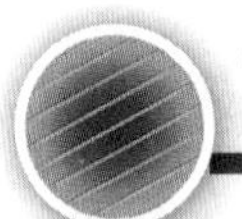

Evidence-Based Practice

Supporting Community Empowerment

In 2008, the Department for Communities and Local Government (Pratchett et al., 2009) commissioned a systematic review of the evidence base supporting community empowerment. The review focused on three aspects of the effects of empowerment initiatives: effects on individual participants, effects on communities, and effects on decision making. Individual effects included development of personal skills in influencing local services. Community effects examined such things as improved levels of political efficacy, social capital, and social cohesiveness. Finally, decision-making effects included the ability of individuals and communities to influence decision making.

The review identified six mechanisms for promoting community empowerment: asset transfer, citizen governance, electronic participation, participatory budgeting, petitions, and redress. Asset transfer referred to a mechanism for promoting community management or ownership of community assets and social enterprises. This particular strategy was found to be effective in achieving public control over decision making and assets, but required ongoing support to prevent setting communities up for failure and overburdening volunteer staff.

Citizen governance strategies involved incorporation of community residents on decision-making boards and forums that make public policy decisions. The success of this strategy depends on the openness of policy makers to attend to citizen input. Electronic participation through e-forums and petitions was an effective means of empowerment for segments of the population who took part in them, but were limited in their ability to effect empowerment at the wider community level.

Participatory budgeting involves citizen participation in the development of budgets and allocation of resources. This strategy is capable of achieving wide levels of empowerment, but requires willingness to engage in transformational political change. Petitions serve to raise policy makers' awareness of community concerns. When petitions are attended to and community members can see specific effects, they can be empowering; when they are ignored, they may become disempowering.

Finally, redress is a mechanism for community members to voice complaints that are investigated and responded to. Because complaints are usually unrelated to formal decision-making processes, they are unlikely to result in widespread community empowerment. Each of the strategies was found to result in some level of empowerment, primarily at the level of the individual citizen. Only the citizen governance and participatory budgeting strategies were consistently associated with a community empowerment effect (Pratchett et al., 2009).

Although there are a number of reports on the results of community empowerment initiatives in resolving community problems, less research has been done on their effectiveness in actually empowering communities and increasing their abilities to be self-determining and self-reliant. This lack limits the evidence base for strategies that work or do not work in promoting community empowerment.

1. What community empowerment strategies, if any, have been initiated in your community?
2. To what extent has the effectiveness of those strategies in promoting empowerment been evaluated?
3. How might you go about evaluating those strategies in terms of their effects on community empowerment, thereby contributing to the evidence base for the effectiveness of community empowerment in helping communities address health disparities?

STRATEGIES FOR PROMOTING COMMUNITY EMPOWERMENT. Implementation of community empowerment activities encompasses the basic principles of implementing any community program. These principles will be discussed in detail in Chapter 15∞. Here, we will briefly address some general strategies to foster empowerment.

Members of the community should be involved in all aspects of community empowerment initiatives from identification of the problem or issue to be addressed, to development of objectives or expected outcomes to be achieved, to development of strategic approaches to achieve those outcomes, to management of everyday implementation of the campaign, and to evaluation of its effectiveness. Table 10-3● indicates some of the skills required of community members in each of these areas of involvement. Population health nurses and other empowering professionals may be instrumental in assisting community members to develop these skills.

Studies of population health nurses in their role of community empowerment have identified the need to work *with* rather than *for* community members (Aston et al., 2009). This requires a shift in perspective for both community members and nurses from seeing the nurse as an expert to viewing him or her as a community resource and partner. Interviews with population health nurses elicited four major strategies for empowering communities employed by the nurses. These included building trusting relationships, building community members' confidence and skill, engaging in empowering educational strategies, and connecting individuals and groups to broader social networks (Aston et al., 2009).

TABLE 10-3 Skills Required for Stages of Involvement in Community Empowerment Initiatives

Activity Stage	Requisite Skills
Problem identification	• Literature review • Analysis of epidemiologic data • Identification of community needs • Appraisal of program design
Objective development	• Development of objectives for problem resolution • Development of empowerment
Strategy development to empower individuals, groups, and communities	• Materials development • Knowledge of relevant models and theories • Interpersonal communication • Workshop/meeting facilitation • Effective group and public presentation
Management by the community	• Fund-raising • Budgeting • Resource procurement • Human resource management • Managing consultant input
Evaluation	• Designing evaluation methodology • Developing evaluation questions • Analyzing evaluation data • Interpreting and presenting findings

Activities involved in building relationships included active listening, belief in the capacity of community members to guide their own destiny, a focus on strengths, and creation of a safe environment that fosters community participation in decision making. The strategy of building confidence and skills involved promoting active participation in decision making by marginalized populations and actively soliciting their input and participation. Other activities related to this strategy included starting from and building on community members' strengths, giving positive feedback and affirmation, and engaging in a constant shifting of roles for the nurse and pulling back as community members became more competent (Aston et al., 2009).

Use of empowering educational strategies involved roles as consultants and as process-focused educators. As consultants, the nurses shared information with community members. In the role of process-focused educators, they asked questions to stimulate thought, provided information, and discussed possible next steps in the resolution of community problems. Finally, the nurses connected community members, both individuals and groups, with broader social networks. Activities related to this strategy included building partnerships among groups, establishing self-help groups, connecting to other agencies, and advocating for community needs. Other activities included linking agencies together and working collaboratively with multiple sectors of the community to assist community members to achieve desired outcomes (Aston et al., 2009).

The nurses also identified constraints to their practice in empowering communities. These included a lack of funding for empowerment efforts, lack of visibility, and lack of understanding of the nurses' role in empowerment by politicians, the general public, and public health nurse managers. Other constraints included competing demands for limited time and conflicting responsibilities for mandated programs such as immunizations, increased paperwork drawing them away from active participation in communities, and a limited presence at planning tables (Aston et al., 2009). Population health nurses may need to actively advocate for their role in community empowerment, study the effects of that role, and discover ways to combine that role with other mandated responsibilities.

Evaluating Community Empowerment

Evaluation of community empowerment is another area that should involve community members as participants in all phases, from conceptualizing the evaluation, to data collection and analysis, to dissemination and use of evaluative findings. Community participation in evaluation helps to continue to build community competence while assessing the outcomes of prior activities. **Participatory evaluation** is a process in which "the stakeholders themselves are responsible for collecting and analyzing the information and for generating recommendations for change" (World Bank, 2011, para. 2). As early as

1997, the United Nations Development Programme (UNDP) recommended participatory evaluation for the assessment of the effectiveness of international programming. In their program evaluation handbook, they noted that "project stakeholders and beneficiaries are the key actors of the evaluation process and not the mere objects of the evaluation" (1997, p. 1).

Participatory evaluation has several benefits. Some of these advantages are presented in the *Highlights* box below.

Considerations in participatory evaluation, a form of participatory action research, include questions of who participates in the evaluation and to what degree, who determines the issues to be addressed, how to engage participation by community members, and the power dynamics between researchers and community members. Obviously, it would be unwieldy for the entire community to participate in the design and conduct of an evaluation of empowerment initiatives, so community leaders and empowering professionals should determine what segments of the community should be involved and what that involvement should constitute. Broad input from community members beyond those actually involved in conducting the evaluation should be solicited, however, in determining what issues or questions should be addressed.

Engaging the participation of community members in participatory evaluation may be difficult for a number of reasons. In their work with youth, Checkoway and Richards-Schuster (n.d.) identified a number of barriers to participation that are applicable to other members of the community as well. First, people may not have time to be involved in the time-consuming process of evaluation, and they may be frustrated by lack of expertise in evaluation methods. Health care professionals and others may view community residents as passive recipients of services rather than as active participants in the development and evaluation of services and the policies that support them. In addition, both community members and professionals may view evaluation as an area that requires special expertise. Finally, local authorities may not want to share the power embodied in evaluation with community members. This last barrier may also be reflected in different perspectives of power and control between community members and researchers assisting with the evaluation. Population health nurses can assist in eliminating these barriers to participation by planning evaluation activities to fit community members' schedules, fostering varying levels of participation, and educating community members in the process of evaluation. In addition, they can advocate with authority figures for community involvement in evaluation.

Steps in participatory or empowering evaluation are similar to those in any evaluation process except that community participation is integral in each step. The basic steps are: (a) framing the scope and focus of the evaluation, (b) developing an organizational structure to support evaluation activities, (c) determining the evaluation questions to be asked, (d) gathering information to address the questions asked, (e) analyzing the information and making some sense of it, (f) sharing information with others, and (g) taking action based on evaluation findings (Checkoway & Richards-Schuster, n.d.; Rabinowitz, 2013). Each of these steps will be explored in more detail in Chapter 15∞. For further information about participatory action research as it relates to community empowerment, see the resources provided in the External Resources section of the student resources site.

In the context of community empowerment, both the outcomes of a specific initiative and the extent of community empowerment achieved should be evaluated. For example, the evaluation might focus on the health outcomes achieved through community activity (e.g., the decrease in accident fatalities resulting from community advocacy for traffic-calming interventions such as speed bumps in residential areas) and the level of community empowerment reached.

The extent of empowerment achieved can be evaluated in terms of each of the four domains of empowerment. These domains and related evaluation questions are presented in Table 10-4•.

A final measure of the effectiveness of community empowerment efforts would be the extent to which community members are included in policy making. The ultimate goal of effective community organizing and empowerment should be the inclusion of community members in every aspect of policy making. Studies of community empowerment initiatives have demonstrated increases in preventive behaviors among

Highlights

Advantages of Participatory Evaluation

- It provides a perspective on the needs of project beneficiaries and the effectiveness of interventions.
- It facilitates information gathering from salient stakeholders.
- It highlights what did and did not work from the perspective of community members.
- It can help to explain why something did or did not work.
- It empowers community members and provides a voice for those who may frequently be unheard.
- It teaches skills useful in other endeavors.
- It fosters self-efficacy and self-confidence in community members.
- It provides an example of ways in which community members can take control of their lives.
- It encourages community ownership of activities and initiatives.
- It can foster creativity in thinking and problem resolution.
- It facilitates collaborative activity.
- It fits into a larger participatory effort and fosters overall community empowerment.

Data from: Rabinowitz, P. (2013). *Participatory evaluation.* Retrieved from http://ctb.ku.edu/en/table-of-contents/evaluate/evaluation/participatory-evaluation/main

TABLE 10-4 Domains of Community Empowerment and Potential Evaluation Questions

Domain	Potential Evaluation Questions
Community activation	• To what extent have community members increased their participation in small groups and organizations designed to take action on community problems? • To what extent have new community participants been engaged in problem resolution? • To what extent have new community networks or or groups been established? • To what extent is the community able to engage in critical assessment of causes of inequities and powerlessness?
Community competence development	• To what extent is the community able to identify community problems and possible solutions? • How effective is the community in disseminating information to improve community members' understanding of issues and potential solutions?
Program management skill development	• To what extent has local community leadership been developed? • To what extent are local leaders able to foster community participation, facilitate problem resolution, resolve conflict, and so on? • To what extent are effective communication strategies used within the community? • To what extent are community members able to identify and evaluate evidence-based solutions to problems?
Supportive environment development	• To what extent has the community developed organizational structures that facilitate participation in decision making, effectively mobilize and allocate resources, and so on? • To what extent is the community able to mobilize both internal and external resources? • To what extent are community members able to effectively lobby and advocate for political support or needed resources? • To what extent are community assets and existing resources brought to bear to solve identified problems? • To what extent have internal links between individuals or organizations within the community been developed or strengthened? • To what extent have links to external organizations been created or strengthened? • To what extent have power relationships with outside entities been equalized? • To what extent has the community been able to exercise control of decisions and resource allocations affecting the welfare of its members?

community members and better intersectoral coordination of health promotion efforts (Sanchez et al., 2009), changes in attitudes and skills at individual levels, improvement in cross-cultural relationships, and awareness of a need for involvement in social leadership at broader levels (Tsey et al., 2010). In addition, some studies have shown changes in the attitudes and behaviors of governmental organizations and agencies. As noted by one group, "just as citizens honed their civic skills and vociferously pressed their views, government developed a culture of responding to and learning from, rather than rejecting, many grassroots initiatives" (Putnam & Feldstein, as quoted in New Laboratories of Democracy, 2009, p. 3).

CHAPTER RECAP

Empowerment is a strategy used by population health nurses and others to promote self-advocacy among individuals, organizations, communities, and populations. The ultimate goal of empowerment is to allow people to assume control over the decisions that affect their health and well-being. Empowerment begins where community members are, moves them toward the goal of political and social action on their own behalf, and involves the development of discreet skills as well as feelings of self-confidence and self-efficacy. Empowerment activities can occur within the context of the nursing process moving from enhancing community assessment capabilities to planning, implementing, and evaluating empowerment activities. Empowerment initiatives often begin with a focus on a discrete issue or problem, but the lessons learned can lead to greater community involvement in wider social and political action.

CASE STUDY Indigent Health Care

You have been given a referral to visit Mrs. Esparza, who lost her baby after a premature delivery. The address you have been given is located in a poor neighborhood that houses a large number of migrant workers. When you arrive at the home, you discover that it is a two-bedroom apartment occupied by three couples and their five children. Both Mrs. Esparza and her husband are present when you arrive, and both are obviously grieving the loss of their third child. In talking with them, you discover that Mrs. Esparza did not receive any prenatal care and was admitted to the delivery unit of the local hospital after going to the emergency room when she experienced heavy contractions in the 29th week of her pregnancy. Mr. Esparza becomes angry when you ask about prenatal care, shouting that they tried to get an appointment at the health department's prenatal clinic but were told there was a 2-month wait for new appointments. At that time Mrs. Esparza was in the fifth month of her pregnancy. In tears, he informs you that they did not have the money to see a private doctor. Even though most of the migrant workers are in the United States legally, they are not eligible for any financial assistance. Your state does not provide Medicaid pregnancy coverage for nonresident women. Mrs. Esparza reminds her husband that they are not alone in their suffering. When you inquire further into her comment, she tells you that seven other women in the apartment complex have lost babies at some point in their pregnancies in the last 2 years. You comfort the family as best you can, make arrangements for Mrs. Esparza to receive a postpartum examination at the health department, and refer the three families to the immunization clinic because all of the children in the home are behind on their immunizations. You explain that both postpartum services and immunizations are free to those who do not have money to pay for them, even for nonresidents.

When you return to the office, fellow population health nurses describe similar visits to families in the area. In checking county vital statistics, you note that the census track where the Esparzas live and two adjacent areas that house large migrant populations have a fetal death rate three times that of the rest of the county.

1. How would you begin to empower the migrant worker community to address the issue of lack of access to prenatal care?
2. What assets might you look for within the migrant community to address the issue?
3. What allies might you find in the nonmigrant community to assist you?
4. How can you motivate participation by community members in the initiative?

REFERENCES

Aston, M., Meagher-Stewart, D., Edwards, N., & Young, L. M. (2009). Public health nurses' primary care practice: Strategies for fostering citizen participation. *Journal of Community Health Nursing, 26,* 24–34. doi:10.1080/07370010802605762

Bailey, N. (2010). Understanding community empowerment in urban regeneration and planning in England: Putting policy and practice in context. *Planning, Practice and Research, 25,* 317–332. doi:10.1080/02697459.2010.503425

Bartle, P. (2008). The human factor and community empowerment. *Review of Human Factor Studies Special Edition, 14*(1), 99–122.

Bartle, P. (2013). *Community Empowerment Collective Society.* Retrieved from http://cec.vcn.bc.ca/cmp/collect.htm

Burkett, I. (2013, Spring). Community to community empowerment: The story of the AusCongo Network. *Practice Insights, 2,* 6–8.

Checkoway, B., & Richards-Schuster, K. (n.d.). *Participatory evaluation with young people.* Retrieved from http://www.ssw.umich.edu/public/current-Projects/youthAndCommunity/pubs/youthbook.pdf

Clark, M. J., Cary, S., Diemert, G., Ceballos, R., Sifuentes, M., Atteberry, I., ..., Trieu, S. (2003). Involving communities in community assessment. *Public Health Nursing, 20,* 456–463.

Conrad, E. (n.d.). *General Tubman.* Retrieved from http://harriettubman.com/tubman2.html

Cooke, I. (2013, Spring). Community ownership: A catalyst for community-led regeneration. *Practice Insights, 2,* 4–5.

Craig, G., & Mayo, M. (2013, Spring). Reflections on two decades of "community empowerment." *Practice Insights, 2,* 16–17.

de Wit, J., & Berner, E. (2009). Progressive patronage? Municipalities, NGOs, CBOs and the limits to slum dwellers' empowerment. *Development and Change, 40,* 927–947. doi:10.1111/j.1467-7660.2009.01589.x

Driggs, M. B. (1980). *They called her Moses: Harriet Tubman.* Retrieved from http://harriettubman.com/callhermoses.html

Hancock, T., & Minkler, M. (2012). Community health assessment or healthy community assessment: Whose community? Whose health? Whose assessment? In M. Minkler (Ed.), *Community organizing and community building for health* and welfare (3rd ed., pp. 153–170). New Brunswick, NJ: Rutgers University Press.

Improvement and Development Agency. (2012). *Useful definitions.* Retrieved from http://www.idea.gov.uk/idk/core/page.do?pageId=16639526

International Association for Community Development. (2014). *About us.* Retrieved from http://www.iacdglobal.org/about

Kasmel, A., & Tanggaard, P. (2011). Conceptualizing organizational domains of community empowerment through empowerment evaluations in Estonian communities. *Societies, 1,* 3–29. doi: 10.3390/soc10100093

Laverack, G. (2005). *Public health: Power, empowerment, and professional practice.* New York: Palgrave Macmillan.

Laverack, G. (2007). *Health promotion practice: Building empowered communities.* New York, NY: Open University Press.

Leech, T. G. J., & Potts, E., Jr. (2010). Community empowerment through an academic product: Implications for the social-justice oriented scholar. *Journal of African American Studies, 14,* 75–86. doi:10.1007/s12111-009-9108-3

Lewis, J. J. (n.d.). *Harriet Tubman: From slavery to freedom.* Retrieved from http://womenshistory.about.com/od/harriettubman/a/tubman_slavery.htm

Maschi, B. (n.d.). *Harriett Tubman: Runaway slave, underground railroad conductor.* Retrieved from http://www.americancivilwar.com/women/harriet_tubman.html

Minkler, M., & Wallerstein, N. (2012). Improving health through community organization and community building. In M. Minkler (Ed.), *Community organizing and community building for health* and welfare (3rd ed., pp. 37–58). New Brunswick, NJ: Rutgers University Press.

Neighbor Works® America. (2014). *Neighbor works community building program.* Retrieved from http://www.nw.org/Network/neighborworksprogs/leadership/default.asp

New laboratories of democracy: How local government is reinventing civic engagement. Part 1: Structure and form. (2009). *National Civic Review, 98*(2), 3–8. doi:10.1002/ncr.245

New York History Net. (n.d.). *The life of Harriet Tubman.* Retrieved from http://www.nyhistory.com/harriettubman/life.htm

Pratchett, L., Durose, C., Lowndes, V., Smith, G., Stoker, G., & Wales, C. (2009). Empowering communities to influence local decision making: A systematic review of the evidence. *Benefits, 17,* 297–299.

Rabinowitz, P. (2013). *Participatory evaluation.* Retrieved from http://ctb.ku.edu/en/table-of-contents/evaluate/evaluation/participatory-evaluation/main

Sahlman, R. (2011). *Harriet Tubman.* Retrieved from http://incwell.com/Biographies/Tubman.html

Sanchez, L., Perez, D., Cruz, G., Castro, M., Kour, G., Shkedy, Z., …, Van der Stuyft, P. (2009). *Tropical Medicine & International Health, 14,* 1356–1364. doi:10.1111/j.1365-3156.2009.02379.x

Scott, T. N. (2009). Utilization of the natural helper model in health promotion targeting African American men. *Journal of Holistic Nursing, 27,* 282–292. doi:10.1177/0898010109339929

Staples, L. (2012). Selecting and cutting the issue. In M. Minkler (Ed.), *Community organizing and community building for health* and welfare (3rd ed., pp. 187–214). New Brunswick, NJ: Rutgers University Press.

Stein, J. (n.d.). *Using the stages of team development.* Retrieved from http://hrweb.mit.edu/learning-development/learning-topics/teams/articles/stages-development

Tsey, K., Whiteside, M., Haswell-Elkins, M., Bainbridge, R., Cadet-James, Y., & Wilson, A. (2010). Empowerment and indigenous Australian health: A synthesis of findings from Family Wellbeing formative research. *Health and Social Care in the Community, 18,* 169–179. doi:10.1111/j.1365-2524.2009.00885.x

United Nations Development Programme. (1997). *Who are the question-makers? A participatory evaluation handbook. Part II: Participatory evaluation.* Retrieved from http://www.undp.org/evaluation/documents/who.htm

Wiggins, N., Johnson, D., Avila, M., Farquhar, S. A., Michael, Y. L., Rios, T., & Lopez, A. (2009). Using popular education for community empowerment: Perspectives of community health workers in the *Poder es Salud*/Power for Health program. *Critical Public Health, 19*(1), 11–22. doi:10.1080/09581590802375855

World Bank. (2011). *Participatory methods.* Retrieved from http://web.worldbank.org/WBSITE/EXTERNAL/TOPICS/EXTPOVERTY/EXTISPMA/0,,contentMDK:20190347~menuPK:412148~pagePK:148956~piPK:216618~theSitePK:384329,00.html

World Health Organization. (2008). *Closing the gap in a generation: Health equity through action on the social determinants of health.* Retrieved from http://whqlibdoc.who.int/publications/2008/9789241563703_eng.pdf

World Health Organization. (2009). *Health Promotion Track 1: Community empowerment.* 7th global conference on health promotion. Retrieved from http://www.who.int/healthpromotion/conferences/7gchp/track1/en/index.html

World Health Organization. (2012). *Prevention and treatment of HIV and other sexually transmitted infections for sex workers in low- and middle-income countries: Recommendations for a public health approach.* Retrieved from http://apps.who.int/iris/bitstream/10665/77745/1/9789241504744_eng.pdf?ua=1

CHAPTER

11 Health Promotion and Education Strategies

Learning Outcomes

After reading this chapter, you should be able to:

1. Define health promotion.
2. Distinguish health promotion from health education.
3. Apply selected models for health promotion practice.
4. Analyze the implications of language and health literacy for health promotion.
5. Identify four strategies for health promotion.
6. Describe the health education process.
7. Discuss the use of social marketing, branding, and tailoring in promoting health.
8. Design and implement a health education program for a selected population.
9. Describe criteria for evaluating health-related websites on the Internet.

Key Terms

community health workers (CHWs)
health care provider control expectations
health education
learning domain
literacy
locus of control
media advocacy
social media

Advocacy Then

Tobacco Control Advocate, John F. Banzhaf III

Advocacy for tobacco control began more than 40 years ago with the filing of a complaint action with the Federal Communications Commission (FCC) by John F. Banzhaf III, a Columbia University law student. Banzhaf first alerted a television station that had broadcast the cigarette commercial that triggered his memories of what he had learned about the "fairness doctrine" and informed them that the FCC policy required broadcasters to provide free airtime for opposing views on controversial public issues. The station refused and Banzhaf lodged his complaint with the FCC. The FCC, in turn, notified the station that the few news stories covering the ills of tobacco use aired by the station did not offset the breadth of its cigarette advertising and required the station to provide considerable time for opposing information. Although the station appealed the ruling, the appeal was overturned in 1968 (Banzhaf, et al. v. Federal Communications Commission, et al., n.d.; Professor John F. Banzhaf, III, n.d.).

As a result, millions of dollars of free airtime was provided from 1967 to 1970, leading to a significant drop in tobacco consumption. In 1970, all radio and television cigarette advertising was banned in the United States (Office on Smoking and Health, 2012).

Banzhaf became director of Action on Smoking and Health (ASH), a nonprofit antismoking organization that uses legal action to advocate for a smoke-free world. Currently ASH is actively involved with the Framework Convention Alliance, a coalition of more than 400 organizations from over 100 countries that was instrumental in the development of the World Health Organization Framework Convention on Tobacco Control, the first-ever treaty related to a global public health issue (ASH, n.d.).

Advocacy Now

Culturally Sensitive Prenatal Care

Advocacy is not always undertaken by professionals for the good of clients. Arnold, Aragon, Shephard, and Van Sell (2011) described advocacy for culturally sensitive prenatal education undertaken by members of the Cherokee Nation and the March of Dimes. A 2006 survey by the Cherokee Nation in Oklahoma indicated that less than 10% of the prenatal literature provided to pregnant American Indian/Alaska Native (AI/AN) women was culturally appropriate. Utilization of prenatal care in this population is low and infant mortality and preterm birthrates are high. March of Dimes staff and volunteer faculty established an AI/AN Women's Committee representing ten tribes to address these issues.

The women conducted focus groups in their communities and eventually decided to write a prenatal education booklet in the way a mother would educate her daughter about pregnancy. The booklet, entitled *The Coming of the Blessing,* incorporated beliefs and life values common across tribes and took more than a year to produce. It incorporated the use of color, positive voice, inclusion of family and community support, photographs, communication of health risks (e.g., alcohol use), and seeking support from family and friends, all of which are reflected in traditional tribal cultures. Factual information was provided by health care professionals and then "translated" into a cultural voice by women in the advisory committee using the concept of the medicine wheel to discuss the childbearing cycle from preconception through three trimesters of pregnancy to delivery. The booklet has been used on reservations throughout the country and has become a major program initiative for the March of Dimes, which continues to advise the agency on AI/AN women's health issues.

Six distinct approaches have been taken to public health over time (Awofeso, 2004). The first approach involved health protection by means of social structures and lasted from ancient times until the 1830s. These social structures included rules of behavior, usually enforced by means of religious, political, or cultural sanctions. "Miasma control" was the second approach to fostering the health of the public. Miasmas were harmful mists or vapors in the air. This era of public health, from the 1840s through the 1870s, was exemplified by the sanitary movement and gained impetus from Chadwick's 1842 *Inquiry into the Sanitary Conditions of the Labouring Population of Great Britain*. From approximately 1880 to 1940, public health practice focused on contagion control based on the germ theory. During the 1940s to 1960s, emphasis was placed on preventive medicine, which expanded the germ theory to consider other disease vectors and nutritive factors in illness. Public health activity in this era was focused on populations at high risk for specific conditions. The 1970s and 1980s saw the rise of the primary health care movement, based on the Declaration of Alma-Ata, and recognized the effects of social factors on health. Finally, from 1990 to the present, the focus has been on the "new public health," which emphasizes health promotion based on the ability of members of the population to make informed health decisions. This new focus retains many of the features of prior eras, including regulation of some aspects of health via legislation, sanitation, immunization, a focus on risk modification, and recognition of the effects of social conditions on health. The eras and foci of public health practice over time are summarized in Table 11-1 ●. The emphasis on health promotion in the new public health focus highlights the importance of this role for population health nurses.

TABLE 11-1 Eras of Public Health Practice and Related Foci

Era	Time Period	Focus
Health protection	Ancient times–1830s	Regulation of behavior reinforced by religious, political, or cultural sanctions
Miasma control	1840s–1870s	Sanitation
Contagion control	1880s–1930s	Immunization, disinfection
Preventive medicine	1940s–1960s	Risk factor modification
Primary health care	1970s–1980s	Modification of social and other factors that influence health
Health promotion	1990s–present	Development of capacity for informed health decisions

Defining Health Promotion

A basic definition of health promotion was provided in Chapter 1∞. Health promotion, as delineated by the *Ottawa Charter for Health Promotion* (World Health Organization [WHO], 1986), and reinforced in the *Bangkok Charter for Health Promotion in a Global World* (WHO, 2005), is a process that fosters people's ability to improve their own health by increasing their control of its determining factors. Health promotion is more than educating people to change their behavior; it also involves public policy formation, development of environments that support health, and promotion of community action to create conditions conducive to good health.

The Ottawa Charter emphasized health as a "resource for living" rather than an end in itself and marked an international shift from disease prevention to capacity building, improving the capability of nations and communities to provide environments that support health and healthy behaviors. The Charter identified three strategies to promote global health: advocacy for conditions favorable to health, development of environments that support health as well as personal information and skills to make health decisions, and mediation between groups (Tones & Green, 2010).

The foci of the Ottawa Charter were further expanded in 1997 in the *Jakarta Declaration on Leading Health Promotion into the 21st Century*. The Jakarta Declaration viewed health promotion as increasing healthy life expectancy by increasing health gains throughout populations, reducing inequities, promoting human rights, and enhancing social capital. The Declaration also established four priorities for health promotion in the 21st century: promoting social and individual responsibility for health, increasing investment in health development, increasing partnerships for health, and developing a global infrastructure for health promotion (Tones & Green, 2010).

In the United States, health promotion efforts tend to continue to be focused on behavior modification and prevention of specific health conditions (termed *vertical health promotion*), rather than on changing broader factors that influence health (*horizontal health promotion*) (Tones & Green, 2010). In 2003, however, the United States Department of Health and Human Services (USDHHS, 2003) launched the *Steps to a Healthier US* initiative, which focused on promoting behavior change and improving policy and environmental conditions that support healthy behavior and illness prevention. The *Steps* initiatives focused on reducing the burden of five specific conditions—asthma, cancer, diabetes, heart disease and stroke, and obesity—and employed both vertical and horizontal health promotion strategies. The vertical strategies focused on behavior modification and prevention of the five conditions. The horizontal strategies addressed the policies and environmental conditions that influence health, such as insurance coverage for smoking cessation and incentives for schools to include physical activity in the curriculum.

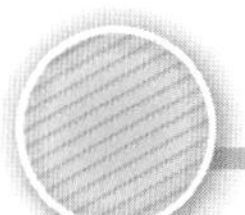

Global Perspectives

Health Promotion Initiatives

Health promotion is an area of international concern and initiative spanning nearly 40 years. In 1974, *The Lalonde Report* in Canada shifted the focus of discussion of gains in population health from biomedical advances to consideration of the influences of other non-health-sector determinants of health. This perspective was solidified in the World Health Organization's 1978 Declaration of Alma-Ata with its focus on primary care and "health for all by 2000." In the United States, the focus on health promotion took the form of a first set of national health promotion and disease prevention objectives promulgated in 1980 (de Salazar & Anderson, 2008).

During the 1980s, the *Healthy Cities* movement of the World Health Organization's European Region, continued the focus on environments that promote health, and the first WHO International Conference on Health Promotion was held in Ottawa, Canada, in 1986. That conference issued the *Ottawa Charter for Health Promotion*, still the definitive international perspective on health promotion. Subsequent conferences broadened the perspective on the varied social and economic determinants that affect health and that must be addressed if health is to be promoted. The 2005 conference resulted in the *Bangkok Charter for Health Promotion*, which forwarded the perspective that health promotion is critical to global development and should be a key focus of communities, societies, and corporate institutions alike (de Salazar & Anderson, 2008).

Despite the long history of health promotion efforts around the world, de Salazar and Anderson (2008), noted the limited scope and success of health promotion initiatives. Rather than dealing with the broader categories of determinants of health, such as social and economic inequities, health promotion initiatives "continue to deal mostly with activities to control and prevent proximal causes of morbidity and mortality. Citizens and communities are not fully participating in the decisions that affect their lives" (p. 20).

The Need for Health Promotion

The U.S. health care system is being overwhelmed by demands for care for myriad chronic diseases, and the system cannot continue to meet those demands. We must do something to motivate the American people to promote and protect their own health and to change the conditions in which people live to foster better health. The need for a focus on health promotion is evident in the information highlighted in the box on the next page. The data reported there led to the conclusion that health promotion is an "economic necessity" (Mathar & Jansen, 2010). It has been estimated that increasing the proportion of the population who engage in 20 health promotion and illness prevention services recommended by the U.S. Preventive Services Task Force to 90% would result in health care cost savings of nearly $22 billion (Maclosek, Coffield, Flottemesch, Edwards, & Solberg, 2010). Similarly, interventions to reduce lifestyle-related risks for diabetes and hypertension have the potential to result in annual savings of $9 billion, increasing to nearly $25 billion when the possible effects on comorbid conditions are considered (Ormond, Spillman, Waldmann, Caswell, & Tereshchenko, 2011).

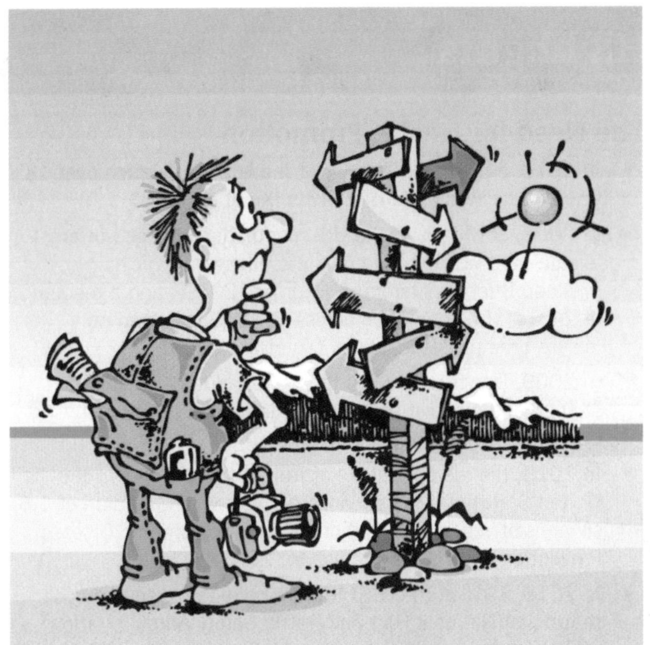

Lack of health literacy can leave clients wandering in a confusing health care system. *(CorelZavr/Fotolia)*

Models for Health Promotion

A number of models have been developed to guide health promotion practice. These include the Precaution Adoption Process model (Weinstein, Sandman, & Blalock, 2008), the Information-Motivation-Behavioral Skills (IMB) Model (Fisher, Fisher, & Shuper, 2009), the Theory of Reasoned Action and the related Theory of Planned Behavior (Eadie, 2014; Fisher, Kohut, Salisbury, & Salvadori, 2013; Southey, 2011), and the Health Belief Model (Tones & Green, 2010). Additional models include the Attitude-Social Influence-Efficacy Model (Verstraeten et al., 2014) and Pender's Health Promotion Model (Pender, Murdaugh, & Parsons, 2010). Each of these and various other models are an attempt to explain why people do or do not engage in health-promoting activity. These explanations assist population health nurses to understand the motivations and factors involved in such decisions and help them to select appropriate strategies for promoting health in the population. Although it is not possible to discuss all of these models here, the reader is referred to the literature

Highlights

The Need for Health Promotion

- In 2010, a median of 17.3% of the U.S. population over 18 years of age was current smokers (Xu et al., 2013).
- In 2009, only 18% of the U.S. population engaged in any leisure-time walking, and only 2% engaged in bicycling (Pucher, Buehler, Merom, & Bauman, 2011), and a median of 24% of the population across all states reported no leisure-time physical activity (Xu et al., 2013).
- In 2009, less than one fourth of U.S. adults engaged in strengthening activities at least twice a week (National Center for Health Statistics, 2011).
- In 2013, the median intake of fruits among adults in the United States was 1.1 servings per day, with a median of 1.6 servings of vegetables (National Center for Chronic Disease Prevention and Health Promotion, 2013).
- In 2013, 13% of the U.S. population did not regularly use seat belts (National Highway Traffic Safety Administration, 2014).
- In 2010, a median of 15.1% of the U.S. population engaged in binge drinking, and 5% reported heavy drinking (Xu et al., 2013).
- The median prevalence of overweight across states in 2010 was 36.2%, and the median prevalence of obesity was 28.5% (Xu et al., 2013).
- In 2009, a median 40% of people across all states reported insufficient rest or sleep for at least 14 days in the prior month (Li et al., 2011).

Data from: Li et al., 2011; National Center for Chronic Disease Prevention and Health Promotion. (2013). *State indicator report on fruits and vegetables, 2013.* Retrieved from http://www.cdc.gov/nutrition/downloads/State-Indicator-Report-Fruits-Vegetables-2013.pdf; National Center for Health Statistics, 2011; National Highway Traffic Safety Administration. (2014). *Seat belt use in 2013—Overall results.* Retrieved from http://www-nrd.nhtsa.dot.gov/Pubs/811875.pdf; Pucher, Buehler, Merom, & Bauman, 2011; Xu, F., Town, M., Balluz, L. S., Bartoli, W. P., Murphy, W., Chowdury, P. P., ... Crawford, C.A. (2013). Surveillance for certain health behaviors among states and selected local areas—United States, 2010. *Morbidity and Mortality Weekly Report, 62*(SS-1), 1–247.

cited for a description of the models. In this chapter, we will briefly explore the Precaution Adoption Process model, the Theories of Reasoned Action and Planned Behavior, the Health Belief Model, and Pender's Health Promotion Model.

The Precaution Adoption Process Model

The Precaution Adoption Process model is a stage model that describes stages in decisions to adopt or not adopt a health-related behavior (whether or not to take a specific precautionary action) (Weinstein et al., 2008). In stage 1, the person is unaware of the health-related issue and the need to adopt any particular health-related behavior. In stage 2, one is aware of the issue but is unengaged by it and is not considering any action. In stage 3, the person is deciding whether or not to act. He or she has considered the possibility of action but has not yet made a decision whether or not to adopt the behavior. Stage 3 may be followed by either stage 4 or stage 5. In stage 4, the person has decided not to act. Conversely, in stage 5, the person has decided to act but has not yet taken action. The process may stop at stage 4 for those who decide not to adopt the behavior in question. People in stages 4 and 5 are more resistant to persuasion than those in stage 3 who have not yet made a decision. Given human tenacity, it is more difficult to influence someone to change his or her mind than it is to persuade someone to act who has not yet made a decision one way or the other. Persons in stage 5 who have decided to adopt the behavior proceed to stage 6, in which they act to engage in the behavior, and hopefully to stage 7, in which the behavior becomes a routine part of their lifestyle. This process explaining the adoption or nonadoption of the health-related behavior of exercise is depicted in Figure 11-1●.

We can apply this model using a community-based example of installing speed bumps in residential areas. The decision to employ speed bumps to slow traffic must be adopted by the

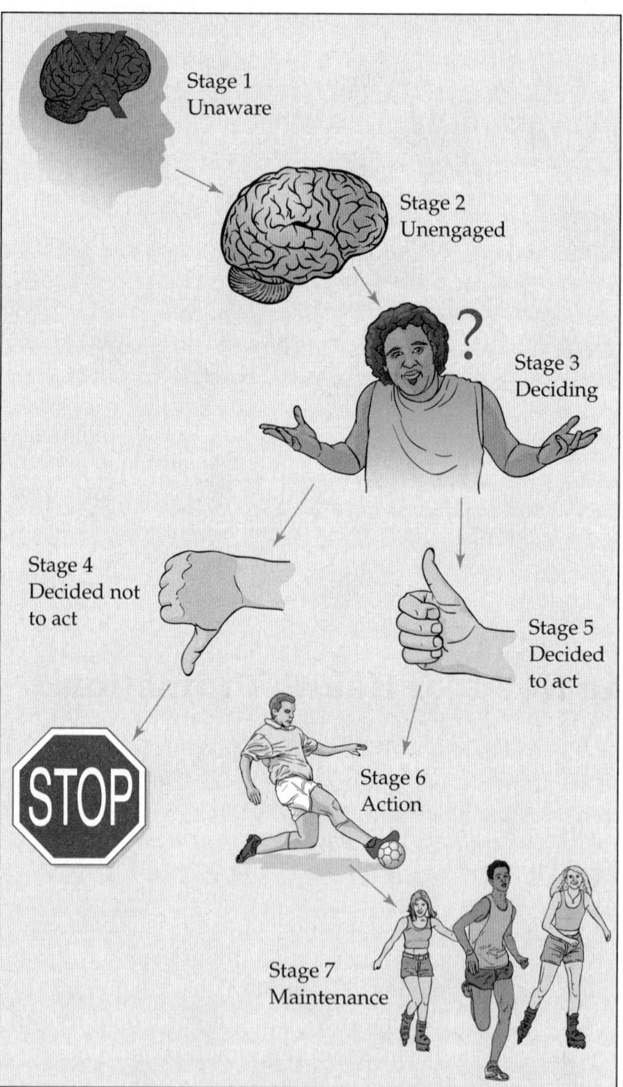

FIGURE 11-1 Stages of Adoption of Exercise Behavior

City Council. In the first stage of the decision adoption process, the Council is unaware of the extent of and potential for injury and death due to drivers exceeding the speed limit in residential areas. In stage 2, Council members may have become aware of the high frequency of pedestrian injuries in these areas, but are not considering taking any action to remedy the situation. At stage 3, the Council may be presented with a petition from local residents for the installation of speed bumps, but has not decided whether or not to authorize their installation. If the City Council proceeds to stage 4, they will decide not to install speed bumps possibly based on the cost of installation, which they believe would outweigh the benefits to be gained in terms of injuries and deaths prevented. If, on the other hand, they vote to install the speed bumps, but have not yet authorized the City Accounting Office to put out bids for their installation, they are in stage 5 of the adoption process. At stage 6, all processes are in place, and speed bumps are being installed in identified residential areas. The City Council may then proceed to stage 7, in which construction of all new residential developments within the city limits must include speed bumps.

The Theories of Reasoned Action and Planned Behavior

The Theory of Reasoned Action, developed by Ajzen and Fishbein, is based on two types of beliefs: behavioral beliefs and normative beliefs. Behavioral beliefs reflect a person's attitudes toward the expected consequences of the behavior. For example, if you expect that exercise will result in a more desirable figure, and if you value that more desirable shape, you are likely to value, and engage in, exercise. Normative beliefs relate to subjective norms influenced by others. In the theory, the intention to act is based on one's perceptions of others' attitudes toward the behavior and the value placed on others' judgments (Fisher et al., 2013). According to the related Theory of Planned behavior, action is also influenced by perceptions of one's ability to control behavior. Behavioral beliefs, normative beliefs, and control beliefs all combine to result in behavioral intention, which is the precursor to actual behavior (Southey, 2011), as depicted in Figure 11-2●. For example, if you want to quit smoking (behavioral belief) and perceive that significant others in your life want you to quit (normative belief), but you think stopping smoking will be too difficult (control belief), you will probably not attempt to quit even though your own attitudes and those of people who matter to you support quitting.

Using the previous population-level example of the speed bumps, if City Council members expect the installation of the barriers to reduce speeds on residential streets and subsequently reduce the frequency of pedestrian injuries and deaths, they may approve their installation. Action to install the speed bumps is even more likely if City Council members believe that failure to take action will anger voters to the point they will not be reelected. Both the perceived consequences of installing speed bumps and perceptions of voters' attitudes will influence

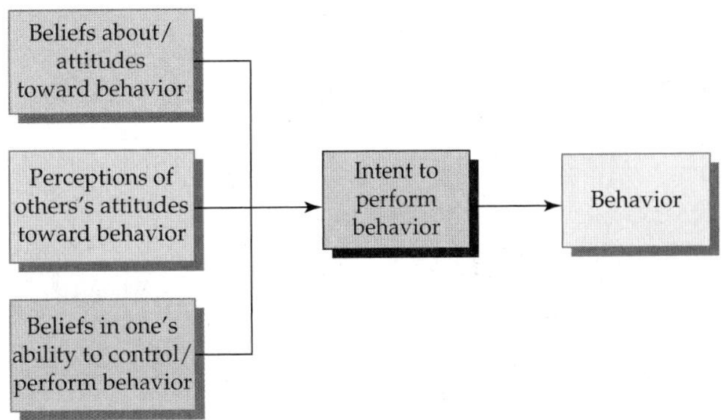

FIGURE 11-2 Elements of the Theories of Reasoned Action and Planned Behavior

their decision to take a health-promoting action on the part of the city. Their intention to act, however, may be further influenced by perceptions of their ability to do so. For example, they might believe that the city budget will not support the installation of speed bumps.

A further extension of these two theories, the Integrative Model of Behavioral Prediction, expands the elements influencing intention and subsequent action to include background influences, such as individual characteristics, culture, emotion, and intervention exposure. Environmental factors and personal skills and abilities related to the desired behavior also influence performance of the behavior (Fishbein, 2009).

The Health Belief Model

The Health Belief Model was developed by Becker, Rosenstock, and their colleagues several years ago and has been widely used in research and program development related to health-promoting behaviors. Elements of the model include individual perceptions of susceptibility and severity, modifying factors (demographic, sociopsychologic, and structural or environmental variables), perceptions of benefits and barriers to action, and cues to action. In the model, health-promotive action is based on four basic premises or beliefs. First, one believes that one is susceptible to, or at risk for, a particular health problem. Second, one believes that the health problem can have serious consequences. Third, one believes that the problem can be prevented and fourth, that the benefits of action outweigh the costs or barriers (Tones & Green, 2010). An additional element, self-efficacy, was added to the model after 1988. *Self-efficacy* is the belief that one is capable of the behavior desired or of achieving change (Martin, Haskard-Zolnierek, & DiMatteo, 2010).

As an example, you may believe that, never having had chickenpox as a child, you are susceptible to chickenpox (perceived susceptibility). You also believe that chickenpox may cause serious consequences (perceived severity). This perception is confirmed when one of your classmates is hospitalized with complications of chickenpox (cue to action). In addition, you know that varicella immunization will virtually

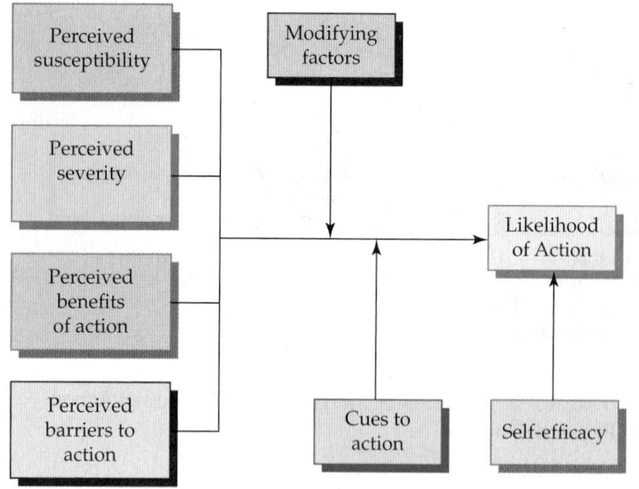

FIGURE 11-3 Elements of the Health Belief Model

eliminate your risk of developing chickenpox (perceived benefit to action). Even though you know the possibility of an adverse reaction to the vaccine exists and you have to skip lunch to visit the student health center (perceived costs), you decide the benefits outweigh the barriers, and you get immunized.

Examining our community-level example of installing speed bumps in the light of this model, perceptions of susceptibility would relate to City Council members' perceptions of the potential for injuries on residential streets. The perceived severity of the problem would reflect their knowledge of the number of deaths and serious injuries that have occurred. Perceived benefits might include reduced frequency of pedestrian injuries and satisfied voters. The cost of installing the speed bumps and, possibly, the loss of revenue from speeding tickets, might constitute perceived barriers to the project. Other successful strategies to minimize injuries, such as enacting helmet laws for bicyclists, might contribute to beliefs in self-efficacy among council members. Finally, the fact that the mayor's son was nearly hit by a speeding car in front of his house may serve as a cue to action that motivates Council members to authorize the installation of speed bumps. Elements of the Health Belief Model are depicted in Figure 11-3•.

Pender's Health Promotion Model

Nola Pender has developed a nursing model that directs nursing intervention for health promotion. In the Health Promotion Model, behavior is influenced by individual characteristics and behavior-specific cognitions and affect (emotion) that result in a commitment to action. Commitment to action results in actual behavior but may be modified by competing demands and preferences (Pender, et al., 2010). Individual characteristics include personal biological, psychological, and sociocultural factors that are relevant to the behavior involved. Prior behavior in this area is another individual characteristic that influences health-promoting behavior. For example, a client who was physically active prior to pregnancy will be more likely to engage in exercise after delivery than one who was not.

Behavior-specific cognitions and attitudes include the perceived benefits of and barriers to health-promoting activity as well as one's perceived self-efficacy. For example, the community that does not perceive itself as able to cope with the problem of inadequate housing will probably not take any action to resolve the problem. Activity-related affect or feeling states related to the behavior, to oneself, or to the situation are also important in motivating health-promoting behavior. Interpersonal and situational influences are additional factors related to cognition and affect that influence behavior. For example, if family members support weight loss, a client is more likely to stick to a diet. Conversely, low income, a situational influence, might adversely affect the client's weight loss options.

Individual characteristics and behavior-specific cognitions and affect may lead to a commitment to health-promoting activity. Commitment includes both the intention to act and a specific plan of action. Commitment to action should lead to performance of the actual health-promoting behavior unless there is interference from competing demands and preferences. For example, the client's intention to diet may be subverted by a family member's serious illness and the need to eat in fast-food restaurants near the hospital.

Although Pender's model was developed to be used to enhance health-promoting behavior with individual clients, it can also be applied to population groups. Using the speed bump example, individual characteristics might relate to members of the City Council or of the community. For example, if members of the City Council have young children or live on busy residential streets, they may be more inclined to take action than if they do not. Conversely, if the area of the city requesting speed bumps is composed largely of immigrants who rarely vote in local elections, Council members may be less likely to respond. Prior action may also have a bearing on the Council's decision. For example, if they have taken other "traffic calming" actions (approaches to traffic control that are self-enforcing) such as installing cameras on traffic lights at busy intersections, they may be inclined to install speed bumps as well. If, however, the City Council perceives itself to have little control over traffic violations, their perceived lack of self-efficacy may lead them to decide that speed bumps will have little impact.

Emotional reactions to the problem may have an influence on the Council's decision as well. If, for example, the most recent death of a child led to rioting or demonstrations outside City Hall, or if one of the Council members has had a child injured by a speeding driver, action may be forthcoming. Again, the City Council would weigh the perceived benefits of installing speed bumps (voter satisfaction and fewer injuries) against the perceived costs (financial costs of installing the speed bumps, need to delay construction of a city park, etc.) to decide whether or not to commit to installing the speed bumps. Even if the Council votes to install the bumps, installation may be sidetracked by a subsequent financial crisis or by

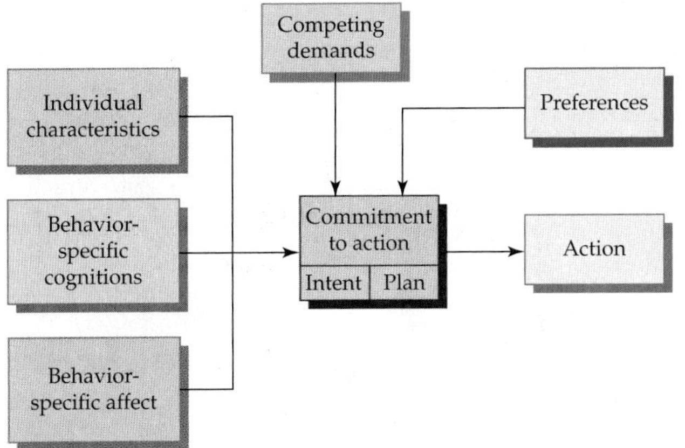

FIGURE 11-4 Elements of Pender's Health Promotion Model

torrential rains that delay construction, both of which would reflect situational constraints that impede action to implement the Council's decision. Elements of Pender's model are depicted in Figure 11-4●.

Population Health Nursing and Health Promotion

Use of a health promotion model permits the population health nurse to identify factors involved in the health promotion situation and to design health promotion programs that address these factors. Use of a model also focuses attention on all of the factors that influence health promotion, not just personal behaviors, and leads to a more horizontal approach to health promotion. The 2011 Institute of Medicine report "The Future of Nursing: Leading Change, Advancing Health" highlighted health promotion as one of the "traditional and current strengths" of the nursing profession. Given their focus on health, health promotion is an even more critical role for population health nurses than for nurses in other specialty areas.

Some research, however, indicates that population health nurses' concept of health promotion is narrowly circumscribed and addressed primarily due to their responsibility for health education. Little attention is given in the practice of some population health nurses to activities related to empowerment of populations and social determinants of health promotion capabilities (Richard et al., 2010). Some authors have found that additional education assists population health nurses to provide behavior change counseling to individual clients (Pfister-Minogue & Salveson, 2010), but further attention is needed to prepare them for the full spectrum of health promotion activities.

Factors Influencing Health Promotion

In executing their role in health promotion, population health nurses must consider a number of important factors that may influence the health promotion situation. Four major influences on health promotion will be considered here: fatalism, readiness for change, health literacy, and the attitudes of health professionals toward health promotion.

FATALISM. Fatalism was defined in Chapter 5∞ as the belief that one's fate is fixed and that personal efforts can do little to affect that fate. Other definitions of fatalism include "a belief in a lack of personal power or control over destiny or fate (Drew & Schoenberg, 2011, p. 164) or "the general belief that all events, and in particular, the actions and occurrences that form an individual life, are determined by fate" (Espinosa de los Monteros & Gallo, 2011, p. 311). Fatalistic beliefs have often been found to be associated with lower rates of participation in health promotion, prevention, and screening activities (Smith-Howell et al., 2011).

Such beliefs have also been linked to an external locus of control orientation. The concept of **locus of control** relates to one's perceptions that one's life and circumstances are primarily under one's personal control (internal locus of control) or under the control of fate or of powerful others (external locus of control). In the past, fatalism has been seen as a stable global belief associated with decisions not to take preventive or health-promotive actions (Keeley, Wright, & Condit, 2009). People with an external locus of control have been found to be more fatalistic and were often perceived as ignorant and in need of educational efforts to change their perceptions of self-efficacy (Drew & Schoenberg, 2011).

More recent research, however, has suggested that fatalism is a complex construct that may reflect a population's response to the realities of their life circumstances (Drew & Schoenberg, 2011). For example, when a population consistently sees its members dying from conditions like AIDS in the absence of access to effective treatment, it is not unreasonable to develop a perception that AIDS is life threatening and that little can be done to avoid it or deal with its consequences. Some authors have even suggested that fatalistic beliefs may serve a variety of functions within a population without interfering with propensities to take action to promote health and prevent illness. Some suggested functions include stress relief, uncertainty management, sense making, and face saving (Keeley et al., 2009).

A somewhat fatalistic attitude of "what will be, will be" can promote acceptance of the future without undue worry thereby relieving stress. Similarly, fatalistic beliefs can help to address the unpredictability and uncertainty associated with disease. For example, it is widely known that smoking is associated with lung cancer, but nonsmokers also develop lung cancer. Relegating those cases of cancer in nonsmokers to fate can serve functions of managing uncertainty and making sense of their occurrence. Getting the disease without smoking makes sense if it was one's fate. Finally, fatalism may serve a face saving function in the presence of existing disease avoiding guilt or blame for the development of an illness. If it was my fate to develop lung cancer, I do not have to fret about actions I might have taken to prevent it but didn't (Keeley et al., 2009). In some recent studies, people have been found to express highly fatalistic perceptions while simultaneously taking action to promote their health suggesting that fatalism is a much more complicated concept than previously thought and its precise influence on health-related behaviors remains largely unknown (Flores et al., 2009).

An external locus of control perspective may even serve to facilitate health-promoting behaviors. For example, people who have strong **health care provider control expectations** or beliefs that health care providers control their health, tend to have an external locus of control and hold fatalistic beliefs. However, they may also be more likely than those with lower health care provider control expectations to follow provider recommendations for health promotion and illness prevention behaviors (Roncancio, Ward, & Berenson, 2011).

Population health nurses engaging in health promotion activities need to consider the potential effects of fatalistic beliefs and locus of control on health-related behavior by members of the population. Do members of the population have a tendency toward fatalism? If so, what is the basis for those fatalistic beliefs and do they impede health-promoting behaviors? When fatalism has a basis in realistic appraisal of life circumstances, efforts to change those circumstances may be more effective in fostering health promotion than attempts to change perceptions of locus of control or belief systems.

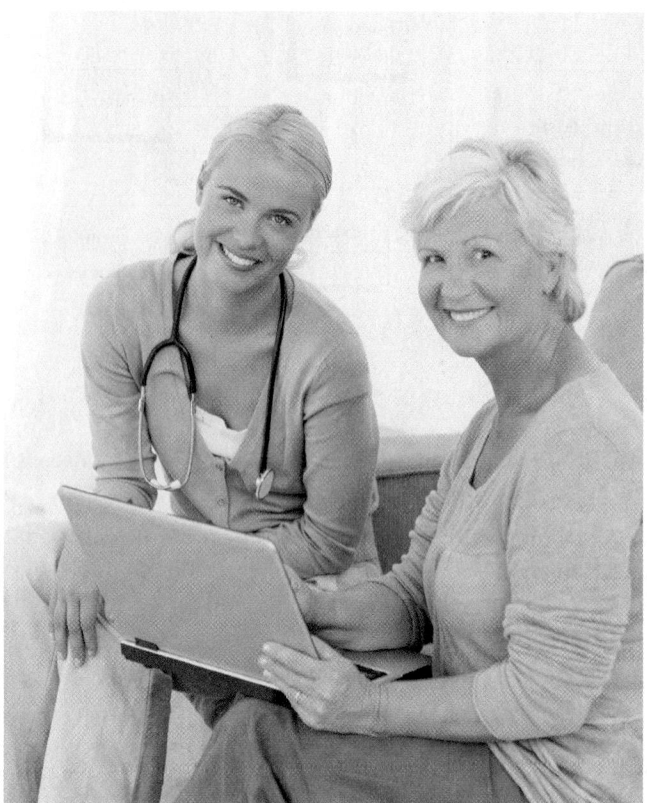

Health education can be provided to individuals or groups of people.
(WavebreakMediaMicro/Fotolia)

READINESS FOR CHANGE. Involvement in health-promoting behaviors often requires a change, either on the part of the individual client or the population. However, people only engage in change when they are good are ready to do so. The smoker, for example, must be ready to quit smoking. Similarly, society must be ready to take the steps needed to provide universal access to health care or to enforce measures to prevent injury, such as seat belt or helmet use. Until the individual or the group is ready for change, change to more healthful behaviors will not occur.

The Transtheoretical Model of Change proposes that readiness for change occurs in a series of stages similar to those described earlier in discussion of the precaution adoption process model. The first stage is one of precontemplation in which one is not even thinking of making a change or aware of the need for change. In the contemplation stage, one is considering change and plans to take action within 6 months. The third stage involves preparation for the change. In the fourth, or action stage, one engages in the new behavior, and in the maintenance stage, one integrates the behavior into one's usual routine (Prochaska, Redding, & Evers, 2008).

Population health nurses can use this model to foster health-promoting behaviors by determining what stage an individual or a population is in and then engaging in strategies to facilitate movement into the next and subsequent stages of change. Different strategies are appropriate for different stages (Martin et al., 2010). For example, consciousness raising techniques highlight the need for change in moving people from the first to the second stage of change. Similarly, emotional support and helpful tips for making a change can facilitate the action stage.

HEALTH LITERACY. Health literacy is another factor that influences health promotion. **Literacy** is defined as "a person's ability to read, write, speak, and solve problems at levels needed to function in society" (Office of Disease Prevention and Health Promotion [ODPHP], 2010, p. 3). Health literacy was defined in Chapter 5∞, as the extent to which an individual is able to obtain, process, and understand health-related information in order to make informed decisions about health issues. A health literate person is able to use health information "generatively" to make decisions in unfamiliar situations. Poor health literacy, on the other hand, is associated with emergency department use, hospitalization, poor self-reported health, and increased mortality. Limited health literacy also affects people's ability to search for health-related information, adopt healthy behaviors, and act on health alerts to take appropriate action (ODPHP, 2012). Only approximately 12% of the U.S. population displays proficiency in health literacy. The rest of the population has some level of difficulty understanding and completing health-related tasks (National Network of Libraries of Medicine, 2013).

Health literacy is assessed at several levels, the highest being "proficient." As noted above, only 12% of the U.S. population falls into this category. Another 52% of the population has intermediate health literacy, while 22% has basic health literacy, and 14% are below the basic level. Seventy-seven million people in the United States display basic or below basic levels of literacy (National Network of Libraries of Medicine, 2013), and

90% of U.S. adults have difficulty understanding routine health information. Health literacy levels are lowest among Hispanics compared to other racial and ethnic groups, persons with low educational levels, and the elderly. In fact, two thirds of persons over 60 years of age are at or below basic literacy levels and 39% has below basic levels (National Patient Safety Foundation, 2011).

One's ability to understand health-related information depends on the complexity or difficulty of the information, the individual's knowledge and skill levels, and his or her motivation to achieve full understanding. Health literacy is diminished with lack of understanding of medical terms or basic physiology, the inability to interpret numbers or determine levels of risk, the fear and confusion generated by receiving a serious diagnosis, and the need for complicated care for complex health conditions (ODPHP, n.d.). For many members of the population, poor health literacy is complicated by limited proficiency in English and the dearth of interpreters in many health care settings (National Patient Safety Foundation, 2011).

Population health nurses would assess the literacy levels of individual clients and population groups and then design health promotion initiatives appropriate to the level of literacy exhibited. Many people today obtain health-related information from media-based, rather than print-based, sources. Disparities in health literacy, however, are compounded for people who do not have access to media such as the Internet and various forms of social media. For those who do have access to these resources, population health nurses can use the strategies outlined in the ODPHP publication, "Health Literacy Online: A Guide to Writing and Designing Easy-to-use Health Web Sites" (ODPHP, 2010). ODPHP has also created a "Quick Guide to Health Literacy" that provides tips for working with individuals and populations with low levels of health literacy. In addition, ODPHP provides access to a number of other resources to address limited health literacy in the population. For further information about the guide and other ODPHP materials, see the resources provided in the *External Resources* section of the student resources site.

HEALTH PROFESSIONALS' ATTITUDES TO HEALTH PROMOTION. Health professionals' attitudes toward and involvement in health promotion activities also influence health promotion behaviors among individual clients and the general public. Although health promotion is the primary focus of public health professionals, health care providers involved in direct care of individuals and families have a role to play as well. Lack of time and reliance on written materials can lead to poor care and ineffective health promotion, particularly among population groups with low literacy levels.

Health care providers may often miss opportunities for health promotion in the care of individual clients. For example, Murray and colleagues (Murray, Lewis, Coleman, Britton, & McNeill, 2009) found that 394 attempts to quit smoking were made among 1805 study respondents, and more than one third of these were unplanned attempts. The reason for attempting to quit for nearly 30% of this group was the advice of a health professional, yet more than half of these attempts received no support in their efforts to stop smoking. Providers of care to individuals should incorporate evidence-based health promotion strategies into their practice on a routine basis. For further information about guidelines for evidence-based strategies from the U.S. Preventive Services Task Force, see the resources provided in the *External Resources* section of the student resources site.

Health system factors beyond the activities of individual health care providers also influence health promotion behaviors by members of the population. A study by the Colorado Department of Health indicated that many health insurance plans operating in the state were not covering health promotion and illness prevention services recommended by the Preventive Services Task Force. For example, considerable variability was noted in coverage of and restrictions on screening for tobacco use and cessation services including pharmacotherapy for nicotine addiction. Variability in coverage was also noted for obesity screening and counseling services (Colorado Department of Public Health and Environment, 2011).

Strategies for Health Promotion

Population health nurses use a variety of strategies to foster health promotion at the population level. Four particular strategies will be discussed here: health education; social marketing, branding, and tailoring; legislation; and the use of community health workers (CHWs). Health education provides the information and skills required to make effective health-related decisions. Social marketing and the related concepts of branding and tailoring emphasize enhancing people's motivation to act and reflects the view of personal agency. Motivating people to actually take advantage of opportunities for physical activity present in the community exemplifies social marketing.

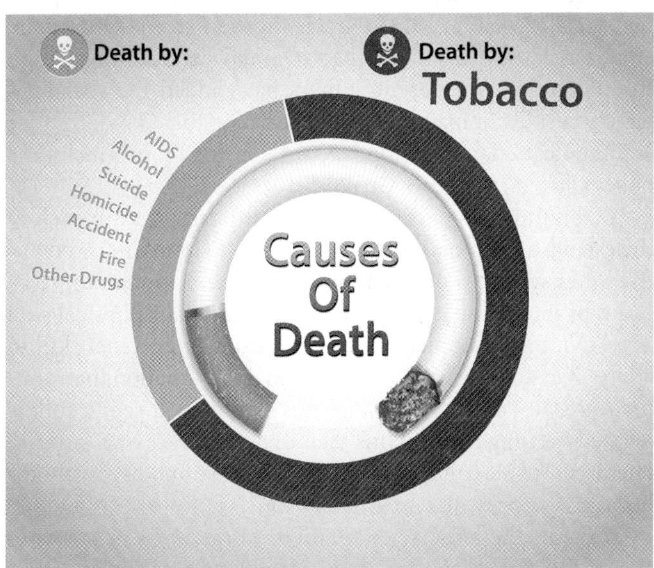

Social marketing promotes health-related messages.
(Harshmunjal/Fotolia)

Legislative action, on the other hand, may mandate health promotion activities, such as motorcycle helmet use, or create conditions conducive to health promotion. Finally, the use of community health workers to promote healthy behavior within the population capitalizes on the influence of trusted members of the community. Often a combination of strategies is most effective in achieving health promotion objectives. Each of the four strategies is briefly addressed below.

HEALTH EDUCATION. The first health promotion strategy to be addressed is health education. Health education is a participatory learning process that enables people to make informed decisions about health. The World Health Organization (2014, para. 1) defined **health education** as the use of learning experiences to improve people's knowledge or change their attitudes for the purpose of fostering health.

The primary purpose of health education is to assist clients in making health-related decisions. Health education may equip clients to make any of three types of health-related decisions: decisions about self-care, decisions about the use of health resources, and decisions about societal health issues.

Domains of health learning. Different types of learning may be required to facilitate health-promotive action. Types of health learning have been classified into four learning domains: the cognitive, affective, psychomotor, and social interaction skills domains (Tones & Green, 2010). A **learning domain** is the category or type of learning desired as a result of the health education encounter. The classic taxonomy of learning domains included the cognitive, affective, psychomotor, and perceptual domains (Bloom, Englehart, Furst, Hill, & Krathwohl, 1956). The cognitive domain encompasses intellectual skills related to factual information and its application. In the affective domain, the focus of learning is on attitudes and values. Emphasis in the psychomotor domain is on the learning of physical manipulative skills (Bastable, 2013). Finally, in the perceptual domain, emphasis is on learning to perceive and extract information from stimuli. More recent authors have added the social interaction skills domain to address learning that is required for communication, persuasion, and influencing others (including policy makers) (Tones & Green, 2010).

Taxonomies of learning tasks classify tasks within each of the established domains in a hierarchical fashion. In the cognitive and psychomotor domains, learning tasks are arranged in order of increasing complexity of intellectual or physical skill involved. For example, it requires greater intellectual skill to apply a fact to a particular decision-making situation than simply to recall the fact. Similarly, less skill is required to follow printed knitting instructions than to create one's own pattern. Hierarchies of learning tasks in the cognitive and psychomotor domains are presented in Table 11-2•.

Tasks in the affective domain are organized in terms of the degree to which an attitude or value has been internalized by the learner (Krathwohl, Bloom, & Masia, 1964). For example, the student who consistently displays empathy for clients is operating at a higher level of internalization than one who merely discusses the importance of empathy in nursing. The taxonomy of the affective domain is also presented in Table 11-2.

Finally, learning tasks in the perceptual domain are arranged in terms of the extent to which the learner is able to extract information from a situation by way of perceptual skills. For example, a nursing student might notice a few salient characteristics of a family during a first home visit (e.g., cleanliness of the home, character of mother–child interactions), whereas an experienced community health nurse would derive much more information from the same encounter. The levels of a proposed taxonomy for the perceptual domain are listed in Table 11-2.

Principles of learning. A number of principles of learning have been identified that apply to health education as well as to other forms of learning encounters. These principles can be grouped as general principles of learning and principles related to the health education message and its delivery. The first, and possibly most important, general principle is that effective teaching and learning is based on a need to know and should be preceded by an assessment of learning needs. The learning assessment should also include an evaluation of readiness to learn. Readiness may be a function of developmental level as well as attention, motivation, and interest. The second overarching principle is one of accountability in which both teachers and learners are accountable for achievement of the desired learning outcomes. Third, learning should occur in a "safe" environment in which the learner is free to make mistakes and to learn from them. In addition, effective learning involves action or doing combined with reflection on what has been learned. Learners need to be actively engaged in the learning process, as learning depends on some form of neural activity: seeing, hearing, smelling, feeling, thinking, physical or motor activity, or some other kind of activity. This means that learning is multi-sensory. People process new information with multiple senses, although some people may prefer one sensory modality (e.g., visual learning) over another (e.g., auditory learning).

Additional principles of learning reflect its incremental, as well as social, nature. Current learning must be integrated into past learning experiences with learning accumulated over time. In this respect, learning is facilitated by association with past learning. Learning is reinforced by repetition, but repetition must occur in circumstances that maintain interest and attention. Retention of learning is also influenced by the recency and frequency of use of learned information and by experiences of success or failure in the learning encounter. Both praise and criticism may affect learning and retention, but may do so differently for different people. For example, research has indicated that constructive criticism may be more effective than effusive praise with confident capable learners, but may actually be harmful for less able learners. Balanced feedback including mild encouragement and occasional mild criticism may be more effective in promoting learning than either fulsome praise or extreme criticism.

TABLE 11-2 Taxonomy of Learning Tasks in the Cognitive, Psychomotor, Affective, and Perceptual Domains

Domain	Learning Tasks and Description
Cognitive	• Knowledge: Recall of facts, methods, or processes *Sample learning objective:* Learners will be able to list elements of the food pyramid. • Comprehension: Basic understanding of the meaning of facts *Sample learning objective:* Learners will be able to describe elements of the food pyramid in terms of recommended servings. • Application: Use of abstractions in concrete situations *Sample learning objective:* Learners will be able to evaluate their diet in light of the servings recommended for elements of the food pyramid. • Analysis: Ability to break concepts down into component parts *Sample learning objective:* Learners will be able to identify the nutrients provided by selected elements of the food pyramid. • Synthesis: Ability to combine parts into a new pattern or whole *Sample learning objective:* Learners will be able to incorporate food preferences of a specific ethnic group into a food pyramid tailored to that group. • Evaluation: Judgment about the value of information and processes for specific purposes *Sample learning objective:* Learners will be able to describe the relative importance of incorporating elements of the food pyramid in diets designed for prevention or treatment of obesity.
Affective	• Receiving: Sensitization to the existence of a phenomenon *Sample learning objective:* Learners will describe protections for the civil rights of gay and lesbian members of the community. • Responding: Low level of commitment to behaviors embodying a value, performance of the behavior because of outside constraint *Sample learning objective:* Learners will adhere to legally mandated protections afforded to gay and lesbian members of the community. • Valuing: Ascribing worth to a thing, behavior, or value accompanied by fairly consistent performance of related behaviors *Sample learning objective:* Learners will usually refrain from actions discriminating against gay and lesbian members of the community. • Organization: Organization of values in hierarchical relationships *Sample learning objective:* Learners will be able to apply the value of nondiscrimination to other segments of the population. • Characterization: Person can be characterized by consistent behavior in keeping with a specific set of values *Sample learning objective:* Learners will consistently refrain from discriminatory actions against "undesirable" segments of the population.
Psychomotor	• Perception: Awareness of objects and the relationships among them *Sample learning objective:* Learners will be able to discuss items needed for insulin injection. • Set: Physical, mental, and emotional readiness to act *Sample learning objective:* Learners will express willingness to learn insulin injection technique. • Guided response: Performance of an action with instructor input and guidance *Sample learning objective:* Learners will demonstrate correct insulin injection technique with instructor coaching. • Mechanism: Performance of task as a habit *Sample learning objective:* Learners consistently demonstrate correct insulin injection technique. • Complex overt response: Performance of task with a high degree of skill *Sample learning objective:* Learners demonstrate correct insulin injection technique smoothly and rapidly. • Adaptation: Ability to adjust the skill to meet the needs of new situations *Sample learning objective:* Learners are able to adjust insulin dosage to accommodate increased exercise. • Origination: Ability to create new acts or ways of manipulating materials *Sample learning objective:* Learners are able to switch to use of an insulin pump with little difficulty.
Perceptual	• Sensation: Awareness of differences, or change, in stimuli *Sample learning objective:* Nursing students can distinguish an abnormal tympanic membrane from a normal one. • Figure perception: Awareness of an object or phenomenon as a distinct entity *Sample learning objective:* Nursing students can identify the light reflex on a tympanic membrane. • Symbol perception: Identification of pattern or form, ability to name or classify an object or phenomenon *Sample learning objective:* Nursing students can distinguish a bulging tympanic membrane from a retracted one. • Perception of meaning: Awareness of significance of symbols, ability to interrelate symbols *Sample learning objective:* Nursing students can recognize a bulging tympanic membrane as evidence of possible middle ear infection. • Perceptive performance: Complex decisions with multiple factors, ability to change behavior based on its effectiveness *Sample learning objective:* Nursing students can combine evidence of a bulging tympanic membrane, loss of typical tympanic membrane landmarks, fever, and ear pain to derive a diagnosis of probable middle ear infection.

Learning is also social in that we learn best with others or from observing the behavior of others. In addition, learning is affected, either positively or negatively, by emotional experiences and relationships in the learning environment. The emotional effect of a specific learning activity can also influence retention of learning. We tend to remember best learning experiences that aroused either highly positive or negative emotions. Relationships within the learning context must be founded on trust. When the audience is a culturally diverse group, health education should be developed and delivered by a culturally diverse team including trusted members of the cultural groups involved. Similarly, when the audience involves members of previously disenfranchised communities, time will be required to create trust and rapport between the target audience and the health educators. Including community members in planning health education programs will enhance the development of trust and rapport as well as make the program more culturally appropriate. In addition, there is a need to recognize the culturally specific history of the group and how it influences health behaviors and readiness for health education.

Learning is also a lifelong endeavor and one continues to learn, whether formally or informally, throughout life. Finally, the ability to learn may be affected by physiologic factors such as fatigue, pain, poor nutrition, and so on. These general principles of learning, as well as self-explanatory principles related to the health education message and its delivery, are summarized in Table 11-3●.

Assessing health education needs. The health education process begins with an assessment of the audience, their health education needs, and the learning environment. When the client is a population group, the first task in assessment is to identify the target audience. Selection of the target audience may be based on level of need, resources available, or probability of success. Assessment then proceeds to identifying characteristics of the audience that influence the learning situation. The assessment can be conducted in terms of the determinants of health in the population health nursing model, addressing biological, psychological, environmental, sociocultural, behavioral, and health system factors that influence the health education situation.

TABLE 11-3 General, Message-Related, and Delivery-Related Principles of Learning

General Principles of Learning	Delivery-Related Principles of Learning
• Effective learning is based on an assessment of learning needs and readiness to learn.	• Information should be linked to existing knowledge.
• Teachers and learners must be accountable for achieving desired learning outcomes.	• Information should be presented in fun and interactive ways to promote integration of concepts.
• Learning should occur in a safe environment in which mistakes have minimal consequences.	• Modes of presentation should allow sufficient time for group members to assimilate and interact with it.
• Effective learning involves active participation in the learning encounter and incorporation of multiple sensory modalities.	• Messages should be presented in clear, simple language, and should avoid professional jargon.
• Learning is incremental and new learning should be associated with and integrated into prior learning.	• Materials should generally be developed at grade levels one to two grades below the highest grade completed in school and should employ short sentences and simple, one- and two-syllable words.
• Learning is reinforced by repetition that occurs in circumstances that maintain interest and attention.	• Information should be reinforced and repeated as needed, using illustrations as appropriate.
• Retention of learning is reinforced by recency and frequency of use as well as by positive and negative feedback.	• Written materials should use large type fonts and a mix of upper- and lowercase letters and should employ ample white space to prevent readers from being overwhelmed by content.
• Learning is social and occurs best in interactions with others.	• Information in written materials should be bulleted when possible.
• Learning is influenced by emotions and requires trust. Time will be required to develop trust with disenfranchised groups before effective learning can occur.	• Written materials should be reinforced verbally.
• Culturally diverse teams should develop health education programs for culturally diverse audiences. Curriculum development should acknowledge and incorporate the distinct culturally specific history of the target audience.	• Multiple approaches should be used to assess understanding of content (e.g., questioning, demonstration, etc.).
Message-Related Principles of Learning	
• Messages personalized to the audience will be more effective than global or generalized messages suitable for mass dissemination.	
• Health education messages should include content most relevant to the target audience, rather than trying to cover all of the related information.	
• The message should highlight important concepts relevant to the audience.	

When members of the target audience participate in conducting the assessment, the accuracy of the assessment and its relevance to their needs are enhanced.

Biological considerations influence both the learning needs and the learning capabilities of individual clients or populations. To learn effectively, clients may need to have reached a certain level of physical or psychological maturation. For example, small children who have not yet developed abilities for abstract thought will need concrete examples of concepts to be learned. Similarly, a child who still has poorly developed eye–hand coordination will have difficulty learning insulin injection techniques, so teaching will most likely involve parents as well. At the other end of the age spectrum, changes associated with aging may lead to sensory impairment that influences learning among older populations. Age or maturation level also affects the client's need for education. For instance, preschool children do not need information about menstruation, but preadolescent girls do. In addition, clients' maturational levels may influence existing knowledge of a particular subject. For example, a group of third graders will probably have a broader knowledge of nutrition concepts than preschoolers.

Assessing aspects of physiologic function in the population may reveal special needs for health education or impediments to learning. For example, a high prevalence of diabetes in the population suggests a need for diabetes prevention or self-care education, whereas high incidence rates for sexually transmitted diseases among adolescents indicate other needs for prevention education. Inadequate physiologic function can also give rise to impediments to learning. For example, the presence of physical disabilities may require specialized approaches to health education. Pain, another biophysical factor, may also impede learning.

Psychological determinants can profoundly influence willingness and ability to learn. Attitudes toward health and health behaviors can either enhance or detract from the motivation to learn. Among clients attending a series of parenting classes, for example, those parents who attend only because of a court mandate related to child abuse usually benefit less than those who attend because they perceive a need for help. Fatalistic beliefs discussed earlier may also influence motivation to learn and to act on health-related information.

Psychological factors such as stress and anxiety can also impede learning, even for those who are motivated to learn. Population health nurses can limit the negative effects of psychological determinants by actions designed to decrease stress and anxiety. For example, the nurse can create a climate in which clients do not feel threatened and in which the nurse educator is seen as a source of support rather than a threat. The nurse who has children and who teaches parenting classes for abusive parents might create such a climate by beginning the first session with a description of the frustration the nurse sometimes feels as a parent.

Environmental factors should also be considered in terms of their effects on learning. Is there adequate lighting for the tasks to be accomplished? Is there too much noise? Will clients be distracted by other activities occurring in the learning environment? During a home visit, for example, the nurse might ask that the television be turned off before attempting to educate a hypertensive client about his or her medication.

Environmental factors may also give rise to the need for health education. For example, population groups affected by natural disasters may need education on how to purify their drinking water to prevent communicable diseases. Similarly, health education efforts might be targeted to persons with chronic respiratory conditions in areas with significant air pollution.

Sociocultural determinants are particularly influential in shaping attitudes about health and health-related behaviors. Examples and attitudes of those around us influence our willingness to engage in self-care behaviors in addition to affecting our attitudes to health issues at the societal level.

Sociocultural factors also influence one's exposure to health-related information. People with lower education levels are less likely than those with more formal education to have been exposed to prior health education. The education level of the population and of specific target audiences essentially influences the nurse's choice of teaching strategies and content to be presented. Health literacy, discussed earlier, is another example of a sociocultural factor that influences the health education situation.

Cultural influences on health education with population groups include typical communication styles, concepts of time and personal space, values, and perceptions of environmental control. Client life roles and role expectations, which are culturally defined, are other factors that may affect interest in health education and motivation to learn. When content is perceived to be relevant to the roles one is expected to fulfill, one's motivation to learn is likely to be high. Roles may also influence one's ability to attend to health messages. For example, if members of the audience are responsible for the care of children, they are unlikely to be able to attend educational presentations unless child care is arranged.

Culture may also influence the effectiveness of health education in terms of the trust placed in health professionals. Many culturally diverse audiences may distrust health professionals as a result of past experiences or cultural misunderstandings. Language is a particularly important sociocultural consideration in health education initiatives in the United States, where in 2010, 21% of the population spoke a language other than English at home and approximately 40% of those spoke English "less than very well" (U.S. Census Bureau, 2011). Research has indicated that non-English-speakers are less likely than their English-speaking counterparts to have a regular source of health care and to receive preventive care and may be at higher risk for medical error.

Occupation is another social factor that can give rise to health education needs. Trash collectors, for example, might require education related to body mechanics and techniques for lifting heavy objects, whereas nurses require information about how to handle contaminated needles and other equipment.

Behavioral factors also influence needs for health education. For example, the extent of obesity in the United States suggests the need for intensive dietary education. Similarly, smokers may need help with smoking cessation and education on alternative ways to meet needs satisfied by smoking. As another example, sexually active clients may need education regarding contraceptives and safe sexual practices.

Preventive and therapeutic recommendations related to health system determinants may precipitate a need for health education. For example, clients may need to be educated on the correct use of medications or how to keep a sprained ankle immobilized to promote healing. Elements of the health care regimen may also influence clients' abilities to learn. For example, pain medication may make a client drowsy and inhibit the ability to learn material presented. As we saw earlier, the degree of emphasis placed on health promotion and health education by health care providers and providers' expertise in using the health education process are other health system determinants that influence clients' health-related knowledge and attitudes. Tips for assessing a health education situation are presented below. In addition, an assessment tool is provided in the *Assessment Guidelines* section of the student resources site. Population health nurses would use these tools to assess the need for health education at individual and population levels and to design health education programs that address those needs.

Planning and implementing health education programs. In the context of health education, planning involves determination of the topic to be addressed, content to be covered, teaching strategies to be employed, and mechanisms to assess learning. Elements of the planning process include prioritizing learning needs, developing goals and objectives, and selecting content and teaching/learning strategies. Other considerations in planning and implementing health education programs include language and health literacy and the use of the Internet as a teaching medium.

FOCUSED ASSESSMENT Assessing the Health Education Situation

Biological Determinants

- What is the age composition of the target audience? What learning needs arise from the age and developmental level of the audience? Will the developmental level of the audience affect the ability to learn or the teaching strategies used?
- Do physical health problems in the population give rise to the need for health education or pose any impediments to learning?

Psychological Determinants

- Is the target population aware of the need for health education? What is the level of motivation to learn? Will population attitudes toward health and health behaviors enhance or detract from learning ability?
- Does the target audience exhibit levels of stress or anxiety that will interfere with learning?
- Do fatalistic beliefs influence learning motivation or ability to learn?

Environmental Determinants

- Are there conditions in the physical environment that give rise to a need for health education? What effects, if any, will the physical environment have on learning?

Sociocultural Determinants

- What effects will the learners' peers have on motivation to learn?
- What is the current education level of the learners? What prior exposure to health information has the population received?
- What is the level of health literacy in the population?
- What is the primary language spoken by members of the target audience?
- Are there cultural beliefs and practices that are likely to influence learning?
- Do the occupations of group members give rise to a need for health education?
- Are there other facets of the social situation (e.g., SES, time for or transportation to educational opportunities) that may influence health education? What effect do these facets have on the health education situation?

Behavioral Determinants

- Do health behaviors prevalent in the population give rise to the need for health education?

Health System Determinants

- Do local health care providers emphasize health promotion and health education? Do members of the population have access to health care services where they might receive health education?
- Does the population have a need for education regarding the use of health care services?
- Do health care recommendations give rise to a need for health education? Are there elements of the health care regimen that may influence learning abilities (e.g., medications)?
- Will attitudes toward health care services and providers influence the ability to learn?

Prioritizing learning needs. Planning health education programs begins with prioritizing learning needs. Generally speaking, a learning needs assessment will indicate several areas of need, not all of which can be addressed in a single health education effort. Prioritization involves determining the relative effects of behaviors and risk factors present in the population and the benefits to be achieved by changing them. Another consideration in prioritizing health education needs is the ease with which contributing factors can be changed. For example, members of the population may not use seat belts, get too little exercise, and fail to obtain periodic mammograms. A change to using seat belts would result in the most immediate and dramatic benefit to the community and be the easiest of the three behaviors to change. For these reasons, the population health nurse might first begin with health education efforts in this area. Members of the community can help determine priorities, ensuring that topics of greatest interest and relevance to the target audience are addressed.

Developing goals and objectives. Goal identification involves specifying the broad purpose of the health education encounter. Some authors distinguish between *program goals*—the intended purpose of the overall health education program—and *educational goals*—the learning outcome expected for the audience. For example, the program goal for a nutrition program might be to prevent obesity in school-age children. The educational goal, on the other hand, might be for parents to become knowledgeable regarding appropriate nutrition for their children.

Objectives describe specific outcomes to be achieved as a result of the health education encounter. An objective related to the nutrition program goal might be that the community incidence (number of new cases) of childhood obesity will decline by 50% within 2 years. An educational objective might be that parents are able to correctly describe the number of servings of each element of the food pyramid required by an elementary school student.

Objectives should be stated in measurable terms that allow one to evaluate whether the expected results have been achieved. Evaluation of outcomes also requires that they be specific. For example, an outcome objective such as "reduce adolescent tobacco use" is somewhat vague. If one adolescent smoker stops smoking, have we met our objective? Similarly, an objective to "stop adolescent tobacco use" is not particularly realistic. No matter what interventions are employed, it is unlikely that we will ever prevent all adolescents from using tobacco. A more realistic, and more measurable, objective for tobacco education might be to "reduce the prevalence of tobacco use among high school seniors by 50% within 1 year." As stated, the objective provides a target measure for accomplishment (a 50% decline in the number of seniors who use tobacco) as well as a time frame for expected accomplishment (1 year from program initiation).

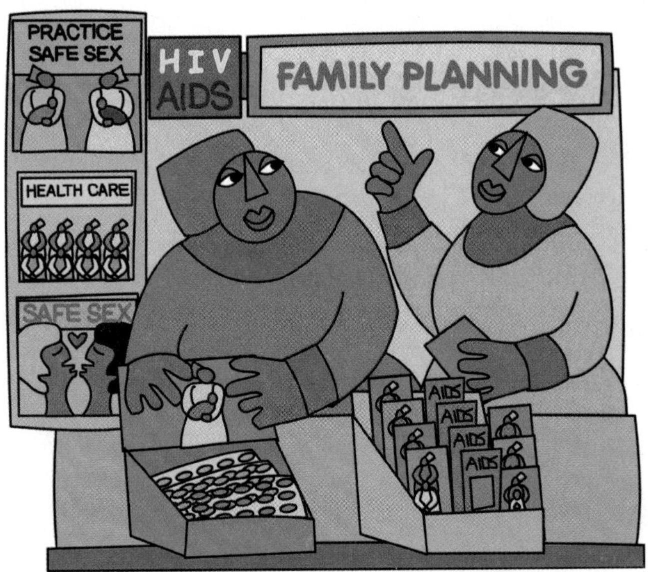

Health promotion messages should be tailored to individual or group risks, attitudes, and values. *(Tntdesigns/Fotolia)*

Selecting content and teaching strategies. The content selected for inclusion in a health education program will depend on its relevance to the target population. Audiences are more likely to attend to information that they perceive as highly relevant to their own situations. One must be selective in planning the content because no audience needs or wishes to learn everything about a particular topic that the health educator may know. Going back to the general principles discussed earlier, an effective educator chooses the content that is most relevant to the target audience.

Selection of teaching strategies will depend on a number of factors, including characteristics of the audience, the content and objectives to be achieved, program budget, time available, cultural appropriateness, and the environment for health education. In educating individual clients, health education messages may make use of tailored or customized communication based on the needs and characteristics of an individual learner or target audience. For example, cancer screening messages that focus on surviving to watch one's children grow and develop will be more effective for parents than for single individuals.

Recently, a number of authors have suggested using highly graphic messages in health education initiatives to motivate healthful behaviors. For example, truth advertising—focusing on making adolescents aware of the tobacco industry's special efforts to target them for smoking initiation—has been associated with an increase in antitobacco attitudes and beliefs among youth (Hopwood & Merritt, 2011).

Much of the work of population health nurses is directed toward educating individuals, families, and population groups regarding health promotion. Population health nurses can use the educational processes described here to promote healthy behavior at all of these levels.

Using media in health education and health promotion. Media portrayal of health-related behavior can influence health promotion either positively or negatively. For example, depiction of smoking in movies has been linked to smoking initiation among youth. In spite of decreases in the extent of smoking depiction in popular movies, approximately 45% of the 137 top-grossing movies in 2010 included on-screen tobacco-related incidents. Six members of the Motion Picture Association of America have policies designed to reduce tobacco use in movies, and among three of these, the number of tobacco-related incidents in youth-rated movies decreased by 96% from 2005 to 2010. Decreases are less noticeable among independent companies and members of the association without tobacco policies (National Center for Chronic Disease Prevention and Health Promotion, 2011).

Media can also be used, however, to support health-promoting behaviors in at least three ways. First, media can be used for public education (Daniels, Glickstein, & Mason, 2012). For example, researchers and community members collaborated on the creation of a *fotonovela*, a type of graphic novel popular with many Latinos, to promote good nutrition in the local Latino population (Hinojosa, et al., 2011).

Second, media can be used for social marketing, creating motivation to change unhealthful behaviors or to engage in healthful ones. Social marketing is discussed in more detail below. Finally, media can be used for **media advocacy**, which is the purposeful use of media messages and approaches to

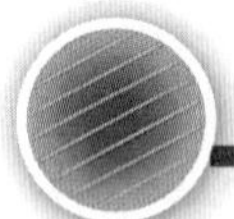

Evidence-Based Practice

Effective Health Promotion Strategies

There is a general lack of evidence for the effectiveness of health promotion initiatives that is compounded by the reliance on randomized clinical trials (RCTs) as the highest and most credible source of evidence. Much of health promotion research, however, is population-based, which makes conducting RCTs difficult. Conversely, the results of RCTs conducted in rigorously controlled settings may or may not be generalizable to the real world of population health. In addition, RCTs focus on individual health-related behaviors and do not account for the myriad social and political factors that influence health-promoting behaviors in the general population (Carter et al., 2011).

In spite of these difficulties, however, there is some indication of the use of evidence-based population level health promotion and illness prevention practices. Much of this evidence has been compiled by the Community Preventive Services Task Force, an independent body appointed by the Director of the Centers for Disease Control and Prevention. The Community Preventive Services Task Force was developed as a complement to the U.S. Preventive Services Task Force, which focuses on health promotion and prevention at the individual client level. Thus far, the Community Preventive Services Task Force has conducted systematic reviews of evidence and compiled recommendations for effective interventions related to topics included in Table 11-4●. For example, community wide campaigns to promote use of folic acid supplements in pregnancy have been found to have a strong evidence base for their efficacy. Similarly, the use of sobriety checkpoints has been found to be an effective strategy to prevent motor vehicle-related injuries (Community Preventive Services Task Force, 2013). For a complete description of evidence-based strategies for population level health promotion and prevention see the resource provided for *The Guide to Community Preventive Services in the External Resources* section of the student resources site.

TABLE 11-4 Topic Areas Addressed by Community Preventive Services Task Force Reviews

Adolescent health	Mental health
Preventing excessive alcohol consumption	Motor vehicle injury prevention
Asthma control	Nutrition
Prevention of birth defects	Obesity
Cancer prevention and control	Oral health
Cardiovascular disease prevention	Physical activity
Diabetes prevention and control	Social environment
Emergency preparedness	Tobacco use
Health communication and social marketing	Vaccination
Health equity	Violence prevention
HIV/AIDS, other STIs and pregnancy	Worksite health promotion

Data from: Community Preventive Services Task Force. (2014). *The Community Guide.* Retrieved from http://www.thecommunityguide.org/index.html

promote a social agenda or policy initiative (Daniels et al., 2012). Media advocacy mobilizes constituents and stakeholders to take action, targets policy makers, and often focuses on changing environmental conditions to promote health. For example, media advocacy has been used to highlight the unhealthful effects of junk food availability in school settings and has led to restrictions on food and drinks available to students. Similarly, a mass media campaign effectively promoted smoking cessation among people exposed to the campaign (Vallone, Duke, Cullen, McCausland, & Allen, 2011).

Media depictions can also be used to understand the insights and motivations of particular groups of people. For example, Black and Peacock (2011) examined depictions of a "strong Black woman script" in media sources popular among African American women. The strong Black woman script represents efforts to live up to cultural expectations to protect their families at the expense of their own needs. They recommended capitalizing on information gleaned from popular depictions to develop alternative approaches and to design culturally tailored interventions to promote health in this population.

The Internet is another medium often used by individual clients, the general public, and health care providers as a source of health-related information. Using the Internet as a medium for health education has both advantages and disadvantages. Two general problems that may be encountered are inaccurate information and biased information. To address these problems, the Health on the Net Foundation (HON, 2013a), a non-government organization designed to promote dissemination of accurate health-related information on the Internet, has developed a code of ethics and criteria for certification of health-related websites. These criteria include elements related to authority, complementarity, confidentiality, attribution, justifiability, transparency, financial disclosure, and advertising (HON, 2013b). The criteria for website certification are described in Table 11-5•. Visitors to a particular Internet site can also look for the display of the HON approval logo or that of other organizations that evaluate health-related websites on the website's home page. For further information about approval organizations, see the resources provided in the *External Resources* section of the student resources site.

The Internet can be an effective mode of health education and health promotion even for persons with low literacy levels. For that reason, the U.S. Office of Disease Prevention and Health Promotion (ODPHP, 2010) has developed guidelines for the creation of easy-to-use health websites described earlier. For further information about the guidelines, see the resources provided in the External Resources section of the student resources site. One should keep in mind, however, that people of lower socioeconomic status or members of some ethnic groups may not have the same access to these modalities as those in the dominant society. It has also been suggested that the Internet may be an effective way of disseminating health promotion messages to people who do not regularly interact with formal health care networks except on an emergency basis (Crilly, Keefe, & Volpe, 2011).

Other forms of social media may also be helpful in fostering health promotion. At the same time, such media may impede successful health promotion activities by disseminating incorrect information. **Social media** include a set of Internet-based tools that enable people to communicate with each other in real time (Stokowski, 2011). Applications like My Space, Facebook, Twitter, Instagram, and blogs are examples of social media. Population health nurses can use social media to disseminate health-related information to a wide segment of the population, but they must also consider these media as potential sources of misinformation. They should also remember that personal postings to social media, if they reflect poorly on the nursing profession, can minimize the public's trust and

TABLE 11-5 Criteria for Health Website Accreditation

Criterion	Description
Authoritative	The website indicates the qualifications of contributing authors.
Complementarity	The website provides information designed to support or complement, rather than replace, the relationship between the user and his or her health care provider.
Privacy	The website respects the privacy and confidentiality of information obtained from users.
Attribution	The website cites the source(s) of information provided and provides modification dates for web pages.
Justifiability	The website provides balanced and appropriate evidence for any claims regarding the benefits or performance of a particular treatment, product, or service.
Transparency	The website provides information on the ownership of the site and provides accessible contact information.
Financial disclosure	The website clearly identifies its source(s) of financial support.
Advertising policy	The website clearly states whether advertising is included in the site and describes its advertising policy. Advertising is clearly differentiated from health-related information.

Data From: Health on the Net Foundation. (2013b). *The HON Code of Conduct for medical and health Web sites (HONcode).* Retrieved from http://www.hon.ch/HONcode/Patients/Conduct.html

impede effective health promotion efforts. For this reason, nurses using social media as avenues for health education and health promotion should take care to present balanced information that has a strong foundation in scientific evidence.

Elements to consider in designing effective health-related websites and other media include the target audience's access to and ability to use the Internet, their ability to read and understand printed material, the complexity of the material to be provided, and the usability of the website. Media designed for people with low literacy levels or limited technology skills will need easily navigated sites that contain clear information. Website and other media designers should consider the following in developing effective health education media:

- People often scan or skip large sections of print, so bullet important points in small, easy to digest segments.
- People may have difficulty spelling search terms, so an alphabetical index of subjects should also be included.
- People tend to focus on the center of the screen so important messages should be positioned above the mid-point, and navigation functions should be positioned in the center or on the left.
- Too much material overwhelms users, so keep content and presentation simple.
- Many people may lack navigational skills, so use step-by-step navigational prompts with active "next" and "back" buttons.
- Media designers should learn as much as possible about potential users and their goals for use. Cultural and motivational characteristics are particularly important areas of information.
- Designers should write "actionable" content that highlights desired behavioral changes and provides specific actions for accomplishing the change. Change is also facilitated by describing the benefits of the change.
- Content should be displayed clearly on the page in a well-organized format that is easy to navigate.
- Engaging users with interactive content maintains interest and attention.
- The effectiveness of the site should be regularly evaluated and revised as needed (ODPHP, 2010).

Population health nurses can use this information to create effective health-related websites to disseminate health promotion information and to influence population and individual health-related behaviors.

SOCIAL MARKETING, BRANDING, AND TAILORING. Decisions regarding health-related behaviors occur within a social and cultural context, and changes in health behavior require an understanding of the influences exerted by that context. These social influences on behavior tend to exist in a hierarchy; one is influenced in turn by one's peer group, one's nuclear and extended family, community norms, and national norms promulgated via mass media (Tones & Green, 2010). Social marketing, as a health promotion strategy, uses information about the factors that influence behavior in specific population groups to promote adoption of health-related behaviors or elimination of unhealthy behaviors. Social marketing is a process designed to change negative behaviors or maintain positive ones for the benefit of the individual and the society (The NMSC, 2010).

Social marketing involves the use of commercial marketing techniques to achieve a health-related goal. The aim is to use commercial marketing principles to address social problems rather than generate profit. In essence, social marketing, as it relates to health promotion, involves conveying a health-related message in a way that is relevant and of interest to a particular target audience. The effectiveness of social marketing is enhanced by "cultural grounding," which involves an appeal based on the values and cultural beliefs and behaviors of the target population. For example, successful antismoking campaigns for young people have been based on social marketing principles grounded in adolescent "culture." Teenagers value being part of the group and being attractive to others. Social marketing campaigns were directed toward making nonsmoking the social norm by emphasizing the unattractive aspects of smoking. Other campaigns focused on the adolescent's need for independence by highlighting the manipulative nature of tobacco industry advertising directed toward teens. The "Truth Campaign," designed to make visible the tobacco industry's manipulative strategies, is credited with preventing 450,000 young people from initiating smoking in its first 4 years (Hopwood & Merritt, 2011).

A social marketing tool kit developed by the Centers for Disease Control and Prevention (CDC, 2010) addresses six phases in the social marketing process. The first phase is describing the problem to be resolved. The second phase involves conducting market research to determine the characteristics of the target audience. The third phase involves creating a marketing strategy or plan of action for the social marketing program. In this phase, the health promotion practitioner identifies the target audience to be reached and influenced by the intervention. More than one target audience may be identified based on market segmentation. Behavioral goals and strategies to achieve them are developed for each target market. For example, the goal of an antitobacco campaign for adults might be smoking cessation by current smokers. This goal might be expanded in a campaign for youth to include cessation by current smokers and non-initiation of smoking by nonsmokers. Similarly, different promotion strategies would be devised for each group based on group characteristics and circumstances that influence smoking behaviors. The last element in creating the marketing strategy is identifying and allocating resources.

In the fourth phase of the social marketing process, the actual intervention is planned. For example, billboards might be designed to convey the message and located where they will be seen by specific targeted audiences. Graphic flyers and posters might be placed in school settings, and so on. The fifth phase involves planning strategies for monitoring and evaluating the intervention, and the sixth phase involves actually implementing the interventions and evaluating their effects. This last phase may also include revising the campaign based on consumer feedback. The phases of social marketing are summarized in Table 11-6●. The focused assessment on the next page can help to guide development of a social marketing plan.

Although they use similar methods, social marketing and commercial marketing differ in a number of respects. The goal of social marketing is to promote health-related behavior, while commercial marketing is designed to promote the purchase of a particular product or service. They also differ in terms of demand. Commercial marketing focuses on "selective demand," the choice of one brand over another competing brand. Social marketing, on the other hand, focuses on "primary demand," the choice of whether or not to engage in a behavior that is often perceived as being counter to one's self-interest and desires. In commercial marketing, the competition is another brand of the same product, while in social marketing, the competing force is an unhealthful behavior, such as smoking. Finally, the two approaches differ in terms of the time involved to witness "delivery" on product promises. For example, smoking can almost instantly enhance one's reputation as "cool," but the beneficial effects of health-promoting behaviors may take decades to be noted (Blitstein, Evans, & Driscoll, 2008).

Social marketing is characterized by the concept of exchange, the use of research to direct action, and the development of a "marketing mix" and positioning strategy. Each of these characteristics will be addressed briefly using the example of smoking among adolescents. In social marketing, adolescents are being asked to exchange something, in this case smoking, for a more healthful behavior, not smoking. The central issue is to determine what exchange will satisfy the target audience, so that the perceived benefits of the change outweigh its costs (Hopwood & Merritt, 2011). For adolescents, being accepted by the group or being more attractive to others might be benefits for which they would exchange smoking.

TABLE 11-6 Phases of the Social Marketing Process

Phase	Description
1. Problem Description	• Identification of the health problem or description of the issue to be resolved, including contributing factors and the target audience for intervention
2. Market research	• Determination of characteristics of the target audience
3. Strategy	• Creation of a tailored marketing development strategy or plan of action for each segment of the target audience
	• Identification and allocation of resources
4. Intervention	• Development of actual marketing design messages
5. Monitoring plan	• Development of strategies for monitoring intervention effectiveness
6. Implementation	• Dissemination of marketing messages
	• Evaluation of the effectiveness of marketing messages

Data from: Centers for Disease Control and Prevention. (2010). CDCynergy lite: Social marketing made simple: A guide for creating effective social marketing plans. Retrieved from http://www.cdc.gov/healthcommunication/pdf/cdcynergylite.pdf

Social marketing is based on research that describes the target population, their attributes, interests, and concerns. Using our adolescent smoking example, researchers would be interested in exploring what motivates smoking behavior in teenagers. The assessment of the target population is followed by research to develop and test marketing messages and strategies with the target population, in this case adolescents. The design of these messages might make use of another marketing research strategy, focus groups of adolescents to develop and/or react to antismoking messages. Finally, research methods are also used to study the application and effectiveness of the marketing interventions. At this point, antismoking messages would be widely disseminated and their effectiveness studied in deterring adolescent smoking.

A marketing mix is based on the four Ps of social marketing: product, price, place, and promotion (Hopwood & Merritt, 2011). The product is the need, service, or desired behavior that the target audience is being asked to adopt (e.g., not smoking). Price reflects the cost of or barriers to adopting the desired behavior or giving up an unhealthy behavior (e.g., possible weight gain, irritability, or being thought "uncool"). The place element of social marketing is the location where the product or service can be obtained (e.g., where smoking cessation programs or nicotine patches are available) as well as the places where members of the target group can be reached. In our adolescent smoking example, this might include junior and senior high schools, sporting events, or rock concerts. Promotion refers to the communication strategies and messages used to motivate members of the target audience to act. This might include posters or radio or television messages that present the less attractive aspects of smoking (e.g., smoker's breath, discolored hands and teeth). Promotion strategies include information related to the product, price, and place where the product or service can be obtained (Hopwood & Merritt, 2011).

Some authors include additional social marketing Ps, such as publics (the different audiences for social marketing strategies), partnerships between social and health agencies to achieve social marketing goals, and policy that addresses environmental changes that promote the desired behavior. A final P involves the "purse strings," or funding to support social marketing strategies (Weinrich, n.d.).

A positioning strategy addresses the price or costs of the behavior vis-à-vis the competing behavior. Developing a positioning strategy involves identifying the benefits of the desired behavior and its costs and comparing them to the benefits and costs of the competing behavior. For example, smoking and nonsmoking are competing behaviors. The primary cost of smoking, of course, is death. However, if the target audience is youth for whom death is a distant event, focusing on this cost will not prove very effective. Focusing on the unattractive aspects of smoking highlights elements of the price of smoking that are apt to get the attention of young people, who are very conscious of personal appearance and attractiveness to others.

Critical elements of social marketing include understanding the competition, understanding the target market, creation of a mutually beneficial exchange, and segmenting the market and targeting interventions to the specific interests of particular market segments. *Segmentation* is the process of identifying subgroups or segments of the population who share certain characteristics that can form the basis for a marketing strategy. For example, knowing the particular communication channels used by a group can help inform appropriate media campaigns. Antismoking information disseminated to young people through Facebook and other social media reflects audience segmentation. Another example is the use of a text messaging service, SEXINFO, to provide sexual health information and referrals to sexually active young people in the San Francisco area (Youth+Tech+Health, 2014). Other nontechnological strategies might be used for other segments of the population, such as older adults who are less computer savvy. Segmentation leads to decisions about the most effective use of resources and promotion strategies for a particular segment of a target population. The *Focused Assessment* below presents some questions to be addressed in designing social marketing campaigns.

Branding is a particular application of social marketing that endeavors to create an image to which consumers can relate and display loyalty. A brand is a set of beliefs or values one associates with a product or service when one encounters a particular name, mark, or symbol (Evans & Hastings, 2008b). For example, the BMW symbol gives rise to connotations of luxury, quality engineering, and so on. Branding has been effectively used in commercial marketing to attract and retain customer loyalty to a particular product. As another example, the Virginia Slims brand of cigarettes and branding communications stating "You've come a long way, baby" conjured visions of strong, independent women who thought for themselves. A branding communication is more than an advertisement; it is a message designed to associate valued benefits with a specific product in the minds of consumers (Blitstein et al., 2008). Because of these associations, the particular "brand" becomes the preferred choice. Public health practitioners have been challenged to develop healthy "brands" or behaviors that become a preferred choice over unhealthy options (Evans & Hastings, 2008a). Public health brands are associations that individuals hold for healthy lifestyles that make them a better option than unhealthy ones (Evans & Hastings, 2008b).

There are three main concepts related to branding: a relationship with the consumer, the value the brand adds to the particular product or service, and an exchange with the consumer. The relationship to the consumer is grounded in a promise of delivery of some good valued by the consumer. For example, branding has been used in youth antitobacco campaigns, promising increased independence through rebellion against manipulation by the tobacco industry. The value added concept includes value beyond the obvious health benefit of the desired behavior. Again, antismoking campaigns have capitalized on values of attractiveness (no "cigarette breath") and "being cool" that are of importance to adolescents. Finally, exchange deals with the concept that the behavior or product is worth the cost or effort involved in obtaining it. Branding involves creating an aspiration to a desirable ideal (being thought attractive), modeling a socially desired behavior, such as exercise, and association with an idealized imagery, such as an attractive and popular person (Evans & Hastings, 2008b).

Branding, attempts to create broad perceptions and associations of the desired behavior within populations. Tailoring, on the other hand, is directed toward the individual. A tailored message is specifically focused on promoting behavior change in an individual and addresses that individual's unique

FOCUSED ASSESSMENT Strategic Questions for Social Marketing Design

- What is the problem to be addressed?
- What behavior change is required to address the problem?
- Who is the audience?
- What are the benefit and barriers to the desired behavior? To competing behaviors?
- What benefits does the audience desire?
- How, when, and where does the behavior occur?
- What would make the behavior easier or more desirable?
- Who has influence with the desired audience?
- What media channels will reach the target audience?

Data from: Centers for Disease Control and Prevention. (2010). CDCynergy lite: Social marketing made simple: A guide for creating effective social marketing plans. Retrieved from http://www.cdc.gov/healthcommunication/pdf/cdcynergylite.pdf

characteristics (Lewis & McCormack, 2008). Tailoring focuses on making the message more relevant to a particular individual or subgroup within the population. For example, your insurance provider may send you health-related information based on the fact that you are of a certain age, ethnicity, and a smoker, information gleaned from your health records.

Population health nurses can use the concept of tailoring to create individualized health messages to promote health in a particular person. This may also be done at a population level by creating tailored message libraries. Creating such libraries involves the development of an assessment tool to identify determinants of health and behavior in a given individual, developing messages related to specific determinants, and creating tailoring algorithms that link specific messages to determinants identified in an assessment. For example, one might use a computerized health-risk assessment that obtains information on age, gender, family history of particular conditions, dietary habits, alcohol and drug consumption, use of safety precautions, and so on. Then on the basis of the person's responses, specific health-promoting messages would be generated. For example, data indicating that one is 16 years old, female, and sexually active, might trigger automated messages related to prevention of pregnancy and sexually transmitted diseases (Lewis & McCormack, 2008).

Population health nurses can use the concepts of social marketing, branding, and tailoring to disseminate health information and promote healthful behaviors. These strategies can also be used to influence policy makers to develop policies that promote health and create conditions conducive to healthful behaviors.

LEGISLATION. Legislation is another approach to health promotion that mandates individual behavior or creates conditions that promote health. For example, a ban on the display of tobacco products in stores in Ontario, Canada decreased tobacco promotion and youth exposure to tobacco marketing (Cohen et al., 2011). Because tobacco has been linked to alcohol use, a similar ban on sales and promotion in places where alcohol is sold might have similar effects (Jiang & Ling, 2011). Legislation with a similar intent was enacted in China mandating that filmmakers limit the extent of on-screen smoking. The legislation also prohibits identifying a cigarette brand and showing smokers in scenes that include teenagers, teens buying cigarettes, or smoking in places where smoking is banned (Currie, 2011).

Legislation has also been used to promote other health-related behaviors. For example, state laws mandating seat belt use were first passed in 1984. As of 2008, all U.S. states except New Hampshire had mandatory seat belt laws. The effects of such laws, however, depend on their enforcement. With respect to seat belt legislation, for example, laws may involve primary or secondary enforcement. Primary seat belt laws permit law enforcement officers to issues tickets solely on the basis of failure to use seat belts. In states with secondary enforcement laws, tickets for nonuse of seat belts can only be issued if drivers are stopped for some other violation. According to data from the 2008 Behavioral Risk Factor Surveillance System, the prevalence of seat belt use was higher in states with primary enforcement laws (National Center for Injury Prevention and Control, 2011). Legislative efforts have also been used to promote healthier diets by limiting trans fats used in restaurants in multiple cities. In 2011, California became the first state to enact a statewide ban on trans fats in food establishments (Assaf, 2014).

On occasion, legislation may undermine health promotion efforts. For example, at the end of 2010, 12 states had legislation that preempted local restrictions on smoking. Preemptive state legislation prohibits local jurisdictions from enacting laws that are more stringent than those of the state. One of the *Healthy People 2020* objectives calls for a reduction in the number of states with preemptive tobacco legislation. From 2000 to 2010, the number of states with preemptive tobacco control laws declined from 18 to 12, and most of the change in such laws dealt with restrictions on smoking in specific places. Laws in several states continue to prohibit local laws related to tobacco advertising and youth access to tobacco products (Office on Smoking and Health, 2011). Legislative mandates may also have unintended consequences. For example, increases in cigarette taxes in some states have led to decreased levels of smoking, but also increased black market sales and decreased tax revenues targeted for smoking cessation programs (Henchman & Drenkard, 2014).

Population health nurses can actively support legislation that promotes health. Using the strategies discussed in Chapter 9∞, they can alert law makers to the need for legislation in a particular area. They can also campaign for and educate the public about such legislative efforts. In addition, population health nurses should keep abreast of legislative attempts to undermine health.

USE OF COMMUNITY HEALTH WORKERS. The final strategy for promoting health in populations is the use of CHWs to disseminate health promotion messages and to foster health-promoting behaviors in the population. Because of the growing shortage of health care professionals, there are not enough personnel to meet the needs for health promotion efforts among the population. CHWs can help to fill this gap. In 2009, the American Public Health Association issued a policy statement on the need to employ CHWs to increase access to care and reduce health-related inequities in the U.S. population. The policy statement called for a systematic approach to the use of CHWs and highlighted the need for policy and practice changes to more fully realize their potential.

Community health workers (CHWs) are "frontline public health workers who are trusted members of and/or have an unusually close understanding of the community served. This trusting relationship enables a CHW to serve as a liaison /link/intermediary between health/social services and the community to facilitate access to service and improve the quality and cultural competence of service delivery" (American Public

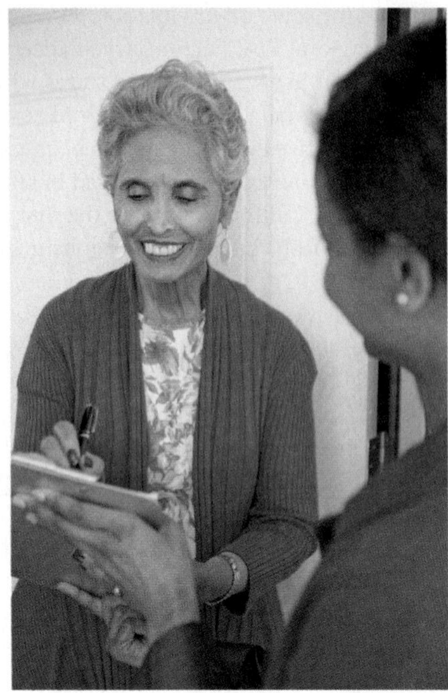

Outreach workers from the community can help to identify and address community member's needs. *(EdBockStock/Shutterstock)*

Health Association, 2009, p. 1). CHWs may be paid staff or volunteers working in concert with local health care professionals. They usually share the ethnicity, language, socioeconomic status, and life experiences of other members of the community (Health Resources and Services Administration [HRSA], 2011). Generally speaking, CHWs enact one or more of several roles and functions as depicted in the *Highlights* box below.

Highlights

Community Health Worker Roles

- Bridging and providing cultural mediation between communities and their members and health and social service systems, particularly by facilitating effective provider–client communication
- Providing culturally appropriate health education and information
- Improving access and continuity of care
- Providing informal counseling and social support
- Monitoring and promoting treatment adherence
- Advocating for individual, family, and community needs
- Providing direct services and conducting screening tests
- Monitoring individual and population health status
- Building individual and community capacity

Data from: American Public Health Association. (2009). *Support for community health workers to increase health access and to reduce health inequities.* Policy Number 20091. Retrieved from http://www.apha.org/advocacy/policy/policysearch/default.htm?id=1393; Balcazar, H., Rosenthal, L. E., Brownstein, N. J., Rush, C. H., Matos, S., & Hernandez, L. (2011). Community health workers can be a public health force for change in the United States: Three actions for a new paradigm. *American Journal of Public Health, 101,* 2199–2203. doi: 10.2105/AJPH.2011.300386

CHWs have been found to be effective in a number of areas. For example, a systematic review of CHW effectiveness found that they contributed to improved disease prevention and cancer screening knowledge, improvement in various health-related behaviors, improved outcomes for conditions such as back pain and asthma, and increased use of some types of health promotion services (Viswanathan et al., 2009). In another study, incorporation of CHWs from multiple community organizations and adding dissemination of immunization information to their other responsibilities was effective in increasing and maintaining immunization rates in New York City (Findley et al., 2009). *Promotores*, Latino CHWs, have also been found to be effective in promoting physical activity; improving blood pressure, fitness, and flexibility; improving community resource use; decreasing depression; and increasing community support for physical activity (Ayala & the San Diego Prevention Research Center Team, 2011). Similarly, peer worker interventions improved rates of eye protection use among migrant citrus harvesters (Monaghan et al., 2011).

Mutual support groups, a strategy related to the use of CHWs, have also been found to be effective in supporting health-promoting behaviors. For example, the AMIGAS program (a Spanish acronym for "friends, Latina women, informing each other, guiding each other, and supporting each other against AIDS") changed gender role perceptions, improved self-efficacy for negotiating safer sex and condom use, and increased HIV knowledge among Latino women in Miami. The program was based on a similar widely disseminated program among African American women, SISTA (Sisters informing sisters about topics on AIDS) (Wingood et al., 2011).

Community health workers have long been used to promote health and prevent illness in international venues and have proven quite effective. For example, Iranian CHWs reported an in-depth understanding of health and factors influencing it and executed a wide range of activities related to health in rural Iran. They noted the importance of trust-based relationships with the communities served and discussed heavy workloads and lack of an effective support system as impeding their effectiveness (Javanparast, Baum, Labonte, & Sanders, 2011). CHWs are often the mainstay of numerous other international health promotion initiatives from use of mosquito netting to water purification efforts.

HRSA has identified six health service models incorporating the use of CHWs. In the first model, the CHWs were lay health workers who advocated for members of the population, educated and mentored them regarding health issues, and served as outreach workers and translators. In the second model, CHWs functioned as members of the health care team completing tasks delegated by the health care team leader.

In the third model, CHWs played the role of health care navigator or care coordinator, assisting clients to negotiate health care systems with a focus on improving access to care and fostering appropriate use of services. The fourth type of model employed CHWs in screening and provision of health education. In the fifth model, CHWs functioned as outreach workers, informing clients of service availability and enrolling them in service programs. Finally, some CHWs functioned as community organizers and capacity builders.

Population health nurses may have a variety of responsibilities with respect to community health workers. As people knowledgeable about local communities, they can identify community members who may be effective CHWs. Population health nurses may also develop and implement curricula to train CHWs for their roles in any given project and may supervise and monitor their performance. Finally, population health nurses may participate in evaluating the effectiveness of CHW initiatives. Population health nurses may advocate for the use of CHWs to participate in health promotion activities in local communities. Likewise, they may use the other strategies described here to foster health-promoting behaviors among population groups and to advocate for policies and conditions that support health promotion.

Evaluating Health Promotion Programs

Like all population health nursing activities, the effectiveness of health promotion initiatives should be evaluated. Several authors have noted the difficulty involved in such an evaluation, primarily because it is difficult to determine, when an event does not occur, if it would have occurred without the intervention. Another area of difficulty lies in the fact that the unit of analysis in community-based health promotion evaluation should be the community, but resource constraints in both programs and program evaluations rarely allow participation by an entire community. Therefore, one has the problem of identifying who in the community was exposed to the program and who was not. In addition, the quasi-experimental nature of most program evaluations leads to selection effects among participants, involving those most interested in a program and possibly more highly motivated regarding the particular topic. Similarly, evaluation measures may focus on complete avoidance of a negative behavior (or always engaging in a positive one) and, thus, may miss small gains (e.g., reduction in the number of cigarettes smoked versus stopping smoking altogether).

In spite of these difficulties, however, health promotion programs can and should be evaluated. This evaluation may occur at different levels. For example, diagnostic evaluation assesses the accuracy of the needs assessment on which the health promotion program was based. Formative evaluation, also called process evaluation, examines the way in which the program was carried out. Finally, summative evaluation may focus on program outcome, impact, or both.

Health promotion programs may also be evaluated in terms of the extent to which they achieve criteria of empowerment, participation, holism, intersectoral collaboration, equity, use of multiple strategies, and sustainability (Tones & Green, 2010). First and foremost, programs should be empowering, allowing beneficiaries to assume control of the program. They should also foster participation of the target population at all stages of development, implementation, and evaluation. Third, they should be holistic, with a focus on multiple aspects of health. They should also involve participation and collaboration by multiple community sectors to achieve desired ends and should be guided by concerns for equity and social justice. Effective health promotion programs also employ a variety of approaches to achieving change. Finally, the results of effective health promotion programs are sustainable, with changes that can be maintained beyond the initial period of funding.

A number of the *Healthy People 2020* objectives reflect health promotion efforts, and the relevant targets can be used to evaluate the effectiveness of specific health promotion initiatives. Many of the objectives related to the leading health indicators emphasize health promotion. For example, objectives related to injury and violence prevention include reductions in pedestrian deaths on public roads, an objective in keeping with our speed bump example earlier in the chapter, as well as increased use of seat belts. Similarly, objectives related to nutrition and obesity include increasing the percentage of people who eat sufficient fruits and vegetables and decreasing fat intake, both of which reflect health promotion. Specific objectives and the degree of progress toward their accomplishment are included in relevant chapters throughout this book. For further information on the *Healthy People 2020* objectives and data on their accomplishment, see the resources provided in the *External Resources* section of the student resources site.

Population health nurses are actively involved in health promotion and health education efforts with individuals, families, and population groups. Table 11-7• describes the elements of a health promotion program and considerations related to assessing the health promotion situation, planning the program, and evaluating its effectiveness. In the table, the assessment of factors influencing the health promotion situation is framed in the context of the determinants of health. The program described is an actual population-based health promotion initiative undertaken by population health nursing students to promote disaster preparedness in a culturally diverse community.

As we have seen, health promotion is more than promoting behavior change among individuals or population groups or providing health-related information. It also involves activity to change the social, political, economic, and/or physical environment in ways that are conducive to health. Achieving changes at these levels requires advocacy and empowerment as well as information giving and motivation.

TABLE 11-7 Elements of a Community Health Promotion Program for Disaster Preparedness

Element	Considerations
Assessment	**Biological Determinants** • Many older people and families with young children live in the community. • There are several disabled community members. **Psychological Determinants** • There is apathy regarding family disaster preparedness among community residents. • Residents do not believe disasters are likely to affect them. **Environmental Determinants** • The community sits on a major geologic fault. • The community is surrounded by dry canyons with potential for wildfires. • The community is in a coastal area that could be subjected to tsunamis. • Many residences are old and might be heavily damaged in an earthquake. • Most of the residences are older homes and rental units. Few of them are equipped with smoke alarms. **Sociocultural Determinants** • The community includes several large groups of Hispanic immigrants and Asian refugees as well as small groups of African Americans, Sudanese and Somali refugees, and older White residents. • Many residents do not speak English. Major languages spoken are English, Spanish, Vietnamese, and Hmong. • Community income levels are low and many community residents have less than a high school education. • Most families in the community have little knowledge of disaster preparedness. • Several homeless individuals live in makeshift shelters in the canyons. • Fire department services are central to the community and respond rapidly to emergency calls. **Behavioral Determinants** • Homeless persons living in the canyons often cook over open fires, posing a wildfire hazard. • Many people in the community smoke, increasing the potential for house fires. • Many of the Hmong population cook over open braziers in their homes, increasing the potential for house fires. • Few families in the community have gathered supplies in the event of potential disasters. **Health System Determinants** • Health care providers in the community do not routinely educate clients regarding disaster preparedness. • The local health department has concentrated on community response to possible bioterrorist attacks and has not actively promoted preparation for other types of disasters.
Purpose/goal	To increase disaster preparedness among families in the community
Objectives	**Affective Domain** • Community residents will demonstrate an understanding of the need for smoke detectors in homes. • Community residents will demonstrate an understanding of the need for disaster preparedness. **Cognitive Domain** • Community residents will be able to identify critical supplies needed for disaster preparedness. • Community residents will demonstrate appropriate responses to specific emergencies.
Content	• Content was chosen to address the two types of disasters most likely to occur in the community: fire and earthquake. • Information about preventing fires, responding to fires and earthquakes, and needed disaster supplies was gathered from a variety of sources (e.g., local fire officials, the Internet, Red Cross, and county health department disaster divisions). • Content was reviewed to pick out the five or six most salient pieces of information.
Teaching strategies/ materials	• The project was planned to be implemented as an exhibit at the multicultural fair held annually in the community. This fair attracts approximately 10,000 people each year, most of whom are community residents. • Because of the fair venue, messages were developed for the limited time people were likely to spend at the booth. • According to community informants, many of the Hmong population were not literate, even in Hmong (which did not have a written form until recently), so information brochures were developed in English, Spanish, and Vietnamese, and pictorial messages were used for the Hmong population. • Pictures and samples of necessary disaster supplies were exhibited. • Fire prevention and response coloring books were obtained from the local fire department and crayons were purchased and wrapped in sets of three to give out with the coloring books. • Posters indicating needed disaster supplies and information families should have were created and hung in the booth. Key information was included on refrigerator magnets given to fair participants. • Donations were solicited for raffle prizes related to disaster prevention and preparedness (e.g., smoke alarms, flashlights) and raffles were held throughout the day to attract fair participants to the booth.

TABLE 11-7 (Continued)

Element	Considerations
Evaluation	• Visitors to the booth were asked to select pictures from a collection of items that they would include in disaster preparedness supplies and attach them to a felt board. This was a highly popular activity and although it was designed primarily for children, many adults participated as well. Most participants were able to select correct items. • Visitors were also asked what they would do in the event of an earthquake (get outside or under a sturdy doorway or table) or a fire (e.g., stop, drop, and roll) and how to prevent fires. Most participants answered correctly. • Ideally, a community survey would be conducted after the fair to determine how many community residents actually collected disaster preparedness supplies or installed smoke detectors, but this was not possible in the time frame available for the project.

CHAPTER RECAP

Health promotion efforts are critically needed to address the increasing cost of health care services for existing illnesses. A number of models have been developed to explain health-promoting behaviors by individuals and population groups and to guide health promotion initiatives. Models presented in the chapter include the Precaution Adoption Process Model, the theories of Reasoned Action and Planned Behavior, the Health Belief Model, and Pender's Health Promotion Model.

Several factors influence the effectiveness of health promotion efforts, including fatalistic behaviors, readiness for change, health literacy, and the attitudes and behaviors of health professionals and health care systems related to health promotion. Four major strategies for health promotion were presented in the chapter: health education; social marketing, branding, and tailoring; legislation; and the use of community health workers to disseminate health promotion messages to selected population groups. The process of health education involves assessment and prioritization of health education needs, developing goals and objectives for health education programs, selecting and implementing health education strategies, and evaluating the effectiveness of health education programs. Population health nursing involvement in health education, social marketing and related activities, legislation, and the use of community health workers in health promotion initiatives were also addressed.

CASE STUDY Promoting Population Health

New legislation in your state has mandated that the majority of funds allocated for public health efforts be devoted to health promotion activities rather than to care of clients with existing health problems. Some of the major health problems encountered in the state at this time include heart disease, family violence, and social isolation among the elderly.

1. Which of these issues would be most amenable to health promotion efforts? Why?
2. Choose one of the three problems and design a set of interventions to address it. How might you employ each of the four health promotion strategies discussed in the chapter to address the problem selected?
3. Discuss the four Ps of social marketing related to the problem selected. How might you segment your target audience?

REFERENCES

Action on Smoking and Health. (n.d.). *Tobacco is a global epidemic.* Retrieved from http://ash.org/globaltc.html

Action on Smoking and Health. (1999). *How Banzhaf's successful antismoking crusade began.* Retrieved from http://www.no-smoking.org/nov99/11-18-99-1.html

American Public Health Association. (2009). *Support for community health workers to increase health access and to reduce health inequities.* Retrieved from http://www.apha.org/advocacy/policy/policysearch/default.htm?id=1393

Arnold, C. M., Aragon, D., Shephard, J., & Van Sell, S. L. (2011). The coming of the blessing: A successful cross-cultural collaborative effort for American Indian/Alaska Native families. *Family & Community Health, 34,* 196–201. doi:10.1097/FCH.0b013e3182196279

Assaf, R. R. (2014). Overview of local, state, and national government legislation restricting transfats. *Clinical Therapeutics, 36,* 3298-332. doi: http://dx.doi.org/10.1016/j.clinthera.2014.01.005

Awofeso, N. (2004). What's new about the new public health? *American Journal of Public Health, 94,* 705–709.

Ayala, G. X., & The San Diego Prevention Research Center Team. (2011). Effects of a promotor-based intervention to promote physical activity: Familias Sanas y Activas. *American Journal of Public Health, 101,* 2261–2268. doi:10.2105/AJPH.2011.300273

Balcazar, H., Rosenthal, L. E., Brownstein, N. J., Rush, C. H., Matos, S., & Hernandez, L. (2011). Community health workers can be a public health force for change in the United States: Three actions for a new paradigm. *American Journal of Public Health, 101,* 2199–2203. doi:10.2105/AJPH.2011.300386

Banzhaf, et al. v. Federal Communications Commission, et al. (n.d.). Retrieved from http://www.tobaccocontrollaws.org/litigation/decisions/us-19681121-banzhaf,-et-al.-v.-federal-com

Bastable, S. B. (2013). *Nurse as educator: Principles of teaching and learning for nursing practice* (4th ed.). Sudbury, MA: Jones and Bartlett.

Black, A. R., & Peacock, N. (2011). Pleasing the masses: Messages for daily life management in African American women's popular media sources. *American Journal of Public Health, 101,* 144–150. doi:10.2105/AJPH.2009.167817

Blitstein, J. L., Evans, W. D., & Driscoll, D. L. (2008). What is a public health brand. In W. D. Evans & G. Hastings (Eds.), *Public health branding: Applying marketing for social change* (pp. 25–41). New York: Oxford University Press.

Bloom, B. S., Englehart, M. D., Furst, E. J., Hill, W. F., & Krathwohl, D. R. (1956). *Taxonomy of educational objectives: The classification of educational goals: Handbook 1: The cognitive domain.* New York: David McKay.

Carter, S. M., Rychetnik, L., Lloyd, B., Kerridge, I. H., Baur, L., Bauman, A., & Hooker, C. (2011). Evidence, ethics, and values: A framework for health promotion. *American Journal of Public Health, 101,* 465–272. doi:10/2105/AJPH.2010.195545

Centers for Disease Control and Prevention. (2010). CDCynergy lite: Social marketing made simple: A guide for creating effective social marketing plans. Retrieved from http://www.cdc.gov/healthcommunication/pdf/cdcynergylite.pdf

Cohen, J. E., Planinac, L., Lavack, A., Robinson, D., O'Connor, S., & DiNardo, J. (2011). Changes in retail tobacco promotions in a cohort of stores before, during, and after a tobacco product display ban. *American Journal of Public Health, 101,* 1879–1881. doi:10.2105/AJPH.2011.300172

Colorado Department of Public Health and Environment. (2011). Health plan implementation of U. S. Preventive Services Task Force A and B recommendations—Colorado, 2010. *Morbidity and Mortality Weekly Report, 60,* 1348–1350.

Community Preventive Services Task Force. (2013). *Annual report to Congress and to agencies related to the work of the task force, 2013.* Retrieved from http://thecommunityguide.org/annualreport/2013-congress-report-full.pdf

Community Preventive Services Task Force. (2014). *The Community Guide.* Retrieved from http://www.thecommunityguide.org/index.html

Cory, S., Ussery-Hall, A., Griffin-Blake, S., Easton, A., Vigeant, J., Balluz, L., . . ., Greenlund, K. (2010). Prevalence of selected risk behaviors and chronic diseases and conditions—Steps Communities, United States, 2006–2007. *Morbidity and Mortality Weekly Report, 59*(SS-8), 1–37.

Crilly, J. F., Keefe, R. H., & Volpe, F. (2011). Use of electronic technologies to promote community and personal health for individuals unconnected to health care systems. *American Journal of Public Health, 101,* 1163–1167. doi:10.2105/AJPH.2010.300003

Currie, D. (2011, April). China tells filmmakers to limit smoking. *The Nation's Health, 21.*

Daniels, J., Glickstein, B., & Mason, D. J. (2012). Using the power of media to influence health policy and politics. In D. J. Mason, J. K. Leavitt, & M. W. Chaffee (Eds.), *Policy & politics in nursing and health care* (6th ed., pp. 88–104). St. Louis, MO: Elsevier Saunders.

de Salazar, L., & Anderson, L. M. (2008). Health promotion in the Americas: Divergent and common ground. In L. Potvin, & D. V. McQueen (Eds.), *Health promotion evaluation practices in the Americas: Values and research* (pp. 13–23). New York: Springer.

Drew, E. M., & Schoenberg, N. A. (2011). Deconstructing fatalism: Ethnographic perspectives on women's decision making about cancer prevention and treatment. *Medical Anthropology Quarterly, 24,* 164–182. doi:10.1111/j.1548-1387.2010.01136.x

Eadie, C. (2014). Health literacy: A conceptual review. *Academy of Medical Surgical Nurses, 23*(1), 1, 10–13.

Espinosa de los Monteros, K., & Gallo, L. C. (2011). The relevance of fatalism in the study of Latina's cancer screening behavior: A systematic review of the literature. *International Journal of Behavioral Medicine, 18,* 310–318. doi:10.1007/s12529-010-9119-4

Evans, W. D., & Hastings, G. (2008a). Preface. In W. D. Evans & G. Hastings (Eds.), *Public health branding: Applying marketing for social change* (pp. vii–xii). New York: Oxford University Press.

Evans, W. D., & Hastings, G. (2008b). Public health branding: Recognition, promise, and delivery of healthy lifestyles. In W. D. Evans & G. Hastings (Eds.), *Public health branding: Applying marketing for social change* (pp. 1–24). New York: Oxford University Press.

Findley, S. E., Sanchez, M., Mejia, M., Ferreira, R., Pena, O., Matos, S., . . ., Irigoyen, M. (2009). REACH 2010: New York City. Effective strategies for integrating immunization promotion into community programs. *Health Promotion Practice, 10*(Suppl. 2), 128S–137S. doi:10.1177/1524839909331544

Fishbein, M. (2009). An integrative model for behavioral prediction and its application to health promotion. In R. J. DiClemente, R. A. Crosby, & M. C. Kegler (Eds.), *Emerging theories in health promotion practice and research: Strategies for improving public health* (2nd ed., pp. 215–234). San Francisco: Jossey-Bass.

Fisher, J. D., Fisher, W. A., & Shuper, P. A. (2009). The information-motivation-behavioral skills model. In R. J. DiClemente, R. A. Crosby, & M. C. Kegler (Eds.), *Emerging theories in health promotion practice and research: Strategies for improving public health* (2nd ed., pp. 21–63). San Francisco: Jossey-Bass.

Fisher, W. A., Kohut, T., Salisbury, C. M. A., & Salvadori, M. I. (2013). Understanding human papillomavirus vaccination intentions: Comparative utility of the theory of reasoned action and the theory of planned behavior in vaccine target age women and men. *Journal of Sexual Medicine, 10,* 2455–2464. doi: 10.1111/jsm.12211

Flores, K., R., Aguirre, A. N., Viladrich, A., Cespedes, A., De La Cruz, A. A., & Abraido-Lanza, A. F. (2009). Fatalism or destiny? A qualitative study and interpretative framework on Dominican women's breast cancer beliefs. *Journal of Immigrant and Minority Health, 11,* 291–301. doi:10.1007/s10903-008-9118-6

Health on the Net Foundation. (2013a). *The commitment to reliable health and medical information on the internet.* Retrieved from http://www.hon.ch/HONcode/Patients/Visitor/visitor.html

Health on the Net Foundation. (2013b). *The HON Code of Conduct for medical and health Web sites (HONcode).* Retrieved from http://www.hon.ch/HONcode/Patients/Conduct.html

Health Resources and Services Administration. (2011). *Community health workers evidence-based models toolbox.* Retrieved from http://www.hrsa.gov/ruralhealth/pdf/chwtoolkit.pdf

Henchman, J., & Drenkard, S. (2014). Cigarette taxes and cigarette smuggling by state. Retrieved from http://taxfoundation.org/article/cigarette-taxes-and-cigarette-smuggling-state

Hinojosa, M. S., Nelson, D., Hinojosa, R., Delgado, A., Witzack, B., Gonzales, M., . . ., Farias, R. (2011). Using fotonovelas to promote healthy eating in a Latino community. *American Journal of Public Health, 101,* 258–259. doi:10.2105/AJPH.2010.198994

Hopwood, T., & Merritt, R. (2011). *The big pocket guide to using social marketing for behavior change.* Retrieved from http://www.thensmc.com/sites/default/files/Big_pocket_guide_2011.pdf

Institute of Medicine. (2011). *The future of nursing: Leading change, advancing health.* Washington, DC: National Academies Press.

Javanparast, S., Baum, F., Labonte, R., & Sanders, D. (2011). Community health workers' perspectives on their contribution to rural health and well-being in Iran. *American Journal of Public Health, 101,* 2287–2292. doi:10.2105/AJPH.2011.300355

Jiang, N., & Ling, P. M. (2011). Reinforcement of smoking and drinking: Tobacco marketing strategies linked with alcohol in the United States. *American Journal of Public Health, 101,* 1942–1954. doi:10.2105/AJPH.2011.300157

Keeley, B., Wright, L., & Condit, C. M. (2009). Functions of health fatalism: Fatalistic talk as face saving, uncertainty, management, stress relief, and sense making. *Sociology of Health & Illness, 31,* 734–747. doi:10.1111/j.1467-9566.2009.01164.x

Krathwohl, D. R., Bloom, B. S., & Masia, B. B. (1964). *Taxonomy of educational objectives: The classification of educational goals: Handbook 1: The affective domain.* New York: David McKay.

Lewis, M. A., & McCormack, L. A. (2008). The intersection between tailored health communication and branding for health promotion. In W. D. Evans & G. Hastings (Eds.), *Public health branding: Applying marketing for social change* (pp. 251–269). New York: Oxford University Press.

Li, C., Balluz, L. S., Okoro, C. A., Strine, T. W., Lin, J.-M. S., Town, M., . . ., Valluru, B. (2011). Surveillance of certain health behaviors and conditions among states and selected local areas—Behavioral Risk Factor Surveillance System, United States, 2009. *Morbidity and Mortality Weekly Report, 60* (SS-9), 1–248.

Maclosek, M. V., Coffield, A. B., Flottemesch, T. J., Edwards, N. M., & Solberg, L. I. (2010). Greater use of preventive services in U. S. health care could save lives at little or no cost. *Health Affairs, 9,* 1656–1660. doi:10.1377/hlthaff.2008.0701

Martin, L. R., Haskard-Zolnierek, K. B., & DiMatteo, M. R. (2010). *Health behavior change and treatment adherence.* New York, NY: Oxford University Press.

Mathar, T., & Jansen, Y. J. F. M. (2010). Introduction: Health promotion and prevention programmes in practice. In T. Mathar & Y. J. F. M. Jansen (Eds.), *Health promotion and prevention programmes in practice* (pp. 9–27). New Burnswick, NJ: Transaction.

Monaghan, P. F., Forst, L. S., Tovar-Aguilar, J. A., Bryant, C., A., Israel, G. D., Galindo-Gonzalez, S., . . ., McDermott, R. J. (2011). Preventing eye injuries among citrus harvesters: The community health worker model. *American Journal of Public Health, 101,* 2269–2274. doi:10.2105/AJPH.2011.300316

Murray, R. L., Lewis, S. A., Coleman, T., Britton, J., & McNeill, A. (2009). Unplanned attempts to quit smoking: Missed opportunities for health promotion? *Addiction, 104,* 1901–1909. doi:10.1111/j.1360-0443.2009.02647.x

National Center for Chronic Disease Prevention and Health Promotion. (2011). Smoking in top-grossing movies—United States, 2010. *Morbidity and Mortality Weekly Report, 60,* 909–913.

National Center for Chronic Disease Prevention and Health Promotion. (2013). *State indicator report on fruits and vegetables, 2013.* Retrieved from http://www.cdc.gov/nutrition/downloads/State-Indicator-Report-Fruits-Vegetables-2013.pdf

National Center for Health Statistics. (2011). Percentage of adults aged > 18 years who engaged in leisure-time strengthening activities at least twice a week, by race/ethnicity and sex—National Health Interview Survey, United States, 2009. *Morbidity and Mortality Weekly Report, 60,* 1429.

National Center for Injury Prevention and Control. (2011). Vital signs: Nonfatal, motor vehicle-occupant injuries (2009) and seat belt use (2008) among adults—United States. *Morbidity and Mortality Weekly Report, 59,* 1681–1686.

National Highway Traffic Safety Administration. (2014). *Seat belt use in 2013 – Overall results.* Retrieved from http://www-nrd.nhtsa.dot.gov/Pubs/811875.pdf

National Network of Libraries of Medicine. (2013). *Health Literacy.* Retrieved from http://nnlm.gov/outreach/consumer/hlthlit.html

National Patient Safety Foundation. (2011). *Health literacy: Statistics at-a-glance.* Retrieved from http://www.npsf.org/wp-content/uploads/2011/12/AskMe3_Stats_English.pdf

The NMSC. (2010). *What is social marketing?* Retrieved from http://www.thensmc.com/content/what-social-marketing-1

Office of Disease Prevention and Health Promotion. (n.d.). *A quick guide to health literacy.* Retrieved from http://www.health.gov/communication/literacy/quickguide/Quickguide.pdf

Office of Disease Prevention and Health Promotion. (2010). *Health literacy online: A guide to writing and designing easy-to-use health Web sites.* Washington, DC: Author.

Office of Disease Prevention and Health Promotion. (2012). *Health literacy overview.* Retrieved from http://health.gov/communication/literacy/Default.asp

Office on Smoking and Health. (2011). State preemption of local tobacco control policies restricting smoking, advertising, and youth access—United States, 2000–2010. *Morbidity and Mortality Weekly Report, 60,* 1124–1127.

Office on Smoking and Health. (2012). *Smoking and tobacco use: Legislation* Retrieved from http://www.cdc.gov/tobacco/data_statistics/by_topic/policy/legislation/

Ormond, B. A., Spillman, B. C., Waldmann, T. A., Caswell, K. J., & Tereshchenko, B. (2011). Potential national and state medical care savings from primary disease prevention. *American Journal of Public Health, 101,* 157–164. doi:10.2105/AJPH.2009.182287

Pender, N. J., Murdaugh, C. L., & Parsons, M. A. (2010). *Health promotion in nursing practice* (6th ed.). Upper Saddle River, NJ: Prentice Hall.

Pfister-Minogue, K. A., & Salveson, C. (2010). Training and experiences of public health nurses in using behavior change counseling. *Public Health Nursing, 27,* 544–551. doi:10.1111/j.1525-1446.2010.00884.x

Prochaska, J. O., Redding, C. A., & Evers, K. E. (2008). The transtheoretical model and states of change. In K. Glanz, B. K. Rimer, & K. Viswanath (Eds.), *Health behavior and health education: Theory, research, and practice* (4th ed., pp. 97–122). San Francisco, CA: John Wiley & Sons.

Professor John F. Banzhaf, III. (n.d.). Retrieved from http://banzhaf.net/

Pucher, J., Buehler, R., Merom, D., & Bauman, A. (2011). Walking and cycling in the United States, 2001–2009: Evidence from the National Household Travel Surveys. *American Journal of Public Health, 100*(Suppl. 1), S310–S317. doi:10.2105/AJPH.2010.300067

Richard, L., Gendron, S., Beaudet, N., Boisvert, N., Sauve, M. S., & Garceau-Brodeur, M.-H. (2010). Health promotion and disease prevention among nurses working in local public health organizations in Montreal, Quebec. *Public Health Nursing, 27,* 450–458. doi:10.1111/j.1525-1446.2010.00878.x

Roncancio, A. M., Ward, K. K., & Berenson, A. B. (2011). Hispanic women's health provider control expectations: The influence of fatalism and acculturation. *Journal of Health Care for the Poor and Underserved, 11,* 482–490. doi:10.1353/hpu.2011.0038

Shelley, D., Cantrell, M. J., Moon-Howard, J., Ramjohn, D. Q., & VanDevanter, N. (2007). The $5 man: The underground economic response to a large cigarette tax increase in New York City. *American Journal of Public Health, 97,* 1483–1488. doi:10.2105/AJPH,2005.079921

Smith-Howell, E. R., Rawl, S. M., Champion, V. L., Skinner, C. S., Springston, J., Krier, C., . . ., Myers, L. J. (2011). Exploring the role of cancer fatalism as a barrier to colorectal cancer screening. *Western Journal of Nursing Research, 33,* 140–141. doi:10.1170/0193945910378810

Social Marketing Institute. (n.d.). *Social marketing.* Retrieved from http://www.social-marketing.org/sm.html

Southey, G. (2011). The theories of reasoned action and planned behavior applied to business decisions: A selective annotated bibliography. *Journal of New Business Ideas and Trends, 9*(1), 43–50. Retrieved from http://www.apha.org/advocacy/policy/policysearch/default.htm?id=1460

Stokowski, L. A. (2011). *Social media and nurses: Promising or perilous?* http://www.medscape.com/viewarticle/753317?src=mp&spon=24.

Tones, K., & Green, J. (2010). *Health promotion: Planning and strategies* (2nd ed.). Thousand Oaks, CA: Sage.

U.S. Census Bureau. (2011). *Language spoken at home by ability to speak English for the population 5 years and over.* Retrieved from http://factfinder2.census.gov/faces/tableservices/jsf/pages/productview.xhtml?pid=ACS_10_1YR_B16001&prodType=table

U.S. Department of Health and Human Services. (2003). *The power of prevention.* Retrieved from http://www.Healthierus.gov/steps

Vallone, D. M., Duke, J. C., Cullen, J., McCausland, K. L., & Allen, J. A. (2011). Evaluation of EX: A national mass media smoking cessation campaign. *American Journal of Public Health, 101,* 302–309. doi:10.2105/AJPH.2009.190454

Verstraeten, R., Van Royen, K., Ochoa-Avilés, A., Penafiel, D., Holdsworth, M., Donoso, S., . . . Kolsteren, P. (2014). A conceptual framework for healthy eating behavior in Ecuadorian adolescents: A qualitative study. *Plos One, 9*(1), e87183. doi: 10.1371/journal.pone.0087183

Viswanathan, M., Kraschnewski, J., Nishikawa, B., Morgan, L. C., Thieda, P., Honeycutt, A., . . ., Jonas, D. (2009). *Outcomes of community health worker interventions.* http://www.ahrq.gov/downloads/pub/evidence/pdf/comhealthwork/comhwork.pdf.

Weinrich, N. K. (n.d.). *What is social marketing?* Retrieved from http://www.social-marketing .com/Whatis.html.

Weinstein, N. D., Sandman, P. M., & Blalock, S. J. (2008). The precaution adoption process model. In K. Glanz, B. K. Rimer, & K. Viswanath (Eds.), *Health behavior and health education: Theory, research, and practice* (4th ed., pp. 123–147). San Francisco, CA: John Wiley & Sons.

Wingood, G. M., DiClemente, R. J., Villamizar, K., Er, D. L., DeVarona, M., Taveras, J., . . ., Jean, R. (2011). Efficacy of a health educator-delivered HIV prevention intervention for Latina women: A randomized controlled trial. *American Journal of Public Health, 101,* 2245–2252. doi:10.2105/AJPH.2011.300340

World Health Organization. (1986). *Ottawa charter for health promotion.* Geneva, Switzerland: Author.

World Health Organization. (2005). *Bangkok charter for health promotion in a globalized world.* Geneva, Switzerland: Author.

World Health Organization. (2014). *Health education.* Retrieved from http://www.who.int/topics/health_education/en/

Xu, F., Town, M., Balluz, L. S. Bartoli, W. P., Murphy, W., Chowdury, P. P., . . ., Crawford, C.A. (2013). Surveillance for certain health behaviors among states and selected local areas—United States, 2010. *Morbidity and Mortality Weekly Report, 62*(SS-1), 1-247.

Youth+Tech+Health. (2014). *SEXINFO.* Retrieved from http://yth.org/projects/sexinfo/

CHAPTER

12 Case Management Strategies

Learning Outcomes

After reading this chapter, you should be able to:

1 Identify client-centered and system-centered goals of case management.

2 Describe models for case management.

3 Discuss standards and principles of case management practice.

4 Analyze legal and ethical issues related to case management.

5 Identify potential criteria for selecting clients or populations in need of case management.

6 Assess the need for case management and factors influencing the case management situation.

7 Discuss aspects of developing and implementing a case management plan.

8 Describe at least three considerations in delegation.

9 Describe the benchmarking process and its use in case management.

Key Terms

abandonment

benchmark

case management

delegation

discharge planning

disease management

negligence

negligent referral

resource file

utilization review

Advocacy Then

Origins of Case Management

Case management originated with the early settlement houses. When community health nursing was initiated at the Henry Street Settlement in 1893, case management became an integral part of the services provided. This focus on case management was continued in the home visiting services provided by the Metropolitan Life Insurance Company, begun in 1911 with the aim of minimizing payment of death benefits and of providing service to the enrolled community. Case management was primarily used to eliminate "useless cases" for which participating Visiting Nurse Associations were not reimbursed. These early efforts at case management, as we know it today, focused on appropriate case selection, early referral to needed services, and discharge when services were no longer needed (Buhler-Wilkerson, 2001). Population health nurses assessed the needs of clients and their families and linked them to available services as needed. When services were not available, particularly to low-income clients, they were often provided by the population health nurses themselves. The nurses also worked with public and private agencies to create systems of care to which clients could be referred.

Advocacy Now

Screening for Perinatal Depression

Federal funding for perinatal care received by a local clinic mandated routine depression screening in pregnant women seen in the clinic. Screening was being provided for English- and Spanish-speaking clients, but not for Arabic-speaking Iraqi Chaldean immigrant women due to language barriers. Dr. Kathy McCarthy, a family nurse practitioner and nurse midwife working in the clinic, arranged to have the depression screening instrument translated into Arabic, using a standard translation and back translation process. She then arranged for the resulting translation to be reviewed by a focus group of Iraqi Chaldean women to assure its meaning and cultural sensitivity. Kathy also arranged for an Arabic-speaking nursing student to administer the screening tool to pregnant Iraqi women seen for perinatal services.

Unsurprisingly, given their history of past repression and immigration, nearly two thirds of the women exhibited significant signs of depression. Unfortunately, there were limited resources available in the community to meet their needs, again primarily due to language barriers. Dr. McCarthy worked with several local providers and a social service agency dealing with the Iraqi immigrant population to create a referral network for those women who screened positive for depression.

Until recently, case management continued to be practiced rather informally as coordination of care provided to clients of population health nurses and a few other health care providers. Now, case management is perceived as a formal discipline with principles that cut across multiple providers and settings. Case management practice in general exhibits two key features: provision of an interface between clients and needed services and assuring that services provided meet reasonable standards of quality and support achievement of important health-related outcomes (Commission for Case Manager Certification, n.d.b). These key features lead to achievement of three related overall goals for case management. The first outcome is the ability of clients and their caregivers to progress toward health-related goals within the constraints of available resources (American Case Management Association [ACMA], 2014).

For individual clients and their families, case management ensures effective coordination of care and helps to reduce the confusion and complexity of the health care system. The case manager can assist the client to obtain needed services in the most acceptable and affordable settings. Case management, if effectively performed, also results in improved client health outcomes in many instances. Effective case management focuses attention on all of the client's health needs to minimize the development of other health problems. In addition, case management provides clients with continuity of care and a regular and consistent source of assistance with health needs.

The second goal of case management operates at a systems level and reflects improvement in the overall effectiveness of health services through collaboration and coordination designed to promote appropriate use of services and reduction of duplication, gaps, and barriers to service (ACMA, 2014). At the health system level, case management emphasizes service delivery in the least expensive setting possible, thereby limiting the overall cost of health care. System-centered goals focus on equitable resource allocation, decreased utilization, and cost containment while maintaining service quality. Additional system-centered goals include decreased fragmentation of care provided in the most efficient manner. Effective case management minimizes hospitalization for needs that can be dealt with in community practice settings. For clients who do need hospitalization, case management may shorten the length of stay and prevent subsequent readmissions by adequately addressing continuing health care needs after discharge. The cost of health care is also minimized when case management eliminates duplication of services. The third goal of case management is to promote the client's right to self-determination (ACMA, 2014). Table 12-1● summarizes client-centered and system-centered goals and benefits of case management.

Defining Case Management

Case management is a collaborative process between the case manager and the client and his or her family designed to identify and meet health care needs through quality, cost-effective services (CMSA, 2010). This definition highlights two key elements of case management: quality and cost-effectiveness. Case management activities are designed to provide quality care to achieve designated health outcomes at the least possible cost.

The definition provided at left implies that case management is necessarily directed toward individual clients and their families. Case management also occurs at the population level, however. When directed toward specific client populations, it is often referred to as population health management, a set of services and interventions that address the health needs of a particular targeted population. Key components of population health management include identification of the population, assessment of population health needs, risk stratification for those most in need of services, engagement and communication, health management interventions, and outcomes measurement. The goal of population health management is to maintain or improve the health of a group of individuals through cost-effective, tailored interventions that address health promotion and illness prevention, risk management, care coordination, and disease management.

Population health management may be viewed from two perspectives. In the public health perspective, population health management refers to promotion and maintenance of health in a geographically defined population. From a health care delivery system perspective, population health management addresses the health needs of the population that receives services from the system (Hacker & Walker, 2013), often those enrolled in a particular delivery system or groups of clients that consume excessive levels of system resources (e.g., people with congestive heart failure or diabetes) (Murphy, McGready, Griswold, & Sylvia, 2014). Case management for groups of people with a common high-cost diagnosis is often referred to as disease management. In both public health and health system perspectives, population health management necessitates a change from an illness orientation to a wellness focus (Hacker & Walker, 2013). Studies have indicated that population health management approaches decrease health spending as well as improve health status in the populations affected (Rust et al., 2011).

TABLE 12-1 Client-Centered and System-Centered Goals and Benefits of Case Management

Client-Centered Goals/Benefits	System-Centered Goals/Benefits
• Access to quality sources of needed care over a continuum of services • Access to acceptable and affordable health care services • Continuity of care and consistent source of assistance • Better coordination of care • Assistance in negotiating a complex health care system • Attention to multiple health needs • Attainment of positive health outcomes • Ability to function independently • Prevention of deterioration • Reduced risk and need for acute care services • Adjustment of client and family to illness states • Improved quality of life • Increased satisfaction with care • Empowerment and self-determination	• Cost containment and cost-efficiency • Minimization of hospitalization and rehospitalization • Reduced duplication and fragmentation of services • Decreased service utilization and elimination of inappropriate care • Effective resource allocation • Earlier discharge • Better communication among agencies and providers • Integrated service delivery and ease of transfer among agencies • Increased access to services • Decreased paperwork • Reduced time for authorization of services • Increased client satisfaction • Increased professional satisfaction • Financial viability

Health maintenance organizations and other managed care systems often engage in population health management to promote the health of their membership and decrease their health care costs. Examples of population health management include risk reduction strategies such as providing smoking cessation services and reminders of the need for mammograms, pap smears, and other screenings designed to promote early detection and prompt treatment of disease. These types of activities are likely to become more salient with Affordable Care Act requirements for health care institutions receiving federal funds to conduct community needs assessments that go beyond an enrolled group of clients and to engage in activities to address those needs (Hacker & Walker, 2013).

Case Management Models

A number of models of case management have been developed and will be briefly discussed here. Two such models or approaches to case management are linked models and intensive case management models. In linked models, case managers make referrals for services to independent services and networks. In intensive case management models, the majority of services needed by clients are offered by a single organization, often the organization that provides the case management services (Vroomen et al., 2012). Case management by population health nurses would typically be based on a linked model, whereas case management services within a hospital system would usually employ an intensive case management approach.

The New York State Department of Health (2013) distinguished two levels of case management services for clients with HIV/AIDS: supportive case management and comprehensive case management. These two levels are also appropriate to groups of people with other conditions such as diabetes, hypertension, and so on. Supportive case management addresses immediate discrete service needs and involves short-term service provision. Comprehensive case management is a proactive model of service for people with complex needs who require long-term service. The goal of comprehensive case management is to decrease the need for extensive services as well as to deal with a broad array of client problems.

Offredy, Bunn, and Morgan (2009) also described a tiered case management system comprised of three levels. The first level is designed to provide self-care support for the bulk of the population needing services (e.g., patients with diabetes, pregnant teenagers). The second level of case management involves high-risk disease management and might be appropriate for brittle diabetics or women with high-risk pregnancies who require more intense services and more frequent monitoring. The third level addresses care of clients with complex needs who require a broad array of services (e.g., a client with diabetes who is also homeless and has a problem with substance abuse).

Another way of distinguishing case management models is in terms of the provider of case management services. Disease-specific case management is often provided by a nurse with expertise in a particular area (e.g., diabetes or cardiovascular disease) who provides both direct care related to management of the disease as well as education, advice, and referral for other needed services. A team-based approach, on the other hand, involves services by a multidisciplinary team with a designated coordinator (who is often a population health nurse) (Offredy et al., 2009). These two approaches may also be referred to as integrated or collaborative models. In an integrated model, a single case manager performs all of the case management functions related to care of clients as well as system-level functions (such as dealing with reimbursement and billing issues). A collaborative practice model separates the clinical and business functions of case management and may incorporate the efforts of multiple providers to meet client needs (Case Management's Day, 2011).

Case management activities may be performed by population health nurses as employees of agencies providing services to clients and population groups, as self-employed case managers, or as employees of case management services. Population health nurses may also function as single case managers or as part of a multidisciplinary case management team, often serving as the coordinator of team activities.

Standards and Principles of Case Management

The Case Management Society of America (CMSA, 2010) has developed a set of standards for case management practice. For further information about the standards document, see the resources provided in the *External Resources* section of the student resources site. In addition, The Commission for Case Manager Certification (CCMC) has developed a "Code of Professional Conduct for Case Managers" (CCMC, 2009) and provides mechanisms for certification for individual case managers (CCMC, n.d.a, n.d.b).

Within the standards document, CMSA has identified guiding principles for case management practice. First and

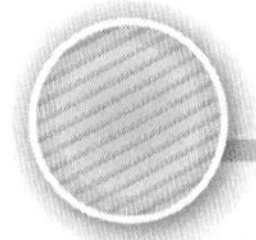

Global Perspectives

Case Management Around the World

Case management is widely practiced by nurses and other professionals in the United States, but is a newer phenomenon in other countries. Examine the international nursing literature. Where is nursing case management being implemented? Who provides case management services? How does its implementation differ from case management in the United States? Are there elements of case management in other countries that might improve U.S. case management services? Some sources included in the reference list for this chapter to get you started include the following: Goga and Muhe (2011); Grange (2011); Klaske, W., Annema, C., De Keyser, J., and Middel, B. (2010); Lam at el. (2010); Olbort et al. (2009); Setoya, Sato, Satake, and Ito (2001); and Thurman et al. (2010).

foremost, case management should be client-centered and collaborative. Case management activities focus primarily on meeting the needs of individual clients and their caretakers or on a specific client population. Collaboration should occur with clients and their families as well as with members of a wide variety of health care disciplines. This involves facilitation of self-determination and self-care on the part of individual clients or populations served as well as incorporation of a determinants of health perspective. Another principle is that case management is comprehensive and holistic, incorporating health promotion, illness, prevention, and risk mitigation as well as care for existing health and psychosocial problems. Case management activities vary with the intensity and type of client needs for service. Effective case management also incorporates cultural competence based on recognition of and respect for diversity. Furthermore, case management strategies and interventions should be evidence-based and creative and should promote optimal client safety.

Case management incorporates principles of behavioral change and requires effective communication between case manager and client and among various providers. Case managers link individuals or populations with needed community resources and assist them in navigating the health care system to promote quality care and to achieve optimal health outcomes. In addition, case management should be based on an ethical framework incorporating client advocacy, as needed, at either the individual client or population level. Case management should promote achievement of quality outcomes as well as the measurement of those outcomes and should foster compliance with federal, state, local, and organizational rules and regulations. Finally, casc management should be undertaken by case managers who pursue excellence and maintain competence in practice. These principles are summarized in the *Highlights* box at right.

Highlights

Principles of Case Management

- Case management is client-centered and collaborative.
- Case management focuses primarily on meeting clients' needs.
- Case management facilitates self-determination and self-care.
- Case management addresses a variety of determinants of health.
- Case management is comprehensive and holistic.
- Case management activities vary with the intensity and type of care needed by clients.
- Case management is culturally competent, based on recognition of and respect for diversity.
- Case management is evidence-based and creative.
- Case management promotes optimal client saftey.
- Case management incorporates principles of behavior change.
- Case management requires effective communication.
- Case management links clients with needed community resources.
- Case management assists with navigating the health care system.
- Case management is based on an ethical framework and incorporates client advocacy as needed.
- Case management promotes achievement and measurement of quality outcomes.
- Case management fosters compliance with federal, state, local, and organizational rules and regulations.
- Case management is performed by case managers who pursue excellence and maintain competence in practice.

Competencies and Functions of Case Managers

Effective case management practice requires possession of certain competencies including expert clinical knowledge and knowledge of available community resources. Case managers must possess the critical thinking skills needed to incorporate evidence-based practice strategies as appropriate to a given situation. They also need to have an understanding of organizational, legal, and professional standards delineating practice and reporting requirements and the ability to operate flexibly and creatively within the constraints of available resources and existing protocols and policies. Additional competencies include cultural sensitivity and the ability to engage in responsible and ethical advocacy that balances joint accountability to clients and to health care systems. Skill in delegation and referral are also required and will be discussed in more detail later in this chapter. Finally, competent case managers exhibit self-awareness and communication skills that enable collaboration at multiple levels. These competencies are summarized in the *Highlights* box on page 292.

The role functions of case managers vary to a certain extent, based on the case management model employed; however, there are some generalizations that can be made regarding the roles played and functions performed by case managers across systems. Typical functions of case managers and examples of related activities for both individual- and population-level case management are summarized in Table 12-2●. General functions delineated by the Case Management Society of America (2010) include conducting a comprehensive needs assessment, including assessment of health literacy; planning to maximize health care responses, quality of care, and cost-effective outcomes; facilitating communication and coordination of care; educating clients and others; empowering clients; and encouraging appropriate health care utilization. Additional functions include assisting clients in care transitions, promoting self-advocacy and self-determination, and advocacy for clients and health care systems.

Highlights

Competencies of Effective Case Managers

- Expert clinical knowledge
- Knowledge of available resources
- Critical thinking skills in the application of evidence-based practice strategies
- Understanding of organizational, legal, and professional standards
- Flexibility and creativity
- Cultural competence
- Advocacy skills
- Ability to balance joint accountability to clients and health care systems
- Delegation skills
- Referral skills
- Self-awareness
- Communication skills that promote collaboration

The Case Management Process

The process of case management is similar to the nursing process with a few additional components (CMSA, 2010). Part of the assessment component in case management involves identification and selection of clients who will benefit from case management services. This process is often referred to as "intake" and involves screening clients, determining priorities, and determining eligibility for case management services. This preliminary assessment is followed by a more in-depth assessment to identify specific client problems, needs, and desired outcomes of service. The next step in the process is the development of a case management plan to provide or arrange for the needed services in the most cost-effective setting. Planning is followed by implementation of services and coordination of an array of services by the case manager. Both implementation and outcomes are evaluated from a patient or population perspective and modifications are made to the plan of care as needed. The case management process concludes with disengagement and termination of services (CMSA, 2010). Elements of the case management process are summarized in the *highlights* box on the next page.

TABLE 12-2 Case Manager Role Functions

Role Function	Description
Needs assessment	Identifies the needs of individual clients or population groups *Individual example:* Identifies the needs of a pregnant teenager from a holistic perspective *Population example:* Identifies the service needs of pregnant teens as a population group
Planning to meet needs	Develops a plan of care in collaboration with the client, caregiver, and other providers to maximize health outcomes and minimize costs of care *Individual example:* Develops an evidence-based asthma management plan that addresses environmental triggers in conjunction with client and family members *Population example:* Assists in the development of comprehensive health promotion, illness prevention, and treatment services for children with asthma
Facilitating communication	Facilitates communication among health team members and between the health care team and the client and family *Individual example:* Explains the plan of care for medical management of a child's asthma to the child and family members *Population example:* Conveys the needs of a client population to local social and health services agencies
Coordinating care	Arranges seamless care across systems and agencies to meet individual client or population needs; makes referrals to needed services; serves as liaison to community agencies *Individual example:* Arranges for transfer of client records from primary care provider and hospital to home health agency *Population example:* Helps to negotiate provision of counseling services by the County Mental Health Agency for clients with HIV/AIDS receiving care at a local hospice
Educating clients and others	Educates clients, families, health care providers, and the public regarding health issues and interventions to promote informed decision making *Individual example:* Educates a child with asthma and his or her family on use of a rescue inhaler *Population example:* Educates teachers and school administrators on the relationship between asthma and exercise and the need for use of inhalers prior to physical activities
Empowering	Empowers individual clients and populations to problem solve and engage in self-advocacy *Individual example:* Assists an elderly woman who is not yet able to function independently to negotiate an extension of home care services *Population example:* Assists a group of low-income elderly in the community to negotiate low-cost assistance with household tasks from students of a local high school

TABLE 12-2 (Continued)

Role Function	Description
Encouraging appropriate use of health services	Educates individual clients and population groups for appropriate use of health care services *Individual example:* Educates parents of a child with asthma on valid indicators for emergency department use *Population example:* Educates a group of clients with diabetes on control measures to prevent unnecessary hospitalizations
Assisting with transitions to other levels of care	Assists with smooth transitions between elements of the health care system *Individual example:* Develops a discharge plan for an elderly woman leaving the hospital after repair of a hip fracture *Population example:* Develops procedures and processes for transferring clients from acute to home care services
Promoting self-advocacy and self-determination	Encourages individual clients and population groups to voice their needs and concerns about care *Individual example*: Encourages a Hispanic client with diabetes to request a referral to a dietician familiar with ethnic food preferences *Population example:* Assists clients of a local health agency who are dissatisfied with services to arrange a meeting with agency administrators to voice their concerns
Joint advocacy	Attempts to balance the needs of clients with those of health care delivery systems, giving priority to clients' needs when conflicts occur *Individual example:* Explains to a client who is capable of attending an out-patient physical therapy program why home therapy is no longer warranted *Population example:* Promotes legislation to mandate insurance coverage of in-home physical therapy for clients who are homebound or lack transportation to access out-patient services

Highlights

Elements of the Case Management Process

- Intake
- Assessment of needs, problems, and outcome goals
- Development of the case management plan
- Implementation of the plan and coordination of activities
- Monitoring and evaluaton of outcomes
- Modification of the plan as needed
- Disengagement and termination of services

Ethical and Legal Issues in Case Management

Ethical issues in case management arise out of limited resources in the face of an increasing need for health care services. Other sources of issues arise from the constraints imposed by restrictions in insurance coverage of health care services needed by individual clients and population groups and restrictions on payment for case management services themselves.

Limited resources lead to concerns with the fair allocation of resources based on elements such as age, gender, socioeconomic status, and so on. A related concern is the appropriate time frame for providing care. For example, case managers may try to minimize service frequency to allow them to provide services over a longer period of time, based on anticipated client needs. Other ethical concerns relate to client autonomy and their right to refuse services or to engage in unhealthful behaviors. Case managers may also be faced with the need to violate system rules to meet clients' needs, providing services appropriate to client needs given resource constraints.

Although many of the legal and ethical issues in case management are common to other aspects of population health nursing, some warrant special attention. These issues include confidentiality, denial of services, abandonment, breach of contract, negligence, and reportable events. With respect to confidentiality, the CMSA (2010) noted that the case manager must comply with all relevant national, state, and local regulations and employer policies regarding patient privacy while acting in the client's best interests. The issue of confidentiality has two aspects in case management. The first is the need for client permission to make contacts and arrangements for services on the client's behalf. The case management plan should be presented to and agreed upon by the client before any further action is taken. The second aspect of confidentiality relates to unauthorized disclosure of information about the client. To avoid a breach of confidentiality in this area, the population health nurse case manager should inform clients of the need to share information with others and obtain client authorization before doing so.

Denial of services includes failure to provide services that are not deemed necessary or for which the client is not eligible. Wrongful denial of services involves decisions not to provide care that are arbitrary and are not based on medical information related to need. Population health nurses often find themselves in the position of advocating for clients who have been denied services. For example, a school nurse may need to convince school officials of the need for a learning disability assessment for a student who is performing poorly in school. At the population level, the same school nurse may advocate for changes in referral procedures that make disability assessment more accessible to all children in need. In the latter instance, the school nurse is engaging in population case management, whereas advocacy for a specific child would be part of individual case management.

Abandonment occurs when a health care provider terminates services to a client with continuing needs without notifying the client or arranging for services from another provider. Although population health nurse case managers may encounter situations in which services need to be terminated (e.g., in the face of client failure to comply with the treatment plan), the nurse should make every effort to avoid abandonment. It may be helpful to develop a contract with clients indicating both case manager and client responsibilities with respect to the case management plan. In addition, the case manager should carefully document both positive and negative aspects of the client's response to case management services and continued efforts to enlist client cooperation. Although *abandonment* is a term that has legal implications in the care of individual clients, the concept of abandonment may also apply to population groups. For example, population health nurses may need to assist communities to find ways to meet the needs of low-income families for child care when after-school program budgets are cut.

Breach of contract occurs when a managed care organization drops a client from the plan without adequate justification or when the system fails to pay for care that should be covered by a plan. Breach of contract, in the legal sense, applies to care of individual clients, although communities might be said to breach an unwritten contract with citizens when they discontinue needed service programs.

Several types of negligence also pose legal and ethical issues in case management. **Negligence** is the failure to act in a situation as a reasonably prudent nurse would if faced with the same situation. Wrongful denial of services could be considered a form of negligence at the system level. Other types of negligence include negligent actions on the part of the case manager or other providers and negligent referrals. Failure of a local health department to provide effective communicable disease control programs could be considered an example of negligence at the population level.

Nurse case managers may also be held legally liable for negligent referrals. A **negligent referral** may be one that is inappropriate and results in harm or injury to the client or a failure to make a referral when one is warranted. Case managers can prevent negligent referrals by investigating the providers or agencies to which they refer clients in terms of licensure and relevant accreditation, client outcomes data, billing practices, insurance coverage, and malpractice information. A second tactic to prevent negligent referrals is to provide the client with several provider options rather than making a single referral. Finally, the case manager should follow up on the outcomes of referrals made.

The last legal issue to be addressed here is reportable events. Like all nurses, nurse case managers have a legal mandate to report the occurrence, or even the suspicion, of certain kinds of events. These include child and elder abuse and, in some jurisdictions, intimate partner violence. Other reportable events include violent injuries, specific communicable diseases, and coroners' cases. Nurse case managers should be aware of what events (particularly what communicable diseases) are considered reportable in their area and should also let clients know of the need to report such events when they occur.

Case Management and Health Care Reform

The focus of the Affordable Care Act on health promotion and illness and injury prevention will make population health management even more important than it currently is. A number of key provisions of ACA address population health. First, ACA expands access to insurance coverage by expanding Medicaid programs, insurance exchanges, and support of community health centers. A second emphasis in the ACA is on improving the quality of care provided by means of quality improvement initiatives and support for patient-centered outcomes research. Third, provisions to promote accountable care organizations (ACOs) that take responsibility for health outcomes in the populations they serve are intended to foster health promotion and illness prevention activities. In addition, expanded coverage of health promotion and prevention activities will have an effect on population health. Finally, there is a set of provisions within ACA that focuses on community-based and population-based activities and worksite wellness initiatives. As noted earlier, the requirement for hospitals to conduct community health needs assessments will help to focus attention on population health needs (Stoto, 2013).

Reimbursement changes in health care funding arising from health care reform legislation will increase the need for case management to reduce the costs of care and assure provision of care in a safe and efficient manner (Case Management's Day, 2011). Other effects on case management services have arisen from previous federal initiatives, such as the Deficit Reduction Act of 2005, which minimized use of Medicaid child welfare funds for case management services. In addition, the Centers for Medicare and Medicaid Services (CMS) Quality Framework for Medicaid Home and Community Based Services promoted quality improvement in services to disabled clients, which are often addressed through case management services. Recognizing the potential impact of these and other health care reform issues, the Case Management Society of America (2009) has developed a case management model legislative act to outline key elements of case management programs for inclusion in state and federal legislation.

Population Health Nursing and Case Management

Population health nurses functioning as individual or population case managers employ the nursing process in designing case management plans and systems of care. Elements of the case management process include assessing the need for case management, planning and implementing case management services, and evaluating the effects of those services.

Assessing the Need for Case Management

Not all clients encountered by population health nurses will need case management services, so the nurse must identify those clients who do need services and can benefit most from them. Case management services are often targeted to certain population groups or individuals who meet specific criteria. Such criteria often include clients or groups of people who are at high risk of hospital admission, who have complex health needs, or who make extensive and costly use of health care services (Abell, Hughes, Reilly, Berzins, & Challis, 2010). Clients with HIV/AIDS, diabetes, and cancer are all examples of populations with high-cost diagnoses. These diseases also result in high-volume resource use that may warrant development of case management services. Case management services might also be developed for pregnant women or children with asthma for whom services are often poorly coordinated and for whom case management has been shown to have significant positive effects.

Individual client indicators of the need for case management can be categorized as personal indicators, health-related indicators, and social indicators. Personal indicators may include diminished functional status, a history of substance abuse or mental illness, poor cognitive abilities, prior noncompliance with treatment plans, age over 65 years, experience of a major life change or significant change in self-image, potential for severe emotional response to illness, or unrealistic expectations of potential outcomes of care. Health-related factors include the presence of specific medical conditions or diagnoses (e.g., Alzheimer's disease, AIDS, eating disorders, severe burns, trauma), multiple diagnoses, history of prolonged recovery or increased potential for complications, recent or frequent hospital readmissions or emergency department use, intentional or unintentional drug overdose, and involvement of multiple health care providers, agencies, or funding sources. Social indicators may include living alone or with a person who is disabled, being uninsured, evidence of family violence, homelessness or an unhealthy home environment, lack of support systems or financial resources, single parenthood, or living in an area where services are lacking. The presence of one or more of these indicators does not necessarily mean that the client is in need of case management services, but it should alert the population health nurse to that possibility. The nurse would then further explore the client situation to determine an actual need for services.

Assessing the Case Management Situation

To develop an effective case management plan for an individual client or a case management system for a specific population group, the population health nurse case manager must assess the client's (or group's) health status and identify factors in the situation that affect health and are likely to affect the case management plan and achievement of planned health outcomes. Assessment should also validate the need for case management and may be organized in terms of the dimensions of health. For example, biophysical considerations such as age and physiological health status or functional ability may indicate problems that need to be addressed by the case manager or constraints that will affect interventions selected. Arthritic deformities may complicate the ability of a diabetic client to draw up and give an insulin injection, so the case management plan will need to account for these limitations. At the population level, extensive cardiovascular comorbidity in a population with diabetes will necessitate the development of a case management system that addresses problems related to both diseases.

Similarly, mental health status, coping abilities, and anxiety are psychological determinants that may affect case management needs and activities with individual clients. In terms of population case management, a high incidence of suicide among disabled residents would be an indication of the need for case management programs. Physical environmental considerations that may influence the case management situation include clients' living conditions or neighborhood social capital, as well as the influences of environmental pollution. For example, population case management for persons with asthma would need to address control of environmental triggers, possibly even at the level of advocating legislation for better control of air pollutants, as well as education for individuals on reducing triggers in the home or work setting.

Sociocultural factors will also influence the types and extent of services to be included in the case management plan. Some factors to consider are the client's education level, support systems, economic status, occupation, transportation, and cultural beliefs and behaviors. Changes in social roles should also be considered in assessing the case management situation. Unemployment and financial status are examples of two sociocultural factors that might influence population case management for persons with HIV/AIDS. Behavioral considerations such as substance abuse, lack of physical activity, or poor diet may also give rise to the need for case management or influence development of the case management plan. Using the HIV/AIDS example, population case management systems might be developed differently for men who have sex with men (MSM) than for heterosexual women.

Considerations related to the health care system include assessment of the types of health care services that the client is likely to need. The nurse case manager assesses the availability of those services in the client's community as well as influences related to the type and level of insurance coverage the client has. Client attitudes toward health services and health care providers are another important element of this dimension affecting case management. At the population level, the nurse case manager might assess the cluster of services available to meet the needs of specific populations (e.g., those with HIV/AIDS). The nurse could also explore existing interactions between service organizations and the need and desire for closer coordination of services. A tool for assessing case management

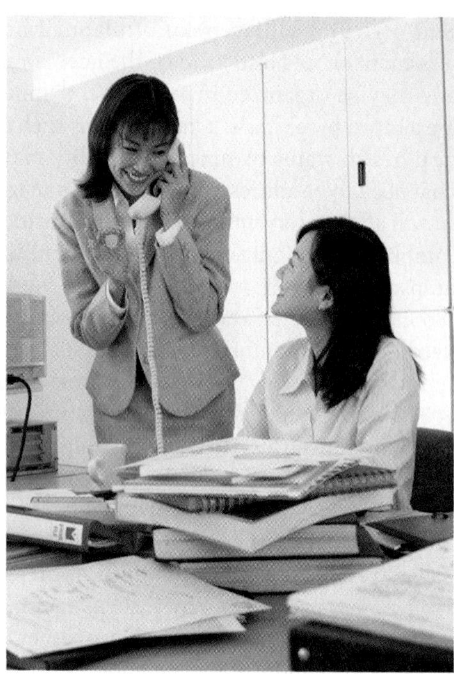

Case management often entails coordination of health care services. *(Sozaijiten/Pearson Education. Inc)*

situations from the perspective of the determinants of health included in the population health nursing model can be found in the student resources site.

Planning and Implementing Case Management Strategies

The population health nurse develops and executes a case management plan for an individual client or plans and implements care management systems for population groups. Specific foci in planning and implementation of case management strategies at individual and population levels include the development of the case management plan, communicating the plan, delegating, initiating referrals, and designing case management systems. Each of these foci is briefly discussed below.

DEVELOPING THE CASE MANAGEMENT PLAN. A case management plan is a series of expected outcomes of care and related activities that address the contribution of each discipline involved in the care of a particular patient or population. Effective case management plans are interdisciplinary and flexible and address clients' needs in a comprehensive fashion.

Activity may reflect case management or disease management. Case management addresses the entire client situation to resolve as many identified needs as possible given the resources available. **Disease management**, on the other hand, is the process of addressing client health needs resulting from a particular disease or condition. Assisting a client with diabetes to control his or her disease is an example of disease management. Assisting the same client to meet a wide variety of health and social needs is case management. A similar distinction can be made at the population case management level. For example, services to a diabetic population that focus on control of their disease involve disease management. Services to the same population that address a wider array of needs, not just those related to diabetes control, exemplify case management.

Case or disease management plans should be based on available evidence-based guidelines. In using evidence-based guidelines, the case manager conducts a generic assessment of the client or population and then determines the applicability of elements of the guidelines based on the assessment. Guidelines may need to be modified or adapted to meet the needs of particular clients or population groups. For example, a guideline for care of populations with HIV/AIDS may be modified for use with a population comprised mainly of MSM.

Discharge planning is a special application of the case management process that involves identification of follow-up needs and arranging care after discharge from a hospital or other institutional setting. Discharge planning is intended to ease the transition from one level of care to another. Indicators of the need for discharge planning are similar to those for case management in general, but studies suggest that, at least for older clients, functional dependence is the best predictor of readmission and a significant indicator of the need for discharge planning.

The Nursing Interventions Classification (NIC) schema (Bulechek, Butcher, Dochterman, & Wagner, 2012) has identified discharge planning as a specific nursing intervention designed to facilitate transitions between health care settings or from institutional settings to the client's home. CMS has noted that discharge planning should be a collaborative endeavor between health care professionals and the client and family. Discharge planning as outlined by CMS includes identification of the client's follow-up care needs, integration of necessary community services and facilities to meet those needs, and cross-disciplinary collaboration in addressing client needs. Discharge planning also involves preparing the client for discharge and beginning to meet the identified discharge needs. The discharge plan should be congruent with the client's health care,

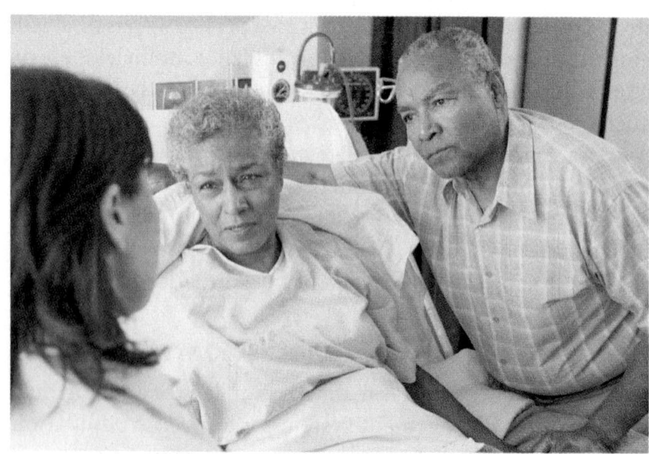

Case management often begins with discharge planning for hospitalized clients. *(Monkey Business Images/Shutterstock)*

social, psychological, and financial needs. CMS has also developed discharge planning guidelines for home health agencies, hospices, psychiatric institutions, and other health care settings. Although discharge planning is not required by CMS for clients seen in outpatient or emergency settings who are not admitted to the hospital, CMS has suggested that such facilities might also benefit from the development of specific discharge planning processes (CMS, 2013). A client discharge assessment tool to facilitate discharge planning is available in the student resources for this book. In addition, the Family Caregiver Alliance (2009) has developed a hospital discharge planning guide for families and caregivers. For further information about the discharge planning guide, see the resources provided in the External Resources section of the student resources site.

Implementation of the case management plan involves communicating the plan, delegating, initiating referrals, and monitoring plan implementation. Each of these aspects of implementing the plan will be discussed briefly.

COMMUNICATING THE PLAN. Clients and their significant others should be involved in the development of the case management plan. Once the plan is in place, they will need to be informed of arrangements made for care and expectations of them in following through on the management plan. For example, clients may need to call to make a specific appointment with a provider even though care has been arranged by the case manager. Clients will also need to know about any payments required and the names of contact persons in agencies to which they have been referred. Additional information to be conveyed to clients relates to the expected duration and outcome of services.

The case manager also needs to communicate the case management plan to the providers who will be giving the necessary care. Client needs and expectations of the provider should be addressed as well as any previous plans and their effects, expectations for continued care, and any other information relevant to the client's situation. The case manager should be careful to obtain the consent of the client before providing such information. Finally, the payer should be informed of and approve the management plan. The nurse case manager should confirm and document that referral agencies and payers have received the information sent. He or she should also confirm that clients and family members understand the information provided.

DELEGATING. In a population health nursing context, **delegation** is transferring responsibility for the completion of nursing and other health care tasks to other competent individuals, such as ancillary nursing personnel, the client, or a family member or caregiver. Delegation of nursing tasks must be done in such a way as to protect the health and safety of the client, family, and, on occasion, the public. Delegation involves specific steps and related activities presented in Table 12-3•.

INITIATING REFERRALS. The case manager and his or her delegatees, may not be able to provide all of the services needed by a client or population group. In this case, the case manager makes referrals to other sources of service to meet client needs. Referral involves directing a client to another source of information or assistance. It differs from delegation in that the nurse case manager relinquishes responsibility for implementation of the portions of the plan of care for which the client is referred, although he or she retains overall responsibility for the quality of care provided. Referrals to a variety of health care and related services may be part of case management for an individual client and his or her family. Similarly, case management systems for groups of clients may make use of an identified set of agencies to address most needs of the population group. Four basic considerations enter into the decision to refer clients to particular providers, agencies, or services: the acceptability of the referral, eligibility for services, constraints operating in the situation, and community resources available.

Acceptability. The first consideration in making a referral is the acceptability of the referral to the client. Some clients may be unwilling to obtain help if they perceive it as "charity." In other cases, clients may have philosophies different from those of the referral resource. For example, a Southern Baptist client may be reluctant to accept assistance from an agency supported by the Roman Catholic Church. Barriers to acceptability of a specific referral may include fear of a strange agency or provider, prior negative experiences, lack of faith in the referral resource, failure to acknowledge a problem requiring referral, and concerns about costs. Finally, reaching out for assistance may be counter to the client's culture or frame of reference, or willingness to follow up on a referral may be hindered by client concerns with higher priorities.

Eligibility. The second consideration in referral is the client's eligibility for the service provided. There are many determinants of eligibility for service. Sometimes eligibility is based on financial need, and clients may need to provide evidence of income and expenditures. In other instances, eligibility might be based on residence within a particular jurisdiction or membership in a particular group. For example, nonresidents are not usually eligible for state-supported medical assistance, or a particular agency may provide services only to members of a specific religious or ethnic group. Eligibility can also be based on age. As an example, senior citizens' groups usually do not provide services for anyone under the age of 55. Finally, eligibility is sometimes based on the existence of a particular condition. For instance, certain shelter services might be available only to abused women rather than to homeless people in general.

Situational constraints. The presence of situational constraints, or factors in the client's situation that would prevent him or her from following through on a referral, is a third consideration. For example, does the client have transportation available to go to the appropriate place of care? If clients do not speak English, will they be able to find an interpreter to help them, or are interpretation services provided by the agency? The nurse making the referral should assess any situational constraints present and then take action to eliminate or minimize the

TABLE 12-3 Steps and Related Activities in the Delegation Process

Steps in the Delegation Process	Related Activities
Define the task	• Identify the task or tasks to be delegated • Identify the skills needed to perform the task • Identify the resources needed • Identify expected outcomes and related measurements of achievement • Determine the extent of supervision needed
Assess the situation	• Assess the complexity, variability, and urgency of care • Identify the level of clinical decision making required • Identify the predictability of the client situation • Examine the range and severity of potential adverse outcomes associated with the task • Determine the range and complexity of actions required in the event of adverse outcomes • Promote client/family involvement in decision making • Identify the therapeutic benefits and risks of delegating the task
Identify potential delegatees	• Assess delegatees' skills in relation to the task requirements
Provide training as needed	• Provide any training needed to perform the task • Allow time to practice the task if needed
Communicate with the delegatee	Inform the delegatee regarding • The purpose of the task • Task importance and priorities for performing the task • Expected results • Expected observations to be reported • Performance standards • Procedures to be followed
Inventory resources	• Inventory resources available against those needed to perform the task • Procure additional resources, if needed
Delegate the task	• Establish timelines and deadlines • Communicate these to the delegatee
Monitor task completion	• Monitor progress in performing the task • Provide feedback on task performance • Provide timely intervention for problems or concerns
Evaluate delegation	Evaluate the delegation process in terms of • Task accomplishment • Outcomes achieved • Timeliness and effectiveness of communication • Need for adjustment of the plan of care • Performance of the delegatee and acknowledgement of task accomplishment

Data from: Delegation. (n.d.). Retrieved from http://www.businessballs.com/delegation.htm#steps; Heathfield, S. M. (2014). *Delegation as a leadership style: Tips for effective delegation.* Retrieved from http://humanresources.about.com/cs/manageperformance/a/delegation.htm; National Council of State Boards of Nursing. (2012). *The four steps of the delegation process.* Retrieved from https://transitiontopractice.org/files/module1/Communication%20-%20Delegation%20Process.pdf; Randall, M. (2013). *6 steps for more effective delegation.* Retrieved from http://www.fastcompany.com/3006643/6-steps-more-effective-delegation; Thakur, S., & Edwards, G. (2010). *Sample of a delegation flowchart.* Retrieved from http://www.brighthub.com/office/project-management/articles/89316.aspx

effects of those constraints. The nurse case manager may also need to coordinate funding benefits among multiple agencies to prevent barriers to timely access to care.

Resource availability. Information related to each of the three previous referral considerations will be readily available if the nurse has thoroughly assessed each of the dimensions of health prior to developing the case management plan. Resource availability information, on the other hand, will be obtained through assessment of the community. The population health nurse case manager needs to be familiar with health care and other services available in the community. Information on community resources can be obtained in a number of ways. Two major sources of information are the local health department and the yellow pages. Other resources are neighborhood information and referral centers, local government offices and chambers of commerce, and police and fire departments. The local library is also a source of information and may even have a directory of local resources.

It is not sufficient for the population health nurse to merely be aware of the existence of community resources. The nurse must know where these resources are located and understand the requirements for referral to each resource. The nurse should systematically collect information on the types of services a referral resource provides, criteria for eligibility for services, and whether any fee is involved. Information to be sought also includes indicators of the quality of services provided and the credentials and competence of providers. The population health nurse case manager may want to establish a **resource file** or database to systematically organize and store

Resource category: Transportation Funding source: Voluntary
Agency name: St. Martha's Catholic Church
Address: 3710 Montebank Rd, Otenada, Mississippi
Phone number: 817-3421 Business hours: Mon-Fri 8-4
Contact person: Mrs. Jefferson Title: receptionist / secretary
Source of referral: self or other
Eligibility: anyone without transportation - need not be members of church
Fee: none
Services: Provides transportation to church services as well as other services such as Dr.'s office, grocery shopping, etc. on periodic basis
Access: call to arrange transportation
Other comments: 1) Do not provide transportation on long-term basis, i.e., to work or school
2) depends upon availability of volunteer drivers
3) drivers trained to assist disabled riders

FIGURE 12-1 Sample Resource File Entry

information on area resources. Figure 12-1● depicts a sample resource file entry. The resource file can be organized by category of services. A particular agency with more than one type of service could be entered in several different categories, or a cross-reference system could be used. The resource described in Figure 12-1 deals with transportation.

Information about the resource's funding source can be useful in tracking service availability. For example, if tax revenues have declined in the area, the population health nurse case manager may want to contact agencies funded by public money to determine whether services have been cut prior to making a specific referral. Also, it may be important to some clients to know that the services they receive from an agency are provided by tax dollars rather than "charity."

Of course, the resource file entry includes the referral resource's full name, address, and telephone number. The business hours notation may refer to when the agency is open or times when a particular service is offered. For example, the entry might read "Family planning: Monday, 9:00 A.M.–noon, Prenatal: Tuesday, 1:00–4:00 P.M."

It is helpful to have the name of a contact person in the agency as well. Referrals are facilitated when agency personnel are familiar with the person making the referral. Unfortunately, situations do occur in which some agency employees are more inclined to accommodate professional colleagues than clients. When the nurse case manager refers a client to an agency and gives that individual the name of a contact person who knows the nurse, the client who mentions nurse's name may get a more prompt response than the client who does not have a specific person to contact. Having a specific contact person within the agency may also facilitate requests for services when the request is made by the nurse case manager rather than the client.

"Source of referral" in Figure 12-1 refers to the preferred originator of the referral. Some agencies accept referrals only from specific persons, frequently physicians. If a professional referral is required, the nurse should specifically inquire about the acceptability of referrals from nurse practitioners, if they are available in the area. In the example in Figure 12-1, no specific referral source is required. Clients may request services on their own or be referred by anyone else.

As noted previously, information related to the eligibility of clients for services is very important. To make appropriate referrals, the nurse must know who is eligible for a particular service and who is not. This helps to minimize client frustration in being referred for services for which they do not qualify.

The importance of a notation regarding fees is obvious. Clients need to know beforehand if they will be charged for services provided by the referral resource. The nurse should also be familiar with the types of insurance coverage accepted by the resource. For example, does the agency accept clients covered by Medicaid but not TriCare? An additional notation might indicate whether the agency can help clients with financial arrangements for out-of-pocket expenses. The nurse should also know whether payment is expected at the time of services or if the client will receive a bill later.

Notation should also be made regarding the types of services provided by the resource. The entry regarding access reflects the means by which the client gains entry to the system. In the example in Figure 12-1, the client needs to call ahead to arrange transportation. Additional information under this entry would indicate any supporting documentation the client must provide to be eligible for services. Should he or she bring health insurance papers, or just the policy number? Will the client need proof of residence, monthly expenditures, or medical expenses?

Finally, the nurse should obtain and store information regarding the competence of providers to whom referrals are made. Information about the credentials of providers, prior client complaints, malpractice actions, and so on can be recorded in the comments section as indicated in the third comment in Figure 12-1.

The type of information included in the sample resource file entry allows the population health nurse case manager to make appropriate referrals that do not waste clients' time and energy. It also allows the nurse to prepare clients for what they will encounter in following through on a referral. The file should be updated on a regular basis and as circumstances in various agencies change. Having a specific contact person in each agency may help to ensure that the nurse is notified of program changes. Experiences and reactions of clients following the use of a particular resource can also be used to update resource information and to evaluate the quality of service provided. A copy of the resource file entry form is included on the student resources site.

MONITORING PLAN IMPLEMENTATION. Monitoring is another important aspect of implementing the case management plan. Once the plan is developed, the population health nurse case manager does not simply let the plan proceed to unfold on its own or close the case to case management services. Rather, the nurse case manager monitors the implementation of the plan and the progress made in achieving identified goals. Specific areas to be addressed at this stage include monitoring changes in the client's medical status (either positive or negative), social circumstances, and the quality of care provided; observing for changes in functional ability or mobility; and identifying evolving education needs. In addition, the nurse will assess the effectiveness of pain management if relevant and monitor changes in client or family satisfaction with services and their outcomes.

Evaluating the Process and Outcomes of Case Management

Evaluation is an integral component of the case management process. The population health nurse case manager focuses on three areas in evaluating case management: client outcomes, quality of care, and system outcomes.

Client outcomes resulting from case management for individual clients may lie in improved health status, better quality of life, or improved ability to manage a chronic condition. Case management services have been found to be effective in achieving client health-related outcomes in a number of situations. For example, a literature review found that nursing case management had significant effects for clients with diabetes, chronic obstructive pulmonary disease, or coronary heart disease. Types of outcomes achieved included improvement in objective clinical measurements, improved functionality and quality of life, increased client satisfaction, better adherence to treatment regimens, and improved self-care (Sutherland & Hayter, 2009). Case management has also demonstrated positive health outcomes for clients with substance abuse disorders (Day et al., 2012), those with HIV/AIDS (Thurman, Haas, Dushimimana, Lavin, & Mock, 2010), women receiving Temporary Assistance for Needy Families (TANF) (Kneipp et al., 2011), and Hong Kong elders with mild dementia (Lam et al., 2010).

As noted earlier, the case manager is responsible for monitoring and evaluating the quality of services provided in implementing the case management plan. To obtain evaluative data in this area, the nurse might periodically visit providers to observe and discuss the quality of care given. For example, the nurse might ask an oncologist about the breadth of options usually presented to women with breast cancer. An oncologist who presents only one option to clients may not be the most appropriate referral for the case manager to make. The population health nurse case manager might also contact clients or family members to obtain their perceptions of the quality of services provided. The nurse should be particularly alert to situations in which clients discontinue services from one or more providers before goals are achieved. Exploration of the client's reasons for discontinuing services may indicate poor quality of care.

Quality of care should also be assessed in population case management. Evaluating the quality of care may involve the use of benchmarks. A **benchmark** is a standard of performance against which the performance of a given system can be judged. Clinical benchmarking reflects the best outcome actually achieved for a group of clients or a diagnosis, as well the best possible achievable outcome. Steps in the benchmarking process using services to clients with hypertension as an example are presented in Table 12-4●.

Evaluation of quality of care may also make use of one or more sets of national quality indicators. Such indicators include the Health Plan Employer Data and Information Set (HEDIS), developed by the National Committee for Quality Assurance, and the Outcome-based Quality Indicators (OBQI) for home health agencies, based on the federal government's Outcome

TABLE 12-4 Steps in the Benchmarking Process Using Hypertension Control Services in a Primary Care Clinic as an Example

Benchmarking Step	Example
Identify a specific area of practice to be evaluated	• Hypertension control
Identify a desired client-focused outcome	• Blood pressure consistently below 140/90 in 90% of clients • Medication adherence of at least 80% in 90% of clients
Identify key factors and processes that affect the outcome	• Medication education
Identify comparison organizations against which to evaluate local clinic performance	• Other similar primary care clinics with effective hypertension control programs
Identify benchmarks for best practice for each factor	• Medication education provided at initial visit for 90% of clients • Medication adherence assessed and reinforced at each subsequent visit
Collect local setting data on performance related to the benchmarks	• Percent of patients who receive medication education at initiation of anti-hypertensive treatment • Percent of patients with documented evidence of medication adherence assessment and reinforcement at each visit
Obtain comparison data from best-performing primary care clinics	• Percent of patients who receive medication education at initiation of anti-hypertensive treatment in comparison clinics • Percent of patients with documented evidence of medication adherence assessment and reinforcement at each visit in comparison clinics
Compare local setting results with identified best practice (benchmark)	• Local setting performance at, above, or below comparison benchmark
Share results with others involved	• Share findings with system providers who care for clients with hypertension
Develop an action plan to improve performance that incorporates best practices from other settings	• Identify factors impeding medication education at initial visit • Develop processes to promote medication education at initial visit • Implement action plan • Evaluate effects of practice change
Implement the action plan	• Develop culturally and linguistically appropriate educational processes for medication education based on clinic clientele • Implement educational processes
Monitor progress in improving outcomes	• Monitor provision of medication education • Monitor medication adherence in clients • Monitor effects on extent of blood pressure control in clinic population with hypertension

Data from: Agency for Healthcare Research and Quality. (2013). *Benchmarking.* Retrieved from http://healthit.ahrq.gov/health-it-tools-and-resources/workflow-assessment-health-it-toolkit/all-workflow-tools/benchmarking; Ettorchi-Tardy, A., Levif, M., & Michel, P. (2012). Benchmarking: A method for continuous quality improvement in health. *Health Policy, 7*(4), e101–119. PMC3359088. Retrieved from http://www.ncbi.nlm.nih.gov/pmc/articles/PMC3359088/

and Assessment Information Set (OASIS). Quality indicators have also been developed by the URAC (formerly the Utilization Review Accreditation Commission) specifically for evaluation of case management services through URAC's accreditation process (URAC, n.d.a, n.d.b). For further information about these sets of quality indicators, see the resources provided in the *External Resources* section of the student resources site.

Systems outcomes should also be evaluated; systems outcomes reflect the effects of case management on the health care system. Elements that might be evaluated in this area include staff or client satisfaction, length of stay (or frequency and duration of care), and costs of care. Other system outcome variables that might be examined include the number of days that clients did not meet established outcome criteria, reimbursement denial amounts or rates, readmissions, emergency department visits, and costs per case for case management versus cost savings resulting from case management services. For example, case management for homeless clients with chronic illness resulted in an average cost saving of more than $6,000 per person served compared to usual care without case management (Basu, Kee, Buchanan, & Sadowski, 2011).

Evaluating system outcomes may also entail utilization review. **Utilization review** is a process of monitoring the use, delivery, and cost-effectiveness of health care services as well as their appropriateness in a given situation. Utilization review also involves monitoring the quality of care provided (*Mosby's Medical Dictionary*, 2012; *Utilization review*, n.d.). According to the current CMS manual, organizations participating in Medicare and Medicaid funded programs are required to engage in utilization review. Areas for review include the necessity and duration of services, the availability and use of needed professional services, timeliness of services, and therapeutic interventions provided (CMS, 2008). Utilization review is frequently used to determine whether or not case management services will be reimbursed by insurers (Professional Services Network, 2010). State Medicaid systems also employ utilization review to restrict provision of unnecessary and inappropriate care examining the medical necessity for care, place of care, length of stay, and prior authorization for certain services (Florida Agency for Health Care Administration, 2011). Similarly, the State of California Department of Industrial Relations (2014) uses a Medical Treatment Utilization Schedule (MTUS) to guide physicians providing services under the workers' compensation system to provide evidence-based care for work-related injuries. Services provided are reviewed in light of the MTUS. California employers or their claims administrators are required by law to have utilization review programs (California Division of Workers Compensation, 2014).

Other approaches to evaluating system outcomes for case management systems include quality outcomes measurement and the development of quality indicators. Quality outcomes measurement involves the identification of measures of quality in system performance and collection of data related to those measures. An example of a quality indicator might be reduction in pain levels in home care clients within a specified number of hours after intervention. Measurement of the indicator would require a follow-up contact with the client within that time frame to determine whether the pain has been controlled at an acceptable level. At the system level, the percentage of clients whose pain is effectively controlled would be the quality indicator. Benchmarking, as discussed earlier, may be used to establish measures for quality indicators.

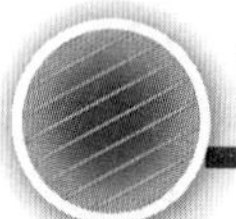

Evidence-Based Practice

Effectiveness of Case Management

In spite of studies that have demonstrated the effectiveness of case management for some categories of clients, some authors contend that there is no overall evidence of the effectiveness of case management as a strategy for addressing chronic illness needs. For example, Offredy et al. (2009) conducted a review of literature and found that, in spite of client and caregiver reports of the benefits of case management, wide variation in outcome measures across studies resulted in inconclusive evidence of its effectiveness across a variety of chronic illnesses. It may be that case management has differential effects with different population groups and different health-related conditions.

1. Select a particular chronic health condition and examine the literature related to case management for clients with that condition.
2. What does the evidence indicate overall regarding the effectiveness of case management for this condition?
3. Are there client- or population-related factors that influence the effectiveness of case management strategies? How might these factors be modified to promote more effective case management?

CHAPTER RECAP

Case management has been shown to be an effective nursing intervention used since the beginning of population health nursing practice. Case management strategies may be employed at individual or population levels. Several models have been developed for case management services including self-determination models, consumer choice of case manager models, coordinated database systems, and tiered management systems. Standards and principles of case management practice have been developed by the Case Management Society of America and can guide the population health nurse in providing individual or population-based case management services that incorporate identified case manager roles and functions.

A variety of ethical and legal issues arise in the context of case management services. Ethical issues include allocation of resources and client autonomy and self-determination. Legal considerations in case management center on client confidentiality and privacy, denial of services, abandonment, breach of contract, negligence, and reportable events.

Provision of case management services may increase with health care reform, but the full effects of reform legislation are yet to be seen following resolution of court challenges to the Affordable Care Act. The case management process involves assessing the need for case management services, planning and implementing case management strategies, and evaluating the effects of case management in terms of client and health care delivery system outcomes. Population health nurses can improve their practice with more systematic use of the case management process with individuals as well as population groups.

CASE STUDY Population Case Management in Action

As a population health nurse working in an elementary school in a small town, you notice a significant increase in both school absences related to asthma and children who are coming to your office with difficulty breathing during the school day. Although each child's situation is unique, they seem to share a number of common characteristics. Most of them are from low-income families in which both parents work. They all live in the neighborhood surrounding the school. There is considerable construction occurring in the neighborhood that keeps everything coated with dust. The school yard is a home for pollen-producing weeds. The school is old and previous water leaks have led to widespread mold and mildew in some of the classrooms and in the heating vents.

Most of the children are using albuterol inhalers when they have difficulty breathing, but few of them are using nasal steroids on a regular basis or using their albuterol prior to activities in the school yard. Many of the children tell you that their doctors have prescribed nasal steroids, but their families cannot afford to have the prescriptions filled. In talking with some of the primary care providers in the community, you find that they are frustrated with their inability to control asthma in many of the children and that their practices are inundated with children with mild to severe attacks.

1. Does this situation warrant development of a case management system? Why or why not?
2. What are the children's health needs in this situation? How do biophysical, psychological, environmental, sociocultural, behavioral, and health system factors influence those needs?
3. What desired outcomes would you establish for a case management system?
4. How would you involve members of the community in developing the case management plan? Who should be involved?
5. What referrals would be appropriate for many of the children? What is the expected outcome of these referrals? How would you go about making the referrals?
6. How would you evaluate the case management system for this population? Be specific about the evaluative criteria you would use and how you would obtain the information to evaluate care.

REFERENCES

Abell, J., Hughes, J., Reilly, S., Berzins, K., & Challis, D. (2010). Targeting in case management. *Care Management Journals, 11*, 11–18. doi:10.1891/1521-0987.11.1.11

Agency for Healthcare Research and Quality. (2013). *Benchmarking*. Retrieved from http://healthit.ahrq.gov/health-it-tools-and-resources/workflow-assessment-health-it-toolkit/all-workflow-tools/benchmarking

American Case Management Association. (2014). *About ACMA*. Retrieved from http://www.acmaweb.org/section.aspx?sID=4&mn=mn1&sn=sn1&wpg=mh

Basu, A., Kee, R., Buchanan, D., & Sadowski, L. S. (2011). Comparative cost analysis of housing and case management program for chronically ill homeless adults compared to usual care. *Health Services Research, 47*(1, Part II), 523–543. doi:10.1111/j.1475-6773.2011.01350.x

Buhler-Wilkerson, K. (2001). *No place like home: A history of nursing and home care in the United States*. Baltimore: Johns Hopkins University.

Bulechek, G. M., Butcher, H. K., & Dochterman, J. M., & Wagner, C. (Eds.). (2013). Nursing interventions classification (6th ed.). St. Louis, MO: Mosby.

California Division of Workers Compensation. (2014). *Answers to your questions about utilization review*. Retrieved from http://www.dir.ca.gov/dwc/factsheets/factsheet_a.pdf

Case Management Society of America. (n.d.). *What is case management?* Retrieved from http://www.cmsa.org/Home/CMSA/WhatisaCaseManager/tabid/224/Default.aspx

Case Management Society of America. (2009). *Case management model act*. Retrieved from http://cmsa.org/portals/0/pdf/PublicPolicy/CMSA_Model_Act.pdf

Case Management Society of America. (2010). *Standards of practice for case management*. Retrieved from http://cmsa.org/portals/0/pdf/memberonly/StandardsOfPractice.pdf

"Case management's day": Health care reform proves CM's importance. (2011). *Hospital Case Management, 19*(1), 1–6.

Centers for Medicare and Medicaid Services. (2008). *CMS manual*. Retrieved from http://www.cms.gov/Regulations-and-Guidance/Guidance/Transmittals/downloads/R37SOMA.pdf

Centers for Medicare and Medicaid Services. (2013). *Discharge planning*. Retrieved from http://www.cms.gov/Outreach-and-Education/Medicare-Learning-Network-MLN/MLNProducts/Downloads/Discharge-Planning-Booklet-ICN908184.pdf

Commission for Case Manager Certification. (n.d.a). *Case management facts.* Retrieved from http://ccmcertification.org/about-us/about-case-management/case-management-facts

Commission for Case Manager Certification. (n.d.b). *Definition and philosophy of case management.* Retrieved from http://ccmcertification.org/about-us/about-case-management/definition-and-philosophy-case-management

Commission for Case Manager Certification. (2009). *Code of professional conduct for case managers with standards, rules, procedures and penalties.* Retrieved from http://ccmcertification.org/sites/default/files/downloads/2012/Code%20of%20Professional%20Conduct%20for%20Case%20Managers.pdf

Day, C. A., Demirkol, A., Tynan, M., Curry, K., Hines, S., Lintzeris, N., & Haber, P. S. (2012). Individual versus team-based case-management for clients of opioid treatment services: An initial evaluation of what clients prefer. *Drug and Alcohol Review, 31,* 499–506. doi:10.1111/j.1465-3362.2011.00347.x

Delegation. (n.d.). Retrieved from http://www.businessballs.com/delegation.htm#steps

Ettorchi-Tardy, A., Levif, M., & Michel, P. (2012). Benchmarking: A method for continuous quality improvement in health. *Health Policy, 7*(4), e101–119. PMC3359088. Retrieved from http://www.ncbi.nlm.nih.gov/pmc/articles/PMC3359088/

Family Caregiver Alliance. (2009). *Hospital discharge planning: A guide for families and caregivers.* Retrieved from https://caregiver.org/hospital-discharge-planning-guide-families-and-caregivers

Florida Agency for Health Care Administration. (2011). *Utilization review – Quality assurance/quality improvement.* Retrieved from http://www.fdhc.state.fl.us/medicaid/Utilization_Review/index.shtml

Goga, A. E., & Muhe, L. M. (2011). Global challenges with scale-up of the integrated management of childhood illness strategy: Results of a multi-country study. *BMC Public Health, 11,* 503–512. doi: 10.1186/1471-2458-11-503

Grange, M. (2011). How community matrons perceive their effectiveness in case management. *Nursing Older People, 23*(5), 24–29. no doi

Hacker, K., & Walker, D. K. (2013). Achieving population health in accountable care organizations. *American Journal of Public Health 103,* 1163–1167. doi: 10.2105/AJPH.2013.301254

Heathfield, S. M. (2014). *Delegation as a leadership style: Tips for effective delegation.* Retrieved from http://humanresources.about.com/cs/manageperformance/a/delegation.htm

Klaske, W., Annema, C., De Keyser, J., & Middel, B. (2010). Design of a randomized controlled trial (RCT) on the effectiveness of a Dutch patient advocacy case management intervention among severely disabled multiple sclerosis patients. *BMC Health Services Research, 10,* 142–151. doi: 10.1186/1472-6963-10-142

Kneipp, S. M., Kairalla, J. A., Lutz, B. J., Pereira, D., Hall, A. G., Flocks, J., ..., Schwartz, T. (2011). Public health nursing case management for women receiving Temporary Assistance for Needy Families: A randomized controlled trial using community-based participatory research. *American Journal of Public Health, 101,* 1759–1768. doi:10.2105/AJPH.2011.300210

Lam, L. C. W., Lee, J. S. W., Chung, J. C. C., Lau, A., Woo, J., & Kwok, T. C. Y. (2010). A randomized controlled trial to examine the effectiveness of case management model for community dwelling older persons with mild dementia in Hong Kong. *International Journal of Geriatric Psychiatry, 25,* 395–402. doi:10.1002/gps.2352

Mosby's Medical Dictionary (9th ed.). (2012). Maryland Heights, MO: Mosby Elsevier.

Murphy, S. M. W., McGready, J., Griswold, M., & Sylvia, M. L. (2014). A method for estimating cost savings for population health management programs. *Health Services Research, 48*(2, part 1), 582–602. doi: 10.1111/j.1475-6773.2012.01457.x

National Council of State Boards of Nursing. (2012). *The four steps of the delegation process.* Retrieved from https://transitiontopractice.org/files/module1/Communication%20-%20Delegation%20Process.pdf

New York State Department of Health. (2013). *Case management definitions.* Retrieved from http://www.health.ny.gov/diseases/aids/standards/casemanagement/definitions.htm

Offredy, M., Bunn, F., & Morgan, J. (2009). Case management in long term conditions: An inconsistent journey? *British Journal of Community Nursing, 14,* 252–257.

Olbort, R., Mahler, C., Campbell, S., Reushcenbach, B., Müller-Tasch, T., Szecsenyi, J., & Peters-Klimm, F. (2009). Doctor's assistants' views of case management to improve chronic heart failure care in general practice: A qualitative study. *Journal of Advanced Nursing, 65,* 799–808. doi: 10.1111/j.1365-2648.2008.04934.x

Professional Services Network. (2010). *Understanding the utilization review process.* Retrieved from http://www.psninc.net/blog/utilization-review/understanding-the-utilization-review-process/

Randall, M. (2013). *6 steps for more effective delegation.* Retrieved from http://www.fastcompany.com/3006643/6-steps-more-effective-delegation

Rust, G., Strothers, H., Miller, W. J., McLaren, S., Moore, B., & Sambamoorthi, U. (2011). Economic impact of a Medicaid population health management program. *Population Health Management, 14,* 215–222. doi: 10.1089/pop.2010.0036

Setoya, Y., Sato, S., Satake, N., & Ito, J. (2001). Care management in Japanese acute psychiatric units: A national study. *International Journal of Mental Health, 40*(3), 41–54. doi: 10.2753/IMH0020-7411400303

State of California Department of Industrial Relations. (2014). Medical treatment utilization schedule (MTUS). Retrieved from http://www.dir.ca.gov/dwc/MTUS/MTUS.html

Stoto, M. A. (2013). *Population health in the Affordable Care Act era.* Retrieved from http://www.academyhealth.org/files/AH2013pophealth.pdf

Sutherland, D., & Hayter, M. (2009). Structured review: Evaluating the effectiveness of nurse case managers in improving health outcomes in three major chronic diseases. *Journal of Clinical Nursing, 19,* 2978–2992. doi:10.1111/j.1365-2702.2009.02900.x

Thakur, S., & Edwards, G. (2010). *Sample of a delegation flowchart.* Retrieved from http://www.brighthub.com/office/project-management/articles/89316.aspx

Thurman, T. R., Haas, L., Dushimimana, A., Lavin, B., & Mock, N. (2010). *Evaluation of a case management program for HIV clients in Rwanda. AIDS Care, 22,* 759–765. doi:10.1080/09540120903443376

URAC. (n.d.a). *Case management.* Retrieved from https://www.urac.org/accreditation-and-measurement/accreditation-programs/all-programs/case-management/

URAC. (n.d.b). *Case management programs.* Retrieved from https://www.urac.org/accreditation-and-measurement/accreditation-programs/case-management-programs/

Utilization review. (n.d.). In *Merriam-Webster's online medical dictionary.* Retrieved from http://www.merriam-webster.com/medical/utilization%20review

Vroomen, J. M., Van Mierlo, L. D., van de Ven, P. M., Bosmans, J. E., van den Dungen, P., Meiland, F. J. M., ... van Hout, H. P. J. (2012). Comparing Dutch case management care models for people with dementia and their caregivers: The design of the COMPAS study. *BMC Health Services Research, 12,* 132–141. doi: 10.1186/1472-6963-12-132

CHAPTER

13 Home Visits as a Population Health Nursing Strategy

Learning Outcomes

After reading this chapter, you should be able to:

1. Describe the advantages of a home visit as a means of providing nursing care.
2. Analyze challenges encountered by population health nurses making home visits.
3. Identify the major purposes of home visiting programs.
4. Describe major considerations in planning a home visit.
5. Identify tasks involved in implementing a home visit.
6. Analyze the effects of potential distractions during a home visit.
7. Discuss the need for both long-term and short-term evaluative criteria for the effectiveness of a home visit.
8. Describe the relationship between home health nursing and population health nursing.
9. Discuss the need for collaboration in home health and hospice nursing.
10. Discuss funding sources for home health and hospice care.
11. Apply evaluative criteria for home health and hospice care services.

Key Terms

certificate of need
certification
conditions of participation
home health care
home health resource groups (HHRGs)
home visit
home visiting program
hospice care
Outcome and Assessment Information Set (OASIS)
palliative care
proprietary agencies

Advocacy Then

The Metropolitan Life Insurance Company Home Visiting Program

Home visits by nurses have been a mainstay of population health nursing since its establishment by Florence Nightingale in England and Lillian Wald in the United States. Begun initially to meet the needs of poor immigrants in New York City, the concept of home visits as a care delivery mechanism expanded to a variety of populations. Lillian Wald advocated for a home-visiting service for policy holders of the Metropolitan Life Insurance Company, the largest life insurance company in the country at that time (Metlife, n.d.b).

In 1909, Metropolitan Life president Henry Fiske touted the company as a "social program" designed to improve the welfare of the public. He hired social worker Lee Frankel who established the company's welfare division. Miss Wald challenged Frankel to incorporate a more humanitarian perspective and argued that home visits would improve the health of policy holders and decrease the company's payment of death benefits as a result of decreased mortality among those served (Buhler-Wilkerson, 2001, 2002/2012). The result was the establishment of the Metropolitan Life Visiting Nurse Service in which Henry Street nurses visited ill industrial policy holders. Company agents, who visited policy holders weekly to collect premiums, encouraged recipients to seek nursing services and provided referrals to the nearest visiting nurse services (Metlife, n.d.a).

Established as a pilot project in New York City in 1909, the program's success led to rapid expansion and by 1911, services were offered to Metropolitan policy holders throughout the country (Buhler-Wilkerson, 2001). The program continued without interruption until 1953. Through its more-than-50-year history, the Metropolitan Life Visiting Nurse Service provided care to more than 20 million policy holders in the United States and Canada. At its peak, in 1935, 35 of every 1,000 policy holders received care for illnesses such as tuberculosis, diphtheria, influenza, and smallpox (Metlife, n.d.a) as well as other services such as health education.

Advocacy Now

Home Visiting Programs in Health Care Reform

Advocacy for home visitation programs continues today. As part of the 2008–2010 efforts to enact health care reform legislation, nursing and other professional groups lobbied extensively to assure that funding for home visit programs for women and children were included. Members of the Home Visiting Coalition (2008, 2009), an organization comprising six agencies that support and provide home visit services to parents and children, wrote letters to then President-elect Obama and influential members of the Congress supporting the inclusion of home visit programs in proposed legislation. Similarly, the Nursing Community (2010), an affiliation of more than 40 professional nursing organizations, included nurse home visitation among its recommendations for health care reform. Other advocacy activities included testimony on the effectiveness of home visitation programs before the U.S. House of Representatives Ways and Means Subcommittee on Income Security and Family Support (U.S. House of Representatives, 2009), numerous letters, and full-page advertisements in *Roll Call* and *Congress Daily* funded by the Nurse-Family Partnership (NFP, 2011d).

As a result of this activity, the Patient Protection and Affordable Care Act (ACA)—H.R. 3590, signed by President Obama in March 2010, included subtitle L, which amended the Social Security Act Title V to mandate provision of grants for early childhood home visitation programs and made appropriations for fiscal years 2010–2014 (H. R. 3590, 111th Congress, 2009–2010). This addition to the ACA resulted in authorization of $1.5 billion over 5 years to support home visiting programs for parents and children (NFP, 2011a). To assist local and state agencies to take advantage of these monies, NFP created a Federal Home Visitation Initiative Tool Kit (NFP, 2011b). For a more in-depth discussion of the activity involved in this extensive and successful advocacy effort, see Thompson, Clark, Howland, and Mueller (2011).

Historical photographs of population health nurses often show them caring for clients in their homes. Indeed, home care was the initial focus of population health nursing. Home visiting as a nursing intervention originated as a result of three movements in the 18th and 19th centuries. The first was a growing social awareness of the needs of the poor and the second was the related recognition that hygiene and living conditions contributed to disease. The third movement was the development of nursing as a profession (Pastor, 2006). Home visits by professional nurses were supported in England by Florence Nightingale (Council on Community Pediatrics, 2009) and began in Canada in the early 17th century with the work of orders of religious nuns. In the United States, nursing home visits were initiated by the nurses of the Henry Street Settlement (Cawthorne & Arons, 2010).

The home was where most clients were to be found and where early population health nurses had to go to reach them. Today, the home is only one setting where population health nurses care for their clients. Home visits permit nurses to gain a clear picture of the health needs of the population, as conditions and needs seen from household to household suggest the broader health status and needs of the larger population. Despite the broadening of population health nursing over the years to encompass many other places and settings, home visits remain a strategic tool for health care delivery. In fact, given the increasing cost of health care services in institutional settings, an aging population with an increasingly long life span, and increases in chronic disease prevalence, home visits are more needed now than in the recent past. In addition, recent technological advances have made it possible to provide a variety of care in the home setting not previously possible.

Defining a Home Visit and Types of Home Visits

A home visit by a nurse is different from a social visit that might be made by friends or relatives. Pastor (2006) conducted an analysis of the concept of "home visit" based on the uses of the term in the professional literature. In her concept analysis, she identified the antecedents (precursor conditions), critical attributes, and consequences of the home visit process. The antecedents included a health-related need, a health professional visitor, a client recipient, and an interaction that takes place within the home setting in a neighborhood context. The critical attributes of a home visit included gaining entrée, "seeing" first hand the client's needs and circumstances, and understanding those needs from the perspective of the client. Consequences of the process included receipt of health information by the client, potentially improved health status, referral for additional services, increased client satisfaction with care, and increased self-care knowledge on the part of the client.

Based on the results of the concept analysis, a **home visit**, as conceptualized in population health nursing, is a formal interaction of a nurse and a client at the client's place of residence designed to provide nursing care related to an identified health need. The place of residence may actually be the client's home (house or apartment), the home of a family member with whom the client resides, or a residential setting such as a group home or an assisted living facility.

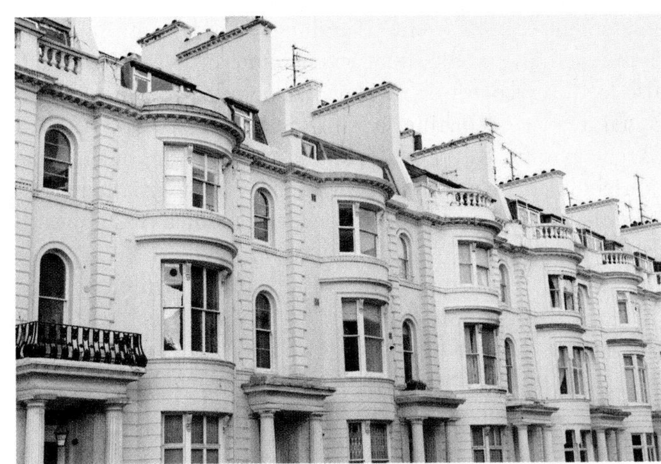

Population health nurses make visits to a variety of homes.
(Stillkost/Fotolia)

Home visits are widely used by population health nurses as an intervention to achieve a number of purposes that generally fit into four potentially overlapping categories. Most population health nursing visits are designed to promote health and prevent illness in specific population groups (e.g., mothers and young children). Home visits may also be made to provide community-based long-term care services designed to foster self-care and allow people to remain in their homes and avoid institutionalization (Riggs, Madigan, & Fortinsky, 2011). Such visits are often targeted at the elderly or persons with chronic illnesses or other conditions requiring complex care or lifestyle changes. The third category includes visits to provide skilled nursing services, usually intended to meet short-term needs (Riggs et al., 2011). Finally, home visits may be made to address the needs of the terminally ill and their families through hospice services. The last two categories of visits will be discussed in more detail in the section dealing with the home health and hospice contexts.

Advantages and Disadvantages of Home Visits

Home visits, as a strategy of care, have both advantages and disadvantages. Some of the advantages of home visits include obtaining a complete picture of the client situation, identification of environmental influences on health, the ability to view relationships among family members and with the larger community, opportunity to see actual performance of activities of daily living, and better evaluation of intervention effects. As noted earlier, home visits give the nurse an opportunity to see the client and family in their natural setting, allow for better assessment of both strengths and needs, and permit tailoring of interventions to the situation encountered. Home visits can also lead to recognition of previously unidentified health and social needs. According to Tinker, Postma, and Butterfield (2011), a home visit provides an "assessment window into the household characteristics" (p. 36), including environmental issues, that would not ordinarily be identified in a typical health care setting.

Home visits also have a few disadvantages. Unfortunately, the poorest-functioning families, who tend to benefit the most from home visiting programs, are also often least responsive to such programs, perhaps because participation entails time that they feel is better spent in meeting higher-priority needs. In many European countries, home visits to pregnant women and young children or to elders are a routine part of health care services provided under national health insurance plans (Council on Community Pediatrics, 2009; Ekmann, Vass, & Avlund, 2010). In the United States, however, home visits tend to be targeted to certain at-risk populations, resulting in stigma or family self-perceptions of incompetence (Thompson et al., 2011).

Home visits are not an inexpensive health care delivery strategy. Nurses and other health care providers can see several clients in clinics or other health care settings in the time required to make one home visit. Generally speaking, however, quality home visit programs that have demonstrable results are cost effective. For example, the cost of the Nurse–Family Partnership program, a home visiting program for first-time pregnant women and their children, is estimated at $7,271 per child served over the two-and-a-half years of the program. However, the program has been credited with estimated cost savings of more than $41,000 per child due to reductions in welfare participation, crime and criminal justice costs, and mental and other health care costs, resulting in a net savings of $5.70 for every dollar spent on the program (Pew Center on the States, 2011).

Home Visiting Programs

Some population health nurses may be involved in the implementation of specific home visiting programs that are designed to achieve particular outcomes with certain targeted populations. Most of the existing large-scale home visitation programs are designed to assist families and children. In this context, a **home visiting program** is defined as "a structured program that strengthens families by 1) expanding parent/caregivers knowledge and skills to nurture child development, 2) promoting growth and health development of young children, and 3) connecting families to resources in the community" (National Human Services Assembly, 2007, p. 2).

In 2007, more than 4,600 program sites provided such programs using one of six models focusing on a combination of parent-centered and child-centered outcomes. These programs are summarized in Table 13-1●. For further information about

TABLE 13-1 National Models for Home Visitation Programs Serving Families and Children

Model	Target Population	Focus
Early Head Start	Low-income pregnant women with infants and toddlers at risk for problems	• Healthy pregnancy • Child health and development • Effective family function
Healthy Families America	Families experiencing stressful lives, at-risk pregnancy, or early postpartum families	• Positive parenting • Child health and development • Prevention of child abuse and neglect
Home Instruction Program for Preschool Youngsters (HIPPY)	Families of preschool children in need of services living in high-risk neighborhoods	• Empowerment of parents as teachers of children • Parental school and community involvement • School success
Nurse-Family Partnership (NFP)	Low-income first-time pregnant women and their children to 2 years of age	• Healthy pregnancy • Child health and development • Improved economic self-sufficiency • Improved maternal life course
Parent-Child Home Program (PCHP)	Low-income families with educationally at-risk preschool children	• Language and literacy development in children • School readiness • Empowerment for effective parenting
Parents as Teachers (PAT)	Families with prekindergarten children at risk for problems	• Early detection of developmental delay or health problems • School readiness and success • Prevention of child abuse and neglect • Parental efficacy and self-confidence • Development of home–school partnerships

Data from: Cawthorne, A., & Arons, J. (2010). *There's no place like home: Home visiting programs can support pregnant women and new parents.* Retrieved from http://www.americanprogress.org/issues/2010/01/pdf/home_visitation.pdf; National Human Services Assembly. (2007). *Home visiting: Strengthening families by promoting parenting success.* [Policy brief No. 23]. Retrieved from http://nationalassembly.org/FSPC/documents/PolicyBriefs/FSPBrief23FINAL.pdf; Thompson, D. K., Clark, M. J., Howland, L. C., & Mueller, M.-R. (2011). The Patient Protection and Affordable Care Act of 2010 (PL 111–148): An analysis of maternal–child health home visitation. *Policy, Politics, & Nursing Practice.* Advance online publication. doi: 10.1177/1527154411424616

Highlights

Characteristics of Effective Home Visiting Programs

- A high level of engagement with families, with frequent visits over a prolonged period of time (2 years or longer)
- A clear set of program goals with appropriate related curricula and program materials
- Assurance of consistency of program design and its implementation
- Use of visitors with qualifications appropriate to achievement of program goals
- A "dual-generation" focus on addressing the needs of both parents and children
- Coordination with other sources of support (e.g., a consistent health care provider or "medical home")
- Interventions tailored to the target population (e.g., cultural, language, or other adaptation, as warranted)

Data from: National Human Services Assembly. (2007). *Home visiting: Strengthening families by promoting parenting success.* [Policy brief No. 23]. Retrieved from http://nationalassembly.org/FSPC/documents/PolicyBriefs/FSPBrief23FINAL.pdf

specific home visiting programs, see the resources provided in the *External Resources* section of the student resources site.

As is evident in the table, each of the programs differs slightly in terms of the population served and the anticipated program outcomes. In addition to these national models, there are numerous "organic" or home-grown programs specific to a particular location or organization. The national models have been shown to be highly effective in achieving their particular sets of outcomes. Local programs may also be effective depending on the extent to which they exhibit the characteristics of high-quality programs. Those characteristics are summarized in the *Highlights* box above.

The Home Visit Process

Home visits, whether a general population health nursing intervention or part of a planned home visitation program, must be focused, purposeful events in order to be effective. Like any other nursing intervention, the home visit should be a planned event with specified goals and objectives. The nursing process provides a framework for systematically organizing the home visit to make it an effective nursing intervention.

Initiating the Home Visit

Home visits by population health nurses are initiated for a variety of reasons. Often, the nurse receives a request for a visit from another health care provider or agency. Reasons for such requests include health care needs related to specific health problems or needs for health-promotive services. For example, many hospital obstetrics units refer all first-time mothers for home visits by population health nurses to provide assistance in parenting and to promote a successful postpartum course and adjustment to parenthood. Similarly, a physician might request a home visit to educate a hypertensive client about prescribed medications.

Clients themselves might also initiate home visits. For example, a mother concerned about her child's recurrent nightmares may call and request a home visit by a population health nurse. Friends and family might also initiate a home visit. A neighbor might inform the nurse that he or she thinks the children next door are being abused, or a mother may request a home visit to help her daughter deal with the loss of a child. Finally, the population health nurse may initiate a home visit. The nurse might note that a child seen in the well-child clinic

Global Perspectives

Promoting Infant Survival

A joint statement by the World Health Organization and the United Nations Children's Fund (UNICEF) in 2009 recommended systematic home visiting programs in the first week of life to reduce neonatal mortality. The report noted that an estimated 3.7 million babies in developing countries die in the first four weeks of life; most of them at home. As indicated in the report, "home visitations after birth is a strategy to deliver effective elements of care to newborns and increase newborn survival" (WHO & UNICEF, 2009, p. 3).

The focus of care in home visiting programs is on both infant and mother. Elements of care for the newborn include promoting early breast-feeding, fostering skin-to-skin care to maintain warmth, promoting hygiene (particularly with respect to umbilical cord care), assessing for problems and making referrals for care as needed, promoting birth registration and immunization, and identifying additional care needs. Maternal care foci include assessment for complications (fever, bleeding, infection), managing breast-feeding problems, counseling on birth spacing, and referral for additional assistance as needed (WHO & UNICEF, 2009).

As of 2012, 30 of 58 countries in Africa and Asia had implemented community-based maternal and child postnatal programs, but only four countries provided home visits to more than 50% of newborns. Home visiting programs have been implemented by government CHWs in some areas and volunteers in others. An informal meeting to address development of home visiting programs generated the following recommendations:

- Advocacy for the development of policies on postnatal home visitation and the provision of resources for implementation
- Technical guidance on the optimal services to be provided, timing and frequency of visits, and implementation in different settings
- Training and incentives for workers
- Development of practical guidelines for program implementation
- Research on models, logistics, and use of technology in home visiting programs, and barriers to implementation (WHO, 2012)

is developmentally delayed and decide to visit the home to see if environmental factors are contributing to the delayed development. Other important aspects of initiating a home visit are communicating the reason for the home visit, creating appropriate expectations for the visit on the part of both the client and the nurse, overcoming fear, and building rapport with the client.

Conducting a Preliminary Health Assessment

Before the home visit, the nurse conducts a preliminary assessment to review existing information about the client and his or her situation. Previously acquired client data should be reviewed and factors influencing client health status identified. If the client is already known to the nurse or the agency, a certain amount of data is available in agency records, notes from previous visits, and other material. Such data can be used by the nurse to refresh his or her memory regarding the client's health status.

If the client is new to an agency, available data will probably be limited to that received with the request for services. In such a case, the nurse needs to look for general cues that suggest client strengths and potential problems. For example, if the home visit is requested for follow-up on a newborn and his adolescent mother, the nurse knows that infant feeding, sleep patterns, maternal knowledge of child care, bonding, uterine involution, maternal coping abilities, and family planning are areas that may need to be addressed during the visit. Similarly, if the referral is for an elderly woman with uncontrolled hypertension, the nurse will identify areas related to diet, medication, safety, and exercise for investigation during the visit.

All aspects of the client's life should be reviewed to detect strengths, existing problems, and potential problems that may need to be addressed during the visit. Using the determinants of health as a framework, the nurse reviews available information on biological, psychological, environmental, sociocultural, behavioral, and health system factors that influence the client's health status. By assessing client factors in each of these areas, the nurse enters the client's residence better prepared to deal with the wide variety of client needs likely to be encountered.

BIOLOGICAL DETERMINANTS. In the biological dimension, the nurse would consider the effects of age and client development level on health status. For example, if the family includes adolescent children, the nurse might focus on sexuality issues, whereas home safety might be more relevant to a family with small children or elderly members. The nurse would also obtain information on existing physical health problems and the presence of disability in clients as well as immunization status and other physiologic factors that influence health.

PSYCHOLOGICAL DETERMINANTS. Considerations related to psychological factors include evidence of family stress and coping. Nurses making home visits may often find themselves called upon to provide emotional support to individual clients or families in crisis, particularly until other services (e.g., counseling) can be obtained. The client with a terminal illness and his or her family are particularly in need of emotional support by the nurse.

ENVIRONMENTAL DETERMINANTS. In the environmental area, the nurse obtains information about the home environment with particular attention to home safety needs, based on the client's and family members' ages, health status, and functional abilities.

Other environmental safety conditions may relate to the client's condition or to therapeutic regimens to be implemented in the home. Continuous chemotherapy infusions, for example, are successfully administered in homes, but they present unique safety hazards. For example, some agents are extremely toxic to skin tissue. Needles and other equipment used to administer these agents also present contamination and injury hazards.

Infection control is another safety issue related to the provision of health care in the physical environment of the home. Infection control in the home has a dual focus: protecting the client and family and protecting the nurse. The nurse should adhere to the agency's standards of practice, incorporate universal precautions for preventing the spread of blood-borne diseases, and educate clients and family members in infection control measures, including universal precautions. In the preliminary assessment, the community health nurse is alert to the potential for problems related to infection control within the client's home environment.

The primary infection control measure in any setting is adequate hand washing before and after giving any direct care to clients. Hands should be thoroughly washed with soap and running water. This may require creativity on the part of nurses or family members in homes without running water. For example, the nurse may wet his or her hands, apply soap, and lather thoroughly, then ask a family member to pour clean water over the hands to rinse them. The nurse can also make a habit of carrying paper towels on home visits to avoid using family towels that were used previously. Many nurses now carry waterless hand-cleansing agents with them on home visits. The nurse may also identify a need to instruct family members in the importance of hand washing in the care of the client and as a general measure for preventing the spread of disease.

Infection control in the home, as in other settings, involves the use of sterile precautions in any invasive procedures, appropriate disposal of bodily secretions and excretions, and isolation precautions as warranted by the client's condition. Nurses working in the home with clients who have blood-borne diseases such as AIDS and hepatitis should use universal blood and body fluid precautions. These precautions apply to any body fluids, including blood, semen, vaginal secretions, cerebrospinal fluid, synovial fluid, pleural fluid, peritoneal fluid, pericardial fluid, and amniotic fluid, and feces, nasal secretions, sputum, sweat, urine, and vomitus that contains visible blood. Identification of the possible need for universal precautions and other infection control measures during the preliminary assessment allows the population health nurse to plan effectively to promote personal safety and that of the client and family. Care should also be taken in the disposal of secretions and excretions of clients with other conditions. For example, sputum from clients with active tuberculosis should be handled with care, and the feces of chronic typhoid carriers should be disposed of in a municipal sewer system.

SOCIOCULTURAL DETERMINANTS. Sociocultural factors to be considered in the assessment include the client's or family's economic status, interactions with the outside world, and occupational or employment considerations. The nurse would also obtain information on cultural or religious factors that influence the client's health as well as the extent of the client's social support system. Client–family interactions are another sociocultural determinant that may influence the client's health. The nurse would also be alert to information about family caretakers' responsibilities and how these might affect the health of both the client and the caretaker.

Cultural factors should also be considered. For example, the client's cultural food preferences or modes of preparation should be considered in planning to meet nutritional needs. Similarly, child-rearing practices may affect the plan of care for a young child. For instance, in some cultural groups even very young children may make independent decisions about taking medications or adhering to other elements of a treatment plan. If this is the case, the nurse will need to work with both the parent and the child to ensure compliance.

BEHAVIORAL DETERMINANTS. Behavioral considerations would include information about the client's consumption patterns and nutritional needs based on age or health status. Information regarding substance use or abuse would also be relevant to the planning of effective nursing interventions.

HEALTH SYSTEM DETERMINANTS. The effects of the health system on the client are also an area to be addressed in the preliminary assessment. What is the source of payment for home health services? Does the client have access to other health promotion and health restoration services? Are these services effectively utilized by the client? The focused assessment on the next page provides tips for assessing each of the six determinants of health in a preliminary assessment in preparation for a home visit.

Deriving Nursing Diagnoses

The diagnostic reasoning process is used to derive nursing diagnoses. The nurse examines available data and then develops diagnostic hypotheses that seem to explain the data. Hypothesis evaluation takes place when the nurse actually makes the home visit and obtains additional data to confirm or disconfirm the diagnostic hypotheses. The diagnostic hypotheses generated from the preliminary assessment, however, give the nurse some direction for planning nursing interventions to be performed during the home visit. Based on the data available in the preliminary assessment, the nurse makes nursing diagnoses related to health conditions to be addressed during the home visit. These diagnoses may be positive diagnoses, problem-focused nursing diagnoses, or health-promotive diagnoses.

Positive nursing diagnoses reflect client strengths identified in the preliminary assessment. For example, available data may indicate "effective coping with the demands imposed by a handicapped child due to a strong family support system." This diagnosis suggests that the nurse will reinforce family support as a factor contributing to effective coping.

Problem-focused nursing diagnoses may reflect potential problems or actual problems for which there is evidence in the preliminary assessment data. For example, an existing problem of "ineffective contraceptive use due to inadequate knowledge of contraceptive methods" may have been documented on a previous home visit. Unless there is also an indication that this problem has been resolved, the nurse will probably address it during the subsequent home visit. Preliminary assessment data may suggest potential problems as well. For example, the request for services might indicate that the client's husband is in the Navy and is due to leave on extended sea duty. This information would suggest a nursing diagnosis of "potential for ineffective coping due to loss of spousal assistance."

Nursing diagnoses might also reflect the need for health-promotive services. For example, there will soon be a "need for routine immunizations" for a newborn child. Similarly, the mother has a "need for postpartum follow-up due to recent delivery."

Planning the Home Visit

Based on the preliminary assessment, the population health nurse makes plans for a home visit to address the health needs most likely to be present in the situation. Tasks to be accomplished in planning the visit include reviewing previous interventions, prioritizing client needs, developing goals and objectives for care, and considering client acceptance and timing. Other tasks of this stage include delineating activities needed to meet client needs, obtaining needed materials, and planning evaluation.

REVIEWING PREVIOUS INTERVENTIONS. The first step in planning is to review any previous interventions related to client health needs and the efficacy of those interventions. This information allows the nurse to eliminate interventions that have been unsuccessful in the past and to identify interventions that have worked.

PRIORITIZING CLIENT NEEDS. The next task is to give priority to identified client needs. Client care needs may be prioritized on the basis of their potential to threaten the client's health, the degree to which they concern the client, or their ease of solution. It is often impossible to address all of the client's health problems in a single visit, so the nurse must decide which

FOCUSED ASSESSMENT Assessing the Home Visit Situation

Biological Determinants

- What are the ages of persons in the home? Do the age and developmental level of persons in the home give rise to specific health needs?
- Do any persons in the home have existing physical health problems?
- Does anyone in the home have difficulty performing activities of daily living?
- Do persons in the home exhibit other physiologic states that necessitate health care (e.g., pregnancy)?

Psychological Determinants

- What is the emotional status of persons living in the home? How effective are the coping strategies used by persons living in the home? Is there a need for respite for family caregivers?
- Is there a history of mental illness in anyone living in the home?
- Do persons in the home interact effectively with one another? What effects do interpersonal interactions have on health? What is the potential for domestic violence in the home?

Environmental Determinants

- Where is the home located? Is the neighborhood safe? Are there environmental conditions in the neighborhood that adversely affect health?
- Are there safety hazards in the home? Does the home environment accommodate the age-related safety needs of persons living there?
- Is the home in good repair? Does it have the usual amenities (e.g., running water, heat, electricity, refrigeration, cooking facilities)?
- Is the home equipped to meet special needs of persons living there (e.g., safe administration of oxygen, mobility aids)?
- Does the home situation pose an infection risk for persons living there?

Sociocultural Determinants

- What are the educational and economic levels of persons living in the home? How do they affect health status?
- What is the extent of social support available to those living in the home? Do they make use of available social support?
- Are persons living in the home employed? How does employment affect health status and health care needs?
- Are there religious or cultural practices in the home that influence health?
- Is there sufficient provision for personal privacy in the home?

Behavioral Determinants

- Does anyone living in the home have special dietary needs? Are those needs being met?
- Does anyone living in the home smoke? What are the potential health effects of smoking on persons living in the home?
- Is there evidence of substance abuse in the home?
- Do any of those living in the home use medications on a regular basis? If so, are they used and stored appropriately?

Health System Determinants

- Is health care utilization by persons living in the home appropriate?
- Are there barriers to access to health care services for persons living in the home?
- How are home care services reimbursed?

needs require immediate attention. For example, if the wife has been admitted to an alcohol treatment center and there is no one to care for the children while the father works, provision of child care and dealing with the children's feelings about their mother's absence may be the only things that can be accomplished on the initial visit. Other problems, such as poor nutritional habits and the need for immunizations for the toddler, can be deferred until a later visit.

DEVELOPING GOALS AND OBJECTIVES. After determining which client needs will be addressed in the forthcoming visit, the nurse develops goals and objectives related to each area of need. Goals are generally stated expectations, whereas objectives are more specific. In the previous example, the nurse's goal might be to enable the family to function adequately in the mother's absence. In this instance, an outcome objective might be that adequate child care will be obtained so the father can return to work.

The health care needs that will be addressed during a home visit may reflect the levels of health care: health promotion, illness and injury prevention, resolution, and restoration. When health care needs occur in the realm of health promotion and illness or injury prevention, goals and outcome objectives reflect positive health states or the absence of specific health problems as expected outcomes of care. For example, a goal for health promotion might be "development of effective parenting skills." A related outcome objective might be that the client "will display effective communication skills in relating to children."

Goals and objectives related to needs for resolution focus on alleviation of specific problems. For example, a goal for a client with hypertension might be "effective control of elevated blood pressure" and the related outcome objective might be a blood pressure that is "consistently below 140/90." Similarly, goals and objectives for restoration reflect client achievement of a prior level of function or the prevention of recurrence of a health problem.

CONSIDERING ACCEPTANCE AND TIMING. In planning a home visit, the nurse should consider the client's readiness to accept intervention as well as the timing of the visit and the introduction of intervention. The nurse may find, for example, that a relatively minor problem with which the client is preoccupied must be addressed before the client is willing to deal with other health needs. Clients may be fearful of home visits, particularly if they are viewed as evidence of poor performance on their part. For this reason, the population health nurse may need to put considerable effort in a first contact into building a level of trust and rapport with the client.

Timing is another important consideration in planning an effective home visit. If the visit interferes with other activities important to the client, the client may not be as open to the visit as would otherwise be the case. Other activities that compete with a home visit for the client's attention might be the visit of a friend, an upcoming doctor's appointment, getting the children ready for an outing, or even something as mundane as a favorite soap opera. Prescheduling or rescheduling home visits can make the visit a more effective intervention if something else is interfering.

Timing also relates to the degree of rapport established between client and nurse. Clients need time to develop trust in the nurse before intimate issues can be addressed. For example, a pregnant adolescent may feel too uncomfortable and threatened by the nurse during early visits to admit to prior drug use and ask about its effects on the baby. The nurse should judge the appropriateness of the timing in bringing up intimate issues for discussion and wait, if possible, until rapport is established with the client. Efforts at cost containment have often limited the number of visits that can be made to a particular client, so population health nurses must work to develop trust and rapport early in their interactions with clients.

IDENTIFYING APPROPRIATE NURSING INTERVENTIONS. The next aspect of planning the home visit is the planning of specific nursing activities for each nursing diagnosis to be addressed. Planned interventions should be based on evidence of their effectiveness and may incorporate practice guidelines. Practice guidelines are available from a number of sources. For further information about practice guidelines, see the resources provided in the *External Resources* section of the student resources site. Agency procedures and protocols and clinical pathways may also be used as guides for planning nursing interventions during a home visit. Protocols and clinical pathways may differ from agency to agency and should be tailored to the goals and resources of the particular agency as well as to the particular client's needs.

The activities planned reflect the nurse's assessment of health care needs and the factors influencing them. In the previous example, referral to a Head Start program may provide assistance with child care, but only if the children involved are of the right ages. If the youngsters are of school age, the appropriate nursing intervention might be to help the father explore the possibility of an after-school program, if one is available, or have the children go home with the parents of a friend until the father can pick them up after work.

Nursing activities can focus on both health promotion and the resolution of health-related problems. For example, the population health nurse might provide the parents of a toddler with anticipatory guidance regarding toilet training or assist parents to discuss sexuality with their preteen daughter. Other positive interventions might focus on providing adequate nutrition for a young child or promoting a healthy pregnancy for a pregnant woman.

Specific interventions employed by the nurse might include referral, education, and technical procedures. For example, the nurse might refer a family to social services for financial assistance, teach a mother about appropriate nutrition for the family, or check a hypertensive client's blood pressure. The interventions selected should be directed toward achieving the goals and objectives established while taking into account the constraints and supports in the individual client situation.

OBTAINING NECESSARY MATERIALS. One aspect of planning the home visit is obtaining materials and supplies that may be needed to implement planned interventions. Because the visit takes place in the client's home, the nurse cannot assume that necessary supplies will be available there. If the nurse plans to engage in nutrition education, he or she might want to leave a selection of pamphlets with the client to reinforce teaching. If planned activities involve weighing a premature infant, the nurse will want to take along a scale.

Equipment and supplies may also be needed for other procedures such as dressing changes, catheterizations, injections, and blood pressure checks. Because the nurse frequently does a physical assessment of one or more clients, additional equipment such as a stethoscope, percussion hammer, tongue blade, flashlight, and otophthalmoscope will need to be obtained prior to setting out for the visit.

PLANNING FOR EVALUATION. As with every other process employed by population health nurses, the planning phase of the home visit process concludes with plans for evaluation. The nurse determines the criteria to be used to evaluate the effectiveness of the home visit. Criteria for evaluating client outcomes are derived from the outcome objectives developed for the visit. Because the outcome of nursing interventions undertaken during a home visit may not be immediately apparent, the nurse needs to develop both short-term and long-term evaluative criteria. Short-term criteria are likely to be based on client response to interventions. For example, the nurse may make a referral for immunizations, but the mother cannot follow through on the referral and receive immunizations on the spot. The nurse, however, can evaluate the mother's response to the referral. Does the mother seem interested? Does she indicate that she will follow through on the referral? On subsequent visits, the nurse would employ long-term outcome criteria to evaluate the effects of interventions. In this instance, the criteria would include whether the client's child received needed immunizations.

Outcome evaluation addresses the level of health care involved in the nursing interventions employed. Evaluative criteria for health promotion and illness and injury prevention measures, for example, reflect health promotion or the absence of specific health problems. For example, criteria for interventions to foster immunity to childhood diseases would include whether immunizations were obtained and the presence or absence of immunizable diseases such as measles. If the client develops measles, prevention of illness obviously was not effective.

Evaluation of resolution measures focuses on the degree to which an existing problem has been resolved. For example, a client's hypertension may have been uncontrolled because of poor medication adherence. Evaluative criteria in this instance would include the degree of adherence achieved and the client's blood pressure measurements. Criteria to evaluate restoration measures reflect the degree to which a client has regained a prior level of health or prevented recurrent health problems. For example, have passive range-of-motion exercises helped a client recovering from a broken arm to regain strength and mobility? Has parenting education by the nurse prevented further episodes of child abuse in an abusive family?

The nurse also develops criteria to evaluate implementation of the planned home visit. These criteria are derived from process objectives developed for the visit. For example, was the nurse adequately prepared to address the health care needs encountered during the visit? Were the appropriate supplies available for implementing planned interventions?

Implementing the Planned Visit

The next step in the home visit process is conducting the visit itself. Several tasks are involved in implementing the planned visit. These include validating the health needs and diagnoses identified in the preliminary assessment, identifying additional needs, mutual goal setting, modifying the intervention plan as needed, performing nursing interventions, and dealing with distractions.

VALIDATING ASSESSMENT AND DIAGNOSES. The first task in implementing the home visit is to validate the accuracy of the preliminary assessment. Problems identified from the available data may or may not exist when the nurse actually enters the home. For example, the nurse may find that the family's poor diet is not the result of lack of knowledge about nutrition, but stems from a lack of money to purchase nutritious foods. Or the nurse may find that what appeared to nurses on the postpartum unit to be poor maternal–infant bonding was not actually the case. Similarly, the nurse may discover that expected strengths or positive nursing diagnoses do not accurately reflect the client's actual health status. For example, a mother who appeared to be coping effectively with her child's handicap may really have been exhibiting denial of the condition. It is particularly important that the nurse involve the client in a reassessment of his or her needs and to modify the plan of care as needed, also in conjunction with the client.

IDENTIFYING ADDITIONAL NEEDS. During the visit, the nurse collects additional data related to biological, psychological, environmental, sociocultural, behavioral, and health system factors to identify additional health care needs. For example, when the nurse arrives to visit a new mother and her infant son, the nurse may find that the client's father recently had a heart attack. The client may be much more in need of assistance in finding child care for her new baby, so she can spend time at the hospital than in discussing immunization and postpartum concerns. Or the nurse may find that, in addition to having a new baby, the client's husband is out of work and the 12-year-old has been skipping school. Again, clients need to be actively involved in determining needs and prioritizing them if nurses are to avoid imposing their preconceived agenda for the visit.

MUTUAL GOAL SETTING. Although the nurse has established tentative goals and objectives for the visit during the planning stage, those goals are revisited during implementation. The nurse shares with the client the initial goals established for addressing health needs identified in the preliminary assessment, as well as additional problems identified, and together they set or revise goals to be achieved during the current visit or throughout a series of visits. This is particularly important when clients will be responsible for implementing interventions designed to achieve those goals. If the client is not in agreement regarding the goals to be achieved, implementation may not occur.

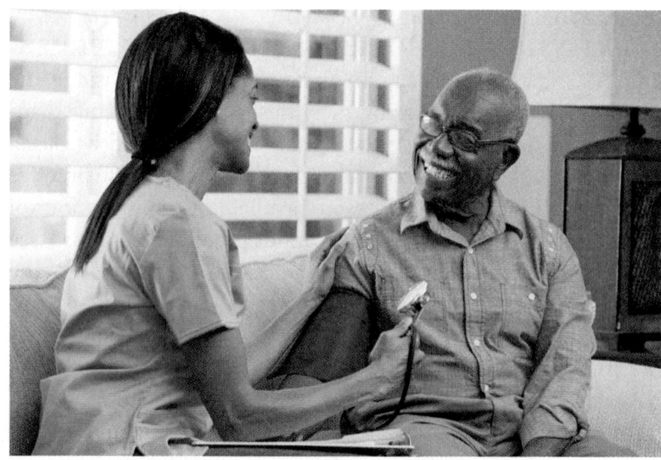

Population health nurses assess clients' physical health status in the home. *(Monkey Business/Fotolia)*

MODIFYING THE PLAN OF CARE. Based on what the nurse finds in the course of the home visit and on input from the client or family, the initial plan of care may need to be modified. In doing this, the nurse may need to restructure priorities based on new data and client input. For instance, if the 2-year-old has cut her arm and is bleeding profusely when the nurse arrives, this problem takes precedence over the nurse's plan to discuss the potential for sibling rivalry. The nurse may either implement interventions as planned or modify the plan as the client's situation and desires dictate.

PERFORMING NURSING INTERVENTIONS. Only after the plan of care has been modified as needed does the nurse perform whatever nursing interventions are warranted by the client situation. As noted earlier, these activities may include health promotion, illness and injury prevention, resolution, and health restoration measures. For example, the nurse working with a new mother might discuss parenting skills as a means of preventing child abuse (injury prevention), give the mother suggestions for dealing with the infant's spitting up (resolution), and discuss options for contraception to prevent a subsequent pregnancy (restoration).

Any or all of the levels can be emphasized, depending on the situation encountered. For example, if the mother is inexperienced and concerned about child care skills in feeding, bathing, and parenting, the emphasis would be on health promotion. Conversely, if the nurse arrives to find a baby screaming with gas pains, emphasis is placed on making the infant more comfortable and relieving the mother's anxiety (resolution). Once this has been accomplished, the nurse can focus on suggestions to prevent a recurrence of the problem (restoration).

DEALING WITH DISTRACTIONS. One important consideration in implementing a home visit is dealing with distractions. Distractions are generally of three types: environmental, behavioral, and nurse-initiated. Environmental distractions arise from both the physical and social environments and may include background noise, crowded surroundings, and interruptions by other family members or outsiders. The occurrence of such distractions during the home visit can give the nurse a clear picture of the client's environment and the way in which the client and family interact among themselves and with others. For example, if mother and child are continually yelling at one another during the visit, this suggests the existence of family communication problems. On the other hand, positive interactions between a mother and her young child provide evidence of effective parenting skills.

Despite the information that can be gleaned from these distractions, their negative effects on the interaction between client and nurse need to be minimized. Requesting that the television be turned off during the visit or moving the client to a more private area can minimize some distractions. Or the nurse may ask an intrusive younger child to draw a picture to allow the parent and nurse to talk with fewer interruptions. If there are too many distractions that cannot be eliminated or overcome, the nurse can ask the client if there is a better time for the visit, when fewer interruptions will occur, and reschedule the visit for a later date. For example, subsequent visits might be planned to coincide with the toddler's nap.

Behavioral distractions consist of behaviors employed by the client to distract the nurse from the purpose of the visit. Again, the use of such distractions can be a cue for the nurse that certain topics are uncomfortable for the client or that the client does not quite trust the nurse or may feel guilty about something. The nurse can benefit from the distraction by exploring the reasons for the client's behaviors and working to establish trust.

The last category of distractions originates with the nurse. These distractions create barriers to relationships with clients. Fears, role preoccupation, and personal reactions to different lifestyles can distract the nurse from the purpose of the home visit. Nurses may fear bodily harm, rejection by the client, or the lack of control that is implicit in a home visit. In today's violent society, fear of bodily harm is understandable, and nurses making home visits should employ the personal safety precautions presented in Table 13-2•.

TABLE 13-2 Personal Safety Considerations in Home Visiting

Appearance
- Wear a name tag and uniform or other apparel that identifies you as a nurse.
- Do not carry a purse or wear expensive jewelry.
- Leave any valuables at home or lock them in the trunk of the car before leaving the office.

Transportation
- Keep your car in good repair and with a full tank of gas.
- Carry emergency supplies such as a flashlight and blanket.
- Always lock your car and carry keys in hand when leaving the client's home.
- Park near the client's home with your car in view of the home whenever possible.
- Avoid the use of public transportation if possible.
- Get complete and accurate directions to the home.

The Situation
- Call ahead to alert the client that you will be coming.
- Ask the client to secure pets before your visit.
- Walk directly to the client's home, without detours to local shops or other places.
- Keep one arm free while walking to the client's home.
- Avoid isolated areas, especially late in the day or at night.
- Knock before entering the client's home, even if the door is open.
- Make joint visits in dangerous neighborhoods or situations or employ an escort service if needed.
- Listen to the client's messages regarding potential safety hazards.
- Make home visits at times when illicit activity (such as drug transactions) is less likely to occur or when potentially dangerous family members will not be present.
- Carry a whistle that is easily accessible.
- Become familiar with personal defense techniques.
- Leave any situation that appears to hold a risk of personal danger.
- Stay alert and observe your surroundings.

Population health nurses may also create distractions by being so preoccupied with their original purpose that they fail to see the need to modify the planned home visit. No planned intervention is so important that it cannot be postponed if more important needs intervene. Nurses who continue to pursue predetermined goals in the light of other client needs reduce their credibility with clients and create barriers to effective intervention. For example, the nurse who insists on talking about infant feeding when the client just had an argument with her husband and fears he will leave her is not meeting the client's needs.

Finally, population health nurses may be put off by the contrast between their own lifestyles and those of the clients they are visiting. In dealing with feelings engendered by such differences, it is helpful to understand that one's own attitudes are the product of one's upbringing and culture and clients derive their attitudes in the same way. In dealing with lifestyle differences, the nurse must be aware of her or his personal feelings and their impact on nursing effectiveness. The nurse must also determine what aspects of the client's lifestyle may be detrimental to health and focus on those, while accepting other differences in attitude or behavior as hallmarks of the client's uniqueness. Being thoroughly informed about cultural and ethnic differences also minimizes negative reactions by the nurse to such differences. Some of these differences were discussed in Chapter 5∞.

Evaluating the Home Visit

Before concluding the visit, the nurse evaluates the effectiveness of interventions in terms of their appropriateness to the situation and the client's response. This evaluation is conducted using criteria established in planning the visit. It may not be possible, at this point, to determine the eventual outcome of nursing care. The nurse can, however, examine the client's initial response to interventions. Was the mother interested in obtaining contraceptives? Is it likely that she will follow through on a referral to the immunization clinic? Did the client voice an intention to reduce fat intake? Could the client accurately demonstrate the correct technique for bottle-feeding the infant?

Evaluating the ultimate outcome of interventions may occur at subsequent visits. For example, on the next visit, the nurse might determine whether the mother obtained contraceptives. If she called but was not able to get an appointment, the nurse would determine the reason. Based on information obtained, there may be a need for advocacy on the part of the nurse. If the client did not seek contraceptive services, the nurse should determine the reason for her behavior. Was the client distracted by crises that occurred in the meantime, but plans to call for an appointment next week? Did she not have transportation to the clinic? Or maybe she does not really want contraceptives. If the client lacks transportation, the nurse might help her explore ways of getting transportation. If the client does not really want contraceptives, the nurse can either explore why or accept the client's wishes.

As noted earlier, evaluation of nursing interventions during a home visit should reflect the level of health care involved. The nurse examines both the short-term and long-term effects of interventions aimed at the health promotion, prevention, resolution, and restoration, as appropriate. For example, if the home visit focused on resolution of existing health problems, evaluation will also be focused at this level. If several levels were addressed during the visit, evaluation will focus on the effects of interventions at each level.

The nurse also evaluates his or her use of the home visit process. Was the preliminary assessment adequate? Was information available that the nurse neglected to review, resulting in unexpected problems during the visit itself? For example, did the nurse ask about the husband's reaction to the new baby when the record indicates the client is not married? Did the nurse miss cues to additional problems during the visit? Was the nurse able to plan interventions consistent with client needs, attitudes, and desires? Was the nurse able to deal effectively with distractions? If not, why not? Answers to these and similar questions allow the nurse to improve his or her use of the home visit process in subsequent client encounters.

Home visitation programs can also be evaluated in terms of their processes and outcomes. Home visits, although less expensive than hospitalization or some other means of service delivery, are not without cost, and the effects of such programs should be evaluated. Many home visiting programs have been found to be highly effective in achieving specific outcomes, but others have not shown any benefit. For example, home visitation programs have been credited with promoting regular prenatal care, smoking cessation during pregnancy, and better prenatal nutrition (Pew Center on the States, 2011). Postpartum visits to low-income mothers also resulted in improved depression scores, better patient satisfaction, and less use of emergency department services for their infants (Christie & Bunting, 2011).

In addition, home visit programs have been shown to support infant development and health, as well as decrease rates of child abuse and neglect and promote parental education, employment, and improved family relationships (Pew Center on the States, 2011). In fact, the Community Preventive Services Task Force (2005) found strong evidence for the effectiveness of home visitation programs in preventing child abuse in at-risk families. Similarly, incorporation of family violence screening into child-health home visits was shown to improve disclosure and identification of abused women (Vanderburg, Wright, Boston, & Zimmerman, 2010). High-quality national home visiting programs for families and young children have been shown to be so consistently effective that the American Academy of Pediatrics supported advocacy for home visiting programs as part of health care reform as early as 1998 (Council on Community Pediatrics, 2009).

Among the elderly, home visits often improve medication adherence and functional status and help keep people at home and improve their quality of life, particularly at the end of life Riggs et al., 2011). Environmental improvements have also been shown to result from home visit interventions (Pastor, 2006).

Documenting Home Visits

Follow-up to a home visit involves documenting what took place. As we will see later in this chapter, accurate documentation is particularly important in ensuring appropriate reimbursement for services. Several aspects of the visit should be documented. The nurse should document the actual (not preliminary) assessment of client health status, health needs identified and goals established, as well as the interventions employed to achieve those goals. Clients' responses to interventions should also be documented, as well as the short- and long-term outcomes of interventions. At the end of each visit, the nurse should also document future plans for care. Finally, at the end of services, the nurse should write a discharge summary of the interventions employed and the client's health status at the close of care. If referrals have been made for continued care from other agencies, these should also be documented.

Termination

Unlike care in other settings, home visiting services may continue over a protracted period of time. This necessitates planning for termination of services. Ideally, preparation for termination should begin with the first visit when the client is informed of the time-limited nature and expected duration of services. Reminders of termination are then provided at each subsequent visit. At the actual time of termination, the nurse would review with the client the degree of achievement of mutual goals and make referrals for continued care as needed. Components of the home visit process are summarized in Table 13-3●.

TABLE 13-3 Components of the Home Visit Process

Initiation	Schedule the home visit with the client, introducing the home visitor and explaining the purpose of the home visit.
Preliminary assessment	Review available client data to determine health care needs related to biological, psychological, environmental, sociocultural, behavioral, and health system determinants of health.
Diagnosis	Develop diagnostic hypotheses based on preliminary assessment.
Planning	Review previous interventions and their effects.
	Prioritize client needs and identify those to be addressed during the visit.
	Develop goals and objectives for visit and identify levels of health care involved.
	Consider client acceptance and timing of visit.
	Identify appropriate nursing interventions to address problems.
	Obtain needed supplies and equipment.
	Plan for evaluation of the home visit.
Implementation	Validate preliminary assessment and nursing diagnostic hypotheses.
	Identify other client needs.
	Engage in mutual goal setting with client to meet identified needs.
	Modify plan of care as needed.
	Carry out nursing interventions.
	Deal with distractions.
Evaluation	Evaluate client response to interventions.
	Evaluate short-term and long-term outcomes of intervention.
	Evaluate the quality of planning and implementation of the home visit.
	Evaluate outcomes and quality of care at the aggregate as well as individual levels.
Documentation	Document client assessment, health needs identified, and goals established.
	Document interventions.
	Document client response to interventions.
	Document outcome of interventions.
	Document future plan of care.
	Document client health status at discharge.
Termination	Plan for termination from the first visit.
	Inform client of the time-limited nature of services and their probable duration.
	Review goal accomplishment with the client.
	Make referrals for continuing care, if needed.

Home Visits in the Home Health and Hospice Contexts

A number of authors distinguish between home health care and population health nursing. The distinction arose from the early split between personal health care services and public health services when official health agencies began to emphasize population-based screening and health promotion services. Authors who make this distinction base it on the fact that home health nursing is primarily illness focused and that it deals with individuals rather than population groups. Other authors, however, point out that home health nurses do deal with aggregate needs. From this perspective, home health nurses identify populations at risk and in need of home health services and define the role of home health nursing in meeting the needs of individual clients and the larger community. The population focus in home health comes in the planning of systems of care based on an assessment of population needs, characteristics, and resources.

Still other authors suggest that illness is both an individual or family problem and a community experience. This was the perspective of early population health nurses who provided personal health services in clients' homes and simultaneously campaigned to improve social conditions. These nurses and their supporters believed that the conditions of the sick in their homes influenced the health of society in general.

Although today home health nurses work primarily with ill individuals, they continue to employ knowledge of environmental, social, and personal health factors. That knowledge is a combination of public health science and nursing practice and is the hallmark of population health nursing. It would seem, then, that the distinction between population health nursing and home health nursing is an artificial one and that home health is actually a subspecialty within population health nursing in which the primary, but not sole, focus is on resolution of existing health problems and health restoration. Effective home health nurses who provide holistic nursing care employ principles of population health nursing within the segment of the population that is ill.

Home health care is defined as "an array of services for people of all ages, provided in the home and community setting, that encompasses health promotion and teaching, curative intervention, end-of-life care, rehabilitation, support and maintenance, social adaptation, and integration and support for the informal (family) caregiver" (Canadian Home Care Association, 2009, pp. 21–22). Home health nursing is characterized by holism, care management, resource coordination, collaboration, and both autonomous and interdependent practice. Interdependent practice involves collaboration with members of other health care disciplines: both professional (e.g., physicians, physical therapists) and nonprofessional (e.g., home health aides), as well as the client and family members.

Home health nurses, like other population health nurses, practice autonomously and are responsible for the achievement of designated outcomes of care. Home health nurses may also specialize in the care of terminally ill clients through the provision of hospice services. Home care services are usually provided under the aegis of a home health agency, and may include a range of care from skilled nursing and therapy services to personal care and homemaking assistance.

Hospice care is a program of palliative care and support services provided to terminally ill clients and their families. **Palliative care** is care provided for the purpose of alleviating symptoms (physical, psychological, or spiritual), associated with terminal or chronic conditions, rather than promoting a cure. Hospice care may be provided in both home and inpatient settings, but we are concerned here only with home hospice services. Hospice care involves not only care for the terminally ill client, but also bereavement services and counseling for family members and others.

Home health and hospice care, as we know them today, originated in the work of voluntary agencies such as the Visiting Nurse Associations (VNAs) and other organizations. One early home health and hospice agency was established in 1883 by the Good Cheer Society, whose members visited sick mill workers and their families in Nashua, New Hampshire. The society hired its first nurse in 1902, later became a VNA, and finally became Home Health & Hospice Care in 1989 with the consolidation of home health, VNA, and hospice organizations (Home Health & Hospice Care, 2012).

Home health care today continues to be focused on the resolution of specific health problems rather than on health promotion. Although health promotion may take place in home health care visits, it is not the initial purpose for the visit as it might be in other types of home visiting programs. The goal of home health care is to provide the services needed to restore the client to an optimal level of function given the constraints of chronic conditions, or in the case of hospice care, to provide for symptom amelioration until death.

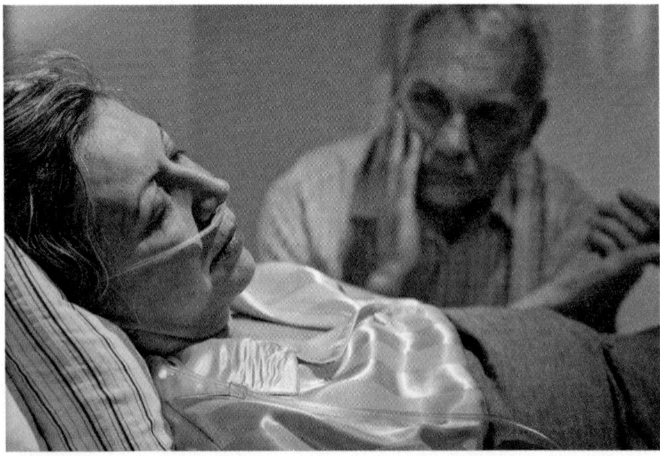

Some population health nurses may provide hospice or palliative care services in the home. *(CandyBox Images/Fotolia)*

From the 1930s to the 1950s, the availability of hospital care decreased the need for home health care for the sick. Then, as hospital costs increased, home care was seen as an effective way to minimize the costs of providing care. In 1965, the Medicare home health benefit was established to provide home care to the elderly and others who qualified for Medicare. This led to the development of many proprietary home care agencies. **Proprietary agencies** are independent home health agencies owned by individuals or corporations that operate on a for-profit basis.

In 2014, the National Association for Home Health & Hospice (NAHC, 2014) listed more than 33,000 home health and hospice agencies in its locator database, and 1,400 agencies provided both home health and hospice services (National Center for Health Statistics [NCHS], 2011). In 2010, 10,914 home health agencies and 3,509 hospices were Medicare certified (NCHS, 2013). According to the most recent National Home Health and Hospice Survey (NCHS, 2007b), on any given day, 1.46 million persons received home health services, and there was a nearly fivefold increase in the number of patients discharged from hospice services (usually due to death) from 1992 to 2007 (NCHS, 2007a).

These figures suggest the enormous amount of health care provided by home health and hospice agencies in the United States. Funding for services is derived from public insurance programs (e.g., Medicare and Medicaid), private insurance, and out-of-pocket spending by recipients of care. In 2010, the Centers for Medicare and Medicaid Services spent $44.3 billion on home health services for Medicare and Medicaid recipients. Similar figures are noted for Medicare-funded hospice services, with Medicare funding $12.9 million for hospice services in 2010. Together home health care and hospice services accounted for 8.2% of all Medicare expenditures in 2010 (CMS, 2011a). In 2009, nearly 42% of all Americans who died had received hospice services (Dose, Rhudy, Holland, & Olsson, 2011).

It is likely that the need for home health services will increase in the future for several reasons. First, acute care settings will continue to attempt to reduce costs by shortening the length of hospital stays. Second, increasing rates of chronic disease in an aging population necessitate assistance to prevent institutionalization. Third, advances in technology make provision of highly technical care possible in the home setting, and finally, the majority of the population would prefer to receive care at home rather than in an institution (Canadian Home Care Association, 2009).

Collaboration in Home Health and Hospice Care

Clients' needs for home health or hospice services must be certified by a primary care provider before reimbursement for services will be forthcoming. Individual clients or families may contract independently for home health services, but unless the need for services is validated by the primary provider, payment will need to be made out of pocket. In other types of home visitation services, on the other hand, clients may self-refer or population health nurses may identify people in need of home visit services while providing other services. In these types of home visiting programs, the decision of whether or not to provide services lies with the nurse and the client, not with a third party.

Because home health services are provided under the auspices of the primary care provider, there is a particular need for close collaboration among client, nurse, and primary care provider. In addition, home health clients often need services provided by other health care professionals, such as physical therapists, dieticians, and so on. Again, it is extremely important for all those participating in the care of the client to be kept informed of the client's health status and to engage in collaborative care planning. A similar need also occurs in the case of hospice care. Physicians or nurse practitioners may need to be actively involved to ensure effective pain management. Similarly, spiritual care advisors and volunteers may be helpful in assisting the client and family members to adjust to the eventuality of death. For both home health and hospice care clients, there may be a need for durable medical equipment (DME) provided by outside vendors, and population health nurses often serve as liaisons to DME vendors, assisting clients to get the best possible care. Like other population health nurses, home health and hospice nurses may also make referrals for additional services to meet identified client needs. Referrals would be made using the process discussed in Chapter 12∞.

Technology and Home Care Services

Another area in which home health care differs from general population health nursing home visitation is that of care involving technology. Basic population health nursing is generally very low-tech care. Home health care, on the other hand, may rely on very sophisticated technology used in the home setting. Many services and procedures that were once only available in the hospital or outpatient setting are now being provided in homes. This requires that home health nurses be knowledgeable about high-tech equipment and procedures to a greater extent than is required of most population health nurses. Some of the more common concerns, such as safety considerations in the use of oxygen in the home and the need for universal precautions in dealing with blood and body fluids, are familiar to population health nurses in general.

Disposal of hazardous wastes in the home setting is another aspect of home care that is different from that in hospital settings. For example, clients who use lancets to check daily blood sugar levels should be educated on their appropriate disposal. Other more specialized equipment, such as infusion pumps or sophisticated monitors, may be less familiar and nurses who encounter clients using these technologies will need to be familiar with them. There is also a movement toward telemedicine with extremely sophisticated monitoring capabilities that will allow more in-depth follow-up for home health clients than typically exists.

Funding Home Health and Hospice Services

Home health and hospice services may be provided by a variety of different types of agencies. The major categories of agencies are for-profit or proprietary agencies, voluntary nonprofit agencies, and government and other agencies. As noted earlier, proprietary agencies provide home health and hospice services in order to generate revenue. Nonprofit agencies may be operated by church groups or other voluntary organizations (e.g., VNAs) and are supported by philanthropic donations as well as third-party payment from insurance or government sources. Some government agencies also provide home health services (e.g., the Veteran's Administration), and services may also be reimbursed under the auspices of pension plans or other organizations.

Whatever the type of home care or hospice agency, funding for services may be derived from private health insurance, government funding through Medicare or Medicaid, or, in some cases, personal out-of-pocket payment. Most home care and hospice agencies derive their funding from all of these sources. To receive reimbursement for services under Medicare or Medicaid, however, agencies must be certified. **Certification** is a process by which an agency is judged to meet specific **conditions of participation**, requirements to be met to qualify for reimbursement under Medicare or Medicaid programs as spelled out in the United States Code, Title 42 (2010). Agencies must be certified separately for participation in each program, although many home health and hospice agencies are certified by both Medicare and Medicaid. Periodic recertification is required and usually entails a visit to the agency by CMS evaluators to assure continued compliance with the conditions of participation. Reviews may also be triggered by certain occurrences, such as excessive fall or infection rates, client complaints, or the death of a client. Many private insurance companies also require home health and hospice agencies to meet the Medicare and Medicaid certification requirements to be eligible for reimbursement for services provided. A similar set of conditions for participation are required for CMS reimbursement for hospice services.

The rate of payment is dependent on three variables related to the client: clinical severity (C) of the client's condition, functional status (F), and anticipated service (S) utilization. Each client is scored on these three variables at the start of care on the basis of 23 questions included in the Start of Care OASIS-C assessment form. **OASIS** stands for **Outcome and Assessment Information Set**, a system of assessment and documentation developed to assess patient needs and subsequent outcomes of care by Medicare home care agencies. The results of a subset of OASIS items are publicly available on the Medicare.gov Home Health Compare website. OASIS data contribute to quality improvement in home health care in five target areas: (a) effectiveness of care, (b) efficiency, (c) equity, (d) patient-centeredness, and (e) safety (CMS 2014a). For further information about OASIS, see the resources provided in the *External Resources* section of the student resources site.

Based on the composite score using responses to OASIS assessment items, the client is placed in one of 80 **home health resource groups (HHRGs)**, reimbursement rate categories for home health services similar to the diagnosis-related groups (DRGs) for Medicare-funded hospitalizations. HHRGs are used to determine the rate of pay for an episode of home health care. The HHRG payment is a flat rate of reimbursement for all needed nursing and home care visits provided during an episode of care. Additional payments may be made for "therapy add-ons" or physical, occupational, or speech therapy services needed by the client. Medicare may also authorize outlier payments for clients with catastrophic care needs. These payments are intended to offset the losses encountered by the agency in serving these clients (CMS, 2013a).

Home health care provided under private insurance may be funded on a fee-for-service, per-visit basis or under capitation arrangements, discussed in Chapter 6∞. Managed care organizations, on the other hand, often fund home care services on a prospective flat-rate basis similar to Medicare.

In addition to the requirements for agency certification, clients who receive services reimbursed under Medicare must meet certain eligibility requirements in addition to being eligible for Social Security benefits. These requirements include certification of the need for care and a care plan developed by the client's physician. Periodically, this plan of care must be reviewed and updated with recertification of the need for services. As of 2010, recertification must include a face-to-face encounter between client and physician or a nurse practitioner, clinical nurse specialist, nurse midwife, or physician's assistant working in collaboration with or under the supervision of the physician. In addition, eligible clients must be homebound and need at least one of the following services: intermittent skilled nursing care; physical, speech, or occupational therapy; skilled observation and assessment; and case management and evaluation (CMS, 2010c). Generally speaking, clients are considered homebound if they cannot leave their homes, except for health provider visits, without great difficulty. Medicaid home care eligibility criteria vary from state to state and usually require clients to "spend down" their assets to become financially eligible for care.

Licensing of Home Health and Hospice Services

Licensure of home health and hospice agencies is state or locally controlled, depending on where the agency is located. In California, for example, licensing is a state regulatory function. Some areas require a certificate of need prior to licensing a home health agency or other types of service organizations (e.g., mental health services). A **certificate of need** is a state process designed to limit health facility proliferation and minimize costs by promoting careful planning of new services and construction (National Conference of State Legislatures, 2013). The trend appears to be toward increasing regulation of licensure for home health agencies; thus, the reader is encouraged to seek out licensing requirements for agencies in his or her own area.

In addition to state licensure, home health agencies may choose to be accredited by the Joint Commission or the Community Health Accreditation Program (CHAP). Accreditation involves meeting more rigorous standards for quality of care and performance than the minimum standards set by state and federal governments. Both home health care and hospice programs can be accredited by the Joint Commission and CHAP (CHAP, n.d.; Joint Commission, 2009). For further information about the accreditation process and standards, see the resources provided in the *External Resources* section of the student resources site.

Standards for Home Health and Hospice Nursing

Individual home health nurses, as well as agencies, should meet established standards. The "Scope and Standards for Home Health Nursing Practice," most recently published by the American Nurses Association (ANA) in 2007 are in the process of revision (Harris, 2013). The revised document will continue to reflect the scope of practice of home health nurses as well as standards of care for individual clients and standards of professional performance for the home care nurse. The standards of care relate to assessment, diagnosis, outcome identification, planning, implementation, and evaluation—in other words, the use of the nursing process in the care of clients. Standards of performance relate to ethical considerations, education, evidence-based practice and research, quality of practice, communication, leadership, collaboration, professional practice evaluation, resource utilization, and environmental health within the home health specialty field. Each of the standards addresses competencies for home health nursing at generalist and advanced levels of practice (Harris, Gorski, & Narayan, n.d.). A similar set of standards for hospice and palliative nursing practice was developed by the ANA and the Hospice and Palliative Nurses Association in 2007 and were revised in 2014 (ANA, 2014). Standards have also been established for home health nursing education, and a model curriculum is available from the Home Healthcare Nurses Association. The association also provides resources for palliative and end-of-life care. For further information about the standards for home health and hospice and palliative care nursing, see the resources provided in the *External Resources* section of the student resources site.

Evaluating Home Health and Hospice Services

Evaluation of home visiting services must be undertaken at both aggregate and individual levels. At the individual level, evaluation would be similar to the evaluation of all home visits discussed earlier. The OASIS system promotes documentation that supports assessment of care outcomes at both individual and aggregate levels (CMS, 2014b). The OASIS documentation suite includes several documents that are required of

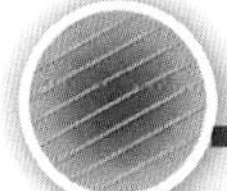

Evidence-Based Practice

The Nurse-Family Partnership Program

Williams and colleagues (2009) commented that in 2003 only 3% of practice guidelines (35 of 1026) included in the National Guideline Clearinghouse addressed home care or home visitation. Although that number had increased 62-fold by 2008, there still remains a significant lack of evidence on which to base home visiting practice.

One exception to this is the extensive evidence base that supports the effectiveness of the Nurse-Family Partnership (NFP) program, a national home visitation program providing services to first-time pregnant low-income women and their children. Services begin during pregnancy and continue until the child is 2 years of age and focus on health-related behaviors, positive parenting, and personal development of the woman (Coalition for Evidence-based Policy, 2012). Randomized, controlled, longitudinal studies of program recipients in three locations, some for as long as 19 years, have reported significant positive results including less abuse and neglect, better vocabulary and intellectual functioning, and fewer behavioral problems among children of mothers enrolled in the program compared to a group of control children. Girl children also had fewer arrests and convictions, fewer pregnancies, and less Medicaid use (Eckenrode et al., 2010). Mothers had fewer births and greater intervals between pregnancies, longer-lasting partner relationships, and spent less time on welfare and receiving food stamps than control mothers. Participating mothers also reported fewer episodes of domestic violence (Coalition for Evidence-based Policy, 2012; Give Well, 2010). Study mothers also experienced better prenatal health, increased employment, and their children had fewer childhood injuries and exhibited better school readiness (NFP, 2011c). Other program effects included less alcohol or drug-related role impairment among the women (Olds et al., 2010) and lower substance abuse rates among the children as well as better mental health and school performance for the children (Kitzman et al., 2010). Overall, the return on investment for the program has been estimated at $5.70 for every dollar spent, amounting to overall cost savings of $41,419 over the lifetime of a child served (Pew Center on the States, 2011). Similar research is needed to provide evidence for the effectiveness of home visiting programs for other population groups.

home health agencies that receive Medicare reimbursement. Components of the suite include: (a) the Start of Care OASIS, a standardized assessment form used at the initiation of care, (b) a reassessment conducted after the 55th day of care and before the 60th day if care continues into another episode, and (c) the Discharge OASIS, completed at the close of care. The Discharge OASIS documents change in the client's health status at the end of care and must be completed within 48 hours of the last visit.

OASIS items address three types of quality measures: outcome measures, process measures, and measures of potentially avoidable events (CMS, 2014d). Outcome measures include end-result outcomes that reflect the client's status as a result of care and utilization measures, measures of the utilization of health services (e.g., rehospitalizations). Process measures evaluate the performance of the home care agency with respect to specific evidence-based care processes of care, such as timeliness of admission, pain assessment and reassessment, fall-risk assessment, immunizations, and depression and pressure ulcer assessment. Potentially avoidable events measures address negative outcomes such as pressure ulcer development, falls (with and without injuries), and so on.

One of the functions of the OASIS documentation suite is to permit home care agencies to assess their care relative to that provided by other home care agencies. This is facilitated by several reports that are generated by the OASIS system. The first type of report involves Outcome-Based Quality Monitoring (OBQM), which generates two types of reports: the Agency Patient-related Characteristics Report, and the Potentially Avoidable Event Report, formerly known as the Adverse Event Outcome report. The Agency Patient-related Characteristics Report provides information about the clients served by the agency including length of service, need for emergency care or hospitalization during service, and so on. The Potentially Avoidable Event Report provides information on the types and frequency of 12 specific adverse events experienced by clients (e.g., falls, medication errors) (CMS, 2014c).

OASIS also enables Outcome-Based Quality Improvement (OBQI) reports. OBQI reports include the Agency Patient-related Characteristics Report described above as well as the OBQI Outcome Report, and the Patient Tally Report. The Outcome Report addresses changes in patients' health status over time for 37 outcome measures included in OASIS (CMS, 2014b). General categories of measures include timeliness of care and care coordination; various aspects of assessment, care planning, and implementation; patient education; and preventive care (e.g., medication error, pressure ulcer, and fall prevention and immunizations) (CMS, 2011b). The Patient Tally Report provides information about each client included in the Outcomes Report data and permits agencies to select clients for process investigation purposes (CMS, 2014b). Data included in the various reports provide comparisons to other home health agencies and to the particular agency's performance over time. CMS also provides process-based quality improvement (PBQI) and outcome-based quality monitoring and quality improvement manuals that assist agencies in the interpretation and use of evaluative data for program improvement (CMS, 2010a, 2010b, 2011b).

As noted earlier, data related to some of the measures included in OASIS are made available to the general public to help them in the selection of quality home health agencies. These findings are available through *Home Health Compare.* Home Health Compare is a federal website provided by Medicare that provides the public with information related to specific home health care agencies. Users can search for agencies operating in their location and make comparisons across a variety of quality-of-care measures as well as patient satisfaction with care (Home Health Compare, 2012). The website also provides a checklist that consumers can use to evaluate potential home health agencies when services are needed (Home Health Compare, n.d.). For further information about *Home Health Compare* and available comparison data, see the resources provided in the *External Resources* section of the student resources site.

CHAPTER RECAP

Home visits, as a form of nursing intervention, have been used by population health nurses since the early days of their practice, and home visits remain a viable alternative to other health care delivery settings. The nursing process provides a context for structuring home visits to provide health care to individuals and their families. Quality home visitation programs that display certain characteristics have been shown to be effective in achieving designated outcomes for families and children, pregnant women, and the elderly. Home visits are also used as a mechanism for service delivery in home health care and hospice care. Both home health care and hospice care are more closely regulated than other home visiting programs because of their ties to reimbursement under Medicare and Medicaid.

CASE STUDY The Home Visit

You are a population health nurse working for the Hastings City Health Department. Your supervisor took the following request for nursing services by phone and passed it on to you because the address is part of your district. You know that this address is in an older residential area with a large Hispanic population.

Hastings City Health Department

Request for Nursing Services

Source of Request: *La Paloma Hospital Maternity Unit*

Date of Request: *7-12-15*

Client: *Maria Flores* Date of Birth: *10-21-99*

Address: *8359 Marlboro Way, Marquette, AR 36019*

Head of Household: *Juan Flores (client's father)*

Reason for Referral: *Delivered 5 lb. 7 oz. baby boy on 7-5-15. Gestational age 32 weeks. Baby remains in NICU with RDS. Prognosis good. Client had no prenatal care. Lives with parents and 2 younger sisters (ages 8 and 13). Both parents work, but family income insufficient to pay hospital bill. Family does not have insurance. Immigration status unknown. Request home assessment prior to anticipated discharge 8-1-15.*

1. Based on the information you have, what health care needs related to biological, psychological, environmental, socio-cultural, behavioral, and health system determinants of health would you identify in your preliminary assessment? List your diagnostic hypotheses.
2. What nursing interventions would you plan for the health needs you are likely to encounter in a visit to this client? Identify your planned interventions as addressing health promotion, illness and injury prevention, resolution, or restoration measures.
3. What supplies and materials might you need on this home visit?
4. How would you go about validating your preliminary assessment and diagnostic hypotheses? How would you include Maria in goal setting and planning for the interaction? Would you include other family members? Why or why not? Would you collaborate with other health care professionals or make any referrals in meeting Maria's needs? If so, with whom would you collaborate? What referrals would you make, and why?
5. What additional assessment data would you want to obtain during your visit?
6. What evaluative criteria would you use to conduct outcome and process evaluation of care provided to this client and her family?
7. On what basis would you make the determination to terminate services to Maria?

REFERENCES

American Nurses Association and Hospice and Palliative Nurses Association. (2014). *Scope and standards of practice: Palliative nursing: An essential resource for hospice and palliative nurses.* Silver Spring, MD: nursesbooks.org.

Buhler-Wilkerson, K. (2001). *No place like home: A history of nursing and home care in the United States.* Baltimore, MD: Johns Hopkins University.

Buhler-Wilkerson, K. (2012). No place like home: A history of nursing and home care in the U.S. *Home Healthcare Nurse, 30,* 446–452. Reprinted from Buhler-Wilkerson, K. (2002). *Home Healthcare Nurse, 20,* 641–647. doi: 10.1097/NHH.0b013e3182651880

Canadian Home Care Association. (2009). *Home care in Canada: From the margins to the mainstream.* Retrieved from http://www.cha.ca/wp-content/uploads/2012/11/Home_Care_in_Canada_From_the_Margins_to_the_Mainstream_web.pdf

Cawthorne, A., & Arons, J. (2010). *There's no place like home: Home visiting programs can support pregnant women and new parents.* Retrieved from http://www.americanprogress.org/issues/2010/01/pdf/home_visitation.pdf.

Centers for Medicare Medicaid Services. (2010a). *Outcome-based quality improvement (OBQI) manual.* Retrieved from http://www.cms.gov/Medicare/Quality-Initiatives-Patient-Assessment-Instruments/HomeHealthQualityInits/Downloads/HHQIOBQIManual.pdf

Centers for Medicare Medicaid Services. (2010b). *Outcome-based quality monitoring (OBQM) manual.* Retrieved from http://www.cms.gov/Medicare/Quality-Initiatives-Patient-Assessment-Instruments/HomeHealthQualityInits/Downloads/HHQIOBQMManual.pdf

Centers for Medicare Medicaid Services. (2010c). *A physician's guide to medicare's home health certification, including the face-to-face encounter.* Retrieved from https://www.cms.gov/Outreach-and-Education/Medicare-Learning-Network-MLN/MLNMattersArticles/Downloads/SE1219.pdf

Centers for Medicare & Medicaid Services. (2011a). *Data compendium, 2011 edition.* Retrieved from http://www.cms.gov/Research-Statistics-Data-and-Systems/Statistics-Trends-and-Reports/DataCompendium/2011_Data_Compendium.html

Centers for Medicare Medicaid Services. (2011b). *Outcome and Assessment Information Set—OASIS-C: Process-based quality improvement (PBQI) manual.* Retrieved from http://www.cms.gov/Medicare/Quality-Initiatives-Patient-Assessment-Instruments/HomeHealthQualityInits/Downloads/HHQIProcessBasedQualityImprovementManual.pdf

Centers for Medicare Medicaid Services. (2013). *Home health PPS.* Retrieved from http://www.cms.gov/Medicare/Medicare-Fee-for-Service-Payment/HomeHealthPPS/index.html

Centers for Medicare Medicaid Services. (2014a). *Home health quality initiative.* Retrieved from http://www.cms.gov/Medicare/Quality-Initiatives-Patient-Assessment-Instruments/HomeHealthQualityInits/index.html

Centers for Medicare Medicaid Services. (2014b). *OASIS OBQI.* Retrieved from http://www.cms.gov/Medicare/Quality-Initiatives-Patient-Assessment-Instruments/HomeHealthQualityInits/HHQIOASISOBQI.html

Centers for Medicare Medicaid Services. (2014c). *OASIS OBQM.* Retrieved from http://www.cms.gov/Medicare/Quality-Initiatives-Patient-Assessment-Instruments/HomeHealthQualityInits/HHQIOASISOBQM.html

Centers for Medicare Medicaid Services. (2014d). *Quality measures.* Retrieved from http://www.cms.gov/Medicare/Quality-Initiatives-Patient-Assessment-Instruments/HomeHealthQualityInits/HHQIQualityMeasures.html

Christie, J., & Bunting, B. (2011). The effect of health visitors' postpartum home visit frequency on first-time mothers: Cluster randomized trial. *International Journal of Nursing Studies, 48,* 689–702. doi:10.1016/j.ijnurstu.2010.10.011

Coalition for Evidence-Based Policy. (2012). *Evidence summary for the nurse-family partnership.* Retrieved from http://toptierevidence.org/wordpress/wp-content/uploads/NFP-updated-summary-for-release-March-2012.pdf

Community Health Accreditation Program. (n.d.). *CHAP accreditation.* Retrieved from http://chapinc.org/Accreditation

Community Preventive Services Task Force. (2005). *Early childhood home visitation to prevent violence.* Retrieved from http://www.thecommunityguide.org/violence/home/homevisitation.html

Council on Community Pediatrics. (2009). The role of pre-school home visiting programs in improving children's developmental health and outcomes. *Pediatrics, 123,* 598–603. doi:10.1542/peds.2008-3607

Dose, A. M., Rhudy, L. M., Holland, D. E., & Olsson, M. E. (2011). The experience of transition from hospital to home hospice: Unexpected disruption. *Journal of Hospice & Palliative Nursing, 13,* 394–402. doi:10.1097/NJH.0b013e318227f8f2

Eckenrode, J., Campa, M., Luckey, D. W., Henderson, C. R., Cole, R., Kitzman, H., et al. (2010). Long-term effects of prenatal and infancy nurse home visitation on the life course of youths: 19-year follow up of a randomized trial. *Archives of Pediatrics & Adolescent Medicine, 164,* 9–15. doi:10.1001/archpediatrics.2009.240

Ekmann, A., Vass, M., & Avlund, K. (2010). Preventive home visits to older home-dwelling people in Denmark: Are invitational procedures of importance? *Health and Social Care in the Community, 18,* 563–571. doi:10.1111/j.1365-2524.2010.00941.x

Give Well. (2010). *The nurse-family partnership program.* Retrieved from http://www.givewell.org/united-states/programs/nurse-family-partnership

Harris, M. D. (2013). We need your input….This is your opportunity to have a voice in the future of your profession. *Home Healthcare Nurse, 31,* 177–181. doi: 10.1097/NHH.0b013e31828bcd88

Harris, M. D., Gorski, L., & Narayan, M. C. (n.d.). American Nurses Association scope and standards of home health nursing practice. Retrieved from http://www.nahc.org/assets/1/7/am13-501.pdf

Home Health & Hospice Care. (2012). *Agency history.* Retrieved from http://www.hhhc.org/history

Home Health Compare. (n.d.). *Home health agency checklist.* Retrieved from http://www.medicare.gov/what-medicare-covers/home-health-care/Home%20Health%20Agency%20Checklist.pdf

Home Health Compare. (2012). *Finding an home health agency.* Retrieved from http://www.medicare.gov/homehealthcompare/search.aspx

Home Visiting Coalition. (2008, December 10). *Letter to the honorable president-elect Barack Obama.* Retrieved from http://otrans.3cdn.net/20b5ce663c69fe213f_ptm6b9939.pdf

Home Visiting Coalition. (2009, May 15). *Letter to the honorable Max Baucus, Edward Kennedy, Charles Grassley, Michael Enzi, George Miller, Howard McKeon, Henry Waxman, Joe Barton, Charles Rangel, & Dave Camp.* Retrieved from http://www.nursefamilypartnership.org/assets/PDF/Policy/HV_Coalition_letter_5-15-09-20

H. R. 3590, 111th Congress. (2009–2010). *Bill summary and status.* Retrieved from http://thomas.loc.gov/cgi-bin/bdquery/z?111:HR03590:@@@D&summ2=3&

Joint Commission. (2009). *Facts about home care accreditation.* Retrieved from http://www.jointcommission.org/assets/1/18/Home_Care_Accreditation_12_09.pdf

Kitzman, H. J., Cole, R. E., Hanks, C. A., Anson, E. A., Arcoleo, K. J., . . . , Holmberg, J. R. (2010). Enduring effects of prenatal and infancy home visiting by nurses on children. *Archives of Pediatrics & Adolescent Medicine, 164,* 412–418. doi:10.1001/archpediatrics.2010.76

MetLife. (n.d.a). *Helping and healing people.* Retrieved from http://global.metlife.com/about/metlife-history/helping-healing-people/index.html

MetLife. (n.d.b). *MetLife begins.* Retrieved from http://global.metlife.com/about/metlife-history/metlife-begins/index.html

National Association for Home Health & Hospice. (2014). *Agency locator.* Retrieved from http://www.nahcagencylocator.com/

National Center for Health Statistics. (2007a). *Home health and hospice care agencies: 2007 National Home and Hospice Care Survey.* Retrieved from http://www.cdc.gov/nchs/data/nhhcs/2007hospicecaresurvey.pdf

National Center for Health Statistics. (2007b). *Home health care patients and hospice care discharges: 2007 National Home and Hospice Care Survey.* Retrieved from http://www.cdc.gov/nchs/data/nhhcs/2007hospicecaredischarges.pdf

National Center for Health Statistics. (2011). Annual number of patients discharged from hospice care by primary diagnosis (cancer versus all other diseases)—United States, National Home and Hospice Care Survey, 1992–2007. *Morbidity & Mortality Weekly Report, 60,* 143.

National Center for Health Statistics. (2013). *Health United States, 2012: With special feature on emergency care.* Retrieved from http://www.cdc.gov/nchs/data/hus/hus12.pdf

National Conference of State Legislatures. (2013). *Certificate of need: State laws and programs.* Retrieved from http://www.ncsl.org/issues-research/health/con-certificate-of-need-state-laws.aspx

National Human Services Assembly. (2007). *Home visiting: Strengthening families by promoting parenting success* [Policy brief No. 23]. Retrieved from http://nationalassembly.org/FSPC/documents/PolicyBriefs/FSPBrief23FINAL.pdf

Nurse-Family Partnership. (2011a). *Federal funding for home visitation.* Retrieved from http://www.nursefamilypartnership.org/public-policy/federal-hv-funding-guidance

Nurse-Family Partnership. (2011b). *Federal home visitation initiative tool kit.* Retrieved from http://www.nursefamilypartnership.org/public-policy/federal-hv-funding-guidance/NFP-Tool-Kit-for-State

Nurse Family Partnership. (2011c). *Proven effective through extensive research.* Retrieved from http://www.nursefamilypartnership.org/proven-results

Nurse-Family Partnership. (2011d). *Securing support to serve greater needs.* Retrieved from http://www.nursefamilypartnership.org/public-policy/legislation-pending—enacted

Nursing Community. (2010, January 6). *Letter to the honorable Nancy Pelosi & Harry Reid.* Retrieved from http://www.npwh.org/files/public/Nursing%20Community%20Letter_HC%20ReformConference%201-6-2010.pdf

Olds, D. L., Kitzman, H. J., Cole, R. E., Hanks, C. A., Arcoleo, K. J., Anson, E. A., …, Stevenson, A. J. (2010). Enduring effects of prenatal and infancy home visiting by nurses on maternal life course and government spending. *Archives of Pediatrics & Adolescent Medicine, 164*, 419–414. doi:10.1001/archpediatrics.2010.49

Pastor, D. K. (2006). Home sweet home: A concept analysis of home visiting. *Home Healthcare Nurse, 24*, 389–394.

Pew Center on the States. (2011). *The business case for home visiting*. Retrieved from http://www.pewstates.org/uploadedFiles/PCS_Assets/2011/The_Business_Case_for_Home_Visiting.pdf

Riggs, J. S., Madigan, E. A., & Fortinsky, R. H. (2011). Home health care nursing visit intensity and heart failure patient outcomes. *Home Health Care Management & Practice, 23*, 412–420. doi:10.1177/1084822311405456

Thompson, D. K., Clark, M. J., Howland, L. C., & Mueller, M.-R. (2011). The Patient Protection and Affordable Care Act of 2010 (PL 111–148): An analysis of maternal-child health home visitation. *Policy, Politics, & Nursing Practice*. Advance online publication, doi:10.1177/1527154411424616

Tinker, E., Postma, J., & Butterfield, P. (2011). Barriers and facilitators in the delivery of environmental risk reduction by public health nurses in the home setting. *Public Health Nursing, 28*, 35–42. doi:10.1111/j.1525-1446.2010.00887.x

United States Code. (2010). *Title 42: The Public Health and Welfare. Part E. Section 1395bbb—Conditions of participation for home health agencies: Home health quality*. Retrieved from http://www.gpo.gov/fdsys/pkg/USCODE-2010-title42/pdf/USCODE-2010-title42-chap7-subchapXVIII-partE-sec1395bbb.pdf

U.S. House of Representatives, 111th Congress. (2009). *Hearing on proposals to provide federal funding for early childhood home visitation programs: Hearing before the ways and means subcommittee on income security and family support, house of representatives, 111th congress*. Retrieved from http://www.gpo.gov/fdsys/pkg/CHRG-111hhrg52502/pdf/CHRG-111hhrg52502.pdf

Vanderburg, S., Wright, L., Boston, S., & Zimmerman, G. (2010). Maternal child home visiting program improves nursing practice for screening of woman abuse. *Public Health Nursing, 27*, 347–352. doi:10.1111/j.1525-1446.2010.00865.x

Williams, P. R., Rachel, M., Cooper, J., Walker, J., Winters, K., Harrington, M., & Askew, R. (2009). Keeping it real: Evidence-based practice in home health care. *Home Health Care Nurse, 27*, 522–531. doi:10.1097/01.NHH.0000361922.20388.80

World Health Organization. (2012). *Informal meeting on provision of home-based care to mother and child in the first week after birth*. Retrieved from http://apps.who.int/iris/bitstream/10665/77742/1/9789241504614_eng.pdf?ua=1

World Health Organization & UNICEF. (2009). *Homevisits for the newborn child: A strategy to improve survival*. Retrieved from http://whqlibdoc.who.int/hq/2009/WHO_FCH_CAH_09.02_eng.pdf?ua=1

UNIT

4

Nursing Care of Special Populations

Chapters

CHAPTER

14 Care of Families

Learning Outcomes

After reading this chapter, you should be able to:

1. Describe the elements of at least one theoretical perspective on families.
2. Describe at least five types of families.
3. Identify biological, psychological, environmental, sociocultural, behavioral, and health system determinants that affect family health.
4. Differentiate between formal and informal family roles.
5. Differentiate among situational, developmental, and structural crises.
6. Discuss family-focused interventions related to health promotion, illness and injury prevention, problem resolution, and health restoration.

Key Terms

blended families
childless family
crisis
ecomap
extended family
family
family resilience
genogram
hardiness
nuclear family
role
role conflict
role overload
single-parent families
system
work–life balance

Advocacy Then

The Whittier Center

Care of families has long been an approach used by population health nurses to improve the overall health of the public. Public health nurses from the Henry Street Settlement provided care to families and endeavored to meet the health promotion and health restoration needs of all family members. Similar efforts were undertaken in other parts of the country. In 1912, for example, the Whittier Center, named after John Greenleaf Whittier, American poet and abolitionist, began its efforts to alleviate the health and social problems of the Black community in Philadelphia (Carthon, 2011).

One of the early initiatives of the center addressed the high tuberculosis (TB) mortality rates in the population served. Black mortality was more than twice that of the White population in the city, in part due to poverty and crowded living conditions, as well as limited availability of treatment services and Black residents' unwillingness to use what treatment services were available because of mistrust (Carthon, 2011).

In 1913, the center hired Elizabeth Tyler, its first Black public health nurse, to visit Black families in their homes, gaining their trust and investigating possible cases of tuberculosis. Within months, Tyler had made visits to more than 1,000 families and made numerous referrals to the Phipps Institute TB treatment services. In the first year of her efforts, the number of Black clients attending the TB clinics was 12-fold higher than in the prior 11 years combined. By 1921, the center's health professional staff had increased to 10 nurses and 12 physicians (Carthon, 2011).

The nurses did more than just identify suspected cases of tuberculosis, but also provided health education for both children and adults. Additional services included prenatal and well-child clinics and home supervision of ill family members (Carthon, 2011).

Advocacy Now

Advocating for Low-Income Renters

Recent international immigrants to a large city in the southwestern United States tend to locate initially in a low-income run-down neighborhood. Housing is at a premium and low-income levels mean that several families usually live in rental units designed for a single nuclear family. Most of the rental units in the area are owned by absentee landlords, who do not maintain the properties. Safety issues and housing code violations are common, but because of language difficulties, lack of other affordable housing, and, in some cases, illegal immigration status, many tenants are reluctant to complain to landlords and ask for repairs. Those who do are often evicted with minimal notice and find it difficult to find other housing.

A county health nurse assigned to the area identified the safety issues and housing code violations as a significant problem in the community. She began to take pictures of the violations, documenting where they occurred, who the landlord was, and any attempts made by tenants or herself to have these issues addressed. She brought her evidence to the community collaborative, an alliance of local health and human services agencies that had a history of advocating for underserved and vulnerable populations. The collaborative initiated a town-hall meeting which was attended by community residents and various city officials, including housing authority administrators. The photographs as well as the findings of focus groups with area residents were presented. As a result, the city created a housing ombudsman position within the community to handle complaints of code violations and to interface among tenants, landlords, and the housing authority. In addition, the law school of a university located in the community provided a series of landlord-tenant educational sessions to acquaint both tenants and landlords with their rights and responsibilities. Subsequent city regulations were also enacted to prevent unwarranted evictions and to protect tenants from unfair treatment by landlords.

According to 2010 census figures, the U.S. population included 78.8 million family households. Each of these households shares some common characteristics, but each is unique. Population health nurses often care for discrete family units, but as always, their primary focus is on the health of the overall population. Care of individual families, however, provides information about the health status and needs of the general population. Families are also frequently the unit of service for programs designed to address the overall health needs of the population.

Theoretical Perspectives on Family

Many disciplines provide care and services to families and have developed theoretical models for dealing with families. Three general categories of models will be discussed here: systems models, life-cycle models, and symbolic interaction models. Other social science family models, such as stress theory and family change theory, are useful in addressing selected family problems, but do not provide the broad scope of understanding required for population health nursing care of families.

Systems Models

Systems models view families as open systems in which the whole of the system is more than the sum of its component parts or members, but also includes the interactions among them. The health of the family as a unit is influenced by interactions among members and between the family system and larger outside systems. The basic concepts of systems theory are derived from biologist Ludwig von Bertalanffy's general systems theory (Dallos & Draper, 2010). Systems theory incorporates basic principles that can be applied to any kind of system from an automobile engine, to the human body, to families, to organizations, to communities, and so on (von Bertalanffy, 1973). A **system** is a set of elements in interaction with each other in which the interaction is ordered rather than random (von Bertalanffy, 1981). From the perspective of systems theory, "families are systems of interconnected and interdependent individuals" (Genopro, n.d.a, p. 1).

The following four basic assumptions underlie systems theory:

- Elements within a system are interconnected; therefore, the focus is on the interactions among its various elements.
- The system interacts with its environment and the effects of this interaction are reciprocal.
- A system must be considered as a whole.
- A system is not a real entity, but is a model or depiction of how a family functions (Dupuis, 2010).

A system is composed of *subsystems*. Systems are hierarchical in nature, with some systems in turn constituting subsystems within more complex systems. For example, the cardiovascular system is a subsystem in the human body, a system that is itself a subsystem in the totality of an individual, who is a subsystem in a family system, and so on. In a family, the subsystems are the family members or combinations of members (Dupuis, 2010). Three possible combined family subsystems are the marital or couple subsystem, parent–child subsystems (e.g., mother–son, father and children, etc.), and the sibling subsystem (Fleming, n.d.).

Another concept of systems theory is the *suprasystem* or the environment in which a given system functions. The next higher-order system in the hierarchy of systems is part of the suprasystem for a lower-order system. For example, one's kin network is part of the suprasystem for one's immediate family system. The community is also a part of the suprasystem with which the family interacts. The concept of hierarchical systems is depicted in Figure 14-1●.

Any system is more than the sum of its parts or the subsystems of which it is composed, also incorporating the reciprocal interactions among its parts. This systems principle means that whatever affects one portion of a system will affect other portions because of their interdependence. The interrelationships between subsystems within the system, between subsystems and the suprasystem, and between the suprasystem and the system as a whole are important determinants of health and are one of the major foci in using a systems approach to family health nursing.

All systems have *boundaries* that define what is part of the system and what is not. For example, a community may have geographic boundaries such as city limits; whereas a family's boundaries are often (but not always) determined by blood and legal ties. The permeability of the system boundary determines whether one is dealing with an open or closed system. An *open*

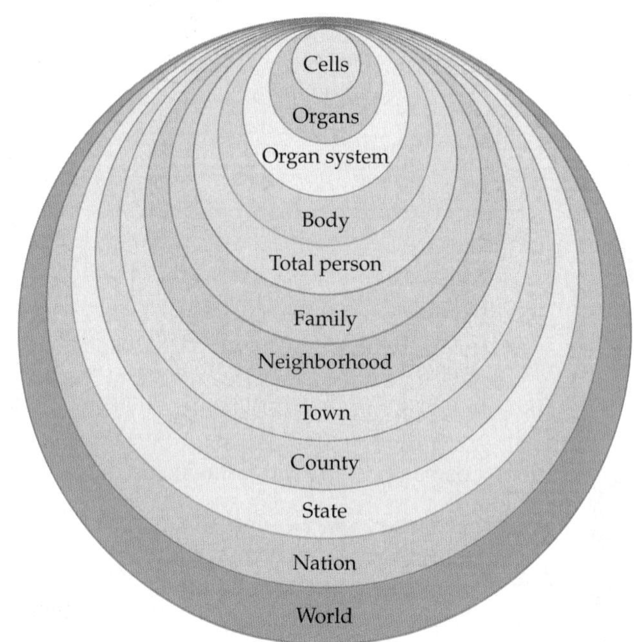

FIGURE 14-1 Hierarchical Systems

system is one that exchanges matter, energy, or information with the environment; a *closed system* does not.

All systems also have two mutual goals: maintenance of a steady state (morphostasis) and system growth in response to change (morphogenesis). The basic premise of family systems theory is that family systems organize themselves in ways that allow them to achieve these two goals (Fleming, n.d.).

Feedback is another important systems concept and consists of "patterns or channels of interaction and communication that facilitate movement toward morphogenesis or morphostasis" (Fleming, n.d., p. 2). Feedback is the process whereby the system output returns as input. Negative feedback indicates that family processes are achieving desired goals and that no change is required. Positive feedback, on the other hand, indicates that discrepancies remain between actual and desired states and that action is required.

Population health nurses use systems theory to identify the component subsystems within the family and to assess the quality of their interactions. For example, the nurse would assess whether or not the couple subsystem functions effectively in meeting the family's needs. Or, is there conflict within this subsystem that jeopardizes the family's ability to meet its needs and those of its members? For instance, if parents cannot agree on issues of discipline, children may not be appropriately socialized. Similarly, if neither member of the couple is employed, the family's ability to meet its financial needs might be compromised. In single-parent families, the lack of a couple subsystem may affect family health depending on how well the family adjusts to this circumstance, how well the single parent is able to carry out the typical activities of this subsystem, and the extent of support available to the single parent.

Family Life Cycle Theory

Life cycle or developmental approaches to family nursing are based on the supposition that human beings and social units, such as families, develop in a logical fashion with predictable stages or milestones along the way. A family stage is defined as a period of time in which the structure of the family and/or interactions of role relationships are markedly different from those in other time periods (White, n.d.). A family life course or career is defined as "all the events and periods of time (stages) between events traversed by a family" (White, n.d., p. 1). Each stage in the family life cycle is accompanied by transitions to which the family must adapt. The quality of family adaptation, however, is influenced by the unique situations of families as they encounter both anticipated and unanticipated transitions (Dallos & Draper, 2010). Some transitions are typical of most families, for example, adjusting to being a couple. Others, such as the death of a family member or unemployment of the primary bread winner, are unanticipated. Both kinds of transitions require changes in family structures and interactions that enable the family to successfully adapt to changing circumstances.

Families generally experience some stress as they pass from one stage to the next, since the transition usually involves one or more role changes. The family needs to negotiate these changes and respond by re-evaluating roles and goals. Initial life cycle theories developed by authors such as Duvall and Miller (1990), posited a set of universal stages through which families progress. These stages included: the beginning family or marital relationship, early childbearing, the family with preschool children, the family with school-age children, the family with adolescent children, and the launching center family, the family of middle years, and the family in retirement and old age.

One of the criticisms of Duvall's developmental model was that it applied primarily to the traditional family structure of husband, wife, and children and was less useful in working with other family forms. More recently, other authors have examined the concept of family transitions from a broader perspective. For example, in the late 1990s, Carter and McGoldrick (1999) identified transitions experienced by divorced families and families resulting from remarriage. A more general set of typical family transitions is presented in Table 14-1●.

TABLE 14-1 Stages and Transitions in a Typical Family Life Cycle

Stage	Transitions
Independence/separation from one's family of origin	• Becoming emotionally, economically, and socially self-supporting • Developing the capacity for intimacy • Developing an individual identity outside one's family • Becoming responsible for one's own health • Establishing one's occupation or career
Coupling/marriage/committed union	• Dealing jointly with financial issues • Developing a joint lifestyle • Developing/modifying relationships with extended kin networks • Adjusting to intimacy/sexuality • Developing friendships • Achieving interdependence
Parenting (babies to adolescents)	• Adapting to role changes • Modifying the couple relationship • Modifying relationships with kin networks • Adjusting to child developmental stages • Letting children go • Refocusing on midlife relationships and career goals
Launching adult children	• Developing adult relationships with children • Accepting new family members • Dealing with increasing health issues • Caring for older parents • Refocusing on the couple relationship • Realigning roles as in-laws and grandparents
Retirement	• Adapting to changes in family structure • Adapting to changes in life style (especially reduced income) • Caring for increasingly frail parents • Adjusting to declining physical abilities • Dealing with the loss of family members • Maintaining personal interests • Conducting life review

Data from: Healthwise. (2013). *Family life cycle – Topic overview.* Retrieved from http://children.webmd.com/tc/family-life-cycle-topic-overview

Not all families encounter all of the stages and transitions included in Table 14-1. For example, some couples may be unable or choose not to have children. Other families, such as blended families, or stepfamilies, experience the stages in a compressed nonlinear fashion, becoming a couple and joint parents simultaneously. Other transitions, such as school transitions, relationship changes (e.g., divorce), job changes, moves, illness, or abuse, may be unanticipated (Berg, Loth, Hanson, Croll-Lampert, & Neumark-Sztainer, 2012). All the transitions, however, require adaptation and renegotiation of member roles. Each transition is marked by the need to deal with the emotional effects of the transition and the need for changes in family relationships. In large part, a family's ability to adjust effectively to a transition lies in its interpretation of the transition. For example, if the family interprets the changed circumstances necessitating transition as a catastrophe, family members usually experience distress. On the other hand, if the stress of transition is perceived as a challenge, the family is more likely to adapt successfully. When the stress engendered by a transition is unable to be addressed using the family's usual coping mechanisms, the result is a family crisis (VanKatwyk, n.d.).

Adaptation to family life cycle transitions may occur at one of three levels of change. Level 1 change is internal to the family and does not result in a change in family structure. For example, retirement may necessitate changes in family interaction patterns, expenditures, and so on, but it does not result in a change in the composition of the family. Level 2 changes, however, result in changes in the actual structure of the family. Divorce and death of a family member are examples of level 2 changes. Level 3 change involves transformation, or a "shift in paradigms, in the basic beliefs and assumptions about life" (VanKatwyk, n.d., p. 9). For example, the woman who has defined herself in terms of her role as a mother may need to transform herself, developing a new vision of herself as a person apart from her children.

In applying a life cycle model to family nursing, the focus of care is on identifying the transitions being experienced by families and the success of family adaptation to changing circumstances and intervening to promote successful transitions. The population health nurse would identify the transitions experienced by the family, the adaptive demands of those transitions, and the extent to which the family is or is not adapting successfully. In the face of unsuccessful adaptation, the nurse would engage in interventions designed to facilitate successful accomplishment of the transition. For example, if a family is unwilling or unable to accommodate to role changes required by the growing independence of an adolescent, the nurse can assist family members to see the adolescent's rebellion as a normal developmental stage and foster strategies to promote independence in a safe environment.

Symbolic Interactionism

Symbolic interaction theory views the family as a group of interacting individuals whose interactions shape the roles and personalities of its members. Like systems theory, it focuses on interaction processes among family members, but also considers the roles performed by each member and the ways in which those roles are defined and shaped through family interactions. A major focus of the theory is on socialization, a reciprocal process that affects the self-concepts of family members (Gecas & Tsushima, n.d.).

Key principles of symbolic interactionism are symbols, acting, and roles. Symbolic interactionism is the process of giving meaning to symbols and words as a result of interactions with others. One's actions then depend on the meaning one ascribes to a particular symbol or word (Carlson, 2013; Milliken & Schreiber, 2012). For example, the word or symbol of mother may have different meanings or connotations in different families. In one family, mother may be associated with loving care; in another it may reflect harsh discipline. One's interactions with one's mother, then, are shaped by one's perception of what a mother is. In the first case, one's response and interactions may reflect mutual love and respect; in the second, interactions may be colored by fear of punishment.

Role is the third basic principle of symbolic interactionism. A **role** is defined as "the rights and duties attached to any given social position" (Carlson, 2013, p. 459). One's family position is one's place in a kinship structure, frequently defined by gender, marriage or blood relationship, and generational relationship (White, n.d.). In a traditional family of husband, wife, and children, the mother role is a gender role played by the female spouse. The character of a relationship may also affect one's role. For example, the relationship of a stepmother to her stepchildren is a marital, rather than a blood relationship, so her mother role is often quite different from that of a biological mother. Generational relationships also influence roles. The role of son, vis-à-vis his father is different from that of a brother with respect to a female sibling because of the generational difference or similarity. The quality of a family member's role performance in his or her multiple roles is contingent on the family's expectations for someone in that role as well as one's perceptions of what is expected by others (Carlson, 2013).

Using symbolic interaction theory, the population health nurse would examine the roles of family members as well as the meaning and expectations related to those roles and how they shape the interactions among family members. When role expectations are inappropriate, the nurse would intervene to promote more appropriate role expectations. For example, interactions between husband and wife may be negatively influenced by differing definitions of the mother and wife roles. If the woman holds emancipated views of the role of the wife as an equal partner, and the man holds more traditional views of a subservient wife subject to his authority, the situation is ripe for conflict. If both spouses hold more traditional expectations of the wife/mother role, conflict would be less likely. In this situation, the nurse would work to assist the couple to identify the differences in their role expectations and come to some sort of compromise if possible. Similarly, a parent may have inappropriate expectations for the behavior of a 2-year-old and perceive the negativity typical of this age as defiance.

In this case, the nurse could educate the parents regarding the normality of this behavior and suggest strategies that promote better behavior on the part of the child but still foster his or her independence.

The Family as a Unit of Care

The family is the oldest and most persistent of all social institutions, but it has changed radically in the last few decades in terms of its structure and role functions. In fact, both the definition of family and the array of types of families have altered drastically in recent years.

Defining Family

Multiple authors have noted the difficulty of even defining what constitutes a family. *Family Ties*, a family support organization, notes that "families are who you love" (n.d.b, p. 1). Yet, this definition and the later description of a "caregiving unit" do not reflect the reality of all families. There are families in which family members do not love each other and do not engage in caregiving for their members. To be useful, a definition of family must be broad enough to apply to all instances of family across multiple cultures.

Until the late 1980s, a "traditional family" was defined as two parents and at least one child (Munro & Munro, n.d.) with the unstated expectation that the parents would be male and female. This configuration was considered the ideal, and any other family form was considered "deviant" (Munro & Munro, n.d.). This traditional definition no longer suffices, nor is it applicable to the majority of U.S. families.

The definition of what constitutes a family often depends on the situation and purpose for the definition. For example, inclusive definitions are highly individualized and are based on who is considered a member of a given family and who is not. In other instances, family is defined from a theoretical perspective to facilitate research. For example, symbolic interaction theory defines a family as a "unit of interacting personalities," while systems theory defines family as a system comprising subsystems in interaction with each other. Situational definitions are often used to guide practice. For instance, child welfare systems might define families "pedifocally" as all the persons, agencies, and other entities interested in the welfare of a particular child. In such a case, a family might consist of biological parents, members of the extended family, foster parents, a case worker, and so on (Munro & Munro, n.d.).

Normative definitions are those based on agreed-upon societal rules and expectations for what constitutes a family in a given society or culture. A unit with at least one parent and one child is the usual normative definition of a family in many societies, but this definition excludes a childless couple or an older couple whose children have died or moved away. In other societies, the larger kinship group is defined normatively as one's family (Munro & Munro, n.d.). Many authors agree that there is no single definition of family and that a family no longer has a fixed form but is free form. Munro and Munro (n.d., p. 1) aptly stated that "The term family has been replaced by families and has become the embodiment of whatever the individual perceives to be family." For our purposes, a **family** is a social system consisting of two or more people who define themselves as a family and work collectively to meet members' needs.

Family Types

Families come in multiple sizes and configurations, and the role and structure of the family has evolved with societal changes. Factors underlying these changes include delayed age at marriage, increased single parenthood, movement of women into the workforce, and delayed and declining fertility and mortality with fewer children born and more older persons living longer. Attributes previously considered integral to the concept of family, such as the presence of children and being related by blood or marriage, may or may not be found in today's varied family structures. Different authors describe the variability among families somewhat differently, but some common family forms include the nuclear family, the extended family, single-parent families, blended families, and childless families (Shelton, 2010).

As we saw earlier, the traditional nuclear family was composed of a husband and wife with one or more biological or adopted children. Today, however, nuclear families may be formed by same-sex couples (who may or may not be married depending on state laws) with children or unmarried heterosexual couples with children. A more current definition of a **nuclear family** is an adult couple with biological or adopted children. In 2009, census figures indicated that about 6% of U.S. households consisted of unmarried partners, 91% of which involved heterosexual male–female couples, 4% male partners, and 4.6% female partners (U.S. Census Bureau, 2012). According to the American Academy of Pediatrics (2014), approximately 2 million children live with gay, lesbian, or bisexual parents.

In terms of family households, an **extended family** involves two or more adults from different generations living in the same household (Family Ties, n.d.a), but not all extended families live together. When they do occupy the same household, the reasons for a multigenerational family are many. In some instances, grandparents join the household to provide care for children or to receive care themselves from members of younger generations. Financial strains experienced by either generation may give rise to intergenerational households. For example, grown children may move back home after loss of employment or retired elders may not be financially able to maintain an independent residence. Worldwide, the prevalence of multigenerational families has increased by 40% in the last 10 years, and such families may consist of three or more generations (Goyer, 2010). Extended families may involve many convoluted interrelationships among members that may give rise to conflict or a variety of other difficulties and issues that may require intervention by the population health nurse.

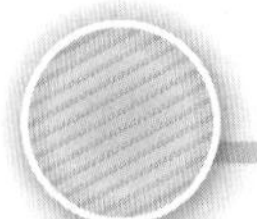

Global Perspectives

Change in Family Structure

Many cultures with traditional extended family structures are moving to more nuclear families rather than multiple generations living together. Examine the international family literature. What are the factors that are contributing to this change in family structure? What effect has this change had on family life and health? On the availability of family support?

Single-parent families, one adult and one or more children living in the same household, are also more numerous today than in the past and are the fastest growing family form in North America. In fact, it is anticipated that half of all U.S. children will spend some portion of their lives in a single-parent family. Single-parent families may occur for a number of reasons. Some single women who get pregnant choose not to marry; other single-parent families result from divorce or the death of a spouse (Family Ties, n.d.a). With the relaxation of adoption regulations in many states, many more single adults, including heterosexual, gay, lesbian, bisexual, and transgender adults, are adopting children. Single-parent families, particularly those headed by women, encounter a number of social stressors that may require assistance from the population health nurse. Among these stressors are poverty and role overload as one parent attempts to fulfill both mother and father roles as well as meet the family's financial needs.

"Grandfamilies," families in which grandparents are raising their grandchildren, may take any of the three family forms discussed thus far. Some grandparents who are responsible for the care of their grandchildren live in an extended family situation in which the children's parents are also present (Goyer, 2010). In other instances, single grandparents or older couples are raising their grandchildren. An estimated 2.5 million grandparents are raising their grandchildren with or without parental involvement (American Association of Retired Persons [AARP], n.d.). Other relatives, such as aunts, uncles, and older siblings, may also take on the responsibilities of raising children whose parents are unwilling or unable to care for them. Such situations create both blessings and burdens for the family members, and may result in financial, health, educational, occupational, and retirement challenges. Population health nurses should be particularly attuned to the needs of both children and adults in these families.

Blended families, or stepfamilies, are composed of a heterosexual or same-sex couple, one or both of whom have been involved in a prior relationship, and children from the prior relationship(s). Like several of the other family forms, blended families may arise in a variety of circumstances. In most instances, a family with children is dissolved by divorce, and one or both of the ex-spouses remarries. On average, 50% of first-time marriages end in divorce, and two thirds of divorced women and three fourths of divorced men choose to remarry. Approximately 65% of those remarriages include children of one or both spouses (Dupuis, 2010). Blended families may also be created when a spouse dies and the widow or widower remarries. Blended families may include younger children living in the household some or all of the time or adult children who have left home.

Blended families have been described as "incomplete institutions" because they do not have societal rules or role models for how interactions within the family should occur. Many people entering blended families anticipate that the rules and relationships from prior nuclear families will apply. However, due to differences in role expectations, culture, traditions, and values, this is unlikely to be the case (Dupuis, 2010). Like the other family types discussed above, blended families encounter a variety of transitions, however, given the lack of prior relationships and rules of interaction developed over time, these transitions may occur simultaneously and be less easy to adjust to than in other families. For example, in many blended families, the spousal couple do not have time to adjust to being a couple before they must address the needs of children (Cornish, 2013a, 2013b). Population health nurses may need to assist blended families to surmount these transitions effectively. Some potential keys to successful blending that can be fostered in these families include sharing feelings without blaming, finding solutions that address the needs of multiple family members, establishing rules and systems that can be modified as indicated by experience, and developing effective conflict resolution mechanisms (Cornish, 2013a).

The final family form to be addressed here is the **childless family**, an adult couple who have never had children (Shelton, 2010) or who live apart from children. In 2010, only 74% of family households included a married couple, and nearly 60% of those households were childless (U.S. Census Bureau, 2012). Childlessness may be voluntary or involuntary, permanent or temporary (Family Ties, n.d.a). Some families may choose not to have children; others are unable to do so. Still other families may plan to have children at some future time, or may have children who have died or no longer live in the home.

Population Health Nursing and Care of Families

Population health nurses work with individual families and with families as an aggregate within the population. In doing so, they examine epidemiologic factors that influence family health status and use the nursing process to assess family health, diagnose needs for care, and plan, implement, and evaluate care for families at both individual and societal levels.

Assessing Family Health Status

Assessment of family health takes place with respect to individual families and the overall health of families within the population. Factors related to each category of health determinants affect the health status and health needs of families. Biological, psychological, environmental, sociocultural, behavioral, and health system determinants of family health will be briefly addressed here.

BIOLOGICAL DETERMINANTS. When the population health nurse first encounters a family, assessment begins with the gathering of data to identify the physical needs of family members. It is important to note that the physical status of each family member should be explored as a biological determinant of overall family health. The physical health status of each member affects how the family functions and how members relate to each other. For example, if a child has a chronic disease, the entire family must make adjustments to accommodate the youngster's special needs. The parents have to adjust their schedules to care for the child and ensure that the child is seen by appropriate health care providers. Siblings may assume household chores or provide some measure of care for their ill brother or sister. Other family members can assist with care and offer emotional support for the parents and children. As another example, chronic back pain due to an occupational injury may result in restructuring of family roles, relationships, and interpersonal interactions, as well as increased family stress.

Knowledge of the age, gender, and race of family members, as well as information related to genetic inheritance, can guide the nurse in identifying problems and planning family care. For example, knowing that there are several young children in the home, the nurse may emphasize safety precautions when interacting with the family. An elderly family is more likely to have members with chronic, debilitating illnesses and may need closer scrutiny for evidence of these problems. The presence of older family members may contribute to *filial crises* in which they and their adult children are faced with acknowledging their mortality and accommodating role reversals. Multiple generations in the household may also result in the *sandwich generation* phenomenon in which younger adult members are responsible for meeting the needs of their children as well as their aging parents. Or, a family's race may increase its members' risks for certain diseases such as sickle cell disease among African Americans and peoples of Eastern Mediterranean descent.

The health status of individual family members, as well as their genetic inheritance, can be reflected in a genogram (Genopro, n.d.b). A **genogram** is a diagram of a family tree incorporating information regarding family members and their relationships over at least three generations that reflects family structure as well as health status. Genograms help identify repeating patterns in families and areas for potential intervention. Information that may be included in a genogram includes dates of births, deaths, marriages, separations, and divorces; health status (including presence of acute and chronic illness); ethnicity; genetic inheritance; occupation or unemployment; retirement; and significant family problems such as trouble with the law, family violence, or incest. Creation of a genogram is an excellent method of family engagement when the population health nurse first encounters the family. A sample genogram is presented in Figure 14-2●.

By convention, certain symbols have certain meanings in a genogram. For example, females are represented by circles and males by squares. Squares and circles marked with an "X" indicate deceased family members. A double circle or square indicates the *index person* or identified client. The lines connecting persons in the diagram indicate the character of relationships between them. A couple is designated by a horizontal line between its members; in a heterosexual couple, the male is traditionally placed to the left. Any children of the couple are included below the couple line, oldest to youngest starting on the left. Biological children are indicated by a solid line, adopted children by a broken line, and foster children by a dotted line. When a couple is divorced, the couple line is double cross-hatched (Genopro, n.d.b, n.d.c, n.d.d).

The developmental status of individual family members is also an important determinant of family health. For example, parents who have not accomplished developmental tasks of adolescence and young adulthood may have difficulty focusing on the needs of their children. Successful adaptation to the transitions typically encountered by families discussed earlier in this chapter will also affect family health status. A *Focused Assessment* related to biological determinants of family health is presented below.

The population health nurse would also collect data regarding biological determinants of family health at the aggregate level. For example, effective health care planning for families requires information about the proportion of elderly families and those with young children in the population and the number of families with disabled members or other individual health problems that may affect overall population health. The questions included in the *Focused Assessment* might be adapted in assessing families as an aggregate within the population.

PSYCHOLOGICAL DETERMINANTS. Psychological determinants are a particularly important component of family health since families are instrumental in the development of the self-concept of family members and their abilities to interact effectively with people inside and outside of the family. Areas for consideration include communication patterns, relationships and dynamics, coping and emotional strengths, child-rearing practices, family goals, the presence or absence of emotional problems, and the existence of family crises.

FOCUSED ASSESSMENT Assessing Biological Determinants of Family Health

- What are the age, gender, and racial/ethnic composition of the family?
- How adequately have individual family members accomplished age-appropriate developmental tasks?
- Do individual family members' developmental stages create stress in the family?
- What developmental stage is the family in? How well has the family achieved the tasks of this and previous developmental stages?
- Do family members have any existing physical health conditions that are affecting family function?
- Is there a family history of genetic predisposition to disease?
- What is the immunization status of family members?

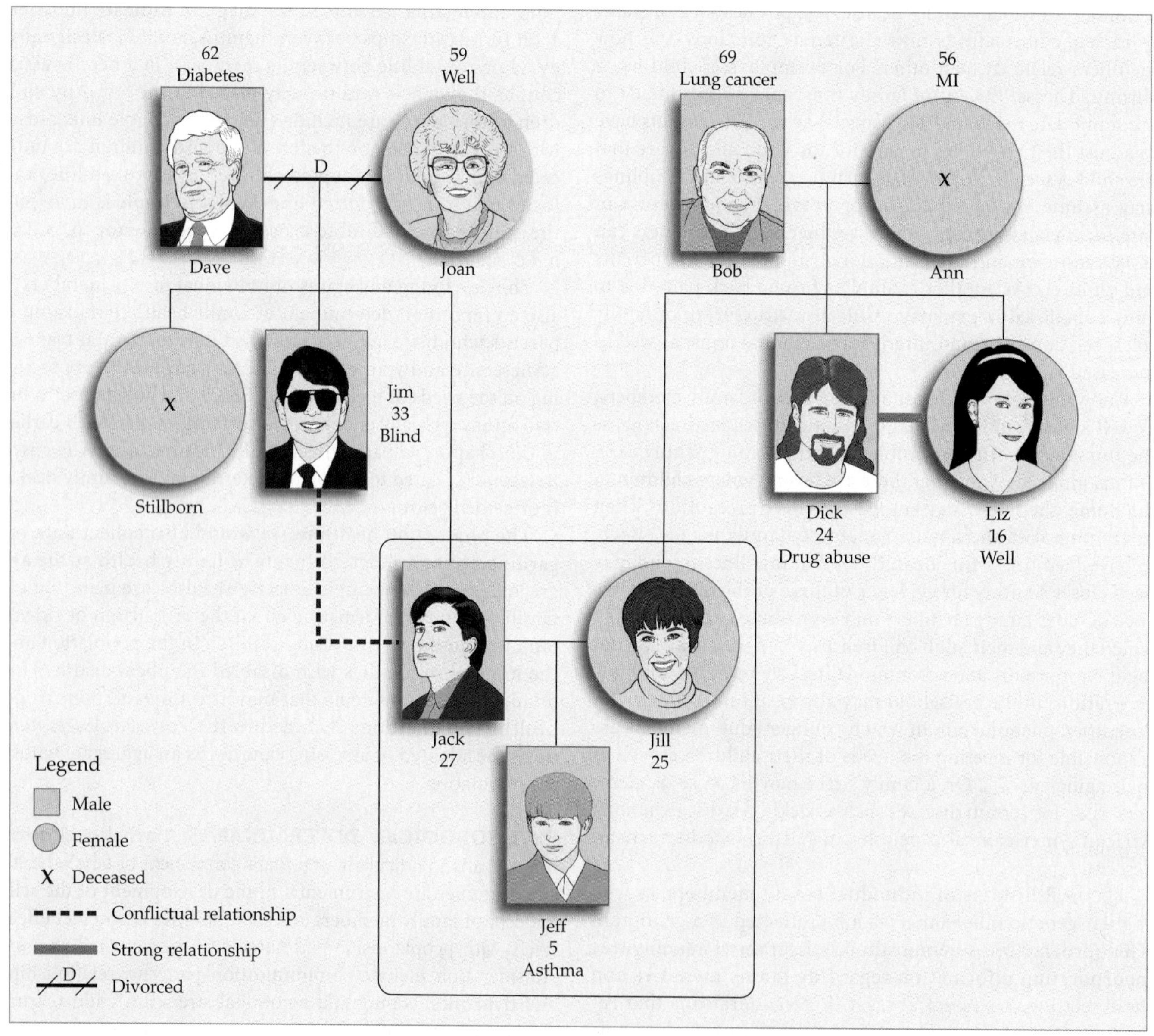

FIGURE 14-2 Sample Family Genogram

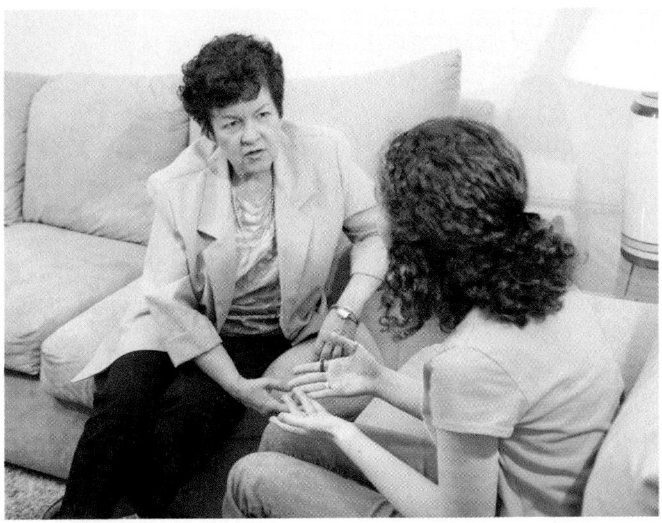

Effective communication is an important factor in family health. *(Lisa F. Young/Fotolia)*

Communication patterns. Communication patterns are an important indicator of psychological function in the family. Family communication occurs both verbally and nonverbally, and family members need to be able to correctly interpret both forms of communication. For example, most parents learn to distinquish, based on the character of an infant's cry, whether the child is tired and fussy, hungry, or has a dirty diaper. Other forms of verbal and nonverbal communication may be more difficult to interpret, based in part on expectations related to what is being communicated as well as the clarity, openness, and honesty of communication. Both verbal and nonverbal communication should be considered in family assessment, as should the listening ability of family members. How do members communicate values and ideas? When one family member talks, do others listen? Do they show anger or boredom while listening?

Communication within dyadic relationships in the family is characterized by degrees of symmetry and complementarity. In a symmetrical relationship, the two parties communicate as equals. In a complementary relationship, they communicate as superior and inferior. Both types of relationships are appropriate in certain situations (Wright & Leahy, 2013). For example, one would expect communication in a parent–child dyad to be complementary when children are young, but to exhibit a greater degree of symmetry as children grow older.

The feeling tone expressed in communication is another indicator of the psychological environment. Family communications may contribute to interpersonal difficulties or facilitate cohesion and problem resolution. Sarcastic and resentful statements could block further communication between family members. For example, "When are you ever going to use your head?" does not facilitate communication. Other types of one-way communication include repeated complaints, manipulation through covert requests, insulting remarks, lack of validation, and inability to focus on an issue.

Communication patterns can influence the effectiveness of parenting, particularly in the area of discipline. Praise enhances the development of self-worth in the child, whereas negative or condescending communications restrict the child's development. More about communications and child discipline can be found in Chapter 16∞.

The nurse should be aware of dysfunctional communication patterns that may be employed within families. For instance, messages may be passed from one family member to another in a chainlike fashion that does not allow for reciprocal discussion; or communication may isolate a family member, as when the mother and children exclude the father from their discussions. Another problematic pattern is the wheel in which a central person directs what communication will be passed between family members. By way of comparison, a successful pattern of communication is the "switchboard" in which there is reciprocal communication among all family members. Figure 14-3● illustrates these patterns of communication.

A final consideration is the degree of communication between the family and the suprasystem. Is the family open to new ideas and opinions from people outside the family? Are outsiders invited to participate in family discussions or are they expected to "mind their own business"?

Family relationships and family dynamics. Family relationships and family dynamics are other areas in the family's psychological environment that influence health. Family relationships are those bonds between family members that create identifiable patterns, such as subgroups and isolated members. Family relationships that are close, cohesive, and supportive of individual members contribute to individual health and to the health of the family as a whole. Excessively close relationships, however, may inhibit individual development and be detrimental to both individual and family health. Distant, nonsupportive, or conflictual relationships increase stress within families and contribute to poor physical and mental health in family members.

Interactions within the family and between the family and its external environment can be depicted in an **ecomap**, a visual representation of relationships within and outside of the family. An ecomap can be used to depict the relationships of family members with each other and with outside forces such as health care providers, employers, and extended family members. Ecomaps also portray resources available to the family, or their absence, and highlight areas of conflict that may require intervention (Missouri Department of Social Services, Children's Division, 2011). The segment of the genogram including the household of interest may be contained within the larger central circle of the ecomap. Outside forces are represented by smaller circles on the periphery. Again, relationships are represented by the types of lines connecting

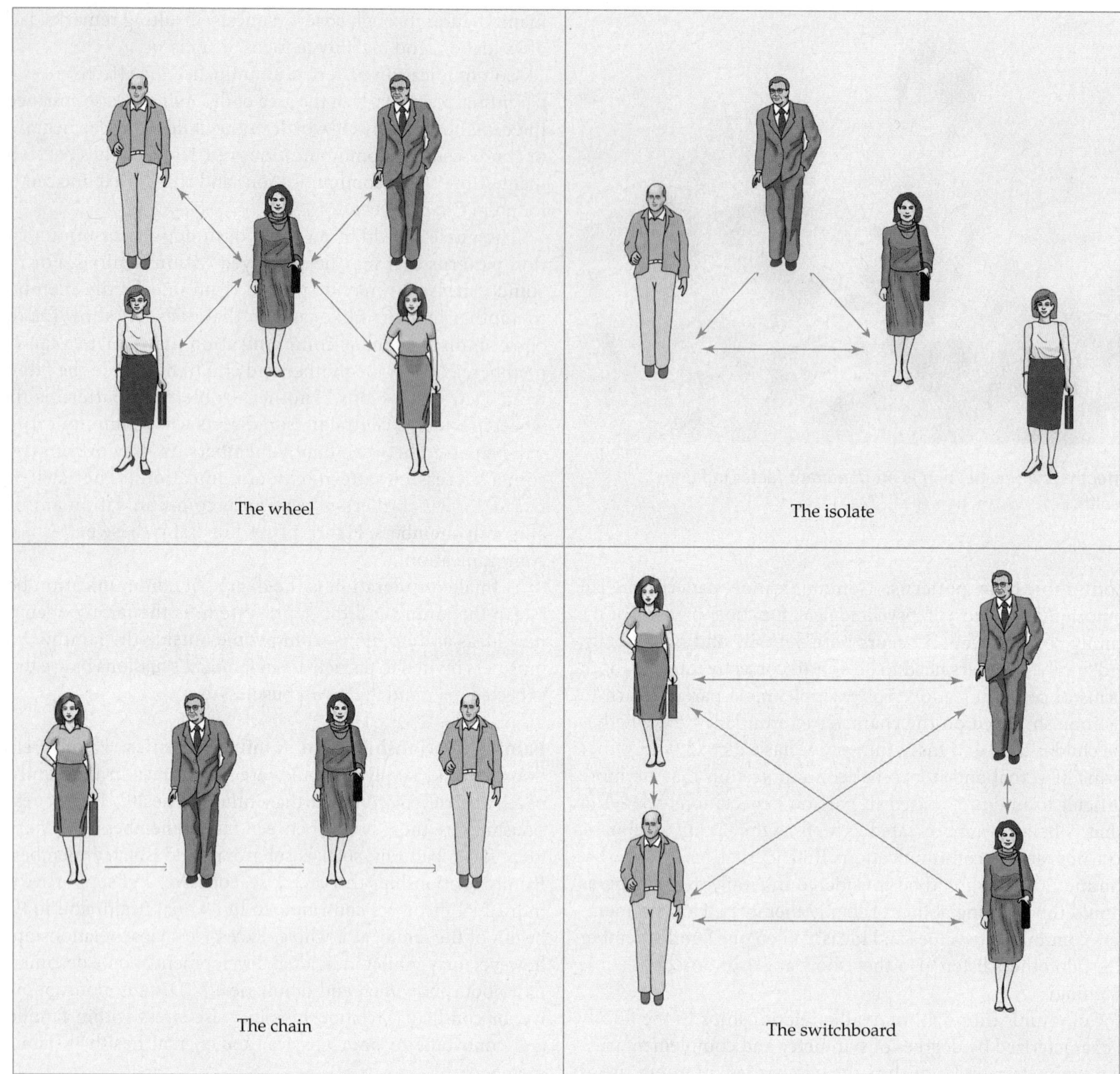

FIGURE 14-3 Family Communication Patterns

the circles in the diagram. Figure 14-4● presents a sample ecomap in which there are strong supportive relationships between the wife and the population health nurse and between the son and his teacher and conflictual relationships between the husband and his employer and between the family and the next door neighbor. There is also a tenuous relationship with the extended family. For further information on constructing a family ecomap, see the resources provided in the *External Resources* section of the student resources site.

Family dynamics involve hierarchical patterns within the family. Power and leadership within the family are central elements of family dynamics. Power should be appropriately distributed within the family based on circumstances. For example, young children generally have little power and influence in families; but as children age, they should have increasing power and influence with respect to family decisions, particularly those that affect themselves. In some families, however, family life may revolve around the needs of one member, often to the detriment of the health of other family members. This may be particularly true in families with disabled members.

Family dynamics are assessed by observing family leadership patterns. Who are the primary decision makers? Who controls conversations? Is there a leader in the family? What leadership style does the leader employ? Do family members respect the leader? Do they respect each other? Respect

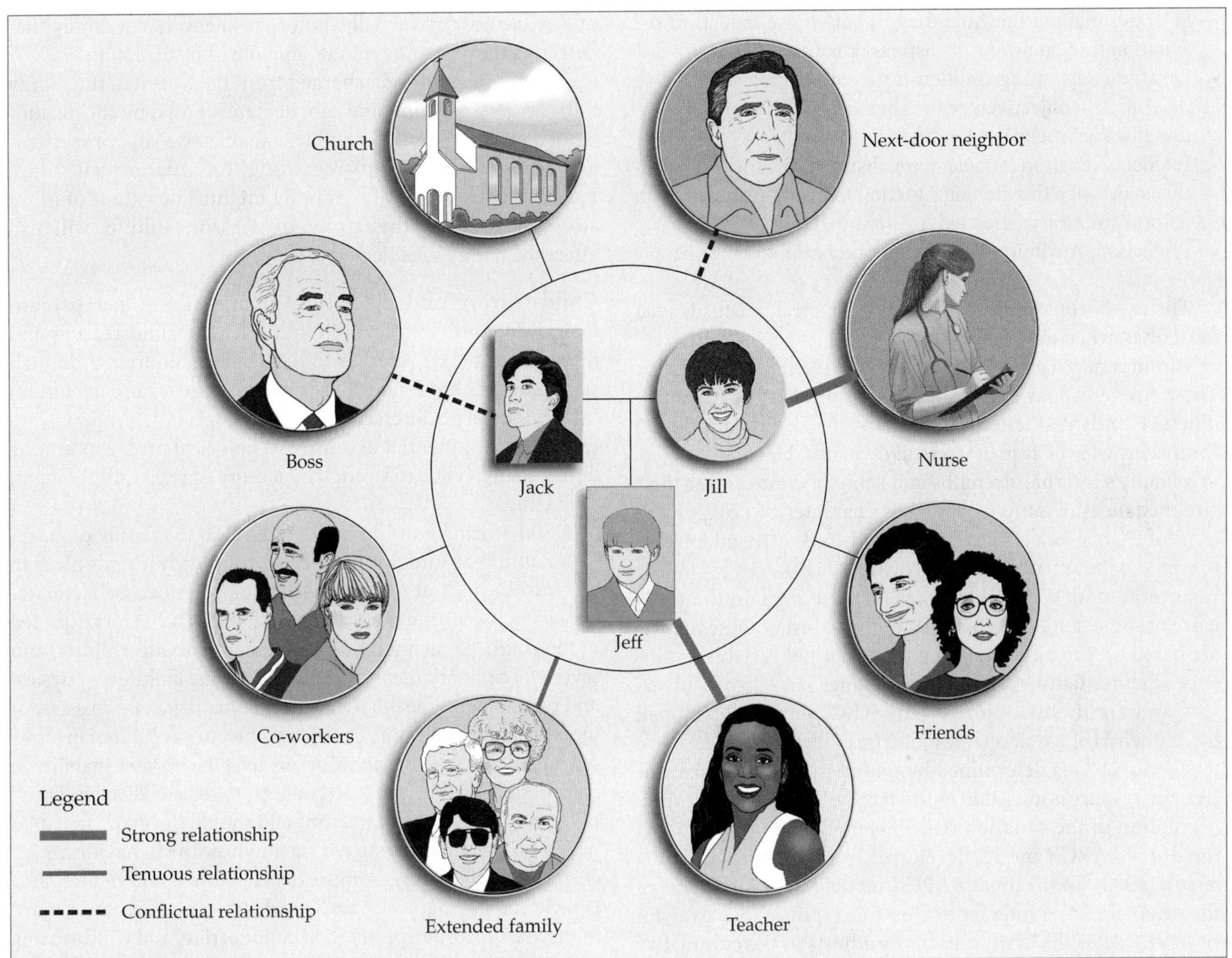

FIGURE 14-4 Sample Family Ecomap

requires that children view parents as individuals as well as parents. Likewise, parents need to learn to respect their children as individuals.

Power within families is often culturally determined. For example, in some cultural groups, adult men hold decision-making power in families. In others, power is equally distributed between husband and wife. The relative power and influence of children will also vary within cultural groups and may even vary among children in the same family (e.g., the eldest son having greater influence in the family than other children). When culturally determined power distribution enhances family health or has no specific impact on health, it is appropriate. If, however, culturally determined power distribution no longer serves the family or impedes the health of the family unit or that of individual members, intervention may be needed. Chapter 5∞ contains more information on the cultural aspects of power and authority in families.

Family coping and emotional strengths. Identifying a family's coping strategies and defense mechanisms enables the nurse to assist families to deal realistically with stress and crisis. Coping strategies are behaviors that help a family to adapt to stress or change and are characterized by positive problem-solving methods that prevent or resolve crisis situations. Coping involves specific actions taken to manage demands on the family and to bring resources to bear on family problems.

Defense mechanisms are tactics for avoiding recognition of problems. They may be used when the family cannot immediately determine how to solve a problem. Defense mechanisms are not considered problematic unless they interfere with coping and may actually be helpful in allowing time to organize resources before facing a problem. Common family defense mechanisms include:

- Denial: Ignoring threat-provoking aspects of a situation or changing the meaning of the situation to make it less threatening
- Rationalization: Giving a "good" or rational excuse, but not the real reason for responding to a situation with a particular behavior

- Selective inattention: Attending to only those aspects of the situation that do not cause distress or pain
- Isolation: Separating emotion from content in a situation so one can deal objectively with otherwise threatening or emotionally overwhelming conditions
- Intellectualization: Focusing on abstract, technical, or logical aspects of a threatening situation to insulate oneself from painful emotions generated by the situation
- Projection: Attributing one's own motivation to other people

The use of coping strategies or defense mechanisms is seen most often when the family is faced with change.

Families may also exhibit strengths in the face of adversity. These strengths may be referred to as family resilience or hardiness. **Family resilience** is the ability of a family to function competently in the face of stressful demands. **Hardiness** refers to a family's internal strengths and sense of control over their circumstances. Family hardiness is characterized by perceptions of change as a challenge to growth and active adaptation to stressful life situations (Chen & Clark, 2010).

Several models have been developed to explain the resilience of some families rather than others. Most of these models are based on the understanding that multiple variables influence whether families are able to "bounce back" from adversity, and are modifications of the ABCX model developed by Reuben Hill (McDonald, n.d.). In Hill's model, response to stressors (X) is determined by the interplay of the stressor (A), the resources available to the family (B), and the family's perception of the situation (C). This model was expanded in the double ABCX model developed by McCubbin and Patterson (1983). In the double ABCX model, the components of the original model interact to create a response to a stressful situation. After the event, the family adjusts to the cumulative effect of multiple stressors (aA) by employing new and existing resources (bB), and by redefining their perception of the original stressful event (cC). The result is a level of postcrisis adaptation (or maladaptation) (xX).

McCubbin and McCubbin (1993) later modified the model to indicate two stages of family response to stress: adjustment and adaptation. In the short-term adjustment stage, the family attempts to manage the stressor without major changes in family functional patterns. Adaptation is a long-term goal in which the family is able to cope with the stressor on an ongoing basis using both new and existing patterns of function. Family resources that facilitate adjustment and adaptation may be internal to the family (e.g., characteristics and capabilities of family members) or external (e.g., social support networks) (McCubbin, Thompson, & McCubbin, 2001). As an example, when a child is hospitalized with a new diagnosis of diabetes, the family must adjust to the hospitalization while still maintaining family function. Parents may alternate staying with the hospitalized child and caring for other children. Grandparents or friends may function as family resources assisting in the maintenance of family function (e.g., picking other children up after school, providing meals). If the family perceives themselves as able to cope with the hospitalization and later with the ongoing demands of the diagnosis, they will be more resilient than a family that perceives the difficulties of the situation as insurmountable.

When the child is discharged from the hospital, the family must adapt to the ongoing care demands posed by the diagnosis of diabetes. A resilient family with effective support systems and positive perceptions regarding the situation will adapt more readily than another family might. The extent of other stressors affecting the family, or stressor buildup, will also affect the family's resilience.

Child-rearing and discipline practices. Another psychological determinant of family health is the child-rearing and discipline practices employed to socialize children. Although such practices are usually derived from culture, a sociocultural factor, they are addressed as a psychological determinant because of their potential to cause psychological problems among family members or to strengthen a sense of right and wrong in each child.

Child-rearing attitudes and practices in the family often reflect cultural attitudes toward children and children's place in the world. Cultural mores also define prescribed behaviors of parents in socializing their children as well as behaviors expected of the child. Harsh and punitive interactions with children and severe disciplinary measures can undermine children's physical and psychological health. On the other hand, lax, permissive, or inconsistent parenting also causes problems for children in terms of confusion regarding appropriate behavior or later inability to control their own behavior to conform to societal dictates. Discipline should be fair and relevant and should be linked to explanations of what was done wrong and how the behavior can be corrected in the future. A more detailed discussion of discipline is included in Chapter 16∞. Knowledge of the cultural groups in the area, their perspectives on child rearing, and child-rearing and discipline practices prevalent within the population can lead to identification of family problems at the aggregate level.

Family goals. Family goals are a function of family values and reflect a family's cultural background. Family goals also vary with a family's developmental stage, economic status, and the physical health of family members. Problems arise when there is disagreement on family goals. For example, an immigrant family may have worked hard to send their son to college (a family goal). Before his sophomore year, the son refused to return to school, preferring instead to work as a plumber's apprentice. The discrepancy between the son's personal goals and those of the family created a stressful situation for all family members.

Conflict may also occur between the goals of the family unit and societal goals and expectations. For example, a common societal goal is to provide children and young people with an education that will allow them to be more productive members of society. Family goals of economic security, however, may conflict with this societal goal when gainful employment by adolescent family members is given higher priority than educational attainment. Similarly, family goals of economic security conflict with societal goals of child safety when young children are left to supervise younger siblings while parents work. At the aggregate level, knowledge of the cultural groups in the area and their perspectives on acceptable family goals also gives population health nurses some insight into possible family goals.

Presence of mental illness. Another psychological determinant of family health to be addressed here is the presence or absence of mental or emotional illness among family members. Such illnesses not only affect the health status of individual family members, but can profoundly influence the health of the family unit. For example, postpartum depression has been linked to poor health outcomes for both mother and baby. Similarly, coping with chronic mental illness or substance abuse disorders take an inordinate toll on the family unit and its individual members. At the aggregate level, population health nurses can develop a picture of psychological determinants that have the potential for affecting the health of families within the population. The incidence and prevalence of family violence or suicide, for example, can suggest potential problems that may be faced by individual families as well as societal attitudes that may contribute to problems. Similarly, the extent of mental illness in the population may suggest psychological factors impinging on family health. The extent of resources available to families dealing with mental health issues is another area for exploration at the aggregate level.

Family crisis. Family exposure to stress may lead to the development of a crisis situation. A family can view any situation as a crisis. What is a crisis for one family may not be a crisis for another. Moreover, some families function and thrive on daily crises and would deteriorate if crisis situations were eliminated from their lives. Crisis assessment and intervention, then, must be based on the family's perception of a crisis event.

A **crisis** is a circumstance in which one encounters a problem that is seemingly unsolvable; none of one's usual method of problem solving works. The problem becomes psychologically overwhelming, and anxiety and tension increase until the family becomes disorganized and unable to cope. A crisis state is unlikely to be sustained over a long period because it is difficult to endure the high stress and tension associated with crisis without breakdown or change. The result of a crisis can be either resolution, resulting in a healthier, more positive state of being, or loss of well-being and a higher potential for recurrent crisis. Temporary relief can be gained from the use of defense mechanisms, environmental action, or both. Resolution and more permanent relief and growth require appropriate coping mechanisms. During periods of crisis, families are more susceptible to change and are usually more open to help when it is offered. This receptivity affords the nurse the opportunity to produce change with modest intervention.

Families experience three types of crises: developmental, situational, and structural (Nelson, 2012). A developmental crisis is viewed as a "normal" transition point where old patterns of communication and old roles must be exchanged for new patterns and roles. Every family experiences developmental crisis points, whether or not a crisis is actually experienced. Examples of transition periods when developmental crises may occur are adolescence, marriage, parenthood, and one's first job. Such periods in life are usually predictable, so families can be prepared to use coping mechanisms that assist them through each transition period.

A situational crisis can occur when the family experiences an event that is sudden, unexpected, and unpredictable. Such events threaten biological, psychological, or social integrity and lead to disorganization, tension, and severe anxiety. Examples include illness, accidents, job loss, death, and natural disasters.

Developmental and situational crises require a change in roles or the addition of new roles, and structural crises occur when a family is unable or unwilling to accept new roles (Nelson, 2012). There may be a history of poor role modeling by parents that leaves children unprepared for new roles and unable to leave home successfully. There may be family members who are unable or unwilling to view one member in a new role. For example, it is sometimes difficult for parents to acknowledge that their teenage children need to make decisions for themselves.

Some crises may arise that contain elements of both situational and developmental crisis events. For example, a young girl may be going through the developmental transition of adolescence and encounter the situational crisis of an unwanted pregnancy. The multiplicity of crisis events further impairs the family's ability to cope.

Why do some families go into crisis while others do not? Four categories of factors seem to play a part in determining whether or not a crisis will occur. These factors relate to: (a) the stressor itself and the family's perceptions of the stressor, (b) other stressors impinging on the family, (c) the family's coping ability, and (d) the extent of family resources. Factors related to the stressor and how it is perceived by the family include the extent of the impact of the stressor on the family and the severity of that impact, the duration of the stressor and whether its onset was sudden or gradual, and the degree of perceived control the family has over the stressor. A stressor that is perceived as manageable is less likely to cause a crisis situation than one that is seen as uncontrollable. The cause and predictability of the stressor may also influence the occurrence of crisis. Stressors with unknown causes or unpredictable effects create greater anxiety and greater potential for crisis.

The family's perception of the stressor may be distorted by previous experience with crises that were not growth producing. For example, there are crisis-prone families who have a chronic inability to perceive or solve existing problems. Their inability to cope with problems results in an exaggerated response to new challenges, and crises occur for them that would be averted by other families.

The extent of other concurrent stressors affecting the family may also be a determining factor in the development of a crisis. Multiple stressors may have additive effects that precipitate crises. As noted earlier, developmental and situational crises may occur simultaneously stretching the family's coping abilities beyond their limits. Existing family problems such as illness, unemployment, and marital strife, may make a seemingly minor stressor a precipitating factor in a crisis. Situational demands created by the stressor may also increase the potential for crisis.

Unfortunately, situational demands created by the health care system may enhance the potential for crisis. For example, the illness of a child is a stressor; if taking the child to the clinic necessitates losing work time and money, this creates an additional burden for the family.

The family's coping mechanisms represent internal family resources important to crisis resolution. Among these resources are cohesion or closeness among family members, open communication, use of humor, control of the meaning of the problem, and role flexibility. The family's ability to cope lessens the impact of any crisis event. It is important to assess what degree of success has been achieved using these mechanisms in the past and whether the family is aware of the mechanisms used.

Situational support arises from external resources such as the extended family, community agencies, churches, neighbors, and friends of the family. The degree of security felt by family members in relationships with these support systems may be sufficient to avert crises. A tool designed to assess family risk for experiencing a crisis is included in the *Assessment Guidelines* section of the student resources site. The assessment guidelines are framed in terms of the determinants of health that influence the occurrence of a crisis for a given family. The *Focused Assessment* included below provides tips for assessing the effects of psychological determinants on family health.

At the aggregate level, there are usually no statistical data available regarding the number of families that are experiencing crises. Population health nurses can, however, get some sense of the magnitude of family crises from interviews with family counselors. These providers should also have some insight into the types of crises most often experienced by families. Police data on the number of calls related to family altercations can also provide some indication of the level of family crises experienced in the community. Population health nurses can also gather data on social conditions that are likely to precipitate family crises. For example, unemployment and poverty levels in the community can provide information on some of the stresses experienced by families.

ENVIRONMENTAL DETERMINANTS. Environmental factors within and outside the home also affect the health of families. Within this setting, the family develops either functional or dysfunctional relationships. A chaotic, crowded, unsanitary, or unsafe home can contribute to physical and psychological health problems among family members. Considerations within the home include space available to family members, both for family interactions and for individual privacy. Another consideration is the presence of safety hazards in the home. What constitutes a safety hazard depends, in part, on the ages and health status of family members. For example, uncovered electrical outlets would be a safety hazard in homes with young children, and dangling cords and loose throw rugs would be safety hazards for both young children and elderly family members.

FOCUSED ASSESSMENT Assessing Psychological Determinants of Family Health

- What are the typical modes of family communication? How effective are family communication patterns? What areas are taboo in family communication?
- How cohesive is the family? Do family members exhibit close supportive relationships?
- How are decisions made in the family? By whom? Which family members have input into decisions? Who is responsible for carrying out family decisions?
- Who is the leader in the family? Does the leader use a leadership style appropriate to the age and abilities of other family members?
- Do family members express respect for each other?
- Is there evidence of violence within the family? What forms of discipline are used in the family? Is the discipline used appropriate?
- What emotional strengths does the family exhibit? How does the family deal with change?
- What coping strategies does the family use? How effective are these strategies?
- What are the family's goals? Do individual goals conflict with or complement family goals? What values are reflected in the family's goals?
- Is there evidence of mental illness in the family? What is the effect of mental illness on family relationships? On family function?
- How well does the family deal with crisis? Is there an existing crisis within the family? If so, what type of crisis is it? What are the hazardous situation and precipitating factors in the crisis?
- What are the perceptions of the family regarding the crisis situation?
- Is there potential for harm to family members as a result of the crisis (e.g., homicide or suicide)?
- What defense mechanisms and coping strategies has the family employed?
- What internal and external sources of support are available to deal with the crisis?
- What options for action are available to resolve the crisis situation? To what extent are family members aware of options? What are the advantages and disadvantages of the options available?

FOCUSED ASSESSMENT Assessing Environmental Determinants of Family Health

- Where does the family live?
- What is the physical condition of the home? Are there safety hazards in the home?
- Is plumbing adequate? Is the amount of available space adequate for the number of persons in the family?
- Does the family have an emergency plan?
- How safe is the neighborhood? Are there environmental hazards in the neighborhood?
- Does the family have access to necessary goods and services (e.g., grocery stores)?

The family's external environment includes the neighborhood in which they live and the larger environment. Physical environmental characteristics at this level include the types of homes in the area, degree of industrialization, crime rate, and level of sanitation. Other important considerations include population density, common occupations of neighbors, and the availability of transportation, shopping facilities, health services, churches, schools, and recreational facilities. Each of these areas is assessed in relation to the specific needs of individual family members and of the family as a whole.

Assessment tips related to environmental determinants of family health are provided in the *Focused Assessment* above. At the aggregate level, the population health nurse would obtain similar information about environmental conditions within the community. What is the proportion of unsafe housing in the community? What sources of pollution are present? What is the disaster potential in the community and how might a disaster affect resident families? The answers to these and other questions will give the population health nurse some idea of the environmental conditions that may be faced by families in general as well as those experienced by specific families.

SOCIOCULTURAL DETERMINANTS. Sociocultural determinants of family health share some of the influences of the psychological environment. For instance, relationships outside the family are the basis for a portion of personality development. The leadership ability of individual family members is developed in school and in cultural, social, and political organizations where family members have the opportunity to interact with others and to contribute to community endeavors. Family discussions of social, cultural, and political issues help to develop social awareness as children grow and encourage the children to become involved in community, county, state, and national politics or social movements. Areas for consideration in the sociocultural dimension include family members' roles, culture and religion, social class and economic status, employment and occupational factors, and external resources. An additional special consideration for some families is their status as refugees, which is discussed later in this chapter.

Family roles. One of the most interesting aspects of sociocultural determinants in family life is role enactment. As we saw earlier, roles are socially expected behavior patterns determined by a person's position or status within a family. Each person in a family occupies several roles by virtue of his or her position. For example, an adult woman in a family may have the roles of child caretaker, cook, and confidante, but these roles may be played by men in some families. Roles can take two forms: formal and informal. Formal roles are expected sets of behaviors associated with family positions such as husband, wife, mother, father, and child. Examples of formal roles are those of breadwinner, homemaker, house repairperson, chauffeur, child caretaker, financial manager, and cook. Informal roles are those expected behaviors not associated with a particular position. Informal roles influence the psychological dimension within the family by determining whether, how, and by whom emotional needs are met.

Family roles may be complementary or conflictual in nature. **Role conflict** is a state in which the demands of a single role are contradictory or when the demands attending several roles contradict or compete with each other. For example, a mother who works will experience role conflict when a business meeting she is expected to attend conflicts with her child's school play. Role conflict can also occur when one individual's definition of a role does not correspond with someone else's definition of the same role. For example, a husband may expect his wife to be responsible for all the cooking for the family, but the wife may work late and expect the husband to prepare an evening meal.

Role overload is another phenomenon that occurs in families when members assume multiple roles. **Role overload** is a situation in which an individual is confronted with too many role expectations at one time, even though these expectations do not contradict each other. For example, a mother with four children who returns to school and also has a part-time job may experience role overload in trying to meet the demands of housekeeping, cooking family meals, performing well on the job, and making straight As. Role overload may give rise to what has been called "spillover stress," stress that accumulates and takes a toll on the person experiencing stress that may then affect relationships with other family members. For example, a single parent experiencing role overload may begin to neglect an elderly parent who depends on his or her care.

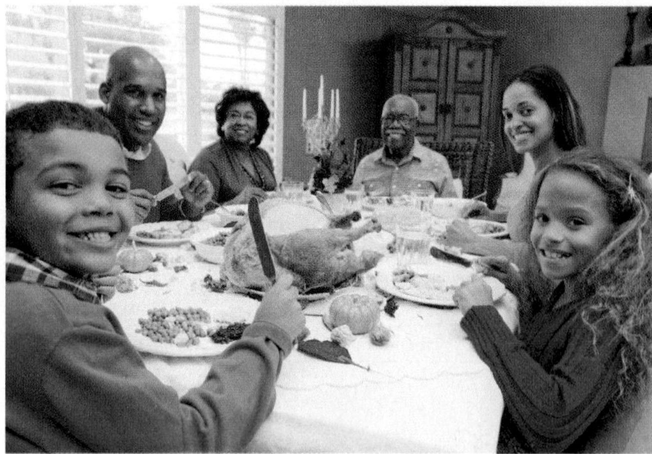

Meals can be a time of sharing. *(Monkey Business/Fotolia)*

Role overload is particularly apparent with respect to family caregiver roles and may result in diminished health for the person caring for ill or disabled family members. In 2009, more than 42 million people provided assistance to adult family members in their performance of activities of daily living. The value of these services was $450 billion, an increase of $75 billion over 2007 figures (Feinberg, Reinhard, Houser, & Choula, 2011). Factors contributing to the increased need for long-term care giving by family members include greater longevity, the increased cost of hospitalization, and shorter length of hospital stays resulting in people being discharged with greater care needs than in the past. By 2040, estimates of the number of people over 85 years of age needing assistance from family range from 8 to 20 million; much of this care will be provided by family members who are themselves over 65 years of age (Anngela-Cole & Hilton, 2009). Potential effects of caregiving for caregivers include social isolation, diminished physical health, depression, anxiety, and both financial and interpersonal strain.

The effects of caregiving may be different based on the overall level of function of the family as well as the characteristics of both caregivers and recipients. For example, caregivers who are themselves in poor physical health are apt to experience greater caregiver stress than those who are more physically healthy. Similarly, the functional abilities of the care recipient influence the amount of care needed and time spent in giving care and the consequent potential for caregiver stress. Beliefs, attitudes, and values held by the caregiver have also been shown to influence the amount of stress experienced (Anngela-Cole & Hilton, 2009). For example, caregivers who view caregiving as an onerous duty may experience more stress than those who see it as a reciprocal return for past care provided to them by older family members. The availability of internal and external support available to the caregiver also influences his or her experience of caregiver strain.

Caregiver employment outside the home may increase or decrease caregiving stress. For some caregivers, outside employment adds to role overload as they try to balance occupational demands with those of caregiving. For others, employment may provide a respite from the concerns of caregiving (Anngela-Cole & Hilton, 2009). Population health nurses should assess the extent of caregiver burden within individual families as well as the extent of family caregiving and available resources in the population.

Flexibility of family roles and mutual respect for individuality are other sociocultural determinants of family health. Family roles often change when a family member is absent, ill, or incapacitated and cannot fulfill his or her usual roles. It is important to assess the ability of family members to take on these unfilled roles and make the necessary role adjustments. When the ill or absent member is ready to resume roles, a readjustment may again be necessary. For example, when Frank had his heart attack, Beth had to go to work and assume the breadwinner role. Now Frank is recovered and can return to work. Beth likes her job and does not want to quit. Assistance in adjusting to changes in roles can alleviate conflict and stress in this and similar situations.

Role adjustments may also be required as the family progresses through its various developmental stages. For example, the parental role should be enacted differently with an adolescent child than with a preschooler.

Culture and Religion. Family cultural information is essential to building relationships and designing family interventions that will not conflict with cultural values. Does the family engage in cultural practices related to health? If so, are these practices helpful or harmful? What cultural factors will affect attempts to resolve family health problems?

Cultural factors may support or impede family abilities to adapt to changing environmental circumstances and may influence the health of individual members. Cultural factors play a large part in determining family caregiver roles, how those roles are performed and by whom, and the effect of those roles on the health of caregivers.

One specific aspect of culture that may influence family health is that of religious affiliation or spirituality. The influence of religious beliefs and practices on the health of the family can be assessed by asking specific questions about the importance of religion in family interactions and decision making and the role of religion for the family as a whole. For example, strong religious beliefs may prohibit the use of contraceptives, or health teaching may need to be modified in keeping with the family's religious convictions. Or religious beliefs and practices may promote health. For example, proscription of alcoholic beverages in some cultures can have positive health effects, but may lead to guilt in family members who drink in defiance of cultural proscriptions. Close affiliation with an organized church may also provide a source of emotional and/or material support for family members in time of need.

Social and economic status. The social class and economic status of a family can profoundly affect its health. Lack of financial resources can mean that the family does not have enough nutritious food, adequate shelter, or access to health care. Social-class delineations involve groupings of people based on financial status, race, occupation, education, lifestyle, and language. In the United States, the lower social class consists of people with less money, less education, and less access to resources such as health care.

The family's social class is important to the extent that it affects lifestyle, interactions with the external environment, and the health-related behaviors of the family. Economic status is closely tied to social class and educational level. At the aggregate level, data on the proportion of families living in poverty and the educational and economic levels of the population or subgroups in the population can provide information on the potential effects of social and economic factors on the health of individual families.

Employment and occupational factors. Job-related factors that influence family health may present in three forms. First, the job might produce stress for a family member that results in illness. Second, the family member might be exposed to hazards that he or she brings home to others. Third, job-related problems and time constraints might interfere with family commitments and contribute to family stress.

Occupational or workplace stress can lead to a number of stress-related illnesses. Safety hazards within the work setting may cause injury and disability to the family breadwinner(s). The financial burden and stress of an occupation-related illness have led to divorce and the dissolution of families, among other problems. Similarly, job-related stress may lead to reduced energy for effective parenting and for maintaining the couple bond if one exists. In single-parent families, job-related stress may contribute to exhaustion and inability to function effectively as a parent.

Sometimes, hazardous substances to which a working family member is exposed not only threaten the individual, but may also inadvertently be brought home to other family members. For example, nurses and other health care workers may transmit some infectious diseases to family members via clothing and shoes. Working with lead or other hazardous substances may also result in exposure of family members through contaminated clothing and other articles worn on the job.

Job-related family problems also might arise if a family member's work commitment conflicts with family commitments. Such work-family conflicts are increasing as a result of several factors. These include increasing female workforce participation and resulting reconceptualized gender roles within families, higher divorce rates that necessitate single parents functioning as both breadwinners and child caretakers, and more family members with both child care and elder care responsibilities (Williams & Boushey, 2010). The ideal situation is one of **work–life balance**, which has been defined as the absence of conflict between work and family roles or failure of role expectations in one setting to interfere with those of the other setting (Slan-Jerusalim & Chen, 2009). However, such balance is not often achieved and most family members experience some degree of work–family conflict with a variety of consequences. Some of these consequences include crossover stress experienced by other family members, spillover to other roles (e.g., to both parental and spousal roles), and emotional exhaustion and burnout (Hall, Dollard, Tuckey, Winefield, & Thompson, 2010).

Conflict between work and family roles may result from several factors and may include time strain, missed work or family activities, and spillover of stress from one setting to the other (Kelly, Moen, & Tranby, 2011). Time-based conflict is a function of role overload, in which the family member does not have sufficient time to effectively perform both work and family role expectations. Spillover stress occurs when strain in one role causes strain in others. For example, conflict with one's supervisor may spill over into one's interactions with spouse, children, or other family members. Behavior-based strain is related to role conflict in that the expected behaviors in work and family roles are incompatible.

Work–family conflict tends to be reciprocal in nature. Work-role strain affects family life, and family stress may also affect one's work performance. These two effects are sometimes differentiated as work–family conflict, in which work roles interfere with effective performance of family roles, and family–work conflict, in which family role strain adversely affects work-role performance. Competition between an important work meeting and a family member's birthday is an example of the former. Lack of concentration at work due to concern for one's aging parents is an example of family–work conflict.

Employment may have other effects on family health status and effective family function. For some family members, employment of one or more family members may result in eligibility for health insurance coverage. Other people are not employed in positions that offer health insurance. Similarly, some jobs allow more flexibility of schedules that permit employees to address family needs; others are less flexible. Some employers may also provide assistance with child care or other family responsibilities or provide counseling to assist employees in dealing with family-related issues. Finally, as we saw earlier, employment may serve as a respite from family caregiving activities.

External resources. As we saw in Chapter 1∞, personal or family social capital and community social capital influence health and illness in the population. Individual family capital may include extended family members, churches, or other social organizations in which a family participates that can provide support in times of need. The form of that support may be emotional, material, or instrumental. For example, being able to discuss one's worries related to one or more children with friends or extended family members may provide a parent with emotional support. Suggestions from the population health nurse on how to handle a rebellious adolescent are an example of instrumental support, and obtaining a short-term loan from one's parents is an example of material support.

External family resources may also be derived from community social capital. This would include the availability of social services to families in need. For example, the availability of the Temporary Assistance to Needy Families (TANF) to some low-income families is one form of community social capital. Other examples include American Red Cross Disaster Relief Services for families affected by natural or human-precipitated disasters and crisis counseling centers for low-income families.

At the population level, the population health nurse should assess conditions that affect the social environment of families as well as the overall availability of social resources for families. What is the level of unemployment in the community? What is the availability of jobs, particularly for families with low education levels? What social and cultural attitudes prevalent in the population may affect family health and function? Similarly, the nurse would assess the resources available to families such as financial assistance, education for parenting, and so on.

Refugee status. One additional sociocultural factor that profoundly affects the health and functional ability of many families is their status as refugees or immigrants. Immigration restrictions may result in lengthy separations for families that create a variety of social and psychological stresses. Family members are not permanently lost, as they would be in death, but the uncertainty regarding the length of separation does not permit families to acknowledge and work through the loss. When family members are reunited, idealization may make it difficult to reincorporate returned individuals who do not conform to one's memories of them. In addition, family roles will have been adapted to their absence and will need to be renegotiated with their return. Individual family members will have changed, and the recognition of those changes (e.g., aging, loss of roles), may affect self-image. In addition, most family members will need to address their emotional responses to the separation (e.g., guilt for leaving others behind, feelings of betrayal and abandonment). Finally, achievement of balance during separation may have necessitated the use of surrogates that may be questioned in family reunification. The effects of family separation and reunifcation may be particularly severe for adolescents (Suarez-Orozco, Bang, & Kim, 2011). For example, an uncle or family friend may have served as a surrogate father in the father's absence, and the appropriateness of this surrogate may be questioned when the father is reunited with the family. Knowledge of the number of refugee families in the community and their countries of origin will assist the population health nurse in identifying some of the potential problems that these families may experience. Assessment tips related to sociocultural determinants of family health are provided in the *Focused Assessment* below.

BEHAVIORAL DETERMINANTS. Health-related behavior is the fifth area for consideration in the epidemiology of family health. Families model patterns of preventive care, diet, exercise, hygiene, and other health-related behaviors that can profoundly affect family health now and in the future. Areas of focus include family consumption patterns, rest and sleep patterns, exercise and leisure activities, safety practices, and considerations related to sexuality and contraception.

Family consumption patterns. As we have seen in other chapters, a large percentage of Americans are obese or overweight. In other parts of the world, many people are malnourished. These dichotomous states of ill health are both related to family consumption patterns, either overconsumption or underconsumption of nutrients. For many Americans, family diets include excessive amounts of fat and calories, but are deficient in many vitamins and minerals due to low intake of fruits and vegetables. Healthy diets are difficult to achieve given the fast-paced nature of American family life. Family members often have little time to spend on food preparation and may rely heavily on fast foods

FOCUSED ASSESSMENT Assessing Sociocultural Determinants of Family Health

- What formal and informal roles are enacted by family members? How flexible and interchangeable are these roles?
- How congruent are family roles with those of the dominant culture?
- Is there evidence of role conflict? Role overload?
- Is the family experiencing conflict between work and family roles? If so, what is the effect on family health?
- Are there special considerations related to family caregiving roles? If so, what are they and how do they affect family health?
- How adequate were family role models?
- Are essential family roles being adequately performed?
- Are there expected changes in family roles? How will the family adapt to these changes?
- What cultural and religious factors influence family health status?
- What is the family's income? Is the family's income sufficient to meet needs?
- Are family members employed? What are the occupations of family members? Do occupational roles conflict with family roles? Do occupational roles present health hazards for family members?
- Is this a refugee family? If so, how have they adapted to their changed environment?

rather than balanced family meals. Other families may have difficulty affording healthful foods.

Cultural patterns evident in food selection, preparation, and consumption may also influence family health status. For example, the excessive use of fried or high-fat foods sometimes seen among Latinos or families in the southern United States contributes to the increased incidence of atherosclerosis, heart disease, and stroke among members of these populations.

Other consumption patterns that affect family health status include the use of tobacco, alcohol, and illicit drugs. According to the 2012 National Health Interview Survey, 18.1% of U.S. adults over 18 years of age were smokers (National Center for Health Statistics, 2014), and a significant number of U.S. children are exposed to cigarette smoke in the home. Drug and alcohol abuse by family members affect health in a number of ways. Substance abuse affects the personal physical and emotional health of the substance abusing member and may result in the inability to carry out necessary family functions adversely affecting the health status of other family members. In addition, substance abuse may contribute to family violence or neglect. Population-level data on consumption patterns, particularly those related to tobacco, drugs, and alcohol, can suggest problems that may be experienced by individual families.

Rest and sleep. Family rest and sleep patterns may also be a source of problems. For example, a new baby may sleep during the day and cry at night. This will adversely affect parents' rest and their subsequent performance the next day.

Another problem frequently encountered with respect to family sleep patterns is that of differing work schedules. If, for example, one parent works days and the other works nights, this situation may limit their opportunities to interact with each other and with their children. A parent's typical rest and sleep schedule may also require children to play at a neighbor's house during the day or find quiet pastimes at home.

Physical activity and leisure. Regular physical activity is necessary for good health. The earlier children are included in such activities, the more likely they are to build lifetime habits of exercise. Research has also indicated that other aspects of family life influence participation in physical activity. For example, the Ways to Enhance Children's Activity and Nutrition (WECAN) program developed by the National Heart, Lung, and Blood Institute (NHLBI) focuses on improving physical activity levels within the entire family as a strategy to combat childhood obesity (NHLBI, 2013). Exercise and leisure activities that include the entire family promote cohesion. At times, it is also helpful to plan leisure activities that are unique to certain members of the family. This allows for individuality among family members and promotes a balance between family togetherness and separateness that is needed for individual development.

The nurse can also help the family identify potential health risks involved in leisure activities. For example, are safety helmets worn by all family members on bike trips? What are the safety rules when the family goes swimming? Is a backyard pool covered when not in use to prevent a child from going in alone or falling in accidentally?

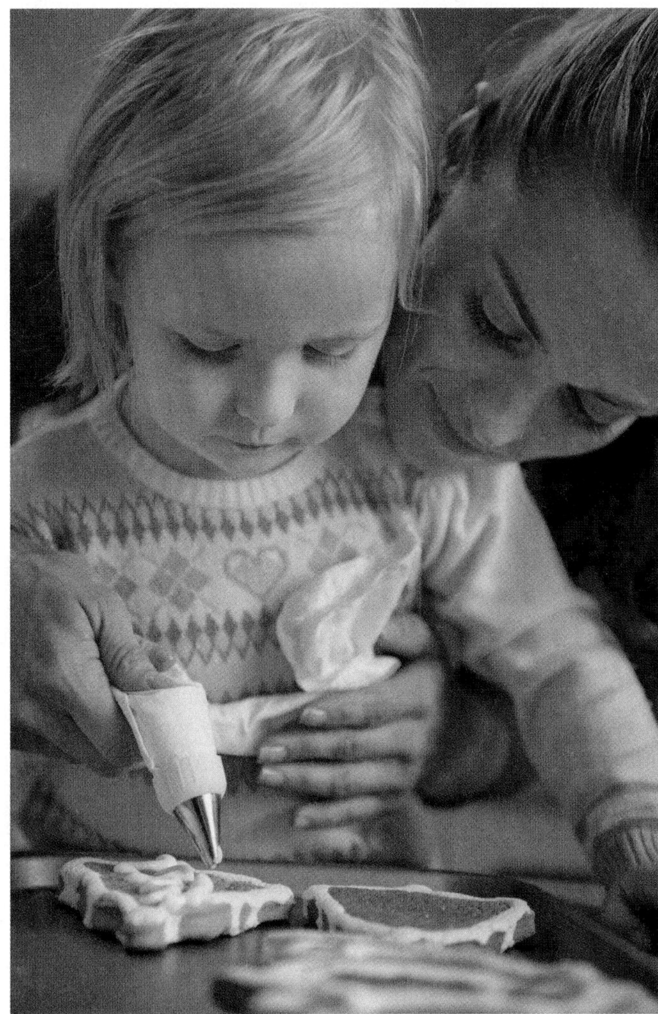

Developing shared traditions promotes family cohesion. *(Alliance/Fotolia)*

High costs and low income may limit the activities that families can do together, but should not eliminate them. At the aggregate level, the nurse can also obtain information on the types of leisure time activities available to families in the community through examination of the telephone book and Internet, personal observation of the community, or interviews with staff at recreational facilities.

Household and other safety practices. Safety practices such as the use of seat belts, infant safety seats, cribs with safe spacing between rails and proper mattress width, proper disposal of hazardous substances, and safety education for children are important considerations in family assessment. Are these behavioral safety factors evident in the household? Who is the person most attentive to family safety issues? What family behaviors contribute to health risks for members? The *Assessment Guidelines* section of the student resources site contains three guidelines for assessing safety issues in families. Two of the guidelines provide tips for assessing home safety for children and older adult family members, respectively, and the third addresses safety education issues for children and adolescents.

Sexuality and contraception. One additional behavioral consideration in assessing family health relates to sexual attitudes and practices and use of contraception. Once sufficient rapport has been established, the population health nurse would explore family needs for contraception or for assistance in discussing sexuality with adolescent family members. The population health nurse can identify family planning needs and make referrals for contraceptive services as needed.

The population health nurse would also explore family attitudes toward sexuality as well as sexual behaviors of family members. Families that have traditional, and particularly religion-based, attitudes toward sexual activity as being confined to marriage and occurring between a man and a woman, may have difficulty accepting and adjusting to an adolescent pregnancy or a gay, lesbian, or bisexual orientation of an individual family member. Similarly, acceptance of a transgendered family member may be difficult. The population health nurse may provide counseling for families dealing with sexuality issues or make referrals for assistance as needed. Nurses may also need to provide help in dealing with instances of sexual abuse within families. Tips for assessing sexuality issues as well as overall assessment of behavioral determinants influencing family health are provided in the *Focused Assessment* below. The questions provided reflect assessment of the individual family, but can be adapted to assess families at the aggregate level as well.

HEALTH SYSTEM DETERMINANTS. Factors related to the health system also affect family health. Two major considerations for individual families are family attitudes to health and response to illness and family use of available services. Aggregate-level considerations include the availability and effectiveness of health services provided to families in the population.

Family attitudes toward health and response to illness. Culturally determined attitudes toward health and illness also influence family health status. Families as a whole may see health promotion and illness prevention as a priority, or these activities may be valued for some family members and not others. For example, parents may make an effort to meet the health promotion needs of their children, but neglect their own needs or those of older family members. Similarly, family members may only seek health care when their ability to perform their respective functions is impaired. In part, this may be the result of cultural definitions of health and illness, but may also arise from lack of access to affordable health care services.

Family response to illness is another important influence on family health. How do family members deal with illness? Part of learning about this aspect of family life is determining who in the family decides when an ill family member should stay home from work or school and whether an ill member should receive health care. For example, in some families the mother decides who is ill and consults the father when she believes that the illness is severe enough to require the services of a health care provider. Family caregivers may themselves be in need of nursing intervention in order to function effectively in their caregiving role. As we saw earlier, family caregivers provide much of the care to ill family members. Unfortunately, they often receive

FOCUSED ASSESSMENT Assessing Behavioral Determinants of Family Health

- What are the food preferences and consumption patterns of the family? How are foods usually prepared? By whom?
- Do family members smoke or use or abuse alcohol or other substances?
- What medications are used by family members? Is medication use appropriate? Are medications stored safely?
- Do family members get adequate rest and exercise?
- What kinds of physical and leisure activities do family members engage in? Do leisure activities pose any health hazards?
- Do family members engage in appropriate safety precautions in the following areas?

  Consistent seat belt use
  Use of safety equipment such as eye and ear protection
  Use of infant safety seats
  Cribs with safe spacing between rails and proper mattress width
  Proper storage and disposal of hazardous substances
  Safety education of children regarding not talking to or going with strangers, crossing the street safely, and using seat belts and safety equipment such as helmets, goggles, and ear protection
  Safe use of appliances and craft equipment such as saws, glues, and drills
- Who in the family engages in sexual activity? Is there a need for contraceptives? What is the attitude of family members toward sexual activity?

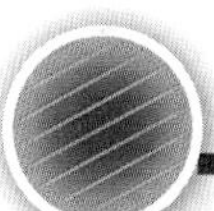

Evidence-Based Practice

Caregiver Burden

Several studies have shown that persons caring for family members with disabilities or chronic illness often experience caregiver burden with consequent physical and psychological health effects. Conduct a literature search for studies related to the positive and negative effects of family caregiving. Based on the literature, can you identify factors that would place family caregivers at particular risk for caregiver burden and its subsequent effects? What interventions have shown evidence of being effective in minimizing caregiver burden? How might population health nurses incorporate these interventions into their care of families?

little support from health care professionals in doing so. Too often, they are expected to accept responsibility for care without the required knowledge or abilities, and increased risk of institutionalization of an ill family may result from deterioration of either the ill member or the family caretaker. Population health nurses should assist family caregivers with the emotional as well as physical and cognitive challenges of caregiving.

Use of health care services. Family functions with respect to illness vary with the type of illness. For example, family functions in the case of acute illness include providing or obtaining health care, reassigning roles, and supporting the sick person. Additional functions in dealing with chronic illness include avoiding or coping with medical crises, preserving the family's quality of life, and arranging treatment modes and mechanisms. In the face of terminal illness, family functions also include dealing with shock and fear and minimizing pain and discomfort.

Do family members have a source of health care? Do they have health insurance? Often, there may be providers available for mothers and children because of federal and state programs. Fathers and other young adult males, however, are often excluded from these programs. The nurse may be asked to help families find health care for excluded family members who become ill.

Health care may be limited because of a lack of funds, language barriers, distance to health care facilities, transportation limitations, and many other problems. The nurse needs to determine these deterrents to access and find resources within the community to help families obtain health care. Occasionally, even when families have health insurance, members are not able to take full advantage of this resource because they do not understand what services are covered (or not covered). The nurse can help them understand insurance benefits or refer families to resources in the community who can explain insurance benefits and how to use them.

At the aggregate level, the population health nurse would assess the availability of health services needed by families in the population. What illness-preventive and health-promotive services are available? Are they accessible to all families in the population or only to certain subgroups? What services are available to resolve health problems or restore health?

Aggregate-level assessment also focuses on the effectiveness of health services provided to families in the population and the extent to which those services are utilized. For example, are prenatal services available but underutilized by families in the community or by certain segments of the community? Local figures on the proportion of pregnancies for which no prenatal care is received are one measure of service utilization. Similarly, the nurse might obtain data on the number of nonemergent visits to emergency departments suggesting inappropriate use of emergency services for routine illness. Accessibility and affordability of services available to families in the community should also be assessed. Again, general information on the types of services available can be gleaned from the telephone directory or Web. Information on costs and other accessibility issues (e.g., hours of operation, types of insurance taken) can best be obtained through interviews or surveys of local providers and health care agencies. Assessment tips related to health system influences on family health are provided in the *Focused Assessment* on page 350. A guideline for assessing overall family health status is included in the *Assessment Guidelines* section of the student resources site.

Diagnostic Reasoning and Care of Families

The data obtained during family health assessment enable the nurse to make informed decisions about the health care needs of families. These needs are stated in the form of nursing diagnoses. The population health nurse may develop nursing diagnoses related to individual families or to families as a group within the larger population. For example, the nurse may diagnose "family exhibiting ineffective coping related to changes in roles and relationships in a newly constituted stepfamily as evidenced by conflict between stepmother and stepchildren." An example of an aggregate family nursing diagnosis might be "families with chronically ill children at risk for increased stress related to lack of adequate community support services."

Planning and Implementing Health Care for Families

Not all families will require population health nursing intervention. Some indications of the need for intervention based on nursing diagnoses derived from the family health assessment include:

- Illness in a family member with a detrimental effect on the family unit

FOCUSED ASSESSMENT Assessing Health System Determinants of Family Health

- How does the family define health and illness? How does the family prioritize health in relation to other family needs and goals?
- How do family members deal with illness?
- Who makes health-related decisions in the family? Who carries out those decisions?
- What health-related behaviors do family members exhibit?
- What is the family's usual source of health care?
- Is the family's use of health care services appropriate?
- Does the family have health insurance? If so, are all family members covered? What services are covered?
- How adequate are health promotion, illness and injury prevention, health problem resolution, and health restoration services available to families?
- How available, accessible, and affordable are health services for families in the community?

- Family factors that contribute to ill health in a family member
- Recent diagnosis of serious illness in a family member
- Marked deterioration in the health status of a family member
- Hospital admission or discharge of a family member
- Missed or delayed developmental milestones
- Death of a family member
- Presence of psychological, environmental, sociocultural, behavioral, or health system factors detrimental to family health and function

When intervention is required, population health nurses plan nursing interventions to address identified needs. These interventions may be directed toward improving the health of specific families or of all families within a population and may take place at the promotion, prevention, resolution, or restoration levels of health care. Population-level interventions will often involve the creation or expansion of an infrastructure that supports effective family function and provides services needed by families in the population.

HEALTH PROMOTION AND ILLNESS/INJURY PREVENTION. Population health nurses can educate family members regarding the need for adequate nutrition, rest, and physical activity to promote health. Safety education and advocating use of safety devices or equipment are some potential approaches to health protection and injury prevention with families. Similarly, the nurse may teach family members how to minimize lead exposure in residential areas with high levels of lead contamination in soil or water or advocate with landlords for removal of lead-based paint or other safety hazards in older housing. Illness prevention may include teaching effective hygiene, referral for immunization, or advocating for access to safe water and food supplies as well as other interventions.

At the aggregate level, health promotion and prevention activities by population health nurses are likely to be directed toward advocacy for environmental protection and social justice or assuring the availability of health promotion and illness prevention services to families. For example, population health nurses may be actively involved in local initiatives to guarantee families a living wage or to assure that immunization and other health promotion and illness prevention services are available to low-income families.

Teaching coping skills and modeling effective communication strategies with adolescents are two interventions that population health nurses might employ to prevent family crises. The population health nurse may advocate for a balance between increasing independence and supervision of adolescents. Advocacy related to financial difficulties (e.g., linking families to available sources of financial support, employment assistance, and so on) may also help alleviate factors that contribute to family crises. Prevention of family crisis also includes providing anticipatory guidance related to common crises of family life and assisting families to develop effective coping strategies to combat the stress of situational crises.

It may be impossible, and sometimes undesirable, to prevent a crisis situation from occurring; however, the nurse can assist the family to prepare for and cope with the event. For example, the birth of a child or change of employment may be a very desirable event. Such an event requires changes in lifestyle and family adaptation that might precipitate a crisis. The nurse can assist the family to explore areas in which change will be required, avenues for accomplishing these changes, and strategies for dealing with the anxiety related to change. Through preventive activities implemented via anticipatory guidance, potential crises may be averted even though stressful events occur.

RESOLVING HEALTH PROBLEMS. Problem-resolution activities with families may be aimed at assisting families to obtain needed care for existing health problems or helping families to deal with these problems. For example, the nurse might facilitate a family meeting to discuss role allocation in order to minimize role overload for a few family members. Similarly, the nurse might refer a family with a substance-abusing member to community resources to help them deal with the problem. In the advocacy role, the nurse may help families explore treatment options or obtain approval for substance abuse treatment coverage under their insurance plan. The population health nurse might even engage in advocacy with an employer to assure access to an available employee assistance program (EAP).

Population health nurses may also be instrumental in linking families with other services needed to resolve existing family health problems. For example, they may encourage a wife and mother to remove herself and her children from an abusive situation as well as provide information where the woman can get help. In this instance, the nurse may need to advocate with local police or court officials for adequate protection for the woman and her children. At a more mundane level, the population health nurse may refer family members to sources of medical assistance to deal with existing illnesses. For example, the nurse may refer a family to a community clinic for treatment of the grandmother's hypertension.

Crisis intervention is an important element of problem resolution in the care of many families. Crisis intervention is directed toward helping members to discuss and define the problem and to express their feelings concerning the crisis situation. The nurse is an active listener and participates attentively, but the family must do the work. The emphasis is on bringing feelings out into the open. The nurse must be truthful, honest, and forthright, and should not give false reassurance about the situation.

Exploration of coping mechanisms already used enables the nurse to help the family examine ways to cope. The nurse's involvement includes helping the family to explore other options for dealing with the situation. The pros and cons of each of these alternatives should be discussed with the family. At this stage, the nurse may need to be fairly directive in assisting family members to implement agreed-upon strategies for resolving the crisis. For example, if the family has decided to confront a substance-abusing member with the need for treatment, the nurse may need to assign specific tasks to certain family members to implement the confrontation.

Advocacy for services to resolve family health problems may be needed at the population level. The population health nurse may be actively involved in alerting health policy makers to the need for family services and in initiating plans for programs to meet those needs. For example, if the nurse's assessment indicates that most families in the population are dual-earner or single-parent families whose needs for child care services are not being met, he or she may initiate community efforts to provide additional child care resources. Similarly, as seen in the *Advocacy Now* feature at the beginning of this chapter, knowledge of widespread violations of housing codes in rental housing for families identified by a population health nurse may lead to involvement of the housing authority and advocacy activities to promote code enforcement.

HEALTH RESTORATION. With respect to health restoration, population health nurses may assist families to cope with long-term health problems or to deal with the consequences of those problems in ways that promote an optimal level of health. For example, a nurse might suggest home modifications that permit a disabled family member to be more functional within the family or help a family coping with Alzheimer's disease to locate respite care. Another example of health restoration for a family is assisting families to deal with the loss of a loved one, particularly during holidays and anniversaries.

After successful resolution of a crisis, health restoration activities might involve following up with the family to help them recognize their use of the problem-solving process, identify how the crisis might have been averted if possible, and engage in activities that will prevent future crises from occurring.

Health restoration activities may also occur at the aggregate level. For example, the population health nurse might advocate for the development of respite services for family caretakers or create support groups for crisis-prone families to help them avoid future crises.

Evaluating Family Care

Evaluation of family care begins as the nurse examines the adequacy of assessment data and continues as he or she evaluates alternative approaches to meeting families' health needs. Post-intervention evaluation focuses on the achievement of mutually agreed-upon objectives for family care and the processes and structures that promote accomplishment of these objectives.

Evaluation will occur at the level of individual families who receive care and at the population level. With respect to the care of individual families, the nurse would examine whether care has resulted in expected family outcomes. Is the family better able to cope with stress? Have communications between parents and adolescent children improved? The nurse would also assess the appropriateness of interventions employed and the quality of their implementation. Were the interventions appropriate to the family's cultural beliefs and practices? To the family's educational level? Did the family experience frustration in following through on referrals because the nurse did not select appropriate resources or did not effectively prepare the family to act on the referral?

At the aggregate level, evaluation will focus on outcomes and processes of care for groups of families rather than individual families. Is respite care readily available to families that need it? Is respite care provided in the most cost-effective manner? What are the effects of respite care on the level of stress experienced by families with disabled members? These and other questions can address outcome and process evaluation of programs designed to serve groups of families within the population.

Much of the work of population health nurses involves care of families in a variety of health care settings. Family care should be based on the principles presented in this chapter and should contribute to the improvement of the overall health status of the population in which the family lives. Use of the nursing process in the context of population-focused care permits population health nurses to meet the health needs of individual families as well as those of the larger community.

CHAPTER RECAP

Population health nurses provide care to individual families and design, implement, and evaluate programs to meet the needs of groups of families within the larger population. Family care may be based on a variety of theoretical perspectives on the family, including systems, life cycle, and symbolic interactionist perspectives.

Provision of care to individual families and groups of families in the population employs the nursing process to direct nursing intervention. Assessment of family health status and of the needs of groups of families within the population addresses biological, psychological, environmental, sociocultural, behavioral, and health system determinants that influence the health of individual families and families in the larger population. Population health nurses plan and implement activities related to health promotion, illness and injury prevention, problem resolution, and health restoration for individual families and at the population level. Similarly, evaluation of the effectiveness of care occurs at both individual and population levels.

CASE STUDY A Family in Need

Alfinia Michaels is a 45-year-old single parent of two children, a boy of 8 years and a girl of 5. She has recently been diagnosed with breast cancer and is scheduled to have a lumpectomy and reconstruction of her right breast in 2 weeks. Ms. Michaels is divorced and is responsible for the care of her 79-year-old father who has mild Alzheimer's disease. Her father is still capable of caring for himself during the day while she works, but cannot be left alone overnight and cannot care for the children. Ms. Michaels has one sister who lives approximately 150 miles away. She states that she and her sister have always been close. Ms. Michaels's former husband lives in the same community. He provides child support and health insurance for the children and takes them every other weekend. Ms. Michaels does not have health insurance because she works two part-time jobs, neither of which includes benefits. She tells the population health nurse she doesn't have any idea how she will pay for her surgery and the chemotherapy that will follow. She is worried about care of her father and her children during her hospitalization and afterward.

- What biological, psychological, environmental, sociocultural, behavioral, and health system factors are influencing this situation?
- Is this a crisis situation? If so, what type of crisis would this be?
- What nursing interventions might the population health nurse employ with this family?
- How might the nurse evaluate the effectiveness of nursing intervention?
- How might your interventions be different if you find that many families in the population are experiencing similar problems?

REFERENCES

American Academy of Pediatrics. (2014). *Different types of families: A portrait gallery.* Retrieved from http://www.healthychildren.org/English/family-life/family-dynamics/types-of-families/Pages/Different-Types-of-Familes-A-Portrait-Gallery.aspx

American Association of Retired Persons. (n.d.). *Grandfacts: State fact sheets for grandparents and other relatives raising children.* Retrieved from http://www.aarp.org/relationships/friends-family/grandfacts-sheets/?MP=KNC-360I-GOOGLE-REL-FRI&HBX_PK=grandparents_raising_children&utm_source=GOOGLE&utm_medium=cpc&utm_term=grandparents%2Braising%2Bchildren&utm_campaign=G_Grandfacts&360cid=SI_308824835_10641909541_1

Anngela-Cole, L., & Hilton, J. M. (2009). The role of caregiver attitudes and culture in family care giving for older adults. *Home Health Care Services Quarterly, 28,* 59–83. doi:10.1080/01621420903014790

Berg, J. M., Loth, K., Hanson, C., Croll-Lampert, J., & Neumark-Sztainer, D. (2012). Family life cycle transitions and the onset of eating disorders. *Journal of Clinical Nursing, 21,* 1355–1363. doi:10.1111/j.1365-2702.2011.03762.x

Carlson, E. (2013). Precepting and symbolic interactionism: A theoretical look at preceptorship during clinical practice. *Journal of Advanced Nursing, 69,* 457–464. doi: 10.1111/j.1365-2648.2012.06047.x

Carter, B., & McGoldrick, M. (1999). Overview: The expanded family life cycle: Individual, family, and social perspectives. In B. Carter & M. McGoldrick (Eds.), *The expanded family, life cycle: Individual, family and social perspectives* (3rd ed., pp. 1–26). Boston, MA: Allyn & Bacon.

Carthon, M. B. (2011). Making ends meet: Community networks and health promotion among Blacks in the City of Brotherly Love. *American Journal of Public Health, 101,* 1392–1401. doi:10.2105/AJPH.2011.300125

Chen, J.-Y., & Clark, M. J. (2010). Family resources and parental health in families of children with Duchenne muscular dystrophy. *Journal of Nursing Research, 18,* 239–248.

Cornish, A. (2013a). *Blending: Is there a right way?* Retrieved from http://www.blendedfamilyfocus.com/a-right-way/

Cornish, A. (2013b). *What is a blended family?* Retrieved from http://www.blendedfamilyfocus.com/what-is-a-blended-family/

Dallos, R., & Draper, R. (2010). *An introduction to family therapy: Systemic theory and practice* (3rd ed.). New York, NY: McGraw-Hill.

Dupuis, S. (2010). Examining the blended family: The application of systems theory toward an understanding of the blended family system. *Journal of Couple & Relationship Therapy, 9,* 239–251. doi:10.1080/15332691.2010.491784

Duvall, E., & Miller, B. (1990). *Marriage and family development* (6th ed.). New York, NY: Harper College.

Family Ties. (n.d.a). *What are the family types?* Retrieved from http://www.edu.pe.ca/southernkings/familytypes.htm

Family Ties. (n.d.b). *What is a family?* Retrieved from http://www.edu.pe.ca/southernkings/familydefinition.htm

Feinberg, L., Reinhard, S. C., Houser, A., & Choula, R. (2011). *Valuing the invaluable: 2011 update on the growing contributions and costs of family caregiving.* Retrieved from http://assets.aarp.org/rgcenter/ppi/ltc/i51-caregiving.pdf

Fleming, W. M. (n.d.). Family systems theory—Basic concepts/propositions. In *Marriage and family encyclopedia.* Retrieved from http://family.jrank.org/pages/597/Family-Systems-Theory-Basic-Concepts-Propositions.html

Gecas, V., & Tsushima, T. (n.d.). Symbolic interactionism—Symbolic interactionism and family studies. In *Marriage and family encyclopedia.* Retrieved from http://family.jrank.org/pages/1677/Symbolic-Interactionism-Symbolic-Interactionism-Family-Studies.html

Genopro. (n.d.a). *Family systems theory.* Retrieved from http://www.genopro.com/genogram/family-systems-theory/

Genopro. (n.d.b). *Introduction to the genogram.* Retrieved from http://www.genopro.com/genogram/

Genopro. (n.d.c). *Rules to build genograms.* Retrieved from http://www.genopro.com/genogram/rules/

Genopro. (n.d.d). *Symbols used in genogram.* Retrieved from http://www.genopro.com/genogram/symbols/

Goyer, A. (2010). *More grandparents raising grandkids.* http://www.aarp.org/relationships/grandparenting/info-12-2010/more_grandparents_raising_grandchildren.html

Hall, G. B., Dollard, M. F., Tuckey, M. R., Winefield, A. H., & Thompson, B. M. (2010). Job demands work-family conflict and emotional exhaustion in police officers. *Journal of Occupational and Organizational Psychology, 83,* 237–250. doi:10.1348/096317908X401723

Healthwise. (2013). *Family life cycle—Topic overview.* Retrieved from http://children.webmd.com/tc/family-life-cycle-topic-overview

Kelly, E. L., Moen, P., & Tranby, E. (2011). Changing workplaces to reduce work-family conflict: Schedule control in a white-collar organization. *American Sociological Review, 76,* 265-209. doi: 10.1177/0003122411400056

McCubbin, H. I., & Patterson, J. M. (1983). The family stress process: The double ABCX model of adjustment and adaptation. *Marriage & Family Review,* 6(1), 7–37. doi:10.1300/J002v06n01_02

McCubbin, H. I., Thompson, A. I., & McCubbin, M. A. (2001). *Family measures: Stress, coping, and resiliency—Inventories for research and practice.* Honolulu, HI: Kamehameha Schools.

McCubbin, M. A., & McCubbin, H. I. (1993). Families coping with illness: The resiliency model of family stress, adjustment, and adaptation. In C. B. Danielson, B. Hamel-Bissell, & P. Winstead-Fry (Eds.), *Families, health and illness: Perspectives on coping and intervention* (pp. 21–63). St. Louis, MO: Mosby.

McDonald, L. (n.d.). *Hill's theory of family stress and buffers: Build the protective factor of social relationships and positive perception with multifamily groups.* Retrieved from http://cecp.air.org/vc/presentations/2selective/3lmcdon/HILL'S_FAMILY_STRESS_THEORY_AND_FAST.htm

Milliken, P. J., & Schrieber, R. (2012). Examining the nexus between grounded theory and symbolic interactionism. *International Journal of Qualitative Methods, 11,* 684–696.

Missouri Department of Social Services, Children's Division. (2011). *Child welfare manual* (Section 7, Chapter 25). Retrieved from http://www.dss.mo.gov/cd/info/cwmanual/section7/ch1_33/sec7ch25.htm

Munro, B., & Munro, G. (n.d.). Definition of family—Related constructs, inclusive definitions, theoretical definitions, situational definitions, normative definitions, conclusion. In *Marriage and family encyclopedia.* Retrieved from http://family.jrank.org/pages/492/Family-Definition.html

National Center for Health Statistics. (2014). *Smoking prevalence.* Retrieved from http://www.cdc.gov/nchs/fastats/smoking.htm

National Heart, Lung, and Blood Institute. (2013). *WE CAN: Ways to enhance children's activity and nutrition.* Retrieved from http://www.nhlbi.nih.gov/health/public/heart/obesity/wecan/get-active/index.htm

Nelson, P. T. (2012). *Surviving a family crisis.* Retrieved from http://extension.udel.edu/factsheet/surviving-a-family-crisis/

Shelton, T. (2010). *The 4 essentials types of family structure.* Retrieved from http://ezinearticles.com/?he-4-Essential-Types-of-Family-Structure&id=4658559

Slan-Jerusalim, R., & Chen, C. P. (2009). Work-family conflict and career development theories: A search for helping strategies. *Journal of Counseling & Development, 87,* 492–499. doi:10.1002/j.1556-6678.2009.tb00134.x

Suarez-Orozco, C., Bang, H. J., & Kim, H. Y. (2011). I felt like my heart was staying behind: Psychological implications of family separations and reunifications for immigrant youth. *Journal of Adolescent Research, 26,* 222–257. doi: 10.1177/0743558410376830

U.S. Census Bureau. (2012). *The 2012 statistical abstract: Population: Households, families, group quarters.* Retrieved from http://www.census.gov/compendia/statab/cats/population/households_families_group_quarters.html

VanKatwyk, P. L. (n.d.). *Family life cycle theory.* Retrieved from http://www.academia.edu/5696061/FAMILY_LIFE_CYCLE_THEORY1

von Bertalanffy, L. (1973). *General systems theory.* New York, NY: George Braziller.

von Bertalanffy, L. (1981). *A systems view of man.* Boulder, CO: Westview.

White, J., M. (n.d.). Family development theory—Basic concepts and propositions. In *Marriage and family encyclopedia.* Retrieved from http://family.jrank.org/pages/515/Family-Development-Theory-Basic-Concepts-Propositions.html

Williams, J. C., & Boushey, H. (2010). *The three faces of work-family conflict: The poor, the professionals and the missing middle.* Retrieved from http://www.americanprogress.org/wp-content/uploads/issues/2010/01/pdf/threefaces.pdf

Wright, L. M., & Leahey, M. (2013). *Nurses and families: A guide to family assessment and intervention* (6th ed.). Philadelphia, PA: F. A. Davis.

CHAPTER

15 Care of Communities and Target Populations

Learning Outcomes

After reading this chapter, you should be able to:

1. Discuss the rationale for engaging members of the population in every phase of population health assessment and health program planning, implementation, and evaluation.
2. Describe factors related to each of the six categories of determinants of health to be addressed in assessing the health of a population.
3. Describe the components of a population nursing diagnosis.
4. Identify five tasks in planning health programs to meet the needs of populations.
5. Analyze the elements of a program theory or logic model and its usefulness in health program planning.
6. Describe four levels of acceptance of a health care program.
7. Describe the six steps in the process of evaluating a health care program.

Key Terms

asset mapping
community assessment
community engagement
comprehensive community engagement strategy (CCES)
empowerment evaluation
geographic information systems (GISs)
key informants
outcome measures
outcome objectives
planning
population
process objectives
program theory
windshield survey

Advocacy Then

Store Front Health Services

In 1965, Nancy Milio, a young White public health nurse working for the Detroit Visiting Nurses Association, was frustrated with her inability to connect with residents of a largely Black neighborhood for which she was responsible. After identifying a need for locally provided prenatal care, she submitted a proposal for a clinic to the mayor's office. Although the proposal was not accepted, it was later funded by the Office of Economic Opportunity, an element of then President Lyndon Johnson's War on Poverty (Milio, 1970).

Recognizing a need for buy-in from local residents, Milio invited several local women to participate in discussions regarding the project's design. As a result of these discussions, the project morphed from a prenatal clinic to include a day-care center eventually named "Moms and Tots." Local residents were hired to do the required renovations for the site, and men and women living in the area were employed as staff, with the only qualification being a commitment to the success of the project. Help was also sought from outside agencies to provide needed follow-up for prenatal clients and to address other needs encountered in the prenatal and child care clientele (Milio, 1970).

As time passed, residents began to expand the services provided by the center to address needs identified in the neighborhood. These included boys and girls clubs, health education, and other services. When a racial incident on the street where the center was located resulted in withdrawal of support from both health and social service agencies, residents were sufficiently empowered to initiate a campaign to find alternate funding, in which they were successful. The restored funding allowed them to increase the day-care hours, provide transportation, and meet other community needs (Milio, 1970).

In July of 1967, racial conflicts resulted in 3 days of riots in and around the neighborhood. The center, located at 9226 Kercheval Street, was one of the few buildings that was not burned or looted.

Advocacy Now

Meeting the Population's Needs

Jeffrey Brenner, a physician, was called to the scene of a shooting near his house in Camden, New Jersey. When he arrived, he was the first person to try to help the victim, although police were already on the scene. Despite his efforts, the man died (Gawande, 2011).

As a medical student, Brenner had volunteered in a free clinic for Hispanic immigrants. Following graduation and a family practice residency, he was employed at a family practice clinic in Camden. Appointed as a citizen member of a police reform commission, he learned about mapping criminal events and centering resources in high-crime areas. When local police refused to create the crime maps, Brenner began mapping data on assaults obtained from emergency department records at three local hospitals. His maps indicated where victims lived in the city. Eventually, he expanded his data collection to include other health-related events, such as falls. Based on the data, he identified two city blocks in Camden that contributed to a large proportion of health care costs, and noted that approximately 1% of the population accounted for 30% of medical costs (Gawande, 2011).

Armed with his cost data, Brenner convinced local emergency department personnel to help him identify their most difficult and expensive patients. He began to follow these individuals and worked with a nurse practitioner to help meet their needs. Much of his effort involved the type of case management a population health nurse would provide. With funding from small grants, he was able to hire a small staff that operated with desk space at a local hospital. The group, called the Camden Coalition of Healthcare Providers, provides services through home visits and telephone calls because there isn't any funding for a clinic. As a result of their efforts, they have improved the health and reduced the health care utilization of "super users," people who use extensive and costly health care services as a result of poor disease management. In fact, they have reduced ED visits for this group by 40% and health care costs by 56%. Overall, the project results demonstrated that concentrating on the most expensive clients within a population can improve population health and decrease health care costs (Gawande, 2011).

Nowhere is the advocacy role of population health nurses more apparent than in the care of population groups. From the beginnings of population health nursing in the United States, population health nurses have been assessing the needs of population groups and planning and implementing programs to meet those needs. As noted several times in earlier chapters, the focus of population health nursing is on the health of population groups or aggregates. In many instances, this focus entails providing care to communities, target groups within communities, or other population groups. For our purposes, a **population** encompasses the human inhabitants of a given geographic area that might be as large as the entire world, a country, or state, or as small as a specific community or neighborhood. A community, as we saw in Chapter 1∞, is a group of people who share common interests, who interact with each other, and who function collectively within a defined social structure to address common concerns. Communities are smaller segments that make up a population. Unlike members of a community, members of a population may or may not share common interests, act collectively, or function within a defined social structure. A target group or target population is a subgroup within the population whose members exhibit particular health needs (such as victims of family violence), are at particular risk for the development of problems (e.g., members of refugee groups), or are the intended audience for a particular health-related initiative.

This care of whole population groups is sometimes referred to as population health management, which was defined in Chapter 1∞. Population health management involves health promotion and illness prevention strategies at the aggregate level designed to improve overall population health status.

Although population health nurses have long been involved in advocacy and program development to address the health needs of population groups, this focus was subsumed within care of individuals and families for many years. For example, a set of objectives for public health nursing developed by the National Organization for Public Health Nursing (NOPHN) in 1931 focused on the care of individuals and families, with community-level initiatives aimed at developing resources to meet their needs. By 1949, a new statement of *Public Health Nursing Responsibilities in a Community Health Program*, also by NOPHN, reflected an expanded focus for public health nursing in population-based program planning. According to this statement, population health nurses were expected not only to participate in planning nursing services but also to address social problems affecting health (Abrams, 2004). Most recently, in 2013, the Quad Council, an association of nursing organizations with a focus on population health, revised the "Public Health Nursing: Scope and Standards of Practice" maintaining this focus on population health, with care of individuals and families within the context of population-level practice (American Nurses Association [ANA], 2013). Today, skills in population assessment and program planning are expected of nurses prepared for beginning level population health nursing.

Community Engagement and Population-Based Health Initiatives

Most population-based health care interventions are developed in collaboration with members of other professions and the population rather than by population health nurses in isolation. In the past, interventions for population groups frequently entailed health professionals' identification of problems and development and implementation of programs to solve them with minimal input from group members. More recently, health professionals have advocated the involvement of members of the population at all stages of intervention, from participation in identifying population needs and capabilities to the development, implementation, and evaluation of programs that enhance local capacity to meet those needs. This involvement is termed **community engagement**, which has been defined as "the actions that agencies take to enable them to consult, involve, listen and respond to communities through ongoing relationships and dialogue" (Local Government Association, 2012, para. 7).

Benefits of Engagement

Incorporating members of the population in the identification of and planning to resolve health-related issues has a variety of advantages that are summarized in the *Highlights* box below. In the past, public health professionals tended to inform members of the population about health issues and programs designed to address them. Community engagement, however, necessitates two-way communication between members of the population and policy makers or health care providers. Effective two-way communication is characterized by collaboration and talking *with*, rather than *to* members of the population, seeking common ground, accepting responsibility rather than exerting authority, and understanding of different points of view. Two-way communication is both top-down and bottom-up and acknowledges values that provide the foundation for attitudes and actions (Minnesota Department of Health, n.d.).

Models for Engagement

A number of models have been developed to promote engagement of populations in the resolution of health-related issues. Among these are the Asset-Based Community Development (ABCD) model (McKnight, 2013), the Association for Community Health Improvement (ACHI) model, the Cultural Complementarity Model (Minnesota Department of Health, n.d.), and the Active Community Engagement (ACE) Continuum (Doggett, 2010). The ABCD model focuses on identifying and using population strengths, assets, and resources to address problems and issues in the population. Rather than focusing on deficits, the model emphasizes using existing strengths to create new opportunities and address issues. Often, populations and communities include a wide variety of resources and skills that are not being effectively mobilized to promote population health. According to the model, community members possess gifts or assets that can be used to meet the needs of other members or to develop solutions to overall community problems. Assets are distributed by means of connections between members of the community and between associations formed by community members (McKnight, 2013).

The ACHI model focuses on education and the development of leadership and other skills within the population along with the dissemination of practical tools to promote engagement and collaboration among multiple sectors of the population. Specific areas of focus of the association include access to care, chronic disease prevention and management, community benefit practices among health care establishments, collaborative strategies, and the use of measurement and evaluation techniques to establish goals and judge progress toward their achievement (Minnesota Department of Health, n.d.).

The Cultural Complementarity Model focuses on the strengths represented by cultural diversity within the population. Within the model, initiatives focus on developing "circle consensus" characterized by shared rights and responsibilities, the concept of *power with* rather than *power over* members of the population, sharing of resources rather than competition for them, an inclusive approach and exchange among all parties, shared learning, and concerted efforts to eliminate racist thinking and attitudes (Minnesota Department of Health, n.d.).

The ACE Continuum conceptualizes engagement as an evolving process of increasing public involvement in health assessment and program development and evaluation processes. In the model, engagement occurs across three levels that reflect progressively greater involvement in decision making and control (Doggett, 2010). The three levels of engagement are consultation, cooperation, and collaboration. At the consultative level, community members provide input regarding needs and program design at the request of an agency. Cooperation is characterized by greater involvement of members of the population in assessment and decision making, while at the collaborative level, officials and members of the public share power and responsibility for needs identification, program design, and evaluation.

Each level of involvement addresses four elements of engagement at progressively increasing levels. The four elements are: (a) involvement in assessment, (b) access to information, (c) inclusion in planning and decision making, and (d) local capacity to advocate with institutions and governing structures (Doggett, 2010). A fifth consideration is the

Highlights

Benefits of Community Engagement

- A focus on social justice: Community engagement results in shared power and resources and incorporates segments of the population that are often voiceless.
- Cultural acceptability of services: Community engagement leads to the development of culturally sensitive and appropriate services that are acceptable to members of the population.
- Development of trust: Incorporating members of the population in identification and intervention related to health issues builds trust in health care authorities and increases their credibility with members of the population.
- Supports outreach: Population members included in planning can serve as ambassadors to others in the population, explaining the need and rationale for services and delivery systems.
- Improved connections: Community engagement strengthens connections among members of the population and social service agencies, creating a greater sense of community.
- Leadership development: Engagement of members of the population enhances their leadership skills in health and other arenas.
- Critical reflection: Community engagement promotes reflection on the knowledge and values that provide a foundation for collaborative efforts (Minnesota Department of Health, n.d.).

TABLE 15-1 Components of the Active Community Engagement (ACE) Continuum

Characteristic of Engagement	Consultation	Cooperation	Collaboration
Involvement in assessment	Population members provide input via community forums to refine programs designed by government agency to address STDs	Population members engage in dialogue with representatives of government agency to identify issues and factors related to STD incidence	Population and agency members share power in determing issues to be addressed related to STD incidence
Access to information	Government agency informs the public about STD issues	Population agents disseminate STD information to the public	Population agents facilitate dialogue with other members of the public regarding STD issues
Inclusion in decision making	Agency members solicit input/ approval from population leaders at start of programs	Population leaders and advisory groups involved in decision making related to STD services	Community-based organizations (CBOs) and groups collaborate in design of STD services
Capacity to advocate	Agency engages in community outreach	Agency builds capacity of local leadership and advisory groups to oversee STD services	Collaborative efforts to build CBO capacity and promote organizational links to address STD issues
Accountability to the public	Agency develops STD services/ policies with minimal population input	Systems exist for citizen participation in policy development	Population members have power equal to agency to determine policy directions and resource allocation

Adapted from: Doggett, E. (2010). *Community engagement in the PEPFAR Special Initiative on Sexual and Gender-based Violence.* Retrieved from http://www.healthpolicyinitiative.com/Publications/Documents/1288_1_PEPFAR_GBV_Community_Engagement_FINAL_acc.pdf

accountability to community members exhibited by the health or governmental organization. Table 15-1● applies the elements of the model to population engagement in addressing the issue of increased incidence of sexually transmitted diseases (STDs) in the population. For further information on the ABCD, ACHI, and ACE models, see the resources provided in the *External Resources* section of the student resources site.

Principles of Engagement

The U.S. federal government has developed principles for engaging populations in health care delivery decisions. These principles, as published by the Clinical and Translational Science Awards Consortium & Community Engagement Key Function Committee Task Force on the Principles of Community Engagement (2011), are presented in the *Highlights* box on the next page. Additional principles derived from experience in engaging communities in health care planning are also included. Although the principles address engagement of communities, they are applicable to engagement efforts with any of the populations with which population health nurses may work.

Developing a Comprehensive Community Engagement Strategy

Because multiple agencies within a population may seek to promote community engagement, it is helpful if some sort of overall engagement strategy can be developed to minimize overlap and prevent exhausting the time and energy resources of members of the population. Public and voluntary agencies within a locality may want to consider developing a comprehensive community engagement strategy. A **comprehensive community engagement strategy (CCES)** is a coordinated approach to community engagement that involves multiple local partners (Improvement and Development Agency for Local Government, 2009). Benefits of a CCES include greater efficiency in service delivery, improved community cohesion, greater accountability among partners, improved public satisfaction with services, better knowledge of the array of available resources, improved relations between members of the population and decision makers, a bottom-up approach to service improvement, and improved health outcomes. Although specific elements of a CCES may vary from group to group, the *Highlights* box on the next page provides some guidelines on features to be included.

Population health nurses may be instrumental in initiating development of a CCES. Because of their intimate familiarity with the population, they can also help to identify partners to be involved in development of the CCES as well as individuals in the population who can be targeted for engagement efforts.

Nursing Care of Populations

As we have seen, the focus of population health nursing practice is the care of entire populations, whether large populations (e.g., residents of a state or nation) or smaller groups (e.g., members of a community, neighborhood, or target group within a larger population). In caring for populations, population health nurses employ the same steps of the nursing process as are used in the care of individuals and families: assessment, diagnosis, planning, implementation, and evaluation. Each of these steps will be discussed in the context of caring for population groups.

Highlights

Principles of Community Engagement

- Establish the purpose of engagement and the populations to be engaged.
- Develop an organizational culture that values and actively pursues engagement of members of the population served. This requires strong organizational leadership in support of engagement.
- Create a locally based planning mechanism that incorporates ongoing input from members of the population. An infrastructure that supports engagement is also needed.
- Learn about the population's culture, economic conditions, social networks, political and power structures, norms and values, history and demographic trends, history, and experience with other engagement efforts. Determine how the population perceives those promoting engagement.
- Establish trusting relationships, work with formal and informal leaders, and seek commitment from community organizations and leaders to create processes for mobilizing the community.
- Accept that collective self-determination is the responsibility and right of all people in a population. No external entity can bestow on a group the power to act in its own self-interest.
- Recognize that partnerships are essential to engagement.
- Recognize and respect diversity and factors affecting diversity within the population.
- Recognize the potential negative effects of external events on population engagement (e.g., shifts in funding priorities of governmental agencies) and work to minimize them as much as possible.
- Incorporate members of the population into all aspects of population assessment, program planning, implementation, and evaluation.
- Link community planning to ongoing operational management of programs established.
- Sustain community engagement by identifying and mobilizing population assets and strengths and by developing the population's capacity and resources to make decisions and take action.
- Create accessible ways for members of the population to become engaged and to track progress on meeting priorities established and plans made.
- Be prepared to release control of actions or interventions to members of the population and be flexible enough to meet changing needs.
- Recognize the need for long-term commitment by all parties.
- Sustain health improvements through policy and system changes.

Data from: Clinical and Translational Science Awards Consortium & Community Engagement Key Function Committee Task Force on the Principles of Community Engagement. (2011). *Principles of community engagement* (2nd ed.). Retrieved from http://www.atsdr.cdc.gov/communityengagement/pdf/PCE_Report_508_FINAL.pdf

Assessing Population Health Status

A **community assessment** is defined as "an effort to identify and prioritize a community's health needs, accomplished by collecting and analyzing data, including input from the community" (Bilton, 2011, p. 21). The assessment forms the basis for health care planning and assists in targeting services, raising community awareness of issues to be addressed, provides benchmarks for determining progress in addressing needs, and promotes collaboration in improving health. The Patient Protection and Affordable Care Act mandates that charitable hospitals conduct an assessment of the health status and needs of the population served by the institution every 3 years in order to retain their tax-exempt status. By law, the assessment by a health organization must include input from persons who "represent the broad interests of its community, including those with special knowledge or expertise in public health"

Highlights

Elements of a Comprehensive Community Engagement Strategy

- Shared values and principles: A statement of explicit commitment to empowering and engaging members of the population in assessment, program planning and implementation, and evaluation.
- Targets and priorities: Identification of key issues for collaboration and the extent and mechanisms of collaboration.
- Roles and responsibilities of partners: Identification of partner roles and responsibilities and mechanisms for monitoring their execution.
- Shared resources: Identification of resources available and how they will be allocated.
- Shared learning programs: Joint expenditures on capacity building and training for members of the population that build the skills needed for engagement and involvement.
- Information sharing: Determination of what information will be shared and how, as well as protocols for disaggregating data in ways that are useful for partners, an overall calendar of engagement activities, and a database of community and volunteer organizations.
- Multi-partner structures: Identification of linkages among organizations and agencies, shared structures, and approaches to development of area councils.
- Coordinated support for community networks.
- Joint actions: Approaches to be taken to engage population members and build social capital.

Data from: Improvement and Development Agency for Local Government, Urban Forum and the National Association for Voluntary and Community Action. (2009). *Developing Your Comprehensive Community Engagement Strategy— A Practical Guide for Local Strategic Partnerships.* Retrieved from http://www.navca.org.uk/existing/NR/rdonlyres/36e222bb-ee81-4c13-b60f-0278db6d4d46/0/cces_guide_2009_03.pdf

(Rosenbaum, 2013, p. 3). In addition, facilities must report to the Internal Revenue Service regarding action plans to address identified population health needs. Several basic principles of community assessment have been identified in the literature. These principles include the following:

- Incorporation of multisector collaboration in all phases of community health improvement, including assessment, planning, investment, implementation, and evaluation
- Broad community engagement in the process
- Use of a sufficiently broad definition of community to allow population-wide interventions and a targeted focus on disparities in the population
- Promotion of maximum transparency and accountability
- Use of high-quality data derived from and shared with diverse sources
- Use of evidence-based and innovative interventions
- Evaluation to promote continuous improvement (Rosenbaum, 2013).

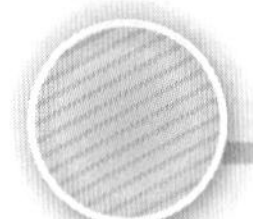

Global Perspectives

Voluntary Nursing Service in Japan

Kenkounippon21 is a national mandate in Japan much like *Healthy People 2020* in the United States. As this mandate for health promotion through individual and social efforts was being developed, the Japanese Nursing Association was developing a new system of community nursing services that included the use of volunteer services. An assessment of community needs indicated a need for education and consultation services for clients with minor health problems. Based on this assessment, community health nursing faculty met with the local nursing association to propose a project to meet this need. They also visited the city office, met with the director of health promotion and local public health nurses, and visited a nursing alumni association and a medical association in the community. All of them agreed to collaborate in initiating a new voluntary nursing service. The local nursing association provided the funds; the city office provided the place; the nursing alumni association recruited volunteer nurses; and the medical association supported the new service. Nursing faculty members wrote grants to purchase equipment to measure bone mass, energy expenditure, blood pressure, and body mass index.

The nursing faculty group established a center to provide volunteer nursing services. The center is open on Saturdays from 2 to 4 p.m. twice a month at a citizens' plaza. The location is easily accessible to community members, and they can choose among a variety of free services, including nursing guidance and education, health measurement, and information and referral services. Through their ability to network with multiple segments of society, these nurses have created a program that meets the needs of both individual clients and the community.

Ariko Noji, PhD, RN Chiba University College of Nursing, Chiba, Japan

THE ASSESSMENT PROCESS. A number of organizations, such as Catholic Health Association of the United States (2013), the Iowa Department of Public Health (2013) and the Association for Community Health Improvement (ACHI, n.d.a, n.d.b; Bilton, 2011) have identified the steps in the community or population health assessment process that are depicted in Table 15-2●. The steps incorporated in the table address both the assessment and diagnosis phases of the nursing process, and the priority setting step sets the stage for planning, which will be discussed later in this chapter.

Usually, a wide variety of data are collected in a population assessment. The breadth and depth of data collected will vary somewhat depending on the scope of the assessment, but for a comprehensive assessment of population health status, data on all aspects of health and factors that affect health are required. Assessment data may be either quantitative or qualitative. *Quantitative* data reflect numbers of people, characteristics, or events within the population. Examples of quantitative data include the number of people in specific age or ethnic groups and the rates of specific diseases and causes of death within the population. *Qualitative* data focus on perceptions of health, attitudes, and health concerns as voiced by members of the population. For example, population members' identification of adolescent pregnancy, substance abuse, and lack of affordable housing as health-related problems reflects qualitative data.

Population assessment data may be obtained in several ways including use of focus groups, key informant interviews, surveys of residents, secondary analysis of existing data, and use of data from geographic information systems (GISs). A focus group consists of people who have personal experience of the topic of interest and who meet to discuss their perceptions of that topic. Perspectives may be formulated or changed in the context of group discussion, and the nature of the interaction among focus group participants is itself considered data.

Assessment team members might also interview members of the community and key informants. **Key informants** are people who, because of their position, possess information and insights about the population. Key informants include both formal and informal leaders. Examples of key informants include public officials, school and health care personnel, prominent businesspeople, and local clergy. Again, it is important not to restrict interviews to these sources, but also to interview typical residents because of the possible differences in perceptions of the population's health needs. General surveys of members of the population may also be used to collect either quantitative or qualitative assessment data.

Population assessment data may already exist in other forms. For example, the local health department will have a variety of data on the incidence of specific communicable diseases and may also collect additional data on a routine basis. Data may also be obtained from the records of health care providers and institutions, service agencies, civic organizations, and other groups. Data from other focused assessments may also be available. For example, a local agency may have collected data related to transportation needs among the elderly.

TABLE 15-2 Steps in the Community/Population Assessment Process

Step	Tasks
Create an infrastructure to support the assessment	• Obtain leadership support • Determine team membership and roles • Create a work plan and time line • Determine resource needs • Develop a budget • Identify and engage community stakeholders
Define the assessment scope and purpose	• Identify the geographic area/population to be assessed • Identify the data needed and possible data sources • Identify users of assessment data and their information needs • Clarify the potential uses of assessment data • Identify data collection tools, strategies, and roles
Profile the population	• Collect data on key characteristics of the population • Collect data related to the health status of the population • Identify positive and negative factors affecting population health status • Identify currently available services • Obtain residents' perspectives on health and health needs • Examine findings in light of local and national priorities for health
Analyze data	• Compare findings with those for other populations • Examine trends over time • Identify discrepancies in data (e.g., statistical findings vs. resident perceptions) • Identify population assets as well as needs
Identify action priorities	• Identify relevant values and criteria for priority setting • Determine whose priorities will be addressed • Determine the number of priority issues that can be addressed initially • Decide on priority issues based on the number of people affected, the impact on their lives, equity, and availability of potential solutions and required expertise
Document and disseminate results	• Create key messages for relevant audiences • Develop plans for dialogue and communication regarding results

Data from: Association for Community Health Improvement. (n.d.a). *Assessment process map.* Retrieved from http://www.assesstoolkit.org/assesstoolkit/introassessment.jsp#; Association for Community Health Improvement. (n.d.b). *Introduction to the Association for Community Health Improvement's Community Health Assessment Toolkit.* Retrieved from http://www.assesstoolkit.org/assesstoolkit/ACHI-CHAT-intro-slides-8-27-10.pdf; Bilton, M. (2011, October). Community health needs assessment (Executive briefing 3). *Trustee,* 21–24; Catholic Health Association of the United States. (2013). *Assessing and addressing community health needs.* Retrieved from http://www.chausa.org/docs/default-source/general-files/cb_assessingaddressing-pdf.pdf?sfvrsn=4; Iowa Department of Public Health. (2013). *Community health needs assessment and health improvement plan (CHNA&HIP) guide.* Retrieved from http://www.idph.state.ia.us/chnahip/Guide.aspx

Asset mapping is another means of collecting data about a community, particularly regarding its resources. **Asset mapping** is a process that identifies the geographic locations or features of the environment that influence population health (Santilli, Caroll-Scott, Wong, & Ickovics, 2011). Asset maps can highlight both population needs and resources and may engage communities in the process of their creation. For example, one community employed high school students to create an asset map locating pharmacies, health care facilities, convenience and grocery stores, liquor stores, fast food and other restaurants, parks, gardens, recreational facilities, and elements of the information environment (e.g., location of billboards with health-related messages). The asset mapping also included a neighborhood "street scan," which rated neighborhoods on 15 items related to safety, walkability, the condition of streets and sidewalks, presence of bicycle lanes, adherence to traffic laws, and accessibility of public transportation (Santilli et al., 2011).

Asset mapping can also identify some elements of the sociocultural and health system environments affecting the health of the population. For example, the type and location of local churches or other organizations or health care facilities can be plotted on the asset map. Asset mapping may also involve door-to-door interviews with residents to determine talents and abilities that might be employed to address population health needs. For example, if child care is an issue within the population, an asset map might help to identify community members who would be interested in providing child care in their homes. The population health nurse could then work with these individuals and others to meet regulatory requirements for in-home child care.

A population assessment may involve the development of several asset maps, each related to a different type of community resource. For example, one asset map might indicate the location and types of educational resources available in the community, whereas another identifies agencies and organizations providing health care services.

A windshield survey is an assessment technique similar to asset mapping. A **windshield survey** is an informal means of collecting population assessment data by driving through an area and observing its visible features. Data elements collected are similar to those in an asset map, but may also include characteristics such as the level of repair of houses, extent of traffic on streets, number of street people visible, and so on. For more information on conducting a windshield survey, see the *External Resources* section of the student resources site.

Asset maps and windshield surveys may make use of geographic information systems to store data. **Geographic information systems (GISs)** are computerized databases that collect and store information and display it in the form of maps and geographic distributions of various factors. In a GIS, data are geocoded by census block to enable specific data to be located on a map of the area. Geographic information systems are useful for identifying areas or segments of the population at risk for specific health problems or targeting interventions to areas of greatest need. In addition, GISs can also identify gaps in services and mislocation of service centers (Dubowitz et al., 2011).

Requirements for effective GISs that can be used to assess the need for and plan health care services include geo-enabled data related to factors such population health outcomes (e.g., locations of major accidents, residents with diabetes), risk factor distribution (e.g., smokers), and services distribution (e.g., locations of health care facilities, police stations). There is also a need for the infrastructure resources and technological capabilities to support GIS technology, including personnel and time for geographic data collection and entry as well as data management software. Finally, local agencies need to have the capacity to use geocoded data and to relocate services in response to identification of areas of need.

ASSESSING THE DETERMINANTS OF POPULATION HEALTH. Factors that influence population health can be conceptualized in various ways. In this chapter, we will use the six categories of determinants of health to frame our discussion of factors affecting the health of population groups.

Biological determinants. Human biological factors influencing a population's health reflect specific physical attributes of its members. The first of these attributes is age. Others reflect the genetic inheritance, physiologic function, and immunization status of the population.

The age composition of the population is an important indicator of probable health needs. Typically, there is a greater need for health services in areas with large numbers of the very young and the very old. Large numbers of women of childbearing age increase the need for prenatal and family planning services. Accident prevention is a major consideration in populations with large numbers of school-age and younger children.

Another population factor related to age composition is the annual birth rate, which provides information on the growth of the younger segments of the population. The annual birth rate is calculated on the basis of the number of live births during the year in relation to the total population. Birth rates are calculated per 1,000 persons. Birth statistics are usually compiled by official local and state health agencies and can be obtained from these sources.

Age-specific death rates also provide valuable information regarding the health status of the population. An age-specific death rate is the number of deaths in a particular age group compared with the population within that group. Because of the relatively small number of deaths in some age groups, the multiplier used in calculating age-specific death rates is 100,000. Excess deaths (deaths over the number that would be expected for that age group in the general population) for any age group in the population would indicate the presence of health problems.

The average age at death also provides an indication of overall population health. If people in the community typically die at a relatively young age, this suggests the existence of health problems that are contributing to these early deaths. Native Americans, for example, have shorter life expectancies than the rest of the U.S. population because of the high incidence of such health problems as chronic disease and alcoholism and high rates of homicide.

The gender composition of the population is one feature of its genetic inheritance. Many health problems such as obesity, hypertension, and various forms of cancer are more prevalent in one gender than in the other. Knowing the composition of the population with respect to gender assists the assessment team to identify health needs and plan programs to meet them. For example, the knowledge that women constitute 79% of a particular population might suggest the need for easily accessible detection programs for cancer of the cervix and breast.

The racial or ethnic composition of a population is another important factor in assessment. Knowledge of the ethnicity and racial origin of the population helps to pinpoint health problems known to be prevalent in certain groups, such as sickle cell disease in African Americans and diabetes in some Native American tribes.

Information about physiologic function in a population is derived from morbidity and mortality data as well as other health status indicators such as immunization levels. Mortality rates of concern to population health nurses include the crude death rate, cause-specific death rates, and death rates among specific segments of the population, such as the elderly, minority groups, and the homeless.

The crude death rate reflects all deaths in the population regardless of age or cause of death. The crude death rate presents a picture of the overall health status of the population but does not suggest the presence of specific health problems that may be contributing to deaths.

Cause-specific death rates, on the other hand, provide information about a population's specific health problems. Cause-specific death rates are the number of deaths in the population attributable to specific conditions, such as diabetes, heart disease, or suicide. They are calculated in proportion to the total population using a multiplier of 100,000. When death rates due to specific causes are higher than those of populations with a comparable age composition, health care programs may be needed to addresses these causes of death.

The majority of health problems are nonfatal, and many existing health problems in the population are not brought to light by examining mortality statistics alone. For this reason, those conducting a population health assessment must consider morbidity as well as mortality rates. Morbidity rates reflect the extent of illness present in the population. The two morbidity statistics of greatest significance in population health assessment are prevalence and incidence rates. Prevalence rates indicate the *total* number of cases of a particular condition at any given time. Incidence rates indicate the number of *new* cases of the condition identified over a specified time period. For example, eight new cases of tuberculosis may have been diagnosed in Buffalo County last month (incidence), but 39 people in the county are currently under treatment for active tuberculosis (prevalence).

Immunity is the final consideration related to biological factors influencing population health. Immunization levels and the overall immune status of the population influence susceptibility to a variety of communicable diseases. Even when specific individuals do not have immunity to a particular disease, if immune levels in the community are high, their chances of being exposed to the disease are diminished. This protective element of general population immunization levels is referred to as "herd immunity."

Information on biological factors influencing health will come from a number of sources. For example, information on the age, gender, and racial/ethnic composition of the population can be obtained from census figures for the census tracts that make up the community. Data on gender and racial composition may also be available from state and local agencies. Birth and death statistics are usually compiled by official local and state health agencies and can be obtained from these sources. Information on mortality may also be available from other sources. For example, insurance companies or trauma centers might be able to provide information on motor vehicle fatalities, and homicide figures may be available from local law enforcement agencies. Information on age at death is compiled by local health agencies, but may also be obtained by a review of death certificates or examination of obituaries published in local newspapers.

Local and state health departments also compile statistics on the incidence and prevalence of certain reportable health conditions. These conditions include many communicable diseases, but may also include other conditions for which special surveillance programs are in place. For example, in some areas information is compiled on newly diagnosed cases of hypertension. Another indicator of population morbidity is the *rate under treatment* or the number of people seeking assistance for specific health problems. For example, the number of people being treated for depression says a great deal about the mental health of the population and may be obtained from local treatment facilities. For other conditions, the assessment team may need to seek other sources of data. Cancer registries may be a source of information about the incidence and prevalence of certain forms of cancer, and local health care facilities and providers may have figures related to the incidence of other conditions. For example, the local hospital may have data on the number of clients hospitalized for diabetes, myocardial infarction, and other conditions.

Immunization levels within the population also provide information on the physiologic function of its members. Information on immunization levels is usually extrapolated from immunization figures derived from school records. In areas where a large number of school-age children are not immunized, there are probably also large numbers of unimmunized younger children, and overall immunization levels in the general population are also likely to be low. School immunization records, however, are not always an accurate indicator of high immunization levels. Because immunization is required for school entry in most places, school-age children may be immunized, while younger children remain unimmunized. For additional data on immunization levels, the assessment team might want to examine the records of public immunization clinics as well as those of private physicians who provide immunization services.

In addition to obtaining information regarding the population being assessed, the assessment team will also want to obtain similar figures for other populations in order to make comparisons. Comparison figures on morbidity and mortality at state and national levels can be obtained from state health departments and from various federal publications, respectively. One publication that contains a great deal of information on morbidity and mortality statistics is the *Morbidity and Mortality Weekly Report* published by the Centers for Disease Control and Prevention (CDC). Such data are also available online at the CDC website. National morbidity and mortality data can also be obtained from health and life insurance companies as well as voluntary agencies concerned with specific health problems, such as the American Cancer Society and the American Heart Association. Comparisons may also be made with prior data for the population being assessed. This trend data can indicate changes in community health problems over time. Tips on assessing biological determinants of population health are included in the *Focused Assessment* on the next page.

Psychological determinants. The psychological environment influences the health of the population by increasing or mediating exposure to stress and affects the ability of the population to function effectively. In addition, elements of the psychological dimension may enhance or impede population-based action to resolve identified health problems. Some of the psychological determinants to be addressed in a population health assessment include the future prospects of the population, significant events in the population's history and the response to those events, communication networks existing within the population, and the adequacy of protective services. Other considerations in this area include evidence of psychological problems such as suicide and homicide rates and identifiable sources of stress within the population.

Learning about a population's prospects helps those conducting the assessment to gain a clearer picture of the psychological climate affecting population health. If a population is growing and productive, for example, apathy regarding health problems is less likely than might be the case if the group is

FOCUSED ASSESSMENT Biological Determinants in Population Health Assessment

- What is the age composition of the population? What is the annual birth rate? What are the age-specific death rates in the population? What is the average age at death of population members?
- What is the racial and ethnic composition of the population? What is the relative proportion of men and women overall and in specific age groups? What genetically determined illnesses, if any, are prevalent in the population?
- What are the cause-specific mortality rates for the population? What physiologic conditions are prevalent? What is the extent of disability within the population? How does the population of interest compare with state and national morbidity and mortality figures?
- What is the overall immunization level in the population?

economically depressed and faltering. Similarly, a community that is in decline or has multiple problems is also more likely to have multiple sources of stress that affect the health of its residents.

Similarly, information about a population's history can provide insight into previous and current health problems and how the population has dealt with them. Historical information may also provide some clue as to how the population will deal with subsequent problems and where strengths lie. For example, historical information on the cohesive response of community members to a past crisis suggests a strength that will enable the population to face future crises.

The psychological environment created by relationships between subgroups within the population should also be explored. Harmonious relations between groups indicate a psychological climate that is conducive to cooperative action to resolve identified problems. Tension and distrust between groups, on the other hand, may make resolution of population health problems more difficult.

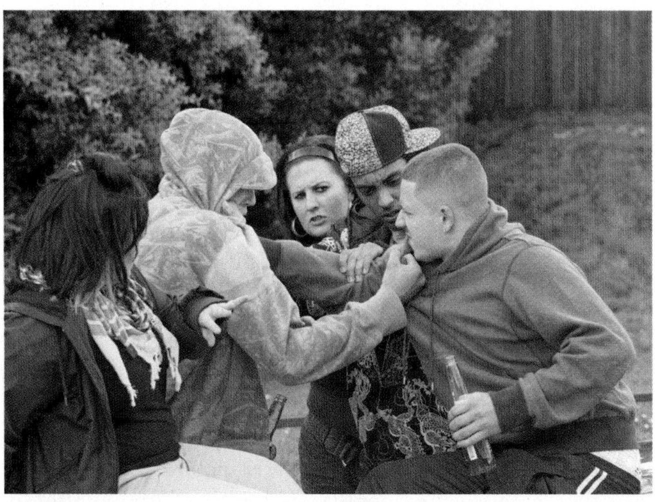

Conflict between groups in the population affects the overall health status of its members. *(Monkey Business/Fotolia)*

The adequacy of protective services provided by law enforcement, fire, and other emergency personnel can profoundly influence the psychological climate of an area. Adequate protective services help to create a psychological environment that enhances feelings of personal safety and security. Where these services are inadequate to meet residents' needs, stress and insecurity are created and can negatively influence the health of the population.

Communication is an important contributing factor in the psychological climate of a population; therefore, the adequacy of communication networks should also be explored. This includes the availability and accessibility of a telecommunication infrastructure in the population. Communication within the population may be formal or informal. Formal channels include media such as radio, television, and newspapers, as well as the form that public announcements may take. Informal communications take place outside of these channels. For example, rumors about a particular religious or ethnic group may serve to exacerbate intergroup tension and strife. The degree of trust placed in official formal communications is another element of the psychological dimension that may enhance or detract from population health.

Other indicators of the psychological environment in a population include annual incidence rates for homicide and suicide. Rates for specific subgroups within the population should also be examined, for there is usually considerable variation among different racial and ethnic groups. For example, both suicide and homicide rates are frequently higher for minority group members than for the general population in most areas. Examination of these figures and their distribution in the population may help to identify factors contributing to poor psychological health in certain subgroups or in the population in general.

Common sources of stress within the environment also influence population health. Widespread unemployment, lack of available housing, and crowded living conditions are sources of stress in a population. These and other sources of stress serve to create a psychological environment that is not conducive to health.

Information on the psychological determinants of population health is obtained primarily through observation and

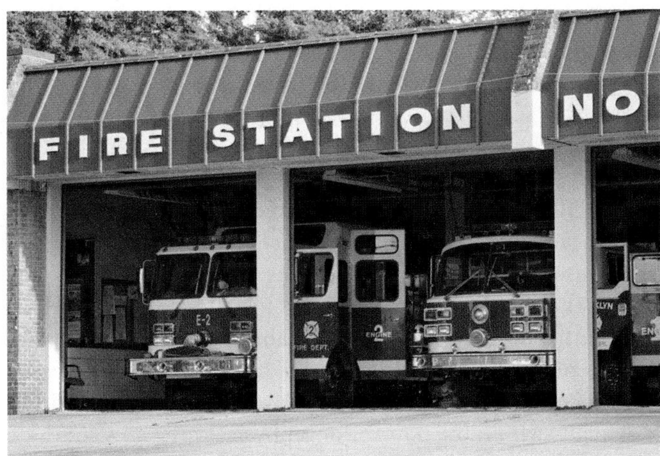

The adequacy of protective services influences a community's psychological health. *(Denise Kappa/Fotolia)*

through interviews with area residents. Again, it is important to get a broad representation of community membership among the people interviewed. The assessment team should be alert to unrest and conflict between groups within the population and the implications of such psychological tensions for the health of the population and its members. Information in this area may be derived from a review of local news articles or from police data regarding civil unrest.

Those assessing the health of a population would obtain information about the availability and quality of police and fire services, as well as information on the availability and adequacy of legal services, services for victims of abuse, and consumer protection services. Residents can be surveyed to determine their perceptions of the quality of these services. Area insurance agencies might also have data on injuries related to violence or fires that would provide indirect evidence of protective services. Information on rates for fire insurance coverage in the area also reflects the quality of services. Data about the psychological environment of a population might be obtained using the *Focused Assessment* provided below.

Environmental determinants. Physical environmental factors affecting a population include its location, its type (e.g., rural, urban, or suburban) and size, topographical features, and climate. Other physical factors to be assessed include the type and adequacy of housing and considerations related to water supply, nuisance factors, and potential for disaster.

The location, climate, and physical geography or topography of the community provide indications of some health problems likely to occur in the population. An area that is heavily wooded, for example, might increase the index of suspicion for problems such as Rocky Mountain spotted fever and Lyme disease. On the other hand, a dry, arid desert area would be more conducive to problems of heat exhaustion.

Size and population density, as well as the type of community, are other factors that influence the types of health problems encountered and resources available to the population. Certain health problems are more prevalent in urban areas than in rural ones and vice versa. Statistics indicate that suicide is more prevalent in urban communities, whereas one would expect a problem like rabies to occur more often in a rural area where wild animals are likely to be infected. Urban dwellers are less likely to encounter rabid animals because of regulations regarding vaccination of pets. Rural and urban areas also have unique strengths. For example, rural communities are often characterized by a tendency for neighbors to help each other, whereas urban areas generally have a greater variety of health care services within close proximity.

Housing is another important physical environmental factor. Inadequate, unsafe, or unsanitary housing conditions contribute to a variety of health problems including higher rates of environmental disease and injury (Jacobs, 2011). Overcrowding has been found to increase the incidence of a number of health concerns. Communicable diseases are spread more rapidly in crowded conditions, and the prevalence of stress-related conditions such as alcohol abuse, suicide, and other forms of violence increases with crowding as well. Adequate housing is characterized by sufficient privacy and space; physical accessibility; structural stability and durability; adequate lighting, heat, and ventilation; infrastructure including adequate

FOCUSED ASSESSMENT — Psychological Determinants in Population Health Assessment

- What stressors affect the health of the population? How do members of the population usually deal with crises? What significant events have occurred in the history of the population? What was the response to those events? What are the population's prospects for the future?
- How cohesive is the population? Is there evidence of tension between groups in the population?
- How adequate are protective services?
- What are the formal communication channels in the population? The informal channels?
- What are the prevalence rates for mental illnesses in the population? What is the homicide rate? Suicide rate?
- What are the rates of crime in the population? What types of crimes are prevalent?

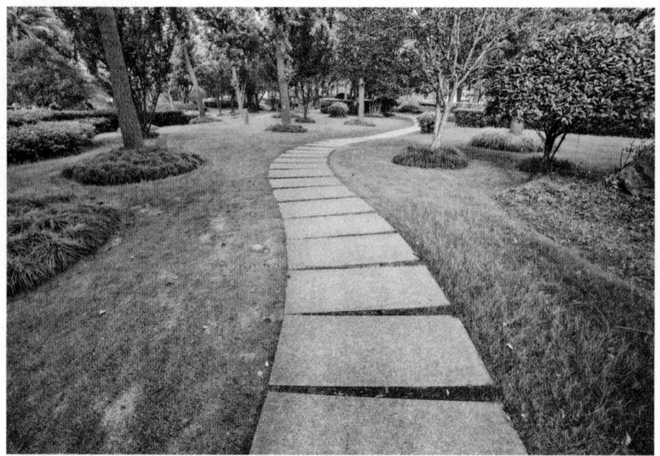

Open space areas can promote physical activity among community members. *(Zhu Difeng/Fotolia)*

water supply, sanitation, and waste management; environmental quality; and accessible location with respect to work and basic facilities. Housing adequacy in a population also relates to its affordability. Healthy housing is defined as "housing that is sited, designed, built, renovated, and maintained in ways that support the health of residents" (Jacobs, 2011, p. S115).

The source of a population's water supply is another important physical environmental consideration. Are most residents supplied by local water systems or do they have independent wells? What is the level of *potability*, or drinkability, of the water? Is the population's water supply safe for drinking, or does it pose biological or chemical hazards to health? The presence or absence of fluoride in the water supply is a possible indicator of dental health.

Large population water systems are regulated by the provisions of the Safe Drinking Water Act. Such systems serve approximately 96% of the U.S. population. Small systems that serve fewer than 15 households or private individual wells are unregulated.

Population health assessment should also address the population's water infrastructure and any contributions it might make to disparities in access to potable water. In the 2007 National Housing Survey, for example, approximately 1% of U.S. households were without piped water, and some whole communities lacked piped water. These figures were higher in *colonias* along the U.S.–Mexico border and among Native Americans (VanDerslice, 2011).

Disposal of wastes is another environmental determinant of population health. Disposal methods for various types of materials, particularly hazardous wastes, should be considered. Do disposal methods ensure adequate safeguards for the health of the public or is there potential for environmental pollution as a result of waste disposal? Concerns about hazardous waste disposal were addressed in Chapter 4∞.

Physical environmental factors may also contribute to accidental injuries. For example, particularly dangerous intersections may be the sites of frequent motor vehicle accidents, or large numbers of swimming pools in the area may contribute to the incidence of drowning.

Nuisance factors such as insects, noxious plants, and other substances may provide additional physical health hazards or prove offensive to the senses, thereby decreasing the quality of life for the population. Nearby dairy farms, for example, might provide insect breeding grounds that contribute to the incidence of insect-borne diseases, or there might be an airport that presents a noise hazard. Another consideration in terms of nuisances is the presence of various pollutants in the environment. The effects of pollution and the population health nurse's responsibility with regard to pollution were discussed in Chapter 4∞.

Finally, within the population's physical environment there may be the potential for either natural or human-caused disasters. Is the population situated on a major fault line and subject to earthquakes? Is there a chemical manufacturing plant close by that presents a potential hazard? Assessment of the potential for disaster and the population health nurse's role in planning for disaster response are addressed in more detail in Chapter 25∞.

Elements of the built environment, in addition to housing, also affect the health of the population. For example, the World Health Organization has found strong evidence for the adverse effects on health of such environmental conditions as secondhand smoke, pollutants, high-rise construction, and multifamily housing (Jacobs, 2011).

Many environmental determinants of population health can be directly observed, as indicated in the discussion of asset maps and windshield surveys. For example, the nurse or other members of the assessment team might drive through the area assessing its geographic features, nuisance factors, and the general adequacy of housing. Information about pollution, water supply, and waste disposal might be obtained from local government bureaus or the nearby public health agency. Data on population size and density are available from census figures or from local government agencies. This information, as well as information on the typical climate and geographic features, may also be available in local publications or from the chamber of commerce. A *Focused Assessment* for environmental conditions affecting a population's health is provided on the next page.

Sociocultural determinants. From the previous discussion it is clear that sociocultural and psychological determinants are closely interrelated. Social and cultural factors influence the psychological dimension and have other effects on health as well. Considerations in assessing sociocultural determinants include information about government and leadership, language, income and education levels, employment levels and occupations, marital status and family composition, and religion. Other areas to be addressed include transportation and the availability of goods and services needed by residents.

A population's government and power structure are important considerations in terms of planning and implementing programs designed to solve population health problems and to make effective use of resources. Who holds the purse strings?

FOCUSED ASSESSMENT Environmental Determinants in Population Health Assessment

- Where is the population located (urban, rural region)? How large is the area occupied by the population? How densely populated? What topographical features could influence the health of population members? What is the local climate like?
- What is the quality of housing in the population? Is affordable housing available? Are dwellings in good repair?
- What is the population's source of water? Is the water supply adequate to meet population needs? Is it safe for consumption? How is waste disposal handled?
- What plants and animals are common in the area?
- Is there evidence of environmental pollution that may affect health?
- Are there nuisance factors present in the area? If so, what are they? How do they affect health?
- Is there potential for disaster in the population? If so, what kind of disasters are likely? What is the extent of disaster preparation in the population?

How are decisions made? Who are the decision makers? Those conducting the health assessment should identify both formal and informal leaders. In one isolated community, for example, no program was successful unless it first received approval from one elderly matriarch. It was she who controlled the community despite the presence of elected officials.

Information on the population's official leadership can be obtained from the local governmental agencies. Informal leaders may be more difficult to identify, but, if they do not already know this information, assessment team members can ask key informants in the population (e.g., school principals, clergy, and official leaders) who the informal leaders are. Other health care providers and business leaders might also provide information on informal leadership within the population.

Language is another important sociocultural factor affecting the health of the population. Language influences interactions among members of the population as well as their ability to obtain needed goods and services. Closely related to language are the cultural affiliations within the population. Major cultural differences between racial and ethnic segments of the population can create stress and increase the potential for civil strife and discord. Information about cultural affiliations also provides insights into health-related attitudes and behaviors and directions for tailoring health service interventions to enhance their effectiveness.

The average income of residents also has bearing on a population's health status. For example, a strong relationship exists between the economic status of the population and certain critical indicators of health. Economic status influences the ability of residents to provide for basic necessities and to gain access to health care services. In addition, the income of residents influences the tax base of the population and the types of services provided. For example, when many residents are unemployed or have low incomes, they have less money to spend. Businesses take in less money and revenues from sales and other taxes are decreased. Consequently, the community is less able to provide essential services for its citizens.

Income is closely related to education level. People who have received a lesser education may have lower-paying jobs. They also tend to have less health-related knowledge, and, consequently, lower levels of health. Both income and education levels are indicators of a population's standard of living and, indirectly, of its health status. The prevalence of several acute and chronic conditions in the population (e.g., tuberculosis, pneumonia, and heart disease) tends to decline as income and education levels rise.

Because large numbers of people within a population are usually employed, it is important to consider the types of occupations and possible health hazards involved. Persons in some occupational groups are at higher risk for certain health problems than those in other groups. For example, histoplasmosis occurs frequently among people who work with birds (e.g., poultry farmers), and black lung (pneumoconiosis) is prevalent among coal miners.

In addition to information about employment, the level of unemployment in the population provides an indication of possible health problems. Unemployment contributes to stress and to decreased income levels that affect access to health care as well as other necessary goods and services.

Religious affiliations within a population can either foster or impede health practices. Religious beliefs may affect health or influence the acceptability of health programs to members of the population. For example, some religious groups may be averse to the idea of providing on-site health care services in high schools because of the fear that contraceptive services will be provided. Similarly, local religious groups may provide significant community resources and should be included in assets assessment.

Marital status and family composition are other social factors that might influence the health of a population. Those conducting a population health assessment would consider the number of single-parent families and older persons living alone. Generally, married individuals have lower death and illness rates than those who are unmarried; therefore, information about marital status in the population can provide clues to overall health status.

Accessibility of transportation is an important factor related to the use of health services and is, therefore, a necessary component of the assessment. Transportation difficulties compound health problems where large numbers of people are poor or elderly, chronically ill or disabled, poorly motivated with respect to health, or who are mothers with small children.

Social norms within the population are other factors that may influence population health. Social norms are "rules that dictate acceptable behavior within a group" (Karasek, Ahern, & Galea, 2012, p. 343). For example, neighborhood social norms related to smoking have been associated with smoking cessation rates among the population.

Public policies are social norms that have been codified as laws or regulations and can have a significant influence on population health. For example, several provisions of the Patient Protection and Affordable Care Act are intended to influence population health. We have already discussed the mandate for periodic community assessment by tax-exempt hospitals. Other provisions intended to affect population health relate to the availability of grants to support medical home and community-based care programs; coverage for preventive health and wellness services; increased funding for community health centers; a focus on outcome measures for chronic disease, wellness care, and prevention; and funds for employer wellness programs for small employers (Larkin, 2010).

The assessment team should assess the degree to which language presents a barrier to health education or to the provision of other health care services. Key informants in the population can provide information about languages spoken. Schoolteachers and principals, for example, are knowledgeable about languages spoken by their students. Those conducting the population assessment may also derive this information from personal observations. For example, they may spend time observing stores where large segments of the population shop or check for newspapers and radio and television broadcasts in languages other than English.

Another aspect of language to be assessed is the use of colloquialisms. Are there unique ways in which members of the population express themselves? Unfortunately, much of this information is gleaned by trial and error on the part of the nurse; however, the nurse can ask key informants about the use of colloquialisms and about their meaning.

Assessment team members also need to identify the host of cultural factors within the population that may affect its health status (see Chapter 5∞). Information on cultural groups in the population can be obtained from key informants and through observation. The presence of ethnic markets and restaurants, as well as non-English newspapers and radio stations can also provide information on the ethnic/cultural composition of the population.

Information on income and education levels, other important sociocultural influences on population health, can be obtained from census figures. This information may also be available from local government agencies or school districts. In addition to determining the education level of the population, education resources should be examined. This information enables the assessment team to make diagnoses regarding the adequacy of resources for meeting identified health needs. The telephone directory and Web are good starting places for obtaining information on education facilities in the area. Assessment team members can then interview administrators of those facilities or review their brochures and other publications to determine the types of education programs offered. Local school personnel can also provide information on education opportunities available to the population.

Information about area businesses and industries is available from the local chamber of commerce or Web. The numbers of people employed in specific occupations can be obtained from major employers in the area. Questions should also be asked about health hazards presented by community occupations. The population health assessment team would address the potential for exposure to hazardous substances (e.g., asbestos and chlorine gas), radiation, noise, or vibration, as well as the potential for injury due to falls or use of hazardous equipment. In addition to determining the potential for occupational injury or illness, the team would obtain figures on the extent to which such conditions occur. This type of information may be obtained from the illness and accident records of major employers or may be available from the state occupational health agency.

Unemployment figures can be obtained from state or local employment offices. Occupational data derived from a population assessment might be based on the *Focused Assessment* included on the next page.

Telephone directories and Internet data can provide a picture of the religious groups represented in the population. Membership rosters of specific houses of worship can provide information on the number of people affiliated with each religious group. The assessment team can also interview members of local religious groups to determine the extent of their influence on health and their level of involvement in health-related activities. For example, some congregations may organize periodic blood pressure screening events or provide health-related education programs for their members.

Information on marriage and family composition is available from census data for the area. Vital statistics collected by the local health department can also provide data on marriages and the frequency of divorce among members of the population.

With respect to transportation, the assessment team can obtain information on the number of families with cars from area census data. Information on other forms of transportation can be gleaned from the telephone directory or Internet and by contacting bus and taxi companies to determine routes and fares.

In addition, the assessment team members would obtain data on the types and adequacy of goods and services available to the population, including recreational programs, local shopping facilities, prices for goods and services, and social service programs. Much of this information can be obtained through participant observation. For example, the nurse might shop in local stores or look for recreational pursuits. Information about the number and types of stores and services is also available in the telephone directory and possibly on the Internet. Newspaper advertisements provide information on local prices. Finally, assessment team members can contact personnel at local social service agencies to obtain information about the services offered. Data related to a population's sociocultural environment might be obtained using the *Focused Assessment* questions provided below.

Behavioral determinants. Behavioral factors influence the health status of a population and its members. Areas to be considered in this dimension include consumption patterns, leisure pursuits, and other health-related behaviors.

Consumption patterns play a major part in the development of health or illness. In assessing consumption patterns in the population, the assessment team would examine dietary patterns and the use of potentially harmful substances.

Information is needed on the general nutritional level of the population and on specific dietary patterns. For example, information would be sought on the prevalence of overweight individuals in the population or the incidence of anemia in school-age children. Another area for consideration is any ethnic nutritional patterns that might influence health either positively or negatively. For example, movement away from traditional foods to typical American dietary practices has contributed to obesity and a variety of chronic diseases among many ethnic cultural groups.

The use of harmful substances is another area to explore. The level of alcohol consumption within the population should be examined, both for the population in general and for specific target groups. The extent of both legal and illegal drug use may also merit investigation, including the types of substances abused and the typical sources of abused substances. The extent of smoking and other forms of tobacco use in the population should also be considered.

Information about leisure activities prevalent in the population can also indicate the potential for certain kinds of health problems. For example, boating, waterskiing, and related recreational activities increase the risk of drowning and similar accidents. On the other hand, if watching television is the primary form of recreation, there may be increased potential for heart disease and other conditions associated with a sedentary lifestyle. The presence or absence of recreational opportunities available to the population may also affect the psychological environment and the ability to deal with stress effectively.

Information on dietary patterns may be obtained by interviews and surveys of residents as well as by observation of foods purchased in grocery stores. The assessment team would determine the number of residents who smoke and whether that number is increasing or decreasing. Indirect indicators of the use of alcohol, drugs, and tobacco include sales of these items. This information can be obtained from interviews with personnel in stores that sell these items or from information about the related taxes collected. Information on substance abuse may be reflected in law enforcement agencies' records of arrests or accidents related to drugs and alcohol. Information can also be obtained on the number of admissions to drug and alcohol treatment facilities. Self-help groups, such as a local chapter of Alcoholics Anonymous, may also provide information on the extent of substance abuse problems. Data reflecting a population's consumption patterns would include information derived from the *Focused Assessment* on page 370.

Information on leisure-related physical activity is usually obtained by means of interviews and surveys. To determine the extent of interest in various forms of exercise, assessment team members might also contact groups that offer exercise-related classes or businesses that sell related equipment. In addition, they can observe for joggers or other exercise enthusiasts as

FOCUSED ASSESSMENT Sociocultural Determinants in Population Health Assessment

- How are community decisions made? Who makes them? Who holds power in the population? How is that power exercised? What is the population's governance structure? How effective is governance? Who are the formal and informal leaders in the population?
- What cultural groups are represented in the population? What languages are spoken? What cultural beliefs and behaviors are prevalent in the population? What is the character of relationships between members of different cultural groups in the population?
- What religious affiliations are represented in the population? What effect do they have on community life and health?
- What is the general education level of the population? What educational resources and facilities are present?
- What is the income level and distribution within the population?
- What is the rate of unemployment in the population? Who are the major employers in the area? What kinds of occupations are represented? What occupational health hazards are present?
- How accessible is transportation in the community?
- What is the marital status of the population? What is the typical family structure in the population?
- How accessible are goods and services to members of the population?
- What are the social norms espoused by members of the population? What effects do these norms have on population health?
- What are the effects of public policies on population health?

they move about the community. Information on recreational opportunities can be obtained from the telephone directory and the Internet, from direct observation, and from events publicized in the newspaper or other means of communication employed by the population.

Members of the population conducting the health assessment should also examine the prevalence of other health-related behaviors. For example, information would be obtained on the extent of seat belt use in passenger vehicles or the use of safety devices in certain occupational settings. Information on failure to use seat belts might be available from policy or insurance records of motor vehicle accidents, and failure to use occupational safety devices would be reflected in Occupational Safety and Health Administration (OSHA) accident reports.

The assessment team would also be interested in such behaviors as the extent of heterosexual and homosexual activity and use of condoms and other forms of protection against conception and sexually transmitted diseases. Two negative indicators of contraceptive use are the proportion of births that are unintended and the population abortion rate. In areas with a high prevalence of injection drug use, assessment team members would also try to obtain information on the extent of needle sharing and other practices that contribute to the spread of HIV/AIDS infection and hepatitis C. Much of this information is available only through observation and through interviews with key informants. The *Focused Assessment* included below provides guidelines for assessing behavioral determinants of population health.

Health system determinants. Health care system factors can profoundly affect the health of a population. Assessment in this area involves identifying existing services, assessing their level of performance, and identifying areas in which services are lacking. Relevant information includes the types of health care services available to members of the population and their effectiveness in addressing population health needs. What levels of health care services are available? How adequate are these services to meet the needs of the people? The availability and accessibility of specific types of services and how effectively they are used can influence population health. For example, the percentage of pregnant women who receive prenatal care and the point in the pregnancy at which care usually begins affect maternal and infant health. The availability and adequacy of services provided by emergency medical personnel and by emergency rooms or trauma centers are other examples of health system determinants that influence population health. Other questions relate to the availability and accessibility of certain types of health care providers. For example, there may be several physicians in town, but none of them provide prenatal services because of malpractice concerns.

The extent to which available health services are overused or underused may also affect the health status of the population, and factors that contribute to overuse and to underuse would be considered. For example, emergency room services might be overused because many people cannot afford a regular source of health care and seek care only in crisis situations. Conversely, the services of clinics and physicians might be underused because they are offered at inconvenient times or places, because people have no means of transportation to such services, or because residents may simply not be aware of the need for or availability of certain services.

Another area for consideration is the financing of health care. Considerations to be addressed include who pays for health care services, the adequacy of funding sources for meeting population health needs, the priority given to health-related concerns in planning budgetary allocations, the extent of health insurance coverage in the population, and the availability of funds to pay for care for the indigent (see Chapter 6∞ for a detailed discussion of economic influences on population health). Financing of health care can also provide an indirect

FOCUSED ASSESSMENT Behavioral Determinants in Population Health Assessment

- What are the usual food preferences and consumption patterns in the population? What is the nutritional level in the population? What percentage of the population is overweight? Underweight?
- What is the extent of drug abuse in the population? How easy is it to obtain drugs?
- What is the extent of alcohol and tobacco sales in the population? What is the prevalence of arrests related to alcohol and other drugs? What is the extent of tobacco use in the population? What is the rate of hospital admissions for health problems related to alcohol, drug, and tobacco use?
- What exercise and leisure opportunities are available to the population? To what extent are they utilized? Do leisure activities pose any health or safety hazards?
- What is the attitude of the population toward sexual activity? Toward homosexuality? What is the prevalence of unsafe sexual practices in the population? What is the extent of contraceptive use in the population?
- To what extent do members of the population engage in safety practices (e.g., seat belt use)?

indication of prevailing attitudes toward health. Adequate health care budgeting indicates that health is considered a public priority.

Other considerations related to the health care system include community definitions of health and illness and the use of culturally prescribed health practices and practitioners. As we saw in Chapter 5∞, culturally determined health behaviors may have both positive and negative effects on a population's health status. For example, herbal remedies used by some cultural groups may have positive effects, but when used in combination with scientific medicine, may impede treatment or create adverse health effects.

In assessing health system determinants, assessment team members would obtain information on the type of health services available to members of the population. Such information can be derived from a variety of sources, such as the telephone directory, the Internet, word of mouth, and personal observation. Referral services provided by professional organizations or agencies such as local senior citizens groups can also supply information on health care providers and facilities. Health care institutions are also a source of information on services provided and fees involved.

Utilization figures for health care services can be obtained from health care facilities and providers. Information on health insurance coverage may be available from insurance agencies or major health care facilities in the area, or through population-based surveys. Health care facility records may also contain data on the percentage of the population without health insurance. Information about recipients of Medicaid and Medicare benefits is available from the agencies that administer these programs. Information on other sources of funding for health care services can be solicited from public officials as well as local health care agencies and institutions.

The *Focused Assessment* questions provided below can help you assess health system factors affecting population health. A tool to guide a comprehensive assessment of the determinants of population health is included in *Assessment Guidelines* section of the student resources site. Table 15-3 provides several sources of population assessment information and examples of data that might be obtained from each source.

TABLE 15-3 Sources of Population Assessment Data

Type of Data	Source	Example
Quantitative	Census figures Local agencies	Age composition of population Racial composition of population Child abuse incidence figures from child protective services Diabetes admissions from hospitals Immunization levels from schools
	Population surveys	Frequency of health services use Common health problems
	Observation	Number and types of educational institutions Number and types of recreational opportunities
	Newspaper reports	Incidence of homicide Incidence of motor vehicle fatalities
	Telephone book	Number and types of health care providers Number and types of churches
Qualitative	Population surveys	Attitudes toward health Attitudes toward specific health issues
	Key informant interviews	Perceptions of population health needs
	Resident interviews	Perceptions of health needs
	Observation	Quality of housing
	Participant observation	Barriers to health care for handicapped individuals

FOCUSED ASSESSMENT Health System Determinants in Population Health Assessment

- What types of health promotion, illness and injury prevention, problem resolution, and health restoration services are available to the population? How accessible are these services? Are the types of services available adequate to meet population health needs? Are available services culturally relevant to members of the population?
- To what extent are available health care services utilized? What barriers to service utilization exist in the population?
- Are there alternative or complementary health services available to the population? To what extent do members of the population use alternative/complementary health services? What is the level and quality of interaction between alternative and scientific health care systems?
- How are health care services financed? What proportion of the population has health insurance? What level of priority is given to health care services in budgeting local funds? What are community attitudes toward health care services and providers?

In addition to determining appropriate data collection methods, the nurse and members of the population preparing to conduct a population health assessment explore methods for organizing and analyzing the data obtained. When modes of data organization and analysis are identified as much as possible prior to data collection, interpretation of the masses of information obtained becomes much easier.

Deriving Population-Level Nursing Diagnoses

The collection of data on factors influencing the health status of a population is the first step in identifying resources and health needs. To be of any value, the data must be interpreted and analyzed to derive nursing diagnoses. In other words, assessment data are used to identify health-related needs amenable to nursing action and the resources that will support action. Population nursing diagnoses should reflect population strengths or competencies, as well as existing, emerging, and potential threats to health.

Diagnostic reasoning in the care of populations involves comparing population assessment data to identified standards to identify health problems and assets available to solve them. One type of standard that may be used by the population health nurse in data analysis is the general health status of the state or the nation. In doing so, the nurse might ask the following questions: How does this group stand in relation to the larger population on a variety of measures of health status? Is the local birth rate higher or lower than that of the state or the nation? How do death rates compare? For example, mortality related to diabetes is considerably higher in U.S. Hispanic and African American populations than in the Caucasian population. Do morbidity rates for various illnesses exceed national and state rates? How do income and education levels compare?

Another standard with which to compare present data is found in the history of the population. How do current rates compare with those of a year ago? Five years ago? Are health status indicators improving or declining?

Population members' perceptions of areas of need are a third type of standard with which to compare the data gathered. What health problems are mentioned in interviews with population members? What problems are perceived by other health care professionals and population leaders? What are the expectations of the population regarding these problems?

Diagnostic reasoning gives rise to statements of risk for specific health problems. Population nursing diagnoses provide a comprehensive picture of the population's health. Diagnoses may be either positive or negative. Positive diagnoses reflect population strengths and may also indicate improvements in the population's health status. Components of a population nursing diagnosis include (a) identification of the population or subgroup at risk, (b) a potential adverse situation or risk, (c) factors or characteristics contributing to the level of risk, and (d) evidence to support the increased or decreased level of risk. The elements of the diagnosis provide information about the causative factors involved and guidance for action as needed. The *Highlights* box below provides a template for a population diagnosis as well as examples of positive and negative diagnoses. As indicated in the negative example, factors related to the risk may be related to an absence of relevant health-related services as well as to other factors or behaviors in the population.

Planning Population-Based Health Initiatives

Whenever a negative diagnosis is made, planning to address the unmet need or risk situation is warranted, and the population health nurse should engage members of the population in planning health care initiatives to meet the identified needs. **Planning** is a collaborative and systematic process used to attain a predetermined goal. Planning is collaborative in the sense that persons who will be affected by the planned program need to be involved in its planning. It is systematic in that change is consciously and deliberately brought about.

Planning should be strengths-based, rather than being focused on health deficits. Deficit-focused planning relies on a traditional problem-solving process of problem identification, cause analysis, and identification of possible solutions by the implementing agency. In contrast, strengths-based planning incorporates existing population resources and strengths, visioning of potential outcomes based on those strengths, and

Highlights

Population Diagnosis Template and Sample Diagnoses

Population Diagnosis Template

[**population at risk**] for [**risk**] related to [**factors contributing to increased/decreased risk**] as evidenced by [**evidence supporting risk assessment**].

Sample Negative Nursing Diagnosis

Large adolescent population [**population subgroup at risk**] at risk for sexually transmitted diseases (STDs) [**risk**] related to self-report of unprotected sexual activity by 75% of high school students, lack of knowledge related to STD transmission, and lack of access to condoms [**factors contributing to increased risk**], as evidenced by: (a) gonorrhea incidence rate of 357 per 1,000 population, (b) 30% increase in number of cases of *Chlamydia trachomatis* infection in last year, and (c) 5% increase in sexually transmitted hepatitis B among adolescents [**evidence of elevated risk**].

Sample Positive Nursing Diagnosis (demonstrating improvement)

Diminished risk of STDs [**risk**] for adolescents [**population subgroup at risk**] related to older age at initiation of sexual activity and 50% increase in condom use by sexually active adolescents [**factors related to decreased risk**], as evidenced by 50% decrease in gonorrhea and *chlamydia* infection rates among adolescents [**evidence of decreased risk**].

dialogue with members of the population regarding possible approaches to resolution of problems. Deficit-focused planning is founded on assumptions that the population does not have the capacity to resolve its own problems and, in fact, may itself be a problem to be solved. A further assumption is that health care experts know best what should be done to resolve health-related problems. Strengths-based planning, on the other hand, is based on the assumptions that the population can fix its own problems and that members of the population know best what will or will not work to resolve those problems.

Planning may occur at two levels: specific health-related programs and development of community-level interventions that involve multiple foci and are coordinated to achieve maximum improvement in population health. Community-level interventions focus on reducing health disparities in the population by promoting the health and welfare of group members and by enhancing the population's capacity to promote its own health and well-being. It is based on the recognition that individual health programs may have interactive effects that may enhance or impede overall support and resource utilization or increase or decrease the population's capacity for future problem solving (Trickett et al., 2011). As a simple example, designing a program to address increased HIV/AIDS incidence may siphon resources from other STD control programs or from programs designed to improve overall population access to care.

Community-level intervention minimizes development of programs in independent silos and focuses on programming to address a variety of population health needs that have been prioritized. Community-level intervention also contributes to the effectiveness of health planning because it considers the overall context in which health care delivery occurs. When members of the population are involved in planning community-level interventions, they address population-identified issues and serve to enhance the population's capacity to resolve those issues. Community-level interventions also make more effective use of scarce resources and result in lessons that can be applied to future population health issues (Trickett et al., 2011). For purposes of promoting understanding of the planning process, however, this chapter focuses on planning discrete health programs rather than on the development of complex community-level interventions or care delivery systems. Population health nurses in practice, however, would be involved in setting priorities and contributing to the development of community-level interventions or systems that address multiple population health issues.

The program planning process may incorporate a variety of steps depending on the planning model used. For our purposes, we will use a five-step model that includes defining and prioritizing the issue to be addressed, creating the planning group, analyzing the issue, developing the program, and setting the stage for evaluation.

DEFINING AND PRIORITIZING POPULATION HEALTH ISSUES. A large-scale population health assessment will usually identify a number of health issues that could be addressed through health program planning. In some cases, several different issues may be addressed simultaneously through the development of separate health care delivery programs. In others, a number of related issues may be combined and addressed by a single, more comprehensive program. In any event, it is unlikely that all of a population's health-related problems, issues, and needs can be addressed at once given the finite resources available. For this reason, it is necessary to examine the issues derived from the assessment, prioritize them, and define the issue or issues to be addressed in program planning.

The criteria used to prioritize population health needs are essentially the same as those used in working with individuals and families: (a) severity of the threat to the population's health, (b) degree of population concern about the issue, and (c) extent to which meeting one need depends on meeting other needs. It is likely that the priorities of the population group involve needs that are easily perceived. Participation of population members in the assessment process helps them become aware of less obvious needs that might have greater priority than other more obvious ones.

The process of assigning priority to the health needs identified in a population health assessment involves developing criteria for decision making, establishing standards for minimally acceptable levels of the criteria, and assigning weights to the criteria. The criteria are based on values held by program planners and members of the population. When the values of population members and health care professionals conflict, dialogue and negotiation are required.

A high-priority problem will usually meet criteria of severity, significant population concern, and high cost to society. A standard for severity might be that a minimum of 20% of the population be affected by the problem; whereas significant population concern would be evident if at least 30% of residents surveyed mentioned a particular problem as needing attention. Possible standards for cost to society might be the number of days of lost school or work attendance or the actual monetary cost for medical treatment for the problem. Each of these three criteria (and others developed) would be given a weight reflecting its relative importance in decisions about priorities. For example, high societal cost might be given greater value than the level of concern expressed about a given problem. All of the problems identified in the population health assessment would be evaluated in terms of the weighted criteria, and those with higher priority scores would be addressed first in efforts to resolve population health problems. At this point, population health nurses may need to advocate for giving population concerns a high priority, even when health care providers may see other problems as more important.

Once health-related issues have been prioritized, the population health nurse and other group members can define the specific problem or set of problems to be addressed by program planning. For example, the group may need to determine whether the issue to be addressed is obesity in the general population or obesity as it occurs in school-aged children. Depending on the way the issue is defined, approaches to its resolution may be quite different.

Definition of the problem or issue to be addressed should also lead to establishment of specific goals for its resolution. Program goals are broad statements of desired outcomes that provide the general direction for program development, in contrast to objectives, which are measurable indicators of program accomplishments. A goal statement should speak to the resolution of the identified issue. For example, if the issue to be addressed is poor nutrition among older members of the population, the goal would be to improve the nutritional status of older persons.

CREATING THE PLANNING GROUP. The group of people who develop a health care program to meet an identified population health need may be the same as those who participated in the population health assessment. More than likely, however, there will be a need to include others in the planning process who have specific expertise or interest related to the issue to be addressed. The population health nurse may need to advocate for the inclusion of specific people in the planning body, particularly members of the target group. Because of their connections in the population, population health nurses are likely to know of people who would be assets to the planning group.

For health program planning to be successful, it is important to determine who should be included in the planning group. Generally speaking, five categories of people should be included: those in authority who must approve or fund the program, people with expertise related to the issue to be addressed, those who will implement the program, those who will benefit from it, and, finally, people who might resist the program. Those with authority to address the issue should be included because they usually control resources that will be required to implement the program and because they may resist the program if they see it as overlapping or competing with other existing programs. People with expertise related to the issue have knowledge of potential solutions to the problem that have been used elsewhere and may be effective in the population of interest. They are also usually in a position to identify alternatives that have been shown to be unsuccessful in the past.

Health care professionals may fall into the expert category, but may also be implementers of the program. Implementers are in a position to implement a program as designed or to sabotage it; their buy-in is essential if the program is to be implemented effectively. Implementers may also have insights into what will and will not work in a given situation. Responsibility for ultimate acceptance and use of a program lies with those who are intended to benefit from it. Potential beneficiaries of a program should be involved in planning to ensure that the program meets their needs and is culturally acceptable to them.

It may seem contrary to common sense to include people who are likely to resist development and implementation of a program in its planning. In reality, however, incorporating resisters into the planning group often converts them into supporters. Their presence during program planning permits incorporation of program elements that will defuse their resistance. When they are satisfied that the program planned is not a threat to their own interests or values, they will then act to convince other potential resisters of the benefits of the program. Given the particular issue to be addressed, there may be additional people who do not fall into any of these categories who should be included in the planning group. For example, if media advocacy will be needed to gain public acceptance of the program, members of the local media should be invited to join the planning group. The *Highlights* box presented below includes considerations in creating a planning group to address the health care needs of prison inmates. In addition to determining who should be involved, other tasks in creating the planning group include developing planning competence among group members and formulating a group philosophy. Group members should also engage in the tasks of group development discussed in Chapter 10∞.

Few health care professionals or consumers have any educational background or experience in program planning. For this reason, the population health nurse or other planning group leader may find it necessary to educate members of the planning group about the planning processes and activities involved. It may also be necessary to prevent the group from engaging in activities for which an adequate foundation has yet to be provided. In doing so, the population health nurse needs to exercise well-developed skills in group dynamics (see Chapter 10∞). Other tasks to be accomplished at this stage of planning include establishing the organizational structure of the group and clarifying the roles and responsibilities of planning group members.

The next task in creating the planning group, formulating a philosophy, is not often carried out as a conscious activity, but is an assumption on the part of group members. For example, there must be some type of commitment to adequate health care for prison inmates before a group would even consider planning a program to meet prisoners' needs. It is, however, important that the philosophies of various members of the planning group be compatible. Therefore, group members should be encouraged to verbalize their philosophies and to identify and deal with areas of conflict between philosophies.

Highlights

Creating a Planning Group to Address the Health Care Needs of Inmates

Those in authority: Corrections officials, elected officials

Experts: Health care providers with experience in correctional settings, corrections experts, financial analysts to determine potential program costs

Implementers: Corrections personnel, health care personnel

Beneficiaries: Inmates and their families

Resisters: Corrections officials and personnel, taxpayers, elected officials

Others: Inmate advocates

ANALYZING THE ISSUE AND CHOOSING AN INTERVENTION. The next task in program planning is to analyze the issue or problem, its contributing factors, and potential alternative solutions. Much of the data required for this analysis may already be available from the population health assessment, but the planning group may find that they need to collect additional information related to the issue. For example, the population health assessment may have identified problems related to adequate housing that include issues of safety, affordability, and landlord intimidation, but the committee may need more information on the kinds of safety risks present in local housing, the extent of those risks, who is affected by housing affordability issues and why, and which tenants are being intimidated by landlords and why. The planning group will then develop methods for collecting the additional information needed for effective planning to address the housing issue.

Analysis of the issue to be addressed also includes determining the level of health care involved in its resolution. Is the issue one that can be addressed through health promotion or illness and injury prevention strategies? Or does problem resolution require intervention at the resolution or restoration level?

Other information to be obtained and analyzed by the planning group may relate to potential solutions to problems identified. What strategies have other communities used to address similar problems? How effective were those strategies? What features of those strategies might be appropriate to this population? Which of the strategies could be implemented in this population or how might the strategies need to be adapted to be appropriate to this population? Some potential solutions have a stronger evidence base for their effectiveness than others. The Community Preventive Services Task Force (2014a) has developed information on a variety of community-based interventions linked to achievement of *Healthy People 2020* objectives. The task force has identified a number of interventions that have strong research support as well as many that have insufficient evidence of their effectiveness to warrant use in many population situations. For more information on the evidence base for an array of community-based interventions, see the *External Resources* section of the student resources site.

Information obtained should be analyzed by the planning group to gain a complete picture of factors contributing to the problem and to assist in identifying or developing a strategy to address those factors and resolve the problem. Usually such an analysis will lead to several alternative approaches to problem resolution that must be evaluated in the light of criteria established by the planning group for acceptable solutions. Examples of critical criteria for solutions to population health problems might be that they fit within available budgetary resources or are acceptable to particular ethnic or religious groups within the population.

Potential solutions to problems should always be evaluated in terms of cost, feasibility, acceptability, availability of necessary resources, efficiency, equity, political advantage, and identifiability of the target group, as well as the quality of evidence for their effectiveness. Generally speaking, an alternative that costs less will be viewed more favorably, other factors being equal, than one that costs more, or one alternative may be selected over another because its implementation is more feasible. For example, it is considerably easier to install a traffic light at an accident-prone intersection than to build a bridge to route one intersecting road over the other.

Potential solutions should also be evaluated in terms of their acceptability to policy makers, implementers, and the population. Policy makers are unlikely to approve an alternative that diminishes their power or authority, and implementers are certainly unlikely to accept a potential solution that requires them to work overtime or without pay if another alternative is available. Similarly, members of the population affected by the

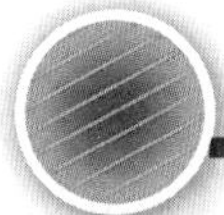

Evidence-Based Practice

Health Communication and Social Marketing

Health communication and social marketing is one type of population health intervention for which the Community Preventive Services Task Force (2014b) has examined the evidence base. Based on their review, several communication strategies are recommended for use in addressing specific population health problems. For example, mass media campaigns have been found effective in preventing motor vehicle-related injury and more circumscribed media campaigns are recommended for cancer prevention and control. Insufficient evidence of efficacy has been found for mass media campaigns, however, in addressing cancer prevention and control, obesity prevention, promotion of physical activity, and tobacco use cessation.

Interpersonal communication, for example, through group education or one-to-one counseling, has been found to be effective and is recommended for cancer prevention and control, motor vehicle accident injury prevention, and violence prevention in schools. The task force found insufficient evidence to recommend interpersonal communication techniques in addressing obesity prevention, enhancement of physical activity, and promotion of immunization, but community-wide interventions incorporating multiple strategies are recommended to address several of these areas (Community Preventive Services Task Force, 2014b).

proposed program may find one alternative more acceptable than another for a variety of reasons.

Alternative solutions may also differ in terms of the resources needed to implement them. Generally speaking, an alternative that requires fewer resources or for which resources are already available is more likely to be endorsed than one that requires extensive or scarce resources. For example, a group seeking to improve the nutritional status of schoolchildren may select an alternative that makes use of existing facilities used to prepare meals for senior citizens rather than one that necessitates providing kitchen facilities in each school. Efficiency is a related criterion on which alternative solutions to a particular problem can be evaluated. An efficient alternative makes better use of available resources and is usually viewed more favorably than an inefficient one. An asset-oriented assessment and positive population diagnoses derived from the assessment can provide a picture of the resources already available within the population and can assist in assessing the relative resource needs of alternative solutions.

Questions of equity also arise in evaluating alternative solutions to a problem. Alternatives that unfairly discriminate against one segment of the population are usually rejected. For example, one alternative to the problem of dealing with teen pregnancy might be to provide contraceptive services in the larger high schools. If, however, these schools tend to serve the upper-middle-class segment of the population while lower-class students attend smaller schools, this alternative would discriminate against a segment of the population also needing service.

Political consequences also need to be considered. For instance, an alternative plan that provides services to a highly vocal voting bloc might be viewed more favorably by politicians than one that serves a less politically involved minority group. Evaluation of alternatives may also involve forecasting regarding the effects of other possible events on the problem or its solution. For example, if a vaccine for HIV infection were likely to be available in the near future, planners may not want to put a lot of resources into a condom promotion program.

Finally, alternative solutions should be evaluated in terms of the identifiability of the target group. One potential solution for preventing the spread of AIDS might be to screen all prostitutes in the population for HIV infection. It is somewhat difficult, however, to identify this group of people, as prostitution is an illegal activity in most places. It might be easier to screen everyone who requests contraceptive services because this group is both sexually active and identifiable.

Consideration of possible sources of opposition also contributes to selection of the most appropriate alternative. If it is known that members of the local PTA would vigorously oppose a "sex fair" as a means of educating adolescents on sexual issues, another less threatening alternative would be more appropriate.

Analysis of alternatives leads to selection of one or more interventions judged to meet the criteria set for acceptable solutions. Once this selection has been made, the planning group can proceed to the tasks involved in developing the actual program.

DEVELOPING THE PROGRAM. The four primary tasks involved in developing the program include identifying program objectives, delineating the program theory, delineating actions to achieve objectives, and identifying and obtaining resources. Each of these tasks will be briefly addressed here.

Identifying objectives. The first step in actually developing the program is to identify the objectives the program is intended to accomplish. Objectives are statements of specific outcomes expected to result from the program that contribute to the realization of the overall goal.

Program developers usually address two kinds of objectives: outcome objectives and process objectives. **Outcome objectives** reflect the expected results of a program for its intended beneficiaries and, in the case of population-level programming, for the overall population. An outcome for a smoking cessation program, for example, might be that 75% of program participants successfully quit smoking within 6 months of starting the program. An outcome objective at the population level might be a 50% reduction in the prevalence of smoking within the population in the year after program implementation.

Outcome objectives may be designed at multiple levels and may include short-term, intermediate, and long-term outcomes. For instance, short-term objectives of a nutrition education program might be that people understand the food pyramid and are able to use the pyramid to select an appropriate number of servings of each category of food. An intermediate objective might be that people change their dietary habits based on the education received. A long-term objective might be a 30% decrease in the prevalence of obesity within the population.

Process objectives are statements of the level of expected performance of program staff in carrying out a program. Using our nutrition education program as an example, a process objective might be that the program is provided to 300 people over the course of a year. Another process objective might be that the program is provided in three different languages.

Effective program objectives reflect the following characteristics:

- **Measurable:** Achievement of the objective can be measured. Measurability involves specification of a benchmark or expected level of achievement (e.g., 75% of smoking cessation program participants will stop smoking).
- **Precise:** The expected outcome is clear and precisely stated.
- **Time specific:** The objective includes a statement of the time within which it should be accomplished.
- **Reasonable or practical:** The objective is practical and able to be met with a reasonable amount of effort and using a reasonable level of available resources.
- **Within group capability:** The objective is within the competence of the planning group to accomplish, given members' expertise and authority.
- **Legal:** The objective can be achieved using legal activities.
- **Congruent with population social norms and values:** The objective is consistent with the values and morals of implementers and members of the population or target group.

- **Carries minimal side effects:** The objective has minimal side effects, and these effects are acceptable to program beneficiaries.
- **Fits budgetary limitations:** The objective can be accomplished within existing budgetary constraints.

Using the long-term outcome objective for our smoking cessation program as an example, the objective is both precise and measurable in that we expect a 50% (measurable) decrease in smoking behavior (not overall tobacco use) in the population. The objective is also time specific in that we expect it to be achieved within 1 year of program initiation. It is also legal, in that it is not illegal for people to stop smoking; however, it may not be reasonable to expect such a dramatic drop in the prevalence of smoking as a result of the program. If the population values health and does not attach religious or cultural value to smoking, the objective is also congruent with population social norms and values. Achieving the objective also carries minimal side effects for the beneficiaries (temporary irritability, potential weight gain), but these side effects are outweighed by the benefits of smoking cessation. At this point, we do not know for sure if the objective fits within the group's capabilities or if it fits budgetary limitations because we do not know what those capabilities or limitations are, but it is reasonable to suspect that the objective also meets these criteria.

Delineating the program theory. To develop effective health care programs for populations, it is helpful to know how the program is supposed to work. A **program theory** or logic model is an explanation of how elements of a program interact to produce the expected outcomes. Program theories usually reflect a series of if/then statements, such as "If we do this, that will occur, and that will lead to a further result, which will eventually lead to the desired outcome." The theory also includes the rationale for the proposed connections between actions and the desired outcome. A logic model is a graphic description of the program theory, or a diagram indicating program inputs and activities and how they should result in the desired program outcome (Wilder Research, 2009). For more information on the program theories and logic models, see the *External Resources* section of the student resources site.

In addition to describing how a program is expected to produce the desired results, program theories or logic models serve several other purposes. Obviously, they identify the theoretical framework underlying the program, but they also provide guidance for organizing program evaluation efforts and determining the program's readiness for evaluation. Finally, they enable program planners to assess the fidelity of the program in meeting its expected outcomes. Figure 15-1 presents a partial program theory for our smoking cessation program.

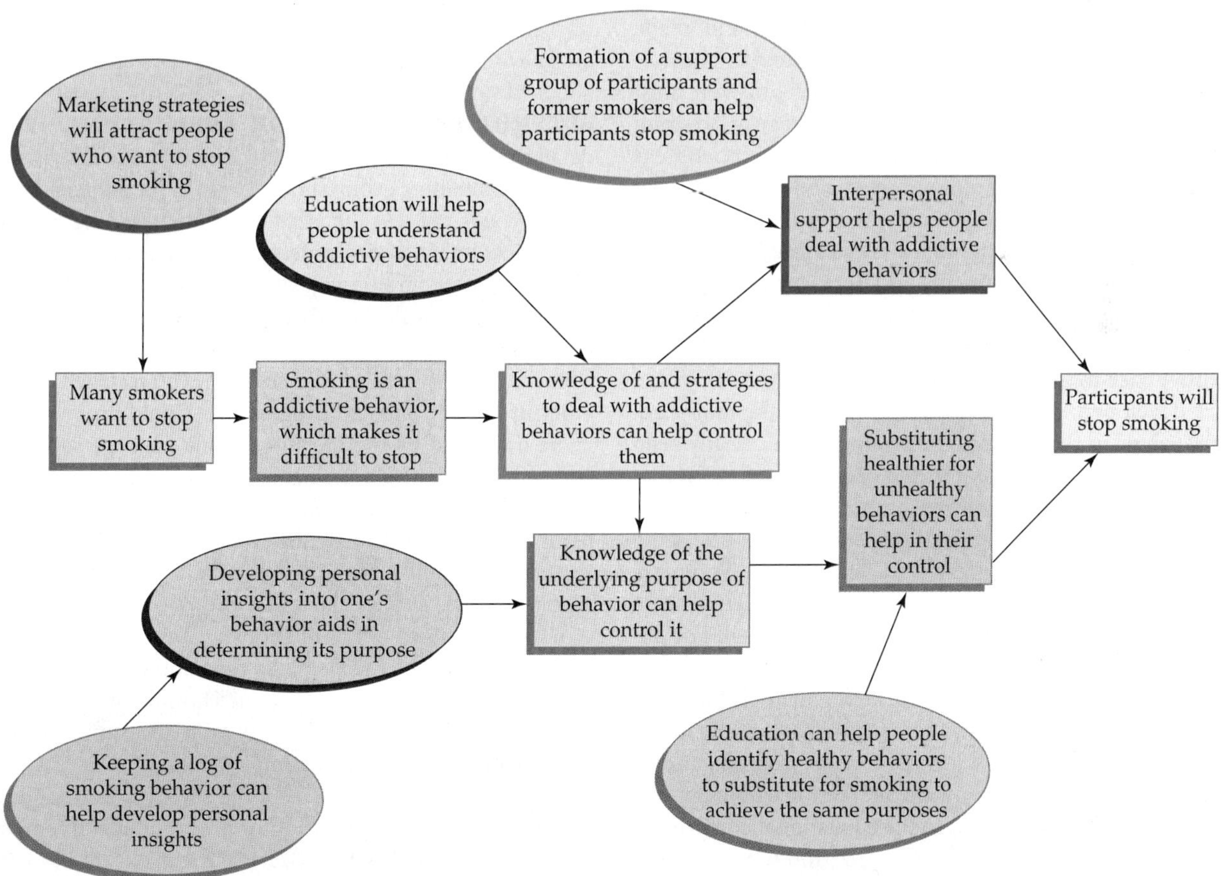

FIGURE 15-1 Partial Program Theory for a Smoking Cessation Program

Rectangles in Figure 15-1 indicate the basic theoretical foundation explaining how a program to promote smoking cessation should work. This is sometimes referred to as the cause-and-effect portion of a program theory. The ovals contain elements of program or intervention activities designed to bring about the desired outcome; smoking cessation among program participants. The theory of cause and effect suggests that although many smokers wish to stop smoking they are unable to do so because of the difficulties involved in stopping an addictive behavior. However, the theory also suggests that knowledge of addictive behaviors as well as one's own motivation for that behavior can help people quit smoking. Knowledge can also assist people to identify substitute behaviors that can achieve the same purpose as smoking. Development of this knowledge occurs through program activities such as education and keeping a log of one's smoking behavior. Since interpersonal support has also been found to help people deal with addictive behaviors, another intervention to be included in the program is the formation of a support group for participants. No one will participate in the program, however, unless they are made aware of it, which suggests that another necessary activity involves recruiting participants through program marketing.

Delineating program activities to achieve outcome objectives. The next step in the planning process is delineating specific activities required to carry out the program. This is usually considered the "nitty-gritty" of planning, and many planning groups mistakenly jump immediately to this phase of activity. For planning to be effective, however, this step must be preceded by those discussed earlier. In this stage of program planning, the population health nurse may need to function as an advocate within the planning group for interventions that are evidence-based and logically connected to the desired outcomes. The population health nurse may also need to advocate for interventions that are culturally and linguistically appropriate to the target population and that consider the population's educational and economic assets.

In this phase of planning, the step-by-step details of the plan are developed. To a large extent, many of the major activities involved in carrying out the program have already been delineated in the development of the program theory. Using the smoking cessation program example, required activities will include developing the educational curriculum, designing a marketing strategy and materials, developing the organizational structure for the support group, and so on. Each of these activities has subactivities that need to be completed. For example, some of the activities related to marketing will include determining whether to employ a marketing firm, deciding on the message and what media will be used to disseminate it, determining how people should register for the program, and so on down to the last detail of how the marketing campaign will be carried out. Activities related to the educational component of the program include determining when and where to hold group sessions, what content should be presented at each session, and what teaching-learning strategies will be used.

Identifying and obtaining resources. Once program activities have been delineated in detail, the resources needed to carry them out can be identified. Resources include personnel, money, materials, and time. To continue with the previous example of smoking cessation, a variety of resources will be needed to implement the program. Personnel resources may include people knowledgeable about smoking, its health effects, and addictive behaviors; people with marketing expertise; and artists and designers to develop attractive marketing and curricular materials. Funds will be needed to produce teaching and recruiting materials and to pay staff. Materials needed include curricular and recruiting materials as well as facilities and equipment for the educational sessions and support group meetings. Many of these resources may have been identified in the course of the asset-oriented population health assessment.

The planning group must not only decide what resources are required but also specify how these resources can be obtained. Will the group write a grant proposal or lobby the local government for funds for the program? Will they hire someone to create marketing materials or design them themselves? Can materials be printed at cost by a local printer? The final consideration with respect to resources is that of time. The time needed to put the program into operation must be determined and specific timelines for various components of program development set. Population health nurses as advocates may assist with grant writing to obtain resources needed for program implementation. They may also assist in linking the planning group with existing resources.

SETTING THE STAGE FOR EVALUATION. When the detailed plan has been constructed and specific activities delineated, the planning group should begin to set the stage for evaluation. At this point in the planning process, setting the stage for evaluation includes two aspects: evaluating the plan itself and planning for program evaluation. With respect to the plan, is it based on identified needs of the target group or population or is it unrelated to those needs? Is the plan flexible enough to adapt to changing circumstances in the foreseeable future? How efficient will the planned program be? Could program efficiency be improved by modification of the plan? Finally, how adequate is the plan? Have all constraints and contingencies been addressed? Answers to these and similar questions enable the planning group to evaluate the plan and to identify the need for any modifications before implementation. Again, the program theory or logic model can assist in evaluating the plan itself. Are the cause-and-effect relationships assumed in the model based on evidence? Are the links clear and direct, or have some necessary activities been forgotten? Have the necessary tasks of program implementation been identified in sufficient detail to prevent any surprises during implementation?

The second aspect in setting the stage for evaluation is beginning to plan for evaluation of program effectiveness. This may seem a bit premature because the program has not even started; however, it is essential. Unless planning for program evaluation is incorporated at this stage, the data needed for evaluating program outcomes and processes may not be available when the time arrives to conduct the actual evaluation.

Planning for evaluation involves four considerations. The first of these is determining criteria on which the program should be evaluated. The second consideration is the types of data to be collected and the means used to collect the data. Determining the resources needed to carry out the evaluation is the third consideration. Finally, the planning group should determine who will evaluate the program. All of these considerations are addressed in greater detail in the section on evaluating population-based health care programs. At this juncture it is sufficient to reemphasize the point that planning for evaluation begins during program planning, not after the program has been implemented.

Effective health program planning involves all of the steps discussed here. When steps are ignored or bypassed, the program planned is likely to be less effective and its implementation may prove more difficult. Steps in the planning process are summarized in the *Highlights* box below.

Implementing Population-Based Health Initiatives

It is not enough for the planning group to plan for a health care program to meet identified population needs. The group must also ensure that the plan is implemented as designed. The goal of implementation is to integrate program activities into existing networks in such a way that the program is sustained as long as the need for it continues. Implementing a health program involves several considerations. These include getting the plan accepted, performing the tasks involved in implementing the program, and using strategies that foster implementation of the program as planned.

PLAN ACCEPTANCE. Acceptance of the planned program occurs at four levels. The first level is acceptance by community policy makers. If policy makers have been represented on the planning group, this level of acceptance should already have been achieved. If not, population health nurses can serve as advocates in presenting the plan to policy makers or in preparing members of the population to present the plan themselves. For example, a group of population health nursing students wanted to present information on STD prevention at their religious-sponsored university. A faculty member assisted the students to couch their prevention message in a way that would be acceptable to the campus population. She then met with the Vice President for Student Affairs to gain his support for the project.

The second level of acceptance involves convincing those who are to carry out the plan to implement it as designed. Again, if program implementers have been adequately represented in the planning effort, this level of acceptance is already partially achieved. All that remains is for the implementers to convert the plan into an operational program.

Acceptance and participation in the planned program by members of the target population is the third level of acceptance. If, for example, the planned program involves providing contraceptive services to sexually active adolescents, the third level of acceptance involves adolescents' participation in the program. Acceptance at this level may require marketing the program to the intended target population.

The fourth level of acceptance involves potential resisters. Resisters, particularly those with influence with any of the prior three groups, can make or break a program. They can influence policy makers to reject the program or withhold required funding. They may also influence participation in the program by members of the target population or convince implementers to sabotage the program. Once again, if potential resisters have been included effectively in the planning group, their influence on program implementation is more likely to be positive than negative. Using the STD example, the Vice President for Student Affairs was a potential resister. Because of the population health nursing faculty member's advocacy, he became a supporter of the program and helped to defuse other sources of resistance on campus.

TASKS OF IMPLEMENTATION. Three basic tasks are involved in program implementation: activity delineation and sequencing, task allocation, and task performance. Necessary activities have been broadly outlined during the program planning phase. Now they must be specifically delineated and sub-activities identified. This involves identifying needed categories of action and the skills required for their performance. At this point, implementers would determine the appropriate sequencing of activities and might establish a specific time frame for

Highlights

Steps in the Planning Process

- Defining and prioritizing population health issues: Identifying population health issues derived from the population health assessment, prioritizing them on the basis of agreed-upon criteria, defining the specific problem or issue to be addressed in program planning, and developing the overall program goal.
- Creating the planning group: Selecting planning group members, developing planning competence in group members, formulating a group philosophy, and developing effective group dynamics.
- Analyzing the issue: Determining needs for and obtaining additional information related to the issue to be addressed in the program, levels of health care involved, and potential solutions. Possible solutions are analyzed in the context of criteria for acceptable solutions and one or more options selected.
- Developing the program: Designing the program, including identifying objectives, delineating the program theory, designing actions to accomplish program objectives, and identifying and obtaining necessary resources.
- Setting the stage for evaluation: Evaluating the adequacy of the plan, revising it as needed, and planning for later program evaluation.

their accomplishment. Returning to the program theory in Figure 15-1, program implementation would entail determining the details of the marketing program and the activities needed to establish the smokers' support group.

Task allocation involves identifying the expertise of program implementers relative to the skills needed to implement the program. At this point, responsibility is assigned for various activities to be performed. Such assignments must be communicated to those involved, who must be provided with whatever education or training is required to implement the program. Finally, the activities themselves are carried out and the planned program is put into operation.

STRATEGIES FOR IMPLEMENTATION. Program implementation can be enhanced if several specific implementation strategies are employed. The first strategy is to assign responsibility for coordination of the total effort to one person. Identifying preparatory steps to each activity and listing them in sequence also fosters implementation of the program as planned.

Another strategy is periodic consultation with those implementing the program to address any difficulties that arise. Finally, the chances of implementing the program as planned are enhanced when everyone involved is clearly informed of expectations and the time frame for meeting expectations.

Members of the planning group, or designated others, must monitor implementation of the program to determine any barriers to implementation or any changes needed in the plan itself. Implementation monitoring can help program personnel and community members determine whether or not the program was implemented as planned, the extent to which the targeted recipients were reached, and any modifications needed to make the program more effective. Other considerations include identification of barriers to implementation and determining factors that may inhibit program effectiveness. Implementation monitoring is discussed in more detail below.

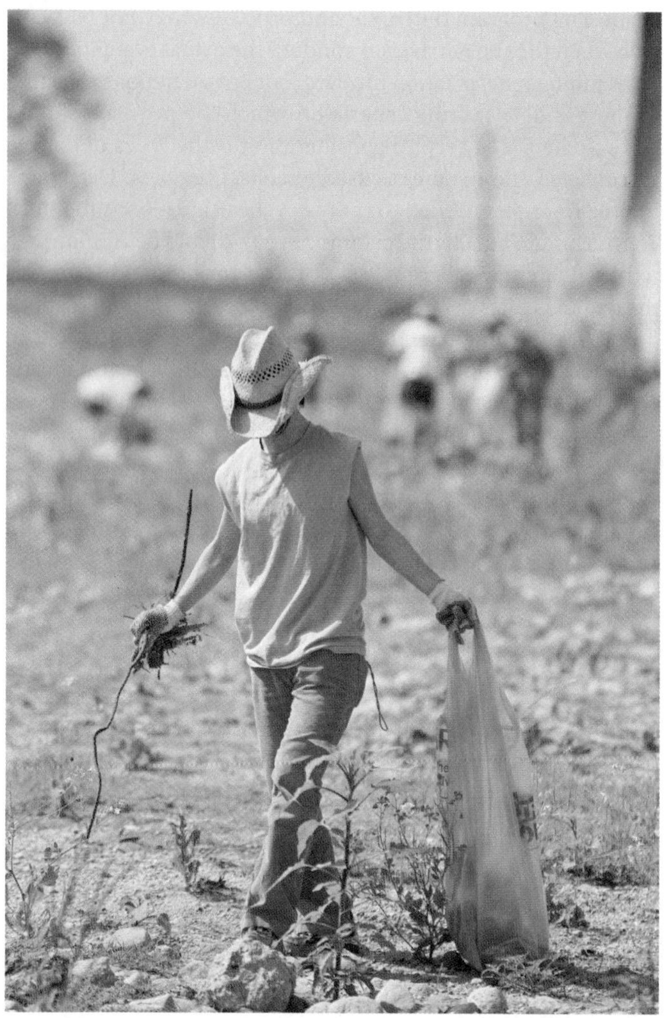

Community clean-up projects promote efforts for a healthy environment. *(Greatbass/Fotolia)*

Evaluating Population-Based Health Initiatives

Evaluating the effects of health-related programs is an essential feature of the care of populations. Program evaluation is needed for many of the same reasons that a systematic process is used in program planning. Health care providers recognize the limitation of available resources and must be accountable to the members of the population who use the program and, particularly, to those who pay for the program. They must be able to justify the program's existence and continuation. This can be done only by documenting the effectiveness of programs in solving the problems they were designed to address.

Evaluation of a particular program may be undertaken for a variety of reasons. Some of these include justifying program continuation or expansion, improving the quality of service provided, determining future courses of action, and determining the impact of the program. Other reasons for evaluation might be to call attention to the program, to assess personnel performance, or to assuage political expectations. The underlying purpose for program evaluation, however, is to make better programmatic decisions.

The CDC has developed a framework for the evaluation of population-based health programs (CDC 2011a, 2011b, 2011c, 2012). This framework poses a series of general questions that can guide program evaluation (CDC, 2012). These questions include the following:

- What will be evaluated?
- What aspects of the program will be considered in judging its performance?
- What standards will be used to judge the program's performance?
- What evidence will be used to compare program performance with the standards selected?
- What conclusions can be drawn from comparing program data with the standards selected?
- How will the evaluation information be used to improve program effectiveness?

The first four questions guide the development of the evaluation plan. The last two address analysis and use of evaluative data. The framework also delineates the steps in the evaluation process and standards for an effective evaluation. Before we discuss the evaluation process and standards, however, we will examine some general considerations in program evaluation.

GENERAL CONSIDERATIONS IN PROGRAM EVALUATION. There are a number of general considerations to be addressed in designing a program evaluation. These include the purpose of the evaluation, who should conduct the evaluation, political considerations, ethical considerations, and considerations regarding the type of evaluation to be conducted.

The evaluation purpose. The purpose of the evaluation influences all other aspects of the process. For example, if the purpose of the evaluation is to justify continuing a program, the evaluation will focus on determining whether the program has a beneficial effect on the health of the population group for which it is designed. On the other hand, if the purpose is to decide whether programs are under- or overused, evaluation will focus on the number of persons served. In other words, the purpose of the evaluation influences the types of data collected and how they are used.

Possible purposes for evaluation include deciding to continue or discontinue the program, improving the program, testing a new idea or approach, comparing two similar programs, making decisions to add or drop an element of a program, determining the feasibility of implementing the program elsewhere, and allocating resources among competing programs. Other potential purposes for program evaluation include justifying program expenditures, determining if the implementation timeline is on target, gaining support for program expansion, drawing attention to the program, and demonstrating the achievements of the program.

Evaluator considerations. Another consideration in planning for evaluation is the question of who will conduct the evaluation. Should the evaluators be people who implement the program? Program beneficiaries? Outside experts? Or someone else? Considerations in selecting who will evaluate the program include trust and credibility, access and cooperation, hidden agendas, and confidentiality. Who will have credibility in evaluating the program? An outside expert might have credibility with policy makers, but less with program participants or members of the population. Program implementers might be trusted by other staff and by program beneficiaries, but be somewhat biased in their approach to data analysis and conclusions drawn. Policy makers might also conduct the evaluation, but might have hidden agendas related to the program, as might program staff.

Program implementers will have access to much of the data needed for the evaluation and may have the cooperation of other staff members and beneficiaries. An outside expert is likely to be relatively objective in his or her evaluation, but is not as well acquainted with possible data sources and may not be trusted by program staff and beneficiaries, which might lead to decreased cooperation on their part. Outside evaluators also tend to be a rather expensive alternative.

Another possibility, and one that is in keeping with population engagement, is empowerment evaluation. **Empowerment evaluation** is an interactive process in which members of the population, in collaboration with the support team, identify issues and evaluation questions to be addressed, the manner in which they will be addressed, and the use to be made of the information obtained.

Empowerment evaluation assists population groups to develop the skills to assess and improve their own quality of life. In empowerment evaluation, the population health nurse evaluator serves as an educator, advocate, and facilitator. Members of the population determine the focus and methods for the evaluation and participate in data collection and analysis and use of the findings. If members of the population are to collect evaluation data, consideration should be given to confidentiality issues if client records are used as a data source. The evaluation team should consider all of these possibilities before determining who will conduct the evaluation.

Political considerations. Program evaluation occurs within a political context, and so political factors should be considered in designing the evaluation. Evaluations, for example, may be undertaken purely for political reasons, such as delaying decisions about the program. For example, some policy makers may be calling for discontinuation of a program. Others who support the program, however, may propose an evaluation of program effects to delay any action taken with respect to the program. Policy makers may also choose to evaluate a program in order to escape pressure from competing interest groups. For example, different segments of the population may support different alternative solutions to an identified problem. In this instance, evaluation of programs based on the different alternatives may give policy makers support for choosing one alternative over another.

Program evaluation may also be conducted to provide legitimacy for prior decisions or to support program expansion. For example, data on the effectiveness of adapting a *Parents as Teachers* program (a national program to promote school readiness in children) specifically for Hmong families were used to support adaptation of the program to Hispanic families in the same community. Finally, program evaluation may be used to promote support for the program. In this instance, there is a risk that those proposing the evaluation may want to highlight only positive aspects of the program rather than conduct a comprehensive evaluation of program effects.

In addition, population health nurses and members of the population engaged in program evaluation may want to consider the political uses to which evaluation findings may be put. For example, positive evaluation findings may be used to support reelection of public officials who supported program initiation. Conversely, negative findings may be used to bolster the candidacy of a political opponent. Negative findings regarding program effectiveness may be used to close programs that provide other benefits for a population (e.g., visibility of cultural minority groups, employment opportunities for community members, and so on).

Ethical considerations. Ethical conflicts must be anticipated in program evaluation. Participation in the evaluation should be voluntary for staff and clients alike. This poses some problems in that staff members are sometimes unwilling to reveal information that reflects poorly on them or on the program that employs them. To circumvent this reluctance, the evaluator needs to have a variety of sources of data that provide an overall picture of the program and its effects.

Confidentiality is another issue. Persons who provide data need to be assured that their individual responses will not be identifiable. There is also the question of who will have access to the findings of the evaluation. Should findings be shared only with those involved in the program? With their supervisors? With funding agencies or regulatory bodies? The use to which findings can be put is also of concern. Can the evaluator publish the information? Will it be used to fire personnel?

Finally, the evaluation team must consider the risks and benefits accruing from the evaluation. Is there potential for harm to the participants, either clients or staff? Do the anticipated benefits of the evaluation outweigh any possible risks?

Type of evaluation. The last major consideration in evaluating a health care program is the type of evaluation to be conducted. Program evaluation may occur either prospectively or retrospectively. In a prospective evaluation, the evaluation is planned and evaluative criteria are determined prior to program implementation. Retrospective evaluation is designed after the program is completed or at least in the process of being implemented. Although prospective evaluation is the recommended approach, there are many occasions in which population health nurses may be involved in retrospective evaluation. For example, population health nurses may be asked to assist in the evaluation of existing programs for which evaluative mechanisms and criteria were not established during program planning. At times, population health nurses will be asked to evaluate programs that do not even have clear expected outcomes. In those instances, the first step in the evaluation process is to determine what the program is expected to achieve.

Whether the approach used in program evaluation is prospective or retrospective, there are three basic types of evaluation that can be conducted: implementation monitoring, process evaluation, and outcome evaluation. Many program evaluations incorporate more than one type of evaluation.

Implementation monitoring. Implementation monitoring involves examining the extent to which the program has been implemented as planned. Has the organizational structure of the program been implemented as designed? Structure reflects the delivery system characteristics of the program including its organization, the types of personnel employed, types of clients served, and so on. Evaluative questions that might be asked in implementation monitoring include the following:

- Do program staff have the education and expertise to carry out the program and meet identified population needs?
- Is the program attracting the anticipated number and type of participants? Are there barriers to access to services for some segments of the population? If so, what are they and how can they be overcome?
- Are program activities being implemented as planned? If not, what factors are impeding planned implementation?
- Is program implementation proceeding within the anticipated time frame? If not, what factors are delaying implementation of various elements of the program?

Process evaluation. The second type of evaluation is process evaluation. Here, one is concerned with the quality of interactions between program implementers and recipients. Process evaluation examines program performance and may take the perspective of quality assurance or quality improvement. The focus in quality assurance is on making sure that the processes by which care is provided meet certain established standards. If the standard has been met, no action is warranted and program operation continues unmodified. Quality improvement, on the other hand, focuses on continuing improvement in program performance. The philosophy behind quality improvement, also referred to as continuous quality improvement (CQI) or total quality management (TQM), is that clients' needs and expectations change over time and that an effective health care program is continually changing to better meet those needs. This can be achieved only if the processes of care are being continually examined and improved as needed. Quality improvement focuses on enhancing the processes of care to create more effective outcomes.

Process evaluation occurs during program implementation (Strickland, Hodge, & Tom-Orme, 2009) and addresses questions of what is working (or not working) within the program and why. Process evaluation also helps to determine why program objectives may not be met (Substance Abuse and Mental Health Services Administration [SAMHSA], n.d.). In addition, process evaluation may be useful in implementing the program in other places. For example, information about processes that worked and did not work in one setting may assist in developing more effective processes in other similar settings.

Process evaluation also examines the context in which the program operates. When the context changes, the program may also need to change to continue to effectively achieve its expected outcomes. For example, an existing community immunization program may have been planned prior to the arrival of a large refugee population. Program processes will need to be changed to incorporate outreach activities, informed consent, and education regarding side effects in other languages to accommodate the cultural background of this new group of beneficiaries.

Additional considerations that may be incorporated in process evaluation include issues of efficiency, cost, equity, adequacy, quality, timeliness, and satisfaction with care received.

Efficiency evaluation addresses the use of resources in relation to the outcomes achieved by the program. Cost reflects the entire cost of the program and its acceptability to implementers, policy makers, and funding sources. Programs may be highly effective, but may be delivered at a cost too high to be supported. Equity concerns the extent to which the needs of the entire target population, rather than only certain segments, are met. Adequacy, on the other hand, addresses the extent to which all of the related needs of the target population are met by the program. Quality evaluation reflects whether the care provided by the program meets established standards. Evaluation of timeliness addresses whether services are provided within an anticipated time frame. Finally, satisfaction with program services is evaluated from the perspectives of the individuals who receive them, providers, and the population at large. Possible process evaluation criteria and potential evaluative questions are provided in Table 15-4• Evaluative questions are considered in the context of an immunization program for vaccine-preventable diseases.

Outcome evaluation. Outcome evaluation focuses on the consequences of the program for the health and welfare of the population, irrespective of how well organized or efficient the program was. Outcome evaluation documents the effects of the program and justifies decisions to continue, modify, or eliminate it. The greatest difficulty in evaluating the effects of population health programs lies in the extended time between interventions and their effects. For this reason, outcome evaluation may focus on short-term, intermediate, and long-term outcomes or on *effect* and *impact.*

A program's effect is the degree to which specific outcome objectives were met. This addresses the achievement of

TABLE 15-4 Process Evaluation Criteria and Related Evaluation Questions

Criterion	Potential Evaluation Questions
Context	• Has the context within which the program operates changed? (e.g., are community members able to get immunizations from other sources, or has there been a change in the population needing program services?) • Is there still a need for the program given the altered program context? • Are changes needed in the program to adapt to changes in the context? (e.g., does the immunization program need to adapt to provide services to non-English-speaking community members?)
Efficiency	• What is the cost of the program per unit accomplishment? (e.g., what is the cost of an immunization program per child fully immunized?) • Are resources (time, personnel, equipment and supplies, funding) being used as efficiently as possible? (e.g., would immunization services in the context of other services, such as Women, Infants, and Children (WIC) services, reach more clients?) • How much waste occurs in the use of program resources? (e.g., how many doses of vaccine expire before they can be used?)
Cost	• What is the overall cost of the program? • Is the cost of the program acceptable given the level of benefits achieved? • What is the cost of the program in terms of lost opportunities? (e.g., what other programs might be funded with that money or implemented with staff time?)
Equity	• Are various segments of the target population benefiting equally from the program? If not, why? (e.g., are Hispanic clients less likely to take advantage of immunization services? If so, why?) • Do some segments of the target population have difficulty obtaining program services? (e.g., does an immunization program provide services to children but not to adults?)
Adequacy	• Does the program address all of the target population's needs in the area to be addressed? (e.g., does an immunization program provide all the required immunizations for school entry or only some of them?)
Quality	• Do the services provided conform to recognized standards? (e.g., are parents given accurate information on which to give informed consent for immunizations? Are they informed of potential reactions and what to do about them?) • Is the performance of staff monitored to determine the quality of services provided? If so, what do results indicate? (e.g., do staff use appropriate immunization techniques for people of different ages?) • What indicators are used to measure quality in the services provided? Are these indicators valid and reliable? (e.g., how is the performance of staff in providing immunizations services evaluated?)
Timeliness	• Are program services received in a timely fashion and within an expected time frame? • Are services available when requested, or do clients have to wait to obtain services? (e.g., can parents get their children immunized when needed, or do they have to wait for an appointment?) • Are expected program results achieved within an expected time frame? (e.g., have community immunization levels increased to the expected level in the anticipated time from program initiation?)
Satisfaction	• What is the level of satisfaction with the program expressed by program beneficiaries? By service providers? By the community? • What are areas of dissatisfaction, if any? What factors contribute to dissatisfaction with the program? • Are program recipients satisfied with the services provided by the program? • Are they satisfied with program outcomes? • Are policy makers satisfied that the program is achieving its intended outcomes at a reasonable cost?

short-term, and possibly intermediate, outcomes. Using the example of the health department immunization program, the effect of the program is evaluated when one determines whether the *Healthy People 2020* objectives of full immunization coverage for 80% of children aged 19 through 36 months and influenza vaccine coverage for 90% of noninstitutionalized adults over age 65 have been achieved (U.S. Department of Health and Human Services [USDHHS], 2013). If the objectives have been achieved, the program can be considered effective. If not, the evaluator must determine to what degree the objective has been met and whether continuation of the program is warranted. For example, if vaccine coverage was achieved for 75% of young children in the population, extending the program would probably be considered. If, on the other hand, only 60% of the children in this age group are fully immunized, alternative approaches may need to be considered. For more information on *Healthy People 2020* objectives that might be used to evaluate population health program outcomes, see the *External Resources* section of the student resources site.

The impact of a program is how well it serves to attain overall goals. If the goal was to decrease the incidence of vaccine-preventable diseases, for example, the achievement of improved immunization rates should contribute to goal achievement. If, however, the goal was to reduce the incidence of communicable diseases in general, increasing immunization rates will only be partially successful, since some communicable disease cannot be prevented with immunization. In this instance, the program was effective in accomplishing its objective, but accomplishing the objective did not lead to achievement of the overall goal.

Health programs can have a number of outcomes. Often, the outcomes arise out of the program's stated objectives as in the examples above. Other outcomes may also be of interest. Usually, however, it is not feasible or even possible to examine all of a program's possible outcomes, so the evaluation team will need to decide which outcomes will be the focus of program evaluation. As noted earlier, members of the population should be intimately involved in the selection of outcomes to be measured.

For each outcome selected, the evaluation team will develop one or more outcome measures to assess that outcome. **Outcome measures** involve the assessment of one or more variables related to expected program results. Immunization rates and incidence rates for vaccine-preventable diseases might be outcome measures to evaluate an immunization program.

In designing a program evaluation, the evaluation team needs to decide which types of evaluation are appropriate—implementation monitoring, process evaluation, or outcome evaluation. A particular program can be evaluated with respect to any one aspect or a combination of several. The aspects selected depend on the purposes of the evaluation and the time and other resources available. Most health program evaluations will incorporate several aspects of evaluation.

EVALUATION STANDARDS. The CDC framework for program evaluation incorporates standards for evaluation adopted from the Joint Committee on Standards for Educational Evaluation. The framework incorporates 30 standards organized in four categories related to the utility of the evaluation, its feasibility, the propriety with which the evaluation is conducted, and its accuracy (CDC, 2011a). The focus of each category of standard and the related elements are presented in Table 15-5 ●.

THE EVALUATION PROCESS. Like any other systematic process, evaluation takes place in a series of specific steps. Some of these steps, such as planning the evaluation, have already been completed as part of the total planning process. Other steps are included in the CDC framework for evaluation. These steps include engaging stakeholders, describing the program, focusing the evaluation, gathering credible evidence, drawing and justifying conclusions, and disseminating and using findings. Each step is briefly discussed below. For more information on the CDC evaluation framework, see the *External Resources* section of the student resources site.

Engaging stakeholders. Stakeholders for a population health program include those served or affected by the program, program implementers, authority figures or regulators, funders, and others who may use the evaluation findings. For population-based programs, members of the general public may also be program stakeholders. Engagement at this level involves fostering input and participation in the design and conduct of the evaluation among those who have an interest in its findings. Stakeholder engagement helps to increase the utility of the evaluation for making decisions about the program, as well as increasing the evaluation's credibility. Engagement also serves to enhance the cultural sensitivity of the evaluation and helps to protect the rights of participants and prevent conflicts of interest that might jeopardize the credibility of findings (CDC, 2011b).

Engagement activities should focus on inclusion of less-powerful members of the population in the design and conduct of the evaluation. Evaluation planners will need to develop mechanisms to coordinate stakeholder input in all phases of the evaluation. Decisions will need to be made on who should be involved in the evaluation and how that involvement should occur (CDC, 2011b).

Describing the program. The second step in the evaluation process involves describing the program being evaluated, its purpose, and the context in which it operates. Description includes information about how the program was designed to function as well as how it actually operates. Contextual information provided may influence evaluation conclusions. For example, if a program was designed primarily to address the health needs of low-income segments of the population, but an economic recession leads to extensive unemployment, resources allocated to the program may not be evaluated as sufficient to meet program needs. In addition, the impact of the program may be less than anticipated because of the increased need for services in the population (CDC, 2011b).

TABLE 15-5 Categories and Related Elements of Evaluation Standards

Category	Focus	Related Elements
Utility standards	Assuring the meeting of information needs of intended evaluation users	• Evaluator credibility • Attention to stakeholders • Purposes negotiated on the basis of the needs of stakeholders • Specification of explicit values underlying the evaluation • Information relevant to the needs of stakeholders • Meaningful processes and products • Timely and appropriate communication and reporting • Concern for consequences and appropriate use of findings
Feasibility standards	Assuring that the evaluation is realistic, prudent, diplomatic, and makes effective use of resources	• Use of effective project management strategies • Use of practical and responsive procedures • Consideration of contextual factors • Effective and efficient resource use
Propriety standards	Assuring that the evaluation is conducted legally, ethically, and with due regard for the welfare of those involved and those affected by the results	• Responsive and inclusive orientation to all stakeholders • Negotiation of formal agreements making expectations explicit and accounting for the needs, expectations, and cultural contexts of those involved • Protection of human rights and respect for dignity • Clarity and fairness in addressing stakeholder needs and purposes • Transparency and disclosure of findings, limitations, and conclusions • Honest disclosure of conflicts of interest • Fiscal accountability for evaluation resources expended
Accuracy standards	Assuring that the evaluation conveys accurate information about features that determine the worth or merit of the program	• Explicitly justified conclusions and decisions • Valid interpretation of findings • Reliable information • Explicit and sufficiently detailed descriptions of programs and their contexts • Use of systematic information management strategies • Sound design and analytic approaches appropriate to the evaluation purpose • Explicitly documented evaluation reasoning • Effective and accurate communication and reporting of findings

Data from: American Evaluation Association. (n.d.). *The program evaluation standards: Summary form.* Retrieved from http://www.eval.org/p/cm/ld/fid=103_; Centers for Disease Control and Prevention. (2011a). *Evaluation standards.* Retrieved from http://www.cdc.gov/eval/standards/index.htm

Elements of the program description include the need for which the program was designed, the goals and objectives to be achieved and criteria for their achievement, the rationale for program activities drawn from the program theory, and the stage of the program's development. Other considerations in describing the program include the context in which it operates and linkages with other initiatives in the population (CDC, 2011b).

Focusing the evaluation. Focusing the evaluation involves determining the evaluation questions to be addressed and developing mechanisms to answer those questions. In developing evaluation questions, the evaluation team reviews the program theory, specifies program objectives (process and outcome) to be addressed, translates the program theory and objectives into evaluation questions, and selects the questions to be addressed in the evaluation process. Goals for the evaluation, evaluative criteria, types of data needed, and appropriate methods of data collection were established as part of the evaluation design process. Evaluative criteria and type of evaluation are based on the purpose of the evaluation and the evaluation questions asked. If the intent of the evaluation is to determine the extent to which outcome objectives are met, evaluative criteria will be derived from those objectives. In the immunization program example, evaluative criteria related to outcome objectives would include immunization levels and disease incidence in the population. If the intent is to assess the efficiency of the program, evaluative criteria might include the number of immunizations given, the length of time people had to wait for immunizations, and the effectiveness of marketing strategies for reaching specific target populations.

Data needed to answer the evaluation questions are determined and data collection procedures established. Designing the evaluation also involves determining the necessary equipment and supplies. If, for example, the evaluation team wanted to know if adequate levels of immunity had been achieved in those immunized, they would need supplies for drawing and testing blood samples. It is more likely, however, that evaluation of the program will involve collecting data on the percentage of the population immunized based on a survey of immunization records and the incidence of disease based on local surveillance strategies.

Gathering credible evidence. The evaluative criteria chosen influence the types of data collected and the manner in which they are collected. Data collection strategies may also need to take into consideration the language of program participants, their ability to read (in which case printed surveys would not be appropriate), or other elements of the program context. For the immunization program, records will need to be kept regarding the number and types of immunizations given, categories of persons to whom they were given (e.g., children, adults, members of ethnic groups). Data collection will also necessitate generating information on the existing immunization rates in the community if that has not already been obtained in the assessment that motivated program planning.

Identification of the type of data needed and appropriate data collection mechanisms should occur collaboratively between members of the population and the evaluation experts. Areas to be considered include the indicators or outcome measures to be evaluated, data collection tools, specific processes and procedures for data collection (e.g., population surveys, focus groups of program recipients, record review, and so on), training those who will collect the data, and approaches to storing and categorizing information obtained. Another important consideration is protecting the confidentiality of information and its sources (CDC, 2011b).

Drawing and justifying conclusions. Once data have been collected, they must be analyzed and interpreted and conclusions drawn. Analysis may involve conducting statistical tests of relationships or identification of concepts and themes from qualitative information. The evaluation team should employ analysis strategies that are consistent with the evaluation questions asked.

Interpreting the findings and drawing conclusions about the program is the next task in the evaluation. At this point, data are compared with the evaluative criteria or benchmarks. In evaluating the achievement of the outcome objectives of an immunization program, the evaluation team would compare the immunization rates achieved to those specified in the program objectives. If the program has achieved an 80% immunization rate for children 19 to 36 months of age and 90% for noninstitutionalized persons over age 65, the program would be judged to be effective and would probably be continued. If the program has only achieved rates of 60% and 75%, respectively, but these rates represent an increase from before the program, the program might be considered somewhat effective. The extent of improvement would need to be considered, however, in deciding whether to continue the program.

Data may also be used to assess the processes by which the program is carried out. For example, in the community focus group project described by Clark and associates (2003), one of the process objectives for the assessment was to include specific segments of the population in the assessment. When the assessment process was evaluated, the steering committee found that focus group participation mirrored community composition in terms of age, ethnicity, and the proportion of residents versus service providers in the community. Thus, the process objective was judged to be met.

In examining data related to the efficient use of supplies, an evaluation team might look at what percentage of vaccines purchased was used and what percentage was wasted. If the criterion derived from process objectives specified that less than 5% of vaccine supplies purchased be wasted and the team finds that closer to 10% was actually wasted, the program processes are not operating as efficiently as planned and program modifications may be warranted.

It is important that the conclusions drawn be congruent with the evaluation findings and are supported by the actual data obtained. In addition, the situations, time periods, and contexts to which the conclusions apply should be made clear (CDC, 2011b). For example, even though a program to reduce childhood obesity was found to be effective with a Hispanic population, to conclude that the program would be equally effective with another ethnic group would be unwarranted.

Disseminating and using findings. To be of use in making program decisions, evaluation findings need to be disseminated to a variety of individuals and groups in the population including program recipients, implementers, policy makers, funders, and so on. Findings may also need to be disseminated to others who are contemplating similar programs. The task of the evaluation team, at this point, is to determine who should be told about the evaluation findings and conclusions and when and how communication of results will occur. Dissemination of interim findings may occur during the evaluation, or dissemination may occur after the evaluation is completed (CDC, 2011b).

Findings need to be translated into language that will be understood by various stakeholder audiences and should be used to derive specific recommendations regarding the program. The team communicates the findings, as well as information about the evaluation process, in appropriate forms to the stakeholder groups. In keeping with empowerment strategies, members of the population should certainly comprise one stakeholder group to whom findings and recommendations are communicated.

The findings of the evaluation should be used as a basis for decisions about the program. Basically, three decisions can be made based on evaluative findings: to continue, to modify, or to discontinue the program. If the evaluation team finds that the program's objectives are being achieved, they may recommend continuing the program. If the team finds that only a few members of the target population are participating in the program, they may recommend either stopping the program or taking steps to increase participation. For example, perhaps marketing strategies need to be changed to target specific ethnic groups with low immunization rates who are not taking advantage of the program. Looking at program efficiency, if the assessment team finds that 10% of the vaccines purchased are being wasted, various waste control practices may need to be instituted.

CHAPTER RECAP

Care of populations or subgroups within a population makes use of the nursing process to assess population strengths and needs, and plan, implement, and evaluate population-based health programs. Members of the population should be engaged in each step along the way to enhance the effectiveness of population-based interventions and local health agencies may want to promote the development of a comprehensive community engagement strategy to foster a systematic approach to public engagement in addressing a variety of issues.

Factors related to each of the six categories of determinants of health are considered in assessing the assets and health needs of population groups. Planning to meet those needs then employs an organized and systematic process involving creation of a planning group, development of planning competence, developing goals and objectives based on program theory, and delineating resources and actions needed to accomplish goals and objectives. Implementation and evaluation of health care delivery programs are also systematic processes employed by population health nurses and others in the population.

CASE STUDY Caring for Copper City

You are a population health nurse assigned to Copper City, a small town in New Mexico with a population of 3,000. You have just arrived in town and have been given the task of assisting community members to assess the health needs of the community and develop a plan to meet those needs. Your assessment committee consists of yourself, one of the local physicians, the elementary school principal, two teachers, the pastors of two local churches, the owner of one of the local copper mines, and five community residents.

During the assessment, the assessment team obtains the following information: Copper City is a small town run by a city council and a mayor. Most of these officials are administrators of the local copper mines or owners of large chicken farms in the area. The town is in a largely rural area, 50 miles from Tucumcari. The surrounding countryside is hot and arid.

The ethnic composition of the town is 80% Caucasian of European ancestry and 20% Latino, primarily of Mexican descent. Fifty percent of the town's population is under 8 years of age. There are very few elderly persons in the community because Copper City is a relatively new town that grew up around copper mines discovered in the last 20 years. The birth rate is 30 per 1,000 population. Approximately 10% of all births are premature, and the neonatal death rate is 50 per 1,000 live births. Only about 10% of the women receive prenatal care during their pregnancies.

The major industries in the area are copper mines and chicken farms, which employ approximately 85% of the adult men and 50% of the women. The majority of the Latino population works on the chicken farms. The remaining 15% of the adult men and another 20% of the adult women are employed in offices and shops in the town. The unemployment level is 0.5%, far lower than that of the state and the nation.

The average annual family income is $8,000, and 75% of the population is below the poverty level. Nearly one third of those below the poverty level receive some form of assistance such as Medicaid or Temporary Aid to Needy Families (TANF).

The predominant religion among the Caucasian population is Methodist, and among the Latino group it is Roman Catholic. There are two Methodist churches in town, one Catholic church, and a small Southern Baptist congregation.

Many of the Latino groups engage in alternative health practices. They frequently seek health care from a local *yerbero* (herbalist). They may also drive to a nearby town to solicit the services of a *curandera* (faith healer). Close to one third of the Latino population speaks only Spanish.

The average education level for the community is 10th grade. For the Spanish-speaking group, however, it is only 3rd grade. Education facilities in the town include a grade school and a high school. The high school also offers adult education classes at night. There is a Head Start program that enrolls 50 children, but no other child care facilities are available.

There is a high incidence of tuberculosis in the community, and anemia and pinworms are common problems among the preschool and school-age children. Several of the men have been disabled as a result of accidents in the mines.

The only transportation to Tucumcari is by car or by train, which comes through town morning and evening. About half of the families in town own cars.

There is one general practice physician and one dentist in the town. The nearest hospital is in Tucumcari, and the funeral home hearse is used as an ambulance for emergency transportation to the hospital. The driver and one attendant have had basic first aid training but have not been educated as emergency medical technicians. The county health department provides family planning, prenatal, well-child, and immunization services 1 day a week in the basement of the larger of the two Methodist churches. In addition to yourself, the staff consists of a physician, one licensed practical nurse, a master's-prepared family nurse practitioner, and a nutritionist. The well-child and immunization services are heavily used, and immunization levels in the community are high among both preschoolers and school-age youngsters.

1. What are the biological, psychological, environmental, sociocultural, behavioral, and health system factors influencing the health of this community?
2. What assets are present in this community that might assist with problem resolution?
3. What population nursing diagnoses might you derive from the assessment team's data?
4. What health problems are evident in the case study? Which do you think are the three most important problems for this community? Why have you given these problems priority over others? Do you think other members of the assessment team would prioritize them differently? Why or why not?
5. Select one of the three top-priority problems and design a health program to resolve it. Be sure to address the following:
   - Level of health care involved (e.g., prevention, promotion, resolution, restoration)
   - Who should be involved in the planning group, why, and how you would obtain community participation in planning
   - Additional information you would need, if any, and where you would obtain that information
   - Goals and objectives for the program
   - Resources needed to implement the program
6. How would you gain acceptance of your program?
7. How would you go about implementing the program?
8. How would you conduct outcome and process evaluation of the program?

REFERENCES

Abrams, S. E. (2004). From function to competency in public health nursing, 1931 to 2003. *Public Health Nursing, 21,* 507–510.

American Evaluation Association. (n.d.). *The program evaluation standards: Summary form.* Retrieved from http://www.eval.org/p/cm/ld/fid=103

American Nurses Association. (2013). *Public health nursing: Scope and standards of practice* (2nd ed.). Silver Spring, MD: Nursesbooks.org.

Association for Community Health Improvement. (n.d.a). *Assessment process map.* Retrieved from http://www.assesstoolkit.org/assesstoolkit/introassessment.jsp#

Association for Community Health Improvement. (n.d.b). *Introduction to the Association for Community Health Improvement's Community Health Assessment Toolkit.* Retrieved from http://www.assesstoolkit.org/assesstoolkit/ACHI-CHAT-intro-slides-8-27-10.pdf

Bilton, M. (2011, October). Community health needs assessment (Executive briefing 3). *Trustee,* 21–24.

Catholic Health Association of the United States. (2013). *Assessing and addressing community health needs.* Retrieved from http://www.chausa.org/docs/default-source/general-files/cb_assessingaddressing-pdf.pdf?sfvrsn=4

Centers for Disease Control and Prevention. (2011a). *Evaluation standards.* Retrieved from http://www.cdc.gov/eval/standards/index.htm

Centers for Disease Control and Prevention. (2011b). *Evaluation steps.* Retrieved from http://www.cdc.gov/eval/steps/index.htm

Centers for Disease Control and Prevention. (2011c). *Hints for conducting strong evaluations.* Retrieved from http://www.cdc.gov/eval/strongevaluations/index.htm

Centers for Disease Control and Prevention. (2012). *A framework for program evaluation.* Retrieved from http://www.cdc.gov/eval/framework/index.htm

Clark, M. J., Cary, S., Diemert, G., Ceballos, R., Sifuentes, M., Atteberry, I., …, Trieu, S. (2003). Involving community in community assessment. *Public Health Nursing, 20,* 456–463.

Clinical and Translational Science Awards Consortium & Community Engagement Key Function Committee Task Force on the Principles of Community Engagement. (2011). *Principles of community engagement* (2nd ed.). Retrieved from http://www.atsdr.cdc.gov/communityengagement/pdf/PCE_Report_508_FINAL.pdf

Community Preventive Services Task Force. (2014a). *Guide to community preventive services.* Retrieved from http://www.thecommunityguide.org/index.html

Community Preventive Services Task Force. (2014b). *Health communication and social marketing.* Retrieved from http://www.thecommunityguide.org/healthcommunication/index.html

Doggett, E. (2010). *Community engagement in the PEPFAR Special Initiative on Sexual and Gender-based Violence.* Retrieved from http://www.healthpolicyinitiative.com/Publications/Documents/1288_1_PEPFAR_GBV_Community_Engagement_FINAL_acc.pdf

Dubowitz, T., Williams, M., Steiner, E. D., Weden, M. M., Miyashiro, L., Jacobsen, D., & Lurie, N. (2011). Using geographic information systems to match local health needs with public health services and programs. *American Journal of Public Health, 101,* 1664–1665. doi:10.2105/AJPH.2011.300195

Gawande, A. (2011, January 24). The hot spotters. *The New Yorker*. Retrieved from http://www.newyorker.com/reporting/2011/01/24/110124fa_fact_gawande

Improvement and Development Agency for Local Government, Urban Forum and the National Association for Voluntary and Community Action. (2009). *Developing your comprehensive community engagement strategy—A practical guide for local strategic partnerships*. Retrieved from http://www.navca.org.uk/existing/NR/rdonlyres/36e222bb-ee81-4c13-b60f-0278db6d4d46/0/cces_guide_2009_03.pdf

Iowa Department of Public Health. (2013). *Community health needs assessment and health improvement plan (CHNA&HIP) guide*. Retrieved from http://www.idph.state.ia.us/chnahip/Guide.aspx

Jacobs, D. E. (2011). Environmental health disparities in housing. *American Journal of Public Health, 101,* S115–S122. doi:10.2105/AJPH.2010.300058

Karasek, D., Ahern, J., & Galea, S. (2012). Social norms, collective efficacy, and smoking cessation in urban neighborhoods. *American Journal of Public Health, 102,* 343–351. doi:10.2105/AJPH.2011.300364

Larkin, H. (2010, October). Managing population health. *H&HN: Hospitals & Health Networks,* 28–32.

Local Government Association. (2012). *Useful definitions*. Retrieved from http://www.local.gov.uk/web/guest/localism-act/-/journal_content/56/10180/3511060/ARTICLE

McKnight, J. (2013). *A basic guide to ABCD community organizing*. Retrieved from http://www.abcdinstitute.org/docs/A%20Basic%20Guide%20to%20ABCD%20Community%20Organizing-1.pdf

Milio, N. (1970). *9226 Kercheval: The storefront that did not burn*. Ann Arbor, MI: University of Michigan Press.

Minnesota Department of Health. (n.d.). *Overview: What is community engagement?* Retrieved from http://www.health.state.mn.us/communityeng/intro/

Rosenbaum, S. (2013). *Principles to consider for the implementation of a community health needs assessment process*. Retrieved from http://nnphi.org/CMSuploads/PrinciplesToConsiderForTheImplementationOfACHNAProcess_GWU_20130604.pdf

Santilli, A., Carroll-Scott, A., Wong, F., & Ickovics, J. (2011). Urban youths go 3000 miles: Engaging and supporting young residents to conduct neighborhood asset mapping. *American Journal of Public Health, 101,* 2207–2210. doi:10.2105/AJPH.2011.300351

Strickland, C. J., Hodge, F., & Tom-Orme, L. (2009). Formative evaluation and community empowerment among American Indian/Alaska Natives. In L. Potvin & D. V. McQueen (Eds.), *Health promotion evaluation practices in the Americas* (pp. 179–190). New York, NY: Springer.

Substance Abuse and Mental Health Services Administration. (n.d.). *Using process evaluation to monitor program implementation*. Retrieved from http://captus.samhsa.gov/access-resources/using-process-evaluation-monitor-program-implementation

Trickett, E. J., Beehler, S., Deutsch, C., Green, L. W., Hawe, P., McLeroy, K., …, Trimble, J. (2011). Advancing the science of community-level interventions. *American Journal of Public Health, 101,* 1410–1419. doi:10.2105/AJPH.2010.300113

U.S. Department of Health and Human Services. (2013). *Immunization and infectious diseases: Objectives*. Retrieved from http://www.healthypeople.gov/2020/topicsobjectives2020/objectiveslist.aspx?topicId=23

VanDerslice, J. (2011). Drinking water infrastructure and environmental disparities: Evidence and methodological considerations. *American Journal of Public Health, 101,* S109–S114. doi:10.2105/AJPH.2011.300189

Wilder Research. (2009). *Program theory and logic models*. Retrieved from http://www.evaluatod.org/resources/evaluation-guides/LogicModel_8-09.pdf

CHAPTER

16 Care of Child and Adolescent Populations

Learning Outcomes

After reading this chapter, you should be able to:

1. Identify determinants affecting the health of children and adolescents.
2. Describe at least five health promotion and five illness/injury prevention measures appropriate to the care of children and adolescents and analyze the role of the population health nurse with respect to each.
3. Identify at least three foci in care to resolve existing health problems among children and adolescents and give examples of population health nursing interventions related to each.
4. Describe three considerations in restorative health care for children and adolescents and analyze the role of the population health nurse with respect to each.

Key Terms

adverse childhood events (ACEs)

anticipatory guidance

attention deficit hyperactivity disorder (ADHD)

binge drinking

child maltreatment

cocooning

development

developmental milestones

growth

herd immunity

immunization information systems (IISs)

menarche

Advocacy Then

Lillian Wald and Child Health

Throughout her nursing career, Lillian Wald, the co-founder of the Henry Street Settlement and U.S. public health nursing, displayed a great deal of concern for the welfare of children. One of the first projects undertaken at Henry Street was the creation of a small playground for neighborhood children in the settlement house's backyard. This interest led to her involvement with the Outdoor Recreation League, an organization dedicated to the development of public parks and playgrounds in New York City. Wald and other members of the League raised funds to improve and maintain Seward Park, which later became New York City's first municipal playground (Jewish Women's Archive, n.d.b).

Wald's concern for the health and welfare of children culminated in her work to curtail child labor and establish the Federal Children's Bureau. Initially begun as a private initiative by the National Child Labor Committee, concerned citizens used $100,000 in private funds to investigate child labor conditions. Committee members realized that effective change needed to occur as a result of federal legislative mandate. From 1905 until the creation of the bureau in 1912, Wald endeavored to influence federal policy, actively campaigning for legislation to protect children and promote their health (Jewish Women's Archive, n.d.a).

Advocacy Now

Policy Change and Environmental Contributors to Childhood Asthma

A variety of individual, genetic, and environmental factors contribute to the incidence and prevalence of asthma in children. Often control efforts are directed toward effective disease management by those affected, and relatively little attention is given to changing environmental factors that contribute to asthma (Krieger, Sargent, Arons, Standish, & Brindis, 2011).

Recognizing that exposure to outdoor asthma "triggers" is more common for children in low socioeconomic groups than in their more affluent counterparts, the California Endowment created the Community Action to Fight Asthma (CAFA) Initiative to influence policies that affect community-based environmental risk factors for asthma. To accomplish their goals, the organization employed an environmental justice framework that incorporated technical assistance providers, input from local and regional community coalitions, and media advocacy to support policy development to minimize environmental risk factors. Policy initiatives included development of standard use of thermographic cameras by housing authorities to improve identification and remediation of housing-related asthma risk factors, creation of legal precedents and regulations to ameliorate substandard housing conditions, training of local community health workers to assess indoor air quality in homes, development of guidelines for school renovation to minimize moisture and improve ventilation, implementation of "anti-idling" regulations for school buses to minimize exhaust emissions, rerouting of major highways away from residential areas in low-income communities, implementing wood burning ordinances to limit particulate emissions, and reducing truck, rail yard, and ship pollution. Other policy outcomes included prohibition of school siting near major highways, education on activity related to air quality status, school district level processes to reduce asthma triggers, replacement of diesel-fueled buses with cleaner burning models, removing pollution exemption regulations for farm equipment, and establishment of statewide greenhouse gas emission standards. Policy initiatives occurred at local, regional, and state levels, and their success was attributed to the incorporation of technical assistance, inclusion of community members, and advocacy training for members of the population (Krieger et al., 2011).

In 2012, the U.S. population included 82.5 million children less than 18 years of age in 2011. This amounts to 26% of the total U.S. population with 6.4% under 5 years of age, and nearly 20% aged 5 to 17 years (U.S. Census Bureau, 2013). Children and adolescents have specific health needs and problems that can be addressed by population health nurses. Population health nursing practice with children and adolescents involves assessing the health status and needs of these populations; deriving community health diagnoses; designing and implementing programs at all levels of health care to meet those needs; and evaluating the effectiveness of these programs.

Health Issues for Children and Adolescents

A number of current issues are of concern in relation to the health of children and adolescents in the United States and worldwide. Trends related to several of those issues, including mortality, preterm birth, injury, communicable and chronic conditions, psychological health problems, developmental disorders, and violence, will be discussed before we move to population health nursing care for this population.

Child and Adolescent Mortality

Infant mortality in the United States is higher than in many other developed nations. In 2014, the United States ranked 55th out of 224 countries in terms of infant mortality at 6.17 deaths per 1,000 live births (Central Intelligence Agency [CIA], 2014). Although this rate has declined considerably from the 100 deaths per 1,000 births in 1900 (MacDorman & Mathews, 2011), it has not kept pace with declining infant mortality in other countries and has only declined slightly in recent years. Even within the United States, infant mortality varies greatly among segments of the population. For example, infant mortality in 2010 was more than twice as high for Black infants as for White infants (Murphy, Xu, & Kochanek, 2013) with similar differences for American Indian and Alaskan Native infants (National Center for Health Statistics, 2011c).

Infants are not the only children to suffer premature death. In 2010, the overall mortality rate for children 5 to 14 years of age was 13 deaths per 100,000 children (Federal Interagency Forum on Child and Family Statistics, 2012). The leading causes of death for infants, children, adolescents, and young adults aged 1 to 24 years are depicted in Table 16-1●.

Preterm Births

Preterm births are a significant contributor to infant mortality. Preterm births also increase the risks for morbidity related to asthma, hypertension, diabetes, stroke, myocardial infarction, and heart disease in later life (Johnson & Schoeni, 2011). In 2011, approximately 12% of U.S. births were preterm (Federal Interagency Forum on Child and Family Statistics, 2013).

Injury

Unintentional injuries are another factor in child and adolescent mortality and morbidity. For example, the death rate for unintentional injuries among children 1 to 4 years of age was 8 per 100,000 in 2011. Among those aged 5 to 14 years, the unintentional mortality rate was 4 per 100,000 children (Federal Interagency Forum on Child and Family Statistics, 2013). Motor vehicle accidents are the leading cause of death in children, accounting for 1,051 deaths in children less than 14 years of age in 2009. Approximately 45% of these children were unrestrained at the time of the accident indicating that many of these deaths were preventable (Centers for Disease Control and Prevention [CDC], 2011). Another 179,000 children were injured in motor vehicle accidents that year, and a CDC study indicated that approximately 618,000 children rode without safety precautions at least some of the time in the prior year. The study also indicated that child restraint use was associated with adult seat belt use and that, when restraints were used, they were used incorrectly 72% of the time (National Center for Injury Prevention and Control [NCIPC], 2014e).

Similarly, many drowning fatalities in children are preventable. About 20% of all drowning deaths occur in children under 14 years of age; for every death, another five children are treated in emergency departments for nonfatal submersion injuries, often resulting in brain damage, long-term disability, learning disability, or permanent functional loss. The highest incidence of drowning deaths occurs in children 1 to 4 years of age, most often in home pools. Risk factors for drowning in children include inability to swim, lack of barriers to access to water, lack of adult supervision, failure to wear life jackets, alcohol use (among adolescents), and seizure disorder (NCIPC, 2014g).

Other major sources of injury among children and adolescents include playground injuries and unintentional poisoning. Approximately 300 children are seen in emergency departments for unintentional poisonings and 2 children die every day (NCIPC, 2012b).

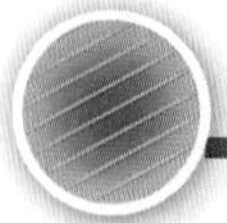

Evidence-Based Practice

Research Regarding Children as Subjects

Evidence-based practice requires that research be conducted with the same types of people to whom findings will be applied. For this reason, the federal government has ruled that all research receiving federal support include children as subjects, if relevant to the study. Why is such a ruling appropriate? What ethical dilemmas might this policy pose? In what types of studies would inclusion of children as subjects not be appropriate?

TABLE 16-1 Leading Causes of Infant, Child, and Adolescent Mortality, United States, 2010

Infants	1–4 years	5–9 years	10–14 years	15–24 years
Congenital anomalies	Unintentional injuries	Unintentional injuries	Unintentional injuries	Unintentional injuries
Short gestation	Congenital anomalies	Malignant neoplasms	Malignant neoplasms	Homicide
Sudden infant death syndrome (SIDS)	Homicide	Congenital anomalies	Suicide	Suicide
Maternal pregnancy complications	Malignant neoplasms	Homicide	Homicide	Malignant neoplasms
Unintentional injury	Heart disease	Heart disease	Congenital anomalies	Heart disease
Placenta cord membranes	Influenza and pneumonia	Chronic low respiratory disease	Heart disease	Congenital anomalies
Bacterial sepsis	Septicemia	Cerebrovascular	Chronic low respiratory disease	Cerebrovascular
Respiratory distress	Benign neoplasms	Benign neoplasms	Benign neoplasms	Complicated pregnancy
Circulatory system disease	Perinatal period	Influenza and pneumonia	Cerebrovascular	Cerebrovascular
Necrotizing enterocolitis	Chronic low respiratory disease	Septicemia	Septicemia	Chronic lower respiratory disease

Data from: Office of Statistics and Programming, National Center for Injury Prevention and Control. (2013). *10 leading causes of death by age group, United States, 2010.* Retrieved from http://www.cdc.gov/injury/wisqars/pdf/10LCID_All_Deaths_By_Age_Group_2010-a.pdf

Another 200,000 children under 14 years of age are injured on playgrounds each year, and 45% of those events result in severe injuries. About three fourths of these injuries occur in public playgrounds. From 1990 to 2000, playground injuries resulted in 147 deaths in this age group of children. Annual costs of playground injuries are estimated at $1.2 billion. The incidence of playground injuries is highest in children aged 5 to 9 years, and, somewhat surprisingly, girls account for 55% of the injuries. Injuries in public playgrounds most often occur on climbing apparatus, but occur more frequently on swings in home play areas (NCIPC, 2012a).

Heat-related injuries and illnesses also occur in adolescents, particularly in conjunction with sports practice and competition, and are the leading cause of death among high school athletes. From 2005 to 2009, for example, 100 schools sampled reported 118 instances of heat illness in which one or more days were lost from practice. Extrapolated nationally, this would amount to more than 9,000 cases per year. This does not account for additional instances in which no practice restrictions resulted (Gilchrist et al., 2010). Sports participation also results in a variety of other injuries among children and adolescents.

Communicable Diseases

In spite of the progress made in the control of communicable disease with the use of a wide variety of vaccines, communicable disease still contributes to signifcant levels of morbidity and mortality in the United States and throughout the world. For example, pertussis (whooping cough) still results in disease and death, particularly in infants under 12 months of age who have not developed sufficient immunity. A mean of 3,055 cases occurred in the United States each year from 2000 to 2004, resulting in an average of 19 deaths per year in this age group. Most of these infections occurred in infants less than 2 months old. For this reason, the Advisory Committee on Immunization Practices (ACIP, 2011b) has recommended **cocooning**, routine immunization of pregnant and postpartum women and others who are in close contact with young infants to prevent exposure to pertussis.

HIV infection and AIDS are other areas of concern with respect to communicable diseases in children. UNICEF (2013) estimated that in 2011, 3.1 to 3.8 million children under 15 years of age were living with HIV worldwide. In addition, millions of children have lost one or more parents to AIDS, and many more are affected by the poverty, homelessness, and discrimination that often accompany a diagnosis of AIDS in the family. In 2011, approximately 330,000 children were newly infected with HIV, and 230,000 deaths occurred in children under 15 years of age.

In the United States, 39% of all new HIV infections occurred in people 13 to 29 years of age, although this age group accounts for only 20% of the population. Slightly more than two thirds of these cases occur in young men and adolescents who have sex with other men. Youth infection with HIV is associated with early sexual activity, unprotected sex, lack of knowledge, substance use, the presence of other sexually transmitted diseases and sexual abuse (Division of HIV/AIDS Prevention, 2011).

According to the most recent CDC fact sheet, most cases of HIV infection and AIDS in young children result from perinatal transmission of the virus either during pregnancy or afterwards (e.g., via breast-feeding). Although perinatal transmission of HIV in the United States declined from 15.2 cases per 100,000 live births in 2007 to 9.9 cases per 100,000, 162 infants were infected perinatally with HIV in 2010 (CDC, 2014).

As we saw in Chapter 8∞, a variety of other communicable diseases affect children throughout the world, including malaria, tuberculosis, rotavirus infection, and so on. Communicable diseases will be discussed in more detail in Chapter 26∞.

Chronic Conditions

Although one frequently associates chronic illness with older members of the population, a whole host of chronic conditions affect children and adolescents as well. As noted by some authors, advances in medical technology have led to a growing number of children and adolescents who are living with complex health needs due to conditions that would have resulted in death in the past. These health needs are ongoing, rather than the result of a single episode of acute illness. In many instances, these children are dependent on some type of medical technology for their survival. Even for children and adolescents who are not dependent on life-sustaining technology, they and their families face a lifelong effort to manage their conditions. The presence of a chronic condition may also limit children's abilities. In 2011, 9% of children aged 5 to 17 years experienced activity limitations due to one or more chronic conditions (Federal Interagency Forum on Child and Family Statistics, 2013). A few examples of the magnitude of the burden of chronic illness in children and adolescents are presented below.

The CDC (2012) estimates that 40,000 U.S. children are born with heart defects each year, requiring lifelong care. Another approximately 30,000 U.S. children and adults are affected by cystic fibrosis (CF), a condition that is most often diagnosed in young children before the age of 2 years. About 1,000 new cases of CF are diagnosed each year. Although the survival time for these children has been extended due to medical advances, the mean survival age still remains at about 30 years (Cystic Fibrosis Foundation, n.d.).

Cancer is another common cause of chronic illness and mortality in children and adolescents. According to the U.S. Cancer Statistics Working Group (2013), the overall invasive cancer incidence in children from birth to 14 years of age is 16.4 per 100,000 children and 17.5 per 100,000 from birth to age 19 years. Leukemia is the most common form of childhood malignancy followed by brain and other nervous system tumors.

Epilepsy also occurs in children as well as in other age groups; in fact the incidence of epilepsy is highest in children under 2 years of age and people over age 65. Approximately 45,000 diagnoses of epilepsy are made in children less than 15 years of age each year, with a current prevalence of 326,000 people under age 15. About 1% of the population will develop epilepsy by the age of 20, and 10% will have experienced a seizure by the time they are 75 years old. The incidence of epilepsy is higher in children with mental retardation and cerebral palsy, and may occur in as much as 50% of those with both conditions. Children whose parents have epilepsy are also at higher risk for developing the disease, although the risk is higher if the mother has epilepsy than the father. Approximately 70% of children with epilepsy enter remission (being seizure free for five or more years without medication), but remission is less likely to occur with children with co-existing conditions such as cerebral palsy or other neurological conditions. Approximately one third of cases of epilepsy cannot be controlled even with medication (Shafer, 2014).

Usually thought of as a disease of the elderly, arthritis also affects the young. The Arthritis Foundation (2014) estimates that 294,000 children under 18 years of age have pediatric arthritis and other rheumatologic conditions. These diseases result in more than 827,000 ambulatory care visits each year and account for $128 billion annually in direct medical costs and indirect costs (e.g., lost parental wages and productivity) (Arthritis Foundation, 2014).

Obesity is a chronic condition that affects thousands of young people and increases their risk of developing a variety of other chronic diseases including diabetes, heart disease, and arthritis. In the 2011 Youth Risk Behavior Surveillance (YRBS) survey, 13% of high school students reported that they were obese, with higher levels of obesity among male students (16.1%) than females (9.8%). In addition, nearly a third of students (29%) described themselves as overweight, with girls more likely to describe themselves as overweight than boys. Close to half (46%) indicated that they were trying to lose weight (Eaton et al., 2012). In 2009–2010, 18% of U.S. children aged 6 to 17 years were considered obese, three times the obesity rate for 1976 to 1980 (Federal Interagency Forum on Child and Family Statistics, 2013).

Diabetes is one of several conditions for which obesity is a risk factor. According to the Division of Diabetes Translation (2011), one of every 400 children and adolescents had type 1 or 2 diabetes in 2010. This amounts to more than 215,000 people under the age of 20 (American Diabetes Association, 2011).

Perhaps the most common chronic condition among children and adolescents is asthma. In the 2011 YRBS, 23% of high school students surveyed indicated that they had been told by a doctor or nurse that they had asthma and nearly 12% reported current asthma (Eaton et al., 2012). Overall, in 2011, an estimated 10% of all U.S. children had a current diagnosis of asthma. For many of these children, their disease was well controlled with medication and environmental modifications, but approximately 60% continued to experience symptoms (Federal Interagency Forum on Child and Family Statistics, 2013).

Psychological and Behavioral Health Problems

Children also experience a variety of psychological and behavioral health problems, the most common of which is **attention deficit hyperactivity disorder (ADHD)**, a chronic condition characterized by poor attention span, impulsive behavior, and/or hyperactivity (National Institute of Mental Health [NIMH], 2012). Based on parental self-report in the National Survey of Children's Health, the incidence of ADHD appears to be increasing, rising from 7.8% of U.S. children in 2003 to 11% in 2011 (National Center for Birth Defects and Disability [NCBDDD], 2014a). ADHD is characterized by age-inappropriate levels of inattention and hyperactivity that contribute to difficulties in school, family, and social interactions (Visser, Bitsko, Danielson, Perou, & Blumberg, 2010).

ADHD may be associated with co-morbidities such as oppositional-defiant disorder, learning disability, conduct disorder, anxiety or depression, bipolar disorder, Tourette syndrome, sleep disorder, or substance abuse (NIMH, 2012). In other instances, these other conditions may be misdiagnosed as ADHD. ADHD is often accompanied by increased risk behavior, particularly related to driving in the teen years that may put the child at greater risk of injury (NIMH, 2012).

Possible contributing factors include genetics, in utero exposure to tobacco or alcohol, and brain injury. There is some thought that certain food additives may also be associated with ADHD, but research findings are inconclusive (NIMH, 2012). Boys are approximately twice as likely as girls to display ADHD (National Center on Birth Defects and Developmental Disabilities [NCBDDD], 2014a), although there is some thought that girls are more likely to exhibit the inattentive form of ADHD and thus be less disruptive and less likely to be diagnosed than boys. The annual cost of ADHD is estimated to be $12,500 to $15,458 per child in 2005 dollar equivalents (NCBDDD, 2014a).

Guidelines from the American Academy of Pediatrics suggest that ADHD should be considered in any child aged 4 to 18 years with academic difficulties or behavioral problems who exhibits inattention, hyperactivity, or impulsivity. Diagnosis should be based on diagnostic criteria in the *Diagnostic and Statistical Manual*—(5th ed.) (DSM-5) of the American Psychiatric Association. These criteria include impairment in more than one setting when alternative causes have been ruled out. Diagnosis should also consider co-occurring conditions such as those listed earlier (NCBDDD, 2013a).

Children and adolescents also experience a variety of other psychological problems. In a 2011 survey, 5% of parents reported that their child experienced serious difficulty in getting along with others or problems with emotions, concentration, or behavior (Federal Interagency Forum on Child and Family Statistics, 2013). This is a slight increase from 5.1% of parents of 4- to 17-year-old children who reported serious emotional or behavioral difficulties between 2004 and 2009 (National Center for Health Statistics, 2011a).

The 2009 National Comorbidity Survey of Adolescents (NCS-A) indicated that nearly 32% of adolescents surveyed reported anxiety disorders, 19% exhibited behavioral disorders, 14% reported mood disorders such as anxiety or depression, and 11% reported a substance abuse disorder. The overall prevalence of severe emotional distress or impairment was 22%, and an estimated one in every 4 or 5 adolescents experiences these conditions at some point in their lives (Merikangas et al., 2010).

There is some evidence that **adverse childhood events (ACEs)**, experiences such as verbal, physical, or sexual abuse or family dysfunction during childhood, may contribute to adverse events in adulthood as well as in childhood. Consequences linked to ACEs include substance abuse, depression, cardiovascular disease, diabetes, cancer, and premature death. In the 2009 Behavioral Risk Factor Surveillance System survey, nearly 60% of adults reported being exposed to ACEs in childhood, with nearly 9% of respondents reporting five or more ACEs as children. These findings highlight the need to prevent adverse childhood events as well as provide trauma-focused services for those children who experience them (Bynum et al., 2010).

Developmental Disorders

Children and adolescents may also experience a number of developmental disorders. Some of the more common disorders include cerebral palsy, fetal alcohol syndrome (FAS) and related disorders, autism spectrum disorders, and Down syndrome. Cerebral palsy (CP) is the most common developmental motor disability in children, affecting the ability to move and maintain balance and posture. It may result from abnormal brain development or damage that affects muscle control (NCBDDD, 2013c).

Fetal alcohol syndrome may occur in 0.2 to 2 infants per 1,000 births, and related fetal alcohol spectrum disorders (FASD) probably occur three times as often. Both FAS and FASD occur as a result of fetal exposure to alcohol when mothers drink during pregnancy. From 2006 to 2010, approximately 8% of pregnant women reported alcohol use during pregnancy and 1.4% reported **binge drinking** (defined as four or more alcoholic drinks in one period of time). The estimated lifetime costs of FAS are about $2 million per person; these costs do not include those associated with FASD. The annual cost for FAS in the United States is estimated at $4 billion (NCBDDD, 2014d). FAS and FASD result in delayed or abnormal brain function and may contribute to a variety of disabling conditions.

Autism spectrum disorders (ASDs) comprise a group of developmental disabilities that interfere with communication and social and behavioral function. As indicated by the term, they occur along a spectrum and affect individuals differently. Three basic types of ASD have been identified: autistic disorders, Asperger syndrome, and pervasive developmental disorder. Autistic disorders are characterized by language delays, difficulties with communication and social interaction, and unusual behaviors and interests. They may also be accompanied by intellectual disability. Children with Asperger syndrome display similar difficulties with social interactions and unusual behavior, but usually lack the language and intellectual manifestations of autistic disorders. Pervasive developmental disorders are those that do not fall into either of the other two categories. Symptoms tend to be similar but are often milder than for the other forms of ASDs (NCBDDD, 2014c).

In 2010, ASDs affected approximately 1 in every 68 children, an increase from 1 in 110 children in 2006. It is unclear whether this increase is the result of an actual increase in incidence or better diagnostic capabilities. Like ADHD, ASDs are far more common in boys than in girls, with a rate of 1 in 42 boys compared to 1 in 189 girls. Most children with ASDs do not have associated intellectual disabilities, but there is a high incidence of other co-occurring developmental, psychiatric, neurological, chromosomal, and genetic disorders. Little is known about the causes of ASDs, but there is evidence of increased risk with prematurity or low birth weight and with older parents. Medical costs for children with ASDs have been estimated at $17,000 to $21,000 per child per year. In addition, ASDs may result in expenditures of $40,000 to $60,000 per child per year for intensive behavioral therapies (NCBDDD, 2014b).

Down syndrome is the result of chromosomal abnormalities and occurs in approximately 6,000 U.S. infants each year. This equates to 1 in every 700 children born. Down syndrome is associated with characteristic facial features of wide spaced eyes with an epicanthic fold that makes the eyes appear slanted, a protruding tongue, and a single crease across the palm of the hand. Down syndrome is most often associated with intellectual difficulties, but may also be accompanied by physical health problems such as increased susceptibility to serious respiratory infections (NCBDDD, 2013b).

Developmental disorders have a variety of effects on mental, physical, and social development in children. In addition, some of these disorders put children at increased risk for other health problems. For example, children with neurological and neurodevelopmental disorders are at greater risk than other children for complications of influenza (DiOrio et al., 2012). Like other children with disabling conditions, they may also be subject to harassment, ridicule, and discrimination.

Violence

Children and youth may be victims or perpetrators of violence, or both. They may also witness violence in their families or at school which may have lasting consequences for all those involved. In 2010, 4,824 homicide victims were between 10 and 24 years of age, and more than 707,000 children and youth are seen in emergency departments each year for injuries related to violence. More than 3 million reports of child maltreatment are received by state and local agencies every year, nearly six per minute (NCIPC, 2012c, 2014b). As was the case with several conditions discussed earlier, boys are more likely to experience violence-related injuries than girls. For example, the rate of injury among 10- to 14-year-olds was 543.7 per 100,000 for boys and 332.4 per 100,000 for girls. For 15- to 19-year olds, the rates were 1,488.6 for boys and 894.8 for girls (NCIPC, 2014h).

Many of these injuries are due to **child maltreatment**, which is defined as "any act or series of acts of commission or omission by a parent or other caregiver (e.g., clergy, coach, teacher) that results in harm, potential for harm, or threat of harm to a child" (NCIPC, 2014a, p. 1). According the the Federal Interagency Forum on Child and Family Statistics (2013), the rate of substantiated reports of child maltreatment in 2010 was 10 per 1,000 children from birth to 17 years of age. The highest incidence rate was seen among children less than 1 year of age at 23 per 1,000. In addition, 8 per 1,000 juveniles aged 12 to 17 years were the victims of serious violent crime.

Violence against children and adolescents may also occur in the school setting. In the Massachusetts Youth Health Survey, for example, nearly 27% of middle school students and 16% of high school students reported being victims of bullying. Both middle school and high school students also self-reported being bullies (7.5% and 8.4%, respectively), and nearly 10% of middle school students and 6.5% of high school students reported being both bullies and victims of bullying at school (McKenna, Mullen, & Hertz, 2011). Victims often had a disability, but bullies were more likely to be obese and to have poor grades than victims. Both groups of children reported considering and attempting suicide.

According to the 2011 YRBS, more than 7% of high school students surveyed had been threatened or injured with a weapon one or more times on school property within the prior year and more than 16% of students reported bringing a weapon to school in the previous 30 days. Twenty percent of the students reported being bullied at school, and more than 16% had experienced electronic bullying. Nearly 6% of students had missed one or more days of school due to fears for their safety, and 26% of the respondents had had their property stolen or damaged at school (Eaton et al., 2012).

Youth violence also occurs in the context of intimate relationships. Data from the NCIPC (2014f) indicate that 20% of women and 14% of men who reported being victims of rape or other violence by an intimate partner first experienced intimate partner violence as teenagers. In the YRBS, more than 9% of students reported being hit, slapped, or purposely physically hurt by a boyfriend or girlfriend (Eaton et al., 2012).

Suicide among youth is another area of growing concern. In 2007, for example, the suicide rate among 10- to 14-year-olds was 0.9 per 100,000 children. The rate increased to 6.9 among those 15 to 19 years of age (Crosby, Ortega, & Stevens, 2011). Suicide, homicide, abuse, and other forms of violence against and by children and adolescents will be addressed in more detail in Chapter 30∞.

Population Health Nursing Care of Child and Adolescent Populations

Population health nurses provide care to individuals and to populations of children and adolescents. Population-based care is framed in the context of the nursing process beginning with an assessment of the health status of child and adolescent populations and identification of positive and negative population health nursing diagnoses and progressing through the planning, implementation, and evaluation of health care programs to meet identified needs in these populations.

Assessing the Health of Child and Adolescent Populations

Factors in each of the six categories of determinants of health influence the health of children and adolescents. We will briefly examine considerations related to biological, psychological, environmental, sociocultural, behavioral, and health system determinants as they affect the health of these populations.

BIOLOGICAL DETERMINANTS. Biological considerations related to the health of children and adolescents include the effects of maturation and aging and factors that affect both, genetic inheritance, and physiologic function. Factors contributing to health and illness among children and adolescents in each of these areas will be briefly addressed.

Age and maturation. Children of different ages are susceptible to different types of health problems. For example, children under 5 years of age are at particular risk for influenza mortality and should receive annual immunizations (Blanton et al., 2011). Similarly, the risk of unwanted pregnancy emerges with developing sexual maturity in the adolescent.

Areas to be assessed with respect to maturation and aging include growth and development. **Growth** is an increase in body size or change in the structure, function, and complexity of body cells until a point of maturity. Overweight and obesity are serious problems related to growth in the U.S. child and adolescent populations, whereas many children in other parts of the world are malnourished and exhibit growth retardation. There may also be significant disparities among subgroups within the population with respect to growth parameters. For example, refugee children are often below their age mates for height and weight due to malnutrition in their countries of origin. Obesity is also more prevalent in some child and adolescent populations than in others. When rates of obesity among children and adolescents in the population are high, population health nurses can identify contributing factors and advocate for programs to prevent or treat obesity. For example, a nurse might advocate for more physical activity and healthier meals in school settings or for the development of recreational opportunities that encourage physical activity among children and adolescents.

Development is a process of patterned, orderly, and lifelong change in structure, thought, or behavior that occurs as a result of physical or emotional maturation. With the individual child or adolescent, the population health nurse would assess the extent to which specific developmental milestones have been met. **Developmental milestones** are critical behaviors expected at specific ages, and their assessment can be accomplished using a variety of tools. Information about a wide variety of developmental screening tools is available on the Internet and through various professional organizations.

At the population level, the population health nurse would focus on the extent of developmental delay in the population. The most common causes of delayed development are the developmental disorders discussed earlier in this chapter. Other causes of developmental delays are acute and chronic illness and lack of an environment that fosters development. When the latter is the case, the population health nurse can advocate with parents and other caretakers for conditions that stimulate appropriate development. For example, in some families, younger children do not develop language skills appropriate to their ages because family members anticipate and address their needs without the child having to voice them in understandable language. In such a case, the population health nurse would encourage parents and older siblings not to meet the child's needs until the child has indicated them verbally. Similarly, population health nurses may need to advocate for a balance between independence and supervision for adolescents so they gradually become independent from their parents. Nurses may also need to reassure parents that testing of family values is a normal part of adolescence, not evidence of rebellion.

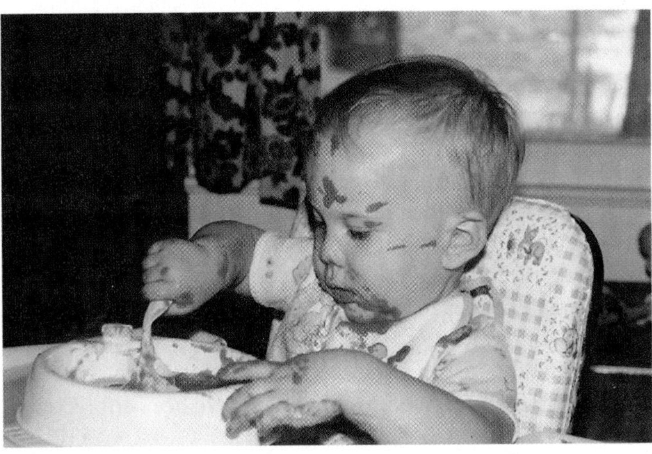

Children need opportunities to develop age-appropriate skills.
((Mary Jo Clark))

Another maturational or developmental consideration for the adolescent population is the usual age at which adolescents become sexually mature, which may differ for different segments of the community. For example, African American adolescents may become sexually mature at an earlier age than their Caucasian or Asian counterparts.

Menarche, the first appearance of menstrual flow in the adolescent girl, usually occurs between 12 and 13 years of age. Menarche that occurs too early (age 8 or younger) is associated with precocious puberty, an anomaly of the endocrine system. Delayed menarche (after age 18) is also a signal that the endocrine system is not functioning properly. Either early or late onset of menses is cause for referral for medical evaluation. Menarche may appear earlier or later than average in some ethnic populations, and the nurse should be familiar with population parameters for the onset of menstruation.

The physical and emotional changes that occur just prior to and with menarche have the potential to create physical or psychological problems for the adolescent girl. Assessment of preadolescent girls should include the extent of sexual changes, knowledge of menstruation, and preparation for the event. If menarche has occurred, other considerations related to menstruation may include menstrual regularity, extent and duration of flow, and the experience of dysmenorrhea, or painful menstruation. The nurse would also inquire about signs and symptoms of premenstrual distress (premenstrual syndrome) such as depression, irritability, nervousness, tension, inability to concentrate, breast tenderness, bloating, edema, fatigue, headache, and food cravings. Symptoms of premenstrual distress may be severe and require medical referral or may be less severe and respond to dietary changes and exercise. Menarche heralds the beginning potential for pregnancy, so the typical age of menarche in the population, or within certain subpopulations, can suggest the age at which sex education should be undertaken. Population health nurses also need to be aware of cultural attitudes to menarche within the population. Menarche in some societies is met with female genital mutilation, and population health nurses should be aware of the extent to which women in the community may have been subjected to this practice.

Physical sexual maturation in the male typically begins between ages 9.5 and 14 years and is completed between ages 14 and 18 years. Adolescent males are typically very concerned with sexual and physical development, often comparing themselves to other males and many times experiencing anxiety about the possibility that their development is delayed or inadequate. In some cases, this anxiety can be sufficient to cause social impairment or serious emotional distress, and the population health nurse should make a special effort to be supportive and accepting. The population health nurse can also assist adolescent male clients by offering information and reassurance about the normal patterns and variations in growth and development. In the majority of adolescent males, a degree of transient gynecomastia (enlargement of the breasts) occurs. This is variable in degree, but can be a source of significant concern to the adolescent; again, reassurance, explanation, and acceptance are of benefit.

During this period, adolescents become increasingly concerned with the values of peers and are increasingly focused on achieving acceptance from the peer group. They are prone to value the opinions of peers over those of parents, and attitudes are more reflective of peers than of family. Adolescent males often experience identity uncertainty, and may engage in a variety of behaviors that, although perhaps disconcerting to family or other adults, are necessary experiments in determining their self-concepts. Hormonal changes result in increased growth and libido, confronting adolescent males with the possibility of new (and perhaps anxiety-provoking) roles; these changes are also mirrored in the behavior of peers, on which the teenager tends to model his own behaviors and choices.

Adolescent males may feel embarrassed about the physical and emotional changes they experience. For example, they may have spontaneous and ill-timed erections or nocturnal emissions. Physical development and social circumstances, coupled with peer pressure and a desire to conform, may lead to varying degrees of sexual activity, presenting the risks of unwanted pregnancy and sexually transmitted diseases. Other adolescent males may begin to discover a same-sex orientation during these years and should be supported as well.

Over time, the adolescent male's preoccupation with sexual performance and activity as the major parameters of a relationship are increasingly replaced by romantic attributes and genuine caring; initially, these romantic views are often stereotypical and exaggerated, but this also changes as he progresses through early adulthood. Again, the nurse's role involves assessing the young male's development relative to existing norms; providing education about growth, development, sexuality, and related risks and safety precautions; and providing reassurance and guidance relative to the changes experienced. Population health nurses can also advocate for appropriate sexuality education for adolescents to help them deal with the many issues surrounding sexual maturation.

Genetic inheritance. Genetic inheritance is another biological determinant to be considered in the assessment of child and adolescent populations. Gender and racial or ethnic background are two intrinsic genetic factors that influence the health of children and adolescents. Male and female children and children of different racial and ethnic groups tend to experience different types of health problems. For example, the nurse might identify the prevalence of urinary tract infections in school-age girls as a community problem because urinary tract infections occur more frequently in girls than in boys in this age group. Similarly, screening tests for sickle cell disease should be routinely conducted on African American children and others at risk.

Genetic factors also play a part in the development of other health problems. For example, an identical twin of a child with an autism spectrum disorder has 36% to 95% chance of also exhibiting an ASD. Similarly, parents who have one child with an ASD have a 2% to 18% chance of having a second child who is affected (NCBDDD, 2014b). Population health nurses would determine the prevalence of conditions with a genetic component in the overall population and work to initiate programs to prevent or address those conditions that have a high prevalence in the population.

Physiologic function. Considerations related to physiologic function include the incidence and prevalence of specific physical health problems in the child and adolescent populations. Information on the leading causes of child and adolescent deaths in the population provides an overview of the health status of these two groups. The top causes of infant and child mortality in the United States were presented in Table 16-1●. The population health nurse would explore relevant mortality figures for the child and adolescent populations in his or her community.

Not all illnesses result in death, and assessment of the child and adolescent population may reveal high prevalence rates of other acute and chronic illnesses. If acute and chronic diseases are prevalent among the child and adolescent population in the community, population health nurses may need to advocate for effective illness prevention programs or services to deal with existing illness. For example, if a large proportion of the school population has asthma, the population health nurse may advocate for creation of school-based asthma management programs. Similarly, if the prevalence of childhood cancers is high, population health nurses may initiate investigation

FOCUSED ASSESSMENT Assessing Biological Determinants Influencing Child and Adolescent Health

- What is the age composition of the child and adolescent population?
- What is the gender composition of the child and adolescent population?
- What is the racial/ethnic composition of the child and adolescent population?
- What are the gender-specific attitudes and expectations regarding boys and girls in the population?
- What is the extent of growth retardation in the child and adolescent population?
- What is the extent of developmental delay in the child and adolescent population? What are the typical causes of delays?
- What are cause-specific child and adolescent mortality rates in the population?
- What are the rates of morbidity for specific acute and chronic health problems in the child and adolescent population?
- What is the level of immunization coverage in the child and adolescent population?

of environmental factors that may be contributing to high prevalence.

Another aspect of physiologic function that should be explored with respect to the child and adolescent populations is immunization. Maintenance of high rates of immunization among children not only protects individual children from disease, but also serves to protect other members of the population via herd immunity. **Herd immunity** is the level of protection provided to unimmunized people when immunization rates are high among the rest of the population. If most children, for example, are immunized against varicella (chickenpox), the chances of an adult without immunity being exposed to the disease are considerably reduced. For further information about recommended immunizations for children and adolscents, see the *External Resources* section of the student resources site.

When immunization levels within the population are low, population health nurses may need to advocate with parents for needed childhood immunizations for individual children or with health care delivery systems to make sure that immunizations are available. For example, the population health nurse might advocate for development of outreach immunization clinics for low-income families in underserved neighborhoods. Elements of a focused assessment of biological determinants affecting the health of children and adolescents are presented above.

PSYCHOLOGICAL DETERMINANTS. A number of psychological determinants influence the health status of child and adolescent populations. These include family dynamics, parental coping and mental health, mental health problems in the child and adolescent population, and the potential for and extent of abuse.

Family dynamics, parental expectations, and discipline. Family dynamics affect the child's or adolescent's interactions with parents and other family members and influence self-image and development of self-esteem. Children who are subjected to denigration, neglect, or harsh discipline may grow up considering themselves unworthy of love or esteem. Children may also internalize feelings and roles based on the dynamics of their families of origin. For example, children of divorced parents may experience feelings of guilt or emotional distress related to the dissolution of their family. Research has also shown consistently that children exposed to hostility and aggressive behaviors by other family members are more likely to display these behaviors themselves.

Parental expectations of children shape children's expectations of themselves and others. Failure to meet parental expectations may contribute to guilt and depression, whereas unrealistic parental expectations may result in inappropriate discipline for behaviors that are normal for a child's or adolescent's developmental stage. For example, parents may expect a 3-year-old child to be toilet trained even at night and punish the child for bedwetting when this is normal behavior at this age. Parental expectations may also stifle adolescent development. For example, in many Asian cultures, adolescents may be expected to choose an occupation that brings benefit or recognition to the family rather than one in which the adolescent may be personally interested. Such expectations may cause conflict within the family or psychological problems for the adolescent. At the population level, there may be societal expectations of children and adolescents that create stress for both the children and their families.

Parental coping and mental health. Parental stress levels affect their ability to parent effectively. The number of women with small children in the population may provide indirect information on coping abilities, since child rearing has been found to contribute to cumulative stress, and the mental health of women with young children tends to be worse than for those without children. Similarly, the level of mental health problems in the adult population can affect parents' abilities to be effective in caring for their children.

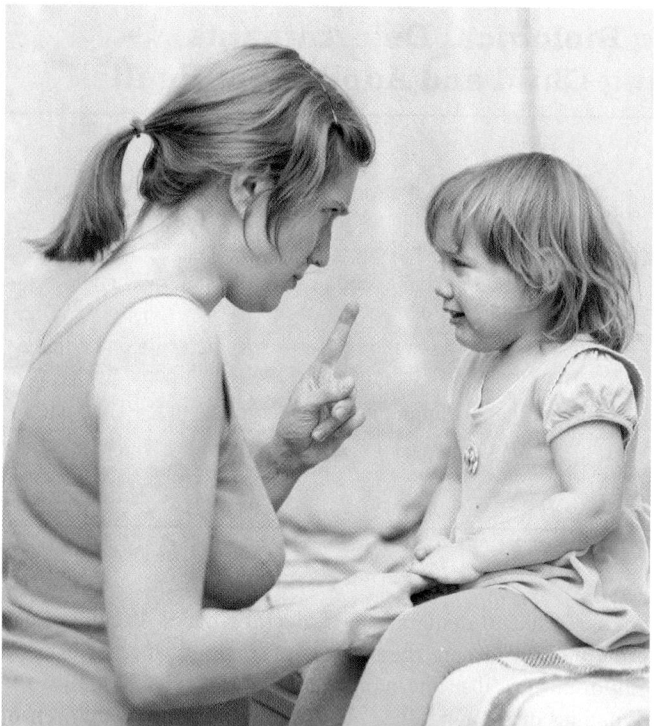

Discipline is frequently a thorny issue in raising children.
(JackF/Fotolia)

Mental health problems in the child and adolescent population. The frequency and types of mental health problems encountered in children and adolescents also provide information about the health status of these populations. For example, from 2004 to 2009 slightly more than 5% of U.S. children 4 to 17 years of age were reported by their parents as having serious mental health problems in the National Health Interview Survey (National Center for Health Statistics, 2011a). In addition, according to the 2011 YRBS, more than 28% of high school students reported feeling so sad or hopeless that they stopped one or more usual activities and nearly 16% had seriously considered suicide in the prior year. Thirteen percent of the respondents had actually made a suicide plan and 2.4% of students nationwide had attempted suicide (Eaton et al., 2012). High rates of mental illness in the child and adolescent population may necessitate population health nursing advocacy for effective treatment services. For example, a population health nurse may assist schoolteachers and counselors to set up a program that facilitates identification and referral of depressed students for treatment services.

Abuse and maltreatment. Physical, sexual, and psychological abuse and neglect are other problems that affect the psychological health of children and adolescents. The effects of childhood abuse are many and varied and may include future prostitution, drug and alcohol abuse, and more unprotected sexual activity. Abused children are at risk for adverse health effects as well as behavior problems as adults.

Risk factors and protective factors for abuse are summarized in Table 16-2●. The problem of child abuse and potential nursing interventions are addressed in more detail in Chapter 30∞. The *Focused Assessment* provided on the next page includes tips on assessing psychological determinants influencing child and adolescent health.

ENVIRONMENTAL DETERMINANTS. Children are more susceptible than adults to a variety of environmental pollutants. For example, because their nervous systems are not yet fully developed, young children are more susceptible than adults or older children to the effects of lead poisoning. According to the National Center for Environmental Health (NCEH), children in 4 million U.S. households are exposed to lead and approximately 500,000 children have elevated blood lead levels (NCEH, 2012). Lead poisoning may be more prevalent in some population groups than others. For instance, refugee children may arrive in the United States with higher blood lead levels than native children or may develop elevated blood lead levels

TABLE 16-2 Risk Factors and Protective Factors for Child Maltreatment

Risk Factors	Protective Factors
Victimization Risk Factors Age under 4 years Special needs that increase caregiver burden **Perpetration Risk Factors** Lack of understanding of children's needs, child development Lack of parenting skills Parental history of maltreatment as a child Parental substance abuse or mental illness Parental characteristics (young age, low education, single parenthood, multiple children, low income) Transient caregivers in the home Parental thoughts that justify maltreatment Social isolation Family disorganization, dissolution, or violence Parenting stress, poor parent–child relationships Community violence Low neighborhood social capital	Supportive family environment Supportive social networks Nurturing parenting skills Stable family relationships Household rules and child monitoring Parental employment Adequate housing Access to needed health care and social services Caring adults outside the family who serve as role models or mentors Communities that support parents and take responsibility for preventing abuse

Data from: National Center for Injury Prevention and Control. (2014d). *Child maltreatment: Risk and protective factors.* Retrieved from http://www.cdc.gov/ViolencePrevention/childmaltreatment/riskprotectivefactors.html

FOCUSED ASSESSMENT Assessing Psychological Determinants of Child and Adolescent Health

- What is the extent of mental illness in the child and adolescent population? Among parents?
- What are the cultural expectations of children and adolescents in the population? To what extent do these expectations create stress for children and adolescents?
- What is the suicide rate among children and adolescents in the population?
- What are the typical approaches to discipline in the population?
- What is the extent of abuse in the child and adolescent population? What forms of abuse are prevalent? What factors contribute to abuse of children and adolescents? What is the attitude of the population to abuse of children and adolescents?

after resettlement due to living in older housing contaminated with lead-based paint. Overall, although more children have been routinely tested for elevated blood lead levels, prevalence has declined significantly in recent years. In 2012, 2.5 million children were tested with elevated levels found in less than 1%, a significant decrease from 7.6% in 1997. The percentage of children tesing positive varied from state to state with the highest prevalence (19.65%) in Louisiana and the lowest (0.15%) in Arizona and Florida (NCEH, 2014).

Lead exposure is only one of several household environmental hazards that the population health nurse may want to assess in the population. Such an assessment can be guided by the U.S. Department of Housing and Urban Development's (HUD) (2008) "Healthy Housing Inspection Manual." In addition to poisoning hazards, such as lead, carbon monoxide, and so on, the manual addresses assessment for a variety of internal and external safety hazards, pests, and other household health risks. For further information about the manual, see the *External Resources* section of the student resources site.

Insecticide exposure and air pollution are other continuing problems for children and adolescents. In 2011, for example, 66% of U.S. children lived in counties with concentrations above recommended levels for one or more air pollutants. This figure represents an increase from 59% of children in 2009, but an overall decrease from 77% in 2003 (Federal Interagency Forum on Child and Family Statistics, 2012, 2013). Population health nurses should be alert to the presence of environmental pollutants and other hazards and their effects on children. See Chapter 4∞ for a more detailed discussion of environmental health hazards.

Safety hazards are another major factor in the physical environment that influences the health of children of all ages. Safety concerns are related to children's physical surroundings and their ability to gain access to dangerous substances. As we saw earlier, injuries account for significant morbidity and mortality among children and adolescents. Safety issues in the home can be assessed using the HUD inspection manual described above.

Playground safety is another area that should be assessed by the population health nurse. The National Program for Playground Safety (2014b) has identified four components of playground safety, creating the acronym SAFE, that should be assessed. These components include supervision, age-appropriate playgrounds, fall surface, and equipment maintenance. Each of these components can be evaluated using assessment kits for child care and school settings developed by the National Program for Playground Safety (2014a). For further information about the tool kits, see the *External Resources* section of the student resources site.

Advocacy for child and adolescent safety is an important aspect of population health nursing for this population. In carrying out this advocacy role, population health nurses might campaign for effective enforcement of seat belt legislation or for gun safety education for local families and youth. Other

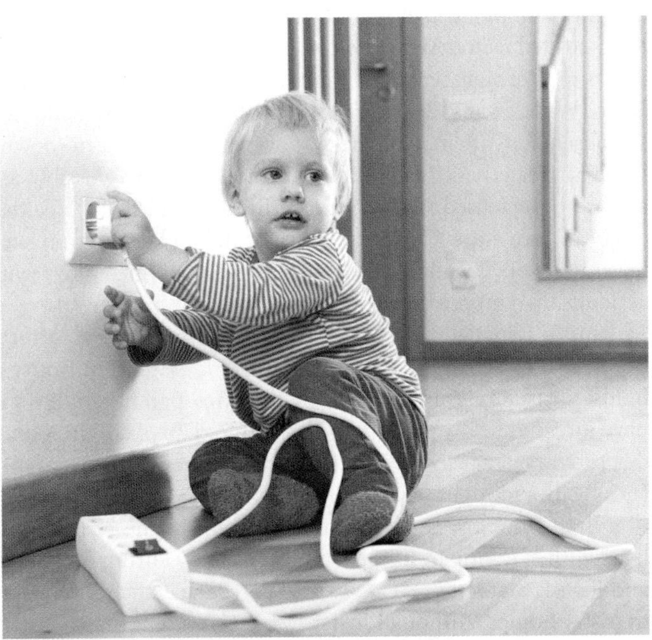

Childproofing a home entails different strategies for children of different ages. *(JackF/Fotolia)*

FOCUSED ASSESSMENT Assessing Environmental Determinants of Child and Adolescent Health

- What pollutants affect the health of the child and adolescent population? What factors contribute to the presence of pollutants? What are the health effects of pollutants for children and adolescents?
- What safety hazards are present in the community? How do they affect the health of the child and adolescent population?
- How adequate is family housing in the community?

environmental initiatives may include housing inspection and advocacy for removal of environmental hazards or elimination of environmental pollutants. Questions for a focused assessment of environmental factors influencing child and adolescent health are provided above.

SOCIOCULTURAL DETERMINANTS. A variety of sociocultural factors affect the health of children and adolescents. As we saw earlier, a number of these factors have implications for childrens' psychological health. In addition, factors such as employment, family income, and education levels affect access to health care services and knowledge of health care needs. For example, in 2011, 16.1 million U.S. children (22%) under 18 years of age lived in poverty, an increase from 16% in 2001. In addition, 22% lived in households that were food insecure at least part of the time during the year (Federal Interagency Forum on Child and Family Statistics, 2013). Poverty has a variety of long-term effects on child health beyond access to care. For example, early childhood poverty has been associated with obesity in childhood and into adulthood that is influenced by cumulative exposures to associated factors such as crowding, noise, substandard housing, family turmoil, separation from parents, and exposure to violence (Wells, Evans, Beavis, & Ong, 2010). In addition, children in households with incomes below poverty level have been shown to be at greater risk for diminished learning ability, possibly as a result of increased stress (National Institute of Mental Health, 2012) and are more likely to have behavioral problems, complete fewer years of education, and have more years of unemployment as adults than more affluent children (Macartney, 2011).

Family structure and living arrangements may also affect the health of children and adolescents. Single-parent households, for example, are more likely than two-parent families to have incomes below poverty level. In 2012, 64% of children under 18 years of age lived with two parents, 28% with one parent (primarily a mother), and 4% with neither parent. Sightly more than half (55%) of those without a parent in the household lived with a grandparent (Federal Interagency Forum on Child and Family Statistics, 2013). A small percentage of children live in foster homes. Although foster home placement may be better than circumstances experienced in their birth families, children in foster homes are at greater risk than other children for both mental and physical health problems as adults (Ziotnick, Tam, & Soman, 2012).

Family function also affects the health of children and adolescents. Parental stress is associated with a variety of adverse effects on children, and in the National Survey on Drug Use and Health, nearly 9% of parenting adults reported serious levels of psychological stress (Russell, Sinclair, Poteat, & Koenig, 2012). The presence of substance abuse, smoking, and violence within the family adversely affect child health and the prevalence of these circumstances in the population should be explored by the population health nurse as an indication of factors that may affect child and adolescent health.

Parental employment and work schedules have also been shown to affect child and adolescent health and welfare. Although employment may improve income levels and access to needed goods and services, it may have other effects on child health. Many parents work nonstandard schedules precisely to allow them to arrange favorable child care; however, child care may be less available at nonscheduled times (e.g., during evening and night shifts). Nonstandard work hours also limit parent availability to children when children are home from school and diminish family time. Parents may be prevented from attending many family and community events involving their children, and nonstandard schedules may affect parental sleep and parenting capabilities.

Parental education level affects income and knowledge of effective parenting. These effects are compounded when one or more parents do not speak the dominant language of the community. In 2010, 22% of U.S. children under 18 years of age lived in homes where a language other than English was spoken. Children who do not speak English at home may face difficulties in school and in later employment (Federal Interagency Forum on Child and Family Statistics, 2013). Immigration and acculturation may have both positive and negative effects on children's health. In one study, for example, Spanish-speaking Hispanic boys in Texas were more likely to consume more milk and fruits than those who spoke English, but were less likely to be aware of the relationship between overweight and health problems (Lino et al., 2012).

Legislation and media are two other important sociocultural factors that influence the health of child and adolescent populations. Legislation may have positive or negative effects. For example, state legislation controlling food options available in California school settings has led to a decrease in childhood obesity prevalence. Similarly, legislation regarding immunization of middle school students has been associated with increased immunity to several childhood diseases.

The United Nations Convention on the Rights of the Child addressed rights of children that should be supported by effective legislation. Among the rights specifically addressed in the convention were the right to education, health care, and protection from execution for crimes committed under the age of 18 years. Although the convention was signed by U.S. delegates, it was not approved by the U.S. Senate due to provisions in many states for trying youth as adults for certain serious crimes. As of 2013, only the United States and Somalia had not ratified the convention (Amnesty International, 2013). In addition, the rights of fetuses are not protected by U.S. law, although in some jurisdictions, fetal rights are protected once a fetus is considered viable. A growing number of states have fetal homicide laws, primarily laws that address the loss of a fetus after intentional injury to the mother (National Conference of State Legislatures, 2013). After birth, a child's rights are recognized, but decision-making rights are generally assigned to parents or to the state in loco parentis until a child reaches the age of majority.

Media coverage and role models are often associated with the assumption of risky behaviors such as smoking, drinking, and sexual activity by adolescents, but media may have beneficial effects as well. For instance, a mass media campaign effectively promoted smoking cessation among smokers exposed to it (Vallone, Duke, Cullen, McCausland, & Allen, 2011).

Prejudice in the social environment may also affect children. For instance, they may be subjected to ridicule by other children at school because of their dress, physical appearance, family culture, or religion. Prejudice may lead to bias-based harassment based on ethnicity, sexual orientation, disability, religion, or gender. Research has indicated that bias-based harassment may be even more detrimental to children's health than generalized harassment related to appearance or speech patterns. Harassment may lead to increased risk for mental illness, substance abuse, and truancy and may result in threats of violence, victimization, or destruction of one's personal property. In studies, 35% to 40% of children have reported harassment based on prejudicial attitudes, and 15.5% related to their sexual orientation (Russell et al., 2012).

Family religious affiliation may provide social support, but can also lead to potential health problems. For example, children who receive exemption from immunization on the basis of religious beliefs may be at greater risk for disease than their immunized counterparts despite the effects of herd immunity. The *Focused Assessment* below provides tips for assessing sociocultural determinants of child and adolescent health.

BEHAVIORAL DETERMINANTS. Several behavioral determinants also affect the health of children and adolescents. Behavioral considerations in assessing these populations may relate to behaviors of children and adolescents themselves and those of their parents. Major areas for consideration in terms of behavioral determinants include nutrition, rest and exercise, exposure to hazardous substances, safety practices, and sexual activity.

Earlier we noted the need for the population health nurse to assess the extent of poverty and hunger in the population. This is particularly important in developing countries, but should not be neglected in the United States and other areas of the developed world where poverty affects certain subgroups within the population. In the United States, however, nutritional deficits are more likely to reflect the lack of specific nutrients or caloric excess.

Population health nurses should be alert to child feeding practices in the population such as the extent to which newborns are breast-fed or bottle-fed, the availability of fast food in the community, and the extent to which families frequent fast-food establishments. Exclusive breast-feeding for the first 6 months is the recommended dietary standard for infants. Based on CDC data, however, only approximately three fourths of mothers initiate breast-feeding at their child's birth and just 49% continue to breastfeed their infants for 6 months

FOCUSED ASSESSMENT Assessing Sociocultural Determinants of Child and Adolescent Health

- What are the culturally defined roles for children and adolescents in the community? What effect do these roles have on health?
- How do social factors such as education level, employment, and income affect the health of the child and adolescent population?
- What is the extent of parental employment outside the home? How does this affect child and adolescent health?
- What is the extent of employment among the child and adolescent population? What effect does employment have on health?
- What is the availability of child care services in the community? How adequate are child care services to meet the needs of working parents?
- How adequate are educational opportunities available to the child and adolescent population?
- How do legislative initiatives affect the health of the child and adolescent population?
- To what extent are members of the child and adolescent population subjected to bias-based harassment? What are the effects of harassment on health?

(CDC, 2013). Less exclusive breast-feeding has been associated with increased asthma and allergies (e.g., atopic dermatitis) in children as well as other adverse effects. Breast-feeding is strongly influenced by cultural beliefs and practices and by a family's degree of acculturation. Cultural influences on breast-feeding were addressed in more detail in Chapter 5∞.

Dietary practices are also important among toddlers and older children and adolescents, and the population health nurse would assess dietary patterns among preschool, school age, and adolescent children in the population. As we saw earlier, obesity is a common problem related to diet and nutrition in the United States and worldwide. According to the National Health and Nutrition Examination Survey (NHANES), the 2009–2010 prevalence of obesity in infants and toddlers was 9.7%, and 16.9% of 2- to 17-year-olds were obese (Ogden, Carroll, Kit, & Flegal, 2012). A tool to assess the nutritional status of individual children and adolescents is available in the *Assessment Guidelines* section of the student resources site.

Problems of obesity can be combated by adequate exercise as well as healthier diets, yet few children and adolescents engage in recommended levels of physical activity. For example, in the 2011 YBRS, just under half of the students surveyed had engaged in any physical activity in the week prior to the survey, and nearly 14% had engaged in no physical activity at all (Eaton et al., 2012). In part, the decline in physical activity among school-age children over the last several years can be attributed to increased television viewing and computer use. In addition to their effects on physical activity levels, these activities have been associated with increased psychological difficulties in some children (de Leeuw, de Bruijin, de Weert-Van Oene, & Schrijvers, 2010).

Many public health professionals have called for an increase in physical education in schools to promote physical activity among school-age children and adolescents. Special attention should be given to the activity needs of children with chronic illness and handicapping disabilities. For example, children with asthma may have reduced activity levels as a result of their reactive airway disease and other children may have impediments to physical activity that limit their participation. Again, population health nurses can advocate for age-appropriate physical activities for children and adolescents, particularly those with special needs.

Exposure of children and adolescents to hazardous substances (e.g., lead) in the physical environment was addressed earlier; however, children and adolescents are exposed to other hazardous substances through their own behavior or that of parents and other family members. For example, from 2006 to 2010, 76% of pregnant women drank alcohol, and 1.4% engaged in binge drinking (Marchetta et al., 2012). Maternal smoking during pregnancy also has significant health effects on their children. Not only are children and adolescents exposed to the effects of smoking in utero, a large percentage of children are also exposed to second-hand smoke in the home setting. In addition, children and adolescents themselves may smoke or use other forms of tobacco. In 2011, for example, 23% of high school students responding to the YBRS reported current cigarette, cigar, or smokeless tobacco use, and nearly 8% of those who smoke, smoked more than 10 cigarettes per day. Nearly half of the smokers had unsuccessfully attempted to quit smoking (Eaton et al., 2012).

As with tobacco, children and adolescents may expose themselves to alcohol and other drugs. In 2011, for example, 40% of high school students in the YRBS reported using marijuana, and 6.8% had used any form of cocaine, while just over 11% had used inhalants. Nearly 71% reported having at least one alcoholic drink in their lifetimes, and roughly 22% of the students reported binge drinking (Eaton et al., 2012).

Use of safety measures is another area that the population health nurse would assess with respect to the child and adolescent population. Use of safety precautions by young children is usually controlled by their parents, but as children get older they should accept greater personal responsibility for their safety. Developmentally, however, adolescents and preadolescents tend to perceive themselves as invulnerable and may fail to use appropriate safety precautions, particularly with respect to safety equipment in recreational pursuits.

Adolescent sexual activity can have a profound influence on health in this population group, particularly in terms of unwanted pregnancy and sexually transmitted diseases (STDs). According to YRBS data, 47% of U.S. high school students in 2011 reported ever engaging in sexual intercourse (Kann, Lowry, Eaton, & Wechsler, 2012), 6% of them prior to age 13 (Eaton et al., 2012). More than a third of the students (37.5%) were currently sexually active, and nearly 19% had had sexual intercourse with more than four partners (Kann et al., 2012). Boys are slightly more likely than girls to report multiple sexual partners (National Center for Health Statistics, 2011b). Only 46% of the sexually active adolescents responding to the YRBS reported using a condom at last intercourse (Kann et al., 2012), and only 13% had been tested for HIV (Eaton et al., 2012).

Sexual activity puts preadolescents and adolescents at risk for STDs and unintended pregnancies. Approximately 400,000 U.S. teenagers 15 to 19 years of age give birth each year—the highest teen birth rate in the world. According to the Pregnancy Risk Assessment Monitoring System (PRAMS), approximately half of adolescents who got pregnant from 2004 to 2008 did not use any form of contraception, and one third of the nonusers thought they could not get pregnant at the time of intercourse, suggesting a significant lack of knowledge on the part of U.S. teens (Harrison, Gavin, & Hastings, 2012). In 2011, the rate of births to adolescent mothers 15 to 17 years of age was 15 births per 1,000 girls (Federal Interagency Forum on Child and Family Statistics, 2013). Although this is a decline from the prior year, adolescent pregnancy remains a significant problem leading to school dropout for the pregnant teen, low birth weight infants, lower academic achievement among the children, and an increased likelihood that girl children will themselves experience adolescent pregnancy (Harrison et al., 2012). Population health nurses should assess the extent of sexual activity in the population as well as the prevalence of STDs and pregnancies in this population and the extent of educational and preventive services available to adolescents.

Consideration should also be given to sexual orientation and sexual identity in the adolescent population. A gay, lesbian, or bisexual orientation or a transgendered identity may lead to a variety of psychological difficulties for those involved, including feelings of guilt and depression. Sexual orientation or transgenderism may also lead to family difficulties as well as victimization by peers or others. From 2001 to 2009, nine sites administering the YRBS incorporated questions on adolescent sexual orientation. A median of 93% of respondents reported a heterosexual orientation, 1.3% reported a same-sex orientation, 3.7% reported a bisexual orientation, and 2.5% were unsure of their sexual orientation. In addition, 12 sites asked about the gender of sexual partners, 40.5% of the students responding reported no sexual encounters, 53.5% reported only heterosexual contacts, 2.5% reported same-sex encounters, and 3.3% reported encounters with both males and females (Kann et al., 2011). There may be a particular need for population health nurses to advocate for services for sexually active students. A focused assessment of behavioral determinants of child and adolescent health is included below.

HEALTH SYSTEM DETERMINANTS. A number of factors in the health care delivery system influence the health of children and adolescents. Some of these factors include attitudes toward health and health care, usual sources of health care, and use of health care services. According to the National Center for Health Statistics (2013), 4.7% of U.S. children under 18 years of age did not have a regular source of care or a "medical home" in 2010–2011. A *medical home* is a regular source of health care that is characterized by access to preventive care, 24-hour availability of ambulatory and inpatient care, continuity, access to subspecialty referrals and interaction between providers and school and community agencies as needed, and maintenance of a central health record for the child.

Poor children, in particular, may lack a regular source of care, relying on emergency departments for care. This practice increases the costs of care and decreases opportunities for basic preventive and health-promotive services. Having a regular source of care is impeded by reimbursement patterns of federal insurance programs for children, and parental job loss has contributed to periods of uninsurance for many low-income families including children.

In 2011, 7 million U.S. children (9%) had no health insurance coverage (Federal Interagency Forum on Child and Family Statistics, 2013). Children without health insurance are 18 times less likely to have a regular source of health care than those with private health insurance and are 14 times less likely than publicly insured children to to have a regular provider (Federal Interagency Forum on Child and Family Statistics, 2013). Tips for assessing health system determinants influencing the health of child and adolescent populations are provided on page 404.

Population health nurses provide services to individual children and adolescents and their families as well as to these populations as aggregates. Whether services are provided to individuals or population groups, population health nurses must first assess their health status and health needs. The focus of this chapter is on meeting the needs of children and adolescents as population groups. A tool for assessing the overall health of an individual child or adolescent is provided in the *Assessment Guidelines* section of the student resources site.

Diagnostic Reasoning and the Health of Child and Adolescent Populations

Based on the data gathered in the assessment of the child or adolescent population, the population health nurse derives diagnoses or statements based on health status and health care needs. Both positive and problem-focused nursing diagnoses may be derived from the data obtained. Diagnoses may reflect

FOCUSED ASSESSMENT: Assessing Behavioral Determinants of Child and Adolescent Health

- What are the dietary patterns typical of children and adolescents in the population?
- What are the physical activity patterns typical of children and adolescents in the population?
- What recreational activities are available to the child and adolescent population? What health benefits and hazards are posed by recreational activities?
- What are the effects of dietary and physical activity patterns on the health of the child and adolescent population?
- What is the extent of child and adolescent exposure to tobacco in the home? To use of other substances?
- What is the extent of tobacco, alcohol, and drug use among the child and adolescent population?
- What is the extent of sexual activity among children and adolescents?
- To what extent is safety instruction (including sexual safety) provided to children and adolescents?
- To what extent do children and adolescents engage in effective safety practices (e.g., seat belt use, protective recreational equipment, condom use).

FOCUSED ASSESSMENT Assessing Health System Determinants of Child and Adolescent Health

- What percentage of the child and adolescent population has a regular source of health care?
- What is the extent of insurance coverage in the child and adolescent population?
- How adequate are available health services in meeting the needs of the child and adolescent population?
- To what extent do health care needs of the child and adolescent population go unmet?
- To what extent does the child and adolescent population make use of available health promotion and illness prevention services?

the need for measures to promote health, prevent injury or illness, resolve existing health problems, or restore health. For example, a positive population nursing diagnosis related to disease prevention is "high immunization levels due to high parental motivation and access to immunization services." On the other hand, a problem-focused nursing diagnosis related to immunizations is "lack of appropriate immunizations for age due to lack of access to low-cost immunizations." Another problem-focused nursing diagnosis for the population related to injury prevention is "increased potential for child abuse due to widespread unemployment and increased community incidence of mental health problems."

Nursing diagnoses related to resolution of existing health problems in the population are necessarily problem focused. An example of a nursing diagnosis for the child population might be "lack of services available in the community to meet the needs of children with developmental problems." For adolescents, a relevant nursing diagnosis might be "increased incidence of adolescent pregnancy due to widespread sexual activity, lack of effective sexuality education, and lack of access to contraceptive services." Nursing diagnoses at the population level might also reflect environmental, psychological, sociocultural, or behavioral considerations affecting children's and adolescents' overall health status.

At the restoration level of health care, nursing diagnoses focus on the need to prevent complications of existing problems or to prevent the recurrence of problems. For example, the nurse might derive nursing diagnoses of "lack of respite for families of children with chronic health problems" or "barriers to effective participation in physical activity by children with handicapping conditions."

Planning and Implementing Health Care for Child and Adolescent Populations

Population health nursing interventions may be planned to address needs for health promotion, illness and injury prevention, resolution of existing problems, or health restoration. Generally speaking, population health nurses will engage in collaborative planning with members of other disciplines as well as parents and other members of the population. Planning groups may also include older children and adolescents expected to benefit from the programs developed.

PROMOTING HEALTH. A number of general interventions may be used to promote the health of children and adolescents. These categories of intervention include assuring access to health care; promoting growth and development; providing adequate nutrition; promoting physical activity; promoting dental care; and supporting effective parenting.

Assuring access to health care. One of the best means of promoting the health of children and adolescents is to ensure that they have access to needed health care services. Population health nurses can be instrumental in linking individual children and adolescents to needed services and in assuring that health services are available to these population groups. This can be accomplished by implementing several strategies that have been recommended for improving child health in general and reducing disparities in health status among subpopulations of children and adolescents. These strategies include the following:

- Assuring that all children and adolescents have a regular source of primary health care that includes health promotion services
- Eliminating co-payments and cost sharing for health promotion services
- Assessing the adequacy of health promotion services available to children and adolescents
- Educating parents and health care providers regarding health promotion, and
- Developing information systems to monitor health promotion activities and detect disparities among subpopulations of children and adolescents

Implementing these strategies at the level of the individual child or adolescent will usually require referral to an effective source of care. Implementation may also involve referral for public insurance programs such as the State Childrens Health Insurance Program (SCHIP) or Medicaid for those children and adolescents who are eligible for these programs. At the population level, implementing these strategies will most likely require population health nurses to be politically active in advocating and planning for services to promote child and adolescent health. For example, nurses may need to advocate for programs that support good nutrition or that promote physical activity among school children.

Promoting growth and development. To develop properly, children need an environment conducive to growth and development. Population health nurses can assist parents and communities in creating such environments. They can educate both the general public and specific families regarding developmental milestones children and adolescents need to accomplish. They can alert parents to the challenges posed by these milestones through **anticipatory guidance**, the provision of information to parents and others regarding behavioral expectations of children and adolescents at a particular age, before they reach that age. Population health nurses can also advocate for community programs and environmental conditions that promote growth and development within safe parameters. For example, they can promote sports appropriate to children's abilities and developmental levels and foster the use of effective safety equipment in such programs. In addition, nurses can advocate for humanistic educational programs that promote emotional and physical, as well as cognitive development. A tool for assessing developmental levels in individual children and adolescents is provided in the *Assessment Guidelines* section of the student resources site.

Providing adequate nutrition. For infants, providing adequate nutrition can best be met by promoting breast-feeding. Population health nurses can encourage pregnant women to consider breast-feeding their infants and provide support with breast-feeding. They may also need to educate mothers on appropriate nutrition while breast-feeding and the need to increase fluid intake. Nurses may also make referrals to a variety of organizations that provide breast-feeding information, support, and assistance. For further information about sources for breast-feeding assistance, see the *External Resources* section of the student resources site. Population health nurses may also need to advocate for conditions that promote breast-feeding, including private areas for breast pumping in work places and places where women can breast-feed their infants in public facilities.

Good nutrition is also an issue for older children and adolescents. As we saw earlier, many U.S. children are overweight or obese and are not eating nutritious diets. Diets tend to be high in calories and carbohydrates and low in fruits and vegetables. Population health nurses can educate the public regarding the efficacy of breast-feeding and the need for and contents of an adequate diet for children and adolescents. In addition, they can advocate for nutritional supplementation programs and for adequate nutrition programs in schools and other institutional settings. Population health nurses can also promote policies that diminish access to "junk foods" for children and adolescents. For example, they can spearhead initiatives to remove candy and soft drink vending machines from schools and recreation areas and promote healthy fast-food alternatives at popular chain restaurants.

Population health nurses should also be alert to the extent of unhealthy dieting practices, particularly among adolescents. In the 2011 YRBS, for example, 12% of students had not eaten for more than 24 hours, 5% had taken diet pills and similar preparations without a doctor's advice, and 4% had vomited or taken laxatives to lose weight or keep from gaining weight (Eaton et al., 2012). Population health nurses may need to assist children and adolescents to develop healthy body images and, for those who are overweight or obese, direct them to healthy approaches to weight loss. Nurses may also need to advocate for realistic media portrayals of appropriate body images.

Promoting physical activity. Promoting physical activity among children and adolescents is another intervention aimed at promoting health and, in particular, preventing obesity. Based on 2011 YRBS data, only 28.7% of high school students surveyed had participated in strenuous physical activity for at least 60 minutes on each of the preceding 7 days. Conversely, approximately a third of the students reported playing video or computer games or watching television more than 3 hours a day on an average school day (Eaton et al., 2012). Population health nurses can help to educate children and adolescents on the need for increased physical activity and advocate for the inclusion of physical activity in school curricula. They can also advocate for neighborhood environments that promote physical activity (e.g., schools within walking or biking distance of homes, bicycle paths, and safe activity areas).

Promoting dental health. Dental hygiene should begin as soon as the child's first tooth erupts. At this time, parents can be encouraged to rub teeth briskly with a dry washcloth. Later, parents can begin to brush the child's teeth with a soft toothbrush. Older children can be taught to brush and floss their own teeth with adult supervision. Use of fluoridated toothpaste should be encouraged in areas with unfluoridated water; parents can give fluoride-containing vitamins to infants in such areas. In addition to instructing parents about the need for preventive dental care, population health nurses can be actively involved in promoting fluoridation of community drinking water.

Population health nurses can educate the public about the need to wean infants from the bottle before a year of age to prevent bottle-mouth syndrome. The use of sugarless snacks and rinsing the mouth after eating—when brushing is not possible—can also be encouraged. Finally, population health nurses should encourage parents to obtain regular dental checkups for children and to get prompt attention for dental problems. Financial assistance may be needed for such services for low-income families. In such cases, the population health nurse may make a referral for Medicaid in those areas where dental care is covered or work to promote the availability of such services in the population.

Supporting effective parenting. Parenting has been described as one of the hardest jobs in the world and the one for which we receive the least preparation. Many parents find their first years as parents overwhelming. Areas of difficulty often include lack of confidence in the parental role, meeting the demands of being parents, finding time for oneself, and feeling exhausted. The availability of support for parenting can assist parents in more effective performance of parental roles. Social support may include information resources, material support (e.g., financial help with health care or nutrition needs, educational needs, and so on), emotional support, or assistance in the actual performance of parenting tasks. Support may come from family members or health care and other professionals.

Social support for parents can be provided by population health nurses. For example, they may provide informational support by educating families regarding the needs of children and adolescents, or emotional support in dealing with the frustrations of parenthood. They may also provide emotional support by giving parents both positive and negative feedback on their performance as parents. Less often, population health nurses may assist parents in finding sources of material support through referrals for financial assistance. They may also assist parents to obtain help with actual parenting by arranging for respite services for a parent, or advocating the presence of such services in the community. Population health nurses may also assist parents to develop effective coping strategies to minimize the effects of parenting and other stresses on their health and that of their children.

Support for parenting for parents of young children may frequently address issues of discipline. Table 16-3● provides several general principles of child and adolescent discipline that population health nurses can use to educate community members.

The converse of promoting effective discipline of children and adolescents is preventing abuse of children and adolescents by their parents and other adults or older siblings. In the United States, the role of the population health nurse in identifying and reporting child abuse is quite clear cut. Population health nurses are part of a group of professionals, including health care providers, teachers, and others, who are required by law to report any suspicion of abuse of a child or adolescent. The role of the nurse may not be as clearly defined in other countries. Identification and reporting of child abuse can foster effective parenting because it gives parents an opportunity to learn more appropriate ways to interact with their children. Population health nurses may also refer parents to sources of information or programs that promote effective parenting. These include programs such as the Nurse Family Partnership (NFP) program discussed in Chapter 14∞ and the Triple P: Positive Parenting Program (n.d.), a program designed to prevent and treat behavioral and emotional problems in children and adolescents. For further information about the Triple P program, see the *External Resources* section of the student resources site.

Additional health promotion measures may be employed in caring for children and adolescents. For example, population health nurses may help to design and implement programs that foster healthy self-concepts and development of effective coping strategies in child and adolescent populations. Special intervention may also be warranted to create a healthy self-image in children with chronic conditions or disabilities. For example, the physically handicapped child can be helped to develop skills such as artistic ability that contribute to a positive self-image. Health promotion interventions employed by population health nurses in caring for children are summarized in Table 16-4●.

TABLE 16-3 Principles of Effective Discipline and Related Considerations

Principle	Disciplinary Consideration
Importance	Employ discipline for important matters Do not automatically say "no" to everything Determine what is unacceptable behavior
Consistency	Maintain consistency in what is considered unacceptable behavior Maintain consistency between and among authority figures If a behavior is acceptable in some situations and not in others, make sure children understand the difference and why it is so
Calm	Never act in anger Employ a "cooling off" period, if needed, and make sure children understand the need to deal with anger appropriately
Time	Allow time for compliance with directions before taking disciplinary action
Limits	Set rules and limits for behavior ahead of time and make sure children are aware of them Make sure limits are within the child's age and developmental capacity to comply Give a warning for unanticipated unacceptable behaviors the first time
Understanding	Make sure children understand the rules and the reasons for them
Prevention	Prevent unacceptable behavior rather than punish it whenever possible Remove sources of temptation from younger children Provide adequate adult supervision of children
Investigation	Ascertain the facts of the situation before taking disciplinary action Ask for the child's explanation of the situation and his or her behavior When the behavior is unacceptable but the child's reasons are appropriate, make sure he or she understands why the behavior should not be repeated
Meaningfulness	Make sure children understand the reason for disciplinary action Explain how the child can improve his or her behavior Use a form of discipline appropriate to the child and the situation

PREVENTING ILLNESS AND INJURY. The second level of health care involves interventions to prevent illness and

TABLE 16-4 Health Promotion Interventions for Child and Adolescent Populations

Focus	Interventions
Assuring access to health care	Making referrals to sources of health care Promoting a regular source of health care for all children and adolescents Advocating health insurance coverage for children and adolescents
Promoting growth and development	Educating parents and the public regarding normal growth and development Advocating environments that promote adequate growth and development of children and adolescents Promoting continued development of adolescent parents as well as their children
Providing adequate nutrition	Promoting breast-feeding Educating parents, children, and the public regarding nutritional needs of children and adolescents Advocating healthy nutrition in schools and day care centers Advocating for healthier food choices in restaurants and other venues
Promoting physical activity	Educating children and adolescents regarding the need for physical activity Advocating for physical activity in school curricula Advocating for environments conducive to physical activity
Promoting dental care	Promoting dental hygiene Advocating for access to dental care services
Supporting effective parenting	Providing support for parents Educating parents for care of children and adolescents Advocating for respite care as needed Assisting parents with discipline issues Educating parents for realistic expectations of their children Taking action to minimize parental sources of stress Promoting effective parental coping strategies
Other health promotion activities	Promoting effective coping strategies among children and adolescents Assisting in the development of healthy self-concepts among children and adolescents Meeting the health promotion needs of children with special needs

injury in the child and adolescent population. General areas for prevention to be addressed here include preventing prematurity, low birth weight, and infant mortality; preventing communicable diseases and chronic conditions; and preventing injury.

Preventing prematurity, low birth weight, and infant mortality. Premature birth and low birth weight (LBW) are two of the major contributors to infant mortality worldwide. Adolescent mothers are more likely than older mothers to have a low birth weight baby, so preventing adolescent pregnancies can reduce the incidence of prematurity and low birth weight. Population health nurses can advocate for and develop programs designed to delay initiation of sexual activity by providing adolescents and preadolescents with effective sexuality education. In addition, nurses can educate sexually active teenagers regarding contraception and make referrals to contraceptive services for individual teens. They can also advocate for the availability of contraceptive services for this population and encourage the use of long-term modes of contraception that do not rely on on-the-spot compliance or motivation for use (e.g., contraceptive implants). In addition, nurses can assist adolescents to develop negotiation skills regarding contraceptive use with their partners (Harrison et al., 2012). Particular attention may be needed to see that adolescent mothers continue to meet their own personal developmental tasks as well as meeting those of their children. This may necessitate advocacy on the part of population health nurses for educational assistance and other support services for adolescent parents.

Mothers who smoke or drink alcohol during pregnancy also have a higher risk of premature delivery and LBW babies than nonsmokers. In addition to contributing to death, prematurity and low birth weight start young children off at a disadvantage that may or may not be overcome in later years. Both prematurity and low birth weight and subsequent infant mortality can be prevented by a group of population health nursing interventions including delayed pregnancy, early and effective prenatal care, adequate prenatal nutrition, and prevention of smoking and use of alcohol during pregnancy. Population health nurses can refer individual clients to prenatal services and engage in political advocacy to make sure that such services are available to all women of childbearing age. They can also educate the public regarding the need for adequate prenatal care.

In addition, population health nurses can promote smoking cessation among pregnant women, discourage the use of alcohol in pregnancy, and promote the use of folic acid (NCBDDD, 2013b). Nurses can educate pregnant women and may refer clients to smoking cessation services or advocate for the availability of low-cost smoking cessation services.

In addition to promoting prenatal care, population health nurses can educate pregnant women regarding the need for good nutrition during pregnancy and make referrals for programs such as the Supplemental Nutrition Program for Women, Infants, and Children (WIC). They can also assist women of childbearing age with diabetes control and prepregnancy weight control to minimize the potential for premature births and low birth weight babies (CDC, 2012).

Preventing Communicable Diseases. The most effective means of preventing many communicable diseases among children and adolescents is, of course, immunization. The *Healthy People 2020* target is to achieve 95% immunization rates among all kindergarteners for polio, diphtheria, pertussis, tetanus, measles, mumps, rubella, hepatitis, and varicella vaccines. In 2011, coverage rates among federal immunization program grantees ranged from 54% for varicella to 95% coverage for DTP, with coverage for most other vaccines above 90% (Stokley, Stanwyck, Avey, & Greby, 2011). Vaccination for human papillomavirus (HPV) is also recommended, initially for girls, but also for boys since 2011 (ACIP, 2011a), but coverage remains relatively low. Low coverage rates are also noted for HIB, hepatitis A, and rotavirus vaccines among U.S. children from 19 to 35 months of age, and only approximately 64% of children in this age group had received all of the recommended vaccine doses in 2009 (Wooten, Kolasa, Singletown, & Shefer, 2010).

Similar targets for immunization have been set by the World Health Organization (WHO). In 1974, WHO and UNICEF developed a Global Immunization Vision and Strategy (GIVS). One of the goals of this strategy was to increase to 90% the extent of coverage with three doses of DTP vaccine by 2010. By that time, however, only 67% of countries had achieved the goal (WHO, UNICEF, & Global Immunization Division, Center for Global Health, 2011).

Effective immunization levels may be hampered by health care provider errors as well as parental failure to get their children immunized. For example, many providers mistakenly believe that the presence of mild fever is a contraindication for immunization and forego many valid opportunities to immunize children and adolescents. There have also been a growing number of errors in giving adult Tdap vaccine to children instead of pediatric DTaP. The lower case letters in the Tdap designation indicate the use of a weaker antigen sufficient to boost immunity in previously immunized individuals but not strong enough to support initial development of immunity. These errors result in underimmunization of young children. The Institute for Safe Medication Practices (2010) recommnends educating parents on the vaccines their children should be receiving and having them double check vaccine appropriateness with providers.

Population health nurses may be actively involved in referring individual children and adolescents for immunizations and in assuring that immunization services are available to these populations. They may also be involved in initiatives to promote immunization. For example, text messages have been found to be effective in reminding parents of the need for immunizations (Stockwell et al., 2012).

Use of immunization services is also facilitated by the development of **immunization information systems (IISs)**, confidential databases that collect and store vaccination data from multiple providers and generate reminders to providers or parents when subsequent immunizations are due. In 2010, the

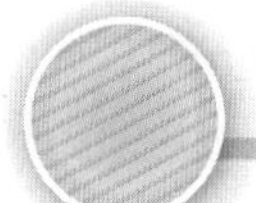

Global Perspectives

Global Vaccination Coverage

In 1974, only 5% of the world's children were fully immunized with the vaccines available at the time. In response to improved, but still low immunization rates, the World Health Organization (WHO) and the United Nations Children's Fund (UNICEF) initiated the Global Immunization Vision and Strategy (GIVS) in 2005. GIVS is designed to decrease vaccine-preventable disease-related mortality and morbidity throughout the world through increased immunization rates (WHO, UNICEF, & Global Immunization Division, 2011).

By 2010, worldwide coverage for three doses of DTP vaccine was 85%, as was the rate for receipt of at least one dose of measles-containing vaccine. Rates for immunization with at least three doses of polio vaccine were slightly higher at 86%, while rates for three doses of hepatitis B vaccine were 75% and three doses of Hib vaccine were lowest at only 42%. Approximately 19.3 million children had not received some or all of the routinely recommended vaccines, leaving them susceptible to disease and death from preventable conditions. Nearly half of these children lived in three nations (India, Nigeria, and the Democratic Republic of Congo), and two thirds of them live in 10 countries (WHO, UNICEF, & Global Immunization Division, Center for Global Health, 2011).

Coverage with newer vaccines is even lower. Rotavirus, for example, is the number one cause of diarrheal morbidity and mortality among young children in Latin America and the Caribbean, contributing to more than 8,000 deaths each year. In 2009, WHO recommended rotavirus immunization for all children less than 32 weeks of age. In 2010, only 66% of Latin American and Caribbean children less than 1 year of age had been immunized. As of June, 2011, rotavirus vaccine had been incorporated in the recommended immunization schedule in 14 of the 32 nations in Latin America and the Caribbean (de Oliveira et al, 2011) placing increased emphasis on prevention of this deadly disease but indicating the need for further efforts.

Task Force on Community Preventive Services recommended that all immunizations be documented in IISs, and the *Healthy People 2020* objectives call for 95% of children under 6 years of age to be included in an IIS. In 2009, however, only 77% of U.S. children's immunizations were recorded in an IIS (Brand, Rasulnia, & Urquhart, 2011). As of 2010, among 54 federal immunization program grantees, more than 11,000 public and 36,500 private immunization providers participated in an IIS, but monitoring of the extent of participation is hampered by lack of knowledge of all vaccine providers in a given jurisdiction and the transient nature of some providers (e.g., settings that provide influenza immunizations only during certain months) (Fath, Ng, & Pabst, 2012).

Population health nurses may also educate the public, particularly adolescents, regarding practices to prevent specific communicable diseases such as HIV/AIDS. UNICEF (2013) has developed four goals to prevent worldwide transmission of HIV infection and development of AIDS in children and adolescents. These include preventing mother-to-child transmission, treating pediatric infection, preventing infection among children and adolescents, and protecting and supporting children affected by AIDS in the family. CDC (2014) has identified several strategies for preventing perinatal transmission of HIV infection including routine testing of pregnant women, repeat screening of women at high risk for infection in the third trimester of pregnancy, antiretroviral treatment for infected women during pregnancy and for their newborns, and elective cesarean sections for women with high viral loads at the time of delivery. Population health nurses can be actively involved in promoting HIV screening for pregnant women and referring individual women for screening. Prenatal care and screening can also help identify women with other STDs (e.g., syphilis, genital herpes, and hepatitis B) that can be transmitted perinatally to their infants. For those women who are infected, population health nurses can provide case management services for diagnosis and treatment as well as educating them and the general public about the dangers of breast-feeding in the presence of HIV infection. They can also arrange for screening of infants born to HIV-infected women and make referrals for treatment as needed.

Population health nurses can also educate sexually active adolescents regarding safe sexual practices to prevent HIV infection and other STDs. They can also advocate for condom availability for this population to prevent transmission and educate adolescents on their use. In addition, population health nurses can help to educate the public and adolescents on the potential for infection with injectable drug use as well as advocate for harm reduction policies and treatment availability for adolescents who use drugs.

Hygiene and protection of food and water supplies are additional measures to prevent communicable diseases in children and adolescents, particularly in developing areas of the world. Population health nurses can educate the public regarding hygiene and preventing contamination of food and water supplies. For example, good hand hygiene, appropriate disposal of soiled tissues, and appropriate coughing and sneezing "etiquette" can minimize disease transmission for a wide variety of airborne and enteric pathogens. Nurses can also advocate for safe water and food supplies at the societal level.

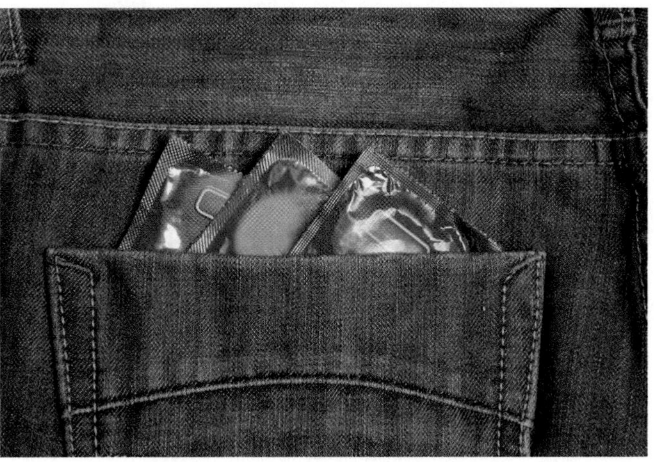

Population health nurses can educate both parents and teens about STDs and pregnancy prevention. *(Arti Om/Fotolia)*

Preventing chronic conditions. Population health nurses may also be actively involved in initiatives to prevent the development of chronic conditions in children and adolescents. Preventing injury that leads to chronic disability is discussed later in this section, but population health nurses can help to prevent chronic and handicapping conditions with a genetic component by making referrals for genetic testing and counseling. They can also assist families in making informed decisions about future pregnancies based on screening results.

Population health nursing activities to prevent or resolve problems of overweight and obesity can help to prevent a variety of chronic conditions in childhood and later in life. Weight control may prevent the development of diabetes as well as cardiovascular disease. Similarly, nurses can advocate for elimination of exposures to environmental toxins such as lead and other heavy metals, air pollution, and pesticides. This may involve advocacy to eliminate toxins in the external environment or for parental smoking cessation to prevent exposure to second hand smoke in the home. Population health nurses may also be involved in the development and implementation of programs to prevent initiation of tobacco use and other harmful substances by children and adolescents.

Preventing injury. As we saw earlier, accidental injuries are a major cause of death and disability among children and adolescents, and population health nurses should be actively involved in promoting safety across the age spectrum. Again, parental and public education are the primary means for accomplishing this objective, but population health nurses can also campaign for safe conditions in play areas as well as the development and enforcement of safety regulations such as seat belt and helmet

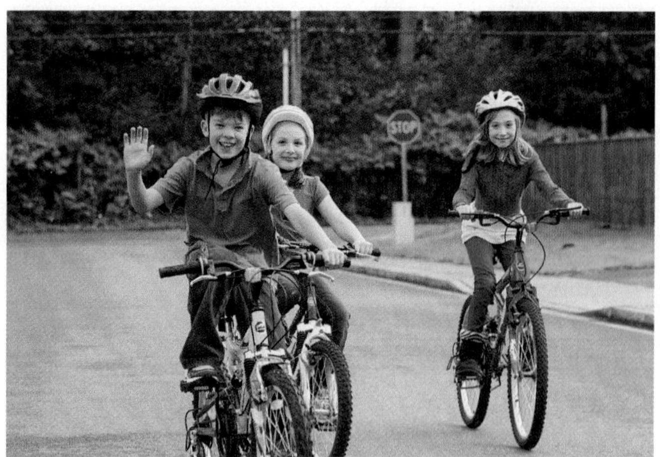

Safety education is an important issue for parents and children. *(Mat Hayward/Fotolia)*

use, effective labeling and storage of household chemicals, and so on.

Population health nurses can promote the use of safety devices and equipment. For example, they can educate individual families and their children, as well as the general public, regarding the correct use of age-appropriate restraints in motor vehicles. In addition, they may campaign for strict enforcement of restraint legislation for all vehicle occupants.

Playground safety is another issue for children and adolescents. The National Program for Playground Safety (2014b) has developed recommendations that can be used by population health nurses to educate parents and the general public regarding playground safety. These recommendations include:

- Adult supervision of children in play activities: Children should be visible to adults in all areas of the playground. This may necessitate the use of see-through walls for crawl spaces and tunnels. Easily understood rules for play should be posted, reviewed with children, and enforced.
- Choice of age and developmentally appropriate play equipment: Playgrounds should be designed with separate areas for children of different ages, with play equipment scaled to child size. Guardrails should be installed to prevent falls off platforms, and standing areas should be provided on platforms more than 6 feet high to permit children to rethink their descent options.
- Provision of safe surfacing below play equipment: Approximately 12 inches of loose fill or unitary surfaces (e.g., resilient mats) should be provided under play structures and for six feet in all directions (with more space in front of slides and swings). Structures should be limited to a height of 6 feet for preschool children and 8 feet for school age children.
- Regular maintenance of all equipment and play surfaces: Gaps or snags in which clothing can catch or body parts be trapped should be eliminated. Broken equipment or equipment with missing parts should be repaired or removed, and rusted metal, broken plastic, or splintered wood should be eliminated or repaired.

Accidental and, among adolescents and preadolescents, intentional poisoning are other areas of concern for population health nurses caring for child and adolescent populations. Nurses can actively promote safety education regarding the use and storage of poisonous materials among the general public. They may also be involved in efforts to promote effective labeling of hazardous substances and in suicide prevention activities with youth. These activities are discussed in more detail in Chapter 30∞. Selected elements of an education program to promote child and adolescent safety are included in Table 16-5•. An assessment tool that population health nurses can use to assess home safety for children and adolescents is included in the *Assessment Guidelines* section of the student resources site.

Preventing violence. The final area to be addressed in the prevention of illness and injury among children and adolescents is prevention of violence. Prevention of abuse of children and adolescents should focus on reducing risk factors and enhancing protective factors as outlined in Table 16-2. NCIPC (2014c) has identified several effective programs to prevent child maltreatment. Strategies for prevention of violence against youth and youth suicide are addressed in detail in Chapter 30∞.

Prevention of violence by youth is also of concern. The National Center for Injury Prevention and Control (2012c) has identified four strategies to minimize youth violence. The first of these strategies is parent- and family-based programs that improve family function and provide parents with strategies for promoting nonviolent conflict resolution among their children. The second strategy is education of children on handling difficult social situations. Such efforts may occur in schools or other settings frequented by children and adolescents. Mentoring programs that pair young people with caring adults can provide effective role models in conflict resolution. Finally, changes in social and economic circumstances that promote violence can be undertaken. Population health nurses may be involved in advocating for, developing, and implementing programs that address each of these four strategies. For example, they may refer parents to existing support programs or assist in the development of such programs. Similarly, they may be actively involved in educating children and youth for nonviolent conflict resolution or in developing mentoring programs for youth. They may also advocate for societal changes that modify social and economic conditions that promote violence, such as school policies on bullying and harassment. Prevention of violence in the school setting will be addressed in more detail in Chapter 22∞. Table 16-6• summarizes population health nursing interventions related to injury and illness prevention for child and adolescent populations.

RESOLVING EXISTING HEALTH PROBLEMS. Population health nursing interventions to resolve existing health problems in child and adolescent populations centers on screening for health problems, caring for minor illness, and caring

TABLE 16-5 Education to Prevent Injury in Children and Adolescents

Age	Safety Education
Infant (birth–1 year)	Not leaving child unattended on elevated surfaces or in bath Use of car seat restraint Use of safety straps in high chairs, strollers, swings, infant seats, etc. Use of flame-retardant sleepwear Crib safety: Narrow spaces between slats, bumper pads, no plastic coverings, nontoxic paint, no soft pillows Toy safety: No sharp edges or small parts, no long strings, siblings' toys out of reach
Toddler (2–3 years)	Not leaving child unattended in bath or pool Use of car seat restraint Adequate adult supervision Home safety: Outlet covers, sharp and poisonous objects locked away, medications out of reach, child-resistant containers, gated stairs, bathroom doors closed, no dangling electrical cords Play equipment: Age-appropriate and in good repair, on appropriate surface Toy safety: Age-appropriate toys, no small parts Fenced yard/swimming pool
Preschool child (4–6 years)	Use of booster seat in vehicle Adequate adult supervision Home safety: Outlet covers, sharp and poisonous objects locked away, medications out of reach, child-resistant containers, gated stairs, bathroom doors closed, no dangling electrical cords Play equipment: Age-appropriate and in good repair, on appropriate surface Toy safety: Age-appropriate toys, no small parts, adult supervision with potentially hazardous toys Safety practices: Education regarding interaction with strangers, crossing the street, fire safety, water safety
School-age child (6–12 years)	Use of booster seat/adult seat belt based on height and weight Sports safety: Age-appropriate sports, use of safety equipment, adequate adult supervision Firearms: Locked separately from ammunition Safety practices: Education regarding stranger interactions, caring for self at home, sports, bicycling and helmet use, water safety, use of medications, swimming instruction
Adolescent (13–18 years)	Safe driving Use of seat belts Sports safety: Age-appropriate sports, use of safety equipment, adequate adult supervision Safety practices: Education regarding use of firearms, caring for self and others at home, use of medications, dangerous situations (e.g., alcohol and driving, fighting), stranger interactions Sexuality: Abstinence, safe sexual practices Use of drugs and alcohol

for children and adolescents with chronic and life threatening conditions. Each of these areas will be briefly addressed here.

Screening for health problems. Screening for conditions at birth is usually employed when treatment soon after birth leads to improved health outcomes. Each state determines the panel of required screenings for newborns born in that state. Screening occurs for core conditions and secondary conditions. Core conditions are those for which routine screening is conducted; secondary conditions are those that may be identified in the process of screening or confirmatory testing resulting from core screenings. Criteria for the selection of mandatory screening tests include the availability of specific and sensitive screening tests, well understood health outcomes of the condition, availability of an effective treatment that minimizes the effects of the condition, and the possible influence of screening outcomes for future family reproductive decisions. Newborn screening categories include a variety of inherited metabolic disorders including several disorders of amino acid metabolism (e.g., maple sugar urine disease, phenylketonuria), disorders of fatty acid metabolism (e.g., dehydrogenase deficiencies, cartinine uptake deficit), and disorders of organic acid metabolism (e.g., cobalamin disorders, glutaric acidemia). Other categories of core conditions include endocrine disorders (e.g., congenital hypothyroidism, adrenal hyperplasia), hemoglobin disorders (e.g., sickle cell anemia, S beta-thalassemia), and other conditions such as cystic fibrosis, galactosemia, hearing loss, and severe combined immunodeficiencies (Chen et al., 2012).

Routine screening for existing conditions takes place at other ages as well as at birth. The U.S. Preventive Services Task Force (USPSTF, 2010) has found sufficient evidence of effectiveness to warrant routine screening of newborns for many of the conditions presented earlier. Evidence has also been found for the efficacy of screening for amblyopia, strabismus, and visual acuity in children under 5 years of age, obesity in children from age 6 years on, and major depressive disorders when there is access to services to address positive screening in children from 12 to 18 years of age. The task force, however, has not found sufficient evidence for other routine screenings that are often employed with children. For example, the task force reported insufficient evidence of the utility of screening children for scoliosis or high blood lead levels in the absence of symptoms, even for children

TABLE 16-6 Illness and Injury Prevention Interventions for Children and Adolescents

Focus	Interventions
Reducing prematurity, low birth weight, and infant mortality	Providing sexuality education Promoting effective contraception to prevent unplanned pregnancies Promoting effective prenatal care and advocating for low-cost pregnancy services Promoting supplemental nutrition programs for pregnant women and children and making referrals to existing programs Encouraging smoking cessation and elimination of alcohol during pregnancy Assisting with prepregnancy weight control and control of diabetes
Preventing communicable diseases	Promoting immunization and referring for immunization services Advocating for development and participation in immunization information systems Promoting cocooning to protect young infants from vaccine preventable diseases Modifying immunization practices or schedules for children with special needs Promoting prenatal care and screening and treatment for HIV and other STDs in pregnant women Promoting condom use and safe sexual practices among adolescents Educating the public and families with respect to good hygiene and protection of food and water supplies Advocating for effective sanitation and safe food and water supplies
Preventing chronic conditions	Preventing or resolving obesity and overweight Preventing exposure to environmental toxins Advocating for elimination of environmental toxins Encouraging parental smoking cessation Preventing or resolving obesity and overweight
Preventing injury	Encouraging provision of adequate supervision of children and adolescents Advocating for strong legislation and strict enforcement to protect children and adolescents Promoting use of effective safety devices Teaching children and adolescents regarding safety issues Advocating for elimination of safety hazards in the environment
Preventing violence by youth	Advocating for, developing, and referring families to parent- or family-based programs to improve parenting and family function Advocating for and providing social development training programs for youth that provide assistance in nonviolent conflict resolution Advocating for and assisting in the development of mentoring programs for youth Advocating for social and economic changes in conditions that promote violence

with multiple risk factors (USPSTF, 2010). Some health insurance organizations, however, continue to recommend a variety of screening measures for children of different ages (Wellmark Blue Cross Blue Shield of Iowa & Wellmark Blue Cross Blue Shield of South Dakota, 2013). Table 16-7• provides information about screening procedures recommended for selected age groups.

Other screening procedures may be warranted for children and adolescents in certain circumstances. For example, children with a family history of diabetes may be screened for this condition. Similarly, children or adolescents who have been exposed to traumatic events (e.g., school violence, natural disaster) should be screened for depression and other mental health problems. Population health nurses may be actively involved in providing routine and specialized screening services or may need to advocate for access to these services for the child and adolescent populations.

Caring for minor illness. Children and adolescents experience a variety of minor health problems. Many of these problems can be addressed effectively at home if parents or other caregivers know how to deal with them. For other problems, or when home care does not resolve the problem, professional care is required. Population health nurses can educate the public regarding appropriate home treatment for minor illness and when professional care is required.

Population health nurses can educate parents and the public on the signs of illness in children, appropriate measures to be taken at home, and when to seek medical intervention. Some approaches to parent education may be more effective than others, for example, a systematic review of related literature found that formal education strategies using mixed educational methods were effective in educating parents about fever control, but semi-formal and informal strategies were not (Young, Watts, & Wilson, 2010).

Caretakers and the public should be acquainted with what is normal and what is abnormal, as well as what home remedies are appropriate and what might be harmful. In addition to providing such information at the population level, population

TABLE 16-7 Screening Procedures for Children and Adolescents

Age	Screening Procedure
Children of all ages	Health history, physical examination, height and weight, development, immunization status
Newborn	Inherited metabolic disorders, endocrine disorders, hemoglobin disorders, other conditions including cystic fibrosis, biotidinase deficiency, galactosemia, hearing loss, and immunodeficiency
Infant	Head circumference (to 24 months), subjective hearing and vision screening (parental report), immunization status, hematocrit/hemoglobin (12 months). Infants at risk should also be screened for low hematocrit or hemoglobin at 4 months, tuberculosis, lead
Early childhood	BMI, blood pressure, objective vision (3 years) and hearing (4 years), autism (24–30 months), amblyopia, strabismus, visual acuity, dental health, and fluoride availability. Young children at risk should be screened for hematocrit/hemoglobin, tuberculosis, cholesterol, lead
Middle childhood	BMI, blood pressure, objective vision and hearing screening, obesity, and fluoride availability. Children at risk should be screened for hemoglobin/hematocrit, tuberculosis, cholesterol, lead
Adolescence	BMI, blood pressure, objective vision and hearing screening, depression, obesity, and fluoride availability. Adolescents at risk should also be screened for hematocrit/hemoglobin; tuberculosis; cholesterol; STDs; drug, alcohol, and tobacco use; pelvic exam

Sources: U.S. Preventive Services Task Force. (2010). *The guide to clinical preventive services 2010–2011.* Retrieved from http://www.ahrq.gov/clinic/pocketgd.htm; Wellmark Blue Cross Blue Shield of Iowa & Wellmark Blue Cross Blue Shield of South Dakota. (2013). *Pediatric screening and prevention guideline.* Retrieved from http://www.wellmark.com/HealthAndWellness/WellnessResources/docs/PediatricPreventiveHealthGuidelines.pdf

health nurses frequently are called on to assess the health status of specific children and recommend appropriate interventions or make referrals for medical assistance.

Caring for children and adolescents with chronic illness. We most often think of chronic illness in the context of caring for elderly clients, but as we saw earlier many children are also affected in some way by chronic illness. Chronic conditions may also affect children's performance or their interactions with others in the school setting. Problems posed by chronic illness in school settings are addressed in more detail in Chapter 22∞. Children and adolescents with chronic conditions are sometimes referred to as children and youth with special needs, defined by the Maternal and Child Health Bureau (n.d., p. 1) as "all children who have, or are at increased risk for, chronic physical, developmental, behavioral, or emotional conditions and who also require health and related services of a type or amount beyond that required by children generally."

Much intervention with families with children experiencing chronic illness has focused on development of family resilience or hardiness discussed in Chapter 14∞. Families dealing with children and adolescents with chronic illnesses encounter a number of needs that population health nurses can assist them with. Some of these needs relate to medical care, education of the parent and/or child for self-management, emotional support, and respite care. Population health nurses also need to help families deal with the disruptions of normal family life caused by the presence of chronic illness in a child, while recognizing the expertise of parents in caring for their own children.

Health system factors that affect family response to chronic illness include fragmentation of care and lack of social support for parental caregivers. Parents may find themselves engaged in frequent battles to obtain needed health and education services for their children. Support programs for families of children with chronic illnesses are usually severely underfunded, if they exist at all. Parents are often unprepared for the demands of their new caregiver role and may view the presence of a population health nurse as both helpful and disruptive of family routine and privacy.

The need for adaptation to a chronic condition in a child begins with the diagnosis of the condition. Warner and Hauser (2011) noted that diagnosis of chronic illness in a child is related to a series of "ambiguous losses." Ambiguity begins prior to diagnosis with uncertainty about what is wrong with the child. Once a diagnosis has been made, there is ambiguity regarding the meaning of the condition and its effects on the life of the child and the family. Finally, there is ambiguity on what the life course of the child will be like and how the chronic illness will affect abilities and the child's identity. The effects of these aspects of ambiguity are seen in at least five areas. The first is how the family should respond to the diagnosis. The second deals with the adaptation of family roles, rules, and rituals required by the child's illness. Ambiguity may also make it difficult for family members to validate their distress and seek assistance due to the lack of visible signs of a loss. Similarly, the ambiguity of the loss may lead to changes in individual views of the world. For example, either parents or child may view the existence of the condition as unfair or unjust. Finally, ambiguity and uncertainty may compound the physical and psychological exhaustion experienced by family members (Warner & Hauser, 2011).

Initial areas of concern for parents of children with a chronic condition include developing specific care skills (e.g., medication administration, suctioning, physical therapy), reorganizing family roles to incorporate care of the affected child, and continuing to meet other family and social responsibilities.

Meeting medical needs may involve coordinating services, juggling appointments, and obtaining needed supplies and equipment as well as learning how to use them. Parents may also experience lack of time for themselves or to maintain family and social relationships, dealing with their own emotional responses and those of the child and other family members, dealing with feelings of guilt or loss or changes in personal identities (e.g., becoming a caregiver versus other roles) (Hewitt-Taylor, 2008a).

Parents often exhibit exhaustion due to the need to be on 24-hour "call." Even when children are involved in school or other activities, parents may be called upon to deal with emergencies or questions that arise. Exhaustion or hopelessness may also arise in the context of thoughts of the long-term nature of care for some conditions. For example, if the child is not expected to be able to fend for him or herself as an adult, parents and other family members may need to engage in long-term planning. Another area of concern is parental abilities to maintain their own health. For example, Chen and Clark (2010) found that the level of family support and parental perceptions of their child's illness were significantly associated with parental health status in families with a child with Duchene muscular dystrophy.

Families with children experiencing a chronic illness may need assistance in developing coping skills that will help them adapt to the burden of care. Families may use three types of coping to help them adjust (Warner & Hauser, 2011). Appraisal-focused coping addresses family members' appraisal of the meaning of the stressor. For example, family members who perceive the stress as a challenge or care as a demonstration of love and caring may adapt better than those who perceive care demands as a burden. Or, family members may cope by comparing themselves favorably to others who "have it much worse." Problem-focused coping is action oriented and involves planning and action to deal with sources of stress. Reorganization of family roles so one parent can stay with the child during an extended hospital stay or to relieve some of the caretaking burden from one parent are examples of problem-focused coping. Finally, emotional coping strategies are designed to regulate emotional responses to stress. For example, parents may adopt meditation, exercise, or journaling to help them deal with negative emotions generated by the situation.

The presence of a child with a chronic condition within the family may also have profound effects on relationships within and outside of the family. There may be changes in a spousal relationship, if one exists, as parents take on roles related to the care of the child. Parents may also have less time to spend with other children, and siblings may need to curtail some activities due to the needs of the ill brother or sister. Family outings or vacations may necessitate intensive planning and logistical arrangements to accommodate the care and equipment needs of the child affected. Similarly, the home environment may need to be rearranged to accommodate equipment and supplies needed (Hewitt-Taylor, 2008a).

The effects of a brother or sister with a chronic condition on siblings may be both positive and negative. Research has suggested that they are often more tolerant of individuals who are "different," but may experience frustration and discrimination when peers react to the ill sibling. Similarly, they may be expected to mature more rapidly than other children their ages and take some responsibility for care of their brothers or sisters (Hewitt-Taylor, 2008a).

The child with a chronic condition also has unique needs that population health nurses can assist the family with. This is particularly true of adolescents with chronic conditions, who need to achieve balance between parental oversight of their disease management (as well as other aspects of life) with autonomy and self-management (Warner & Hauser, 2011). Population health nurses can assist adolescents and their parents to achieve realistic compromises that promote development of adult responsibility. They can also assist parents to recognize that risk taking is a normal part of adolescent development, but make sure that the adolescent is fully aware of the potential consequences of typical risk-taking behavior. For example, the nurse may need to impress upon youth the potential for interactive effects between alcohol and medications taken for a chronic condition. Adolescents may also need help with sexual identity development and sexual expression which is often dependent on the reaction of others to one's condition (Hewitt-Taylor, 2008b). Population health nurses can also help adolescents to accept more responsibility for management of their own illness (O'Donohue & Tolle, 2011).

In addition, population health nurses may need to be active advocates for transition care for adolescents approaching adulthood. For example, access to many supportive services for children with chronic conditions may cease when they reach their majority. Population health nurses can advocate for supportive care for these young adults as well as advocate for social conditions that help meet the needs of younger children with chronic illness and their families. For example, they may need to work for transportation access for children and adolescents with mobility difficulties or changing rooms in stores that accommodate wheelchairs (Hewitt-Taylor, 2008b).

Both the *Healthy People 2010* and *Healthy People 2020* national objectives call for access to comprehensive services for children and youth with special needs. In 2005–2006, however, less than 18% of children with special needs received care in a health care delivery system that met all the quality indicators for comprehensive services. These indicators include family involvement in decision making, availability of a medical home, adequate health insurance coverage that assures continuity and comprehensiveness of services, provision of screening and surveillance as well as preventive medical and dental services, ease of use, and effective planning for successful transitions into adulthood (Strickland et al., 2011).

Caring for children and adolescents with terminal illness. Families with children with terminal illnesses face many of the same challenges as those whose children have chronic illnesses.

A review of studies of parents with children with cancer indicated four common themes which may characterize families dealing with any life-threatening illness in a child (da Silva, Jacob, & Nasciemento, 2010). Parents reported changes in their relationships, some positive and some negative, that occurred over the course of the child's illness. A second theme was that of communication difficulties when parents found it difficult to discuss their feelings about their child's impending death. Such communication difficulties may also affect others in the family, such as the ill child and siblings. Parents also often found themselves unable to provide mutual support, and gender differences were noted in parental stress and the ability to identify the other's stress. Mothers usually experienced higher levels of stress than fathers, probably due to greater assumption of caretaking roles.

Another theme was that of role changes. Mothers often traded the wife role for the mother role, although many fathers assumed greater caretaking roles over time. In the caretaking role, mothers were often absent from the home to be with the child during extended hospitalizations. This absence resulted in their inability to fulfill roles in relation to other members of the family, with these roles often assumed by the father or other children. Sometimes the fatigue accompanying these role changes meant that neither parent was able to effectively fulfill household and family roles. A final concern voiced by parents was the frequent inability to get input from a co-parent in care decisions due to the time sensitive nature of many of those decisions (da Silva et al., 2010).

All of these issues may lead to deteriorating health in other family members, particularly adult caretakers of the ill child. A longitudinal study of parents of children with terminal illness in Canada found the health of parents worsened in conjunction with the increasing complexity of the child's condition (Brehaut et al., 2011).

The two primary functions of population health nurses in the care of children and adolescents with terminal illnesses are palliative care and assisting families with grieving. WHO (2014) has noted that palliative care for children is "active total care of the child's mind, body, and spirit, and also involves giving support to the family" (para. 1). The goal of palliative care is to enhance the quality of life of the child and his or her family through control of symptoms and alleviation of other conditions (e.g., loneliness, depression) that may diminish quality of life. Palliative care also seeks to ensure continued effective functioning of the family unit. Population health nurses may be involved in the provision of palliative care for individual children or adolescents or refer clients for palliative and hospice care services. At the aggregate level, they can work to assure the availability of pediatric palliative and hospice care services in the community and their accessibility to all those in need of them.

Assisting families to deal with grief is another important function of the population health nurse in caring for children and adolescents with terminal illnesses. These families engage in anticipatory grieving that may be characterized by feelings of despair, hopelessness, and worthlessness. Such feelings have been found to be more intense in families whose child is newly diagnosed (Al-Gamal & Long, 2010), but may resurface throughout the trajectory of the child's illness. Population health nurses can assist family members, including the child affected, to discuss their feelings and to seek mutual support. The nurse can also refer families to hospice services, or to religious counselors, if desired by the family. Nurses can also link family members with support groups to help them deal with their grief before and/or after the child's death.

One innovative and effective approach to providing mutual support is the use of computer technology. Population health nurses can refer families to existing services or may be involved in their development and implementation. In addition, population health nurses may advocate for the availability of bereavement services for families of children with terminal illnesses. Table 16-8• summarizes potential population health nursing interventions for resolving problems related to the care of children and adolescents with terminal illnesses as well as other physical and mental health problems experienced by children and youth.

RESTORING HEALTH AND MANAGING LONG-TERM CONDITIONS. Health restoration addresses the particular health problems experienced by children or adolescents. Generally, there are three aspects to health restoration with children and adolescents: promoting self-management, preventing further consequences, and promoting adjustment.

Promoting self-management. Population health nurses may assist parents and older children and adolescents to develop self-management expertise related to care of chronic conditions or to engage in other self-management activities. For example, resolving an existing problem of teenage pregnancy may involve referral for prenatal care and education to promote a healthy pregnancy, but restoring a state of health and promoting self-management may involve educating the adolescent parent on child care and promoting further development for the teenager as well as for the newborn. Self-management in this instance may also involve assisting the family to adjust to the presence of a new member and modifying family roles to allow the teenager to assume the parenting role while providing adequate support for that role.

In the case of chronic illness, self-management may involve assisting an older child or adolescent to take increasing responsibility for medication compliance, adherence to dietary restrictions and so on. The population health nurse may also help the child to maintain as normal a lifestyle as possible in the face of the chronic condition.

At the population level, the population health nurse might be involved in the development of programs that promote self-management by families and children affected by a variety of health problems. For example, he or she might initiate educational programs and self-help groups for families of children with asthma. The nurse may also need to advocate for insurance coverage for such services and for their availability and accessibility in the community.

TABLE 16-8 Interventions to Resolve Existing Health Problems in Child and Adolescent Populations

Focus	Interventions
Screening for health problems	• Providing routine screening services for children and adolescents • Interpreting screening test results for families and making referrals for follow-up diagnosis and treatment • Advocating for available and accessible screening services • Planning and implementing population-based health screening programs for children and adolescents
Caring for minor illness	• Educating families and the public to recognize signs of minor illness in children and adolescents • Educating families and the public regarding home care of minor illness and how to know when professional care is needed • Providing or referring for treatment for minor illness for individual children/adolescents, when needed • Advocating available and accessible services for minor illness care
Caring for children and adolescents with chronic illnesses	• Educating families and the public regarding signs of chronic illness in children and adolescents • Referring individual children and adolescents for diagnosis and treatment of chronic illness • Providing case management services for children and adolescents with chronic illness • Assisting families to adapt to the care needs of a child or adolescent with chronic illness • Teaching children and adolescents and their families for self-management of chronic illness • Referring caretakers of children and adolescents with chronic illnesses for respite services • Promoting normal growth and development in children with chronic illness • Advocating environmental changes to minimize disabilities due to chronic illness • Advocating available and accessible diagnostic and treatment services for children and adolescents with chronic illness
Caring for children and adolescents with terminal illness	• Providing or referring families for palliative care and hospice services • Assisting families with the grief process • Referring children and adolescents and their families for support services as needed • Initiating bereavement care • Advocating available and accessible palliative and bereavement care for children and adolescents and their families • Developing technology-mediated mutual support groups for families of children with terminal illnesses

Preventing consequences. Health restoration also involves maintaining health by preventing further consequences of health problems. For example, the child with diabetes requires attention to diet, exercise, and medication to control the diabetes and prevent physical consequences of the disease itself. At the same time, attention must be given to promoting the child's adjustment to the condition and normalizing his or her life as much as possible. Nursing interventions would be geared toward convincing the child to stick to his or her diet and promoting social interactions with peers.

The nurse might also need to intervene to prevent or minimize the consequences of a child's condition for the rest of the family. For example, the nurse might need to point out to parents that in their concern for the child with a chronic heart condition, they are neglecting the needs of siblings. Health restoration for an infant with AIDS may entail educating parents on the disposal of bodily fluids and excreta to prevent infection of other family members. Health restoration may entail a wide variety of activities on the part of the nurse, from education on how to deal with specific conditions to referral for assistance with major medical expenses. Nurses may also need to act as advocates for children with chronic conditions. The example that most readily comes to mind is the need for advocacy for children with AIDS who are still well enough to attend school.

Emotional support by the nurse is a very important part of health restoration for children with chronic conditions and their families. Parents' and children's feelings about the condition need to be acknowledged and addressed. The nurse can also reinforce positive activities on the part of parent or child. Again, this support may need to be extended as families go through the grieving process. Grieving will probably occur with most chronic illnesses, even those that are not terminal, and the nurse should be prepared to reassure families that their feelings of grief are normal and to support them through this process.

Again, advocacy may be needed at the population level to assure access to needed services that prevent consequences of health problems. For example, the population health nurse may need to advocate for special education arrangements for adolescent parents that permit them to continue their education while fulfilling their parental responsibilities.

Promoting adjustment. The population health nurse may also engage in activities that are designed to return the child and family to a relatively normal state of existence. For children or adolescents with chronic illnesses or disabilities, this means restoring function as much as possible, preventing further loss of function, and assisting the child and his or her family to adapt lifestyles and behaviors to the presence of a chronic condition. The population health nurse might accomplish this by encouraging the family to discuss problems posed by the child's condition and to view the condition in the most positive light possible. The nurse should also encourage the family to normalize family life as much as possible. For example, if the Little League activities of a sibling have been curtailed because of an exacerbation of the child's illness, parents should make an attempt to reinstitute those activities as soon as the youngster's condition is stable, or the family can be encouraged to call on members of their support network to take the sibling to baseball practice and games. Interventions that might be used by population health nurses in health restoration with children and adolescents and their families are presented in Table 16-9•.

Evaluating Health Care for Child and Adolescent Populations

The effectiveness of nursing interventions for the individual child or adolescent is assessed in the same manner that care of any specific client is evaluated. Has intervention fostered the child's growth and development? Is the child's nutrition adequate to meet his or her needs? Is the child up to date on his or her immunizations? Have physical or psychological hazards been eliminated from the child's environment? Is the child receiving health care as needed? Have acute health care problems been resolved?

The population health nurse would also examine the extent to which care has contributed to the adjustment of the child and family to an existing chronic disease or disability. Are parents comfortable and adequately prepared to parent a child with special needs? Do they perform this role adequately? Have complications of the child's condition been prevented?

The population health nurse may also be involved in evaluating the effects of interventions at the aggregate level. This might entail evaluating the extent to which national objectives for the health of children and adolescents have been achieved. The *Healthy People 2020* objectives on pages 418 to 420 address selected issues related to child and adolescent health. Current data for these and other related objectives for child and adolescent health are available from the U.S. Department of Health and Human Services *Healthy People 2020* website. Population health nurses might be involved in gathering data related to the status of these objectives in their own communities to evaluate the effectiveness of child and adolescent care. They may also be involved in activities to evaluate the effects of other initiatives related to child and adolescent health.

TABLE 16-9 Health Restoration Interventions for Child and Adolescent Populations

Focus	Interventions
Promoting self-management	• Educating children, adolescents, their families, and the public to promote self-management related to health problems • Advocating for societal and environmental changes needed to promote self-management of health issues among children and adolescents and their families • Advocating for, planning, and implementing accessible services that promote self-management
Preventing consequences	• Monitoring and promoting effective disease management for children and adolescents with chronic conditions • Advocating for support services for children and adolescents with chronic conditions • Promoting development of children and adolescents with chronic conditions • Providing or referring for counseling for children and adolescents and their families as needed • Providing emotional support for children, adolescents, and their families • Referring caretakers for respite care as needed
Promoting adjustment	• Promoting lifestyle changes consistent with effective disease management • Promoting normal family life as much as possible • Promoting communication within the family and between the family and health care providers • Initiating or referring families to existing support groups • Advocating for societal and environmental changes necessary for effective adjustment to a chronic illness

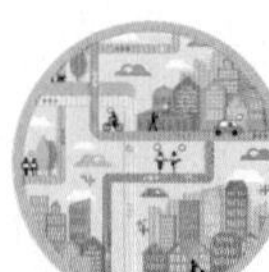

Healthy People 2020

Selected Objectives Related to Child and Adolescent Health

OBJECTIVE	BASELINE (YEAR)	TARGET	CURRENT DATA (YEAR)	DATA SOURCE
MICH-1 Reduce the rate of fetal and infant deaths MICH-1.3 All infant deaths	6.7 infant deaths per 1,000 live births (2006)	6.0 infant deaths per 1,000 live births	6.4 (2009)	National Vital Statistics System (NVSS), CDC, NCHS
MICH-3 Reduce the rate of child deaths MICH-3.1 Children aged 1–4 years MICH-3.2 Children aged 5–9 years	29.4/100,000 (2007) 13.8/100,000 (2007)	26.5/100,000 12.4/100,000	26.5 (2010) 11.4 (2010)	National Vital Statistics System (NVSS), CDC, NCHS
MICH-4 Reduce the rate of adolescent and young adult deaths MICH-4.1 Adolescents 10–14 years MICH-3.1 Adolescents 15–19 years	16.5/100,000 (2007) 60.3/100,000 (2007)	14.8/100,000 54.3/100,000	14.3 (2010) 49.4 (2010)	National Vital Statistics System (NVSS), CDC, NCHS
MICH-8.2 Reduce very low birth weight	1.5% of live births (2007)	1.4% of live births	1.4% (2010)	National Vital Statistics System (NVSS), CDC, NCHS
MICH-10-2 Increase the proportion of pregnant women who receive early and adequate prenatal care	70.5% (2007)	77.6%	NDA	National Vital Statistics System (NVSS), CDC, NCHS
MICH-11.3 Increase abstinence from cigarette smoking among pregnant women	89.6% (2007)	98.6%	NDA	National Vital Statistics System (NVSS), CDC, NCHS
MICH-21.5 Increase the proportion of infants who are breast-fed exclusively through 6 months	14.1% (2006)	25.5%	14.6% (2008)	National Immunization Survey (NIS), CDC, NCIRD, and NCHS
MICH-25 Reduce the occurrence of fetal alcohol syndrome (FAS)	3.6//10,000 live births (2006)	N/A*	NDA	Fetal Alcohol Syndrome Surveillance Network (FASSnet), CDC, NCBDDD
MICH-30.1 Increase the proportion of children who have access to a medical home	57.5% of children under age 18 years (2007)	63.3%	54.4% (2011–2012)	National Survey of Children's Health (NSCH), HRSA, MCHB and CDC, NCHS
MICH-30.2 Increase the proportion of children with special health care needs who have access to a medical home	47.1% of children under age 18 years	51.8%	43% (2009–2010)	National Survey of Children with Special Health Care Needs (NSCSHCN), HRSA, MCHB and CDC, NCHS
AH-5.6 Decrease school absenteeism among adolescents due to illness or injury	5% missed 11 or more whole school days (2008)	TBD	5.3% (2011)	National Health Interview Survey (NHIS), CDC, NCHS
AH-10 Decrease the proportion of public schools with a serious violent incident	17.2% of public schools (2007–2008)	15.5%	NDA	School Survey on Crime and Safety (SSOCS), ED, IES, NCES

Healthy People 2020 (Continued)

OBJECTIVE	BASELINE (YEAR)	TARGET	CURRENT DATA (YEAR)	DATA SOURCE
AH-11.1 Decrease the rate of minor and young adult perpetration of violent crimes	444/100,000 adolescents and young adults aged 10 to 24 years (2008)	399.6 arrests/ 100,000 population aged 10 to 24 years	NDA	Violent Crime Index, Uniform Crime Reporting Program, DOJ, FBI, CJIS
IID-8 Increase the proportion of children aged 19 to 35 months who receive the recommended doses of DTaP, polio, MMR, Hib, hepatitis B, varicella and PCV vaccines	44.3% of children (2009)	80%	68.5% (2011)	National Immunization Survey (NIS), CDC, NCIRD, and NCHS
IID-18 Increase the proportion of children under 6 years of age whose immunization records are in fully operational, population-based immunization information systems	75% (2008)	95%	83.6% (2011)	Immunization Program Annual Reports, CDC, NCIRD
NWS-2.1 Increase the proportion of schools that do not sell or offer calorically sweetened beverages to students	9.3%	21.3%	NDA	School Health Policies and Programs Study, CDC
NWS-10 Reduce the proportion of children and adolescents 2–19 years who are considered obese	16.1% (2005–2008)	14.5%	16.9% (2009–2010)	National Health and Nutrition Examination Survey (NHANES), CDC, NCHS
NWS-12 Eliminate very low food security among children	1.3% of households with children (2008)	0.2%	1% (2011)	Food Security Supplement to the Current Population Survey, U.S. Department of Commerce, Bureau of the Census
NWS-14 Increase the contribution of fruits to the diets of the population aged 2 years and older	0.5 cup equivalents of fruits per 1,000 calories (2001–2004)	0.9 cup equivalents per 1,000 calories	NDA	National Health and Nutrition Examination Survey (NHANES), CDC, NCHS and USDA, ARS
NWS-18 Reduce consumption of saturated fat in the population aged 2 years and older	11.3% of total calorie intake (2003–2006)	9.5%	11% (2007–2010)	National Health and Nutrition Examination Survey (NHANES), CDC, NCHS and USDA, ARS
PA-5 Increase the proportion of adolescents who participate in daily school physical education	33.3% (2009)	36.6%	31.5% (2011)	Youth Risk Behavior Surveillance System (YRBSS), CDC, NCCDPHP
PA-8.2.3 Increase the proportion of adolescents in 9th through 12th grade who view television, videos, or play video games for no more than 2 hours a day Comparable objectives for preschool and school-age children	67.2% (2009)	73.9%	67.6% (2011)	National Health and Nutrition Examination Survey (NHANES)

Continued on next page

Healthy People 2020 (Continued)

OBJECTIVE	BASELINE (YEAR)	TARGET	CURRENT DATA (YEAR)	DATA SOURCE
SA-2.3 Increase the proportion of high school seniors never using substances—Alcoholic beverages	27.7% of high school seniors (2009)	30.5%	NDA	Monitoring the Future Survey (MTF), NIH
SA-2.4 Increase the proportion of high school seniors never using substances—Illicit drugs	53.3% (2009)	58.6%	NDA	Monitoring the Future Survey (MTF), NIH
FP-8.1 Reduce the pregnancy rate among adolescent females aged 15 to 17 years	40.2 pregnancies/ 1,000 females (2005)	36.2 pregnancies/ 1,000	39.5 (2008)	Abortion Provider Survey, Guttmacher Institute; Abortion Surveillance Data, CDC, NCCDPHP; National Vital Statistics System–Natality (NVSS–N), CDC, NCHS; National Survey of Family Growth (NSFG), CDC, NCHS
FP-11.3 Increase the proportion of sexually active females aged 15 to 19 years who use a condom and hormonal or intrauterine contraception at last intercourse	18.3% (2006–2010)	20.1%	NDA	National Survey of Family Growth (NSFG), CDC

NDA = No data available

*Some data are being collected for information purposes only, so no targets have been set.

Data from: U.S. Department of Health and Human Services. (2013). *Topics and objectives index.* Retrieved from http://www.healthypeople.gov/2020/topicsobjectives2020/default.aspx

CHAPTER RECAP

Population health nursing services for children and adolescents are one of the most effective means of enhancing the health of the overall population. Population health nurses can educate the public, parents, and children on health-promoting and illness and injury preventing behaviors and engage in early intervention and health restoration for existing health problems to minimize their effects on the health of individual children and on the population during childhood and adolescence and on into adulthood.

CASE STUDY Protecting Children's Health

You are a population health nurse in a small town on the Arizona-Mexico border. The pediatric nurse practitioner in the local well-child clinic comes to you with concerns about the high blood lead levels he has encountered in a number of school-age children in the community. When you look at past figures for lead poisoning in the area, you find that the incidence has steadily increased until it is about twice that of other nearby communities. The community is bisected by a major interstate highway and new cases of lead poisoning seem to be clustered along the interstate and in a part of town that houses a large population of Hispanic migrants and their families. Epidemiologic investigation indicates that there are high levels of lead in the soil adjacent to the highway and deteriorating lead-based paint in a large portion of the older homes in low-income areas of town. In addition, the investigation finds that several small stores in the Hispanic part of town sell a brand of candy imported from Mexico that has high levels of lead contamination. The candy is inexpensive and very popular with local children.

1. What biological, psychological, environmental, sociocultural, behavioral, and health system factors are contributing to the high incidence of elevated blood lead levels in children in the community?
2. In addition to yourself, who should be involved in planning programs to decrease the incidence of lead poisoning?
3. What evidence-based interventions might the planning group employ to address the problem?
4. What level(s) of health care would be involved in addressing the problems of lead poisoning incidence and prevalence?
5. How might the effectiveness of the interventions be evaluated?

REFERENCES

Advisory Committee on Immunization Practices. (2011a). Recommendations on the use of quadrivalent human papillomavirus vaccine in males. *Morbidity and Mortality Weekly Report, 60,* 1705–1708.

Advisory Committee on Immunization Practices. (2011b). Updated recommendations for use of tetanus toxoid, reduced diphtheria toxoid, and acellular pertussis vaccine (Tdap) in pregnant women and persons who have or anticipate having close contact with an infant aged < 12 months. *Morbidity and Mortality Weekly Report, 60,* 1424–1426.

Al-Gamal, E., & Long, T. (2010). Anticipatory grieving among parents living with a child with cancer. *Journal of Advanced Nursing, 66,* 1980–1990. doi:10.1111/j.1365-2648.2010.05381.x

American Diabetes Association. (2011). *Diabetes statistics.* Retrieved from http://www.diabetes.org/diabetes-basics/diabetes-statistics/?loc=DropDownDB-stats

Amnesty International. (2013). *Convention on the rights of the child.* Retrieved from https://www.amnestyusa.org/our-work/issues/children-s-rights/convention-on-the-rights-of-the-child

Arthritis Foundation. (2014). *Juvenile arthritis fact sheet.* Retrieved from http://www.arthritis.org/ja-fact-sheet.php

Blanton, L., Dhara, R., Brammer, L., Bresee, J., Cox, N., Finelli, L., & Wong, K. K. (2011). Influenza-associated pediatric deaths—United States, September 2010–August 2011. *Morbidity and Mortality Weekly Report, 60,* 1233–1238.

Brand, W., Rasulnia, R., & Urquhart, G. (2011). Progress in immunization information systems—United States, 2009. *Morbidity and Mortality Weekly Report, 60,* 10–12.

Brehaut, J. C., Garner, R. E., Miller, A. R., Lach, L. M., Klassen, A. F., Rosenbaum, P. L., & Kohen, D. E. (2011). Changes over time in the health of caregivers of children with health problems: Growth-curve findings from a 10-year Canadian population-based study. *American Journal of Public Health, 101,* 2308–2316. doi:10.2015/AJPH.2011.300298

Bynum, L., Griffon, T., Ridings, D. L., Wynkoop, K. S., Anda, R. F., Edwards, V. J., & Croft, J. B. (2010). Adverse childhood experiences reported by adults—Five states, 2009. *Morbidity and Mortality Weekly Report, 59,* 1609–1613.

Central Intelligence Agency. (2014). *World fact book.* Retrieved from https://www.cia.gov/library/publications/the-world-factbook/rankorder/2091rank.html

Centers for Disease Control and Prevention. (2011). National child passenger safety week—September 18–24, 2011. *Morbidity and Mortality Weekly Report, 60,* 1252.

Centers for Disease Control and Prevention. (2012). National birth defects prevention month and folic acid awareness week – January 2012. *Morbidity and Mortality Weekly Report, 60,* 1746.

Centers for Disease Control and Prevention. (2013). *Breastfeeding report card – United States, 2013.* Retrieved from http://www.cdc.gov/breastfeeding/pdf/2013breastfeedingreportcard.pdf

Centers for Disease Control and Prevention. (2014). *HIV among pregnant women, infants and children.* Retrieved from http://www.cdc.gov/hiv/risk/gender/pregnantwomen/facts/

Chen, B., Mei, J., Kalman, L., Shahangian, S., Williams, I., Gagnon, M., …, Zehnbauer, R. (2012). Good laboratory practices for biochemical genetic testing and newborn screening for inherited metabolic disorders. *Morbidity and Mortality Weekly Report, 61*(RR2), 1–44.

Chen, J.-Y., & Clark, M. J. (2010). Family resources and parental health in families of children with Duchene muscular dystrophy. *Journal of Nursing Research (Taiwan), 18,* 239–248. doi:10.1097/JNR.0b013e3181fbe37b

Crosby, A. E., Ortega, L., & Stevens, M. R. (2011). Suicides—United States, 1999–2007. *Morbidity and Mortality Weekly Report, 60*(Suppl.), 56–59

Cystic Fibrosis Foundation. (n.d.). *About cystic fibrosis.* Retrieved from http://www.cff.org/AboutCF/

da Silva, R. M., Jacob, E., & Nasciemento, L. C. (2010). Impact of childhood cancer on parents' relationships: An integrative review. *Journal of Nursing Scholarship, 42,* 250–261. doi:10.1111/j.1547-5069.2010.01360.x

de Leeuw, J. R. J., de Bruijin, M., de Weert-van Oene, G. H., & Schrijvers, A. J. P. (2010). Internet and game behavior at a secondary school and a newly developed health promotion programme: A prospective study. *BMC Public Health, 10,* 544. doi:10.1186/1471-2458-10-544

de Oliveira, L. H., Sanwogou, J., Matus-Ruiz, C., Tambini, G., Want, S. A., Agocs, M., … Desai, R. (2011). Progress in the Introduction of Rotavirus Vaccine—Latin American and the Caribbean, 2006-2010. *Morbidity and Mortality Weekly report, 60,* 1611–1614.

DiOrio, M., de Fijter, S., Schwartz, M., Page, S. L., Jhung, M. A., Finelli, L., …, Graitcer, S. (2012). Severe influenza among children and young adults with neurologic and neurodevelopmental conditions—Ohio, 2011. *Morbidity and Mortality Weekly Report, 60,* 1729–1733.

Division of Diabetes Translation. (2011). *National diabetes fact sheet, 2011.* Retrieved from http://www.cdc.gov/diabetes/pubs/pdf/ndfs_2011.pdf

Division of HIV/AIDS prevention. (2011). *HIV among youth.* Retrieved from http://www.cdc.gov/hiv/youth/pdf/youth.pdf

Eaton, D. K., Kann, L., Kinchen, S., Shanklin, S., Flint, K. H., Hawkins, J., ..., Wechsler, H. (2012). Youth risk behavior surveillance—United States, 2012. *Morbidity and Mortality Weekly Report, 61*(SS4), 1 162

Fath, J., Ng, T. W., & Pabst, L. J. (2012). Progress in immunization information systems—United States, 2010. *Morbidity and Mortality Weekly Report, 61*, 464–467.

Federal Interagency Forum on Child and Family Statistics. (2012). *America's children in brief: Key national indicators of well-being, 2012.* Retrieved from http://www.childstats.gov/pdf/ac2012/ac_12.pdf

Federal Interagency Forum on Child and Family Statistics. (2013). *America's children: Key national indicators of well-being, 2013.* Retrieved from http://www.childstats.gov/americaschildren/index.asp

Gilchrist, J., Haileyesus, T., Murphy, M., Comstock, R. D., Collins, C., & McIlvain, N. (2010). Heat illness among high school athletes—United States, 2005–2009. *Morbidity and Mortality Weekly Report, 59*, 1009–1013.

Harrison, A. T., Gavin, L., & Hastings, P. A. (2012). Prepregnancy contraceptive use among teens with unintended pregnancies resulting in live births—Pregnancy risk assessment monitoring system (PRAMS), 2004–2008. *Morbidity and Mortality Weekly Report, 61*, 25–29.

Hewitt-Taylor, J. L. (2008a). *Children with complex and continuing health needs: The experiences of children, families, and care staff.* Philadelphia, PA: Jessica Kingsley.

Hewitt-Taylor, J. L. (2008b). *Providing support at home for children and young people who have complex health needs.* Chichester, UK: John Wiley & Sons.

Institute for Safe Medication Practices. (2010). *DTaP-Tdap mix-ups now affecting hundreds of patients.* Retrieved from http://www.medscape.com/viewarticle/726330?src=mp&spon=24

Jewish Women's Archive. (n.d.a). *History makers—Federal Children's Bureau—Lillian Wald, 1867–1940.* Retrieved from http://www.jwa.org/historymakers/wald/federal-childrens-bureau

Jewish Women's Archive. (n.d.b). *History makers—Lillian Wald—Outdoor Recreation League.* Retrieved from http://www.jwa.org/historymakers/wald/outdoor-recreation-league

Johnson, R. C., & Schoeni, R. F. (2011). Early-life origins of adult disease: National Longitudinal Population-Based Study of the United States. *American Journal of Public Health, 101*, 2317–2324. doi:10.2015/AJPH.2011.300252

Kann, L., Olsen, E. O., McManus, T., Kinchen, S., Chyen, D., Harris, W. A., & Wechsler, H. (2011). Sexual identity, sex of sexual contacts, and health risk behaviors among students in grades 9–12—Youth Risk Behavior Surveillance, selected sites, United States, 2001–2009. *Morbidity and Mortality Weekly Report, 60*(SS1), 1–133

Kann, L., Lowry, R., Eaton, D., & Wechsler, H. (2012). Trends in HIV-related risk behaviors among high school students—United States, 1991–2011. *Morbidity and Mortality Weekly Report, 61*, 556–560.

Krieger, M., Sargent, K., Arons, A., Standish, M., & Brindis, C. D. (2011). Creating an environmental justice framework for policy change in childhood asthma: A grassroots to treetops approach. *American Journal of Public Health, 101*(Suppl. 1), S208–S216. doi:10.2015/AJPH.2011.300188

Lino, C., Mirchandani, G. G., Castrucci, B. C., Chavez, N., Handler, A., & Hoeslscher, D. M. (2012). The effect of acculturation on healthy lifestyle characteristics among Hispanic fourth-grade children in Texas public schools, 2004–2005. *Journal of School Health, 82*, 166–174. doi: 10.1111/j.1746-1561.2011.00682.x

Macartney, S. (2011). *Child poverty in the United States 2009 and 2010: Selected race groups and Hispanic origin—American Community Survey briefs.* Retrieved from http://www.census.gov/prod/2011pubs/acsbr10-05.pdf

MacDorman, M. F., & Mathews, T. J. (2011). Infant deaths—United States, 2000–2007. *Morbidity and Mortality Weekly Report, 60*(Suppl.), 49–51.

Marchetta, C. M., Denny, C. H., Floyd, R. L., Cjeal, N. E., Sniezek, J. E., & McKnight- Eily, L. R. (2012). Alcohol use and binge drinking among women of childbearing age—United States, 2006–2010. *Morbidity and Mortality Weekly Report, 61*, 534–538.

Maternal and Child Health Bureau. (n.d.). *Division of Services for Children with Special Health Needs (DSCSHN) fact sheet.* Retrieved from http://mchb.hrsa.gov/about/factsheets/dschcnfacts.PDF

McKenna, M., Mullen, J., & Hertz, M. (2011). Bullying among middle school and high school students—Massachusetts, 2009. *Morbidity and Mortality Weekly Report, 60*, 465–471.

Merikangas, K. R., He, J., Burstein, M., Swanson, S. A., Avenevoli, S., Cui, L., ..., Swendsen. J. (2010). Lifetime prevalence of mental disorders in U.S. adolescents: Results from the National Comorbidity Study-Adolescent Supplement (NCS-A). *Journal of the American Academy of Child and Adolescent Psychiatry, 49*, 980–989. doi:10.1016/j.jaac.2010.05.017

Murphy, S. L., Xu, J., & Kochanek, K. D. (2013). Deaths: Final data for 2010. *National Vital Statistics Reports, 61*(4), 1–118.

National Center for Environmental Health. (2012). *Lead.* Retrieved from http://www.cdc.gov/nceh/lead/

National Center for Environmental Health. (2014). *Number of children tested and confirmed EBLLs by state, year, and BLL Group, Children < 72 months old.* Retrieved from http://www.cdc.gov/nceh/lead/data/StateConfirmedByYear1997-2012.htm

National Center for Health Statistics. (2011a). Percentage of children with serious emotional or behavioral difficulties, by age group and family income group—National Health Interview Survey, United States, 2004–2009. *Morbidity and Mortality Weekly Report, 60*, 555.

National Center for Health Statistics. (2011b). Percentage of teens aged 15–19 years who had opposite-sex sexual partners in the past 12 months, by number of partners—United States, 2006–2010. *Morbidity and Mortality Weekly Report, 60*, 1460.

National Center for Health Statistics. (2011c). Term infant mortality rates, by race/ethnicity—United States. *Morbidity and Mortality Weekly Report, 69*, 1396.

National Center for Health Statistics. (2013). *Health, United States, 2012: With special feature on emergency care.* Retrieved from http://www.cdc.gov/nchs/data/hus/hus12.pdf

National Center for Injury Prevention and Control. (2012a). *Playground injuries: Fact sheet.* Retrieved from http://www.cdc.gov/HomeandRecreationalSafety/Playground-Injuries/playgroundinjuries-factsheet.htm

National Center for Injury Prevention and Control. (2012b). *Protect the ones you love.* Retrieved from http://www.cdc.gov/safechild/poisoning/index.html

National Center for Injury Prevention and Control. (2012c). *Understanding teen dating violence: Fact sheet.* Retrieved from http://www.cdc.gov/ViolencePrevention/pdf/TeenDatingViolence2012-a.pdf

National Center for Injury Prevention and Control. (2014a). *Child maltreatment: Definitions.* Retrieved from http://www.cdc.gov/ViolencePrevention/childmaltreatment/definitions.html

National Center for Injury Prevention and Control. (2014b). *Child maltreatment prevention.* Retrieved from http://www.cdc.gov/ViolencePrevention/childmaltreatment/index.html

National Center for Injury Prevention and Control. (2014b). *Child maltreatment: Prevention strategies.* Retrieved from http://www.cdc.gov/ViolencePrevention/childmaltreatment/prevention.html

National Center for Injury Prevention and Control. (2014d). *Child maltreatment: Risk and protective factors.* Retrieved from http://www.cdc.gov/ViolencePrevention/childmaltreatment/riskprotectivefactors.html

National Center for Injury Prevention and Control. (2014e). *Child passenger safety: Fact sheet.* Retrieved from http://www.cdc.gov/MotorVehicleSafety/Child_Passenger_Safety/CPS-Factsheet.html

National Center for Injury Prevention and Control. (2014f). *Teen dating violence.* Retrieved from http://www.cdc.gov/violenceprevention/intimatepartnerviolence/teen_dating_violence.html

National Center for Injury Prevention and Control. (2014g). *Unintentional drowning: Get the facts.* Retrieved from http://www.cdc.gov/HomeandRecreationalSafety/Water-Safety/waterinjuries-factsheet.html

National Center for Injury Prevention and Control. (2014h). *Violence prevention: Data & statistics.* Retrieved from http://www.cdc.gov/ViolencePrevention/data_stats/index.html

National Center on Birth Defects and Developmental Disabilities. (2013a). *Attention deficit hyperactivity disorder (ADHD): Recommendations from the American Academy of Pediatrics.* Retrieved from http://www.cdc.gov/ncbddd/adhd/guidelines.html

National Center on Birth Defects and Developmental Disabilities. (2013b). *Birth defects: Down syndrome.* Retrieved from http://www.cdc.gov/ncbddd/birthdefects/DownSyndrome.html

National Center on Birth Defects and Developmental Disabilities. (2013c). *Facts about cerebral palsy.* Retrieved from http://www.cdc.gov/ncbddd/cp/facts.html

National Center on Birth Defects and Developmental Disabilities. (2014a). *Attention deficit hyperactivity disorder (ADHD): Data & statistics.* Retrieved from http://www.cdc.gov/ncbddd/fasd/data.html

National Center on Birth Defects and Developmental Disabilities. (2014b). *Autism spectrum disorders: Data & statistics.* Retrieved from http://www.cdc.gov/ncbddd/autism/data.html

National Center on Birth Defects and Developmental Disabilities. (2014c). *Autism spectrum disorders: Facts about ASDs.* Retrieved from http://www.cdc.gov/NCBDDD/autism/facts.html

National Center on Birth Defects and Developmental Disabilities. (2014d). *Fetal alcohol spectrum disorders: Data & Statistics.* Retrieved from http://www.cdc.gov/ncbddd/fasd/data.html

National Conference of State Legislatures. (2013). *Fetal homicide laws.* Retrieved from http://www.ncsl.org/research/health/fetal-homicide-state-laws.aspx

National Institute of Mental Health. (2012). *Attention deficit hyperactivity disorder (ADHD).* Retrieved from http://www.nimh.nih.gov/health/publications/attention-deficit-hyperactivity-disorder/adhd_booklet.pdf

National Program for Playground Safety. (2014a). *Assessment kits.* Retrieved from http://www.playgroundsafety.org/products/assessment-kits

National Program for Playground Safety. (2014b). *S.A.F.E.* Retrieved from http://www.playgroundsafety.org/safe

O'Donohue, W., & Tolle, L. W. (2011). Introduction—Adolescents with chronic illnesses: Issues and answers. In W. T. O'Donohue & L. W. Tolle (Eds.), *Behavioral approaches to chronic disease in adolescents: A guide to integrative care* (pp. 3–14). New York, NY: Springer.

Office of Statistics and Programming, National Center for Injury Prevention and Control. (2013). *10 leading causes of death by age group, United States, 2010.* Retrieved from http://www.cdc.gov/injury/wisqars/pdf/10LCID_All_Deaths_By_Age_Group_2010-a.pdf

Ogden, C. L., Carroll, D., Kit, B. K., & Flegal, K. M. (2012). Prevalence in obesity and trends in body mass index among US children and adolescents, 2009–2010. *Journal of the American Medical Association, 305,* 483–490. doi:10.1001/jama.2012.40

Russell, S. T., Sinclair, K. O., Poteat, V. P., & Koenig, B. W. (2012). Adolescent health and harassment based on discriminatory bias. *American Journal of Public Health, 102,* 493–495. doi:10.2015/AJPH.2011.300430

Shafer, P. O. (2014). *About epilepsy - The basics.* Retrieved from http://www.epilepsy.com/learn/about-epilepsy-basics

Stockwell, M. S., Kharbanda, E. O., Martinez, R. A., Lara, M., Vawdrey, D., Natarajan, K., & Rickert, V. I. (2012). Text4Health: Impact of a text message reminder-recalls for pediatric and adolescent immunizations. *American Journal of Public Health, 102,* e15–e21. doi:10.2105/AJPH.2011.300331

Stokley, S., Stanwyck, C., Avey, B., & Greby, S. (2011). Vaccination coverage among children in kindergarten—United States, 2009–10 school year. *Morbidity and Mortality Weekly Report, 60,* 700–704.

Strickland, B. B., Van Dyck, P. C., Kogan, M. D., Lauver, C., Blumberg, S. J., Bethell, C. D., & Newacheck, P. W. (2011). Assessing and ensuring a comprehensive system of services for children with special health care needs: A public health approach. *American Journal of Public Health, 101,* 224–231. doi:10.2105/AJPH.2009.177915

Triple P: Positive Parenting Program. (n.d.). *Triple P in a nutshell.* Retrieved from http://www.triplep.net/glo-en/find-out-about-triple-p/triple-p-in-a-nutshell/

UNICEF. (2013). *Statistics by area / HIV/AIDS.* Retrieved from http://www.childinfo.org/hiv_aids.html

U.S. Cancer Statistics Working Group. (2013). *United States Cancer Statistics: 1999–2008 incidence and mortality web-based report.* Retrieved from http://apps.nccd.cdc.gov/uscs/childhoodcancerbyprimarysite.aspx

U.S. Census Bureau. (2013). *The 2012 statistical abstract of the United States.* Retrieved from http://factfinder2.census.gov/faces/tableservices/jsf/pages/productview.xhtml?src=bkmk

U.S. Department of Health and Human Services. (2013). *Topics and objectives index.* Retrieved from http://www.healthypeople.gov/2020/topicsobjectives2020/default.aspx

U.S. Department of Housing and Urban Development. (2008). *Healthy housing inspection manual.* Retrieved from http://www.cdc.gov/nceh/publications/books/inspectionmanual/Healthy_Housing_Inspection_Manual.pdf

U.S. Preventive Services Task Force. (2010). *The guide to clinical preventive services 2010–2011.* Retrieved from http://www.ahrq.gov/clinic/pocketgd.htm

Vallone, D. M., Duke, J. C., Cullen, J., McCausland, K. L., & Allen, J. A. (2011). Evaluation of EX: A national mass media smoking cessation campaign. *American Journal of Public Health, 101,* 302–309. doi:10.2105/AJPH.2009.190454

Visser, S. N., Bitsko, R. H., Danielson, M. L., Perou, R., & Blumberg, S. J. (2010). Increasing prevalence of parent-reported attention-deficit/hyperactivity disorder among children—United States, 2003 and 2007. *Morbidity and Mortality Weekly Report, 59,* 1439–1443.

Warner, D. E., & Hauser, S. T. (2011). Unique considerations when treating adolescents with chronic illness. In W. T. O'Donohue & L. W. Tolle (Eds.), *Behavioral approaches to chronic disease in adolescents: A guide to integrative care* (pp. 3–14). New York, NY: Springer.

Wellmark Blue Cross Blue Shield of Iowa & Wellmark Blue Cross Blue Shield of South Dakota. (2013). *Pediatric screening and prevention guideline.* Retrieved from http://www.wellmark.com/HealthAndWellness/WellnessResources/docs/PediatricPreventiveHealthGuidelines.pdf

Wells, N. M., Evans, G. W., Beavis, A., & Ong, A. D. (2010). Early childhood poverty, cumulative risk exposure, and body mass index trajectories through young adulthood. *American Journal of Public Health, 100,* 2507–2512. doi:10.2015/AJPH.2009.184291

Wooten, K. G., Kolasa, M., Singleton, J. A., & Shefer, A. (2010). National, state, and local area vaccination coverage among children aged 19–35 months—United States, 2009. *Morbidity and Mortality Weekly Report, 59,* 1171–1177.

World Health Organization. (2014). *Palliative care.* Retrieved from http://www.who.int/cancer/palliative/en/

World Health Organization, United Nations Children's Fund, & Global Immunization Division, Center for Global Health. (2011). Global routine vaccination coverage, 2010. *Morbidity and Mortality Weekly Report, 60,* 1520–1522.

Young, M., Watts, R., & Wilson, S. (2010). The effectiveness of educational strategies in improving parental/caregiver management of fever in their child: A systematic review. *JBI Library of Systematic Reviews, 8,* 826–868. JBL000399.

Ziotnick, C., Tam, T. W., & Soman, L. A. (2012). Life course outcomes on mental and physical health: The impact of foster care on adulthood. *American Journal of Public Health, 103,* 534–540. doi:10.2015/AJPH.2011.300285

CHAPTER

17 Care of Men

Learning Outcomes

After reading this chapter, you should be able to:

1. Describe major considerations in assessing biophysical, psychological, environmental, sociocultural, behavioral, and health care system determinants affecting men's health.
2. Identify major considerations in health promotion and illness/injury prevention for men and analyze the role of the population health nurse with respect to each.
3. Describe areas of focus in resolving existing health problems among men and related population health nursing roles.
4. Describe considerations in restorative health care for men and analyze the role of the population health nurse in each.

Key Terms

erectile dysfunction (ED)
infertility
joblessness
masculinity
reframing
unemployment

Advocacy Then and Now

Advocating for Men's Health and Men in Nursing

Nurses themselves often need advocacy to be assured fair treatment. This has been no less true for male nurses than for females. Although early nursing outside of the family was primarily a masculine endeavor carried out by male religious orders, nursing in the 19th and 20th centuries became a largely feminine profession. Men were frequently denied admission to schools of nursing and were not eligible to become members of the Army Nurse Corps until 1955 and the Navy Nurse Corps until 1965 (Tranbarger, 2007).

Recognizing the need for advocacy for the rights of male nurses, Steve Miller, a nurse, established a "Men in Nursing in Michigan" organization in 1971. After some initial setbacks, the organization was reorganized in 1974 as the Male Nurses Association and became the American Assembly for Men in Nursing (AAMN) in 1981. The initial aim of the assembly was to recruit men to the nursing profession, but this focus was later expanded to provide networking and mentorship opportunities and address issues that concerned men in nursing. The organization also promotes research and education regarding men's health issues (Tranbarger, 2007).

Today, AAMN is a national organization with myriad local chapters (AAMN, 2011). Recent activities include promotion of gender-neutral language in nursing education (AAMN Board of Directors, 2010) and a position statement on the development of a men's health curriculum in schools of nursing to address the health needs of the male population (AAMN, 2010).

What does it mean to be a man? Relevant literature distinguishes between being male and masculinity. Maleness is perceived as a biological phenomenon, while **masculinity** is a personal and social construct that varies within individuals and across cultural groups (Synnott, 2009). Some authors propose five different conceptualizations or models of gender as depicted in Table 17-1●.

According to 2010 census data (U.S. Census Bureau, 2012a), men over 20 years of age constituted 48% of the U.S. adult population. This amounted to nearly 109.2 million men. By 2015, men over age 18 are expected to comprise 48.7% of the adult population (U.S. Census Bureau, 2012b). The worldwide male population amounts to 3.3 billion (Synnott, 2009). Although health care services have traditionally been designed around men's health care needs, U.S. men encounter a number of health disparities when compared to women. Failure to attend to men's health as a population group is attested to by the fact that only in the two most recent sets of national health objectives, have issues unique to men's health, such as prostate cancer mortality, been addressed (U.S. Department of Health and Human Services [USDHHS], 2013), whereas uniquely female health problems (e.g., maternal and cervical cancer mortality) have been addressed in multiple sets of objectives.

TABLE 17-1 Models of Gender Conceptualization

Model	Characteristic Features
Romantic	Men and women are different but complementary and equal opposites, united by mutual interdependence
Patriarchal	Men are superior to women and dominate women. Males sacrifice themselves to protect women and women are privileged in some ways (e.g., not being subject to military service).
Misandric	Women are superior to men. Men are viewed as villains, and women, as a group, are engaged in a war against men.
Postmodern	Gender is a continuum rather than a dichotomy. Humans are biologically and psychologically bisexual, and there are multiple fluid sexualities. Gender roles are cultural rather than biological and are based on behavioral performance (e.g., how one dresses or one's mannerisms). There are greater differences within traditional male/female genders than between them.
Multiple conflict/ identity	Gender relations are predicated on power. Men and women are not the same, nor are they opposite. They are not usually equal in all respects; nor is one gender always powerful and the other powerless. Gender differences are interwoven with power differences in other societal aspects including class, race, religion, ethnicity, language, and political affiliation.

Data from: Synnott, A. (2009). *Rethinking men: Heroes, villains, and victims.* Burlington, VT: Ashgate.

Men differ from women in their patterns of physical health disorders and health-related needs. These differences are attributable to (a) physiologic differences between men and women, (b) differences in health-related habits and health-seeking behavior, and (c) differences in social roles, stress, and coping. A great deal of health-related literature has been written about specific problems that influence men's health status (e.g., cardiovascular disease, lung cancer, etc.). Very little, however, is written about the overall health needs of men. The health care of men has been fragmented, approached from an episodic perspective, and little effort has been made to provide comprehensive, holistic health services.

Evidence of health disparities between men and women is seen in differences in life expectancy, mortality, and rates of illness and injury. Men die younger than women and overall have higher incidences of most chronic diseases than women. Average life expectancy for U.S. men at birth in 2010 was 76 years compared to 81 years for women, and the all-cause mortality rate for males of all ages was 887.1 per 100,000 population versus 634.9 per 100,000 women. Years of productive life lost due to death before age 75 came to 8,735 for men and only 5,195 for women (National Center for Health Statistics [NCHS], 2013). Life expectancy for men is less than for women in all regions of the world, and men are more likely than women to die between ages 15 and 60 years (World Health Organization, 2013).

These differences do not seem to be solely a product of differences in gender socialization or roles. Some authors have suggested that the universal disparity in longevity between men and women may be the result of innate biological differences. For example, it is known that female hormones have a protective effect with respect to cardiovascular disease. This and other biological differences may play a significant role in differences in longevity between men and women.

Chronic disease incidence also tends to be higher among men than women. For example, 2008 cancer incidence was higher for men than women for all sites except reproductive cancers. Likewise, diabetes incidence is higher for men than women (Beckles, Zhu, & Moonsinghe, 2011). In addition, diabetes is less likely to be controlled among men than women (NCHS, 2013). Similar differences in the incidence and degree of control of hypertension are noted between men and women (Keenan & Rosendorf, 2011). HIV infection rates for men are three times those for women and climbing, whereas infection rates for women have declined slightly since 2005 (Hall, Hughes, Dean, Mermin, & Fenton, 2011).

Men are also more likely than women to be victims of war, crime, homicide, suicide, and accidental injury and death, particularly in occupational settings (Synnott, 2009). For example, in 2007 motor vehicle accident mortality was higher among men than women for all racial and ethnic groups (West & Naumann, 2011). In addition, suicide rates are nearly four times higher for men than for women (NCHS, 2013).

Three explanatory paradigms have been advanced to explain these disparities. These include personal behaviors, cultural factors, and health system factors (Synnott, 2009). Personal behaviors include elements of risk taking as well as lack of personal health care activities. Cultural factors include gender socialization, occupational exposures to hazardous conditions, and so on, and health system factors include the lack of attention to men's health issues presented above as well as lack of access to health care services. Factors related to each of these three paradigms are addressed below in terms of behavioral, sociocultural, and health systems determinants of health, respectively.

Population Health Nursing and Care of Men

Population health nursing activities in care of the male population involve use of the nursing process at both the individual and population levels. Assessment of men's health status addresses each of the categories of determinants of health to identify factors contributing to health and illness among men. Planning and implementation of interventions geared toward health promotion and illness/injury prevention, resolution of existing health problems, and restoration of health are also part of the population health nurse's role with respect to men. Finally, population health nurses evaluate the effects of care on men's health status at individual and population levels.

Assessing the Health Status of Men

Factors related to each of the six categories of determinants of health affect men's health status. We will briefly consider major factors related to biological, psychological, environmental, sociocultural, behavioral, and health system determinants and their influence on the health of the male population. Assessment of the male population can be conducted using the *Population Health Assessment and Intervention Guide* included in the *Assessment Guidelines* for Chapter 15∞. A tool to assess the health of an individual male client is included in the *Assessment Guidelines* section of the student resources site.

BIOLOGICAL DETERMINANTS. Considerations in assessing biological determinants of men's health are presented in the focused assessment on the next page. Areas to be addressed include the demographics of the population, as well as morbidity and mortality related to physical health conditions, and levels of immunity. Much of this information is available from data collected by official health agencies and health care facilities and providers in the area. Local emergency departments may be able to provide statistics on accidental injuries among men. Similarly, local police departments may have data on accident-related calls and the injuries suffered. For other conditions, such as erectile dysfunction, extent of disability, and immunization levels among men, there are often no statistical data available, and information may be best obtained by means of community surveys.

Men experience a variety of physical health conditions, many of which can be prevented or their effects ameliorated

FOCUSED ASSESSMENT Assessing Biological Determinants of Men's Health

- What is the age composition of the male population?
- What is the racial/ethnic composition of the male population?
- What are the main causes of mortality in the male population?
- What acute and chronic illnesses are prevalent in the male population? What factors contribute to the prevalence of these conditions?
- What is the prevalence of sexual dysfunction in the male population?
- What is the level of immunity to specific communicable diseases among the male population?

by effective population health nursing intervention. Table 17-2● provides a comparison of male and female mortality for selected causes of death in the United States in 2008. As indicated in the table, only for Alzheimer's disease, are female mortality rates higher than those for males, with the greatest differences in suicide and homicide mortality.

Men also experience higher levels of morbidity for many health problems than do women (Table 17-3●). For example, men tend to develop coronary heart disease (CHD) 10 to 15 years earlier than women and account for 70% of premature mortality (before age 65) from CHD. In addition to being more likely than women to be overweight or obese, men tend to have more abdominal obesity that is associated with coronary heart disease (Salzman & Wender, 2006). Generally, men are likely to report less difficulty seeing with corrective lenses but have greater difficulty hearing with advancing age and are slightly less likely than women to report themselves as in poor health (NCHS, 2012a).

Men also have higher rates of sexually transmitted diseases (STDs) than women. For example, the incidence of HIV infection in men is more than three times that in women. Men also experience other reproductive conditions, such as breast cancer (although at a much lower rate than women) and prostate cancer. Prostate cancer is the most common cancer diagnosis in men. In 2009, 206,640 men in the United States were diagnosed with prostate cancer, and 28,088 U.S. men died from prostate cancer. The overall incidence rate was 137.7 per 100,000 men (U.S. Cancer Statistics Working Group, 2013). One in every six men will develop prostate cancer in his lifetime. Prostate cancer may result in feelings of inadequacy that lead to changes in relationships, feelings of lost manhood, and changes in sexual feelings, as well as to erectile dysfunction. Although prostate cancer is frequently not life threatening, its implications for men's quality of life cannot be underestimated. Prostate cancer and benign prostatic hyperplasia or hypertrophy (BPH) may both obstruct urinary flow, resulting in reduced urinary flow, increasing frequency, and nocturia. Approximately half of men over 60 years of age experience BPH (Deters & Kim, 2011).

TABLE 17-2 Male and Female Mortality from Selected Causes, United States, 2008 (per 100,000 population)

Cause of Mortality	Men	Women	Ratio Men to Women
Overall	900.6	643.4	1.4 to 1
Heart disease	232	150.4	1.5 to 1
Malignant neoplasms	213	148.5	1.4 to 1
Unintentional injury	53.6	25.1	2.1 to 1
Chronic lower respiratory disease	51.4	39.1	1.3 to 1
Cerebrovascular disease	40.9	39.9	1.02 to 1
Diabetes mellitus	25.6	18.8	1.4 to 1
Alzheimer's disease	20.1	26.7	0.75 to 1
Suicide	18.9	4.8	3.9 to 1
Chronic liver disease and cirrhosis	12.7	6.0	2.1 to 1
Homicide	9.3	2.4	3.9 to 1
HIV disease	4.8	1.9	2.5 to 1

Data from: National Center for Health Statistics. (2012a). *Health, United States, 2011: With special feature on socioeconomic status and health.* Retrieved from http://www.cdc.gov/nchs/data/hus/hus11.pdf

TABLE 17-3 Male and Female Morbidity from Selected Causes, United States

Cause of Morbidity	Men	Women	Ratio Men to Women
HIV infection (per 100,000)	35.9	11.5	3.1 to 1
Hypertension	30.6%	28.7%	—
Diabetes mellitus (per 100,000)	8.1	7.7	1.05 to 1
Colorectal cancer (per 100,000)	49.2	37.1	1.3 to 1
Prostate cancer (per 100,000)	137.7	—	—
Lung cancer (per 100,000)	78.2	54.1	1.4 to 1
Malignant melanoma	24.7	15.8	1.6 to 1
Pancreatic cancer (per 100,000)	13.5	10.3	1.3 to 1
Asthma (current)	6.2%	10%	—
Arthritis (per 100,000)	4.1	9.8	0.42 to 1
Basic activity limitation	53.8%	63.6%	—
Elevated blood cholesterol	32.5%	31%	—
Overweight	43%	27%	—
Obesity	27%	23%	—
Injury (per 100,000)	10,285	8,622	1.19 to 1

Data from: Beckles, G. L., Zhu, J., & Moonsinghe, R. (2011, January 14). Diabetes—United States, 2004 and 2008. *Morbidity and Mortality Weekly Report, 60*(Suppl), 90–93; Centers for Disease Control and Prevention. (2012a). *Arthritis.* Retrieved from http://www.cdc.gov/arthritis/basics/rheumatoid.htm#5; Centers for Disease Control and Prevention. (2012b). *Cholesterol facts.* Retrieved from http://www.cdc.gov/cholesterol/facts.htm; Centers for Disease Control and Prevention. (2013). *Cancer among men.* Retrieved from http://www.cdc.gov/cancer/dcpc/data/men.htm; Hall, H. I., Hughes, D., Dean, H. D., Mermin, J. H., & Fenton, K. A. (2011, January 14). HIV infection—United States, 2005 and 2008. *Morbidity and Mortality Weekly Report, 60*(Suppl), 87–89; Keenan, N. L., & Rosendorf, K. A. (2011, January 14). Prevalence of hypertension and controlled hypertension—United States, 2005–2008. *Morbidity and Mortality Weekly Report, 60*(Suppl), 94–97; National Center for Health Statistics. (2012a). Percentage of men aged 25–64 years with activity limitation, by age group and veteran status—United States, National Health Interview Survey (NHIS), 2007–2010. *Morbidity and Mortality Weekly Report, 61,* 845; National Center for Health Statistics. (2012b). *Vital and health statistics: Summary health statistics for U.S. adults: National Health Interview Survey, 2011.* Retrieved from http://www.cdc.gov/nchs/data/series/sr_10/sr10_256.pdf; National Center for Injury Prevention and Control. (2013). *Unintentional all injury causes nonfatal injuries and rates per 100,000.* Retrieved from http://webappa.cdc.gov/sasweb/ncipc/nfirates2001.html; Salzman, B. E., & Wender, R., C. (2006). Male sex: A major health disparity. In C. A. Haines & R. C. Wender (Eds.), *Primary care: Clinics in office practice: Men's health, 33,* 1–16. doi: 10.1016/j.pop.2005.11.014

Erectile dysfunction is another reproductive problem common among men. **Erectile dysfunction (ED)**, formerly called impotence, occurs when a man cannot achieve or maintain an erection sufficient for satisfactory sexual activity. ED may result in total or periodic inability to achieve an erection or the inability to sustain an erection. As many as 30 million U.S. men may be affected, and the incidence of ED increases with age. ED may occur as a result of diabetes, atherosclerosis, hypertension, obesity, or nerve damage or as a side effect of many medications or surgery (e.g., following prostatectomy). ED may also be associated with lifestyle factors, such as smoking and alcohol consumption, or with stress and fear of sexual failure. Occasionally, ED is the result of low testosterone levels. In addition to its psychological effects on men's health, ED may also signal undiagnosed chronic conditions and should not be ignored. Unfortunately, many men are reluctant to admit to erectile dysfunction and may not seek help (National Kidney and Urologic Diseases Information Clearinghouse, 2012).

Infertility also poses significant threats to men's self-image. **Infertility** is the inability to become pregnant or to impregnate one's female partner after at least a year of intercourse without using contraceptives. In approximately one third of couples unable to get pregnant, the difficulty lies with the male partner (American Academy of Family Physicians, 2014). Possible causes of infertility include prior surgeries, pelvic trauma, sexually transmitted disease, genetic causes such as Klinefelter's syndrome, medication use, and toxic exposures.

Another area to be addressed in assessing men's physiologic function is the presence of long-term consequences of accidental injury. Males at all ages have higher rates of unintentional injuries than females. In 2012, for example, U.S. men over 20 years of age sustained more than 10.6 million unintentional injuries for an incidence rate of 10,285 injuries per 100,000 men, compared to only 13.7 million injuries in women (8,622 per 100,000). Male–female differences are particularly evident with respect to unintentional firearms injuries (9.5 per 100,000 men versus 1.41 per 100,000 for women) and injuries resulting from assault (672.71 and 449.75 per 100,000 population for men and women, respectively) (National Center for Injury Prevention and Control, 2013). As we will see later in this chapter, many of these differences arise from risk behaviors engaged in by men. Other factors that may contribute to accidental injuries and should be assessed by the population health nurse are sensory impairments. These impairments, if undetected and uncorrected, may contribute to a variety of physical and psychological health problems.

The last aspect of physiologic function to be considered in assessing the health status of men is immunization levels. Men, as well as women, should be immunized against tetanus, diphtheria, and pertussis (Tdap), influenza, and pneumococcal disease, and susceptible men should also receive varicella vaccine. Although men may be more likely than women to have received tetanus vaccines in the last 10 years, they are less likely to have received influenza vaccine in the past year or to ever have received pneumococcal vaccine. *Healthy People 2020* objectives have not been achieved for either men or women, however. For example, in 2011–2012, only 35% of men and 43% of women aged 18 years of age and older had received influenza vaccine, far below the 2020 target of 70%. Similarly, only 15% of men and 18% of women had received pneumococcal vaccination targeted at 60% of the population (USDHHS, 2014a).

PSYCHOLOGICAL DETERMINANTS. Several psychological determinants are of concern to population health nurses caring for men. These elements include socialization, stress, and coping abilities, as well as suicide as an outcome of ineffective coping. Other considerations related to psychological determinants of health include the incidence and prevalence of mental illness in the population. The *Focused Assessment* below provides questions that can be used to assess this aspect of men's health. Information to address some of the questions may be available from official health agencies and mental health providers in the area, but much of it may need to be solicited from members of the population through surveys and other data collection methods.

Men, like women, have several basic psychological needs. These include the needs to know and be known to others, to be mutually interdependent, to love and be loved, and to live meaningful lives. Society, however, has socialized both men and women to accept a stereotypical male role that makes it difficult to meet these needs. General dimensions of this stereotyped role include a need to actively differentiate oneself from women and refrain from behaviors ascribed to women (such as demonstrating affection or seeking help) and a need to see oneself as superior to others. Other dimensions include the need to be strong and self-reliant and to be more powerful than others, even if this means resorting to violence to demonstrate one's power.

Because of this stereotyped view of the masculine role, men experience social pressures to conform that sometimes conflict with health. Socialized to view the male role as strong or invulnerable, a man may have difficulty admitting health-related frailties to a population health nurse or seeking health care. Similarly, men who believe that taking physical risks is fundamental to their masculinity may experience more frequent health impairment from trauma. Pressure to assert one's manliness also contributes to early initiation of sexual activity by young men, putting them at risk for STDs and unintended fatherhood. As can be seen in these examples, when societal messages about male roles are internalized by men, they become psychological factors influencing health-related behaviors.

Men may also have a stronger psychological need than women to see themselves as healthy and even invulnerable. Because men tend to value strength and endurance more than women, they are more likely to conceal or suppress pain and other perceived indicators of frailty. An example of this state of mind can be seen in the male post–myocardial infarction client who resumes shoveling snow against the recommendations of health care professionals and his family, and who continues the activity despite the return of the now-familiar angina. As a result of this need for strength in his self-image, the male client minimizes the importance of the problem. Consequently, when shoveling snow causes further angina, he may seek health care less readily and use it less effectively than would a female client in a similar situation.

Similar responses may occur with mental health problems. Traditional American culture prohibits men from expressing emotions other than anger and aggression, and men may be unable to express grief, sadness, or powerlessness, allowing these emotions to fester and contributing to depression. Based on data from the National Center for Health Statistics (NCHS, 2013) for 2010–2011, men less frequently reported serious psychological distress in the prior 30 days than women (2.8% and 3.7%, respectively).

Postpartum depression is a mental health concern that is not often acknowledged with respect to men. Postpartum depression is normally associated with women. Research suggests, however, that 24% to 50% of men whose wives experience postpartum depression may experience it themselves.

FOCUSED ASSESSMENT Assessing Psychological Determinants of Men's Health

- What are the primary sources of stress to which men in the population are exposed?
- What are the incidence and prevalence of mental illness in the male population? What specific mental health problems are prevalent in the population?
- How are mental health problems viewed by men in the population? Are there cultural differences in how mental illness is viewed?
- What is the extent of postpartum depression among men in families with young infants?
- What is the rate of suicide in the male population?
- How are men socialized in the population? Does socialization contribute to health problems among men? How does male socialization affect coping abilities?

Overall, 10% of new fathers may experience this condition. Postpartum depression in men may arise from worsening symptoms in their wives or changes in the marital relationship and may be compounded by economic concerns or substance abuse. Depression in new fathers affects father–infant interaction, and infants with two depressed parents are at high-risk for poor development. Again, male socialization may influence men's willingness to seek help, and many men may have difficulty identifying sources of professional and social support that are often available only to women (Letourneau, Duffett-Leger, Dennis, Stewart, & Tryphonopoulos, 2010). Population health nurses dealing with families with a new infant should be alert to the potential for postpartum depression in fathers as well as mothers.

Male values of strength and endurance do not always adversely affect a male client's health. Some men who value strength actually may be more motivated to exercise and maintain a higher level of general fitness and to seek preventive health care to preserve their sense of themselves as strong and invulnerable. For example, men are slightly less likely than women to be physically inactive (NCHS, 2012b).

Another psychological barrier to men's health is the male client's conflicting response to feelings regarding a health problem. For example, a man who values strength may exercise regularly, but he may avoid having a swelling in his groin examined because he cannot cope effectively with the fear that the swelling may represent a threat to his sexuality.

Men and women are exposed to different types of stress and cope with stress in different ways. For example, men may be more likely than women to engage in avoidant coping strategies. Similarly, post-traumatic stress disorder (PTSD) arises from different types of events and manifests differently in men and women. Although previously thought a condition primarily affecting men, more women actually experience PTSD than men (National Institute of Mental Health [NIMH], 2009). PTSD will be addressed in more detail in Chapter 28∞, but the population health nurse should be alert to its potential appearance among individual men clients and its incidence in the male population. PTSD and other mental health problems may contribute to suicide. As we saw in Table 17-2, suicide incidence is nearly four times higher in men than in women. Suicide claims more lives among men annually than many of the diseases that health care professionals combat so effectively. Because suicide is such a frequent cause of mortality for men, it is important that population health nurses assess individual men and the male population for the presence of suicide risk factors, including bereavement, social isolation, unemployment, depression or other psychiatric disorders, substance abuse, risk-taking or avoidance behaviors, and reluctance to seek help. Protective factors against suicide include social and peer support and a stable domestic situation (Centre for Suicide Prevention, 2011).

ENVIRONMENTAL DETERMINANTS. With the exception of the occupational environment, which is addressed in the discussion of sociocultural factors, the effects of the physical environment on men's health are much the same as they are on women's health; pollution, overcrowding, and safety hazards adversely affect both. Men, however, may have increased exposure to environmental hazards due to occupational and leisure activity choices. In addition, there is some evidence that climate may have differential effects on mortality among men and women. For example, some research has indicated that differences in gender mortality rates are greater at extreme latitudes, suggesting that men may be more adversely affected by climate extremes than women (Salzman & Wender, 2006).

One's living environment also influences health status. In 2009, nearly 5% of male householders lived in inadequate housing units (those with plumbing, heating, electrical, and upkeep deficiencies), only slightly less than women at 5.5%. In addition, 22.5% of male householders lived in unhealthy housing with rodents, leaks, peeling paint, and lack of smoke detectors in addition to the criteria of inadequate housing noted above (Raymond, Wheeler, & Brown, 2011). Questions to assess environmental determinants of men's health are provided in the *Focused Assessment* below. Much of the related assessment data will be obtained through observation of environmental conditions to which men are exposed. Information on occupations and occupational hazards may be available from a local Chamber of Commerce or area businesses or from injury and disability claims filed with insurance companies.

SOCIOCULTURAL DETERMINANTS. Many influences on men's health arise from sociocultural determinants. We have

FOCUSED ASSESSMENT — Assessing Environmental Determinants of Men's Health

- To what environmental health hazards are men in the population exposed?
- What environmental hazards are posed by occupational settings? By recreational pursuits among men?
- What environmental hazards are posed by housing conditions for men in the population?
- To what extent does the physical environment promote or impede healthy behaviors by men (e.g., physical activity)?

already discussed the influences of gender socialization, a sociocultural factor, on men's psychological health. Other considerations in the sociocultural dimension affecting men's health include family interactions, economic and occupational issues, and issues related to violence. Much of the assessment data related to sociocultural determinants of men's health will be obtained from area statistics, observation, and surveys and interviews with men in the population. Questions to guide the assessment are presented in the *Focused Assessment* included below.

Family interactions. By far, the largest proportion of men lives within a family situation, which may create both positive and negative health effects. Worldwide, most men are married by the time they are in their 30s, but delayed marriage is associated with higher educational levels. By their 40s to mid-50s, most men have been married, some of them several times. In 2011, 58% of U.S men over 15 years of age were married, 35% had never married, approximately 2% were widowed, and more than 9% were divorced (U.S. Census Bureau, 2011).

Marriage has been shown to have a protective health effect for both men and women; however, because of socialization to a stereotyped male role and gender communication styles discussed earlier, men may have difficulty interacting within the family in ways that effectively meet their psychological needs. Differing role expectations between spouses may lead to marital conflicts and, in some cases, spouse or child abuse. Family violence and its effects on health are discussed in more detail in Chapter 30∞. It is, however, important for the population health nurse dealing with male clients to assess the marital status of the male population.

Parenting is another aspect of family interaction that may affect men's health. Young men in the United States are delaying initiation of sexual activity to a slightly older age than in previous years; however, by age 19 approximately 71% of young men and 36% of women are sexually active. The rate of adolescent fatherhood declined from 1991 to 2010 (25 per 1,000 males 15 to 19 years of age to 16 per 1,000), but adolescent males continue to father children (Guttmacher Institute, 2014). Population health nurses should be alert to the needs of individual adolescent fathers as well as the population of teen fathers.

Approximately one fourth of U.S. men have had a child by 20 years of age and 50% by age 30. Approximately 13% of sexually active males 15 to 19 years of age reported being involved in a pregnancy. Younger age at initiation of sexual activity contributes to risk of pregnancy, with 22% of adolescent males who have sex prior to age 15 involved in a pregnancy. Conversely, use of contraceptives during the first sexual experience decreases the risk of pregnancy from 18% to 12% (Planned Parenthood Federation of America, 2012). Early parenthood is more likely among minority men and those with lower educational levels (Guttmacher Institute, 2014).

More than half (56%) of teenage fathers are not living in the same household at the time of the child's birth (Scott, Steward-Streng, Manlove, & Moore, 2012), but often continue to be involved with their children, providing significant levels of informal support (e.g., transportation to and from school, help with school work, child care) (Resilience Advocacy Project, 2012). In addition, teen fathers frequently have additional children by the time they are 22 to 24 years of age. In one study, for example, 49% of those who fathered children as

FOCUSED ASSESSMENT Assessing Sociocultural Determinants of Men's Health

- What are the social roles expected of men? What effects do these role expectations have on men's health? What differences in men's roles are present within different cultural groups in the population?
- What opportunities for social interaction are available to men in the population? How do men in the population typically interact with others?
- To what extent are men perpetrators or victims of violence? What are the health effects of exposure to violence?
- What is the extent of social support available to men in the population?
- What is the percentage of single-parent families headed by men in the population?
- What is the typical educational level of men in the population?
- What is the economic status of men in the population? What is the average income of men in the population?
- What effects do economic, educational, and employment levels have on men's health?
- What transportation opportunities are available to men in the population?
- To what extent do men in the population function as caretakers for other family members? To what extent do these men experience caretaker burden?
- What percentage of men in the population is employed? What are the typical occupations for men in the population? What effects do occupation and employment setting have on men's health? What support do employers provide for men's other roles and responsibilities?
- What child care services are available to working single male parents? What is the cost of these services?

adolescents had more than one child by this age, and 17% had three or more children (Scott et al., 2012), often by different women, compounding difficulties in interactions with children and financial support.

Like adolescent mothers, teenaged fathers are at increased risk for low educational attainment and low-income levels. In some studies, 38% of young fathers do not complete high school, and less than 30% continue beyond a high school education. The lack of education and income further impair their abilities to provide child support. Teen fathers are also disadvantaged by the complexity of family court systems and lack of access to legal assistance (Resilience Advocacy Project, 2012).

Child health and development is fostered by interactions with both parents, even when one is functioning in a noncustodial role. Fatherless children, particularly boys, have higher rates of incarceration, suicide, behavioral disorders, dropping out of high school, delinquency, and juvenile detention rates than those whose fathers are actively involved in their lives. They may also receive less family support for educational attainment and display worse scholastic performance than children from two-parent households (Parker, n.d.). Divorce may also separate many men from their children. According to census data, in 2010, slightly more than 23% of U.S. children under 18 years of age were living in homes without their father present. Conversely, 3.4% were living with their fathers alone (U.S. Census Bureau, 2012c).

Roles related to fatherhood differ among cultural groups and are changing in many societies. In more traditional cultures emphasis tends to be placed on indirect parental care among fathers, for example, provision of family resources. The amount of time fathers spend with children also differs from group to group. In polygynous societies, for example, men are more focused on their mates than on their children. In most societies, however, fatherhood often entails elements of socialization or discipline of children. The amount of time that men in many social groups are spending in child care activities is increasing, however (Gray & Anderson, 2010).

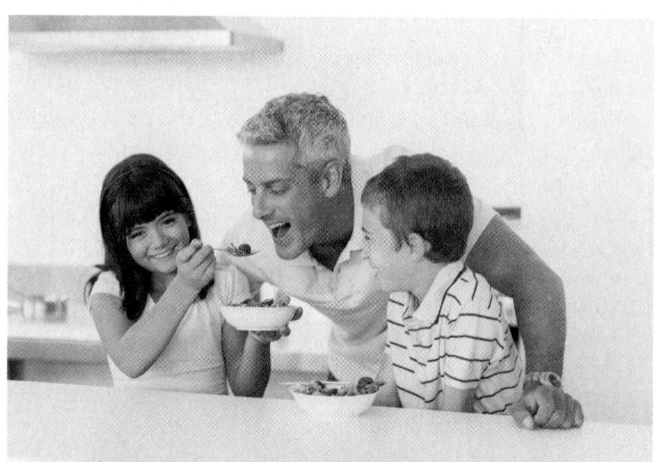

More men are raising children as single parents.
(WavebreakmediaMicro/Fotolia)

Because of typical male socialization, many men have little or no child care experience, yet the increase in the number of working women has led to greater assumption of child care duties by men. Many men may find themselves single parents as a result of divorce or the death of their wives. Others may have partial custody of children as a result of divorce. Population health nurses should be alert to the needs of adolescent and adult fathers and engage in advocacy to assure that these needs are met at both individual and population levels.

Changes in family interactions within cultural groups also influence marital relationships and role expectations. Many men who have been socialized to more traditional gender roles, may find it difficult to adapt to changing expectations of their family roles. In addition to assuming greater responsibility for child care, men may encounter expectations of their engagement in other household activities such as cooking and housekeeping. Similarly, men, whose models for women's roles were their more traditional mothers may have difficulty adapting to women's growing expectations for equality in decision making within the family as well as their participation in careers and employment outside the home. Changes in gender roles and power differentials between men and women have been likened to other transfers of power that have occurred throughout history, such as the transfer of power from master to slave, from employer to employee, and from monarchs and government to the general public (Synnott, 2009).

Divorce constitutes another aspect of family relations that may influence men's health status. Divorce is one of the most significant stressors a person can experience, and it may have a profound effect on the physical and psychological health of all family members. Divorced men, in particular, have been shown to experience increased morbidity and mortality as compared with married men. Men may respond to divorce or its aftermath with intense anger, a profound sense of loss, or significant depression. Suicidal behavior occasionally occurs as the man reacts to the divorce as an assault against his self-image and self-worth, or homicidal behavior if he directs his anger toward his ex-spouse. Widowed men also tend to fare less well than widowed women.

Economic and occupational issues. In most cultures, men are the primary breadwinners for the family, although more and more women throughout the world can be found in the workforce. Worldwide poverty and poor employment prospects undermine men's ability to fulfill their provider roles. Unemployment may be high in many developing countries and urbanization may lead young men to leave their families for extended periods of time to seek employment where it can be found. In the United States, men fare better than women in terms of their economic status, yet economic influences can have profound effects on their health status.

Economic status is closely linked to employment and unemployment. Some authors make a distinction between the societal experience of unemployment and the individual experience of "joblessness." From this perspective, **unemployment**

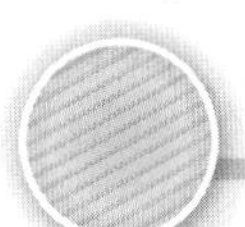

Global Perspectives

WHO: A Gender and Health Development Program

In every region of the world, men have a lower life expectancy at birth than women, with the greatest difference in life expectancy (8 years) seen in the European region. Men also have a higher probability than women of dying between the ages of 15 and 60 years. In addition, men have higher rates of elevated blood pressure and smoking and other tobacco use (World Health Organization [WHO], 2013). There is obviously a need for gender equity in health care services. The WHO Eastern Mediterranean Regional Office (EMRO) (n.d.) has initiated a Gender and Health Development Program. Although the program is designed to address many gender inequities related to women's health, it emphasizes the need for overall gender-based data analysis and health care planning. EMRO has designed the following test of one's knowledge of gender as it relates to health status.

Circle T for "true" or F for "false" for each question to test your knowledge on gender and health.

1. A gender-responsive workplan recognizes the differences between women's and men's health needs and vulnerabilities and includes actions to ensure these differential needs are addressed. **T / F**
2. Gender norms are standards set by society that determine what roles and responsibilities men and women should assume in society. **T / F**
3. Time, money, information, transportation, and social support networks are all resources that impact health outcomes. **T / F**
4. A women who is unable to see a doctor without head of house hold permission is an example of a gender issue in health. **T / F**
5. Women and men always have the same access to time, money, information, transportation, and social support networks. **T / F**
6. Gender mainstreaming is concerned only with integrating perspectives and realities of female populations groups. **T / F**
7. Sex disaggregated health data enables identification of differences between men, women, boys and girls. **T / F**
8. Gender in health refers only to reproductive health and conditions related to hormonal changes, and genetic or hereditary conditions. **T / F**
9. Fairness and justice in the distribution of benefits, power, resources, and responsibilities between women and men according to their needs is called gender discrimination. **T / F**
10. Health policies that do not distinguish between the needs of male and female population groups are called "gender blind." **T / F**

Correct answers: T, T, T, T, F, F, T, F, F, T

is the proportion of the workforce that is not employed at a specific point in time and is a statistical measure reflecting the general state of the economy. **Joblessness**, on the other hand, is the personalized experience of being out of work when one desires employment. Joblessness can have significant implications for both physical and mental health among men since men often base their self-worth on occupational performance and success. Although joblessness affects the mental health of both men and women, its mental health effects may be worse for men than women. In 2010, 71% of the U.S. adult male population was employed, and 10.5% of those in the workforce were unemployed (U.S. Census Bureau, 2012d). Among men who lost their jobs between 2007 and 2009, 39% remained unemployed in January 2010 (U.S. Census Bureau, 2012e) suggesting implications for their mental health.

The median weekly income for all men in 2010 was $824 (U.S. Census Bureau, 2012f). More than 19 million men (13% of all U.S. men) had incomes below poverty level in 2009 (U.S. Census Bureau, 2012g). Poverty is one of several reasons that men are more likely than women to be homeless. Despite the differences in the incidence of homelessness among men and women, homeless shelter systems are often better designed to meet the needs of women and children than those of men. Issues related to homelessness will be addressed in more detail in Chapter 21∞.

Men are more likely than women to be employed in jobs that entail physical health risks. In 2011, for example, men experienced 11 times more occupational fatalities than women. The highest rates of death occurred as a result of transportation incidents in the course of employment (Bureau of Labor Statistics, 2012).

Violence and trauma. Earlier, we discussed the implications of PTSD for men's psychological health. PTSD and other health problems arise from exposure to a variety of forms of violence and trauma. Men are more likely than women to be exposed to societal violence in many forms. With few exceptions, men constitute the bulk of homicide victims throughout the world (United Nations Office on Drugs and Crime, 2013). For example, in 2010, the global homicide rate for men was 8.4 per 100,000 men, down from 16.6 in 1980, but still nearly three-and-a-half times that of women (4.3 per 100,000) (NCHS, 2013). Men are also exposed to slightly higher rates of physical assault than women. In 2012, the serious violent crime victimization rate for men was 9.4 per 1,000 males over 12 years of age compared to 6.6 per 1,000 females (Langton, Planty, & Truman, 2013).

Violence also occurs in families, and men, as well as women, are subjected to intimate partner violence (IPV). More than 35% of women and 28% of men report being subjected to IPV at some point in their lives, but the number of men who are victims may be inaccurate due to many men's unwillingness to admit to victimization by their partner. Men are less likely than women to be injured as a result of IPV (Black et al., 2011). IPV is addressed in more detail in Chapter 30∞.

Overall, men in 2007 were nearly four times more likely than women to sustain a violence-related injury. Trauma also results from unintentional injury, and a consistent pattern in male–female differences in unintentional injuries has been seen, with men more than twice as likely as women to be injured (Sorenson, 2011). Legal and educational systems are other sociocultural determinants that may result in health status disparities between men and women. For example, laws are more often enacted to protect women than men, and men are more likely than women to be incarcerated. In the educational system, boys may be "treated as defective girls" (Synnott, 2009, p. 228) because of their frequently rowdy behavior. In addition, boys are more likely than girls to have learning disabilities and most elementary school teachers are women. There has also been a tendency to "criminalize" school discipline problems, calling the police for minor infractions (Synnott, 2009).

Men may also have less extensive social networks than women and may be less likely to call on members of social networks for assistance, again related to the idea of masculine strength and the weakness perceived in needing help. Aside from the psychological effects of an adequate social network, the extent of one's social network has also been shown to be associated with other health-related behaviors, such as engaging in physical activity (Shelton et al., 2011).

BEHAVIORAL DETERMINANTS. Behavioral factors seem to make a greater contribution to men's health status than to that of women. Because of their gender socialization, men are more inclined to engage in high-risk behaviors and less apt to perform healthful behaviors (Sorenson, 2011). Some behavioral considerations to be addressed in assessing men's health include consumption patterns, exercise and leisure, sexual activity, and other behavioral risk factors. Questions to guide assessment of behavioral determinants influencing men's health are provided in the *Focused Assessment* below. Some population level behavioral data may be available from government health agencies (e.g., smoking, alcohol use, seat belt use); other information may be gleaned through police records (e.g., arrests for illegal drug use or driving while intoxicated) or through community surveys.

Consumption patterns. Consumption patterns include diet as well as substance use and abuse. As we saw earlier, U.S. men are more likely than women to be both overweight and obese. A healthy weight is defined as one that is appropriate to one's height and body type. Healthy weight is most often determined on the basis of body mass index (BMI) and waist circumference. BMI is an indicator of the extent of body fat and is based on the relationship between height and weight (Centers for Disease Control and Prevention [CDC], 2011).

Waist circumference is related to BMI, but is also an independent predictor of risk for many chronic diseases, including type 2 diabetes, hypertension, and cardiovascular disease (National Heart, Lung and Blood Institute, n.d.). For more information on assessing waist circumference and calculating BMI, see the *External Resources* section of the student resources site.

Men may be somewhat less likely than women to eat a healthy diet. Looking at targets for specific nutrients included in the *Healthy People 2020* objectives, men are farther from achieving objectives related to fruit, vegetable, and sodium consumption. Men and women are essentially equal in terms of solid fat and added sugar consumption. Neither men nor women, however, have achieved the targets for any of these nutrients (Health Indicators Warehouse, n.d.a, n.d.b, n.d.c, n.d.d).

With respect to substance use and abuse, men 18 to 64 years of age were more likely than women to be current cigarette smokers in 2011 (23.6% and 18.8%, respectively). Among those over 12 years of age, men were more likely than women to use any illicit drug (nearly 3% and 2.5%, respectively). Male-female differences in use of alcohol are similar, with 57.4% of men and 46.5% of women using any alcohol. Men, however, are nearly twice as likely as women to engage in binge drinking and nearly

FOCUSED ASSESSMENT

Assessing Behavioral Determinants of Men's Health

- What are the dietary consumption patterns typical of men in the population? How do these patterns differ within subgroups within the population?
- What is the prevalence of smoking among men in the population?
- What is the extent of alcohol and other drug use in the population?
- To what extent do men in the population engage in safety practices (e.g., seat belt use)?
- To what extent do men who are sexually active engage in safe sexual practices?
- To what extent do men engage in health screening or health promotion/illness prevention practices such as colorectal screening, routine dental care, or annual influenza immunizations?

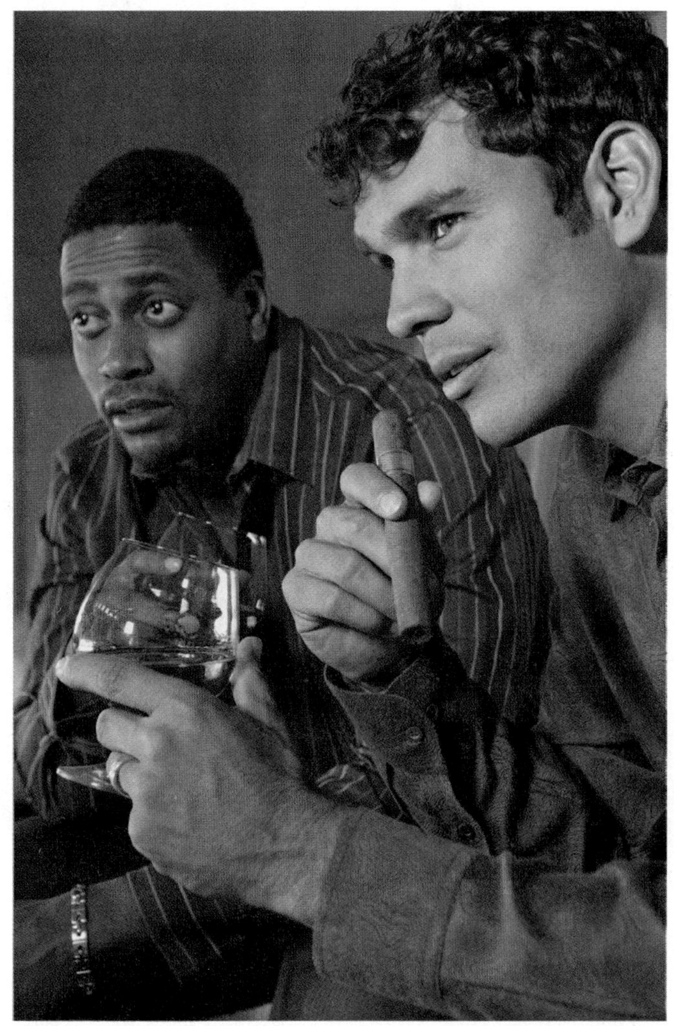

Tobacco and alcohol use are more common among men than among women. *(Bst2012/Fotolia)*

three times more likely to report heavy drinking (NCHS, 2013). In addition, drug-induced mortality rates are higher for men (15.8 per 100,000 population in 2007) than for women (9.3 per 100,000) (Paulozzi, 2011).

Exercise and leisure. Men are more likely than women to engage in leisure-time physical activity. In 2010, for example, just over 25% of men, but only 16.5% of women over 18 years of age met both aerobic and muscle strengthening targets for *Healthy People 2020.* On the negative side, however, nearly 44% of men met neither target (NCHS, 2012a).

Men and women increasingly share similar leisure patterns in American culture. Nevertheless, men still tend to be more active in competitive contact sports and, more often than women, to choose leisure activities involving some degree of physical risk (skydiving, white-water rafting, rock climbing). Participation in athletic sports is closely linked with images of masculinity and reinforces tendencies to aggressiveness and violence, increasing the potential for injury. Expectations of masculinity may also lead men to downplay the severity of injuries, delay treatment, and take insufficient time for healing. Men also tend to choose leisure activities associated with alcohol consumption. For these reasons, men experience relatively greater incidence of recreation-related trauma.

Other behavioral risk factors. Sexual activity among men was addressed earlier in this chapter, but population health nurses should assess the extent of sexual activity and number of partners for individual men as well as for the male population in general. Other assessment considerations include the extent of sexuality education among young men, knowledge and use of contraceptives, and use of condoms to prevent sexually transmitted infections.

Use of seat belts and other safety devices is another behavior that can significantly affect men's health. Because of masculine socialization to risk as an element of manliness, men are less likely than women to engage in a variety of safety practices, including seat belt or helmet use. They are also more likely to engage in high-risk recreational activities, particularly in the context of alcohol or drug use. In addition, media portrayals of men engaged in unhealthy behaviors contribute to risk taking and negative health effects in men.

Men may also be less likely than women to engage in health-related behaviors, such as screening for disease. For example, 2008 figures indicated that only 65% of men had received colorectal cancer screening (Rim, Joseph, Steele, Thompson, & Seeff, 2011). Similarly, in 2010, only 49% of men over 50 years of age received influenza immunizations (NCHS, 2013). Population health nurses should assess the extent to which men in the population engage in relevant screening and preventive activities, such as colorectal cancer screening, preventive dental visits, and so on.

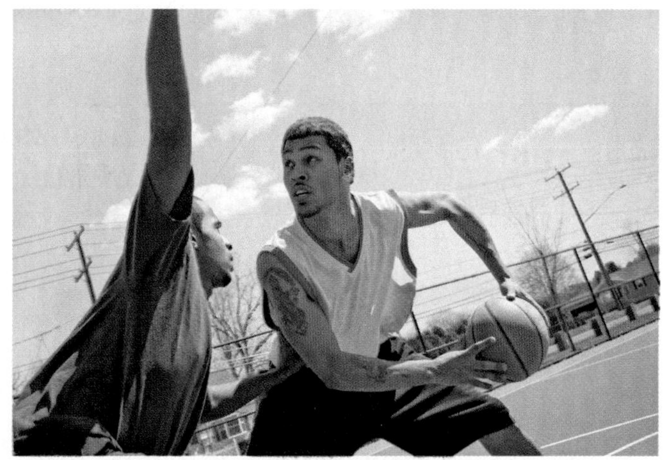

Men are somewhat more likely than women to engage in vigorous leisure-time physical activity. *(ArenaCreative/Fotolia)*

HEALTH SYSTEM DETERMINANTS. Population health nurses also assess determinants within the health system that influence men's health status. The *Focused Assessment* below provides guidelines for assessing these determinants. Generally speaking, men define health as the ability to be employed and to be economically independent, and, in some cases, to have adequate sexual function. Despite unhealthy lifestyles and shorter lives than women, most men consider themselves to be in good health. As noted earlier, gender socialization may lead men to "tough out" pain and delay seeking help until conditions interfere with their ability to work.

Factors other than gender socialization may also prohibit men from seeking health care. Some of these factors include lack of trust in providers, language barriers, lack of health insurance, financial difficulties, and difficulty relating to providers. Lack of health insurance and cost of care are particularly salient factors in men's failure to access health care services. In 2011, for example, 13% of men aged 18 to 64 years did not get, or delayed, health care due to costs, and men who did seek care had average out-of-pocket expenses of $219 per person in 2009. In addition, nearly 9% of men did not get prescription drugs and 14.5% did not receive needed dental care due to costs in 2011(NCHS, 2013).

Men are more likely than women to be uninsured and less likely than women to have Medicaid coverage. For example, in 2011, nearly 19% of men under 65 years of age had no health insurance coverage, compared to less than16% of women. Medicaid coverage for men was just over 16% versus 19.3% for women. Women also have a larger proportion of health care expenditures covered by private insurance than men (NCHS, 2013).

Another factor in men's failure to use health care services on a level commensurate with women is their perceived lack of a need for health care. Women routinely enter the health care system through services related to pregnancy, contraception, and routine screenings (e.g., Papanicolaou smears). These services serve as avenues for other health promotion activities as well as for detection of illness. Men do not routinely access any health-promotive services that would provide a similar door to other needed health care. Health care services are not crafted to target men, nor are many providers educated specifically to address the health care needs and motivations (or lack thereof) of men.

Diagnostic Reasoning and Men's Health

Based on factors in each of the categories of determinants of health that affect the health of individual male clients or men as a population group, the population health nurse would develop relevant nursing diagnoses, and plan and implement interventions to improve men's health. Nursing diagnoses may reflect positive or negative health states or increased risk for disease. A positive diagnosis might be "high prevalence of adequate physical activity due to presence of multiple low-cost opportunities for exercise." An example of a negative diagnosis might be "increased risk of sexually transmitted diseases among young adult men due to unprotected sexual activity." Based on the diagnoses derived from the assessment of men's health status and health needs, the population health nurse would collaborate with other segments of the population to plan, implement, and evaluate health care delivery programs to meet the identified health needs of men.

Planning to Meet the Health Needs of Men

Interventions to improve the health status of men in the population may focus on health promotion, illness and injury prevention, health restoration, or rehabilitation. The level of health care at which intervention occurs depends on the status of health problems to be addressed.

HEALTH PROMOTION. Although it is difficult to generalize about male clients' attitudes toward health promotion activities, there are some commonly encountered patterns of health behavior among men. One such behavior is a tendency to view exercise as sufficient to compensate for unhealthy behaviors such as a high intake of fats in the diet. Men also tend to attribute greater significance to health changes they can sense

FOCUSED ASSESSMENT — Assessing Health System Determinants of Men's Health

- What percentage of the male population has a regular source of health care?
- What are the attitudes of men to health and health care services? How do they define health and illness?
- What percentage of the male population has health insurance coverage?
- What health services are available to men in the population? Are health care services needed by men available to all segments of the population?
- What barriers to obtaining health care do men encounter?
- What are the attitudes of health care providers to care of men? To care of nonheterosexual men? How do these attitudes affect health care utilization by men?

than to those they cannot (e.g., they can sense pain but not elevated blood pressure). Because men tend to rate their health as very good or excellent more often than women, they may feel they do not need to be actively involved in health promotion activities. They may also err in their health appraisal efforts, stemming from a tendency to believe that their past athletic or current work activities may provide for their present health needs ("When I was a teenager I would run all day." "I work hard all day in the fresh air. What could be healthier than that?"). Population health nurses may need to advocate among men for changing attitudes to health and health-related behaviors through health education initiatives and reframing approaches.

Reframing, which focuses on helping clients to see the same situation in a different light, is one technique that can be used to promote positive behavioral change. A second technique for promoting change involves emphasizing alternate ways of coping with anxiety or fearfulness. Education, of course, is a crucial aspect of any health promotion strategy. Education is perhaps most effective when teaching is initiated with school-age male youngsters, as this is the stage when lifelong health values and habits are forming. Health promotion by family members is known to be a significant motivator and predictor of client compliance and outcomes, and involvement of family members in educational efforts and treatment planning is usually of significant benefit.

General approaches to promoting health among men are included in the HEALTH program, a six-point program intended to facilitate creation of health care services that better meet the health promotion needs of men. HEALTH is an acronym that stands for **H**umanize, **E**ducate, **A**ssume, **L**ocate, **T**ailor, and **H**ighlight (Courtenay, 2004). Health services for men should humanize the experience of illness by emphasizing the normality of experiencing and acknowledging pain, weakness, fear, and similar emotions to defuse the "macho" gender socialization to which men are subjected. Population health nurses can advocate for realistic health-related messages that emphasize the normality of these experiences and assist men to see them in the light of catalysts for health-related behaviors. Population health nurses working with men should educate them regarding the need for screening, health promotion, and risk reduction. It may also be helpful in working with men to assume the worst and to over exaggerate risks to make the point of the need for change in health-related behaviors. Population health nurses and other health care providers should also support men's health through follow-up telephone calls and advocate return visits for health promotion purposes after acute care needs have been met. Health care services for men should also be tailored to their specific needs with input from those involved. Population health nurses, in particular, are in a position to advocate for the inclusion of men in planning health services relevant to their needs. For example, a population health nurse might identify men who are single parents and encourage them to be involved in the development of support services for men who are parenting alone. Finally, effective health care services for men highlight strengths and lay out the costs and benefits of health-promoting behaviors such as exercise, diet, and so on, in terms that are relevant to men. Population health nurses can help to draft health-related messages in language that is meaningful to men, addressing consequences and benefits in meaningful terms. For example, a population health nurse might approach the need for health promotion and illness prevention among men in terms of their continued ability to work or support their families, both elements of male gender socialization.

Health promotion interventions for men should focus on the development of healthy lifestyles related to diet and physical activity as well as the promotion of effective coping skills. For example, population health nurses may advocate for environments that promote physical activity among men as well as engagement in physical activity by individual men. Promoting coping strategies among men would focus primarily on moving men from a reliance on avoidant coping mechanisms to more confrontive types of coping. This may necessitate specific education for coping as early as grade school and continuing on throughout the educational process. Coping education can also be employed in settings where men experience considerable stress such as the workplace. Population health nurses can advocate for and develop coping skills training programs tailored to men in both school and work settings. Table 17-4• summarizes major foci in health promotion for men and provides examples of related population health nursing interventions.

INJURY AND ILLNESS PREVENTION. Injury and illness prevention concerns specific to men focus on chronic disease prevention behaviors, immunization, safety practices, and elimination of high-risk behaviors. Chronic diseases in men can be prevented through adequate nutrition, physical activity and weight control, and elimination of behaviors such as smoking. Education for the prevention and control of other underlying

TABLE 17-4 Health Promotion Interventions in the Care of Men

Focus	Sample Interventions
Reframing	• Creating health care systems tailored to address men's needs and health-related perceptions
Promoting healthy lifestyles	• Promoting healthy diet • Promoting physical activity
Promoting coping	• Enhancing coping through teaching of confrontive coping strategies
Advocacy	• Advocating for environmental modifications to promote health • Advocating for access to health promotion education and services for men

diseases can also help to prevent chronic disease. For example, compliance with hypertension treatment can minimize the risk of developing cardiovascular disease. More information on prevention of chronic illnesses is provided in Chapter 27∞.

Environmental modification can also help to prevent chronic diseases and injuries. For example, population health nurses can be advocates for elimination of hazardous exposures in work and other settings that put men at risk for environmentally caused diseases.

Immunizations for men should focus on prevention of diseases such as tetanus, hepatitis A and B, influenza, and pneumonia for those at highest risk of disease due to occupational exposure (e.g., working outdoors or around animals) or high-risk behaviors such as oral-anal intercourse or injection drug use. Men with chronic conditions, particularly chronic respiratory conditions, or who work with susceptible populations should routinely receive immunizations for influenza and pneumonia. Because most adult men are part of the workforce, population health nurses may need to advocate for immunization services at times and locations that fit busy schedules. In addition, they can advocate for workplace policies that promote immunization, particularly in settings where risk of infectious disease is high. For example, a population health nurse might promote development and enforcement of a policy mandating regular tetanus boosters among construction workers. The nurse working in this setting might also monitor immunization status among employees and provide tetanus immunizations as needed.

Prevention interventions for men would also focus on injury prevention and safe sexual practices. Because of men's socialization to accept personal risk and their tendency to engage in high-risk behaviors, injury prevention often depends on legislation and regulation. Population health nurses can advocate for the passage and enforcement of legislation related to use of seat belts and other protective devices. Population health nurses can also monitor and report occupational safety hazards that put men at risk for injury or toxic exposures. Legislative advocacy may also be required in this area. Groups of men can also be educated regarding the need for effective injury prevention and the possible long-term consequences of injury.

Education may also need to focus on safe sexual practices. The U.S. President's Emergency Plan for AIDS Relief (PEPFAR, n.d.) has recommended an ABC approach for sexual health promotion for men: **A**bstinence, **B**eing faithful to one partner, and **C**ondom use. Specific services are needed for men's reproductive health needs as well as women's. In addition, the U.S. Preventive Services Task Force (USPSTF, 2012) has recommended high-intensity counseling on STI prevention for sexually active adolescents and adults. Again, population health nursing advocacy may be required before such programs for men are developed.

Another approach to illness and injury prevention in men is the elimination of high-risk behaviors. Elimination of high-risk sexual behaviors has already been addressed, but attention should also be given to smoking cessation and prevention or cessation of illicit drug use. Population health nurses can educate men about the need for smoking cessation and make referrals to smoking cessation services. They can also advocate for smoke-free workplace legislation to limit places where smoking is permitted or for coverage of smoking cessation assistance under health insurance plans. They can engage in similar interventions related to drug use, which is discussed in more detail in Chapter 29∞. Population health nurses may also need to advocate for the availability of such services and for their coverage under health insurance.

Table 17-5• summarizes illness/injury prevention foci for men as well as examples of population health nursing interventions related to each focus.

RESOLUTION OF EXISTING HEALTH PROBLEMS. Resolving health problems among men involves the earliest possible detection of health needs through effective screening. Resolution of existing problems also encompasses the actual treatment of the health needs or disorders themselves.

Population health nurses may participate in health screening activities by providing or encouraging the client's use of such health measures as blood pressure screening and cardiovascular risk-assessment programs in public, educational, or occupational settings. Men are more likely than women to have multiple risk factors for heart disease and stroke, and population health nurses can design, implement, and promote participation in risk assessments for the male population.

TABLE 17-5 Illness and Injury Prevention Interventions in the Care of Men

Focus	Sample Interventions
Control of disease risk factors	• Referring for treatment of underlying conditions that contribute to chronic illness (e.g., hypertension) • Promoting smoking cessation • Promoting safe sexual practices • Promoting and providing immunization services
Injury prevention	• Promoting safety behaviors (e.g., seat belt and helmet use) • Monitoring and eliminating environmental safety hazards and exposures
Advocacy	• Advocating for available and accessible prevention services • Advocating for safety legislation and enforcement • Advocating insurance coverage of adult immunizations

Nurses can also facilitate the offering and use of screening examinations by other health care professionals within the community, such as rectal examinations and screening for type 2 diabetes in men with blood pressures over 135/80 (USPSTF, 2012).

Routine screening procedures for men include tobacco use and alcohol misuse, colorectal cancer, hypertension, lipid disorders, and obesity. Other screening tests are recommended for men at particular risk for certain conditions. Recommendations of the U.S. Preventive Services Task Force (2012) for screening in men are presented in Table 17-6●. Population health nurses may need to advocate for access to routine screening services, particularly among low-income men and those without health insurance. Of note are the changes in prostate and testicular cancer screening recommendations based on scientific evidence described below.

Population health nurses may refer men with existing health problems for medical evaluation and treatment. They may also participate in the treatment of illnesses experienced by male clients. In the case of ischemic and certain other cardiac disorders, for example, stress has been shown to impact negatively on treatment outcomes, in some cases leading to a threefold increase in mortality (e.g., in post–myocardial infarction clients). Treatment programs that identify high-stress clients during hospitalization, track and reduce their stress levels after discharge, and provide prompt assistance from nurses in the community when episodes of increased stress occur can result in significant reduction of the stress-related mortality experienced by post–myocardial infarction clients.

TABLE 17-6 Routine Screening Recommendations for Men

Type of Screening	Recommendation
Abdominal aortic aneurysm	One time for men aged 65 to 75 years who have ever smoked tobacco
Alcohol misuse	All adult men
Colorectal cancer	Men 50 to 75 years of age by fecal occult blood, sigmoidoscopy, and/or colonoscopy
Depression	Adult men in practice settings where follow-up is available
Diabetes	Adult men with blood pressures >135/80 mm Hg
Hypertension	All men over 18 years of age
HIV infection	All adult and adolescent men at risk of infection
Lipid disorders	All men over 35 years of age and men 20 to 35 years of age at risk of CHD
Obesity	All adult men
Syphilis	All men at risk
Tobacco use	All adult men

Data from: U.S. Preventive Services Task Force. (2013). *Recommendations for adults.* Retrieved from http://www.uspreventiveservicestaskforce.org/adultrec.htm

Again, advocacy may be required to assure access to diagnostic and treatment services for men. For example, a population health nurse might assist in the development of stress-reduction programs in the workplace or coping skills training programs in school and work settings.

HEALTH RESTORATION. Health restoration services for men are directed at those disorders that influence men's health in some ongoing manner or that have a likelihood of recurrence. The goals of rehabilitation are to assist men in coping with the continuing manifestations of illness and to reduce the likelihood of future episodes of an illness. To this end, it is useful to group rehabilitation measures into care directed toward those disorders that affect men's sexual functioning or sexual identity or as they present a threat to notions about masculinity and male strength. Restoration measures also would be directed at supporting compliance with long-term therapy.

One area for restoration intervention by the population health nurse involves those disorders that affect the male client's sexual functioning or sexual identity, such as testicular cancer and ED. Male clients with testicular cancer may face significant emotional distress owing to the effects of treatment on their sexuality. Treatment for testicular cancer is surgical removal of the affected testes followed by hormonal therapy. These treatments, along with their side effects (loss of fertility, emasculation), can have a profound impact on the client's self-image and psychosocial functioning. Similarly, long-standing ED may have implications for men's psychological health and population health nurses may need to refer men for assistance in creating healthier self-images that are not based on sexual prowess. Population health nurses may need to advocate for development of and access to services dealing with sexual dysfunction. They may also be instrumental in changing men's attitudes to sexual dysfunction and their willingness to seek help.

An important intervention in this regard involves encouraging men to join support groups. Interaction with other men who have experienced the same problems can be very effective in facilitating adjustment to treatments that so tangibly affect men's sense of masculinity. On a one-to-one basis, the nurse can be accepting, supportive, and facilitative of the male client's expression of his feeling of loss. Population health nurses may also be instrumental in initiating supportive groups for these men or in advocating their availability in the community.

Some disorders may affect men's sense of strength; this is particularly true of cardiovascular disorders. The heart is a symbol of masculine strength for some men. Consequently, cardiovascular disorders not only can leave residual symptoms and physiological impairment, but can also threaten a man's self-image. Men with cardiovascular disease often benefit from interventions that support their self-image as masculine and from discussing their feelings about their illness. As

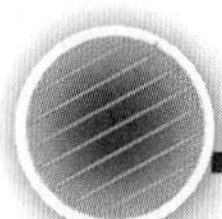

Evidence-Based Practice

Prostate and Testicular Cancer Screening

In spite of the relatively common practice of routine screening for prostate cancer using prostate-specific antigen (PSA testing), the U.S. Preventive Services Task Force (2010, 2013) has found insufficient evidence for screening men under 75 years of age. In addition, the task force has recommended against screening men over age 75. This recommendation is based on lack of evidence of the need for and effectiveness of treatment when prostate cancer is detected. The conclusion of the task force was that routine screening benefits only a few men and may cause harm to many men due to unnecessary treatment, treatment side effects, and mental suffering for them and their families.

In addition, the USPSTF has recommended against screening for testicular cancer in adolescent or adult males noting that there is inadequate evidence that early detection through either testicular self-examination or clinical examination influences cure rates. In fact, the evidence reviewed indicates that 90% of testicular cancer will be cured regardless of stage at diagnosis. The task force also noted the potential for harm related to false positive results, anxiety, or the results of diagnostic tests or treatments (USPSTF, 2011a, 2011b).

noted elsewhere, stress management training also can have a significant positive effect on outcomes for men who have cardiovascular disease. These interventions are essential to promote adjustment and compliance with treatment.

Of course, population health nurses should also support and reinforce men's positive responses to cardiac rehabilitation efforts initiated in other treatment settings. Foremost among these would be weight control, limited intake of saturated fats, regular exercise, compliance with follow-up examinations and medications, and control of other disorders that exacerbate cardiovascular disease (hypertension, diabetes).

In the case of some chronic disorders, especially those producing no overt symptoms, men tend to be lax about complying with long-term treatment recommendations. This is especially true for male clients with hypertension. Interventions that help men understand the importance of controlling this disorder and that build on their perceptions of masculinity are very helpful. Maintaining a regimen of antihypertensive medications may be especially difficult for men when side effects interfere with necessary masculine roles. Examples of such side effects could include impotence, dizziness, and decreased tolerance for physical activity. Nurses can assist men by teaching ways to compensate for these side effects, thereby helping them to maintain a sense of control over circumstances. In cases in which the side effects are not manageable and are affecting clients' masculinity (impotence), collaborating with the client's physician or assisting the client to discuss the problem with the physician can lead to acceptance of the treatment for hypertension.

Preventing recidivism, or rehospitalization, in instances of substance abuse is a major rehabilitation intervention in working with men. Interventions that decrease the likelihood of recidivism include encouraging the use of therapeutic support groups (Alcoholics Anonymous) and education regarding factors that predispose one to continued substance abuse (poor coping skills, co-dependent relationships, maintaining social contacts with abusers). It is also important for the population health nurse to consider the client's family and significant others when caring for substance-abusing men. Families and significant others can be either enablers of substance abuse or corrective forces leading to its elimination. Education of family and support persons regarding behaviors that produce improvement and those that permit further substance abuse is essential, and referrals to family treatment and support services are also of value.

The Internet may be a particularly valuable tool for educating men regarding rehabilitation and self-management of chronic illnesses as well as for motivating primary prevention activities by men. More and more, the U.S. population is turning to the Internet as a source of information. Population health nurses can help to create websites to provide such information as well as monitor existing sites for their accuracy and credibility.

Evaluating Health Care for Men

As in working with other population groups, population health nursing plans and interventions are evaluated by determining the degree to which population health goals have been met. It is also important to determine whether interventions were efficient. Could the same results have been accomplished with less expense of time or other resources?

The effects of interventions for men at the aggregate level can be assessed in terms of the accomplishment of national health objectives (USDHHS, 2014b). Selected objectives related to men's health are presented in the *Healthy People 2020* feature on pages 441 and 442. Information about objectives related to men's health and their current status is available on the *Healthy People 2020* website.

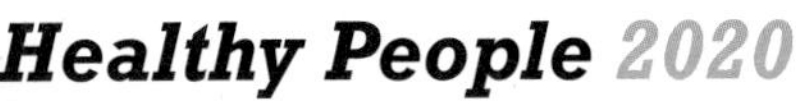

Healthy People 2020

Selected Objectives Related to Men's Health

OBJECTIVE	BASELINE (YEAR)	TARGET	CURRENT DATA (YEAR)	DATA SOURCES
AHS-1.1 Increase the proportion of men with medical insurance	83.2% (2008)	100%	81.2 (2011)	National Health Interview Survey (NHIS), CDC, National Center for Health Statistics (NCHS)
AHS-3 Increase the proportion of men 18–64 years of age with a usual primary care provider	75.5% (2008)	83.9%	72.9% (2010)	NHIS, CDC, NCHS
AHS-5 Increase the proportion of men with a source of ongoing care	74.3 (2010)	89.4	76.6% (2010)	NHIS, CDC, NCHS
AHS-6 Reduce the proportion of men unable to obtain or delay obtaining medical care, dental care, or prescription medications	9.1% (2007)	9%	8.8% (2010)	Medical Expenditure Panel Survey (MEPS), AHRQ
AOCBC-2 Reduce the proportion of men with Dr. diagnosed arthritis who experience a limitation in activity due to arthritis or joint symptoms	37.6% (2008)	35.5%	37.9% (2011)	NHIS, CDC, NCHS
AOCBC-12 Reduce activity limitation due to chronic back conditions per 1,000 men	28.8% (2008)	26.6	34.4% (2011)	NHIS, CDC, NCHS
C-1 Reduce cancer deaths per 100,000 men	218.8 (2007)	161.4	209.9 (2010)	National Vitals Statistics System–Mortality (NVSS-M), CDC, NCHS
C-2 Reduce lung cancer deaths per 100,000 men	64.9 (2007)	45.5	60.3 (2010)	NVSS-M, CDC, NCHS
C-5 Reduce colorectal cancer deaths per 100,000 men	20.4	14.5	19.1 (2010)	NVSS-M, CDC, NCHS
C-7 Reduce prostate cancer deaths per 100,000 men	24.2 (2007)	21.8	21.9 (2010)	NVSS-M, CDC, NCHS
C-8 Reduce melanoma cancer deaths per 100,000 men	4.0 (2007)	2.4	4.1 (2010)	NVSS-M, CDC, NCHS
C-16 Increase the proportion of men who receive colorectal cancer screening	52.2% (2008)	70.5%	59.3% (2010)	NHIS, CDC, NCHS
D-3 Reduce diabetes deaths per 100,000 men	88.8 (2007)	65.8	86.1 (2010)	NVSS-M, CDC, NCHS
HDS-2 Reduce coronary heart disease deaths per 100,000 men	169.2 (2007)	103.4	151.3 (2010)	NVSS-M, CDC, NCHS
HDS-3 Reduce stroke deaths per 100,000 men	43.7 (2007)	34.8	39.3 (2010)	NVSS-M, CDC, NCHS

Continued on next page

Healthy People 2020 (Continued)

OBJECTIVE	BASELINE (YEAR)	TARGET	CURRENT DATA (YEAR)	DATA SOURCES
HDS-5.1 Reduce the proportion of men with hypertension	30.6% (2005–2008)	26.9%	NDA	National Health and Nutrition Examination Survey (NHANES), CDC, NCHS
HDS-6 Increase the proportion of men who have had their blood cholesterol level checked in the past 5 years	72.2% (2008)	82.1%	NDA	NHIS, CDC, NCHS
HDS-7 Reduce the proportion of men with high blood cholesterol levels	13.5% (2005–2008)	13.5%	NDA	NHANES, CDC, NCHS
HIV-4 Reduce new cases of AIDs per 100,000 adult and adolescent men	20.6 (2007)	12.4	20 (2010)	HIV Surveillance System, CDC, NCHHSTP
IVP-1.3 Reduce emergency department visits for nonfatal injuries per 100,000 men	9156.7 (2007)	7453.4	10,441.1 (2010)	National Hospital Ambulatory Medical Care Survey (NHAMCS), CDC, NCHS
IVP-11 Reduce unintentional injury deaths per 100,000 men	55.9 (2007)	36	51.5 (2010)	NVSS-M, CDC, NCHS
IVP-29 Reduce homicides per 100,000 men	9.7 (2007)	5.5	8.4 (2010)	NVSS-M, CDC, NCHS
NWS-9 Reduce the proportion of adult men who are obese	32.5% (2005–2008)	30.5%	35.5% (2009-2010)	NHANES, CDC, NCHS
PA-1 Reduce the proportion of adult men who engage in no leisure time physical activity	33.9% (2008)	32.6%	29.8% (2011)	NHIS, CDC, NCHS
SA-12 Reduce drug-induced deaths per 100,000 men	16 (2007)	11.3	15.9 (2010)	NVSS-M, CDC, NCHS
TU-1.1 Reduce cigarette smoking by adult men	20.6% (2008)	12%	19% (2011)	NHIS, CDC, NCHS
TU-4.1 Increase smoking cessation attempts by adult men smokers	48.3% (2008)	80%	48.9% (2011)	NHIS, CDC, NCHS

NDA = No data available

Data from: U.S. Department of Health and Human Services. (2014b). *Topics and objectives index: Healthy people.* Retrieved from http://www.healthypeople.gov/2020/topicsobjectives2020/

CHAPTER RECAP

Men have a variety of health care needs that they may or may not acknowledge. Population health nurses identify factors related to biological, psychological, environmental, sociocultural, behavioral, and health system determinants of health and use this information to develop population level or individual nursing diagnoses. They then engage in health promotion, illness and injury prevention, health restoration, and rehabilitation interventions to address the needs identified. Population health nurses can be actively involved in fostering health promotion and illness/injury prevention activities by men and encouraging men to seek health care as needed. They may also provide direct services to male clients, particularly with respect to education for promotion, prevention, and disease management. In addition, population health nurses may be involved in advocacy activities to assure the availability and accessibility of needed services to improve men's health status.

CASE STUDY Promoting Sexual Health in Men

There is a high rate of sexually transmitted diseases among men in the community where you are employed as a population health nurse. Particularly high incidence rates are noted for *Chlamydia trachomatis* and gonorrhea. Significant disparities are noted in incidence rates among Caucasian, African American, and Latino men, with incidence higher among young African American and Latino men than among Caucasians, although incidence among all three groups is high. STD incidence does not seem to be associated with sexual orientation since high rates are noted for both exclusively heterosexual men and those who have sex with other men.

1. How might you address the problem of STD incidence at the population level?
2. What additional information might you need to determine appropriate interventions for the problem?
3. What other segments of the community would you involve in developing your interventions?

REFERENCES

AAMN Board of Directors. (2010). *Gender neutral nursing education.* Retrieved from http://aamn.org/docs/GenderNeutralDraft5July2011.pdf

American Academy of Family Physicians. (2014). *Male infertility.* Retrieved from http://familydoctor.org/familydoctor/en/diseases-conditions/male-infertility.html

American Assembly for Men in Nursing. (2010). *Position statement on men's health curriculum in schools of nursing.* Retrieved from http://aamn.org/docs/Men_Health_Curriculum_Final_Version_5-6-2010.pdf

American Assembly for Men in Nursing. (2011). *AAMN: Advancing men in nursing.* Retrieved from http://aamn.org/aamn.shtml

Beckles, G. L., Zhu, J., & Moonsinghe, R. (2011, January 14). Diabetes - United States, 2004 and 2008. *Morbidity and Mortality Weekly Report, 60*(Suppl.), 90–93.

Black, M. C., Basile, K. C. Breiding, M. J., Smith, S. G., Walters, M. L., Merrick, M. T., ... Stevens, M. R. (2011). *The National Intimate Partner and Sexual Violence Survey: 2010 summary report.* Retrieved from http://www.cdc.gov/violenceprevention/pdf/nisvs_report2010-a.pdf

Bureau of Labor Statistics. (2012). *2011 census of fatal occupational injuries (preliminary data). Table A-7. Fatal occupational injuries by worker characteristics and event or exposure, all U.S., 2011.* Retrieved from http://www.bls.gov/iif/oshwc/cfoi/cftb0265.pdf

Centers for Disease Control and Prevention. (2011). *Assessing your weight.* Retrieved from http://www.cdc.gov/healthyweight/assessing/index.html

Centers for Disease Control and Prevention. (2012a). *Arthritis.* Retrieved from http://www.cdc.gov/arthritis/basics/rheumatoid.htm#5

Centers for Disease Control and Prevention. (2012b). *Cholesterol facts.* Retrieved from http://www.cdc.gov/cholesterol/facts.htm

Centers for Disease Control and Prevention. (2013). *Cancer among men.* Retrieved from http://www.cdc.gov/cancer/dcpc/data/men.htm

Centre for Suicide Prevention. (2011). *Men and suicide: A high-risk population?* Retrieved from http://suicideinfo.ca/LinkClick.aspx?fileticket=n5ZgwCH83L8%3D&tabid=563

Courtenay, W. H. (2004, Fall). Best practice for improving college men's health. *New Directions for Student Services, 107,* 59–74.

Deters, L. A., & Kim, E. D. (2011). *Benign prostatic hypertrophy.* Retrieved from http://emedicine.medscape.com/article/437359-overview

Gray, P. B., & Anderson, K. G. (2010). *Fatherhood: Evolution and paternal behavior.* Cambridge, MA: Harvard University Press.

Guttmacher Institute. (2014). *Facts on American teen's sexual and reproductive health.* Retrieved from http://www.guttmacher.org/pubs/FB-ATSRH.pdf

Hall, H. I., Hughes, D., Dean, H. D., Mermin, J. H., & Fenton, K. A. (2011, January 14). HIV infection = United States, 2005 and 2008. *Morbidity and Mortality Weekly Report, 60*(Suppl.), 87–89.

Health Indicators Warehouse. (n.d.a). *Fruit consumption.* Retrieved from http://www.healthindicators.gov/Indicators/Fruitconsumption_1217/Profile/Data

Health Indicators Warehouse. (n.d.b). *Sodium consumption.* Retrieved from http://www.healthindicators.gov/Indicators/Sodiumconsumption_1222/Profile/Data

Health Indicators Warehouse. (n.d.c). *Solid fats and added sugar consumption.* Retrieved from http://www.healthindicators.gov/Indicators/Solidfatandaddedsugarconsumption_1238/Profile/Data

Health Indicators Warehouse. (n.d.d). *Vegetable consumption.* Retrieved from http://www.healthindicators.gov/Indicators/Totalvegetableconsumption_1218/Profile/Data

Keenan, N. L., & Rosendorf, K. A. (2011, January 14). Prevalence of hypertension and controlled hypertension = United States, 2005–2008. *Morbidity and Mortality Weekly Report, 60*(Suppl.), 94–97.

Langton, L., Planty, M., & Truman, J. (2013). *Crime victimization, 2012.* Retrieved from http://www.bjs.gov/content/pub/pdf/cv12.pdf

Letourneau, N., Duffett-Leger, L., Dennis, C.-L., Stewart, M., & Tryphonopoulos, P. D. (2010). Identifying the support needs of fathers affected by post-partum depression: A pilot study. *Journal of Psychiatric and Mental Health Nursing, 18,* 41–47. doi:10.1111/j.1365-2859.2010.01627.x

National Center for Health Statistics. (2012a). Percentage of men aged 25–64 years with activity limitation, by age group and veteran status—United States, National Health Interview Survey (NHIS), 2007–2010. *Morbidity and Mortality Weekly Report, 61,* 845.

National Center for Health Statistics. (2012b). *Vital and health statistics: Summary health statistics for U.S. adults: National Health Interview Survey, 2011.* Retrieved from http://www.cdc.gov/nchs/data/series/sr_10/sr10_256.pdf

National Center for Health Statistics. (2013). *Health, United States, 2012: With special feature on emergency care.* Retrieved from http://www.cdc.gov/nchs/data/hus/hus12.pdf

National Center for Injury Prevention and Control. (2013). *Unintentional all injury causes nonfatal injuries and rates per 100,000.* Retrieved from http://webappa.cdc.gov/sasweb/ncipc/nfirates2001.html

National Heart, Lung and Blood Institute. (n.d.). *Guidelines on overweight and obesity: Electronic textbook.* Retrieved from http://www.nhlbi.nih.gov/guidelines/obesity/e_txtbk/txgd/4142.htm

National Institute of Mental Health. (2009). *Anxiety disorders.* Retrieved from http://www.nimh.nih.gov/health/publications/anxiety-disorders/nimhanxiety.pdf

National Kidney and Urologic Diseases Information Clearinghouse. (2012). *Erectile dysfunction.* Retrieved from http://kidney.niddk.nih.gov/KUDiseases/pubs/ED/index.aspx

Parker, W. (n.d.). *Statistics on fatherless children in America.* Retrieved from http://fatherhood.about.com/od/fathersrights/a/fatherless_children.htm?p=1

Paulozzi, L. J. (2011, January 14). Drug-induced deaths—United States, 2003–2007. *Morbidity and Mortality Weekly Report, 60*(Suppl.), 60–61.

Planned Parenthood Federation of America. (2012). *Pregnancy and childbearing among U.S. teens.* Retrieved from http://www.plannedparenthood.org/files/PPFA/pregnancy_and_childbearing.pdf

Raymond, J., Wheeler, W., & Brown, M. J. (2011, January 14). Inadequate and unhealthy housing, 2007 and 2009. *Morbidity and Mortality Weekly Report, 60*(Suppl.), 21–27.

Resilience Advocacy Project. (2012). *Who cares about teen dads? How family court can help break a cycle of poverty.* Retrieved from http://resiliencelaw.org/wordpress2011/wp-content/uploads/2012/06/Teen-Father-White-Paper-FINAL-VERSION.pdf

Rim, S. H., Joseph, D. A., Steele, C. B., Thompson, T. D., & Seeff, L. C. (2011). Colorectal cancer screening ? United States, 2002, 2004, 2006, and 2008. *Morbidity and Mortality Weekly Report, 60*(Suppl.), 42–46.

Salzman, B. E., & Wender, R., C. (2006). Male sex: A major health disparity. In C. A. Haines & R. C. Wender (Eds.), *Primary care: Clinics in office practice: Men's health, 33,* 1–16. doi:10.1016/j.pop.2005.11.014

Scott, M., Steward-Streng, N. R., Manlove, J., & Moore, K. A. (2012). *The characteristics and circumstances of teen fathers: At the birth of their first child and beyond.* Retrieved from http://www.childtrends.org/wp-content/uploads/2013/03/Child_Trends-2012_06_01_RB_TeenFathers.pdf

Shelton, R. C., McNeill, L. H., Puleo, E., Wolin, K. Y., Emmons, K. M., & Bennett, G. G. (2011). The association between social factors and physical activity among low-income adults living in public housing. *American Journal of Public Health, 101,* 2102–2110. doi:1-.2105/AJPH.2010.196030

Sorenson, S. B. (2011). Gender disparities in injury mortality: Consistent, persistent, and larger than you'd think. *American Journal of Public Health, 101,* S353–S358. doi:10.2105/AJPH.2010.300029

Synnott, A. (2009). *Rethinking men: Heroes, villains, and victims.* Burlington, VT: Ashgate.

Tranbarger, R. E. (2007). The American Assembly for Men in Nursing (AAMN): The first 30 years as reported in *Interaction.* In C. E. O'Lynn & R. E. Tranbarger (Eds.), *Men in nursing: History, challenges, and opportunities* (pp. 67–81). New York, NY: Springer.

United Nations Office on Drugs and Crime. (2013). *Global study on homicide, 2013.* Retrieved from http://www.unodc.org/documents/gsh/pdfs/2014_GLOBAL_HOMICIDE_BOOK_web.pdf

United States President's Emergency Plan for AIDS Relief. (n.d.). *Defining the ABC approach.* Retrieved from http://www.pepfar.gov/reports/guidance/75837.htm

U.S. Cancer Statistics Working Group. (2013). *2009 top ten cancers.* Retrieved from http://apps.nccd.cdc.gov/uscs/toptencancers.aspx

U.S. Census Bureau. (2011). *American fact finder: Sex by marital status for the population 15 years and over.* Retrieved from http://factfinder2.census.gov/faces/tableservices/jsf/pages/productview.xhtml?pid=ACS_11_1YR_B12001&prodType=table

U. S. Census Bureau. (2012a). *Statistical abstract of the United States, Table 7. Resident population by sex and age: 1980 to 2010.* Retrieved from http://www.census.gov/compendia/statab/2012/tables/12s0007.pdf

U. S. Census Bureau. (2012b). *Statistical abstract of the United States, Table 9. Resident population projections by sex and age: 2010 to 2050.* Retrieved from http://www.census.gov/compendia/statab/2012/tables/12s0009.pdf

U.S. Census Bureau. (2012c). *Statistical abstract of the United States, Table 69. Children under 18 years old by presence of parents: 2000–2012.* Retrieved from http://www.census.gov/compendia/statab/2012/tables/12s0069.pdf

U.S. Census Bureau. (2012d). *Statistical abstract of the United States, Table 588. Civilian population—Employment status by sex, race and ethnicity: 1970–2009.* Retrieved from http://www.census.gov/compendia/statab/2012/tables/12s0588.pdf

U.S. Census Bureau. (2012e). *Statistical abstract of the United States, Table 614. Displaced workers by selected characteristics, 2010.* Retrieved from http://www.census.gov/compendia/statab/2012/tables/12s0614.pdf

U.S. Census Bureau. (2012f). *Statistical abstract of the United States, Table 648. Full-time wage and salary workers—Number and earnings, 2000 to 2010.* Retrieved from http://www.census.gov/compendia/statab/2012/tables/12s0649.pdf

U.S. Census Bureau. (2012g). *Statistical abstract of the United States, Table 713. People below poverty level by selected characteristics: 2009.* Retrieved from http://www.census.gov/compendia/statab/2012/tables/12s0713.pdf

U.S. Department of Health and Human Services. (2013). *Cancer.* Retrieved from http://www.healthypeople.gov/2020/topicsobjectives2020/objectiveslist.aspx?topicId=5

U.S. Department of Health and Human Services. (2014a). *Immunizations and infectious diseases.* Retrieved from http://www.healthypeople.gov/2020/topicsobjectives2020/objectiveslist.aspx?topicId=23

U.S. Department of Health and Human Services. (2014b). *Topics and objectives index: Healthy people*. Retrieved from http://www.healthypeople.gov/2020/topicsobjectives2020/default.aspx

U.S. Preventive Services Task Force. (2011a). *Screening for testicular cancer*. Retrieved from http://www.uspreventiveservicestaskforce.org/uspstf/uspstest.htm

U.S. Preventive Services Task Force. (2011b). *Screening for testicular cancer: Clinical summary of U.S. Preventive Services Task Force reaffirmation recommendation*. Retrieved from http://www.uspreventiveservicestaskforce.org/uspstf10/testicular/testicupsum.pdf

U.S. Preventive Services Task Force. (2012). *The guide to clinical preventive services 2010-2011*. Retrieved from http://www.ahrq.gov/professionals/clinicians-providers/guidelines-recommendations/guide/guide-clinical-preventive-services.pdf

U.S. Preventive Services Task Force. (2013). *Recommendations for adults*. Retrieved from http://www.uspreventiveservicestaskforce.org/adultrec.htm

West, B., & Naumann, R. B. (2011, January 14). Motor vehicle-related deaths – United States, 2003–2007. *Morbidity and Mortality Weekly Report, 60*(Suppl.), 52–55.

World Health Organization. (2013). *World health statistics 2012*. Retrieved from http://www.who.int/gho/publications/world_health_statistics/EN_WHS2012_Full.pdf

World Health Organization, Regional Office for the Eastern Mediterranean. (n.d.). *Gender in health and development: Gender and health questions*. Retrieved from http://www.emro.who.int/gender/infocus/gender-health-test.html

CHAPTER

18 Care of Women

Learning Outcomes

After reading this chapter, you should be able to:

1. Identify at least two factors in each category of determinants of health that influence the health of women.
2. Identify health problems common to women.
3. Identify concerns in health promotion for women and analyze the role of the population health nurse with respect to each.
4. Discuss strategies for illness and injury prevention for women and related population health nursing interventions.
5. Describe areas of health problem resolution for women and design population health nursing interventions related to each.
6. Describe considerations in health restoration for women.

Key Terms

bioidentical hormone replacement therapy (BHRT)

dysmenorrhea

gender

gestational diabetes mellitus (GDM)

menopause

osteoporosis

perimenopause

postmenopause

premenopause

premenstrual dysphoric disorder (PMDD)

premenstrual syndrome (PMS)

sex

Advocacy Then

Margaret Sanger and Contraceptive Services for Women

As a result of exposure to the health effects of multiple pregnancies on her mother's health, Margaret Sanger, one of the early nurses of the Henry Street Settlement was particularly sympathetic to the plight of poor women in New York City who were affected by multiple unwanted pregnancies. Distribution of contraceptive devices and information was prohibited by the Comstock Act passed in 1873, putting women at risk for multiple pregnancies or illegal abortions in unsafe conditions (Lewis, 2010).

Sanger founded the American Birth Control League, which eventually became the Planned Parenthood Foundation, to provide birth control information and services to women. She also started the first birth control clinic in the United States. Sanger dedicated herself to providing contraceptive information to women and was subjected to prosecution and imprisonment for "mailing obscenities" and "creating a public nuisance." In large part, her arrests and the resulting public outcry led to legal changes permitting contraceptive availability for women (Margaret Sanger, 2013).

Sanger was also instrumental in the development of birth control pills, or a "magic pill" that women could take as easily as aspirin. She recruited a reproductive specialist, Gregory Pincus, to begin development of a hormonal contraceptive and found funding for the project through Katherine McCormick, widow of the International Harvester magnate. This project eventually resulted in FDA approval of the first birth control pill in 1960 (Margaret Sanger, 2013). Sanger died in 1966, just after the U.S. Supreme Court ruled that private use of contraceptives by married couples was legal (Margaret Sanger Papers Project, 2010).

Sanger's contributions to women's health are not uncontroversial, and she is reviled by some as being racist because of her eugenicist beliefs. Those beliefs are used by some as evidence of a conspiracy to limit the African American population (Goldberg, 2012). Her grandson, however, noted that Sanger saw women as "natural eugenicists" striving to improve the health of their children (and subsequently the overall gene pool) by limiting their number through birth control (Margaret Sanger, 2013). In addition, in a 1957 interview with TV commentator, Mike Wallace, archived by the University of Texas at Austin's Harry Ransom Center, Sanger herself cited her motivation as the need to prevent the pain and suffering of women forced by legal sanctions to bear child after child (*Mike Wallace Interview,* 1957). She also voiced her concern about population control. Finally, the point is made that recognition of racism on Sanger's part would have precluded Martin Luther King, Jr.'s acceptance of Planned Parenthood's Margaret Sanger award in 1966, and his praise of her for launching "a movement which is obeying a higher law to preserve human life under humane conditions" (Goldberg, 2012, p.6).

Some of Sanger's beliefs, for example the desirability of involuntary sterilization of the mentally incompetent, are admittedly appalling and foreign to today's nursing advocacy for the rights of the disenfranchised, and should not be upheld; however, her contribution to access to contraceptive information and services for all women in the face of extreme opposition should be recognized.

Advocacy Now

Dorothy Irene Height and Women's Rights

For much of her 98 years of life, Dorothy Irene Height fought for the rights of African Americans, women, and the underprivileged. Encouraged by her mother to obtain an education, Height was denied admission to Barnard College, although accepted, because the institution had already filled its quota of African American students. Instead she earned her undergraduate degree in psychology and social work at New York University, then went on to earn a master's in Educational Psychology and finally a doctoral degree (Williams, 2011).

A victim of both racial and gender-based discrimination herself, Height was actively involved in the National Council of Negro Women, which she headed for more than 20 years. Initiatives of the organization focused on women's rights, including equal employment and education for women.

Height was the only woman included in the United Council of Civil Rights Leaders and supported a campaign to register African American voters through a "Wednesdays in Mississippi" initiative bringing northern women to Jackson, Mississippi to promote voting rights (Shulman, 2012). She later extended her human rights activities on an international basis through the Women's Federation of the World Council of Churches (NASW Foundation, 2004).

At her 2010 memorial service in Washington, DC, speakers noted her ability to build coalitions to direct attention to the needs of all disadvantaged individuals and for "fighting against all our nation's evil isms: racism, sexism, classism, and ageism" (Cosby as quoted in Williams, 2011, p. 8). Similarly, President Barrack Obama praised Height's ability "to make us see the drive for civil rights and women's rights not as a separate struggle, but as part of a larger movement to secure the rights of all humanity, regardless of gender, regardless of race, regardless of ethnicity" (as quoted in Williams, 2011, p. 8).

Women's health encompasses the health status of women as well as the factors that promote or impede health. Population health nursing has long been involved in strategies and interventions to improve the health of individual women and of women as a population group.

In 2010, women constituted 51.5% of the U.S. population over 18 years of age (U.S. Census Bureau, 2012a). By 2015, women are projected to comprise a similar proportion of the population (51.3%) (U.S. Census Bureau, 2012b). About 64% of U.S. women in 2010 were between the ages of 20 and 64 years, and 10% were over 65 years of age (Howden & Meyer, 2011). The health care needs of this latter group are addressed in Chapter 19∞. In this chapter, we will focus on the care of young and middle adult women.

Distinctions are made between the terms sex and gender as they relate to men and women. **Sex** is an individual characteristic determined by biological parameters, the differential possession of X and Y chromosomes. **Gender**, on the other hand, is a social construction encompassing behavioral expectations that are loosely associated with one's biological sex but are culturally defined and vary from one cultural group to another. Two perspectives on gender have been suggested: an equality perspective and a difference perspective (Annandale, 2009). In the equality perspective, women should have parity with men and have equal access to valued spheres of life such as education, employment, and so on. The focus in an equality perspective is on overall health status. The difference perspective views men and women as equal but different as a result of biological differences. Emphasis is on control of one's own body and the focus is more on reproductive health than health in general.

Some authors point to the paradox in the health status of men and women. Women live longer than men, but experience greater levels of illness and disability. In part, the difference lies in the types of health problems experienced by men and women. Men tend to experience more acute life-threatening conditions, while women have more chronic debilitating conditions that do not result in death. Worldwide, the average life expectancy for women in 2011 was 72 years compared to only 68 years for men, with a slightly larger longevity advantage for women in the Americas (79 years for women and 73 years for men) (World Health Organization [WHO], 2013). In 2010, a 65-year-old man in the United States could expect to live another 17.7 years, compared to 20.3 years for a woman of 65 (National Center for Health Statistics [NCHS], 2013).

The importance of improving the health of women in the United States is reflected in the national health objectives for the year 2020. Multiple objectives specifically target the health needs of women (U.S. Department of Health and Human Services [USDHHS], 2014). These objectives can be viewed by accessing the *Healthy People 2020* website; selected objectives are included at the end of this chapter.

Population Health Nursing and Women's Health

Population health nursing care of women involves use of the nursing process at both individual and population levels. Assessment of women's health status addresses each of the categories of determinants of health to identify factors contributing to health and illness in this population. Planning and implementation of interventions geared toward health promotion and illness/injury prevention, resolution of existing health problems, and restoration of health are also part of population health nurses' care of women. Finally, population health nurses evaluate the effects of care on women's health status at individual and population levels.

Assessing the Health Status of Women

Factors influencing women's health status occur in each of the six categories of health determinants. In this chapter, we will briefly examine factors in the biophysical, psychological, environmental, sociocultural, behavioral, and health system dimensions that contribute to health and illness among women. Assessment of the female population can

Global Perspectives

Addressing Women's Health Issues

A 2009 report by the World Health Organization (WHO, 2009a) contended that women are significantly disadvantaged with respect to health status and health care throughout the world. In part, disparities between men and women are due to lack of attention to some problems that affect only women, differential impact of some health conditions on men and women and the subsequent need to tailor services specifically to women's needs, differential access to health care services, and women's more limited ability to wield resources needed to protect and promote their health. The WHO report delineates concerns for disparities throughout women's life spans from childhood through adolescence, childbearing years, and old age (WHO, 2009a).

Differences in women's health status also occur from one nation to another. The table below indicates the top causes of mortality for females of all ages in low-, middle-, and high-income countries. These findings suggest that different strategies are needed in different parts of the world to effectively address women's health issues.

WHO recommendations for improving women's health status worldwide include the following:

- Developing strong leadership that incorporates participation of women in setting health priorities and agendas that go beyond maternal mortality and reproductive health.
- Promoting "gender mainstreaming" to minimize male-female inequities that affect health. *Gender mainstreaming* is a process of considering the implications of all actions, including legislation, policies, and health care delivery programming, for the health of both men and women. It involves "making women's as well as men's concerns and experiences an integral dimension of the design, implementation, monitoring, and evaluation of policies and programmes in all political, economic, and societal spheres, so that women and men benefit equally and inequality is not perpetuated" (United Nations Economic and Social Council, as quoted in WHO 2009a, p. 74).
- Building accountability in government systems by tracking and monitoring indicators of health.
- Developing health services and programs that
  - Respond specifically to women's health needs.
  - Promote women's autonomy and participation in decision making related to their health.
- Promoting universal access to care.
- Removing gender-based differentials in public policy, particularly with respect to property rights; employment accessibility, promotion, and compensation; education; health promotion services; economic opportunity; access to resources, including technology; gender-based discrimination, norms, and policies; violence; and opportunities for older women to contribute productively.
- Tracking progress toward achievement of health-related goals and targets. (WHO, 2009a)

Differences in Female Causes of Death in Low-, Middle-, and High-income Countries

Low-income Countries	Middle-income Countries	High-income Countries
Lower respiratory infections	Stroke	Ischemic heart disease
Ischemic heart disease	Ischemic heart disease	Stroke
Diarrheal diseases	Chronic obstructive pulmonary disease	Alzheimer's and other dementias
Stroke	Lower respiratory infections	Lower respiratory infections
HIV/AIDS	Hypertensive heart disease	Breast cancer
Maternal conditions	Diabetes mellitus	Trachea, bronchus, and lung cancer
Neonatal infections	HIV/AIDS	Colon and rectal cancers
Prematurity and low birth weight	Breast cancer	Chronic obstructive pulmonary disease
Malaria	Stomach cancer	Diabetes mellitus
Chronic obstructive pulmonary disease	Trachea, bronchus, and lung cancer	Hypertensive heart disease

Source: World Health Organization. (2009b). *Women's health.* Retrieved from http://www.who.int/mediacentre/factsheets/fs334/en/index.html

be conducted using the *Population Health Assessment and Intervention Guide* included in the *Assessment Guidelines* for Chapter 15∞. A tool to assess the health of an individual woman is also included in the *Assessment Guidelines* on the student resources site.

BIOLOGICAL DETERMINANTS. Biological factors are of concern to the population health nurse working to improve the health of women in the community. Specific areas for consideration include genetic inheritance, maturation and aging, and physiologic function.

Genetic inheritance. Women are prone to a number of genetically related or genetically linked conditions. For example, cancers of the breast have been shown to occur more frequently among women whose mothers, sisters, aunts, or grandmothers have had similar cancers. Similarly, diseases of the thyroid gland seem to occur more frequently among women than men, as do diabetes, asthma, various forms of dermatitis, and hay fever–type allergies, all of which may involve genetic predisposition to disease.

Maturation and aging. In general, physical maturation of females follows the developmental schedule typical of children. Sexual maturation, however, follows a unique trajectory in women. Stages of sexual maturation and the relevant time periods are presented in Table 18-1 ●. As we saw in Chapter 16∞, menarche occurs at slightly different ages in different racial and ethnic groups.

Premenopause is the period of a woman's life in which she is most likely to become pregnant, the years of fertility. These childbearing years generally last from menarche to age 44, when women enter the perimenopausal period. In 2008, approximately 61.7 million U.S. women were of childbearing age (Dye, 2010).

Menstruation during premenopause is usually free of medical complications. Some women, however, experience dysmenorrhea or premenstrual syndrome. **Dysmenorrhea** is painful menstruation, usually manifested in abdominal cramping. **Premenstrual syndrome (PMS)** includes a variety of physical or emotional symptoms that occur 7 to 10 days prior to menstruation and disappear shortly after menstruation starts (Gallenberg, 2012). In addition, 3% to 8% of women may be affected by **premenstrual dysphoric disorder (PMDD)**, a condition of depressed mood and irritability severe enough to interfere with interpersonal relationships and everyday activities. Both PMS and PMDD may be related to hormonal changes that occur during the menstrual cycle. Other possible contributing factors include alcohol abuse, being overweight, excessive caffeine intake, a family history of PMDD, or lack of exercise (*Premenstrual dysphoric disorder*, 2013).

Perimenopause is a transition period between premenopause and menopause, when the physical and hormonal changes that herald cessation of menstruation occur. Perimenopause may begin as early as the 30s in some women, but more typically begins in the 40s (Mayo Clinic Staff, 2012). Perimenopause is characterized by less predictability regarding menstrual cycles in terms of frequency, duration, and amount of bleeding. Perimenopause may also be associated with a variety of vasomotor symptoms, sleep disturbance, anxiety, and depression. Hormone replacement therapy may be effective in addressing the discomforts of the perimenopausal period. Some herbal preparations, such as black cohosh and plant phytogens, may also be used to deal with the symptoms associated with perimenopause. Population health nurses should be aware of the extent to which these preparations are used by women in the community, as well as their knowledge about potential adverse effects. There is some evidence to suggest that the discomforts experienced by some women during perimenopause are, at least in part, a function of cultural expectations. For this reason, population health nurses should also explore cultural beliefs, attitudes, and behaviors related to perimenopause and

TABLE 18-1 Stages of Female Sexual Maturation

Sexual Characteristic	Stage Description	Related Ages
Pubic hair development	1. Prepubertal: similar to hair on the abdomen	Childhood
	2. Sparse growth of long, pigmented, straight or slightly curly hair	9.4 years–10.6 years
	3. Sparsely distributed, longer, darker, more curly hair	10.5 years–11.8 years
	4. Coarser adult type hair not yet spread to medial thighs	11.9 years–13.1 years
	5. Adult quality hair in classic triangular distribution, may extend to medial aspects of thighs	14.7 years–16.3 years
Breast development	1. Prepubertal: No breast tissue, slightly elevated nipple	Childhood
	2. Wider, darker, elevated areola, palpable bud of glandular tissue below areola	9.4 years–10.3 years
	3. Further enlargement of breast and areola, rounded contour, no contour change between areola and breast	10.7 years–11.7 years
	4. Projection of papilla and areola as secondary mound above breast	12.2 years–13.2 years
	5. Mature adult breast, loss of secondary mound	13.9 years–15.4 years (may never occur in some women)

Data from: American Academy of Pediatrics. (2012). *Sexual maturity stages.* Retrieved from https://www.pediatriccareonline.org/pco/ub/view/PPP/312032/all/Sexual%20 Maturity%20Stages%20?amod=aapea&login=true&nfstatus=401&nftoken=00000000-0000-0000-0000-000000000000&nfstatusdescription=ERROR%3a+No+local+token

menopause among women in the community. The effects of perimenopause may also arise from socioeconomic factors in women's lives, but it is at present unknown how much psychological distress is the result of hormonal changes and how much derives from socioeconomic and cultural influences.

Menopause is defined by WHO as "the permanent cessation of menstruation resulting from the loss of ovarian follicular activity or follicle depletion" (Weismiller, 2009, p. 199). Menopause has occurred when the woman has been without menses for 12 months (Mayo Clinic Staff, 2012). The average age for menopause is 51 years, but normal menopause can occur as early as age 40. Some women experience menopause as a result of surgical interventions such as hysterectomy. Early menopause may be associated with increased health problems such as osteoporosis and increased mortality risk. Hormonal treatments commonly used to treat the discomforts of menopause have also been linked to increased risk of heart attack, breast cancer, stroke, and blood clots (NCCAM, 2012).

Postmenopause is the period of time that extends from menopause until death and may cover as much as one third of women's lives. Because of the hormonal changes that occur with menopause, the postmenopausal period is a time of increased risk for a number of health problems. Several of these, such as osteoporosis and heart disease, are discussed in the section addressing physiologic function. Population health nurses may engage in advocacy to change negative social attitudes toward perimenopausal and menopausal women. Conversely, they may assist women to deal effectively with the effects of these negative attitudes as well as the physical discomforts of menopause. Finally, population health nurses can be actively involved in educating women to minimize the negative effects of menopausal changes (e.g., bone loss) on their health.

Other areas for consideration with respect to maturation and aging include the effects of aging in general on health status (which will be addressed in Chapter 19∞) and women's emotional maturation.

Physiologic function. Physiologic function is another biological determinant influencing the health of women as a population group. Specific considerations related to physiologic function include the incidence and prevalence of specific illnesses and functional limitations, reproductive issues of pregnancy and infertility, and immunization levels.

Physical illness and disability. Women are affected by a variety of acute and chronic illnesses that may not occur in men (e.g., uterine cancer), have different risk factors and manifestations than for the same diseases in men, or may require different approaches to treatment than the same diseases in men. Women are more likely than men to experience multiple chronic diseases and to be disabled as a result of them. In addition, physiologic differences in drug metabolism between men and women lead to differences in treatment effects. Several conditions and their effects on women will be discussed here. In addition, women are more likely to experience disability with chronic conditions than men, so the prevalence and effects of disability in women are also examined. The leading causes of mortality in U.S. women in 2010 were compared to those for men in Chapter 17∞ and included heart disease; malignant neoplasms; cerebrovascular disease; chronic lower respiratory diseases; Alzheimer's disease, unintentional injury; diabetes mellitus; influenza and pneumonia; nephritis, nephrotic syndrome, and nephrosis; and septicemia (NCHS, 2013).

Heart disease accounts for 25% of deaths among U.S. women. In addition, women more often experience uncommon symptoms of heart attack and are less likely than men to seek care (Division for Heart Disease and Stroke Prevention, 2013). Women are less likely than men to have heart disease, but are almost as likely to have hypertension and more likely than men to experience stroke (NCHS, 2012). Overall breast cancer mortality among women in 2010 was 22.1 per 100,000 women and increased with age. Homicide mortality among women of all ages in the same year was 2.3 per 100,000 population and suicide mortality was 5 per 100,000 women (NCHS, 2013).

Other conditions affecting women may not cause death but contribute to significant morbidity. For example, women are more likely than men to have emphysema, asthma, hay fever, sinusitis, and chronic bronchitis, as well as ulcers, kidney disease, diagnosed arthritis, and other chronic joint symptoms (NCHS, 2012).

Women are slightly less likely than men to have diabetes, but are more likely to have their diabetes under control (NCHS, 2013). Similarly, approximately 28% of women have hypertension compared to more than 30% of men, but nearly half of the women affected have their blood pressure under control

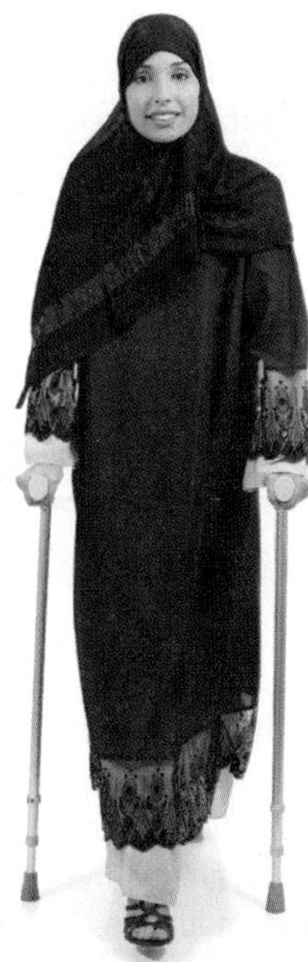

Women are more likely than men to experience disability.
(Antonioguillem/Fotolia)

(Keenan & Rosendorf, 2011). The prevalence of overweight and obesity among women, however, is less encouraging. After 20 years of age, approximately 29% of women become obese compared to only 26% of men. Overweight prevalence among women increases with age to 37% of those aged 40 to 59 years (Freedman, 2011).

Human immunodeficiency virus (HIV) infection and acquired immune deficiency syndrome (AIDS) are other diseases that affect large numbers of women. Although initially considered a disease of gay men, the proportion of women affected has steadily risen. Between 1990 and 2010, for example, the proportion of new AIDS cases involving women increased from 11% to 21% (Division of HIV/AIDS Prevention, 2014). Advocacy by population health nurses is needed to increase efforts to protect women from HIV infection, particularly in cultural groups where women are not empowered to insist on condom use by their partners. Population health nurses may also advocate for available screening and treatment services for women.

Osteoporosis is another physiologic condition of concern for women during the perimenopausal and postmenopausal years. **Osteoporosis** is a "systematic skeletal disorder characterized by low bone mass and microarchitectural deterioration of bone tissue predisposing to an increased risk for fracture" (Lash, Nicholson, Velez, Harrison, & McCort, 2009, p. 182). Approximately 8 million U.S. women and 2 million men have osteoporosis, which results in 1.5 million fractures annually, including 300,000 hospitalizations and 180,000 nursing home placements for hip fractures alone. More than half of postmenopausal women in the United States have decreased bone mineral density, and 16% of them have osteoporosis. Like many conditions, the prevalence of osteoporosis increases with age, with women over age 80 having a rate of disease 10 times higher than those in their 50s. Approximately 20% of people with osteoporotic fractures require long-term care, and the estimated annual cost for hip fractures alone amounts to $15 billion (Lash et al., 2009).

Osteoporosis has a variety of causes, including long-term use of certain medications (e.g., glucocorticoids and other immunosuppressants, hormonal and anti-hormonal agents, and some anti-convulsants), renal failure, hypogonadism, and alcoholism. Osteoporosis may also occur as a result of cancer therapies or organ transplant (Lash et al., 2009).

In addition to causing mortality and morbidity in the population, many of the conditions discussed above, as well as others, contribute to disability among women. Disability results from an interaction between a person's functional abilities and the environment and tends to increase with increasing age. Women are more likely than men to have difficulty with all types of physical activity. In addition, women are more likely to have vision problems and to be edentulous (NCHS, 2012). In 2011, for example, nearly 15% of women needed assistance with personal care activities compared to roughly 10% of men, and women were in need of more physical assistance in all physical activity categories (NCHS, 2011). In addition, nearly two thirds of women, versus just over half of men, have difficulty with at least one basic activity. Similarly, more women than men have difficulty with at least one complex activity related to self-care, have difficulty seeing even with corrective lenses, and are more likely to rate their health as fair or poor (NCHS, 2013).

Pregnancy. Pregnancy and related issues are unique to women and should be considered in assessing biological determinants of women's health. Half of all U.S. pregnancies (51%) are unintended often leading to abortion. In 2008, for example, 40% of unintended pregnancies were aborted. For unintended pregnancies ending in birth, 65% were funded by public insurance. The overall public cost for unintended pregnancy was $12.5 billion (Guttmacher Institute, 2013b).

U.S. rates of unintended pregnancy are higher than many other developed nations, and approximately 30% of U.S. women become pregnant before the age of 30 (Planned Parenthood Federation of America, 2012). Unintended pregnancy is related to poverty, cohabitation, membership in minority groups, lower educational level, and younger age. Unintended pregnancy is also associated with delayed prenatal care, premature birth, and physical and mental effects for both mother and child (Guttmacher Institute, 2013b). *Healthy*

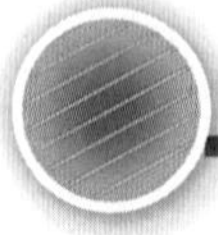

Evidence-Based Practice

Contraceptive Options

Women with chronic health conditions are often limited in the use of various forms of contraception in the mistaken belief that particular methods are contraindicated. To eliminate these mythical contraindications, the Centers for Disease Control and Prevention (CDC) has developed evidence-based guidelines for providers to use in joint contraceptive decision making with women clients. Use of these guidelines is intended to reduce the high rate of unintended pregnancy among American women. The guidelines were published in 2010 and were based on medical eligibility criteria established by WHO in 2009. The guidelines are based on recent evidence-based data and should supercede what is included in product information inserts that are often outdated (Turok, Wysocki, Grimes, & Deal, 2011).

The guidelines are updated periodically. In fact, in 2012, revised guidelines were published related to the use of hormonal contraceptives for HIV-infected women and those at high risk for infection (CDC, 2012). For more information about the most recent guideline, see the *External Resources* section of the student resources site.

People 2020 objectives include the goal of reducing unintended pregnancies to 10% of all pregnancies.

More than half of unintended pregnancies are the result of failure to use contraceptives. Approximately two thirds of women at risk for an unintended pregnancy use contraception consistently and correctly (Guttmacher Institute, 2013b); those who use contraceptives consistently and correctly account for only 5% of unintended pregnancies. As of 2012, approximately 11% of women at risk for unintended pregnancies did not engage in regular use of contraceptives. Rates of nonuse are highest among adolescents (18%) and lowest among women 40 to 44 years of age. Lack of access to and promotion of long-acting contraceptive options (e.g., hormonal implants, intrauterine devices) also contribute to the problem, particularly among women without a steady sexual partner. Use of such options addresses the unplanned nature of many sexual encounters. Based on 2009 data, 8.5% of women using contraceptives used long-acting reversible methods, up from 2.4% in 2002. Use of emergency contraception after unprotected intercourse is also low (Guttmacher Institute, 2013a).

Even when pregnancy is intended and desired, it gives rise to needs for care and poses risks to the health of the woman and fetus. Early prenatal care promotes mother and child health, but is often lacking. In 2011, for example, not quite 74% of U.S. women received care in the first trimester of pregnancy, and 6% began care in the third trimester or received no care at all. Teenagers and members of ethnic minority groups were least likely to receive early care (Maternal and Child Health Bureau [MCHB], 2013).

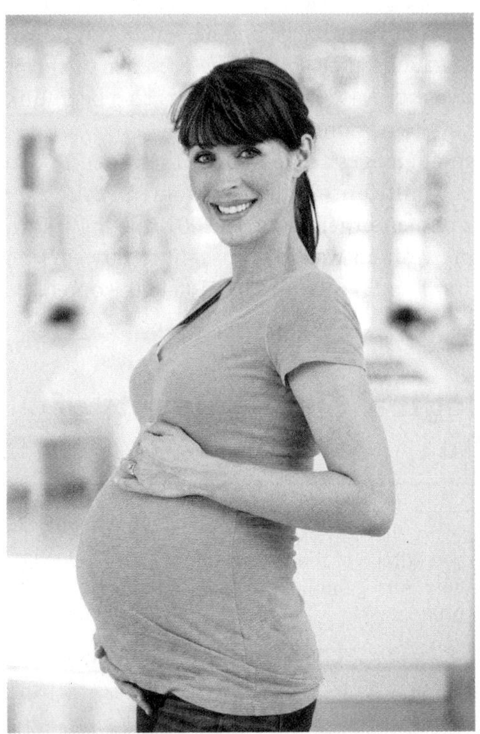

Health promotion for women and their children should begin before conception. *(Monkey Business/Fotolia)*

Lack of prenatal care is a significant contributor to complications of pregnancy such as gestational diabetes mellitus, preeclampsia, and toxemia. **Gestational diabetes mellitus (GDM)** is a condition characterized by increased blood glucose levels resulting from the body's inability to meet the increased insulin needs posed by pregnancy (National Diabetes Information Clearinghouse [NDIC], 2013). Anywhere from 2% to 10% of pregnant women develop GDM, but new diagnostic criteria have suggested incidence as high as 18% of pregnant women. One to two thirds of these women will go on to develop type 2 diabetes in 10 to 20 years (NDIC, 2013). GDM can be prevented through attention to diet and exercise, and population health nurses can assist prepregnant women to lose extra weight and promote adequate diet and physical activity among those who are pregnant.

Preeclampsia and eclampsia are other pregnancy-related conditions that may affect maternal and child health. Preeclampsia and eclampsia are sometimes referred to as pregnancy-induced hypertension (PIH) and are characterized by a rapid elevation in blood pressure that may result in seizures, stroke, organ failure, and death. Risk factors include early teenage years or age over 40 years, first pregnancy, obesity, multiple pregnancies, connective tissue diseases, and chronic hypertension, diabetes, and kidney disorders. Preeclampsia occurs in approximately 5% to 8% of pregnancies worldwide. Eclampsia accounts for 13% of maternal deaths (18% of maternal deaths in the United States) and 15% of premature deliveries. In addition, it is the most common reason for the decision to perform a cesarean section. Signs and symptoms of preeclampsia and eclampsia include sudden weight gain, elevated blood pressure, edema, headache, changes in vision, and proteinuria, all of which are monitored closely by population health nurses caring for pregnant women (Preeclampsia Foundation, n.d.).

Pregnancy may also complicate control of other health conditions, for example, diabetes and thyroid disorders. Hormonal changes that occur in pregnancy may have differential effects on several autoimmune diseases, improving some and worsening others. For example, lupus erythematosis may become worse during pregnancy, or after delivery, and common symptoms of pregnancy must be distinguished from a flareup (Khurana & Isaacs, 2014). Conversely, rheumatoid arthritis may improve (Temprano & Chelmow, 2013).

Some women must cope with fetal or infant death. As noted earlier, culture plays a significant role in the response to the death of an infant. Fetal loss also leads to depression and anxiety in subsequent pregnancies for both partners, but more so for women than men. Population health nurses can assist women who have lost infants to cope with their grief. For example, nurses may link these women to support groups or counseling services. They may also need to advocate for time to grieve with family members or friends who expect the woman to "grieve, and then get on with her life."

Even a pregnancy with a normal course and favorable outcome may result in problems for the mother. For example, some women may experience postpartum depression that has significant health effects for them and their children. Postpartum or postnatal depression (PND) is characterized by dysphoric mood, feelings of guilt, inadequacy in the maternal role, anxiety, poor sleep and appetite, excessive fatigue and emotional lability (Wylie, Martin, Marlands, Martin, & Rankin, 2011). Overall incidence of PND has been estimated at 13% of women within 1 month of delivery (Letourneau, Duffet-Leger, Dennis, Sewart, & Tryphonopoulos, 2010). Postpartum depression in mothers has been associated with delayed language development and behavior problems in their children. In addition, a depressed mother is less likely to be able to effectively care for and nurture her infant.

Development of postpartum depression appears to be mediated by social support and cultural factors. The postpartum period is characterized by major changes and adjustments in women's lives. During this time women need to recover from the physical stresses of pregnancy and delivery, while meeting the needs of their newborn infants and often maintaining other responsibilities as well. Refugee women may be particularly susceptible to PND due to the stress of immigration, social isolation and lack of social support, and lack of financial resources (O'Mahony & Donnelly, 2010).

Immunizations are the last aspect of physiologic function to be considered in relation to women's physiologic health status. Women's immunization rates, like those for all adults, are lower than recommended. Immunizations of particular concern for women include rubella and tetanus vaccine, as well as other vaccines that create antibodies that can cross the placental barrier and provide protection for newborn infants. Women should also receive HPV, influenza, and other immunizations as appropriate. Some questions that can assist the population health nurse to assess biological determinants of women's health are provided in the *Focused Assessment* below.

PSYCHOLOGICAL DETERMINANTS. Psychological factors can have a profound effect on women's health. Areas of particular concern are stress and coping abilities and mental health and illness in the female population.

Stress and coping. The first area for consideration related to psychological determinants of women's health is the extent of women's exposure to stress and their abilities to cope with that stress. It is well known that stress contributes to a variety of illnesses in both men and women. For example, stress plays a part in the development of tuberculosis and hypertension. Severe life events and the stress that accompanies them have also been shown to be related to breast cancer in women. Women, in general, have been found to be less happy and to experience more stress than men. Although women tend to experience more stress than men, they often have better coping skills and are more likely than men to seek social support to deal with stress.

Sources of stress for women include stresses related to interpersonal relationships, financial status, children, and family health. Women generally tend to use confrontive, rather than avoidance, coping strategies.

Mental health and illness. Women often internalize emotional stress, leading to internalized disorders such as depression and anxiety. In one national study, nearly 4% of women over the age of 18 reported experiencing serious psychological distress in the past 30 days, compared to less than 3% of men (NCHS, 2013). Incidence rates for depression are 50% to 100% higher in women than in men. In addition, women experience longer episodes of depression, more frequent recurrences, and more chronic depression than men. Depressed women are also more likely than men to have co-morbid anxiety and other psychiatric disorders (Anxiety and Depression Association of America, n.d.). General risk factors for depression include genetic predisposition, hormonal factors, previous episodes of depression, poor coping, poverty, negative life events and psychosocial stressors, and substance abuse. The presence of chronic illness, particularly cardiovascular disease, has also been linked to the incidence of depression.

Women at all ages are less likely than men to commit suicide, but a significant number of women each year succumb to despair and end their lives. In 2007, the highest rate of suicide among women was for those 40 to 60 years of age, and ranged from 8 to 8.8 suicides per 100,000 women. Population

FOCUSED ASSESSMENT

Assessing Biological Determinants of Women's Health

- What is the age composition of the female population?
- What is the racial/ethnic composition of the female population?
- What are the main causes of mortality in the female population?
- What acute and chronic illnesses are prevalent in the female population? What factors contribute to the prevalence of these conditions?
- What percentage of the female population is of childbearing age? What is the annual birth rate in the population? What is the fertility rate?
- What is the level of immunity to specific communicable diseases among the female population?

estimates of depression in women as well as rates for attempted and completed suicide are important data for an aggregate assessment of women's health.

Other mental health problems that are prevalent among women include eating disorders, post-traumatic stress disorder (PTSD), and chronic fatigue syndrome. As many as 24 million people in the United States experience eating disorders, including anorexia nervosa, bulimia, and binge eating. The vast majority of these people (85% to 90%) are women. Eating disorders tend to manifest most often in adolescence, but can last for a lifetime (National Association of Anorexia Nervosa and Associated Disorders [ANAD], 2014).

Research on women and trauma exposure and its effects suggests that, although women are slightly less likely to be exposed to trauma than men, they are more likely to develop chronic PTSD. Estimates from the National Comorbidity Survey indicate that 50% of women and 60% of men experienced at least one traumatic life event. Rape and sexual assault, parental neglect, childhood physical abuse, domestic violence, and sudden death of a loved one are the most common traumatic events experienced by women. Lifetime estimates of the prevalence of PTSD are twice as high for women as for men (10% vs. 5%) (U.S. Department of Veterans Affairs, 2014). Gender differences in the incidence and prevalence of PTSD in response to traumatic events may stem from women's tendency to blame themselves for the event and the relative importance of interpersonal relationships in women's lives.

Chronic fatigue syndrome (CFS) occurs four times more often in women than in men and most often manifests between 40 and 50 years of age (CDC, 2013). CFS can have severe debilitating effects that profoundly affect one's mental health.

Women also experience schizophrenia, which tends to occur at a later age in women than in men, but symptoms rarely begin after age 45 (National Institute of Mental Health, 2009). Tips for assessing psychological determinants of health for the female population are presented in the *Focused Assessment* below.

ENVIRONMENTAL DETERMINANTS. Physical environmental factors also influence the health of women. They are exposed to physical environmental hazards both at home and in the work setting. In the home, environmental hazards include household chemicals used to clean, inhalants such as powders and sprays, and the potential for falls related to stools, stairs, and throw rugs. The effects of the workplace on women's health are covered later in this chapter during the discussion of the occupational component of the sociocultural dimension. Environmental determinants are particularly evident in rates for accidental injuries. Although women have far lower injury rates than men, significant morbidity and mortality are related to unintentional injuries in women. Another area for consideration is the reproductive effects of environmental pollutants, and the population health nurse should be alert to connections between environmental conditions and adverse pregnancy outcomes in the population. In addition, lack of exposure to sunlight in the physical environment may lead to vitamin D deficiency. Since vitamin D is required for calcium absorption, this physical environmental factor may increase the potential for osteoporosis and fracture injuries. The *Focused Assessment* on the next page provides questions that can guide the population health nurse's assessment of environmental determinants affecting women's health.

SOCIOCULTURAL DETERMINANTS. Many sociocultural factors affect the health status of women. Sociocultural determinants of health appear to be more relevant for women than men and appear to contribute significantly to disparities in health status, self-rated health, functional ability, and chronic conditions between men and women. Some of the more influential factors among these are societal pressures regarding roles and relationships, occupational and economic issues, and violence and abuse.

Roles and relationships. Women often define themselves in terms of relationships with others. Women's roles in these relationships are culturally defined by the society in which they live. Society even specifies how women should look. U.S. entertainment media, in particular, promote a strong cultural value for thinness, often leading women to engage in poor health behaviors and resulting in eating disorders and depression.

Many of women's relationships entail caregiving roles in which they have primary responsibility for the care of children,

FOCUSED ASSESSMENT Assessing Psychological Determinants of Women's Health

- What are the sources of stress to which women in the population are exposed?
- What are the incidence and prevalence of mental illness in the female population? What specific mental health problems are prevalent in the population?
- What is the societal attitude toward women? Does this attitude contribute to stress for women in the population?
- What is the extent of nonheterosexual orientation in the female population? What are the societal attitudes toward nonheterosexual orientation? How does this affect the level of stress experienced by women in the population?

FOCUSED ASSESSMENT Assessing Environmental Determinants of Women's Health

- To what environmental health hazards are women in the population exposed?
- What environmental hazards are posed by occupational settings?
- Are women engaged in recreational pursuits that pose physical environmental hazards?
- To what extent does the physical environment promote or impede healthy behaviors by women (e.g., physical activity)?
- What are the reproductive effects of environmental conditions?

spouses, aging parents, and ill family members that compound the stresses of daily life. In 2010, for example, 55% of U.S. women were married, and more than 20% were divorced or widowed (U.S. Census Bureau, 2012c). In 2009, nearly 30% of all U.S. households with children were headed by single parents (U.S. Census Bureau, 2012g), and in 2012, 84% of more than 12 million single-parent families were headed by women. Approximately half of these female-headed families had incomes below poverty level (Single Mother Guide, 2013).

Women are often responsible for caring for the home and children as well as older family members. In addition, women are often employed outside the home. For example, in 2010, women constituted more than 47% of the U.S. workforce (U.S. Census Bureau, 2012d), but women continue to provide the bulk of family caregiving, caring for both children and aging parents. About 70% of all families with children have adults in the workforce and 25% of U.S. workers also have elder care responsibilities.

Women often need to take time from work to care for family members during major life events, such as the birth of a child or serious illness. The Federal Family and Medical Leave Act provides some coverage for working men and women with family responsibilities, but covers only about half of the workforce. As of 2009, only California and New Jersey had comprehensive paid family leave policies for care of a family member and eight other states had proposed family leave policies. Several other states had more restrictive policies (Weber, 2009).

Child care responsibilities have been shown to pose a cumulative burden for women due to chronic strain that is exacerbated by low levels of resources and low socioeconomic status. Idealized concepts of motherhood, for example, include ideals of sacrifice and may lead to guilt and stigmatization when women choose to work outside the home (Zoellner & Hedlund, 2010). Parenting stress may contribute to lower levels of mental health in mothers of young children that is often compounded by problems with child care and stressful working situations, which results in adverse effects for both parents and children. For example, in one study, maternal depression was associated with parenting stress and limited ability to engage in positive child bedtime routines (Zajicek-Farber, Mayer, & Daugherty, 2012). Suicide rates are highest among middle-aged women 40 to 60 years of age, those most likely to experience multiple stressors related to family responsibilities. In 2007, for example, the suicide rate for women in this age group ranged from 8.0 to 8.8 per 100,000 women (Crosby, Ortega, & Stevens, 2011).

These effects may be mitigated by social support from family and friends. In general, women tend to have larger social networks than men, providing them with more sources of support. For some women, this support comes in the form of electronic social media interactions (Dare & Green, 2011). The assistance of spouses also mitigates the stress of caretaking burdens for married women.

In spite of access to more sources of interpersonal support than men, women often experience inequalities in access to other resources as a result of constraints on the choices within society. These choices may be constrained at any of three levels. At the social policy level, societies may choose to treat men and women equally or differently. For example, decisions could be made to increase social security payments to older women because of wage inequalities experienced during their working lives. Conversely, women may receive lower levels of resources due to continuing perceptions of men as the "family breadwinners." Population health nurses should advocate for examination of the effects of social policy decisions on the health of both women and men.

Women's choices may also be constrained by the extent of their exposure to the hassles of daily life. For example, in a two-parent household, mothers, more often than fathers, are expected to stay home from work with an ill child or to care for aging parents. Similarly, they may be expected to integrate multiple aspects of their lives, for example, combining shopping trips with their daily work commute. Finally, women's choices are constrained by the need to balance work and family responsibilities and the "family unfriendly" nature of many work cultures. These constraints arise because men's and women's work and family roles have not changed as rapidly as changes in social opportunities.

Cultural expectations also define communication patterns in terms of gender. Gender determines appropriate topics of conversation as well as the words and phrases that may appropriately be used. Gender differences lead to the lack of a common language between men and women and contribute to miscommunication, particularly in the area of sexuality, but also in other aspects of life. Cultural factors and related expectations may also lead women to "self-silence" and sacrifice

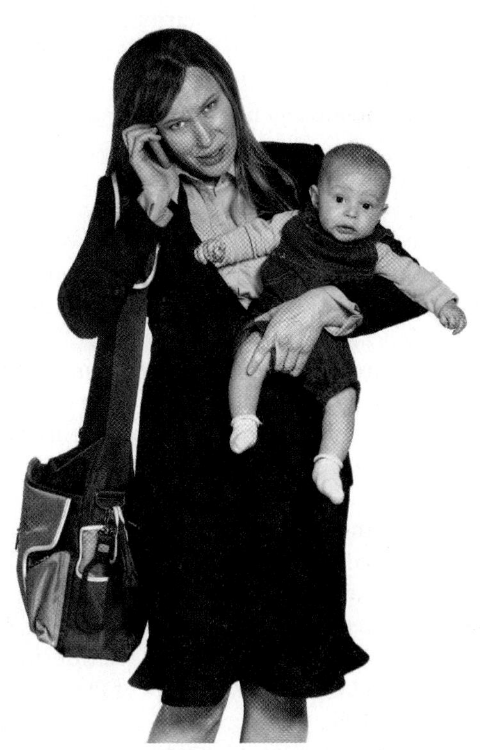

Women may find it difficult to balance work and family roles.
(Scott Griessel/Fotolia)

their own desires to meet social expectations. Self-silencing is often done to avoid conflict, maintain a relationship, or to promote one's physical or psychological safety, but may lead to inner anger and confusion and result in depression (Jack & Ali, 2010). In fact, some authors have noted that risk factors for depression in women "might, more accurately, be conceptualized as proxy variables for a range of rights violations" (Astbury, 2010, p. 23). Some of these often violated rights were delineated by the 1948 United Nations General Assembly Universal Declaration of Rights and include rights to liberty and personal security; freedom from slavery, servitude, torture, or degrading treatment; equality and equal protection before the law; freedom of movement; just and favorable working conditions (including equitable pay); and a standard of living that supports health and well-being (Astbury, 2010).

Other authors have noted that women are disadvantaged by a variety of social justice issues including constraints on reproductive decisions and disproportionate effects of poverty and violence. Causes of social injustice derive from an assumption of a male social norm that leads to gender discrimination in multiple areas (e.g., research, underrepresentation in academic, medical, business, policy formation, government arenas).

Occupational and economic issues. Both occupational and economic issues can have direct and indirect effects on women's health. More than 15% of adult women in the United States lived in poverty in 2009, and employed women earned just 80% of men's income for the same jobs. Salary discrepancies are worse for women with baccalaureate degrees or higher levels of education (U.S. Census Bureau, 2012e, 2012f).

Economic status also influences one's housing adequacy. Women are generally less likely than men to experience homelessness. In 2009–2010, for example, roughly one third of sheltered homeless individuals were women (Substance Abuse and Mental Health Services Administration [SAMSHA], 2011). Women, however head up nearly two thirds of homeless families with children (National Coalition for the Homeless, 2011). In large part, the increasing numbers of homeless women with children arises from low-wage employment and welfare reform that has minimized support to low-income families (National Coalition for the Homeless, 2012). Even when women are housed, they are more likely than men to live in inadequate housing. For example, in 2009, 4.9% of men lived in inadequate housing units (those with plumbing, heating, electrical, or upkeep deficiencies) compared to 5.5% of women. Similarly, 24.6% of female householders lived in unhealthy housing units with rodents, leaks, peeling paint, and no smoke alarms, in addition to the characteristics of inadequacy noted above, compared to 22.5% of men (Raymond, Wheeler, & Brown, 2011).

Lower income is frequently associated with higher incidence of disability, chronic disease, and generally poor health; and women's health status has been shown to decline as their income declines.

Many women in the paid labor force continue to work in traditional "women's jobs" such as nursing, teaching, the garment industry, and secretarial/clerical and service jobs. Although considered "women's work," these jobs are not without health risks. Physical risks arise from chemicals, radiation, infectious disease, noise, vibration, and repetitive movements. Employed women may also experience a higher incidence of musculoskeletal problems than men, possibly due to repetitive work, poor ergonomic work design, and reduced opportunity to rest and exercise at home as a result of family obligations outside of work.

As more women enter the world of "men's work," such as heavy industry, construction, mining, and factory work, they face a different set of physical hazards. Health risks arise from heavy lifting, use of dangerous machinery, and tools that were designed for larger men rather than smaller women. Minority women are at higher risk than White women for job-related injury because they often take jobs that others will not. Their economic need prevents them from saying no or quitting. Women are also more likely than men to work in small companies that do not provide health insurance benefits.

High-tech employment, once touted as safe, also entails health risks. The scrupulously clean area needed to produce a computer chip or to work with computers contains potential threats to human reproduction posed by radiofrequency or microwave radiation, video display terminal radiation, and arsine and chlorine gases. Working women today face essentially the same physical hazards as working men. They have the same risks for reproductive failure, respiratory ailments, skin disorders, and cancer. The health risks of the work setting are discussed in more detail in Chapter 24∞.

The psychological environment of the workplace can be as detrimental to women's health as its physical hazards. For example, studies have shown that it is not the female administrator who suffers the most from stress and depression, but women in the more traditional positions of secretary and clerk. It is postulated that stress is intensified by the lack of freedom to control one's work that secretaries and clerks experience. The "dead-end" quality of these jobs with little possibility of advancement may decrease incentive. In addition, the low salaries available for secretaries and clerks add stresses related to financial insecurity.

Labor force participation by women increases their access to both material and social support, but adds to the burden of their work when combined with family responsibilities. In addition, work increases the potential for toxic exposures and other occupational risks. Women, more often than men, are employed in low-income, high-risk jobs. Even women who work at home are exposed to more risks from the use of hazardous cooking fuels and pesticides.

Social factors in the work environment also affect women's health. The world of work for women differs from that for men in several ways. First, more jobs are open to men than to women. In addition, those jobs that are open to women often provide unequal pay and levels of benefits compared with similar jobs among men. Finally, until a 1991 Supreme Court ruling, women were more often barred from work based on reproductive capacities than were men. Childbearing has also been blamed for women's late entry into the workforce and women's lack of training and education.

Child care is another social environmental factor that creates problems for the working woman. Employer or community assistance with child care is practically nonexistent. Invariably, women must find quality child care on their own. If children are sick, it is usually the mother who stays home, often without pay, to care for them. Work may also interfere with child care responsibilities in other ways. For example, although breastfeeding is encouraged, few places of employment offer private spaces or time for mothers to pump their breasts.

Disproportionate pay between traditional women's jobs and such "men's work" as road construction is a strong incentive for women to seek such jobs. Women who enter male-dominated jobs often feel pressure to prove they are equal to men in ability. They may not speak out against safety hazards because they do not want to appear weak or "unable to take it." Sexual harassment is another problem that may be encountered by women in the work setting. Although there are laws prohibiting such abuse, women may not complain because they need work so badly.

Social factors related to approaching retirement may affect the health status of the middle-aged woman. The woman who is nearing retirement needs to be aware of and plan for the financial shortfalls that are likely to occur with retirement. Leaving the workforce means living in poverty for many older people. Retirement assets are usually tied to lifetime income. Women who worked for low pay and poor benefits will have neither pensions nor full Social Security benefits. A divorced woman may draw Social Security from her ex-husband's account if they were married at least 10 years, but widows face declining incomes following the death of a spouse.

Violence and abuse. Abuse of women is the product of many psychological and sociocultural determinants, and it fosters a psychological environment detrimental to women's health. Because it is primarily social and cultural conditions that allow abuse to occur, the issue is addressed as a sociocultural determinant of women's health.

Women are subjected to a variety of abusive situations throughout the world. These may include abuse during war and social upheaval, sex-selective abortion of female fetuses, honor killings, trafficking, genital mutilation, sexual harassment, objectification in advertising, and restricted educational opportunities (Synnott, 2009). Women may also experience sexual and reproductive coercion, which is defined as "behavior intended to maintain power and control in a relationship related to reproductive health by someone who is, was, or wishes to be involved in an intimate or dating relationship with an adult or adolescent" (American College of Obstetricians and Gynecologists [ACOG], 2013, p. 1). Coercion may involve attempts to impregnate a woman who does not wish to become pregnant, to control pregnancy outcomes (e.g., by urging or forbidding abortion), to force unprotected sexual activity, or to interfere with contraceptive use (ACOG, 2013).

In addition, more than 35% of U.S. women will be subjected to physical abuse, rape or stalking by an intimate partner in their lifetimes (Black et al., 2011). Each year more than 324,000 pregnant women are abused by their partners (ACOG, 2012). According to U.S. Department of Justice statistics, women are four times more likely than men to be victims of rape or assault (Truman, Langton, & Planty, 2013). In addition, the 2012 nonfatal sexual assault injury rate was 49.44 per 100,000 women compared to 5.2 per 100,000 men (National Center for Injury Prevention and Control, 2013). Physical abuse of women often results in death, with the highest rate occurring among women 20 to 24 years of age (4.2 per 100,000 women) and declining with advancing age (Logan, Smith, & Stevens, 2011). Exposure to abuse and to other stressors may also contribute to suicide among women.

Psychological dependence on males and poor self-esteem on the part of both the victim and the abuser are some of the psychological factors resulting in abuse. Feelings of shame and worthlessness may hamper the woman's ability to seek help while in an abusive situation. Societal attitudes toward abused women often compound the problems of abuse for victims. Assessment of violence and other sociocultural determinants affecting women's health can be guided by the questions included in the *Focused Assessment* on the next page.

BEHAVIORAL DETERMINANTS. Behavioral factors also affect the health of women clients. Areas of particular concern include dietary consumption patterns; tobacco, alcohol, and

FOCUSED ASSESSMENT Assessing Sociocultural Determinants of Women's Health

- What are the social roles expected of women? What effects do these role expectations have on women's health?
- What opportunities for social interaction are available to women in the population?
- What is the extent of social support available to women in the population?
- What is the percentage of single-parent families headed by women in the population?
- What is the typical educational status of women in the population?
- What is the economic status of women in the population? Are women allowed to own property in their own names? Are they allowed to control money and other family resources?
- What transportation opportunities are available to women in the population?
- To what extent do women in the population function as caretakers for other family members? To what extent do these women experience caretaker burden?
- What percentage of women in the population is employed? What are the typical occupations for women in the population? What effects do occupation and employment setting have on women's health? What support do employers provide for women's other roles and responsibilities?
- What child care services are available to working women? What is the cost of these services?
- What are the incidence and prevalence of abuse of women in the population? What are the societal attitudes toward abuse of women? What resources are available to abused women in the population?

drug use; physical activity and exercise, and health screening behaviors. Unprotected sexual activity, another behavioral consideration, was addressed in the context of issues related to contraception and pregnancy earlier in the chapter.

Consumption patterns. Dietary concerns may be particularly problematic among women, many of whom are obese or overweight or who engage in fad diets to attain or maintain a fashionably slim figure. Fad dieting is especially prevalent among adolescent females who also have high incidence rates for eating disorders such as bulimia and anorexia nervosa.

Women are more likely than men to be underweight (NCHS, 2012), but slightly less likely to be obese and more likely to eat healthier diets. Unfortunately, women still fail to achieve dietary indicators delineated by *Healthy People 2020*. For example, women eat fewer than the recommended number of servings of fruits and vegetables, and their average sodium and fat intake is higher than recommended (Health Indicators Warehouse, n.d.i, n.d.p, n.d.q, n.d.t).

Smoking is another consumption pattern that is problematic for some women. Although the number of male smokers has declined rather dramatically in the last few years, the number of women who smoke has not declined as rapidly, leading to corresponding increases in lung cancer and heart disease among women. In 2011, approximately two thirds of women were non-smokers, compared to less than half of men (NCHS, 2012). In 2011, 21.2% of men were current smokers, but only 16.8% of women smoked (NCHS, 2013). Several factors contribute to the continued prevalence of smoking among women. These include attempts to control weight, perceptions that smoking controls negative mood, extensive targeting of women by tobacco company advertising, and the dependence of the media on tobacco revenue and sponsorship of women's fashions, athletics, and other events by tobacco companies that stifle media coverage of the negative effects of smoking.

Substance use and abuse among women is another area of concern related to consumption patterns. Although women still tend to abuse alcohol and drugs less often than men, the incidence of such problems among females is increasing. In 2011, roughly one quarter of women abstained from alcohol use, but 43% were engaged in regular use (NCHS, 2012), and a median 17.2% reported binge drinking in 2012 (National Center on Birth Defects and Developmental Disabilities, 2014). In addition, from 2006 to 2010 76% of pregnant women reported alcohol use during pregnancy, and 1.4% reported binge drinking (Marchetta et al., 2012). In general, men tend to have higher rates of alcohol and drug abuse, while women, particularly younger women, are more likely than men to engage in all forms of nonmedical use of prescription drugs (Volkow, 2010).

Women also engage in the use of other drugs. In 2009, for example, 6.8% of women over 12 years of age used any illicit drug, 4.7% used marijuana, and 2.5 made nonmedical use of psychotherapeutic drugs (NCHS, 2013). Drug-induced mortality rates for women were approximately two thirds those of men in 2007 (9.3/100,000 women vs. 15.8/100,000 men) (Paulozzi, 2011). Problems of substance abuse are addressed in Chapter 29∞.

Physical activity and exercise. Another major behavioral determinant that influences women's health is physical activity and exercise. An active lifestyle promotes overall health and is associated with a variety of positive health effects. In spite of the benefits of physical activity, however, less than half of U.S. women engage in sufficient physical activity to meet *Healthy People 2020* goals. In 2011, for example, more than

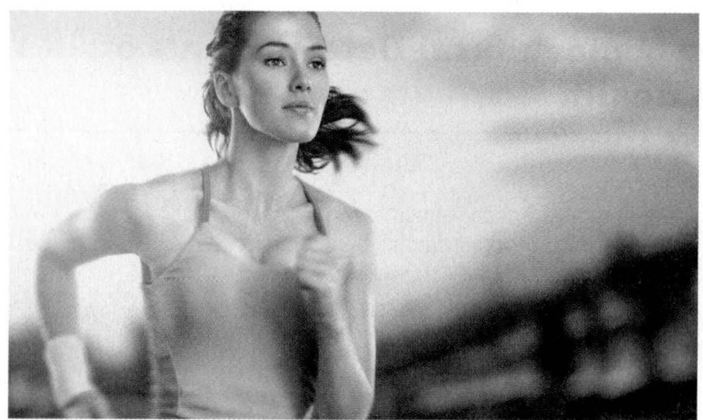

Physical activity is an important aspect of health promotion for women of all ages. *(Konstantin Yuganov/Fotolia)*

half of women (51.5%) met neither aerobic exercise nor muscle strengthening recommendations, and only 17.2% of women met the recommendations for both areas (NCHS, 2013). Women report a number of constraints for physical activity, including job and family demands, fatigue, illness, and lack of facilities and opportunities for physical activity. Other barriers included economics, safety concerns, weather, and the hassles associated with personal care (e.g., showering) after physical activity.

Other health-related behaviors. The final behavioral determinant to be addressed includes behaviors related to health promotion, illness prevention, and screening. Some of these behaviors include health promoting behaviors such as getting sufficient sleep. Others are related to prevention of specific health problems, like immunization and skin cancer prevention, while others reflect women's participation in screening behaviors such as mammography. Table 18-2• presents information on the extent of selected health promotion, illness prevention, and screening behaviors among U.S. women. Questions to guide assessment of behavioral determinants affecting women's health are provided in the *Focused Assessment* on the next page.

HEALTH SYSTEM DETERMINANTS. Lack of attention to women's health needs, lack of illness prevention and health

TABLE 18-2 Women's Use of Selected Health Promotion, Illness and Injury Prevention, and Screening Services

Service	Percentage Use	Data Year
Blood pressure screening	93.5%	2008
Cervical cancer screening	82.8%	2010
Cholesterol screening—in last 5 years	76.8%	2008
Colorectal cancer screening—50–75 years of age	59.1%	2010
Condom use by unmarried females—15–44 years of age	35.1%	2006–2010
Contraceptive use at most recent sexual encounter	83%	2006–2008
Depression screening by primary care provider	2.8%	2010
Flu vaccination—18–64 years of age	28.7%	2008
Flu vaccination—pregnant women	27.6%	2008
HIV testing—pregnant women	72%	2006–2010
HIV status awareness	84.7%	2009
HPV vaccination—girls 13–15 years of age	30%	2011
Mammography—50–74 years of age	72.4%	2010
Oral and pharyngeal cancer early detection	41.5%	2009
Skin cancer protective measures	73.4%	2010
Sufficient sleep	68.8%	2012
Tobacco screening in physican office visits	68.3%	2010

Data from: Health Indicators Warehouse. (n.d.a). *Blood pressure screening: Adults (percent).* Retrieved from http://healthindicators.gov/Indicators/Blood-pressure-screening-adults-percent_883/Profile/Data; Health Indicators Warehouse. (n.d.b). *Cervical cancer screening: Women 21–65 years (percent).* Retrieved from http://healthindicators.gov/Indicators/Cervical-cancer-screening-women-21-65-years-percent_505/Profile/Data; Health Indicators Warehouse. (n.d.c). *Cholesterol screening: Adults (percent).* Retrieved from http://healthindicators.gov/Indicators/Cholesterol-screening-adults-percent_886/Profile/Data; Health Indicators Warehouse. (n.d.d). *Colorectal cancer screening: Persons 50-75 years (percent).* Retrieved from http://healthindicators.gov/Indicators/Colorectal-cancer-screening-persons-50-75-years-percent_506/Profile/Data; Health Indicators Warehouse. (n.d.e). *Condom use: Unmarried females 15–44 years (percent).* Retrieved from http://healthindicators.gov/Indicators/Condom-use-unmarried-females-15-44-years-percent_940/Profile/Data; Health Indicators Warehouse. (n.d.f). *Depression screening by primary care providers: Adults (percent).* Retrieved from http://healthindicators.gov/Indicators/Depression-screening-by-primary-care-providers-adults-percent_1120/Profile/Data; Health Indicators Warehouse. (n.d.g). *Flu vaccination: Adults 18-64 years (percent).* Retrieved from http://healthindicators.gov/Indicators/Flu-vaccination-adults-18-64-years-percent_1033/Profile/Data; Health Indicators Warehouse. (n.d.h). *Flu vaccination: Pregnant women (percent).* Retrieved from http://healthindicators.gov/Indicators/Flu-vaccination-pregnant-women-percent_1038/Profile; Health Indicators Warehouse. (n.d.j). *HIV infection status awareness (percent).* Retrieved from http://healthindicators.gov/Indicators/HIV-infection-status-awareness-percent_942/Profile; Health Indicators Warehouse. (n.d.k). *HIV testing: Pregnant women (percent).* Retrieved from http://healthindicators.gov/Indicators/HIV-testing-pregnant-women-percent_946/Profile/Data; Health Indicators Warehouse. (n.d.l). *HPV vaccination: Girls 13–15 years (percent).* Retrieved from http://healthindicators.gov/Indicators/HPV-vaccination-girls-13-15-years-percent_1013/Profile/Data; Health Indicators Warehouse. (n.d.m). *Mammography: Women 50–74 years (percent).* Retrieved from http://healthindicators.gov/Indicators/Mammography-women-50-74-years-percent_507/Profile/Data; Health Indicators Warehouse. (n.d.n). *Oral and pharyngeal cancer early detection (percent).* Retrieved from http://healthindicators.gov/Indicators/Oral-and-pharyngeal-cancer-early-detection-percent_1264/Profile/Data; Health Indicators Warehouse. (n.d.o). *Skin cancer protective measures: Adults (percent).* Retrieved from http://healthindicators.gov/Indicators/Skin-cancer-protective-measures-adults-percent_504/Profile/Data; Health Indicators Warehouse. (n.d.r). *Sufficient sleep: Adults (percent).* Retrieved from http://healthindicators.gov/Indicators/Sufficient-sleep-adults-percent_1472/Profile/Data; Health Indicators Warehouse. (n.d.s). *Tobacco screening in physician office visits: Adults (percent).* Retrieved from http://healthindicators.gov/Indicators/Tobacco-screening-in-physician-office-visits-adults-percent_1557/Profile/Data

FOCUSED ASSESSMENT Assessing Behavioral Determinants of Women's Health

- What are the dietary consumption patterns typical of women in the population?
- What is the prevalence of smoking among women in the population?
- What is the extent of alcohol, tobacco, and other drug use in the population?
- To what extent do women in the population engage in safety practices (e.g., seat belt use)?
- To what extent do women who are sexually active engage in safe sexual practices?
- What is the extent of contraceptive use in the population?
- To what extent do women engage in health promotion, illness and injury prevention, and screening practices?

promotion resources, and health insurance discrimination are health care system factors that adversely affect women. The medical system tends to focus on female reproductive problems, frequently to the exclusion of other health problems faced by women. Failure to recognize and deal with physical abuse is just one example of failure of the health care system to meet the needs of women. By and large, the health care system has only recently come to recognize the special health needs of the female client.

Services provided by the health care system tend to focus on problem resolution and health restoration following injury or illness. Few efforts are made to provide preventive health care, particularly for women, and those preventive health services that are available are not always offered at a time when busy working women can take advantage of them. Compounding this problem is the lack of provision for child care while women seek preventive health care services.

In a periodic review of state policies affecting women's health, the National Women's Law Center (2010) grades the nation and each state with respect to the achievement of policy goals related to health. For the most part, these goals reflect the *Healthy People 2020* objectives. States are graded F – failing, U – unsatisfactory, S- not quite satisfactory, or S – satisfactory. Table 18-3 summarizes the extent to which some of these major policy goals for women's health have been met by the states.

The cost of health care is a barrier to health service utilization for women. Women are less likely than men to have employment-based health insurance, and they are more likely to work in part-time jobs or jobs that do not offer this benefit. Single women are also less likely to be able to pay the monthly insurance premiums. This situation is particularly hard on divorced and separated women with children who are already faced with financial difficulties. According to NCHS (2013) figures, in 2011, 15.6% of women under 65 years of age had no health insurance and another 19.3% were covered by Medicaid.

Having a regular source of health care is the greatest predictor of the use of preventive services, yet from 2010 to 2011, nearly 15% of women had no regular source of care (NCHS, 2013). By 2011, this figure had decreased slightly to 11% of U.S. women (NCHS, 2012). For many women who do have insurance coverage, it is often as spousal dependents, increasing their loss of insurance in the case of spousal job loss, divorce, or widowhood. Only about a third of women (35%) are covered by their own employment-based insurance plan (Kaiser Family Foundation, 2013). Discontinuous insurance coverage increases lack of access to care due to the inability to develop a relationship with a consistent health care provider. Many uninsured women rely on emergency departments or hospital clinics for care, thereby increasing societal expenses for care.

Even when women do have health insurance coverage, many essential services are not covered or out-of-pocket costs prohibit them from receiving needed services. For example, in 2010, nearly 16% of women aged 18 to 64 years did not get or delayed needed care due to costs. Similarly, 13.5% of women did not get prescriptions filled, and nearly 20% did not receive needed dental services. In 2008, annual mean out-of-pocket costs for services that were received were higher for women than men ($285 and $258, respectively). Lack of access to services is particularly noticeable for preventive care. For instance, only two thirds of women over 40 years of age had received a mammogram in the prior 2 years in 2010, and roughly 74% received a pap smear within the last 3 years (NCHS, 2013).

Prior to recent legislation such as the Affordable Care Act (ACA) and the Health Care and Education Affordability Reconciliation Act of 2010, insurance companies could engage in gender discrimination in premiums, eligibility, and services covered. For example, under some insurance plans, pregnancy could be considered a preexisting condition, which was not covered. Similarly, women could be charged higher premiums than men or be excluded from coverage altogether based on a prior cesarean section. The two pieces of legislation prohibit gender differences in premiums in the individual and small group insurance markets, but continue to allow "gender rating" of premiums in the large group insurance market. For example, at age 25 women in large group employer-sponsored insurance programs could expect to pay 6% to 45% higher premiums than men. Two other provisions of ACA benefit women

TABLE 18-3 Selected Indicators for Women's Health and Their Achievement in the United States

Indicator	Number of States Rated*				National Rating
	S	S-	U	F	
Health insurance		1	14	36	F
Pap smear in the last 3 years		1	39	11	F
Mammogram in the last 2 years	44		2	5	S
Colorectal cancer screening	51				S
Cholesterol screening	23	11	12	5	S-
Leisure time physical activity	4	17	11	19	U
Percentage of obesity		3	13	35	F
Five fruits and vegetables a day			1	50	F
Binge drinking	5	9	9	28	F
Smoking	2	17	12	20	U
Annual dental visit	51				S
Coronary heart disease mortality	1	9	18	23	F
Stroke mortality	1	5	16	29	F
Lung cancer mortality	1	1	5	44	F
Breast cancer mortality	13	27	10	1	S-
High blood pressure		3	17	31	F
Diabetes incidence		1	13	37	F
AIDS rate/100,000	6	44		1	S-
Chlamydia		8	23	20	U
Maternal mortality rate	4	30	13	4	U
Life expectancy		4	21	26	F
Living below poverty level			4	47	F
Eliminate gender wage gap			1	50	F
High school completion	24	11	6	10	U

* Includes District of Columbia

Data from: National Women's Law Center. (2010). *Health care report card: Making the grade on women's health: A national and state by state report card.* Retrieved from http://hrc.nwlc.org/

by mandating preventive screenings for women without higher premiums or co-payments and prohibiting lack of coverage for victims of domestic violence (Pearsall, 2011). The *Focused Assessment* questions below can be used to identify health system determinants affecting the health of the female population.

Diagnostic Reasoning and Women's Health

Based on information obtained during assessment, population health nurses develop nursing diagnoses that direct further interventions. These diagnoses reflect both positive health states and potential or existing health problems and the factors

FOCUSED ASSESSMENT — Assessing Health System Determinants of Women's Health

- What percentage of the female population has a regular source of health care?
- What are the attitudes of women toward health and health care services?
- What percentage of the female population has health insurance coverage?
- What health services are available to women in the population? Are health care services needed by women available to all segments of the population?
- What barriers to obtaining health care do women encounter?
- What are the attitudes of health care providers to care of women? To the care of nonheterosexual women?

contributing to them. Nursing diagnoses might relate to health problems experienced by an individual woman such as "role overload due to employment, single parenthood, and lack of a social support network." Or diagnoses may be made at the aggregate level regarding the health needs of groups of women. An example of a nursing diagnosis at this level might be a "need for adequate and inexpensive child care due to the number of single-parent working women and a lack of affordable child care."

Planning to Meet the Health Needs of Women

In planning to meet the identified health needs of the female population, population health nurses incorporate the general principles of planning discussed in Chapter 15∞. It is important to keep in mind the unique needs of female clients. Participation by women in planning health care services is particularly important in view of the passive and dependent role expected of female clients by health care providers of the past. Women need to be encouraged to be active participants in health care decision making.

Planning and implementing care for groups of women also need to be based on women's unique circumstances. Services should be offered at times when women, especially working women, can take advantage of them. Provision for transportation and child care services during appointments might also need to be considered. Financing of such programs can be problematic, given the lower earning capacity of many women, and political activity to ensure program funding may need to be part of the planning process. Meeting the health needs of female clients may involve planning and implementing health promotion, illness and injury prevention, problem resolution, and health restoration interventions.

HEALTH PROMOTION. Planning and implementing health promotion services for women focus on four main goals:

- Promoting healthy behaviors
- Developing and maintaining healthy relationships and living conditions
- Developing adequate coping strategies
- Promoting healthy pregnancy outcomes

Health promotion measures related to each of the goals will be briefly discussed.

Promoting healthy behaviors. Although women are more likely than men to engage in health promoting behaviors, they still may need assistance in developing and sustaining these behaviors. For example, population health nurses may need to educate women on the elements of a healthy diet or the need for adequate rest and physical activity. Given women's multiple roles, they may also need help in integrating these activities into their busy schedules.

Women may also need encouragement to focus on meeting their own needs and to balance those needs with those of others for whose care they may be responsible. Intervention in this area may be particularly important for single women with children who may be fulfilling both parental roles as well as the breadwinner role. Women caretakers may also need respite from continual demands on their time and energy. Population health nurses can refer to or advocate for the availability of needed supports and services for women. For example, they might assist in the development of respite services for women who care for young children or disabled family members. Or they might advocate with the women themselves, encouraging them to take needed time for themselves and to delegate some of their responsibilities to others if possible.

Developing and maintaining healthy relationships and living conditions. Population health nurses may also assist women to develop and maintain healthy interpersonal relationships. For example, they may help women to develop healthy self-images that contribute to satisfying relationships. This may be particularly true for young women in their development of sexual intimacy. Population health nurses can educate women about sexuality as well as how to resist sexual advances or negotiate contraceptive use. In one study, for example, interviews with 10 young women indicated that none of them attempted to initiate condom use by their partners. In many cases, this failure was based on reliance on the male partner to protect them, being in an abusive situation, or believing they were involved in a monogamous relationship, sometimes even after being informed of a diagnosis of a sexually transmitted infection. In large part, these young women indicated they did not feel empowered to negotiate condom use (East, Jackson, O'Brien, & Peters, 2011).

Sexuality education is needed by women throughout the world. To promote effective education, there is a need for political and social leadership that recognizes women's needs. Resources needed and available for such education as well as social and economic constraints should be identified. In addition, there is a need for preparation of qualified teachers and incorporation of women in the planning of such educational services (Boonstra, 2011).

Young girls approaching menarche, women experiencing perimenopause and menopause, and infertile women may also be in particular need of interventions to assist them to develop or maintain strong self-images. Working women who are entering retirement or mothers who are experiencing the departure of children from the home may need help coming to grips with changes in their roles without feeling devalued or useless. Similarly, women who have decided to leave an abusive situation or obtain a divorce may need assistance in dealing with feelings of guilt, loss, and depression. Population health nurses can provide anticipatory guidance regarding all of these changes and assist women to work through them effectively without diminished self-esteem. In addition, nurses can provide assistance with the practical aspects of change (e.g., menstrual education, referral for hormone replacement therapy [HRT], financial assistance, etc.).

Women can be assisted to develop assertiveness skills as well as to believe in their own self-worth. These skills may help women to refrain from developing unhealthy relationships with men or with others in their environments. There may also be a need to assist women to achieve healthy relationships in the work setting. The population health nurse may work to change the psychosocial environment of the work setting by means of several strategies. These strategies include educating and socializing women to expect wage equity and to believe that their work is as important as a man's, promoting legislation to prevent job discrimination, educating women about their rights, and encouraging women to challenge sexual harassment. The population health nurse working in the occupational setting can provide effective care for women by identifying and understanding stressors affecting women in the work setting, counseling them regarding work options, and assisting them with child care resources. Additional strategies include supporting women running for political office, influencing the legislative process, and promoting collective bargaining, mentoring, and networking among women.

Another major contribution can be made by population health nurses who have clients experiencing role proliferation. These nurses can assist clients to plan efficient use of time, to use outside help when possible, and to let go of minor household duties that can wait. Single women with children may particularly need help in this area.

Population health nurses can also assist women to create healthful living conditions. In 2009, for example, more than 5% of U.S. women lived in inadequate housing, and nearly 25% lived in unhealthy housing units (Raymond et al., 2011). Population health nurses can advocate for healthy housing and other environmental conditions that promote health (e.g., the presence of walking or biking trails in the community). They can also refer women experiencing substandard housing to housing authorities for assistance or to social resources for assistance with rent and so on.

Developing adequate coping strategies. Health promotion for female clients may also involve assistance in the development of coping skills and assertiveness. Interventions can be designed to improve women's self-esteem and to teach them how to cope with life stress in effective ways. Development of coping skills and self-esteem not only assists women in maintaining balance in their lives, but also assists in the development of healthy relationships.

Promoting healthy pregnancies. One health promotion strategy specific to women is provision of prenatal care. Population health nurses can educate women prior to and during pregnancy regarding adequate diet and physical activity and can refer pregnant women for prenatal care services. In addition, they can provide antenatal care monitoring women for risk factors and engage in strategies to modify those risk factors. They can also help women with anticipatory guidance regarding child birth and infant care as well as help them adapt to the changes in interpersonal relationships that occur with the advent of a child. Population health nurses may also need to educate the public regarding the need for early prenatal care and advocate for access to prenatal care services for all segments of the population. Population health nursing strategies for health promotion among women are summarized in Table 18-4●. A prenatal care inventory is included among the *Assessment Guidelines* included on the student resources site. For more information

TABLE 18-4 Health Promotion Strategies for Women

Focus	Strategies
Promoting healthy behaviors	• Educate women regarding the need for nutrition and physical activity • Assist women to integrate healthy diet and exercise behaviors into their schedules • Encourage women to balance their own needs with those of others • Refer women to support and respite services as needed • Advocate for support/respite services
Developing and maintaining healthy relationships and living conditions	• Assist women to develop assertiveness skills • Assist women to develop healthy self-images • Advocate for and provide sexuality education • Assist women to negotiate for safe sexual practice • Provide anticipatory guidance for life transitions • Advocate for changes in psychosocial environments in the work setting • Promote equitable working conditions • Help women with time management skills • Refer women for housing assistance as needed
Developing effective coping strategies	• Teach and model effective coping skills
Promoting healthy pregnancies	• Educate women regarding diet and physical activity before and during pregnancy • Refer pregnant women for prenatal care • Advocate for prenatal services • Provide anticipatory guidance for pregnancy, childbirth, and infant care as well as changes in relationships

on assessing waist circumference and calculating BMI, see the *External Resources* section of the student resources site. A postpartum newborn care inventory is also provided.

ILLNESS AND INJURY PREVENTION. Population health nurses are also actively involved in preventing illness and injury among women.

Illness prevention. Illness prevention interventions focus primarily on screening for and elimination of risk factors and immunization. Population health nurses can provide services to prevent such risk behaviors as smoking, binge drinking, and unprotected sexual activity. Nurses can also refer women who are current smokers to smoking cessation programs to prevent the development of a host of tobacco-related health problems.

Osteoporosis prevention is another important aspect of illness and injury prevention for women, and population health nurses can educate women regarding calcium and vitamin D intake and the need for physical activity as well as the contributions of tobacco and heavy alcohol use to osteoporosis (Lash et al., 2009). They may also refer women with existing osteoporosis for treatment to prevent fractures and subsequent disability.

There is considerable controversy regarding the use of HRT to prevent osteoporosis or treat symptoms of menopause. Growing evidence of possible breast cancer and cardiovascular disease risks related to HRT have led many women to choose natural remedies or bioidentical hormone replacement therapy to deal with menopausal discomforts. A number of botanical preparations, including black cohosh, red clover, *don quai*, ginseng, kava, and soy have been used to treat various menopausal symptoms, but most have been shown to be ineffective or to cause potential harm. For example, black cohosh and kava use may result in liver problems, and *don quai* interacts with warfarin (National Center for Complementary and Alternative Medicine [NCCAM], 2012).

Bioidentical hormone replacement therapy (BHRT) involves the use of laboratory manufactured compounds similar to natural hormones to combat symptoms of menopause. These preparations are not approved by the Food and Drug Administration and can vary widely in their composition. Because their safety and effectiveness have not yet been demonstrated, clients should be cautioned against their use. There is some evidence, however, that mind and body therapies such as yoga, tai chi, qi gong, and acupuncture may provide relief for menopausal symptoms (NCCAM, 2012).

Prevention of sexually transmitted infections (STIs) may involve education regarding condom use or referral for access to condoms and other services. Similarly, preventing unwanted pregnancies may include educating women on contraceptive options and referring them for available services as well as advocating for access to publicly funded family planning services. In 2008, for example, a $1.9 million expenditure on contraceptive services saved more than $7 billion in costs related to unwanted pregnancies. Without public funding for contraceptive services, the costs for unwanted pregnancies could increase to as much as $18 billion per year (Guttmacher Institute, 2013b).

Immunization is another strategy for disease prevention among women. CDC (2014) recommendations for immunization of women are summarized in Table 18-5●. As indicated in the table, women should be routinely immunized for certain conditions and women at high risk for disease should receive additional immunizations.

Injury prevention. Attention should also be given to injury prevention through personal behaviors such as the use of seat belts and other safety devices. In the work setting, population health nurses can encourage women to report safety hazards (or the nurse can report them personally) and foster personal preventive measures such as the use of safety gear and protective devices. With respect to physical activity, women should also be educated regarding prevention of exercise-related musculoskeletal injury and encouraged to be realistic in goal setting and injury prevention.

Prevention of violence against women is another strategy for injury prevention. Women can be educated to identify and avoid dangerous situations. When women are in situations in

TABLE 18-5 Recommended Immunizations for Women 19 to 59 Years

Immunization	Age Group	Comments
Influenza	All ages	1 dose annually
Td/Tdap	All ages	1 dose Tdap, followed by Td booster every 10 years
Varicella	All ages	2 doses (contraindicated in pregnancy)
Human papillomavirus (HPV)	19–26 years	3 doses
Measles, Mumps, Rubella	19–55 years	1 or 2 doses (contraindicated in pregnancy)
Pneumococcal polysaccharide (PPSV23)	19–59 years	1 or 2 doses for women at risk
Pneumococcal 13-valent conjugate (PCV13)	19–59 years	1 dose for women at risk
Meningococcal	19–59 years	1 or more doses for women at risk
Hepatitis A	19–59 years	2 doses for women at risk
Hepatitis B	19–59 years	2 doses for women at risk

Data from: Centers for Disease Control and Prevention. (2014). *Recommended adult immunization schedule – United States – 2014.* Retrieved from http://www.cdc.gov/vaccines/schedules/downloads/adult/adult-schedule.pdf

which the potential for abuse is high, population health nurses can refer them to safe houses and assist them with obtaining physical and legal protection. Nurses can also work for public policies that promote the safety of women and preservation of their rights. Strategies for illness and injury prevention among women are summarized in Table 18-6●.

TABLE 18-6 Illness and Injury Prevention Strategies for Women

Focus	Strategy
Illness Prevention	• Screening for and elimination of risk factors for disease • Osteoporosis prevention through diet and physical activity • STD prevention through monogamous relationships and condom use • Prevention of unwanted pregnancies through access to and use of contraceptive services • Immunization
Injury Prevention	• Promoting safe environments at home and work • Promoting use of safety devices and practices • Advocacy for policies and services that prevent abuse of women

RESOLUTION OF EXISTING HEALTH PROBLEMS. Resolution of existing health problems in the female population focuses on screening, diagnosis, and treatment.

Screening. Several organizations make recommendations for routine screening procedures among women. For example, the American Cancer Society has made recommendations for breast and cervical cancer screening in women. Similarly, the U.S. Preventive Services Task Force has examined evidence regarding the effectiveness of specific screening procedures in different population groups (e.g., men, women, children, adults, and people with specific risk factors) and developed an extensive set of recommendations for routine screening practices. Routine screening procedures specifically recommended for women are summarized in Table 18-7●. Individual women should, of course, also be screened for other health problems for which they may be at risk.

USPSTF (2013b) has recommended screening of women of childbearing age for IPV. As noted earlier, the American

TABLE 18-7 Recommendations for Routine Screening for Women

Type of Screening	Recommendation
Alcohol misuse	All adult women (including pregnant women)
Bacteruria	Pregnant women on the first visit or at 12 to 16 weeks gestation
Breast cancer	Biannual mammography for women aged 50 to 74 years, individualized decision after age 75
Cervical cancer	Papanicolau smear every 3 years age 21 to 65 years or with cytological testing and HPV testing every 5 years in women aged 30 to 35 to extend the screening interval
Chlamydia	Sexually active or pregnant women under 24 years of age and those over 24 who are at risk
Colorectal cancer	Women 50 to 75 years of age by fecal occult blood, sigmoidoscopy, and/or colonoscopy
Depression	Adult women in practice settings where follow-up is available
Diabetes	Adult women with blood pressures >135/80 mm Hg
Gonorrhea	All sexually active women at risk of infection
Hepatitis B	Pregnant women at the first prenatal visit
Hypertension	All women over 18 years of age
HIV infection	All adult and adolescent women at risk of infection, all pregnant women
Intimate partner violence	Women of childbearing age
Iron deficiency anemia	Pregnant women
Lipid disorders	All women over 45 years of age and those 20 to 45 years of age at risk of CHD
Neural tube defects and preeclampsia	Screening recommendations are currently being updated
Obesity	All adult women
Osteoporosis	Women over 65 years of age and those with fracture risk equal to a 65-year-old woman with no additional risk factors
Rh incompatibility	All pregnant women on the first prenatal visit, repeated at 24 to 28 weeks gestation for women who are unsensitized Rh-negative unless the father is known to be Rh-negative
Rubella	Screening recommendations are currently being updated
Syphilis	All women at risk, all pregnant women
Tobacco use	All adult women

Data from: U.S. Preventive Services Task Force. (2013a). *Recommendations for adults.* Retrieved from http://www.uspreventiveservicestaskforce.org/adultrec.htm

College of Obstetricians and Gynecologists (2013) has also recommended screening women for sexual or reproductive coercion.

Population health nurses can educate the public regarding the need for routine screening procedures and can advocate for the availability of screening services for all segments of the female population. Population health nurses may also be involved in case management for women whose screening tests are positive. These women may need assistance in accessing further diagnostic and treatment services.

Treatment. Population health nurses refer women for medical or social assistance with any identified health problems. Problems unique to female clients for which treatment may be required include infertility, fertility control, menopause, and physical abuse. Intervention may also be required for existing acute and chronic health conditions.

Treatment for infertility generally requires referral to a fertility specialist. The role of the population health nurse, with respect to infertility, focuses on case finding, referral, and support during a fertility workup. The nurse can also assist the client and her significant other in considering alternative options such as adoption, artificial insemination, and in vitro fertilization. The nurse may also refer couples to self-help groups for assistance in dealing with psychological problems of infertility. In addition, the population health nurse may assist infertile women to deal with the psychological ramifications of their condition. This may be particularly needed for women from cultural groups in which a woman's identity or worth is based on her ability to have children. At the population level, population health nurses can work with other elements of the health and social systems to assure that infertility services are available to those who need them.

During perimenopause, population health nurses may refer clients to a physician or nurse practitioner for discomfort related to hot flashes or other symptoms. Population health nurses can also educate clients and the general public on lifestyle approaches to the treatment of menopausal symptoms, such as dressing in layers, using a fan, consuming cold foods and beverages, exercise, weight loss, nonsmoking, and relaxation techniques (Weismiller, 2009). Similarly, nurses can assist patients with osteoporosis to make lifestyle changes related to weight bearing physical activity, fall prevention, and use of hip protector pads as well as refer them for pharmacologic treatment with calcium, vitamin D, biophosphonates, raloxifene, and possibly estrogen replacement therapy barring other contraindications (e.g., a history of breast cancer) (Lash et al., 2009).

Menopause may cause vaginal dryness and discomfort during sexual intercourse. The nurse can counsel women concerning longer foreplay and the use of vaginal lubricants to relieve the problem.

Some women also experience decreased sexual desire. The population health nurse can help clients explore contributing factors in this experience such as depression, a feeling of being at the end of the reproductive years, and acceptance of a new phase of life. Self-help groups for women who are having similar problems are extremely beneficial during this stage of life. If there is no such group in the local community, the nurse might start one by inviting clients to meet and begin discussions.

Intervention related to physical abuse of women has two dimensions. The first of these is dealing with the physical and psychological effects of physical abuse, and the second is dealing with the source of the problem itself. Recognizing the problem is a prerequisite to either dimension of treatment. Female clients should be asked in a caring and sensitive manner about any violence in their lives. Careful recording of the history and of information regarding old and new injuries is important in the diagnosis of abuse. Such a record may reveal a pattern the woman is unwilling or unable to admit to the nurse. If there is evidence of abuse, it is unethical for the nurse not to confirm this diagnosis with the client. Allowing the woman to describe what is happening to her through open-ended questions is therapeutic and can serve as the first step in stemming the cycle of abuse.

It is important that the nurse convey to the client that she does not deserve to be abused and that the nurse is concerned about her. These critical statements are needed to convey to the client that someone cares and that she is not worthless, helpless, or deserving of abuse.

It is not easy for a population health nurse to intervene in an abusive relationship. Inherent in such situations are reasons to fear that intervention will not be successful, that the woman may become depressed and suicidal or resent the nurse for interfering in a private family matter, or that the abuser may punish the woman or the nurse. Such fears have kept health care professionals from pursuing evidence and attempting to help women in abusive situations.

When the nurse is able to work through and conquer personal fear and is able to identify a client in an abusive relationship, the nurse should encourage the client to discuss the circumstances of her abuse. It is important that the client realize the danger inherent in her situation.

Once the diagnosis of abuse is made, the primary goal is to assist the woman to reestablish a feeling of control and to empower her to change the situation. Supportive counseling and reassurance are essential. The nurse should let the woman work out her problems at her own pace. Each woman has the capacity to change when she is ready. The nurse must realize that the victim will feel ambivalence in the relationship she has with her partner. The nurse should support realistic ideas for change and assist the client in altering unrealistic ideas. The nurse should help the client to clarify her beliefs about the situation. The nurse should also help to identify myths about abuse that the client may have internalized. For example, if the victim believes that she deserves the beatings, the nurse can assure the client that her partner is totally responsible for his or her own actions.

The nurse can help the client explore alternative plans for solutions to her problem. What are her personal supports? Is there anyone to whom she can go for help? The client may want to go home. If the client can do this without risk of suicide or homicide, the nurse can help her plan strategies for managing at home and provide her with resources for assistance or escape should the need arise. If necessary, however, the population health nurse can also help the woman to plan a quick getaway. The client needs to accumulate extra money, collect necessary documents like birth certificates and immunization records for children, pack a change of clothing, and carry a few emergency supplies. If the client has children, she should take them with her if she leaves or risk losing them to the abuser if he or she should claim that the client abandoned them.

The nurse should avoid becoming another controller in the life of the client. The physically abused woman needs every opportunity to develop independence. Nurses tend to want to rescue victims to stop the violence, but they cannot make decisions for the woman. Although nurses can provide information on shelters and other resources, they must allow the woman to make her own decisions.

Nurses should be familiar with the resources they recommend. Are they reliable? Will they assist the woman to become independent while providing a safe haven for her and her children? If the client is a lesbian, bisexual, or transgender woman, will her needs be effectively met in the shelter? Or will she be subjected to hostility and further abuse?

Population health nurses can also provide assistance in referrals for medical care for injuries and for counseling to deal with contributing factors and psychological effects of abuse. Such services may be needed for children as well as the woman. The woman should also be cautioned that her children may resist being removed from their home and other family members. If this should be the case, the population health nurse can help the client cope with grief and hostility on the part of the children. The client may also need help in dealing with her own grief over the loss of a significant relationship.

When adequate treatment facilities to meet the needs of women are not available, population health nurses can become actively involved in advocating for these services and in developing and implementing them. Population health nurses may also need to advocate for the availability of services for certain specific segments of the population, for example, low-income women or lesbian women.

HEALTH RESTORATION. As with all clients, health restoration interventions in the care of women focus on rehabilitation and preventing the recurrence of health problems. Areas in which interventions are particularly warranted for the female client include pregnancy, abuse, and STDs. Health restoration services may also be needed to deal with some of the effects of menopause, chronic illness, or abuse. Dealing with the long-term management of chronic illness is another feature of health restoration that will be addressed in more detail in Chapter 27∞.

Health restoration with respect to pregnancy involves the use of an effective contraceptive to prevent subsequent pregnancies. Again, the nurse may be involved in education, counseling, and referral for contraceptive services. Health restoration might also involve assisting women and their families to adjust to the advent of a new baby or to deal with the psychological effects of a negative pregnancy outcome.

In the case of abuse, restoration necessitates the rebuilding of the woman's life and that of her family. This may involve developing new financial resources as well as ways of coping with problems. The woman needs to become self-sufficient. Again, referrals to a variety of agencies to help with employment skills and provide counseling may be of assistance. Nurses may also need to collaborate with other segments of the community to assure enforcement of protections for abused women and availability of services to assist them in rebuilding their lives.

Women can also be helped to prevent recurrence of STDs or to cope with the life changes necessitated by a diagnosis of HIV/AIDS or chronic hepatitis B or C. Health restoration related to STDs is discussed more fully in Chapter 26∞. Other restoration measures may be warranted for existing chronic health problems. For example, women may need to be assisted to adapt to lifestyle changes necessitated by chronic illness or to manage symptoms such as pain. Health restoration related to chronic physical and mental health conditions are addressed in Chapters 27∞ and 28∞, while issues of restoration related to substance abuse and violence are addressed in Chapters 29∞ and 30∞, respectively.

Evaluating Health Care for Women

Health care provided to women should be evaluated using the evaluative process described in Chapter 15∞. Once more, it is important to evaluate both the quality of the care given and its outcomes. Because of the dependent role of many women, it is particularly important that they play an active role in evaluating the health care they are given. At the national level, the 2020 objectives for the health of women can provide criteria for evaluating women's health care services. Evaluative information on selected national objectives related to women's health is presented in the *Healthy People 2020* feature on the next page. Information on other objectives that relate to women, as well as to other segments of the population, is included in relevant chapters of this book.

Women's health care needs are many and varied and are often poorly addressed by existing health care systems. Population health nurses may provide health care for women at all four levels of health care: health promotion, illness and injury prevention, resolution of existing health problems, and health restoration. Care may also be provided to individual women or to groups of women within the population, and often involves advocacy for services to meet women's needs.

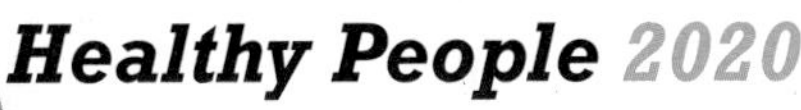

Healthy People 2020

Selected Objectives Related to Women's Health

OBJECTIVE	BASELINE (YEAR)	TARGET	CURRENT DATA (YEAR)	DATA SOURCES
AHS-1.1 Increase the proportion of women with health insurance	84.6% (2008)	100%	82.8% (2011)	National Health Interview Survey (NHIS), CDC, National Center for Health Statistics (NCHS)
AHS-3 Increase the proportion of women 19–64 years with a usual primary care provider	79.9% (2007)	83.9%	80.5% (2010)	NHIS, CDC, NCHS
AHS-5.3 Increase the proportion of women 19–64 years with a source of ongoing care	87% (2008)	89.4	85.8% (2011)	NHIS, CDC, NCHS
AHS-6.1 Reduce the proportion of women unable to obtain or delay obtaining medical care, dental care, or prescription medications	10.8% (2007)	9%	11.7% (2010)	Medical Expenditure Panel Survey (MEPS), AHRQ
AOCBC-2 Reduce the proportion of women with doctor-diagnosed arthritis who experience a limitation in activity due to arthritis or joint symptoms	40.6% (2008)	35.5%	42.7% (2011)	NHIS, CDC, NCHS
AOCBC-10 Reduce the proportion of women with osteoporosis	8.9% (2005--2008)	5.3%	NDA	NHANES, CDC, NCHS
AOCBC-12 Reduce activity limitation due to chronic back conditions per 1,000 women	32.2 (2008)	27.6	34.9 (2011)	NHIS, CDC, NCHS
C-1 Reduce cancer deaths per 100,000 women	152.3 (2007)	161.4	146.7 (2010)	National Vitals Statistics System–Mortality (NVSS-M), CDC, NCHS
C-3 Reduce the female breast cancer death rate per 100,000 women	23.0 (2007)	20.7	22.1 (2010)	NVSS-M, CDC, NCHS
C-4 Reduce the cervical cancer death rate per 100,000 women	2.4 (2007)	2.2	2.3 (2010)	NVSS-M, CDC, NCHS
C-5 Reduce colorectal cancer deaths per 100,000 women	14.6 (2007)	14.5	13.4 (2010)	NVSS-M, CDC, NCHS
C-8 Reduce melanoma cancer deaths per 100,000 women	1.7 (2007)	2.4	1.7 (2010)	NVSS-M, CDC, NCHS
C-16 Increase the proportion of women who receive colorectal cancer screening	52.1% (2008)	70.5%	59.1%%	NHIS, CDC, NCHS
D-3 Reduce diabetes deaths per 100,000 women	62.9 (2007)	66.6	58.9 (2010)	NVSS-M, CDC, NCHS
FP-1 Increase the proportion of pregnancies that are intended	51% (2002)	56%	51.3% (2006)	Guttmacher Institute Abortion Provider Survey, National Survey of Family Growth (NSFG), NVSS-N, CDC, NCHS

Continued on next page

Healthy People 2020 (Continued)

OBJECTIVE	BASELINE (YEAR)	TARGET	CURRENT DATA (YEAR)	DATA SOURCES
FP-6 Increase the proportion of females at risk of unintended pregnancy who used contraceptives or whose partners used contraceptives at last sexual intercourse	83.3% (2006–2010)	91.6%	NDA	Guttmacher Institute Abortion Provider Survey, National Survey of Family Growth (NSFG), NVSS-N, CDC, NCHS
HDS-2 Reduce coronary heart disease deaths per 100,000 women	98.8 (2007)	103.4	84.9 (2010)	NVSS-M, CDC, NCHS
HDS-3 Reduce stroke deaths per 100,000 women	42.7 (2007)	34.8	38.3 (2010)	NVSS-M, CDC, NCHS
HDS-5.1 Reduce the proportion of women with hypertension	28.7% (2005–2008)	26.9%	NDA	National Health and Nutrition Examination Survey (NHANES), CDC, NCHS
HDS-6 Increase the proportion of women who have had their blood cholesterol level checked in the past 5 years	76.8% (2008)	82.1%	NDA	NHIS, CDC, NCHS
HDS-7 Reduce the proportion of women with high blood cholesterol levels	16.1% (2005–2008)	13.5%	NDA	NHANES, CDC, NCHS
HIV-4 Reduce new cases of AIDs per 100,000 adult and adolescent women	7.3 (2007)	12.4	6.4 (2010)	National HIV Surveillance System, CDC, National Center for HIV/AIDS, Viral Hepatitis, STD, and TB Prevention (NCHHSTP)
HIV-8.2 Reduce new cases of perinatally acquired AIDS	34 (2007)	31	18 (2010)	National HIV Surveillance System, CDC
HIV-17.1 Increase the proportion of sexually active unmarried females aged 15–44 years who use condoms	35.1% (2006–2010)	38.6%	NDA	National Survey of Family Growth (NSFG), CDC, NCHS
IVP-11 Reduce unintentional injury deaths per 100,000 women	26.1 (2007)	36.4	25.6 (2010)	NVSS-M, CDC, NCHS
IVP-29 Reduce homicides per 100,000 women	2.5 (2007)	5.5	2.3 (2010)	NVSS-M, CDC, NCHS
MICH-5 Reduce maternal mortality rate per 100,000 live births	12.7 (2007)	11.4	NDA	NVSS-M, NVSS-N, CDC, NCHS
MICH-6 Reduce maternal illness and complications due to pregnancy	31.1% (2007)	28%	NDA	National Hospital Discharge Survey (NHDS), CDC, NCHS
MICH-10.1 Increase the proportion of pregnant women who receive prenatal care in the first trimester	70.8% (2007)	77.9%	NDA	NVSS-N, CDC, NCHS
NWS-9 Reduce the proportion of adult women who are obese	35.3% (2005–2008)	30.5%	35.8% (2009–2010)	NHANES, CDC, NCHS

Continued on next page

Healthy People 2020 (Continued)

OBJECTIVE	BASELINE (YEAR)	TARGET	CURRENT DATA (YEAR)	DATA SOURCES
NWS-21.3 Reduce iron deficiency anemia among females aged 12–49 years	10.4% (2005–2008)	9.4%	NDA	NHANES, CDC, NCHS
PA-1 Reduce the proportion of adult women who engage in no leisure time physical activity	38.2% (2008)	32.6%	33.1% (2011)	NHIS, CDC, NCHS
SA-12 Reduce drug-induced deaths per 100,000 women	9.3 (2007)	11.3	10 (2010)	NVSS-M, CDC, NCHS
TU-1.1 Reduce cigarette smoking by adult women	18.5% (2008)	80%	16.8% (2011)%	NHIS, CDC, NCHS
TU-4.1 Increase smoking cessation attempts by adult women smokers	51.5% (2008)	80%	49.5% (2011)	NHIS, CDC, NCHS

NDA = No data available

Data from: U.S. Department of Health and Human Services. (2014). Retrieved from http://healthypeople.gov/2020/topicsobjectives2020/default.aspx

CHAPTER RECAP

Women have unique health needs that arise from biological, psychological, environmental, sociocultural, behavioral, and health system factors that influence health. Population health nurses can influence the health of the female population by assessing their health needs, developing relevant population health nursing diagnoses, and planning, implementing, and evaluating programs of care that address those needs. Such programs of care may focus on health promotion, illness and injury prevention, resolution of existing health problems, and health restoration. Health promotion focused interventions include promoting healthy behaviors, promoting healthy interpersonal relationships, creating living conditions and work environments that foster health, assistance in developing effective coping strategies, and promoting healthy pregnancies. Foci for illness and injury prevention among women include elimination of risk factors for disease, preventing osteoporosis, STD prevention, contraception, and immunization. Additional emphases in injury prevention include eliminating safety hazards at home and at work, promoting use of safety devices and practices, and preventing abuse. Resolution of existing health problems involves screening, diagnosis, and treatment for illnesses and other conditions including addressing psychosocial issues, such as poverty, that influence access to health care. Finally, health restoration foci include dealing with the long-term consequences of illness and injury and preventing recurrent health problems.

CASE STUDY Preventing Gestational Diabetes Mellitus

You are a population health nurse in a small town in rural New Mexico. In conducting a comprehensive assessment of health needs in the area, you noted that the incidence of GDM is quite high. Nationwide incidence of GDM is about 2%, but approximately 6% of pregnant women in this community develop GDM each year. Approximately 10% to 15% of these women go on to develop type 2 diabetes. The local population is about 60% Hispanic, 30% Anglo, and 10% Asian. Many of the Hispanic population are undocumented migrant families who work on the local farms and ranches. The Asian population tend to be recent arrivals to the community who work in a local high-tech industry. GDM is most prevalent among the Hispanic population who often receive late or no prenatal care. Overweight and obesity are significant problems in the Hispanic and Anglo populations, but not in the Asian population.

1. What factors related to biological, psychological, environmental, sociocultural, behavioral, and health system determinants are influencing GDM (either positively or negatively)? What additional information would you want to obtain related to each category of determinants?
2. How would you word a related population health nursing diagnosis?
3. What evidence-based practice guidelines are available for preventing GDM?
4. What type of intervention, based on the evidence, might be implemented to decrease the incidence of GDM in this community?
5. What would be the target population for the intervention? How might the intervention need to be tailored to the target population?
6. What other segments of the community might you collaborate with in resolving this problem?
7. How would you evaluate the effectiveness of your intervention?

REFERENCES

American Academy of Pediatrics. (2012). *Sexual maturity stages*. Retrieved from https://www.pediatriccareonline.org/pco/ub/view/PPP/312032/all/Sexual%20Maturity%20Stages%20?amod=aapea&login=true&nfstatus=401&nftoken=00000000-0000-0000-0000-000000000000&nfstatusdescription=ERROR%3a+No+local+token

American College of Obstetricians and Gynecologists. (2012). *IPV—An under-recognized public health epidemic*. Retrieved from http://www.acog.org/About_ACOG/News_Room/News_Releases/2012/IPV_An_Under-Recognized_Public_Health_Epidemic?p=1

American College of Obstetricians and Gynecologists. (2013). *Reproductive and sexual coercion*. Retrieved from http://www.acog.org/~/media/Committee%20Opinions/Committee%20on%20Health%20Care%20for%20Underserved%20Women/co554.pdf?dmc=1&ts=20130207T1447181754

Annandale, S. (2009). *Women's health and social change*. New York, NY: Routledge.

Anxiety and Depression Association of America. (n.d.). *Facts*. Retrieved from http://www.adaa.org/living-with-anxiety/women/facts

Astbury, J. (2010). Social causes of women's depression: A question of rights violated? In D. C. Jack & A. Ali (Eds.), *Silencing the self across cultures: Depression and gender in the social world* (pp. 19–45). New York, NY: Oxford University Press.

Black, M. C., Basile, K. C. Breiding, M. J., Smith, S. G., Walters, M. L., Merrick, M. T., … Stevens, M. R. (2011). *The National Intimate Partner and Sexual Violence Survey: 2010 summary report*. Retrieved from http://www.cdc.gov/violenceprevention/pdf/nisvs_report2010-a.pdf

Boonstra, H. D. (2011). Advancing sexuality education in developing countries. *Guttmacher Policy Review, 14*(3), 17–23. Retrieved from http://www.guttmacher.org/pubs/gpr/14/3/gpr140317.pdf

Centers for Disease Control and Prevention. (2012). *United States Medical Eligibility Criteria (USMEC) for contraceptive use*. Retrieved from http://www.cdc.gov/reproductivehealth/UnintendedPregnancy/USMEC.htm

Centers for Disease Control and Prevention. (2013). *Chronic fatigue syndrome—Who's at risk?* Retrieved from http://www.cdc.gov/cfs/causes/risk-groups.html

Centers for Disease Control and Prevention. (2014). *Recommended adult immunization schedule—United States—2013*. Retrieved from http://www.cdc.gov/vaccines/schedules/downloads/adult/adult-schedule.pdf

Crosby, A. E., Ortega, L., & Stevens, M. R. (2011). Suicides—United States, 1999–2007. *Morbidity and Mortality Weekly Report, 60*(Suppl.), 56–59.

Dare, J., & Green, L. (2011). Rethinking social support in women's midlife years: Women's experiences of social support in online environments. *European Journal of Cultural Studies, 14*, 473–490. doi: 10.1177/1367549411412203

Division for Heart Disease and Stroke Prevention. (2013). *Women and heart disease fact sheet*. Retrieved from http://www.cdc.gov/dhdsp/data_statistics/fact_sheets/fs_women_heart.htm

Division of HIV/AIDS Prevention. (2014). HIV among *women*. Retrieved from http://www.cdc.gov/hiv/risk/gender/women/facts/index.html?utm_source=feedburner&utm_medium=feed&utm_campaign=Feed%3A+pkidshivnews+(PKIDs'+HIV%2FAIDS+News)

Dye, J. L. (2010). *Fertility of American women*. Retrieved from http://www.census.gov/prod/2010pubs/p20-563.pdf

East, L., Jackson, D., O'Brien, L., & Peters, K. (2011). Condom negotiation: Experiences of sexually active young women. *Journal of Advanced Nursing, 67*, 77–85. doi:10.1111/j.1365-2648.2010.05451.x

Freedman, D. S. (2011). Obesity = United States, 1988–2008. *Morbidity and Mortality Weekly Report, 60*(Suppl.), 73–77.

Gallenberg, M. M. (2012). *Premenstrual syndrome (PMS)*. Retrieved from http://www.mayoclinic.com/health/pmdd/AN01372

Goldberg, M. (2012). *Awakenings: On Margaret Sanger*. Retrieved from http://www.thenation.com/print/article/166121/awakenings-margaret-sanger

Guttmacher Institute. (2013a). *Contraceptive use in the United States*. Retrieved from http://www.guttmacher.org/pubs/fb_contr_use.html

Guttmacher Institute. (2013b). *Facts on unintended pregnancy in the United States*. Retrieved from http://www.guttmacher.org/pubs/FB-Unintended-Pregnancy-US.pdf

Health Indicators Warehouse. (n.d.a). *Blood pressure screening: Adults (percent)*. Retrieved from http://healthindicators.gov/Indicators/Blood-pressure-screening-adults-percent_883/Profile/Data

Health Indicators Warehouse. (n.d.b). *Cervical cancer screening: Women 21–65 years (percent)*. Retrieved from http://healthindicators.gov/Indicators/Cervical-cancer-screening-women-21-65-years-percent_505/Profile/Data

Health Indicators Warehouse. (n.d.c). *Cholesterol screening: Adults (percent)*. Retrieved from http://healthindicators.gov/Indicators/Cholesterol-screening-adults-percent_886/Profile/Data

Health Indicators Warehouse. (n.d.d). *Colorectal cancer screening: Persons 50–75 years (percent)*. Retrieved from http://healthindicators.gov/Indicators/Colorectal-cancer-screening-persons-50-75-years-percent_506/Profile/Data

Health Indicators Warehouse. (n.d.e). *Condom use: Unmarried females 15–44 years (percent).* Retrieved from http://healthindicators.gov/Indicators/Condom-use-unmarried-females-15-44-years-percent_940/Profile/Data

Health Indicators Warehouse. (n.d.f). *Depression screening by primary care providers: Adults (percent).* Retrieved from http://healthindicators.gov/Indicators/Depression-screening-by-primary-care-providers-adults-percent_1120/Profile/Data

Health Indicators Warehouse. (n.d.g). *Flu vaccination: Adults 18–64 years (percent).* Retrieved from http://healthindicators.gov/Indicators/Flu-vaccination-adults-18-64-years-percent_1033/Profile/Data

Health Indicators Warehouse. (n.d.h). *Flu vaccination: Pregnant women (percent).* Retrieved from http://healthindicators.gov/Indicators/Flu-vaccination-pregnant-women-percent_1038/Profile

Health Indicators Warehouse. (n.d.i). *Fruit consumption.* Retrieved from http://www.healthindicators.gov/Indicators/Fruitconsumption_1217/Profile/Data

Health Indicators Warehouse. (n.d.j). *HIV infection status awareness (percent).* Retrieved from http://healthindicators.gov/Indicators/HIV-infection-status-awareness-percent_942/Profile

Health Indicators Warehouse. (n.d.k). *HIV testing: Pregnant women (percent).* Retrieved from http://healthindicators.gov/Indicators/HIV-testing-pregnant-women-percent_946/Profile/Data

Health Indicators Warehouse. (n.d.l). *HPV vaccination: Girls 13–15 years (percent).* Retrieved from http://healthindicators.gov/Indicators/HPV-vaccination-girls-13-15-years-percent_1013/Profile/Data

Health Indicators Warehouse. (n.d.m). *Mammography: Women 50–74 years (percent).* Retrieved from http://healthindicators.gov/Indicators/Mammography-women-50-74-years-percent_507/Profile/Data

Health Indicators Warehouse. (n.d.n). *Oral and pharyngeal cancer early detection (percent).* Retrieved from http://healthindicators.gov/Indicators/Oral-and-pharyngeal-cancer-early-detection-percent_1264/Profile/Data

Health Indicators Warehouse. (n.d.o). *Skin cancer protective measures: Adults (percent).* Retrieved from http://healthindicators.gov/Indicators/Skin-cancer-protective-measures-adults-percent_504/Profile/Data

Health Indicators Warehouse. (n.d.p). *Sodium consumption.* Retrieved from http://www.healthindicators.gov/Indicators/Sodiumconsumption_1222/Profile/Data

Health Indicators Warehouse. (n.d.q). *Solid fats and added sugar consumption.* Retrieved from http://www.healthindicators.gov/Indicators/Solidfatandaddedsugarconsumption_1238/Profile/Data

Health Indicators Warehouse. (n.d.r). *Sufficient sleep: Adults (percent).* Retrieved from http://healthindicators.gov/Indicators/Sufficient-sleep-adults-percent_1472/Profile/Data

Health Indicators Warehouse. (n.d.s). *Tobacco screening in physician office visits: Adults (percent).* Retrieved from http://healthindicators.gov/Indicators/Tobacco-screening-in-physician-office-visits-adults-percent_1557/Profile/Data

Health Indicators Warehouse. (n.d.t). *Vegetable consumption.* Retrieved from http://www.healthindicators.gov/Indicators/Totalvegetableconsumption_1218/Profile/Data

Howden, L. M., & Meyer, J. A. (2011). *Age and sex composition: 2010–2010 census briefs.* Retrieved from http://www.census.gov/prod/cen2010/briefs/c2010br-03.pdf

Jack, D. C., & Ali, A. (2010). Introduction: Culture, self-silencing, and depression: A contextual-relational perspective. In D. C. Jack & A. Ali (Eds.), *Silencing the self across cultures: Depression and gender in the social world* (pp. 3–17). New York: Oxford University Press.

Kaiser Family Foundation. (2013). *Health reform: Implications for women's access to coverage and care.* Retrieved from http://kaiserfamilyfoundation.files.wordpress.com/2012/03/7987-03-health-reform-implications-for-women_s-access-to-coverage-and-care.pdf

Keenan, N. L., & Rosendorf, K. A. (2011, January 14). Prevalence of hypertension and controlled hypertension = United States, 2005–2008. *Morbidity and Mortality Weekly Report, 60*(Suppl.), 94–97.

Khurana, R., & Isaacs, C. (2014). *Systemic lupus erythematosus and pregnancy.* Retrieved from http://emedicine.medscape.com/article/335055-overview

Lash, R. W., Nicholson, J. M., Velez, L., Harrison, R. V., & McCort, J. (2009). Diagnosis and management of osteoporosis. *Primary Care: Clinics in Office Practice, 36,* 181–198. doi:10.1016/j.pop.2008.10.009

Letourneau, N., Duffett-Leger, L., Dennis, C.-L., Stewart, M., & Tryphonopoulos, P. D. (2010). Identifying the support needs of fathers affected by post-partum depression: A pilot study. *Journal of Psychiatric and Mental Health Nursing, 18,* 41–47. doi:10.1111/j.1365-2859.2010.01627.x

Lewis, J. J. (2010). *Margaret Sanger.* Retrieved from http://womenshistory.about.com/od/sangermargaret/p/margaret_sanger.htm.

Logan, J. E., Smith, S. G., & Stevens, M. R. (2011). Homicides—United States, 1999–2007. *Morbidity and Mortality Weekly Report, 60*(Suppl.), 67–70.

Marchetta, C. M., Denny, C. H., Floyd, R. L., Cjeal, N. E., Sniezek, J. E., & McKnight- Eily, L. R. (2012). Alcohol use and binge drinking among women of childbearing age—United States, 2006–2010. *Morbidity and Mortality Weekly Report, 61,* 534–538.

Margaret Sanger. (2013). *The Biography Channel website.* Retrieved from http://www.biography.com/people/margaret-sanger-9471186

Margaret Sanger Papers Project. (2010). *About Margaret Sanger.* Retrieved from http://sangerpapers.wordpress.com//?s=About+Margaret+Sanger&search=Go

Maternal and Child Health Bureau. (2013). *Child health USA 2013: Prenatal care.* Retrieved from http://mchb.hrsa.gov/chusa13/dl/pdf/chusa13.pdf

Mayo Clinic Staff. (2012). *Perimenopause.* Retrieved from http://www.mayoclinic.org/diseases-conditions/perimenopause/basics/definition/con-20029473

The Mike Wallace interview: Margaret Sanger. (1957, September 21). Retrieved from http://www.hrc.utexas.edu/multimedia/video/2008/wallace/sanger_margaret.html

NASW Foundation. (2004). *NASW social work pioneers: Dorothy Irene Height.* Retrieved from http://www.naswfoundation.org/pioneers/h/height.htm

National Association of Anorexia Nervosa and Associated Disorders. (2014). *Eating disorders statistics.* Retrieved from http://www.anad.org/get-information/about-eating-disorders/eating-disorders-statistics/

National Center for Complementary and Alternative Medicine. (2012). *Menopausal symptoms and complementary health practices.* Retrieved from http://nccam.nih.gov/health/menopause/menopausesymptoms

National Center for Health Statistics. (2011). Percentage of noninstitutionalized adults aged >80 years who need help with personal care, by sex—United States, 2008–2009. *Morbidity and Mortality Weekly Report, 60,* 819.

National Center for Health Statistics. (2012). *Vital and health statistics: Summary health statistics for U.S. adults: National Health Interview Survey, 2011.* Retrieved from http://www.cdc.gov/nchs/data/series/sr_10/sr10_256.pdf

National Center for Health Statistics. (2013). *Health, United States, 2012: With special feature on emergency care.* Retrieved from http://www.cdc.gov/nchs/data/hus/hus12.pdf

National Center for Injury Prevention and Control. (2013). *Sexual assault all injury causes nonfatal injury and rates per 100,000, 2012.* Retrieved from http://webappa.cdc.gov/sasweb/ncipc/nfirates2001.html

National Center on Birth Defects and Developmental Disabilities. (2014). *State-specific alcohol consumption rates for 2012.* Retrieved from http://www.cdc.gov/ncbddd/fasd/monitor_table.html

National Coalition for the Homeless. (2011). *Who is homeless?* Retrieved from http://www.nationalhomeless.org/factsheets/who.html

National Coalition for the Homeless. (2012). *Homeless families with children.* Retrieved from http://www.nationalhomeless.org/factsheets/families.html

National Diabetes Information Clearinghouse. (2011). *National diabetes statistics, 2011.* Retrieved from http://diabetes.niddk.nih.gov/dm/pubs/statistics/#Gestational

National Diabetes Information Clearinghouse. (2013). *What I need to know about gestational diabetes.* Retrieved from http://diabetes.niddk.nih.gov/dm/pubs/gestational/#1

National Institute of Mental Health. (2009). *Schizophrenia: What is schizophrenia?* Retrieved from http://www.nimh.nih.gov/health/publications/schizophrenia/index.shtml

National Women's Law Center. (2010). *Health care report card: Making the grade on women's health: A national and state by state report card.* Retrieved from http://hrc.nwlc.org/

O'Mahony, J., & Donnelly, T. (2010). Immigrant and refugee women's post-partum depression help-seeking experiences and access to care: A review and analysis of the literature. *Journal of Psychiatric and Mental Health Nursing, 17,* 917–928. doi:10.1111/j.1365-2850.2010.01625.x

Paulozzi, L. J. (2011, January 14). Drug-induced deaths—United States, 2003–2007. *Morbidity and Mortality Weekly Report, 60*(Suppl.), 60–61.

Pearsall, B. (2011). Health care: The high cost of being a woman. *Outlook: The Magazine of AAUW, 105*(1), 8–11.

Planned Parenthood Federation of America. (2012). *Pregnancy and childbearing among U.S. teens.* Retrieved from http://www.plannedparenthood.org/files/PPFA/pregnancy_and_childbearing.pdf

Preeclampsia Foundation. (n.d.). *Preeclampsia fact sheet.* Retrieved from http://www.preeclampsia.org/pdf/Preeclampsia%20Fact%20sheet%20v2.pdf

Premenstrual dysphoric disorder. (2013). Retrieved from http://www.nlm.nih.gov/medlineplus/ency/article/007193.htm

Raymond, J., Wheeler, W., & Brown, M. J. (2011). Inadequate and unhealthy housing, 2007 and 2009. *Morbidity and Mortality Weekly Report, 60*(Suppl.), 21–27.

Shulman, H. C. (2012). *Dorothy Irene Height: Civil rights activist.* Retrieved from http://iipdigital.usembassy.gov/st/English/publication/2010/07/20100713175927ihecuor0.9198376.html#axzz2KdFJQFtI

Single Mother Guide. (2013). *Single mother statistics.* Retrieved from http://singlemotherguide.com/single-mother-statistics/

Substance Abuse and Mental Health Services Administration. (2011). *Current statistics on the prevalence and characteristics of people experiencing homelessness in the United States.* Retrieved from http://homeless.samhsa.gov/ResourceFiles/hrc_factsheet.pdf

Synnott, A. (2009). *Rethinking men: Heroes, villains, and victims.* Burlington, VT: Ashgate.

Temprano, K. K., & Chelmow, D. (2013). *Rheumatoid arthritis and pregnancy.* Retrieved from http://emedicine.medscape.com/article/335186-overview

Truman, J., Langton, L., & Planty, M. (2013). *Criminal victimization, 2012.* Retrieved from http://www.bjs.gov/content/pub/pdf/cv12.pdf

Turok, D. K., Wysocki, S. J., Grimes, D. A., & Deal, M. A. (2011). *Contraceptive update: CDC medical eligibility criteria for women with chronic conditions.* Retrieved from http://www.medscape.org/viewarticle/742950

U.S. Census Bureau. (2012a). *Statistical abstract of the United States, Table 7. Resident population by sex and age: 1980 to 2010.* Retrieved from http://www.census.gov/compendia/statab/2012/tables/12s0007.pdf

U.S. Census Bureau. (2012b). *Statistical abstract of the United States, Table 9. Resident population projections by sex and age: 2010 to 2050.* Retrieved from http://www.census.gov/compendia/statab/2012/tables/12s0009.pdf

U.S. Census Bureau. (2012c). *Statistical abstract of the United States, Table 57. Marital status of the population by sex and age.* Retrieved from http://www.census.gov/compendia/statab/2012/tables/12s0058.pdf

U.S. Census Bureau. (2012d). *Statistical abstract of the United States, Table 616. Employed civilians by occupation, sex, race, and Hispanic origin, 2010.* Retrieved from http://www.census.gov/compendia/statab/2012/tables/12s0616.pdf

U.S. Census Bureau. (2012e). *Statistical abstract of the United States, Table 648. Full-time wage and salary workers—Number and earnings, 2000 to 2010.* Retrieved from http://www.census.gov/compendia/statab/2012/tables/12s0649.pdf

U.S. Census Bureau. (2012f). *Statistical abstract of the United States, Table 713. People below poverty level by selected characteristics: 2009.* Retrieved from http://www.census.gov/compendia/statab/2012/tables/12s0713.pdf

U.S. Census Bureau. (2012g). *Table 1337. Single-parent households: 1980–2009.* Retrieved from http://www.census.gov/compendia/statab/2012/tables/12s1337.pdf

U.S. Department of Health and Human Services. (2014). *Topics and objectives index: Healthy people.* Retrieved from http://www.healthypeople.gov/2020/topicsobjectives2020/

U.S. Department of Veterans Affairs. (2014). *PTSD: National Center for PTSD: How common is PTSD?* Retrieved from http://www.ptsd.va.gov/public/PTSD-overview/basics/how-common-is-ptsd.asp

U.S. Preventive Services Task Force. (2013a). *Recommendations for adults.* Retrieved from http://www.uspreventiveservicestaskforce.org/adultrec.htm

U.S. Preventive Services Task Force. (2013b). *Screening for intimate partner violence and abuse of elderly and vulnerable adults.* Retrieved from http://www.uspreventiveservicestaskforce.org/uspstf/uspsipv.htm

Volkow, N. D. (2010). *Prescription drug abuse.* Retrieved from http://www.drugabuse.gov/about-nida/legislative-activities/testimony-to-congress/2010/09/prescription-drug-abuse

Weber, J. (2009). *Paid family leave: One solution to helping today's working families meet their family responsibilities at critical times.* Retrieved from http://workfamily.sas.upenn.edu/sites/workfamily.sas.upenn.edu/files/imported/pdfs/policy_makers17.pdf

Weismiller, D. G. (2009). Menopause. *Primary Care: Clinics in Office Practice, 36,* 199–126. doi:10.1016/j.pop.2008.10.007

Williams, L. E. (2011). Dorothy Irene Height: A life well-lived. *Phi Kappa Phi Forum, 91*(2), 8–11.

World Health Organization. (2009a). *Women and health: Today's evidence, Tomorrow's agenda.* Retrieved from http://whqlibdoc.who.int/publications/2009/9789241563857_eng.pdf

World Health Organization. (2009b). *Women's health.* Retrieved from http://www.who.int/mediacentre/factsheets/fs334/en/index.html

World Health Organization. (2013). *World health statistics 2013.* Retrieved from http://apps.who.int/iris/bitstream/10665/81965/1/9789241564588_eng.pdf?ua=1

Wylie, L., Martin, C. J., Marlands, G., Martin, C. R., & Rankin, J. (2011). The enigma of post-natal depression: An update. *Journal of Psychiatric and Mental Health Nursing, 18,* 48–58. doi:10.1111/j.1365-2850.2010.01626.x

Zajicek-Farber, M. I., Mayer, L. M., & Daugherty, L. G. (2012). Connections among parental mental health, stress, child routines, and early emotional behavioral regulation of preschool children in low-income families. *Journal of the Society for Social Work and Research, 3*(1), 31-50. doi: 10.5243/jsswr.2012.3

Zoellner, T., & Hedlund, S. (2010). Women's self-silencing and depression in the socio-cultural context of Germany. In D. C. Jack & A. Ali (Eds.), *Silencing the self across cultures: Depression and gender in the social world* (pp. 107–127). New York, NY: Oxford University Press.

CHAPTER

19 Care of the Older Population

Learning Outcomes

After reading this chapter, you should be able to:

1. Describe three categories of perspectives on aging.
2. Describe biological, psychological, environmental, sociocultural, behavioral, and health system determinants influencing the health of older populations.
3. Identify major considerations in health promotion in the care of older adults and analyze population health nursing roles related to each.
4. Discuss major foci for illness and injury prevention among older adults and describe related population health nursing roles.
5. Describe measures designed to resolve common health problems among older populations.
6. Identify at least three foci for health restoration with older clients and give examples of related population health nursing interventions.
7. Identify considerations that may influence population health nurses' approach to health education for older clients.
8. Identify foci for evaluating the care of older populations.

Key Terms

advance directives

advanced activities of daily living (AADLs)

ageism

aging

aging in place

balanced aging

basic activities of daily living (BADLs)

comorbidity

dementia

elder maltreatment

elderly support ratio

encore careers

functional status

incontinence

instrumental activities of daily living (IADLs)

life-sustaining treatment

old-age dependency ratio

respite

social network

successful aging

transnationalism

validation therapy

Advocacy Then

Promoting End-of-Life Care

Although the elderly are not the only ones to need end-of-life care, one often thinks of death as it relates to the culmination of a long life. Research indicates that many people experience significant pain. This is particularly true for patients with chronic illnesses and those who are approaching death. For example, an estimated 75% of patients with terminal illnesses experience pain as they approach death (Fink & Gates, 2010). One of nursing's primary functions is to address relief of such symptoms, yet for much of our history, there was no organized approach to addressing this function. Care of the dying and symptom relief received little attention until two women, Dame Cicely Saunders and Florence Wald, began movements to address these issues.

Dame Cicely Saunders was educated as a nurse, social worker, and physician (Cicely Saunders International, n.d.). She began her work with dying patients in 1948 and in 1967 founded the first hospice, radically altering approaches to care for the dying and their families (St. Christopher's Hospice, 2013). The mission of St. Christopher's and other hospices is to combine symptom management and compassionate care for the dying and their families, going beyond the commonly held belief of the time that there is nothing that can be done for the dying. Dame Cicely also pioneered research on interventions to control pain at the end of life. Her work led to the establishment of hospices around the world.

Beginning her nursing career at New York's Visiting Nurse Service (American Nurses Association, n.d.), which grew out of the Henry Street Settlement founded by Lillian Wald, Dr. Florence Wald believed that nurses should be community-focused and address the needs of patients across the lifespan from birth to death (Connecticut Women's Hall of Fame, n.d.). In 1965, Dr. Wald attended a presentation on palliative care by Dame Cicely at Yale University, where Wald was Dean of the Mental Health and Psychiatric Nursing Program. Frustrated with the conventional focus of medical care on cure, Wald incorporated concepts of end-of-life care into the nursing curriculum at Yale and founded the first U.S. hospice in Branford, Connecticut (Connecticut Women's Hall of Fame, n.d.). The hospice's services were based on a study of the needs of terminally ill patients. Wald went on to become a major proponent of end-of-life and palliative care in the United States (Adams, 2010).

Advocacy Now

Meeting the Needs of Elders in the Community

Located in central Taiwan, Fu-Kang Community Care Center's mission is "Health promotion and improved life style for people." In keeping with this mission, the staff have designed programs and activities to promote people's knowledge and health-related behaviors. A community assessment revealed diagnoses related to fall risk, insomnia, and chronic disease management. A retired nursing supervisor from the Health Bureau, the head nurse of the local health center, nursing professors from the local university, the pharmacist of a community drug store, and local seniors were invited to participate in designing programs to address these needs. These programs include: a tour to Ho-Li, a small town, and music therapy designed to promote body exercise matched to musical rhyme schemes. Other program foci include healthy eating, sleeping well, fall prevention using Tai Chi exercise, and coping with chronic disease. Blood pressure monitoring is included with each activity, and case management services are provided as needed.

Shin was one of the program participants. The first time she came to our care station, she was an 83-year-old woman in a wheelchair accompanied by her caretaker. She asked us for any elderly activity, and we invited her and facilitated her participation. Initially, she sat quietly in a corner, being assisted with all of her care.

Shin had been the midwife for Ho-Li, a small town in Taichung, Taiwan. People there are hardworking and simple. In the 1970s, most women chose to deliver their baby at home. Shin was the only midwife in the small town, and she had delivered most of its residents. She worked hard to take care of mothers and babies, sometimes day and night. Time passed, and she paid for her care with her health, at the age of 80, she had a stroke, and her husband passed away in the same year. She became a lonely old woman. Her children hired an assistant to care for her.

Although she was now confined to a wheelchair, she will never forget her career as a midwife. While talking with people delivered by her, her eyes brightened, and she would say "The value of a midwife is to create new lives and resources in this town. . . . The career of a midwife gave me a meaningful life. . . . Most of the people in Ho-Li were delivered by me. I can recognize every person in this town." We could see the pride in her face when she talked about her career, but somehow, she still seemed shrunken and lonely. Her wheelchair emphasized the effects of the years on her body.

Each time, Shin was pushed by an assistant. She enjoyed her interactions with the other participants and volunteers. Sometimes, she made paper flowers, and she enjoyed the trips and the music therapy. She became more interactive, particularly when she would ask others: "Were you delivered by me?" Recently, Shin came into our care station through the front door. She asked for no wheelchair; she wanted to walk into the station. With our support, she walked in. And, we saw a brave new life in our town—Ho-Li.

Chen Chien Tzu-Chuan,
Hung Kuang University

According to U.S. Census Bureau figures (2013), people over the age of 65 years comprised 13.4% of the U.S. population in 2012. Nearly 6% of this group was over 75 years of age, and there were more than 53,000 people over 100 years of age in the United States in 2010 (Werner, 2011). By 2050, the elderly are expected to comprise more than 20% of the population. Similar figures are noted worldwide. In 1990, for example, people over 60 years of age constituted only 9% of the world's population. By 2013, this figure had risen to 11.7% and is expected to climb to 21% by 2050. It is anticipated that developing countries will experience a faster aging process among their populations than developed countries, further burdening already strapped social, economic, and health resources (United Nations, Department of Economic and Social Affairs, Population Division, 2013).

Increased longevity and decreasing fertility are continuing to change the proportion of elderly people in relation to other age groups in the population. Worldwide life expectancy is anticipated to increase from 42 to 65 years in various parts of the world in 1950 to 68 to 78 years by 2015. By 2045 to 2050, life expectancy in more developed countries is expected to be 83 years, with a mean life expectancy of 78 years in less developed regions. Similarly, fertility is expected to decline from 6.6 children per adult woman in 1950–1955 to 2.2 by 2050 (United Nations, Department of Economic and Social Affairs, Population Division, 2013).

As the world's population ages, there will be a growing demand for health care services that improve the quality of life as well as longevity. This emphasis on quality of life can be seen in the national health objectives for 2020 addressing the health needs of the elderly. A major thread throughout these objectives is to reduce activity limitations that impair the quality of life for older persons. These objectives can be viewed on the *Healthy People 2020* website and selected objectives are included at the end of this chapter. Concern for the health of the older population of the world also stems from a desire to minimize health care expenditures. Because of the prevalence of multiple chronic illnesses, the elderly account for a significant percentage of all health care expenditures worldwide. For example, based on Medical Expenditure Survey data, in 2010 people over 65 years of age had mean health care expenditures 2.6 times higher than those under 65. Medicare funded 63% of health care for those over 65 at a cost of $6.9 billion (Agency for Healthcare Research and Quality [AHRQ], 2013a, 2013b). Similarly, mean prescription medication costs for the elderly in 2010 were more than twice as high as those for people under 65 years of age (AHRQ, 2013c), and the elderly accounted for more than $19,000 per person in hospitalization costs, nearly 81% of which were funded by Medicare (AHRQ, 2013d).

Nurses have long provided care to individual older clients and to the elderly as a population group. The American Association of Colleges of Nursing and the John A. Hartford

Foundation Institute for Geriatric Nursing (2010) have developed a set of competencies required of baccalaureate nursing preparation for care of the elderly in the United States. For further information about the competencies, see the *External Resources* section of the student resources site. These competencies primarily address knowledge required for care of individual elderly clients, but can be adapted to the care of the elderly as a vulnerable population. This latter application to the health of the elderly population is the thrust of this chapter.

Theoretical Perspectives on Aging

From the perspective of gerontologic care, **aging** is defined as a complex set of physical, emotional, and social changes that contribute to increased risk for health problems and functional decline. Aging involves a gradual and progressive loss of function over time and is not a product of disease, although the effects of aging may place older people at higher risk for disease.

As many as 300 theoretical perspectives have been advanced to explain how and why aging occurs. Generally speaking, these perspectives can be divided into three categories: biological perspectives, psychological perspectives, and sociological perspectives. Biological theories posit that aging is a phenomenon experienced by all members of a given species, that it is a process of physical decline, that it is progressive and gradual, and that it is irreversible.

Some of the current biological perspectives on aging include the cross-linking/glycation hypothesis, the evolutionary senescence theory, the genome maintenance hypothesis, the neuroendocrine hypothesis, the replicative senescence hypothesis, the oxidative damage/free radical hypothesis, and the rate of living theory. Table 19-1 ● summarizes the basic premises of each of these perspectives.

Psychological theories of aging focus on psychological changes that occur with age and propose that effective aging requires development of effective coping strategies over time. Major theories in this area include Jung's theory of individualism, in which the individual's mental focus changes from the external to the internal world, and the developmental theories. Erik Erikson's stage theory of development proposed eight stages of life in which the individual needed to accomplish specific developmental tasks that would facilitate task accomplishment in later stages (Harder, 2012). Peck took Erikson's last two stages, which encompass the last 40 to 50 years of life, and subdivided them into seven more discrete stages that cover middle age and older adult life (Saxon & Etten, 2010). In Peck's final stage, the individual engages in life review in preparation for death. Table 19-2 ● presents an overview of developmental theories and associated foci for task accomplishment.

TABLE 19-1 Underlying Premises of Selected Biological Perspectives on Aging

Theoretical Perspective	Underlying Premise
Cross-linking/glycation hypothesis	Proteins, DNA, and other structural molecules develop inappropriate affinities over time that decrease molecular mobility or elasticity inhibiting protein breakdown by proteases. Glycation is one form of cross-linking in which glucose molecules adhere to proteins inhibiting their normal function. Cross-linking has been shown to be related to wrinkling and other dermatologic changes in aging as well as cataract formation.
Evolutionary senescence theory	Aging may result from genetic mutations that manifest only after reproductive years and can be passed from one generation to another. Genetic effects that may enhance reproductive capacity may have negative effects later in life. This may reflect a need for balance between cell maintenance and reproduction.
Genome maintenance hypothesis	Regular damage to DNA that does not lead to cell death or is not corrected by normal physiologic processes may result in genetic mutations that may be passed on to future generations of cells. These insults may accumulate with age and lead to cellular functional decline. Similarly, cellular repair functions may deteriorate with age.
Neuroendocrine hypothesis	Declining function in the hypothalamus reduces hormonal control of major endocrine functions and regulatory systems for blood pressure, sleep, and sugar metabolism.
Oxidative damage/free radical hypothesis	Normal cell metabolism results in the production of free radicals that can damage DNA. Generally, the body eliminates free radicals, but over time missed radicals accumulate and result in cell changes related to aging.
Rate of living theory	Energy consumption may limit longevity and increased metabolic rates may influence the deleterious effects of free radicals.
Replicative senescence hypothesis	Cell reproduction is limited by the length of telomeres that must be split evenly with a full complement of genetic material going to each daughter cell. Small portions of telomeres are lost with each replication until a cell is no longer able to reproduce effectively.

Source: American Federation for Aging Research. (2011). *Theories of aging.* Retrieved from http://www.afar.org/docs/migrated/111121_INFOAGING_GUIDE_THEORIES_OF_AGINGFR.pdf

TABLE 19-2 Stages and Foci of Erikson's and Peck's Developmental Theories

Life Stage	Erikson's Stages	Focus
Infancy	Stage 1: Trust vs. mistrust	Erikson: Development of a sense of trust in self and others
Childhood	Stage 2: Autonomy vs. shame and doubt	Erikson: Development of the ability to express oneself and cooperate with others
Childhood	Stage 3: Initiative vs. guilt	Erikson: Development of purposeful behavior and the ability to evaluate one's own behavior
Childhood	Stage 4: Industry vs. inferiority	Erikson: Development of belief in one's own abilities
Adolescence	Stage 5: Identity vs. role confusion	Erikson: Development of a sense of self and plans to actualize one's potential
Adolescence/early adulthood	Stage 6: Intimacy vs. isolation	Erikson: Development of one's capacity for reciprocal relationships
Middle age	Stage 7: Generativity vs. stagnation	Erikson: Promotion of creativity and productivity and development of the capacity to care for others Peck: Development of the ability to value wisdom over physical competence Shifting relationships to emphasize friendship and companionship over sexual satisfaction Development of flexibility in roles and relationships Development of mental and intellectual flexibility
Late adulthood	Stage 8: Ego identity vs. despair	Erikson: Acceptance of one's life as unique and worthwhile Peck: Development of the ability to value one's self outside of work roles Development of abilities to adapt to physical changes and effects of aging Maintenance of an active interest in the external world

Sources: Corie. (2010). *Theories of aging.* Retrieved from http://aginginalabama.org/2010/05/default.aspx; Harder, A. F. (2012). *The developmental stages of Erik Erikson.* Retrieved from http://www.support4change.com/index.php?view=article&catid=35%3Awho-you-are&id=47%3Aerik-eriksons-developmental-stages&tmpl=component&print=1&layout=default&page=&option=com_content&Itemid=108

Sociological theories of aging focus on changes in roles and relationships that occur with advancing age and are strongly influenced by cultural values and attitudes toward the aged and aging (Fung, 2013). Theories in this group tend to be mutually exclusive. For example, disengagement theory proposes that individuals disengage from life as a means of making way for a younger generation in preparation for death. Simultaneously, society stops providing useful roles for elders to play. Older persons may disengage, however, not because of their own desires but because they are forced to do so by societal expectations resulting from **ageism**, which is prejudice or discrimination based on chronological age or appearance of age. In activity and continuity theories, however, older persons maintain their interest in life, but their specific interests change. In activity theory, successful aging is dependent on one's ability to stay active and to find meaningful substitutes for prior roles. Successful aging, from the perspective of continuity theory, involves maintaining a balance between continuity and change in one's life. According to this theory, older people are often happiest in activities similar to those experienced in the past (VickyRN, 2013). Socioemotional selectivity theory suggests that the elderly have internalized sociocultural values that inform their actions as they age, and that this internalization accelerates with age. In this theory, older people prioritize goals that contribute to development of emotional meaning in life, adjusting personal goals to fit situational constraints (Fung, 2013).

Population Health Nursing and Care of Older Populations

Population health nurses use the elements of the nursing process to identify needs for, plan, implement, and evaluate care for older populations. Each of these aspects of care will be addressed here.

Assessing the Health Status and Needs of Older Populations

Factors related to each of the six categories of health determinants influence the health of the older population, often with greater effects than on the health of people in younger age groups. Population health nurses would identify determinants that influence the health of specific older populations, assessing health status and needs and developing population health nursing diagnoses. Assessment of an older population can be conducted using the *Population Health Assessment and*

Intervention Guide included on the student resources site. A second tool to assess the health of an individual older client is also included on the site.

BIOLOGICAL DETERMINANTS Major biological determinants of health in the elderly include those related to gender and aging and physiologic function, including immunization status.

Gender and Aging. Gender and the effects of aging are two biological determinants in assessing the health status of older populations. According to 2012 census figures, 56% of the U.S. population over 65 years of age is female. Approximately 12% of U.S. men and nearly 15% of women are over 65 years of age. The ratio of women to men is 1.26 women to every man at age 65, but increases to 1.46 to 1 after age 75 (U.S. Census Bureau, 2013). Because of lower incomes and other sociocultural factors that we will discuss later, older women may be at greater risk for poor health than men.

Although it may affect individual clients somewhat differently, aging results in a number of universal changes in physical structure and function. Normal changes occur in all body systems, but at different rates for different people. They may, however, increase the older client's risk of developing illness and disability. Physical changes related to aging and their possible implications for health are summarized in Table 19-3●.

TABLE 19-3 Common Physical Changes of Aging and Their Implications for Health

System	Changes Noted	Possible Health Implications
Integumentary		
Skin	Decreased turgor, sclerosis, and loss of subcutaneous fat, leading to wrinkles	Lowered self-esteem
	Increased pigmentation, cherry angiomas	
	Cool to touch, dry	Itching, risk of injury, insomnia
	Thinning, compromised thermoregulation	Hypothermia, hyperthermia
	Decreased perspiration	Hyperthermia, heatstroke
Hair	Thin, decreased pigmentation	Lowered self-esteem
Nails	Thickened, ridges, decreased rate of growth	Difficulty trimming nails, potential for injury
Cardiovascular	Less efficient pump action and lower cardiac reserves result in decreased ability to respond to increased cardiac demand	Decreased physical ability, fatigue, exercise intolerance, shortness of breath, intolerance of volume depletion
	Thickening of vessel walls, replacement of muscle fiber with collagen	Elevated blood pressure, varicosities, venous stasis, pressure sores, cool skin
	Valvular stenosis	Murmurs, arrhythmias, atrial fibrillation
	Impaired baroreceptor function	Postural/orthostatic hypotension
Respiratory	Decreased elasticity of alveolar sacs, skeletal changes of chest	Decreased gas exchange, decreased physical ability, dyspnea
	Slower mucus transport, decreased cough strength, dysphagia	Increased potential for infection or aspiration
	Postnasal drip	
Gastrointestinal	Wearing down of teeth	Difficulty chewing
	Decreased saliva production	Dry mouth, difficulty digesting starches
	Loss of taste buds sense of smell	Decreased appetite, malnutrition
	Muscle atrophy of cheeks, tongue, etc.	Difficulty chewing, slower to eat
	Thinned esophageal wall	Feeling of fullness, heartburn after meals
	Decreased peristalsis	Constipation, altered drug absorption
	Decreased hydrochloric acid and stomach enzyme production	Pernicious anemia, frequent eructation, increased risk of infection
	Decreased lip size, sagging abdomen	Change in self-concept
	Atrophied gums	Poorly fitting dentures, difficulty chewing, potential for mouth ulcers, loss of remaining teeth
	Weakening of the bowel wall	Diverticulosis and diverticulitis
	Changes in carbohydrate metabolism	Manifestation of a genetic predisposition to diabetes
	Decreased gallbladder function	Potential for gallstones
	Decreased bowel sounds	Potential for misdiagnosis
	Fissures in tongue	
	Increased or decreased liver size (2–3 cm below costal border)	Potential for misdiagnosis

TABLE 19-3 (*Continued*)

System	Changes Noted	Possible Health Implications
Renal	Decreased number of nephrons and decreased ability to filter or concentrate urine	Fluid and electrolyte imbalance, drug toxicity, nocturia, increased potential for falls
Reproductive		
Female	Atrophied ovaries, uterus	Ovarian cysts
	Atrophy of external genitalia, pendulous breasts, small flat nipple, decreased pubic hair	Lower self-esteem
	Scant vaginal secretions	Dyspareunia
	Vaginal mucosa thinned and friable	
Male	Decreased size of penis and testes, decreased pubic hair, pendulous scrotum	Lowered self-esteem
	Enlarged prostate	Difficulty urinating, incontinence
Musculoskeletal	Decreased muscle size and strength	Decreased physical ability, increased weakness, fatigue
	Decreased range of motion in joints, affecting gait, posture, balance, and flexibility	Increased risk of falls, decreased mobility
	Kyphosis	Lowered self-esteem
	Joint instability	Increased risk of falls, injury
	Straight thoracic spine	
	Breakdown of chondrocytes in joint cartilage	Osteoarthritis, joint pain, reduced abilities for activities of daily living
	Osteoporosis	Increased risk of fracture
Neurological	Diminished hearing, vision, touch, and increased reaction time	Increased risk for injury, social isolation
	Diminished pupil size, peripheral vision, adaptation, accommodation	Potential for falls and other injuries
	Diminished sense of smell, taste	Decreased appetite, malnutrition
	Decreased balance	Increased risk of injury
	Decreased pain sensation	Increased risk of injury
	Decreased ability to problem-solve	Difficulty adjusting to new situations
	Diminished deep tendon reflexes	
	Decreased sphincter tone	Incontinence (fecal or urinary)
	Diminished short-term memory	Forgetfulness
Endocrine		
Thyroid	Irregular, fibrous changes	
Female	Decreased estrogen and progesterone production	Osteoporosis, menopause
Male	Decreased testosterone production	Fatigue, weight loss, decreased libido, erectile dysfunction, lowered self-esteem, depression

Aging also results in changes in patterns of disease that may make diagnosis or treatment of illness more difficult. These changing disease patterns include subtle symptoms such as anorexia, incontinence, changes in functional or mental status, and blunting or absence of fever as an indicator of infection (Smith & Cotter, 2012). The presence of comorbidities may also complicate diagnoses. **Comorbidity** is the coexistence of many chronic physical and/or mental illnesses in the same person at the same time. Drug therapies for one condition, for example, may interact with treatment of another condition, interfering with therapeutic effects or causing adverse effects. In addition, older people may not present with classic symptoms of a given condition, making diagnosis more difficult. For example, many older people do not experience the chest pain typical of myocardial infarction. Finally, older clients, family members, and health care providers may inaccurately interpret abnormal symptoms as facets of normal aging (e.g., many people believe that pain and stiffness are normal concomitants of age).

Other effects of aging involve normal changes in sensory modalities. Changes related to vision include lagging eyelids, slowed pupillary accommodation, decreased lens elasticity leading to visual disturbances and possibly to falls or other injuries. Tear production diminishes causing dry itchy eyes and potential for infection, and diminished pupil size inhibits the ability to adjust to glare. Finally, visual fields are reduced increasing the potential for injury in complex environments (Cacchione, 2012).

Hearing changes include decreased cerumen removal and protection of the ear canal resulting in diminished hearing or potential for infection and contributing to social isolation.

Other changes include thickening of the ear drum and loss of high-frequency hearing as well as the ability to process sounds (Cacchione, 2012). The prevalence of hearing loss doubles with each decade of age, and an estimated two thirds of Americans 70 years of age and older have experienced significant hearing loss (Lustig & Olson, 2014).

Decreased sense of smell may diminish the ability to identify odors and reduce the ability to taste food, which may lead to decreased appetite and poor nutrition. Similarly, decreased numbers of taste buds decrease the ability to detect flavors and enjoy food. As noted in Table 19-3, decreased saliva production may impair digestion and lead to dry mouth, inhibiting swallowing. Tactile and temperature sensation may also decrease, as do the sense of balance and proprioception ability leading to increased injury potential. Finally, changes in pain sensation may also result in injury due to diminished protective reactions (Cacchione, 2012).

The goal of population health nursing in the care of the elderly is to foster healthy aging. The role of the population health nurse is to assist the elderly population to mitigate the adverse effects of aging, prevent unnecessary deterioration in function, and promote quality of life. This may be referred to as **successful aging**, which has been defined as continued physical, mental, and spiritual health and functional ability through middle and later adulthood. Elements of successful aging include absence of disease, continued physical activity, and the ability to live independently with good mental health and effective coping. A related concept is that of **balanced aging**, which is achievement of a balance between needs and abilities by adapting effectively to the exigencies of aging (Butler, Fujii, & Sasaki, 2011).

Physiologic Function. Older populations experience increased mortality and morbidity rates relative to younger groups of people. They also experience higher rates of many other problems that affect their quality of life, such as acute and chronic illnesses, falls and injuries, disability, pain, and incontinence. Immune levels are another consideration with respect to physiologic function in the elderly.

With respect to mortality, age-specific death rates increase with age for most diseases. For example, the U.S. coronary heart disease mortality rate in 2010 was 85 per 100,000 persons aged 45 to 64 years, but increased almost ninefold to 754.3 per 100,000 for all those over 65 years of age, rising to 2,598.6 per 100,000 people over age 85. Similar escalation with age is noted in mortality rates for cerebrovascular disease, malignancies, chronic lower respiratory diseases, and other chronic illnesses (U.S. Department of Health and Human Services [USDHHS], 2014).

Acute and chronic illnesses. Older populations are even more prone to morbidity from acute and chronic illness than to death, and the bulk of the burden of many of these conditions is borne by the older segments of the population. Older adults experience a variety of chronic health problems. The 2012 American Association of Retired Persons (AARP, 2012b) member survey indicated that 28% of those surveyed had at least one chronic health problem, and 25% reported declining physical health. These figures probably underrepresent the extent of chronic health problems in the elderly population, since many low-income seniors and those with low education levels are unlikely to be members of AARP. Table 19-4 presents information on the incidence of some of the more common chronic conditions among the elderly in the United States. Overall, only about half of the population 65 to 74 years of age reported themselves as in excellent or very good health in 2012, and that percentage dropped to only 40% of those older than 75. On the other hand, nearly one fifth (18.4%) of those 65 to 74 years of age and 25% of those over 75 rated their health as fair or poor (National Center for Health Statistics [NCHS], 2014b).

According to the 2009 Behavioral Risk Factor Surveillance System (BRFSS), nearly 23% of people over age 65 were obese (CDC, Administration on Aging [AoA], AHRQ, & Centers for Medicare and Medicaid Services [CMS], 2011). In addition, the elderly are the fastest growing segment of the population with epilepsy. Elderly clients experience longer periods of confusion following seizures and have higher epilepsy-related mortality rates than younger people. Late adult onset seizures are often related to cerebrovascular disease, and treatment is complicated by a variety of comorbidities experienced by the elderly (Acharya & Acharya, 2014). Hypertension is another common chronic disease in the elderly. More women than men experience hypertension (77% and 63%, respectively), and men are more likely than women to have their blood pressure controlled (CDC, AoA, AHRQ, & CMS, 2011).

TABLE 19-4 Percentage of Adults over 65 Years of Age with Selected Health Conditions, 2012

	Percentage of U.S. Older Adults Affected	
Condition	**Age 65–74 Years**	**Over 75 Years of Age**
Coronary heart disease	16.2%	25.8%
Hypertension	52.3%	59.2%
Stroke	6.3%	10.7%
Current asthma	7.8%	6.0%
Emphysema	4.7%	4.7%
Diabetes mellitus	21.1%	19.8%
Kidney disease	3.1%	5.3%
Liver disease	2.1%	1.1%
Arthritis	46.8%	49.4%

Source: National Center for Health Statistics. (2014b). *Vital and health statistics: Summary health statistics for U.S. adults: National health interview survey, 2012.* Retrieved from http://www.cdc.gov/nchs/data/series/sr_10/sr10_260.pdf

Older people tend to experience chronic conditions at higher rates than younger people. For example, roughly 10% of the population over 65 years of age is affected by osteoporosis, compared to less than 2% of those aged 50 to 64 years. The proportion of people affected climbs to more than 20% of those over age 85.

Even for chronic diseases that do not have a higher incidence among older adults, the effects of disease may be more pronounced with age. For instance, only 24% of people aged 45 to 64 years with chronic obstructive pulmonary disease experience resulting activity limitations compared to 32% of those over 65 years of age and 46% of those over 85 (USDHHS, 2013).

Influenza and pneumonia are two acute health conditions that disproportionately affect the elderly. From 2008 to 2010, the U.S. mortality rate for influenza and pneumonia was 7.7 per 100,000 people 45 to 64 years of age, but rose to 110.1 per 100,000 for those over 65. The rate quadrupled for the population over 85 years of age (456.6 per 100,000) (Health Data Interactive, 2014).

HIV infection is also a consideration in the health status of older populations. Although a smaller proportion of the population is affected than in other age groups, the rate of diagnosis for HIV infection in 2011 was 2.3 per 100,000 people 65 years of age and older. In addition, nearly 900 older people were diagnosed with stage 3 AIDS. Older people with HIV infection are more likely than their younger counter parts to advance to stage 3 AIDS within a year of diagnosis of infection. In 2010, 1,886 older people with HIV infection in the United States died and nearly 20,000 people in this age group had died since the beginning of the epidemic (Division of HIV/AIDS Prevention, 2013). Although these figures are less than for other age groups, they are significant because many health care providers do not think of AIDS in the older population and because of the added complication posed by AIDS in the control of other health problems among the elderly.

Falls and injuries. In addition to increased risk related to acute and chronic illnesses, older populations often experience frequent falls and injuries. Worldwide, an estimated 28% to 35% of people over 65 years of age fall each year, and these figures increase to 32% to 42% for those over 70 years of age. Falls account for 40% of international injury mortality (World Health Organization [WHO], 2014).

Fall-related mortality increases with age. In 2010, for example, the rate of fall-related deaths was only 4 per 100,000 population for people aged 45 to 64 years but rose to 53.8 per 100,000 for those over 65 and to 207.7 per 100,000 for people over 85 years of age. Nonfatal injury data shows a similar increase with age. In 2008, the U.S. rate for emergency department visits for nonfatal injuries was 6,540.2 per 100,000 for the 45 to 64 age group, climbing to 7,201.8 per 100,000 for all persons over 65 and nearly doubling to 13,065 for those over 85 years of age (USDHHS, 2014).

One third of older U.S. adults fall each year, and nearly a third of those who fall require medical assistance or experience activity limitations as a result (CDC, 2013a). In 2010, the overall nonfatal injury rate from falls in the elderly was 43 per 1,000 population but jumped to 115 per 1,000 in those over 75 years of age (CDC, 2012). Bathrooms are one of the most common locales for falls, and the 2008 rate of bathroom falls was 112.1 per 100,000 people aged 65 to 74 years, climbing to 241 per 100,000 for those aged 75 to 84 and 515.3 per 100,000 for those over 85 years of age (Stevens & Haas, 2011).

Falls increase the risk of death and disability. For example, 20% to 30% of falls result in moderate to severe injury, and fall-related traumatic brain injury accounts for 46% of fall fatalities. In 2010, falls resulted in 258,000 hip fractures. Falls also increase the risk of nursing home placement, particularly in people over 75 years of age. In addition, experiencing a fall may result in fear of falling, leading to reduced mobility and fitness and greater risk of a subsequent fall. Despite the number of falls that occur among elders each year, only about half of those involved inform their providers of the incident (CDC, 2013a) making it difficult for providers to engage in corrective education and action.

Falls also result in inordinate health care costs. In 2010, for example, the direct medical care costs for falls in the elderly amounted to $30 billion. Costs are expected to rise to $67.7 billion by 2020. The average cost for a fall-related hospitalization is $34,924, and hip fractures account for a large proportion of fall-related hospitalization costs (CDC, 2014a). Costs increase with age, and in 2005, the cost of falls for women over 85 years of age was more than $100 million. In the same year, the cost of falls among men over 65 years of age was $160 million and $189 million for women (CDC, 2012).

Disability. Chronic disease and injury in the elderly often lead to functional limitations and disability. **Functional status** reflects one's ability to perform tasks and fulfill expected social roles. Assessment of functional status includes exploration of abilities at three levels of task complexity: basic, intermediate or instrumental, and advanced activities of daily living. **Basic activities of daily living (BADLs)** are personal-care activities and include the ability to feed, bathe, and dress oneself, and toileting and transfer skills (getting in or out of a chair or bed). In 2011, 28% of Medicare beneficiaries living in community settings reported difficulty in at least one BADL. Activities most commonly affected included walking and bathing (Administration on Aging [AoA], 2013a).

Intermediate or **instrumental activities of daily living (IADLs)** are tasks of moderate complexity, including household tasks such as shopping, laundry, cooking, and housekeeping, as well as abilities to take medications correctly, manage money, and use the telephone or public transportation. In 2012, 12% of Medicare beneficiaries reported difficulties with one or more IADLs (AoA, 2013a). **Advanced activities of daily living (AADLs)** involve complex abilities to engage in voluntary social, occupational, or recreational activities.

The incidence of disability in the elderly increases with the number of chronic conditions. In 2012, 28% of people aged

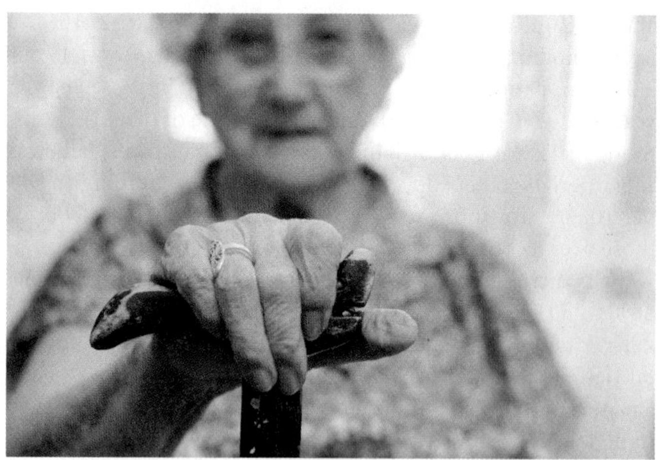

Disability may result in social isolation for many older clients.
(Hunor Kristo/Fotolia)

65 to 74 years in the United States had difficulty with at least one physical activity, and the percentage increased with age to 45% of those 75 years and older (NCHS, 2014b). Based on the 2010 National Health Interview Survey, more than 23 million Americans over 65 years of age (nearly 59%) had at least one basic activity limitation. Just over 3% of the noninstitutionalized population 65 to 74 years of age needed help with personal care, and that figure rose to 10.5% of those over age 75. An additional 21.5 million older adults had vision problems, and 37% had difficulty hearing (CDC, 2014b).

Research has shown that hearing loss, in particular, is associated with lower quality of life and physical and social dysfunction, but that these effects can be ameliorated with the use of hearing aids. Unfortunately, only 20% to 25% of those with hearing impairments use hearing aids (Fischer et al., 2011).

Population health nurses would assess for disability in individual older clients as well as the extent and types of disability prevalent in older populations. The *Focused Assessment* below provides guidance for assessing the extent of functional limitations and disabilities in the elderly population. The data included in the assessment will be collected primarily through community surveys. The guide can also be used to assess disability in individual elderly clients. A more detailed guide for assessing functional status in the elderly is included in the *Assessment Guidelines* on the student resources site.

FOCUSED ASSESSMENT Assessing Disability in the Older Population

Basic Activities of Daily Living

What proportion of the population over 65 years of age has difficulty with

- Feeding (feeding self, chewing, or swallowing)?
- Bathing (getting into or out of a bathtub or shower, manipulating soap or washcloth, washing hair, effectively drying all body parts)?
- Dressing (remembering the order in which clothes are put on, dressing self, bending to put on shoes and socks, manipulating fasteners, putting on and removing sleeves, combing hair, applying makeup)?
- Toileting (ambulating to the bathroom, urinary urgency, removing clothing, positioning self on toilet, lifting from a sitting position on toilet, cleaning self after urination or defecation, replacing clothing)?
- Transfer (getting from lying to sitting position, standing from a sitting position, lying or sitting down)?

Instrumental Activities of Daily Living

What proportion of the population over 65 years of age has difficulty with

- Shopping (transporting self to shopping facilities, navigating within shopping facilities, lifting products from shelves, handling money, carrying purchases to and from car, storing purchases)?
- Laundry (collecting dirty clothing, sorting clothes to be washed or dry-cleaned, accessing laundry facilities, manipulating containers of soap, etc., lifting wet clothing into dryer, hanging or folding clean clothes, putting clean clothing away)?
- Cooking (planning well-balanced meals, safely operating kitchen appliances and utensils, reaching dishes and pots and pans, cleaning and chopping foods, carrying food to the table)?
- Housekeeping (identifying the need for housecleaning, light housekeeping, doing heavy chores, doing yard maintenance)?
- Taking medication (remembering medications, opening medication bottles, swallowing medications, giving injections, etc.)?
- Managing money (budgeting effectively, writing checks, balancing checking account, remembering to pay, and recording payment of bills)?

Advanced Activities of Daily Living

What proportion of the population over 65 years of age has difficulty with

- Social activity (maintaining a group of people with whom to socialize, transporting self to social events, seeing and hearing well enough to interact with others, tiring easily, being fearful of incontinence or embarrassed over financial difficulties)?
- Occupation (carrying out occupational responsibilities, if any)?
- Recreation (having the physical strength and mobility to engage in desired recreational activities, maintaining a group of people with whom to pursue recreation, transporting self to recreational activities)?

Pain. Pain is a significant contributing factor in disability that accompanies a wide variety of acute and chronic illnesses and is a common problem among the elderly. Experience of daily pain has been reported by 35% to 48% of older adults, often resulting from conditions such as arthritis, back pain, cancer, and postherpetic neuralgia (Bruckenthal, Reid, & Reisner, 2009).

Unrelieved pain can diminish quality of life for the elderly through its functional, cognitive, emotional, and social effects. The normal effects of aging may lead to a slightly higher pain threshold for the elderly or differing descriptions of pain, making diagnosis more difficult. Pain is, however, prevalent and is often undertreated in older persons.

Barriers to effective pain management include lack of access to care or treatment, lack of use of adaptive resources, emotional distress and its effects on pain and pain management, knowledge deficits regarding pain management, age-related perceptions by clients and providers that pain is normal in old age, and poor communication with providers. Some patients, for example those with cognitive impairment, may be unable to express pain verbally.

Population health nurses would assess the extent of pain in individual clients as well as the adequacy of pain management for the older population in general. A variety of tools is available for assessing pain in individual clients (refer to Chapter 27∞ student resources). While verbal patients can be asked about their pain or to rate the level of pain experienced, nurses may need to rely on nonverbal indications of pain in nonverbal patients. Such indicators my include increased or diminished body movements; rigidity; changes in sleep and rest or dietary patterns; agitation, aggressiveness, or withdrawal; facial expression; changes in mental status or mood; and vocalizations such as grunting, gasping, calling out, sighing, moaning or groaning, and verbal abusiveness (Bruckenthal et al., 2009). Assessment of pain control at the aggregate level may rely on community surveys or other mechanisms for data gathering.

Incontinence. Incontinence is another common problem among the elderly that may lead to social disability. **Incontinence** is defined as involuntary leakage of urine or feces that may affect personal hygiene or social interaction. As many as 10% of community-dwelling older men and women may experience both fecal and urinary incontinence (International Foundation for Functional Gastrointestinal Disorders, 2013a), with 31% to 70% of those in residential care affected (Roe et al., 2011).

Possible causes of urinary incontinence include aging, bladder cancer or stones, neurological disorders, obstruction, smoking, chronic cough, kidney disease, and diabetes. Additional causes in men include prostatic enlargement due to benign prostatic hypertrophy (BPH) or prostate cancer, while past pregnancy may be a factor for women (Mayo Clinic Staff, 2011b). Older clients may experience several different types of urinary incontinence as indicated in Table 19-5●.

Fecal incontinence may also result from a variety of causes. Some possible contributors include muscle damage or weakness, nerve damage, diarrhea or constipation, pelvic floor dysfunction, loss of bowel storage capacity (e.g., as a result of bowel surgery), and irritable bowel syndrome with scarring of the bowel (International Foundation for Functional Gastrointestinal Disorders, 2014).

Incontinence may contribute to falls when those affected try to hurry to reach the toilet. Other physical consequences may include skin breakdown and urinary problems (Mayo Clinic Staff, 2011b). In addition, either urinary or fecal incontinence may lead to embarrassment and social isolation. Incontinence engenders feelings of incompetence and shame that is fostered by the stigma attached to being unable to control one's bodily functions. Stigma has also been attached to related symptoms such as urgency and frequency (Elstad, Taubenberger, Botelho, & Tennstedt, 2010).

Both fecal and urinary incontinence are distressing to older clients because of the loss of control and feelings of reversion back to babyhood. Clients with incontinence may isolate themselves from others and become virtually housebound due to feelings of embarrassment and incompetence. They may also be reluctant to share problems of incontinence with health care providers. Population health nurses may need to advocate with older clients themselves to encourage them to seek treatment as well as assist them to minimize the effects of incontinence on their lives. They may also need to educate the public regarding incontinence and the potential for treatment.

Immune status. The immune status is another aspect of physiologic function that would be addressed in assessing the health status of individual clients or that of older populations. The Advisory Council on Immunization practices (ACIP) has made

TABLE 19-5 Types of Urinary Incontinence and Distinguishing Features

Type of Incontinence	Distinguishing Features
Stress incontinence	Periodic urine leakage due to pressure on the bladder (e.g., with coughing, sneezing, heavy lifting)
Urge incontinence	A sudden intense need to urinate followed by involuntary urination
Overflow incontinence	Inability to empty the bladder completely with subsequent leakage
Mixed incontinence	A combination of several types of incontinence
Functional incontinence	Physical or mental inability to get to the toilet in time
Total incontinence	Continuous leakage
Temporary incontinence	Due to alcohol use, overhydration, caffeine, bladder irritation (e.g., from coffee, tea, carbonated drinks, artificial sweeteners, acid juices, etc.), medication, urinary tract infection, constipation

Source: Mayo Clinic Staff. (2011b). *Urinary incontinence.* Retrieved from http://www.mayoclinic.com/health/urinary-incontinence/DS00404/

recommendations for the use of several vaccines for people over 65 years of age. Routine recommendations include annual influenza immunization; booster doses for tetanus, diphtheria, and pertussis; two doses of varicella vaccine, herpes zoster vaccine (HZV), and pneumococcal vaccine. For persons at high risk for disease, immunization for meningococcal disease, hepatitis A, and hepatitis B are also recommended (CDC, 2014d). For further information on immunization recommendations for the elderly, see the *External Resources* section of the student resources site. In spite of these recommendations, immunization coverage among older adults in the United States remains relatively low. Table 19-6● presents immunization coverage for selected agents as of 2011.

The immune status of the older population is also influenced by other physiological characteristics that may impede development of immunity following immunization. For example, malnutrition, low basal metabolic rate (BMR), loss of 5% or more of weight in 6 months, reduced upper arm circumference, and reduced ability to perform ADLs have all been associated with reduced vaccine efficacy in the elderly (Sagawa, Kojimahara, Otsuka, Kimura, & Yamaguchi, 2011). For this reason, population health nurses would also explore the extent of these traits in the older population as well as vaccination rates.

TABLE 19-6 Immunization Coverage Among U.S. Adults, 2011

Immunizing Agent	Coverage	Data Year
Tetanus	54.4%	2011
Pneumococcal	62.3%	2011
Herpes zoster	15.8%	2011
Influenza	72%	2009–2010

Sources: Serse, R., Euler, G. L., Gonzalez-Feliciano, A. G., Bryan, L. N., Furlow, C., Weinbaum, W., & Singleton, J. A. (2011). Influenza vaccination coverage—United States, 2000–2010. *Morbidity and Mortality Weekly Report, 60*(Suppl), 38–41; Williams, W. W., Lu, P. J., Greby, S., Bridges, C. B., Ahmed, F., Liang, J. L, ..., Hales, C. (2013). Noninfluenza vaccination coverage among adults—United States, 2011. *Morbidity and Mortality Weekly Report, 62,* 66–72.

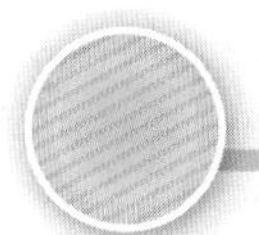

Global Perspectives

Influenza Immunization Rates Among Elders

Influenza immunization rates among elders throughout the world are less than desired. In 2009, for example, Mexico had the highest rate for influenza immunization among Organization for Economic Co-operation and Development (OECD) countries at only 88%. The lowest rate (1.4%) was noted in Estonia. Only 13 of the 21 countries reporting had immunization rates of 50% or more of the elderly population. The United States ranked 6th highest at 66.8% far below the *Healthy People 2020* target of 90% of community-dwelling elders (National Center for Health Statistics, 2012; USDHHS, 2013).

Population health nursing assessment of biological determinants influencing the health of the elderly may occur at either individual or population levels. The *Focused Assessment* below provides some questions that might be used in such assessments.

PSYCHOLOGICAL DETERMINANTS Psychological considerations that particularly influence the health of the older population include dementia and stress, coping, and depression. Although dementia has a number of biophysical causes and effects, it is addressed here because the majority of its effects are mental, with physiological effects arising from the mental deficits caused. Some other psychiatric illnesses will be noted in the elderly population, some of which may be superimposed on other physical illnesses or may result from physical illness.

Dementia. Dementia is a degenerative neurological condition that results in progressive loss of cognitive function leading to the inability to care for oneself and eventually to death. Given

FOCUSED ASSESSMENT Assessing Biological Determinants Influencing the Health of Older Populations

- What is the age and gender composition of the elderly population?
- What are the primary causes of death in the elderly population?
- What is the incidence and prevalence of acute and chronic disease in the elderly population?
- What is the extent of disability in the elderly population? What types of disability are prevalent? What effect does disability have on other aspects of elder health?
- What is the prevalence of conditions such as pain and incontinence? How and to what extent do they influence the health status of the older population?
- What is the immune status of the elderly population? What proportion of the elderly population has received pneumonia vaccine? What proportion has received recent influenza, tetanus, and HZV immunizations? What is the extent of immunity to other diseases in the elderly population (e.g., pertussis, diphtheria)?

the current lack of definitive treatment, the average survival time for someone with severe cognitive impairment is 3.3 years (Mehta, Fung, Kistler, Chang, & Walter, 2010).

In 2011, Behavioral Risk Factor Surveillance System data indicated that nearly 12% of people 65 to 74 years of age in 21 U.S. states reported increased confusion or memory loss, rising to more than 15% of those over age 85 (Adams, Deokar, Anderson, & Edwards, 2013). Among those affected, 29% and nearly 38%, respectively, reported consequent functional difficulties. Alzheimer's disease (AD) is the leading cause of dementia. In 2013, there were an estimated 5 million Americans affected by AD, with projections of 13.8 million affected by 2050 without adequate intervention. Costs of care were $203 billion in 2013 (Alzheimer's Association & CDC, 2013) and are projected to increase to $1.1 trillion by 2050. In addition to the costs of personal care for those affected who cannot care for themselves, people with dementia are three times more likely than those with normal cognitive function to experience a preventable hospitalization (National Center for Chronic Disease Prevention and Health Promotion [NCCDPHP], 2011).

The Centers for Disease Control and Prevention (CDC) has developed the "Healthy Brain Initiative" in an effort to decrease the incidence of dementia in the U.S. population. The initiative has identified 44 action items, 10 of which have priority for immediate implementation. Foci of the initiative include surveillance for risk and incidence, support of policy change, advancing communication and awareness of dementia, and guiding applied prevention research. Additional areas of emphasis include improving the health of caregivers for persons with dementia and addressing depression in those affected (Alzheimer's Association & CDC, 2013; NCCDPHP, 2011). For further information about the initiative, see the *External Resources* section of the student resources site.

Population health nurses may assess cognitive function in individual elderly clients or in the overall older population. The *Focused Assessment* on the next page contains questions to guide assessment of cognitive function in individual clients. At the population level, the nurse would collect data regarding the extent of cognitive impairment within the older population as well as its effects on the overall health of the population and on society as a whole. A tool for assessing cognitive function in the elderly is also available on the student resources site.

Stress, Coping, and Depression. Like people in other age groups, older clients experience stress and have a broad range of abilities to cope with stress. Unlike others, however, older people may have fewer resources to allow them to cope effectively with stress. In 2012, for example, 2% of older community-dwelling elderly people expressed feelings of sadness, and another 2% reported feeling hopeless (NCHS, 2014b). Coping with the helplessness and loss of power often associated with chronic illness may be particularly difficult for older persons, who often need to achieve a balance between assistance and independence.

When older people cannot cope with the stress encountered in their lives, they may become depressed. Depression occurs in more than 6.5 million Americans over age 65. Depression in the elderly may go unrecognized because it is mistaken for the effects of other chronic illnesses. For example, problems with memory and slowed thought processes that may occur with depression might be interpreted as early dementia. Other people may interpret their feelings as sadness or fatigue and not equate them with depression (National Alliance on Mental Illness [NAMI], 2009).

Many older clients with depression have a previous personal history of depressive disorders; others develop depression for the first time late in life. Symptoms of depression in the elderly are often vague and nonspecific and may include lasting sadness or long-term anxiety, sleeping too much or too little or frequent awakening, decreased or increased appetite, loss of interest in previously valued activities, fatigue, restlessness, or difficulty concentrating. Additional symptoms may include thoughts of death or suicide and feelings of hopelessness or guilt (Madden-Baer, 2011).

In addition to diminished quality of life, depression in the elderly has been associated with diminished immunity and increased risk of substance abuse as a means of coping with depression. Depression increases health care use and costs and may lead to functional decline and dependence as well as self-neglect.

Depression may be difficult to diagnose in the elderly for several reasons. Comorbid depression is often missed in the presence of critical illness or undertreated when it is recognized. Providers and family members may miss symptoms of depression, attributing them to aging. At the same time, older clients may feel shame related to their perceived inability to cope and not voice their feelings of depression, or may fail to recognize them for what they are (Madden-Baer, 2011). Many medications used to treat chronic illness in the elderly may also contribute to feelings of depression. Depression may also contribute to lack of adherence to treatment regimens for other chronic health problems.

At its extreme, depression may lead to suicide, which is a significant problem among the elderly, particularly among older men. Suicide rates increase with age and are higher in older men than women (Crosby, Ortega, & Stevens, 2011). Older adults may be more successful in suicide attempts than younger people. In part, this is because suicide is more deliberate and carefully planned, whereas it tends to be more impulsive in younger persons (Demirçin, Akkoyun, Yilmaz, & Gökdoğan, 2011). Overall, older adults account for 16% to 20% of U.S. suicides each year (Madden-Baer, 2011).

Population health nurses would assess for the presence of dementia, depression, and other mental health problems as well as levels and sources of stress and coping skills in individual clients. They would also assess the prevalence of these conditions in the older population. A *Focused Assessment* related to psychological determinants of health in the elderly is

FOCUSED ASSESSMENT Assessing Cognitive Function in Older Clients

Attention Span
- Does the client focus on a single activity to completion?
- Does the client move from activity to activity without completing any?

Concentration
- Is the client able to answer questions without wandering from the topic?
- Does the client ignore irrelevant stimuli while focusing on a task?
- Is the client easily distracted from a subject or task by external stimuli?

Intelligence
- Does the client understand directions and explanations given in everyday language?
- Is the client able to perform basic mathematical calculations?

Judgment
- Does the client engage in action appropriate to the situation?
- Are client behaviors based on an awareness of environmental conditions and possible consequences of action?
- Are the client's plans and goals realistic?
- Can the client effectively budget income?
- Is the client safe driving a car?

Learning Ability
- Is the client able to retain instructions for a new activity?
- Can the client recall information provided?
- Is the client able to correctly demonstrate new skills?

Memory
- Is the client able to remember and describe recent events in some detail?
- Is the client able to describe events from the past in some detail?

Orientation
- Can the client identify him- or herself by name?
- Is the client aware of where he or she is?
- Does the client recognize the identity and function of those around him or her?
- Does the client know what day and time it is?
- Is the client able to separate past, present, and future?

Perception
- Are the client's responses appropriate to the situation?
- Does the client exhibit evidence of hallucinations or illusions?
- Are explanations of events consistent with the events themselves?
- Can the client reproduce simple figures?

Problem Solving
- Is the client able to recognize problems that need resolution?
- Can the client envision alternative solutions to a given problem?
- Can the client weigh alternative solutions and select one appropriate to the situation?
- Can the client describe activities needed to implement the solution?

Psychomotor Ability
- Does the client exhibit repetitive movements that interfere with function?

Reaction Time
- Does the client take an unusually long time to respond to questions or perform motor activities?
- Does the client respond to questions before the question is completed?

Social Intactness
- Are the client's interactions with others appropriate to the situation?
- Is the client able to describe behaviors appropriate and inappropriate to a given situation?

presented on the next page and can be used to assess related factors in either individuals or population groups.

ENVIRONMENTAL DETERMINANTS. Conditions in the physical environment also affect the health of older populations. For example, living in neighborhoods with problems of traffic, noise, crime, trash and litter, poor lighting, and inadequate public transportation has been associated with increased risk of functional loss among elderly residents. Neighborhood factors have also been linked to problems of social isolation, hearing impairment, cognitive impairment, and depression in the elderly.

Physical environmental conditions may also have a direct effect on physical health status. For example, many older persons in the United States live in areas with high levels of pollution. Both ozone and particulate matter pollution have an adverse effect on respiratory function, particularly in people with chronic respiratory diseases.

FOCUSED ASSESSMENT Assessing Psychological Determinants Influencing the Health of Older Populations

- What sources of stress is the elderly population exposed to? What is the extent of their coping abilities?
- What is the prevalence of dementia and other forms of cognitive impairment in the elderly population? What levels of dementia are represented in the population (e.g., mild confusion, vegetative states)?
- What is the extent of depression and mental illness in the elderly population? What mental illnesses are prevalent in the population? What are the rates of suicide and attempted suicide in the elderly population?

Safety hazards are another major consideration with respect to the physical environment of the elderly. Older clients may live in older housing with multiple safety hazards. Or, given recent energy prices, older persons on fixed incomes may have significantly more difficulty heating or cooling their homes than in the past. Both heat and cold have more profound effects on elderly persons than on younger ones due to changes in heat-regulating mechanisms that occur with aging. For example, heat wave mortality has been associated with increasing age. The student resources site includes an inventory for assessing home safety for older clients.

Conversely, older people may live in settings that promote health and independence. Residential areas that provide opportunities for safe exercise by the elderly or assist with accomplishment of routine tasks can delay functional deterioration. Unfortunately many U.S. elderly do not live in such situations. The *Focused Assessment* below provides tips on assessing environmental determinants of health in older populations.

SOCIOCULTURAL CONSIDERATIONS. Sociocultural considerations that have a major impact on the health of the elderly population include living arrangements and family responsibilities; cultural considerations; social support; and education, economic, and employment factors. Abuse and violence are other sociocultural factors that have a profound influence on the health of this vulnerable population.

Living arrangements and family responsibilities. Living arrangements and family responsibilities both have significant influence on the health of the older population. Family configurations and the resulting roles and responsibilities change over time. Children grow up and marry or move away; spouses divorce or die. Older clients may need to adjust to a variety of changes in family roles and responsibilities, some of which are looked forward to and some of which are not. Older men are more likely than older women to be married due to greater longevity among women and the greater size of the older female population. More elders are living alone than in the past. Approximately three fourths of older persons live with other family members in developing countries, compared to only one fourth in developed nations. Even when children live close by, older people are more likely to need outside assistance than in the past due to the number of middle adult women in the workforce. In 2010, 4% of people over 65 years of age in the United States had never married, 72% were living with a spouse, and 27% were living alone (U.S. Census Bureau, 2012a, 2012b). Older women are more than twice as likely as older men to live alone (AoA, 2013a).

Most older Americans (81%) live in their own homes and 19% live in rental units. Nearly half of the older population in the United States spend more than a fourth of their income on housing costs. This is more likely to be true among renters, among whom 74% spent more than a quarter of their monthly income on housing in 2011. Older people

FOCUSED ASSESSMENT Assessing Environmental Determinants Influencing the Health of Older Populations

- How adequate is housing available to the elderly population? What is the extent of home ownership in this population? What safety hazards are presented by housing for the elderly? Are rentals and taxes within the budgetary limitations of most of the elderly population?
- Does the physical environment of the community promote or impede physical activity in the elderly population?
- What health effects does environmental pollution have for the elderly population?

also tend to live in housing that is slightly older than that of the rest of the population with a median construction year of 1970 compared to 1976 for the general population. In addition, more than 3% of homes of the elderly had physical problems (AoA, 2013a).

Older people are accepting greater responsibility for raising grandchildren than in the past. In 2010, for example, an estimated 881,000 people over 60 years of age assumed at least partial responsibility for caring for their grandchildren (U.S. Census Bureau, 2012c). In a 2012 member survey, 12% of respondents were the primary caretakers for at least one grandchild (AARP, 2012a). These responsibilities often devolved on grandparents when their adult children died, were divorced, were mentally ill, or were incarcerated.

Caregiving responsibilities may also be undertaken by older persons in the care of aging spouses. In 2009, 42.1 million people in the United States provided care to an adult with functional limitations at any given point, and 61.6 million provided care at some time during the year. Most of these caregivers were women, and 85% were caring for someone over 50 years of age. The average number of hours of care per week was 20 hours, and the estimated economic value of this care was $450 billion, almost as much as the total Medicare expenditure. Caregiving activities include providing companionship, helping with household tasks, personal care, dealing with financial concerns, administering medications, coordinating services, providing transportation, and communicating with professionals (Feinberg, Reinhard, Houser, & Choula, 2011).

A survey of elderly caregivers for family members with dementia revealed a concept of "role captivity," a feeling of being trapped by the burdens of the caretaker role. Feelings of entrapment were associated with higher levels of depression (Givens, Mezzacappa, Heeren, Yaffe, & Fredman, 2014). In other studies, caregivers with higher perceived burdens have reported worse physical and mental health than non-caregivers (Buyck et al., 2011). Similarly, persons with hip fractures whose caregivers expressed needs for information achieved better long-term outcomes than those whose caregivers did not. Conversely, those whose caregivers reported greater needs for social services were less likely to recover their ability to walk and engage in ADLs (Shyu, Chen, Wu, & Cheng, 2010).

Caregiving by older people also imposes financial burdens on caregivers. Approximately one fourth of older caregivers experience moderate to severe financial hardships due to lost wages and out-of-pocket costs. For example, an estimated 42% of caregivers spend more than $5,000 a year for unreimbursed expenses related to caregiving. As a result, caregivers may cut back on expenditures for their own needs further compounding the negative effects of caregiving on their health (Feinberg et al., 2011).

Social support. Social support is another major sociocultural influence on the health of the elderly population. Social support occurs at societal, neighborhood, and individual levels. At the societal level, social support is a function of the sense of solidarity felt by subsegments of the population with other segments. In many European countries, for example, there is greater solidarity in which younger people feel a greater responsibility for the welfare of older generations than is usually the case in the United States. In stable neighborhoods, opportunities for social interaction increase social support available from neighbors who can be called upon at short notice because of their propinquity.

Social support may arise from either informal or formal social networks. A **social network** is the web of social relationships within which one interacts with other people and from which one receives social support. Social support includes emotional, instrumental, or financial assistance from the social network. The informal social network consists of friends, family members, and neighbors, whereas the formal network comprises health and social service providers. Religious affiliation may provide a form of social support that often bridges the formal and informal networks. For example, many congregations provide material and emotional support to their members.

Some authors have noted that examination of the health of elderly populations should include consideration both of the social support available and perceptions of its adequacy among recipients. Most older persons seek social support most often from family members, particularly spouses. The quality of support provided, however, is affected by several factors, including propinquity and past relationships. Provision of support may be reciprocal among family members, for example, when adult children provide assistance to aging parents and parents provide child care for grandchildren.

For immigrant families, intergenerational support may be transnational in nature, where some family members live in one country and some in another. **Transnationalism** is defined as a process by which family members living in different countries maintain ties and avenues of social support. Transnational social support may be made more difficult by monetary exchanges, immigration laws, and other forces that regulate movement of people and objects across international borders. Some refugee immigrant families may not even have transnational support available. Many refugee families have been separated or have had family members killed. In addition, family members left in the country of origin may not have the freedom to contact immigrant members or may have little in the way of support to offer. Population health nurses can be actively involved in linking these clients to other sources of support (e.g., churches or other organizations). They may also advocate for the availability of necessary support services for these older clients.

Education, employment, and economic status. Many older people are more likely than younger ones to have limited education. In 2009, 8.5% of people in the United States 65 to 79 years of age had not completed high school. This figure nearly doubled to 16.6% for those over 85 years of age (Beckles & Truman, 2011). Progress has been made, however, in the educational level of older Americans, with high school graduation rates increasing from 28% in 1970 to 81% in 2012. In addition, nearly a fourth of those over 65 years of age had attained a bachelor's or higher degree in 2012 (AoA, 2013a).

Although older age is often believed to be a time of retirement, many older people in the United States are continuing to work beyond retirement age. In 2002, workers over 55 years of age constituted 14% of the U.S. workforce (Hughes et al., 2011); in 2009, this figure had risen to 19% (Wuellner et al., 2011). By 2015, those over age 55 years are expected to constitute 30% of the workforce (Hughes et al., 2011). In March of 2013, more than a third of people over 55 years of age were employed, and another 5.8% were unemployed and seeking employment (AARP Public Policy Institute, 2013).

Many older workers are forgoing retirement due to better health or a desire to enter another career field. A 2008 survey (MetLife Foundation & Civic Ventures, 2008) found that significant numbers of persons aged 40 to 70 years were involved in or hoped to pursue "encore careers." **Encore careers** involve occupational changes in the second half of life focusing on meaningful work that makes a difference in the world. Between 6% and 9.5% of people between 40 and 70 years of age were already involved in encore careers, and nearly half of those not currently engaged in such work expressed interest in an encore career.

In other cases different factors are at work in continued employment among the elderly. For example, policy changes, such as the elimination of mandatory retirement ages for many occupations, may permit working into one's later years. At the same time, the age for drawing Social Security benefits has been advanced, prohibiting retirement for many individuals who had planned to retire at age 65. Economic need and a lack of replacement workers are other factors contributing to the postponement of retirement for many older adults. Continuation of older workers in employment settings raises concerns for worker safety. Although older workers experience fewer injuries than younger ones, they may lose more work time when they are injured (Wuellner et al., 2011). In addition, absenteeism due to illness is higher in older than in younger workers (Hughes et al., 2011).

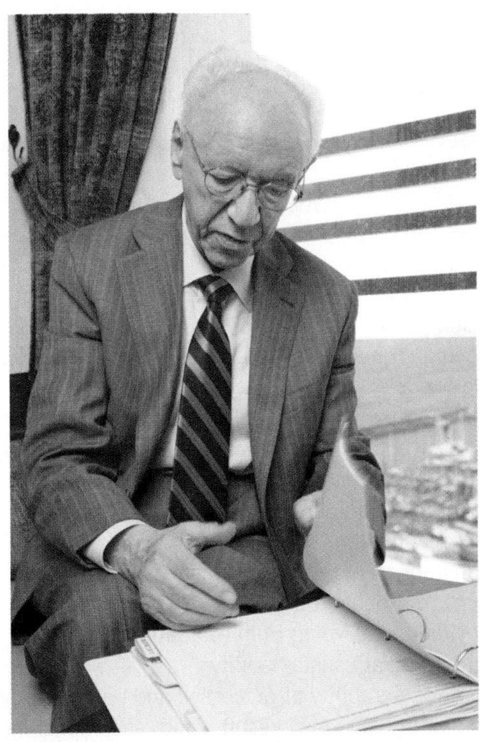

Older individuals may continue to be successfully employed beyond the typical retirement age. *(Eldadcarin/Fotolia)*

Both education level and employment affect the economic status of the older population. In 2012, using the traditional federal definition of poverty, an estimated 9.1% of people over 65 years of age in the United States had incomes at or below poverty level (Social Security Administration [SSA] 2014b). A revised supplemental poverty measure (SPM) has been developed, however, that better accounts for both income and necessary expenditures including resources from public assistance programs and geographic differences in housing costs, out-of-pocket medical costs, and so on (U.S. Census Bureau, 2011). When this revised measure is applied, the percentage of those over 65 years of age who live in poverty rises to 15.1% (Short, 2012). In 2012, 2.8% of people over 65 years of age in the United States had no income beyond Social Security, and the median household income for those over 65 was $39,196 compared to annual incomes of $65,000 for those 55 to 61 years of age and $57,350 for the 62- to 64-year-old group (SSA, 2014b). In 2011, the largest group of U.S. elderly (24%) reported incomes of $15,000 to $24,999 (AoA, 2013a). The median Social Security benefit for people over 65 years of age in 2012 was $16,799, with older persons (e.g., over 80 years of age) earning slightly less than younger ones (SSA, 2014b).

Approximately 90% of the U.S. older population receives at least a portion of their income from Social Security. Overall 39% of the income for this age group derives from Social Security funds. In 2013, more than half (52%) of older married couples and nearly three fourths (74%) of unmarried individuals over 65 years of age derived at least half of their income from Social Security, and nearly one quarter and one half, respectively relied on Social Security for 90% of their income (SSA, 2014a). Some older persons also receive income from other sources. For example, continued employment earned persons over 65 years of age a median of $30,000 in addition to Social Security earnings in 2012 (SSA, 2014b).

Whatever the source of their income, many seniors do not have enough money to live on. In fact, approximately 16% of U.S. seniors over 60 years of age were food insecure in 2011. This amounts to 4.8 million people, more than twice as many as in 2001 (National Foundation to End Senior Hunger, 2013). An estimated one third of senior households have no money left after paying for essential expenses. In 2012 the average credit card debt among those over 65 years of age was more than $9,283. A significant proportion of elders spend more than 30% of their income on housing and an estimated 16%

of older homeowners owe more on their homes than they are worth (National Council on Aging, 2014).

A growing proportion of the elderly cannot afford housing at all, and the number of elderly homeless persons is increasing. Contributing factors for homelessness in this population include poverty and lack of affordable housing. There are an estimated nine elders for every affordable senior housing unit, and the waiting list for subsidized housing may be as long as 3 to 5 years (National Coalition for the Homeless, 2009).

There is a great deal of concern lately about retirement funding. Much has been written in the United States about the Social Security and Medicare systems in particular. At present, most countries have set 65 years of age as the minimum age for drawing public pension benefits, and many employers have mandatory retirement at a specific age. Only Australia and the United States prohibit mandatory retirement except in certain age-dependent occupations. Because of increased longevity, many people can expect to spend a significant portion of their lives in retirement. The **old-age dependency ratio**, or the number of workers to nonworking elders, is expected to increase as the population continues to age. Another related concept is the **elderly support ratio** or the number of people over 65 years of age per 100 people aged 20 to 64 years. Changes in these two ratios result in a declining tax base from which to fund services to the elderly as well as other segments of the population. For example, in 2012, there were 2.8 workers for every Social Security beneficiary in the United States; by 2033, that ratio is expected to decrease to 2.1 workers per beneficiary (SSA, 2014a). Solvency in retirement was one of several concerns voiced by AARP members in a 2012 member survey. Other areas of concern were increasing taxes, consumer fraud, continuing independence (e.g., being able to drive), and being able to age at home (AARP, 2012c)

Empowerment. Empowerment of older adults requires changes in attitudes toward aging and the elderly as well as affirmation of their rights. Disempowerment may stem from loss of autonomy and the ability to make decisions for oneself as well as assumptions that older people are incapable of decision making (Beales, 2012).

Empowerment is affected by both agency and an opportunity structure. Agency refers to the capacity of the individual to make meaningful decisions. Opportunity structure, on the other hand, involves the formal and informal contexts in which decisions are made. Empowerment results from a confluence of the existence of an opportunity to make choices, use of that opportunity by the individual, and the outcome of the choice.

Strategies that promote empowerment of the elderly include age-specific policies and budgets that support their rights and independence, maintenance of physical and mental health, incentives and opportunities for participation in decision making including political participation, age-friendly design of facilities and social structures, and legal recognition of rights. Empowerment is also fostered by access to knowledge of services and information providers, avenues to redress concerns and grievances, policies that promote income and health security, recognized societal roles, and capacity for self-advocacy (Beales, 2012).

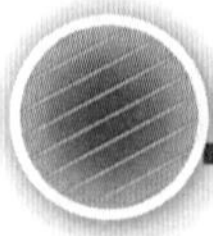

Evidence-Based Practice

Promoting Health in the Elderly

The healthProelderly project conducted a review of best practices in health promotion among the elderly in 11 European countries (Lis, Reichert, Cosack, Billings, & Brown, 2008). The project began with a review of literature on health promotion for older people. The review was followed by identification of 170 best practice programs in participating nations, from which a set of 16 quality criteria were derived. These quality criteria were used to develop best practice guidelines, which were then used to evaluate three health promotion programs in each country. Evaluation results were used to create best practice guidelines for practitioners working with older clients.

The guidelines include recommendations for addressing the following aspects of health promotion program development:

- Identifying and accessing target groups for health promotion programs
- Addressing diversity in the target population
- Involving older people in program development
- Empowering participants and motivating them to take charge of their own health
- Designing evidence-based interventions
- Developing multifaceted and holistic interventions
- Employing strategies and methods appropriate to the target population
- Planning the setting for health promotion activities and assuring easy access
- Involving all stakeholders in planning and implementation
- Using an interdisciplinary approach
- Involving volunteers
- Ensuring effective financial management, quality assurance, and organizational structure
- Employing and learning from evaluation findings
- Ensuring program sustainability
- Making transferability of processes and outcomes evident
- Disseminating program results and accomplishments (Lis et al., 2008)

Abuse and violence. One final sociocultural consideration that affects the health of the older population is that of violence and abuse. The increase in the older population has been accompanied by a disproportionate increase in elder abuse or maltreatment. **Elder maltreatment** is defined as "any abuse and neglect of persons age 60 and older by a caregiver or other person in a relationship involving an expectation of trust" (National Center for Injury Prevention and Control [NCIPC], 2014a, para 1).

In a 2009 report to the Institute of Justice, a study of more than 5,000 persons over 60 years of age indicated that nearly 5% had experienced emotional mistreatment, 1.6% reported physical maltreatment, 0.6% reported sexual maltreatment, 5% reported neglect, and 5.2% reported financial exploitation (Acierno, Hernandez-Tejada, Muzzy, & Steve, 2009). Table 19-7 presents the percentage of elders reporting specific types of abuse and the most common perpetrators of each type. One additional type of elder maltreatment is self-neglect or failure or refusal of the older person to care for his or her own basic needs (NCIPC, 2014a).

At its extreme, elder maltreatment results in death. The 2008 homicide rate among people 65 years of age and older was 2.1 per 100,000 population. Elder abuse is discussed in more detail in Chapter 30. The *Focused Assessment* included below provides tips on assessing violence directed at the elderly as well as other sociocultural determinants of elder health.

TABLE 19-7 Categories of Elder Maltreatment and Common Perpetrators

Maltreatment Category	Percent Affected	Common Perpetrators
Emotional mistreatment	4.6% (overall) 14% (since age 60)	• Spouse/partner (25%) • Child/grandchild (19%)
Physical maltreatment	1.6%	• Spouse/partner (57%) • Child/grandchild (10%)
Sexual abuse	0.6%	• Spouse/partner (40%) • Acquaintance (40%)
Neglect	5.1%	• Child/grandchild (39%) • Spouse/partner (28%)
Financial exploitation	5.2%	Multiple possible perpetrators, no specific data available

Source: Acierno, R., Hernandez-Tejada, M., Muzzy, W., & Steve, K. (2009). *National elder mistreatment study.* Retrieved from https://www.ncjrs.gov/pdffiles1/nij/grants/226456.pdf

BEHAVIORAL DETERMINANTS. Sociocultural and behavioral lifestyle factors can profoundly affect the health of older populations. Behavioral factors, such as diet and other consumption patterns, physical activity, sexuality, and medication use, have important influences on the health of the older population. Factors in each of these areas will be briefly addressed.

Diet. Diet figures significantly in many health problems experienced by older clients. Conversely, health problems such as

FOCUSED ASSESSMENT Assessing Sociocultural Determinants Influencing the Health of Older Populations

- What are societal attitudes toward the elderly? To what extent does the society provide support services for its older members?
- What is the ethnic composition of the elderly population? What languages are spoken among the elderly population? How does culture influence the health of the elderly population?
- What religious affiliations are represented among the elderly population? What health and social services are provided to the elderly population by religious organizations in the community?
- What is the level of economic support available to the elderly population? What is the income distribution within the elderly population? What are the typical sources of income for members of the elderly population? What is the proportion of elderly living in poverty or near poverty?
- What is the typical education level in the elderly population? How does education level influence health?
- What proportion of the elderly population is working? What are the occupations typical of elderly members of the population?
- What retirement planning and assistance are available to older members of the population?
- What proportion of the older population is engaged in caretaking for other family members? What is the effect of caretaking on their health?
- What transportation resources are available to the elderly population? Are they accessible to older clients with mobility limitations? Are they affordable?
- What shopping facilities and other services are available to older members of the population? Are they accessible and affordable?
- What is the extent of social isolation in the elderly population? What resources are available in the community to limit social isolation?
- What is the level of empowerment among members of the older population? What societal factors promote or impede participation in decision making for older adults?
- What is the extent of violence and abuse against elders in the population? What factors are contributing to violence and abuse?

loss of teeth may affect dietary intake. Based on National Health Interview Survey data, in 2010 to 2012, 7.4% of the total U.S. population was edentulous (without any teeth), but this percentage increased to 23.1% of those over 65 years of age and to 32.2% over 85 years (CDC, n.d.). Presence or absence of teeth, diminished gastric secretion and motility, and diminished sense of taste or smell may affect older clients' ability or desire to eat a nutritious diet.

Some of the nutrition-related problems experienced by the older population include malnutrition, obesity, elevated cholesterol levels, dehydration, and deficiencies in certain specific nutrients. Approximately 1.1% of the U.S. population 65 to 74 years of age and more than twice as many (2.6%) of those age 75 and older were underweight in 2013 (NCHS, 2014b). As many as 1 million homebound community dwelling elderly may be malnourished (National Resource Center on Nutrition, Physical Activity, and Aging, n.d.a), and an estimated 3,000 U.S. adults die of malnutrition each year (Dray, 2011). Contributing factors include decreased appetite or difficulty eating, dietary restrictions that limit food choices, poverty, reduced social contact, dementia, depression, and substance abuse. Consequences of malnutrition include diminished immune system function and greater risk for infection, poor wound healing, and muscle weakness that may contribute to falls and injuries (Mayo Clinic Staff, 2011a).

In 2012, nearly 41% of the U.S. population aged 65 to 74 years was overweight, and another 29% was obese. Overweight and obesity prevalence among those over 75 years of age were slightly lower at 30% and 18%, respectively (NCHS, 2014b). Older individuals with disabilities are even more likely to be obese. Obese and overweight individuals may forgo health care due to embarrassment regarding their weight.

Chronic dehydration is another dietary problem that occurs frequently in older populations. Dehydration leads to loss of muscle function, depression, altered states of consciousness, renal failure, and increased potential for medication toxicity, hypo- or hyperthermia, and infection. Dehydration is often unrecognized in the elderly, and mortality may be as much as seven times higher in dehydrated elders than in the general elderly population.

Finally, older clients may be lacking in specific nutrients such as iron, protein, and calcium. Calcium, in particular, is needed to prevent or ameliorate the effects of osteoporosis. Many older women, however, do not know that they should continue calcium intake into their older years. Population health nurses would assess the nutritional status of individual clients as well as that of the general elderly population, including factors contributing to malnutrition, dehydration, and overweight/obesity in the population.

Other consumption patterns. Other consumption patterns that affect the health status of the older adult population include tobacco, alcohol, and drug use. In 2012, more than 11% of people aged 65 to 74 years in the United States reported current smoking, and 40.5% reported being former smokers. The percentages of current and former smokers were slightly lower among people over 75 years of age at 5.7% and 41%, respectively (NCHS, 2014b). Elderly smokers are more likely than their younger counterparts to have health-related effects due to diminished respiratory function as a result of aging. Many older clients believe that smoking cessation will not make much difference with respect to their health. Smoking cessation at any age, however, can have beneficial effects, and population health nurses should promote smoking cessation among elderly clients who smoke.

Alcohol consumption may also affect the health of the older adult population. In 2012, current regular alcohol use was reported by 41.6% of Americans aged 65 to 74 years and 30% of those over 75 (NCHS, 2014b), and in 2009, binge drinking was reported by nearly 4% of those over age 65 (Kanny, Liu, & Brewer, 2011).

Misuse of other drugs may also occur among the elderly, and the negative effects of drug use accumulate over time. Opioids and benzodiazepines are among the mostly commonly abused drugs in the older population. Prescription drug abuse in the U.S. elderly is expected to increase by 190% from 911,000 people affected in 2001 to 2.7 million by 2020. Ten percent of people who sought treatment for substance abuse disorders in 2005 were over 50 years of age (Johns Hopkins Medicine, 2010). An estimated 4.4 million U.S. seniors are expected to need substance abuse treatment by 2020 compared to only 1.7 million in 2000. Treatment needs are expected to double in Europe (Roe, Beynon, Pickering, & Duffy, 2010). Unfortunately, treatment programs for older adults are often lacking and detoxification programs pose special hazards for the older population. Population health nurses would assess the older population for levels of substance use and abuse as well as the availability of smoking cessation and substance abuse treatment services targeted at this population.

Physical activity. As with their perceptions of the need for continued calcium intake, many older people do not believe they need to engage in much physical activity. Physical activity by older adults, however, has been shown to prevent disability and improve overall health and functional ability.

Physical activity provides both physical and psychological benefits for older clients. In the physical realm, exercise contributes to improved cardiovascular function, better control of hypertension and hyperlipidemia, and prevention of osteoporosis. Additional physical benefits include reduction in diabetes risk; increased muscle, bone, and joint strength; and decreased risk of falls. Psychologically, physical activity contributes to emotional well-being and improved self-assurance and self-concept and may be linked to improvements in cognition.

In spite of evidence regarding the benefits of physical activity, many older adults remain sedentary. According to 2012 figures, large numbers of people over 65 years of age failed to engage in recommended levels of physical activity. More than half met neither aerobic activity nor strengthening activity goals outlined in *Healthy People 2020* (NCHS, 2014b). In fact, research

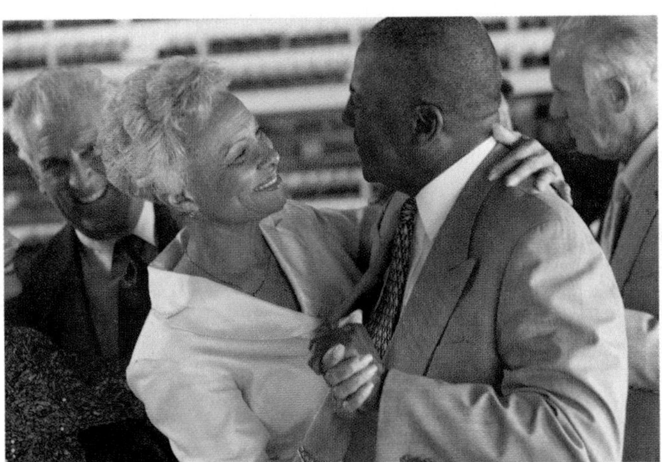

Physical activity is an important element of physical and mental health. *(Monkey Business/Fotolia)*

suggests that older people engage in purposive self-limitation of activity, more often spending time socializing, relaxing, reading, or watching television than in physical activity such as sports, exercise, and recreational activities (Guo & Phillips, 2010).

Sexuality. Sexuality considerations related to the older population include knowledge, attitudes, values, and behaviors, as well as changes in anatomy and physiology due to the aging process. Primary health care providers often assume that older clients are asexual and rarely discuss sexual issues with members of the older adult population. Evidence suggests that, despite these perceptions, sexuality continues to be an area of importance for many older people.

Older clients may also have concerns regarding sexual dysfunction. Because most older people grew up in an era when sexuality was not a topic for discussion, they may find it difficult to talk about such concerns with health care providers. As we saw in Chapter 17∞, many of the medications used to treat chronic diseases common in the elderly cause impotence in men. Similarly, aging may decrease vaginal secretions, making intercourse painful for older women (Chapter 18∞). Both older men and women may experience diminished sexual interest, which may interfere with marital intimacy.

Medication use. Medication use and misuse are significant factors in the health of the older adult population. Medication use is increasing among the elderly. National data indicate that nearly 90% of all people over 65 years of age use at least one prescription drug, with greater use among women than men. In 2007–2010, 47.5% of people over 65 years of age used five or more prescription drugs. The most commonly used drug categories among the elderly were cardiovascular and cholesterol lowering medications (NCHS, 2014a).

In addition to taking multiple prescription medications, older adults may also use a variety of over-the-counter (OTC) medications and herbal therapies, compounding the potential for drug interactions and adverse reactions. A 2010 survey by AARP and the National Center for Complementary and Alternative Medicine (NCCAM) indicated that half of respondents over 50 years of age had used some form of complementary or alternative medicine (CAM) at some point in their lives, and 47% had used CAM in the prior year. Among these people, 37% reported using herbal preparations. Frequent reasons given for CAM use included health promotion and illness prevention, pain relief, treatment of specific diseases, or to supplement conventional medicine. More than two thirds of the respondents did not inform their primary health care providers about their CAM use often because providers did not ask about CAM use and clients did not think to bring it up or feared provider disapproval (AARP & NCCAM, 2011).

In addition to the combination of multiple drugs, OTC medications, and herbal remedies, medication use in the elderly is complicated by the effects of aging. As age increases, changes occur in drug metabolism that increase the risk of adverse reactions and overdose.

Older clients may also have difficulty taking medications as recommended. An estimated 50% of the elderly have difficulty adhering to medication regimens. Medication misuse and nonadherence have been linked to poor control of many chronic health conditions and preventable hospital admissions and emergency department visits (American College of Preventive Medicine, 2011). Possible reasons for lack of adherence to treatment regimens are presented in Table 19-8● .

The *Focused Assessment* provided on page 499 can guide evaluation of medication use in elderly clients.

Other health-related behaviors. Population health nurses should also assess the extent of other health-related behaviors by individual clients and within the older population. Behaviors of particular interest include safety practices, driving, and obtaining immunizations. Population health nurses would assess the extent of use of safety devices and practices. For example, do older clients wear good fitting footwear to help prevent falls? Similarly, do they use assistive devices as appropriate to foster mobility while minimizing the risk of falls?

As noted earlier, continued ability to drive a car is an area of concern for many older people. Driving helps older adults maintain their independence. In 2009, there were 33 million drivers over the age of 65 on U.S. streets and highways. Older adults are more likely than younger ones to sustain injuries in motor vehicle accidents, and in 2008, vehicular accidents killed 5,500 U.S. elders and injured another 183,000 (NCIPC, 2013a). Fortunately, most older adults engage in safe driving habits, wearing seatbelts, and driving only in safe weather conditions. In addition, older drivers are less likely to drive while under the influence of alcohol. Older people may not, however, recognize the risks posed by many medications in terms of drowsiness or dizziness. Population health nurses should assist older clients and their families to determine when continued driving is no longer safe. They can also assist older people in finding alternate forms of transportation and advocate for the availability of transportation services for this population.

TABLE 19-8 Categories of Factors Influencing Nonadherence Among Older Clients

Category	Influencing Factors
Patient-related factors	• Visual, hearing, or cognitive impairment (including developmental disability or dementia) • Limited dexterity • Difficulty swallowing • Difficulty remembering • Lack of disease knowledge and understanding of need for therapy • Denial of condition or need for therapy • Level of self-efficacy • Motivation • Fear or experience of adverse/side effects • Fear of dependence • Feelings of stigmatization • Anxiety, stress • Depression/mental health disorder • Substance abuse
Social factors	• Language barriers • Low health literacy • Lack of social support • Difficulty incorporating compliance into daily schedules • Lack of pharmacy access • Cultural beliefs and attitudes • Elder abuse
Economic factors	• Medication/copayment costs • Lack of health insurance/drug coverage
Condition-related factors	• Absence of symptoms • Lack of immediate benefit • Need for unwanted behavioral changes
Therapy-related factors	• Complexity of regimen • Need to master certain cognitive or psychomotor skills (e.g., dosage calculation, use of monitoring devices) • Duration of therapy • Frequent changes in therapy • Perceived social stigma attached to therapy
Health system-related factors	• Quality of relationships with providers • Extent of provider communication skills • Lack of positive reinforcement • Lack of educational capacity in health system • Failure to tailor educational materials to client literacy or education level, culture • Client frustration with quality of care, wait times, etc. • Lack of continuity of care

Source: American College of Preventive Medicine. (2011). *Medication adherence—Improving health outcomes: A resource from the American College of Preventive Medicine.* Retrieved from http://c.ymcdn.com/sites/www.acpm.org/resource/resmgr/timetools-files/adherenceclinicalreference.pdf

As noted earlier, population health nurses assessing the health of older populations should assess the immune levels within the population. They should also examine the extent to which older people avail themselves of recommended immunizations. In 2011, national coverage for pneumococcal disease among people over 65 years of age was only 62% (Williams et al., 2013), and during the 2012–2013 influenza season, only 66.7% of this population were immunized (National Center for Immunization and Respiratory Diseases, 2013). Similarly, only slightly over half of older Americans were up to date on tetanus immunizations (Williams et al., 2013). Behavioral determinants affecting the health of the older population can be assessed using the questions posed in the *Focused Assessment* on the next page.

HEALTH SYSTEM DETERMINANTS. The demand for health care services increases significantly in older people. Most of this increase is due to the multiple chronic illnesses experienced by older adults. For this reason, early diagnosis and effective treatment of chronic illness can help decrease the societal burden of care for the elderly.

The concept of "aging in place" was conceived as a way of improving the quality of life for older adults and of decreasing the cost burden of their care by maintaining older individuals in their homes whenever possible and providing care in the least expensive setting. **Aging in place** means being able to remain in one's home despite challenges posed by aging or health-related conditions (MetLife, 2010). Based on a Metropolitan Life

FOCUSED ASSESSMENT Assessing Medication Use in Older Clients

- Is the client taking prescribed medications?
- Is the client taking over-the-counter (OTC) medications?
- Is the client using any complementary or alternative therapies? If so, is there potential for interactions with prescription medications?
- Are any of the client's medications contraindicated by existing health conditions?
- Do OTC medications potentiate or counteract prescription medications?
- Do prescription medications potentiate or counteract each other?
- Does the client take prescription and OTC medications as directed (e.g., correct dose, route, time)?
- Does the client comply with other directions regarding medications (e.g., not taking with dairy products)?
- Is the client aware of potential food–drug interactions or drug–drug interactions?
- Are medications achieving the desired effects?
- Is the client experiencing any medication side effects?
- What is the client doing about medication side effects, if any?
- Is the client exhibiting symptoms of any adverse medication effects?

Insurance Company Mature Market Institute report (MetLife, 2010), three foci are required for effective aging in place in the United States. The first is a focus on maintaining the independence of the older person. The second requires more economical use of available resources, and the third addresses the need for coordinated, comprehensive, collaborative relationships between providers and businesses to support aging in place. Provision of comprehensive coordinated services will require access to health care and other services, mechanisms for funding prescription and other coverage to meet health-related needs, and the availability of infrastructure support that allows older people, even those with multiple health problems to remain in their own homes. An additional health system determinant that influences the health of the older populations is the quality of interactions with health care providers.

Health care access. Access to health care services for older Americans has improved significantly since the advent of Medicare in the 1960s. In 2012, Medicare provided health insurance coverage for 93% of the U.S. population over 65 years of age, and 9% of the population also received Medicaid funded services. Overall, 98% of the population 65 years of age and older had some form of health insurance (AoA, 2013a).

The costs of health care to those without insurance can be prohibitive. Even with insurance, costs of care may impede access. For example, in 2011, the average out-of-pocket expenditure for health-related expenses was $4,769, an increase of 40% from 2000 figures (AoA, 2013a). A couple retiring at age 65 in 2013 will need an estimated $240,000 to cover health-related expenses over the remainder of their lives, and this figure does not even account for possible long-term care

FOCUSED ASSESSMENT Assessing Behavioral Determinants Influencing the Health of Older Populations

- What are the typical dietary patterns among the elderly in the population? What is the extent of obesity in the elderly population? What nutritional deficits are prevalent in the elderly population?
- What is the extent of smoking, alcohol, and drug use in the elderly population? What are the treatment rates for alcohol and drug abuse?
- To what extent do members of the elderly population engage in health-related behaviors such as testicular self-examination, mammography, and so on?
- To what extent do members of the elderly population employ safety precautions such as seat belt use?
- What proportion of the elderly population drives? What is the incidence of motor vehicle accidents among this population?
- What prescription and OTC medications are typically taken by elderly clients? What is the incidence of adverse events due to inappropriate medication use in the population?

expenses (Hamilton, 2013). More than three fourths of AARP members surveyed in 2012 indicated that paying for health care expenses was one of their biggest concerns (AARP, 2012b).

Some older adults also have no regular source of health care. In 2012, for example, nearly 4% of those aged 65 to 74 years and 2.8% of those over 75 had no usual source of care. Emergency departments were relied on for routine health care for 1.6% of those 65 to 74 years of age and 1.5% of those over age 75 (NCHS, 2014b). In 2012, 2.4% of older Americans reported failing to obtain needed health care services due to costs (AoA, 2013a).

Prescription drugs. Two elements of the health care system related to prescription drugs affect the health of older populations. The first is prescription of inappropriate drugs, and the second is the cost of medications.

A recent systematic review of related research (Opondo et al., 2012) indicated that more than 20% of prescriptions provided to elderly patients in primary care settings were inappropriate. Inappropriate medications most often prescribed included propoxyphene, doxazosin, diphenhydramine, and amitriptyline. The latter two medications have the greatest potential for adverse effects. The authors suggested that computerized clinical decision support systems could reduce the prevalence of inappropriately prescribed medications. Table 19-9● provides information on selected drugs that should be used with caution among older clients.

The cost of prescription drugs is one of the impediments to medication compliance among the elderly. Overall the cost of drugs per Medicare beneficiary in the United States increased almost fourfold from 1992 to 2008, to an average per person cost of $2,834 in 2008. Much of this increase can be attributed to increased prices of medications rather than increased numbers of prescriptions.

Drug costs vary significantly among older clients, with 6% of U.S. elders incurring no costs in 2008 and 15% incurring costs of $5,000 or more. Costs also vary by health status. For example, in 2008 the average drug cost for persons with no chronic conditions was $1,230, compared to $5,300 for those with five or more chronic conditions (Federal Interagency Forum on Aging-Related Statistics, 2012).

Prior to 2006, prescription drug costs were born out-of-pocket by most elderly. In January 2006, however, Medicare Part D was initiated to subsidize prescription medications for part D subscribers. Part D included two options: enrollment in a stand-alone drug plan or enrollment in a Medicare Advantage managed care program that includes prescription drug benefits (Centers for Medicare and Medicaid Services [CMS], 2014). For further information about Medicare Part D drug coverage, see the *External Resources* section of the student resources site.

The advent of Medicare Part D prescription drug coverage substantially reduced out-of-pocket costs for medications, from 60% of costs in 1992 to 23% of costs in 2008. From June of 2006 to October 2011, the number of Medicare beneficiaries enrolled in Part D prescription drug plans increased from 18.2 million to 23.8 million people or 38% of all Medicare beneficiaries (Federal Interagency Forum on Aging-related Statistics, 2012).

TABLE 19-9 Hazardous Medications for Older Clients

Drug Classification	Specific Medications	Potential Hazard
Analgesics	Meperidine, pentazocine, propoxyphene	Confusion, hallucinations
Anticholinergics/antihistamines	Chlorpheniramine, diphenhydramine, hydroxyzine, cyproheptadine, promethazine, tripelennamine, dexchlorpheniramine	Confusion, delirium, blurred vision, constipation, dry mouth, lightheadedness, urinary difficulty or incontinence, hallucinations, tachycardia
Anticoagulants	Warfarin, Coumadin	Bleeding, particularly with malnutrition, low albumin levels, interactions with Cipro, phenytoin, amiodarone, cephalosporins, high-dose penicillins, aspirin, barbiturates, cholestryamine, Lovenox, herbals (Ginkgo biloba, garlic), and high vitamin K foods Increased risk of serious injury with falls
Antihypertensives	Alpha-blockers, beta-blockers, diuretics	Orthostatic hypertension, sedation and depression, confusion, impotence, constipation
Cardiotonics	Digoxin	Increased risk of toxicity, arrhythmias
Diuretics	Potassium losing diuretics	Hypokalemia
Hypoglycemics	Insulin, Metformin	Hypoglycemia, vision changes
Nonsteroidal anti-inflammatory drugs (NSAIDS)	Naproxen, oxaprozin, piroxicam	GI bleeding, renal failure, high blood pressure, heart failure
Psychoactive drugs	Sedative/hypnotics, antidepressants, anxiolytics, antipsychotics, psychoactive stimulants	Increased risk of falls and other injuries, GI effects

Data from: Zwicker, D. A., & Fulmer, T. (2012). Reducing adverse drug events. In M. Boltz, E. Capezuti, T. Fulmer, & D. Zwicker (Eds.) *Evidence-based geriatric nursing protocols for best practice* (4th ed., pp. 324–362). New York, NY: Springer.

Initiation of Medicare Part D prescription drug coverage did not entirely eliminate the problem of high drug costs for seniors, however. Coverage provisions created a "doughnut hole" in which clients paid the bulk of the costs of prescription coverage. The doughnut hole was entered when the beneficiary had incurred $2,250 in annual drug costs. Once total costs had exceeded $5,100 in a year, Part D benefits resumed with a small copayment of approximately 5% of costs. In 2010 the Affordable Care Act (ACA) was enacted, provisions of which are intended to gradually reduce the effects of the doughnut hole and eliminate it entirely by 2020 (AARP, n.d.). From the passage of the act until October 2011, ACA resulted in more than $464 million in savings on prescription drug costs for the American elderly (Reid, 2011). For 2014, Part D enrollees paid the basic premium for their specific Part D plan plus a maximum deductible amount of $310, as well as a copayment (a flat fee for each prescription) or co-insurance (a percentage of the cost of the prescription) until total drug costs for the year reached $2,850. From that point until drug costs for the year totaled $4,550, the beneficiary paid 47.5% of the cost of brand-name drugs and 72% of the cost of generic drugs. Beyond the doughnut hole, the beneficiary pays only a small copayment for each prescription (CMS, 2014).

Infrastructure support. Infrastructure support factors that affect the health of older populations arise out of environment, sociocultural, and health system determinants. For example, housing modifications that accommodate diminished functional status (e.g., ramps versus stairs, home safety features) are environmental factors that can allow people to remain at home and continue to be independent. Similarly, transportation systems that meet the needs of the elderly who are no longer able to drive and policies that support in-home assistance are sociocultural determinants that foster aging in place. Within the health care system, the availability of home health and care management services, durable medical equipment, home telehealth services, and respite services for caretakers are examples of factors that can support aging in place (MetLife, 2010).

Client–provider interactions. Another major health system consideration that affects the health of older populations is the quality of interactions with health care providers. These interactions are shaped by knowledge and attitudes on the part of providers as well as clients. As reflected in the discussion of inappropriate prescriptions given to older adults, some providers do not have the knowledge or expertise to provide effective care to this population.

Difficulties in client–provider interactions may also arise from communication barriers and lack of empowerment of older persons. Health care providers may be particularly prone to attempting to make decisions for older clients based on perceptions of what is "in their best interests." Empowerment of older clients was addressed earlier as a sociocultural determinant of health in older clients.

Barriers to effective communication between older clients and health care providers may stem from client attitudes and abilities or from provider characteristics. Client attributes that may impede communication include diminished communication abilities due to declining hearing, vision, or cognitive ability; diminished self-worth; and lack of knowledge about health-related issues. Provider-related barriers may include ageist attitudes and discrimination, as well as lack of knowledge and expertise regarding the needs of and interventions appropriate to older clients. Lack of health literacy on the part of clients and failure of providers to consider literacy issues may also impede communication.

Differences may also arise from the primary foci of providers and clients. Providers tend to focus on disease and its treatment, whereas the primary focus of many older clients is on quality of life. An additional barrier to communication between health care providers and older clients is a phenomenon called "elder speak." Elder speak is an approach to communication with the elderly that conveys a message of incompetence and control and may take one of two forms: excessively nurturing communication and controlling communication. Elder speak may be characterized by a slow rate of speech, exaggerated intonation, elevated pitch and volume, frequent repetition, and the use of simple vocabulary and grammar. Other characteristics may include use of inappropriate terms of endearment (e.g., "honey" or "sweetie"), use of the plural pronoun "we," and use of questions that prompt a specific answer (e.g., "you want to wear this pretty blue sweater, don't you?") such as one might use with a child. Research has indicated that a significant proportion of communication occurring in nursing home settings involves elder speak, and older clients in both institutional and home settings report they perceive the use of such speech as demeaning, patronizing, or implying incompetence. In one study, the use of elder speak was closely related to resistiveness to care among patients with dementia, while normal speech was related to cooperation with care (Williams, Herman, Gajweski, & Wilson, 2009).

Information on access to health care as well as use of health care services can be obtained from local providers as well as community surveys of the elderly population. Community surveys and health institutions can also provide information on the extent or lack of health care insurance in the older population. Information on the quality of interactions between providers and older clients, however, is likely to be available only through community surveys or small-scale qualitative studies involving participant observation or interviews. *Focused Assessment* questions related to the health system determinants of health in older populations are provided on the next page.

Diagnostic Reasoning and Care of Older Populations

Once the population health nurse has determined the extent to which factors in each category of determinants of health are affecting the health of the older population and determined what those effects are, he or she would derive population nursing diagnoses related to the population's health status. These

FOCUSED ASSESSMENT Assessing Health System Determinants Influencing the Health of Older Populations

- What proportion of the elderly population has a regular source of health care?
- What is the level of insurance coverage among the elderly population (e.g., Medicare A and B, supplementary insurance)?
- To what extent are medication needs covered by insurance plans among the elderly population?
- What preventive and restorative health care services are available to members of the elderly population? To what extent are these services used by the population? How adequate are these services in meeting the needs of the elderly population?
- To what extent are palliative services, end-of-life care, and hospice services available and accessible to the elderly population?

diagnoses would reflect the problems identified in the elderly population as well as the availability of resources within the community to address these problems.

Nursing diagnoses may be either positive or negative. An example of a positive diagnosis might be: "community ability to maintain older clients in their own homes due to the availability and accessibility of assistance with ADLs." Positive diagnoses usually indicate that no further nursing intervention is needed, but that the health status of the population in this area should continue to be monitored. A negative diagnosis might be "lack of assistance with ADLs for older persons with functional disabilities." In this instance, the diagnosis would indicate the need for intervention by nurses and others in the community to resolve the identified problem.

Planning to Meet the Health Needs of Older Populations

Planning to meet the health care needs of older clients may involve health promotion, illness and injury prevention, resolution of existing health problems, or health restoration services. Major emphases in planning health care for older clients should be on successful aging and promotion of self-care. As noted earlier, aging can result in loss of functional abilities, stamina, and so on, but these losses can be balanced to achieve successful aging. Health care for older clients should be based on the standards for gerontological nursing practice developed by the American Nurses Association (2010). For further information about the standards, see the *External Resources* section of the student resources site.

General recommendations for addressing the health needs of the older population in the United States have been delineated in the *Guide to Community Preventive Services*. These recommendations include the following: (CDC, AoA, AHRQ, & CMS, 2011):

- Reducing out-of-pocket costs for care
- Increasing annual wellness visits
- Providing routine reminders for immunizations and recommended screening tests
- Using "small" media (e.g., newspapers, radio) to raise health awareness
- Tailoring health-related messages to individual needs and risk factors
- Initiating standing orders to prevent missed opportunities for preventive services
- Reducing structural barriers to access to care (e.g., distance, hours of operation, availability of respite services)
- Expanding access to care beyond traditional health care sites to community locations
- Providing "one-stop shopping" for health care services

Considerations related to each specific level of health care are discussed below.

HEALTH PROMOTION. Health promotion among the elderly is imperative for several reasons. First, they are the fastest-growing segment of the population. In addition, they exhibit the highest prevalence of chronic illness, and finally, they use the majority of health care services. Increasing longevity necessitates a focus on health promotion and illness prevention; however, these aspects of care are often neglected among the elderly in the mistaken belief that there is little benefit to be gained for people who may already have multiple chronic illnesses.

Health promotion often depends on changes in health-related behaviors. Although we often think about behavioral change as occurring at the individual-client level, behavior-related interventions should actually occur at three levels: individual, community, and national. Population health nurses can be particularly active in promoting activity at each of these levels. At the individual level, population health nurses can educate clients to take steps to modify dietary and physical activity behaviors to promote health. At the community level, initiatives can be undertaken to change environmental factors that influence health-related behaviors. These initiatives may include public policy interventions such as designing communities to promote safe opportunities for physical activity by all age groups, but particularly for the elderly. At the national level, comprehensive campaigns can be undertaken to address widespread behavior change among either clients (e.g., the recent campaign on weight control and physical activity) or health care providers (e.g., the development of national guidelines for preventive activities).

Population health nurses may need to actively advocate for the availability of health promotion services to older clients. They may also need to advocate among the elderly population to foster use of these services. General aspects of health promotion in the older population include maintaining independence and life resolution. More specific considerations include nutrition, rest and physical activity, and health promotion for caregivers.

Maintaining independence. Because of physical and economic limitations, it is sometimes difficult for older persons to maintain their independence. Decreased income and physical inability to care for themselves sometimes force older clients to give up their own residence and live with family members. Whatever the living arrangements of older clients, population health nurses should assist them to maintain the highest degree of independence possible. Some older clients may be able to continue to live alone if referred to supportive services such as homemaker aides, transportation services, and Meals-on-Wheels.

Maintaining independence may demand new approaches to doing things. For example, when physical limitations prohibit typical self-care activities, such as bathing or washing dishes, due to inabilities to turn on stubborn taps, population health nurses can suggest replacing twist-type faucet controls with lever taps or using a dishcloth or nonslip material to grip the tap handle. Developing new approaches to self-care first involves identification of the underlying problem and development of alternative techniques to achieve one's goals. Elders should be encouraged to do as much as possible for themselves and have outside assistance provided only when needed. Modifications in storage facilities to place frequently used items in handy locations may help as will the use of assistive devices such as "grabbers." In other cases it may be helpful to simplify tasks (e.g., putting all tooth brushing needs in the same place). Decluttering areas and placing items in the sequence in which they are usually used may also be helpful. In addition, spreading active tasks throughout the day or week with ample time for rest or when pain is at a minimum may help to conserve client's energy and minimize discomfort. Environmental adaptations such as raised toilet seats, ramps rather than stairs, or moving to single-level housing may also promote continued independence (Swann, 2010).

When older persons are living with family members, the nurse can encourage family members to foster independence in the client. This may mean encouraging families to assign specific roles within the household to the older family member. Population health nurses can also be actively involved in designing and implementing programs intended to assist older clients to age in place.

Life resolution. Creating meaning for one's life is one of the developmental tasks to be accomplished by older adults. This entails developing a personal set of goals and the ability to view one's life as having been productive. Reminiscence is one way of accomplishing life resolution and achieving positive feelings about one's own life. The population health nurse must recognize and foster older clients' need to reminisce and should encourage family members to do so as well. This is sometimes difficult given the nurse's busy schedule and the number of clients who need to be seen; however, nurses should be able to find some time during interactions with older clients to listen to these reminiscences and to help clients reflect on their lives. In spite of cognitive losses, reminiscence or "life review" has also been shown to be effective with some clients with Alzheimer's disease (Chao, Chen, Liu, & Clark, 2008).

Nutrition. Adequate nutrition is important for the older population to maintain health, prevent disease, and prevent further effects of existing chronic conditions. Adequate nutrition for health promotion frequently entails a reduction in caloric intake. Despite reduced caloric needs, older adults continue to require a balance of all other nutrients. Nutritional deficits are most frequently noted for calcium; iron; vitamins A, D, and C; the B vitamins riboflavin and thiamine; and dietary fiber. Population health nurses can promote the health of older clients by educating this population regarding their nutritional requirements.

Other, more general interventions may also be needed to improve older clients' nutritional status by eliminating impediments to good nutrition. For example, social isolation may need to be addressed because people tend to eat better in company with others. Older clients can be referred to senior nutrition centers, or family members can be encouraged to drop by at mealtimes to eat with older clients who live alone. Interventions may also be required to deal with nausea, poorly fitting dentures, or other factors that may impede good nutrition. Population health nurses may also need to be active in the development and implementation of programs to meet the nutritional needs of the older population where these services do not already exist, or in increasing access to existing services for underserved segments of the population.

As noted earlier, a significant proportion of the U.S. elderly population is obese and another group is undernourished. Worldwide, malnutrition is a common problem among seniors. The Older Americans Act nutrition program has been designed to provide an integrated diet and exercise program for the older population. The program serves a threefold purpose: to reduce hunger and food insecurity among older Americans, to promote socialization, and to promote health and well-being through access to nutrition and other health promotion and illness prevention services (AoA, 2013b).

The Older Americans Act (OAA) funds three types of nutrition programs for the elderly: congregate nutrition services (e.g., lunches in senior centers or other locales), home-delivered services, and the Nutrition Services Incentive Program (NSIP) that provides additional funds to states and territories and eligible tribal organizations for the purchase of food for senior nutrition programs. NSIP funds can be used only for food purchase and not for preparation or other nutrition-related services, such as nutrition education (AoA, 2013b). The National Resource Center on Nutrition, Physical Activity, and Aging (n.d.b) has developed a two-part guideline to assist communities in developing senior nutrition programs. For further information about the guidelines, see the *External Resources* section of the student resources site.

Physical activity and rest. Many people believe that the need for exercise decreases with age; however, older people need exercise as much as their younger counterparts. CDC (2014c) recommendations for physical activity among older adults include muscle strengthening that works all major muscle groups on 2 or more days a week and either 150 minutes of moderate intensity aerobic activity or 75 minutes of vigorous-intensity aerobic activity or an equivalent combination of moderate and vigorous activity per week. Older clients can be encouraged to spread their activity over the day or week to avoid fatigue and discomfort.

Unfortunately, members of the older adult population often fail to engage in recommended physical activity. Barriers to physical activity among the elderly include lack of time, pain, boredom, fatigue, unsafe environments, fear of injury, lack of awareness of the need to exercise, environments not conducive to physical activity, and failure to set reasonable exercise goals. Population health nurses can help design and provide physical activity programs for older adults that address these barriers. Community-based exercise programs can have positive effects on physical activity among older clients.

The quality of rest is another consideration in caring for the older adult population. Many older adults experience insomnia that may be due to underlying disease states, medications, or use of alcohol, tobacco, or caffeine. Interventions that may assist clients with insomnia include treating underlying diseases, keeping a sleep log to determine possible triggers to wakefulness, adjusting medication regimens as needed, and promoting good sleep hygiene. The last can be accomplished by promoting exercise (particularly outdoor activity); increasing exposure to light; avoiding alcohol, tobacco, and caffeine after midafternoon; avoiding daytime naps if possible; and not working in bed. Other possible interventions include developing a relaxing bedtime routine, promoting pain control, and reducing ambient lighting an hour or so before bed (Hulisz & Duff, 2009). Population health nurses can educate clients with sleep problems regarding these strategies. They should also caution clients regarding the potential adverse effects of the use of over-the-counter sleep aids and herbal supplements because of their interactions with many prescription medications. Nurses may also refer clients for medical care of underlying diseases or for changes in medications that may be contributing to wakefulness.

Caregiver health promotion. Health promotion interventions may also be required for caregivers of older clients. The Family Caregiver Alliance (2012) has developed several foci and action steps to enhance caregiver health and well-being as presented in Table 19-10●. Population health nurses can assist caregivers to attend to their own needs and engage in the suggested activities. Population health nursing interventions related to health promotion for caregivers as well as for the older population are summarized in Table 19-11●. For information on sources of assistance for caregivers, see the *External Resources* section of the student resources site.

ILLNESS AND INJURY PREVENTION. The second level of health care involves strategies to prevent specific illnesses and injuries. Several barriers to illness and injury prevention in older populations have been identified (Ogden, Richards, & Shenson, 2012). These include lack of insurance coverage and out-of-pocket costs for preventive services, although this has been somewhat minimized by preventive health provisions of the Affordable Care Act. For example, in 2011, 17 million older Americans received preventive services funded without copayments under ACA (Reid, 2011). Other barriers to preventive services include lack of providers knowledgeable about geriatric prevention needs, lack of coordination of services, and low health literacy and education levels including language difficulties. Another barrier is the existence of multiple comorbidities that require complex management (Ogden et al., 2012). For example, limited ability to stand and move makes it difficult to obtain a mammogram without specialized equipment. Major considerations in illness and injury prevention for the elderly to be addressed here include elimination or modification of risk factors and prevention of specific diseases, injury and abuse prevention, prevention of incontinence, and immunization.

Risk factor modification. Population health nurses assist older individuals and population groups to modify or eliminate risk factors for disease. This may involve interventions like

TABLE 19-10 Activities to Promote Caregiver Health

Caregiver Health Promotion Activities
• Reduce personal stress • Set achievable goals • Seek solutions to problems • Communicate constructively • Ask for and accept help • Share personal concerns with primary care providers • Engage in exercise • Get adequate rest and nutrition • Accept and deal with emotions • Attend to personal health needs • Participate in nurturing activities • Change negative views • Seek counselling as needed

Source: Family Caregiver Alliance. (2012). *Taking care of you: Self-care for family caregivers.* Retrieved from https://caregiver.org/taking-care-you-self-care-family-caregivers

TABLE 19-11 Health Promotion Strategies for Older Populations

Area of Focus	Health Promotion Strategies
Maintaining independence	Participate in the development of services that allow clients to live independently as long as possible. Promote environments that support independent living by the older population.
Life resolution	Encourage reminiscence.
Diet and nutrition	Educate public regarding nutritional needs of older adults. Assure access to nutritional foods. Eliminate social and environmental barriers to good nutrition.
Physical activity and rest	Educate the older population on the need for exercise. Participate in the development of physical activity programs that address the most common barriers to exercise among older clients. Develop programs to deal with insomnia in the elderly.
Caregiver health promotion	Assist caregivers with adjustment to caregiving. Promote caregiver independence and personal life. Educate caregivers for needed skills. Educate and encourage caregivers regarding nutrition, physical activity, and rest. Educate and assist caregivers to adapt to the effects of aging on their own abilities. Educate caregivers regarding fall prevention and medication safety. Refer caregivers for hearing and vision checks and correction services. Promote social interaction by caregivers. Refer caregivers to social support networks. Advocate for and initiate caregiver support networks. Advocate for and refer to respite care. Assist caregivers with stress management, referring for professional care as needed. Assist caregivers to develop good coping skills. Provide positive reinforcement for caregiver activities. Assist caregivers with emergency planning and execution of power of attorney. Assist caregivers in navigating the Internet and judging the credibility of information found; refer for assistance with computer literacy skills.

smoking cessation or effective management of existing health conditions, such as obesity, diabetes, or hypertension, that are risk factors for other conditions like cardiovascular disease and stroke. Treatment for diseases that increase older adults risk of subsequent health problems will be addressed in the section on resolution of existing health problems.

Smoking cessation may be beneficial for the older population in preventing smoking-attributable health problems. In fact, the U.S. Preventive Services Task Force (USPSTF, 2013) has recommended asking all adults about tobacco use and referring current users to tobacco cessation programs. In addition to the obvious cardiovascular and respiratory effects, not smoking has been associated with decreased risk for colorectal and other cancers. A 5As model has been developed to assist with smoking cessation in older adults. Elements of this model include:

1. **A**sking about smoking behaviors
2. **A**dvising clients regarding the need to stop smoking
3. **A**ssessing clients' willingness to stop smoking
4. **A**ssisting them with smoking cessation strategies or referral to smoking cessation programs
5. **A**rranging for follow-up to support smoking cessation and monitor its effectiveness (AHRQ, n.d.).

Research in nine HMOs has indicated that incorporating more than just advising clients to stop smoking is associated with better success rates. Unfortunately, older clients are frequently not even advised to stop smoking much less assisted with referrals or pharmacotherapy to assist cessation. From 2002 to 2007, for example, 24% of men and 30% of women over 65 years of age reported not being counseled to stop smoking (CDC, AoA, AHRQ, & CMS, 2011). Population health nurses can refer older clients who smoke to smoking cessation programs or assist in the development of such programs. They can also campaign for access to such programs and coverage of smoking cessation under health insurance plans.

USPSTF has also made a few other recommendations for preventive interventions among older clients (as well as screening recommendations, which will be discussed later in this chapter). Preventive recommendations include the use of aspirin to prevent myocardial infarction in men 45 to 79 years of age, and women aged 55 to 79 years. Similarly, all sexually active adults should be counseled regarding prevention of sexually transmitted diseases (STDs) whatever their age. In addition, exercise or physical therapy has been recommended along with the use of vitamin D in people over 65 years at risk for falls, but the task force recently rescinded its long-standing recommendation to combine supplemental calcium and vitamin D to prevent fractures citing a lack of sufficient evidence of efficacy. Other recommendations include dietary counseling for adults with hyperlipidemia. Finally, USPSTF has recommended against the use of hormone replacement therapy to prevent osteoporosis and cardiovascular disease in postmenopausal women (USPSTF, 2013). Recommendations change, however, with advances in knowledge. For information on current prevention recommendations for the elderly, see the *External Resources* section of the student resources site.

Injury and abuse prevention. Safety and injury prevention are areas of significant concern in the care of the older population. As we saw earlier, falls and other injuries are major contributors to disability in older populations. Risk factors for falls in the elderly include arthritis, problems with gait or balance, poor muscle strength, and vision problems. The risk of falls also increases with the number of medications taken.

Fall prevention education alone has not been particularly effective in reducing falls in the elderly. One reason is that, while older people may accept fall prevention messages, they often do not view them as relevant to themselves. Instead, older clients may be more receptive to messages that emphasize health and independence. Elements of fall prevention programs include assessment for fall risk and tailored interventions based on risk factors identified; exercise, such as tai chi; medication review for drugs that cause dizziness, drowsiness, or postural hypotension, and use of corrective lenses for vision problems (CDC, 2013a). Tai chi and other similar exercise programs for older populations have been shown to reduce falls by as much as half (NCIPC, 2013b). Elimination of safety hazards also serves to prevent falls and may include installing handrails and lights on stairs and grab bars and nonslip mats in showers and tubs; removing throw rugs, cords, and other trip hazards; providing adequate lighting; using shades and curtains to reduce glare; and wearing sturdy shoes, rather than slippers, inside and outside (CDC, 2013b).

Safe driving is another area of concern among older clients, particularly those with sensory impairments or diminished reaction times. Strategies for motor vehicle accident prevention in this age group include exercise to promote flexibility and strength, medication review, and vision assessment. Population health nurses can also encourage older clients to drive during the day and in good weather, find and plan the safest routes ahead of time, and avoid distractions while driving. They can also encourage unsafe drivers to use public transit or ride with others (NCIPC, 2013a). Unfortunately, transportation services for the elderly are often lacking, leaving older populations with decreased mobility and diminished opportunities for social interaction.

Motor vehicles are also problematic when older people are pedestrians. In many areas, the bulk of pedestrian fatalities occur among elderly individuals. In areas where there are large numbers of elderly, nurses can campaign for traffic signals at heavily used crossings, strict enforcement of speed limits, and public awareness of the presence of older adults.

Population health nurses can initiate and participate in education campaigns related to safety issues for the older population. In addition, they can support initiatives that promote safe environments for the elderly. Finally, they may need to engage in activity to promote access to public transportation to meet the needs of the elderly, particularly those with disabilities that may limit their ability to use existing transportation systems.

Home and neighborhood safety and prevention of elder abuse are two other safety concerns with older populations. Population health nurses can be active in promoting police activity to make neighborhoods safe for older clients to move about in them. They may also be involved in the development of neighborhood watch programs and in programs to alert public safety officials that older clients are residing in particular places. This is particularly important for older disabled individuals in the community. For example, nurses can participate in the development of programs to identify homes with older residents so fire and police personnel can meet their special needs in the event of an emergency.

The last area of concern in promoting the safety of older clients is preventing abuse and neglect. Risk factors for abuse occur at the individual, relationship, community, and societal level. Individual level factors related to perpetrators of abuse include the presence of mental illness, substance abuse, high levels of hostility, poor preparation for caregiving activities, assumption of caregiving responsibilities at an early age, inadequate coping, and exposure to maltreatment as a child. Relationship factors include financial or emotional dependence on the elder, disruptive behavior on the part of the elder, and lack of formal and informal support systems. At the community level, limited or unavailable formal support services may contribute to abuse. Finally, societal factors include social tolerance for aggressive behavior, a culture in which individuals are given great freedom to make decisions for others, social expectations related to family caregiving responsibility, stoic beliefs, philosophies, and negative attitudes toward aging and elders (NCIPC, 2014b). Population health nurses can assess for the presence of these risk factors in individual situations as well as their prevalence within the population. They can also make referrals for assistance to modify risk factors and advocate for the availability of services to prevent abuse. Specific interventions for preventing abuse are discussed in more detail in Chapter 30∞.

Immunization. The Advisory Committee on Immunization Practices (ACIP) currently recommends one dose of tetanus toxoid, reduced diphtheria toxoid, and acellular pertussis

(Tdap) vaccine for all adults, followed by tetanus and diphtheria toxoid (Td) boosters every 10 years. Other vaccines recommended for routine administration for people over 65 years of age include annual influenza immunization, two doses of chickenpox vaccine, one dose of herpes zoster vaccine (HZV) after 60 years of age to prevent shingles, and one dose of pneumococcal vaccine. Additional recommendations for older adults at particular risk of disease include meningococcal, hepatitis A, and hepatitis B immunization (CDC, 2014d). Immunization recommendations are updated, and population health nurses can obtain the most recent ACIP recommendations from the CDC website.

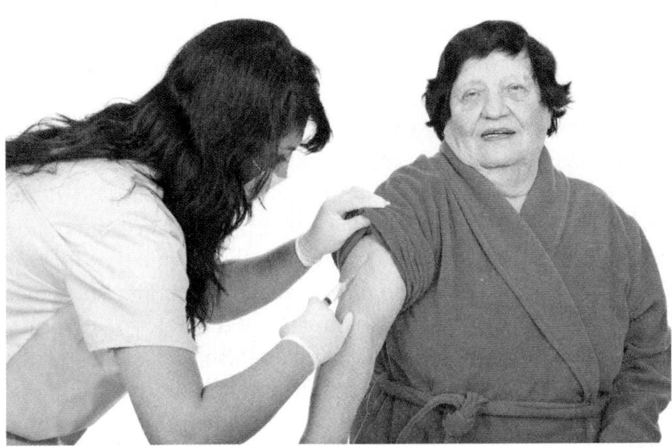

Immunization is an important component of prevention for older adults. *(Gabriel Blaj/Fotolia)*

Population health nurses can be active in providing immunization services for older adults as well as in educating the older population regarding the need for immunizations. Nurses may also be involved in the design of programs and services to meet the immunization needs of the older population, making sure that all segments of the population have access to services. Such services may be provided under standing orders in nontraditional settings, such as pharmacies, senior centers, and so on, improving the proportion of the older population that has access to immunization services.

Incontinence prevention. The last aspect of prevention to be addressed here is prevention of incontinence. Urinary incontinence may be prevented by maintaining a healthy weight, refraining from smoking, performing Kegel exercises to strengthen pelvic floor muscles, preventing constipation, and avoiding bladder irritants such as alcohol or caffeine (Mayo Clinic Staff, 2011b). Preventing fecal incontinence may involve ingesting adequate fiber and preventing constipation, avoiding foods that irritate the gastrointestinal tract, establishing a regular time for defecation, and stimulating bowel emptying on a regular basis (International Foundation for Functional Gastrointestinal Disorders, 2013b). Interventions for preventing incontinence, as well as other illness and injury prevention strategies are summarized in Table 19-12●.

RESOLUTION OF EXISTING PROBLEMS. Resolution of existing health problems in the older population involves screening, diagnosis, and treatment of disease. Because of the prevalence of chronic illness, self-management of disease is another important area of emphasis in health problem resolution.

TABLE 19-12 Illness and Injury Prevention Strategies for Older Populations

Area of Focus	Strategy
Risk factor modification	Educate the older population on the need for and benefits of smoking cessation. Assist in the development of programs to assist older clients with smoking cessation.
Injury and abuse prevention	Educate public regarding safety issues for older adults. Promote exercise to strengthen muscles, bones, and joints. Eliminate environmental safety hazards. Educate older drivers regarding the hazards of driving. Promote alternative forms of transportation for older adults. Initiate or promote programs to alert fire and police personnel to older clients in specific residences. Promote family coping abilities and relieve stress to prevent abuse of older persons.
Immunization	Educate older populations regarding the need for immunizations. Provide immunization services and assure their accessibility to all segments of the older population. Develop immunization programs in places where older clients are frequently found.
Incontinence prevention	Educate older populations regarding diet and physical activity to maintain healthy weight. Encourage smoking cessation. Refer for smoking cessation assistance. Teach clients to perform Kegel exercises. Encourage avoidance of bladder irritants such as alcohol and caffeine. Encourage fiber consumption to prevent constipation.

Screening. Screening is another aspect of care that is often neglected among older clients. Many people believe that it is not necessary to engage in early detection of disease because the benefits of treatment are minimal among the elderly. A number of disease conditions can still be effectively treated in the older population, however, if found early enough. For example, older adults are perceived to have a poor prognosis for colorectal cancer, yet surgery is quite effective following early detection of disease. Screening procedures recommended by USPSTF (2013) for older adults are summarized in Table 19-13•.

Population health nurses can educate older clients regarding the need for routine screening and refer them for screening services. Clients with particular risk factors or symptoms of possible disease should also be referred for screening and diagnostic services as appropriate. For example, a population health nurse might refer an older immigrant woman with a persistent productive cough for tuberculosis screening or refer a client with an elevated blood pressure for possible diagnosis and treatment of hypertension. Population health nurses may also need to advocate for access to screening services for older clients. For example, a nurse might advocate expanding breast cancer education and screening programs to target older women.

Other authorities recommend additional screening for the older population. For example, although the USPSTF has found insufficient evidence for the effectiveness of in-depth fall risk assessment, geriatric specialists have recommended a brief routine screening for fall risk, followed by in-depth assessment in those who are deemed at risk. Risk factor modification is then directed toward individual risk factors. Medicare includes fall risk screening in annual preventive care visits (Renfro & Fehrer, 2011). A tool for fall risk screening and other screening tools for use with older clients have been developed by the Hartford Institute for Geriatric Nursing (2013). For information about geriatric fall risk assessment and other best practice interventions, see the *External Resources* section of the student resources site.

Dealing with common health problems. As noted earlier, older clients experience a variety of health problems related to the effects of aging. They are also subject to problems stemming from chronic and communicable diseases. Resolution of problems related to communicable diseases and chronic conditions is addressed in detail in Chapters 26∞ and 27∞. Here we will address interventions for some of the routine health problems commonly found in older populations. Population health nurses can assist individual clients in dealing with these problems or educate the older population in general. Some of the common problems encountered in caring for older clients include skin breakdown, constipation, urinary and fecal incontinence, sensory loss, mobility limitations, pain, and cognitive impairment. Additional problems that may be encountered by population health nurses working with this population include depression, social isolation, abuse and neglect, and substance abuse. Inadequate financial resources and the need for advocacy at individual and population levels are also areas that may be addressed by means of population health nursing interventions.

Some problems, like fecal and urinary incontinence, chronic pain, and cognitive impairment, are particularly distressing to clients and their caregivers and warrant specific consideration. Generally speaking, behavioral approaches have proven more

TABLE 19-13 Routine Screening Recommendations for Older Populations

Type of Screening	Recommendation
Abdominal aortic aneurysm	One-time screening in men aged 65 to 75 years who have ever smoked
Alcohol misuse	All adults, with referral for those with drinking problems
Colorectal cancer	All adults aged 50–75 years (fecal occult blood, sigmoidoscopy, and/or colonoscopy)
Depression	Older adults in practice settings where follow-up is available
Diabetes mellitus	Older adults with blood pressures > 135/80
Elder abuse	Insufficient evidence for or against routine screening
Hearing impairment	Insufficient evidence for routine screening of asymptomatic persons
Hypertension	All older adults
Lipid disorders	Men over age 35 and women over age 45 if at risk (total cholesterol and HDL-C)
Mammogram	Every 2 years for women aged 50–74 years Insufficient evidence for routine screening after age 75
Obesity	All older adults with referral for those with BMIs over 30 kg/m^2
Osteoporosis	Women over age 65
Papanicolaou smear	Not recommended for women over age 65 with prior normal smears and no risk factors
Prostate cancer	Not recommended because potential harm outweighs possible benefit of early detection
Tobacco use	All adult men

Source: U.S. Preventive Services Task Force. (2013). *Recommendations for adults.* Retrieved from http://www.uspreventiveservicestaskforce.org/adultrec.htm

effective than medication in reducing urinary incontinence. Recommended interventions include decreasing fluid intake after the evening meal, Kegel exercises, and eliminating constipation. Additional approaches may include treatment of underlying physical causes, use of prescription drugs, or modification of existing drug regimens. Bladder training may also be helpful, including withholding urination to build bladder capacity, double voiding (urinating once and then trying to urinate again a short while later) to assist with complete emptying of the bladder, and scheduled toileting. More invasive therapies are also available, such as urethral inserts and vaginal pessaries, injection of bulking agents into tissues surrounding the urethral meatus, and nerve stimulators to strengthen pelvic muscles, as well as surgical intervention (Mayo Clinic Staff, 2011b). Population health nurses may refer individual clients to such services or advocate for their availability to members of the older population.

Population health nurses may also engage in interventions to prevent consequences of urinary incontinence, such as use of absorbent pads and protective garments. Additional considerations include skin protection through good hygiene and use of barrier creams (e.g., petroleum jelly), maintaining a clear path to the toilet, and using an elevated toilet seat. In some cases structural modifications to living arrangements may be needed, such as the addition of another bathroom, or widening the bathroom doorway to permit wheelchair or walker access (Mayo Clinic Staff, 2011b).

Treatment of fecal incontinence may also employ a variety of strategies depending on its cause and severity. Population health nurses should encourage clients with incontinence to be examined by their primary care provider to identify any underlying medical conditions. In addition, population health nurses can suggest several dietary changes that may improve continence. For example, if incontinence is due to watery stools or constipation, increasing bulk in the diet may contribute to stools that are more formed and easier to control. Conversely, for some people, high-fiber diets may have a laxative effect, increasing the problem of incontinence. Specific foods that relax the internal anal sphincter (e.g., caffeine-containing beverages and foods such as coffee, tea, and chocolate) may need to be avoided. Other food and that may contribute to fecal incontinence include fatty meats, fried foods, alcohol, dairy products, cured or smoked meat, some fruits and fruit juices (e.g., apples, pears, peaches), and artificial sweeteners (National Digestive Diseases Information Clearinghouse [NDDIC], 2013; Norton, 2011).

Keeping a food diary may also allow the client to identify other foods that cause problems. Population health nurses can educate clients about other dietary strategies that may help, including ingesting an appropriate amount of fiber and drinking approximately 64 ounces of fluid per day unless fluids are otherwise contraindicated. Fluid intake should consist primarily of water; milk and drinks with caffeine, alcohol, or carbonation should be avoided (National Digestive Diseases Information Clearinghouse, 2013).

Medications may also be used in the control of fecal incontinence, but clients should be encouraged to consult their primary care providers rather than use over-the-counter remedies. Bowel training, involving development of regular bowel patterns and going to the bathroom when the urge is felt, has also been found to be helpful in dealing with fecal incontinence (Norton, 2011). Other procedures similar to those described for urinary incontinence may also be used, and population health nurses can refer clients for evaluation for these procedures as needed. They can also advocate for their availability to older clients.

Population health nurses can also assist older clients with fecal or urinary incontinence to address the psychological effects of these problems. Some easy suggestions are to carry a backpack with cleanup supplies and a change of clothing whenever one leaves the house, locate restrooms before they are needed, use the toilet before leaving home, wear disposable undergarments or sanitary pads if needed, or use oral fecal deodorants for frequent episodes of incontinence.

Chronic pain in the elderly is often overlooked or undertreated. As we saw earlier, a significant proportion of older clients experience ongoing pain that is perceived by them and by their providers and caretakers to be a normal part of aging. Others experience pain as a result of a variety of chronic illnesses. A number of barriers exist to effective pain control in the older population. These barriers may relate to providers, to clients and/or their families, or to the health system in general. Provider-related barriers include lack of expertise in pain assessment and management with older clients, concerns related to potential addiction, inability to assess pain in clients with cognitive impairment, and the previously mentioned perception that pain is normal in the aged. Client/family barriers include fear of medication side effects and addiction, reluctance to complain of pain, and, again, the fatalism exemplified in the belief that pain is a part of aging that must be accepted. Health system barriers include the cost of pain medication, insufficient time to adequately assess pain and its management during client encounters, and cultural biases in the health professions against opioid use.

Population health nurses can help educate the general public, as well as health care providers, regarding the need for appropriate pain control in the elderly. In addition, they can assist in the development of alternative options for pain control (e.g., development of and insurance coverage for acupuncture, guided imagery, and other pain relief services). Population health nursing advocacy may be required with health care providers, with family members, or within the health system to develop attitudes and services that support effective pain control for older clients. For example, the population health nurse might educate family members, or even clients themselves, regarding the improbability of addiction. Or, the nurse may need to advocate for access to pain-control services for low-income elderly clients.

Shortness of breath characteristic of advanced COPD can also be very disabling for older clients. In addition to referring clients for medical evaluation and possible therapy with bronchodilators, steroids, and oxygen, population health nurses can assist clients with COPD in implementing a variety of strategies that may improve lung function and limit disability. The primary intervention among smokers is, of course, smoking cessation. Population health nurses can refer clients who smoke to smoking cessation programs. They may need to advocate with insurance plans for coverage of such services as necessary therapy for COPD. Other foci for COPD care include avoiding lung irritants, such as second-hand smoke, air pollution, and dust; medication compliance and follow-up care, recognizing and preparing for respiratory emergencies, and emotional support from family, friends, and health care professionals (National Heart, Lung and Blood Institute [NHLBI], 2013a, 2013b).

Population health nurses can also suggest that clients refrain from excessive use of cough medicines to control the chronic cough characteristic of COPD because they decrease clearance of secretions, making clients more susceptible to respiratory infection (Rennard, 2014). The nurse can also refer clients for pneumonia vaccine as well as annual influenza immunization to prevent infection. Nutrition is another important aspect of COPD control. Suggestions for improving the nutritional status of clients with COPD include the following:

- Resting before meals
- Eating slowly and taking small bites that are chewed thoroughly
- Choosing foods that are easy to prepare and to chew
- Asking family members to help with meal preparation
- Eating smaller, more frequent meals
- Drinking fluids at the end of the meal instead of before or with food
- Sitting up straight while eating and using pursed-lip breathing during the meal
- Obtaining meals from a local Meals-on-Wheels program
- Eating the main meal early in the day to provide energy for the rest of the day (Cleveland Clinic, 2011).

Pulmonary rehabilitation is another approach to controlling the debilitating effects of COPD. Comprehensive pulmonary rehabilitation may include education, exercise, psychosocial support, and the use of specific breathing techniques such as pursed-lip breathing, diaphragmatic breathing, and controlled coughing (Cleveland Clinic, n.d.). For information on easy-to-follow client instructions for these breathing techniques, see the *External Resources* section of the student resources site. Population health nurses can teach these strategies to clients with COPD as well as advocate for access to necessary diagnostic and treatment services.

As we saw earlier, the number of older adults with cognitive impairment is expected to increase significantly in the next few decades. In older clients, it is particularly important to distinguish among depression, dementia, and delirium, as each of these conditions may produce similar effects. Depression, as we will see in Chapter 30∞, can be effectively treated in most older clients. Treatment goals for depression in the elderly include reduction of suicide risk, improved level of function, and improved quality of life. Older antidepressant medications (e.g., tricyclic antidepressants, or TCAs) are cardiotoxic and may be less well tolerated in the elderly than newer drugs, leading to increased risk of overdose and mortality. For this reason, these drugs should not be routinely used to treat depression in older clients. Instead, "novel antidepressants" (e.g., selective serotonin reuptake inhibitors, SSRIs) are recommended with close monitoring of treatment and adverse effects. Older clients may also be more likely than younger ones to experience "discontinuation syndrome," a temporary condition that may include severe cognitive impairment, so they should be cautioned against abruptly stopping their medications. Population health nurses may advocate with health care providers for recognition and treatment of depression in elderly clients. They may also engage in political advocacy to assure access to treatment services for the older population. The principles of political advocacy were discussed in Chapter 9∞.

Delirium is usually characterized by a sudden onset and is generally reversible if the underlying cause is identified and treated. Some possible causes of delirium in the elderly include drug toxicity, infectious diseases, problems with elimination, exacerbation of chronic illness, or development of new disease processes. Other potential causes of delirium include changes in the psychosocial context such as a recent loss, a move to a new residence, or hospitalization. Dementia, on the other hand, is characterized by a gradual onset, progressive decline, and irreversibility.

Recently, there has been progress in the development of drug therapies to retard the progression of Alzheimer's disease. Until a truly effective treatment is found, however, early detection and advance planning for progressive decline are the best modes of control for this condition. The most effective approaches to care of individual clients with Alzheimer's disease combine medication, lifestyle changes, and supportive services for both clients and their families.

The goal of treatment in the face of cognitive impairment is to maintain the client's quality of life as much as possible. Some medications may be helpful in slowing cognitive decline in clients with Alzheimer's disease, particularly when initiated early in the disease process. Antidepressants, mood stabilizers, and antipsychotics may also be warranted for some clients although, as we saw earlier, use of these medications may lead to accidental injury in some clients. Activities that enhance cognitive capabilities may also be of some help (Chao et al., 2008; Spector, Orrell, & Woods, 2010; Yuill & Hollis, 2011). Consistent routines, reduction of environmental stimulation and triggers for agitated or aggressive behavior, and adequate rest are other interventions that may assist the cognitively impaired client.

In the past, reality orientation was recommended as a strategy for dealing with confusion in older people, particularly those with dementia. Reality orientation was a practice of reminding the client of "reality" when they strayed too far from it. For example, the nurse might persistently inform a client with dementia that her husband would not be coming to visit her because he died 3 years ago or that she cannot find the closet because she is no longer living in her old home. Research has indicated, however, that reality orientation may result in anxiety and distress.

A more recent approach is termed **validation therapy**, a therapeutic approach to dealing with dementia by *validating* and accepting what the client perceives as reality, focusing on the emotional foundation for the belief or behavior (National Health Service, 2013). Validation therapy is based on the theory that people attempt to resolve unfinished life issues and that retreat into a specific *unreality* is an attempt to do that. It also presupposes that there is a reason for the behavior exhibited. Validation classifies dementia behaviors into four progressive stages: malorientation, time confusion, repetitive motion, and vegetation (Validation Training Institute, 2013b). In the malorientation stage, the client expresses past conflicts in "disguised forms." For example, a client may believe that her daughter is her mother and reenact conflicts from the past. In the time confusion stage, the client retreats inward and may not be in touch with reality, but still attempts to resolve old life issues. In the repetitive motion stage, movements replace words in the attempt to resolve past conflicts, and finally, in the vegetation stage, the client gives up trying to resolve life issues and retreats from the world. In the validation approach, the caregiver (nurse or family member) accepts what the client perceives as reality and tries to redirect them without engaging in confrontations aimed at orienting them to reality. For example, a confused client may be asking when her dead husband will arrive. Rather than reminding her that he will never arrive because he is dead, the caretaker might just say, "It sounds like you really miss him," thus exploring the emotion underlying the question.

Although validation therapy was developed between 1963 and 1980, there has been limited research examining its effectiveness in addressing the problems of dementia until recently. In the last few years, several studies have demonstrated its effectiveness in dealing with elders with dementia (Validation Training Institute, 2013a).

Advocacy may be required to be sure that treatment and supportive services are available in the community for older clients with impaired cognitive function and their families. Advocacy is also needed to support continuing research on the effectiveness of therapeutic approaches in dealing with the issues of dementia and cognitive impairment in the elderly.

Support for caregivers is another area for intervention in dealing with cognitive impairment and other problems in the elderly. A number of policy recommendations have been formulated to address the needs of caregivers. These include caregiver friendly workplace policies that promote flexibility in hours worked and time to deal with care recipients' needs, modifying family medical leave legislation to provide better coverage, and providing funding for support services, including respite services. Additional recommendations address the need to modify Social Security requirements for persons who leave work to care for ill family members, paying family members for care, integrating them into care planning, developing a standard definition of family care giving, and promoting research on caregiving (Feinberg et al., 2011). Population health nurses may be actively involved in advocating for these policy changes at local, state, and national levels.

The National Family Caregiver Support Program (NFCSP), funded by the Administration on Aging, has identified five core services needed by caregivers. These include information on available resources; referral to needed services; counseling, group support, and caregiver training; respite; and supplemental services (AoA, 2012). Caregivers need information regarding the older client's condition and treatment regimen as well as the availability of services in the local community and how to obtain them. Information may also be needed on managing life changes and on dealing with financial and legal issues, particularly in the face of increasing cognitive impairment in the recipient of care. Caregivers may also benefit from counseling services that help them to cope with the physical and emotional burdens of caregiving. Counseling may prevent caregivers from being "entrapped" by their caregiving role as noted earlier. **Respite**, the provision of temporary relief from caregiving responsibilities, is often lacking for many caregivers who have 24-hour, 7-day-a-week responsibilities for the care of their aging family members. When available, respite may be provided by informal (other family members and friends) or formal support networks. Finally, caregivers may need help with obtaining needed supplies and assistive devices or in dealing with the financial burden of caregiving.

Specific intervention to address the psychological stress experienced by caregivers may also be needed. A systematic review of research on dealing with stress among caregivers identified two general approaches to dealing with caregiver stress: psychoeducational skill building and psychotherapy or counseling. Psychoeducational skill building may involve development of skills to reduce stress, behavior management skills training, depression management, anger management, or progressive lowering of caretakers' stress threshold. Psychotherapy programs tended to focus on the use of cognitive behavioral therapy. Programs targeted toward promoting caregiver quality of life and providing combinations of skill building, education, and support services were found to be more effective than single focus programs (Gallagher-Thompson, & Coon, 2007).

Disease self-management. Effective chronic disease control requires a combination of supportive care, self-management, maintenance of function, and prevention of further disability. Over time, chronic illness requires an increasing burden of self-management.

Self-management of chronic disease requires the presence of physical, environmental, mental, and socioeconomic factors that promote effective disease management. For example, one must have the cognitive ability, economic resources, and knowledge of and access to a variety of community services needed to manage the chronic condition. Depression is an emotional factor that may preclude an environment conducive to self-management of disease.

Effective self-management of disease is also dependent on possessing the knowledge and skills required to engage in self-management behaviors. For example, the client with hypertension will need to monitor his or her blood pressure as well as correctly take medications prescribed.

Self-management of chronic disease involves a number of activities, including symptom response and monitoring, compliance with complicated medical and lifestyle regimens, and developing the skills needed for self-management. Effective self-management of disease among older clients includes establishing treatment goals, identifying alternative methods to achieve these goals, planning short-term interventions to achieve goals, implementing the plan, and evaluating and revising the plan.

Managing medications is an important element of self-management of chronic illness. Adherence to medication regimens is affected by a variety of factors related to the condition and the complexity of therapy, physical and emotional client-related factors, social and economic factors, and health system factors. Physical client-related factors may include visual or cognitive impairment, impaired dexterity, or difficulty swallowing. Perceptions of risk and consequences and depression are examples of emotional factors that may influence adherence. Social and economic factors may include low health literacy, language difficulties, or the inability to afford medications or fit treatment elements into one's daily schedule. Finally, examples of health system factors include provider lack of effective communication skills or restricted formularies that preclude ordering medications that foster adherence (e.g., monthly injections for osteoporosis rather than daily pills or injections) (American College of Preventive Medicine, 2011).

The American College of Preventive Medicine (2011) has developed the mnemonic SIMPLE to reflect several adherence promoting strategies that can be used to foster adherence. The elements of the system and examples of related strategies are presented below:

S—Simplify the regimen as much as possible, breaking it into simple steps that fit with the client's lifestyle. Use adherence aids such as pill dispensers or organizers.

I—Impart knowledge that will foster adherence, such as the purpose of the regimen, potential consequences of nonadherence, and so on, and involve the client and family in decision making.

M—Modify client beliefs and behaviors if possible, focus on positive benefits of adherence and address fears and concerns honestly. Provide positive reinforcement.

P—Provide communication and trust. Make sure that clients understand the treatment regimen and related instructions and provide emotional support for needed lifestyle changes. Engage in active listening and allow time for questions.

L—Leave one's bias aside. Examine attitudes toward clients of different backgrounds and their effects on provider–client relationships. Develop an understanding of clients' cultural beliefs and attitudes. Use culturally appropriate interventions.

E—Evaluate adherence. Ask about adherence at each encounter and identify and address barriers to adherence. Periodically review medication containers and prescription renewal dates (American College of Preventive Medicine, 2011).

Population health nurses may assist with this task by encouraging providers to simplify medication regimens as much as possible for older adults. Targeted interventions that assist older adults with medication adherence may also be helpful. Technological interventions such as prompting devices, electronic dispensers, monitoring devices, and data management systems may be effective for clients who can afford them, but research is needed to test their effectiveness in practice. Unfortunately, many elderly clients cannot afford these technological advances. Other, less expensive, strategies include pill organizers and telephone reminders, and population health nurses can advocate the use of such strategies with low-income clients.

With increasing drug advertising, clients may request specific drugs, and population health nurses need to be knowledgeable in answering clients' questions about drugs for their conditions. Population health nurses can also refer clients to websites that provide comparisons of the effectiveness of specific medications. Effectiveness comparisons for multiple categories of drugs can be made using an online tool developed by AARP (n.d.). For more information about the tool, see the *External Resources* section of the student resources site.

Clients may also have questions about Medicare part D prescription drug coverage benefits, and population health nurses can either educate clients themselves or refer them to other sources of information. Population health nurses may also need to advocate for effective drug coverage for older clients and assist them to select prescription drug plans that best meet their personal needs. At the national level, population health nurses also need to advocate coverage for a set of drugs most commonly used by older clients under all Medicare-approved prescription drug plans. The provisions of Medicare part D were discussed in more detail in Chapter 7∞.

The effectiveness of self-management of chronic illness may be evaluated based on symptom assessment and physical examination, direct indicators of disease processes (e.g., blood glucose levels), or indirect indicators of medication compliance (e.g., pill counts, prescription refills). Additional measures of effectiveness include subjective reports of clients or family members or the frequency of visits to primary health care providers or emergency departments. Interventions for addressing disease self-management and resolving other problems common among older clients are presented in Table 19-14•.

HEALTH RESTORATION. Health restoration activities for older clients include restoring health and functional status as much as possible and providing palliative and end-of-life care.

Rehabilitation. Health restoration for the individual client may involve rehabilitation services, but the type of service

TABLE 19-14 Strategies for Resolving Existing Health Problems in Older Populations

Client Problem	Resolution Strategies
Screening	Refer for routine screening procedures. Refer for additional screening as needed. Advocate for coverage for disease screening. Interpret screening results and refer for diagnostic and treatment services as needed.
Skin breakdown	Inspect extremities regularly for lesions. Keep lesions clean and dry. Apply skin protectants to prevent irritation with fecal or urinary incontinence. Eliminate pressure by frequent changes of position. Refer for treatment as needed.
Constipation	Encourage fluid and fiber intake. Discourage ignoring urge to defecate. Encourage regular exercise. Encourage regular bowel habits. Use mild laxatives as needed; discourage overuse. Administer enemas as needed; discourage overuse. Administer bulk products or stool softeners as indicated.
Urinary incontinence	Refer for urological consult or treatment of underlying physical causes. Refer for modification of medication regimen as needed. Encourage frequent voiding and double voiding. Teach Kegel exercises. Decrease fluids after the evening meal. Assist with bladder training. Encourage use of sanitary pads, panty liners, etc., with frequent changes of such aids. Keep skin clean and dry; change clothing and bed linen as needed. Offer bedpan or urinal frequently or assist to bedside commode at frequent intervals.
Fecal incontinence	Refer for medical treatment of underlying causes as needed. Educate for dietary changes to address contributing factors. Encourage avoidance of caffeinated beverages and chocolate. Suggest smaller, more frequent meals. Suggest eating and drinking at different times. Encourage consumption of soluble fiber. Encourage sufficient fluid intake. Teach Kegel exercises or assist with bowel training. Suggest strategies to decrease embarrassment.
Sensory loss	Provide adequate lighting. Keep eyeglasses clean and hearing aids functional. Eliminate safety hazards. Use large-print books or materials. Use multisensory approaches to communication and teaching. Avoid using colors that make discrimination difficult. Speak clearly and slowly, at a lower pitch, avoid "elderspeak." Eliminate background noise. Assist clients to obtain voice enhancers for phone. Use additional herbs and spices in food, but use with discretion. Purchase small amounts of perishable foods. Check pilot lights on gas appliances frequently. Encourage the use of smoke detectors.

(Continued)

TABLE 19-14 (*Continued*)

Client Problem	Resolution Strategies
Mobility limitation	Provide assistance with ambulation, transfer, etc. Assist clients to obtain equipment such as walkers and wheelchairs. Install ramps, tub rails, etc., as needed. Promote access to public facilities for older persons. Assist clients to find alternative sources of transportation. Make referrals for assistance with personal care or instrumental activities as needed.
Pain	Plan activities for times when pain is controlled. Encourage warm soaks. Encourage adequate rest and exercise to prevent mobility limitations. Encourage effective use of analgesics. Refer for assistance with alternative pain control measures.
COPD (shortness of breath)	Refer for medical therapy (e.g., bronchodilators, steroids, oxygen), as needed. Educate regarding safety precautions with oxygen therapy. Encourage smoking cessation, as needed. Advocate for coverage of smoking cessation under health insurance plans. Encourage and refer for pneumonia and influenza immunization. Promote adequate nutrition. Encourage small, easily prepared and eaten meals or ask for assistance in meal preparation from family members. Discourage use of cough suppressants. Suggest taking fluids at the end of the meal rather than before or with foods. Refer to Meals-on-Wheels, if appropriate. Suggest sitting upright to eat. Educate client for pursed-lip breathing, diaphragmatic breathing, and controlled coughing. Promote physical activity as tolerated. Advocate for access to necessary diagnostic and treatment services.
Cognitive impairment	Apply principles of validation therapy, if helpful. Refer for Alzheimer's drug therapy as indicated. Refer for antidepressant, mood-stabilizing, or antipsychotic medications as needed. Promote exercise (register wanderers with national registry if appropriate). Promote activities to enhance memory (e.g., discussion of current events, games, puzzles, etc.). Educate families and caregivers regarding the progression of disease. Provide hand massage or therapeutic touch services or teach these interventions to caregivers. Establish consistent daily routines. Reduce environmental stimulation and triggers for aberrant behavior. Provide adequate rest. Promote reminiscence therapy.
Depression	Accept feelings and reflect on their normality; encourage client to discuss feelings. Refer for counseling or medications as needed.
Social isolation	Compensate for sensory loss; enhance communication abilities. Improve mobility; provide access to transportation. Assist clients to obtain adequate financial resources. Refer clients to new support systems. Assist clients to deal with grief over loss of loved ones.
Abuse or neglect	Assist caretakers to develop positive coping strategies. Assist families to obtain respite care or day care for older members. Refer families for counseling as needed. Arrange placement in temporary shelter. Assist families in making other arrangements for safe care of older clients. Advocate for laws and protective services systems that protect older clients from abuse.

TABLE 19-14 (Continued)

Client Problem	Resolution Strategies
Substance abuse	Identify problem drinking by older clients. Refer for therapy, Alcoholics Anonymous, or Al-Anon as appropriate. Observe for toxic effects of alcohol ingestion. Maintain hydration and nutrition.
Inadequate financial resources	Refer for financial assistance. Assist with budgeting and priority allocation. Educate for less expensive means of meeting needs. Function as an advocate as needed.
Caregiver stress	Educate for needed caregiving skills. Promote behavior management skills. Promote coping skills. Refer for counseling as needed. Refer for or promote availability of respite services. Advocate policy changes and legislation to support family caregiving.
Disease self-management	Educate older clients/caregivers for disease self-management (procedures, medication management, etc.). Promote symptom management and educate for appropriate response. Promote adherence to therapeutic regimens. Promote lifestyle modification, as needed. Educate clients to recognize the need for professional assistance.

needed depends on the problems experienced by the client. For example, intervention for an abused older client may include long-term counseling for family members to prevent subsequent abuse as well as counseling for the older client to address the psychological effects of abuse. Restoration related to financial inadequacies may involve assistance with budgeting. Rehabilitation following a fracture may involve physical therapy, while recovery from a myocardial infarction will require cardiac rehabilitation. Similarly, pulmonary rehabilitation for clients with COPD may involve education for exercise training, social support, and teaching breathing techniques (Rennard, 2014). The role of the population health nurse with respect to rehabilitation for individual clients may involve referral for rehabilitation services, encouraging clients to participate fully in rehabilitation programs, and monitoring the effects of rehabilitation. At the aggregate level, population health nurses may need to advocate for the availability of or assist in designing rehabilitation services needed by members of the community as well as for adequate funding for such services.

Palliative care. Palliative care is another important consideration in health restoration with the older adult population. Because of the incurability of many chronic conditions, the only avenue open for intervention is symptom management. Palliative care addresses pain and symptom relief and maintenance of quality of life without attempting to cure an underlying disease process. The intent of palliative care is to decrease suffering and improve quality of life for both clients and families (Meier, 2010). Although often viewed in the context of end-of-life care, palliative care is also warranted when symptom control is the primary goal of care. Important features of palliative care include relief of pain and other symptoms, effective communication with health care providers, and achievement of a sense of completion. Characteristics of palliative care include a client-centered perspective, focus on symptom relief, safety, and decreased resource utilization. Palliative care focuses on meeting the needs of clients and their families, particularly on minimizing the experience and effects of distressing symptoms such as pain, anxiety, confusion, and so on. Such care is safe in that it does not hasten death, but promotes physical and psychological comfort as death approaches. Finally, palliative care decreases resource utilization by minimizing the use of expensive technologies that offer little potential benefit for the client (Meier, 2010). Palliative care services need to be initiated in a timely fashion irrespective of disease prognosis.

Unfortunately, such services are not equitably available to older clients in the population. Population health nurses can refer individual clients to palliative care services and monitor their effectiveness. They also need to advocate for the availability and affordability of such services for all segments of the population.

Palliative care often takes place in hospice settings. Unfortunately, Medicare's requirement for hospice care includes forgoing all further curative measures and a projected life expectancy of less than 6 months (Centers for Medicare and Medicaid Services, 2012a). The need for palliative care services affects a broader population than those in the terminal stages of life-threatening illnesses. Medicare Part B and Medicaid also cover some palliative medications and treatments (Caring Connections, n.d.; CMS, 2012b). Some hospices, particularly those in managed care systems, are now instituting separate palliative services that may be initiated prior to actual hospice care. Some managed care organizations also cover the cost of palliative care.

Population health nurses may be involved in providing palliative care to older clients and others with incurable conditions but more often provide referrals to palliative care services and monitor their effectiveness. Population health nurses may be actively involved in developing palliative care services and in advocating coverage of these services under both public and private health insurance programs.

End-of-life care. Three specific considerations must be addressed in providing effective end-of-life care to older clients. These include formulation of advance directives, personal preparation for death, and actual care of the dying client.

Advance directives are legal statements of one's wishes regarding health care in the event of incapacitation. Advance care planning may result in specific documents such as living wills or health-related powers of attorney. These documents specify circumstances in which life-sustaining treatment is or is not to be provided and appoint a surrogate to make decisions regarding life-sustaining treatments in the event of the client's incapacitation. **Life-sustaining treatment** is medical intervention to forestall death that has no appreciable effect on underlying disease processes or injuries.

To be effective, advance care planning documents must be supported by state policies, usually legislation, that promotes their implementation. The National Hospice and Palliative Care Organization (2013) provides information on the development of advance directives and its website contains links to information on execution of advanced directives in specific states. For more information about advance directives, see the *External Resources* section of the student resources site.

Population health nurses may need to encourage older clients and their families to engage in advance health care planning and to execute the appropriate documents. They may also need to advocate for compliance with advance directives by family members or health care providers when these directives have been written.

Preparation for death usually also entails a number of practical activities involved in getting one's affairs in order. Older clients may need to make decisions about funeral arrangements or the disposition of their belongings. Both nurses and family members should be encouraged to listen to clients in their reflections on such matters, rather than put them off with assurances that they "won't die for a long time yet." Population health nurses may need to advocate with family members to encourage them to address older clients' concerns about dying. Nurses may also need to refer clients for legal assistance with wills, burial plans, and other financial arrangements. Many communities have low-cost legal aid services available to elderly clients. Population health nurses should keep in mind, however, that clients may exhibit cultural differences in their preparation for death. For example, in many cultures, such decisions are believed to be the responsibility of children, and the dying client should not be bothered. In others, discussion of death is believed to hasten its occurrence, so clients are not willing to explore plans related to their deaths.

End-of-life care begins when the focus of care shifts from cure and restoration of health to promoting a peaceful death and may occur over differing periods of time based on the "dying trajectory" in a particular situation. Dying trajectories may be of three general types. In the first trajectory the client experiences a short period of rapid decline followed shortly by death. The second trajectory involves a slow decline with periodic acute crises requiring medical intervention. In the third trajectory, the client experiences a prolonged decline and lingering death (Gabrielle, 2011).

Major considerations in end-of-life care include dealing with preparatory grief, management of pain and other symptoms, dealing with anxiety and depression, meeting spiritual needs, and assisting family members with mourning (Strada, 2013). Both clients with terminal conditions and their families engage in preparatory or anticipatory grief as a natural preparation for approaching death. At this time, population health nurses may need to assist clients and family members to deal with feelings of guilt and focus on positive aspects of life. As noted earlier, clients may also need help in getting their affairs in order. Pain management may involve both pharmacologic and nonpharmacologic therapies, and clients and families may need to be encouraged to use analgesics and other modalities to promote comfort. Similarly, medications and counseling may be needed to address issues of anxiety and depression, and population health nurses can make referrals for these services as needed. Meeting spiritual needs may mean referring client and family members to religious counselors or assisting them to address spirituality in their own ways. Finally, family members may need assistance to deal with grief after the death, again possibly requiring referral to counseling or bereavement groups. Interventions for end-of-life care and other aspects of health restoration for older adult populations are summarized in Table 19-15.

Implementing Care for Older Populations

Two major considerations in implementing care for older populations are health education directed at this group and political advocacy. Health education initiatives are based on the general principles of teaching and learning discussed in Chapter 11, but there are also some unique considerations in implementing education programs for the older adult population.

Older adults may exhibit some decline in linguistic skills with age. Auditory communication may be too fast-paced for comprehension or contain too much information to be easily comprehensible. As we saw earlier, many older adults experience hearing and vision impairments as well as cognitive impairments that may impede learning. Strategies to circumvent hearing loss include using a lower-pitched voice; facing

TABLE 19-15 Strategies for Health Restoration and End-of-Life Care in Older Populations

Area of Focus	Intervention Strategy
Rehabilitation	Refer clients for rehabilitation services. Encourage clients to participate fully in rehabilitation programs. Monitor the effects of rehabilitation. Advocate for available and affordable rehabilitation services. Advocate for adequate insurance coverage of rehabilitation services.
Palliative care	Provide palliative care to individual clients or refer them to palliative care services as needed. Monitor the effectiveness of palliative care. Advocate for the availability and affordability of palliative care services.
End-of-life care	Assist individual clients and families with advance care planning. Advocate for adherence to advance directives within health care systems. Assist clients and families to deal with preparatory grief. Assist clients and families to deal with feelings of guilt. Help dying clients come to some life resolution. Assist dying clients to get their lives in order. Refer for legal or other assistance as needed. Provide culturally sensitive and appropriate end-of-life care to individual clients. Provide or refer for pharmacologic and nonpharmacologic pain management. Assist with management of other symptoms. Refer for assistance with anxiety and depression. Refer for spiritual counseling if desired. Refer survivors to counseling or bereavement groups as needed. Advocate for effective state and national policies related to advance directives. Advocate for access to hospice and other end-of-life services. Advocate for changes in reimbursement for end-of-life services.

the listener while speaking; employing nonverbal teaching techniques; using clear, concise terminology; and having the client use a hearing aid if needed. The effects of hearing loss can also be minimized by limiting background noise, reemphasizing important points, and supplementing verbal with written materials.

The use of glasses, a magnifying glass, and large print may help to minimize visual deficits. Learning can also be enhanced by visual materials using black lettering on white or yellow paper, providing adequate lighting, and eliminating glare in the learning environment.

In implementing health education plans for older adults, the nurse may need to repeat material more frequently. Because of decreases in short-term memory, it may take longer for some older clients to learn new material. Once material is learned, however, older clients retain it as well as younger ones. Multisensory presentation, multiple repetitions, reinforcement of verbal content with written materials, and use of memory aids (e.g., a calendar for taking medications) may also assist learning in older clients.

Because response times are longer for older people than for their younger counterparts, lessons should proceed at a slower pace, and the nurse should allow more time for responses on the part of the client. Self-paced instruction is helpful. Motivation to learn can be heightened by increasing client participation in the lesson and by setting easily attainable, progressive goals that enhance success and satisfaction. Irrelevant material can confuse clients and should be eliminated from the presentation.

Endurance may be somewhat limited in older clients, so teaching sessions should be kept short (10 to 15 minutes per session). Lessons should be scheduled at times of the day when learners are rested and comfortable. Health education for older clients should not be time limited, as they may need more or less time to learn specific material. Again, learning should be broken down into small, progressive steps so that periodic success will continue to motivate older learners. The teaching-learning process should also allow for rest periods as needed.

Political advocacy may be needed to implement strategies at all levels of care. Political advocacy is based on the general principles discussed in Chapter 9∞ but may require more effort than advocacy for other population groups in countries like the United States that are affected by pervasive ageism. Advocacy efforts may need to start at local levels, with research that documents the cost savings of health promotion strategies and effective end-of-life care. For example, it has been demonstrated that money spent on hospice services decreases hospitalization costs. Similarly, the cost savings associated with family caregiving versus formal care can be used as justification for services to support caregivers.

Evaluating Health Care for Older Populations

Evaluating the effectiveness of health care for older members of the population can occur at the individual or aggregate level. At the individual level, the population health nurse would assess the client's health status and the effects of interventions at each level of health care (promotion, prevention, resolution, and restoration) in improving health status. On occasion, the effectiveness of care would be measured in terms of a peaceful death and the physical and emotional health of family members and caregivers.

At the aggregate level, evaluation of the effects of care on the health of the elderly can be measured, in part, by the level of accomplishment of relevant national health objectives. The status of selected national objectives for the year 2020 related to the health of older clients is found in the *Healthy People 2020* feature below.

Another approach to evaluating health care for older populations is to examine the achievement of key indicators of well-being among the elderly developed by the Federal Interagency Forum on Aging-Related Statistics (2012). Areas of focus within the indicators include population composition, health status, health risks and behaviors, health care (including access, utilization, cost, residential services, and personal assistance and equipment), and end-of-life issues. For more information about indicators, see the *External Resources* section of the student resources site.

Healthy People 2020

Selected Objectives for the Health of Older Adults (65 years or older unless otherwise indicated)

OBJECTIVE	BASELINE (YEAR)	TARGET	CURRENT DATA (YEAR)	DATA SOURCES
AHS-3 Increase the proportion of people over 65 with a usual primary care provider	90.6% (2007)	83.9%	90.2% (2010)	National Health Interview Survey (NHIS), CDC, National Center for Health Statistics (NCHS)
AHS-6 Reduce the proportion of people over 65 unable to obtain or delay obtaining medical care, dental care, or prescription medications	8.6% (2007)	9%	10.3 (2010)	Medical Expenditure Panel Survey (MEPS), AHRQ
AOCBC-2 Reduce the proportion of older adults with Dr. diagnosed arthritis who experience a limitation in activity due to arthritis or joint symptoms	48.5% (2008)	35.5%	46.7% (2011)	NHIS, CDC, NCHS
AOCBC-10 Reduce the proportion of older adults with osteoporosis	10.3% (2005–2008)	5.3%	NDA	NHANES, CDC, NCHS
AOCBC-11 Reduce hip fracture hospitalizations among older adults 11.1 per 100,000 women 11.2 per 100,000 men	823.5 (2007) 464.9 (2007)	741.2 418	NDA NDA	National Hospital Discharge Survey (NHDS), CDC/NCHS
AOCBC-12 Reduce activity limitation due to chronic back conditions per 1,000 older adults	54.0 (2008)	27.6	63.3 (2011)	NHIS, CDC, NCHS
C-1 Reduce cancer deaths per 100,000 older adults	1030.3 (2007)	161.4	985.1 (2010)	National Vitals Statistics System –Mortality (NVSS-M), CDC, NCHS

Healthy People 2020 (Continued)

OBJECTIVE	BASELINE (YEAR)	TARGET	CURRENT DATA (YEAR)	DATA SOURCES
C-3 Reduce the female breast cancer death rate per 100,000 older women	107.8 (2007)	20.7	103.7 (2010)	NVSS-M, CDC, NCHS
C-4 Reduce the cervical cancer death rate per 100,000 older adults	6.3 (2007)	2.2	5.7 (2010)	NVSS-M, CDC, NCHS
C-5 Reduce colorectal cancer deaths per 100,000 older adults	101.3 (2007)	14.5	90.9 (2010)	NVSS-M, CDC, NCHS
C-8 Reduce melanoma cancer deaths per 100,000 older adults	12.9 (2007)	2.4	13.6 (2010)	NVSS-M, CDC, NCHS
C-16 Increase the proportion of adults 65–75 years who receive colorectal cancer screening	60.4% (2008)	70.5%	67.8% (2010)	NHIS, CDC, NCHS
C-18.1 Increase the proportion of women aged 65–74 years counseled regarding mammograms	69.6% (2008)	76.8%	NDA	NHIS, CDC, HCHS
D-3 Reduce diabetes deaths per 100,000 older adults	466.5 (2007)	66.6	439.8 (2010)	NVSS-M, CDC, NCHS
DH-17 Increase the proportion of older adults with disabilities who report sufficient social and emotional support	76.6% (2008)	76.5%	76.1% (2010)	Behavioral Risk Factor Surveillance System (BRFSS), CDC, PHSPO
ENT-VSL 4.2 Increase the proportion of adults 70 years or older who have had a hearing exam in the last 2 years	38.5% (2003–2004)	42.4%	NDA	NHANES, CDC, NCHS
HDS-2 Reduce coronary heart disease deaths per 100,000 older adults	867.9 (2007)	103.4	745.3 (2010)	NVSS-M, CDC, NCHS
HDS-3 Reduce stroke deaths per 100,000 older adults	306.6 (2007)	34.8	273.1 (2010)	NVSS-M, CDC, NCHS
HDS-5.1 Reduce the proportion of older adults with hypertension	70.3% (2005–2008)	26.9%	NDA	National Health and Nutrition Examination Survey (NHANES), CDC, NCHS
HDS-6 Increase the proportion of older adults who have had their blood cholesterol level checked in the past 5 years	94.6% (2008)	82.1%	NDA	NHIS, CDC, NCHS
HDS-7 Reduce the proportion of older adults with high total blood cholesterol levels	15.3% (2005–2008)	13.5%	NDA	NHANES, CDC, NCHS
HDS-11 Increase the proportion of older adults with hypertension taking medication to lower their blood pressure	79.4% (2005–2008)	69.5%	NDA	NHANES, CDC, NCHS
IID-4.4 Decrease the rate of invasive antibiotic pneumococcal infection per 100,000 older adults	12.2 (2008)	9	10.9 (2010)	Active Bacterial Core Surveillance, CDC,NCIR
IID-13.1 Increase the percentage of older adults who receive pneumococcal vaccine	60.1% (2008)	90%	NDA	NHIS, CDC, NCHD

Continued on next page

Healthy People 2020 (Continued)

OBJECTIVE	BASELINE (YEAR)	TARGET	CURRENT DATA (YEAR)	DATA SOURCES
IID-14 Increase the percentage of adults 60 years and older who receive zoster vaccine	6.7% (2008)	30%	NDA	NHIS, CDC, NCHD
IVP-1.1 Reduce the rate of fatal injuries per 100,000 older adults	118.6 (2007)	53.7	120.6 (2010)	NVSS-M, CDC, NCHS
IVP-1.2 Reduce the rate of hospitalization for nonfatal injury per 100,000 older adults	1,878.4 (2007)	555.8	1,991.9 (2010)	National Hospital Discharge Summary (NHDS), CDC, NCHS
IVP-11 Reduce unintentional injury deaths per 100,000 older adults	101.2 (2007)	36	102.6 (2010)	NVSS-M, CDC, NCHS
IVP-23.2 Reduce the rate of fall related deaths per 100,000 older adults	47.0 (2007)	47.0	52.4 (2010)	NVSS-M, CDC, NCHS
IVP-29 Reduce homicides per 100,000 older adults	2.0 (2007)	5.5	2.0 (2010)	NVSS-M, CDC, NCHS
IVP-41 Reduce the rate of nonfatal intentional self-harm injuries per 100,000 older adults	23.5 (2008)	112.8	24.0 (2010)	NVSS-M, CDC, NCHS
NWS-9 Reduce the proportion of older adults who are obese	37.8% (2005–2008)	30.5%	37.8% (2009–2010)	NHANES, CDC, NCHS
OA-2 Increase the proportion of older adults who are up to date on a core set of clinical preventive services 2.1 Men 2.2 Women	46.3% (2008) 47.9% (2008)	50.9% 52.7%	48.5% (2010) 48.5% (2010)	BRFSS, CDC, PHSPO
OA-5 Reduce the proportion of older adults with moderate to severe functional limitations	29.3% (2007)	26.4%	30.8% (2010)	Medicare Current Beneficiary Survey (MCBS), CMS
OA-11 Reduce the rate of emergency department visits due to falls per 100,000 older adults	5,235.1 (2007)	4,711.6	6,083.2 (2010)	National Hospital Ambulatory Medical Care Survey (NHAMCS), CDC, NCHS
OH-3.2 Reduce the proportion of adults 65–74 years with untreated coronal caries	17.1% (1999–2004)	15.4%	NDA	NHANES, CDC, NCHS
OH-3.3 Reduce the proportion of adults 75 years and older with untreated root surface caries	37.9% (1999–2004)	34.1%	NDA	NHANES, CDC, NCHS
OH-4.2 Reduce the proportion of adults 65–74 years who have lost all of their natural teeth	24% (1999–2004)	21.6%	15.3% (2009–2010)	NHANES, CDC, NCHS
PA-1 Reduce the proportion of older adults who engage in no leisure time physical activity	50.4% (2008)	32.6%	45.2% (2010)	NHIS, CDC, NCHS
RD-1.3 Reduce asthma deaths per 100,000 older adults	43.4 (2008)	21.5	37.7 (2010)	NVSS-M, CDC, NCHS

Healthy People 2020 (Continued)

OBJECTIVE	BASELINE (YEAR)	TARGET	CURRENT DATA (YEAR)	DATA SOURCES
RD-10 Reduce COPD deaths per 100,000 older adults	283.1 (2007)	102.6	287 (2010)	NVSS-M, CDC, NCHS
SA-12 Reduce drug-induced deaths per 100,000 older adults	4.4 (2007)	11.3	4.9 (2010)	NVSS-M, CDC, NCHS
TU-1.1 Reduce cigarette smoking by older adults	9.3% (2008)	12%	7.9% (2011)	NHIS, CDC, NCHS
TU-4.1 Increase smoking cessation attempts by older adult smokers	41.6% (2008)	80%	41.6% (2011)	NHIS, CDC, NCHS
V-5.4 Reduce the rate of visual impairment due to cataracts per 1,000 older adults	110.0 (2008)	99	NDA	NHIS, CDC, NCHD
V-5.5 Reduce the rate of visual impairment due to age-related macular degeneration per 1,000 older adults	34.0 (2008)	14	NDA	NHIS, CDC, NCHD

Data from: U.S. Department of Health and Human Services (2014). *Healthy People 2020 topics and objectives.* Retrieved from http://healthypeople.gov/2020/topicsobjectives2020/default.aspx

CHAPTER RECAP

Myriad theories attempt to explain aging, but these theories can be grouped into three main categories. Biological theories address physiologic changes that occur over time leading to the physical changes exhibited in older adults. Psychological theories focus on psychological changes that occur with age and propose that effective aging requires development of effective coping strategies over time. Sociological theories of aging focus on changes in roles and relationships that occur with advancing age.

Factors related to each of the six categories of determinants of health influence the health of older individuals and populations. Biological determinants include the age and gender composition of the older population, physical effects of aging, chronic conditions, and resulting functional limitations, as well as the immune status of the population. Some important psychological determinants include the prevalence and effects of dementia, sources of stress, coping abilities, and depression and other mental health problems. Environmental determinants reflect the fit of older individuals and populations with their environment and include housing and physical safety hazards, neighborhood characteristics, environmental pollution, and so on. Several sociocultural determinants affect the health of older populations including living arrangements and family responsibilities; social support; education, employment, and economic status; level of empowerment, and the prevalence of abuse and violence against the elderly. Behavioral determinants to be considered in assessing the health of the older population include diet and other consumption patterns, physical and sexual activity, medication use, and other health-related behaviors, such as safety practices and use of preventive services. Finally, health system determinants affecting the health of older populations include access to and use of health care services, prescription drug use, infrastructure support, and relationships with providers.

Population health nursing interventions for older clients and populations address health promotion, illness and injury prevention, resolution of existing health problems, and health restoration. Health promotion foci include maintaining independence, fostering life resolution, promoting a healthy diet and adequate physical activity and rest, and fostering caregiver health. Illness and injury prevention center on risk factor modification, injury and abuse prevention, immunization, and preventing incontinence. Resolution of health problems may involve a wide variety of population health nursing interventions depending on the problems experienced, but can be grouped into strategies related to screening, care for common health problems in the older population, and disease self-management strategies. Intervention foci in health restoration may involve return to a prior state of health or preparation for dying and address rehabilitation, palliative care, and end-of-life care for older clients and their families.

Special considerations in implementing care for older clients focus on strategies for health education that address the characteristics of the older population and advocating for policies that support the health and well-being of the elderly. Finally, evaluation of the effectiveness of care for older populations addresses resulting changes in health status for individual clients as well as determination of population level effects. Either *Healthy People 2020* objectives or key indicators of well-being can be used to frame evaluation at the aggregate level.

CASE STUDY Promoting Physical Activity in Older Adults

A small non-profit community center in a large metropolitan area strives to meet the needs of its population of approximately 70,000 people. About 6% of the population is elderly, and like most of the community, they have very low incomes. The community is home to people who speak more than 30 different languages, and providing care for seniors in the community is a challenge. Fortunately, the agency staff include a number of multilingual individuals, so translation is not often a problem. For several years, the community center has provided a senior lunch program and employed a population health nurse who assists elderly clients with a variety of health needs.

One of the nurse's routine tasks is blood pressure monitoring for the seniors who attend the lunch program. Over time, the nurse became aware of the high prevalence of hypertension and obesity in the population. As a result, in addition to the lunch program, the center added an exercise program for seniors several days a week. Grant funds were obtained to hire an exercise coach and now 50 to 60 seniors gather for each session. The exercise program has provided another avenue for social interaction for often isolated seniors as well as for improving their weight, flexibility, and blood pressures.

1. What biological, psychological, environmental, sociocultural, behavioral, and health system determinants are evident in this situation? What additional factors in each category might be influencing the health of these seniors?
2. What levels of health care are represented by the exercise program, the senior lunch program, and blood pressure monitoring activities?
3. How might you evaluate the effects of the exercise program? Of the nutrition program?

REFERENCES

Acharya, J. N., & Acharya, V. J. (2014). Epilepsy in the elderly: Special considerations and challenges. *Annals of the Indian Academy of Neurology, 17*(S1), S18–S26. doi: 10.4103/0972-2327.128645

Acierno, R., Hernandez-Tejada, M., Muzzy, W., & Steve, K. (2009). *National elder mistreatment study*. Retrieved from https://www.ncjrs.gov/pdffiles1/nij/grants/226456.pdf

Adams, C. (2010). Dying with dignity in America: The transformational leadership of Florence Wald. *Journal of Professional Nursing, 26*, 125–132. doi:10.1016/j.profnurs.2009.12.009

Adams, M. L., Deokar, A. J., Anderson, L. A., & Edwards, V. J. (2013). Self-reported increased confusion or memory loss and associated functional difficulties among adults aged > 60 years—21 states, 2011. *Morbidity and Mortality Weekly Report, 62*, 345–350.

Administration on Aging. (2012). *National Family Caregiver Support Program*. Retrieved from http://www.aoa.gov/aoa_programs/hcltc/caregiver/index.aspx

Administration on Aging. (2013a). *A profile of Older Americans: 2012*. Retrieved from http://www.aoa.gov/Aging_Statistics/Profile/2012/9.aspx

Administration on Aging. (2013b). *Nutrition services (OAA Title IIIC)*. Retrieved from http://www.aoa.gov/AoA_programs/HCLTC/Nutrition_Services/index.aspx

Agency for Healthcare Research and Quality. (n.d.). *Five major steps to intervention (The "5 A's")*. Retrieved from http://www.ahrq.gov/professionals/clinicians-providers/guidelines-recommendations/tobacco/5steps.html

Agency for Healthcare Research and Quality. (2013a). *Table 1, Total health services—Mean and median expenses per person with expense and distribution of expenses by source of payment: United States, 2010*. Retrieved from http://meps.ahrq.gov/mepsweb/data_stats/tables_compendia_hh_interactive.jsp?SERVICE=MEPSSocket0&_PROGRAM=MEPSPGM.TC.SAS&File=HCFY2010&Table=HCFY2010%5FPLEXP%5F%40&VAR1=AGE&VAR2=SEX&VAR3=RACETH5C&VAR4=INSURCOV&VAR5=POVCAT10&VAR6=MSA&VAR7=REGION&VAR8=HEALTH&VARO1=4+17+44+64&VARO2=1&VARO3=1&VARO4=1&VARO5=1&VARO6=1&VARO7=1&VARO8=1&_Debug=

Agency for Healthcare Research and Quality. (2013b). *Table 1.1, Total health services—Mean and median expenses per person with expense and distribution of expenses by source of payment: United States, 2010*. Retrieved from http://meps.ahrq.gov/mepsweb/data_stats/tables_compendia_hh_interactive.jsp?SERVICE=MEPSSocket0&_PROGRAM=MEPSPGM.TC.SAS&File=HCFY2010&Table=HCFY2010%5FPLEXP%5F%40&VAR1=AGE&VAR2=SEX&VAR3=RACETH5C&VAR4=INSURCOV&VAR5=POVCAT10&VAR6=MSA&VAR7=REGION&VAR8=HEALTH&VARO1=4+17+44+64&VA

RO2=1&VARO3=1&VARO4=1&VARO5=1&VARO6=1&VARO7=1&VARO8=1&TCOPT1=1.1&_Debug=

Agency for Healthcare Research and Quality. (2013c). *Table 2, Prescription medicines—Mean and median expenses per person with expense and distribution of expenses by source of payment: United States, 2010.* Retrieved from http://meps.ahrq.gov/mepsweb/data_stats/tables_compendia_hh_interactive.jsp?SERVICE=MEPSSocket0&_PROGRAM=MEPSPGM.TC.SAS&File=HCFY2010&Table=HCFY2010%5FPLEXP%5FA&VAR1=AGE&VAR2=SEX&VAR3=RACETH5C&VAR4=INSURCOV&VAR5=POVCAT10&VAR6=MSA&VAR7=REGION&VAR8=HEALTH&VARO1=4+17+44+64&VARO2=1&VARO3=1&VARO4=1&VARO5=1&VARO6=1&VARO7=1&VARO8=1&_Debug=

Agency for Healthcare Research and Quality. (2013d). *Table 5, Hospital inpatient services—Mean and median expenses per person with expense and distribution of expenses by source of payment: United States, 2010.* Retrieved from http://meps.ahrq.gov/mepsweb/data_stats/tables_compendia_hh_interactive.jsp?SERVICE=MEPSSocket0&_PROGRAM=MEPSPGM.TC.SAS&File=HCFY2010&Table=HCFY2010%5FPLEXP%5FD&VAR1=AGE&VAR2=SEX&VAR3=RACETH5C&VAR4=INSURCOV&VAR5=POVCAT10&VAR6=MSA&VAR7=REGION&VAR8=HEALTH&VARO1=4+17+44+64&VARO2=1&VARO3=1&VARO4=1&VARO5=1&VARO6=1&VARO7=1&VARO8=1&_Debug=

Alzheimer's Association & Centers for Disease Control and Prevention. (2013). *The healthy brain initiative: The public health road map for state and national partnerships 2013–2018.* Retrieved from http://www.cdc.gov/aging/pdf/state-aging-health-in-america-2013.pdf

American Association of Colleges of Nursing & Hartford Institute for Geriatric Nursing at New York University College of Nursing. (2010). *Recommended baccalaureate competencies and curricular guidelines for the nursing care of older adults: A supplement to "The Essentials of Baccalaureate Education for Professional Nursing Practice."* Washington, DC: Author.

American Association of Retired Persons. (n.d.). *Drug $avings tool.* Retrieved from http://drugsavings.aarp.org/?cmp=RDRCT-DRGSVG_OCT18_010

American Association of Retired Persons. (2012a). *2012 member opinion survey: Issue spotlight—Grandparenting.* Retrieved from http://www.aarp.org/content/dam/aarp/research/surveys_statistics/general/2013/2012-Member-Opinion-Survey-Issue-Spotlight-Grandparenting-AARP.pdf

American Association of Retired Persons. (2012b). *2012 member opinion survey: Issue spotlight—Health.* Retrieved from http://www.aarp.org/content/dam/aarp/research/surveys_statistics/general/2012/2012-Member-Opinion-Survey-Issue-Spotlight-Health-AARP.pdf

American Association of Retired Persons. (2012c). *2012 member opinion survey: Issue spotlight—Home and family life.* Retrieved from http://www.aarp.org/content/dam/aarp/research/surveys_statistics/general/2013/2012-Member-Opinion-Survey-Issue-Spotlight-Home-and-Family-AARP.pdf

American Association of Retired Persons, Public Policy Institute. (2013). *Fact sheet: The employment situation, March 2013: Discouraging news for the older workforce.* Retrieved from http://www.aarp.org/content/dam/aarp/research/public_policy_institute/econ_sec/2013/the-employment-situation-march-2013-AARP-ppi-econ-sec.pdf

American Association of Retired Persons & National Center for Complementary and Alternative Medicine. (2011). *Complementary and alternative medicine: What people aged 50 and older discuss with their health care providers.* Retrieved from http://nccam.nih.gov/sites/nccam.nih.gov/files/news/camstats/2010/NCCAM_aarp_survey.pdf

American College of Preventive Medicine. (2011). *Medication adherence—Improving health outcomes: A resource from the American College of Preventive Medicine.* Retrieved from http://c.ymcdn.com/sites/www.acpm.org/resource/resmgr/timetools-files/adherenceclinicalreference.pdf

American Federation for Aging Research. (2011). *Theories of aging.* Retrieved from http://www.afar.org/docs/migrated/111121_INFOAGING_GUIDE_THEORIES_OF_AGINGFR.pdf

American Nurses Association. (n.d.). *Florence S. Wald (1917–2008) 1996 inductee.* Retrieved from http://www.nursingworld.org/FlorenceSWald

American Nurses Association. (2010). *Gerontological nursing: Scope and standards of practice.* Silver Spring, MD: Author.

Beales, S. (2012). *Expert group meeting on "Promoting people's empowerment in achieving poverty eradication, social integration, and productive and decent work for all": Empowerment and older people: Enhancing capacities in an ageing world.* Retrieved from http://www.un.org/esa/socdev/egms/docs/2012/SylviaBeales.pdf

Beckles, G. L., & Truman, B. I. (2011). Education and income—United States, 2005 and 2009. *Morbidity and Mortality Weekly Report, 60*(Suppl.), 13–17.

Bruckenthal, P., Reid, C., & Reisner, L. (2009). Special issues in the management of chronic pain in older adults. *Pain Medicine, 10*(S2), S67–S78. doi:10.1111/j.1526-4637.2009.00667.x

Butler, J. P., Fujii, M., & Sasaki, H. (2011). Balanced aging or successful aging? *Geriatrics & Gerontology International, 11,* 1–2. doi:10.1111/j.1447-0594.2010.00661.x

Buyck, J.-F., Bonnaud, S., Boumendil, A., Andrieu, S., Nonenfant, S., Goldberg, M., …, Ankri, J. (2011). Informal caregiving and self-reported mental and physical health: Results from the Gazel cohort study. *American Journal of Public Health, 10,* 1971–1979. doi:10.2105/AJPH.2010.300044

Cacchione, P. Z. (2012). Sensory changes. In M. Bolz, E. Capezuti, T. Fulmer, & D. Zwicker (Eds.), *Evidence-based geriatric nursing protocols for best practice* (4th ed., pp. 48–73). New York, NY: Springer.

Caring Connections. (n.d.). *Palliative care questions and answers.* Retrieved from http://www.caringinfo.org/i4a/pages/index.cfm?pageid=3355

Centers for Disease Control and Prevention. (n.d.). *Edentulism (loss of all natural teeth), ages 18+, US, 1998–2012.* Retrieved from http://205.207.175.93/HDI/TableViewer/tableView.aspx?reportId=110

Centers for Disease Control and Prevention. (2012). *Older adult falls data and statistics.* Retrieved from http://www.cdc.gov/homeandrecreationalsafety/Falls/data.html

Centers for Disease Control and Prevention. (2013a). *Falls among older adults: An Overview.* Retrieved from http://www.cdc.gov/HomeandRecreational-Safety/Falls/adultfalls.html

Centers for Disease Control and Prevention. (2013b). *Focus on preventing falls.* Retrieved from http://www.cdc.gov/Features/OlderAmericans/

Centers for Disease Control and Prevention. (2014a). *Cost of falls among older adults.* Retrieved from http://www.cdc.gov/HomeandRecreationalSafety/Falls/fallcost.html

Centers for Disease Control and Prevention. (2014b). *Disability and functioning (adults).* Retrieved from http://www.cdc.gov/nchs/fastats/disable.htm

Centers for Disease Control and Prevention. (2014c). *How much physical activity do older adults need?* Retrieved from http://www.cdc.gov/physicalactivity/everyone/guidelines/olderadults.html

Centers for Disease Control and Prevention. (2014d). *Recommended adult immunization schedule—United States—2014.* Retrieved from http://www.cdc.gov/vaccines/schedules/downloads/adult/adult-schedule.pdf

Centers for Disease Control and Prevention, Administration on Aging, Agency for Healthcare Research and Quality, & Centers for Medicare and Medicaid Services. (2011). *Enhancing use of clinical preventive services among older adults—Closing the gap.* Retrieved from http://www.cdc.gov/Features/PreventiveServices/Clinical_Preventive_Services_Closing_the_Gap_Report.pdf

Centers for Medicare and Medicaid Services. (2012a). *Medicare benefit policy manual.* Chapter 9—Coverage of hospice services under hospital insurance. Retrieved from http://www.cms.gov/Regulations-and-Guidance/Guidance/Manuals/downloads/bp102c09.pdf

Centers for Medicare and Medicaid Services. (2012b). *Medicare general information, eligibility, and entitlement.* Chapter 1—General overview. Retrieved from http://www.cms.gov/Regulations-and-Guidance/Guidance/Manuals/downloads/ge101c01.pdf

Centers for Medicare and Medicaid Services. (2014). *Costs for Medicare drug coverage.* Retrieved from http://www.medicare.gov/part-d/costs/part-d-costs.html

Chao, S.-Y., Chen, C.-R., Liu, H.-Y., & Clark, M. J. (2008). Meet the real elders: Reminiscence links past and present. *Journal of Clinical Nursing, 17,* 2647–2653.

Cicely Saunders International. (n.d.). *Dame Cicely biography.* Retrieved from http://www.cicelysaundersfoundation.org/about-us/dame-cicely-biography

Cleveland Clinic. (n.d.). *COPD: Chronic obstructive pulmonary disease fundamentals.* Retrieved from http://my.clevelandclinic.org/disorders/chronic_obstructive_pulmonary_disease_copd/pul_overview.aspx

Cleveland Clinic. (2011). *Nutritional guidelines for people with COPD.* Retrieved from http://my.clevelandclinic.org/disorders/Chronic_Obstructive_Pulmonary_Disease_copd/hic_Nutritional_Guidelines_for_People_with_COPD.aspx

Connecticut Women's Hall of Fame. (n.d.). *Florence Wald.* Retrieved from http://www.cwhf.org/inductees/science-health/florence-wald/

Corie. (2010). *Theories of aging.* Retrieved from http://aginginalabama.org/2010/05/default.aspx

Crosby, A. E., Ortega, L., & Stevens, M. R. (2011). Suicides—United States, 1999–2007. *Morbidity and Mortality Weekly Report, 60*(Suppl.), 56–59.

Demirçin, S., Akkoyun, M., Yilmaz, R., & Gökdoğan, M. R. (2011). Suicide of elderly persons: Towards a framework for prevention. *Geriatrics & Gerontology International, 11,* 107–113. doi:10.1111/j.1447-0594.2010.00660.x

Division of HIV/AIDS Prevention. (2013). *HIV Surveillance Report, 2011 (vol. 23).* Retrieved from http://www.cdc.gov/hiv/pdf/statistics_2011_HIV_Surveillance_Report_vol_23.pdf

Dray, S. (2011). *Malnutrition in adults.* Retrieved from http://www.livestrong.com/article/482199-malnutrition-in-adults/

Elstad, E. A., Taubenberger, S. P., Botelho, E. M., & Tennstedt, S. L. (2010). Beyond incontinence: The stigma of other urinary symptoms. *Journal of Advanced Nursing, 66,* 2460–2470. doi:10.1111/j.1365-2648.2010.05422.x

Family Caregiver Alliance. (2012). *Taking care of you: Self-care for family caregivers.* Retrieved from https://caregiver.org/taking-care-you-self-care-family-caregivers

Federal Interagency Forum on Aging-Related Statistics. (2012). *Older Americans 2012: Key indicators of well-being.* Retrieved from http://www.agingstats.gov/Main_Site/Data/2012_Documents/docs/EntireChartbook.pdf

Feinberg, L., Reinhard, S. C., Houser, A., & Choula, R. (2011). *Valuing the invaluable: 2011 update on the growing contributions and costs of family caregiving.* Retrieved from http://assets.aarp.org/rgcenter/ppi/ltc/i51-caregiving.pdf

Fink, M. J., & Gates, R. A. (2010). Pain assessment. In B. R. Ferrell & N. Coyle (Eds.), *Oxford textbook of palliative nursing* (pp. 137–160). New York: Oxford University Press.

Fischer, M. E., Cruickshanke, K. J., Wiley, T. L., Klein, B. E. K., Klein, R., & Tweed, T. S. (2011). Determinants of hearing aid acquisition in older adults. *American Journal of Public Health, 101,* 1449–1550. doi:10.2105/AJPH.2010.300078

Fung, H. H. (2013). Aging in culture. *The Gerontologist,* 33, 369–377. doi: 10.1093/geront/gnt024

Gabrielle, M. S. (2011). Trajectories of chronic illnesses. In S. H. Qualls & J. E. Kasl-Godley (Eds.), *End-of-life issues, grief, and bereavement: What clinicians need to know* (pp. 26–42). Hoboken, NJ: John Wiley & Sons.

Gallagher-Thompson, D., & Coon, D. W. (2007). Evidence-based psychological treatments for distress in family caregivers of older adults. *Psychology and Aging, 22,* 37–51. doi:10.1037/0882-7974.22.1.37

Givens, J. L., Mezzacappa, C., Heeren, T., Yaffe, K., & Fredman. (2014). Depressive symptoms among dementia caregivers: Role of mediating factors. *American Journal of Geriatric Psychiatry, 22,* 481–488. doi: 10.1016/j.jagp.2012.08.010

Guo, G., & Phillips, L. R. (2010). Conceptualization and nursing implications of self-imposed activity limitation among community-dwelling elders. *Public Health Nursing, 27,* 353–361. doi:10.1111/j.1525-1446.2010.00863.x

Hamilton, M. M. (2013, January–February). Have you saved enough for your health care? *AARP Bulletin, 16,* 18–19.

Harder, A. F. (2012). *The developmental stages of Erik Erikson.* Retrieved from http://www.support4change.com/index.php?view=article&catid=35%3Awho-you-are&id=47%3Aerik-eriksons-developmental-stages&tmpl=component&print=1&layout=default&page=&option=com_content&Itemid=108.

Hartford Institute for Geriatric Nursing. (2013). *Assessment tools—Try This ® and How to Try This resources.* Retrieved from http://consultgerirn.org/resources

Health Data Interactive. (2014). *Mortality by underlying cause, ages 18+: US/State, 2001–2010.* Retrieved from http://205.207.175.93/HDI/TableViewer/tableView.aspx?eportId=673

Hughes, S. L., Seymour, R. B., Campbell, R. T., Shaw, J. W., Fabiyi, C., & Sokas, R. (2011). Comparison of two health-promotion programs for older workers. *American Journal of Public Health, 101,* 883–890. doi:10.2105/AJPH.2010.300082

Hulisz, D., & Duff, C. (2009). Assisting seniors with insomnia: A comprehensive approach. *U.S. Pharmacist, 34*(6), 38–43.

International Foundation for Functional Gastrointestinal Disorders. (2013a). *Prevalence of bowel incontinence.* Retrieved from http://www.aboutincontinence.org/site/about-incontinence/prevalence/

International Foundation for Functional Gastrointestinal Disorders. (2013b). *Treatment of incontinence.* Retrieved from http://www.aboutincontinence.org/site/about-incontinence/treatment/

International Foundation for Functional Gastrointestinal Disorders. (2014). *Common causes of incontinence.* Retrieved from http://www.aboutincontinence.org/site/about-incontinence/causes-of-incontinence/

Johns Hopkins Medicine. (2010). *Prescription drugs special report: Drug abuse and the elderly.* Retrieved from http://www.johnshopkinshealthalerts.com/reports/prescription_drugs/3363-1.html

Kanny, D., Liu, Y., & Brewer, R. D. (2011, January 14). Binge drinking = United States, 2009. *Morbidity and Mortality Weekly Report, 60*(Suppl.), 101–104

Lis, K., Reichert, M., Cosack, A., Billings, J., & Brown, P. (Eds.). (2008). *Evidence-based guidelines on health promotion for older people.* Retrieved from http://www.healthproelderly.com/pdf/HPE-Guidelines_Online.pdf

Lustig, T. A., & Olson, S. (Rapporteurs). (2014). *Hearing loss and healthy aging.* Retrieved from http://www.nap.edu/download.php?record_id=18735

Madden-Baer, R. (2011). *The depression epidemic in the elderly.* Retrieved from http://www.huffingtonpost.com/rose-maddenbaer/elderly-depression_b_1022468.html

Mayo Clinic Staff. (2011a). *Senior health: How to prevent and detect malnutrition.* Retrieved from http://www.mayoclinic.com/health/senior-health/HA00066/METHOD=print

Mayo Clinic Staff. (2011b). *Urinary incontinence.* Retrieved from http://www.mayoclinic.com/health/urinary-incontinence/DS00404/

Mehta, K., M., Fung, K. S., Kistler, L., Chang, A., & Walter, L. C. (2010). Impact of cognitive impairment on screening mammography us in older US women. *American Journal of Public Health, 100,* 1917–1923. doi:10.2105/AJPH.2008.158485

Meier, D. E. (2010). The development, status, and future of palliative care. In D. E. Meier, S. L. Isaacs, & R. G. Hughes (Eds.), *Palliative care: Transforming the care of serious illness* (pp. 3–76). San Francisco, CA: Jossey Bass.

MetLife Foundation & Civic Ventures. (2008). *Encore career survey*. Retrieved from http://www.civicventures.org/publications/surveys/encore_career_survey/Encore_Survey.pdf

MetLife Mature Market Institute. (2010). *The MetLife report on aging in place 2.0: Rethinking solutions to the home care challenge.* Retrieved from https://www.metlife.com/assets/cao/mmi/publications/studies/2010/mmi-aging-place-study.pdf

National Alliance on Mental Illness. (2009). *Depression in older persons: Fact sheet.* Retrieved from http://www.nami.org/Template.cfm?Section=By_Illness&template=/ContentManagement/ContentDisplay.cfm&ContentID=7515

National Center for Chronic Disease Prevention and Health Promotion. (2011). *Executive summary progress report on the CDC Healthy Brain Initiative, 2006–2011.* Retrieved from http://www.cdc.gov/aging/pdf/hbisummary_508.pdf

National Center for Health Statistics. (2012). *Health, United States, 2011: With special feature on socioeconomic status and health.* Retrieved from http://www.cdc.gov/nchs/data/hus/hus11.pdf

National Center for Health Statistics. (2014a). *Health United States 2013 with special feature on prescription drugs.* Retrieved from http://www.cdc.gov/nchs/data/hus/hus13.pdf

National Center for Health Statistics. (2014b). *Vital and health statistics: Summary health statistics for U.S. adults: National Health Interview Survey, 2012.* Retrieved from http://www.cdc.gov/nchs/data/series/sr_10/sr10_260.pdf

National Center for Immunization and Respiratory Diseases. (2013). *Flu vaccination coverage, United States, 2012–13 influenza season.* Retrieved from http://www.cdc.gov/flu/fluvaxview/coverage-1213estimates.htm

National Center for Injury Prevention and Control. (2013a). *Older adult drivers: Get the facts.* Retrieved from http://www.cdc.gov/Motorvehicle-safety/Older_Adult_Drivers/adult-drivers_factsheet.html

National Center for Injury Prevention and Control. (2013b). *Saving lives and protecting people from violence and injuries.* Retrieved from http://www.cdc.gov/injury/overview

National Center for Injury Prevention and Control. (2014a). *Elder maltreatment: Definition.* Retrieved from http://www.cdc.gov/ViolencePrevention/eldermaltreatment/definitions.html

National Center for Injury Prevention and Control. (2014b). *Elder maltreatment: Risk and protective factors.* Retrieved from http://www.cdc.gov/ViolencePrevention/eldermaltreatment/riskprotectivefactors.html

National Coalition for the Homeless. (2009). *Homelessness among elderly persons.* Retrieved from http://www.nationalhomeless.org/factsheets/Elderly.pdf

National Council on Aging. (2014). *Economic security for seniors: Fact sheet.* Retrieved from http://www.ncoa.org/assets/files/pdf/FactSheet_Economic-Security.pdf

National Digestive Diseases Information Clearinghouse. (2013). *Fecal incontinence.* Retrieved from http://digestive.niddk.nih.gov/ddiseases/pubs/fecalincontinence/index.aspx#eating

National Foundation to End Senior Hunger. (2013). *Spotlight on senior hunger executive summary.* Retrieved from http://www.nfesh.org/wp-content/uploads/2013/05/Senior-Hunger-Research.pdf

National Health Service. (2013). *How is dementia treated?* Retrieved from http://www.nhs.uk/Conditions/dementia-guide/Pages/dementia-treatment.aspx

National Heart, Lung and Blood Institute. (2013a). *How is COPD treated?* Retrieved from http://www.nhlbi.nih.gov/health/health-topics/topics/copd/treatment.html

National Heart, Lung and Blood Institute. (2013b). *Living with COPD.* Retrieved from http://www.nhlbi.nih.gov/health/health-topics/topics/copd/livingwith.html

National Hospice and Palliative Care Organization. (2013). *Planning ahead.* Retrieved from http://www.caringinfo.org/i4a/pages/index.cfm?pageid=3289

National Resource Center on Nutrition, Physical Activity, and Aging. (n.d.a). *Malnutrition and Older Americans.* Retrieved from http://nutritionandaging.fiu.edu/aging_network/malfact2.asp

National Resource Center on Nutrition, Physical Activity, and Aging. (n.d.b). *You can!: Steps to healthier aging.* Retrieved from http://nutritionandaging.fiu.edu/You_Can/index.asp

Norton, W. F. (2011). *Medical treatment and management of incontinence.* Milwaukee, WI: International Foundation for Functional Gastrointestinal Disorders.

Ogden, L. L., Richards, C. L., & Shenson, D. (2012). Clinical preventive services for older adults: The interface between personal health care and public health services. *American Journal of Public Health, 102,* 419–425. doi:10.2105/AJPH.2011.300353

Opondo, D., Eslami, S., Visscher, S., de Rooij, S. E., Verheij, R., Korevaar, J. C., & Abu-Hanna, A. (2012). *Inappropriateness of medication prescriptions to elderly patients in the primary care setting: A systematic review.* Retrieved from http://www.plosone.org/article/info%3Adoi%2F10.1371%2Fjournal.pone.0043617

Reid, H. (2011, October). The new law works. *AARP Bulletin, 34.*

Renfro, M. O., & Fehrer, S. (2011). Multifactorial screening for fall risk in community-dwelling older adults in the primary care office: Development of the fall risk assessment & screening tool. *American Physical Therapy Association, 34,* 174–183. doi:10.1519/JPT.0b013e31820e4855

Rennard, S. I. (2014). *Patient information: Chronic obstructive pulmonary disease (COPD) treatments (Beyond the basics).* Retrieved from http://www.uptodate.com/contents/chronic-obstructive-pulmonary-disease-copd-treatments-beyond-the-basics?source=search_result&search=copd+management&selectedTitle=1%7E14

Roe, B., Beynon, C., Pickering, L., & Duffy, P. (2010). Experiences of drug use and aging: Health, quality of life, relationship and service implications. *Journal of Advanced Nursing, 66,* 1968–1979. doi:10.1111/j.1365-2648.2010.05378.x

Roe, B., Flanagan, L., Jack, B., Barrett, J., Chung, A., Shaw, C., & Williams, K. (2011). Systematic review of the management of incontinence and promotion of continence in older people in care homes: Descriptive studies with urinary incontinence as primary focus. *Journal of Advanced Nursing, 67,* 228–250. doi:10.1111/j.1365-2648.2010.05481.x

Sagawa, M., Kojimahara, N., Otsuka, N., Kimura, M., & Yamaguchi, N. (2011). Immune response to influenza vaccine in the elderly: Association with nutritional and physical status. *Geriatrics & Gerontology International, 11,* 63–68. doi:10.1111/j.1447-0594.2010.00641.x

Saxon, S. V., & Etten, M. J. (2010). *Physical change & aging: A guide for the helping professions* (5th ed.). New York, NY: Springer.

Serse, R., Euler, G. L., Gonzalez-Feliciano, A. G., Bryan, L. N., Furlow, C., Weinbaum, W., & Singleton, J. A. (2011). Influenza vaccination coverage—United States, 2000–2010. *Morbidity and Mortality Weekly Report, 60*(Suppl.), 38–41

Short, K. (2012). *The research supplemental poverty measure: 2011.* Retrieved from http://www.census.gov/hhes/povmeas/methodology/supplemental/research/Short_ResearchSPM2011.pdf

Shyu, Y.-I. L., Chen, M.-C., Wu, C.-C., & Cheng, H.-S. (2010). Family caregivers' needs predict functional recovery of older care recipients after hip fracture. *Journal of Advanced Nursing, 66,* 2450–2459. doi:10.1111/j.1365-2648.2010.05418.x

Smith, C. M., & Cotter, V. T. (2012). Age-related changes in health. In M. Bolz, E. Capezuti, T. Fulmer, & D. Zwicker (Eds.), *Evidence-based geriatric nursing protocols for best practice* (4th ed., pp. 23–47). New York, NY: Springer.

Social Security Administration. (2014a). *Fact sheet social security*. Retrieved from http://www.ssa.gov/pressoffice/factsheets/basicfact-alt.pdf

Social Security Administration. (2014b). *Income of the population 55 and older, 2012*. Retrieved from http://www.socialsecurity.gov/policy/docs/statcomps/income_pop55/2012/incpop12.pdf

Spector, A., Orrell, M., & Woods, B. (2010). Cognitive stimulation therapy (CST) effects on different areas of cognitive function for people with dementia. *International Journal of Geriatric Psychiatry, 25,* 1253–1258.

St. Christopher's Hospice. (2013). *Dame Cicely Saunders: Her life and work*. Retrieved from http://www.stchristophers.org.uk/about/damecicelysaunders

Stevens, J. A., & Haas, E. N. (2011). Nonfatal bathroom injuries among persons aged > 15 years—United States, 2008. *Morbidity and Mortality Weekly Report, 60,* 729–733.

Strada, E. A. (2013). *The helping professional's guide to end-of-life care*. Oakland, CA: New Harbinger.

Swann, J. (2010). Ways of doing things differently to maintain independence. *British Journal of Healthcare Assistants, 4,* 294–298.

United Nations, Department of Economic and Social Affairs, Population Division. (2013). *World population ageing 2013*. Retrieved from http://www.un.org/en/development/desa/population/publications/pdf/ageing/WorldPopulationAgeing2013.pdf

U.S. Census Bureau. (2011). *Special tabulation of supplemental poverty measure estimates*. Retrieved from http://www.census.gov/hhes/povmeas/methodology/supplemental/research/SpecialTabulation.pdf

U.S. Census Bureau. (2012a). *Statistical abstract of the United States, Table 34. Persons 65 years old and over—Characteristics by age: 1990 to 2010*. Retrieved from http://www.census.gov/compendia/statab/2012/tables/12s0034.pdf

U.S. Census Bureau. (2012b). *Statistical abstract of the United States, Table 35. Persons 65 years old and over—Living arrangements and disability status, 2009*. Retrieved from http://www.census.gov/compendia/statab/2012/tables/12s0035.pdf

U.S. Census Bureau. (2012c). *Statistical abstract of the United States, Table 70. Grandparents living with grandchildren by race and sex: 2009*. Retrieved from http://www.census.gov/compendia/statab/2012/tables/12s0070.pdf

U.S. Census Bureau. (2013). *The older population in the United States: 2012. Table 1. Population by age and sex, 2012*. Retrieved from http://www.census.gov/population/age/data/2012.html

U.S. Department of Health and Human Services. (2013). *Immunization and infectious diseases objectives*. Retrieved from http://healthypeople.gov/2020/topicsobjectives2020/objectiveslist.aspx?topicId=23

U.S. Department of Health and Human Services (2014). *Healthy People 2020 topics and objectives*. Retrieved from http://healthypeople.gov/2020/topicsobjectives2020/default.aspx

U.S. Preventive Services Task Force. (2013). *Recommendations for adults*. Retrieved from http://www.uspreventiveservicestaskforce.org/adultrec.htm

Validation Training Institute. (2013a). *Research on validation*. Retrieved from https://vfvalidation.org/web.php?equest=research_on_validation

Validation Training Institute. (2013b). *What is validation?* Retrieved from https://vfvalidation.org/web.php?equest=what_is_validation

VickyRN. (2013). *Theories of aging (Part 3): Sociological theories*. Retrieved from http://allnurses-breakroom.com/geriatrics-aging-elderly/theories-aging-part-412760.html

Werner, C. (2011). *The older population: 2010—2010 census briefs*. Retrieved from http://www.census.gov/prod/cen2010/briefs/c2010br-09.pdf

Williams, K. N., Herman, R., Gajweski, B., & Wilson, K. (2009). Elderspeak communication: Impact on dementia care. *American Journal of Alzheimer's Disease and Other Dementias, 24*(1), 11–20. doi:10.1177/1533317508318472

Williams, W. W., Lu, P. J., Greby, S., Bridges, C. B., Ahmed, F., Liang, J. L., …, Hales, C. (2013). Noninfluenza vaccination coverage among adults—United States, 2011. *Morbidity and Mortality Weekly Report, 62,* 66–72.

World Health Organization. (2014). *Falls prevention in older age*. Retrieved from http://www.who.int/ageing/projects/falls_prevention_older_age/en/

Wuellner, S. E., Walters, J. K., St. Louis, T., Leinenkugel, K., Rogers, P. F., Lefkowitz, D., …, Castillo, D. N. (2011). Nonfatal occupational injuries and illness among older workers—United States, 2009. *Morbidity and Mortality Weekly Report, 60,* 503–510.

Yuill, N., & Hollis, V. (2011). A systematic review of cognitive stimulation therapy for older adults with mild to moderate dementia: An occupational therapy perspective. *Occupational Therapy International, 18,* 163–186.

Zwicker, D. A., & Fulmer, T. (2012). Reducing adverse drug events. In M. Boltz, E. Capezuti, T. Fulmer, & D. Zwicker (Eds.), *Evidence-based geriatric nursing protocols for best practice* (4th ed., pp. 324–362). New York, NY: Springer.

CHAPTER

20 Care of Gay, Lesbian, Bisexual, and Transgender Populations

Learning Outcomes

After reading this chapter, you should be able to:

1. Discuss concepts related to gender identity and sexual orientation.
2. Identify determinants of health affecting gay, lesbian, bisexual, and transgender individuals.
3. Describe health promotion and illness/injury prevention measures appropriate to the care of the GLBT population and population health nursing roles in each.
4. Identify areas of focus in resolving existing health problems in the GLBT population and related poulation health nursing roles.
5. Describe considerations relevant to restorative health care for the GLBT population and the population health nursing roles related to each.

Key Terms

biphobia
cisgender
coming out
disclosure
gender dysphoria
gender expression
gender identity
gender nonconforming individual
gender role conformity
hate crimes
heterosexism
homophobia
minority stress
second-parent adoption
serosorting
sexual orientation
syndemic
transgender individuals
transphobia
transsexuals

Advocacy Then

Lesbian Health Care

The 1970s saw an emphasis on gay liberation, coming out, and demands for equitable treatment. Access to culturally sensitive health care for lesbians (and other members of the gay, lesbian, bisexual, and transgender [GLBT] population) lagged significantly behind other social changes. Joan Waitkevicz, a lesbian physician, teamed with several other lesbian health activists to establish the St. Mark's Women's Health Collective. The intent of the clinic was to provide a source of safe comfortable care for lesbians in New York City. Subsequently, Dr. Waitkevicz became involved in the Gay Women's Focus at Beth Israel Medical Center, the first hospital-based health center for lesbian women (Labaton, 2012).

Advocacy Now

Winning Freedom from Discrimination

Members of the GLBT population have been subjected to continuing discrimination in large and small ways. For years, the Boy Scouts of America (BSA) expressly forbade gay boys from membership in the organization. In May of 2013, however, a grassroots coalition of organizations campaigned for and won a removal of the prohibition on gay scouts. Petitions were initiated on websites such as change.org and were signed by more than 300,000 people and the campaign was covered by major news media and magazines. Contacts were made with prominent BSA board members who were CEOs of major U.S. companies. In addition, major corporate donors to BSA, such as Intel and UPS, were convinced to suspend their funding to the organization until the ban was lifted, and *National Geographic* called for change. Gay Eagle Scouts also persuaded the band Train to refuse to perform at a scheduled Boy Scout concert. In addition, seven members of the U.S. House of Representatives signed a letter advocating for the reform. Despite this success, however, BSA still prohibits GLBT adults from functioning as Boy Scout leaders, and further advocacy is needed to achieve complete equality within the organization (Scouts for Equality, 2013).

Variations in sexual orientation and gender identity have been present throughout recorded human history, but, until recently, they have been deemed aberrations and have rarely been considered in terms of their implications for health and health care delivery. Collectively, people who exhibit these variations are referred to as the GLBT community or population. Despite some similarities among different elements of the GLBT population, they are display a diverse range of age, racial/ethnic, and socioeconomic characteristics as well as variation in sexual orientation (Institute of Medicine [IOM], 2011). Members of this population experience health issues that are both similar to and different from their heterosexual or "straight" counterparts, and population health nurses must be prepared to provide health care to effectively meet their needs. In addition, population health nurses may be actively involved in advocacy to assure provision of service to this population.

Sexual Orientation and Gender Identity

Before examining the health-related needs of the GLBT population, it is important to define some related concepts. **Sexual orientation** refers to one's preferred choice of sexual or romantic partners or the gender(s) of people to whom one is attracted. Attraction may be to people of one's own sex, the opposite sex, or both sexes. Sexual orientation comprises three aspects: attraction, behavior, and identity (IOM, 2011, p. 27). Commonly used terms for different sexual orientations include *heterosexual*, *homosexual*, and *bisexual*. Heterosexual or straight individuals are primarily attracted to members of the opposite biological sex, while homosexual individuals are attracted primarily to members of their own biological sex. Bisexual individuals are attracted to members of both sexes. These preferences constitute the attraction aspect of sexual orientation. The behavioral aspect reflects one's actual sexual behavior or activity with members of one sex or the other. The identity aspect of sexual orientation reflects one's sense of self as a member of a particular social group based on a shared orientation (IOM, 2011). For example, women who identify themselves as lesbian share a sexual or romantic preference for other women, while gay men prefer other men.

There is no general consensus on the use of the terms *heterosexual, homosexual,* and so on, primarily because the terms are defined differently by different groups. Sexual orientation is culturally defined, and what is considered homosexual in one culture may not be in another, even if it involves same-sex sexual activity (Martinez-Donate et al., 2010). For example, some men who self-identify as straight have sexual intercourse with other men, and are commonly referred to as "men who have sex with men" or MSM. Sometimes such same-sex behavior is situational, as in the case of prisoners who do not have access to members of the opposite sex. In other cases, it may involve casual sexual encounters with members of the same sex.

Similar lack of clarity occurs in definitions of bisexuality. For instance, men who self-identify as gay may also have sexual interactions with women, but do not consider themselves bisexual. Similarly, women who self-identify as lesbian may also have sexual encounters with men. For the purposes of this book, self-identification as a gay, lesbian, bisexual, or transgender individual will be used as the primary means of distinguishing membership in these groups. Readers should be aware, however, that different definitions have been used in some of the research that will be reported here. Where relevant, the terms "men who have sex with men" (MSM) or "women who have sex with women" (WSW) will be used since they encompass both gay/lesbian and bisexual individuals as well as some who self-identify as straight despite occasional same-sex sexual activity.

Synnott (2009) described four perspectives on sex or gender: anatomical, chromosomal, hormonal, and psychological. The anatomical perspective relies on sex-specific internal and external organs (e.g., a uterus, penis, prostate, etc.); the chromosomal perspective is based on the number of X and Y chromosomes one possesses. In the hormonal perspective, one's sex is defined by the balance of male and female hormones. The final perspective involves one's felt identity or gender identity.

Gender identity differs from sexual orientation in that it reflects one's perception of self as a man or woman, boy or girl. One's gender identity may or may not correspond to one's biological sex. Transgender individuals are born anatomically one gender, but identify with the other, with both genders (bigender individuals), or neither (Synnott, 2009; Wilson et al., 2010). Transgender individuals are a diverse group whose members do not conform to culturally defined gender expectations (Bockting, Miner, Romine, Hamilton, & Coleman, 2013). They may differ in terms of their gender identity, gender presentation or expression, or sexual orientation. Transgender individuals may or may not exhibit **gender role conformity,** the extent to which one adheres to cultural norms for his or her anatomical sex. Depending on circumstances, they may conform to their birth sex, their self-perceived gender, or both at different times. **Cisgender** refers to an individual whose self-perceived gender is congruent with his or her assigned birth gender (National Coalition of Anti-Violence Programs, 2013). **Gender expression** is how one presents oneself as masculine or feminine (or possibly neither) in terms of personality, appearance, and behavior (IOM, 2011). A **gender-nonconforming individual** is one who by nature or choice does not conform to societal gender expectations (Parents, Families, and Friends of Lesbians and Gays [PFLAG], n.d.a). **Transgender individuals** are persons whose gender identity does not match their assigned birth gender (PFLAG, n.d.b). Members of the transgender community view this as an all-encompassing term that includes cross-dressers, drag kings and queens, and transsexuals although not all of these individuals self-identify as members of the other gender. For example, a drag queen may be a biological male who dresses as a female, but still considers himself male. **Transsexuals** are persons who believe they were born into the "wrong" body and are actually members of the opposite gender. Transsexual is sometimes used to distinguish those who have undergone sexual reassignment surgery (SRS) to change their anatomical appearance to that of members of the opposite gender. In the transgender community, the preferred term for this surgical procedure is "gender recognition surgery" denoting recognition of their appropriate gender identity. Women who have surgical procedures to become men

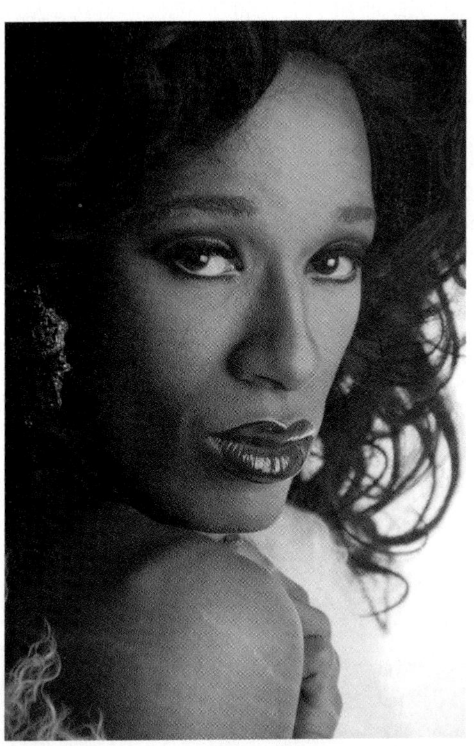

Transgender individuals identify as members of the opposite gender and dress and act accordingly. *(Karen Struthers/Fotolia)*

are known as female-to-male (FTM) transgenders, transmen, or transguys. Men who undergo SRS may be known as male-to-female (MTF) transgendered individuals or transwomen (UC Berkeley Gender Equity Resource Center, n.d.). Transgender individuals may exhibit different sexual orientations as well. For example, MTF transgender persons may be attracted to men, other women, or both. On occasion, MTF transgender individuals may be labeled as MSM, although they consider themselves women who have sex with men. Similarly, FTM transgender individuals who have sex with transwomen consider themselves straight.

Additional definitions describing the diversity of gender identity and sexual orientation are presented in Table 20-1 ●.

Determining the Size of the GLBT Population

Although differences in sexual orientation and sexual identity are becoming more socially acceptable, continuing stigma may preclude many people from living openly or acknowledging membership in the GLBT population. This makes it difficult to accurately determine the size of the gay, lesbian, bisexual, and transgender populations. Inferences regarding the extent of sexual and gender diversity are often drawn from related data. For example, 2005 Census Bureau data included more than 770,000 same-sex couples in households throughout the United States, many of whom are probably gay or lesbian couples. Census data, however, probably underrepresent the GLBT population due to fear of exposure or differences in definitions. In an American Community Survey, an estimated 8.8% of the U.S. residents self-identified as gay or bisexual. In other estimates, as many as 7% of women may self-identify as lesbian, and 8% of men as gay or bisexual (Buffie, 2011). In the 2010 National Survey of Sexual Health and Behavior, 6.8% of men, and 4.5% of women self-identified as homosexual, gay, lesbian, or bisexual, while the estimated size of the transgender population varies from 1 person per 2,900 men in Singapore to 1 per 100,000 in the United States. Comparable ratios for women are 1:8,300 for Singapore and 1:400,000 U.S. women (IOM, 2011).

TABLE 20-1 Definitions of Terms Related to Gender Identity and Sexual Orientation

Gender Identity Terminology	Definition
Bigender person	One who identifies as both man and woman. May take hormones and live part-time in the cross-gender role.
Cisgender/gender-straight/gender-normative	A person who by nature or choice conforms to social gender-based expectations for his or her anatomic sex.
Cross-dresser (previously transvestite)	One who adopts the clothing and behaviors of the opposite sex for emotional or sexual gratification. May live part-time in the cross-gender role.
Drag kings or queens	Persons who dress in the clothing of the opposite gender and adopt a hyperfeminine or hypermasculine presentation. May live part-time in the cross-gender role often in the context of a performance. Does not necessarily indicate sexuality or gender identity.
Gender diverse	One who does not conform to societal gender-based expectations
Gender fluid	One whose gender identification shifts with time and circumstances.
Gender nonconforming individual	One who, by nature or by choice, does not conform to normative gender expectations
Gender queer/two spirit	One who possesses both masculine and feminine characteristics, who may or may not desire hormones or surgery and may or may not live full- or part-time in the cross-gender role.
Pangender	One whose gender identity involves multiple gender expressions.
Transgenderists	Persons who live full-time in the cross-gender role. They may take hormones, but do not desire surgery.
Transsexuals	Persons who desire to or actually engage in masculinization or feminization of the body by means of hormones and/or surgery and live full-time in the cross-gender role.

Sexual Orientation Terminology	Definition
Asexual	One who is not sexually attracted to either gender.
Bisexual	One who is sexually or romantically attracted to two sexes (man and woman, transsexual, or any combination of them). The attraction may not be simultaneous or of equal intensity.
Gay/gay man	A man who is sexually or romantically attracted to other men.
Homosexuality	Sexual, emotional, or romantic attraction to persons of one's same sex.
Lesbian	A woman who is sexually or romantically attracted to other women.
Pansexual	One whose sexual orientation or gender identity is fluid.
Straight	One attracted to a gender other than his or her own.

Based on: Institute of Medicine. (2011). *The health of lesbian, gay, bisexual, and transgender people: Building a foundation for better understanding.* Washington, DC: National Academies Press; UC Berkeley Gender Equity Resource Center. (n.d.). *Definitions of terms.* Retrieved from http://geneq.berkeley.edu/lgbt_resources_definiton_of_terms

From 2001 to 2009, only nine sites participating in the Youth Risk Behavior Surveillance System asked questions about sexual orientation, with a median of 93% of teens reporting a heterosexual orientation, 1.3% gay or lesbian, and 3.7 bisexual. An additional 2.5% of youth were unsure regarding their sexual orientation. Twelve sites assessed only sexual contact, for which 53.5% reported intercourse with the opposite sex only, 2.5% with the same sex only, and 3.3% with both sexes (Kann et al., 2011). The Guttmacher Institute (2014), on the other hand, has reported estimates of 3% of 18- to 19-year-old males and 8% of females self-identifying as homosexual or bisexual. The number of women who have sex with women may be particularly hard to determine as they tend to be a more hidden population than
likely to be viewed in
circumstances.

Population
Care of GL

Population health n
and implement heal
GLBT population in
advocating for this
international levels.
ments of the nursin
lation, planning an
effects of interventio

Assessing the

Assessing the healt
gender populations
six categories of de
pede health and hea

BIOLOGICAL D
related to the healt
tion and aging and
GLBT culture em
population among
estimated 1 to 3
bers in the United
2012), and the old
to 6 million mem
tus in society, old
than others in obt
lation of particula
the health proble
stress of sexual minority status and resulting stigmatization and discrimination (IOM, 2011). Older gay men, who lived through the early stages of the HIV epidemic, may be at particular risk of lack of social support in old age due to having outlived many of their peers. Similarly, GLBT adolescents may experience more health problems than their straight counterparts due to the added stress of stigma and discrimination.

Members of the GLBT population also tend to be at greater risk for a number of physical health problems than the general population. In part, this is due to the greater prevalence of high-risk behaviors in this population, as well as to reluctance to seek medical care. Much of the attention given to health issues in this population to date has focused on the extent of sexually transmitted infections (STIs). For example, MSM account for most of the new syphilis diagnoses in many health department jurisdictions (Mayer, 2011). Many MSM with primary and secondary syphilis are co-infected with HIV (Cohen et al., 2012), but MSM often do not perceive themselves to be at risk for HIV infection. For example, in the 2008 National Health Behavior Survey, the prevalence rate of HIV infection among
g MSM in 21 cities was 19%, yet nearly half of these men
) were unaware of their infection. Lack of awareness was
more likely in young MSM from ethnic minority groups
th et al., 2010). From 2001 to 2006 there was a 93% in-
e in new HIV infections among young Black MSM in 33
s and a 144% increase in the state of Wisconsin between
and 2008 (Biedrzycki et al., 2011). More recently, up
3% of African American MSM have been reported to be
-positive compared to 16% of White MSM, and the rate
cidence among this group is growing faster than among
r high-risk groups (Fields et al., 2013). MSM accounted
53% of all new HIV diagnoses in 2006 (Parsons, Grov, &
ub, 2012). HIV incidence is also high among MTF trans-
der women (Wilson et al., 2010). Women who have sex
women and bisexual women have also been found to be
reater risk for *Chlamydia trachomatis* infection than those
are exclusively heterosexual (Singh, Fine, & Marrazzo,
1).

Members of the GLBT population experience other health
blems at higher rates than the general population. For ex-
ple, lesbian women have been found to be twice as likely to
obese as other women, placing them at greater risk for car-
vascular and other weight-related problems (Boehmer et al.,
1). Similarly, transgender individuals have higher rates of
esity than the general population (Conron, Scott, Stowell, &
nders, 2012). Gay men, on the other hand, are less likely than
eir straight counterparts to be obese or overweight (Conron,
miaga, & Landers, 2010). In addition, lesbian women are
s likely than other women to bear children, increasing their
k of breast cancer (Allina, 2012).

Membership in dual minority groups may also adversely af-
ct physical health status. For example, Hispanic lesbian and
sexual women were found in one study to have higher rates of
thma and disability, and Hispanic bisexual women reported
ore arthritis and poorer overall health than either Caucasian lesbian and bisexual women or straight Hispanic women (Kim & Fredriksen-Goldsen, 2012). Based on Behavioral Risk Factor Surveillance System (BRFSS) data for Massachusetts, members of sexual minority groups, in general, were more likely than others to report activity limitations, tension, smoking, drug use, and asthma. No differences were noted, however, with respect to the incidence of diabetes or heart disease (Conron et al., 2010).

In addition to higher rates of disability, gay, lesbian, and bisexual individuals have been found to experience disability at younger ages than the general population (Fredriksen-Goldsen, Kim, & Barcan, 2012). Mortality rates, however, are no higher for MSM than for other men, when HIV-related mortality is excluded (Cochran & Mays, 2011).

For transgender individuals, measures to modify anatomical structures may have health consequences as well as benefits. For example, feminizing hormones may increase one's risk of venous thrombosis and pulmonary embolism. Other potential adverse effects include gallstones, liver disease, pancreatitis, and glucose intolerance. Conversely, although estrogen therapy may increase stroke and coronary heart disease risk in straight women, it does not seem to do so in transgender MTF women and may actually shift lipid profiles to a more typical female pattern resulting in a protective effect. Masculinizing hormones used by FTM transgender individuals may lead to acne, weight gain, possible polycythemia, liver disease, insulin resistance, fluid retention and edema, and increased risk of cardiovascular disease due to a shift to a typically masculine lipid profile. Finally, FTM transgender individuals may experience bone mineral loss following oophorectomy without regular testosterone use (Gender Centre, 2013). Population health nurses should be alert to these problems in individual transgender clients and to increased incidence in the transgender population. Another problem is that hormones may be perceived as a cause of medical problems when there is some other underlying disease process involved.

Immunity is another consideration related to biological determinants of health in the GLBT population. In addition to routine immunizations suggested for adults, sexually active gay, bisexual, and transgender men and women should also receive immunization for hepatitis A and B. Population health nurses should assess immunity among individual clients as well as levels of immunity in the gay, bisexual, and transgender population at large.

PSYCHOLOGICAL DETERMINANTS. Homosexuality,or same-sex attraction, was considered a psychiatric disease by the American Psychiatric Association from 1952 until 1973. The 1952 *Diagnostic and Statistical Manual of Mental Disorders* (DSM) included homosexuality as a sociopathic personality disorder leading to widespread laws that criminalized homosexuality activity and prohibited employment and licensure in several occupations. Although homosexuality was removed as a psychiatric disorder from later versions of the DSM, gender identity disorder and gender dysphoria were added as psychiatric diagnoses (IOM, 2011). **Gender dysphoria** has been defined as serious discomfort or distress related to one's biologically defined sex. Gender dysphoria has been retained as a diagnosis in the DSM-5 (American Psychiatric Association, 2013), but has been separated from the sexual dysfunction section of the manual. The reported intent of the diagnosis and related chapter is to promote care for individuals who experience severe distress related to the incongruence between their self-perceived gender identity and their biological sex. Relabeling of the diagnosis as gender dysphoria versus gender identity disorder is also intended to diminish the perception of pathology related to gender-atypical behavior (Moran, 2013). Generally, gender dysphoria is diminished in most individuals who experience sexual reassignment surgery. In the interim, however, population health nurses may need to be particularly alert to suicidal ideation in individuals who exhibit severe gender dysphoria.

Although GLBT individuals do not appear to be any more intrinsically susceptible to mental illness than their straight counterparts, there is some evidence to suggest that they have a slightly higher prevalence of mental illness, possibly as a result of "minority stress." **Minority stress** is the stress associated with being a member of any stigmatized minority group (Buffie, 2011). Many mental health problems in the GLBT population are linked to the discrimination experienced in interactions with the straight world. For example, meta-analysis of related research has indicated a lifetime prevalence of depression and anxiety disorders one-and-a-half times higher in gay, lesbian, and bisexual individuals than in the straight population (Choi, Paul, Ayala, Boylan, & Gregorich, 2013).

A person who realizes that he or she is gay, lesbian, bisexual, or transgender has three basic choices. She or he can live openly as a member of a sexual minority group risking potential rejection by family, loss of one's job or professional reputation, and societal labeling and abuse. Denial is a second option that requires considerable expenditure of energy in fulfilling the accepted gender. Finally, he or she can live a sexually diverse life but maintain a straight appearance.

GLBT individuals who do not live their identities openly must deal, on a daily basis, with the fear that others will discover who they really are. This involves the complex task of vigilance about how they look and act, where they are, who they are with, and what they say. This may mean constantly monitoring responses and changing pronouns to misrepresent the identity of partners. They must hide from coworkers, family, or friends important life events such as a new relationship or the breakup of an old one. Although they grieve such losses, their grief is not sanctioned by society and is another source of hidden stress. Transgender individuals also run the risk of rejection and physical assault if their biological gender is discovered or, if they continue to maintain a cross-gender role in some venues, if their transgender activities are discovered. Recently, members of the GLBT community have also had to deal with increased fears of being "outed" by other, more militant individuals. *Outing* involves publicizing another's sexual orientation without their consent.

GLBT individuals may internalize societal discrimination and prejudice leading to low self-esteem and depression. The phenomenon of internalization is supported by findings that enactment of legislation limiting marriage to a man and a woman in 14 states resulted in significant increases in the incidence of psychiatric problems in the GLBT population in those states, compared to no increase in states without such bans (Buffie, 2011). Internalization among young MSM may lead to risky sexual behaviors and increased potential for sexually transmitted infections (Halkitis et al., 2013).

Members of the GLBT population are subject to overt discrimination as well as to the stress of inadvertent or insensitive comments by others who do not recognize them as gay, lesbian, bisexual, or transgender individuals. Due to the stigma of membership in a sexual minority group and the potential for retaliation, they are also faced with the quandary of whether to actively work for equality or remain hidden from public view (Buffie, 2011). Data from the National Transgender Discrimination Survey, for example, indicated that transgender individuals were routinely subjected to discrimination in educational, employment, public service, and health care settings (Grant et al., 2011). Mental health problems are also associated with stigmatization among transgender individuals. In one study, for example, 44% of transgender individuals reported depression, 33% reported clinical anxiety, and 27.5% reported somatization (Bockting et al., 2013).

Members of sexual minorities are more likely than the general population to be exposed to violence and traumatic events at earlier ages and may be at greater risk for posttraumatic stress disorder (Roberts, Austin, Corliss, Vandermorris, & Koenen, 2010). Suicide is a significant problem in GLBT populations, particularly among youth. The lifetime risk of suicide for gays, lesbians, and bisexuals is nearly two-and-a-half times greater than that of the straight population (Choi et al., 2013), and risks are even higher for ethnic minority gay, lesbian, and bisexual youth (O'Donnell, Meyer, & Schwartz, 2011). Similarly, three fourths of Caucasian transgender individuals reported suicidal ideation, and 64% of those had attempted suicide (Nemoto, Böedeker, & Iwamato, 2011). Population health nurses should be alert to the presence of mental health problems in GLBT individuals as well as to a high incidence of problems in this population. As we will see later, they can make referrals for mental health services as needed as well as work to minimize factors that contribute to mental health problems among GLBT individuals.

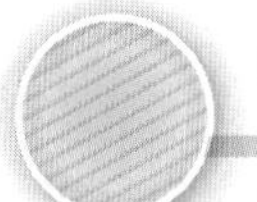

Global Perspectives

Protecting the Rights of Sexual Minorities

In December of 2008, Senegal hosted the International Conference on AIDS and Sexually Transmitted Infections in Africa. Later that same month nine members of a nongovernmental agency focused on HIV prevention and support for those with AIDS were convicted of homosexuality and given 5-year prison terms (Moody, 2009). Although the convictions were later overturned due to international outcry, they are representative of the circumstances faced by GLBT individuals throughout the world.

Several authors have noted the need for both research and policy formation related to global issues of sexual minority populations. The Global Research and Advocacy Group (2013) has included sexual minority issues as one element of its global research agenda. Similarly, Fabrice Houdart, the country officer for the Central Asia arm of the World Bank, has called for research into the economic and societal costs of homophobia and transphobia as a precursor for action to support development to assist poor sexual minority group members, and has suggested mobile telephone applications as a means of collecting data from, educating, and mobilizing sexual minorities throughout the world (Houdart, 2012a, 2012b).

With respect to global policy, a diverse group of human rights experts developed the Yogyakarta Principles, applying the principles of international human rights law to the support of members of sexual minority groups. These principles and their application to the GLBT population are summarized in the following table.

Application of International Human Rights Law to Sexual Orientation and Gender Identity

Principle	Application to Sexual Orientation and Gender Identity
1. The right to universal enjoyment of human rights	• Incorporate GLBT rights into national constitutions • Amend legislation that impinges on human rights for GLBT individuals • Educate people to promote enjoyment of human rights irrespective of sexual orientation or gender identity • Recognize all aspects of human identity including sexual orientation or gender identity in policy making
2. The right to equality and nondiscrimination	• Embody principles of nondiscrimination based on sexual orientation or gender identity in national constitutions • Repeal criminal or other legal provisions that prohibit consensual same-sex activity • Prohibit or eliminate discrimination based on sexual orientation or gender identity • Take measures to ensure equal advancement of persons of diverse sexual orientation or gender identity • Take action to eliminate prejudicial or discriminatory attitudes or behaviors based on sexual orientation or gender identity

(Continued)

Principle	Application to Sexual Orientation and Gender Identity
3. The right to recognition before the law	• Assure abilities of GLBT persons to enter contracts or own property • Take legal measures to respect and recognize each person's self-defined gender identity • Take legislative action to assure that legal documents reflect the person's self-defined gender identity • Ensure that such procedures respect the privacy of GLBT individuals • Ensure that changes to identity documents are recognized in all contexts where gender identification is required by law • Provide social support for persons undergoing gender transition or reassignment
4. The right to life	• Repeal all legislation that prohibits consensual sex, and in the interim refrain from imposing the death penalty for such actions • Remit existing death sentences for consensual same-sex activity • Cease state condoned attacks on the lives of persons based on sexual orientation or gender identity and assure that such attacks are vigorously investigated and prosecuted
5. The right to security of the person	• Prevent and provide protection from harassment and violence based on sexual orientation or gender identity • Enact legislative measures to impose appropriate criminal penalties for violence and harassment based on sexual orientation or gender identity, including within the family • Investigate and prosecute all allegations of violence against persons based on sexual orientation or gender identity and provide support for victims • Educate the public to combat the prejudices underlying such actions
6. The right to privacy	• Ensure the right to privacy of actions, including same-sex consensual activity without undue interference • Repeal any law that prohibits or criminalizes gender expression in dress, speech, or mannerisms or through bodily changes • Ensure the right to decide when, how, and to whom to disclose information related to sexual orientation or gender identity and protect individuals from unwanted disclosure
7. The right to freedom from arbitrary deprivation of liberty	• Assure that sexual orientation or gender identity is not used as a basis for arrest or detention • Educate police accordingly • Maintain accurate records of arrests motivated by sexual orientation or gender identity
8. The right to a fair trial	• Prohibit or eliminate prejudicial criminal or civil judicial treatment based on sexual orientation or gender identity • Protect persons from prosecution based on sexual orientation or gender identity • Train judges and other court personnel on international human rights
9. The right to treatment with humanity while in detention	• Avoid further marginalization or violence against detained persons based on sexual orientation or gender identity • Provide access to medical care and counseling for detained GLBT individuals • Put protective measures in place to prevent violence against prisoners based on sexual orientation or gender identity • Where permitted, ensure equal conjugal visits for same-sex couples in detention settings • Provide for independent monitoring of detention facilities with respect to treatment of GLBT individuals • Train detention facility staff regarding international human rights
10. The right to freedom from torture and cruel, inhuman, or degrading treatment or punishment	• Prevent or protect GLBT individuals from torture and cruel, inhuman, or degrading treatment or punishment based on sexual orientation or gender identity • Identify persons subjected to torture and cruel, inhuman, or degrading treatment or punishment based on sexual orientation or gender identity and offer support, redress, and reparation
11. The right to protection from all forms of exploitation, sale, and trafficking of human beings	• Prevent or protect individuals from sexual exploitation based on actual or perceived sexual orientation or gender identity • Establish measures to protect vulnerable individuals from trafficking or exploitation based on sexual orientation or gender identity

Principle	Application to Sexual Orientation and Gender Identity
12. The right to work	• Eliminate and prohibit employment discrimination based on sexual orientation or gender identity • Provide training to counter discriminatory attitudes based on sexual orientation or gender identity in employment settings
13. The right to social security and other social protection measures	• Ensure equal access to social security and other social benefits to all regardless of sexual orientation or gender identity
14. The right to an adequate standard of living	• Ensure equal access to food, safe drinking water, adequate sanitation, and clothing without regard for sexual orientation or gender identity
15. The right to adequate housing	• Ensure security of tenure and access to affordable, habitable, accessible, culturally appropriate, and safe housing, including shelter accommodation, regardless of sexual orientation or gender identity • Prohibit evictions not in conformity with international human rights that are based on sexual orientation or gender identity • Ensure equal rights to land and home ownership and inheritance regardless of sexual orientation or gender identity
16. The right to education	• Ensure equal access to education and equal treatment by teachers regardless of sexual orientation or gender identity • Ensure that education is directed to respect for human rights including those of GLBT individuals • Provide protection for staff, students, and teachers from violence and harassment based on sexual orientation or gender identity • Ensure that discipline is enacted without regard for sexual orientation or gender identity
17. The right to the highest attainable standard of health	• Provide access to health care goods and services without regard for sexual orientation or gender identity • Facilitate access to competent gender reassignment services • Ensure that health care providers treat all clients and their partners without discrimination based on sexual orientation or gender identity • Train health care personnel to provide quality care regardless of sexual orientation or gender identity
18. Protection from medical abuses	• Ensure that no child's body is irreversibly changed to impose a gender identity without free, full informed consent by the child • Protect persons from involuntary participation in research on the basis of sexual orientation or gender identity • Ensure that medical or psychological treatment does not expressly treat sexual orientation or gender identity as a condition to be treated, cured, or suppressed
19. The right to freedom of opinion and expression	• Promote full freedom of expression and opinion without regard for sexual orientation or gender identity • Ensure that notions of public morality, health, or security do not restrict expression of opinion regarding sexual orientation or gender identity • Ensure that exercise of the right to freedom of expression does not violate the rights of GLBT individuals • Ensure that all persons, regardless of sexual orientation or gender identity, have access to information and participation in public debate
20. The right to freedom of peaceful assembly and association	• Ensure rights to organize around and advocate for sexual orientation or gender identity issues • Ensure that notions of public morality, health, or security are not used to restrict freedom of assembly related to sexual orientation or gender identity issues
21. The right to freedom of thought, conscience, and religion	• Ensure that the expression, practice, and promotion of different opinions and beliefs regarding sexual orientation or gender identity is not undertaken in a manner incompatible with human rights
22. The right to freedom of movement	• Ensure that the right of freedom of movement and residence is guaranteed regardless of sexual orientation or gender identity

(*Continued*)

Principle	Application to Sexual Orientation and Gender Identity
23. The right to seek asylum	• Ensure that a well-founded fear of persecution based on sexual orientation or gender identity is accepted as grounds for granting asylum • Prohibit discrimination regarding asylum based on sexual orientation or gender identity • Prohibit extradition to a country or state where one could be subjected to torture, persecution, or cruel and inhuman treatment or punishment based on sexual orientation or gender identity
24. The right to found a family	• Ensure the right to found a family through adoption or assisted procreation regardless of sexual orientation or gender identity • Ensure that laws and policies recognize diverse family forms and protect families from discrimination based on sexual orientation or gender identity • Prohibit consideration of a parent's sexual orientation or gender identity as incompatible with a child's best interests in court proceedings • Permit children who are capable of exercising decisions to make decisions on their own behalf • Where same-sex marriage is recognized, ensure that same-sex couples have equal benefits to different-sex couples • Ensure that marriages and other legally recognized partnerships are entered only voluntarily
25. The right to participate in public life	• Ensure full enjoyment of the right to participate in public life and levels of government service regardless of sexual orientation or gender identity • Take measures to eliminate stereotypes and prejudices that prevent or restrict participation in public life based on sexual orientation or gender identity • Ensure the right of each person to participate in policy formation that affects his or her life regardless of sexual orientation or gender identity
26. The right to participate in cultural life	• Ensure opportunities to participate in cultural life regardless of sexual orientation or gender identity • Foster dialogue among cultural groups, including groups that hold different views of sexual orientation or gender identity
27. The right to promote human rights	• Take measures to combat activities or campaigns against human rights defenders working on issues of sexual orientation or gender identity • Ensure the protection of human rights defenders working on sexual orientation or gender identity issues from violence, threat, or discrimination • Support recognition and accreditation of human rights organizations that work on sexual orientation or gender identity issues at national and international levels
28. The right to effective remedies and redress	• Establish legal procedures that ensure victims of human rights violations based on sexual orientation or gender identity have full redress • Ensure that remedies are enforced and implemented in timely fashion • Establish effective institutions for redress of violations of human rights based on sexual orientation or gender identity and effectively train personnel • Ensure access to knowledge of procedures for redress of violations based on sexual orientation or gender identity • Ensure financial aid for persons unable to afford legal processes related to redress
29. Accountability	• Establish criminal, civil, and administrative procedures and monitoring mechanisms to ensure accountability of perpetrators of human rights violations based on sexual orientation or gender identity • Ensure that allegations of violations of rights based on sexual orientation or gender identity are thoroughly investigated and when substantiated, penalties enacted • Establish independent institutions and procedures to monitor formation and enforcement of laws to eliminate discrimination based on sexual orientation or gender identity • Remove obstacles preventing perpetrators of human rights violations based on sexual orientation or gender identity from being held accountable

Data from: The Yogyakarta Principles: Principles on the application of international human rights law in relation to sexual orientation and gender identity. (2007). Retrieved from http://www.yogyakartaprinciples.org/principles_en.pdf

ENVIRONMENTAL DETERMINANTS. Members of the GLBT population are exposed to many of the same environmental health hazards as the general population. In addition, environmental factors, such as population density, may affect the availability of support services. For example, rural areas may lack access to services and to health care providers who are comfortable dealing with GLBT individuals. Rural populations have also been shown to be less accepting of sexual diversity and may contribute to diminished family support of GLBT individuals. Urban settings, particularly those with large GLBT populations, may provide more supportive environments and better access to needed services (IOM, 2011).

SOCIOCULTURAL DETERMINANTS. Sociocultural factors have a profound impact on the health status and health-related behaviors of GLBT individuals. Sociocultural elements that may negatively affect the health and well-being of the GLBT population include homophobia and heterosexism, stigmatization, discrimination, and violence. Social relationships and socioeconomic status are additional areas for consideration in assessing sociocultural determinants of health in GLBT populations.

Homophobia and heterosexism. Discrimination and violence against gay men, lesbians, bisexuals, and transgender individuals has been attributed to **homophobia**, an irrational fear or hatred of people who exhibit a nonheterosexist sexual orientation or rejection of one's own homosexual feelings. Related terms include **biphobia**, which is defined as fear and intolerance of persons who are bisexual (UC Berkeley Gender Equity Resource Center, n.d.), and **transphobia**, defined as fear or hatred of people who do not conform to traditional gender norms (Trans Respect Versus Transphobia, n.d.). Some authors note, however, that the use of the term *homophobia* restricts responses to gay men and lesbians to an individual phenomenon, when it is evident that it is in reality a societally constructed entity that influences many aspects of the sociocultural environment. For that reason, many authors prefer the term **heterosexism**, which is defined as the assumption that all people are heterosexual and belief that heterosexuality is "normal" and superior to other sexual orientations (UC Berkeley Gender Equity Resource Center, n.d.). Heterosexism results in oppression, stigmatization, discrimination, and violence against members of GLBT populations.

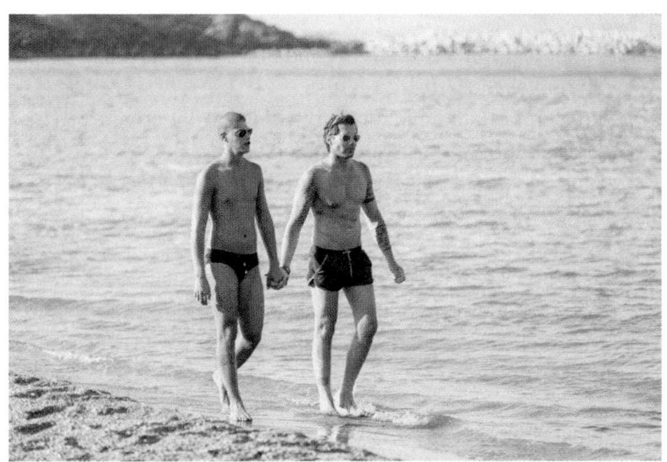

Same-sex couples may experience discrimination in a variety of settings, including health care settings. *(Francesco83/Fotolia)*

Heterosexism is a cultural phenomenon in which opposite sex attraction and behavior are the expected cultural norms. Heterosexism may be more deeply embedded in some cultures than others. MSM who are members of cultural minority groups with strong heterosexist beliefs may be faced with less tolerance than others. For example, some authors have noted that Latino gay and bisexual men in Southern California are simultaneously exposed to more relaxed attitudes to homosexual behavior in the majority culture and strict cultural attitudes. Similarly, many Asian cultures attach significant stigma to sexually diverse individuals as well as to their families.

Among young urban, African American men, a subculture exists among persons who have sex with other men and women, but do not consider themselves either gay or bisexual. This subcultural group is sometimes referred to as "down low." Members of the group tend to divorce sexual behavior from sexual identity and pride themselves on their masculinity (Heath & Goggin, 2009). For these reasons, health promotion and illness campaigns designed to reach gay and bisexual men may not be effective in this subpopulation.

Cultural conflicts similar to those experienced by Latinos and Asians may also be encountered by older gay men who developed their sexual identities in an age when it was more prudent to keep one's sexual orientation hidden. This group may be at particular disadvantage in dealing with the effects of societal heterosexism as well as ageism (Wight et al., 2012).

Stigmatization and discrimination. Societal attitudes toward what many consider deviant behavior may lead to prejudice, discrimination, harassment, and victimization. As noted by the Institute of Medicine (2011), members of the GLBT community have a common experience of stigmatization and have historically been marginalized by a heterosexual society.

In various studies, two thirds to three fourths of sexual minority group members report lifetime experience of discrimination (Choi et al., 2013; McCabe, Bostwick, Hughes, West, & Boyd, 2010), and more than 20% reported experiencing discrimination in the prior year (Choi et al., 2013). Similarly, approximately two thirds of transgender individuals report being subjected to gender-identity-based discrimination, which is compounded when people are members of more than one stigmatized group. In one study, 56% of transgender individuals had experienced verbal harassment, 37% reported employment discrimination, and 19% reported being subjected to physical violence (Bockting et al., 2013). Multiple sources and experiences of discrimination have an additive effect on psychological health in GLBT populations (McCabe et al., 2010).

Stigmatization and discrimination are linked to psychological distress and psychopathology for members of minority groups, including those of sexual minorities. Experience of discrimination has been associated with mood, anxiety, and substance abuse disorders. Discussion of experiences of discrimination, however, seems to have a protective effect (McLaughlin, Hatzenbuehler, & Keyes, 2010), and population health nurses can encourage GLBT individuals to reveal and discuss their experiences, providing both emotional support and assistance in redressing discriminatory practices.

Responses to stigmatization and discrimination are varied among the GLBT population. Some individuals may resist "coming out" or disclosure. **Coming out** involves openly living as a gay, lesbian, bisexual, or transgender individual, while **disclosure** involves revelation of one's sexual orientation or gender identity to selected individuals in one's life. Both responses bring the risk of discrimination and rejection by family and friends. Being "out" may relieve internal stress at the risk of the loss of important social connections.

Other GLBT individuals strive to create new relationships with people who will accept their sexual diversity. Some GLBT youth turn to the Internet to meet other sexual minority group members. Initial interaction online provides a sense of anonymity and safety from the associated stigma. A review of research from the 1990s through 2013 provided evidence of increasing use of the internet for making sexual connections. Some studies indicated increased sexual risk behaviors related to use of the Internet to meet other GLBT individuals and some did not find such associations. The Internet has also been used increasingly to conduct research with GLBT populations and to disseminate health-related information (Grov, Breslow, Newcomb, Rosenberger, & Bauermeister, 2014).

In addition to individual experiences of discrimination, GLBT individuals as a group are discriminated against by societal policies. One major area of societal discrimination lies in bans on same-sex marriage that exist in many states. Being married conveys a number of advantages not available to members of same-sex relationships. For example, employment-based partner health insurance benefits are often restricted to married individuals. Similarly, tax breaks afforded by joint tax returns are available to married couples, but not to those in relationships that do not have the legal status of marriage. Differences also occur for both partners and children in terms of survivor benefits under Social Security (Buffie, 2011). In fact, denial of Social Security spousal benefits costs same-sex couples an estimated $124 million annually (Fredriksen-Goldsen, 2012).

Due to the general lack of recognition of same-sex marriages, same-sex couples are not eligible for more than 1,000 benefits accorded by the federal government to married couples. For example, in addition to the tax and survivorship benefits noted above, the federal Medical Leave Act does not

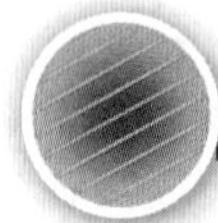

Evidence-Based Practice

Basing Evidence on Real People

To be of use in directing practice, evidence derived from research needs to reflect the population targeted for care. Unfortunately, with many stigmatized conditions such as membership in sexual minority groups, members of the target population may be difficult to reach using traditional approaches to subject recruitment. Some authors have suggested peer ethnography as a means of targeting special populations of interest for whom evidence-based interventions are lacking.

Ethnography is a research methodology in which the researcher becomes immersed in the population being studied and derives information from direct observation and face-to-face interactions with members of the target population. Gaining entrée to specific groups may be difficult for outsiders, particularly when the group has a history of discrimination. In peer ethnography, however, members of the target group are trained in ethnographic methods and can provide an insider's view of group member's beliefs and behaviors (Mutchler, McKay, Davitt, & Gordon, 2013). In what other stigmatized groups might peer ethnography be of use in developing a sound evidence base for practice?

Additional recommendations for research to build an evidence base for care of the GLBT population have been advanced by the Institute of Medicine (2011). These recommendations include the following:

- Development of a research agenda by NIH to advance understanding of GLBT health issues.
- Inclusion of data collection regarding sexual orientation and gender identity in federally funded surveys.
- Inclusion of data on sexual orientation and gender identity in electronic health records.
- Development of standardized measures of sexual orientation and gender identity.
- Support of methodological research related to GLBT health.
- Comprehensive research training related to GLBT health at NIH.
- Encouragement of NIH grant applicants to explicitly address inclusion or exclusion of sexual and gender minorities in study samples.

cover domestic partners or same-sex relationships, although some employers extend coverage to all employees. In 2011, only nine states and the District of Columbia included same-sex spouses and domestic partners under state medical leave legislation. Similarly, same-sex couples are not protected from loss of their home in order to spend down to be eligible for long-term care services under Medicaid. Heterosexual spouses, however, are protected from home loss in these circumstances (Fredriksen-Goldsen, 2012).

In the recent past, there has been considerable legislation designed to foster or impede bans on same-sex marriage. California's proposition 8 and other similar legislation legally defined marriage as occurring between a man and a woman. The 9th U.S. Circuit Court of Appeals ruled proposition 8 unconstitutional, and in July 2013, the U.S. Supreme Court failed to rule on the issue, thus upholding the unconstitutionality of the act and its provisions and supporting federal benefits for same-sex married couples in the states that permit same-sex marriage. It remains unclear, however, if federal marriage benefits will be based on the ruling only in states that legalize same-sex marriage, or will apply throughout the country. The ruling also fails to settle the question of whether or not any state has the right to ban marriage between same-sex couples. As of mid-2013, 12 states plus California permit same-sex marriage, and public opinion has slowly been turning in favor of same-sex marriage (Mintz, 2013).

In June of 2013, the U.S. Supreme court ruled that provisions of the Defense of Marriage Act that deny same-sex couples the same federal legal protections as any other married couple are unconstitutional. At its inception, the ruling applied to states and territories that recognize same-sex marriages. For those living in states that do not recognize their marriages, additional work is needed to promote equity (Freedom to Marry, 2013). Population health nurses can advocate for changes in state laws that promote equity for all married couples.

Some authors have maintained that same-sex marriage is another facet of the ongoing evolution of the societal concept of marriage. They cite as evidence former laws and social mores that defined marriage as occurring between a man and woman of the same race, social status, or religion (Buffie, 2011). Legalization of same-sex marriage has been associated with improved health among gay and lesbian individuals. For example, in one study, legalization was associated with a decrease in medical and mental health care visits and lower health care costs among gay men, both those who had committed relationships and those who did not, again suggesting population as well as individual benefits of minimizing stigma and discriminatory practices (Hatzenbuehler et al., 2012).

A number of groups and organizations have been established to advocate for policies and legislation that prohibit discrimination against members of the various GLBT populations. For example, the Transgender Law Center in San Francisco works on behalf of transgender individuals to create a society that recognizes freedom of gender expression as a basic right of the individual (Transgender Law Center, 2013). Similarly, the New England-based Gay & Lesbian Advocates & Defenders organization (GLAD) works through litigation, public policy advocacy, and education to eliminate discrimination related to gender identity and expression, sexual orientation, or HIV status (GLAD, 2013).

Social relationships. Interactions within families beyond the legality of marriage are another element of the sociocultural dimension that affects the health of the GLBT population. Disclosure of a nonheterosexual orientation or transgenderism to family members and their response, homosexual relationships, and homosexual parenting are the three primary aspects of family interaction to be assessed by the population health nurse.

Two different themes occur in families' responses to disclosure of a family member's homosexuality: loving acceptance or rejection. All families who come to know of GLBT members need to deal with feelings of grief, guilt, and fear for their child or sibling. GLBT youth who experience family rejection are more likely to experience a variety of psychological and behavioral problems. Family acceptance, on the other hand, has been strongly correlated with higher levels of self-esteem, social support, and overall health in GLBT adolescents and young adults. Acceptance also seems to be a protective factor for depression, substance abuse, suicidal ideation, and lifetime

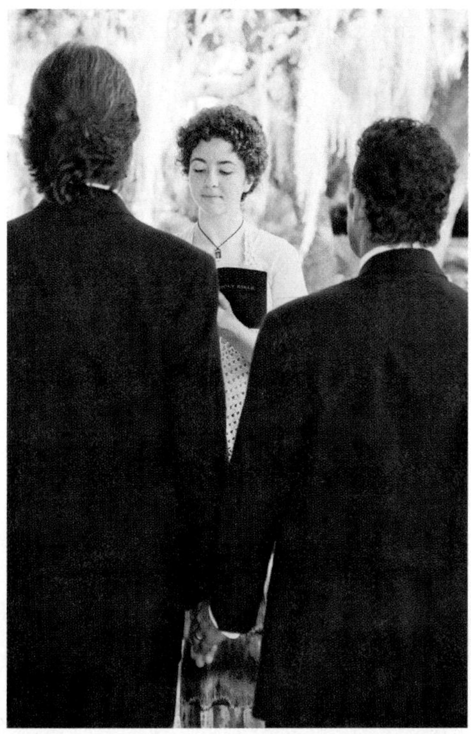

Marriage between same-sex couples should entail the same rights and responsibilities as those accorded to heterosexual couples.
(Lisa F. Young/Fotolia)

suicide attempts (Ryan, Russell, Huebner, Diaz, & Sanchez, 2010).

For those families that are able to accept homosexuality, bisexuality, or transgenderism in one of their members, acceptance appears to come about in stages similar to the stages of grief experienced with the loss of a loved one. The first stage is one of grief, followed by a period of denial during which parents may see their child's professed sexual identity as a "phase" that he or she will grow out of. This stage is followed successively by stages characterized by guilt and anger and, finally, loving acceptance. For some families, acceptance is followed by advocacy (Broad, 2014). Unfortunately, some families never achieve the stage of acceptance of their loved one's sexual orientation or gender identity.

Parental response to the disclosure of homosexuality is strongly influenced by a variety of factors: the strength of traditional gender role conceptions, perceptions of the probable attitudes of significant others in the family's social network, and parental age and education level. Affiliation with conservative religious ideologies and intolerance of other stigmatized groups are other factors that affect parental resolution of grief over the lost image of their child (Broad, 2014).

GLBT individuals may face decisions about disclosure to spouses and friends as well as parents and siblings. Many GLBT individuals are or have been involved in committed heterosexual relationships, and many of them have children. Some individuals do not become aware of or accept their sexual diversity until after marriage. Others marry in an attempt to deny or hide their sexual orientation or gender identity. Responses of spouses to the disclosure of homosexuality, bisexuality, or transgenderism vary considerably and may include feelings of living with a "stranger," guilt, development of an asexual friendship or a semi-open relationship in which partners are free to take outside lovers, or a desire for divorce. Transgender identity changes can be particularly devastating to marital relationships, as the spouse questions not only the partner's sexual identity but his or her own as well. Population health nurses should assess the extent of clients' disclosure of their sexual identities and the effects of the responses received. Nurses should also assess the needs of family members for assistance in dealing with the disclosure. The Family Acceptance Project has created a screening tool to identify GLBT youth who are experiencing serious family rejection. Information and training on the screening tool are available at the website, and a source for further information is included in the *External Resources* section of the student resources site. Table 20-2• provides examples of accepting and rejecting behaviors that population health nurses can share with families of GLBT individuals.

Disclosure to family members is usually not a one time event. As families grow and change, both the GLBT family member and others face decisions regarding disclosure to other family members and friends. In other words, families engage in their own "coming out" regarding the sexual diversity of family members, although this process is framed somewhat differently than the coming out experienced by members of the GLBT population (Broad, 2014). Disclosure of one's sexual orientation or gender identity to children is another dilemma faced by gay, bisexual, and transgender men. Depending on when and how disclosure occurs, children may exhibit the same range of responses shown by other family members. Some considerations in disclosure of sexual orientation or gender identity to children are provided on the student resources site.

TABLE 20-2 Accepting and Rejecting Behaviors by Families of GLBT Individuals

Accepting Behaviors	Rejecting Behaviors
Discussing with a GLBT family member their identity and feelings	Engaging in physical punishment of expressions of GLBT identity
Expressing affection for the GLBT family member	Engaging in verbal abuse or name-calling related to a family member's GLBT identity
Supporting the GLBT family member's identity	Excluding GLBT member from family activities
Advocating for fair treatment of the GLBT family member	Prohibiting access to GLBT friends, information, or support resources
Requiring respect of the GLBT family member by other family members	Blaming GLBT family members when they are subjected to discrimination related to their identity
Connecting the GLBT family member with relevant resources and organizations	Attempting to change a GLBT family member's appearance or behavior
Assisting the GLBT family member to identify appropriate GLBT role models	Informing a GLBT family member of their "sinfulness" and likelihood of divine punishment
Welcoming the GLBT family member's friends and partners	Indicating that you are ashamed of the GLBT family member or the unwanted attention they draw to the family
Supporting the GLBT family member's gender expression	Refusing to allow a GLBT family member to disclose or discuss their identity with others
Expressing the belief that a GLBT family member can have a happy and productive life	

Based on: Ryan, C. (2009). *Supportive families, healthy children: Helping families with lesbian, gay, bisexual & transgender children.* Retrieved from http://familyproject.sfsu.edu/files/English_Final_Print_Version_Last.pdf

Parenting by GLBT families brings its own stresses, many of them similar to those experienced by straight parents. GLBT individuals may become parents in a number of ways: in heterosexual relationships prior to coming out, as foster parents or through adoption, or in cooperation with a sperm donor or surrogate mother. Data cited in the IOM (2011) report on the health of the GLBT population indicated that 35% of lesbians, 8% of gay men, 67% of bisexual women, and 36% of bisexual men had at least one child. In addition, key findings of a study by the Urban Institute and Williams Institute indicated that half of gay men and 41% of lesbian women want to have children, and approximately 2 million GLBT individuals are interested in adopting children. In 2010, 65,000 children had been adopted by a gay or lesbian parent, and gay/lesbian parents were caring for an estimated 14,000 foster children (Sudol, 2010).

Adoption or foster parenting by GLBT individuals may pose more difficulties than for straight couples. Although 60% of adoption agencies surveyed in a national study accepted applications from prospective GLBT parents, only 40% had actually placed children in GLBT households, and only 19% of agencies actively sought out GLBT individuals as adoptive parents. Federal law does not address adoption by GLBT individuals, and some states, particularly those that do not recognize same-sex marriage, prohibit adoption by members of the GLBT population. In 2010, only six states had laws prohibiting adoption discrimination against GLBT individuals, three had laws restricting GLBT adoption, and three others had laws or policies that restricted adoption. Even fewer states (only four) have laws or legislation that prohibit exclusion of GLBT individuals from serving as foster parents, and one state (Nebraska) actively prohibited foster parenting by gay individuals. A study by the Children's Bureau and AdoptUSKids recommended inclusive practices by all adoption and foster child agencies that emphasize sexual orientation and gender identity in their nondiscrimination policies, include information about GLBT families in recruiting materials, and use inclusive language on paperwork (Sudol, 2010). GLBT families have been described as an untapped resource for foster and adoptive families and assessment guidance for agencies considering placement of a child in a GLBT family have been developed (Mallon, 2011). Population health nurses can assess state and local policies and legislation related to adoption and fostering by GLBT families and advocate for equitable treatment of these populations. For further information about GLBT foster parenting, adoption, and family life, see the *External Resources* section of the student resources site.

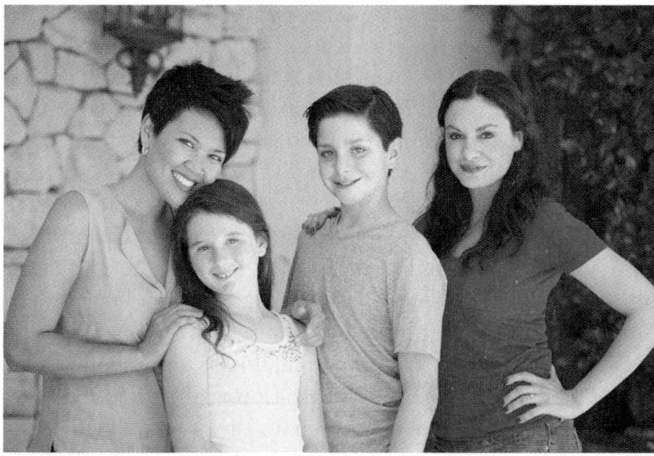

More same-sex couples are choosing to have and raise children.
(Zoomyimages/Fotolia)

Other GLBT individuals may choose to have children through surrogate parent arrangements in which a woman is impregnated either through intercourse or artificial insemination by sperm from a donor male. Conversely, a gay or bisexual man, or an FTM transgender individual who has not had an orchiectomy may impregnate a surrogate mother or a female partner. Both arrangements have the potential for legal risks and challenges, particularly if the donor or surrogate is known. For example, sperm donors may later sue for access to interaction with the child or be held liable for child support. Similarly, surrogate mothers may sue for custody. Such eventualities can be minimized by being knowledgeable regarding state laws related to donor status and surrogacy, working with a physician or women's health practitioner, and having an attorney execute a detailed contract regarding the rights and responsibilities of all parties (Forman, n.d.).

The parental rights of same-sex partners may also be called into question if a same-sex partnership dissolves or with the death of the biological or adoptive parent of any children. This can be forestalled by a second-parent adoption. **Second-parent adoption** is a legal procedure in which a same-sex parent formally adopts his or her partner's biological or adoptive child as a second, legally recognized parent. As of 2014, 23 states and the District of Columbia provided for second-parent adoption by same-sex couples; in 8 states various obstacles exist with respect to adoption by same-sex couples or unmarried individuals. In the remaining states, decisions are made on a case-by-case basis, but in Florida legislation prohibiting adoption by "homosexuals" was declared unconstitutional in 2010 (Human Rights Campaign, 2014).

The mistaken societal view that sexual orientation or transgenderism can be transmitted to children has motivated a great deal of research on the effects of GLBT parenting on children. Research has indicated, however, that being raised by a GLBT parent does not have adverse effects for children. They have not been shown to face greater stigma and are not more likely to be abused or to exhibit sexual diversity than other children. In addition, they seem to develop more secure parental attachments and grow up as successfully as children in heterosexual families (Sudol, 2010).

GLBT couples' relationships are subjected to the same kinds of stress as straight relationships, but this stress may be exacerbated by the absence of social support for the marital role. Therapists who work with gay and lesbian couples have identified several additional issues that threaten the stability of their relationships. These issues include differences in the stages of coming out between partners, differences with respect to extended family involvement, inequalities of power, and financial conflict and disparity in income. With the exception of the stage of coming out, these same issues may also affect the stability of relationships among straight couples.

Another aspect of family relationships that affects GLBT individuals more so than straight members of the population is that of informal caregiving. Societal and health system policies often create restrictions on who can provide family caregiving that do not recognize the rights of same-sex partners, particularly in states that do not recognize same-sex marriages or formal unions. For example, partners may be restricted from visiting, being involved in care decisions, and making funeral arrangements. In addition, as noted earlier, partners may face challenges to or denial of fiscal rights related to Social Security, property ownership, and custody of minor children. In one study, 13% of people caring for sick or disabled spouses or partners were in same-sex relationships, yet these individuals are frequently not eligible for caregiving assistance and lack legal protections to support caregiving (Fredriksen-Goldsen, 2012).

When the support of a GLBT individual's family of origin is lacking, many people turn to associations with other GLBT individuals for support. Affinity with the GLBT community has been linked to better health and, in the past, to safer sexual practices among MSM. This may be changing, however, as younger MSM engage in more socially acceptable practices such as unprotected sexual intercourse (Halkitis et al., 2013). In some studies, for example, condom use is less likely in interactions with one's main partner than with casual sexual partners (Wilson et al., 2010), and in one study in New York City, 19% of MSM reported unprotected anal intercourse (Halkitis et al., 2013).

Socioeconomic status. Some members of the GLBT community tend to be of higher socioeconomic status than the general population, and some are of lower status. Sexual minority youth tend to leave home earlier and are more likely to be homeless than other young people. For example, in one study of Massachusetts high school students, 25% of lesbian and gay teens and 15% of bisexual teens were homeless compared to only 3% of heterosexual students. Homelessness may be a result of victimization and abuse at home and places GLBT youth at high risk for violence, substance abuse, and mental health problems (Corliss, Goodenow, Nichols, & Austin, 2011). Similarly, transgender individuals have been found to be more likely to be unemployed and poor than nontransgender people (Conron et al., 2012). Some transgender individuals lack education and career training or may be discriminated against with respect to employment. For many of them, sex work becomes an economic alternative that is linked to high risk situations and behaviors, such as substance abuse, unsafe sexual practices, and the potential for physical and sexual abuse. In addition, the stigma and social isolation associated with sex work may increase their vulnerability to mental illness and sexually transmitted infections (Nemoto et al., 2011). Older GLBT individuals are at particular risk for poverty and its effects on health (LGBT Movement Advancement Project [MAP] & Services and Advocacy for Gay, Lesbian, Bisexual and Transgender Elders [SAGE], 2010).

Conversely, California Health Interview survey data indicated that lesbian women tend to be better educated and have higher incomes than women in general. The same is true for gay men, but bisexual men tended to have lower incomes than straight men (Boehmer, Miao, Linkletter, & Clark, 2012). Socioeconomic status has implications for health. For example, although self-reported health status does not differ between people with same-sex partners and those with different-sex partners in general, people with same-sex partners with lower incomes, particularly young women, in one study rated their health as worse than those with different-sex partners (Thomeer, 2013). Similarly, financial concerns and independence issues have been associated with depression in older gay men (Wight et al., 2012).

Violence and hate crimes. One additional sociocultural factor that has implications for health in the GLBT population is that of violence and hate crimes. **Hate crimes**, also known as bias crimes, involve criminal violence based on sexual minority or other stigmatized status (e.g., race, religion). In 2009, 1,482 victims were subjected to hate crimes related to gender orientation in the United States, a number that probably far underrepresents actual occurrence since not all jurisdictions report hate crimes. Hate crimes against gay men are more common than among lesbian women or bisexuals (U.S. Census Bureau, 2012). A meta-analysis of studies of sexual minority adolescents published in 2011 indicated they were 3.8 times more likely to experience sexual abuse, 1.2 times more likely to be subjected to parental physical abuse, 1.7 times more likely to be assaulted at school, and 2.4 times more likely to miss school due to fear than straight youth (Friedman et al., 2011).

A systematic review and meta-analysis indicated that men who have sex with men who experience sexual abuse as children were at higher risk for HIV infection and engaged in several high-risk sexual behaviors. Such behaviors included having multiple partners and frequent casual partners, engaging in unprotected sexual activity, and having sex while under the influence of alcohol or other drugs (Lloyd & Operario, 2012). Risk for violence is also high among transgender individuals. A report on hate-related violence by the National Coalition of Anti-Violence Programs indicated that half of hate-motivated homicides were perpetrated against transgender women. Similarly, transgender individuals were more likely than others to be subjected to discrimination, threats, intimidation, and police violence. Violence victimization was even more likely for GLBT individuals of color than for the overall GLBT population (National Coalition of Anti-Violence Programs, 2013).

GLBT families may also experience intimate partner violence (IPV) just as heterosexual couples do. Bureau of

Justice Statistics data (Catalano, Smith, Snyder, & Rand, 2009) indicated that approximately 7% of IPV against men is perpetrated by other men, and 1% of women are subjected to IPV by other women. A review of literature indicated that IPV among men who have sex with men is at least as high or higher than in the heterosexual population (Finneran & Stephenson, 2012).

Most IPV-related social services are designed to assist abused women, so men may not be able to find assistance when needed. Victimization may not even be acknowledged as IPV in jurisdictions that do not recognize same-sex marriage, making it difficult for abused men to obtain protective orders. In addition, GLBT individuals may be reluctant to report IPV for fear that it will be used as ammunition against same-sex relationships and support for prejudicial attitudes.

BEHAVIORAL DETERMINANTS. Behavioral factors are also important influences on the health of the GLBT population. Specific areas to be assessed include sexual practices, substance use and abuse, and health-promoting and illness preventive behaviors.

Sexual practices. Unsafe sexual practices exhibited by some GLBT individuals include unprotected anal intercourse (UAI) or failure to use condoms and sexual activity for pay. Some MSM and transgender individuals may engage in sex work and may also engage in substance use during sex to "clock coin," exchanging sexual favors for money or substances (Mutchler et al., 2013). A far more common practice, however, is unprotected anal intercourse, which increases the risk of spread of STIs.

Some GLBT individuals may engage in **serosorting**, limiting sexual partners to persons of the same HIV status or use of condoms with HIV discordant partners (Eaton, Cherry, Cain, & Pope, 2011; Wilson et al., 2010). Many gay and bisexual men are less likely to use condoms with their primary partners than with casual or commercial partners. Failure to use condoms with main partners may reflect a sense of intimacy and safety or partners' negative attitudes toward condom use (Wilson et al., 2010). In addition, some MSM may use female insertive condoms for anal intercourse. Insertive condoms, however, have only been approved by the Food and Drug Administration for vaginal intercourse, and their effectiveness in preventing STI with anal intercourse is unknown (Kelvin et al., 2011).

Although serosorting may have a protective effect, its effectiveness is undermined if the partner's serostatus is unknown, if either party has relationships outside of the main partnership, or with frequent changes in main partners or multiple serial partnerships over time (Halkitis et al., 2013). In one large survey of MSM, 54% reported UAI with a male partner, 37% with their main partner, and 25% with casual partners. UAI has been associated with use of Viagra and other sex-related drugs, a greater number of partners, use of crystal methamphetamine and amyl nitrites, and a belief that HIV infection is less of a threat now due to effective treatment (Schwarcz et al., 2007). Chronic alcohol use and use of marijuana, cocaine, and club drugs have also been linked to UAI (Mutchler et al., 2013). Unsafe sexual practices among MSM have been predicted to result in the possibility that as many as 40% of MSM may be HIV-infected by 40 years of age (Parsons et al., 2012). Use of sex toys and group sex as well as UAI have also been implicated in increased risk of hepatitis C among MSM (Fierer et al., 2011).

Bisexual women may also be at risk for STIs. In one study, bisexual women had a greater number of male partners, were less likely to use condoms, and engaged in more drug and alcohol use than women with only male partners. WSW and bisexual women may also have more new partners, more than one partner, or symptomatic sexual partners than straight women (Singh et al., 2011).

Unsafe sexual practices such as UAI may, in some individuals, be part of a "syndemic" that increases HIV risk in sexual minority populations. A **syndemic** is a situation in which multiple epidemics interact to enhance the adverse effects of each. Elements of a suggested syndemic related to sexual risk taking include compulsive sexual behavior, depression, childhood sexual abuse, intimate partner violence, and polydrug use, all of which (except childhood sexual abuse) have been linked to HIV seropositivity (Parsons et al., 2012). Population health nurses will assess GLBT individuals for unsafe sex practices. They will also assess the extent of such practices or evidence of a syndemic in the population.

Substance use and abuse. Generally speaking, members of the GLBT population are more likely to smoke, drink, and use drugs than the general population. For example, in the California Health Interview Survey, lesbians and bisexual women were found to be twice as likely as straight women to be current smokers and 2.5 times more likely to engage in binge drinking. Gay and bisexual men were more likely to be current smokers, but less likely to engage in binge drinking than straight men. Differences in findings for many behaviors included in the survey varied by age group, suggesting that interventions should be age-specific (Boehmer et al., 2012).

Similarly, Massachusetts Behavioral Risk Factor Surveillance System data from 2001 to 2008 suggested that sexual minority group members were more likely to report smoking and drinking than the rest of the population. Bisexual women were also more likely to engage in binge drinking. On a positive note, gay, lesbian, and bisexual individuals were also more likely to participate in HIV testing. Transgender individuals in Massachusetts also reported greater prevalence of smoking (Conron et al., 2012). Smoking is approximately twice as prevalent among GLBT individuals as in the overall population, partly due to specific targeting of the GLBT community by tobacco marketing strategies (Levinson, Hood, & Mahajan, 2012).

Illicit drug use may also be more prevalent in some GLBT populations than in the general public. For example, sexual minority youth have been found to be more likely than other youth to use a number of illicit drugs (Newcomb, Birkett, Corliss, & Mistanski, 2014). An area of growing concern among gay men is the use of methamphetamines. Heavy methamphetamine use began in this population in the 1970s and has escalated to become the most common illicit drug used by gay and bisexual men (Rozsa, 2013).

Many factors contribute to extensive substance use, both licit and illicit. The stress of being part of a stigmatized and marginalized population may be a significant contributing factor. With respect to methamphetamine, some people use it to heighten sexual pleasure or as part of social interactions. Methamphetamine use among HIV-infected individuals is of particular concern because it contributes to increased viral load and decreased immune response, and decreases medication adherence (Parsons, Kowalczyk, Botsko, Tomassilli, & Golub, 2013). Population health nurses should assess the extent of tobacco, alcohol, and drug use in GLBT populations and the prevalence of related health problems.

Other health-related behaviors. Members of the GLBT population may also engage in other behaviors that support health or contribute to health problems. For example, some MTF transgender individuals may resort to injecting silicon oil, often in the buttocks or hips, to create a more feminine body image. Such injections were banned by the Food and Drug Administration (FDA), but are still provided by "black market" providers, who may or may not adhere to appropriate infection control measures. The silicon itself may contribute to pulmonary emboli or pneumonia, and facial injections may result in cellulitis and loss of vision. In addition, silicon is gravity dependent and may migrate within the body, causing deformity and disability (Sanchez-Ponte et al., 2012).

Transgender individuals may also self-inject nonprescription hormones, often at higher than usual treatment doses. For example, large proportions of transgender individuals in Washington, DC, San Francisco, Chicago, Virginia, and Ontario, Canada reported use of hormones from nonmedical sources. In addition, a few respondents in the Canadian study reported attempting surgical orchiectomies or mastectomies on themselves (Rotondi et al., 2013). The health effects of high-dose hormone injections are not yet known, but needle sharing for both hormone injection and intravenous drug use pose health risks for the transgender population.

GLBT individuals may also engage in health promoting and illness preventive behaviors. For example, according to the 2008 National HIV Behavioral Surveillance System (NHBS), 90% of MSM had been tested for HIV in their lifetimes and 62% were tested in the prior year. Similarly, 35% had been tested for syphilis, and 51% received hepatitis vaccine (Finlayson et al., 2011). In addition, based on California Health Interview Survey data, bisexual men have been found to be more likely than their gay or straight counterparts to eat five or more fruits and vegetables per day; however, lesbian and bisexual women are less likely to do so. Lesbians, gays, and bisexual individuals were more likely than straight individuals to engage in vigorous physical activity and muscle strengthening, and gay men were more likely than straight or bisexual men to obtain colon cancer screening (Boehmer et al., 2012).

HEALTH SYSTEM DETERMINANTS. Factors related to the health care system also influence the health of the GLBT population. Two main assessment considerations in this area are barriers to health care and the availability of culturally sensitive health care services.

Barriers to health care. Members of the GLBT population may encounter homophobia and heterosexism among health care workers and care delivery systems. In addition, the perception of homophobia represents a significant barrier to health care that may lead people to forego health care unless absolutely necessary.

According to the Institute of Medicine (2011), barriers to health care may be personal or structural. Personal barriers include enacted stigma on the part of providers, felt stigma, and internalized stigma. Enacted stigma involves explicit behaviors on the part of health care providers that express stigma, such as denial of care, provision of inadequate care, or verbal abuse. Felt stigma is a perception that stigma is likely to be experienced in a given situation (IOM, 2011) that may lead to delay in seeking care, failure to disclose sexual orientation or gender identity, or concerns for confidentiality and disclosure of one's status through employment-based health insurance. Internalized stigma may be expressed by straight individuals in the health care system as prejudice against sexual minority group members, or by members of the GLBT population who have internalized homophobic attitudes as described earlier (IOM, 2011).

Structural barriers to health care are the result of institutional stigma, which is the manifestation of stigma within social institutions. Failure to provide health insurance coverage for same-sex spouses and lack of legal recognition of partners and inclusion in health decision making are examples of institutional stigma. Another example of institutional stigma is insurance companies that discontinue coverage of transgender individuals when their gender identity is disclosed. Such practice will be prohibited under the Affordable Care Act. Lack of health care provider knowledge and expertise in addressing the needs of sexual minority group members is another structural barrier to effective health care (IOM, 2011).

In one study, roughly 4% of gay, lesbian, and bisexual respondents reported discrimination in obtaining health care and in their treatment by health care providers (McLaughlin et al., 2010). In the California Health Interview Survey, bisexual men and women were less likely than straight individuals to have health insurance, yet gay and bisexual men utilized health care services more often than straight men. Gay, lesbian, and bisexual individuals were also more likely to make emergency department visits than their straight counterparts (Boehmer et al., 2012). Transgender individuals have also reported lack of access to health care as well as transphobia among providers (Nemoto et al., 2011).

Even when individual health care providers are devoid of homophobia, various circumstances may threaten GLBT clients and act as health barriers. For example, assessment questions about birth control practices, if answered truthfully, might have the effect of requiring that a client disclose his sexual identity. For the client who fears loss of health care benefits (due to assumed higher risk of HIV/AIDS), this is a situation to be avoided. Confidentiality issues may also prevent GLBT individuals at risk for HIV infection from being tested, and when HIV infection is diagnosed, provisions of the Ryan White Care Act HIV/AIDS program vary from state to state, so access to necessary care may be restricted.

Health care providers are often poorly educated with respect to the needs of and care for members of GLBT populations. Although major health professional organizations, such as the American Medical Association (AMA, n.d.), American Psychiatric Association (2014), and American Psychological Association (2009), have developed policy statements affirming the normality of same-sex sexual orientations and the right of GLBT individuals to quality health care, incorporation of GLBT issues in health professional education is often confined to discussion of HIV infection and other STIs. The World Professional Association for Transgender Health (2011), however, has established standards that can assist professionals in the care of transgender individuals. For further information about the standards, see the *External Resources* section of the student resources site.

Culturally sensitive health care. The Institute of Medicine (2011) has recommended education of health care professionals to effectively provide culturally sensitive health care to GLBT individuals and groups. Health care systems should also be revamped to remove sources of institutional stigma. For instance, substituting gender-neutral pronouns for gender-specific terms on all forms has been suggested. Examples of gender-neutral pronouns are provided in Table 20-3•. Gender-neutral pronouns, however, have not been widely endorsed or adopted in the transgender community.

The Transgender Law Center (2011) has developed a set of principles for designing health care services to meet the needs of the transgender community that can be adapted to creating culturally sensitive services for the GLBT population in general. These principles are as follows:

- Involve a diverse group of leaders from the GLBT community in designing effective services to assure that they meet the needs of the target population.
- Build leadership from all elements of the community, particularly hidden segments that are often underrepresented and underserved.
- Focus on the motivations of the community.
- Recruit people for specific activities and functions.
- Clarify roles and responsibilities that respect the expertise of community members and minimize the role of officials or providers.
- Enlist the support of policy makers.
- Assess the health care issues of the GLBT community and fully understand the underlying factors.
- Analyze the policy environment and its effects on health care for GLBT individuals.
- Develop specific goals for care and policy formulation.
- Develop systems that provide routine primary care and also address GLBT-specific health care issues.
- Create culturally tailored literature for the GLBT population.

Common issues to be addressed in developing culturally sensitive health care delivery programs for the GLBT population include training providers for cultural competency, using inclusive terminology in intake forms, promoting a medical home, and funding access to care. An additional, often neglected issue is the provision of gender-neutral bathrooms (Transgender Law Center, 2011).

Population health nurses should assess factors related to each of the six areas of determinants of health as a precursor to planning and implementing health care services for this population. The comprehensive target group assessment tool included on the student resources site can be used as the basis for such an assessment.

TABLE 20-3 Substituting Gender-neutral for Gender-specific Pronouns

Gender-specific Pronoun	Gender-neutral Pronoun
She/he	Ze (pronounced "zee")
Her/him	Hir (pronounced "here")
Her/his	Hir (pronounced "here")
Hers/his	Hirs (pronounced "heres")
Herself-himself	Hirself (pronounced "herself")

Based on: UC Berkeley Gender Equity Resource Center. (n.d.). *Definitions of terms.* Retrieved from http://geneq.berkeley.edu/lgbt_resources_definiton_of_terms

Planning and Implementing Health Care for the GLBT Population

Health care services to address the needs of the GLBT population will occur at each of the four levels of health care. Selected population health nursing interventions related to health promotion, illness and injury prevention, resolution of existing health problems, and health restoration will be addressed here.

HEALTH PROMOTION. Members of the GLBT population are in need of the same health promotion interventions as the general public. For example, adequate nutrition and physical activity can be promoted in this population. Because of the potential exposure to minority stress, members of the GLBT population may need assistance in developing effective coping strategies. Population health nurses can teach coping strategies to individual members of the GLBT population. They can also advocate for equitable treatment to reduce the potential for minority stress. For example, improved mental health can be promoted through advocacy for recognition of same-sex marriage for gay and lesbian couples and promoting access to hormone therapies and sexual reassignment surgery for transgender individuals.

ILLNESS AND INJURY PREVENTION. Effective illness and injury prevention strategies for the GLBT population include measures to prevent HIV infection and other STIs as well as immunization for illnesses such as hepatitis A and B for those at risk of infection. Population health nurses can promote safe sexual practices, including strengthening partner relationships and norms for monogamy, elimination of unprotected anal intercourse, use of condoms, and promotion of serosorting strategies. In addition, nurses can assist members of the GLBT population to develop skills related to discussion of HIV status and negotiation for safer sexual practices. Other illness and injury prevention strategies would be similar to those for the general population and include promoting safety and eliminating risk behaviors (e.g., use of safety devices, smoking cessation, and so on).

Programs to prevent UAI among men who have sex with men have yielded mixed results. For example, a social marketing strategy targeted toward men who self-identified as straight, but engaged in sex with men was successful in motivating condom use (Martinez-Donate et al., 2010). In other populations, however, campaigns to promote condom use have not been very effective (Halkitis et al. 2013). Population health nurses can be actively involved in educating MSM for safer sexual practices and in advocating these practices in venues that reach MSM. For example, a population health nurse might advocate for a condom dispenser in a prominent location in a gay bar or convince gay publications to include articles advocating safer sexual practices. Nurses might even volunteer to write health-related articles for these publications. Table 20-4• summarizes relevant health promotion and illness and injury prevention strategies for GLBT populations.

TABLE 20-4 Health Promotion and Illness/Injury Prevention Strategies for GLBT Populations

Focus	Strategy
Health promotion	Promote adequate nutrition Promote physical activity Promote effective coping Advocate for environments that promote health Advocate for equitable treatment
Illness/Injury prevention	Promote safe sexual practices Strengthen relationships and promote monogamy Encourage routine and risk-specific immunizations Promote general safety practices Assist with development of abilities to discuss HIV status and negotiate safer sexual practices Promote serosorting strategies and condom use Discourage unprotected intercourse Encourage risk factor elimination

RESOLVING EXISTING HEALTH PROBLEMS. As with the general population, resolution of existing health problems in the GLBT population focuses on screening and treatment. Lesbian and bisexual women require the same screening interventions as straight women (e.g., mammography, cervical cancer screening). Similarly, gay and bisexual men should receive the screenings recommended for all men. Transgender individuals, however, may require screening services related to both genders. For example, MTF transgender individuals need regular mammograms due to the use of female hormones and risk of breast cancer, but they will usually still need regular prostate examinations as well. Similarly, most FTM transgender individuals continue to need regular cervical cancer screening. Because lesbian women typically do not use contraceptive services (a common route to health care services for straight women), they may miss opportunities for routine breast and cervical cancer screening.

Members of the GLBT population at risk for sexually transmitted infections such as HIV infection, syphilis, gonorrhea, *Chlamydia trachomatis*, or hepatitis should also be screened for these conditions. In addition, because of the greater prevalence of smoking, problem drinking, and drug use in the GLBT population, sexual minority group members may need to be screened and referred for problems in these areas. Depression screening may also be warranted. Population health nurses may provide or make referrals for relevant screening services. They may also need to advocate for provision of needed services and their coverage under health insurance plans.

Treatment strategies will depend on the type of health problems experienced by members of the GLBT population. General considerations in treatment of existing health problems among GLBT individuals include assuring access through health insurance coverage, reforming the health insurance market to cover needed services, promoting trusting relationships and disclosure of sexual orientation and gender identity to health care providers, educating providers to give effective care, developing GLBT-friendly health care systems, and ensuring confidentiality.

Effective treatment for transgender individuals often involves feminizing or masculinizing genitoplasty as well as hormone therapy. Feminizing genitoplasty for MTF transgenders usually includes orchiectomy, penectomy, vaginoplasty, and volvoplasty and may also include breast augmentation and electrolysis of facial and body hair. Surgery for FTM transgender individuals often includes chest reconstruction or reduction mammoplasty (reduction of breast tissue) and creation of an artificial penis. Feminizing genitoplasty is often quite successful, but no completely satisfactory techniques have yet been developed for masculinizing surgery, and both may result in possible surgical complications. Population health nurses may refer clients for sexual reassignment surgery and/or hormone therapy and may also advocate for coverage for these services under health insurance plans. Surgical procedures are often not covered under health insurance plans and many transgender individuals have to pay for surgery out-of-pocket and attempt to get reimbursement or forgo surgery.

Another area for resolution of existing health care problems is the need for assistance and support for caregiving in the GLBT population (Fredriksen-Goldsen, 2012). There is also a need to recognize and make referrals for treatment related to intimate partner violence among same-sex couples and bisexual and transgender individuals. Population health nurses may refer individual GLBT clients for treatment services or assist in the development of services available to this population. They may also need to advocate for available services or for insurance coverage of needed services. For further information about sources of assistance to which population health nurses might refer GLBT clients, see the *External Resources* section of the student resources site.

HEALTH RESTORATION. Health restoration services for members of the GLBT population would be similar to those for the general population. In addition, transgender individuals may need assistance in recovering from sexual reassignment surgery and with legal issues surrounding gender identification (e.g., legal name changes, change of gender on identification or birth certificates, etc.). Population health nurses can monitor the effects of surgery and recovery. In addition, population health nurses should help monitor transgender individuals for effects related to hormone therapy such as increased risk of heart disease, stroke, and breast cancer. If clients are dissatisfied with the results of surgery, nurses can refer them for psychological assistance in dealing with their disillusionment. Population health nurses can also refer transgender clients for assistance with legal issues. Strategies for resolution of existing health problems and health restoration for GLBT populations are summarized in Table 20-5●.

Evaluating Health Care for the GLBT Population

Healthy People 2020 includes two developmental objectives related to GLBT health. The first objective is to increase the number of population-based data systems that include questions related to the health of the gay, lesbian, and bisexual population. The second is similar and reflects the needs for data about the health status of the transgender population (U.S. Department of Health and Human Services [USDHHS], 2013). No current status data is available for either objective so they are not useful in evaluating the effects of care on the health of the GLBT population.

Another approach to evaluating care for the GLBT population lies in the Healthcare Quality Index created by the Human Rights Campaign Foundation (Snowden, 2013). Although the index does not provide information on health status, it does provide data related to the quality of health care provided to members of the GLBT population by 718 health care establishments in 2013, a 153% increase over participation in 2012.

TABLE 20-5 Strategies for Resolving Existing Health Problems and Health Restoration in the GLBT Population

Focus	Strategy
Resolving existing health problems	Provide or refer members of the GLBT population for relevant screening services Provide or refer for STI screening (including HIV screening) for members of the GLBT population at risk for STIs Conduct brief screenings for smoking, problem drinking, and drug use behaviors as needed Conduct or refer for screening for depression Assist in the design and implementation of culturally appropriate screening and treatment services for members of the GLBT population Advocate for the availability of needed screening services (particularly dual gender screenings for transgender individuals) Advocate for insurance coverage for needed screening services Refer members of the GLBT population for needed treatment services Advocate for the availability and coverage of necessary treatment services (particularly for SRS and hormone therapy for transgender individuals) Advocate for access to and funding for necessary treatment services Refer transgender individuals for SRS and/or hormone therapies as needed Advocate for the availability and coverage of treatment services for transgender individuals Refer for treatment of psychological health problems (including substance use and abuse)
Health restoration	Assist with and monitor recovery after SRS Monitor effects of hormone therapy Refer for assistance in dealing with legal issues related to transgenderism

Areas addressed include four core criteria such as inclusion of sexual orientation and gender identity in patient and employee nondiscrimination policies, explicit GLBT-inclusive visitation policies, and provision of staff training in GLBT-centered care. Information is also obtained about 31 additional best policies and practices related to areas such as GLBT patient services and support, transgender-specific services and support, options for patient self-identification, medical decision making, employee benefits and policies, and community engagement (Snowden, 2013). Table 20-6 ● provides some of the major findings from 2013. As indicated in the table, some progress has been made in the creation of GLBT-friendly health care organizations, particularly with respect to the core criteria. Much work remains to be done, however, especially in regard to the additional best practices and policies.

With respect to evaluation of health care effects on the health of GLBT populations, population health nurses will need to obtain locality-specific data. The same data categories included in the *Assessment Guidelines* on the student resources site can be used to collect evaluative data.

TABLE 20-6 Findings from the 2013 Healthcare Quality Index

Criterion	2013 Findings	2012 Findings
Inclusion of sexual orientation in patient nondiscrimination policies	93%	90%
Inclusion of gender identity in patient nondiscrimination policies	87%	76%
Explicit GLBT-inclusive visitation policy	90%	75%
Inclusion of sexual orientation in employee nondiscrimination policies	97%	96%
Inclusion of gender identity in employee nondiscrimination policies	85%	75%
Staff training in GLBT patient-centered care	80%	67%
Communication of nondiscrimination policies Equal visitation policies	91% 90%	
Provision of information regarding GLBT services and issues on organization's website	21%	
Publication of GLBT-specific educational material	18%	
Potential for identification of data from GLBT clients in: Care surveys Satisfaction surveys	 9% 6%	
Review of services to identify GLBT-related gaps	25%	
Provision of transgender-focused staff training	42%	
Creation of unisex bathrooms	59%	
Explicit communication to patients regarding possible designation of a same-sex partner as a medical decision maker	81%	
Provision of health care benefits to same-sex spouses of benefits-eligible employees	55%	
Provision of at least one health insurance plan option that covers medically necessary health services for transgender employees, including gender transition–related treatment	6%	
Provision of opportunities to record same-sex marital relationships in medical records	30%	
Inclusion of different gender identity options in medical records	15%	
Inclusion of sexual orientation options in medical records	13%	
Explicit staff training regarding confidentiality of patient sexual orientation/gender identity information	30%	
Conduct of a formal needs assessment of the GLBT population served by the organization	11%	
Inclusion of an openly GLBT person on a governing or advisory board	50%	

Based on: Snowden, S. (2013). *Healthcare quality index 2013.* Retrieved from http://www.hrc.org/files/assets/resources/HEI_2013_final.pdf

CHAPTER RECAP

Members of the GLBT population have health needs similar to those of other men and women, but they also have many unique health needs that are frequently not met by the health care system due to personal and structural barriers to health care access. Personal barriers may derive from enacted stigma, perceived stigma, or internalized stigma. Structural barriers are created by discriminatory social and institutional policies that reflect the dominant heterosexism of society.

Factors related to each of the six determinants of health affect the health status of the GLBT population. Population health nurses may employ health promotion, illness and injury prevention, resolution, or health restoration strategies to deal with the effects of determinants on the health of the GLBT population. Evaluation of care for members of sexual minority groups focuses on resulting group health status as well as the quality of health care provided. Health care quality may be evaluated using criteria included in the Healthcare Quality Index.

CASE STUDY Access to Health Care

In the course of investigating an outbreak of hepatitis B in a group of young ethnic minority men who have sex with men in a large city, you discover that the majority of them have not seen a health care provider in the past 2 years. Many of them have health insurance, but some do not. Similarly, those affected vary widely in terms of their educational levels.

1. What biological, psychological, environmental, sociocultural, behavioral, and health system factors might be contributing to their failure to use health care services?
2. What population health nursing interventions might promote more effective use of services?

REFERENCES

Allina, A. (2012). Lesbian health gains long due attention from Institute of Medicine. Reprinted in B. Seaman & L. Eldridge (Eds.), *Voices of the women's health movement* (Vol. 1, pp. 387–389). New York, NY: Seven Stories Press.

American Medical Association. (n.d.). *AMA policies on LGBT issues*. Retrieved from https://www.ama-assn.org/ama/pub/about-ama/our-people/member-groups-sections/glbt-advisory-committee/ama-policy-regarding-sexual-orientation.page

American Psychiatric Association. (2013). *DSM-5*. Retrieved from http://www.psychiatry.org/dsm5

American Psychiatric Association. (2014). *LGBT-Sexual orientation*. Retrieved from http://www.psychiatry.org/lgbt-sexual-orientation

American Psychological Association. (2009). *Report of the American Psychological Association Task Force on Appropriate Therapeutic Responses to Sexual Orientation*. Retrieved from http://www.apa.org/pi/lgbt/resources/therapeutic-response.pdf

Biedrzycki, P., Vergeront, J., Gasiorowics, M., Bertolli, J., Oster, A., Spikes, P. S., …, Nielsen, C. F. (2011). Increase in newly diagnosed HIV infections among young black men who have sex with men—Milwaukee County, Wisconsin, 1999–2008. *Morbidity and Mortality Weekly Report, 60,* 99–102.

Bockting, W. O., Miner, M. H., Romine, R. E. S., Hamilton, A., & Coleman, E. (2013). Stigma, mental health, and resilience in an online sample of the US transgender population. *American Journal of Public Health, 103,* 943–951. doi:10.2105/AJPH.2013.301241

Boehmer, U., Mertz, M., Timm, A., Glickman, M., Sullivan, M., & Potter, J. (2011). Overweight and obesity in long-term breast cancer survivors: How does sexual orientation impact BMI? *Cancer Investigation, 29,* 220-228. doi: 10.3109/07357907.2010.550664

Boehmer, U., Miao, X., Linkletter, C., & Clark, M. A. (2012). Adult health behaviors over the life course by sexual orientation. *American Journal of Public Health, 102,* 292–300. doi:10.2105/AJPH.2011.300334

Broad, K. L. (2014). Coming out for parents, families, and friends of lesbians and gays: From support group grieving to love advocacy. *Sexualities, 14,* 399–415. doi: 10.1177/1363460711406792

Buffie, W. C. (2011). Public health implications of same-sex marriage. *American Journal of Public Health, 101,* 986–990. doi:10.2105/AJPH.2010.300112

Catalano, S., Smith, E., Snyder, H., & Rand, M. (2009). *Female victims of violence*. Retrieved from http://www.bjs.gov/content/pub/pdf/fvv.pdf

Choi, K.-Y., Paul, J., Ayala, G., Boylan, R., & Gregorich, S. E. (2013). Experiences of discrimination and their impact on the mental health among African American, Asian and Pacific Islander, and Latino men who have sex with men. *American Journal of Public Health, 103,* 688–874. doi:10.2105/AJPH.2012.301052

Cochran, S. D., & Mays, V. M. (2011). Sexual orientation and mortality among US men aged 17 to 59 years: Results from the National Health and Nutrition Examination Survey III. *American Journal of Public Health, 101,* 1133–1138. doi:10.2105/AJPH.2010.300013

Cohen, S. E., Chew, R., A., Katz, K. A., Bernstein, K. T., Samuel, M. C., Kerndt, P. R., & Bolan, G. (2012). Repeat syphilis among men who have sex with men in California, 2002–2006: Implications for syphilis elimination efforts. *American Journal of Public Health, 101,* e1–e8. doi:10.2105/AJPH.2011.300383

Conron, K. J., Mimiaga, M. J., & Landers, S. J. (2010). A population-based study of sexual orientation identity and gender differences in adult health. *American Journal of Public Health, 100,* 1953–1960. doi:10.2105/AJPH.2009.174169

Conron, K. J., Scott, G., Stowell, G. S., & Landers, S. J. (2012). Transgender health in Massachusetts: Results from a household probability sample of adults. *American Journal of Public Health, 1021,* 118–122. doi:10.2105/AJPH.2011.300315

Corliss, H. L., Goodenow, C. S., Nichols, L., & Austin, S. B. (2011). High burden of homelessness among sexual minority adolescents: Findings from a representative Massachusetts high school sample. *American Journal of Public Health, 101,* 1683–1689. doi:10.2105/AJPH.2011.300155

Eaton, L. A., Cherry, C., Cain, D., & Pope, H. (2011). A novel approach to prevention for at-risk HIV-negative men who have sex with men: Creating a teachable moment to promote informed sexual decision-making. *American Journal of Public Health, 101,* 539–545. doi:10.2105/AJPH.2010.191791

Fields, E. L., Bogart, L. M., Galvan, F. H., Wagner, G. J., Klein, D. J., & Schuster, M. A. (2013). Association of discrimination-related trauma with sexual risk among HIV-positive African American men who have sex with men. *American Journal of Public Health, 103,* 875–880. doi:10.2105/AJPH.2012.300951

Fierer, D. S., Factor, S. H., Uriel, A. J., Carriero, D. C., Dieterich, D. T., Mullen, M. P., ..., Holmberg, S. D. (2011). Sexual transmission of hepatitis C virus among HIV-infected men who have sex with men—New York City, 2005–2010. *Morbidity and Mortality Weekly Report, 60,* 945–950.

Finlayson, T. J., Le, B., Smith, A., Bowles, K., Cribbin, M., Miles, I., ..., DiNenno, E. (2011, October 28). HIV risk, prevention, and testing behaviors among men who have sex with men—National HIV Behavioral Surveillance Systems, 21 U.S. cities, United States, 2008. *Morbidity and Mortality Weekly Report, 60*(SS-14), 1–34.

Finneran, C., & Stephenson, R. (2012). Intimate partner violence among men who have sex with men: A systematic review. *Trauma, Violence, & Abuse, 14,* 168–185. doi: 10.1177/1524838012470034

Forman, D. (n.d.). *Using a known sperm donor: Understanding the legal risks and challenges.* Retrieved from http://www.theafa.org/article/using-a-known-sperm-donor-understanding-the-legal-risks-and-challenges/

Fredriksen-Goldsen, K. I. (2012). Informal caregiving in the LGBT communities. In T. M. Witten & A. E. Eyler (Eds.), *Gay, lesbian, bisexual, and transgender aging* (pp. 59–83). Baltimore, MD: Johns Hopkins University Press.

Fredriksen-Goldsen, K. I., Kim, H. J., & Barcan, S. E. (2012). Disability among lesbian, gay, and bisexual adults: Disparities in prevalence and risk. *American Journal of Public Health, 102,* e9–e15. doi:10.2105/AJPH.2011.300379

Freedom to Marry. (2013). *The Defense of Marriage Act.* Retrieved from http://www.freedomtomarry.org/states/entry/c/doma

Friedman, M. S., Marshal, M. P., Guadamuz, T. E., Wei, C., Wong, C. F., Saewyc, E. M., & Stall, R. (2011). A meta-analysis of disparities in childhood sexual abuse, parental physical abuse, and peer victimization among sexual minority and sexual nonminority individuals. *American Journal of Public Health, 101,* 1481–1494. doi:10.2105/AJPH.2009.190009

Gay & Lesbian Advocates & Defenders. (2013). *About GLAD.* Retrieved from http://www.glad.org/about/mission

Gender Centre. (2013). *Surgery: A guide for F.T.M.s.* Retrieved from http://www.gendercentre.org.au/resources/polare-archive/archived-articles/surgery-a-guide-for-ftms-2.htm

Global Research and Advocacy Group. (2013). *Gender and sexual minorities.* Retrieved from http://www.globalresearchandadvocacygroup.org/es/issues/gender-and-sexual-minorities

Grant, J. M. Mottet, L. A., Tanis, J., Harrison, J., Herman, J. L., & Keisling, M. (2011). *Injustice at every turn: A report of the National Transgender Discrimination Survey.* Retrieved from http://www.transequality.org/PDFs/NTDS_Report.pdf

Grov, C., Breslow, A. S., Newcomb, M. E., Rosenberger, J. G., & Bauermeister, J. A. (2014). Gay and bisexual men's use of the internet: Research from the 1990s through 2013. *Journal of Sex Research, 51,* 390–409. doi: 10.1080/00224499.2013.871626

Guttmacher Institute. (2014). *Fact sheet: American teen's sexual and reproductive health.* Retrieved from http://www.guttmacher.org/pubs/FB-ATSRH.pdf

Halkitis, P. N., Kapadia, F., Siconolfi, D. E., Moeller, R. W., Figueroa, R. P., Barton, S. C., & Blachman-Forshay, J. (2013). Individual, psychosocial, and social correlates of unprotected anal intercourse in a new generation of young men who have sex with men in New York City. *American Journal of Public Health, 103,* 889–895. doi:10.2105/AJPH.20121.300963

Hatzenbuehler, M. L., O'Cleirigh, C., Grasso, C., Mayer, K., Safren, S., & Bradford, J. (2012). Effect of same-sex marriage laws on health care use and expenditures in sexual minority men: A quasi-natural experiment. *American Journal of Public Health, 102,* 285–291. doi:10.2105/AJPH.2011.300382

Heath, J., & Goggin, K. (2009). Attitudes toward male homosexuality, bisexuality, and the down low lifestyle: Demographic differences and HIV implications. *Journal of Bisexuality, 9,* 17–31. doi:10.1080/15299710802659997

Houdart, F. (2012a). *Estimating the global cost of homophobia and transphobia.* Retrieved from http://blogs.worldbank.org/voices/estimating-the-global-cost-of-homophobia-and-transphobia

Houdart, F. (2012b). *The tremendous potential of mobile applications for sexual minorities.* Retrieved from http://blogs.worldbank.org/ic4d/the-tremendous-potential-of-mobile-applications-for-sexual-minorities

Human Rights Campaign. (2014). *Parenting laws: Second parent or stepparent adoption.* Retrieved from http://hrc-assets.s3-website-us-east-1.amazonaws.com//files/assets/resources/Second-parent_5-2014.pdf

Institute of Medicine. (2011). *The health of lesbian, gay, bisexual, and transgender people: Building a foundation for better understanding.* Washington, DC: National Academies Press.

Kann, L., Olsen, E. O., McManus, T., Kinchen, S., Chyen, D., Harris, W. A., & Wechsler, H. (2011). Sexual identity, sex of sexual contacts, and health risk behaviors among students in grades 9–12—Youth Risk Behavior Surveillance, selected sites, United States, 2001–2009. *Morbidity and Mortality Weekly Report, 60*(SS1), 1–133.

Kelvin, E. A., Mantell, J. E., Candelario, N., Hoffman, S., Exner, T. M., Stackhouse, W., & Stein, Z. A. (2011). Off-label use of the female condom for anal intercourse in New York City. *American Journal of Public Health, 101,* 2233–2244. doi:10.2105/AJPH.2011.300260

Kim, H. J., & Fredriksen-Goldsen, K. I. (2012). Hispanic lesbians and bisexual women at heightened risk for health disparities. *American Journal of Public Health, 102,* e9–e15. doi:10.2105/AJPH.2011.300378

Labaton, V. (2012). Putting lesbian health in focus. Reprinted in B. Seaman & L. Eldridge (Eds.), *Voices of the women's health movement* (Vol. 1, pp. 386–387). New York, NY: Seven Stories Press.

Levinson, A. H., Hood, N., & Mahajan, R. (2012). Smoking cessation treatment preferences, intentions, and behaviors among a large sample of Colorado gay, lesbian, bisexual, and transgendered smokers. *Nicotine & Tobacco Research, 14,* 910–918. doi: 10.1093/ntr/ntr303

LGBT Movement Advancement Project (MAP) & Services and Advocacy for Gay, Lesbian, Bisexual and Transgender Elders (SAGE). (2010). *Improving the lives of LGBT older adults.* Retrieved from http://www.americanprogress.org/issues/2010/04/pdf/lgbt_elders.pdf

Lloyd, S., & Operario, D. (2012). HIV risk among men who have sex with men who have experienced childhood sexual abuse: Systematic review and meta-analysis. *AIDS Education and Prevention, 24,* 228–241. doi: 10.1521/aeap.2012.24.3.228

Mallon, G. P. (2011). The home study assessment process for gay, lesbian, bisexual, and transgender prospective foster and adoptive families. *Journal of GLBT Family Studies, 7,* 9–29. doi: 10.1080/1550428X.2011.537229

Martinez-Donate, A. P., Zellner, J., A., Sañudo, F., Fernandez-Cerdeño, A., Hovell, M. F., Sipan, C. L., …, Carrillo, H. (2010). Hombres sanos: Evaluation of a social marketing campaign for heterosexually identified Latino men who have sex with men and women. *American Journal of Public Health, 100,* 2532–2540. doi:10.2105/AJPH.2009.179648

Mayer, K. H. (2011). Sexually transmitted diseases in men who have sex with men. *Clinical Infectious Diseases, 53*(S3), S79–S83. doi: 10.1093/cid/cir696

McCabe, S. E., Bostwick, W. B., Hughes, T. L., West, B. T., & Boyd, C. J. (2010). The relationship between discrimination and substance abuse disorders among lesbian, gay, and bisexual adults in the United States. *American Journal of Public Health, 100,* 1946–1952. doi:10.2105/AJPH.2009.163147

McLaughlin, K. A., Hatzenbuehler, M. L., & Keyes, K. M. (2010). Responses to discrimination and psychiatric disorders among black, Hispanic, female, and lesbian, gay, and bisexual individuals. *American Journal of Public Health, 100,* 1477–1484. doi:10.2105/AJPH.2009.181586

Mintz, H. (2013). *Prop. 8: Supreme Court ends California ban on gay marriage but fight remains.* Retrieved from http://www.mercurynews.com/samesexmarriage/ci_23542472/gay-marriage-prop-8-supreme-court-ruling.

Moody, K. (2009). *Ensuring human and sexual rights for men who have sex with men living with HIV.* Retrieved from http://www.who.int/bulletin/volumes/87/11/09-071175/en/

Moran, M. (2013). *New gender dysphoria criteria replace GID.* Retrieved from http://psychnews.psychiatryonline.org/newsArticle.aspx?articleid=1676226.

Mutchler, M. G., McKay, T., McDavitt, B., & Gordon, K. K. (2013). Using peer ethnography to address health disparities among urban black and Latino men who have sex with men. *American Journal of Public Health, 103,* 849–852. doi:10.2105/AJPH.2012.300988

National Coalition of Anti-Violence Programs. (2013). *Lesbian, gay, bisexual, transgender, queer, and HIV-affected hate violence in 2012.* Retrieved from http://www.avp.org/storage/documents/ncavp_2012_hvreport_final.pdf

Nemoto, T., Böedeker, B., & Iwamoto, M. (2011). Social support, exposure to violence and transphobia, and correlates of depression among male-to-female transgender women with a history of sex work. *American Journal of Public Health, 101,* 1980–1988. doi:10.2105/AJPH.2010.197285

Newcomb, M. E., Birkett, M., Corliss, H. L., & Mistanski, B. (2014). Sexual orientation, gender, and racial differences in illicit drug use in a sample of US high school students. *American Journal of Public Health, 104,* 304–310. doi: 10.2105/AJPH.2013.301702

O'Donnell, S., Meyer, I. H., & Schwartz, S. (2011). Increased risk of suicide attempts among black and Latino lesbians, gay men, and bisexuals. *American Journal of Public Health, 102,* 156–162. doi:10.2105/AJPH.2011.300284

Parents, Families, and Friends of Lesbians and Gays. (n.d.a). *Our daughters and sons: Questions and answers for parents of lesbian, gay, bisexual, and transgender youth and adults.* Retrieved from http://community.pflag.org/page.aspx?pid=316

Parents, Families, and Friends of Lesbians and Gays. (n.d.b). *What does it all mean?* Retrieved from http://community.pflag.org/page.aspx?pid=316

Parsons, J. T., Grov, C., & Golub, S. A. (2012). Sexual compulsivity, co-occurring psychosocial health problems, and HIV risk among gay and bisexual men: Further evidence of a syndemic. *American Journal of Public Health, 101,* 1055–1059. doi:10.2105/AJPH.2010.300032

Parsons, J. T., Kowalczyk, W. J., Botsko, M., Tomassilli, J., & Golub, S. A. (2013). Aggregated versus day level association between methamphetamine use and HIV medication non-adherence among gay and bisexual men. *AIDS Behavior, 17,* 1478–1487. doi:10.1007/s10461-013-0463-7

Roberts, A. L., Austin, B., Corliss, H. L., Vandermorris, A. K., & Koenen, K. C. (2010). Pervasive trauma exposure among US sexual orientation minority adults and risk of posttraumatic stress disorder. *American Journal of Public Health, 102,* 2433–2441. doi:10.2105/AJPH.2009.168971

Rotondi, N. K., Bauer, G., Scanlon, K., Kaay, M., Travers, R., & Travers, A. (2013). Nonprescribed hormone use and self-performed surgeries: "Do-it-yourself" transitions in transgender communities in Ontario, Canada. *American Journal of Public Health, 103,* 1830–1836. doi: 10.2105/AJPH.2013.301348

Rozsa, M. (2013). *Crystal meth and its use among gay men.* Retrieved from http://www.addictionpro.com/print/article/crystal-meth-and-its-use-among-gay-men.

Ryan, C. (2009). *Supportive families, healthy children: Helping families with lesbian, gay, bisexual & transgender children.* Retrieved from http://family-project.sfsu.edu/files/English_Final_Print_Version_Last.pdf.

Ryan, C., Russell, S. T., Huebner, D., Diaz, R., & Sanchez, J. (2010). Family acceptance in adolescence and the health of LGBT young adults. *Journal of Child and Adolescent Psychiatric Nursing, 23,* 205–203. doi:10.1111/j.1744-6171.2010.00246.x

Sanchez-Ponte, A., Marti, E., Rubio, J., Montes, T., Yanguas, C., Sant, F., & Culell, P. (2012). Illegal injection of industrial silicone oil for breast augmentation: Risks, solutions, and results. *The Breast Journal, 18,* 174–176. doi: 10/1111/j.1524-4741.2011.01212

Schwarcz, S., Schemer, S., McFarland, W., Katz, M., Valero, L., Chen, S., & Catania, J. (2007). Prevalence of HIV infection and predictors of high-transmission sexual risk behaviors among men who have sex with men. *American Journal of Public Health, 97,* 1067–1075. doi:10.2105/AJPH.2005.072249

Scouts for Equality. (2013). *Landmark resolution ends discrimination of gay scouts.* Retrieved from http://www.scoutsforequality.com/campaign-news/scouts-for-equality-glaad-and-the-inclusive-scouting-network-applaud-the-boy-scouts-of-America-for-passage-of-non-discrimination-resolution/

Singh, D., Fine, D. N., & Marrazzo, J. M. (2011). Chlamydia trachomatis infection among women reporting sexual activity with women screened in family planning clinics in the Pacific northwest, 1997–2005. *American Journal of Public Health, 101,* 1284–1290. doi:10.2105/AJPH.2009.169631

Smith, A., Miles, I., Le, B., Finlayson, T., Oster, A., & DiNenno, E. (2010). Prevalence and awareness of HIV infection among men who have sex with men—21 cities, United States, 2008. *Morbidity and Mortality Weekly Report, 59,* 1202–1207.

Snowden, S. (2013). *Healthcare quality index 2013.* Retrieved from http://www.hrc.org/files/assets/resources/HEI_2013_final.pdf

Sudol, T. (2010). *LGBT adoptive and foster parenting.* Retrieved from http://www.hunter.cuny.edu/socwork/nrcfcpp/info_services/download/TSudol_LGBT%20Issues_InfoPacket.pdf.

Synnott, A. (2009). *Rethinking men: Heroes, villains, and victims.* Burlington, VT: Ashgate.

Thomeer, M. B. (2013). Sexual minority status and self-rated health: The importance of socioeconomic status, age, and sex. *American Journal of Public Health, 103,* 881–888. doi:10.2105/AJPH.2012.301040

Trans Respect Versus Transphobia. (n.d.). *Working definitions.* Retrieved from http://www.transrespect-transphobia.org/en_US/tvt-project/definitions.htm

Transgender Law Center. (2011). *Organizing for transgender health care: A guide for community clinic organizing and advocacy.* San Francisco, CA: Author.

Transgender Law Center. (2013). *Mission, vision, and values.* Retrieved from http://transgenderlawcenter.org/about/mission

UC Berkeley Gender Equity Resource Center. (n.d.). *Definitions of terms.* Retrieved from http://geneq.berkeley.edu/lgbt_resources_definiton_of_terms

U.S. Census Bureau. (2012). *2012 Statistical abstract of the United States: Law enforcement, courts, & prisons: Crimes and crime rates, Table 322. Hate crimes—number of incidents, offenses, victims, and known offenders, by bias motivation, 2000–2008.* Retrieved from http://www.census.gov/compendia/statab/2012/tables/12s0322.pdf

U.S. Department of Health and Human Services. (2013). *Lesbian, gay, bisexual, and transgender health.* Retrieved from http://healthypeople.gov/2020/topicsobjectives2020/overview.aspx?topicid=25

Wight, R. G., LeBlanc, A. J., de Vries, B., & Detels, R. (2012). Stress and mental health among midlife and older gay-identified men. *American Journal of Public Health, 102,* 503–510. doi:10.2105/AJPH.2011.300384

Wilson, E. C., Garofalo, R., Harris, R., Belter, M., Transgender Advisory Committee, & Adolescent Medicine Trials Network for HIV-AIDS Interventions. (2010). Sexual risk taking among transgender male-to-female youths with different partner types. *American Journal of Public Health, 100,* 1946–1952. doi:10.2105/AJPH.2009.160051

World Professional Association for Transgender Health. (2011). *Standards of care for the health of transsexual, transgender, and gender non-conforming people (version 7).* Retrieved from http://admin.associationsonline.com/uploaded_files/140/files/Standards%20of%20Care%20V7%20-%202011%20WPATH.pdf

The Yogyakarta Principles: Principles on the application of international human rights law in relation to sexual orientation and gender identity. (2007). Retrieved from http://www.yogyakartaprinciples.org/principles_en.pdf

CHAPTER

21 Care of Poor and Homeless Populations

Learning Outcomes

After reading this chapter, you should be able to:

1. Analyze factors contributing to poverty and homelessness.
2. Identify biological, psychological, environmental, sociocultural, behavioral, and health system determinants that influence the health of poor and homeless populations.
3. Describe approaches to health promotion among poor and homeless populations and related population health nursing roles.
4. Discuss interventions related to the prevention of homelessness and illness and injury prevention in poor and homeless populations. Analyze potential roles of population health nurses with respect to each.
5. Identify strategies to resolve the problems of homelessness and poverty and analyze the roles played by population health nurses.
6. Identify restoration strategies for poor and homeless populations.
7. Identify potential foci for evaluating care for poor and homeless populations.

Key Terms

affordable housing
criminalization
deindustrialization
deinstitutionalization
gentrification
homeless individual
means-tested income transfers
poverty
safe havens
single room occupancy unit (SRO)
structural unemployment
worst-case needs households

Advocacy Then

Promoting the Health of New York City's Poor

Organized health services for the poor in New York City were initiated by Lillian Wald and her cohorts at the Henry Street Settlement; however, in the early days of this effort African American nurses were actively involved in improving the lot of poor Black residents of New York. In 1900, Jessie Sleet Scales was hired as the first Black community health nurse in the city by the Charity Organization Society. Her role was to promote tuberculosis treatment in the Black community of New York City. Her appointment as a district nurse was controversial and was only made on the condition that her salary not be paid by the Society, but by a private philanthropist. A trial period of 2 months was agreed upon. In addition to her identified role of tuberculosis care, Scales provided direct care, dressing wounds, bathing patients and newborns, and caring for their mothers. She identified and dealt with numerous other diseases and provided education for hygiene and health promotion. She was so successful that her position was made permanent and she is credited with opening the field of community health nursing to African American nurses (Mosely, 1996).

Another African American nurse, Elizabeth Tyler, was hired by the Henry Street Settlement as the first Black nurse in the organization. Because the Settlement had no Black clients at the time, Tyler actively sought out those in need by soliciting referrals from apartment house janitors. Within 3 months, she had acquired a sufficient clientele to require the employment of another Black nurse, Edith Carter. Tyler later established the Stillman House Branch of the Henry Street Settlement to meet the needs of the Black community in the San Juan Hill area, so named because of fighting between Blacks and Irish and among U.S.- and foreign-born Black residents (Mosely, 1996).

Tyler's and Carter's efforts were initially viewed as intrusive by area residents, and they tended not to be receptive, so the nurses solicited referrals from local physicians. They also visited churches, following obviously ill members to their homes and attempting to persuade them to accept care. Tyler later was employed by the Delaware State Health and Welfare Commission where she was instrumental in developing child health and tuberculosis clinics. Both Tyler and Carter struggled to correct misconceptions and lack of health knowledge, particularly in efforts to combat harmful traditional health practices and the allurements of quack practitioners in the community. Carter, in particular, was well known for her success with patients deemed "incurable" by the medical establishment. According to a supervisor at Henry Street, "to the people in this area Miss Carter *is* Henry Street" (Mosely, 1996, p. 78).

Advocacy Now

Providing Permanent Housing for the Chronically Homeless

The aim of the 100,000 Homes Campaign in communities throughout the nation is to provide permanent housing for the more than 110,000 chronically homeless individuals in the United States. The chronically homeless are those who are without housing for extended periods of time or experience multiple episodes of homelessness. The approach taken is one of "housing first" which focuses first on providing permanent housing and then on addressing factors that contribute to homelessness such as mental illness or substance abuse.

Such strategies are actually less expensive and more effective than traditional approaches such as temporary shelters and transitional housing. The average cost of housing first strategies is about $15,000 per person per year, far cheaper than a year's stay in a shelter. In addition, approximately 85% stayed housed rather than returning to the street. Since 2010, more than 12,000 people have been served by the campaign (Tucker, 2012).

As we have seen in several previous chapters, sociocultural factors play a significant role in determining the health status of population groups. The health- related effects and population health nursing roles with respect to two interrelated sociocultural factors, poverty and homelessness, are explored in detail in this chapter.

Overview of Poverty and Homelessness

In 1948, the United Nations General Assembly adopted the Universal Declaration of Human Rights, Article 25 of which indicates that all people have rights to a standard of living that promotes health and includes access to food, clothing, housing, health care, and necessary social services and security in the event of adversity (United Nations, 1948). The following year, in the United States, the Housing Act of 1949 proposed the achievement of decent housing for every American family (Choldin, n.d.). To further the objectives of these two pieces of legislation, the World Health Organization developed the 11 *Health Principles of Housing* presented in the *Highlights* box at right.

Unfortunately, many of the world's societies do not achieve these principles of justice in housing. United Nations (UN) estimates include more than 100 million homeless people worldwide and another 1 billion people (17% of the world's population) living in inadequate housing (U.N., n.d.). Adequate housing is of concern because of its effects on the health of the population. These effects occur in three ways: through poor physical conditions of housing, through the absence of affordable housing, and through location of housing in unhealthy places.

Defining Poverty and Homelessness

Both poverty and homelessness are defined in multiple ways. **Poverty** is having an income or means of support insufficient to meet one's basic needs; what is considered *sufficient* may vary from one definition to the next. In the United States, poverty is defined in terms of a household income less than the identified threshold based on the number of persons in the household. This official definition of poverty is based on monetary income before taxes, but excluding capital gains and noncash benefits (such as food stamps, Medicaid, or housing subsidy) (U.S. Census Bureau, 2013).

In 2014, the poverty threshold for a single individual was an annual income of $11,670 or less; for a family of four the threshold was an annual income of $23,850 (U.S. Department of Health and Human Services [USDHHS], 2014a). The "near poor" have incomes 100% to 199% above the federal poverty level, while middle-income and high-income levels are 200% to 399% of the poverty threshold and greater than 400% of the poverty threshold (National Center for Health Statistics [NCHS], 2014).

Highlights

The World Health Organization's Health Principles of Housing

1. "Adequate housing provides protection against exposure to agents and vectors of communicable diseases through safe water supply, sanitary excreta disposal, disposal of solid wastes, drainage of surface water, personal and domestic hygiene, safe food preparation, and structural safeguards against disease transmission" (World Health Organization, 1989, p. 2).
2. "Adequate housing provides protection against injuries, poisoning and thermal and other exposures that may contribute to chronic disease and malignancies; special attention should be paid to structural features and furnishings, indoor air pollution, chemical safety, and use of the home as a workplace" (World Health Organization, 1989, p. 9).
3. "Adequate housing helps people's social and psychological development and reduces to a minimum the psychological and social stresses connected with the housing environment" (World Health Organization, 1989, p. 14).
4. "Suitable housing environments provide access to places of work, essential services and amenities that promote good health" (World Health Organization, 1989, p. 15).
5. "Only if residents make proper use of their housing can its health potential be realized to the full" (World Health Organization, 1989, p. 18).
6. "Housing should reduce to a minimum hazards to the health of groups at special risk from the conditions they live in, including women and children, those who live in substandard housing, displaced and mobile populations, and the aged, chronically ill and disabled" (World Health Organization, 1989, p. 20).
7. "Health advocacy, carried out by health authorities and bodies in related fields, should be an integral part of public and private decisions about housing" (World Health Organization, 1989, p. 24).
8. "Economic and social policies that affect the state of housing should support the use of land and housing resources to maximize physical, mental and social health" (World Health Organization, 1989, p. 27).
9. "Economic and social development, as it affects human shelter, should be based on appropriate processes of planning, the formulation and implementation of public policy, and the provision of services, with intersectoral collaboration in: development planning and management; urban and land use planning; housing legislation and standards and their enforcement; the design and construction of housing; the provision of community services; and monitoring and surveillance of the situation." (World Health Organization, 1989, p. 29).
10. "Education—public and professional—should actively foster the provision and use of housing to promote health" (World Health Organization, 1989, p. 36).
11. "In dealing with the needs and problems of the human habitat, community involvement at all levels should support the processes of self-help, help between neighbors, and communal co-operative activities" (World Health Organization, 1989, p. 38).

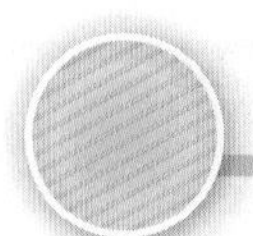

Global Perspectives

World Poverty

Poverty and its consequences are not unique to the United States, and incomes at poverty level would be considered wealth in many nations throughout the world. According to World Health Organization (WHO) figures, more than one fifth of the world's population has an income equivalent to one U.S. dollar per day, and more than half of the populations of 10 countries have incomes at this level. The extent of poverty ranges from less than 2% of the population of many affluent countries to 83.7% of Liberia's total population. The African region has the greatest percentage of people in poverty at 42.6%, followed by the South-East Asian region at 38.4%. Gross national per capital income in 2011 ranged from $1,313 per year in the lowest income countries to $38,690 in the most affluent countries (WHO, 2013).

Poverty may also be defined in terms of the percent of one's income spent on essential goods and services (e.g., food, shelter, and clothing) or one's income relative to the median income in the local area. In the context of the U.S. Rural Rental Housing Loan Program, very low income is defined as an income 50% below the area median income (AMI), and low-income households are below 50% to 80% of the AMI (National Coalition for the Homeless, 2012e). Measurable definitions of poverty are important because they often determine clients' eligibility for assistance programs. For example, eligibility may be restricted to individuals or families with incomes at or below the defined poverty level. In some programs, eligibility may be set at 100% or 150% above poverty level.

Homelessness also has multiple definitions, depending on the purpose of the definition. One of the most commonly used definitions is that posed by Title 42 of the Stewart B. McKinney Homeless Assistance Act of 1987, the first federal legislation in the United States dealing with the problem of homelessness. In a 2009 revision of the McKinney Act, a **homeless individual** is defined as (a) an individual or family without a regular, adequate nighttime residence; (b) an individual or family sleeping in public or private places not designed as a regular sleeping accommodation (c) an individual or family living in a publicly or privately operated shelter; (d) a previously homeless individual who is being discharged from an institution where he or she has been housed; (e) an individual or family who are about to lose their housing with no subsequent residence identified and without the resources or needed to obtain housing; (f) homeless youth or families with children who have a history of housing instability and are likely to continue in this state due to physical, emotional, or social circumstances; and (g) individuals fleeing situations of abuse or dangerous housing conditions (U.S. Department of Housing and Urban Development [HUD] 2009).

The McKinney-Vento Act expands on this definition with respect to homeless children as follows:

> Homeless child and youth (A) means individuals who lack a fixed, regular, and adequate nighttime residence . . . and (B) includes: (i) children and youth who lack a fixed, regular, and adequate nighttime residence, and includes children and youth who are sharing the housing of other persons due to loss of housing, economic hardship, or a similar reason; are living in motels, hotels, trailer parks, or camping grounds due to lack of alternative adequate accommodations; are living in emergency or transitional shelters; are abandoned in hospitals; or are awaiting foster care placement; (ii) children and youth who have a primary nighttime residence that is a private or public place not designed for or ordinarily used as a regular sleeping accommodation for human beings . . . (iii) children and youth who are living in cars, parks, public spaces, abandoned buildings, substandard housing, bus or train stations, or similar settings, and (iv) migratory children . . . who qualify as homeless for the purposes of this subtitle because the children are living in circumstances described in clauses (i) through (iii). (U.S. Department of Education, n.d.)

Other federal agencies include persons on the streets, those in shelters, and those who face imminent eviction (within a week) from a private dwelling or institution (National Coalition for the Homeless, 2011b). The United Nations Committee on Human Rights defined absolute homelessness as "the condition of people without any physical shelter who sleep outdoors, in vehicles, or in abandoned buildings or other places not intended for human habitation" (Substance Abuse and Mental Health Services Administration, n.d., para 1). Other related terms are the "unsheltered homeless" and chronic homelessness. The unsheltered homeless are people living in places not meant for human habitation. Chronic homelessness is defined as having a disability and being continually homeless for more than a year or experiencing four or more episodes of homelessness in the prior three years (Henry, Cortes, & Morris, 2013). Unfortunately, these definitions fail to recognize the large

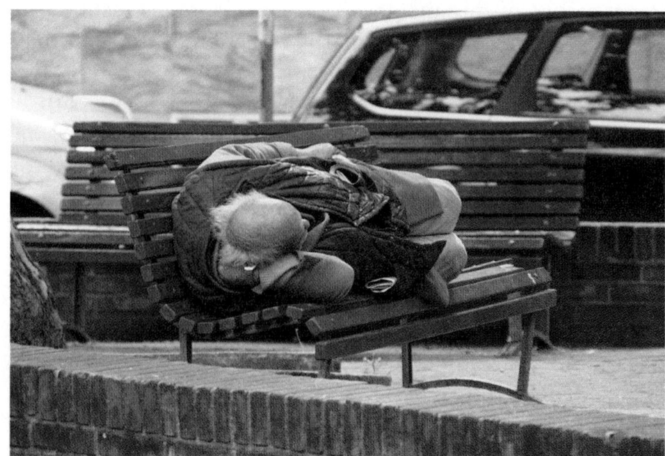

Due to overcrowding in shelters, many homeless individuals have no choice but to sleep outside. *(Giuseppe Porzani/Fotolia)*

segment of the population who are virtually homeless but are living doubled and tripled up with friends or family or who are living in substandard housing (National Coalition for the Homeless, 2012i).This situation is sometimes referred to as "relative homelessness" (SAMHSA, n.d.).

The Magnitude of Poverty and Homelessness

There are no exact figures on the number of poor or homeless persons in the United States. From 2010 to 2011, the median household income in the United States declined by 1.3%, and the national poverty rate increased from 15.3% to 15.9% of households. In 2011, more than 48 million individuals had incomes below the poverty level (National Alliance to End Homelessness, 2013). In 2009, nearly 15% of families and 18.7% of individuals were considered near poverty, at 125% of the poverty level (U.S. Census Bureau, 2012a, 2012e). Also in 2009, 14.7 million children, more than 20% of U.S. children and youth, were living in poverty (U.S. Census Bureau, 2012b).

Both individual poverty among adults and poverty among children is more common among ethnic minority groups than among White Americans. For example, Black children were more than twice as likely as White children to live in poverty. Hispanic children also experience high levels of poverty (U.S. Census Bureau, 2012b). Among individual adults, Blacks had slightly higher poverty rates than Hispanics (25.8% vs. 25.3%), and both had higher rates than Whites (12.3%) or Asians (12.5%) (U.S. Census Bureau, 2012c). American Indian and Alaska Native populations also experienced high rates of poverty at 20.4% (Beckles & Truman, 2011).

The relationship between poverty and homelessness is well established and is best conveyed by the following statement: "If you are poor, you are essentially an illness, and accident, or a paycheck away from living on the streets" (National Coalition for the Homeless, 2011c, p. 1). As with poverty, the exact number of homeless persons is unknown and, in fact, varies from one day to the next. The best estimate is that approximately 13.5 million people in the United States will be homeless at some point in their lives, and on any given night 250,000 to 3.5 million people are homeless (O'Connell et al., 2010). These figures probably underrepresent the true extent of homelessness, since homeless counts are often based on the number of people in shelters or seeking assistance from homeless service providers. Due to shelter overcrowding, fear, and other factors, many homeless people may not seek assistance, and, as noted earlier, many virtually homeless individuals and families are living temporarily with family members or friends (National Coalition for the Homeless, 2011a).

On one night in January 2013, 610,042 homeless people were identified (Henry et al., 2013); this "point-in-time" estimate includes those in shelters and transitional housing or on the streets, but does not include persons in family households (SAMHSA, 2011). From 2011 to 2012, the size of the homeless population in the United States decreased by 0.4% or slightly more than 2,000 people. The rate of homelessness in the general population was 20 homeless per 10,000 people, with a higher rate among veterans (29 per 10,000 veterans) (National Alliance to End Homelessness, 2013). Approximately 85% of the homeless population in the United States in 2013 consisted of single individuals and 15% was homeless as part of a family constellation. In addition, nearly 18% are chronically homeless. Overall, the extent of homelessness declined by nearly 4% from 2012 to 2013, and unsheltered homelessness declined by 7%. Declines in homelessness occurred for all population subgroups (individuals, families, the chronically homeless, and veterans. Most homeless people were staying in shelters or transitional housing, but 35% were "unsheltered," living on the street, in vacant buildings, in cars, or other places not intended for human habitation (Henry et al., 2013).

Although homelessness occurs throughout the nation, five states (California, New York, Florida, Texas, and Georgia) account for more than half of the homeless population. California alone accounts for 22% of the U.S. homeless population (Henry et al., 2013). Families with children make up one of the fastest growing segments of the homeless population, and the effects of homelessness are particularly severe for children and adolescents. An estimated 1.3 million people from 600,000 families will experience homelessness over time, and an additional 3.8 million families live in "precarious housing" and are at high risk for homelessness. Among children, three of every 200 U.S. children will be homeless at some point and more than twice as many will be at risk of homelessness (National Coalition for the Homeless, 2012c). As indicated by these and other figures, the risk for homelessness in the U.S. population is higher than previously thought (National Coalition for the Homeless, 2011a).

Another rapidly increasing, but often overlooked, segment of the homeless population is the elderly. For example, in 2008, 16.8% of the homeless population was over 50 years of age. There is some debate regarding the age at which a homeless person should be considered elderly. Generally, however, 50 years of age is used as a cut-off because homeless people tend to age faster than the general population and a 50-year-old homeless individual may have a health status similar to that of a 70-year-old in the general population (National Coalition for the Homeless, 2012l). The increase in homelessness among the elderly is due, in large part, to the loss of affordable housing in the context of fixed incomes.

Older householders and poor families have a high probability of being part of *worst-case needs households.* **Worst-case needs households** are defined by HUD as "very low income renters who do not receive government housing assistance and who either paid more than one half of their income for rent or lived in severely inadequate conditions or who faced both these challenges" (HUD, 2013, p. 1). Worst-case needs are the result of excessively high rents relative to household income. Approximately 48 million U.S. households were in worst-case situations in 2011, a figure that increased 43.5% from 2007 to 2011. Very low-income households with disabled members were even more likely to be considered worst-case needs households (HUD, 2013).

Population Health Nursing and Care of Poor and Homeless Populations

Population health nurses may encounter homeless clients in a number of venues. They may work in or with shelters for homeless people. Or they may encounter virtually homeless people during home visits to other clients with whom homeless individuals may be staying. Population health nurses may also encounter homeless clients who seek services from other agencies where nurses are employed. Finally, homeless clients may be referred to population health nurses by other agencies and providers.

Homeless individuals may be reluctant to admit to their homelessness for a variety of reasons. They may feel embarrassed about their condition or may want to forestall intrusion into what they may feel is their own affair. Population health nurses should be alert to indicators of possible homelessness in clients they encounter. For example, a population health nurse may note that a client has not taken a shower or washed his or her clothes in some time. Or the client may be hesitant when asked for a home address or may give the address of a known homeless shelter. Clients who report living with other family members or friends may also be virtually homeless. When faced with these indicators, the population health nurse can tactfully explore if the client is indeed homeless and if assistance is desired.

In other instances, clues may be more subtle. For example, in a hearing related to a college academic integrity violation related to plagiarism, the student explained his purchase of a paper from an Internet source as a result of not being able to work in his dorm room because his roommate was using drugs and he was afraid to be associated with him. When a population health nurse faculty member, who happened to be a member of the hearing committee, asked where the student was staying if he was not living in the dorm, he reported that he was living in one of the student lounges on campus. In addition to dealing with the academic integrity violation, the committee took immediate steps to obtain adequate housing for the student. However, his homeless plight would not have been identified if the population health nurse had not caught the cue buried in his defense of plagiarism.

Assessing the Health of Poor and Homeless Populations

The first step in the care of poor and homeless segments of the population is assessing their health status and identifying the factors that influence their health. The population health nurse examines factors that contribute to homelessness in the population as well as the effects of homelessness on health. Factors related to each of the six categories of determinants of health should be examined.

BIOLOGICAL DETERMINANTS. Biological factors, in conjunction with factors in other areas, may lead to poverty and homelessness. Conversely, poverty and homelessness have serious consequences for physical health that vary with gender, age, and prior health status.

With respect to gender, the majority of single homeless individuals are men (67.5%). Women, on the other hand, make up a similar proportion of heads of homeless families, often as a result of domestic violence (National Coalition for the Homeless, 2011b). Among homeless veterans, the bulk of the population is male. In addition, this population is apt to be younger than the rest of the homeless population with 50% of homeless veterans under 51 years of age. Approximately 40% of homeless veterans are African American or Hispanic (National Coalition for Homeless Veterans, n.d.).

People of certain age groups may be more likely than other groups to become homeless or have more negative consequences as a result of homelessness. As we noted earlier, significant numbers of young children are homeless or at risk for homelessness. As many as one in 50 U.S. children may be homeless at any given time, amounting to 800,000 to 1.2 million homeless children, at least half of whom are under 5 years of age (National Coalition for the Homeless, 2012i). Poverty and housing insecurity among children has been associated with poor health, lower weight, and risk for developmental delays (Cutts et al. 2011), and homeless children are at higher risk for increased mortality and lead poisoning than housed children (Kerker et al., 2011). Asthma prevalence rates are also higher for poor children than for the near poor and nonpoor child populations (Moorman, Zahran, Truman, & Molla, 2011). In addition, homeless children with asthma are more likely than their housed counterparts to have severe disease and frequent emergency departments for care and less likely to be on controller medications (Cutuli, Herbers, Rinaldi, Masten, & Oberg, 2010).

There are generally two categories of children among the homeless population, children who are part of homeless families and unaccompanied minors (Corliss, Goodenow, Nichols, & Austin, 2011). Unaccompanied minors may make up as much as 2% of the homeless population (National Coalition for the Homeless, 2011a). Unaccompanied minors are youth under 18 years of age without parental, foster parent, or institutional supervision (National Coalition for the Homeless, 2012k). Reasons for homelessness among adolescents tend to fall into three categories: family problems, economic problems within the family, or residential instability. Family problems may include strained relationships with parents, addiction in a family member, or parental neglect or outright abuse (National Coalition for the Homeless, 2012k). In some studies, sexual minority youth, who often leave home due to abuse or other family problems, may range from 4 to 5% to 50% of homeless unaccompanied youth (Corliss et al., 2011).

Economic problems in the family that may lead to youth homelessness include housing foreclosure leading to separation of adolescents, particularly boys, from other family members due to shelter rules or child welfare policies. Residential instability among youth usually stems from a history of foster care and outgrowing foster care with no other place to go. In some studies, one in five unaccompanied youth arrived at homeless shelters directly from foster care, and one in four had been in foster care within the prior year. In addition to other health risks, homeless youth have been found to be 2 to 10 times more likely to be HIV-infected than their housed age mates as a result of sexual abuse and exploitation and the practice of engaging in sex for money (National Coalition for the Homeless, 2012k).

Certain health conditions may contribute to poverty and homelessness due to limited ability to work. For example, people with HIV/AIDS are at greater risk for homelessness than the general population for a number of reasons. Hospitalization and excessive fatigue may interrupt employment, leading to loss of income and consequent inability to pay for housing. They may also experience discrimination and job loss due to their condition. For other individuals, serious illness, with the attendant medical bills may precipitate homelessness for individuals or families. For example, approximately 40% of people evicted by foreclosures indicated that medical problems played a role in the foreclosure (National Coalition for the Homeless, 2012f). Approximately half of all personal bankruptcies in the United States are the result of serious health problems. As noted by the National Coalition for the Homeless (2012h), serious illness or disability can precipitate loss of employment and savings, eventually resulting in homelessness.

Being poor or homeless also contributes to or complicates other health problems. Homeless individuals are sick more often and have 1.5 to 3.5 times the risk of mortality of their housed counterparts (National Coalition for the Homeless, 2012h; O'Toole et al., 2010). Life expectancy for homeless individuals is approximately 30 years less than for those who do not experience homelessness (National Coalition for the Homeless, 2012f). Mortality rates for HIV/AIDS and substance abuse deaths in New York City were three and five times higher, respectively, in homeless individuals than in the general population and substance abuse deaths were also higher than in the housed low-income population (Kerker et al., 2011). Health problems common among homeless adults include asthma, bronchitis, hypertension, heart disease, cancer, liver and kidney disease, diabetes, and sexually transmitted infections and other infectious conditions. Skin infections and pneumonia are also common.

Other frequently noted problems include malnutrition, TB, and other respiratory diseases resulting from the lack of housing and overcrowding in shelters (National Coalition for the Homeless, 2012h). In addition, homeless individuals are more likely to self-report poor health than either the housed poor or non-poor.

As we can see from this list of common conditions, poor and homeless persons often suffer multiple acute and chronic conditions that require long-term treatment and monitoring that is difficult in circumstances of poverty and homelessness (National Coalition for the Homeless, 2012h). Inadequate diet and lack of access to medications and health care supplies make disease management difficult. For example, hypertension is less likely to be controlled among the poor than the non-poor. Paradoxically, control may be even worse among the near poor (Keenan & Rosendorf, 2011); perhaps because they are less likely than the truly poor to have publicly funded health insurance. Similarly, diabetes prevalence is higher among the poor than the non-poor (Beckles, Zhu, & Moonesinghe, 2011), and glycemic control among diabetics is considerably less likely in the poor than in higher income individuals (NCHS, 2012).

Poor and homeless individuals are also more likely to have physical disabilities (National Coalition for the Homeless, 2011a) and activity limitations. For example, in 2012, 42% of people aged 18 to 64 years in poverty experienced basic activity limitations compared to 21% of those with incomes 400% of poverty level or higher. Similarly, complex activity limitations were found in 28% of the poor versus 8% of high-income individuals. Differences in activity limitations by income level were even more striking among the elderly (NCHS, 2014). In 2012, limitations in activities of daily living (ADLs) and in instrumental activities of daily living (IADLs) were three times more common among the poor than the non-poor (Adams, Kirzinger, & Martinez, 2012). In addition, survival stress experienced by many homeless persons may lead them to put health needs at a lower priority than basic survival needs (O'Connell et al., 2010).

The elderly are at particular risk of health problems stemming from poverty and homelessness. All of the usual problems of the elderly discussed in Chapter 19∞ are intensified by poverty and homelessness. The homeless elderly are particularly susceptible to the effects of communicable diseases, exposure, burns, and trauma due to alcohol use, physical or mental impairment, or assault. The elderly homeless population is also more likely than younger groups to experience chronic disability due to physical, mental, or emotional impairment.

PSYCHOLOGICAL DETERMINANTS. Psychological problems can stem from poverty and homelessness. In 2011–2012, for example, more than 8% of people with incomes below 100% of the federal poverty level reported experiencing severe psychological distress in the prior 30 days, compared to 4.9% of the near poor, 2.6% of middle-income individuals, and only 1.1% of those with incomes more than 400% above the poverty threshold (NCHS, 2014).

Psychological factors can lead to homelessness when people are unable to cope with the demands of daily life and have limited support systems. Mental illness, in particular, is associated with homelessness. An estimated 20% to 25% of the homeless experience severe mental illness and mental illness is the third most common cause of homelessness for single adults (National Coalition for the Homeless, 2012m). In one study 15% of all the people in the California mental health system reported being homeless at one point in their lives. Mental illness may disrupt one's ability to care for oneself, including managing a residence. In addition, mental illness may prevent formation or maintenance of interpersonal relationships or contribute to paranoia and mistrust of others. Mental illness also makes it difficult to obtain and keep a job and may also impede care of one's physical needs. Many mentally ill homeless individuals may attempt to self-medicate themselves in an effort to deal with their symptoms, and many have resulting dual diagnoses of substance abuse and mental illness (National Coalition for the Homeless, 2012m).

Homeless veterans, in particular, have a history of mental illness, with up to 50% of this population affected. Post-traumatic stress disorder (PTSD) is a common diagnosis among homeless veterans, and an estimated 70% have substance disorders (National Coalition for Homeless Veterans, n.d.; National Coalition for the Homeless, 2012j).

In the past, many authors cited the move to deinstitutionalize the mentally ill in the 1950s and 1960s as the cause of increasing homelessness among this population. **Deinstitutionalization** was the process of discharging large numbers of mentally ill persons from mental institutions in an attempt to enable them to live in the least restrictive environment possible. This move was prompted by recognition of the appalling conditions prevalent at the time in many institutions for the mentally ill. Although the intent of deinstitutionalization was laudable, the results were not. Unfortunately, there was no concurrent move to provide the community services needed for the mentally ill to live in noninstitutional settings, leaving them to fend for themselves. Other authors, however, point out that the increase in homeless mentally ill persons did not actually occur until the 1980s, when income and housing assistance programs for this population were withdrawn. Most mentally ill persons do not need to be institutionalized, but they do require access to a variety of supportive services, including housing support, in order to function effectively in society and maintain residential status (National Coalition for the Homeless, 2011c).

Some homeless persons without preexisting mental illness exhibit psychological problems as a result of their homelessness. For example, housing insecurity and frequent moves have been associated with mental health and behavior problems, substance abuse, poor school performance, and increased risk of pregnancy in adolescents (Cutts et al., 2011). Homeless youth have also been found to have higher rates of depression, anxiety, low self-esteem, and conduct disorder than their housed age mates. In addition, rates of PTSD are three times higher in this population than among adolescents who are not homeless (National Coalition for the Homeless, 2012k). Younger children's mental health is also affected by homelessness, and homeless children are more likely than their housed age mates to experience anxiety, depression, and behavior problems.

ENVIRONMENTAL DETERMINANTS. Environmental factors also contribute to the effects of homelessness on health. Exposure to cold, even in the mildest climates, can lead to hypothermia. This is particularly true when people are lying on concrete or are clothed in wet garments. Increased exposure risk for frostbite, immersion foot, and hypothermia occurs primarily in persons who are homeless and living on the streets. Immersion foot, also known as trench foot, occurs when the feet are wet for prolonged periods of time. Although these conditions do not, of themselves result in death, they may contribute to an eightfold increased risk of mortality from other causes (National Coalition for the Homeless, 2012h). Another weather-related environmental phenomenon that has been found to affect migrant farmworkers is the heat index in their often substandard housing. For example, one study of 170 North Carolina farmworker camps found dangerously high heat indexes in most housing units (barracks-style housing, trailers, and houses). High heat indexes in housing units limit recovery from the negative effects of heat exposures during daily work in hot, humid conditions contributing to a high incidence of heat-related deaths in the migrant farmworker population (Quandt, Wiggins, Chen, Bischoff, & Arcury, 2013).

Overcrowding and poor sanitary conditions in homeless shelters contribute to the spread of communicable diseases among a population that is already debilitated by exposure and poor nutritional status. TB, in particular, is rapidly spread in overcrowded shelters (Dobbins et al., 2012; Samuel et al., 2012) and other settings where homeless individuals may congregate. For example, TB transmission in one outbreak also involved two local bars frequented by shelter residents and a local jail, suggesting the potential for spread of the disease to the general public as well as to other shelter residents (Samuel et al., 2012). Crowding in shelter environments is also associated with poor mental health, diminished coping ability, poor parent–child interactions, stressful social relationships, and difficulty sleeping. Crowding has also been associated with food insecurity in shelter residents, particularly homeless families (Cutts et al., 2011).

Another environmental aspect of shelter life lies in the actual physical structure of some shelter facilities. Many shelters are located in older buildings that may have stairs, making it difficult for the elderly and others with limited mobility to access emergency shelter and other services. Access to services in other organizations may also entail long periods of standing in line, which may be difficult for elderly and disabled individuals (National Coalition for the Homeless, 2012l).

Unsafe physical environments also present health hazards for young children. In addition to the potential for physical injury, the restrictions placed by parents on children's activities in unsafe surroundings may result in developmental delays. Prolonged sun exposure and the attendant risk for skin cancer are other environmental factors affecting the homeless of all ages.

Aspects of rural versus urban environments also affect homelessness and access to assistance for poor and homeless individuals. Several authors have noted that even the definition of homelessness "does not fit well with the rural reality" (National Coalition for the Homeless, 2012n, p. 1). Because of the unavailability of shelters in many rural areas, homeless individuals are more likely than their urban counterparts to move in with family members or friends in crowded and substandard conditions. These individuals, however, do not qualify for assistance, and the rural communities that house them are not eligible for federal funding for homeless services (National Coalition for the Homeless, 2012n), leading to a need for a more flexible definition of rural homelessness (National Coalition for the Homeless, 2012f). Based on current definitions, approximately 9% of homelessness in the United States occurs in rural areas, and an estimated 70,000 rural individuals may be homeless on any given night (National Coalition for the Homeless, 2011a).

Even the factors contributing to homelessness differ substantially between urban and rural environments. For example, rural states experience significantly more foreclosures, a frequent cause of homelessness, than urban areas (National Coalition for the Homeless, 2012f). Rural homeless populations are more likely to consist of families, particularly single women with children, with a larger proportion of Native Americans and migrant workers than urban populations (National Coalition for the Homeless, 2012n). Homeless veterans, on the other hand, are more likely to be found in urban than suburban or rural areas (68% and 32%, respectively) (National Coalition for Homeless Veterans, n.d.).

Domestic violence and poverty are also more common precursors to homelessness in rural than urban environments. In fact, rural residents are 1.2 to 2.3 times more likely to be poor than their urban counterparts, and 20% of nonmetropolitan counties are classified as high poverty counties compared to only 5% of metropolitan counties. One third of rural renters (1.9 million households) are "cost burdened," spending more than 30% of their incomes for housing (National Coalition for the Homeless, 2012e).

More rural homelessness is found in agricultural areas and those with declining extractive industries (e.g., coal mining). Paradoxically, increased homelessness in rural areas is also linked to rural areas experiencing economic growth as burgeoning industry and outsiders earning higher incomes create a demand for scarce housing that drives housing costs beyond the budgets of long-time residents.

The greater visibility and population density of urban than rural homeless populations leads to inequities in the availability of and access to needed services, and rural housing needs are often overlooked in policy formation. Even when housing is available in rural areas, it is often substandard, and 30% of nonmetropolitan households experience at least one problem, including high costs, physical deficiencies, or overcrowding (National Coalition for the Homeless, 2012e). In fact, homelessness is often precipitated by substandard housing conditions that make structures uninhabitable. In such cases, relocation to safer housing is often more expensive and beyond the ability of many rural families to afford it. For these reasons, many authors have suggested redefining rural homelessness to include people living in substandard housing, making them eligible for services available to those living on the streets or in shelters (National Coalition for the Homeless, 2012f).

Other contributing factors in rural homelessness include distances between affordable housing and work settings, lack of transportation, restrictive land use regulations and housing codes, rising rent burdens, and insecure tenancy due to changes in real estate markets. For example, inexpensive trailer parks may be replaced by more expensive upscale housing unaffordable to local residents (National Coalition for the Homeless, 2012n).

Homelessness in urban areas brings its own set of difficulties, and some authors have suggested that homeless individuals are "warehoused" in densely populated urban areas. Although temporary shelter and other assistance services may be more accessible in urban than rural areas, there may be a lack of affordable housing and widespread economic distress in the community that limits the availability of work and other supports (Eitzman, Pollio, & North, 2013).

SOCIOCULTURAL DETERMINANTS. Sociocultural factors play a major role in the development of poverty and homelessness and in their effects on health. Lack of affordable housing and available shelter; poverty, inadequate social support and welfare reform; employment; and housing assistance are some of the societal conditions that influence poverty and homelessness. Other considerations to be addressed include education, homelessness among military veterans, domestic violence, mega events and their effects on housing and homelessness, and considerations related to criminal justice, civil rights, and violence against homeless individuals.

Lack of affordable housing and available shelter. Housing is a basic human need. The World Health Organization incorporates four aspects into its definition of housing: house, home, neighborhood, and community. A house is a physical structure or dwelling used, or intended to be used, for human habitation (WHO, 2010). A house, in this context, may include a freestanding dwelling, apartment, condominium, or single room occupancy unit. A **single room occupancy unit (SRO)** is a building that provides single rooms as sleeping accommodations for individuals (City of South San Francisco, n.d.). Bathrooms, kitchens, and other living spaces are shared by tenants in SROs (National Coalition for the Homeless, 2012e). The term "home" encompasses the economic, social, and cultural structure established by a given household. The neighborhood aspect includes streets, shops, places of worship, recreation, green space and transportation surrounding where people actually live, and the community includes those living, working, and providing services in the neighborhood (WHO, 2010). Interventions to address population housing needs must address all four aspects of this definition.

Lack of affordable housing is one of two trends that have contributed to the alarming rise in homelessness in the United States (National Coalition for the Homeless, 2011b). **Affordable housing** is defined as housing that costs no more than 30% of one's income (National Coalition for the Homeless, 2012d). In the United States, approximately

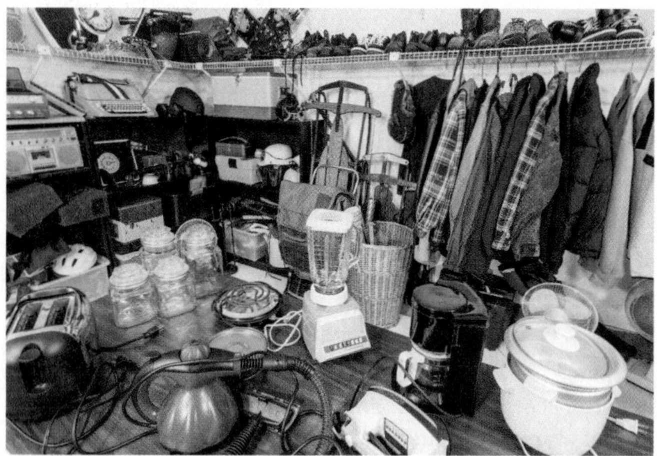

Thrift stores help the poor and homeless to stretch their resources, but still may not meet all their needs. *(rekandphoto/Fotolia)*

6.5 million families spent more than 50% of their income on housing in 2011 (National Alliance to End Homelessness, 2013). Housing costs have escalated tremendously making housing unaffordable for many individuals and families. For example, there was a 41% increase in the fair market rent for a two-bedroom apartment between 2000 and 2009 resulting in high rent burdens—rents that take a large proportion of one's income (National Coalition for the Homeless, 2011c). High rent burden is the result of the lack of affordable adequate housing units relative to the population demand for housing, creating increased competition for available housing, which is worse among low-income individuals and families than those with higher incomes (HUD, 2013). Subsequent increases in the average fair market rents have also occurred. For example, average rents rose by 1.5% just from 2010 to 2011, and the number of rental vacancies also decreased (National Alliance to End Homelessness, 2013).

In 2011, there were an estimated 65 housing units available for every 100 low-income renters and 35 units per 100 extremely low-income renters. From 2011 to 2009, the median renter income decreased by 1.5% whereas the median rent increased by 4.1%. Conversion of formerly resident-owned properties to rental units increased the affordable housing by 3.33 million units, but this gain was offset by the advent of 3.47 million new renter households resulting in a continuing dearth of affordable housing for low-income households (HUD, 2013). In 2009, a worker would have needed to earn $14.97 per hour to be able to afford a one-bedroom apartment and $17.84 per hour for two bedrooms, nearly twice the minimum wage (National Coalition for the Homeless, 2011c).

In addition to low-income workers, the elderly are at an economic disadvantage with respect to affordable housing. The majority of older adults live on fixed incomes and for many, Social Security income, even when augmented by Supplemental Security Income, a subsidy for low-income seniors and disabled persons, is insufficient to afford housing. There are an estimated nine seniors waiting for every occupied unit of affordable elderly housing, and the waiting list for housing assistance may be 3 to 5 years. In addition, households headed by elderly individuals have a one in three chance of being worst-case needs households (National Coalition for the Homeless, 2012l).

Part of the loss of affordable housing stems from **gentrification**, which is defined as a process in which deteriorated low-income housing and businesses are renovated and occupied by higher income individuals (Briney, 2013). It usually involves displacement of low-income housing by higher-income space use such as luxury apartments, condominiums, or office buildings. When gentrification occurs, the ethnic composition of neighborhoods often changes with in-migration of middle-income White families, younger individuals, and couples seeking to be closer to their work. Renovation of older, run-down housing leads to increased rents and property taxes for former residents who choose to remain in the neighborhood. Because of these changes, gentrification may also significantly alter the character and culture of an area (Briney, 2013).

Some authors have described attempts at "positive" gentrification, which often involves the demolition of deteriorating public housing and its replacement by mixed-income housing in which people from different socioeconomic groups buy or rent in the same area. The intent of such efforts is to "deconcentrate" poverty, by placing the poor among others of higher socioeconomic status (Chaskin & Joseph, 2013). Such redevelopment often greatly improves the local infrastructure in terms of open space and streets. It may also result in cultural clashes regarding what constitutes acceptable behavior (e.g., parking cars on the road, accumulation of unused items in yards, and so on) in the reconstituted community (Drew, 2011). In addition, the demolition and rebuilding process forces prior residents to find other housing, and may result in their not returning to their prior neighborhood. In some redevelopment initiatives, efforts are made to enforce inclusion of a certain percentage of low-income housing, but in many jurisdictions, developers can buy their way out of such requirements by paying nominal fines, resulting in many more high-priced than low-income units. In reality, rather than returning to the new and improved housing, many former residents relocate in other nearby disadvantaged neighborhoods. National estimates are that no more than 14% to 25% of former residents return to gentrified neighborhoods. Relocation often disrupts social ties among neighbors, thus decreasing the social capital available to the displaced residents (Goetz, 2010).

Another aspect of the problem is the loss of many SROs, or residential hotel units in inner city areas. Much of this loss is the result of gentrification and conversion of SROs and rooming houses to upscale rentals.

People who are homeless require shelter, and the first step to meeting their needs is the provision of emergency shelter. Shelter, however, may not be available. According to 2012 HUD data, there were 476,119 total shelter beds across the nation in 2012, only 90% of which were available year round (HUD, 2012b). 2012 housing inventory counts (HICs) from

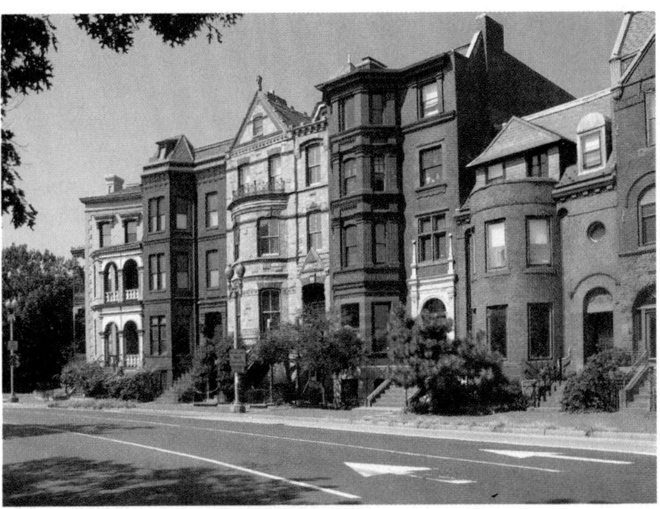

Gentrification of older neighborhoods reduces housing availability for low-income groups. *(Kim Seidl/Fotolia)*

continuums of care, local planning agencies throughout the country that coordinate services in geographic areas, indicated a total of 114,237 units available for families including emergency shelter units, safe havens, transitional housing units, rapid rehousing units, and permanent supportive housing units. An additional 349,277 family beds and 376,318 adult-only beds were available. In addition, slightly more than 28,000 overflow vouchers were available for use at local hotels when other forms of shelter were not available (HUD, 2012a). Despite these numbers, however, on a given night in January as many as 1,740 people could not be provided emergency shelter, and 1,422 could not be provided transitional shelter (National Coalition for the Homeless, 2012b).

Lack of affordable housing and lack of shelter space have led to an increase in the size of the literally homeless population as well as those living doubled-up in the homes of friends and families. From 2010 to 2011, for example, the number of doubled-up households increased by 9.4% (National Alliance to End Homelessness, 2013).

Poverty, social support, and welfare reform. Poverty is the second most major cause of homelessness in the United States, and increasing poverty is the result of eroding employment opportunities and the decreased availability and value of public assistance (National Coalition for the Homeless, 2011b, 2011c). The relationship of employment to poverty and homelessness is addressed later in this chapter.

A large percentage of the homeless are people who are employed, but employment does not protect them from poverty. In 1967, the minimum hourly wage was sufficient to raise a family of three above the federal poverty level. However, the minimum wage was frozen at $3.35 per hour from 1981 to 1990, while the cost of living increased by 48%, resulting in a far from livable wage. As of July 24, 2009, the minimum hourly wage in the United States was set at $7.25 (U.S. Department of Labor, Wage and Hour Division, n.d.). As of June 2014, 22 states and the District of Columbia had minimum wage levels above that set by the federal government, with the highest set at $9.32 per hour (National Conference of State Legislatures, 2014).

The federal minimum wage has not changed since 2009, although a few states have automatic adjustments to their minimum wage rate based on the consumer price index, the local average wage, or some other cost of living formula (National Conference of State Legislatures, 2014). At the minimum wage, a full-time 40-hour-per-week worker would earn $13, 624, which is 25% below the 2009 poverty level for a family of three and even further below the current poverty threshold. A household of that size would need to include more than one minimum wage worker to be able to afford a two-bedroom apartment at fair market rent anywhere in the country. In states with the median fair market rent, a minimum wage worker would need to work 87 hours per week to be able to afford a two-bedroom apartment. Because of high rates of inflation, the real purchasing power of the minimum wage has decreased by 26% since 1979, and the current $7.25 minimum wage is actually worth only $4.42 in buying power. In addition, rising costs for food and gasoline take a greater percentage of household income than in the past, further limiting the funds available for housing (National Coalition for the Homeless, 2012d). The poor simply cannot afford most housing without assistance.

Assistance to low-income individuals and families, however, may not be available or is insufficient to meet their basic needs. In the past, low-income families received cash assistance through the Aid to Families with Dependent Children (AFDC) program. The AFDC program was repealed in 1996 and replaced by the Temporary Assistance to Need Families (TANF) program as part of a sweeping welfare reform program. The intent of welfare reform was to assist persons on the welfare rolls to become employed and fend for themselves. In 2005, however, TANF assisted only half of the families formerly receiving AFDC, and federal appropriations for TANF have not kept up with inflation levels, leading to significant increases in extreme poverty, particularly among young children. In addition, federal support for housing assistance declined by 49% from 1980 to 2003, while approximately 200,000 low-income housing units were destroyed each year (National Coalition for the Homeless, 2011c). In the end, welfare reform was successful in getting many families off the welfare rolls and into paying jobs, but these jobs often do not pay sufficient wages to afford available housing. In addition, there is little assistance to these families for expenses related to work, such as transportation or child care (National Coalition for the Homeless, 2012i).

Financial assistance is available to some segments of the poor population. For example, many low-income senior citizens are eligible for Supplemental Security Income (SSI) in addition to Social Security. For most of these individuals, even the addition of SSI does not raise them above the poverty level (National Coalition for the Homeless, 2012l). Housing subsidies have been shown to assist the poor to remain housed, but many people do not receive subsidies.

Foreclosure is another effect of the current economic crisis that contributes to homelessness. A survey of organizations providing services for the homeless indicated that approximately 10% of their clients were homeless as a result of foreclosure. More than 342,000 foreclosures occurred in the single month of April 2009, an increase of 32% from the same month in 2008. Although one usually thinks of foreclosures affecting home owners who fall behind on mortgage payments, 20% of foreclosures in 2008 were on rental properties, and 40% of families facing eviction due to foreclosures were renters. Many of these families found shelter with family or friends, in homeless shelters, and in hotels or motels, but 26% were reduced to living on the street (National Coalition for the Homeless, 2012f).

A small proportion of low-income individuals and families and some other groups receive federal housing assistance. Housing assistance programs exist for disabled persons and the elderly, as well as veterans, and those in rural areas. Some public housing is also available to low-income individuals and families. Federal housing assistance programs are summarized in Table 21-1●. Unfortunately, these assistance programs may have long waiting lists or lengthy selection processes, and all of them are underfunded to meet the needs of the homeless population. For example, the average waiting period for Section 8 vouchers is 35 months, and only about a third of poor renter households ever receive housing assistance (National Coalition for the Homeless, 2011c). In addition, housing vouchers, if obtained, may not be of much use in areas where low-income housing is scarce.

Employment and homelessness. Unemployment and underemployment are other major social factors contributing to homelessness. Although many people remain employed, there has been a shift in the job market from relatively well-paid manufacturing jobs to lower-paid employment in service indus-

TABLE 21-1 Federal Housing Assistance Programs

Program	Focus	Eligibility/Requirements
Section 811. Supportive Housing for Persons with Disabilities Program	• Small group homes, independent living projects, multifamily housing developments	• Very low-income persons 18 years of age or older with physical or developmental disabilities
Section 202. Supportive Housing for the Elderly Program	• Provision of housing with supportive services for low-income elderly	• Very low-income persons aged 62 years and older • 20% to 25% of funding mandated for nonmetropolitan areas
Section 8. Housing Choice Voucher Program	• Rental assistance through a voucher system administered by state, regional, or local housing authorities that permits renters access to privately owned housing • Recipients find their own housing that meets criteria • Also provides a homeowner's voucher that assists with the purchase of a home by first-time very low-income persons	• Very low-income families, elderly, and disabled individuals • Income cannot exceed 50% of median income of area • Renters pay 30% of monthly income for rent and utilities, voucher covers difference in rental costs
Section 8. Single-Room Occupancy	• Rehabilitation of existing structures to provide SRO units • Rental assistance to meet difference between housing costs and 30% of income • Rental assistance provided for a 10-year period • Provides a single room with communal bathrooms, kitchen, living spaces, laundry facilities, possibly meeting rooms	• Very low-income homeless individuals (income below 50% of area median income) • Renters pay approximately 30% of income for rent, public housing agencies pay landlord the difference in cost
HOPE VI	• Provision of funds to local public housing agencies to destroy and replace or dramatically rehabilitate deteriorated public housing units, including physical and managerial changes and some social and community services • Integration of low-income renters in middle-income areas • Provision of employment support services	• Intensive screening • Agreement to counseling and employment services
Public Housing	• Provision of federally owned and administered rental housing to low-income families and individuals	• Low-income family, elderly, or disabled individual

TABLE 21-1 (Continued)

Program	Focus	Eligibility/Requirements
HOME: Home Investment Partnerships Program	• Funding grants to states or communities to build, buy, or rehabilitate housing units for rental or ownership • Provision of rental assistance for occupants	• Local jurisdictions must contribute 25% match for funds • Income below 80% of area median
Section 502. Rural Home Ownership Direct Loan Program	• Loans to build, repair, renovate, or relocate houses (including mobile/manufactured homes) • Assistance with site purchase and water and sewage disposal arrangements	• Low-income and very-low-income rural families without adequate housing (below 80% of area median) • Able to afford mortgage payments, taxes, and insurance • 40% of funds must be used to serve families with incomes less than 50% of area median income
Section 515. Rural Rental Housing Loans	• Competitive mortgage loans to provide affordable rental housing • Provision of funds to buy and improve land and water and waste disposal systems	• Very low-, low-, and moderate-income families, elderly, and disabled individuals • Renters pay higher of 30% of income or basic rent
Veterans Administration	• Temporary housing funding including emergency shelter and transitional housing, long-term care, and skills training	• Low-income military veterans
HUD-VA Supportive Housing Program	• Vouchers for housing subsidization	• Low-income military veterans
VA Compensated Work Therapy/Transitional Residence Program	• Supervised group home residence • Recipients work for the VA about 33 hours/week and receive salary and maintenance payment	

Data from: National Coalition for the Homeless. (2012e). *Federal housing assistance programs.* Retrieved from http://www.nationalhomeless.org/factsheets/federal.html; National Coalition for the Homeless. (2012j). *Homeless veterans.* Retrieved from http://www.nationalhomeless.org/factsheets/veterans.html

tries (e.g., janitorial work). This phenomenon is referred to as **structural unemployment**, which is unemployment caused by a mismatch between the skills and abilities of persons available to work and the jobs needing to be filled, rather than an absence of jobs. Deindustrialization is a related phenomenon that contributes to structural unemployment. **Deindustrialization** is a shift in economic and occupational structure from a heavy focus on manufacturing to service, technology, and other forms of employment. In structural unemployment, jobs may be available, but those who are unemployed do not have the skills needed to qualify for them. The emergence of high-technology occupations requires new sets of skills that many displaced workers do not have. Such changes in the structure of the job market have resulted in the current relatively high levels of unemployment.

The percentage of homeless people who are jobless varies from group to group. Overall, 44% of the homeless are employed, but many homeless individuals work at low-paying jobs that do not provide sufficient income to meet basic survival needs. Many poor and homeless individuals are underemployed, a measure of those who are unemployed plus those who desire full-time work, but can only find part-time employment. Using this measure, in 2009, 15.8% of the U.S. workforce was underemployed (National Coalition for the Homeless, 2012d). Others who worked full-time remained below the poverty level (U.S. Census Bureau, 2012d).

In addition to declining real wages noted earlier, job security and stability have also declined, and displaced workers may have difficulty finding another job. Even when they do find work, however, many take jobs that pay an average of 13% less than former salaries. People are experiencing more long-term unemployment than in prior years, and the unemployed includes those formerly employed in professional and managerial jobs as well as unskilled workers. These workers often engage in what is termed non-standard work, such as temporary work, day labor, and part-time employment. For example, temporary work has increased by 11% since 1972, but even temporary jobs are being lost, with about 73,000 temporary positions lost per month in 2009 (National Coalition for the Homeless, 2012d). Non-standard work usually does not provide health insurance and other benefits that accompanied many people's prior employment.

Finding employment is difficult for most homeless individuals. Those with mental illness find it hard to maintain a job, if they can get one, because of their instability. Homeless single women with children, who account for almost half of homeless families, have problems of child care while they work. Former prisoners are also at a disadvantage in seeking employment as are young people who often have few employable skills. Similarly, employment is unlikely among elderly homeless people (National Coalition for the Homeless, 2012d, 2012k, 2012l)

Even homeless persons with employable skills in areas where jobs are available may have difficulty negotiating the employment process. Lack of transportation may make it difficult to go to an interview or to get to work when a job is found. In addition, job application and interviews take time, which may prevent the individual from securing food or shelter for the night when these are obtained only after long waits in line in competition with many other homeless persons. Moreover, the homeless person may also find that he or she is penalized for working by reduction or even loss of assistance benefits and publicly financed health care coverage. Homeless individuals who cannot find regular work may engage in day labor or "shadow work." Shadow work may involve selling junk, personal possessions, or plasma; begging or panhandling; scavenging for food, salable goods, or money; and theft, all of which may carry criminal penalties in some jurisdictions.

Other sociocultural factors. Education, veteran status, domestic violence, "mega events," and considerations related to criminal justice, civil rights, and violence are other sociocultural factors related to poverty and homelessness. Education both contributes to and is affected by poverty and homelessness. Many of the poor are from low socioeconomic backgrounds. For example, a third of adults with incomes below poverty level did not complete high school, compared to 29% of those below 125% of the poverty threshold and only 10% of those 150% above poverty level (Beckles & Trumann, 2011). Lack of education results in an absence of employable skills in today's job market, which contributes to poverty and eventually leads to homelessness for many people.

Homelessness also influences educational performance among children and youth. As noted by the National Coalition for the Homeless (2012c), schools provide one of the few avenues for poor and homeless children to develop the skills needed to escape poverty. Unfortunately, the stability of the school environment is complicated by residency requirements, delay in the transfer of records, lack of transportation, and, often, lack of immunization records. Additional problems lie in getting children and youth assessed for special education needs, providing counseling, and promoting participation in before- and after-school activities. Unaccompanied youth also face problems with guardianship and liability. Homeless children are less likely than their housed counterparts to be enrolled in school. An estimated 87% of homeless children are enrolled in school, and only 77% of those attend school regularly. Some effort has been made to promote education among this population. For example, the McKinney Act's Education of Homeless Children and Youth program provides grants to state education agencies to support the education of homeless children, including preschool education. This initiative resulted in a 17% increase in school enrollment from the 2006–2007 academic year to 2007–2008.

Multiple factors, however, continue to impede school attendance by homeless children and youth. Residency requirements to attend local schools, lack of immunization records, delay in transfer of school records, and lack of transportation make school enrollment and attendance difficult. Poor health and lack of food, clothing, and school supplies are other impediments to attendance and good school performance. Although the reauthorization of the McKinney Act in 2001 addressed some of these issues, funding for homeless education programs has not kept up with the need or with the inflation in costs of ancillary services such as food and school supplies. At one point, for example, states receiving funds were unable to provide assistance to 41% of enrolled homeless students. Finally, family mobility due to shelter time limits, domestic violence, or the search for work or affordable housing leads to frequent changes of schools. Students who change schools frequently are nine times more likely to repeat a grade, four times more likely to drop out of school, and three times more likely to be put in special education classes (National Coalition for the Homeless, 2012c), and adolescents with more than two school changes are 50% less likely to graduate than other teens (Cutts et al., 2011).

Military veterans comprise 12% of the homeless population (National Coalition for Homeless Veterans, n.d.). As many as 130,000 to 200,000 veterans may be homeless at any given time, with estimates of 400,000 homeless veterans in the course of a year. As many as three times more veterans experience heavy rent burdens and are at high risk for homelessness. Veterans with disabilities, particularly related to PTSD and traumatic brain injury, are more likely than other veterans to become homeless (National Coalition for the Homeless, 2012j).

Compared to other homeless individuals, veterans are likely to be younger and better educated (National Coalition for the Homeless, 2012j). They are also twice as likely to be hospitalized as homeless individuals who are not veterans (O'Toole et al., 2010). Homeless veterans tend to be found in central city areas (79%) rather than suburban or rural areas (16% and 5%, respectively) (National Coalition for the Homeless, 2012j). In addition to the mental health problems common among homeless veterans, unemployment is a contributing factor in their homelessness. Many veterans are discharged from the military without employable skills useful in the civilian economy making them less able to compete for available jobs (National Coalition for Homeless Veterans, n.d.).

Some efforts have been made to address the needs of homeless veterans. In addition to the programs described in Table 21-1, the Veterans Administration (VA) provides a variety of services to veterans, including those who are homeless. For example, the VA provides health care to 150,000 veterans and other services to 112,000 people annually. In addition, partnerships with community service providers have provided 15,000 residential rehabilitation and transitional beds and more than 30,000 permanent beds, reducing the number of homeless veterans by 70% since 2005 (National Coalition for Homeless Veterans, n.d.). Despite these successes, however, the VA serves only about 25% of the veterans in need, leaving approximately 300,000 veterans without assistance (National Coalition for the Homeless, 2012j). Homeless veterans need a wide variety of coordinated services related to housing, nutrition, health care, substance abuse and mental health treatment, and personal development and job training and placement services (National Coalition for Homeless Veterans, n.d.).

Domestic violence is another factor that contributes to homelessness, particularly among women and children. An estimated 63% of homeless women are victims of domestic abuse and 28% of families are homeless as a result (National Coalition for the Homeless, 2012b). Homeless youth may also be fleeing physical or sexual abuse. Some studies have reported 46% of runaway and homeless youth as physically abused and 17% as sexually abused (National Coalition for the Homeless, 2012k).

Many homeless women and youth have minimal resources and face the choice of remaining in an abusive situation or becoming homeless. They often have nowhere to go. Homeless youth have few employable skills and abused women may have poor work histories and credit ratings as a result of abuse. Homeless women with children often stay in shelters, transitional housing, or permanent supportive housing longer than single homeless men and women because it is often harder for them to find permanent housing. In addition, landlords may discriminate against abused women if they have protective orders in place and may evict families if violence occurs in rental properties (National Coalition for the Homeless, 2012b). Cash assistance, housing, job training, child care, and transportation are some of the needs of abused homeless women with children.

The effect of "mega events" on housing and homelessness is another factor that is often overlooked in an assessment of poor and homeless populations. A special report to the United Nations General Assembly (Rolnik, 2009) highlighted the effects of such mega events in the context of the right to adequate housing. Mega events are large, one time events, often large sporting events that prompt changes in local infrastructure and economies. Examples are the summer and winter Olympic Games and the World Cup of soccer. Such events have both positive and negative effects for the poor and homeless.

On the positive side, mega events lead to the rapid construction of housing as well as improvements in waste management and sanitation capabilities, cleansing of contaminated areas, beautification and environmental upgrading, transportation improvement, and so on. After the event, the surplus housing may be available for local residents. In the interim, however, massive redevelopment initiatives often lead to displacement of the poor and demolition of low-income housing. In many instances, the wealthy developers and governments benefit from increased revenue, tourism, and increased tax revenues, but little of this money filters into programs for the local poor. Evictions are often not accompanied by plans for relocation of displaced individuals and families, and those displaced rarely return to the renovated areas (Rolnik, 2009).

Residents of "informal settlements," such as shanty towns or tent cities, are frequently among the first to be displaced when land is required for redevelopment or construction of enhanced sports facilities. Frequently, these communities are disrupted with community ties broken and people displaced to areas far from employment opportunities or other services. Preparation for mega events also frequently entails cleaning up "unsightly" elements of the city's image through removal and relocation of homeless individuals and criminalization of homelessness. **Criminalization** is the development of laws and regulations and application of criminal penalties to activities such as sleeping on the streets, begging, and so on, that would be perfectly acceptable if performed in private. Criminalization may also affect other activities such as prostitution or sidewalk vending. Offenders may be jailed, and in some instances, may be relocated to large camps with minimal facilities out of sight of event participants and fans (Rolnik, 2009).

Population health nurses may be actively involved in advocacy for human rights in cities where mega events are planned. They and others in the environment should assure that sufficient attention has been given to meeting the needs of the populations most likely to be negatively affected by the event. For example, they should insist on protection of vulnerable populations from forced evictions and on community participation in event planning and decision making (Rolnik, 2009).

Criminalization of homelessness and related activities is only one aspect of criminal justice as it applies to the poor and homeless. Homelessness and lack of basic necessities to support life may lead to crime, as well as prostitution, to obtain money. More often, however, homeless individuals are arrested for actions that, if conducted in private, would be perfectly acceptable. The homeless are overrepresented in jail, and recently released prisoners are at high risk of homelessness due to disruption of family and community ties. Mentally ill inmates have an even more difficult time reintegrating into society and have an even higher risk of homelessness.

Earlier, we saw that the number of available shelter beds is insufficient to meet the need in many jurisdictions. Another barrier to shelter that keeps people on the street and vulnerable to arrest for *nuisance* crimes is the cost of shelter, which may be beyond the means of the most destitute homeless. Fines imposed for *illegal* activities further deplete the money available to homeless individuals for obtaining housing. In addition, mental health and drug courts may also reserve shelter beds for sentencing purposes, further restricting the availability of shelter for many homeless individuals.

Many communities have laws against camping or sleeping in public areas, yet most of these communities lack sufficient shelter beds to meet local needs. Police often conduct sweeps of areas where homeless people congregate prior to major political, entertainment, or sports events, and homeless people are banned outright from some high-income residential and tourist areas. In many places, public parks have been designated as "family" parks, making them off-limits for people without children. Similarly, bars have been placed in the center of public benches to prevent people from lying down on them. Increased policing of gentrified areas and tourist centers effectively removes the homeless from the sight of the more affluent members of the community.

Discrimination in terms of civil rights violations is not the only form of discrimination encountered by homeless individuals and families. In some cases, discrimination in housing markets may actually cause homelessness. Despite legislation to the contrary, Black individuals and families, elderly poor, people with HIV/AIDS, and those with psychiatric disorders frequently encounter discrimination in their efforts to obtain housing. In addition, exclusionary zoning ordinances prohibit construction of multifamily units or high-density housing in many high-income neighborhoods. Requirements for significant acreage upon which to build further restrict development of affordable housing and increase the price of what housing is available.

Discrimination against the poor and homeless, at its extreme, results in violence and victimization in the form of hate crimes. The National Coalition for the Homeless (2012g) identified three types of perpetrators of *hate crimes*: mission offenders, scapegoat offenders, and thrill seekers. Mission offenders perceive themselves to be on a mission to cleanse the world of certain types of undesirable people. Scapegoat offenders engage in violence in response to feelings of frustration with circumstances (e.g., unemployment) that they attribute to members of a particular group. Thrill seekers act violently to derive pleasure from hurting others. The Coalition noted that most violence against homeless persons is committed by thrill seekers, most of whom are young people. In fact, 72% of hate crimes against homeless persons in 2010 were perpetrated by people under 30 years of age and 50% be people under age 20 (National Coalition for the Homeless, 2012g). The elderly and homeless youth are most likely to be victimized (National Coalition for the Homeless, 2012k, 2012l).

Some actions have been taken in many jurisdictions to deter hate crimes against the homeless. For example, several states have added homelessness to their hate crime legislation. Other jurisdictions have initiated training programs for local police in dealing with hate crimes against the homeless and education in schools regarding homelessness. Finally, in some locales, sanctions for intimidation and harassment have been made more severe if these activities are directed against homeless individuals (National Coalition for the Homeless, 2012g).

BEHAVIORAL DETERMINANTS. Behavioral considerations that are particularly relevant to poor and homeless populations include diet and nutrition, rest, substance abuse, and sexual activity. Inadequate nutrition among poor and homeless individuals is a lifestyle factor leading to ill health. As housing and heating costs increase for poor families, food expenditures tend to decrease. One in ten U.S. adults and one in four children are considered food insecure. Food insecurity is defined as a lack of affordable food that supports health (Bruening, MacLehose, Loth, Story, & Neumark-Sztainer, 2012). Family food insecurity is associated with parental overweight, consumption of less health foods, and higher rates of binge eating than in non-insecure families. Food insecure families are particularly likely to be unable to afford fruits and vegetables.

The homeless, even those housed in shelters, rarely have access to kitchen facilities. Some shelters do provide meals, but they are rarely adequate to meet the nutritional needs of those served. This is particularly true in the case of homeless children, who frequently exhibit anemia or serious growth failure, and who often go hungry. The poor and homeless may also have difficulty meeting special dietary needs posed by chronic illness and pregnancy.

Homeless individuals may also have difficulty obtaining adequate rest. Because of increased crime and victimization at night, many homeless individuals may attempt to sleep in the daytime when they are less vulnerable to attack. This further limits their ability to obtain many services that are offered only during the day. The inability to rest frequently places homeless individuals at greater risk for a variety of health problems and worsens existing health conditions. For example, the inability to lie down to rest may lead to venous stasis and contribute to leg and foot ulcers. These adverse effects on circulation are made worse if the homeless individual smokes. Smoking also intensifies the effects of respiratory infections contracted from others in crowded shelters.

Substance abuse is a behavioral factor that may contribute to homelessness when the abuser is unable, because of his or her addiction, to meet, or even care about, needs for shelter. Substance abuse may also lead to expenditure of money for alcohol or drugs that could be used for shelter. On the other hand, homelessness may lead to use and abuse of alcohol and drugs as a form of escape, or alcohol or drugs may be used to relieve symptoms of psychiatric illness. The precise connection between homelessness and substance abuse, however, is unclear. Competition for scarce housing resources may put those with drug and alcohol abuse problems at a disadvantage relative to other homeless individuals. An estimated 38% of homeless individuals are alcohol dependent, and 26% abuse other drugs. Alcohol and drug abuse among the homeless tend to vary with age, with older individuals more likely to abuse alcohol and younger ones to have problems with other substances. Many substance abusing individuals, not surprisingly, put greater emphasis on survival than on treatment for addictions. Continued sobriety is difficult on the streets where substances are widely used. In addition, many substance abuse treatment programs focus on abstinence only strategies rather than harm-reduction strategies that might be more effective in homeless populations. Another barrier to treatment lies in the fact that many treatment facilities for substance abuse do not accept those who are mentally ill and vice versa. Given the prevalence of dual diagnoses in this population, these restrictions make improvement difficult (National Coalition for the Homeless, 2012o). Homeless veterans are particularly likely to suffer from dual diagnoses of mental illness and substance abuse disorders, with 70% being affected by substance abuse (National Coalition for Homeless Veterans, n.d.).

High rates of substance abuse do not explain the overall increase in homelessness. However, substance abuse increases the risk of displacement and homelessness among precariously housed individuals (National Coalition for the Homeless, 2011c). Distinct differences are found in the drinking behavior between high-income (over $50,000 a year) and low-income individuals (less than $15,000). For example, overall binge drinking is more prevalent among higher income individuals, but the frequency of episodes of binge drinking and the number of drinks consumed per episode are higher for low-income persons (Kanny, Liu, & Brewer, 2011).

Smoking is another behavioral determinant that affects the health of poor and homeless populations. According to the Office on Smoking and Health (2014), smoking prevalence was highest among people with incomes below the federal poverty threshold, 29% compared to 17% for adults at or above poverty level.

Sexual minority group membership may be a precursor to homelessness, particularly among young people. Sex trading, or the exchange of sex for money or food, is a lifestyle that may arise as a result of homelessness. Sex trading is particularly prevalent among adolescent runaways who find no other way to earn enough money to support themselves. Sex trading and injection drug use among some members of the homeless population place this group at risk for communicable diseases such as HIV infection and hepatitis B and C.

Homelessness and poverty may also affect other health-related behaviors. For example, homeless children are less likely than other children to have been tested for lead poisoning, but are more likely to have elevated blood lead levels (Kerker et al., 2011). Poverty and homelessness may also make it more difficult for people to engage in health-promoting and illness-preventing activities. Similarly, in 2012 people in poverty were less likely to obtain influenza immunization, pneumococcal vaccine, and colorectal screening than those with higher incomes (NCHS, 2014). For example, people with incomes over $75,000 per year were roughly one-and-a-half times more likely than those with annual incomes under $15,000 to obtain colorectal cancer screening (Rim, Joseph, Steele, Thompson, & Seeff, 2011). In addition, poor women are less likely to receive mammograms and Papanicolaou smears (NCHS, 2014).

HEALTH SYSTEM DETERMINANTS. Health system factors may contribute to homelessness or limit access to care for poor and homeless persons. For example, medical bills for catastrophic illness, particularly for those who do not have health insurance, may catapult individuals and families into homelessness. Catastrophic illness in this population could easily lead to depletion of any existing savings, inability to make rent or mortgage payments, and eventually homelessness.

Lack of treatment services and supportive housing and other services for the mentally ill and substance abusers may also contribute to homelessness. Often, particularly in urban areas, people with mental illness or substance abuse disorders do not receive treatment until they have deteriorated to the point where they are a danger to themselves or others. Such tolerance of deviant behavior prevents these individuals from obtaining help when they need it and when they could most easily benefit from it. Long waits for treatment may prevent individuals with mental illness or substance abuse disorders from obtaining help in a timely fashion and may lead to subsequent homelessness as they become less and less able to cope with life. Even when treatment becomes available, homeless individuals with no contact address cannot be reached and may be dropped from long waiting lists.

More often than causing homelessness, however, health care system factors make it more difficult for poor and homeless individuals to obtain health care and to prevent or resolve health problems. Financial costs are one barrier to health care for this population. In the 2011 National Interview Survey, 19.9 million people or 6.5% of the U.S. population did not receive

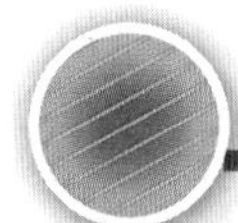

Evidence-Based Practice

Dealing with Homelessness Among the Mentally Ill and Substance Abusers

A systematic review of the literature examining 16 studies of housing and support interventions for people with mental illness who have been homeless indicated that interventions that combined permanent housing, assertive community treatment, and intensive case management support resulted in significant reduction in homelessness and hospitalization, and improved well-being (Nelson, Aubry, & Lafrance, 2007). Unfortunately, many assistance programs for persons with mental illness or substance abuse are predicated on enrollment and completion of psychiatric therapy or substance abuse treatment. More recent studies, however, are indicating that "housing first" programs that focus on providing stable housing for this population without such requirements result in sustained housing as well as reduction in alcohol use and participation in therapy (Tucker, 2012).

Project-based Housing First initiatives provide immediate permanent housing in a single housing project. Despite concerns that such programs enable alcohol or drug use, findings of one study indicated that participants actually decreased their alcohol use. In addition, longer residence in the project was correlated with additional decreases in alcohol use (Collins et al., 2012). Another housing first project resulted in 97% housing retention in the first year and 84% in the second year among chronically homeless individuals with co-occurring mental health and substance abuse diagnoses. Other results included a decrease in psychiatric symptoms and a reduction in the demand for assertive community treatment services (Tsemberis, Kent, & Respress, 2012).

needed medical care due to cost, and another 27.3 million delayed obtaining care. Not surprisingly failure to receive care occurs more often among the poor than the non-poor (13.6% versus 3.7%) (Adams et al., 2012). Similar differences in access to dental care and ability to fill prescriptions were noted between poor and non-poor individuals (NCHS, 2014). For example, in 2011, 12.6 million people aged 18 to 64 years did not take a prescription due to costs. Figures are somewhat lower among those over age 65 (5.8%) due to Medicare prescription benefits. Poor individuals also reported skipping doses, taking less medication than prescribed, using alternative therapies, delaying filling a prescription, and purchasing drugs from other countries (Cohen, Kirzinger, & Gindi, 2013). The latter practice has implications for drug purity and effective dosing. From 2003 to 2012, the number of people who did not seek needed medical care or who failed to fill a prescription increased from 63 million to 80 million people (Stempniak, 2013).

In 2011, more than 10% of the poor, 11% of the near poor, and 4.2% of the non-poor lacked health insurance coverage at some point in the year, and more than 30% of the poor had been without health insurance for more than 36 months (Adams et al., 2012). Provisions of the Affordable Care Act have improved matters somewhat. For example, 48% of people 19 to 64 years of age in 2013 had health insurance compared to only 41% a few years earlier (Stempniak, 2013), but a significant proportion of the population remains uninsured.

Lack of health insurance coverage and frequent moves among the poor and homeless population limits their ability to establish a medical home and to receive health promotive and illness preventive services (Cutts et al., 2011). For example, from 2011 to 2012, roughly a third of persons with incomes below 100% of the poverty threshold had no regular source of care compared to only 10% of those with high incomes (NCHS, 2014). In general, the poor and homeless use more health care services than their housed counterparts, but do so in more expensive venues such as emergency departments. For example, 55% of homeless women, including those with health insurance, reported emergency service use. Percentages were even higher among women with a history of intimate partner abuse (Vijayaraghavan et al., 2012). In another study, homeless children with asthma were more likely than housed children to use emergency department services for exacerbations of their disease (Cutuli et al., 2010).

Some assistance is provided to help homeless individuals and families obtain needed health care. Under the Health Care for the Homeless (HCH) program, for example, more than 740,000 homeless people received services in 2008, but the need far outstrips capability (National Coalition for the Homeless, 2012h). Some homeless individuals, particularly children, may also be eligible for Medicaid; however, enrollment processes are complex, and lack of a permanent address or personal identification may make enrollment difficult. Homeless individuals and families may also lack the expertise or the energy to complete the processes involved in registration or application for services. In 2012, for example, just over half of people with incomes below poverty level were covered under Medicaid (NCHS, 2014).

In addition, health care often takes lower priority than meeting daily survival needs among the poor and homeless. For example, in Toronto, with universal health insurance coverage, competing priorities and barriers like lack of transportation, long waits for services, and feelings of stigmatization and embarrassment were found to prevent use of health care services among the homeless (Hwang et al., 2010). Other problems include lack of personal identification, lack of medical records, fragmentation of services, and lack of continuity of care (National Coalition for the Homeless, 2012h). Lack of child care for other children may also prevent homeless parents from obtaining care for themselves or their children. Provider barriers include insensitivity to the needs and circumstances of the homeless and unwillingness to provide care to those with no means of payment.

Compliance with treatment recommendations may also be difficult. Homeless clients may be unable to afford prescribed medications or may not have a watch to time doses correctly. They may not have access to water to take oral medications, and syringes for insulin may be lost, sold, or stolen. Other difficulties include retaining potency in medications exposed to frequent temperature changes and obtaining prescription refills. Treatment for HIV/AIDS and tuberculosis is particularly difficult among the homeless due to the complexity of treatment regimens (National Coalition for the Homeless, 2012h).

Mental health services for poor and homeless populations are also lacking. Some observers have noted a mismatch between traditional community mental health services and the needs of the homeless population. Comprehensive services are seldom offered at one location, and mental health services seldom address the social factors contributing to homelessness. Availability of integrated mental and physical health services with assistance with social needs, on the other hand, has been found to promote access to behavioral and medical care and foster treatment compliance among the homeless mentally ill and those with substance abuse disorders (Colorado Coalition for the Homeless, 2013).

Population health nurses assess factors related to each of the six categories of determinants of health in identifying the health status and needs of poor and homeless populations. The *Focused Assessment* on the next page provides some questions that can be used in assessing the health of the poor and homeless populations. The assessment tools related to Chapters 16∞, 17∞, 18∞, and 19∞ included in the student resources site can be used to assess the health of poor and homeless children, men, women, and older persons, respectively.

Assessment data for poor and homeless populations may be somewhat more difficult to obtain than data about other, more easily observed populations. Population health nurses working with poor and homeless individuals or groups of people would be particularly alert for commonly encountered health problems. In addition, they would assess individual clients for the presence of any other chronic or communicable diseases, as well as for high prevalence rates for these conditions in the poor and homeless populations. Information regarding prevalent conditions can be sought from health professionals and agencies that care for poor and homeless people. Some data on the age, gender, and ethnic composition of the homeless population may be available from shelter sites and social service agencies. Local churches may also have a sense of the number and types of homeless people served. Local government agencies may also have data on the extent of the homeless population and its composition.

FOCUSED ASSESSMENT Assessing Poor and Homeless Populations

Biological Determinants

- What is the age composition of poor/homeless populations? The ethnic and gender composition?
- What developmental effects have poverty and/or homelessness had on members of the population? What acute and chronic health problems are prevalent? What is the prevalence of pregnancy?
- What is the immunization status of the poor/homeless populations (particularly children)?

Psychological Determinants

- What is the extent of mental illness in the poor/homeless population? What is the extent of depression, anxiety, and suicide?
- What stresses are experienced by this population? How does the poor/homeless population cope with stress?
- What are individual and group responses to poverty/homelessness? To seeking help?

Environmental Determinants

- What are the effects of climatic conditions on the poor/homeless population?
- Where do homeless individuals in the community seek shelter? How adequate are shelter facilities? What hygiene facilities are available to homeless persons?
- Do environmental conditions pose other health hazards for poor/homeless individuals (e.g., flooding under bridges used for shelter)?

Sociocultural Determinants

- What is the community attitude to homelessness? To poor or homeless individuals?
- What is the extent of family support available to the poor/homeless individual? What is the extent of community support available to the poor/homeless population?
- To what extent does family violence contribute to homelessness in the community?
- What effects do education, economic, and employment factors have on poverty/homelessness in the community? What proportion of the eligible poor/homeless population is receiving financial assistance? What proportion of the poor/homeless is employed? In what kind of work?
- What child care resources are available to poor/homeless women with children?
- What education programs are available for homeless children?
- What transportation resources are available to the poor/homeless population?
- What is the availability of low-cost housing in the community? What is the availability of shelter for homeless persons? For individuals with special needs?
- What proportion of the poor/homeless population consists of families? What proportion of poor/homeless families are headed by women?
- What is the extent of crime victimization among homeless individuals?

Behavioral Determinants

- What food resources are available in the community for poor/homeless individuals? What nutritional deficits do poor/homeless individuals exhibit? What is the nutritional value of food available to poor/homeless individuals and families?
- What is the extent of drug and alcohol abuse in the poor/homeless population?
- What is the prevalence of smoking in the poor/homeless population?
- Are there facilities available in the community for homeless individuals to rest during the day? What health effects does lack of rest have on the homeless individual?
- What is the extent of prescription medication use among the poor/homeless population? Do poor/homeless individuals have access to resources to help with medication expenses?
- What is the extent of sex trading and unsafe sexual activity in the population?

Health System Determinants

- What health care services are available to poor/homeless persons in the community? To what extent are these services integrated with other services needed by the population? What is the availability of mental health services for poor/homeless individuals? Drug and alcohol treatment services? To what extent are preventive health services available to and utilized by the poor/homeless population?
- Where do poor/homeless persons usually obtain health care? What are the attitudes of health care providers toward poor/homeless individuals?
- How is health care for poor/homeless persons financed?

Information on the prevalence of specific conditions and immunization status can be obtained in surveys of the poor and homeless population. Surveys of homeless individuals will need to be conducted in places where they congregate. For example, a population health nurse might survey individuals living in a shelter or those who take advantage of community meal programs. Because of the time needed to complete surveys, the lack of resources available to them (e.g., pens or pencils for completing written surveys), and varied levels of education among the homeless population, surveys will be most effective if conducted verbally in the context of other services. For example, the nurse might survey clients as they wait in line at a local soup kitchen or approach them for a few minutes of their time after they finish a meal. Privacy is often lacking in the lives of homeless individuals, and population health nurses should refrain from asking for highly personal information in public settings. Homeless individuals with substance abuse problems may also be wary of admitting these and other illicit behaviors (e.g., theft of food) unless assured of confidentiality. Population health nurses should endeavor to ask survey questions in language appropriate to the client's understanding and in ways that do not imply value judgments. Homeless individuals themselves may be involved in the development of survey tools that address their perceived needs in a sensitive and culturally appropriate manner. Population health nurses can also advocate for the involvement of poor and homeless individuals in data collection and analysis and payment for temporary employment in these activities.

Surveys can also be a mechanism for collecting information on the extent of mental illness and the level of coping skills in the population. Psychiatric treatment facilities may also have data on the number of homeless individuals served and the types of diagnoses seen.

Environmental conditions and their effects on the poor and homeless are often best assessed through observation. What is the local weather and how does it affect the population, particularly the homeless? The adequacy of shelter facilities can be observed by visits to existing shelters. Other places where homeless people congregate can also be observed. At the same time, observations in public places can provide some information on the attitude of others toward obviously homeless individuals as well as on the extent of police activities related to the homeless. Local police records can also provide information on arrests for nuisance crimes.

The extent of family violence as a precursor to homelessness can best be determined by surveys of homeless individuals, particularly women and youth. Police and other protective services agencies are another source of information on family violence. These agencies may also provide information on the availability of shelters for victims of abuse. Shelter personnel can likewise be a source of information on the homeless population.

Educational and employment information can be obtained in a similar manner. Local social service agencies or employment offices may have information on places where poor and homeless individuals may go to seek day labor. Observation and questioning of people in these locations can provide information on the kinds of jobs available and wages paid, as well as potential job hazards faced by the population. Perusal of the local newspaper can also provide a sense of the job opportunities that may be available to poor and homeless individuals. General community employment and economic data may be available from local chambers of commerce or government employment offices. Census data also include this information but may be outdated, depending on the recency of data collection.

Social service agencies and telephone books are potential sources of data regarding child care availability. In addition, the population health nurse can contact local child care providers to determine the availability of care for children in low-income families. Similarly, school districts can provide information on the availability of public preschool programs. School districts can also provide information on the number of homeless children enrolled in local schools, as well as the services available to meet their needs.

Information on shelter availability would most likely be obtained from social service agencies, local churches, or local government offices. These organizations may also have information regarding food resources and other services available to poor and homeless populations. Information on specific nutritive intake, however, is best obtained by observation in shelters or surveys of poor and homeless individuals. Surveys could also be used to determine the extent of health-related behaviors such as smoking, alcohol and drug use, and sex trading, as well as the use of prescription medications. Crime victimization data would be available from local police departments.

General information on the availability of health services can be obtained from telephone directories and the Web, and specific agencies can be contacted to determine the type and extent of services provided to poor and homeless individuals. Emergency departments (EDs), in particular, may have information on the frequency with which uninsured poor and homeless individuals use ED services as a substitute for primary care. Local officials and health care agencies can also be contacted to determine how health care services for poor and homeless individuals are funded.

Diagnostic Reasoning and Care of Poor and Homeless Populations

Based on the assessment of the health status of poor and homeless individuals and populations and factors contributing to that status, nursing diagnoses may be derived at several levels. At the individual client level, the population health nurse may make diagnoses related to the existence of poverty or homelessness. As discussed before, the diagnostic statement includes underlying factors if identifiable, for example, "homelessness due to inability to pay for shelter" or "homelessness due to mental illness and inability to care for self."

Other kinds of diagnoses made at the individual or family level might relate to specific health problems resulting from or intensified by poverty or homelessness. As an example, the nurse might make a diagnosis of "stasis ulcers due to excessive walking and standing and inability to lie down at night" or "malnutrition due to inability to afford food and lack of access to cooking facilities."

Nursing diagnoses may also be made at the population level. For example, the population health nurse may diagnose a significant problem of homelessness in the community. Such diagnoses might be stated as "an increase in the homeless population due to recent closure of major community employer" or "an increase in the number of homeless families due to unemployment and reductions in public assistance programs." Diagnoses may also be made at the aggregate level relative to specific problems engendered by poverty or homelessness, for example, "increased prevalence of tuberculosis due to malnutrition and crowding in shelters for the homeless" or "increased incidence of anemia among poor and homeless children due to poor nutrition."

Planning and Implementing Health Care for Poor and Homeless Populations

Planning to meet the needs of poor and homeless populations should focus on long-term as well as short-term solutions to problems. Planning should also reflect the factors contributing to the needs of the poor and homeless in a particular locale. For example, if most of the homelessness in one community is due to unemployment, long-term interventions would most likely be directed toward improving employment opportunities in the area or increasing the employability of those involved. If, on the other hand, a significant portion of homelessness in the area is due to mental illness and inability to care for oneself, attention would be given to providing supportive services for the mentally ill.

Planning should address the underlying factors contributing to poverty and homelessness as well as their health consequences. For example, providing shelter on a nightly basis may decrease the risk of exposure to cold for homeless persons but does nothing to relieve homelessness. In planning to meet the health needs of individual poor and homeless clients, population health nurses may work independently or in conjunction with other health care and social service providers. When planning to address factors contributing to poverty and homelessness, however, the population health nurse frequently is part of a group of government officials and concerned citizens who have assumed responsibility for dealing with the overall problems of poverty and homelessness. The principles of coalition building, discussed in Chapter 9∞, will be helpful to population health nurses working with others to address problems of homelessness and poverty in the community.

Efforts to alleviate homelessness and its consequences may take place at the promotion, prevention, resolution, or restoration levels of care. Population health nurses may be involved in activities at any or all of these levels. As is true in caring for any client, planning care for a poor or homeless client or population begins with prioritizing health needs. In many instances, the first priority would be obtaining shelter, a measure related to resolution of an existing problem of homelessness. Other health needs could then be addressed in terms of their priority. For each of the health care needs identified for the homeless client or population, the population health nurse would develop specific outcome objectives and design relevant interventions. Planning efforts should be a joint function of the population health nurse, poor or homeless clients, who best know their situation and the kinds of interventions that are likely to be successful in that situation, and other concerned organizations and individuals.

HEALTH PROMOTION. Health promotion for poor and homeless individuals or populations involves the same strategies that might be used with any person or group. Population health nurses might be involved in educating clients or populations regarding good nutrition, rest, and exercise as well as the development of effective coping strategies. At the aggregate level, population health nurses might need to advocate for health promotion services for poor and homeless populations and encourage their use. In addition, they might need to advocate for health insurance and coverage of health promotion services for poor and homeless individuals and populations.

PREVENTION. Prevention strategies for poor and homeless individuals and populations occur at two levels: prevention of poverty and/or homelessness and prevention of illness and injury among poor and homeless individuals and populations.

Preventing poverty and homelessness. Preventing poverty requires the ability to earn incomes sufficient to meet basic human needs, including the need for housing and shelter. Population health nurses can advocate for increases to minimum wage limits to create livable wages. In addition, they may refer individual clients for financial assistance and job training and employment services.

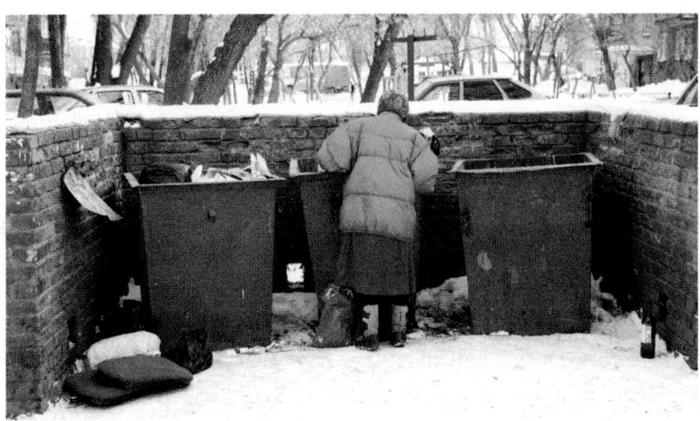

Some homeless individuals may be reduced to scavenging in trash cans for food or items to sell. *(rus09/Fotolia)*

Prevention of homelessness can occur at the individual or family level or at community levels. Population health nurses can help prevent individuals and families from becoming homeless by assisting them to eliminate factors that may contribute to homelessness. For example, if a family is threatened with eviction because of a parent's unemployment, the nurse can assist family members to obtain emergency rent funds from local social service agencies. The nurse can also encourage the family to apply for ongoing financial aid programs or assist the parent to find work.

As noted earlier, some people become homeless because of underlying psychiatric illness and an inability to deal with the requirements for maintaining shelter. Severely disturbed people may just wander away from home and take up residence on the streets. Homelessness in this group can be prevented by referrals for psychiatric therapy and counseling. Case management in the transition from hospital or prison to community may help to prevent homelessness in mentally ill or inmate populations. Nurses may also provide support services to families caring for mentally ill members to prevent these persons from becoming part of the homeless population. Placement in a sheltered home might also be an approach to preventing homelessness in the mentally disturbed person when family members either cannot or do not wish to care for the client. In addition, the population health nurse can monitor the effectiveness of therapy and watch for signs of increasing agitation or disorientation that may precede wandering. The nurse can also assist the disturbed person by giving concrete direction in such tasks as paying rent.

Runaway children and teenagers are another segment of the homeless population for whom homelessness may be prevented through intervention. Efforts of population health nurses to promote effective communication in families and enhance parenting skills may prevent young people from feeling a need to run away. Similarly, efforts to prevent or deal with child abuse may prevent runaways.

Prevention strategies to reduce the incidence of poverty and homelessness at the community level require major changes in societal structure and thinking. Some suggested avenues for intervention include federal support for low-cost housing, increases in the minimum wage, and access to supportive services for the mentally and physically disabled to allow them to function effectively in society. Another suggestion aimed at reducing the incidence of poverty in families with children to prevent their homelessness is to provide child care assistance and paid parental occupational leaves as needed.

Creating employment opportunities and programs to train people in employable skills is another possible preventive measure for both poverty and homelessness. Current public job training programs, however, have been criticized for their failure to facilitate job placement for those who complete the programs. Job training programs directed specifically toward the local job market have been suggested as more appropriate approaches to unemployment. Another societal intervention could be to provide a guaranteed annual income to all citizens. Such an approach is exemplified in part by social insurance programs such as Social Security and unemployment insurance that are not restricted to the poor but available to all eligible participants. Other social programs that may help to prevent homelessness include legal assistance to prevent evictions as well as increased housing subsidies (National Coalition for the Homeless, 2012f, 2012g). Strategies that might prevent evictions and foreclosures or mitigate their effects include counseling to prevent foreclosure, free or pro-bono legal assistance, cash assistance with housing costs, relocation assistance, and purchase of properties by communities for use by low-income persons (National Coalition for the Homeless, 2012f). Changes in housing codes and tax laws to prevent loss of welfare benefits or allowing tax credits in shared housing situations may also be helpful. There is also a need for "discharge planning" for housing assistance for people displaced by building condemnation or renovation or release from prisons and other institutions.

Population health nursing involvement in such activities occurs primarily through advocacy and political action. As advocates, population health nurses can make policy makers aware of the needs of the poor and homeless and can contribute to efforts to plan programs that prevent homelessness. Nurses can also engage in political activities such as those described in Chapter 9∞ to influence policies that help to eliminate conditions that contribute to poverty and homelessness. For example, comprehensive legislation was introduced before the U.S. Congress in November 2005 as part of the Bringing America Home Act (H.R. 4347). Defeated several times, the Bringing America Home Act is being reintroduced. This legislation addresses four main areas of concern: housing security, economic security, health security, and civil rights (National Coalition for the Homeless, 2012a).

Housing security provisions of the act include increasing Section 8 housing vouchers by more than 1.5 million over 10 years, dedicating a proportion of vouchers for special populations such as homeless veterans and youth, authorizing use of surplus federal properties for permanent housing, requiring that federal dollars used for demolition result in the creation of an equal number of low-income housing units, and establishing a Rent Relief Fund within the U.S. Department of the Treasury for emergency assistance to tenants facing eviction. Additional provisions address protection for tenants facing eviction due to foreclosures, providing tax credits for rehabilitation of homes owned by low-income individuals, preventing discrimination by landlords against persons receiving federal housing assistance, and provision of community development block grants to enforce housing codes and provide relocation assistance to people living in uninhabitable dwellings (National Coalition for the Homeless, 2012a).

Economic security provisions of the Bringing America Home Act include establishing a universal livable income indexed to the cost of living, providing the same economic protections enjoyed by permanent workers to temporary workers, establishing training and apprenticeship programs for those with barriers to employment and establishing apprenticeships in skilled trades for homeless persons, repealing statutes that limit SSI income for shelter residents, increasing the allowable asset limit for SSI to $3,000 for an individual or $4,500 for a couple, and providing homeless individuals with access to food stamps. The health security provisions of the act would establish universal health insurance under a single-payer model and strengthen homeless access to mainstream addiction and mental health service programs. Finally, the proposed civil rights provisions would remove barriers to obtaining personal identification for people with no fixed residence, require communities receiving homeless assistance funds to certify that they do not criminalize homelessness or related activities, and add the homeless as a protected category to hate crime legislation (National Coalition for the Homeless, 2012a). Population health nurses can be actively involved in promoting passage of this and similar legislation. For further information about the Bringing American Home Act, see the *External Resources* section of the student resources site.

Population health nurses can also work to promote adoption of sound housing policies and advocate for the creation of more affordable housing and provision of housing assistance for low-income individuals and families.

Preventing illness and injury. Illness and injury prevention strategies may also be undertaken with respect to specific health problems experienced by poor and homeless persons. Here, population health nurses may work with individuals, families, or groups of people. For example, population health nurses working with homeless substance abusers might advocate a program providing clean syringes to injection drug users. If such an approach is not successful, the nurse might provide a simple bleach solution for injection equipment to minimize the risk of blood borne diseases such as hepatitis and HIV/AIDS. Similarly, nurses may provide assistance to families with budgeting and meal planning to provide nutritious meals on limited incomes.

Community-based avenues for preventing homelessness among the mentally ill include providing access to services within the community that enable these persons to care for themselves adequately without institutionalization. Efforts may also be needed to ensure hospitalization for those persons who cannot be adequately maintained in the community. Treatment for substance abuse and secure places for convalescence after hospital discharge might also serve to prevent homelessness in this subgroup.

Also at the group level, nurses may engage in prevention of specific problems by encouraging community groups to provide shelters for homeless individuals. Nurses may also provide basic health care for the homeless, focusing particularly on preventive measures such as influenza vaccine and routine immunizations for children. For example, immunization and other health-related services may be provided in nontraditional settings such as soup kitchens, shelters, and so on. Adequate ventilation, reduced crowding, and use of ultraviolet lights in shelters may also help to prevent the spread of communicable disease.

Another area for prevention of the health consequences of homelessness is adequate nutrition. Population health nurses can advocate for food programs for the needy, including the homeless. They can also serve as consultants to existing food programs to ensure that meals are nutritionally adequate to meet the needs of the population served. Population health nursing activities in this area may also include attempts to arrange diets for homeless clients with special needs (e.g., assisting a diabetic client to select foods from those prepared in a shelter that approximate a diabetic diet as closely as possible).

Population health nurses can also work with other concerned citizens to initiate programs to provide adequate clothing and shoes for homeless clients. Efforts may also be needed to arrange for the homeless to bathe and wash their clothing. In some cities, day shelters that do not provide sleeping accommodations often provide homeless individuals an opportunity to shower and wash their clothing. These shelters may also provide a clean change of clothing on a periodic basis.

Another aggregate approach to preventing specific health problems among the homeless is providing universal access to health care through national health insurance or similar programs at the state level. Nurses can promote such programs through political activity and advocacy and may also be involved in implementing them by providing direct services to the homeless.

In addition, population health nurses can advocate against regulations that criminalize homelessness. They can also campaign for the addition of homelessness to existing hate crimes legislation and advocate for strict enforcement of such laws. Population health nurses may also be involved in educating local law enforcement, youth, and the general public about homelessness to prevent bias, discrimination, and hate crimes against the homeless. Foci and related population health nursing strategies associated with health promotion and prevention for poor and homeless populations are summarized in Table 21-2●.

RESOLUTION OF EXISTING PROBLEMS. Resolving existing health problems among poor and homeless individuals involves addressing both poverty and homelessness. As indicated by the National Coalition for the Homeless provision of housing constitutes "treatment" for homeless persons with health problems, and eliminating homelessness will require the development of affordable housing that fits people's incomes (National Coalition for the Homeless, 2012d; 2012h). Population health nurses working with homeless individuals must first address their priority concerns for shelter and basic necessities before other health needs can be addressed. At the individual level, interventions may include referral for financial assistance via "means-tested income transfers." **Means-tested income transfers** involve the distribution of cash or noncash assistance to individuals and families who meet a test of need based on income and assets. Population health nurses may need to function as advocates to assist clients through the bureaucratic process frequently involved. This is particularly true for elderly

TABLE 21-2 Health Promotion and Prevention Strategies for Poor and Homeless Populations

Focus	Strategy
Health promotion	Promote adequate nutrition Advocate for access to healthy and nutritious foods for low-income and homeless individuals Refer individuals and families to sources of food supplementation Promote physical activity and rest Advocate for the provision of facilities that allow effective rest Promote effective coping Advocate for insurance coverage for health promotion services for poor and homeless populations
Preventing homelessness	Advocate for a livable minimum wage Refer poor individuals and families to sources of financial assistance Make referrals for legal assistance with foreclosures and evictions Advocate for safeguards for individuals and families facing foreclosure and eviction Refer individuals and families for relocation assistance Refer individuals for job training and employment assistance and advocate for the availability of such services as needed Advocate for or refer to mental health or substance abuse treatment services Provide or refer clients to case management services for transitions from hospital or prison to community. Advocate for the availability of such services as needed Promote effective parenting and prevent child abuse and runaways Support the Bring Home America Act and similar legislation Promote adequate consideration of the effects on poor and homeless populations of mega event planning.
Preventing illness and injury	Educate poor and homeless clients for injury and illness prevention Provide or make referrals for preventive services (e.g., immunizations) Advocate for access to preventive services Educate poor and homeless substance abusers for harm reduction Advocate for appropriate ventilation and ultraviolet light in shelter settings Assist poor and homeless individuals in obtaining special dietary requirements Assist homeless clients to meet hygiene needs (e.g., bathing and clean clothes) Advocate against laws and regulations that criminalize homelessness or related activities Advocate for expansion of hate crime legislation to include victimization of the homeless

clients and those with mental health problems. At the community level, nurses can advocate a review of eligibility criteria for means-tested income transfer programs so that a greater proportion of the poor and homeless population is served.

Shelter is an immediate need for homeless individuals. The population health nurse can assist the homeless client to locate temporary shelter. This may be accomplished by means of referrals to existing shelters. If the nurse is not aware of homeless shelters provided in the community, he or she can contact a local YMCA or YWCA, a Salvation Army service center, or local churches for information on shelter availability. When organized shelter facilities are not available, the nurse may try contacting local houses of worship to see if members of religious congregations can provide shelter for a homeless person on a short-term basis. In making a referral for emergency shelter, the population health nurse would consider the needs of the particular client. Ideally, for example, the elderly and women and children would be referred to shelters where they are protected from victimization. Similarly, homeless persons with chronic health problems should be referred to shelters where health services are available and their conditions can be monitored on an ongoing basis.

At the aggregate level, population health nurses can work with government officials and other concerned citizens to develop shelter programs for homeless individuals or families. Avenues that might be pursued include school gymnasiums, churches, and public buildings. Many cities have used these and other buildings as temporary nighttime shelters for the homeless during cold weather. Plans might also be developed for more adequate shelters that provide other services as well as a place to sleep. In designing a shelter program, the population health nurse and other concerned individuals would employ the principles of program planning presented in Chapter 15∞.

For homeless persons with significant mental health problems, it may be necessary to create specialized shelters called **safe havens**, which are secure stable places of residence that place few demands on those receiving help. Many mentally ill homeless individuals are not able to deal with the behavioral restrictions and other policies imposed by many typical homeless shelters. They need a place with limited restrictions that offers the same bed each night, a place to stay during the day, and a place to store their belongings. Because of the special needs of this segment of the homeless population, safe havens do not limit the length of stay for those served. Safe havens then become a stage in clients' progressive movement toward permanent housing in which they can learn to trust and relearn skills needed to maintain a permanent residence while unlearning the distrust required for survival on the streets. Safe havens serve the same function for abused women, allowing them to remain in a secure environment unknown to the abuser where they are protected from abuse by, and often from interaction with men.

Integrated programs that provide shelter with a variety of other needed services have been shown to be more effective in resolving the problems of homelessness, than those that focus on limited aspects of the situation (e.g., the provision of shelter). A comprehensive program for the homeless in Boston incorporates the three core functions and essential services of public health in efforts to address the problems of homelessness in the city. For example, in addition to providing housing assistance and other services for homeless clients, the program has been credited with obtaining health insurance for 75% of its clientele (O'Connell et al., 2010). Similarly, a population-focused primary care approach has been shown to be effective in meeting the needs of homeless veterans. The program provided open access to primary care services as well as on-site integration of housing and benefits assistance, job referral, and so on. In addition to helping resolve the immediate problem of homelessness, the program increased primary care service use and resulted in improved health outcomes such as improved hypertension and diabetes control (O'Toole et al., 2010). Another program that focuses on "Vets helping Vets" provides an integrated set of services in the context of transitional housing. The program includes role modeling of successful coping by formerly homeless veterans and provides the camaraderie previously enjoyed by many former military personnel (National Coalition for Homeless Veterans, n.d.).

Shelters are an emergency resource, not a solution to the problem of homelessness. Population health nurses should help homeless clients find ways to meet long-term shelter needs. For individual clients, this may mean referrals for employment assistance or other services to eliminate factors that resulted in homelessness. At the community level, nurses can participate in planning long-term solutions to the problems of homelessness. Unfortunately, such planning has not often been the focus of community attempts to deal with the problem. Population health nurses can advocate and participate in planning efforts to provide low-cost housing, employment assistance, job training, and other services needed to resolve community problems of homelessness. Initiating these planning activities may require political activity on the part of the population health nurse.

Planning for long-term resolution of the problem of homelessness for runaways involves a different set of strategies. The population health nurse can explore with the youngster his or her reasons for running away from home. Nursing interventions are then directed toward modifying factors that led the child to run away. For example, if the child was abused, the nurse can institute measures to prevent further abuse if the youngster returns to the home, or foster home placement can be arranged. If problems stem from poor family communication, the nurse can make a referral for family counseling or other therapeutic services. The nurse can also serve as a liaison between the child and his or her family, negotiating for changes that make the child's return possible.

Particular care should be taken to involve the child in planning interventions to resolve his or her situation. A child returned to his or her family unwillingly will probably run away again. In addition, such actions on the part of the population health nurse may also destroy any faith the child may have had in health care providers as a source of assistance.

At the aggregate level, population health nurses should alert community policy makers to the need for coordinated services for the homeless offered in a single location to meet the health and social needs of homeless clients. They should also make sure that planning groups in which they participate plan services to address the needs of the homeless for housing, food, clothing, employment, child care services for working parents, and adequate preventive and therapeutic health care services. Planning should also include avenues for outreach and follow-up services, particularly for the homeless who may be lost to service. Such comprehensive programs require changes in health care and social systems that may necessitate legislation and public policy formation that can be guided by nursing input.

Population health nurses can also provide curative services for a variety of health problems experienced by the homeless. For example, they may make referrals for food supplement programs or provide treatment for skin conditions or parasitic infestations. They will also be actively involved in educating clients for self-care. Homeless clients may have difficulty with simple aspects of treatment regimens. For example, if the homeless client does not have access to a clock or watch, it may be difficult to take medications as directed. Nurses can suggest the use of medications that can be taken in conjunction with set activities, such as on arising or at bedtime. As another example, outbreaks of tuberculosis in shelters have been contained, in part, by a new process of a 12-week course of therapy for asymptomatic residents with latent tuberculosis infection as opposed to the traditional therapy prolonged over 6 months (Dobbins et al., 2012). Population health nurses will probably be responsible for such treatment programs for tuberculosis in the future.

The special needs of homeless children and older persons require particular attention. One suggestion is age-segregated shelters or services specifically designed for older persons and families with children to prevent their victimization by other subgroups within the homeless population. Special attention also needs to be given to meeting the nutritional needs of these vulnerable groups as well as those of pregnant women.

HEALTH RESTORATION. Health restoration strategies may be aimed at preventing a recurrence of poverty and homelessness for individuals, families, or groups of people affected. Conversely, the emphasis may be placed on preventing the recurrence of health and social problems that result from conditions of poverty and homelessness. Interventions may also be geared toward long-term maintenance of housing status as well as management of chronic conditions among the poor and formerly homeless.

Population health nursing involvement in health restoration may entail political activity to ensure the provision of services to relieve poverty and homelessness on a long-term basis. This means involvement by nurses in efforts to raise minimum wages or to design programs to educate the homeless for employment in today's society. Advocacy and political activity may also be needed to ensure the adequacy of community services for the mentally ill to allow them to care for themselves or to support their families as caregivers.

At the individual or family level, population health nurses may be involved in referral for employment assistance or for educational programs that allow homeless clients to eliminate the underlying factors involved in their homelessness. Moreover, nurses might assist clients to budget their incomes more effectively or engage in cooperative buying efforts to limit family expenses. Population health nurses may also be actively involved in monitoring the status of mentally ill clients in the home and in assisting families of these clients to obtain respite care and other supportive services needed to prevent the mentally ill client from returning to a state of homelessness. In such cases, nurses also monitor medication use and encourage clients to receive counseling and other rehabilitative services. Strategies for resolving existing health problems and for health restoration in poor and homeless populations are summarized in Table 21-3●.

TABLE 21-3 Strategies for Resolving Existing Health Problems and Health Restoration in Poor and Homeless Populations

Focus	Strategy
Resolving homelessness	Refer for emergency shelter and advocate for needed shelter and transitional beds and permanent housing
	Refer to housing assistance for permanent housing
	Advocate for housing assistance for poor and homeless individuals and families
	Advocate for means-tested income transfer programs for the poor and homeless
	Assist homeless individuals and families to obtain housing subsidies and other services
	Assist in the development of community resources for the poor and homeless, including integrated emergency shelter, transitional housing, job training and placement, mental health and substance abuse treatment, etc.
	Refer homeless individuals and families to safe havens, as needed
	Advocate for affordable housing
	Mediate between homeless youth and their families, as needed
	Advocate for incorporation of poor and homeless people into service and resource planning
Resolving existing health problems	Provide or refer poor and homeless individuals and families for relevant screening services
	Provide or refer for treatment services for existing health problems tailored to the circumstances of the poor and homeless population
	Advocate for the availability of screening and treatment services for the poor and homeless
	Advocate for insurance coverage for needed screening and treatment services
	Refer for treatment of psychological health problems (including substance use and abuse)
Health restoration	Refer poor and homeless individuals for maintenance therapy for mental health problems
	Educate poor and homeless clients for self-management of chronic health conditions
	Monitor mental health status and medication use in poor and homeless populations
	Monitor treatment effectiveness for chronic physical health conditions
	Refer for job training and employment services
	Assist with money management and budgeting skills development

Evaluating Care for Poor and Homeless Populations

Evaluating the effects of nursing interventions with poor and homeless clients can take place at two levels: the individual level and the population level. At the individual level, evaluation of the effectiveness of interventions reflects the client care objectives developed by the nurse and client in planning care. For example, if an objective for a homeless family was to provide them with an income sufficient to meet survival needs, the nurse and family would determine whether this objective has been achieved. Does the family now have sufficient income to provide adequate housing, appropriate nutrition, and other needs? If the objective was to find employment for the mother or father, has this been accomplished?

Evaluation of aggregate-level interventions must also be undertaken. For example, nurses and other concerned individuals will want to determine whether the extent of poverty and homelessness in the population has decreased or whether shelter programs are sufficient to meet the needs of the homeless population. Evaluation of health restoration programs focuses on the extent to which interventions prevent people from returning to poverty and again becoming homeless. Are job training programs effective in increasing the income of participants above the poverty level? Criticism of current welfare programs seems to indicate that such programs do not effectively relieve the problems of the poor and homeless. If current programs are not effectively alleviating the problem, other solutions must be sought; population health nurses must be actively involved in developing those solutions.

One approach to evaluating care for poor and homeless populations is the achievement of national health objectives as they relate to low-income individuals and families. The current status of some of the *Healthy People 2020* objectives for people with incomes less than 100% of poverty is presented below. As we can see from the data, none of the objectives have reached the targets and little progress has been made with respect to many of them. Some of the objectives have actually moved away from the target, indicating that considerable work yet remains to protect the health of the poor. No national objectives have been developed for the homeless population, but objectives related to the poor can also be used to evaluate the effectiveness of care for homeless populations.

Healthy People 2020

Selected Objectives Related to the Health of the Poor

OBJECTIVE	BASELINE (YEAR)	TARGET	CURRENT DATA (YEAR)	DATA SOURCES
AHS-1.1 Increase the proportion of people under 65 years of age <100% of poverty with medical insurance	71% (2008)	100%	71.6% (2011)	National Health Interview Survey (NHIS), CDC/NCHS
AHS-3 Increase the proportion of people <100% of poverty with a usual primary care provider	70.5% (2007)	83.9%	70.8% (2010)	Medical Expenditure Panel Survey (MEPS), AHRQ
AHS-6.1 Reduce the proportion of persons <100% of poverty who are unable to obtain or delay obtaining necessary medical care, dental care, or prescription medications	14.7% (2007)	9%	15% (2010)	Medical Expenditure Panel Survey (MEPS), AHRQ
AOCBC-2 Reduce the proportion of adults <100% of poverty with diagnosed arthritis who experience an activity limitation due to arthritis or joint symptoms	57.8% (2008)	35.5%	61.5% (2011)	NHIS, CDC/NCHS
CDK-1 Reduce the proportion of the U.S. population <100% of poverty with chronic kidney disease	19.8% (1999–2004)	13.6%	NDA	National Health and Nutrition Examination Survey (NHANES), CDC/NCHS
D-5.1 Reduce the proportion of persons with diabetes <100% of poverty with A1c values >9	23.7% (2005–2008)	16.1%	23.5% (2009–2010)	NHANES, CDC/NCHS

Continued on next page

Healthy People 2020 (Continued)

OBJECTIVE	BASELINE (YEAR)	TARGET	CURRENT DATA (YEAR)	DATA SOURCES
DH-17 Increase the proportion of adults <100% of poverty with disabilities who report sufficient social and emotional support	54.2% (2008)	76.5%	NDA	Behavioral Risk Factor Surveillance System (BRFSS), CDC/PHSPO
HC/HIT-6.1 Increase the proportion of persons with incomes <$20,000 who have access to the Internet	43% (2007)	75.4%	63.9% (2012)	Health Information National Trends Survey (HINTS), NIH/NCI
IID-8 Increase the proportion of children aged 19–35 months <100% of poverty who receive recommended doses of DTaP, polio, MMR, Hib, hepatitis B, varicella, and PCV	41.9% (2009)	80%	63.9% (2011)	National Immunization Survey (NIS), CDC, NHS, NCIRP
MDMH-9.1 Increase the proportion of adults aged 18 and over <100% of poverty with serious mental illness who receive treatment	58.7% (2008)	64.6%	60.2% (2011)	National Survey on Drug Use and Health (NSDUH), SAMHSA
NWS-12 Eliminate very low food security among children <100% of poverty	4.1% (2008)	0.2%	2.8% (2011)	Current Population Survey (CPS), Census & DOL/BLS
NWS-13 Reduce household food insecurity in those with incomes <100% of poverty and in so doing reduce hunger	42.2% (2008)	6%	41.1% (2011)	Current Population Survey (CPS), Census & DOL/BLS
NWS-21.1 Reduce iron deficiency anemia among children <100% of poverty aged 1–2 years	19,9% (2005–2008)	14.3%	NDA	NHANES, CDC/NCHS
NWS-22 Reduce iron deficiency among pregnant women <100% of poverty	19.7% (2003–2006)	14.5%	NDA	NHANES, CDC/NCHS
OH-2.1 Reduce the proportion of children aged 3–5 years <100% of poverty with untreated dental decay in their primary teeth	35% (1999–2004)	21.4%	25.3% (2009–2010)	NHANES, CDC/NCHS
SA-8.2 Increase the proportion of persons <100% of poverty who need alcohol and/or illicit drug treatment and receive specialty treatment for abuse or dependence in the last year	16.8% (2008)	10.9%	17.3% (2011)	NSDUH, SAMHSA
TU-1 Reduce cigarette smoking by adults <100% of poverty	31.9% (2008)	12%	29.4% (2011)	NHIS, CDC/NCHS
TU-4.1 Increase smoking cessation attempts by adult smokers	48.5% (2008)	80%	50.8% (2011)	NHIS, CDC/NCHS
V-2 Reduce blindness and visual impairment in children and adolescents age 17 and under <100% of poverty	44.3% (2008)	25.4%	47.1% (2011)	NHIS, CDC/NCHS

NDA = No data available

Data from: U.S. Department of Health and Human Services. (2014b). *Healthy people 2020 topics and objectives.* Retrieved from http://healthypeople.gov/2020/topicsobjectives2020/default.aspx

CHAPTER RECAP

Poverty and homelessness are growing problems in the United States and throughout the world, and population health nurses may encounter poor and homeless individuals and families in a variety of settings. Factors related to each of the six categories of determinants of health contribute to poverty and homelessness and to their effects on health. Population health nurses can provide direct health care services to poor and homeless individuals and families. They may also be actively involved in identifying and collaborating with others to deal with factors that contribute to poverty and homelessness at the population level.

CASE STUDY Preventing Homelessness

An assessment of the health needs of a center city community in a large metropolitan area revealed that the number one concern of area residents was eviction and lack of affordable housing. The majority of area residents are immigrants with limited English capabilities. Housing in the area is generally more than 60 years old and is often in poor repair, not meeting city codes. Housing units, particularly for low-income renters, are scarce, and families are often doubled-up in small apartments. Most rental units are owned by absentee landlords, who give little attention to repairs or elimination of safety hazards. If tenants complain to landlords about deficiencies, they are evicted and new tenants easily found.

Because many of the area residents are refugees from repressive regimes in Southeast Asia, they mistrust government and are afraid to report code violations to the local housing authority. Others, who might report deficiencies, are discouraged by the paperwork involved. The local public health nurse has assisted some residents to file complaints and has begun to take pictures of housing code violations in the homes of many of her clients. She has shared these pictures with the local Community Collaborative, which is working to improve the health status of community members. Lack of functional smoke and carbon monoxide detectors in apartments is a big concern, particularly since large numbers of adults in the community smoke, and much ethnic cooking is done over charcoal braziers inside the apartments.

The community has the lowest mean income level in the county, and although most heads of household are employed, their jobs usually do not include health or other benefits. Part-time employment is common, and even in dual wage-earner families incomes are often still not sufficient to meet basic needs.

Because the area is close to the city's downtown, local developers have begun to buy up deteriorated rental properties and replace them with upscale rental properties and condominiums. Although local housing codes require all new developments to include a certain proportion of low-income housing, developers can circumvent these requirements by paying a minimal fine, which is far exceeded by the potential income from high-income rental units.

Most residents cannot afford to move to other parts of the city because rents would be much higher. Even those who might be able to afford higher rents resist leaving ethnic enclaves that provide them with needed emotional and material support. In addition, residents are close to their jobs and relocation would add travel expenses. Also, a large proportion of the population is children, and parents do not want to uproot them from schools where they fit in and are doing well.

1. What biological, psychological, environmental, sociocultural, behavioral, and health system determinants are influencing the health status of this population? How might these factors contribute to homelessness in the population?
2. What health promotion, prevention, resolution, and restoration strategies might be warranted in this situation? What might be the role of the population health nurse in planning and implementing these strategies?

REFERENCES

Adams, P. F., Kirzinger, W. K., & Martinez, M. E. (2012). *Summary health statistics for the U.S. population: National Health Interview Survey, 2011.* Retrieved from http://www.cdc.gov/nchs/data/series/sr_10/sr10_255.pdf.

Beckles, G. L., & Truman, B. I. (2011, January 14). Education and income—United States, 2005 and 2009. *Morbidity and Mortality Weekly Report, 60*(Suppl.), 13–17

Beckles, G. L., Zhu, J., & Moonesinghe, R. (2011, January 14). Diabetes—United States, 2004 and 2008. *Morbidity and Mortality Weekly Report, 60*(Suppl.), 90–93

Briney, A. (2013). *Gentrification: The controversial topic of gentrification and its impact on the urban core.* Retrieved from http://geography.about.com/od/urbaneconomicgeography/a/gentrification.htm?p=1

Bruening, M., MacLehose, R., Loth, K., Story, M., & Neumark-Sztainer, D. (2012). Feeding a family in a recession: Food insecurity among Minnesota parents. *American Journal of Public Health, 102,* 679–685. doi:10.2105/AJPH.2011.300390

Chaskin, R. J., & Joseph, M. L. (2013). "Positive" gentrification, social control and the "right to the city" in mixed-income communities: Uses and expectations of space and place. *International Journal of Urban and Regional Research, 37,* 480–502. doi:10.1111/j.1468-2427.2012.01158.x

Choldin, H. (n.d.). *Chicago Housing Authority.* Retrieved from http://www.encyclopedia.chicagohistory.org/pages/253.html

City of South San Francisco. (n.d.). *Single room occupancy units.* Retrieved from http://www.ssf.net/index.aspx?NID=319

Cohen, R. A., Kirzinger, W. K., & Gindi, W. M. (2013, April). *Strategies used by adults to reduce their prescription drug costs.* NCHS Data Brief No. 119. Hyattsville, MD: National Center for Health Statistics.

Collins, S. E., Malone, D. K., Clifasefi, S. L., Ginzler, J. A., Garner, M. D., Burlingham, B., . . . , Larimer, M. E. (2012). Project-based housing first for chronically homeless individuals with alcohol problems: Within subjects analyses of 2-year alcohol trajectories. *American Journal of Public Health, 102,* 511–519. doi:10.2105/AJPH.2011.300403

Colorado Coalition for the Homeless. (2013). *Developing an integrated health care model for homeless and other vulnerable populations in Colorado.* Retrieved from http://www.coloradocoalition.org/!userfiles/Library/CCH.SIM.2013.pdf

Corliss, H. L., Goodenow, C. S., Nichols, L., & Austin, S. B. (2011). High burden of homelessness among sexual minority adolescents: Findings from a representative Massachusetts high school sample. *American Journal of Public Health, 101,* 1683–1689. doi:10.2105/AJPH.2011.300155

Cutts, D. B., Meyers, A. F., Black, M. M., Casey, P. H., Chilton, M., Cook, J. T., . . ., Frank, D. A. (2011). US housing insecurity and the health of very young children. *American Journal of Public Health, 101,* 1508–1514. doi:10.2105/AJPH.2011.300139

Cutuli, J. J., Herbers, J., Rinaldi, M., Masten, A. S., & Oberg, C. N. (2010). Asthma and behavior in homeless 4- to 7-year-olds. *Pediatrics, 125,* 145–151. doi: 10.1542/peds.2009-2013

Dobbins, C., Marishta, K., Kuehnert, P., Arbisi, M., Darnall, E., Conover, C., ..., Haddad, M. (2012). Tuberculosis outbreak associated with a homeless shelter—Kane County, Illinois, 2007–2011. *Morbidity and Mortality Weekly Report, 61,* 186–189.

Drew, E. M. (2011). "Listening through white ears": Cross-racial dialogues as a strategy to address the racial effects of gentrification. *Journal of Urban Affairs, 34,* 99–115. doi:10.1111/j.1467-9906.2011.00572.x

Eitzman, B. A., Pollio, D. E., & North, C. S. (2013). The neighborhood context of homelessness. *American Journal of Public Health, 103,* 679–685. doi:10.2105/AJPH.2012.301007

Goetz, E. (2010). Gentrification in black and white: The racial impact of public housing demolition in American cities. *Urban Studies, 48,* 1681–1604. doi:10.1177/0042098010375323

Henry, M., Cortes, A., & Morris, S. (2013). *The 2013 point-in-time estimates of homelessness: Volume 1 of the 2013 Annual Homeless Assessment Report.* Retrieved from https://www.onecpd.info/resources/documents/ahar-2013-part1.pdf

Hwang, S. W., Ueng, J. J. M., Chiu, S., Kiss, A., Tolomiczenko, G., Cowan, L., . . . , Redelmeier, D. A. (2010). Universal health insurance and health care access for homeless persons. *American Journal of Public Health, 100,* 1454–1461. doi:10.2105/AJPH.2009.182022

Kanny, D., Liu, Y., & Brewer, R. D. (2011, January 14). Binge drinking = United States, 2009. *Morbidity and Mortality Weekly Report, 60*(Suppl.), 101–104

Keenan, N. L., & Rosendorf, K. A. (2011, January 14). Prevalence of hypertension and controlled hypertension ? United States, 2005-2008. *Morbidity and Mortality Weekly Report, 60*(Suppl.), 94–97

Kerker, B., Bainbridge, J., Kennedy, J., Bennani, Y., Agerton, T., Marder, D., . . . , Thorpe, L. (2011). A population-based assessment of the health of homeless families in New York City, 2001–2003. *American Journal of Public Health, 101,* 546–553. doi:10.2105/AJPH.2010.193102

Moorman, J. E., Zahran, H., Truman, B. I., & Molla, M. T. (2011, January 14). Current asthma prevalence—United States, 2006–2008. *Morbidity and Mortality Weekly Report, 60*(Suppl.), 84–86

Mosely, M. O. P. (1996). Satisfied to carry the bag: Three black community health nurses' contributions to health care reform, 1900–1937. *Nursing History Review, 4,* 65–82.

National Alliance to End Homelessness. (2013). *The state of homelessness in America 2013.* Retrieved from http://b.3cdn.net/naeh/bb34a7e4cd84ee985c_3vm6r7cjh.pdf

National Center for Health Statistics. (2012). *Health, United States, 2011: With special feature on socioeconomic status and health.* Retrieved from http://www.cdc.gov/nchs/data/hus/hus11.pdf

National Center for Health Statistics. (2014). *Health, United States, 2013: With special feature prescription drugs.* Retrieved from http://www.cdc.gov/nchs/data/hus/hus13.pdf

National Coalition for Homeless Veterans. (n.d.). *Background and statistics.* Retrieved from http://nchv.org/index.php/news/media/background_and_statistics/

National Coalition for the Homeless. (2011a). *How many people experience homelessness?* Retrieved from http://www.nationalhomeless.org/factsheets/How_Many.html

National Coalition for the Homeless. (2011b). *Who is homeless?* Retrieved from http://www.nationalhomeless.org/factsheets/who.html

National Coalition for the Homeless. (2011c). *Why are people homeless?* Retrieved from http://www.nationalhomeless.org/factsheets/why.html

National Coalition for the Homeless. (2012a). *Bring America home act.* Retrieved from http://www.nationalhomeless.org/advocacy/baha.html

National Coalition for the Homeless. (2012b). *Domestic violence and homelessness?* Retrieved from http://www.nationalhomeless.org/factsheets/domestic.html

National Coalition for the Homeless. (2012c). *Education of homeless children and youth.* Retrieved from http://www.nationalhomeless.org/factsheets/education.html

National Coalition for the Homeless. (2012d). *Employment and homelessness.* Retrieved from http://www.nationalhomeless.org/factsheets/employment.html

National Coalition for the Homeless. (2012e). *Federal housing assistance programs.* Retrieved from http://www.nationalhomeless.org/factsheets/federal.html

National Coalition for the Homeless. (2012f). *Foreclosure to homelessness: The forgotten victims of the subprime crisis.* Retrieved from http://www.nationalhomeless.org/factsheets/foreclosure.html

National Coalition for the Homeless. (2012g). *Hate crimes and violence against people experiencing homelessness.* Retrieved from http://www.nationalhomeless.org/factsheets/hatecrimes.html

National Coalition for the Homeless. (2012h). *Health care and homelessness.* Retrieved from http://www.nationalhomeless.org/factsheets/health.html

National Coalition for the Homeless. (2012i). *Homeless families with children.* Retrieved from http://www.nationalhomeless.org/factsheets/families.html

National Coalition for the Homeless. (2012j). *Homeless veterans.* Retrieved from http://www.nationalhomeless.org/factsheets/veterans.html

National Coalition for the Homeless. (2012k). *Homeless youth.* Retrieved from http://www.nationalhomeless.org/factsheets/youth.html

National Coalition for the Homeless. (2012l). *Homelessness among elderly persons.* Retrieved from http://www.nationalhomeless.org/factsheets/elderly.html

National Coalition for the Homeless. (2012m). *Mental illness and homelessness.* Retrieved from http://www.nationalhomeless.org/factsheets/Mental_Illness.html

National Coalition for the Homeless. (2012n). *Rural homelessness.* Retrieved from http://www.nationalhomeless.org/factsheets/rural.html

National Coalition for the Homeless. (2012o). *Substance abuse and homelessness.* Retrieved from http://www.nationalhomeless.org/factsheets/addiction.html

National Conference of State Legislatures. (2014). *State minimum wages.* Retrieved from http://www.ncsl.org/research/labor-and-employment/state-minimum-wage-chart.aspx

Nelson, G., Aubry, T., & Lafrance, A. (2007). A review of the literature on the effectiveness of housing and support, assertive community treatment and intensive case management interventions for persons with mental illness who have been homeless. *American Journal of Orthopsychiatry, 77,* 350–361. doi:10.1937/0002-9432.77.3.350

O'Connell, J. J., Oppenheimer, S. C., Judge, C. M., Taube, R. L., Blanchfield, B. B., Swain, S. E., & Koh, H. K. (2010). The Boston Health Care for the Homeless Program: A public health framework. *American Journal of Public Health, 100,* 1400–1408. doi:10.2105/AJPH.2009.173609

Office on Smoking and Health. (2014). *Adult cigarette smoking in the United States, Current estimates.* Retrieved from http://www.cdc.gov/tobacco/data_statistics/fact_sheets/adult_data/cig_smoking/

O'Toole, T. P., Buckel, L., Bourgault, C., Blumen, J., Redihan, S. G., Jiang, L., & Friedman, P. (2010). Applying the chronic care model to homeless veterans: Effect of a population approach to primary care on utilization and clinical outcomes. *American Journal of Public Health, 103,* 2493–2499. doi:10.2105/AJPH.2009.179416

Quandt, S. A., Wiggins, M. F., Chen, H., Bischoff, W. E., & Arcury, T. A. (2013). Heat index in migrant farmworker housing: Implications for rest and recovery from work-related heat stress. *American Journal of Public Health, 103,* e24–e226. doi:10.2105/AJPH.2012.301135

Rim, S. H., Joseph, D. A., Steele, C. B., Thompson, T., D., & Seeff, L. C. (2011, January 14). Colorectal cancer screening = United States, 2002, 2004, 2006, and 2008. *Morbidity and Mortality Weekly Report, 60*(Suppl.), 42–46

Rolnik, R. (2009). *Report of the Special Rapporteur on adequate housing as a component of the right to an adequate standard of living, and on the right to non-discrimination in this context.* Retrieved from http://www.un.org/wcm/webdav/site/sport/shared/sport/pdfs/Resolutions/A-HRC-13-20/A-HRC-13-20_EN.pdf

Samuel, V., Benjamin, C., Renwick, O., Hilliard, A., Arnwine, S., Spike, D., . . . , Dantes, R. (2012). Tuberculosis cluster associated with homelessness—Duval County, Florida, 2004–2012. *Morbidity and Mortality Weekly Report, 61,* 539–540.

Stempniak, M. (2013). *Affordable care act helps shrink population of young uninsured.* Retrieved from http://www.hhnmag.com/hhnmag/HHNDaily/HHNDailyDisplay.dhtml?id=450006575.

Substance Abuse and Mental Health Services Administration. (n.d.). *Absolute homelessness.* Retrieved from http://homeless.samhsa.gov/Search.aspx?search=absolute+homelessness&tagString=absolute+homelessness

Substance Abuse and Mental Health Services Administration. (2011). *Current statistics on the prevalence and characteristics of people experiencing homelessness in the United States.* Retrieved from http://homeless.samhsa.gov/ResourceFiles/hrc_factsheet.pdf

Tsemberis, S., Kent, D., & Respress, C. (2012). Housing stability and recovery among chronically homeless persons with co-occurring disorders in Washington, DC. *American Journal of Public Health, 102,* 13–16. doi:10.2105/AJPH.2011.300320

Tucker, A. (2012). A roof of one's own. *Smithsonian.com, 43*(3), 14.

United Nations. (n.d.). *Cities of today, Cities of tomorrow. Unit 5: What is wrong with cities?* Retrieved from http://www.un.org/cyberschoolbus/habitat/units/un05hous.asp

United Nations. (1948). *Universal declaration of human rights.* Retrieved from http://www.un.org/en/documents/udhr/

U.S. Census Bureau. (2012a). *Statistical abstract of the United States: 2012: Table 711: People below poverty level and below 125 percent of poverty level by race and Hispanic origin: 1980 to 2009.* Retrieved from http://www.census.gov/compendia/statab/2012/tables/12s0711.pdf

U.S. Census Bureau. (2012b). *Statistical abstract of the United States: 2012: Table 712: Children below poverty level by race and Hispanic origin: 1980–2009.* Retrieved from http://www.census.gov/compendia/statab/2012/tables/12s0712.pdf

U.S. Census Bureau. (2012c). *Statistical abstract of the United States: 2012: Table 713: People below poverty level by selected characteristics: 2009.* Retrieved from http://www.census.gov/compendia/statab/2012/tables/12s0713.pdf

U.S. Census Bureau. (2012d). *Statistical abstract of the United States: 2012: Table 714: Work experience of people during 2009 by poverty status, sex, and age.* Retrieved from http://www.census.gov/compendia/statab/2012/tables/12s0714.pdf

U.S. Census Bureau. (2012e). *Statistical abstract of the United States: 2012: Table 715: Families below poverty level and below 125% of poverty level by race and Hispanic origin: 1980 to 2009.* Retrieved from http://www.census.gov/compendia/statab/2012/tables/12s0715.pdf

U.S. Census Bureau. (2013). *Poverty: Definitions.* Retrieved from http://www.census.gov/hhes/www/poverty/methods/definitions.html

U.S. Department of Education. (n.d.). *McKinney-Vento Homeless Education Assistance Improvements Act of 2001.* Section 725(2). Retrieved from http://www2.ed.gov/policy/elsec/leg/esea02/pg116.html#sec725

U.S. Department of Health and Human Services. (2014a). *Annual update of the HHS poverty guidelines.* Retrieved from http://www.gpo.gov/fdsys/pkg/FR-2014-01-22/pdf/2014-01303.pdf

U.S. Department of Health and Human Services. (2014b). Healthy people 2020 topics and objectives. Retrieved from http://healthypeople.gov/2020/topicsobjectives2020/default.aspx

U.S. Department of Housing and Urban Development. (2009). *McKinney-Vento Homeless Assistance Act as amended by S 896 the Homeless Emergency Assistance and Rapid Transition to Housing (HEARTH) Act of 2009.* Retrieved from https://www.hudexchange.info/resources/documents/homelessassistanceactamendedbyhearth.pdf

U.S. Department of Housing and Urban Development, Office of Policy Development and Research. (2013). *Worst case housing needs 2011: Report to congress.* Retrieved from http://www.huduser.org/Publications/pdf/HUD-506_WorstCase2011.pdf

U.S. Department of Housing and Urban Development. (2012a). *HUD's 2012 continuum of care homeless assistance programs: Housing inventory county report.* Retrieved from https://www.onecpd.info/reports/CoC_HIC_NatlTerrDC_2012.pdf

U.S. Department of Housing and Urban Development. (2012b). *PIT and HIC data since 2007.* Retrieved from https://www.onecpd.info/resource/3031/pit-and-hic-data-since-2007/

U.S. Department of Labor, Wage and Hour Division. (n.d.). *Minimum wage.* Retrieved from http://www.dol.gov/whd/minimumwage.htm

Vijayaraghavan, M., Tochterman, A., Hsu, E., Johnson, K., Marcus, S., & Caton, C. L. M. (2012). Health, access to health care, and health care use among homeless women with a history of intimate partner violence. *Journal of Community Health, 37,* 1032–1039. doi: 10.1007/s10900-011-9527-7

World Health Organization. (1989). *Health principles of housing.* Retrieved from http://whqlibdoc.who.int/publications/1989/9241561270_eng.pdf

World Health Organization. (2010). *International workshop on housing, health, and climate change: Meeting report.* Retrieved from http://www.who.int/hia/house_report.pdf

World Health Organization. (2013). *World health statistics.* Retrieved from http://www.who.int/gho/publications/world_health_statistics/EN_WHS2013_Full.pdf

CHAPTER

22 Care of School Populations

Learning Outcomes

After reading this chapter, you should be able to:

1. Identify the overall goal of a school health program.
2. Describe the components of a coordinated school health program.
3. Describe considerations in assessing biological, psychological, environmental, sociocultural, behavioral, and health system determinants influencing the health of the school population.
4. Identify areas of emphasis in health promotion in the school setting and analyze the role of the population health nurse in each.
5. Discuss facets of illness and injury prevention in the school population and describe population health nursing roles related to each.
6. Describe considerations in resolving existing health problems in the school setting and analyze related population health nursing roles.
7. Describe areas of emphasis in health restoration with the school population and analyze the role of the population health nurse with respect to each.
8. Identify approaches to evaluating the effectiveness of health services for the school population.

Key Terms

active transportation
bullying
competitive foods
coordinated school health program
corporal punishment
cyberbullying
hazard
mainstreaming
mitigation
school-based health centers (SBHCs)
school climate
school-linked health centers
school nursing
sexual harassment

Advocacy Then

Meeting a Community Need

In 1902, thousands of children were being excluded from New York City schools by physician medical inspectors because of communicable conditions such as eye infections, head lice, and so on. A particularly severe outbreak of infectious eye disease led Lillian Wald, founder of the Henry Street Settlement, to offer nurses to treat the infected children (Robert Wood Johnson Foundation [RWJF], 2010). Wald convinced the New York City Board of Health to allow her to assign a nurse, Lina Rogers, to four schools on an experimental basis. Rogers began her work in October of 1902 and was responsible for the health of 10,000 students across the four schools (Hanink, n.d.). The experiment was so successful that Rogers was given an official appointment by the Board of Health in November 1902, and by December another 12 school nurses had been appointed with Rogers serving as the Superintendent of School Nurses.

In the month prior to Rogers's initial appointment, 10,567 children were excluded from school for health reasons. In the same month the following year, only 1,101 students were excluded (RWJF, 2010). As noted by Rogers, "a sensible nurse, with good judgment, discretion, and enthusiasm, may be a powerful factor in the general improvement of a community" (Rogers, as quoted in Hanink, n.d., p. 1). School nursing services based on the New York City model were soon initiated in multiple cities across the nation.

Advocacy Now

American Association of the Deaf-Blind: Achieving Maximum Potential

Individuals with disabilities often require specific services and support for learning. The American Association of the Deaf-Blind (AADB) is a self-advocacy group comprising deaf-blind Americans and their supporters that advocates for conditions that promote the independence and productivity of deaf-blind people and their full integration into society (AADB, 2012). The organization provides information, referral, and technical assistance related to deaf-blindness focusing on such areas as technology support and interpreter support.

In 2009, AADB sponsored advocacy training for a group of young deaf-blind adults. Group participants identified key legislative issues related to deaf-blind issues, researched the issue, and spoke with legislators and legislative assistants to acquaint them with these issues. They also met with President Barack Obama to discuss technological and educational issues for this population (AADB, 2009).

In 2011, 83 million people 3 years of age and older in the United States were enrolled in school. This figure included 5 million nursery school children, 4 million children in kindergarten, 33 million students in grades 1 through 8, 17 million high school students (grades 9 through 12), and 24 million people in college (Davis & Bauman, 2013). The 50 million children in elementary and secondary schools spend a minimum of 6 hours a day in school settings year in and year out, making the school an obvious place to educate people for healthier lives (Division of Adolescent and School Health [DASH], 2011).

The relationship between health and education is a reciprocal one. Health influences one's ability to learn, and health-related factors may result in poor school performance. By the same token, poor educational achievement contributes to poverty and increased health risks. In addition, one's education affects the ability to engage in healthful behaviors (DASH, 2013f). Approximately one third of U.S. students do not graduate from high school, and failure to graduate contributes to lifelong health risks and increased costs. In addition, students who do not graduate are less likely than others to be employed and have health insurance; they are also likely to earn lower salaries. Adolescent pregnancy is particularly associated with failure to earn a high school diploma, with only half of teenage mothers earning their diploma by age 22 (Center for School, Health and Education, 2011).

Schools with effective health programs can capitalize on existing resources to improve the health of the community, and school curricula, policies, and environments can promote healthy behaviors and attitudes for later life. In fact, school health is now seen as a critical component of international efforts to achieve the goal of education for all (Bundy, 2011).

In a 2010, the Health Resources and Services Administration reported that 73,697 registered nurses provided care to students across the United States (NASN, 2014). Most of these school nurses are population health nurses practicing in school settings. Given their population health preparation, school nurses retain their concern for the health of the overall population and apply the principles of population health nursing to the needs of the overall community as well as to the needs of the school population. This multilevel approach reflects the original public health nursing model espoused by the nation's first school nurses. In this model, school nurses cared for individual children during the school day, but engaged in home visits to families and provided health education and health services after school hours and during school vacations (Hawkins & Watson, 2010).

The importance of the school health program as an avenue for improving the health of the population is evident in the number of national health objectives for the year 2020 that reflect health measures in schools. A number of these objectives are directed toward improving the health of young people and target school settings for their achievement. Several of these objectives are addressed later in this chapter.

Historical Perspectives

School nursing is one of several traditional roles for population health nurses. It originated in the United States with compulsory school attendance and a concern for the number of children being excluded from school because of communicable diseases. Health activities in schools were initiated in New York City in 1897, when 150 physicians were hired to inspect students for communicable diseases for 1 hour per

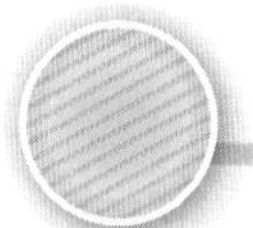

Global Perspectives

Fostering Education for All

In 1990, the World Conference on Education for All adopted the "World Declaration on Education for All: Meeting Basic Learning Needs" in Jomtien, Thailand. The declaration is a commitment to achieving basic education for all people throughout the world (World Conference on Education for All, 1990). In 2000, the World Education Forum expanded on the declaration, creating an action plan laid out in the "Dakar Framework—Education for All: Meeting Our Collective Commitments." The Dakar Framework included six fundamental goals for education throughout the world:

- Expanding and improving comprehensive early childhood care and education, especially for the most vulnerable and disadvantaged children;
- Ensuring that by 2015 all children, particularly girls, children in difficult circumstances, and those belonging to ethnic minorities, have access to complete, free, and compulsory primary education of good quality;
- Ensuring that the learning needs of all young people and adults are met through equitable access to appropriate learning and life-skills programmes;
- Achieving a 50% improvement in levels of adult literacy by 2015, especially for women, and equitable access to basic and continuing education for all adults;
- Eliminating gender disparities in primary and secondary education by 2005, and achieving gender equality in education by 2015, with a focus on ensuring girls' full and equal access to and achievement in basic education of good quality;
- Improving all aspects of the quality of education and ensuring excellence of all so that recognized and measurable learning outcomes are achieved by all, especially in literacy, numeracy, and essential life skills. (World Education Forum, 2000, p. ii)

More recently, world leaders have recognized the inextricable interrelationships between health and educational achievement. As noted in the report, Rethinking School Health: A Key Component of Education for All, effective education of children can only occur if they are ready and able to learn (Bundy, 2011). Children's health profoundly influences both readiness and ability to learn. The report suggests school health programs as efficient and inexpensive mechanisms to improve children's health status and educational achievement, and recommends providing health services in schools related to nutrition and treatment for common conditions that affect children's ability to learn. Treatment might include therapy for worm infestation, correction of vision problems, and resolution of other health problems affecting children's learning ability (Bundy, 2011). Both nationally and globally, educators and health care providers need to recognize and capitalize on the opportunity to improve the health of the overall population offered by educational institutions. At the same time, the reciprocal realization of the influence of health on learning needs to be addressed by adequate levels of health care for school populations.

day (Hanink, n.d.). Children who were found to have communicable diseases or parasitic infestations such as head lice were sent home. Because they received no treatment for their conditions, these children were excluded from school for extended periods of time and continued to serve as reservoirs of infection for friends and family members still in school (Hawkins & Watson, 2010). As noted above, Lillian Wald assigned nurses from the Henry Street Settlement to four New York City schools in a pilot project in school nursing. During that first year, the number of school exclusions declined 90%.

Similar events were occurring elsewhere as well. In 1901, the Chicago Board of Education asked the Visiting Nurses Association to send nurses to visit crippled children in four city schools. In 1905, Jane Adams, founder of Hull House (a settlement house similar to Henry Street, although without a specific nursing focus) provided school nurses for a 10-week trial in Chicago public schools. Again, the success of the trial led to a formalized school nurse role in Chicago in 1908, and employment of school nurses shifted to the Chicago Board of Health in 1910 (Hawkins & Watson, 2010).

Early responsibilities of school nurses included care of sick children, identification of disabilities that made learning difficult, visits to families, and health promotion and illness prevention education. School nurses also provided first-aid services and checked students for head lice and other ailments (Hanink, n.d.; Hawkins & Watson, 2010). Some nurses also provided well-child and prenatal services. In fact, one nurse even initiated sex education in the school, which was accepted by area residents because of the trust they placed in her. As noted earlier, this trust was built by the incorporation of a public health nursing model with services to the larger community as well as students in the school. Because the nurse was well known to members of the community, her intervention was accepted without protest (Hawkins & Watson, 2010).

The potential of schools as avenues for promoting health and dealing with social ills was recognized considerably earlier than the advent of specific health-related services in the school setting. For example, Benjamin Franklin advocated physical exercise as part of the school curriculum, and the report of the Massachusetts Sanitary Commission emphasized the importance of health education and the role of schools in providing it. In 1870, smallpox vaccination was required for school entry as a means of increasing immunization levels in the population, and in 1899 Connecticut made vision screening of schoolchildren mandatory.

Early school nursing focused on preventing the spread of communicable disease and treating ailments related to compulsory school attendance. By the 1930s, however, the focus had shifted to preventive and promotive activities, including case finding, integration of health concepts into school curricula, and maintenance of a healthful school environment. Treatment of any health problems by the nurse was discouraged to prevent infringement on the private medical sector.

School health nurses, dissatisfied with such a minimal role, continued to provide clandestine diagnostic services and treatment of minor ailments in addition to engaging in classroom teaching related to health. More recently, school nurses have begun to return to activities related to the diagnosis and treatment of health problems. Several factors account for current changes in the school nurse role. Among these is the number of families of school-age children in which both parents work. In these families, neither parent may have time to deal with their children's routine health problems. Other factors include increasing student diversity, higher incidence of mental health problems in school-age children, lack of access to care, and homelessness.

Mainstreaming is another major influence on the current role of school nurses in the United States. **Mainstreaming** is the practice of integrating children with serious illnesses or handicapping conditions in regular school settings and classrooms whenever possible. According to the Federal Register (Rules and Regulations, 2006), Section 300.101(c) of the Individuals with Disabilities Education Act specified that "a free appropriate public education (FAPE) must be available to any individual child with a disability who needs special education and related services" (p. 46541).

Mainstreaming has created some difficulties for school health nurses. They now spend a considerable portion of their time caring for children with special needs, which may decrease the time available to meet the needs of other children in the school setting. Population health nurses in school settings may need to advocate for a balance between caring for the special-needs population and other children. They may also need to advocate for effective funding, personnel, facilities, and equipment to provide health care for children with special needs.

The School Health Team

Health problems identified in individual children or in the community served by the school are frequently beyond the capabilities of the population health nurse acting independently. To meet the needs of the school population and the community, the school health nurse often needs to participate as a member of a team. Here we will discuss the school nurse as a member of the team as well as other typical school health team members.

The School Nurse

The National Association of School Nurses (NASN) has defined **school nursing** as specialized area of practice that fosters the health of students as well as their academic achievement (NASN, 2011b). The five main components of the school nurse's role, as defined by NASN, include facilitating normal development, promoting student health and safety and a healthy school environment, providing quality care for potential and identified health problems, providing case management services based on sound clinical judgment, and collaborating with others to enhance student and family capabilities (NASN, 2011b).

The California Commission on Teacher Credentialing (2012), which credentials nurses for school nursing practice as required in the state, indicates that school nurses are authorized by state law to perform the following functions:

- Conduct immunization programs
- Assess the health and developmental status of students and interpret assessment findings
- Interpret health and developmental assessments to parents, teachers, administrators, and others
- Design and implement individual school health maintenance plans
- Refer students, parents, or guardians to needed community resources
- Maintain communication to promote needed treatment
- Interpret medical and nursing findings
- Consult with, conduct in-service training for, and serve as a resource person for school personnel;
- Develop and implement the school health education curriculum and participate in health instruction
- Counsel and assist students and parents in health-related adjustments, and
- Teach health-related subjects under the supervision of a classroom teacher

Additional functions of school nurses in carrying out the designated roles include providing episodic care, management of chronic illness, communicable disease surveillance, health promotion, first-aid and emergency care, screening for a variety of health conditions, administering medications, and preparing for and responding to school and community emergencies (RWJF, 2010). Nurses in specific schools may take on additional roles and functions depending on local needs. A scope and standards statement for school nursing has been developed by NASN and the American Nurses Association (2011). For further information about the standards, see the *External Resources* section of the student resources site.

Unfortunately, approximately half of U.S. schools lack a full-time school nurse (RWJF, 2010). In keeping with the *Healthy People 2020* objectives, NASN (2012a) has recommended nurse-to-student ratios of one nurse to every 750 students in the general population. Ratios decrease for school populations with students who require more intensive nursing care. Suggested ratios are depicted in Table 22-1●.

Preparation for school nursing should include a minimum of a baccalaureate degree in nursing due to the need for autonomous practice and the advanced skills needed to meet the needs of school children with complex conditions. In addition to the recommendation for a baccalaureate degree, NASN supports state school nurse certification requirements and encourages national certification. As noted by NASN (2012b),

TABLE 22-1 Recommended School Nurse to Student Ratios

Recommended Ratio	School Population
1:750	General student population
1:225	Populations of students that may require daily professional service or intervention
1:125	Populations of students with complex health care needs
1:1	Individual students who require daily and continuous professional nursing services

Data from: National Association of School Nurses. (2012a). *Chronic health conditions managed by school nurses.* Retrieved from http://www.nasn.org/Portals/0/positions/2012pschronic.pdf

certification provides recognition of an advanced level of practice in a particular specialty.

State certification may require postbaccalaureate education for school nursing, and requirements vary from state to state. For example, California requires that a school nurse hold a state-issued School Nurse Services Credential. School nurses can obtain a preliminary credential after graduation from a bachelor's or higher degree program in nursing and becoming registered as a nurse in California. Nurses must obtain a "clear" credential within 5 years. The clear credential requires 2 years of experience as a school nurse and successful completion of a state-approved school nurse education program, often at the master's level. The preliminary credential is not renewable, but the clear credential must be renewed every 5 years after meeting practice and continuing education requirements (California Commission on Teacher Credentialing, 2012).

National certification is obtained through the National Board for Certification of School Nurses (NBCSN). Certification requirements include appropriate state RN licensure, 1,000 hours of clinical practice as a school nurse, and successful completion of the certification examination. Elements of the examination address health appraisal, health problems and nursing management, health promotion and disease prevention, special health issues in school settings, and professional issues related to school nursing (NBCSN, 2013). For further information on national certification as a school nurse, see the *External Resources* section of the student resources site.

Other Team Members

Because identified health problems may be the consequence of factors beyond the control of health care professionals, the school health team often consists of a variety of individuals, not all of whom have a health or medical background. The team acts to design a school health program that meets the health needs of students and of the larger community.

The school health team should use the group development strategies discussed in Chapter 10∞ to create an effective team that can address the health needs of the school population and surrounding community. One of the critical features of group development for the school health team is negotiating member roles. Group members should clarify for themselves the roles that each will play so that infringement on anyone's professional territory is avoided.

Specific members of the team will vary with the identified needs of the population, but some of those who may be involved, in addition to the nurse, are parents, teachers, administrators, counselors, psychologists, social workers, physicians and dentists, a health coordinator, food service personnel, janitorial and secretarial staff members, public health officials and other public officials, and students. Additional team members in some school settings include nurse practitioners; unlicensed assistive personnel (UAPs); physical, occupational, and respiratory therapists; and speech pathologists. If unlicensed assistive personnel provide health services in the school setting (e.g., to assist in the care of students with special needs), the school nurse is responsible for delegating appropriate activities and supervising their performance. The school nurse may also assist in educating UAPs for activities as warranted. For example, the nurse may educate a parent volunteer about positioning a child with limited mobility to prevent pressure ulcers or suctioning a child with a tracheostomy. In educating UAPs, the school nurse would be sure to emphasize when the nurse or other provider needs to be notified of changes in a child's condition. The nurse may also educate other school personnel or volunteers in routine first-aid and other simple health-related procedures (e.g., taking a temperature, assisting with height and weight screening).

Parents, of course, have the primary responsibility for the health of their children. With respect to the school health program, parents have a responsibility to reinforce health teaching at home and to follow up on referrals for assistance with health problems identified in their children. They should also provide input into the planning and evaluation of the school health program. Parents may also provide volunteer services for first aid or "sick room duty" when there is not a nurse employed full time. Population health nurses working in school settings may need to advocate for parent involvement in the development and design of school health services as well as evaluation of their effectiveness.

Teachers have a variety of responsibilities for the health of their students, such as motivating students in the development of good health habits, encouraging student responsibility for health, and observing students for signs of health problems. Teachers also have a responsibility to model healthy behavior and provide health instruction. Other responsibilities include assisting with screening efforts and measures to control the spread of disease and helping to identify factors in the physical, psychological, and social environments that are detrimental to the health status of students and coworkers. In addition, teachers may counsel students with health problems and may make referrals for assistance as appropriate.

School administrators include principals, district superintendents, and school board members. Administrators are responsible for the implementation of the school health program and should provide both material and nonmaterial support. They also function as liaisons between the school and the larger community. In collaboration with other team members, administrators participate in planning and evaluating the school health program. Other administrative responsibilities include hiring and evaluating health service employees and fostering collegial relationships among school health team members. Finally, administrators have the ultimate responsibility for the creation of a healthy and safe environment.

Some schools employ counselors, psychologists, or social workers or contract for their services as consultants. Counselors may provide emotional counseling or assistance to students in career decisions. Psychologists may also be involved in counseling for emotional problems. In addition, they may conduct psychological testing on selected youngsters to identify emotional problems or learning disabilities, or they may be called on to administer tests of school readiness to incoming children. Social workers may likewise counsel students regarding problems and may provide referrals for students and families to assist with socioeconomic problems. When the services of these specialists are not available in a particular school setting, many of these functions may be assumed by the school nurse, if he or she is educationally prepared to carry them out, or the nurse might make a referral to an outside source of assistance.

Physicians and dentists usually are not employed by a school system, but they may provide services on a contract or referral basis. Under a contractual arrangement, physicians and dentists may spend a certain amount of time in the school assessing health and dental needs or making treatment recommendations. In other instances, students may be referred to their own physicians or dentists for follow-up treatment of identified health problems. Physical, occupational, or respiratory therapists may be employed in some school systems that provide comprehensive health services or may serve as outside consultants in the care of individual children. School systems may also have similar kinds of interactions with speech pathologists.

The school nurse may function as the school's health coordinator, or the school health team may include a health coordinator who is not a nurse. The health coordinator may be a parent, teacher, or other person with some health-related preparation. Responsibilities of the health coordinator include serving as a liaison with families and with the community, arranging in-service education for staff, facilitating team relationships, and coordinating the health instruction program. Other areas of responsibility include planning for speakers on health topics, arranging health-related learning experiences such as field trips or health fairs, and reviewing materials for use in health education.

In schools where meals are provided, food service personnel are responsible for preparing and serving nutritious meals. They may also be responsible for planning menus, depending on their background and knowledge of the nutritional needs of school-age children. School nurses may provide consultation on healthy diets appropriate to the age of children in a particular school. They may also need to advocate for the availability of foods to meet special dietary needs of children with specific health conditions (e.g., diabetes, difficulty swallowing).

The janitorial staff is usually responsible for maintenance of the physical environment. Remediation of physical health hazards usually comes under their jurisdiction as well. They also ensure the cleanliness of kitchen and sanitary facilities to prevent the transmission of disease.

Clerical personnel are responsible for maintaining student records and for processing family notification of screening test results and recommendations. They may also be responsible for notifying families in the case of student injury or illness.

Public health officials are not employed by the school, but still form part of the school health team in that they are responsible for inspection of school sanitation, cooking facilities, and immunization status. They also act to establish local health policy related to schools and other institutions and to safeguard the health of the overall community. Other public officials may also be involved in planning a school health program to meet the needs of the school's population. Fire or police personnel might be involved, for example, in designing safety education programs for children and their parents.

In older age groups, students within the school may also be part of the school health team. Student responsibilities include helping to maintain a healthful and safe environment and providing input regarding student health needs and planning to meet those needs. Older students should also be involved in evaluating the effectiveness of the school health program.

Population Health Nursing and Care of School Populations

Population health nurses working in school settings apply the nursing process to the care of individual students and their families, to the school population, and to the larger community. In the remainder of this chapter, we will explore the application of the nursing process to nursing care in school settings.

Assessing the Health of School Populations

Use of the nursing process in the school setting begins with an assessment of health needs. The school nurse may assess the health status and needs of individual students or of the school population. In this chapter, we focus on assessing the health needs of the school population and identifying the factors influencing those needs. Areas for consideration include biological, psychological, environmental, sociocultural, behavioral, and health system determinants that influence the health of the school population.

BIOLOGICAL DETERMINANTS. Areas for consideration related to the biological determinants of health include maturation and aging as they affect health and health behaviors, genetic inheritance, and physiologic function.

Maturation and aging. School nurses work with students in preschool, elementary school, junior high and high school, and college and university settings. Consequently, the age of the client population influences the types of health problems that may be present. For example, prevention of childhood communicable diseases would receive greater emphasis in the preschool population, and sexuality issues and substance abuse would be of greater concern with adolescent populations. For college students, substance abuse and sexuality issues are also pertinent, as are stress-related problems stemming from academic pressures and being away from home.

Client maturation also influences the content and process of the health education component of the school health program. Basic hygiene conveyed via cartoon films is appropriate to the preschool or early elementary-age child; a frank discussion of sexuality and sexually transmitted diseases is appropriate with older groups of schoolchildren.

Genetic inheritance. Aspects of genetic inheritance of particular interest to the school nurse are the gender and racial or ethnic composition of the population. A predominance of females in a preschool or an elementary school increases the frequency with which the nurse will encounter students with symptoms of urinary tract infection as these are more common in girls than boys in all age groups except infants. In adolescent girls, there is increased risk of unwanted pregnancy, and sexually transmitted diseases are common among both girls and boys. Boys of all ages tend to have more sports-related injuries with which the nurse must deal.

The racial and ethnic composition of the school population also influences the types of health problems encountered. For example, in schools with large African American populations, sickle cell screening might be included as a routine part of the school health program. The nurse must also be alert to the prevalence of other diseases that exhibit genetic predispositions, such as thalassemia and diabetes.

Physiologic function. An important aspect of the human biological component of the assessment is the physiologic function of the school population. School nurses may encounter students or staff with self-limiting health problems or chronic conditions that affect their abilities to function effectively in the school setting.

Examples of self-limiting conditions include communicable diseases such as the common cold, influenza, and chickenpox and injuries such as a fractured arm or leg. Diabetes, seizure disorders, and minor visual or hearing problems are examples of chronic conditions that may have health and educational implications. Many of these conditions can be controlled if properly diagnosed and treated and do not necessarily interfere with the child's ability to function in school. Other chronic and handicapping conditions do interfere with school function. Examples are blindness, deafness, developmental delay, attention-deficit hyperactivity disorder (ADHD), and long-term effects of fetal drug exposure. Conditions related to environmental or psychological stress may or may not affect physiologic function, although they may affect the child's ability to function effectively in the school situation.

The kinds of physical health problems seen by school nurses among students and staff are many and varied. Both acute and chronic conditions are commonly encountered in the school setting. Acute conditions include a variety of communicable diseases and injuries. Population health nurses may be involved in providing care to individual students (or staff) who are ill or injured. They may also identify trends in illness or injury that require changes in environmental conditions, policies, and so on. Chronic health problems are encountered with greater frequency in today's schools than in the past. In part, this is the effect of mainstreaming children with disabilities and in part, an actual increase in chronic disease incidence in children. The number of school children and adolescents with chronic health conditions increased from 1.8% in the 1960s to 25% in 2007 and continues to climb. Chronic conditions among children in school settings include both physical and mental illnesses. The Rehabilitation Act and the Individuals with Disabilities Education Act (IDEA) protect the right of children with selected conditions to attend school and to be integrated, to the extent possible, into regular classrooms (NASN, 2012a). IDEA mandates special education and related health services for children with specifically designated mental and physical disabilities (RWJF, 2010). NASN (2012a) recommends, however, that schools use a noncategorical approach to identifying children with specific needs for service and risk for school failure rather than a disease specific approach. In 2011, 5.2 million U.S. children received special education or early intervention services. This represents nearly 7% of all children under 18 years of age (Adams, Kirzinger, & Martinez, 2012). School nurses need to be conversant not only with care of minor illness and injury but also with the complex care of children with special needs.

Asthma and overweight are two of the most common chronic problems seen by today's school nurses. Asthma in children is often poorly controlled, and results in millions of lost school days and millions of dollars in lost work time for their caretakers each year. As we saw in Chapter 16∞, overweight and obesity are other significant problems among school-age children.

Immunity is another important consideration related to physiologic function in the school population. The population health nurse working in the school setting monitors the immunization status of students and school employees. For example, maintenance personnel are at risk for tetanus because of the potential for dirty injuries, and their immunization status should be monitored. For female teachers and other school personnel of childbearing age, the risk of rubella during pregnancy is increased by working with children, and they should also be adequately immunized.

A final health problem frequently encountered in the school population that may have a physiologic basis is ADHD. ADHD was discussed in Chapter 16∞.

In addition to assessing the physiologic health status of the school population as a whole, the population health nurse working in a school setting will also assess the health status and needs of individual children. Both entry and periodic assessments may be performed by school nurses. At entry into the school system, all children should receive a comprehensive medical history and assessment of preschool experiences; language, motor, social, and adaptive development; and immunization status, as well as a complete physical examination.

Periodic assessments should be based on age-appropriate guidelines and individual needs and should address new problems, medications, changes in status, and school progress. Assessment should also include screening at appropriate ages for vision, hearing, and dental problems, as well as emotional maturity, language, and motor skills. Assessments for sports participation should also include endurance and muscle strength assessment. All assessments performed in the school setting should include anticipatory guidance for children and/or parents and problem identification and referral as needed. Biological considerations in the school health setting are included in the *Focused Assessment* below.

FOCUSED ASSESSMENT: Assessing Biological Determinants of Health in School Populations

- What is the age composition of the school population (staff and students)? Do any of the students exhibit developmental delays? Are there specific developmental issues related to the age of the student population (e.g., sexual development)?
- What is the relative proportion of males and females in the school population? What is the racial/ethnic composition of the school population?
- What chronic or communicable conditions are prevalent in the school population?
- What are the immunization levels in the school population?

PSYCHOLOGICAL DETERMINANTS. School climate and the presence of mental illness among the population are two of the psychological determinants of concern in assessing health in this setting. Each of these factors will be briefly discussed here.

School climate. Although school climate might also be considered as a sociocultural determinant of health in school settings, it is addressed here because of its psychological implications for health and well-being. **School climate** is defined as the social and educational environment in which students experience learning and social activities designed to meet designated outcomes (Thomas-Presswood & Presswood, 2008). Three elements of a healthy school climate include positive relationships among members of the population, an orientation to personal growth for all members, and elements of system maintenance and system change that support clarity in expectations and their enforcement (Thomas-Presswood & Presswood, 2008).

Positive school climates establish clear behavioral and academic expectations, encourage parental involvement, and engage in activities, programs, and staff development initiatives to prevent bullying and promote social skills and conflict mediation (Thomas-Presswood & Presswood, 2008). The elements of school climate can be seen in relationships between and among students, between teachers and students, among school personnel, and between families and school and the school and the larger community. Other elements include performance expectations and grading practices.

Characteristics of positive school climates are as follows:

- All members of the population perceive the school staff as warm, caring, and concerned.
- Teachers, staff, and administrators see students as valuable and treat them with respect.
- Policies (e.g., grading, discipline policies) are administered to promote personal and educational achievement.
- Educational programs and curricula are ethnically, culturally, linguistically, and socioeconomically inclusive.
- Educators recognize students' accomplishments and encourage them to achieve their potential.
- There is stability among teachers, who display common goals.
- There are clearly defined curricular components and expectations.
- Schoolwide celebrations recognize stakeholder accomplishments.
- Staff are recognized for their contributions to the school.
- Open communication is encouraged.
- Administrators offer tangible support for maintaining a positive school climate (Thomas-Presswood & Presswood, 2008).

Conversely, elements of school climate that have negative effects on members of the school population include poor instruction leading to school failure, reliance on punitive behavior management or discipline strategies, provision of few opportunities for students to learn and practice interpersonal and self-management skills, and unclear and inconsistent rules and expectations or inconsistent correction of violations and failure to reinforce adherence to rules and expectations. Other characteristics of negative school climates include failure to recognize and accommodate to individual differences, failure to help at-risk students connect to the educational process, and lack of agreement among teachers, staff, and administrators regarding implementation of disciplinary strategies (Thomas-Presswood & Presswood, 2008).

Discipline is a particularly knotty problem in the school setting and school personnel should incorporate the general principles of effective discipline presented in Chapter 16∞. NASN (2011a) has adopted a position statement indicating that corporal punishment in schools should be legally prohibited. Similar position statements have been issued by the American Academy of Pediatrics, National Parent Teacher Association, National Association of School Psychologists, and the American Academy of Family Physicians. **Corporal punishment** is the intentional use of physical pain to motivate a change in behavior (NASN, 2011a). Research has indicated that, rather than modifying behavior, corporal punishment has negative effects on student self-image and school performance. As of 2011, corporal punishment has been prohibited in public schools in 29 states. Instead, schools need to employ a multifaceted approach to behavior management in schools that supports parents and teachers and that alters the school climate or classroom environment to minimize problem behaviors (NASN, 2011a).

Mental illness and the school setting. A significant number of school-age children in the United States suffer from mental health problems. According to surveillance data compiled by the Centers for Disease Control and Prevention (CDC), for example, more than 8% of elementary school-age children and nearly 12% of high school-age children in 2011 had ever received a diagnosis of attention deficit hyperactivity disorder. Slightly smaller percentages of students had current behavior or conduct problems in 2007 (3.8% and 4.2%, respectively). Similarly, in 2009–2010, approximately 1.4% of both age groups had received diagnoses of autism or autism spectrum disorders. A far larger percentage of high school-age students (7.8% to 8.5%) reported a major depressive episode in the past year in 2010 to 2011. For elementary-age students, the most recent data for current depression were from 2007 at 1.0% to 1.8%. Finally, between 2005 and 2010 an average of 8.3% of adolescents reported more than 14 mentally unhealthy days in the past month (Perou et al., 2013).

These data suggest the magnitude of mental health problems experienced by students in elementary and high school settings. Mental health problems severely impair students' abilities to be successful in school. For example, about half of students with mental illness fail to complete high school (National

Alliance on Mental Illness [NAMI], 2010). College students are also affected by mental health issues. According to a 2010 NAMI survey, 27% of college students responding reported experiencing depression, and 24% had bipolar disease. Severe anxiety was reported by 11% of students and schizophrenia by 6%. The prevalence of PTSD and ADHD were 6% and 5%, respectively. Among respondents who indicated they were no longer in college, 64% indicated their leaving was due to mental health issues, often as a result of loss of financial aid due to low grades or shifting to part-time study. In addition, 73% of students reported experiencing a mental health crisis while in college, but 35% indicated that their school was not aware of the crisis (NAMI, 2012).

More than half (62%) of the college students surveyed knew how to access learning accommodations, but 57% did not do so, most often because they did not realize that accommodations were available for mental as well as physical disabilities. Half of the students with mental illnesses did not disclose the illness to the institution, often out of fear of consequences of disclosure and concerns regarding confidentiality (NAMI, 2012).

Population health nurses serving in school nursing roles are ideally positioned to identify mental health problems among students at all grade levels, as are other personnel in school-based health centers (Broussard, Chrestman, & Arceneaux, 2012; Center for School, Health and Education, 2011). For example, a study of school nurses in the United Kingdom indicated the vast majority of nurses (93%) dealt with mental health issues among students and over half of them (55%) indicated that mental health problems took more than a quarter of their work time (Haddad, Butler, & Tylee, 2010). Unfortunately, few school nurses (in the United States or the United Kingdom) have received specialized training in addressing such problems, particularly after major traumatic events such as disasters (Broussard et al., 2012; Haddad et al., 2010).

It is not only students' mental health problems that affect their performance and level of achievement in school. Children whose parents have addictive disorders have been found to have higher incidence of a variety of health problems. They are more apt to be late to school, have a higher incidence of learning disability, and receive less assistance with homework than other children. In addition, these children are more likely to experience interpersonal difficulties, social isolation, and school performance problems. Children with parents who have addictive disorders are at higher risk for psychiatric disorders than other children and may be more likely to be abused or to develop substance abuse problems themselves. School nurses should be alert to children whose parents have addictive behaviors and should endeavor to provide them with the psychological and social assistance needed to circumvent the effects of parental disability on health and school performance. The *Focused Assessment* below lists areas for consideration in assessing the psychological dimension of health in the school setting.

ENVIRONMENTAL DETERMINANTS. Factors in the physical environment of the school and the surrounding community influence student safety and other health-related considerations. For example, the distance from school influences the ability of students to engage in active transportation (Kohl & Cook, 2013). **Active transportation** is the use of active means, such as walking and bicycling, to travel to and from school. The use of active transportation declined from 41% of school

FOCUSED ASSESSMENT: Assessing Psychological Determinants of Health in School Populations

- What is the quality of the school climate? What is the quality of relationships among various members of the school population? Between families and the school? Between the school and the larger community?
- What is the extent of connectedness to the school exhibited by students?
- How do peer relationships within the school affect health? Are there students who are harassed by others? What is the effect of this harassment?
- What is the overall character of teacher–student relationships within the school? Do these relationships support connectedness? Do they promote or impede student mental health?
- What is the character of relationships among teachers and between teachers and other school staff? What effect, if any, do these relationships have on the health of students? Of staff?
- What is the character of relationships between the school and parents? Between the school and the larger community? How do these relationships affect the health of the school population?
- What are the discipline policies and procedures in the school setting? Are they implemented fairly? What health effects do discipline policies have on students?
- What are the grading policies of the school? Are they implemented fairly?
- What is the extent of mental illness in the school population? To what extent does mental illness in family members affect the health of students?

students in 1969 to 13% in 2001 (Physical Activity Guidelines for Americans Midcourse Report, 2012). Both school and neighborhood environments influence physical activity. For example, a study in New Zealand found that schools with high levels of sports team participation and communities characterized by high levels of social connection were associated with increased physical activity among students (Utter, Denny, Robinson, Amerantunga, & Milfont, 2011).

School environments may also include conditions that pose safety hazards for students and others in the setting. For example, storing supplies in stairwells may hamper building evacuation in the event of an emergency. Similarly, inappropriate storage of flammable items or inappropriate use of caustic agents for cleaning or in laboratory courses may lead to injury. In addition, architectural features of the school can influence health in multiple ways, both positive and negative. For example, architectural features such as play areas and equipment can influence physical activity. Environmental factors also affect stress, appetite, food choices, and so on (Huang et al., 2013). Similarly, solid perimeter walls (brick or concrete block) are more effective than chain link fences in preventing unauthorized entry and possible danger to students from terrorists or other potential assailants. Similarly, overlapping areas for picking up and dropping students off create the potential for pedestrian injuries (National Clearinghouse for Educational Facilities [NCEF], 2008).

Schools should engage in systematic identification of environmental hazards. A **hazard**, in this context, is any circumstance that has the potential to result in harm or damage to the school or the school population (NCEF, 2008). Risk then is the probability that such a loss will occur. School health nurses and others in the school setting should conduct an in-depth assessment of the hazards present in the setting and surrounding community. The Environmental Protection Agency (2014) has developed a *Healthy School Environments Assessment Tool (Healthy SEAT)* that can be used to assess multiple areas within the school environment. For further information about the tool, see the *External Resources* section of the student resources site.

Once safety hazards in the environment have been identified, members of the school health team can engage in mitigation efforts. The Federal Emergency Management Administration (FEMA) has defined **mitigation** as action taken to prevent or minimize the potential risk to life or property resulting from a hazardous circumstance (NCEF, 2008). Mitigation efforts may include both passive and active safety measures. Passive safety measures are those that are directed at the physical structure or layout of the school, for example, installing traffic calming features, such as speed bumps and stop signs in heavily traveled areas of campus with high risk for accidents and providing a soft surface below play equipment. Active safety measures involve changes in behavior, such as enforcing the use of sports safety equipment or increasing adult supervision during recess. Hiring security guards to prevent unauthorized persons from gaining access to the school is another example of an active safety measure, while installing metal detectors at entrances would be a passive safety measure (NCEF, 2008). The school nurse and other members of the school health team would develop a mitigation plan to address identified hazards. There is also a need for a systematic school safety plan that details how to respond to safety issues (Safe Havens International, n.d.). For information on a tool developed by Safe Havens International to evaluate the quality and comprehensiveness of the school safety plan, see the *External Resources* section of the student resources site.

The nurse and others assess both the internal and external physical environment of the school. The external environment includes the area surrounding the school. Assessment considerations here include traffic patterns, water hazards, use of pesticides, and rodent control in the area. The proximity of hazardous waste dumps or nuclear power plants, industrial hazards, and the presence of various forms of pollution are other environmental concerns in school settings. (See Chapter 4∞ for a discussion of environmental health issues.)

Several aspects of the school's internal environment, such as fire hazards and sanitation, are the responsibility of official agencies such as the fire department and health department; however, other aspects of the physical environment are rarely adequately assessed. The school health nurse needs to be alert to other hazards to physical safety that may be present in the school setting. Examples of these hazards are toxic art supplies, scientific equipment in laboratories, kitchen appliances in home economics classrooms, and chemical substances used either in chemistry labs or by maintenance and janitorial staffs. Animals in classrooms may also present safety hazards in terms of the potential for scratches and bites or disease transmission. Other conditions that may jeopardize safety include asbestos used in building materials, inadequate maintenance of fire hoses and extinguishers, and inoperable communications systems in the event of an emergency.

Other areas of concern are the safety of industrial arts classrooms, the gymnasium, and play areas. As noted in Chapter 16∞, the safety of outdoor play equipment should be inspected on a regular basis and repairs made as needed. A similar need exists for periodic assessment of sports equipment and practices. Other hazards associated with play areas include broken glass and other refuse on the playground. Hard surfaces below play equipment increase the potential for injuries stemming from falls. Weather is another element of the physical environment that affects the health of students. For example, heat illness brought on by sports practice or competition is the leading cause of death in high school athletes. From 2005 to 2009, more than 9,000 heat-related events were estimated among high school students (Gilchrist et al., 2010). Similarly, playing outdoors on days with pollutant levels that exceed safety recommendations can result in asthma exacerbations and other respiratory conditions.

Other assessment considerations with respect to the school's internal physical environment include noise levels within and outside of classrooms and the adequacy of lighting, ventilation, heating, and cooling. Food sanitation should also be assessed. If hot meals are provided at school, cooking facilities should be inspected regularly. Such inspections are usually the official responsibility of the local health department, but the population health nurse should also assess these facilities periodically. If students bring their lunches, the potential for food poisoning from spoiled foods should be appraised.

Assessing sanitary facilities in the school is another area for consideration. Here, the nurse would examine the adequacy of toilet facilities for the size of the school population. The nurse would also periodically inspect sanitary facilities to make sure they are in good working order and do not pose hazards for the transmission of communicable diseases. Again, this area is usually the responsibility of health department personnel, but official inspections may occur only at lengthy intervals and the nurse should be aware of hazards that might arise in the interim.

Another area of concern with respect to sanitation is the use and cleaning of shower facilities. The nurse should assess that showers are adequately cleaned to prevent transmission of communicable conditions such as tinea pedis (athlete's foot).

Physical facilities for preventing the spread of disease by infected children should also be assessed. Are there places within the school where students with infectious conditions can be isolated? All too often, these children are merely kept in the nurse's office until a parent can come for them. This presents opportunities for exposure of all those who visit the nurse while the child is there.

Special consideration should be given to the physical environment as it relates to children with disabilities. Many physical barriers may exist, particularly in older schools, which limit the ability of disabled students to benefit from the education setting. Areas of concern include the presence of ramps, easily opened doors and windows, nonslip flooring, elevators, and curb modifications to eliminate the need to step up. Another consideration is access to toileting facilities. Are toilets accessible to wheelchairs? Are sinks placed so that a wheelchair can be maneuvered beneath them? The placement and height of mirrors, drinking fountains, and telephones are also of concern. Other considerations with respect to the environment of handicapped children are the adequacy of storage for wheelchairs and other special equipment, wheelchair space in classrooms and auditoriums, modification of laboratory and library carrels for wheelchair use, and the adequacy of evacuation plans for the disabled in case of emergency. The intent is to create a school that is barrier-free so that all students, staff, and community members who may use the premises after school hours have access to facilities and equipment. Population health nurses may need to actively advocate for modifications in the school setting that address the needs of students (or employees) with disabilities.

Finally, the school nurse should assess the level of preparation in the school setting for disaster events or terrorist activities. Elements of an effective disaster response plan include personnel organization, forms, specific considerations, and the role of the nurse.

The role of the school nurse with respect to disaster events or terrorist activities includes participation in developing the disaster plan. In the event of an actual disaster, the nurse assists in maintaining calm, triages injuries, and addresses the physical and psychological effects of the disaster. After a disaster event, the nurse helps to address the fears and grief of students and other staff members. In addition to meeting ongoing health care needs, the nurse should provide realistic and reliable information, facilitate referrals for support, and educate staff regarding the psychological effects of such events. Disaster response will be addressed in more detail in Chapter 25∞. Elements of a *Focused Assessment* of physical environmental considerations in the school setting are summarized below.

FOCUSED ASSESSMENT Assessing Environmental Determinants of Health in School Populations

- Are there health hazards present in the school or the surrounding neighborhood?
- Are food sanitation practices adequate to prevent communicable diseases, vermin infestation, and so on?
- Are school facilities adequate and in good repair? Are there adequate facilities for students or staff with physical disabilities?
- What is the character of the environment surrounding the school? What health effects, if any, does the external environment have on the school population?
- What is the potential for disaster within the school setting? Is the school adequately prepared to respond to a disaster event?
- What physical barriers are in place to prevent unauthorized access to school grounds?
- What are the positive and negative health effects of building architecture and school grounds?

SOCIOCULTURAL DETERMINANTS. Sociocultural factors also play a part in influencing the health status of members of the school community. Areas to be addressed in this dimension include culture and ethnicity, economic resources, policy and legislation, abuse and violence, and the potential for terrorism.

Culture and ethnicity. Cultural factors in the school setting may affect educational priorities as well as health-related behaviors. What is the racial or ethnic composition of the school population? Are racial tensions present? Do religious beliefs influence the health of the school population? For example, if there are large numbers of children whose parents object to immunization on religious grounds, the nurse needs to be particularly alert to signs of outbreaks of childhood diseases such as measles, rubella, and diphtheria.

Another area for consideration is the cultural backgrounds of students and school personnel. Are they similar? Do cultural practices influence students' health? Do differences in cultural practices create tension among students or between students and staff? Cultural factors may also lead to inappropriate diagnoses of ADHD for behavior considered perfectly normal in the child's culture or child abuse in the face of cultural health practices such as dermabrasion or cupping. (See Chapter 5 for a discussion of various cultural health practices.) Children whose primary language is not English may also have difficulties in school, and the nurse should work to achieve culturally and linguistically appropriate education for these children. Similarly, children of migrant or homeless families of whatever cultural or ethnic background may have their education disrupted by frequent moves.

Economic resources. The level of resources available to the school is one element in assessing the sociocultural dimension of the school setting. The nurse also needs to assess the community's attitudes toward education because these attitudes determine the allocation of funds for both school and health programs. What level of priority is given to school funding in the community? Do community members support bond issues for school renovation or specific school-based programs? Population health nurses may need to advocate with school boards and other local officials for sufficient funding for school health services. Political advocacy may also be needed at state and national levels to assure adequate funding for education, particularly for school-based health services.

The economic levels of individual students and their families also influence the health status of the school population. Homelessness is an extreme socioeconomic factor that can have a profound effect on the health of school-age children. As we saw in Chapter 21, homeless children often perform poorly in school or fall behind because of frequent moves. As a result of the McKinney Homeless Assistance Act, homeless children are guaranteed access to free and public education. Under this act, homeless children may be eligible for other services that must be provided by schools receiving assistance funds. These services may include clothing, a place to bathe and change clothes, free or reduced-cost meals, school supplies, tutorial assistance, and access to medical care.

Homelessness is often the result of divorce or violence within families. Children may be homeless because their mothers are fleeing an abusive situation. In such circumstances and in disputes over child custody, the school system needs to be alert to the potential for abduction of schoolchildren by the other parent. Similarly, abduction and mistreatment by strangers is an area of concern, and the school nurse should assess school policies designed to prevent such occurrences for their adequacy and the extent to which they are enforced.

Another factor closely related to family economic status is the prevalence of families in which both parents work. Unfortunately, children in dual wage-earner families are often sent to school when they are ill because there is no one at home to care for them. The nurse should assess the number of students who come to school ill and explore with parents their reasons for sending sick children to school. It may be a lack of awareness on the part of parents of the signs and symptoms of illness or the absence of other options.

The nurse should also assess before- and after-school care of children whose parents work. Many so-called *latchkey* children stay at home alone before and after school until parents return from work. Population health nurses can assess the availability of programs for children who are not mature enough to stay home alone and make referrals to these programs if they do not already exist within the school. In addition, nurses can assist parents to determine children's readiness to stay home alone and help to educate both parents and children on conditions that promote the safety of latchkey children.

Policy and legislation. State and federal policy that affects the health of school populations is often provided in legislation. As we saw earlier, legislation related to education for children with disabilities has profoundly influenced the role of school nurses in caring for these children, many of whom have multiple health care needs.

Other policy initiatives may also influence school health. Many policies that affect the health of school populations arise in the Office of Safe and Healthy Students (OSHS) and its three subordinate units: the Safe and Supportive Schools Group, the Healthy Students Group, and the Center for School Preparedness (OSHS, 2014). Individual states also develop laws and regulations related to school health. For further information about laws, rules, regulations, and guidelines related to school health, see the *External Resources* section of the student resources site.

Other federal and state agencies and nonprofit organizations also develop policies that influence health in school populations. For example, the Institute of Medicine (IOM) has developed nutrition standards for schools that address the fat, sugar, and sodium content of foods available in schools. The standards also address nonnutritive food items such as the availability of sweetened and caffeinated beverages, as well as food standards for the school day and for after-school activities (National Center for Chronic Disease Prevention and Health Promotion [NCCDPHP], 2012).

Finally, the standards deal with the availability of "competitive foods." **Competitive foods** are foods sold or available in schools that are outside of federally reimbursable school meal programs and that compete with the more healthful foods offered with the nutrition programs (NCCDPHP, 2012). Similar policies exist within states. As of 2010, 39 states had policies related to the nutritive value of competitive foods (NCCDPHP, 2012). A study of state laws related to nutrition policies in schools indicated little progress from 2003 to 2008, in that the vast majority of states did not have laws related to the quality of school meals for elementary to high schools, competitive foods, or for food and beverage items used for school fund-raising (Mâsse, Perna, Agurs-Collins, & Chriqui, 2013). Federal and state standards and policies also address recommendations for health education and physical education in school settings (DASH, 2013a, 2013e). School districts and individual schools also have numerous policies that influence health in the school population. The population health nurse assesses the myriad policies and their effects on the health of the population. Some authors have suggested the employment of a school "wellness nurse" dedicated to assisting schools to develop and implement policies that promote health and to promote the incorporation of health promotion and illness prevention guidelines in the school setting (Avery, Johnson, Cousins, & Hamilton, 2013).

Bullying, harassment, and violence. A particular need in today's society is to prevent bullying, harassment, and violence in and around the school setting. **Bullying** is "unwanted, aggressive behavior among school-aged children that involves a real or perceived power imbalance" (U.S. Department of Health and Human Services [USDHHS], n.d., para 1). School bullying includes any form of bullying that occurs on school property, on the way to or from school (e.g., on the school bus), or at school-related events. School bullying may involve peer-to-peer interactions, bullying of younger children by older children, or bullying by or of a teacher. Bullying can be differentiated by the number of bullies, the mode of bullying, or the medium used for bullying. *Pack bullying* is perpetrated by a group of individuals as opposed to one-on-one bullying by an individual. Pack bullying is more often seen in high school populations, while individual bullying is more common in elementary school. Both pack bullying and individual bullying can be physical or emotional and can be perpetrated in person or electronically. Bullying can also be differentiated by its intended target, based on homophobia, disability, racism, or religious beliefs (Bullying Statistics, 2013).

In 2011, roughly 28% of students 12 to 18 years of age reported being bullied at school. Bullying included being made fun of or called names, being the subject of rumors, threats of harm, and attempts at coercion. Other manifestations of bullying included being excluded from activities, damage to personal belongings, and being pushed, shoved, tripped, or spit on (National Center for Education Statistics [NCES], 2013).

Sexual harassment is one specific form of bullying that occurs in school populations. **Sexual harassment** is unwelcome behavior with sexual overtones perpetrated in person or electronically (Hill, 2012). In a national survey of students in grades 7 to 12 conducted by the American Association of University Women (AAUW), 48% of participants reported some form of sexual harassment in the prior year, 30% via electronic media. Boys reported being less negatively affected by sexual harassment than girls, but were more likely to be harassers. In the report, sexual harassers were described as often being "misguided comedians" who have no concept of the damage caused by their behaviors (Hill, 2012). Sexual harassment often involves a verbal attack on the victim's sexuality or appearance, for example, spreading rumors that one is gay or lesbian or sexually promiscuous, making suggestive comments, or making sexual threats.

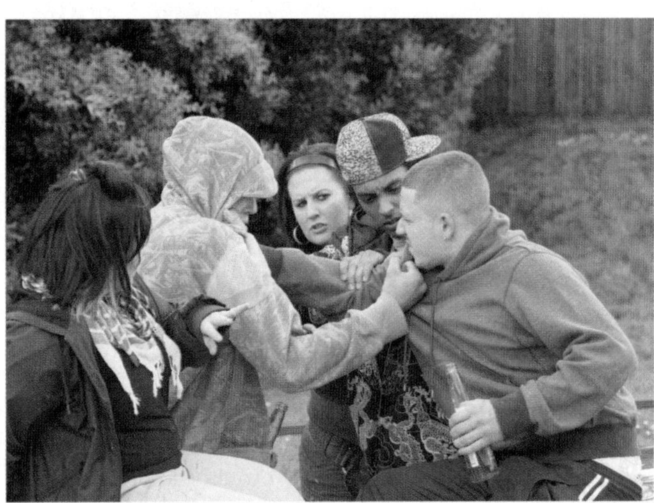

Violence is a significant problem in many school settings.
(Monkey Business/Fotolia)

Bullying that occurs by means of electronic media (e.g., social media postings, telephone calls, texting) is often referred to as cyberbullying or cyber-harassment. **Cyberbullying** is defined as "cruelty to others by sending or posting harmful material using the Internet or cell phone" (National Conference of State Legislatures, 2014, para. 3). In the AAUW survey, 36% of 7th to 12th grade girls and 24% of boys reported experiencing cyberbullying in the prior year (Smolinski, 2012). In another study in Massachusetts, 25.9% of students reported being bullied at school in the last year and 15.8% reported cyberbullying. Most of the students experienced bullying in both formats, which was associated with the highest levels of distress (Schneider, O'Donnell, Stueve, & Coulter, 2012). Nationally, about 9% of 12- to 18-year-old students reported being cyberbullied in 2011 (NCES, 2013). At its worst, bullying in any form may result in suicide or homicide. Suicide by victims of bullying is sometimes referred to as "bullycide," and being a victim of bullying is one of the primary causes of homicide in school settings. Of 31 school-associated violent deaths in elementary and secondary schools during the 2010–2011 school year, just over 80% were homicides, and the remainder were suicides (NCES, 2013).

Violence of all kinds is found in school settings. In 2011, for example, nearly 33% of a nationally representative sample of American 9th to 12th graders reported being in a physical fight in the past year (12% on school premises). Nearly 17% of students reported carrying a weapon to school, and more than 7% reported being threatened or injured with a weapon in the last year. In addition, approximately 160,000 K–12 students go home from school early due to bullying and violence and 5% report skipping school due to fear of violence (Center for School, Health and Education, 2011; National Center for Injury Prevention and Control, 2012). Finally, a full third of high school students report that violence is a big problem in their schools (Center for School, Health and Education, 2011).

Data compiled by the Bureau of Justice Statistics and the National Center for Education Statistics indicate that 31 school-associated violent deaths occurred from July 2010 through June 2011. Of the 31 deaths involving students, school personnel, and nonstudents, 25 were homicides and 6 were suicides. Eleven of these homicides involved children and youth 5 to 18 years of age, and half of the suicides were among students. This is a decrease from 19 violent student deaths the previous year (Robers, Kemp, Truman, & Snyder, 2013).

In addition, 597,500 instances of nonfatal violence ranging from simple assault to serious violence occurred among 12- to 18-year-old students in 2011. More victimizations (theft and violence) in this age group occurred at school than away from school at a rate of 49 victimizations per 1,000 children at school compared to 38 per 1,000 away from school. No differences were noted by locale among serious violent victimization. Violence is pervasive across schools with 74% of public schools experiencing at least one violent crime in the 2009–2010 school year and 16% experiencing one or more serious violent incidents (Robers et al., 2013). All of these figures suggest the magnitude of violence in school settings and population health nurses assessing the health of school populations should be alert to the presence of all forms of bullying, harassment, and violence within the population.

Violence within the school environment can be addressed by explicit codes of conduct that are clearly communicated to students and consistently and uniformly enforced. Weapons should be strictly banned from school campuses and the ban stringently enforced. Peer counseling and off-campus counseling sites to address interpersonal problems have been effective means of reducing violence. The population health nurse in the school setting can assess the level of violence on campus as well as the effectiveness of steps taken to prevent violence. The nurse can also examine the inclusion of conflict resolution strategies and content on interpersonal relations in the school's health education curriculum.

School children may also be subjected to violence and abuse outside of the school setting. Children may suffer physical, emotional, or sexual abuse or neglect within their families. Children with disabilities are nearly twice as likely to be abused as other children, and, although boys and girls are abused with equal frequency, girls are more likely to experience sexual abuse. School nurses should be alert to signs of abuse and neglect in individual children. Child abuse is addressed in more detail in Chapter 30∞.

The extent of crime in the school neighborhood is another aspect of the social environment to be assessed. Is violence a problem for children going to and from school? Is drug dealing going on in the area, and will youngsters be pressured to experiment with drugs? Similarly, the nurse would assess the extent of gang activity in and around the school and its effects on the health of the school population. Questions for a *Focused Assessment* of sociocultural determinants of health in the school setting are presented below.

BEHAVIORAL DETERMINANTS. Enrollment in school is itself a lifestyle factor that influences health. School attendance increases one's risk of exposure to a variety of communicable diseases. Children generally experience an increase in the number of acute illnesses during the first few years of school, whether at the day care/preschool level or with admission to elementary school.

The rigidity of the school day may also affect the health status of students. The nurse determines whether the organization

FOCUSED ASSESSMENT Assessing Sociocultural Determinants of Health in School Populations

- What is the ethnic and cultural composition of the school population? How do ethnicity and culture affect the health of members of the school population?
- What are the community attitudes toward education? Toward the school? To what extent does the community support the school program?
- What economic resources are available to the school?
- What is the economic status of members of the school population? How does economic status affect access to health care?
- How do legislative and policy initiatives affect the school and the health of the school population?
- What are the effects of local school and district policies on health services and health status of the school population?
- What is the extent of violence in the school population? What are the factors underlying episodes of violence? What are the school's policies with respect to violence?
- To what extent are members of the school population subjected to violence and abuse outside the school setting?
- What is the potential for Internet exploitation of students?

of the school day is conducive to health. Assessment areas to be addressed include the extent to which periods of strenuous physical activity are alternated with periods of quiet study and the extent of opportunities for developing a variety of psychomotor as well as academic skills. The nurse also assesses whether mealtimes are arranged so that students have the energy reserves to handle the tasks of the school day. For younger children, this usually means providing a snack time. Another area for assessment is the scheduling of time for toileting activities. The nurse should determine whether children are given time to go to the lavatory or permitted to go when necessary to prevent chronic constipation or urinary tract infection. There should also be opportunities for children to obtain drinks of water. Such opportunities should increase in frequency with hot weather. Other behavioral determinants to be addressed include physical activity, diet and nutrition, substance use and abuse, safety practices, and sexual behavior.

Physical activity. Physical activity affects cognitive skills, attitudes, and academic behavior. Improving physical activity in school students, particularly in time spent in physical education, may increase academic performance (DASH, 2011). With the advent of television and computer game systems, however, children are much less physically active than they were a generation or two ago. Only about 60% of youth met recommendations for physical activity, and the percentage decreased with increasing age and grade level. Boys tend to be more physically active than girls, and this disparity also increases with age. Overall, students from elementary to high school get an average of only 4 minutes of physical activity per day during school time (Kohl & Cook, 2013). Despite these low figures, however, a subcommittee of the President's Council on Fitness, Sports, and Nutrition has noted that, "School settings hold a realistic and evidence-based opportunity to increase physical activity among youth and should be a key part of a national strategy to increase physical activity" (Physical Activity Guidelines for Americans Midcourse Report Subcommittee, 2012).

According to the most recent school health policies and practices study conducted in 2006, only 80% of states required physical education (PE) classes at the elementary school level, increasing to 93% of middle schools and high schools. Even in those states that required PE, only 4% required daily sessions at the elementary level, 8% at the middle school level, and 2% at the high school level. In addition, 37% of states and 90% of school districts recommended or required a regular recess period in elementary school, although approximately 97% of schools included recess in the school day. Policies related to active transportation were even more infrequent, with 14% of states, 18% of school districts, and 44% of schools promoting active transportation (Kohl & Cook, 2013).

In addition to assessing the extent of physical education and recess time, the population health nurse can examine per capita school expenditures for education. States vary widely in the amount of money spent per pupil per year, ranging from a low of $6,612 in Utah to a high of $19,698 in Washington, DC. Only a small percentage of these funds are allocated for physical education and other health-related services (Kohl & Cook, 2013).

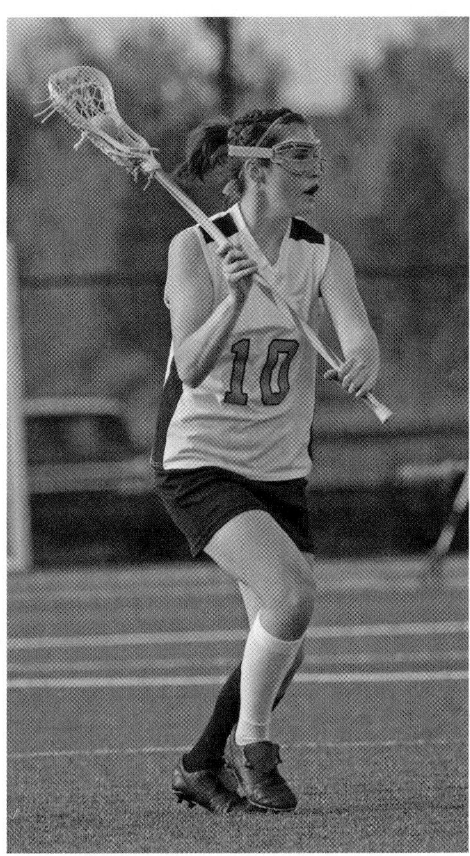

Physical education is an important component of school health.
(Jim/Fotolia)

Recreational activities should also be assessed. Recreational and sports equipment should be examined for safety hazards, and the nurse should be aware of the types of recreational and competitive activities engaged in by students. Are activities adequately supervised? Are sports and recreational programs appropriate to children's ages and developmental levels? For example, contact sports are not appropriate for children in lower elementary grades because of the increased risk of injury. Another question is whether recreational activities are suited to children's interests. Are various opportunities available, or must all children engage in the same activity, whether they choose to or not? Is a gender bias evident in the recreational opportunities provided? For example, is soccer restricted to boys whereas girls are expected to play hopscotch or jump rope? Attention should also be given to the recreational needs of teachers. Are teachers given a break from classroom and playground duties?

The physical education curriculum of the school will also influence students' exercise behaviors. Many schools do not include the exposure to physical education activities required to meet the national health objectives. Research has indicated that features of the school environment such as physical improvements and supervision influence physical activity by students before and after school and at lunch. For example, the presence of permanent grounds improvements such as the installation of basketball and tennis courts and football and soccer goals increases the extent of physical activity by students. Similarly, the availability of recreational equipment influences activity. The school nurse should assess the extent to which the school physical education curriculum and the physical and social environments of the school promote physical activity.

Diet and nutrition. Nutrition is another behavioral determinant that should be assessed in the school population. In one national study, 60% of teachers said that they taught students who came to school hungry. Approximately 21 million students receive free school lunches through federal meal programs, but less than half of them receive breakfast. Research has indicated that eating breakfast improves academic performance. For example, students who eat breakfast tend to score higher on standardized tests, are less likely to experience school absences, and are more likely to graduate than those who do not. Recommendations have been made to move school breakfasts out of the cafeteria and into the classroom, making them a part of the official school day and increasing the number of children who participate (Deloitte, n.d.).

Schools have been criticized for lack of nutrition in foods served and providing access to junk food. Evidence for this criticism lies in the fact that students with improved school nutrition experienced smaller increases in BMIs during the school year than during the summer. This was particularly true for students who were already overweight (von Hippel, Powell, Downey, & Rowland, 2007). In schools without a dietary consultant, the nurse should appraise the nutritional quality of school lunch and/or breakfast programs. Too often, food for such programs is purchased with an eye toward economy rather than nutritional value.

The adequacy of lunches brought from home should also be examined, as should evidence of poor nutrition of meals eaten at home. For example, the nurse would assess children for evidence of anemia, poor growth, and development or overweight and obesity. School nurses may also encounter students who exhibit eating disorders and can assist with referrals for diagnostic and treatment services for these children. The type and prevalence of any food allergies among either students or staff are other considerations for assessment in this area. Population health nurses may need to educate food service personnel regarding food allergies and the need to avoid particularly allergenic foods (e.g., peanuts or use of peanut products in other foods) as a routine precaution.

Other lifestyle behaviors. Other health-related behaviors should also be assessed, particularly among older students. The extent of tobacco use or use of alcohol or other drugs by students or staff should be explored, as should the extent of sexual activity among preadolescent and adolescent students. Approximately half of all high school students have had sexual intercourse (Kann, Brener, McManus, & Wechsler, 2012), yet only 5% of U.S. schools make condoms available to sexually active students (Guttmacher Institute, 2012). Similarly, although a median 90% of public secondary schools across 45 states taught HIV prevention as part of a required course in 2010, only 43% of schools addressed all 11 recommended HIV prevention topics in grades 6 through 12, and the percentages of schools that did so actually declined from 2008 to 2010 (Kann et al., 2012). The nurse should assess the extent of substance use and sexual activity in the school population as well as policies that hinder preventive activities. School nurses should also be alert to signs of pregnancy and sexually transmitted diseases in individual students as well as the potential for sexual assault in the school population. The school nurse should assess the extent of substance use and abuse in the school population, ease of access to these substances in the community, and the adequacy and enforcement of school policies and community regulations regarding their sale and use. The nurse should also be alert to signs of substance use and abuse in individual students and school personnel.

Safety practices should also be assessed in the school setting. Many U.S. school children are engaged in sports activities,

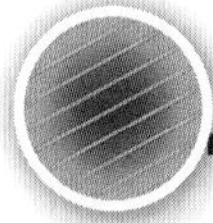

Evidence-Based Practice

Building the Evidence Base for School Health

Interventions

There is considerable evidence that physical activity initiatives in school settings improve student participation in physical activity. However, the Physical Activity Guidelines for Americans Midcourse Report Subcommittee of the President's Council on Fitness, Sports, & Nutrition (2012) identified several research gaps that should be addressed to further develop this evidence base. In particular, research is needed to determine the long-term effects of such initiatives and whether or not such initiatives vary in their effectiveness with particular subgoups within the school population (e.g., differences related to ethnicity, sociocultural status, geographic region, and health status). There is also need to evaluate the effects of school policies related to physical activity.

1. What, if any, research is being done in schools in your area to further this evidence base?
2. How might population health nurses foster such research?

resulting in the potential for serious injury. Risk behaviors associated with injury include failure to use protective gear or seat belts, alcohol use, and access to weapons. Other behavioral risks that should be assessed include unprotected sexual intercourse, piercing, and gambling. Gambling among students often occurs on the Internet and is an increasingly common addiction among high school and college-age students. The *Focused Assessment* below provides questions for assessing behavioral considerations in the health of school populations.

HEALTH SYSTEM DETERMINANTS. Health services within schools have been described as "hidden systems" of care (RWJF, 2010) or as a "patchwork of policies and programs with differing standards, requirements, and populations to be served" (DASH, 2013f). Health system determinants influencing the health of school populations are assessed at both the individual and population levels. At the individual level, the population health nurse assesses the usual source of health care for individual children and their families. Do children have a regular source of health care? Do they make use of health-promotive and illness-preventive services as well as curative services? Or is health care for children crisis oriented, focusing only on treatment of acute conditions? Do children have unmet health needs because their families cannot afford care? The two main considerations at the population level are the presence or absence of a coordinated school health program and school-based health centers.

The coordinated school health program. A coordinated school health program has been defined by a number of organizations and agencies. One of the clearest and most useful definitions, however, is that of the Institute of Medicine. A **coordinated school health program** is "an integrated set of planned, sequential, school-affiliated strategies, activities, and services designed to promote the optimal physical, emotional, social, and educational development of students" (IOM, as quoted in DASH, 2014, p. 1).

Coordinated school health programs serve to eliminate gaps and overlaps in services and funding streams. They also build collaborative relationships among health and education professionals in schools and enhance communication and collaboration of the school, the public health system, and health and education professionals in the community. The focus in a coordinated school health program is on aiding students to protect and promote their own health and to avoid risk behaviors (DASH, 2013f). To that end, the goals of a coordinated school health program are as follows:

- To increase health-related knowledge, attitudes, and skills among members of the school population
- To increase positive health behaviors and outcomes and decrease risk behaviors
- To improve education outcomes
- To improve social outcomes, such as self-discipline and respect for and tolerance of others (DASH, 2013c)

The components of a coordinated school health program are depicted in Figure 22-1● and include health education; physical education; health services; nutrition services; counseling, psychological, and social services; a healthy and safe school environment; health promotion for staff; and family and community involvement (DASH, 2013b). Each component will be briefly addressed.

FOCUSED ASSESSMENT — Assessing Behavioral Determinants of Health in School Populations

- What is the extent of physical activity in the school population? Does the school setting provide opportunities for safe physical activities to meet the needs and interests of all members of the school population?
- To what extent do students walk or bike to school? What factors support or impede "active transportation"?
- What recreational opportunities are available to the school population? Do recreational activities pose health hazards? Are appropriate safety equipment and devices used (e.g., in sports)?
- What are the dietary practices of the school population? To what extent do school food choices support or deter good nutrition? What is the nutritional value of school meals?
- What percentage of students participate in school meal programs? Is school breakfast a routine part of the school day?
- What is the prevalence of food allergies among the school population? What types of food allergies are represented? Do school food services avoid particularly allergenic foods?
- What is the extent of substance use and abuse in the school population? What are the school policies with respect to substance use (e.g., tobacco and alcohol)?
- Do any members of the school population use prescription medications on a regular basis? Are medications used, stored, and dispensed as directed?
- To what extent do members of the school population engage in other health and safety-related practices (e.g., seat belt use and condom use)?
- What is the extent of gambling among the school population?
- What is the extent of piercing and tattooing among the school population? To what extent do these practices influence health?

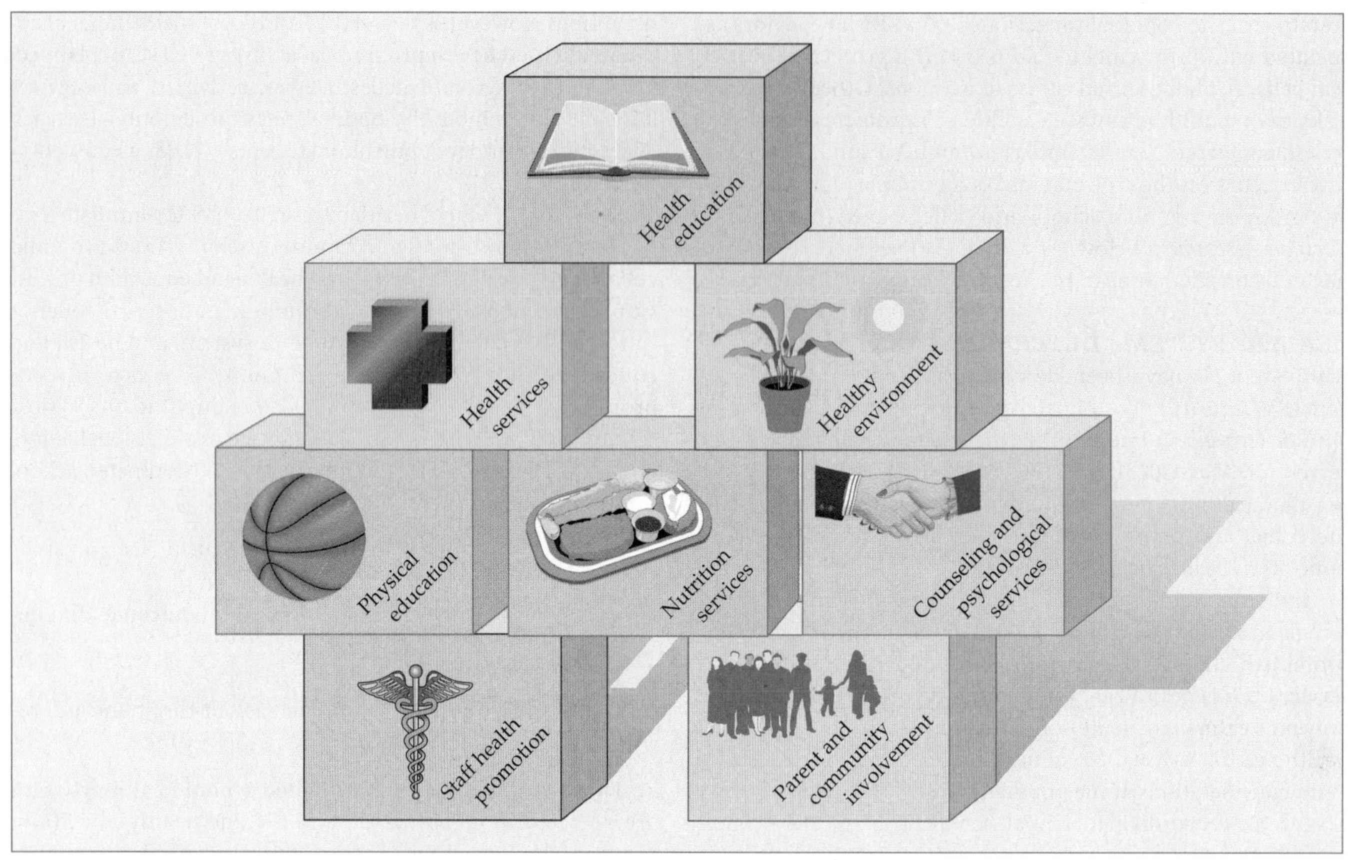

FIGURE 22-1 Components of a Coordinated School Health Program

Health education. The foci for health education in school settings include providing esssential knowledge, shaping values and beliefs to support healthy behavior, shaping group norms to foster healthy behavior, and developing health-related skills. Table 22-2● presents national standards developed to guide health education programs in U.S. schools.

Effective health education curricula in schools focus on achieving clear health-related goals and behavioral outcomes; are research based and theory driven; address individual values, attitudes, and beliefs and motivate students to critically examine related perspectives; address group norms that underlie behaviors; and focus on reinforcing protective behaviors and increasing perceptions of harm from unhealthy behaviors based on realistic personal risk assessments. In addition, effective curricula provide strategies to address social pressures and influences for unhealthy behavior and build personal and

TABLE 22-2 National Standards for Health Education Programs in Schools

Standard	Description
1	Students will comprehend concepts related to health promotion and disease prevention to enhance health
2	Students will analyze the influence of family, peers, culture, media, technology, and other factors on health
3	Students will demonstrate the ability to access valid information, products, and services to enhance health
4	Students will demonstrate the ability to use interpersonal communication skills to enhance health and avoid or reduce health risks
5	Students will demonstrate the ability to use decision-making skills to enhance health
6	Students will demonstrate the ability to use goal-setting skills to enhance health
7	Students will demonstrate the ability to practice health-enhancing behaviors and avoid or reduce health risks
8	Students will demonstrate the ability to advocate for personal, family, and community health

Source: Division of Adolescent and School Health, Centers for Disease Control and Prevention. (2013e). *National health education standards.* Retrieved from http://www.cdc.gov/healthyyouth/sher/standards/index.htm

social competence and self-efficacy, developing skills in communication, refusal, assessing the credibility of health-related information, decision making, planning and goal setting, and self-control and self-management. Other characteristics of effective health education curricula include provision of accurate functional health knowledge; use of strategies that personalize information and interest and engage students; incorporation of age- and developmentally appropriate information, strategies, methods, and materials; and adoption of culturally inclusive strategies, methods, and materials. Finally, effective curricula provide time for instruction and opportunities to practice and reinforce health-related skills and behaviors, as well as opportunities to connect with influential others who affirm and reinforce healthy behaviors. In addition to their focus on students, effective health education programs provide for professional development of teachers to promote their knowledge, comfort, and skill in teaching health-related content (DASH, 2013a).

The population health nurse in the school setting would assess the school health education curriculum in light of the standards and criteria for effectiveness. They would also be involved in developing and implementing effective health education programs in school settings at all levels. CDC (2013a) provides an assessment tool for analyzing health education curricula, the "Health Education Curriculum Analysis Tool" (HECAT). For further information about the tool, see the *External Resources* section of the student resources site.

Physical education. We have already addressed the need for and general lack of physical activity in school populations. The Institute of Medicine has recommended taking a whole-school approach to physical activity, so that activity is threaded throughout the school day, rather than just in the physical education curriculum. Additional recommendations include considering access to and provision of physical activity in school policy decisions at multiple levels (federal and state government, school districts, and individual schools) and creating a mandate for physical education as part of the core curriculum in all schools across the nation. In addition, educational and public health agencies should develop systems to monitor policies and behaviors related to physical activity in schools, and training and development should be provided for teachers to promote physical activity beyond physical education and recess. Finally, all concerned should work to eliminate disparities in physical activities among students groups, particularly those related to access to facilities and opportunities for physical activity (Kohl & Cook, 2013).

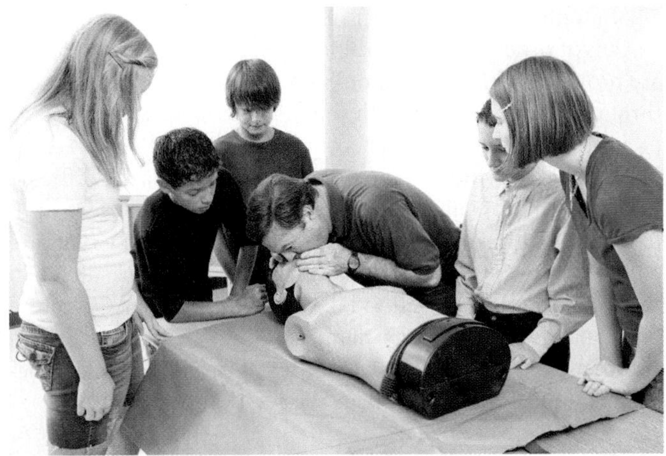

Population health nurses are actively involved in health education in school settings. *(Lisa F. Young/Fotolia)*

As we saw earlier, elements of a whole-school approach to physical activity include an enhanced PE program, classroom physical activity, recess and other activity breaks, intramural and extramural sports, and active transportation to school. The bulk of physical activity during the school day should come from an enhanced PE program. An enhanced PE program can be achieved by increased amount of time in PE classes spent in vigorous physical activity, adding more PE classes to the curriculum, lengthening the time of existing PE classes, meeting the physical activity needs of all students, including those with disabilities, and including activities that are enjoyable and emphasize acquisition of knowledge and skills for lifetime use (Physical Activity Guidelines for Americans, 2012).

Components of a high-quality physical education program include the curriculum itself, related policies and a supportive environment, instruction, and student assessment. Requirements for achieving a high-quality PE program include adequate instructional time (150 minutes per week for elementary students and 225 minutes per week for middle and high school students), provision of instruction by qualified PE specialists, reasonable class sizes, and the availability of appropriate equipment and facilities. An effective PE program makes use of instructional strategies that are inclusive of all students, is adaptable for students with disabilities, expends most of class time in actual physical activity, incorporates well-designed lessons, includes out-of-class assignments that support learning (e.g., calculating calories burned in specific activities), and refrains from using physical activity as punishment for inappropriate behavior. Effective programs also focus on student achievement of measurable goals using appropriate assessment tools, self-assessment of performance by students, feedback to students and parents, and clarity regarding elements used to grade performance (CDC, 2006).

CDC (2013b) has created a tool that can be used by the population health nurse and other school personnel to evaluate the physical education curriculum. For further information about the "Physical Education Curriculum Analysis Tool" (PECAT), see the *External Resources* section of the student resources site.

Health services. The health services component of the coordinated school health program consists of services at all four levels of health care: health promotion, illness and injury prevention, resolution of existing health problems, and health restoration.

These services are provided to students and, on occasion, school personnel. In some school settings, health services may be provided to students' families as well. School health services may be provided on campus by health personnel employed by the school or school district, by outside providers on contract to the school, or by volunteer health professionals. In other instances, services are provided by the students' own primary care providers or by school-linked health centers upon referral by school health personnel. **School-linked health centers** are off-campus agencies that have formal agreements with schools to provide specific services to students (California School Health Centers Association, 2011).

The use of school-linked health centers allows for the provision of services that may be prohibited in the school setting itself (e.g., contraceptive services) or that require a level of expertise not held by school health personnel, such as drug abuse treatment. These centers also have the advantage of an economy of scale, providing specialty services to several schools when it would be cost-prohibitive to have specialized personnel available in each school (Advocates for Youth, n.d.).

The population health nurse assesses the availability of health care services to meet the needs of the school population. Are health-promotive and illness-preventive services easily accessible in the community? Are services available for youngsters with special health needs (e.g., handicapped children)? Are specific pediatric or adolescent services available? Is there access to contraceptive services or treatment of sexually transmitted diseases for the adolescent population?

Nutrition services. The nutrition services component of the coordinated school health program encompasses the quality of food available through and outside of school meal programs, policies and practices related to school nutrition, and the availability of feeding programs beyond the school day (Society of State Leaders of Health and Physical Education, n.d.). This component also includes education to promote good nutrition in children and their families as well as the adoption of innovative programs, such as farm-to-school programs and school gardens, to foster nutrition knowledge and healthy eating (American Dietetic Association, et al., 2010).

Best practices for school nutrition programs recommended by the Society of State Leaders of Health and Physical Education (n.d.) include:

- Creating a school health advisory council to review nutrition services in the school
- Reviewing district and school wellness policies for their effects on nutrition services
- Reviewing the school nutrition education program and integrating instruction with provision of healthy food choices
- Strengthening school nutrition services by providing breakfast in the classroom, demonstrating the relationship of nutrition and physical activity, including more fresh fruits and vegetables in school meals, providing nutrition information to families, increasing enrollment in school meal programs, ensuring healthy options in vending machines, exploring innovative programs, and increasing the availability of affordable, healthy food at school and in the community, and
- Providing recess before lunch.

The final recommendation is based on research indicating that holding recess before lunch prevents children from rushing through meals to get out and play. More is eaten, with fewer foods wasted, and transitioning back to the classroom is easier than from recess (Society of State Leaders of Health and Physical Education, n.d.).

Population health nurses can assess the quality of school meal programs, cleanliness of preparation areas, and the extent of nutrition education in the school setting. In addition, they can help to identify students eligible for free meals and work to enroll them. Hunger among children does not stop when the school year ends, and population health nurses may also assist low-income children and their families to access existing summer food service programs supported by the U.S. Department of Agriculture (2013). If no program exists locally, nurses can assist schools or other local organizations to develop them.

Counseling, psychological, and social services. Another component of the coordinated school health program is the provision of counseling services for psychological or social problems experienced by students and their families. Population health nurses can assess the need for and availability of such services in the school population and among individual students.

Students with disabilities may need special accommodations that allow them to be successful in the educational setting. The most commonly sought accommodations are for learning disabilities, but students with other documented physical and emotional disabilities are eligible for accommodations as well. For students suspected of learning or other disabilities, school nurses can make referrals for testing and can ensure that the appropriate accommodations are made.

Students and school staff may also need counseling for a variety of other personal problems. Sometimes such services are provided within the school, but they may also be available through school-linked health centers described earlier. Suicide prevention is an area in which counseling is urgently needed, yet identification of students contemplating suicide may be difficult. SOS, the Signs of Suicide Prevention Program, is one approach to identifying these students. In the SOS program, students are taught to recognize signs of depression and possible suicide in themselves and peers and to take action using the ACT rubric of Acknowledging feelings, demonstrating Caring, and Telling a responsible adult (Screening for Mental Health, 2010; U.S. Department of Health and Human Services [USDHHS], 2012).

Healthy and safe school environment. Elements of a safe school environment were addressed earlier. Population health nurses would assess the extent of physical safety hazards in the environment as well as the potential for disasters affecting the school population. Another assessment consideration is school policies related to safety. In addition, the nurse would examine the school climate and any factors that threaten the psychological health of students or staff.

Health promotion for staff. Effective school health programs attend to the health needs of school personnel as well as students. The population health nurse would assess the health services (including counseling and nutrition services) available to staff beyond the basic provision of health insurance coverage. Services to school employees serve several purposes, including reduction in illness and absenteeism, enhancement of interest in health issues and willingness to address them with students, and role-modeling healthy behaviors.

Family and community involvement. The final component of the school health program is directed toward fostering partnerships among school, family, and community that enhance the health of the overall community. Family involvement in their children's education has been associated with better school performance. A current policy brief of the National Education Association (2008) notes that involvement occurs in several ways: school support and assistance with parenting, two-way communication between schools and families, volunteering, learning at home (e.g., assistance with homework, goal setting, and other activities), decision making, and community collaboration by coordinating school and community resources and initiatives. The National Parent Teacher Association (NPTA, n.d.) has developed a set of standards for family–school partnerships that include the following:

- Families are active, welcomed, and valued participants in all aspects of school life.
- Families and school staff communicate regularly and in meaningful ways about student learning.
- Families and school staff collaborate to support students' learning and development.
- Families are empowered to advocate for their own and other children to ensure access to learning opportunities that support succcess.
- Families and school staff are equal partners in decisions that affect children and families and collaborate in policy development.
- Families and school staff collaborate with community members to expand learning opportunities, services, and civic participation (NPTA, n.d.).

In addition, the organization has developed an assessment guide that can be used to evaluate the quality of school–family interactions. The guide includes specific indicators for each standard that are rated from "not there yet" through levels 1 (emerging), 2 (progressing), and 3 (excelling), with descriptors for each level (NPTA, 2008). For further information about the guide, see the *External Resources* section of the student resources site.

The population health nurse can use the guide to assess school–family relationships as well as the relationship between the school and the health care community. Are private physicians conversant with regulations for excluding children with communicable conditions from school? Do physicians and other health care providers work cooperatively with school personnel to meet the health care needs of individual youngsters? Do health care providers in the community provide a resource for augmenting school health services?

School-based health centers. In some schools, some of the elements of a coordinated school health program, such as school health services, counseling, and health promotion for staff, are provided through school-based health centers. Under the Affordable Care Act program of grants for school-based health center development, a **school-based health center (SBHC)** is defined as a health clinic located in or near a school facility that is organized through school, community, and health provider relationships, administered by a sponsoring facility, and provides primary health services to children in accord with state requirements for such clinics. Sponsoring facilities can include hospitals, public health departments, community health centers, nonprofit health care agencies, schools or school systems, or a program administered by the Indian Health Service, Bureau of Indian Affairs, or an Indian tribe or tribal organization (Catalogue of Federal Domestic Assistance, n.d.). Common features of SBHCs include written parental consent for student enrollment; an advisory board of community members, parents, youth, and family organizations; clinical services by a multidisciplinary team of qualified professionals; and a comprehensive range of services that meets the identified needs of young people in the community (Center for Health and Health Care in Schools, 2013).

A 2010 study by the Robert Wood Johnson Foundation (RWJF) found 1,900 SBHCs located in 45 states, Washington, DC, and Puerto Rico. These centers provide care to more than 2 million students each year, and 84% of them are led by nurse

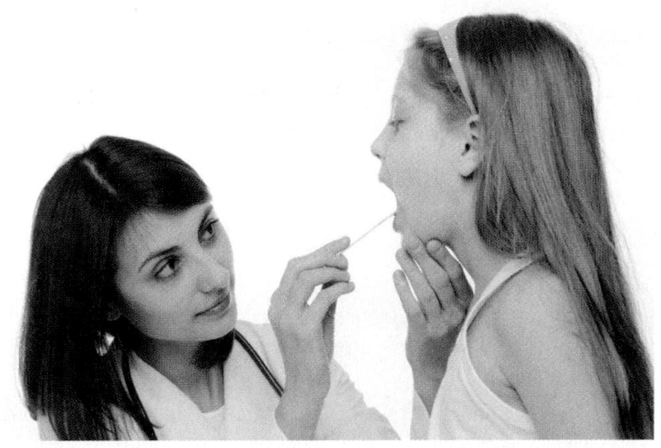

School-based health centers may be the only source of health care for many students. *(Mykola Velychko/Fotolia)*

practitioners. SBHCs do not duplicate the work of the school nurse, but provide primary care and screening services for the school population. Nearly three fourths of them also provide mental health services (RWJF, 2010). Additional services may include immunizations and reproductive services (Walker, Kerns, Lyon, Bruns, & Cosgrove, 2010).

Students with access to SBHCs have been found to be 10 to 21 times more likely to seek mental health services than other students (RWJF, 2010). In addition, students who use SBHCs have been shown to have better grade point averages than nonusers, are less likely to drop out of school, and have less absenteeism. Other outcomes have included decreased hospitalizations and better attendance among students with asthma (Center for School, Health and Education, 2011). SBHCs increase access to medical care for students without a medical home. In some school systems, SBHCs also provide health care services to family members (RWJF, 2010).

Population health nurses may be involved in planning SBHCs or in evaluating their effectiveness. School nurses work collaboratively with SBHC staff to meet the needs of individual students in the school setting. In addition, as much as 20% of SBHC activity is devoted to health education activities and interactions with parents and staff, which may also involve the school nurse (Center for School, Health and Education, 2011).

Tips for assessing health system determinants in a school setting are provided in the *Focused Assessment* below. A specific guideline for conducting a population-based health assessment in the school setting is provided on the student resources site.

Diagnostic Reasoning and Care of School Populations

The second aspect of the use of the nursing process in the school setting is deriving nursing diagnoses from assessment data. Diagnoses can be derived at two levels, in relation to individual students and in relation to the school population. Examples of diagnoses related to an individual student are "difficulty in participating in vigorous physical exercise due to exercise-induced asthma" and "need for referral to child protective services due to suspected physical abuse by father." Diagnoses related to a population group might be "safety hazard due to placement of play equipment on asphalt surface" and "need for drug abuse education due to high prevalence of drug abuse in the surrounding community."

Each of the sample diagnoses provided above contains a statement of the probable underlying cause of the problem. Such a statement provides direction for efforts to resolve the problem. With the individual examples, measures might be taken to provide a tailored physical activity program for the child with asthma and encourage use of a steroid inhaler or to make a referral for child protective services in the abuse situation. One approach to the playground safety hazard might be to relocate play equipment to a sandy area.

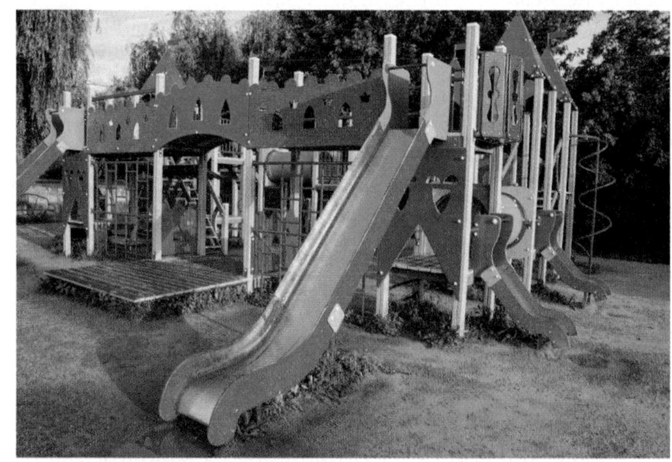

Monitoring the safety of play areas is part of the population health nurse's role in the school setting. *(ksena32/Fotolia)*

FOCUSED ASSESSMENT

Assessing Health System Determinants of Health in School Populations

- What health services are offered in the school setting? How are school health services funded? Is funding adequate to meet health needs?
- Are all of the components of a coordinated school health program in place? How effectively are the components implemented?
- How are school health services organized? Is there a school-based or school-linked health center associated with the school?
- What is the availability of mental health services in the school setting? Are referrals made to outside sources of care as needed?
- How accessible are needed health services in the community? To what extent does the school population use available health services?
- To what extent are school health services coordinated with primary providers and community health services?

Planning and Implementing Services to Meet the Health Needs of School Populations

Several general recommendations have been made for improving health care in school settings. The first of these is to increase the ratio of school nurses to students as identified in *Healthy People 2020* to one nurse to every 750 students. When this was done in New Jersey public schools, improvements were noted in immunization rates, identification of asthma and other life-threatening conditions, and screening rates. In addition, employment of more school nurses resulted in a return of more than 2 hours per day to other personnel who no longer had to deal with students' health problems (RWJF, 2010).

In addition, the Healthy Schools Campaign has made recommendations to both the U.S. Department of Education (USDOE) and the Department of Health and Human Services (USDHHS). Education recommendations included providing grant funding to support health-related training for teachers and principals, developing best practices related to school health, and integrating health measures into data tracking and school accountability systems. A further recommendation was the inclusion of health measures into criteria for the Blue Ribbon Schools program (Healthy Schools Campaign, 2012). The Blue Ribbon Schools program is a national award program that recognizes schools where students perform at the highest levels or that have made significant advances in student academic achievement (USDOE, 2013). Recommendations to USDHHS included reducing barriers to school health services, particularly by regularizing Medicaid payments for services provided to eligible students in school settings, and supporting schools in creating conditions that promote health and prevent illness (Healthy Schools Campaign, 2012).

Planning to meet health needs identified in the school setting takes place at two levels: the macro level, at which the general approach to providing health services in the school is planned, and the micro level, at which plans are made to meet specific health needs of the school population. The population health nurse working in the school setting participates in planning efforts at both levels.

IMPLEMENTING A COORDINATED SCHOOL HEALTH PROGRAM. At the macro level, the population health nurse will be an integral player in the development and implementation of a coordinated school health program if one does not already exist. A school health committee should plan each of the components of the school health program using the program planning process described in Chapter 15∞. Elements to be considered in developing the plan include the population to be served including the age range of students and the extent of services to be provided to staff. The type of services to be provided is another consideration. Typical services are summarized in Table 22-3●. Other planning considerations presented in the table include personnel, resources needed and their availability, budget, record system development, planning for family and community involvement, and approaches to be taken in evaluating the program. Once the plan has been developed,

TABLE 22-3 Considerations in Planning a Coordinated School Health Program

Area for Consideration	Related Elements
Population served	Ages and grades of students involved Extent of service to be provided to staff Provision of services to families
Services provided	Assessment/screening services First aid/emergency response Acute care services Problem management services Immunizations Safety education Health education Physical activity opportunities Nutrition services/education Counseling services Reproductive services Substance abuse services
Personnel	Categories of health and other personnel needed Qualifications of health and other personnel Functions and responsibilities Staff development needs
Resources	Facilities Equipment Supplies/postage Health records Telephone
Record system	Clinical health records for individuals seen Administrative records Immunization records Absenteeism records Program evaluation records Physical activity participation records School meal participation records
Budgetary considerations	Personnel salaries Facility construction and maintenance Equipment and supply costs Record-keeping costs Staff development costs
Family/community involvement	Strategies for promoting parent involvement Roles of parent and other volunteers Strategies for promoting community involvement Availability of shared resources
Program evaluation	Focus of evaluation Data collection procedures Data analysis procedures

implementation can occur. Table 22-4● summarizes the steps in developing and implementing a coordinated school health program. For information on funding sources for coordinated school health programs, see the *External Resources* section of the student resources site.

The health services component of the coordinated school health program also includes planning for specific activities or programs at each of the four levels of health care: health promotion, illness and injury prevention, resolution of existing health problems, and health restoration. Considerations and population health nursing roles at each level are discussed below.

HEALTH PROMOTION. Health promotion in the school setting involves many of the same planning considerations as those used with children in general. Primary areas of focus include health education for lifelong health habits and promoting physical activity and good nutrition. Other concerns in health promotion include developing a strong self-image, positive coping skills, and good interpersonal skills in students.

Health education in the school setting provides a foundation for healthy behaviors in adulthood. Most states and school districts require some form of health education at the elementary and junior and senior high school level. At the elementary level, health education is most likely to be incorporated into the total curriculum. Specific health courses are more likely at the junior and senior high level.

The principles of health education discussed in Chapter 11∞ are particularly relevant to population health nursing in the school setting. The nurse may serve as a resource for teachers on health content, provide health education classes, or both. The school nurse is also involved in the development of the health education curriculum. Activities involved in curriculum development include the assessment of needs and resources, review of health curricula from other school systems, development of goals and objectives, and design of specific learning activities. In addition, the nurse may be involved in preparing teachers to participate in the health education program. Finally, the nurse participates in the implementation and evaluation of the program. School nurses may also be involved in the provision of health education to school staff to enable them to promote their own health as well as serve as role models for healthy behavior for students.

With respect to physical activity, population health nurses working in school settings can assist school personnel in developing a multicomponent school-based activity program. School nurses can assist in the creation of a balanced plan that includes a variety of physical activity opportunities, including arrangements for activities before and after school,

TABLE 22-4 Steps in Planning and Implementing a Coordinated School Health Program

Step	Related Tasks
Secure and maintain administrative support for the program	Incorporate a coordinated school health program into the mission and vision statements of the school district/school Appoint an overseer for the program Obtain and allocate necessary resources Model healthy behavior among all personnel Develop relevant health-related policy Regularly communicate the importance of health to administrators, staff, students, and parents
Establish a school health council	Incorporate representation from all eight components of the coordinated school health program Include parents, community members, and older students
Identify a school health program coordinator	Select a coordinator with both organizational and interpersonal skills
Focus on students	Optimize health status Develop lifelong healthy behaviors Enhance educational performance
Develop a plan for a coordinated school health program using the program planning process	Develop priorities based on identified student needs Determine available resources and other needed resources Develop an action plan with realistic goals and measurable objectives Establish an implementation timeline Evaluate goal achievement
Implement multiple strategies and components	Use innovative strategies appropriate to situational constraints
Address priority health-enhancing and risk behaviors	Focus on age-appropriate health promotion and risk reduction concerns
Provide staff professional development	Educate all personnel on the overall health care program Provide discipline-specific professional education for staff who will implement specific elements of the program

Data from: Division of Adolescent and School Health, Centers for Disease Control and Prevention. (2013d). *How schools can implement coordinated school health.* Retrieved from http://www.cdc.gov/healthyyouth/cshp/schools.htm

incorporation of activity breaks in the classroom, promoting physical activity at recess and lunch breaks, and development of an enhanced physical education program that addresses the standards discussed earlier. In addition, population health nurses can assist schools and communities in the development of mechanisms for active transportation to and from school. For example, nurses may assist in identification of safe biking and walking routes to school or advocate for traffic calming strategies (speed bumps, traffic signals, stop signs, patrolled crossings, etc.) on routes used by students.

Nurses may also assist schools and communities in developing strategies like the "walking school bus," which is a group of children walking to school with one or more adults. Strategies for creating a walking school bus include selecting a neighborhood within walking distance, inviting parents and children to participate, identifying a safe route (or routes) to school, walking the route without children initially to determine its safety, identifying responsible adults to supervise the walk, and developing the logistics (e.g., timing, days of operation, where to meet, etc.). Nurses may also be involved in safety training for students and adult volunteers. CDC recommendations for adult supervision are one adult to six children with more adults for younger children and fewer adults for older groups (Pedestrian and Bicycle Information Center, n.d.).

Nutrition is another important aspect of health promotion with the school population. As noted earlier, when this function is not performed by a dietitian or nutritionist, school nurses assess the nutritional status of children and monitor the nutritional value of school lunches. When nutritional offerings are inadequate, the nurse works with school administrators and food service personnel to improve the nutritional quality of meals served. The nurse may also educate children and their parents regarding nutrition and good dietary habits.

The Division of Adolescent and School Health (DASH, 2011) has developed guidelines and associated strategies for promoting physical activity and nutrition in school populations. Those guidelines and strategies are summarized in Table 22-5•.

Health promotion in the school population includes fostering mental as well as physical health. Mental health education should be provided and should address, at a minimum, self-image development, coping skills, and interpersonal skills. Sound mental health is promoted by a strong self-image developed throughout childhood. Mental health promotion in the school setting should focus on the development of a healthy self-image as well as a healthy physical self. School nurses can foster self-image development by serving as role models in their dealings with children. They can also suggest to teachers learning activities that enhance development of a positive self-image.

Another aspect of health promotion in schools is the development of coping skills. Students and personnel can be assisted to develop active problem-solving strategies that promote their abilities to cope with adverse circumstances. School health nurses can serve as role models in this respect and can also provide counseling that assists students and their families or staff to engage in positive problem solving. Nurses can also reinforce evidence of positive coping by making others aware of their abilities to cope. In addition, the nurse can present information on stress and offer strategies for dealing with stress that enhance the development of sound coping skills.

The ability to interact effectively with others is essential to civilized society. Such abilities are not innate and must be learned. Education for effective interpersonal skills is another aspect of health promotion for the school population. Again, the nurse can serve as a role model for effective interpersonal skills and can educate students, parents, and staff regarding interpersonal interactions and the development of communication skills. The nurse can also provide information on group dynamics and communication skills that can enhance interpersonal skills within groups. For example, the nurse might promote role-play in a class to which a handicapped child will soon be admitted or help youngsters learn how to express anger at a teacher in an appropriate manner. Population health nurses working with school populations may assist individual students in developing these skills. They may also be involved in the creation and support of peer support groups for students with special needs (NAMI, 2012). Aspects of health promotion in the school setting and related population health nursing responsibilities are summarized in Table 22-6•.

ILLNESS AND INJURY PREVENTION. There are two main foci for prevention in school populations: preventing illness and other health-related conditions and preventing injury, including injury resulting from violence. Both foci will be discussed in terms of the population health nurse's role.

Preventing illness and other health-related conditions. Major considerations in preventing illness and other conditions in school populations include immunization, preventing the spread of communicable diseases, HIV and STI prevention, preventing pregnancy, and skin cancer prevention. Students in school settings at all levels are at particular risk for a variety of communicable diseases for which immunization is possible. Immunizations against measles, mumps, rubella, diphtheria, pertussis, tetanus, and polio are required for school entry. School immunization requirements were initiated in 1885 in Massachusetts with a mandate for smallpox immunization for school entry. Immunization for school entry has been assessed by state and local health departments since 1978 (Stokley, Stanwyck, Avey, & Greby, 2011) although specific requirements may vary among jurisdictions. In many states, immunization for *Haemophilus influenzae* B, varicella, and hepatitis B are also required. Immunizations are also available for hepatitis A and influenza. These diseases are discussed in more detail in Chapter 26∞.

The school nurse may be involved in referring individuals who are not immunized for appropriate services or may provide immunizations in the school setting. In addition to providing for routine immunizations, school nurses may also suggest other immunizations in the event of exposure to certain diseases, such as hepatitis A. Population health nurses may need to keep local school boards up to date on recommended

TABLE 22-5 Guidelines and Selected Strategies to Promote Healthy Eating and Physical Activity

Guideline	Related Strategies
Use a coordinated approach to develop, implement, and evaluate healthy eating and physical activity policies and practices	Coordinate healthy eating and physical activity policies through a school health council and coordinator Assess healthy eating and physical activity policies and practices Use a systematic approach to develop, implement, and monitor healthy eating and physical activity policies Evaluate healthy eating and physical activity policies and practices
Establish school environments that support healthy eating and physical activity	Provide access to healthy foods and physical activity opportunities and to safe spaces, facilities, and equipment Establish a climate that encourages and does not stigmatize healthy eating and physical activity Create a school environment that encourages a healthy body image, shape, and size among all students and staff members, is accepting of diverse abilities, and does not tolerate weight-based teasing
Provide a quality school meal program and ensure that students have only appealing, healthy food and beverage choices offered outside of the school meal program	Promote access to and participation in school meals Provide nutritious and appealing school meals that comply with the *Dietary Intake Guidelines for Americans* Ensure that all foods and beverages sold or served outside of school meal programs are nutritious and appealing
Implement a comprehensive physical activity program with quality physical education as the cornerstone	Require K–12 students to participate in daily physical education using a planned and sequential curriculum and instructional practices consistent with national or state physical education standards Provide a substantial percentage of students' recommended daily amount of physical activity in physical education class Use instructional strategies that enhance students' behavioral skills, confidence, and desire to adopt and maintain a physically active lifestyle Provide ample opportunities for all students to engage in physical activity outside of physical education classes Ensure that physical education and other physical activity programs meet the needs and interests of all students
Implement health education that provides students with the knowledge, attitudes, skills, and experiences needed for healthy eating and physical activity	Require health education from prekindergarten through grade 12 Implement a planned and sequential health education curriculum that is culturally and developmentally appropriate, addresses a clear set of behavioral outcomes that promote healthy eating and physical activity, and is based on national standards Use curricula that are consistent with scientific evidence of effectiveness Use classroom instructional methods and strategies that are interactive, engage all students, and are relevant to their daily lives and experiences
Provide students with health, mental health, and social services to address healthy eating, physical activity, and related chronic disease prevention	Assess student needs related to physical activity, nutrition, and obesity, and provide counseling and other services to meet those needs Ensure students have access to needed health, mental health, and social services Provide leadership in advocacy and coordination of effective school physical activity and nutrition policies and practices
Partner with families and community members in development and implementation of healthy eating and physical activity policies, practices, and programs	Encourage communication among schools, families, and community members to promote adoption of healthy eating and physical activity behaviors among students Involve families and community members in the school health council Develop and implement strategies for motivating families to participate in school health programs and activities that promote healthy eating and physical activity Access community resources to help provide healthy eating and physical activity opportunities for students Demonstrate cultural awareness in healthy eating and physical activity practices throughout the school
Provide a school employee wellness program that includes healthy eating and physical activity services for all school staff members	Gather data and information to determine the nutrition and physical activity needs of school staff and assess the availability of existing school employee wellness activities and resources Encourage administrative support for and staff involvement in school employee wellness Develop, implement, and evaluate healthy eating and physical activity programs for all school employees
Employ qualified persons and provide professional development opportunities for physical education, health education, nutrition services, and health, mental health, and social services staff members, as well as staff members who supervise recess, cafeteria time, and out-of-school-time programs	Require the hiring of physical education teachers, health education teachers, and nutrition services staff members who are certified and appropriately prepared to deliver quality instruction, programs, and practices Provide school staff members with annual professional development opportunities to deliver quality physical education, health education, and nutrition services Provide annual professional development opportunities for school health, mental health, and social services staff members and staff who lead or supervise out-of-school-time programs, recess, and cafeteria time

Source: Division of Adolescent and School Health. (2011, September 16). School health guidelines to promote healthy eating and physical activity. *Morbidity and Mortality Weekly Report, 60*(Suppl), 1–76.

TABLE 22-6 Health Promotion Strategies for School Populations

Area of Emphasis	Population Health Nursing Responsibilities
Health education	Participate in designing health education curricula Provide consultation to teachers on health education topics Provide in-service for teachers related to health education Provide health education in the classroom Arrange for other health education experiences (e.g., field trips or guest speakers) Arrange for or provide health education for staff and/or families
Physical activity	Educate students, staff, and families regarding the need for physical activity Assist schools in developing multicomponent physical activity programs Assist schools in promoting active transportation programs Assist in the development of walking school bus programs Help in identifying safe routes to and from school Advocate for traffic calming measures on routes Provide safety training for adults and students
Nutrition	Assess the nutritional quality of school meals Consult on healthy school meal planning Consult on special nutrition needs for specific students Assist in developing a nutrition education program Educate students, staff, and families on good nutrition
Mental health promotion	Advocate for a school climate that promotes mental health Assist in the development of the mental health education curriculum Assist individual students and staff in the development of problem-solving, stress management, and coping skills Teach students and staff problem-solving, stress management, and coping skills Role model effective problem-solving, stress management, and coping skills Assist students and staff to develop effective interpersonal and communication skills Role model effective interpersonal and communication skills Assist in the development of peer support groups for students and staff

immunizations and advocate for changes in immunization requirements to accommodate new national guidelines. Political advocacy may also be needed at the state level to change immunization requirements. At the same time, nurses may need to advocate for immunization waivers for specific children on the basis of religious beliefs or medical contraindications.

School exclusion is another strategy for preventing the spread of disease in the school population. One of the earliest responsibilities of the school nurse was to determine when children should be excluded from school because they had communicable illnesses. Children were also excluded from school as part of an effort to stop the spread of scabies, lice, and other parasites among a highly susceptible population. This responsibility still requires the school nurse to be knowledgeable of the signs and symptoms of communicable disease and infestation and to be aware of state and local regulations regarding school exclusion. Several conditions that usually warrant exclusion and guidelines for readmission of individual students are listed in Table 22-7●.

The responsibility of the nurse does not stop with excluding the affected child from school. The nurse should also educate parents and children regarding the need to stay home from school when they are ill and about care during illness. The nurse may also make referrals for medical care as needed. In addition, the nurse follows up on children excluded from school to make sure that they are receiving appropriate care and that they are able to return to school when there is no longer any danger of exposure to others.

Exclusion may also occur when schools are closed in the event of emergencies or communicable disease outbreaks. Population health nurses working in school settings should be actively involved in monitoring communicable disease incidence and in decisions to close schools. They should also be involved in the development and implementation of emergency response plans. Nurses may be one of several personnel responsible for notifying parents and explaining the situation, particularly in the event of disease outbreaks. They may also be involved in making sure that appropriate parties pick children up from school in an emergency situation and in helping to make sure that all children are accounted for. They may also assist working parents to plan alternative child care arrangements in the event of school closures. In one study of a school closure in response to an outbreak of H1N1 influenza, most parents were accepting of the school dismissals, although 20% reported missing work as a result of having to stay home with children, 2% of whom indicated that this was a major problem (Steelfisher et al., 2010). Assisting parents with preplanning for days when their own childen are ill or in the face of school closures can help to avoid such problems.

Preventing HIV infection and AIDS and other sexually transmitted infections (STIs) involves educating students regarding these diseases and their transmission, promoting abstinence or delayed sexual activity when possible, and promoting condom use for students who are sexually active. As we saw earlier, although most school jurisdictions mandate some form of HIV education, it often occurs after sexual activity has been

TABLE 22-7 Conditions Typically Warranting Exclusion from School and Guidelines for Readmission

Condition	Readmission Guidelines
Bacterial conjunctivitis	After acute symptoms subside
Chickenpox	5 days after eruption of the first vesicles or after lesions are dried
Diphtheria	When negative cultures of nose and throat are obtained at least 24 hours after discontinuing antibiotics
Hepatitis A	One week after onset of jaundice
Impetigo (staphylococcal)	24 hours after treatment is initiated
Influenza	After acute symptoms subside
Measles	4 days after onset of the rash
Meningococcal meningitis	24 hours after chemotherapy is initiated or when the child is sufficiently recovered
Mononucleosis, infectious	After acute symptoms subside. Delay resumption of strenuous physical activity until spleen is nonpalpable.
Mumps	9 days after onset of swelling
Pediculosis	24 hours after application of an effective pediculocide
Pneumonia, pneumococcal and *Mycoplasma*	48 hours after initiation of antibiotics or when child is sufficiently recovered
Pertussis	After 5 days of antibiotic therapy or when child is sufficiently recovered
Respiratory disease (viral) and upper respiratory infection	After acute symptoms subside
Rubella	7 days after onset of the rash
Scabies	24 hours after treatment
Streptococcus (strep throat, scarlet fever, impetigo)	24 hours after treatment is initiated or when child is sufficiently recovered
Tinea corporis	Excluded only from gym, swimming pool, or other activities where exposure of other individuals may occur; activities resume after treatment is completed

initiated. The National HIV/AIDS Strategy, on the other hand, recommends education about HIV and STIs prior to the initiation of sexual activity (Kann et al., 2012). In essence, this means that education should occur in middle school rather than high school. Recommended topics for HIV and other STIs include the difference between HIV and AIDS, STI transmission, diagnosis and treatment information, health consequences, the benefits of abstinence, prevention strategies, and how to access reliable sources of information. Other topics to be addressed include the influence of peers, parents, and the media on sexual risk taking, communication and negotiation skills, goal-setting and decision-making skills, and compassion related to those living with AIDS.

Population health nurses may be involved in the development of HIV and STI education programs and may either teach them or support educational personnel who do so. They are also frequently involved in one-to-one counseling of sexually active students regarding risks and prevention strategies such as condom use. They may also assist students in communication and negotiation strategies to forestall unwanted sexual activity or to promote condom use. Nurses may also need to advocate for the availability of condoms to sexually active students.

Similar strategies are needed to prevent unwanted pregnancies in school populations. Such strategies occur at the individual, school, and outside-of-school levels. At the individual level, school nurses may assist students in making sound decisions for condom use. They may also provide or make referrals for reproductive services such as contraceptives. At the school level, nurses are involved in pregnancy prevention programs and education, assisting students to develop realistic views of sexual activity and the consequences of pregnancy. Finally, population health nurses may need to advocate outside of the school setting for policies that permit provision of reproductive services as part of the coordinated school health program (Center for School, Health and Education, 2011).

Recommended topics for education programs related to pregnancy prevention include reproductive anatomy and physiology, puberty and adolescent development, identity formation, pregnancy and reproduction, and HIV and other STIs. Other areas to be discussed include healthy relationships with family, peers, and intimate partners, with particular attention to the use and impact of technology and media in relationships, and personal safety (Future of Sex Education Initiative, 2012).

Recommendations have also been made for school-based strategies to prevent skin cancer. These recommendations include adoption of policies to minimize ultraviolet exposure in school settings, provision of an environment conducive to sun-safety practices, and health education on skin cancer prevention. Other strategies include encouraging the use of sunscreen and protective clothing and minimizing sun exposure (CDC, n.d.). A final recommendation is to modify school environments to provide more shade through the use of shade structures and planting trees (Division of Cancer Prevention and Control, n.d.). The Arizona Department of Health Services (2013) has developed a "SunWise" program to promote skin cancer prevention in schools. For further information about the program, see the *External Resources* section of the student resources site.

One final aspect of illness prevention in the school population involves prevention of heat-related illnesses. Population health nurses can educate coaches, teachers, students, and parents regarding heat illness, particularly in the context of sports participation. They can also encourage adequate hydration and advocate for implementation of acclimatization guidelines that limit the duration and intensity of summer practice sessions with gradual increases over a 2-week period. Fluid recommendations in hot weather include 200 to 300 mL every 10 to 20 minutes during vigorous physical activity. In addition, nurses can advocate for policies and systems that monitor ambient air temperatures leading to adjustment of physical activities as needed (Gilchrist et al., 2010).

Preventing injury. Elements of injury prevention for school populations include elimination of safety hazards, encouragement of safety practices, prevention of bullying and other forms of violence, and suicide prevention. Part of the school nurse's responsibility is to identify safety hazards and report them to those responsible for eliminating them. Safety education may also be the responsibility of the school nurse. In addition, the nurse might collaborate with others within and outside the school setting to reduce safety hazards in the surrounding area. Moreover, the nurse and other school personnel might become involved in cooperative efforts with local police to reduce drug traffic in the neighborhood.

Specific strategies for preventing violence and bullying in school settings include fostering a culture of respect for all, creating connections between students and adults in the school setting, and breaking the code of silence among students with respect to plans for school violence. Tasks involved in creating a safe, connected school environment where violence is prevented include assessing the school's emotional climate, emphasizing the need to listen to others, adopting a strong but caring stance against the code of silence, and preventing or intervening in bullying. Other tasks include involving members of the school population, parents, and the community in developing a culture of respect and safety, developing trusting relationships between students and at least one adult in the school setting, and creating mechanisms for sustaining safe schools. Population health nurses can advocate for policies related to bullying and violence, including cyberbullying, and educate parents in monitoring and enforcing proper online behavior. Legislation proposed under the Safe Schools Improvement Act would require schools receiving federal aid to have comprehensive anti-harassment and anti-bullying policies and programs to prevent such behaviors. Such legislation would also require schools to report harassment data (Long, 2012). Defeated in 2012, the proposed legislation was reintroduced in 2013, but the bill had not been passed as of June, 2014 (Human Rights Campaign, 2014).

Strategies for preventing sexual harassment in schools include sensitivity training for students and staff and changing the culture of the school so that victims of and witnesses to harassment speak out. Population health nurses can advocate for and assist in implementing such programs. They can also teach school personnel how to recognize and respond to harassment and convey to students that harassment of any kind is not funny (Kearl, 2012).

Schools are also in a position to identify abuse of students or staff and to engage in educational programs to prevent abuse. Students can be taught personal safety, coping and resiliency skills, decision making, impulse control, and anger management. Other curricular topics include conflict resolution and stress management. Parenting education can also be provided to parents to prevent abuse.

Health services should also be provided for children who have been abused, and counseling and psychological and social services provided to address underlying factors. School personnel, including school nurses, are mandated by state law in all states to report suspected abuse to the appropriate authorities. In addition to reporting the situation, however, the nurse has a responsibility to provide counseling or referral for assistance to those involved and to serve as a support person for both victim and abuser. In such cases, referrals may also be needed to address socioeconomic problems that may be contributing to the situation. Finally, schools can participate in community-wide efforts to prevent abuse. Schools and school nurses can also be involved in collaborative efforts with other community groups and agencies to address issues of drug trafficking and gang activity that may contribute to violence on or near schools.

Suicide prevention is another area of concern in injury prevention for school populations. Strategies for prevention involve identifying students at risk for suicide and providing mental health treatment. The Substance Abuse and Mental Health Services Administration (SAMHSA) has identified Signs of Suicide (SOS) prevention programs as an evidence-based suicide prevention strategy (Screening for Mental Health, 2010). This program involves educating students and teachers to identify signs of depression and potential suicide risk in themselves or others and respond using the ACT format discussed earlier. Acknowledging feelings validates and recognizes feelings of depression. Acknowledgment is followed by expressions of caring for the person involved, and by telling a responsible adult about signs of depression and the potential for suicide. Suicide prevention and other aspects of illness and injury prevention in the school setting and related population health nursing responsibilities are summarized in Table 22-8•.

RESOLVING EXISTING HEALTH PROBLEMS. School students and staff may experience existing health problems that require resolution. There are four main approaches for dealing with existing health conditions: screening, referral, counseling, and treatment.

Screening is a major facet of most school health programs and an important responsibility of the school nurse. Screening can be used to detect health conditions that are amenable to treatment and that can be resolved with appropriate therapy.

TABLE 22-8 Illness and Injury Prevention Strategies for School Populations

Area of Emphasis	Population Health Nursing Responsibilities
General illness prevention	Teach effective hygiene, particularly hand washing Advocate for good hygiene in meal preparation
Immunization	Educate students, staff, and families regarding the need for immunization Provide or refer for routine immunization of students and staff as needed Recommend and arrange for additional immunizations as warranted by circumstances (e.g., an outbreak of hepatitis A) Advocate for modifications in immunization requirements as indicated for evidence-based practice
School exclusion	Identify students with communicable conditions and arrange for exclusion from school Notify parents and explain the need for school exclusion Refer for treatment services as needed Educate students and parents on preventing the spread of disease Follow-up on excluded students to ensure appropriate care
HIV/AIDS and other STI prevention	Assist in development and implementation of HIV/AIDS/STI education programs Provide and encourage use of condoms by sexually active students Advocate for condom availability in school settings
Pregnancy prevention	Assist in development and implementation of pregnancy prevention programs Assist students in developing negotiation skills for refusing sexual activity or insisting on safe sexual practices
Skin cancer prevention	Assist in incorporation of sun safety into school curricula Educate students, staff, and families on the importance of sun protection Advocate for sun safety policies in school Encourage use of sunscreen by students and staff for all outdoor activities Encourage wearing of protective clothing (hats, sunglasses, etc.) Encourage use of shaded areas for outdoor activities Advocate for architectural and environmental changes to increase shade on school campuses Role model sun safety practices
Heat illness prevention	Educate coaches, teachers, students, and parents regarding heat illness Encourage adequate hydration Encourage modification of physical activities based on ambient temperatures Advocate implementation of acclimatization guidelines for summer sports practices
Unintentional injury prevention	Identify and report safety hazards to appropriate school authorities Assist in developing and implementing safety education programs for students and staff Collaborate in the development of school policies that promote safety Advocate for environmental modifications that promote safety (e.g., changes in traffic patterns on school grounds, restricted access to school grounds, classroom doors that lock from the inside, safe surfaces under playground equipment) Advocate use of safety equipment in classrooms and sports activities
Bullying and violence prevention	Advocate for development and enforcement of policies against bullying, weapons carrying, and violence at school Foster effective interpersonal relationships among students Foster effective relationships between students and school personnel Teach interpersonal communication and conflict resolution strategies and assist in their incorporation in school curricula Assist in creating a culture of respect for all members of the population Educate students and staff on signs of child abuse
Suicide prevention	Educate students and staff on signs of depression and suicidal ideation Assist in development and implementation of suicide prevention programs Advocate for provision of mental health services on campus Refer depressed students for evaluation and treatment

For example, vision screening is used to identify children with visual problems, the majority of whom can benefit from corrective lenses. Screening may also help to identify children with particular needs that necessitate adjustments in the education program. For example, developmental screening may help to identify youngsters with learning disabilities who will benefit from special education programs.

A screening program also provides an opportunity to stress the importance of health promotion and illness prevention. Dental screening, for example, provides an excellent opportunity to educate students on the need for good dental hygiene. Finally, screening efforts provide one measure of the effectiveness of current preventive efforts. For example, hematocrit screening can provide evidence of one aspect of the efficacy of a school lunch program or nutrition education program in promoting good nutrition.

Screening is a cost-effective approach to the identification of health problems. Typical costs of a screening program include those of the screening procedure itself and of retesting those with positive results, time spent by the nurse in referral, costs of diagnostic and treatment services, special education costs, and costs of corrective maintenance (e.g., for hearing aids or replacing eyeglasses). These costs tend to be far lower than the costs incurred when diagnoses are made later, after problems become more pronounced.

Screening programs typically undertaken in the school setting include screening of vision and hearing, dental screening, height and weight measurements (including BMI), and screening for mental health problems (NASN, 2011b). Other screening tests may also be employed, depending on the needs of the population served by the school. For example, tuberculosis, lead, sickle cell, and diabetes screening may be conducted in communities with high prevalence of these conditions.

The population health nurse in the school setting may perform a variety of roles with respect to screening programs. The nurse might arrange for the screening to be done, conduct the screening tests, or train volunteers to perform certain screening procedures. Moreover, the nurse is usually responsible for informing students and parents of the results of screening tests and for interpreting those results. The nurse may also need to make referrals for follow-up diagnostic or treatment services. In addition, the nurse follows up on these referrals to make sure that students are receiving appropriate health care services.

School health nurses make a number of referrals. In addition to referrals for following up on positive screening test results, the nurse may make referrals for a variety of other services. For example, the nurse might refer children who are not immunized to the local health department for immunizations, or a referral for counseling might be needed for a child with behavior problems. School personnel may also be referred for health problems that require medical attention. In making these and other referrals, the school nurse uses the principles of referral discussed in Chapter 12∞. If services to which children have been referred involve costs to the family, the nurse may need to assist the family to find sources of funding for these services.

Counseling is another important role for the school nurse in resolving existing health problems. As noted in Chapter 1∞, counseling involves assisting clients to make informed health decisions. Nurses may counsel individual students regarding personal problems, or they may assist students, families, and staff to engage in problem solving. They may also be involved in development of counseling services within the coordinated school health program.

School nurses may also be involved in the actual treatment of existing health conditions. Treatment can involve emergency care in the event of illness or injury. School nurse practitioners might even engage in medical management of minor illnesses such as antibiotic treatment of otitis media.

Nurses may also be involved in providing specific treatments designed to minimize the effects of acute and chronic conditions. For example, the nurse may need to dispense prescribed medications or engage in specific technical procedures. The need for expertise in the use of medical technology in the school setting has increased dramatically and derives from the inclusion of children with a variety of physical, mental, and emotional health problems in the school population. The school nurse may also be involved in assisting students and staff with chronic illnesses such as diabetes or asthma to effectively manage their conditions.

School nurses may assist with physical therapy or perform procedures such as tracheostomy suctioning or catheterization. They may also be involved in programs for bowel or bladder training. Population health nurses working with children with disabilities in the school setting may also find it necessary to educate other school personnel in procedures required and deal with the fears experienced by school staff regarding the child's condition.

Caring for children with special health needs in the school setting entails the development of an Individualized Healthcare Plan (IHP). Components of the IHP include a health history, identification of special care needs (e.g., required procedures), an overview of the child's basic health status, and information about medications, including who dispenses them, timing, dosages, routes of administration, and so on. Additional elements of the plan include special dietary or nutritional needs, transportation needs, requirements for specialized equipment, identification of possible problems and strategies to solve them, and a plan for emergency action and transportation. Finally, the IHP should indicate review by the nurse, physician, parent, and school administrator and be incorporated in an easily retrievable location in the student's record. According to the NASN (2012a), IHPs should be developed for students who have multiple health needs, require lengthy care or multiple health care contacts, have daily health care needs, or other identified needs for care.

In addition to planning care for students with special needs, the population health nurse monitors the therapeutic effects and side effects of medications and other treatments. Treatment may also involve monitoring self-medication by students. For conditions such as asthma, the ability to self-medicate may mean a difference between adequately controlled and uncontrolled disease. Unfortunately, some schools have policies that prohibit self-medication by students. The American Academy of Pediatrics (AAP) has recommended that responsible students be allowed to carry and self-administer medications that do not require refrigeration and do not carry the potential for abuse or sale to others. School nurses would be actively involved in determinations of a students' ability to self-administer medications (AAP, 2013).

The Council on School Health of the AAP has issued a policy statement on medication administration in school settings (AAP, 2013). The statement recommends development of medication administration policies in all schools, and

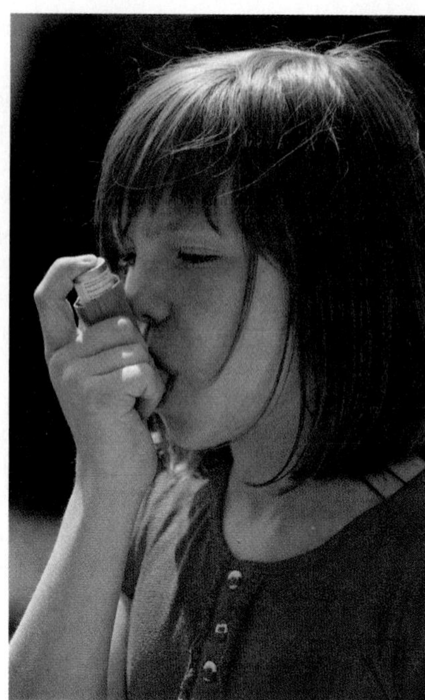

Students may need to carry and self-administer some medications. *(petert2/Fotolia)*

population health nurses can be actively involved in the development of such policies. The ideal situation is to have medications administered by a full-time school nurse; in the nurse's absence, however, administration may be performed by trained unlicensed assistive personnel (UAP) with appropriate supervision from a registered nurse in accord with relevant state laws, regulations, and guidelines. It is recommended that the UAP be a regular employee of the school. General principles of medication administration in the school setting include the following:

- Protecting student safety and preventing errors.
- Identifying the licensed health professional responsible for safe keeping, accessibility, and administration of medications and documentation of their use (including use by students who self-administer medications).
- Conducting regular systematic review of medication administration records.
- Providing ongoing training for UAPs who administer medications.
- Establishing and following effective communication systems related to medication administration.
- Requiring a written medication form signed by both the authorized prescriber and parent.
- Requiring written parental permission for administration of over-the-counter (OTC) medications and limiting the duration of use of OTC medications.
- Protecting student confidentiality.
- Providing training, delegation, and supervision of UAPs who administer medications.
- Permitting responsible students to carry and self-administer emergency medications authorized by school policies
- Encouraging parents to provide spare life-saving emergency medications in the health office.
- Making provision for secured and immediate access to emergency medications at all times, including before and after school and during off-campus school-sponsored activities.
- Storing medications in original, appropriately labeled containers in appropriate locations.
- Returning excess medication to parents or appropriately disposing of it at the end of the school year (AAP, 2013).

Strategies for resolving existing health problems in school settings are summarized in Table 22-9●.

HEALTH RESTORATION. Health restoration services are undertaken to prevent the recurrence of a health problem or to minimize its long-term effects on health. To a large extent, health restoration measures depend on the problems experienced by the student or staff member. Generally speaking, however, there are seven aspects of restoration with which the school nurse is concerned: rehabilitation, preventing the recurrence of acute problems, preventing complications, fostering adjustment to chronic illness and disability, dealing with learning disabilities, sustaining school-based health services, and promoting recovery after a disaster or emergency event.

Students with injuries or serious illness may require rehabilitation services. For example, a student with a severe sports injury may need physical therapy, or a staff member recovering from a heart attack may need assistance with cardiac rehabilitation. School nurses may make referrals for rehabilitative services or encourage active participation in rehabilitation activities. In some cases, they may assist students or staff with physical therapy regimens, or they may monitor the progress and effects of rehabilitation.

Preventing the recurrence of acute health problems depends on adequate treatment for existing problems and elimination of conditions that might lead to recurrence. For example, the school nurse might need to educate parents and children regarding the need to complete the course of therapy for otitis media, or education might be needed related to toileting hygiene (e.g., wiping from front to back) to prevent a recurrent urinary tract infection. The nurse might also engage in efforts to help an abusive parent or unduly harsh teacher find other ways to vent frustrations, or might make a referral to help alleviate financial difficulties that are taxing coping abilities.

Health restoration interventions are also directed toward preventing complications of either acute or chronic health problems. For example, the school nurse might encourage parents of a child with strep throat to complete a course of antibiotics to prevent cardiac and urinary complications. Similarly, the nurse might suggest a cushion and frequent changes of position to prevent pressure sores in a student confined to a wheelchair.

TABLE 22-9 Strategies for Resolving Existing Health Problems in School Populations

Area of Emphasis	Population Health Nursing Responsibilities
Screening	Conduct screening tests or arrange for screening by others Train volunteers in screening procedures Interpret screening test results Notify parents of screening test results Make referrals for further tests or treatments as needed Follow up on referrals to determine outcomes and to ensure appropriate care for identified conditions
Referral	Refer children and families for health care and other services as needed Refer other school personnel for needed services
Counseling	Assist students, staff, or families to make informed health decisions Counsel students, staff, or families regarding personal problems Assist students, staff, or families to engage in problem solving Advocate for access to professional mental health services as needed Encourage students to disclose mental health and other stigmatized conditions to school personnel Encourage students in need of them to request teaching/learning accommodations Work to eliminate the stigma attached to mental health and other stigmatizing conditions Assure that school policies on confidentiality are known and enforced Provide or arrange for targeted mental health support services for special populations (e.g., children with disabilities, GLBT youth, veterans at the college level)
Treatment	Provide first aid for illness or injury Dispense medications prescribed for acute or chronic illnesses Monitor self-medication by students Develop the IHPs for care of children with special health needs Perform special treatments or procedures warranted by identified conditions Teach others to perform special treatments or procedures Monitor therapeutic effects and side effects of medications and other treatments

Health restoration measures for children with chronic or handicapping conditions involve assisting them to adjust to their condition and preventing complications. Specific measures depend on the condition involved. For example, special arrangements for physical education might be needed to prevent recurrent attacks of exercise-induced asthma, and special attention to diet might be required for the diabetic child or staff member. School-based health centers are ideally situated to monitor the effects of chronic disease management in the school population. Easy access to providers allows for drop-in visits to address questions and deal with treatment side effects or concerns (Clayton, Chin, Blackburn, & Escheverria, 2012).

Major considerations in dealing with children with chronic illness in the school setting involve money, transportation and facilities, and equipment. Additional considerations include nutrition and psychological well-being. The school nurse may need to refer students and parents to sources of financial assistance as a way to deal with the long-term care requirements of chronic and disabling conditions.

Transportation and facility considerations in the school setting include issues of physical access to facilities discussed earlier in this chapter. Another area for consideration is transportation to and from school and on field trips. The nurse identifies barriers to access in the school setting and serves as an advocate for the removal of those barriers. Likewise, the nurse attempts to arrange transportation and other circumstances so that students with chronic or disabling conditions can participate in as many regular school activities as possible, including field trips. Advocacy in this area might also be needed with overly protective parents of children with disabilities.

There may also be a need for special equipment to be used either at home or at school. The school nurse makes referrals to obtain such equipment or sees that it is provided by the school itself.

Nutrition may be particularly problematic for schoolchildren with chronic diseases or handicapping conditions. Youngsters with diabetes, for example, may need assistance in adapting a school meal program to a diabetic diet. Severely disabled children may need assistance with eating or may need to be fed. The school nurse assesses the special nutritional needs of children with these and similar conditions and then assists the child, family, and other school personnel to meet those needs. Again, advocacy may be required to assure the availability of special diets for children with particular nutritional needs.

The final consideration for children who have chronic illnesses or disabling conditions is their psychological well-being. These children should be helped to adjust to their conditions and to participate as normally as possible in the school routine. Parents, teachers, and other students may need to be discouraged from undermining the child's independence by "doing for" them. Values clarification exercises can help other children understand the problems of disabled or chronically ill children rather than make fun of them or pity them.

Children with ineffective immune systems may also need interventions to protect them from infection. The need to use universal precautions when dealing with blood and body fluids may heighten these children's sense of isolation and alienation.

Because there does not seem to be any form of prevention available for learning disability, work with learning-disabled children focuses on minimizing the effects of their disability. Some of the interventions that may be planned to assist learning-disabled children are learning by activity, involving multiple senses in learning activities, using repetition, providing direction in small steps, and giving directions without irrelevant detail. Teaching at the appropriate level, a level that creates a challenge but does not lead to frustration, may also be helpful. Other useful strategies include avoiding drastic changes in activities, limiting distractions, and creating a climate in which success is ensured and reinforced as often as possible.

The nurse is involved in development of individualized education plans (IEPs) that allow children with learning disabilities, as well as those with other chronic or handicapping conditions, to learn as easily as possible. Again, attention must be given to the psychological effects of being labeled as *learning disabled*. The nurse may need to function as an advocate with parents, teachers, and other children to avoid the application of labels that undermine the child's self-esteem. The nurse can also function as a role model in providing positive reinforcement for the child's strengths and accomplishments.

Another intervention at this level includes sustaining school-based health services through continued funding. One suggestion for sustaining services involves converting school-based health centers to federally qualified health centers (FQHCs). FQHCs are "community-based and patient-directed organizations that serve populations with limited access to health care" (Health Resources and Services Administration [HRSA]. n.d., p. 1). FQHCs are located in medically underserved communities and have governing boards that include consumers as 51% of the board. They are funded by HRSA and provide comprehensive primary care services on a sliding fee scale as well as supportive services such as education, transportation, and translation as needed (HRSA, n.d.). Population health nurses can help schools explore the ramifications of becoming FQHCs and negotiate the application process. For further information about FQHCs, see the *External Resources* section of the student resources site.

Another aspect of health restoration at the population level is assisting members of the school population to recover from a disaster or a traumatic event, such as a school shooting. School nurses are ideally placed to recognize the psychological after effects of major psychological trauma and for assisting members of the school population to cope with and recover from such events. For example, after Hurricane Katrina, a School Nurse Disaster Response Training Program was initiated to provide school nurses with additional expertise in recognizing and dealing with psychological problems among students and staff. Training included signs and symptoms of negative effects as well as information on local resources and how to access them. The training also addressed school nurse resiliency and dealing with their own responses to the disaster and its aftermath (Broussard et al., 2012). Students and members of the staff may also need assistance in dealing with the long-term physical effects of a disaster or emergency situation. School nurses can make referrals for needed treatment services and can also assist with rehabilitation following injury.

In addition to dealing with physical and psychological issues, population health nurses can refer students, staff, and their families to sources of financial and other assistance to promote recovery. Population health nursing roles in natural and man-made disasters are addressed in more detail in Chapter 25∞. Aspects of health restoration in the care of school populations and related population health nursing roles are summarized in Table 22-10•.

Evaluating Health Care for School Populations

Evaluating the effectiveness of care in the school setting focuses on the outcomes of that care. Evaluation can occur at two levels: the individual child or the total school population. Evaluative criteria for the care of the individual child reflect the effects of nursing care on the student's health status. For example, if a child is no longer abused by his parent, no longer has recurrent ear infections, or is now able to interact effectively with peers, the interventions of the nurse have probably been effective.

Evaluation of population level effects will also depend on the problems for which intervention was provided. Fewer adolescent pregnancies following a pregnancy prevention program or fewer absences among students with asthma after adhering to asthma care guidelines by school-based providers would be examples of the effects of population-based elements of the school health program.

As we noted earlier, various elements of the coordinated school health program can be evaluated using tools such as HECAT and PECAT. The overall coordinated school health program can also be evaluated. The processes used in evaluating the school health program are those discussed in Chapter 15∞. Specific evaluation tools have been developed for assessing the adequacy of the coordinated school health program. These include the *School Health Index* (SHI) developed by CDC (2012) and a similar tool, the *Healthy School Report Card*, developed in Canada (Lohrmann, Vamos, & Yeung, 2011).

Both tools are based on the eight components of the CDC model of a coordinated school health program. The SHI is a self-assessment guide incorporating modules related to each component that schools can use to evaluate their performance. Each module includes several criteria related to a specific component

TABLE 22-10 Health Restoration Strategies for School Populations

Area of Emphasis	Population Health Nursing Responsibilities
Rehabilitation	Refer students or staff for rehabilitative services Encourage active participation in rehabilitation activities Assist with rehabilitation measures (e.g., physical therapy) as needed Monitor rehabilitation progress and effects
Preventing recurrence of acute conditions	Eliminate risk factors for the condition Teach students, staff, or parents how to prevent recurrence of problems Make referrals that can assist in eliminating risk factors
Preventing complications of and promoting adjustment to chronic conditions and disabilities	Assist parents with finding sources of financial aid to deal with chronic conditions and disabilities Advocate for educational accommodations as needed Facilitate meeting special nutritional needs Assist with meeting special needs for transportation and facilities Provide for special equipment needs Promote psychological well-being Assist students, families, and staff to deal with the eventuality of death in terminal illnesses Refer for counseling as needed Function as an advocate as needed
Preventing adverse effects of learning disabilities	Provide consultation for teachers in dealing with children's learning disabilities Participate in the design of IEPs for children with disabilities Function as an advocate for the learning-disabled child as needed Serve as a role model in positively reinforcing the child's accomplishments
Sustaining school-based health services	Assist with identification of mechanisms for continued funding of school-based health services Assist with the development of plans to apply for FQHC status if warranted Conduct research to document the outcomes of school-based health care services
Disaster/Emergency recovery	Assist in identification of students and staff with long-term physical and psychological consequences Assist students and staff in coping with the aftermath of a disaster or emergency Refer students and staff for treatment of physical consequences of an emergency or disaster event Assist students or staff with rehabilitation following injuries sustained in a disaster or emergency event Refer students and staff for counseling for psychological consequences of an emergency or disaster event Refer students, staff, and families to other sources of assistance in disaster recovery

that are rated by school evaluators from "not in place," through "under development" and "partially in place," to "fully in place." The index also addresses several topics of particular interest in assessing the performance of the school health program, such as physical activity and physical education, nutrition, tobacco use prevention, asthma, safety, and sexual health. Separate versions of the tool are available for the elementary school level and middle and high school level. For further information about the tools and guidelines for their use, see the *External Resources* section of the student resources site. A source for information regarding the Healthy School Report Card is also provided.

A similar Continuous Quality Improvement Tool for School-based Health Centers is available for evaluating SBHC performance. Data address comprehensive annual risk assessments and biennial physical examinations for students seen in the SBHC, as well as "sentinel events" typical of various student age groups (Juszczak, Pastore, & Reif, 2013). Sentinel events are similar to the key indicators used for monitoring progress toward achievement of the *Healthy People 2020* objectives in the United States. Separate tools are available for elementary, middle, and high school settings. Some sentinel events, such as annual risk assessments and biennial physical examinations, poor school performance, and treatment for ADHD, are common to all three levels. Additional sentinel events for middle school assessment include tobacco use, pregnancy risk, parent/child conflict, and depression. Sentinel events for the high school version also include alcohol use, risk for violence, STI risk, and depression risk (Juszczak et al., 2013). For more information about the tool, see the *External Resources* section of the student resources site.

The school nurse collaborates with other members of the school health team in designing and implementing an evaluation of a coordinated school health program or an SBHC. The nurse may also be involved in collecting data related to the evaluation and interpreting those data. Finally, the nurse should be actively involved in decisions made on the basis of evaluative data.

At the national level, national objectives for the year 2020 related to school health can provide additional evaluative criteria. Selected objectives related to school health are included on the next page.

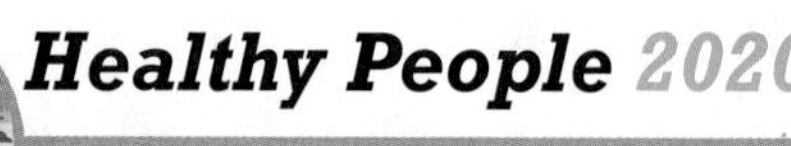

Healthy People 2020

Selected Objectives Related to the Health of School Populations

OBJECTIVE	BASELINE (YEAR)	TARGET	CURRENT DATA (YEAR)	DATA SOURCES
AH-2 Increase the proportion of adolescents who participate in extracurricular and/or out-of school activities	82.4% (2007)	90.6%	82.7% (2011–2012)	National Survey of Child Health (NSCH), CDC, HRSA/MCN
AH-5.1 Increase the proportion of students who graduate with a regular diploma in 4 years	74.9% (2007–2008)	82.4%	NDA	Common Core of Data (CCD), ED/NCES
AH-5.2 Increase the proportion of students served under the Individuals with Disabilities Education Act who graduate high school with a diploma	59.3% (2007–2008)	65.2%	NDA	Common Core of Data (CCD), ED/NCES
AH-5.6 Decrease absenteeism among adolescents due to illness or injury	5% (2008)	TBD	5.3% 2011	National Health Interview Survey (NHIS), CDC/NCHS
AH-6 Increase the proportion of schools with a school breakfast program	68.6% (2006)	75.5%	NDA	School Health Policies and Practices Study (SHPPS), CDC/ NCCDPHP
AH-7 Decrease the proportion of adolescents offered, sold, or given illegal drugs on school property	22.7% (2009)	20.4%	25.6% (2011)	Youth Risk Behavior Surveillance System (YRBSS), CDC/ NCCDPHP
AH-8 Increase the proportion of adolescents whose parents consider them safe at school	86.4% (2007)	95%	90.9 (2011–2012)	NSCH, CDC/ HRSA/ MCN
AH-10 Decrease the proportion of public schools with serious violence incidents	17.2% (2007–2008)	15.5%	NDA	School Survey on Crime and Safety (SSOCS), ED/ NCES
C-20.5 Increase the proportion of adolescents who use protective measures to prevent skin cancer	9.3% (2009)	11.2%	10.8% (2011)	YRBSS, CDC/ NCCDPHP
DH-14 Increase the proportion of children with disabilities who spend at least 80% of their time in a regular education program	56.8% (2007–2008)	73.8%	59.4% (2009–2010)	Data Accountability Center (DAC), ED/ OSERS
EMC-4.3.1 Increase the proportion of elementary schools that require health education that meets U.S. national health education standards*	7.5% (2006)	11.5%	NDA	SHPPS, CDC/ NCCDPHP
ECBP-2.1 Increase the proportion of elementary, middle, and senior schools that provide comprehensive school health education to prevent problems in all priority areas	25.6% (2006)	28.2%	NDA	SHPPS, CDC/ NCCDPHP
ECBP-5.1 Increase the proportion of elementary, middle, and senior schools with a full-time registered nurse school nurse to student ratio of at least 1:750	40.6% (2006)	44.7%	NDA	SHPPS, CDC/ NCCDPHP

Healthy People 2020 (Continued)

OBJECTIVE	BASELINE (YEAR)	TARGET	CURRENT DATA (YEAR)	DATA SOURCES
ECBP-6 Increase the proportion of the population that complete high school	89% (2007)	97.9%	89.8% (2009)	Current Population Survey (CPS), Census, DOL/BLS
FP-12.3 Increase the proportion of females who receive formal instruction on birth control before age 18#	70.5% (2006–2010)	77.6%	NDA	National Survey of Family Growth (NSFG), CDC/ NCHS
IVP-27.1 Increase the proportion of public and private schools requiring students to wear appropriate protective gear in school-sponsored physical education	76.8% (2006)	84.5%	NDA	SHPPS, CDC/ NCCDPHP
IVP-34 Decrease physical fighting among adolescents	31.5% (2009)	28.4%	32.8% (2011)	YRBSS, CDC/ NCCDPHP
IVP-35 Decrease bullying among adolescents	19.9% (2009)	17.9%	20.1% (2011)	YRBSS, CDC/ NCCDPHP
IVP-36 Decrease weapons carrying by adolescents on school property	5.6% (2009)	4.6%	5.4% (2011)	YRBSS, CDC/ NCCDPHP
NWS-2.1 Increase the proportion of schools that do not sell or offer calorically sweetened beverages	9.3% (2006)	21.3%	NDA	SHPPS, CDC/ NCCDPHP
NWS-2.2 Increase the proportion of school districts that require schools to make fruits and vegetables available when food is offered or sold	6.6% (2006)	18.6%	NDA	SHPPS, CDC/ NCCDPHP
OH-9.2 Increase the proportion of SHBCs with oral health components that offer dental care	10.1% (2007–2008)	11.1%	NDA	School-based Health Care Census (SBHCC), National Association of School-based Health Centers (NASBHC)
PA-4.1 Increase the proportion of the nation's public and private elementary schools that require daily PE for all students*	3.8% (2006)	4.2%	NDA	SHPPS, CDC/ NCCDPHP
PA-6.2 Increase the proportion of school districts that require regular recess in elementary schools	57.1% (2006)	62.8%	NDA	SHPPS, CDC/ NCCDPHP
TU-15.2 Increase tobacco-free environments in middle schools including all school facilities, properties, vehicles, and events@	58.7% (2006)	100%	NDA	SHPPS, CDC/ NCCDPHP

NDA—No data available

TBD—To be determined

*Similar objectives have also been developed for middle and high school levels with slightly different baseline data and targets.

Similar objectives have also been developed for males and for HIV/AIDS and STI education with slightly different baseline data and targets.

@ Similar objectives have also been developed for junior and senior high school levels with slightly different baseline data and targets.

Data from: U.S. Department of Health and Human Services. (2014). *Healthy people 2020: Topics and objectives.* Retrieved from http://healthypeople.gov/2020/topicsobjectives2020/default.aspx

CHAPTER RECAP

Population health nursing in schools provides an opportunity for promoting health and preventing illness in children and their families. Population health nurses working in school settings from preschool to college can also assist students and staff with existing health problems, as well as designing school health programs that promote the health of the general public. School nursing requires an advanced level of expertise due to the autonomy and level of responsibility involved, and certification as a school nurse is strongly recommended. School nurses work collaboratively with other members of the school health team and with professionals in the community to promote health and prevent injury and illness in the school population. They are also involved in resolving existing health problems and health restoration in individual students and staff and in the population in general.

Biological, psychological, environmental, sociocultural, behavioral, and health system determinants influence the health of the school population, and the coordinated school health program is designed to address factors in each area. Elements of a coordinated school health program include health education; physical education; health services; nutrition services; a healthy and safe environment; health promotion for school staff; family and community involvement; and counseling, psychological, and social services. Health promotion in the school setting focuses on health education, physical activity, nutrition, and mental health promotion. Prevention of illness and other health conditions in this population addresses immunization and school exclusion, HIV/AIDS and STI prevention, pregnancy prevention, and prevention of skin cancer and heat-related illness. Injury prevention strategies focus on safety and unintentional injury prevention, prevention of bullying and violence, and suicide prevention.

Resolution of existing health problems occurs for individuals and for the population as a whole. Areas of emphasis include screening, referral, counseling, and treatment. Health restoration strategies encompass rehabilitation, preventing recurrence of health problems, preventing complications and promoting adjustment to chronic illness, and preventing adverse effects of learning disabilities. At the population level, health restoration also includes sustaining school health services and recovery from disasters or emergency events.

A variety of approaches are available for evaluating the effectiveness of school health services. These include tools to evaluate the coordinated school health program and the performance of school-based health centers as well as achievement of national health objectives related to schools.

CASE STUDY Dealing with Bullying

The mother of a fifth grade student spent some time volunteering for playground duty during lunch at her son's private religiously affiliated school. During her supervision rotations, she witnessed some cruel treatment of overweight children who could not run as fast as others. Not only were they the last ones chosen for teams during recess, denigrating comments were often made like, "You take him, we don't want him." She had attempted to tactfully remonstrate with the students involved when she witnessed this behavior, but was met with blank and hostile stares. Conversations with her son and other members of the parent organization suggested that verbal and physical aggression were common in the school, but were particularly notable in this fifth grade class. In fact, her son told her, "Mom, if you're not one of the bullies, you'll be one of the victims."

"School nurse" services were provided by non-health-professional volunteers, who did not feel that they could interfere in the situation. The mother, a population health nurse, went to the school principal with her observations and offered to conduct some sensitivity training for her son's class. The principal declined saying that this was just typical behavior of students at that age.

1. What biological, psychological, sociocultural, behavioral, and health system determinants are operating in this situation?
2. What interventions might you employ to resolve the situation? What allies might you seek in your resolution efforts?
3. How would you evaluate the effectiveness of your intervention?

REFERENCES

Adams, P. F., Kirzinger, W. K., & Martinez, M. E. (2012). *Summary health statistics for the U.S. population: National Health Interview Survey 2011*. Retrieved from http://www.cdc.gov/nchs/data/series/sr_10/sr10_255.pdf

Advocates for Youth. (n.d.). *The school-linked health center: A promising model of community-based care for adolescents*. Retrieved from http://www.advocatesforyouth.org/index.php?option=com_content&task=view&id=543&Itemid=177

American Academy of Pediatrics, Council on School Health. (2013). *Policy statement—guidance for the administration of medication in school*. Retrieved from http://pediatrics.aappublications.org/content/124/4/1244.full?sid=a3b63ab1-529b-45e3-906f--8e3181ea8357

American Association of the Deaf-blind. (2009). *Deaf-blind young adults in action*. Retrieved from http://www.aadb.org/advocacy/2009/db_young_adult_in_action.html

American Association of the Deaf-blind. (2012). *About AADB*. Retrieved from http://www.aadb.org/aadb/about_aadb.html

American Dietetic Association, School Nutrition Association, & Society for Nutrition Education. (2010). Position of the American Dietetic Association, School Nutrition Association, & Society for Nutrition Education: Comprehensive school nutrition services. *Journal of the American Dietetic Association, 110*, 1738–1749. doi:10.1016/j.jada.2010.08.035

Arizona Department of Health Services. (2013). *SunWise skin cancer prevention school program*. Retrieved from http://www.azdhs.gov/phs/sunwise/

Avery, G., Johnson, T., Cousins, M., & Hamilton, B. (2013). The school wellness nurse: A model for bridging gaps in school wellness programs. *Pediatric Nursing, 39*(1), 13–18.

Broussard, M., Chrestman, S. K., & Arceneaux, C. K. (2012). Training school health nurses to recognize and refer student behavioral and mental problems in a post-Disaster setting. In J. W. Richardson & T. D. Wright (Eds.), *School-based health care: Advancing educational success and public health* (pp. 65–73). Washington, DC: American Public Health Association.

Bullying Statistics. (2013). *School bullying*. Retrieved from http://www.bullyingstatistics.org/content/school-bullying.html

Bundy, D. (2011). *Rethinking school health: A key component of education for all*. Retrieved from https://openknowledge.worldbank.org/bitstream/handle/10986/2267/600390PUB0ID171Health09780821379073.pdf?sequence=1

California Commission on Teacher Credentialing. (2012). *School nurse services credential*. Retrieved from http://www.ctc.ca.gov/credentials/leaflets/cl380.pdf

California School Health Centers Association. (2011). *School health centers in California*. Retrieved from http://www.ncg.org/s_ncg/bin.asp?CID=19728&DID=56136&DOC=FILE.PDF

Catalogue of Federal Domestic Assistance. (n.d.). *Affordable Care Act (ACA) grants for school-based health center capital expenditures*. Retrieved from https://www.cfda.gov/index?=program&mode=form&tab=core&id=79d4eebead370e109d0bdfa55881d33a

Center for Health and Health Care in Schools. (2013). *Definition of a school-based health center*. Retrieved from http://www.healthinschools.org/en/Health-in-Schools/Health-Services/School-Based-Health-Centers/Caring-for-Kids/definition-of-sbhc.aspx

Center for School, Health and Education. (2011). *The health, well-being and educational success of school-age youth and school-based health care*. Retrieved from http://www.schoolbasedhealthcare.org/wp-content/uploads/2011/09/APHA4_article_Health_Rev_9_14_FINAL2.pdf

Centers for Disease Control and Prevention. (n.d.). *Childhood sunburns can cause skin cancer. What can you do?* Retrieved from http://www.cdc.gov/cancer/skin/pdf/sunsafety_v0908.pdf

Centers for Disease Control and Prevention. (2006). *Physical education curriculum analysis tool (PECAT)*. Retrieved from http://www.cdc.gov/healthyyouth/PECAT/pdf/PECAT.pdf

Centers for Disease Control and Prevention. (2012). *School Health Index: A self-assessment and planning guide*. Elementary school version. Retrieved from http://www.cdc.gov/healthyyouth/shi/pdf/Elementary.pdf

Centers for Disease Control and Prevention. (2013a). *Health education curriculum analysis tool (HECAT)*. Retrieved from http://www.cdc.gov/healthyyouth/HECAT/index.htm

Centers for Disease Control and Prevention. (2013b). *Physical education curriculum analysis tool (PECAT)*. Retrieved from http://www.cdc.gov/healthyyouth/pecat/index.htm

Clayton, S., Chin, T., Blackburn, S., & Escheverria, C. (2012). Different setting, different care: Integrating prevention and clinical care in school-based health centers. In J. W. Richardson & T. D. Wright (Eds.), *School-based health care: Advancing educational success and public health* (pp. 15–25). DC, Washington: American Public Health Association.

Davis, J., & Bauman, K. (2013). *School enrollment in the United States: 2011*. Retrieved from http://www.census.gov/prod/2013pubs/p20-571.pdf

Deloitte. (n.d.). *No kid hungry starts with breakfast: Ending childhood hunger: A social impact analysis*. Retrieved from http://www.nokidhungry.org/pdfs/school-breakfast-brochure.pdf

Division of Adolescent and School Health. (2011, September 16). School health guidelines to promote healthy eating and physical activity. *Morbidity and Mortality Weekly Report, 60*(Suppl.), 1–76.

Division of Adolescent and School Health, Centers for Disease Control and Prevention. (2013a). *Characteristics of an effective health education curriculum*. Retrieved from http://www.cdc.gov/healthyyouth/sher/characteristics/index.htm

Division of Adolescent and School Health, Centers for Disease Control and Prevention. (2013b). *Components of coordinated school health*. Retrieved from http://www.cdc.gov/healthyyouth/cshp/components.htm

Division of Adolescent and School Health, Centers for Disease Control and Prevention. (2013c). *Goals of coordinated school health*. Retrieved from http://www.cdc.gov/healthyyouth/cshp/goals.htm

Division of Adolescent and School Health, Centers for Disease Control and Prevention. (2013d). *How schools can implement coordinated school health*. Retrieved from http://www.cdc.gov/healthyyouth/cshp/schools.htm

Division of Adolescent and School Health, Centers for Disease Control and Prevention. (2013e). *National health education standards*. Retrieved from http://www.cdc.gov/healthyyouth/sher/standards/index.htm

Division of Adolescent and School Health, Centers for Disease Control and Prevention. (2013f). *The case for coordinated school health*. Retrieved from http://www.cdc.gov/healthyyouth/cshp/case.htm

Division of Adolescent and School Health, Centers for Disease Control and Prevention. (2014). *Coordinated school health FAQs*. Retrieved from http://www.cdc.gov/healthyyouth/cshp/faq.htm

Division of Cancer Prevention and Control. (n.d.). *Shade planning for America's schools*. Retrieved from http://www.cdc.gov/cancer/skin/pdf/shade_planning.pdf

Environmental Protection Agency. (2014). *Healthy School Environments Assessment Tool (Healthy SEAT)*. Retrieved from http://www.epa.gov/schools/healthyseat/index.html

Future of Sex Education Initiative. (2012). *National sexuality education standards: Core content and skills, K-12 [a special publication of the Journal of School Health]*. Retrieved from http://www.futureofsexeducation.org/documents/josh-fose-standards-web.pdf

Gilchrist, J., Haileyesus, T., Murphy, M., Comstock, R. D., Collins, C., & McIlvain, N. (2010). Heat illness among high school athletes—United States, 2005-2009. *Morbidity and Mortality Weekly Report, 59,* 1009–1013.

Guttmacher Institute. (2012). *Facts on American teen's sexual and reproductive health.* Retrieved from http://www.guttmacher.org/pubs/FB-ATSRH.pdf

Haddad, M., Butler, G. S., & Tylee, A. (2010). School nurses' involvement, attitudes and training needs for mental health work: A UK-wide cross-sectional study. *Journal of Advanced Nursing, 66,* 2471–2480. doi:10.1111/j.1365-2648.2010.05432x

Hanink, E. (n.d.). *Lina Rogers: The first school nurse.* Retrieved from http://www.workingnurse.com/articles/Lina-Rogers-the-first-school-nurse.

Hawkins, J. W., & Watson, J. C. (2010). School nursing in the Iron Range in a public health nursing model. *Public Health Nursing, 27,* 571–578. doi:10.1111/j.1525-1446.2010.00897.x

Health Resources and Services Administration. (n.d.). *What is a health center?* Retrieved from http://bphc.hrsa.gov/about/

Healthy Schools Campaign. (2012). *Health in mind: Improving education through wellness.* Retrieved from http://healthyschoolscampaign.org/content/uploads/Programs/Health%20in%20Mind/Documents/Health_in_Mind_Report.pdf

Hill, C. (2012). When school harassment crosses the line. *AAUW Outlook, 106,* 8–11.

Huang, T. T.-K., Sorenson, D., Davis, S., Frerichs, L., Brittin, J., Celetano, J., …, Trowbridge, M. J. (2013, February 28). Healthy eating design guidelines for school architecture. *Preventing Chronic Disease, 10,* 120084. doi:10.5888/pcd10.120084

Human Rights Campaign. (2014). *Safe schools improvement act.* Retrieved from http://www.hrc.org/laws-and-legislation/federal-legislation/safe-schools-improvement-act

Juszczak, L., Pastore, D., & Reif, C. J. (2013). *A continuous quality improvement toolforschool-basedhealthcenters.* Retrievedfromhttp://www.healthinschools.org/en/Health-in-Schools/Health-Promotion/Prevention-Programs/Continuous-quality-improvement-for-SBHCs.aspx#tool.

Kann, L., Brener, N., McManus, T., & Wechsler, H. (2012). HIV, other STD, and pregnancy prevention education in public secondary schools—45 states, 2008–2010. *Morbidity and Mortality Weekly Report, 61,* 222–228.

Kearl, H. (2012). What schools can do about sexual harassment. *AAUW Outlook, 106,* 12–15.

Kohl, H. W. III, & Cook, H. D. (Eds.), Committee on Physical Activity and Physical Education in the School Environment. (2013). *Educating the student body: Taking physical activity and physical education to school.* Retrieved from http://www.nap.edu/download.php?record_id=18314

Long, E. (2012). Putting school safety on the books. *AAUW Outlook, 106,* 16–19.

Lorhmann, D. K., Vamos, S., & Yeung, P. (2011). *Creating a healthy school: Using the Healthy School Report Card* (Canadian 2nd ed.). Alexandria, CA: ASCD.

MâsseMâsse, L. C., Perna, F., Agurs-Collins, A., & Chriqui, J. F. (2013). Change in school nutrition-related laws from 2003 to 2008: Evidence from the School Nutrition-Environment State Policy Classification System. *American Journal of Public Health, 103,* 1597–1603. doi:10.2105/AJPH.2012.300896

National Alliance on Mental Illness. (2010). *Facts on children's mental health in America.* Retrieved from http://www.nami.org/Template.cfm?section=federal_and_state_policy_legislation&template=/ContentManagement/ContentDisplay.cfm&ContentID=43804

National Alliance on Mental Illness. (2012). *College students speak: A survey report on mental health.* Retrieved from http://www.nami.org/Content/NavigationMenu/Find_Support/NAMI_on_Campus1/collegereport.pdf

National Association of School Nurses. (2011a). *Corporal punishment in the school setting.* Retrieved from http://www.nasn.org/PolicyAdvocacy/PositionPapersandReports/NASNPositionStatementsFullView/tabid/462/ArticleId/20/Corporal-Punishment-in-the-School-Setting-Revised-2011

National Association of School Nurses. (2011b). *Role of the school nurse.* Retrieved from http://www.nasn.org/portals/0/positions/2011psrole.pdf

National Association of School Nurses. (2012a). *Chronic health conditions managed by school nurses.* Retrieved from http://www.nasn.org/Portals/0/positions/2012pschronic.pdf

National Association of School Nurses. (2012b). *Education, licensure, and certification of school nurses.* Retrieved from http://www.nasn.org/portals/0/positions/2012pseducation.pdf

National Association of School Nurses. (2014). *Frequently asked questions.* Retrieved from http://www.nasn.org/AboutNASN/FrequentlyAskedQuestions

National Association of School Nurses & American Nurses Association. (2011). *School nursing: Scope and standards of practice* (2nd ed.). Washington, DC: American Nurses Association.

National Board for Certification of School Nurses. (2013). *School nursing certification.* Retrieved from http://www.nbcsn.org/examination

National Center for Chronic Disease Prevention and Health Promotion. (2012). *Competitive foods and beverages in U.S. schools: A state policy analysis.* Retrieved from http://www.cdc.gov/healthyyouth/nutrition/pdf/compfoodsbooklet.pdf

National Center for Education Statistics. (2013). *Fast facts: School crime.* Retrieved from http://nces.ed.gov/fastfacts/display.asp?id=49

National Center for Injury Prevention and Control. (2012). *Youth violence: Facts at a glance.* Retrieved from http://www.cdc.gov/ViolencePrevention/pdf/YV-DataSheet-a.pdf

National Clearinghouse for Educational Facilities. (2008). *Mitigating hazards in school facilities.* Retrieved from http://www.ncef.org/pubs/mitigating_hazards.pdf

National Conference of State Legislatures. (2013). *School bullying: Overview.* Retrieved from http://www.ncsl.org/issues-research/educ/school-bullying-overview.aspx

National Education Association. (2008). *Parent, family, community involvement in education.* Retrieved from http://www.nea.org/assets/docs/PB11_ParentInvolvement08.pdf

National Parent Teacher Association. (n.d.). *National standards for family-school partnerships.* Retrieved from http://www.pta.org/files/National_Standards.pdf

National Parent Teacher Association. (2008). *National standards for family-school partnerships: Assessment guide.* Retrieved from http://www.pta.org/files/National_Standards_Assessment_Guide.pdf-

Office of Safe and Healthy Students. (2014). *About us.* Retrieved from http://www2.ed.gov/about/offices/list/oese/oshs/aboutus.html

Pedestrian and Bicycle Information Center for the Partnership for a Walkable America. (n.d.). *Starting a walking school bus.* Retrieved from http://www.walkingschoolbus.org/

Perou, R., Bitsko, R. H., Blumberg, S. J., Pastor, P., Ghandour, R. M., Gfroerer, …, Huang, L. N. (2013, May 17). Health surveillance among children—United States, 2005-2011. *Morbidity and Mortality Weekly Report, 62*(Suppl.), 1–35

Physical Activity Guidelines for Americans Midcourse Report Subcommittee of the President's Council on Fitness, Sports & Nutrition. (2012). *Physical activity guidelines for Americans midcourse report: Strategies to increase physical activity among youth.* Retrieved from http://www.health.gov/paguidelines/midcourse/pag-mid-course-report-final.pdf

Robers, S., Kemp, J., Truman, J., & Snyder, T. D. (2013). *Indicators of school crime and safety: 2012.* Retrieved from http://www.bjs.gov/content/pub/pdf/iscs12.pdf

Robert Wood Johnson Foundation. (2010, August). Unlocking the potential of school nursing: Keeping children healthy, in school, and ready to learn. *Charting Nursing's Future,* 1–8.

Rules and Regulations. (2006, August 14). *Federal Register, 71*(156), 46539–46845.

Safe Havens International. (n.d.). *School safety plan evaluation tool for K12 schools.* Retrieved from http://www.washoe.k12.nv.us/docs/pdf/K-12PlanEvaluationTool-SafeHavensIntl.pdf

Schneider, S. K., O'Donnell, L., Stueve, A., & Coulter, R. W. S. (2012). Cyber-bullying, school bullying, and psychological distress: A regional census of high school students. *American Journal of Public Health, 102,* 171–177. doi:10.2105/AJPH.2011.300308

Screening for Mental Health. (2010). *SOS Signs of Suicide Prevention Program (SOS).* Retrieved from http://www.mentalhealthscreening.org/programs/youth-prevention-programs/sos/

Smolinski, J. (2012). Cyber-harassment: When home isn't a haven. *AAUW Outlook, 106,* 20–21.

Society of State Leaders of Health and Physical Education. (n.d.). *School nutrition services.* Retrieved from http://www.thesociety.org/pdf/MTC-school-nutrition.pdf

Steelfisher, G. K., Blendon, R. J., Bekheit, M. M., Liddon, N., Kahn, E., Schieber, R., & Lubelt, K. (2010). Parental attitudes and experiences during school dismissals related to 2009 Influenza A (H1N1)—United States, 2009. *Morbidity and Mortality Weekly Report, 59,* 1131–1134.

Stokley, S., Stanwyck, C., Avey, B., & Greby, S. (2011). Vaccination coverage among children in kindergarten—United States, 2009–10 school year. *Morbidity and Mortality Weekly Report, 60,* 700–704.

Thomas-Presswood, T. N., & Presswood, D. (2008). *Meeting the needs of students and families from poverty.* Baltimore, MD: Paul H. Brookes.

U.S. Department of Agriculture, Food and Nutrition Service. (2013). *Summer food service program.* Retrieved from http://www.fns.usda.gov/sfsp/frequently-asked-questions-faqs

U.S. Department of Education. (2013). *National Blue Ribbon Schools Program.* Retrieved from http://www2.ed.gov/programs/nclbbrs/index.html

U.S. Department of Health and Human Services. (n.d.). *Bullying definition.* Retrieved from http://www.stopbullying.gov/what-is-bullying/definition/

U.S. Department of Health and Human Services. (2012). *School-based intervention reduces suicide attempts.* Retrieved from http://healthypeople.gov/2020/implement/sharinglibrary.aspx?storyID=12

U.S. Department of Health and Human Services. (2014). *Healthy people 2020: Topics and objectives.* Retrieved from http://healthypeople.gov/2020/topicsobjectives2020/default.aspx

Utter, J., Denny, S., Robinson, E., Ameratunga, S., & Milfont, T. L. (2011). Social and physical contexts of schools and neighborhoods: Associations with physical activity among young people in New Zealand. *American Journal of Public Health, 101,* 1690–1695. doi:10.2105/AJPH.2011.300171

von Hippel, P. T., Powell, B., Downey, D. B., & Rowland, N. J. (2007). The effect of school on overweight in childhood: Gain in body mass index during the school year and during summer vacation. *American Journal of Public Health, 97,* 696–702.

Walker, S. C., Kerns, S. E. U., Lyon, A., Bruns, E. J., & Cosgrove, T. J. (2010). Impact of school based health center use on academic outcomes. *Journal of Adolescent Health, 46,* 251–257. doi:10.1016/jadohealth/2009.07.002

World Conference on Education for All. (1990). *World declaration on education for all: Meeting basic learning needs.* Retrieved from http://www.unesco.org/education/wef/en-conf/Jomtien%20Declaration%20eng.shtm

World Education Forum. (2000). *The Dakar framework for action—Education for all: Meeting our collective commitments.* Retrieved from http://unesdoc.unesco.org/images/0012/001211/121147e.pdf

CHAPTER

23 Care of Employee Populations

Learning Outcomes

After reading this chapter, you should be able to:

1. Describe advantages of providing health care in work settings.
2. Identify types of health and safety hazards encountered in work settings.
3. Identify biological, psychological, environmental, sociocultural, behavioral, and health system determinants that influence health in work settings.
4. Describe areas of emphasis in health promotion, illness and injury prevention, resolution of existing health problems, and health restoration in work settings and analyze the role of the population health nurse with respect to each.
5. Describe approaches to evaluating health care for the working population.

Key Terms

emotional labor
employee assistance program (EAP)
ergonomics
hazard analysis
health indicators
job control
job demands
job strain
occupational health nursing
Occupational Safety and Health Administration (OSHA)
organizational justice
paraoccupational exposure
postexposure prophylaxis (PEP)
presenteeism
reasonable accommodation
screening
work–family balance
work–family conflict
work movement index
workplace aggression

Advocacy Then

Women Workers

As should be obvious, based on prior advocacy accounts in this book, Lillian Wald was involved in much more advocacy than that represented by her work at Henry Street. In addition to campaigning for the Children's Bureau and founding both public health nursing and school nursing, Wald was actively involved in a variety of endeavors to promote the safety of workers. She lobbied for health-related inspections of workplaces and endeavored to convince employers that healthy employees were more productive, encouraging them to prevent injury and illness and to employ nursing or medical professionals in the work setting.

Wald was particularly concerned about the plight of working women, and in 1903, she helped found the Women's Trade Union League. The intent of the league was to investigate the working conditions of women and promote women's trade unions. Wald was a member of the executive committee of the New York City league and was an active advocate and fund raiser (Jewish Women's Archive, 2010). The involvement of Wald and several other WTUL supporters in the National Association of Colored People (NAACP) was instrumental in thwarting employers' plans to bring in Black workers to break the Shirtwaist Strike (Lewis, n.d.) in 1909.

In addition, Wald raised public awareness for unions through her fund-raising and picketing efforts. Wald served on the Joint Board of Sanitary Control, an agency established to monitor environmental conditions in factories. She also advocated for a minimum wage for women and served as a representative to President Woodrow Wilson's Industrial Conference (Jewish Women's Archive, n.d.). Held in October 1919, the conference brought together employer groups, labor unions, and the public. Unfortunately, management representatives refused to agree to a provision endorsing the right of collective bargaining, causing labor representatives to withdraw from the conference. A second, smaller conference was held in 1920 (U.S. Department of Labor, n.d.a).

Advocacy Now

Promoting Breast-feeding at Work

Murtagh and Moulton (2011) described a variety of benefits for mothers, children, and employers when breast-feeding and/or breast pumping are encouraged in the work setting. Breast-feeding promotes child development, better immune system function, and decreased risk of a variety of acute and chronic conditions in children. Mothers experience decreased postpartum bleeding, diminished menstrual blood loss, earlier return to prepregnancy weight levels, and decreased risk of breast and ovarian cancer. Benefits for employers include reduced absenteeism and higher productivity, retention of experienced workers, and improved employee morale and company image. Additional benefits include reduced family expenditures for formula and a projected savings of $3.6 billion in health care costs if targeted breast-feeding rates identified in *Healthy People 2020* were achieved (Murtagh & Moulton, 2011).

Unfortunately, federal law only addresses the availability of reasonable break time to permit breast pumping, and few states have legislation that promotes breast-feeding at work. What is the policy regarding breast-feeding in your nursing education institution? Is breast-feeding of infants encouraged? Permitted? Is privacy provided for breast-feeding or breast pumping? Are there different policies related to breast-feeding by students and faculty/staff members? How might you and your classmates promote development of conditions on campus that foster breast-feeding by students and faculty/staff?

In 2010, 153.8 million people 16 years of age and older were employed in the U.S. civilian work force , and the following year, U.S. workers logged more than 258 trillion work hours (BLS, 2013c; U.S. Census Bureau, 2012a). By 2020, the number of employed people in the United States is expected to grow to more than 164.3 million (Toosi, 2012). Because of the large number of people involved, the work setting is an important place for promoting the health of the general population (Sorenson et al., 2011). Although the work environment contributes to a wide variety of health problems, it also provides opportunities to influence a major segment of the population regarding personal health behaviors and to modify the potential for exposure to hazardous circumstances.

Schulte, Pandalai, Wulsin, and Chun (2012) described four potential patterns or models of interaction between personal characteristics of employees and risk factors present in the occupational setting. In the first model, personal factors and occupational factors operate independently to result in a particular health problem. For example, a person with a substance abuse problem might be required, as part of his or her job, to operate hazardous machinery. In this case, substance abuse may combine with job requirements to lead to serious injury. In the second model, personal risk factors modify the effects of occupational risk factors to produce health-related effects. An example might be smoking on the part of an employee that makes him or her more susceptible to the carcinogenic effects of workplace exposures to coal dust and other substances. The third model posits the reverse relationship, in which workplace factors modify the effects of personal characteristics to affect health. For example, exposure to some respiratory agents in the work setting may exacerbate asthma in employees with this condition. Finally, personal and occupational factors may operate independently leading to different health problems that then interact. For example, being overweight may lead to hypertension and job strain may create stress, both of which may contribute to myocardial infarction.

The effects of work on health were noted by Bernardino Ramazzini, considered the father of occupational medicine, as early as the 1700s. In 1713, Ramazzini wrote about the occupational effects on musculoskeletal health and the effects of sedentary occupations and toxic exposures. Of particular note, Ramazzini addressed the health effects of typical women's occupations as well as those of men (Franco, 2012). Similarly, cutaneous anthrax was first associated with the handling of wool in 1837, although the disease itself was not diagnosed until 1880 (Bell, 2002). Henry Bell, a British physician who attended a man dying of anthrax, sent the death certificate to the police maintaining that the employer had caused the death due to his failure to disinfect the wool the deceased was working with. Bell's actions led to an inquiry and the institution of voluntary guidelines for the wool industry that were in effect until 1899 (Bell, 1902). In the early 20th century, Germany instituted *krankenhaussen*, sickness insurance funds for the working class, which prompted U.S. sociologists to promote occupational disease surveys. The first such survey was conducted in 1910 and focused on "occupational poisons," specifically occupational lead exposure (Hamilton, 2001). Despite this long history of knowledge of the effects of working conditions on health, thousands of workers are injured or develop occupational illnesses every year.

Over the years, however, employers have come to better appreciate that healthy employees are more productive and that it is in the employer's interest to promote and maintain employee health. Moreover, the escalating cost of health insurance makes health promotion increasingly cost-effective. One way that some companies have chosen to decrease health-related costs is to provide on-site health care for employees.

The importance of health care in the occupational setting can be seen in the national health objectives for the year 2020. In fact, one entire section of the objectives deals with health and safety in occupational settings (U.S. Department of Health and Human Services [USDHHS], 2014). The status of selected objectives is addressed later in this chapter. The importance of achieving these objectives is underscored by the fact that the direct and indirect costs of work-related injuries and illnesses are approximately $170 billion per year (Council of State and Territorial Epidemiologists, n.d.). Given the preventable nature of most of these events, health care focusing on the working population makes eminent sense.

Occupational Health Nursing

Not all nurses who practice in occupational settings are population health nurses. The population health nurse, however, is uniquely prepared to meet the health needs of the working population because of his or her knowledge of population health principles. Occupational health nursing is not a new role for the population health nurse. Nurses may have been employed in U.S. work settings as early as 1888, when a group of coal mining companies employed Betty Moulder to provide care for sick miners and their families (Roy, 2013). Organized industrial nursing, as it was then called, began in 1913 with the establishment of an industrial nurse registry (Committee to Assess Training Needs, 2000), and in 1914, the U.S. Public Health Service established the Office of Industrial Hygiene (Roy, 2013). By 1918, more than 800 businesses employed nurses, and colleges and universities began to offer short courses in industrial hygiene to support occupational health nursing practice (Committee to Assess Training Needs, 2000). Since that time, the role of the occupational health nurse has been expanded along with other nursing roles.

The Occupational Safety and Health Administration (OSHA) of the U.S. Department of Labor described occupational health nurses as "registered nurses who independently observe and assess the worker's health status with respect to job tasks and hazards. Using their specialized experience and education, these registered nurses recognize and prevent health effects from hazardous exposures and treat workers' injuries/illnesses" (OSHA, n.d.b, para 1). This definition does not, however, fully describe today's population health nursing role in work settings. It concentrates on the treatment aspects of care and the nurse's dependent functions and does not acknowledge the promotional and preventive aspects that are paramount in this practice setting. In its 2012 *Standards of Occupational and Environmental Health Nursing*, the American Association of Occupational Health Nurses (AAOHN, 2012e) defined **occupational health nursing** as a specialized area of nursing practice focused on health promotion, illness and injury prevention, and restoration in the work environment.

Educational Preparation for Occupational Health Nursing

Several types of nursing personnel may be found in occupational settings, including registered nurses prepared in associate degree and diploma programs in nursing as well as in baccalaureate degree programs; licensed practical nurses; and nurses prepared at the master's level. Because of the need to apply principles of population health nursing, nurses who engage in the full scope of the occupational health nurse's role should be prepared at least at the baccalaureate level in nursing. As noted by OSHA (n.d.b), the educational preparation of occupational health nurses may vary "from entry level to PhD work." Graduate level preparation might be in occupational health nursing, in community or population health nursing, or as a nurse practitioner. According to an Institute of Medicine (IOM) report, graduate preparation for occupational health nursing typically encompasses nursing, medical, and occupational health science; epidemiology; business and economics content; social and behavioral sciences; environmental health; and legal, regulatory, and ethical issues relevant to occupational health (Committee to Assess Training Needs, 2000).

Advanced preparation in occupational health nursing may result in certification by the American Board of Occupational Health Nurses (ABOHN). Established in 1972, the organization's first certification examination was given in 1974; in 2012, ABOHN celebrated its 40th anniversary as a specialty certification body (ABOHN, 2012).

Nurses in other settings may also be involved in providing care for health conditions related to work. This fact suggests that nurse practitioners working in ambulatory care settings where occupational conditions may be seen should have a basic grounding in the principles of occupational health.

Standards and Competencies for Occupational Health Nursing

Like other nursing specialties, occupational health nursing should be practiced in accordance with established standards. The AAOHN (2012e) has established 11 standards for competent occupational and environmental health nursing practice. These standards are focused primarily on the care of individuals in work settings and address both basic and advanced levels of practice. Areas of emphasis within the standards include assessment, diagnosis, outcome identification, planning, implementation, evaluation, resource management, professional development, collaboration, research, and ethics. For further information about the standards, see the *External Resources* section of the student resources site.

In addition, AAOHN (2012a) has developed a code of ethics for nursing practice in occupational health settings. The code addresses respect for human dignity, duty to society, privacy, collaboration, and personal competence and responsibility on the part of the occupational health nurse. (AAOHN, 2012).

Occupational Health Nursing Roles

As noted earlier, the role of the occupational health nurse has undergone significant change since the initial development of the specialty. Some of the factors contributing to those changes include an increased emphasis on evidence-based practice, greater focus on wellness initiatives in the work setting, and growing interest in alternative provider models. Additional factors include a focus on cost reduction, which may result in outsourcing of services and competition for funding, and a proliferation of other professionals who provide care for the employed population (AAOHN, 2012c).

The overall role of the occupation health nurse encompasses health and productivity management, which involves coordination of a variety of programs and services to promote, maintain, or restore the health of the employee population (AAOHN, 2012d). This role requires the occupational health nurse to collaborate with others to identify health and safety needs, prioritize interventions, plan and implement interventions and programs for the working population, and to evaluate care and service delivery systems (AAOHN, 2012c). As noted by AAOHN, occupational health nurses are in ideal positions to identify determinants affecting employee health, promote health-related behaviors, foster cost-saving interventions, and align health services with business goals. They also address legal issues in the work setting, safeguard privacy, and promote collaboration among departments of the employing organization, health care professionals, and outside vendors and organizations (AAOHN, 2012d).

The specific role functions of an occupational health nurse may vary somewhat from setting to setting, but there are some general commonalities among settings. These functions typically include direct primary care services for occupational and nonoccupational illnesses and injuries; case management, health hazard assessment and surveillance; monitoring of illness and injury trends; assuring compliance with regulatory mandates for privacy; health promotion, prevention, early recognition, and treatment of illness and injury; counseling, coaching, and training of employees; and research (AAOHN, 2012c). Additional role functions include crisis intervention, risk reduction, assuring compliance with legal and regulatory mandates for workplace conditions (AAOHN, 2012e), interpretation of medical diagnoses to workers and their families (OSHA, n.d.b), management and administration of the occupational health unit, and the development and maintenance of partnerships with community organizations and agencies (Committee to Assess Training Needs, 2000).

Specialized occupational health nurse consultants, whether internal or external to a particular business or industry, may carry out several additional functions. These may include assessment and identification of the need for occupational health services; development and marketing of health and wellness programs to industry; development of programs to address specific problems within a given setting; provision of direct care in the absence of an occupational health nurse employed in the setting; coordination of services from outside agencies and organizations; orientation of nurses new to occupational health; assistance with research grants and publications; and certification in specialty areas (Roy, 2013).

Population Health Nursing and Care of the Working Population

Nursing care in work settings is based on the use of the nursing process and includes assessment of the health of the population; development of nursing diagnoses; and planning, implementation, and evaluation of interventions to promote, protect, and restore health.

Assessing the Health Status of the Working Population

Assessment of employee health status and health needs is undertaken from the perspective of biological, psychological, environmental, sociocultural, behavioral, and health system determinants that influence health and illness in the working population.

BIOLOGICAL DETERMINANTS. Human biological factors to be addressed in assessing employee health status include those related to maturation and aging, gender, genetic inheritance, and physiologic function.

Maturation and aging. The age composition of a company's workforce affects its health status. If employees are primarily young adults or adolescents, health conditions that may be noted with some frequency include sexually transmitted diseases, hepatitis, and pregnancy. Younger employees may also be at increased risk of injury due to limited job training and skills. In 2012, U.S. labor force statistics indicated that just under 4% of the U.S. workforce was 16 to 19 years of age (5.8 million youth) (BLS, 2013b). The number of youth in the workforce is expected to increase slightly by 2020, but they will make up a smaller percentage of the overall workforce due to increases in the number of people who choose to remain in the workforce after typical retirement age. The percentage of youth in the workforce varies seasonally, ranging from approximately 33% in July 2013 to 24% in February 2014 when school was in session (Office of Disability Employment Policy, 2014).

Younger and older workers are more likely to be fatally injured on the job than middle-aged workers. For example, preliminary data for 2012 indicated a fatal injury rate of 2.9 per 100,000 full-time equivalent workers among 18- to 19-year-old workers. The rate decreases for workers aged 20 to 44 years and then begins to climb at age 45 to reach a peak of 9.8 per 100,000 among workers 65 years of age and older (Bureau of Labor Statistics [BLS], 2012a).

The health needs of older employees should also be considered. Because of prohibitions on forced retirement at specific ages in many occupations, many employees are continuing in the workforce beyond the time when they would have retired. Economic need and a desire for continued productivity are two factors that may influence this trend. Lack of skilled workers to replace them and the desire to embark on new careers are other factors that lead to the retention of older workers in the workforce (Wuellner et al., 2011). The number of workers over 65 years of age doubled from 1997 to 2007 (Sorenson et al., 2011). Based on Bureau of Labor Statistics data, there were more than 30 million people over age 55 in the U.S. workforce in 2010 and this group constituted 19.5% of those employed. This is the fastest growing age group in the workforce (Wuellner et al., 2011), and by 2020, an estimated 25.2% of U.S. employees or 41.4 million workers will be over 55 years of age (Toosi, 2012).

Although older workers bring valued skills and experience, declining physical ability and stamina and increasing sensory impairments place them at higher risk for occupational injury and illness. Although younger workers experience a higher rate of injury, older workers are at greater risk for occupational death as indicated earlier. For example, workers over 65 years of age are more than three times as likely as those in the age range of 18 to 54 years to experience occupational highway transportation fatalities and are twice as likely to die in traffic accidents as those 55 to 64 years of age (Pratt & Rodriguez-Acosta, 2013).

Because of diminished physical capacity, older workers consistently score lower on work ability measures than younger workers, but workplace modifications can improve the workability index for these older employees (Sorenson et al., 2011). In general, older employees tend to have fewer occupational injuries than younger workers, and illness rates are comparable (Wuellner et al., 2011), but older workers typically have more days away from work when illness or injury do occur. For example, the median number of days away from work for nonfatal injuries and illness among workers 65 years of age and older is more than four times that for workers aged 16 to 19 years (12 days and 3 days, respectively) (BLS, 2012b). Older workers are also more likely to experience falls on level surfaces and sustain fractures than younger workers, although they tend to have lower rates for many other types of injuries (Wuellner et al., 2011).

Another effect of aging as it affects occupational health lies in the effects of shiftwork. After age 45 or 50, people have more difficulty adjusting their sleep–wake cycles to accommodate changes in working hours, leading to fatigue, decreased productivity, and increased risk for accidental injury in hazardous working conditions (Smith, Folkard, Tucker, & Evans, 2011).

In addition to the risk for illness, injury, and death, older workers planning to retire in the near future may need assistance with retirement planning and in dealing with retirement issues (see Chapter 19∞ for a discussion of these issues). Older workers may also face discrimination in the workplace due to inaccurate perceptions regarding disability, cognitive decline, and diminished ability to learn new skills. Older workers are a definite asset in many businesses and industries experiencing a lack of younger workers to replace those who retire. In addition, older workers often possess experience and skills lacking in younger employees. Many older workers would remain in the work setting if their needs and preferences were accommodated.

Population health nurses working in occupational settings may find themselves advocating for the special needs of both younger and older workers. For example, they may need to encourage employers to arrange schedules to accommodate school schedules for younger employees. Similarly, they may need to advocate for equipment to assist with heavy lifting or other strenuous activities for older workers.

Gender. Gender is another biological determinant that influences the health of the working population. As noted by Ramazzini in his 18th-century treatise on occupational effects on health, women are not spared from adverse effects of occupational conditions (Franco, 2012). In 2010, women made up nearly half (47.2%) of the U.S. workforce (U.S. Census Bureau, 2012b), and in 2011 women accounted for 43% of all the hours worked (BLS, 2013a).

In spite of having less physical strength than men, women tend to have fewer injuries and account for only 8% of workplace fatalities (BLS, 2013a). In part, this is a result of men being employed in generally more hazardous occupations. These figures are likely to change, however, with more women moving into occupational fields traditionally reserved for men (e.g., construction, agriculture, transportation).

Women also face unique hazards in the work setting. For example, women often experience more difficulty in reconciling work and family roles leading to greater work–family conflicts. Some toxic exposures may also have differential effects for men and women, particularly women of childbearing age, and population health nurses may need to monitor the potential for teratogenic exposures (those that can cause damage to a fetus) in the work setting. There may also be a need to assist working women with contraceptive services or to provide prenatal care and monitor pregnancies. Population health nurses may also need to advocate for work modifications to accommodate pregnancy or to provide opportunities for breast-feeding or pumping breast milk.

Genetic inheritance. Both men and women experience the interaction of genetic inheritance factors with occupational conditions that may lead to illness. Genetic inheritance factors likely to be of greatest importance in the workforce are those related to race and family history of chronic illness. For example, in a largely African American labor force, hypertension may be prevalent. In an Asian population, particularly if large numbers are refugees, communicable diseases such as tuberculosis and parasitic diseases may be common.

Employees may also enter the workforce with a genetic predisposition to a variety of chronic conditions that can interact with occupational environmental risks to cause disease. Population health nurses can identify these genetic risks for chronic health problems and assist employees to engage in risk reduction strategies to prevent illness or to mitigate its effects. For example, workers with a family history of breast or other cancers can be referred for appropriate screening services or assistance with smoking cessation, if needed.

Physiologic function. Elements of physiologic function to be addressed in assessing the health of employees are the extent of injury and illness suffered by the population as well as immunization levels. In 2011, nearly 3 million nonfatal occupational injuries and illnesses occurred in the U.S. private employment sector for an incidence rate of 3.5 events per 100 full-time equivalent (FTE) workers. This represents a decrease in incidence from 5 events per 100 FTE workers from 2003. More than half of the events reported in 2011 required days away from work, job transfer, or restriction of job activities. Most (94.8%) of the events reported involved injuries, three fourths of which occurred in service-providing industries, such as health care, restaurants, and so on, and only one fourth in goods-producing industries. The rate of illness and injury among the additional 18.5 million public workers in federal and state agencies was 5.7 cases per 100 FTE workers, for an overall rate of 20.6 per 10,000 FTE workers (BLS, 2012d).

A total of 4,628 work-related fatalities or 3.4 deaths per 100,000 full-time equivalent workers occurred in 2012 (BLS, 2014), and another 2.9 million injuries were treated in emergency departments, 150,000 resulting in hospitalization (Centers for Disease Control and Prevention [CDC], 2013c). Transportation incidents accounted for 41% of these fatalities; falls, slips, and trips accounted for 15%; being struck by an object or equipment 10%, and other contact with an object or equipment 5%. Mortality rates are higher in some industries than others. For example, the highest rate of fatality occurred in industries related to agriculture, forestry, fishing, hunting (BLS, 2013a), followed by the construction industry (CDC, 2013b). Falls alone accounted for 4,693 fatalities overall and for 35% of deaths in the construction industry (BLS, 2013a; CDC, 2013b, 2013c), and the National Institute for Occupational Safety and Health (NIOSH) has initiated a campaign to prevent falls and reduce fall-related injuries and fatalities (CDC, 2012a). Similarly, fatality rates for both offshore and onshore oil and gas extraction industries are extremely high at 27.1 per 100,000 workers (Gunter, Hill, O'Connor, Retzer, & Lincoln, 2013).

Mortality figures have decreased by approximately 34% from 6, 217 deaths in 1992 to 4,628 in 2012 (Bureau of Labor Statistics, 2014). Estimated societal costs for fatal injuries are $6 billion per year, with an additional cost of $186 million for nonfatal injuries (CDC, 2012b). Musculoskeletal injuries alone, which affect more than 1 million workers each year, have an annual cost estimated at $45 billion to $54 billion (Sorenson et al., 2011). In 2010, for example, 3.1% of the total U.S. workforce experienced carpal tunnel syndrome, a musculoskeletal condition resulting from repetitive wrist movement or pressure, and its incidence increased with age (National Center for Health Statistics, 2011). Musculoskeletal injuries in general account for one third of time lost from work (Tarawneh et al., 2013). Cost figures, coupled with the costs in mortality, lost productivity, and diminished quality of life for those affected suggest the need for concerted efforts to prevent injuries and injury-related fatalities in the occupational setting. Nursing, for example, has a high prevalence of back injuries. Risks for occupational back pain include overexertion, vibration, and increased body mass index. An increased **work movement index**, or the extent of bending, stooping, twisting, and extended reach involved in a job, is also associated with increased risk of back injury.

Occupational illnesses include acute and chronic conditions that may affect an employee's ability to work as well as his or her quality of life. Population health nurses in occupational settings must be prepared to recognize and deal with the multitude of illnesses and injuries likely to arise from workplace conditions.

Illnesses in employees may be either work-related or nonwork-related. Work-related illnesses are acquired as a result of exposure to factors in the work setting. For example, workers in the coal mines are exposed to coal dust that may cause a variety of respiratory conditions (Laney, Wolfe, Petsonk, & Halldin, 2012). Similarly, workers exposed to diacetyl, a chemical compound used to flavor popcorn, are at risk for bronchiolitis obliterans, a severe lung condition with long-term consequences (Feldman, 2011).

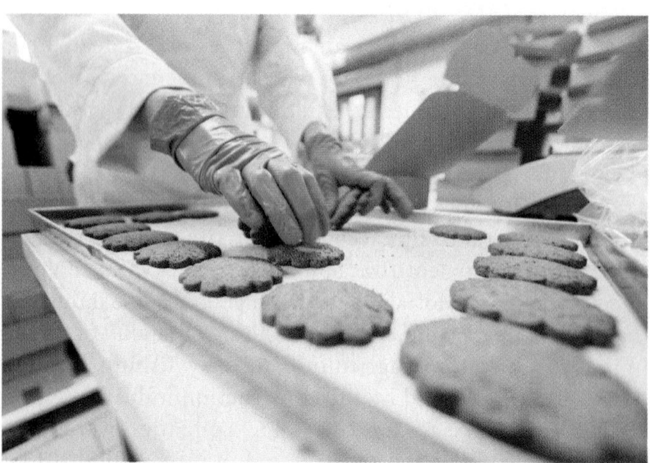

Repetitive movements can contribute to carpal tunnel syndrome.
(Goran Bogicevic/Fotolia)

Between 49,000 and 50,000 U.S. workers die of occupationally acquired illnesses every year (CDC, 2012b; Murray, 2011). Cancers related to occupational exposures are the leading cause of these deaths, and the World Health Organization estimates that 8% to 16% of all cancer deaths worldwide are due to workplace exposures. Occupational risk factors have also been shown to be associated with cardiovascular disease and may account for 15% to 35% of associated mortality (Sorenson et al., 2011). Occupational illness mortality costs the United States approximately $26 billion per year, and nonfatal conditions account for an additional $12 billion in annual costs (CDC, 2012b). Skin diseases are the most commonly encountered occupational illness, followed by respiratory conditions, poisoning, and hearing loss (BLS, 2012b).

Obesity, another common chronic condition, also interacts with workplace factors to create problems. For example, obesity has been hypothetically linked to cardiovascular disease, vibration-induced injury, and asthma in employee populations. Similarly, obesity may modify responses to workplace stress by fostering poor eating habits such as use of high-sugar and high-fat foods. The risk of obesity may also be higher in high-demand jobs over which the employee has little control or that require long working hours. Obesity has also been associated with carpal tunnel syndrome and osteoarthritis in work settings (National Institute of Neurological Disorders and Stroke [NINDS], 2012).

The health care industry poses particular risks for occupational illness. Health care professionals are exposed to a wide variety of pathogenic organisms as well as to stress and job strain and workplace violence.

Chronic conditions, whether occupationally acquired or not, may affect employees' ability to work and their productivity while at work. These conditions may also be exacerbated by working conditions. Approximately 90 million people in the United States suffer from some type of chronic illness, and a significant number of them are included in the workforce. One of the *Healthy People 2020* • objectives (objective DH-9) focuses on reducing barriers to work participation among people who are disabled. A related objective (DH-16) focuses on increasing employment among people who are disabled, and a third (AOCBC-6) addresses reducing the effects of arthritis on the working age population. A similar objective (RD-5) addresses the occupational effects of asthma (USDHHS, 2014). Other *Healthy People 2020* objectives specifically related to occupational health and safety are addressed later in this chapter.

Work-related asthma is a growing concern in occupational settings. Millions of Americans have asthma that may be affected by their working conditions. Asthma, whether in oneself or in a family member, particularly a child, is one of the greatest causes of missed work days. For example, in 2008, 33% of the people who experienced an asthma episode in the prior year had missed work (USDHHS, 2014). Even when workers are not absent due to these conditions, their productivity may be diminished.

Neurotoxic conditions are another concern in occupational health. Some of the conditions encountered include heavy metal poisoning, behavior changes related to chemical exposure, and difficulty concentrating and performing one's job. Specific neurodegenerative disorders, such as presenile dementia, Alzheimer's disease, Parkinson's disease, and motor neuron disease, have also been associated with occupational factors. High prevalence of each of these conditions has been found among teachers, medical personnel, machinists and machine operators, scientists, writers, entertainers, and clerical workers. Selected conditions are also noted with some frequency among workers exposed to pesticides, solvents, and electromagnetic fields.

Noise-induced hearing loss and infectious diseases are other biological considerations in occupational settings. For example, first responders (fire fighters, emergency medical technicians) and health care personnel are at increased risk of bloodborne diseases, whereas employees in manufacturing, construction, and other high-noise occupations are at greater risk for hearing loss.

With respect to dermatologic conditions arising from occupational factors, occupational health nurses are again in a position to assess the health status of employees. As with other types of health problems, the nurse should be aware of outbreaks of dermatologic conditions that indicate the presence of hazards in the environment and a need for control measures. Conditions encountered include a variety of rashes, pruritus, chemical burns, and desquamation.

Occupational injuries and illnesses do not occur only among people who work for pay. Volunteer workers are also subject to occupational risks. An estimated 64.5 million people in the United States volunteered a median of 50 hours per person in 2012. This amounts to 26.5% of the U.S. population over 16 years of age (BLS, 2012c). Australia has developed guidelines to protect the health and safety of volunteer workers. The guidelines include a checklist that volunteer workers or nurses can use to assess the safety of their working conditions (Safe Work Australia, n.d.). For further information about the guidelines, see the *External Resources* section of the student resources site. Similarly, the Ontario Ministry of Labour (2013) has developed information for youth completing volunteer hours for high school graduation. In the United States, some states, such as California, have created programs to provide workers compensation benefits for registered disaster volunteer workers (California Governor's Office of Emergency Services, 2012). Population health nurses, armed with knowledge of injury risks and rates among both employed and volunteer workers, can advocate for safer work environments. They can also educate both employees and volunteers to minimize injury risks.

The extent and type of disability among members of the working population is another biological determinant of health and related health care needs.

Immunization is the final physiologic consideration in assessing health needs in the workplace. The nurse assesses the immunization status of employees, with special emphasis on groups of employees who may be at increased risk for certain diseases preventable by immunization. For example, employees who may be at risk for dirty injuries should be assessed for immunity to tetanus, whereas women of childbearing age should be assessed for immunity to rubella. Health care workers, on the other hand, should be particularly assessed for immunity to hepatitis B, influenza, and other infectious diseases to which they may be exposed. Elements to be considered in an assessment of biological determinants influencing health in the work setting are included in the *Focused Assessment* questions provided below.

FOCUSED ASSESSMENT Assessing Biological Determinants Influencing Health in the Work Setting

- What are the age, gender, and ethnic composition of the employee population? What effects do these factors have on health in the work setting?
- What is the extent of injury in the population? What types of injuries occur? What factors contribute to injuries in the employee population?
- What occupation-related illnesses are common in the population?
- What other illnesses are experienced by the employee population? What is the level of disability in the population? What types of occupational limitations are caused by disability?
- What is the effect of chronic illness or disability on the ability of employees to function effectively in the work setting? Do employees have preexisting health conditions that put them at greater risk for the toxic effects of workplace exposures?
- What are the immunization levels in the employee population?

PSYCHOLOGICAL DETERMINANTS. Assessment of psychological considerations in the work setting involves examination of two major areas: the work climate as it affects health and the presence of mental illness in the workplace.

Workplace climate. Work climate includes the totality of factors in the psychological environment of the work setting. Some major considerations with respect to work climate include job security or insecurity, job strain, and social support. The increasing need for businesses to respond flexibly to market demands has led to greater use of part-time, temporary workers, or contract workers that allows companies to adjust the workforce to meet demands. The need for flexibility results in companies retaining only a small cadre of full-time employees. Part-time and temporary or contract workers are thus faced with increasing job insecurity in which they may be employed today, but out of work tomorrow. Reliance on a large group of part-time or temporary workers also places greater strain on full-time employees who must shoulder the tasks involved in the day-to-day running of the operation. All of this results, not only in an increased work pace, but has been shown to increase conflict and negative relationships within the workplace as employees compete for hours and even possibly for continued employment (Lundberg & Cooper, 2011).

Other elements that contribute to a poor work climate include long hours, shift work, employer surveillance, and sanctions or incentives. Perceptions of organizational injustice also foster an adverse work environment (Sorenson et al., 2011). **Organizational justice** refers to perceptions of fair treatment in the organizational setting. Perceived workplace discrimination, particularly among ethnic minority or immigrant workers, is an example of workplace injustice that has negative health effects. Low perceived organizational justice may give rise to negative emotional reactions to perceptions of unfair treatment.

Job strain is a situation that occurs when one's ability to control one's job is low and job demands are high (Smith & Bielecky, 2012). **Job demands** are the elements of a job that require physical or mental effort (Demir & Rodwell, 2012). The adverse effects of high job demands can be offset by **job control**, or the extent of autonomy one has in decisions regarding how and when one's job will be performed (Demir & Rodwell, 2012). The extent of an employee's social support within the work setting (e.g., from coworkers or supervisors) or from family and friends outside of work can help offset the effects of job strain.

A second model relating psychological factors in the work setting to employee health is the effort–reward imbalance (ERI) model. In this model, the amount of effort expended in one's work is perceived to outweigh the rewards gained (Stansfeld, Shipley, Head, & Fuhrer, 2012). Rewards are not always monetary, but may include psychological rewards, such as personal satisfaction in a job well done, or social rewards, such as recognition for one's efforts or contributions.

Another area in which employees may have minimal control is what is referred to as "emotional labor." **Emotional labor** has been defined as management of one's feelings to conform to organizational expectations (Wharton, 2009). An example of emotional labor in nursing is not allowing the anger caused by a cantankerous patient's verbal insults to show in your face or to affect the quality of care given. In the retail world, emotional labor is exemplified by the old adage, "The customer is always right." Emotional labor occurs in the context of service occupations when the employee cannot afford to display his or her true emotions for fear of alienating a client or customer. Jobs that require emotional labor are characterized by contact with the public, the necessity for producing a favorable emotional state in the customer, and the opportunity for employers to control the emotional activities of their employees.

Some employers purposefully foster employees' control over facets of their jobs. A 2008 study by the U.S. Census Bureau (2012a) addressed the percentage of responding employers that engaged in specific practices to promote job control. The most frequently reported practice was giving leave to employees who provide care to newborn biological or adopted children and allowing them to gradually return to work (57% of employers surveyed), followed by policies allowing employees to determine when to take a break (55%), permitting career breaks for caregiving or other personal or family reasons (47%), allowing personal or family time off without pay (45%), and using paid or unpaid time for education or job training (40%). Other less frequently noted strategies to promote job control included being able to change starting and quitting times, working from home, control over the shift worked, control over paid and unpaid overtime hours, movement from full-time to part-time employment and back, job sharing, working part of the year, personal or family time off without loss of pay, compensatory time off, the ability to do volunteer service during work time, phased retirement options, and sabbatical leaves.

Poor work climate and job strain have been associated with a variety of negative health effects. For example, work stress has been associated with obesity, alcohol use, lack of exercise, anxiety, and burnout (Sorenson et al., 2011). These factors are believed to account for the frequent association between job strain and cardiovascular disease (Nyberg, et al., 2013). Among nurses, burnout due to work stress has been linked to hospital-acquired urinary tract infections in patients (Cimiotti, Aiken, Sloane, & Wu, 2012). Work stress and job strain have also been associated with depression (Sorenson et al., 2011; Stansfeld et al., 2012).

Because of the position of trust that occupational health nurses usually have with employees, they may be among the first to recognize symptoms of stress in individual employees or the work group. With this knowledge, nurses can explore the sources of stress and advocate for improvements in working conditions. Even when the stress might be the result of misperceptions among employees (e.g., rumors that massive layoffs will take place or that the company is being sold), the effects on employee health and work ability can be significant. Population health nurses can help to identify these sources of stress and motivate employers to make changes to reduce stress levels.

Mental health and illness in the workplace. Population health nurses are also in a position to identify employees with mental health problems or to recognize a high prevalence of these problems in the workforce. The sources of workplace stress discussed above may contribute to the development of actual psychiatric diagnoses, or employees may enter the workforce with one or more psychiatric illnesses. Depression, in particular, is a growing problem in the work setting and is the chronic illness most likely to lead to work absences in the United States (Okechukwu, Ayadi, Tamers, Sabbath, & Berkman, 2012). Similarly, in Europe, the Organisation for Economic Cooperation and Development (OECD, 2011) has estimated that 20% of the working population in OECD countries has a clinical mental disorder and that the lifetime prevalence may approach 50%.

Mental illness can be differentiated between mild or moderate illness, frequently referred to as common mental disorders (CMDs), and severe mental disorders (SMDs). CMDs include mood disorders, such as depression, neurotic disorders, such as anxiety, and substance abuse disorders. Without treatment, all of these disorders can evolve into SMDs (OECD, 2011). A variety of stresses contribute to depression in the work setting. For example, lack of job control or job security, job-related conflict, high physical demands or physically uncomfortable work, and hazardous work environments have all been linked to employee depression.

CMDs are generally less debilitating than SMDs, but still have considerable consequences for quality of life and work abilities (OECD, 2011). Changes in job demands in a changing society, such as higher demands for social skills and cognitive competencies, can make it difficult for people with mental illnesses to function effectively in the work setting. In addition, people with mental health problems encounter stigma and fears among coworkers and supervisors.

Depression leads to a number of health-related consequences. For example, depression is a major risk factor for heart disease, high cholesterol, and elevated blood pressure, and depressed employees contribute to health care costs roughly twice those of nondepressed employees. A significant proportion of people with major depression commit suicide. Depression also affects the morale and productivity of coworkers, and the cost to society has been conservatively estimated at 3% to 4% of the gross domestic product of entities like the European Union (OECD, 2011).

There is a need to intervene early in the trajectory of mental illness. Unfortunately, few worksites have programs to address mental illness in employees. Because of the lack of attention to this problem, only a small fraction of people receive the care needed.

Population health nurses are strategically placed to identify employees with both common and severe mental disorders but should keep in mind several legal parameters related to psychiatric illness in the work setting. For example, employers are not permitted to ask about psychiatric illness in hiring decisions, and employees are not required to disclose such diagnoses unless they are requesting accommodations. Employers are also required by the Americans with Disabilities Act to make reasonable accommodations for employees with psychiatric disorders, particularly depression. Population health nurses working with employees with mental health problems may need to ensure access to needed treatment and advocate for accommodations in the work setting. They may also be involved in coordinating care, evaluating the functional ability of employees, and monitoring their use of psychotropic medications.

In assessing psychological determinants influencing the health of clients in work settings, population health nurses identify psychological health problems prevalent in the population and assess factors contributing to those problems. The nurse can assess individual clients or the work group for the following indicators of psychological health problems:

- Increased absenteeism (especially on Mondays, Fridays, and the day after payday)
- Mood changes or changes in relationships with others (especially with health care providers)
- Increased incidence of minor accidents on and off the job
- Complaints of fatigue, weakness, or a general decrease in energy
- Sudden weight loss or gain
- Increased blood pressure
- Frequent stress-related illnesses
- Bloodshot or bleary eyes
- Facial petechiae (especially over the nose)

The *Focused Assessment* on the next page provides guidelines for assessing psychological determinants affecting the health status of the working population.

ENVIRONMENTAL DETERMINANTS. Physical environmental factors contribute to a variety of health problems encountered in work settings. In 2011, for example, 9% of workplace fatalities resulted from environmental conditions and exposures (BLS, 2013a). Categories of health hazards in the physical environment include chemical hazards, physical hazards (radiation, noise, vibration, and exposure to heat and cold), electrical and magnetic field hazards, fire, heavy lifting and uncomfortable working positions, and potential for falls. Additional hazards that may be present in the workplace include exposure to metallic compounds and allergens and molds.

Poor lighting and high noise levels may adversely affect vision and hearing, respectively. In addition, exposure to artificial light during the hours when melatonin production is affected has been linked to incidence of a variety of health

FOCUSED ASSESSMENT Assessing Psychological Determinants Influencing Health in the Work Setting

- To what extent does the work environment contribute to stress? What are the sources of stress in the work environment?
- How do employees cope with stress in the work environment?
- What is the extent of job security or insecurity experienced by members of the workforce?
- Does the work setting require emotional labor? How do employees in the setting approach emotional labor?
- What is the extent of job strain experienced in the work setting? What are the sources of job strain? What measures, if any, does the organization employ to increase job control and minimize job strain?
- To what extent is social support available within and outside of the work setting?
- What is the prevalence of mental illness among employees? What types of mental disorders are present in the workforce? What are the attitudes toward employees with mental health disorders in the work setting? How does the presence of mental illness affect employees' ability to work?

problems that will be addressed in more detail later in the discussion of shiftwork.

Each year, millions of workers are exposed to excessive noise levels, and noise-induced hearing loss is one of the most common occupational health problems in the United States. High noise levels are a particularly significant occupational hazard among members of the military, and military veterans are approximately 30% more likely to experience severe hearing impairment than nonveterans. Among recent veterans of Operation Enduring Freedom and Operation Iraqi Freedom, hearing loss is more than four times more common than for members of the civilian population of similar ages (Greenwald, Tak, & Masterson, 2011). Heavy objects that must be moved or repetitive motion in job tasks may result in musculoskeletal injuries (NINDS, 2012). Awkward work postures, vibration, and temperature are other environmental factors that may contribute to musculoskeletal disorders (Sorenson et al., 2011). In addition, there is a high risk for falls or exposure to excessive heat or cold in many workplaces. All of these physical environmental factors contribute to the risk of occupational injury and illness.

The use of toxic substances in work performance is another source of possible health problems related to the physical environment. Toxic substances may be encountered as solids, liquids, gases, vapors, dust, fumes, fibers, or mists. For example, workers in nail salons experience chronic exposure to a variety of toxic chemicals used in personal care products, for which there is little regulation. Approximately, 90% of more than 10,000 chemicals used in cosmetics have not been tested for safety (Quach et al., 2011). Similarly, the relationship between exposure to soot and scrotal cancer among chimney sweeps has been known since the late 1700s, but chimney soot is now being linked to ischemic heart disease, nonmalignant respiratory diseases, alcoholism, liver disease, and a variety of other cancers in this occupational group (Hogstedt, Jansson, Hugosson, Tinnerberg, & Gustavsson, 2013). Pneumoconiosis and other advanced lung diseases can result from long-term exposure to coal dust (Laney et al., 2012).

Produce inspectors working in enclosed areas have been exposed to high concentrations of pesticides used as fumigants to protect stored produce from infestations (O'Malley et al., 2011), and lab workers, animal caretakers, and health care personnel are also at risk for toxic exposures. For example, a university researcher was infected with *Yersinia pestis*, the causative organism for plague, through contact with an attenuated strain (Ritger et al., 2011). Similarly, a phlebotomist was infected with salmonella in drawing lab samples (Smith et al., 2013). As another example, four veterinary personnel were poisoned by phosphine gas after working on dogs that had ingested a pesticide that interacts with stomach acid to produce the toxic gas (Schwartz, Walker, Sievert, Calvert, & Tsai, 2012).

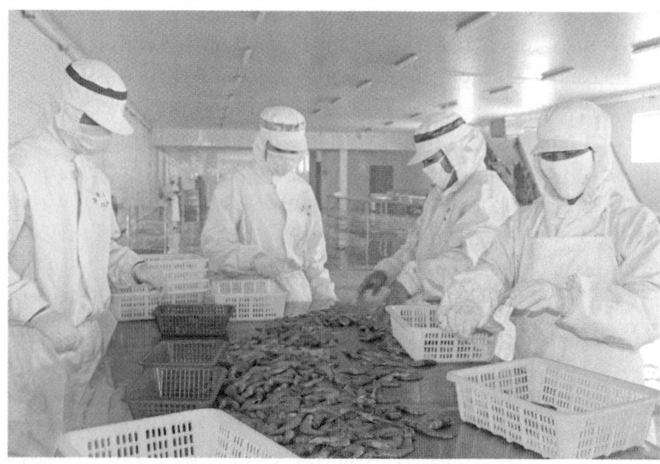

Employees may need protective clothing to prevent toxic exposures. *(Inzyx/Fotolia)*

Health care personnel not only experience exposures to hazardous chemicals (e.g. anesthetists in surgery), but are also exposed to infectious materials from bodily substances, contaminated medical supplies and equipment, contaminated surfaces, or contaminated air (Shefer et al., 2011). In another instance of unanticipated exposure, 23 workers at a metal recycling plant became ill after exposure to chlorine gas from a ruptured salvage tank believed to be empty (Kelsey et al., 2011). Similarly, use of methylene chloride to strip paint from old bathtubs led to cases of fatal poisoning; such results have also been experienced by furniture strippers and other industries that use this chemical (Chester, Rosenman, Grimes, Fagan, & Castillo, 2012). In addition to the potential for exposure to diacetyl in the production of popcorn addressed earlier, bronchiolitis obliterans has been diagnosed on workers exposed to the chemical in coffee flavoring processes (Huff et al., 2013). Finally, workplace exposure to tobacco smoke has been linked to a variety of health problems even among nonsmokers (American Lung Association, 2014). As can be seen in the variety of examples presented here, the work environment can result in exposure to a wide array of conditions hazardous to employees' health.

Population health nurses in occupational settings engage in **hazard analysis**, or an assessment of the vulnerability of workers to workplace contaminants, the probability of exposure, and the severity of potential consequences (AAOHN, 2012e). In addition, they would monitor the frequency of exposures as well as their health effects and provide care to address the results of exposure.

Areas to be assessed relative to the potential for toxic exposures in the workplace include substances used in the setting and their level of demonstrated toxicity, portals of entry into the human body, established legal exposure limits, extent of exposure, potential for interactive exposures, and the presence of existing employee health conditions that put the individuals affected at greater risk for exposure-related illnesses. The nurse and other personnel would also assess the extent and adequacy of controls to prevent or limit exposures and the availability of and compliance with recommended screening and surveillance procedures.

For some people, seemingly innocuous substances may have toxic effects. For example, health care providers may be allergic to the latex gloves used in many settings. Similarly, the presence of food allergens in meals prepared in the work setting can have severe consequences for those with allergies. Population health nurses can be alert to the presence of people with specific allergies in the work setting and assist the company to eliminate the most common allergens. For example, the nurse might work with staff in an employee dining room to eliminate recipes that use peanuts or peanut oil. Similarly, the nurse can advocate for the use of nonlatex gloves in health care settings and other workplaces where gloves are used (e.g., by hotel cleaning staff members).

Equipment may also constitute an occupational health hazard. The use of heavy equipment or sharp tools can result in injury. There is also the potential for hand–arm vibration syndrome in the use of tools that vibrate or visual disturbance related to the use of computer display terminals. Another relatively recent physical hazard generated by widespread computer use is the potential for tendonitis and other similar conditions. The nurse in the occupational setting identifies the presence of any hazards in the physical environment that contribute to health problems. In addition, the nurse monitors the status of known hazards and their effects on the health of employees. The presence of modifiable hazards should lead to advocacy on the part of the nurse to change the physical work environment to eliminate or reduce the potential for exposure to these hazards. Some potential questions for evaluating hazardous conditions in work settings are included in the *Focused Assessment* presented on the next page.

SOCIOCULTURAL DETERMINANTS. The social environment of the work setting can influence employee health status either positively or negatively. The quality of social interactions among employees, attitudes toward work and health, and the presence or absence of racial or other tensions can all affect health status as well as employee productivity.

Assessment of sociocultural considerations affecting health in work settings focuses on five major areas. These include the effects of policy and legislation, the interactive effects of work and family life, the type of work done, immigration, and workplace aggression.

Policy and legislation. In the United States, health-related policy and legislation have a significant impact on the workforce. The three most influential pieces of legislation are the Occupational Safety and Health Act of 1970 (OSH Act), workers' compensation, and the Americans with Disabilities Act. Other state, local, and business-specific policies and regulations also affect the health of employees. The Occupational Safety and Health Act established the **Occupational Safety and Health Administration (OSHA)**, the federal agency charged

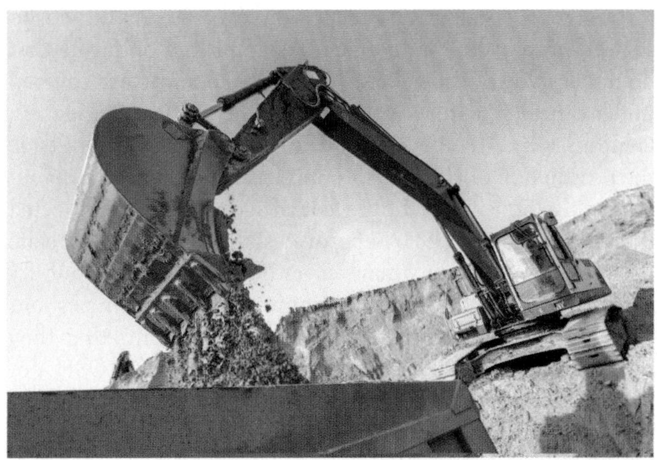

A variety of injuries may occur as a result of heavy equipment operation. *(dima266f/Fotolia)*

FOCUSED ASSESSMENT Assessing Environmental Determinants Influencing Health in the Work Setting

- Does the physical environment of the work setting pose any health hazards?
- What potentially hazardous substances or conditions are associated with production processes (e.g., toxic chemicals, heat)?
- What potentially hazardous substances or conditions are associated with clerical processes (e.g., repetitive movements)? With other office processes (e.g., cleaning products, pesticides)?
- What is the typical extent and duration of exposure to hazardous substances or conditions?
- What are the designated exposure limits for substances and conditions in the work setting?
- What research evidence is there for adverse human health effects (e.g., toxicity, teratogenicity, potential for injury) associated with substances used or conditions existing in the work setting?
- Do low levels of exposure have a cumulative effect?
- What is the usual portal of entry or mechanism of exposure for a specific toxic agent or condition?
- What organ systems are typically affected by specific toxic agents or hazardous conditions?
- What are the usual signs and symptoms of toxicity/health effects?
- Are there synergistic effects among substances or between substances and other conditions (e.g., heat) or health-related behaviors (e.g., smoking)?
- What are the recommended control practices to prevent or minimize potential for exposure?
- Are the recommended practices in place in a given occupational setting (e.g., ventilation, other engineering controls)?
- What are the recommended surveillance practices for monitoring environmental conditions and hazardous exposures? Are there surveillance systems in place for monitoring the presence or extent of hazardous conditions in the environment?
- Are food sanitation practices adequate to prevent communicable diseases, vermin infestation, and so on?
- Are there adequate facilities for handicapped employees?
- Are workstations designed to prevent injury and fatigue?
- Is there potential for a disaster in the work setting? Is there a disaster plan in place?

with protecting the health and welfare of the U.S. private-sector workforce. OSHA was intended to develop and enforce safety standards in work settings to protect U.S. workers from harm (OSHA, 2011). In addition, the legislation established the National Institute for Occupational Safety and Health (NIOSH) to conduct occupational research and make recommendations for safeguarding employee health (NIOSH, 2013a).

OSHA covers all private-sector employees except those who are self-employed, family members employed on farms that do not employ outside workers, and workers who are covered under other regulatory agencies (e.g., the Nuclear Regulatory Commission). Members of the military forces are also outside the jurisdiction of OSHA. State and local government employees are also not covered by the federal agency, but are protected if their state has an OSHA-approved state program. Most state occupational and safety plans cover both private- and public-sector employees. OSHA also monitors federal agencies, but these agencies are regulated under requirements that they meet the same employee protections as required by OSHA of private-sector employers (OSHA, n.d.c). Table 23-1 ● presents the OSHA-mandated employee rights and employer responsibilities related to occupational safety and health.

OSHA is charged with performing periodic inspections of worksites to determine whether standards are being enforced. Inspections may be conducted on a routine basis or may be triggered by certain specific events such as an employee death, hospitalization of three or more employees for work-related occurrences, employee complaints, or referrals from the media or other individuals. Inspections may also be conducted in the event of an imminent danger situation (e.g., possible rupture of a holding tank for hazardous materials). Unfortunately, the number and frequency of OSHA inspections and penalties for violation of standards have been steadily decreasing. In addition, OSHA has been criticized for the excessive length of time required to develop new exposure standards for hazardous substances, which may take as long as 5 to 10 years from proposal to enactment and in one case took 31 years. Finally, the Congressional Review Act of 1996 allows congress to overturn any federal agency's regulations, but to date only the ergonomics standards promulgated by OSHA in 2001 have ever received a congressional veto. In addition, executive orders have permitted the President of the United States to interfere in occupational safety regulations usually through the Office of Management and Budget, which has no related scientific or health care expertise (Feldman, 2011). Most often, such interference has come as a result of pressure from major employer organizations and lobbying groups.

TABLE 23-1 Employee Rights and Employer Responsibilities Under OSHA

Employees Have the Right to:	Employers Must:
Working conditions that do not pose a risk for harm	Follow all relevant OSHA safety and health standards
Receive information and training, in a language they can understand, about chemical and other hazards, measures to prevent harm, and OSHA standards that apply to their workplace	Find and correct safety and health hazards
Review records of work-related injuries and illnesses	Inform employees about chemical hazards through training, labels, alarms, color-coded systems, chemical information sheets, and other methods
Get copies of test results done to find and measure hazards in the workplace	Notify OSHA within 8 hours of a workplace fatality or when three or more employees are hospitalized
File a complaint with OSHA asking for an inspection of their workplace if they believe there is a serious hazard or their employer is not following OSHA rules	Provide required personal protective equipment at no cost to employees
Use their rights under the law without retaliation or discrimination and file complaints with OSHA if retaliation or discrimination occurs	Keep accurate records of work-related injuries and illnesses
	Post OSHA citations, injury, and illness summary data, and the OSHA "Job Safety and Health—It's the Law" poster in the workplace where workers will see them
	Not discriminate or retaliate against any worker for using their rights under the law

Source: Occupational Safety and Health Administration. (2011). *At-a-glance: OSHA.* Retrieved from https://www.osha.gov/Publications/3439at-a-glance.pdf

In spite of these failings, OSHA regulations have been credited with saving the lives of more than 410,000 U.S. workers and preventing countless injuries and illnesses. Recommendations for shoring up the agency's performance include increasing fines for violation of standards to meaningful levels, increasing the capacity of the agency to conduct inspections as mandated in its charge, enacting criminal as well as monetary penalties for failing to safeguard employee health, and basing regulation on updated scientific findings (Murray, 2011). Additional recommendations include expanding coverage to currently unprotected groups and changing the federal regulations so they also cover farm children working on family farms.

Population health nurses working in occupational settings may occasionally find themselves in the position of needing to report OSHA violations in order to protect employee health and safety. In addition, they may need to become politically active to advocate for federal and state enforcement of health and safety regulations.

Workers' compensation legislation is designed to provide for the needs of workers injured or made ill at work and their families. At the federal level, workers' compensation addresses wage replacement benefits, medical treatment, vocational rehabilitation, and some other benefits for federal employees. Other specific groups are also covered under federal legislation and include energy workers with occupational illnesses, longshore and harbor workers, and those who suffer from black lung disease, primarily as a result of mining (U.S. Department of Labor, n.d.b). Nonfederal employees may receive workers' compensation benefits under state legislation, but coverage varies from state to state. The National Conference of State Legislatures (2013) provides an annual update on worker's compensation legislation in specific states. For further information about the report, see the *External Resources* section of the student resources site.

Prior to the establishment of the workers' compensation system, employees were required to prove employer responsibility for an illness or injury before they could claim recompense for lost wages or the cost of medical care. Workers' compensation provides protection for both employee and employer. Under the program, employees are guaranteed wage replacement and medical care costs if they are injured on the job. The system also protects employers from lawsuits by employees to recover lost wages or health care costs. Occupational health nurses are often responsible for tracking and administering workers' compensation for injured employees. They may also need to assist employees to obtain workers' compensation benefits.

The third piece of legislation that affects the workplace is the Americans with Disabilities Act (ADA). The implications of the act for the school setting were discussed in Chapter 22∞ and are similar for occupational settings. ADA was designed to ensure equitable occupational opportunity for those with disabilities (U.S. Department of Justice, n.d.). Under the law, employers are not required to give preferential treatment to disabled job applicants or employees, but are expected to give them the same opportunities for employment or advancement as those without disabilities. Employers are required to provide **reasonable accommodations**, or "modification or adjustment to a job or the work environment that will enable a qualified applicant or employee with a disability to participate in the application process or to perform essential job functions" (Job Accommodation Network, n.d., para. 9). A reasonable accommodation is one that does not impose an undue burden on the employer (Rutkow, Vernick, Tung, & Cohen, 2013). The legislation does not define what constitutes a disability that is covered under the law, but consultants at the Office of Disability Employment Policy's Job Accommodation Network can assist employers with determining whether or not a specific condition in a particular individual employee constitutes a disability that requires reasonable accommodation (JAN, n.d.).

Similar legislative efforts have been undertaken internationally. For example, the United Nations (2006) "Convention on the Rights of Persons with Disabilities" includes the right to employment for individuals with disabilities. According to the convention, adopting nations recognize the right of all individuals, including those with disabilities to gainful employment in open, inclusive, and accessible work environments (Article 27). Most nations throughout the world, including the United States, have adopted the convention (United Nations, 2013).

On occasion, ADA provisions may be in conflict with OSHA regulations designed to limit risks to which employees are exposed. Recent Supreme Court rulings have favored the right of employers to prevent people from working when a particular job would place the person him- or herself at risk due to limitations imposed by a disability. These rulings run contrary to prior decisions that only possible danger to others justified employer decisions not to employ someone in a particular capacity. Population health nurses may need to advocate for disabled workers when such decisions are made in the workplace. They may also assist applicants or employees with disabilities in requesting accommodations. Nurses, employers, and employees can find additional information and assistance with accommodations on the Job Accommodation Network website. For further information about the report, see the *External Resources* section of the student resources site.

State and local laws and policies within specific business organizations have also been found to influence health and safety. For example, by the end of 2010, 26 states and the District of Columbia had smoke-free laws that covered indoor areas of work, restaurants, and bars. An additional 19 states had laws prohibiting smoking in one or two of the three areas. Interestingly, no southern state had enacted any smoke-free legislation, but many communities in the south had local laws prohibiting smoking. Such laws have been shown to reduce nonsmokers' exposure to second-hand smoke, promote smoking cessation among smokers, and change norms related to the acceptability of smoking in public. In addition, they have contributed to reduced incidence of heart attack and asthma hospitalizations in the general public and the workforce (Tyman, Babb, MacNeil, & Griffin, 2011).

Other legislation and policies may also affect health, either positively or negatively. For example, policies that permit breast-feeding of infants or breast pumping are helpful for both mothers and infants. On the other hand, the absence of sick leave policies encourage employees to come to work when ill, jeopardizing their health and that of coworkers.

The work–family interface. Although employees spend considerable time in the work setting, they do have lives outside of work. Interrelationships between work and family may support or impede employee and/or family health. The work–family interface for any given employee may be one of balance or conflict. Balance may be viewed from a variety of perspectives: as the absence of conflict between roles, as full engagement in all roles, as high levels of satisfaction across roles, and as congruence with the relative value attached to multiple roles. Given these multiple perspectives, **work–family balance** can be defined as the extent to which one's work and family roles are balanced and are congruent with one's life values (Greenhaus & Allen, 2011).

Positive effects result from work–life balance. These may include positive spill-over, enrichment, and facilitation (Greenhaus & Allen, 2011). Spill-over involves the transfer of positive feelings, skills, behaviors, and values from one domain to the other. For example, effective interpersonal communication skills demonstrated at work may improve interpersonal interactions in the family. Enrichment relates to the extent to which experiences in one role improve the quality of life or performance in the other. For example, social support from coworkers may help an employee get through a difficult family situation. In facilitation, involvement in one domain contributes to enhanced function in another domain. Engagement in multiple roles may foster enhanced efficiency or improved delegation skills in each. For example, nursing students who are married, have children, and work, as well as going to school, are often better organized than those who are single and not working while in school.

Work–family conflict, on the other hand, is role interference that occurs when work and family roles are incompatible with each other and the resulting conflict makes effective execution of one or both roles difficult (Greenhaus & Allen, 2011). Such conflicts may be time-based, in which work and family roles compete for the limited time available, strain-based, in which strain in one role affects performance in the other, or behavior-based, in which the behaviors required in one role are incompatible with those required in the other (Slan-Jerusalem & Chen, 2009).

Work–family conflict or interference may be bidirectional. Family roles may interfere with work performance when a parent is distracted at work because he or she has a sick child at home. This situation is often referred to as FIW or family interference with work. Conversely, work responsibilities may interfere with family roles (WIF). For example, a mandatory meeting at work may conflict with a celebration of a couple's anniversary. Because of the expanding use of technology in work realms, many employees have what are virtually 24/7 responsibilities leading to greater interference with family life (Sorenson et al., 2011).

Women are more often affected by FIW than men, but both have multiple negative effects for the individuals involved. WIF frequently leads to job dissatisfaction, intentions to leave the job, overload, work distress, and difficult relationships within the family. FIW more often results in family and marital dissatisfaction, parental overload, family distress, and poor work performance. Work–family interference has also been shown to affect employees' overall physical and psychological well-being and health-related behaviors such as alcohol use and smoking (Nelson, Li, Sorenson, & Berkman, 2012). Work–family conflict in either direction also has implications for the employing organization in the form of reduced job and career satisfaction and turnover, reduced employee morale, lower productivity, and increased absenteeism (Slan-Jerusalem & Chen, 2009).

A final aspect of the relationship between work and family relates to paraoccupational exposure to hazardous substances. **Paraoccupational exposure** occurs when family members or others outside the work setting are exposed to hazardous substances transferred from the work setting by an employee. These exposures may involve metals, chemicals, or biological agents. For example, paraoccupational exposure to lead frequently occurs via contaminated clothing. Health care workers, on the other hand, may expose their families to infectious disease agents. Occupational health nurses can be particularly influential in teaching employees how to minimize paraoccupational exposures and in advocating employment policies that minimize the potential for exposure (e.g., through providing protective clothing and changing areas for employees working with hazardous materials). They may also assist employees in dealing with work–family conflicts or advocate working conditions and policies that minimize conflict and promote balance.

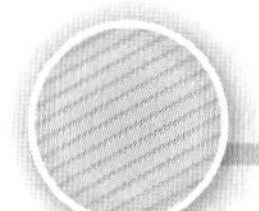

Global Perspectives

Transitioning from an Agricultural Economy to an Industrial Economy

Approximately one third of the world's workforce is employed in agriculture-related occupations, compared to only 10% of the workforce in developed nations (Marucci-Wellman et al., 2011). Many formerly third-world countries, however, are moving rapidly from an agricultural to an industrial economy. As such changes occur, many workers will move from agricultural employment to higher paying jobs in the industrial sector. Many others will combine work in both sectors. Continued agricultural work may be used to supplement income from work in industry. Both movements toward a new occupational sector and combined employment in both sectors pose unique new risks.

In one rural Vietnamese commune for example, nearly half of the workforce continues to work part-time in agriculture, while working full- or part-time in industry. A study by Marucci-Wellman and colleagues (2011) found occupational injury rates for those working fewer than 500 hours per year in the agricultural sector and as much as full-time (2,000 hours/year) in industry four times higher than rates for the overall workforce and persons working only in the industrial sector. These findings held true for both men and women working in dual sectors, but were more pronounced for men who work at more dangerous jobs in both sectors.

Fatigue from working two jobs might be one explanation of the higher injury rates. An alternative explanation might be inexperience in one sector or the other (Marucci-Wellman et al., 2011). The study's findings suggest that workers employed in both agricultural and industrial sectors may need to be particularly targeted for injury prevention programs. The findings also highlight the need to consider the health effects of major occupational shifts in society and the effects of employment in multiple jobs.

Type of work. The type of work performed and specific job demands are other sociocultural factors influencing the health of the working population. For example, agricultural work is one of the most dangerous occupations, with an overall mortality rate seven times higher than that of all other workers in the United States (Marucci-Wellman et al., 2011). Employees' socioeconomic position may influence the type of work performed and thus their level of exposure to hazardous job conditions. Socioeconomic position has also been shown to interact with work stressors to have differential effects on health. For example, people in blue-collar positions who experience job strain have been found to have a greater risk of hypertension and heart attack than white-collar workers, possibly due to the relative lack of options for dealing with stress. In addition, employees of lower socioeconomic status tend to receive less in the way of health promotion services than those of higher status (Sorenson et al., 2011).

Increased job demands and competition for jobs in today's society lead to a faster work pace and more stressful working conditions. In manufacturing areas, higher productivity demands may increase the risk of injury if short cuts are taken. As noted earlier, the use of technology in the workplace makes possible work in different locations and at different times, possibly leading to increased expectations for responses even during one's off time leading to a 24-hour, 7-days a week schedule that interferes with family interactions, leisure, and rest. In addition, the option of telework from home may increase the workload for those who stay in traditional worksites who have the added burden of dealing with the daily needs of the organization as well as meeting the needs of telecommuters (Lundberg & Cooper, 2011).

Some authors have noted a "global trend toward a 24-hour society" (Smith et al., 2011, p. 189). This trend has led to an increase in the proportion of the workforce that works nonstandard hours and may result in irregular schedules or in shiftwork. Shiftwork has been shown to result in a variety of health effects. For example, there is a strong association between shiftwork and coronary heart disease. Shiftwork also interferes with normal circadian rhythms and sleep–wake cycles, with about 10% of shiftworkers experiencing shift work sleep disorder leading to poor sleep, chronic fatigue, anxiety, nervousness, and depression. Frequent association with gastrointestinal disorders and interference with female reproductive cycles have also been found. The fatigue and other effects caused by shiftwork may lead to errors and injury, particularly at night; however, data are difficult to interpret, since the intensity of work and potential for high stress events may vary from shift to shift (Smith et al., 2011). Finally, an expert group within the International Agency for Research on Cancer has concluded that the disruption of circadian rhythms involved in shift work may very well be carcinogenic (Smith et al., 2011).

Population health nurses most probably will not be able to change the operating hours of a business or industry, but they can be alert to the health effects of shiftwork on specific employees and assist them to minimize the effects (e.g., by promoting good sleep hygiene) or advocate for a change in shifts. They can also advocate for shift changes that minimize disruption of circadian rhythms, such as rotation from evening to night shift rather than the reverse (Luckhaupt, 2012). In addition, they should be familiar with the types of work performed in a given occupational setting and the potential effects on the health of employees.

Immigration and work. Immigration is one of three factors that influence the size of the U.S. workforce, the other two factors being fertility and birth rates and mortality in the working age population. Immigration may stem from efforts to escape adverse conditions in one's homeland or the desire for greater opportunity, particularly employment opportunities. Immigration contributes to both growth in the overall workforce and to diversity within the working population. Based on projections from the U.S. Census Bureau, immigration is expected to add 1.4 million people to the workforce each year through 2020, a significant increase over 2004 projections (Toosi, 2012).

Because of their typically low socioeconomic status and frequent lack of highly employable skills, many immigrants are forced into low-paying hazardous occupations. Educated immigrants may also encounter difficulties in obtaining employment in their own fields. For example, nurses educated in other countries may need to take jobs as nursing assistants until they can meet the licensing requirements for a specific state. Similar educational and licensing difficulties might be experienced by other immigrating professionals, such as physicians, lawyers, and teachers.

Among the 2.5 million farm workers in the United States, 78% are immigrants who often move around the country as agricultural labor demands wax and wane. Migrant farm workers may come to the United States alone or may be accompanied by their families. Approximately 20% of them live in employer-provided housing or camps that lack basic amenities. In addition, they often live at a distance from health care and social services or do not have adequate time to address health care needs. Working conditions may also be substandard, and they frequently do not receive federally mandated safety training specific to the hazards of their jobs. In addition, farmworkers do not have the same right-to-know protections as other employees covered by OSHA regulations regarding communication about hazards in the work setting and their potential health effects (Farmworker Justice, 2014).

These conditions are compounded for a growing number of indigenous workers, native peoples of Mexico and other Central and South American countries who are not Latino. These workers tend to be discriminated against by both the U.S.-born farm workers and other migrant workers. Their language and cultures differ significantly from Latino workers and any safety training they may receive may be in English or Spanish, limiting their ability to understand it. Population health nurses should be alert to the presence of immigrant workers in specific work settings as well as the cultural and language barriers they experience in adapting to life and work in the United States. They may need to provide referrals for assistance for individual employees, modify safety and other health-related education to meet their needs, or advocate for equitable treatment and appropriate policies in the work setting.

Workplace aggression. Violence or aggression in the workplace is another sociocultural factor that can profoundly affect health and safety in the occupational setting. **Workplace aggression** involves actions that result in physical, psychological, or emotional harm as perceived by the recipient (Fujishiro, Gee, & de Castro, 2011). Types of workplace aggression may include verbal abuse, bullying, and intimidation; threat of physical harm; physical assault; sexual assault; and homicide. Aggression tends to involve four types of perpetrators: persons in pursuit of criminal activity (e.g., a robbery), customers or other recipients of services (e.g., patients or students), coworkers, or persons who have a personal relationship with the victim, such as spouses or intimate partners (AAOHN, 2013).

Although workplace aggression occurs in many work settings, nurses are at particular risk for victimization because they often work alone, have access to drugs that may be sought by perpetrators, care for people under stress, and have frequent close contact with patients and their families (Magnavita & Heponiemi, 2011). According to U.S. Bureau of Labor statistics, more than 25,000 physical assaults were reported in health care settings in 2007 for an incidence of 158.4 events per 100,000 workers, much higher than in any other industry. Reports of nursing risk for workplace aggression vary from 63.5% to 95% in some settings (Demir & Rodwell, 2012). In other studies, the rate is as high as 13 of every 100 employees. One third to a half of the incidents reported involved nonphysical aggression such as bullying, intimidation, or harassment (Fujishiro et al., 2011). Like bullying in the school setting addressed in Chapter 22∞, workplace bullying often involves intimidation and social isolation. It has been suggested that increased job demands and low job control may lead to violations of existing social norms leading to increased risk of being bullied. For example, high job demands may result in frequent errors leading coworkers to perceive one as incompetent and engage in disparagement and bullying (Demir & Rodwell, 2012).

In a study among health care workers in the Philippines, verbal abuse and bullying were associated with poor general health and work-related injury and illness, while physical assault was associated with missed workdays. In addition, coworker conflicts were often associated with work-related injury (Fujishiro et al., 2011). Similarly, a study of Italian nurses and nursing students indicated that 43% of the nurses and 34% of the students had experienced at least one episode of verbal or physical violence in their clinical lifetimes. Nurses reported being assaulted or harassed most often by patients and their families and friends. Nursing students also reported being subjected to verbal and physical violence by colleagues, staff, and others including teachers, physicians, and supervisors (Magnavita & Heponiemi, 2011). In the United States, a recent study of more than 1,400 early career registered nurses found that nearly half reported verbal abuse from colleagues, with 49% being abused at least once in the prior 3 months, and 5% reported more than 5 episodes of abuse in the same period. Being spoken to in a condescending manner and being ignored were the most commonly reported forms of verbal abuse (Budin, Brewer, Chao, & Kovner, 2013).

Nursing home personnel in Switzerland also reported high levels of aggression (81%). Reports varied by education of the victim with nonstudents being more likely to be victimized than students and RNs more likely than ancillary staff. In part, these results may stem from the practice of reserving assignment of difficult patients to experienced nurses. The authors noted a need for caregivers to understand the factors underlying patient aggression in a more comprehensive way to enable them to deal with aggression more effectively (Zeller, Dassen, Kok, Needham, & Halfens, 2012).

In 2011, 17% of workplace fatalities were the result of violence or other injuries by persons or animals in the work setting, and 10% of those fatalities were homicides. In that same year, a total of 468 workplace homicides were reported; the majority (83%) involving male victims. Among female victims, homicide perpetrators were most often relatives or domestic partners, whereas men were more likely to be killed in robberies. Coworkers or work associates were implicated in 11% of male and 6% of female homicides. Fourteen percent of women employees and 12% of men were killed by a student, patient, client, or customer, and 6% of women and 12% of men were killed by an inmate, detainee, or unapprehended suspect (Bureau of Labor Statistics, 2013a).

Workplace violence has negative effects for both the victim and the employing organization. Consequences for victims may include increased stress and fear of victimization, anxiety, feelings of guilt and self-blame, carrying weapons for self-defense, decreased trust of management and coworkers, decreased job satisfaction, and the intention to leave the job. For employers, workplace aggression results in increased health care and workers' compensation claims, increased legal and security costs, increased employee turnover and absenteeism, and decreased productivity (AAOHN, 2013).

Occupational health nurses may be faced with evidence of workplace violence or bullying and may be forced to advocate for clients. When the perpetrator is also the nurse's supervisor, this may place the nurse in an awkward position. When harassment is based on discrimination because of an employee's gender, ethnicity, or membership in another protected category, someone who reports harassment is protected from employer retaliation. Unfortunately, however, this is not the case when the harassment cannot be linked to discrimination. Despite this disadvantage and the potential for retribution, nurses who are aware of bullying are ethically obligated to report it to the appropriate person or group and to advocate for the safety and security of the employee or employees affected.

OSHA (2004) has recommended conducting a workplace violence risk assessment to identify risk factors for violence in the setting. The assessment would focus on an analysis of incidents of violence and the types of violence perpetrated, perpetrators and clientele characteristics that might contribute to violence (e.g., patients withdrawing from psychoactive substances, persons under significant stress), and elements of the internal and external environment that may contribute to the risk for violence. In addition, OSHA has developed specific guidelines for preventing workplace violence against health care and social services personnel. For further information about the guidelines, see the *External Resources* section of the student resources site.

Additional sociocultural factors that may affect health in the work setting include languages spoken and cultural beliefs and behaviors. For example, employers may provide the traditional Western or Christian holidays but give no consideration for important occasions in other cultural groups. Ethnic and cultural factors may also be the basis for discrimination in the work setting. For example, employees may be harassed by colleagues because of an accent, or employers may prohibit the wearing of culturally prescribed clothing, such as head scarves, in some employment settings. In other settings, such as India and Italy, businesses may close during the hottest part of the day, but stay open late into the evening.

Guidelines for assessing sociocultural determinants influencing health in occupational settings are presented in the *Focused Assessment* on the next page.

BEHAVIORAL DETERMINANTS. Health-related behaviors engaged in by employees also influence the health status of the working population. Behavioral factors to be considered here include consumption patterns related to diet, smoking, and other substance use and abuse, patterns of rest and activity, use of protective measures, immunization, and presenteeism.

FOCUSED ASSESSMENT Assessing Sociocultural Determinants Influencing Health in the Work Setting

- Do OSHA regulations apply to the work setting? Are there other regulations that apply to the setting? If so, what are they, and how do they affect employee health or the role of the occupational health nurse?
- What is the extent of workers' compensation claims in the work group? For what types of problems is compensation provided?
- How do provisions of the Americans with Disabilities Act affect the work setting?
- What effects, if any, does work in this setting have on family relationships? Do employees work nonstandard hours?
- What assistance, if any, is provided to employees relative to child care or care of other family members?
- What is the educational, economic, and cultural background of employees? What languages are spoken by the employee population? How do cultural factors affect work, if at all?
- Does the work pose a high risk for crime victimization?
- Are there intergroup conflicts in the employee population? What is the potential for violence in the work setting?
- What is the extent of social support among employees? To what extent do coworkers support healthful behaviors?
- What is the extent of other forms of workplace aggression in the work setting? What risk factors for workplace violence are present in the setting? To what extent do the physical environment and organizational policy facilitate or impede violence in the workplace?

Consumption patterns. Consumption patterns of interest to the occupational health nurse include those related to food and nutrition, smoking, and drug and alcohol use. The influence of nutrition on health is well established, and the occupational health nurse assesses the nutritional patterns of employees with whom he or she works. In addition, the nurse assesses how the work environment affects eating habits. For example, sufficient opportunity may not be provided for employees to eat despite OSHA regulations regarding time and place for breaks and meals.

The nurse also determines whether food service is available to employees. If there is an employee cafeteria, the nurse may need to assess the nutritional quality of the food provided. If no food services are available in the workplace, the nurse would determine whether they are available nearby, or whether adequate storage facilities exist for employees who bring meals from home.

Another issue that may affect health and productivity in the work setting is the growing use of energy drinks. The amount of caffeine in such drinks is equivalent to one to three cups of coffee or caffeinated soda. Energy drink consumption has been linked to sleep problems, daytime sleepiness, decreased productivity, and risk for injury. Use of energy drinks has been found to be particularly prevalent among deployed military members, nearly 45% of whom reported consuming one such drink per day. An additional 13% of respondents reported drinking three or more drinks and getting less than 4 hours of sleep per night (Toblin, Clark-Walper, Kok, Sipos, & Thomas, 2012).

The prevalence of eating disorders in the workforce is another consideration related to dietary consumption. Occupational health nurses may identify employees (primarily, but not exclusively, young women) who have eating disorders. When employees with eating disorders are identified, the occupational health nurse would usually make a referral for diagnostic confirmation and treatment. Eating disorders are addressed in more detail in Chapter 28∞.

Smoking is another consumption pattern of concern to the occupational health nurse. The most recent National Survey on Drug Use and Health indicated that approximately 28% of full-time employees and nearly a quarter of part-time employees were current smokers (Garrett, Dube, Trosclair, Caraballo, & Pechacek, 2011). Smoking is harmful to health in and of itself. In addition, smoking may increase the adverse effects of other environmental hazards in the work setting, particularly those that affect respiration. Many employers have recently begun to prohibit smoking except in carefully controlled areas in the workplace and have been active in promoting programs to help employees quit smoking. In addition to the health implications, such efforts cut employer expenses. For example, occupational exposure to second-hand smoke may be grounds for employee lawsuits, worker's compensation claims, or a claim of disability discrimination in failure to provide "reasonable accommodation" to protect workers with asthma and other respiratory conditions from the effects of second-hand smoke. Voluntarily creating smoke-free workplaces can save employers from potential costs in all of these situations (Zellers, Graff, & Tobacco Control Legal Consortium, 2008).

Some employers, particularly health care organizations, have gone so far as to implement nonsmoking requirements for employment and to require pre-employment nicotine testing of job applicants. Such policies have ethical implications in curtailing smokers' employment opportunities. In addition, nicotine tests do not distinguish among current smokers, persons exposed to second-hand smoke, and those using assistive devices (e.g., nicotine patches) to stop smoking. Such policies also raise concerns related to social justice since smoking is more common among lower socioeconomic groups (Voigt, 2012). In addition, it is conceivable that nicotine addiction might, at some point, be considered a disability that would require accommodations under ADA.

The population nurse assesses the extent of smoking in the employee population as well as the specific implications of smoking in that particular environment. He or she might educate and assist employees with smoking cessation, but might also need to advocate for the rights of smokers to employment (but not for a right to smoke in the work environment).

Employees may also have problems with substance abuse. For example, an estimated 10% to 15% of nurses may be impaired or recovering from substance abuse disorders (Thomas & Siela, 2011), and other occupational groups may have similar high incidence rates for abuse. The prevalence of these problems should be monitored and the population health nurse in a work setting should be alert to signs and symptoms of substance abuse in employees and engage in interventions to address these problem consumption patterns. Worksite interventions have been shown to be successful in decreasing smoking and other drug use and in reducing fat intake and increasing consumption of fruits, vegetables, and fiber.

Rest and activity. Work places many physical and psychological demands on people. Sometimes these demands result in inadequate rest and recreation, as with the executive who works constantly or the blue-collar worker who holds two jobs in an attempt to make ends meet. Conversely, work may also lead to too much sitting and too little physical activity. Based on 2010 National Health Interview Survey results, 30% of U.S. civilian employees get less than 6 hours of sleep per night, when the recommended amount of sleep is 7 to 9 hours. Insufficient sleep was most common among manufacturing employees (34%) and was particularly prevalent in nightshift workers in the transportation and warehousing industries (70%) and among health care and social assistance personnel (52%) (Luckhaupt, 2012). As we saw earlier, insufficient sleep is detrimental to health and may increase risk for injury or errors.

Problems encountered in the work setting may also interfere with employees' ability to rest when off the job. The nurse in the work setting assesses the amount of activity engaged in by employees and the balance between rest and exercise. He or she also obtains information on the types of recreation used by employees and any potential health hazards posed by recreational choices.

Many companies are recognizing the benefits of exercise in terms of both the physical and psychological health of employees. These companies are promoting physical exercise and may even provide facilities for exercise and recreation in the workplace. If this is the case, the nurse should be alert to potential health hazards and the possibility of too much exercise. For example, if there is a company pool, an employee with epilepsy who swims to relieve tension should be cautioned against swimming alone. Similarly, an overweight executive should engage in physical activity cautiously to lessen the risk of heart attack or injury.

Another factor related to rest and leisure time activity is the extent of multiple jobs held by employees, each of which presents its own unique risks and hazards. In addition, multiple-job holders have less time to rest and recover from the physical

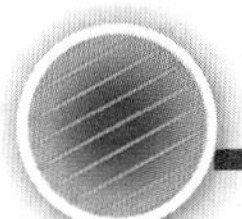

Evidence-Based Practice

Advocating Smoke-free Workplaces

Smoking contributes to substantial morbidity and mortality throughout the world, not only for smokers, but also for those exposed to second-hand smoke. Internationally, an estimated 1.3 million people smoke, about 80% of whom live in low- to middle-income countries. In a given year, 600,000 deaths and 10.9 million disability-adjusted life years are attributable to the effects of second-hand smoke. Individuals with severe disabling respiratory conditions are particularly susceptible to the adverse health effects of second-hand smoke (Rutkow et al., 2013).

Some authors have suggested that legislation mandating work accommodations for persons with disabilities can be used as leverage for promoting smoke-free workplace policies. In the United States, the Americans with Disabilities Act mandates reasonable accommodations for employees with disabilities. Internationally, the United Nations Convention on the Rights of Persons with Disabilities, adopted by numerous countries around the world, has similar provisions (United Nations, 2006), and the WHO Framework Convention on Tobacco Control calls for protection of individuals from second-hand smoke exposure in public places and in work settings (Rutkow et al., 2013).

Arguments for not instituting smoke-free workplace policies often revolve around potential loss of revenue (e.g., in restaurants) or the expense of the change in policy. Evidence has consistently demonstrated that smoking bans have not resulted in decreased revenues or have actually increased revenue slightly. Similarly, research has indicated decreases in hospital admissions for asthma and other respiratory conditions with smoking ban implementation. In addition, studies have demonstrated conclusively that less restrictive policies are not effective in protecting nonsmokers from second-hand smoke (Rutkow et al., 2013). This strong evidence base, coupled with legal mandates to protect employees with disabilities, provide significant ammunition for advocating smoke-free workplace policies in all businesses and industries.

demands of the job as well as less time for family interactions. In August 2013, 4.7% of employed workers in the United States held multiple jobs (BLS, 2013c).

Use of protective measures. Another behavioral factor that is particularly relevant to health in the occupational setting is the use or nonuse of safety and protective measures. Hazards present in the workplace frequently can be mitigated by the use of appropriate safety equipment; however, this can occur only if employees use these devices consistently and appropriately.

The population health nurse identifies the need for safety equipment and also monitors the extent to which it is used. For example, do individuals working in high-noise areas wear earplugs? Are those earplugs correctly fitted? Do people involved in heavy lifting wear weight belts, or do they ignore the potential for injury? Are heavy shoes or gloves worn in areas with dangerous equipment? Again, the attitude of management toward health promotion and illness prevention strongly influences employee behaviors. When administrators, for example, fail to use hearing protection in high-noise areas, they convey an attitude of disinterest in health, which frequently filters down to employees.

Use of sunscreen by employees chronically exposed to sunlight is another protective measure that can influence health and should be encouraged by population health nurses. Outdoor workers sustain six to eight times the sun exposure of employees working indoors, but they frequently fail to use sunscreen as a protective measure against skin cancer. For example, in one Canadian study, only 29% of people who worked more than 4 hours per day in the sun used sunscreen (Marrett, Pichora, & Costa, 2010).

Another aspect of protective measures relates to ergonomics, formerly known as human factors. **Ergonomics** is a scientific discipline that applies an understanding of human–environmental interactions to design work systems to foster human well-being and optimal performance (International Ergonomics Association [IEA], 2014). In essence, it is the practice of making a job fit the employee rather than the other way around. Properly applied, ergonomics improves employee productivity by eliminating barriers to effective work. It also results in greater physical and emotional comfort in the work setting and leads to fewer musculoskeletal injuries due to elements of work such as awkward postures, repetitive movements, and so on (American Psychological Association, 2014; OSHA, n.d.a).

Three aspects of ergonomics should be considered in assessing the health status of the working population: physical ergonomics, cognitive ergonomics, and organizational ergonomics (IEA, 2014). Physical ergonomics address human anatomical, anthropometric (e.g., height and weight), physiologic, and biomechanical characteristics as they relate to physical activity. Consideration of the placement of a computer keyboard in relation to the flexion and extension capabilities of the human wrist is an example of an anatomical characteristic, while the appropriate height of a chair addresses an individual's anthropometric characteristics. Appropriate measures for handling toxic substances would reflect human physiologic responses to specific material, and measures to prevent back strain in lifting would be based on biomechanical characteristics of human musculature.

Cognitive ergonomics is concerned with cognitive processes such as memory, perception, and motor response as they affect the performance of work. Strategies to reduce mental workload and stress reflect cognitive ergonomics. Finally, organizational ergonomics reflects organizational structures that promote or impede work. For example, telecommuting and logical work flow may improve organizational ergonomics.

In the cognitive realm, the population health nurse in an occupational setting would assess the degree to which employees are qualified to perform their particular job function and their interest in that job. Employees who work at jobs that do not interest them, that are beyond their capabilities, or that do not provide sufficient challenge may be at greater risk for both emotional and physical health problems than those who are better suited to their jobs.

Population health nurses working in occupational health settings may be responsible for assessing the ergonomic features of a setting or a particular job. Ergonomic evaluation is frequently done when several employees develop work-related musculoskeletal disorders, but could be employed in a general assessment of the workplace to prevent musculoskeletal injuries. When possible, employees are observed performing their usual job duties. The evaluator also asks injured employees to identify tasks that are most difficult to accomplish. The difficult tasks frequently lead to the identification of specific factors that promote injury and that are amenable to change. In addition to changing features of the job or work environment, ergonomic analysis may lead to employee education in better work techniques to prevent injury.

Another aspect of ergonomic evaluation is an assessment of tools and equipment used in the job and their potential for injury. This may include both power equipment and hand tools and mechanical processes. Ease of use and appropriateness for human anatomical function are considered.

Immunization. Population health nurses in occupational settings would also assess appropriate immunizations among the employee population. For example, health care workers and teachers need a variety of immunizations to keep them from becoming ill and from transmitting infectious diseases to their charges. During the 2011–2012 influenza season, however, only 67% of U.S. health care personnel received influenza vaccine. Immunization levels were considerably higher in hospitals and health systems that mandated immunization—95% compared to only 68% in facilities where it was not mandatory (Ball et al., 2012). In 2009, New York state issued a vaccination mandate for all health care personnel. The mandate was subjected to a number of law suits on grounds of violating individual liberties. Before the suits were heard, however, the mandate was dropped due to a shortage of vaccine (Ottenberg et al., 2011).

Population health nurses can be involved in designing immunization campaigns to promote voluntary immunization. Such campaigns would include educating employees on the need for immunization and planning delivery programs that are convenient and free of cost to employees.

Presenteeism. A final behavioral factor that influences the health of employees in the work setting is working while ill, also called sickness **presenteeism** (Kumar, Grefenstette, Galloway, Albert, & Burke, 2013). CDC recommends that employees stay home for 24 hours after a fever subsides, yet many people either cannot afford to take the time from work or are concerned about being thought of as "slackers." In these conditions and faced with the extent of job insecurity in today's job market, many people choose to continue working when ill. An estimated 42% of the U.S. workforce would not get paid if they stayed home from work, and 33% of the labor force, particularly low-wage employees, lack paid sick days. A computer simulation indicated that nearly 12% of the attack rate for disease transmission can be attributed to workplace exposures and that providing 1 or 2 days of paid sick time would reduce infections by 25% and 39%, respectively (Kumar et al., 2013).

In addition to the lost productivity from employees whose performance is impaired by symptoms of illness, presenteeism is harmful to the ill employee as well as to others in the work setting. When an employee has a communicable disease, for example, coming to work while ill increases the risk of exposure for coworkers and clients. In addition, presenteeism may increase overall risk of premature mortality. The effects of presenteeism are seen with mental as well as physical illness. In one study, for example, mental illness presenteeism cost employers nearly twice as much as absenteeism related to mental health issues. Going to work while ill not only exposes others, but may lengthen the eventual time lost when illness becomes worse (Lundberg & Cooper, 2011).

Population health nurses working in occupational settings assess behaviors affecting the health of individual employees in the work setting as well as the prevalence of harmful behaviors in the work group. The *Focused Assessment* below provides some guidelines for assessing this aspect of health in the work setting.

HEALTH SYSTEM DETERMINANTS. Health system factors influencing employee health relate to both external and internal health care systems. The external system reflects the availability and accessibility of health care services outside the workplace, whereas the internal system consists of those services offered within the workplace.

The external system. In assessing employee health status, the population health nurse in the occupational setting gathers information about the use of health services in the community at large. The nurse examines the type of services used and the reasons for and appropriateness of their use. The nurse also assesses the availability of services needed by company employees in the external health care system.

One of the work-related factors influencing use of outside health services is the availability of insurance coverage. Health insurance is an employment benefit for many, but large segments of the working population do not have health insurance coverage. Many of these uninsured workers do not have sufficient income to afford health insurance themselves or out-of-pocket health care expenses. For example, in 2012, 148.6 million people in the United States had health insurance coverage through their own or a family member's employment (NCHS, 2014). During 2011, 51% of U.S. firms offered health

FOCUSED ASSESSMENT Assessing Behavioral Determinants Influencing Health in the Work Setting

- What behavioral factors influence health in the work setting?
- Do any members of the employee population use prescription medications on a regular basis? Are medications used, stored, and dispensed as directed?
- What is the extent of substance use and abuse by members of the work group? How does substance use and abuse affect employee performance?
- Are safety policies and procedures in place in the work setting? Are they enforced? Do employees use appropriate safety equipment and procedures? Do employees use sunscreen and other protective measures against damaging effects of sunlight?
- Do employees engage in other behaviors (e.g., smoking) that increase their risk of toxic effects from workplace exposures?
- Do employees get sufficient rest and exercise to promote their health? What opportunities are provided for physical activity in the work setting?
- What is the nutritional status of the employee population? What foods are available in the work setting? Does food availability promote good nutrition in the employee population?
- To what extent do employees obtain appropriate immunizations?
- To what extent does sickness presenteeism occur in the employee population? What are the effects of presenteeism for the sick employee, for coworkers, and for the organization?

insurance coverage to their employees (Henry J. Kaiser Family Foundation, 2013). As of 2013, 72% of the overall U.S. civilian workforce had access to medical care benefits, but only 54% chose to obtain coverage, and only 23% of those with wages in the lowest 25% were covered (BLS, 2013d). A substantial proportion of employees who are eligible for health insurance through their workplaces choose not to be insured due to high premiums. In 2012, for example, employers paid an average of 80% of health insurance premiums for coverage for a single individual, but only 69% of the premiums for family coverage (BLS, 2012c). From 2002 to 2012, premiums for employment-based family coverage increased by 97%, but employee contributions to those premiums increased by 102% in the same time frame. Due to the high costs of insurance, many employees who do have coverage choose high deductible plans, particularly in small firms with few employees. In fact the number of employees choosing high deductible plans increased from 10% in 2006 to 26% in 2012. This means that more people have to pay larger amounts out of pocket (up to $1,000 for a single individual and more for a family) before their health insurance coverage begins (Kaiser Family Foundation & Health Research & Educational Trust, 2012).

Some employers are requiring employees to complete health risk assessments. Approximately 11%, of large firms that do so, impose financial penalties on employees with health risks who do not complete wellness programs, and another 9% reward or penalize employees based on achieving biometric outcomes (e.g., weight control, smoking cessation) (Kaiser Family Foundation et al., 2012).

The occupational health nurse should become familiar with the insurance status of employees in the company and with the kinds of benefits covered under group policies, where they exist. Occupational health nurses may also need to advocate for affordable personal and family health insurance coverage for employees in the work setting.

The internal system. The internal health care system consists of those health services and programs provided to employees in the work setting itself. Internal health services may relate to each of the four levels of health care. Programs may reflect attempts to promote employee health and health-related behaviors, environmental modification to prevent illness and injury, care to resolve existing health problems, or care designed to promote rehabilitation and restoration of health. Specific work settings will vary with respect to the extent of services provided in each of these areas. For example, small businesses may not provide any on-site services other than care for emergencies such as might be provided in any setting. Large or multi-site companies, on the other hand, might provide an array of services across the spectrum of care. A few companies also provide health care services for employees' family members. Even in occupational settings that do not provide care to family members, nurses may be asked by employees for assistance in dealing with family health issues. The nurse may counsel the employee regarding resolution of family problems or may provide referrals to outside sources of assistance.

According to a group of experts involved in the Working Group on Worksite Chronic Disease Prevention, for example, health promotion and illness prevention in the worksite tends to have three foci: promoting individual behavior change, promoting change in the work environment, and promoting work–family balance (Sorenson et al., 2011). Services in these three areas might involve employee education for healthy behaviors, such as smoking cessation or weight control; modifications in the work environment or work processes that promote health and prevent illness and injury, such as minimizing employee exposure to toxic substances; or consideration of work schedules and their effects on family interactions and employee physical and mental health.

Services to resolve existing health problems, whether work-related or not, may be provided in the work setting by health care professionals. Alternatively, employees may be referred to outside sources for needed care. For example, an occupational health nurse may provide routine prenatal care for pregnant employees in the work setting or refer them to existing community services. Resolution of existing problems may address immediate stabilization of an injury, or in a large facility, involve X-rays, casting, and so on. Similarly, health care professionals may be actively involved in treating and monitoring treatment effects for chronic diseases or refer employees to their primary providers or other sources of care in the community. Generally speaking, rehabilitations services are not directly provided in the work setting, but occupational health professionals may monitor the effects of rehabilitation and determine when an employee is able to return to work. Each of these categories of services will be addressed in more detail in the discussion of planning and implementing services to meet the needs of the working population.

In assessing those needs, however, the population health nurse in an occupational setting would identify the internal and external health system resources available to employees and determine gaps in services required to address identified health needs in the population. In addition, the nurse would assess the extent of use of available resources as well as their quality and adequacy in meeting the employee population's needs.

A *Focused Assessment* addressing health system considerations in the work setting is presented on the next page. The *Population Health Assessment and Intervention Guide* provided on the student resources site can be used to assess an employee population. In addition, a specific tool for assessing health in work settings is provided.

Diagnostic Reasoning and Care of Working Populations

Population health nurses working in occupational settings derive nursing diagnoses from assessment information related to individuals or groups of employees. For example, the nurse might diagnose "inability to sleep due to work pressures" for an employee who works night shift or "poor employee morale due to increased tension and stress in the work setting." Other nursing diagnoses related to individual employees are a "need

FOCUSED ASSESSMENT Assessing Health System Determinants Influencing Health in the Work Setting

- What health services are offered in the work setting? How are health care services funded? Is funding adequate to meet health needs?
- How accessible are needed health services in the community? To what extent does the employee population use available health services?
- What is the extent of health insurance coverage in the employee population?
- What is the quality of interaction between internal and external health care services?
- To what extent are health promotion and illness/injury prevention emphasized in the work setting?
- What systems are in place to control and monitor toxic exposures in the work setting?
- Are surveillance procedures implemented in a systematic way to periodically assess all employees at risk for exposure?
- What health services are available to resolve existing health problems?
- What emergency response services are available in the health setting?
- What health services related to restoration of health are available?

for referral for counseling due to heavy drinking" and "moderate hearing loss due to failure to use hearing protection in high-noise areas." Nursing diagnoses at the group level might include a "potential for exposure to hepatitis B due to frequent contact with blood" for a group of laboratory technicians in a hospital, and the "potential for falls due to work in elevated areas" for a group of construction workers.

Planning and Implementing Care for Working Populations

Interventions may be developed by the occupational health nurse alone or in conjunction with others in the work setting to address the health needs identified. In the case of individual clients, interventions would be tailored to individual needs and circumstances. When identified health problems affect groups of employees, planned interventions are likely to be more complex. Planning to meet the needs of groups in the workplace will employ the principles of health programming discussed in Chapter 15∞. Whether the client is an individual, a group of employees, or the total population in the work setting, interventions may be planned to address health promotion, illness and injury prevention, resolution of existing health problems, or health restoration.

HEALTH PROMOTION. AAOHN defined health promotion in the employment context as the design of health education initiatives to foster employee responsibility for their own health (Yap & James, 2010). Worksite health promotion, however, involves more than educating employees and changing their health-related behaviors. Characteristics of effective worksite health promotion programs include ongoing education and monitoring, team-based interventions versus individual delivery, a single-disease focus, goal setting, increasing employee knowledge, and self-monitoring. Effective programs also incorporate consistent reminders, initiatives to address barriers to health promotion, and rewards for employee accomplishments (Yap & James, 2010).

Federal programs in the United States can assist businesses with the development of worksite health promotion programs. For example, the National Healthy Worksite Program (NWHP) is intended to assist employers in implementing evidence-based health promotion and wellness programs to reduce chronic disease incidence. NWHP provides funding for employers to establish comprehensive worksite health programs to support physical activity, nutrition, and tobacco-use cessation (CDC, 2013a). Similarly, the Affordable Care Act has created incentives for employers to develop wellness initiatives that reward employees for participation in wellness and/or achievement of specific health-related goals (e.g., weight loss, normal cholesterol levels). Additional rewards, up to 50% of the cost of health coverage, may be provided specifically for programs that prevent or reduce tobacco use (U.S. Department of Labor, 2012).

As noted earlier, health promotion efforts go beyond motivating individual behavior to changing the work environment to promote health, and modifying work–family interactions to foster health (Sorenson et al., 2011). Health promotion initiatives may focus on both individual behavior and organizational strategies that promote health. For example, one program to address stress management encompassed both individual strategies and organizational strategies. Individual strategies included stress awareness and education, relaxation techniques, cognitive coping strategies, and approaches such as meditation and biofeedback, as well as lifestyle changes, such as increased physical activity, healthier diets, smoking cessation, and diminished alcohol intake. Additional strategies at the individual level included interpersonal skill development, promotion of adequate sleep, equalization of gender workload within the family, and focusing on life priorities (Lundberg & Cooper, 2011).

At the organizational level, strategies to promote effective stress management included task redesign and redesign of the work environment to minimize stress, use of flexible work schedules, analysis of work roles and goal establishment, and including employees in participating management and career development activities. Additional organizational strategies focused on ensuring variation in work, providing social support and building cohesive work teams, and establishing fair work policies. Creation of "restorative environments" incorporating green spaces and recreational opportunities were also suggested as organizational strategies to promote stress management. Such environments are believed to decrease the need to constantly engage in "executive brain functions" and allow people to unwind (Lundberg & Cooper, 2011).

There is a particular need for health promotion for older workers in occupational settings. Targeted health promotion programs for older employees include the COACH program and the RealAge program, both of which include in-depth risk assessments and suggested action plans. The RealAge program is a web-based program, whereas the COACH program involves a personal coach who assists employees in developing a risk reduction plan and then provides monthly monitoring. In one study of the interventions, older employees were twice as likely to use the COACH program, and those who did were more likely to engage in more behavior changes than those who used the web-mediated program (Hughes et al., 2011).

A similar program combined weekly personally tailored e-mail messages from an occupational health nurse focused on specific risk behaviors and supplemental website information to motivate physical activity among employees. The weekly messages were found to move people further through the stages of change and resulted in greater increases in physical activity than general e-mail broadcasts (Yap, Davis, Gates, Hemmings, & Pan, 2009a, 2009b).

Population health nurses in occupational settings educate employees to lead healthier lives. They also advocate for company policies that promote health. An organizational culture that supports health conveys to employees that their health is a priority for the company. This message must be supported by company efforts to promote health within the organization. For example, some companies may promote exercise among employees, but an organizational culture that truly supports physical activity may allow time for exercise during the workday or provide facilities (e.g., weight rooms, walking paths) that actually promote physical activity. Similarly, an organizational culture that supports health will take steps to ban all forms of tobacco use in the work setting and will provide tobacco use cessation assistance for those employees who use tobacco. Another feature of an organizational culture that supports health is positive attitudes toward health-promoting behaviors among employees. For example, in such a culture employees who engage in physical activity are the norm, and those who do not are in the minority. Employees support each other in positive health-related behaviors. Population health nurses can be instrumental in promoting an organizational culture that supports health by convincing employers of the value of health promotion in terms of increased productivity, better morale, and reduced absenteeism. They can also help to develop positive attitudes to health promotion among employees by making health-promotion activities relevant to the goals and motivations of the employee group. For example, they might approach smoking cessation from the perspective of the benefits for employees' children if that is a strong motivator for members of the work group. Or they might plan physical activities that fit easily into the workday. Table 23-2● summarizes health promotion strategies and related population health nursing roles in work settings.

ILLNESS AND INJURY PREVENTION. Preventing illness and injury is the second level of health care in the workplace. Population health nursing activities related to both are briefly addressed below.

Illness prevention. Preventing communicable diseases in occupational settings can involve prevention of specific illnesses through immunization or employee behaviors that prevent the spread of infection. Population health nurses would identify categories of employees at risk for specific communicable diseases and provide related immunization services. For example, personnel in health care facilities should receive a variety of immunizations, including influenza, hepatitis B, measles, mumps,

TABLE 23-2 Health Promotion Strategies for Working Populations

Emphasis	Strategies
Promoting individual health behaviors	• Educate employees for healthy behaviors (e.g., physical activity, nutritious diet) • Assist employees to eliminate unhealthy behaviors (e.g., smoking cessation) • Teach effective coping skills • Assist employees to balance work and family roles • Promote adequate sleep and educate employees on sleep hygiene
Fostering an organizational culture to promote health	• Assist in development of worksite policies that promote health (e.g., physical activity breaks and opportunities) • Advocate for development of work environments that promote health • Advocate for healthy food options in the workplace • Advocate strategies that foster job control
Promoting work–family balance	• Advocate for flexible work schedules • Advocate for family care leaves and support services

rubella, pertussis, and varicella (Shefer et al., 2011). Immunization is particularly important for personnel in long-term care facilities due to the vulnerability of residents (Kimura, Nguyen, Higa, Hurwitz, & Vugia, 2007). Similarly, farm workers and others who work outdoors or are at risk for dirty injuries should be adequately immunized against tetanus. Nurses in occupational settings may provide these immunizations or refer employees to outside sources of vaccine, monitoring immunization levels among the population at risk. If outside services are used, the occupational health nurse may need to advocate for cost reimbursement for employees (Ottenberg et al., 2011). When workplace exposures to certain pathogens occur, disease development can be prevented through postexposure prophylaxis. **Postexposure prophylaxis (PEP)** is treatment for a communicable disease following a potential occupational exposure to the infectious agent. For example, health care providers caring for clients with known cases of hepatitis B or C or HIV infection may receive prophylactic treatment to prevent them from developing the disease. Occupational health nurses may be involved in actually providing employees with prophylactic treatment or in referring them for needed services. Prophylaxis will be addressed in more detail in Chapter 26∞.

Prevention of the spread of communicable diseases in the work setting can also be accomplished through effective hygiene, adequate cleaning, and disinfection of contaminated surfaces and equipment (Smith et al., 2013), and, in the case of health care personnel, use of universal precautions (Materna et al., 2010). Strategies to minimize presenteeism can also serve to reduce the spread of many communicable diseases in the workplace. Presenteeism can be discouraged through provision of paid sick days (Kumar et al., 2013), and population health nurses may need to advocate for sick leave policies as well as educate employees regarding the need to stay home when ill. For selected occupational groups, for example, laboratory employees, use of adequate safety precautions in handling specimens would be emphasized (Ritger et al., 2011).

Another aspect of illness prevention involves modifying personal risk factors, particularly those involved in the development of noncommunicable conditions. Risk factors are personal or group characteristics that predispose one to develop a specific health problem. For example, it is well known that smoking increases one's risk of developing heart disease and lung cancer, so smoking is a risk factor for both of these problems.

Some risk factors can be modified or eliminated, thus decreasing one's chances of developing specific health problems. Again, using smoking as an example, people who quit smoking lower their risk of developing lung cancer. Occupational health nurses can be instrumental in assisting employees to modify risk factors, thereby helping them to prevent health problems. Some risk factors that receive particular attention in the occupational setting are smoking, elevated blood pressure, sedentary lifestyle, stress, and overweight.

Occupational health nurses can work on risk factor modification with individuals or groups of employees. They can also engage in risk factor modification efforts at the company level. One example of this would be efforts to convince company policy makers that a no-smoking policy should be instituted and enforced within the workplace. Nurses can also develop weight standards for certain job categories in which being overweight is particularly hazardous.

At the individual level, the nurse can counsel employees regarding the hazards of smoking, particularly in conjunction with occupational exposure to respiratory irritants. She or he can also provide assistance to individuals who wish to quit smoking.

Environmental risk factor modification can also prevent the development of many occupational conditions. For example, work stations can be redesigned to be more ergonomic to prevent musculoskeletal injuries (OSHA, n.d.a). Similarly, exposure to toxic substances in the workplace can be minimized through engineering controls, use of safety precautions and protective gear, or replacement with safer substances and processes. For example, recommendations for preventing the fumigant poisoning of produce inspectors discussed earlier included prolonged aeration of products, conducting inspections in well-aerated areas, and improving airflow in produce storage areas (O'Malley et al., 2011). Similarly, farm workers can be educated regarding correct application of pesticides (Schwartz et al., 2012). Metal recycling plants can implement policies of only accepting containers that have been cut open to prevent release of toxic substances and exposure of workers. Such facilities and others that work with potential hazardous compounds should also develop hazardous gas release evacuation plans (Kelsey et al., 2011).

Population health nurses may be involved in developing protocols for handling of hazardous substances, but they are more likely to educate employees on their implementation as well as on emergency measures to minimize the effects of exposures. For example, they may educate employees on the correct use of ear plugs in high-noise areas or in the use of breathing equipment in high-dust areas (Laney et al., 2012). Education regarding sunscreen use and protective clothing for employees who work outdoors is another important strategy for preventing skin cancer.

Population health nurses can also advocate for measures to minimize job strain that can contribute to a variety of physical and mental health problems (Stansfeld et al., 2012). Restructuring the work environment can help in minimizing occupational stress as a risk factor for health problems. Efforts in this direction include developing flexible schedules to minimize conflicts with employees' outside responsibilities. The nurse can also facilitate employee input into work-related decisions and strive to minimize role overload and role ambiguity. The nurse can also promote opportunity for social interaction, job security, and career development.

As is obvious, many of these efforts must be undertaken by management, but the nurse can provide management with evidence of related research and can provide the impetus for change in these areas. At the individual level, the occupational health nurse can be aware of the stressors experienced by employees in various jobs in the work setting. The nurse is also in a position to monitor the effects of stress on the individual employee and to counsel employees in stress management.

Injury prevention. Injury prevention in the work setting may entail employee education or environmental modification. Physical hazards are the most important cause of occupational morbidity and mortality (Lundberg & Cooper, 2011), and employees need to be acquainted with safety procedures to prevent accidents. For example, there is a need to prevent needlesticks in health care settings, and staff may need to be educated regarding the appropriate disposal of sharps. Similarly, periodic reminders regarding good body mechanics in lifting patients may be needed in the health care setting. There may also be a need to educate employees in the correct use of safety equipment. For example, individuals working in some areas should wear protective clothing or use breathing apparatus. As noted earlier, safety education should be provided to both paid and volunteer employees. The nurse should explain the need for safety equipment and be responsible for monitoring its use. This may entail planning periodic visits to certain areas of the workplace to determine whether employees are indeed using safety equipment as directed.

Employees may also be in need of education in other areas related to injury prevention. Handling of hazardous substances, proper use of machinery, need for fluid replacement in high-heat areas, and good body mechanics are all educational topics that may be appropriate in certain industrial settings. There is also a need for transportation safety measures, particularly for older employees. For example, vehicles may be selected or adapted to promote maximum safety. Company policies can also limit driving, particularly at night, as much as possible and encourage route and trip planning to reduce stress and fatigue. Refresher driver training may also be helpful as is education on chronic health conditions and medications that can affect driving safety. Finally, measures may be needed to compensate for perceptual or cognitive deficits in older people working in heavy traffic zones (e.g., road workers) (Pratt & Rodriguez-Acosta, 2013). There is also a need for stringent transportation safety guidelines for aircraft use. For example, aircraft operations guidelines in the oil and gas industries exceed Federal Aviation Administration guidelines, and nurses can encourage adherence to these guidelines (Gunter et al., 2013). For further information on the guidelines established by the International Association of Oil and Gas Producers, see the *External Resources* section of the student resources site.

Prevention of musculoskeletal injuries may entail redesign of work stations and processes to provide more ergonomic conditions. OSHA (n.d.a) has developed guidelines for the redesign process that include development of management support for redesign, involvement of workers, employee and management training, identification of specific problems, early reporting of symptoms, implementing ergonomic solutions, and evaluating the outcome of redesign efforts. In addition, OSHA and NIOSH have developed ergonomic guidelines for specific industries, such as meat packing, foundries, nursing homes, shipyards, retail grocery stores, and so on. Similarly, guidelines for creating ergonomically appropriate computer work stations have been developed by the U.S. Department of Defense Computer/Electronic Adaptations Program (n.d.). For further information about the these guidelines, see the *External Resources* section of the student resources site.

Another aspect of injury prevention in which the nurse may be involved is monitoring hazardous conditions in the workplace. The nurse should be aware of potential hazards and their appropriate management. In the absence of an industrial hygienist, the nurse may plan and conduct environmental testing to detect hazardous levels of chemicals, heat, or noise.

The nurse may need to acquaint management with the occurrence of injuries due to hazardous conditions and advocate changes designed to protect employees from injuries. Recommendations for dealing with the problem of noise-induced hearing loss, for example, include engineering efforts to minimize noise production, use of properly fitted hearing protection devices, education of employees and managers in the use of protective devices and their importance, and periodic audiometric screening. The occupational health nurse may be actively involved in planning and executing the majority of these recommended activities, particularly in screening for hearing loss, fitting protective devices, and educating employees and supervisors. Control of noise-related hearing loss requires commitment on the part of employees and management to the proper use of protective devices. Motivating employees to use these devices and monitoring their use are crucial functions of the occupational health nurse.

Minimizing the effects of shift work. Occupational health nurses can also help to prevent or minimize the negative effects of shiftwork. Some authors have suggested four general approaches

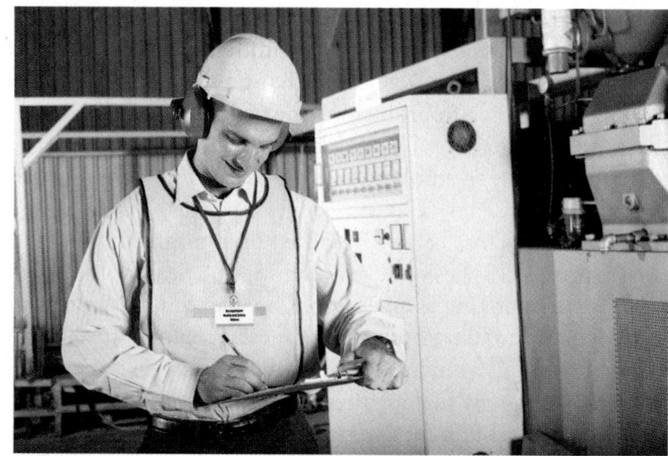

Use of hearing protection in high-noise areas can prevent hearing loss. *(Michaeljung/Fotolia)*

to addressing the effects of shift work: pharmacologic intervention, bright light exposure, education and counseling, and shift-work legislation (Smith et al., 2011). Pharmacologic intervention may involve agents to promote alertness and diminish fatigue on the job or to support adequate sleep. Many agents used for both purposes may have long-term negative effects such as dependence or sleep disruption discussed earlier in relation to the use of energy drinks. Newer sleep enhancing or wakefulness-promoting agents, such as melatonin or modafinil, have been found to have fewer negative effects than hypnotics or stimulants, respectively, but the effects of long-term use are not yet known (Smith et al., 2011).

Exposure to bright light, at approximately five times the usual indoor lighting levels, assists with adjustment of circadian rhythms, but requires a strict schedule of exposure over time (including rest days) that may be difficult for some employees or settings to achieve. Education and counseling on measures to promote adequate sleep have been used, but results are inconsistent. Finally, many European countries have adopted the European Directive related to shiftwork, mandating employee assessment prior to nightshift assignment, regular reassessment, and specific reassessment with possible change in shift in the light of health problems experienced (Smith et al., 2011). Although such assessments are not mandated in the United States, occupational health nurses can advocate for their implementation in the work setting. They can also monitor employees on non-daytime shifts for health problems, particularly sleep problems, and advocate for reassignment as needed.

Preventing workplace aggression. Prevention of workplace aggression begins with an assessment of risk. Population health nurses can help to create workplace violence surveillance systems and analyze data on incidents of violence to discover patterns and areas of risk (AAOHN, 2013). They would then be actively involved in measures to prevent violence and aggression in the workplace. NIOSH has developed a course to assist occupational health nurses to recognize and address workplace violence (NIOSH, 2013b). For more information about the course, see the *External Resources* section of the student resources site.

Initiatives to prevent workplace aggression have several foci including developing a workplace culture that does not tolerate violence, implementing engineering controls, establishing administrative controls, and educating employees to minimize violence. Development of a work culture that does not support violence involves creating management commitment to employee safety and willingness to engage in a variety of measures to promote that safety. Population health nurses in occupational settings can assist in the development of no-tolerance policies that encourage prompt reporting of aggression, prevent reprisals against reporting, and promote rapid and thorough investigation of reports (OSHA, 2004). Occupational health nurses can also educate employees to increase awareness of aggression and to promote reporting of minor events or suspicious behavior that may escalate to violence (AAOHN, 2013).

Engineering controls to prevent or minimize violence may include physical adaptations of the workplace to minimize risk. Such adaptations might include arranging furniture in rooms to prevent entrapment, installing security systems and monitoring systems, and providing sufficient lighting and visibility of employees, particularly at night. Other adaptations might include physical barriers (e.g., glass partitions) between employees and members of the public and easy telephone access.

Administrative controls might include approaches such as background checks on applicants, establishing visitor sign-in procedures, controlling access to specific work areas, and practices that discourage employees working alone, use of identification badges, and so on. Developing and implementing a security plan that includes interface with local law enforcement agencies and providing support to employees who are victims of workplace aggression are other aspects of administrative control. Occupational health nurses can advocate for these and other similar administrative controls in the workplace. They can also educate employees and management regarding workplace aggression policies and procedures and on specific safety measures (e.g., not wearing necklaces or chains that might be used for strangulation, walking to cars in groups, conducting interviews with volatile clients in pairs, etc.). Nurses may also provide education on anger management, conflict resolution, and nonviolent crisis intervention (AAOHN, 2013).

Disaster prevention and preparedness. One final aspect of injury and illness prevention in the occupational setting deals with prevention of and preparedness for disaster events. Many occupational settings pose particular risks for disasters due to the presence of volatile or toxic chemicals and other conditions. AAOHN (2012b) recommends an all-hazards approach to disaster planning in which general approaches to all types of disaster situations are identified, rather than developing different response plans for different types of disasters. Population health nurses can assist in the identification of disaster risks and in planning to mitigate those risks. They may also be involved in planning for evacuation to prevent toxic exposures or other potential for harm in the event of a disaster. Mitigation of disaster risk and the role of the population health nurse in disaster response are addressed in more detail in Chapter 25∞. Table 23-3• summarizes the foci and population health nursing interventions related to illness and injury prevention in occupational settings.

RESOLVING EXISTING HEALTH PROBLEMS. Resolution of existing health problems in work setting may focus on individual workers or the employee population in general. General areas of involvement for occupational health nurses include screening and surveillance, treatment for existing conditions, and emergency care.

Screening and surveillance. Screening activities can take any of three directions. Screening efforts begin with preemployment assessment of potential employees. Screening may also

TABLE 23-3 Illness and Injury Prevention Foci and Intervention Strategies for Working Populations

Focus	Strategies
Illness prevention	• Provide or refer for appropriate immunizations • Provide postexposure prophylaxis for communicable disease exposures • Promote use of effective hygiene (e.g., hand washing) and universal precautions as warranted • Advocate for modification or elimination of risk factors for chronic diseases in the work environment • Educate employees regarding risk factor modification (e.g., smoking cessation, weight reduction) • Provide stress reduction/management education for employees • Advocate for paid sick days and educate employees to minimize presenteeism • Encourage strict attention to laboratory safety procedures
Injury prevention	• Provide safety education for employees (e.g., body mechanics, universal precautions for bloodborne pathogens) • Advocate for availability of adequate safety equipment • Monitor effective use of safety equipment • Assist in development of policies and procedures that prevent injury (e.g., comprehensive driver safety policies) • Advocate for modification or elimination of injury risk factors in the work setting • Advocate for work station or work process redesign to prevent injury • Advocate for replacement of hazardous materials or processes with safer alternatives if possible • Advocate for administrative processes and environmental changes to minimize the negative effects of shift work • Advocate for development of adequate management support for injury prevention policies and procedures
Violence prevention	• Assist in development of workplace no-tolerance policies that create a culture of safety • Advocate for installation of engineering controls that minimize risk for violence (e.g., barriers, restricted access, security systems) • Advocate for administrative controls that minimize risk of violence (e.g., access badges, visitor sign-in processes) • Assist in development of processes and procedures for handling workplace violence or potential for violence • Assist in development of reporting and follow-up procedures for workplace aggression, including disciplinary action • Educate employees and management on personal safety, violence prevention, anger management, conflict management, recognition of potentially violent situations, and crisis management
Disaster prevention and preparedness	• Assist in the identification of disaster risk in the work setting • Assist in planning to eliminate or mitigate disaster risk • Assist in the development and implementation of evacuation plans to minimize injury and illness in the event of a disaster

be conducted at periodic intervals to monitor employee health status. Finally, the work environment may be screened periodically for the presence or absence of hazardous conditions. The population health nurse would be involved in planning and implementing screening efforts at all three levels. **Screening** involves testing individuals for indicators of disease or for risk factors that increase the potential for disease. Screening may occur prior to employment, when considering a job transfer, or on an employee's return from an illness or injury, or when considering retirement for health reasons. Periodic screening may also be employed to monitor employee's health status during employment (Palmer & Brown, 2013). Surveillance, on the other hand, involves the analysis of group data to identify trends and problems in the work setting rather than in individual employees.

Preemployment screening. For many employees, their first interaction with an occupational health nurse is the preemployment screening examination. The purpose of this initial screening is to facilitate employee selection and placement. Hiring an employee for a particular job is in part dependent on his or her physical, mental, and emotional capabilities for performing that job. A similar process may be needed when considering an employee for a change of job. These capabilities can be determined in an initial screening examination. At this time, the nurse usually obtains a complete health history from the employee and conducts a battery of routine screening tests. Nurse practitioners in the occupational setting may also conduct the physical examination.

For certain categories of jobs, preemployment screening may entail criminal background checks and/or drug screening. For example, a security guard who works for a firm that designs and builds equipment for use by the armed services would probably need to have a security clearance. Similarly, a school teacher may be required to undergo a criminal background check related to child abuse or molestation. Occupational health nurses will probably not be involved in a security check for a prospective employee, but they may be responsible for collecting specimens for drug screening tests. They may also be subject to screening themselves as health care institutions and other employers become more careful regarding the background of their employees.

Based on the information derived from the screening, the nurse may make determinations regarding the person's employability in a particular capacity. To make such determinations, the nurse must be familiar with the types of activities involved and stressors encountered in a particular job. The preemployment screening also provides baseline data for determining the effects of working conditions on the health of employees. The questions included in the *Focused Assessment* provided below are designed to help determine an employee's fitness for a specific job. A work fitness inventory is also included on the student resources site.

Periodic screening. The nurse in the occupational setting also plans periodic screening activities to monitor employees' continuing health status. This is particularly true of employees working under hazardous conditions. For example, monitoring

FOCUSED ASSESSMENT Evaluating Fitness for Work

General Considerations

- Does the employee have the necessary training and expertise for the job?
- How will the employee's general health affect job performance?
- What is the employee's gender? Will gender affect job performance and employee health and safety risks?
- What is the employee's body size? Will size affect work performance or risks?
- What is the employee's age? Will age affect work performance or risks?
- What is the employee's nutritional status? Will nutritional status affect work performance or health and safety risks?

Functional Considerations

- Does the employee have the physical stamina required?
- Does the employee have any mobility limitations that would interfere with performance?
- Does the employee have sufficient joint function to do the job?
- Does the employee have any postural limitations that would interfere with performance?
- Does the employee have the required strength for the job?
- Does the employee have the level of coordination required?
- Does the employee have problems with coordination or balance that would interfere with performance?
- Does the employee have any cardiorespiratory limitations?
- Is there a possibility for unconsciousness that would create a safety hazard?
- Does the employee have the required level of sensory acuity?
- Does the employee have communication and speech capabilities required by the job?
- Does the employee have the requisite level of cognitive function (e.g., memory, critical thinking)?
- Will the employee's mental or emotional state (e.g., depression) interfere with performance?
- Does the employee have the required motivational level?
- Does the employee have a substance abuse problem that would interfere with performance?
- Does the employee have effective stress management skills?
- Is there any possibility that the employee might endanger self or others?

Health Care Considerations

- Are there treatment effects that will interfere with performance (e.g., drowsiness from medications)?
- Will subsequent treatment plans interfere with performance (e.g., nausea due to future chemotherapy)?
- What is the employee's prognosis? Will existing conditions improve or deteriorate further?
- Does the employee have any special health needs to be met in the work setting (e.g., diabetic diet)?
- Are any assistive aids or appliances used or required? Will work processes or setting need to be adapted to accommodate these aids (e.g., space for a wheelchair)?

Task/Setting Considerations

- What are the physical and emotional demands of the job?
- Are there risk factors in the work setting that would adversely affect the employee?
- What is the level of stress involved in the job?
- Will the employee be working with others or alone? What health effects might this have?
- What are the temporal aspects of the job and how will they affect health (e.g., shift work, early morning or late evening work, length of shift)?
- Is there travel involved in the job? How will this affect employee health?
- Is the workstation ergonomically designed to minimize injury?

Data from: Palmer, K. T., & Brown, I. (2013). A general framework for assessing fitness for work. In K. T. Palmer, I. Brown, & J. Hobson (Eds.), *Fitness for work: The medical aspects* (5th ed., Chapter 1). Oxford, UK: Oxford University Press.

devices are used by personnel working with radiation and are periodically checked for exposure limits. Likewise, blood chemistries may be done at periodic intervals to test for exposure to toxic substances. Periodic blood pressure screenings and pulmonary function tests may also be warranted. In some occupational groups, such as the armed forces, employees are routinely screened for overweight and for physical capacity.

The types of screening done depend on the type of job performed, the risks involved, and the capabilities required. Some screenings are routinely performed on all employees in a particular setting. For example, employees may receive a routine physical examination at periodic intervals. Other screening tests are performed only on specific employees. For example, lead screening may be done routinely on individuals who work on a plant assembly line, but not on clerical personnel.

Nurses may also be actively involved in providing or promoting routine health screenings that are not related to employees' jobs. For example, the nurse may educate employees regarding the need for colon cancer screening or mammography.

Occupational health nurses are frequently responsible for conducting these and other screening tests on employees. They may also interpret test results, explain them to employees, and take action when warranted by positive test results.

Environmental screening and surveillance. Periodic screening of the environment and surveillance for negative occupational effects may also be warranted, and, in the absence of industrial hygienists or safety engineers, the nurse may be responsible for planning and conducting environmental screenings. For example, the nurse may measure noise levels in various work areas at specific intervals to determine areas in which hearing protection is required. Similarly, measurements of volatile chemicals or radiation might be done in high-risk areas.

Surveillance involves monitoring the employee population for trends in health problems. For example, AAOHN (2013) recommends surveillance for instances of workplace aggression and violence. Similarly, the nurse may note an increase in absences related to gastrointestinal problems among employees who eat in company dining rooms or increases in specific kinds of injuries.

Treatment of existing conditions. The second area of focus in resolving existing health problems in the work setting is the diagnosis and treatment of illness or injury. Population health nurses are actively involved in planning health interventions for individual employees and should also participate in planning health programs to meet the needs of groups of clients.

Many employers go beyond treating only job-related illnesses and conditions to treating a variety of major and minor conditions. The rationale for the extension of services to non-job-related conditions is that any health problem, physical or emotional, can serve to impair an employee's performance. Also, treatment of these conditions within the work setting limits time lost in pursuing outside treatment, saving the company money in the long run.

Depending on the capabilities of the occupational health unit, employees with existing health problems may be referred to the external health care system for problem resolution, or treatment may be provided within the workplace itself. Those occupational health nurses who are nurse practitioners may treat illness in the work setting. Even nurses who are not nurse practitioners may treat minor conditions on the basis of protocols established in conjunction with medical consultation.

Occupational health nurses also need to plan to monitor the effectiveness of therapy, whether or not that therapy is provided by the occupational health unit. For example, an employee with hypertension might be followed by his or her primary care provider, but the occupational health nurse will monitor medication compliance and effects on the employee's blood pressure. In addition, the nurse will educate the employee regarding the condition and its treatment.

In the case of employees with problems related to substance abuse or stress, the population health nurse usually initiates a referral to an appropriate source of assistance. The nurse may also need to function as an advocate for impaired employees, encouraging employers to provide coverage for treatment of psychological as well as physical illness. Nurses may also find it necessary to report substance abuse to supervisory personnel when either the health or the safety of other employees is threatened.

Population health nurses in occupational settings may also be involved in planning and implementing employee assistance programs for employees with psychological problems. An **employee assistance program (EAP)** is a program within the occupational setting designed to counsel employees with psychological problems and assist them in dealing with those problems. EAPs usually focus on motivating individuals to seek help and referring them for needed services. Substance abuse disorders and eating disorders are two types of problems addressed by EAPs. Generally, the occupational health nurse refers an employee to another source of services rather than providing care for these problems within the work setting. However, the nurse may be involved in the development and support of self-help groups within the employment setting to assist employees with these and other problems. For example, guided self-help and cognitive behavioral group therapy may assist employees with eating disorders. Similarly, an occupational health nurse might help to establish a bereavement group to assist employees who have experienced significant losses. Occupational settings also frequently sponsor chapters of Alcoholics Anonymous.

Emergency response. Responding to emergency situations is another aspect of resolving existing problems. Nurses may find themselves dealing with both physical and psychological emergencies and should have a basic plan for dealing with various types of emergencies that may arise. Physical emergencies may result from serious accidents or from physical conditions such as heart attack, stroke, seizure disorder, and hypoglycemia. Treatment for these emergencies is usually based on established protocols.

With respect to emergencies due to illness, it is helpful if the nurse has prior information related to the employee's condition.

For example, if the nurse has prior knowledge that the client is diabetic, the diagnosis of hypoglycemic reaction will be reached and treatment initiated more rapidly than would otherwise be the case. For this reason, occupational health nurses should be well acquainted with employees' health histories.

Psychological emergencies may result in homicide, suicide, or both. Although businesses may have generalized protocols for dealing with such emergencies as threatened homicide or suicide, the nurse faced with such situations will probably need to exercise a great deal of creativity in planning to address a psychological emergency. General considerations include remaining calm and removing others from the immediate vicinity. The nurse *should not* plan any heroic measures that may endanger him- or herself, the employee, or others. Additional interventions are dictated by the situation. Again, prior identification of employees under excessive stress may help to prevent psychiatric emergencies.

Another psychological emergency with which occupational health nurses may need to deal is sexual assault. Most victims of sexual assault in the workplace are women, and most assaults occur at night when women are working in isolation from coworkers or the public. The nurse who encounters a female employee who has been sexually assaulted should address immediate physical and psychological needs, assess the client for suicidal tendencies, and refer her for counseling. The nurse should also alert the appropriate authorities and may need to act as an advocate with the legal and criminal justice systems and provide emotional support.

One further type of emergency that requires an occupational health nursing response is the emergency that affects large numbers of people. Examples of mass emergencies are fires or explosions, radiation exposure, and hazardous substance leaks. In addition to providing treatment for those injured in such emergencies, the nurse may be responsible for assisting in evaluating affected areas and in organizing to provide needed care. Occupational health nurses should be involved in planning the overall company response to such situations as well as in planning health care in such an eventuality. The role of the nurse in disaster preparedness is discussed in greater detail in Chapter 25∞. Major emphases in resolving existing health problems in work settings are summarized in Table 23-4●.

HEALTH RESTORATION. Health restoration or rehabilitation was identified as an element of the occupational health nursing role by the World Health Organization as early as 1982. Rehabilitation in the context of the occupational health setting is a process designed to return the employee, as much as possible, to his or her prior level of function.

Health restoration interventions in work settings are directed toward preventing recurrence of health problems, limiting their consequences, and promoting and maintaining independence. In occupational health settings, health restoration enables the employee to return to work, and the goal is to remove obstacles to a return to productive work or to adapt the workplace to facilitate that return. In some instances, when return to an employee's former position is precluded by the long-term consequences of health problems or the nature of job demands, health restoration may involve preparing him or her for a new role.

The types of intervention strategies employed depend on the problems to be prevented. For example, engineering measures may be used to prevent subsequent leakage of a toxic chemical if a leak has already occurred.

Generally speaking, health care at this level is geared toward preventing the spread of communicable diseases, preventing recurrence of other acute conditions, and preventing complications of chronic conditions. Sick-leave policies and employee immunization are examples of measures that might be taken to stop the spread of influenza in the employee population. As noted earlier,

TABLE 23-4 Strategies for Resolving Existing Health Problems in Working Populations

Focus	Strategies
Screening	• Conduct preemployment screenings • Determine work capacity • Make recommendations regarding work conditions or accommodations • Conduct periodic employee screening • Conduct periodic environmental screening and surveillance • Report and interpret screening findings and make referrals for care or environmental modification as needed
Treatment of existing conditions	• Provide treatment for work-related illness or injury • Provide immediate first aid • Refer for outside medical assistance as needed • Develop health care delivery programs to address high prevalence problems in the occupational setting • Advocate for adequate employee health insurance coverage • Advocate for accessible internal or external health care services to meet employee health needs
Emergency response	• Assist in the development of individual and disaster emergency response plans for the work setting • Respond to individual physical or emotional emergencies • Refer employees for continued treatment as needed • Respond to care needs in an occupational disaster • Evaluate the health effects of occupational disasters

by encouraging employees to take advantage of sick-leave benefits when they or family members are ill, the nurse can minimize exposure of others in the occupational setting to communicable diseases and can control the spread of disease. Safety education might prevent a recurrence of accidental injuries due to hazardous equipment, and use of hearing protection might prevent further deterioration of an employee's hearing after noise exposure has already caused some damage. Similarly, treatment of an employee's hypertension can prevent further health problems.

Another aspect of health restoration in an occupational setting may be assessing an employee's fitness to return to work after an illness or injury. Assessment considerations in this case would be similar to those in preemployment assessment. The occupational health nurse would determine the job demands and assess the employee's ability to meet the requirements of the job. Sometimes this can be facilitated by modifications in job processes or responsibilities to fit an employee's reduced capabilities. Occupational health nurses may need to educate the employee, employer, supervisor, and coworkers regarding capabilities and accommodations needed. Based on the UN convention (2006), the right to work also applies to persons who acquire a disability as a result of employment and appropriate measures should be taken to protect that right.

Health restoration interventions by occupational health nurses may also involve assisting employees to adapt to chronic illness or monitoring the status of workers' compensation claims. Dealing with chronic illness or disability in the work setting may be facilitated by the development of worksite disability management programs. Such programs provide disease management services in the work setting and have been shown to result in cost savings for the organization by preventing days lost to work due to exacerbations or for follow-up appointments in the external health care system.

Occupational health nurses may assist individual employees to cope with chronic illness in a number of ways. They may educate the client to enhance personal coping abilities (e.g., through medication management, self-monitoring skills, etc.) or advocate with management or coworkers for support for self-care. For example, the nurse might arrange for flexible break or meal times to permit employees with diabetes to better manage their diets. Nurses may also advocate for working conditions that accommodate limitations or prevent further deterioration. For example, they may see that the workstation for an employee with chronic back pain is ergonomically evaluated and any needed accommodations made. Occupational health nurses may also connect employees to sources of support, such as self-help groups, outside of the work setting. Finally, they may advocate for adequate health care provider support and insurance coverage to address the costs of needed care.

Another focus in health restoration might be the provision of health care and assistance for both victims and perpetrators of workplace aggression (AAOHN, 2013). Employee assistance programs, for instance, might address anger management issues or deal with posttraumatic stress disorder resulting from an assault in the workplace. Assistance with legal claims or in processing worker's compensation claims might also be needed.

Finally health restoration interventions might be required in the aftermath of a workplace disaster. Population health nurses in occupational settings are ideally placed to identify employees suffering from physical or psychological consequences of a disaster and refer them for assistance. They can also be involved in assessing the emergency response and in improving future responses. Population health nursing roles in disaster recovery are discussed in more detail in Chapter 25∞. Health restoration foci and related strategies in occupational settings are summarized in Table 23-5●.

TABLE 23-5 Health Restoration Strategies for Working Populations

Focus	Strategies
Preventing the spread of communicable diseases	• Provide employee immunization • Educate on infection control procedures • Encourage use of sick days and advocate for sick days for employees
Preventing the recurrence of other acute conditions	• Educate employees to prevent recurrent health problems • Advocate for environmental modifications to prevent recurrent problems
Preventing complications of chronic conditions	• Monitor treatment effects and disease status • Educate employees for disease self-management • Modify the work environment to accommodate limitations due to disability
Assessing fitness to return to work	• Follow up on workers' compensation claims • Assess recovery status • Modify work environment as needed to facilitate return to work • Educate employees, employers, supervisors, and coworkers regarding requirements for a return to work
Assisting victims and perpetrators of workplace aggression	• Make referrals for assistance as needed • Assist with legal or workers' compensation claims • Provide emotional support
Disaster recovery	• Identify employees experiencing physical or psychological consequences of disasters and provide or refer for assistance • Assist in assessing the adequacy of emergency response and in planning for future responses

Implementing nursing interventions in work settings frequently involves collaboration with others. Most often, collaboration occurs between the nurse and the employee. In other instances, the nurse may collaborate with health care providers and others within or outside of the occupational setting. For example, the nurse might collaborate with a pregnant employee's primary health care provider to monitor her progress throughout the pregnancy. Implementing the plan of care for an employee with carpal tunnel syndrome might involve collaboration with the primary care provider and with a supervisor to facilitate movement to a job that does not necessitate repetitive wrist movements or to promote ergonomic redesign of an employee's work station and work processes.

When health problems affect groups of employees, implementing the plan of care might involve collaboration with other health care providers and with company management and other personnel. For example, the nurse who has documented an increased incidence of respiratory conditions due to aerosol exposures will advocate plans to resolve the problem. These plans need to be approved by management and implemented by engineering personnel, if engineering controls are required, or by company purchasing agents, if special respiratory protective devices are needed. In the latter instance, the nurse may be involved in determining the types of protective devices needed and recommending their purchase to management.

Evaluating Health Care in Work Settings

As in all other settings for nursing practice, the effectiveness of health care in work settings must be evaluated. Evaluation can focus on the outcomes of care either for the individual employee or for the total employee population. Evaluation is conducted on the basis of principles discussed in Chapter 15∞ and focuses on the achievement of expected outcomes and the processes used to achieve those outcomes. For example, the occupational health nurse may evaluate the effectiveness of body mechanics education in decreasing the incidence of back injuries. At the individual level, evaluation might focus on the impact of no-smoking education on an individual employee's smoking behavior.

Selected aspects of occupational health and safety programs can also be evaluated using a set of 20 health and exposure surveillance indicators developed by the Council of State and Territorial Epidemiologists (n.d.). **Health indicators** are measures of health (injury or illness) or factors associated with health (exposures, hazards, or interventions) that allow comparisons over time and help guide priorities for prevention and intervention. The indicators are generally used at the state level to monitor occupational health statewide, but could be used in a particular occupational setting. Areas of focus include the demographic profile of the worker population; occupationally acquired illnesses, injuries, and related hospitalizations and days off work; workers' compensation claims; employment in high-risk occupations and industries; and federal or state OSHA inspections and their outcomes (Council of State and Territorial Epidemiologists, n.d.).

Achievement of national objectives related to occupational health can also be used to evaluate efforts in the local occupational setting or at regional, state, and national levels. The status of selected national objectives is summarized below.

Healthy People 2020

Selected Objectives Related to Occupational Health

OBJECTIVE	BASELINE (YEAR)	TARGET	CURRENT DATA (YEAR)	DATA SOURCES
ECBP-8. Increase the proportion of worksites with more than 50 employees that offer an employee health promotion program	Dev	Dev	Dev	National Survey of Employer-sponsored Health Plans, Mercer
ECBP-9. Increase the proportion of employees that participate in employer-sponsored health promotion activities	Dev	Dev	Dev	National Survey of Employer-sponsored Health Plans, Mercer
IID-15.3. Increase hepatitis B vaccine coverage among health care personnel	64.3% (2008)	90%	NDA	National Health Interview Survey (NCHS) CDC/NCHS
OSH-1.1. Reduce deaths from work-related injuries in all industries (per 100,000 workers)	4.0 (2007)	3.6	3.6 (2010)	Census of Fatal Occupational Injuries (CFOI), DOL/BLS, Current Population Survey (CPS) Census & DOL/BLS

Continued on next page

Healthy People 2020 (Continued)

OBJECTIVE	BASELINE (YEAR)	TARGET	CURRENT DATA (YEAR)	DATA SOURCES
OSH-2.1. Reduce work-related injuries in private sector industries resulting in medical treatment, lost work time, or restricted work activity, as reported by employers (per 100 full-time equivalent workers)	4.2 (2008)	3.8	3.5 (2010)	Survey of Occupational Injury and Illness (SOII), DOL/BLS
OSH-3. Reduce the rate of injury and illness due to over-exertion or repetitive motion (per 10,000 workers)	29.6 (2008)	26.6	NDA	SOII, DOL/BLS
OSH-5. Reduce deaths from work-related homicides (per 10,000 full-time equivalent workers	628 (2007)	565	518 (2010)	CFOI, DOL/BLS
OSH-6. Reduce work-related assault (per 10,000 full-time equivalent workers)	8.4 (2007)	7.6	10.4 (2009)	CPS, Census and DOL/BLS, National Electronic Injury Surveillance System—Work Supplement (NEISS-WORK), CDC/NIOSH, CPSC
OSH-7. Reduce the number of persons who have elevated blood lead levels from work exposures (per 100,000 employed adults)	22.5 (2008)	20.2	NDA	Adult Blood Lead Epidemiology and Surveillance Program (ABLES), DCD/NIOSH
OSH-8. Reduce occupational skin diseases or disorders among full-time workers (per 10,000 full-time workers)	4.4 (2008)	4.0	3.3 (2011)	SOII, DOL/BLS
OSH-9. Increase the proportion of employees with access to workplace programs that prevent or reduce stress	Dev	Dev	Dev	Quality of Worklife Module, CDC/NIOSH and NSF
OSH-10. Reduce new cases of work-related noise-induced hearing loss (per 10,000 workers)	2.2 (2008)	2	2.1 (2011)	SOII, DOL/BLS
TU-12. Increase the proportion of persons covered by indoor work policies that prohibit smoking	75.3% (2006–2007)	100%	NDA	CPS, Census and DOL/BLS
V-3.1. Reduce occupational eye injuries resulting in lost work days (per 10,000 full-time workers)	2.9 (2008)	2.6	NDA	SOII, DOL/BLS

NDA = No data available
Dev = A developmental objective for which data and targets have not yet been determined
Data from: U.S. Department of Health and Human Services. (2014). *Healthy people 2020 topics and objectives.* Retrieved from http://healthypeople.gov/2020/topicsobjectives2020/default.aspx

CHAPTER RECAP

Occupational settings contribute to a wide variety of health problems in individuals and in population groups, yet they also provide an ideal setting for influencing health-related behaviors and environmental conditions. Population health nurses employed in occupational settings can do much to promote the health of individual employees, work groups, and the general public.

Factors related to biological, psychological, environmental, sociocultural, behavioral, and health system determinants influence the health of working populations. Population health nurses working in occupational settings assess the positive and negative effects of these factors on the health of the employee population. They also plan, implement, and evaluate interventions to promote health, prevent illness, resolve existing health problems, and restore health and promote return to work in this population.

CASE STUDY Nursing in the Work Setting

You are a population health nurse employed by a large manufacturing plant. On Wednesday you see several employees complaining of abdominal cramping and diarrhea. They all state that their symptoms started at home during the night. You get word from one of the plant supervisors that several of her employees called in sick this morning because of similar symptoms. In checking with other departments, you find that there are a number of absences throughout the plant. Two of the older employees and one who you know has AIDS have been hospitalized with severe dehydration. All of the people with cramps and diarrhea eat regularly in the cafeteria.

1. What biological, psychological, environmental, sociocultural, behavioral, and health system factors are operating in this situation? What additional information would you want to gather?
2. What are your nursing diagnoses?
3. What outcome objectives do you hope to achieve through intervention?
4. What measures will you employ to resolve the identified problems? Why? What illness prevention measures might have prevented the occurrence of these problems? What health restoration measures are warranted to prevent the recurrence of problems or complications?
5. How will you evaluate the effectiveness of your interventions?

REFERENCES

American Association of Occupational Health Nurses. (2012a). *Code of ethics*. Retrieved from http://www.aaohn.org/component/content/article/12-practice/10-code-of-ethics.html

American Association of Occupational Health Nurses. (2012b). *Position statement: All-hazard preparedness: The occupational and environmental nurse role*. Retrieved from http://www.aaohn.org/practice/position-statements.html

American Association of Occupational Health Nurses. (2012c). *Position statement: Delivery of occupational and environmental services*. Retrieved from http://www.aaohn.org/practice/position-statements.html

American Association of Occupational Health Nurses. (2012d). *Position statement: Health and productivity: The occupational and environmental nurse role*. Retrieved from http://www.aaohn.org/practice/position-statements.html

American Association of Occupational Health Nurses. (2012e). *Standards of occupational and environmental nursing*. Retrieved from http://www.aaohn.org/practice/standards.html

American Association of Occupational Health Nurses. (2013). *Position statement: Preventing workplace violence: The occupational and environmental nurse role*. Retrieved from http://www.aaohn.org/practice/position-statements.html

American Board of Occupational Health Nurses. (2012). *History*. Retrieved from http://www.abohn.org/history.cfm

American Lung Association. (2014). *Second hand smoke*. Retrieved from http://www.lung.org/stop-smoking/about-smoking/health-effects/secondhand-smoke.html

American Psychological Association. (2014). *Ergonomics: The science for better living and working*. Retrieved from http://www.apa.org/about/gr/issues/workforce/ergonomics.aspx

Ball, S. W., Walker, D. K., Donahue, S. M. A., Izrael, D., Zhang, J., Euler, G. L., …, MacCannell, T. F. (2012). Influenza vaccination coverage among health-care personnel—2011-12 influenza season, United States. *Morbidity and Mortality Weekly Report, 61*, 753–757.

Bell, J. H. (1902). Anthrax: It's relation to the wool industry. In T. Oliver (Ed.), *Dangerous trades: The historical, social, and legal aspects of industrial occupations as affecting health, by a number of experts* (pp. 634–643). London: John Murray.

Bell, J. H. (2002). Anthrax and the wool trade. *American Journal of Public Health, 92,* 754–757.

Budin, W., C., Brewer, C. S., Chao, Y. Y., & Kovner, C. (2013). Verbal abuse from nurse colleagues and work environment of early career registered nurses. *Journal of Nursing Scholarship, 45,* 3-8-316. doi:10.1111/jnu.12033

Bureau of Labor Statistics. (2012a). *Census of fatal occupational injuries charts, 1992–2012.* Retrieved from http://www.bls.gov/iif/oshwc/cfoi/cfch0011.pdf

Bureau of Labor Statistics. (2012b). *Nonfatal occupational injuries and illnesses requiring days away from work, 2011.* Retrieved from http://www.bls.gov/news.release/pdf/osh2.pdf

Bureau of Labor Statistics. (2012c). *Volunteering in the United States, 2012.* Retrieved from http://www.bls.gov/news.release/volun.nr0.htm

Bureau of Labor Statistics. (2012d). *Workplace injuries and illnesses, 2011.* Retrieved from http://www.bls.gov/news.release/archives/osh_10252012.pdf

Bureau of Labor Statistics. (2013a). *Census of fatal occupational injuries, 2011.* Retrieved from http://www.bls.gov/iif/oshwc/cfoi/cfch0010.pdf

Bureau of Labor Statistics. (2013b). *Employment status of the civilian noninstitutional population by age, sex, and race.* Retrieved from http://www.bls.gov/cps/cpsaat03.pdf

Bureau of Labor Statistics. (2013c). *Table A-9. Selected employment indicators.* Retrieved from http://www.bls.gov/news.release/empsit.t09.htm

Bureau of Labor Statistics. (2013d). *National Compensation Survey: Employee benefits in the United States.* Retrieved from http://www.bls.gov/ncs/ebs/benefits/2013/ebbl0052.pdf

Bureau of Labor Statistics. (2014). *Revisions to the 2012 Census of Fatal Occupational Injuries (CFOI) counts.* Retrieved from http://www.bls.gov/iif/oshwc/cfoi/cfoi_revised12.pdf

California Governor's Office of Emergency Services. (2012). *Disaster service worker volunteer program.* Retrieved from http://www.calema.ca.gov/planningandpreparedness/pages/disaster-service-worker-volunteer-program.aspx

Centers for Disease Control and Prevention. (2012a). Campaign to prevent falls in construction—United States, 2012. *Morbidity and Mortality Weekly Report, 61,* 292.

Centers for Disease Control and Prevention. (2012b). Workers Memorial Day—April 28, 2012. *Morbidity and Mortality Weekly Report, 61,* 281.

Centers for Disease Control and Prevention. (2013a). *About NHWP.* Retrieved from http://www.cdc.gov/nationalhealthyworksite/about/index.html

Centers for Disease Control and Prevention. (2013b). National campaign to prevent falls in construction—United States, 2013. *Morbidity and Mortality Weekly Report, 62,* 317.

Centers for Disease Control and Prevention. (2013c). Workers' Memorial Day—April 28, 2013. *Morbidity and Mortality Weekly Report, 61,* 119–121.

Chester, D., Rosenman, K. D., Grimes, F., K., & Castillo, D. N. (2012). Fatal exposure to methylene chloride among bathtub refinishers—United States, 2000–2011. *Morbidity and Mortality Weekly Report, 62,* 301.

Cimiotti, J. P., Aiken, L. H., Sloane, D. M., & Wu, E. S. (2012). Nursing staff burnout and health care-associated infection. *American Journal of Infection Control, 40,* 486–490. doi:10.1016/j.ajic.2012.02.029

Committee to Assess Training Needs for Occupational Safety and Health Personnel in the United States, Board on Health Science Policy, Institute of Medicine. (2000). *Safe work in the 21st century: Education and training needs for the next decade's occupational safety and health personnel.* Retrieved from http://www.nap.edu/download.php?record_id=9835

Council of State and Territorial Epidemiologists. (n.d.). *Occupational health: Indicators.* Retrieved from http://www.cste.org/group/OHIndicators

Demir, D., & Rodwell, J. (2012). Psychosocial antecedents and consequences of workplace aggression for hospital nurses. *Journal of Nursing Scholarship, 44,* 376–384. doi:10.1111/j.1547-5069.2012.01472.x

Farmworker Justice. (2014). *Pesticide safety.* Retrieved from http://www.farmworkerjustice.org/content/pesticide-safety

Feldman, J. (2011). *OSHA inaction: Onerous requirements imposed on OSHA prevent the agency from issuing lifesaving rules.* Retrieved from http://www.citizen.org/documents/osha-inaction.pdf

Franco, G. (2012). Bernardino Ramazzini and women workers' health in the second half of the XVIIth century. *Journal of Public Health, 34,* 305–308. doi:10.1093/pubmed/fds029

Fujishiro, K., Gee, G. C., & de Castro, A. B. (2011). Associations of workplace aggression with work-related well-being among nurses in the Philippines. *American Journal of Public Health, 101,* 861–867. doi:10.2105/AJPH.2009.188144

Garrett, B. E., Dube, S. R., Trosclair, A., Caraballo, R. S., & Pechacek, T. E. (2011, January 14). Cigarette smoking = United States, 2003–2007. *Morbidity and Mortality Weekly Report, 60*(Suppl.), 109–113

Greenhaus, J. H., & Allen, T. D. (2011). Work-family balance: A review and extension of the literature. In J. C. Quick & L. E. Tetrick (Eds.), *Handbook of occupational psychology* (2nd ed., pp. 165–183). Washington, DC: American Psychological Association.

Greenwald, M. R., Tak, S., & Masterson, E. (2011). Severe hearing impairment among military veterans—United States, 2010. *Morbidity and Mortality Weekly Report, 61,* 753–757.

Gunter, M. M., Hill, R., O'Connor, M. B., Retzer, K. D., & Lincoln, J. M. (2013). Fatal injuries in offshore oil and gas operations—United States, 2003–2010. *Morbidity and Mortality Weekly Report, 60,* 955–958.

Hamilton, A. (2001). The health of immigrants. *American Journal of Public Health, 91,* 1765–1767. (Reprinted from *Exploring the dangerous trades: The autobiography of Alice Hamilton, MD,* by A. Hamilton, 1943, Boston: Little, Brown.)

Henry J. Kaiser Family Foundation. (2013). *Percent of private sector establishments that offer health insurance to employees.* Retrieved from http://kff.org/other/state-indicator/percent-of-firms-offering-coverage/

Hogstedt, C., Jansson, C., Hugosson, M., Tinnerberg, H., & Gustavsson, P. (2013). Cancer incidence in a cohort of Swedish chimney sweeps, 1958–2006. *American Journal of Public Health, 103,* 1708–1714. doi:10.2105/AJPH.2012.300860

Huff, S., Stocks, J. M., Saito, R., Bilhartz, P., Levin, J., Glazer, C., …, McCague, A.-B. (2013). Obliterative bronchiolitis in workers in a coffee-processing facility—Texas, 2008–2012. *Morbidity and Mortality Weekly Report, 62,* 305–307.

Hughes, S. L., Seymour, R. B., Campbell, R. T., Shaw, J. W., Fabiyi, C., & Sokas, R. (2011). Comparison of two health-promotion programs for older workers. *American Journal of Public Health, 101,* 883–890. doi:10.2105/AJPH.2010.300082

International Ergonomics Association. (2014). *Definition of ergonomics.* Retrieved from http://www.iea.cc/whats/index.html

Jewish Women's Archive. (n.d.). *Factory reform: Lillian Wald, 1867–1940.* Retrieved from http://jwa.org/womenofvalor/wald/factory-reform

Jewish Women's Archive. (2010). *History makers—Lillian Wald—Women's Trade Union League.* Retrieved from http://jwa.org/historymakers/wald/Womens-trade-union-league

Job Accommodation Network, Office of Disability Employment Policy, U.S. Department of Labor. (n.d.). *Frequently asked questions.* Retrieved from http://askjan.org/links/faqs.htm

Kaiser Family Foundation & Health Research & Educational Trust. (2012). *Employer health benefits: 2012 summary of findings*. Retrieved from http://kaiserfamilyfoundation.files.wordpress.com/2013/03/8346-employer-health-benefits-annual-survey-summary-of-findings-0912.pdf

Kelsey, K., Roisman, R., Kruetzer, R., Materna, B., Duncan, A., Orr, M., ..., Choudry, E. (2011). Chlorine gas exposure at a metal recycling facility—California, 2010. *Morbidity and Mortality Weekly Report, 60,* 951–954.

Kimura, A. C., Nguyen, C. N., Higa, J. I., Hurwitz, E. L., & Vugia, D. J. (2007). The effectiveness of Vaccine Day and educational interventions on influenza vaccine coverage among health care workers at long-term care facilities. *American Journal of Public Health, 97,* 684–690. doi:10.2105/AJPH.2005.082073

Kumar, S., Grefenstette, J. J., Galloway, D., Albert, S. M., & Burke, D. S. (2013). Policies to reduce influenza in the workplace: Impact assessments using an agent-based model. *American Journal of Public Health, 103,* 1406–1411. doi:10.2105/AJPH.2013.301269

Laney, A. S., Wolfe, A. L., Petsonk, E. L., & Halldin, C. N. (2012). Pneumoconiosis and advanced occupational lung disease among surface coal miners—16 states, 2010–2011. *Morbidity and Mortality Weekly Report, 61,* 431–434.

Lewis, J. J. (n.d.). *Women's Trade Union League—WTUL.* Retrieved from http://womenshistory.about.com/od/worklaborunions/a/wtul.htm.

Luckhaupt, S. E. (2012). Short sleep duration among workers—United States, 2010. *Morbidity and Mortality Weekly Report, 61,* 381–385.

Lundberg, U., & Cooper, C. L. (2011). *The science of occupational health: Stress, psychobiology and the new world of work.* Ames, IA: Wiley-Blackwell.

Magnavita, N., & Heponiemi, T. (2011). Workplace violence against nursing students and nurses: An Italian experience. *Journal of Nursing Scholarship, 43,* 203–210. doi:10.1111/j.1547-5069.2011.01392.x

Marrett, L. D., Pichora, E., & Costa, M. L. (2010). Work-time sun behaviours among Canadian outdoor workers: Results from the 2006 National Sun Survey. *Canadian Journal of Public Health, 101,* 119–122.

Marucci-Wellman, H., Leamon, T. B., Willetts, J. L., Binh, T. T., Diep, N. B., & Wegman, D. H. (2011). Occupational injuries in a commune in rural Vietnam transitioning from agriculture to new industries. *American Journal of Public Health, 101,* 854–860. doi:10.2105/AJPH.2010.300019

Materna, B., Harriman, K., Rosenberg, J., Shusterman, D., Windham, G., Atwell, J., ..., Zipprich, J. (2010). *Morbidity and Mortality Weekly Report, 59,* 1480–1483.

Murray, L. R. (2011, April 20). Now is the time to strengthen our occupational health protections. *The Nation's Health,* p. 3.

Murtagh, L., & Moulton, A. D. (2011). Working mothers, breastfeeding, and the law. *American Journal of Public Health, 101,* 217–223. doi:10.2105/AJPH.2009.185280

National Center for Health Statistics. (2011). Percentage of employed adults aged 18-64 years who had carpal tunnel syndrome in the past 12 months, by sex and age group—National Health Interview Survey, 2010. *Morbidity and Mortality Weekly Report, 60,* 1680.

National Center for Health Statistics. (2014). *Health, United States, 2013: With special feature on prescription drugs.* Retrieved from http://www.cdc.gov/nchs/data/hus/hus13.pdf

National Conference of State Legislatures. (2013). *2013 enacted workers compensation legislation.* Retrieved from http://www.ncsl.org/research/labor-and-employment/2013-enacted-workers-compensation-legislation.aspx

National Institute of Neurological Disorders and Stroke. (2012). *Carpal tunnel syndrome.* Retrieved from http://www.ninds.nih.gov/disorders/carpal_tunnel/carpel_tunnel_FS.pdf

National Institute for Occupational Safety and Health. (2013a). *About NIOSH.* Retrieved from http://www.cdc.gov/niosh/about.html

National Institute for Occupational Safety and Health. (2013b). NIOSH course for nurses on workplace violence. *Morbidity and Mortality Weekly Report, 62,* 705.

Nelson, C. C., Li, Y., Sorenson, G., & Berkman, L. F. (2012). Assessing the relationship between work-family conflict and smoking. *American Journal of Public Health, 102,* 1767–1772. doi:10.2105/AJPH.2011.300413

Nyberg, S. T., Fransson, E. I., Heikkila, K., Alfredsson, L., Casini, A., Clays, E., ... IPD Work Consortium. (2013). Job strain and cardiovascular disease risk factors: Meta-analysis of individual-participant data from 47,000 men and women. *PLoS One, 8*(6), e67323. doi:10.1371/journal.pone.0067323

Occupational Safety and Health Administration. (n.d.a). *Ergonomics.* Retrieved from https://www.osha.gov/SLTC/ergonomics/

Occupational Safety and Health Administration. (n.d.b). *Nursing in occupational health.* Retrieved from https://www.osha.gov/dts/oohn/ohn.html

Occupational Safety and Health Administration. (n.d.c). *OSHA—We can help.* Retrieved from https://www.osha.gov/workers.html#3

Occupational Safety and Health Administration. (2004). *Workplace violence: Guidelines for preventing workplace violence for health care & social service workers.* Retrieved from https://www.osha.gov/Publications/osha3148.pdf

Occupational Safety and Health Administration. (2011). *At-a-glance: OSHA.* Retrieved from https://www.osha.gov/Publications/3439at-a-glance.pdf

Office of Disability Employment Policy. (2014). *Youth employment rate.* Retrieved from http://www.dol.gov/odep/categories/youth/youthemployment.htm

Okechukwu, C. A., Ayadi, A. M., Tamers, S. L., Sabbath, E. L., & Berkman, L. (2012). Household food insufficiency, financial strain, work-family spill-over, and depressive symptoms in the working class: The Work, Family, and Health Network Study. *American Journal of Public Health, 102,* 126–133. doi:10.2105/AJPH.2011.300323

O'Malley, M. A., Fong, H., Mehler, L., Farnsworth, G., Edmiston, S., Schneider, F., ..., Calver, G. M. (2011). Illness associated with exposure to methyl bromide—Fumigated produce—California, 2010. *Morbidity and Mortality Weekly Report, 60,* 913–927.

Ontario Ministry of Labour. (2013). *Information for volunteers.* Retrieved from http://www.worksmartontario.gov.on.ca/scripts/default.asp?contentID=6-1-1&

Organisation for Economic Cooperation and Development. (2011). *Sick on the job? Myths and realities about mental health and work.* Retrieved from http://www.oecd.org/els/emp/49227343.pdf

Ottenberg, A. L., Wu, J. T., Poland, G. A., Jacobson, R. M., Koenig, B. A., & Tilburt, J. C. (2011). Vaccinating health care workers against influenza: The ethical and legal rationale for a mandate. *American Journal of Public Health, 101,* 212–216. doi:10.2105/AJPH.20009.190751

Palmer, K. T., & Brown, I. (2013). A general framework for assessing fitness for work. In K. T. Palmer, I. Brown, & J. Hobson (Eds.), *Fitness for work: The medical aspects* (5th ed., Chapter 1). Oxford, UK: Oxford University Press.

Pratt, S. G., & Rodriguez-Acosta, R. L. (2013). Occupational highway transportation deaths among workers aged >55 years—United States, 2003–2010. *Morbidity and Mortality Weekly Report, 62,* 653–657.

Quach, T., Gunier, R., Tran, A., Von Behren, V., Doan-Billings, P.-A., Nguyen, K.-D., ..., Reynolds, P. (2011). Characterizing workplace exposures in Vietnamese women working in California nail salons. *American Journal of Public Health, 101,* S271–S276. doi:10.2105/AJPH.2010.300099

Ritger, K., Black, S., Weaver, K., Jones, J., Gerber, S., Conover, C., ..., Medina-Marino, A. (2011). Fatal laboratory-acquired infection with an attenuated *Yersinia pestis* strain—Chicago, Illinois, 2009. *Morbidity and Mortality Weekly Report, 60,* 201–205.

Roy, D. R. (2013). Consulting in occupational health nursing. *Workplace Health and Safety, 61*(1), 43–49. doi:10.3928/21650799-20121217-27

Rutkow, L., Vernick, J. S., Tung, G. J., & Cohen, J. E. (2013). Creating smoke-free places through the UN Convention on the Rights of Persons with Disabilities. *American Journal of Public Health, 103,* 1748–1753. doi:10.2105/AJPH.2012.301174

Safe Work Australia. (n.d.). *Volunteers: The essential guide to work health and safety for volunteers.* Retrieved from http://www.safeworkaustralia.gov.au/sites/SWA/model-whs-laws/guidance/volunteers/Documents/Volunteers_Guide.pdf

Schulte, P. A., Pandalai, S., Wulsin, V., & Chun, H. (2012). Interaction of occupational and personal risk factors in workforce health and safety. *American Journal of Public Health, 102,* 434–448. doi:10.2105/AJPH.2011.300249

Schwartz, A., Walker, R., Sievert, J., Calvert, G. M., & Tsai, R. J. (2012). Occupational phosphine gas poisoning at veterinary hospitals from dogs that ingested zinc phosphide—Michigan, Iowa, and Washington, 2006–2011. *Morbidity and Mortality Weekly Report, 61,* 286–288.

Shefer, A., Atkinson, W., Friedman, C., Kuhar, D. T., Mootrey, G., Bialck, S. R., ..., Wallace, G. (2011). Immunization of health-care personnel: Recommendations of the Advisory Committee on Immunization Practices. *Morbidity and Mortality Weekly Report, 60*(RR7), 1–44.

Slan-Jerusalem, R., & Chen, C. P. (2009). Work-family conflict and career development theories: A search for helping strategies. *Journal of Counseling and Development, 87,* 492–499.

Smith, C. S., Folkard, S., Tucker, P., & Evans, M. S. (2011). Work schedules, health, and safety. In J. C. Quick & L. E. Tetrick (Eds.), *Handbook of occupational psychology* (2nd ed., pp. 185–204). Washington, DC: American Psychological Association.

Smith, K., E., Danila, R., Scheftel, J., Fowler, H., Westbrook, A., Dobbins, G., et al. (2013). Occupationally acquired salmonella I 4, 12:i:1,2 infection in a phlebotomist—Minnesota, January, 2013. *Morbidity and Mortality Weekly Report, 62,* 525.

Smith, P. M., & Bielecky, A. (2012). The impact of changes in job strain and its components on the risk of depression. *American Journal of Public Health, 102,* 352–358. doi:10.2105/AJPH.2011.300376

Sorenson, G., Landsbergis, P., Hammer, L., Amick, B. C., Linnan, L., Yancey, A., ..., The Workshop Working Group on Worksite Chronic Disease Prevention. (2011). Preventing chronic disease in the workplace: A workshop report and recommendations. *American Journal of Public Health, 101,* S196–S207. doi:10.2105/AJPH.2010.300075

Stansfeld, S. A., Shipley, M. J., Head, J., & Fuhrer, R. (2012). Repeated job strain and the risk of depression: Longitudinal analysis from the Whitehall II study. *American Journal of Public Health, 102,* 2360–2366. doi:10.2105/AJPH.2011.300589

Tarawneh, I., Lampl, M., Robins, D., Wurzelbacher, S., Bertke, S., Bell, J., & Meyers, A. (2013). Workers' compensation claims for musculoskeletal disorders among wholesale and retail trade industry workers—Ohio, 2005–2009. *Morbidity and Mortality Weekly Report, 62,* 437–442.

Thomas, C. M., & Siela, D. (2011). The impaired nurse. *American Nurse Today, 6*(8). Retrieved from http://www.medscape.com/viewarticle/748598_print

Toblin, R. L., Clark-Walper, C., Kok, B. C., Sipos, M. L., & Thomas, J. L. (2012). Energy drink consumption and its association with sleep problems among U.S. service members on a combat deployment—Afghanistan, 2010. *Morbidity and Mortality Weekly Report, 61,* 895–898.

Toosi, M. (2012, January). Employment outlook: 2010-2020, Labor force projections to 2020: A more slowly growing workforce. *Monthly Labor Review,* 43–64.

Tyman, M., Babb, S., MacNeil, A., & Griffin, M. (2011). State smoke-free laws for worksites, restaurants, and bars—United States, 2000–2010. *Morbidity and Mortality Weekly Report, 60,* 472–475.

United Nations. (2006). *Convention on the rights of persons with disabilities.* Retrieved from http://www.un.org/disabilities/convention/conventionfull.shtml

United Nations. (2013). *CRPD and optional protocol signatures and ratifications.* Retrieved from http://www.un.org/disabilities/documents/maps/enablemap.jpg

U.S. Census Bureau. (2012a). *Statistical Abstract of the United States 2012. Table 607. Type of work flexibility provided to employees: 2008.* Retrieved from http://www.census.gov/compendia/statab/2012/tables/12s0607.pdf

U.S. Census Bureau. (2012b). *Statistical Abstract of the United States 2012. Table 620. Employment by industry: 2000 to 2010.* Retrieved from http://www.census.gov/compendia/statab/2012/tables/12s0620.pdf

U.S. Department of Defense, Computer/Electronic Accommodation Program. (n.d.). *Workplace ergonomics reference guide* (2nd ed.). Retrieved from http://cap.mil/Documents/CAP_Ergo_Guide.pdf

U.S. Department of Health and Human Services. (2014). *Healthy people 2020 topics and objectives.* Retrieved from http://healthypeople.gov/2020/topicsobjectives2020/default.aspx

U.S. Department of Justice, Civil Rights Division. (n.d.). *Introduction to the ADA.* Retrieved from http://www.ada.gov/ada_intro.htm

U.S. Department of Labor. (n.d.a). *Chapter 1: Start-up of the Department and World War I, 1913–1921.* Retrieved from http://www.dol.gov/oasam/programs/history/dolchp01.htm

U.S. Department of Labor. (n.d.b). *Workers' compensation.* Retrieved from http://www.dol.gov/dol/topic/workcomp/

U.S. Department of Labor. (2012). *Fact sheet: The Affordable Care Act and wellness programs.* Retrieved from http://www.dol.gov/ebsa/pdf/fswellnessprogram.pdf

Voigt, K. (2012). Nonsmoker and "nonnicotine" hiring policies: The implications of employment restrictions for tobacco control. *American Journal of Public Health, 102,* 2013–2018. doi:10.2105/AJPH.2012.300745

Wharton, A. S. (2009). The sociology of emotional labor. *Annual Review of Sociology, 35,* 147–165. doi:10.1146/annurev-soc-070308-115944

Wuellner, S. E., Walters, J. K., St. Louis, T., Leinenkugel, K., Rogers, P. F., Lefkowitz, D., ..., Castillo, D. N. (2011). Nonfatal occupational injuries and illness among older workers—United States, 2009. *Morbidity and Mortality Weekly Report, 60,* 503–510.

Yap, T. L., Davis, L. S., Gates, D. M., Hemmings, A. B., & Pan, W. (2009a). The effect of tailored e-mails in the workplace: Part 1. Stage movement toward increased physical activity levels. *AAOHN Journal, 57,* 267–273. doi:10.3928/08910162-20090617-02

Yap, T. L., Davis, L. S., Gates, D. M., Hemmings, A. B., & Pan, W. (2009b). The effect of tailored e-mails in the workplace: Part II. Increasing overall physical activity levels. *AAOHN Journal, 57,* 313–319. doi:10.3928/08910162-20090716-01

Yap, T. L., & James, D. M. B. (2010). Tailored e-mails in the workplace: A focus group analysis. *AAOHN Journal, 58,* 425–432. doi:10.3928/08910162-20100928-05

Zeller, A., Dassen, T., Kok, G., Needham, I., & Halfens, R. J. G. (2012). Factors associated with resident aggression toward caregivers in nursing homes. *Journal of Nursing Scholarship, 44,* 249–257. doi:10.1111/j.1547-5069.2012.01459.x

Zellers, L., & Graff, S. K., Tobacco Control Legal Consortium. (2008). *Workplace smoking: Options for employees and legal risks for employers.* Retrieved from http://ucanr.edu/sites/tobaccofree/files/175147.pdf

CHAPTER

24 Care of Correctional Populations

Learning Outcomes

After reading this chapter, you should be able to:

1. Discuss the impetus for providing health care in correctional settings.
2. Differentiate between basic and advanced nursing practice in correctional settings.
3. Describe biological, psychological, environmental, sociocultural, behavioral, and health system factors that influence health in correctional settings.
4. Identify major aspects of health promotion in correctional settings and analyze the role of the population health nurse in each.
5. Describe major foci in illness and injury prevention in correctional settings and related population health nursing strategies.
6. Describe approaches to resolving existing health problems in correctional settings and analyze population health nursing roles with respect to each.
7. Discuss considerations in health restoration in correctional settings and analyze related population health nursing roles.

Key Terms

assisted outpatient treatment (AOT)
compassionate release
correctional nursing
crisis intervention teams (CITs)
detainees
diversion
forensic nursing
jails
juvenile detention facilities
lockdown
lockup
parolee
prisons
probationer
recidivism
reentry
search and seizure
self-injurious behavior
status offenses
TB prophylaxis

Advocacy Then

Misguided Reform

As we will see in Chapter 29∞, Dorothea Dix was highly successful in initiating prison reform, but her efforts were primarily directed toward removing the mentally ill from jails and prisons and providing them with treatment facilities. In so doing, she also improved some conditions in jails and prisons throughout several states (*Prison and asylum reform, n.d.*). Unfortunately, other attempts at advocacy and reform may have done more harm than good.

In 1787, Philadelphia citizens formed the Philadelphia Society for Alleviating the Miseries of Public Prisons in response to appalling conditions in the local jail. The group investigated prison conditions and presented their findings to the Pennsylvania legislature recommending solitary confinement and hard physical labor as an alternative to previous severe physical punishments such as whipping, hanging, and pillorying (being locked in wooden stocks and subjected to public ridicule). Following passage of the legislation, Pennsylvania established "model" prisons in which inmates were confined to individual cells in a model later known as the "Pennsylvania system." The system called for the complete separation of inmates for their entire sentence to decrease the potential for exposure to bad companions. Each cell, which inmates rarely left, included space for a work area in which the inmate worked at contract labor, a private exercise yard, central heating, a flush toilet, and shower bath. Inmates were fed and worked in their cells and received some vocational instruction. The Auburn system, instituted at the Auburn Penitentiary in New York, was similar except that inmates were fed and worked communally in strict silence during the day and returned to their individual cells as night. Both systems were widely emulated in the United States and Europe. An extensive rash of suicides in the Auburn Penitentiary, however, called attention to the deleterious psychological consequences of "solitary confinement" and these practices were abandoned except for punishment of uncontrolled and recalcitrant inmates. Society members in Philadelphia and a similar organization in Boston, the Prison Discipline Society, did, however, continue to visit prisons, providing independent oversight and perhaps ameliorating some of the more common abuses of prisoners and assuring provision of basic necessities (Johnston, n.d.; Morse, 2007).

Advocacy Now

Incorporating Health into a Public Defender's Office

Recent arrestees often have health issues that have been neglected over significant periods of time. If incarcerated, these needs will be attended to at some point, but many arrestees are freed until their trials. At that point, matters dealing with their court date may make health care a low priority. They are often tied up with multiple appointments with public defenders planning for their trials (Venters et al., 2008).

A collaborative effort between medical residents at Montefiore Medical Center and a public defender's office in a low-income area of New York City was initiated. Originally, social workers at the defender's office made referrals to medical residents at a local community clinic, but few clients accepted referrals, and none of them kept their appointments. As a result, a resident was stationed at the public defender's office on specific days. The resident saw clients at the time of their appointment at the defender's office if he was available and ascertained health care needs. Some encounters addressed questions and others led to appointments at the community clinic. Because of their level of comfort with the defender's office, clients often came there prior to their appointments and were walked to the clinic by staff. Kept appointment rates increased to 66%, higher than the usual rate for the clinic (Venters et al., 2008).

Challenges to the program lay in the limited time the resident was available in the defender's office and a backlog for clinic appointments, so future plans include possible provision of health care services on site in the defender's office (Venters et al., 2008).

The concept of prisons as a place to contain wrongdoers began as early as the 1600s with workhouses that were used to punish people who violated the law. Unfortunately, workhouses were also used to confine family members who were likely to impugn the family's honor through their activities, whether or not those activities were actually criminal in nature (Fagan, 2003). As we saw in Chapter 21∞, criminalization still occurs within populations that society would prefer to ignore, such as the homeless.

Correctional populations may be particularly vulnerable to a variety of health problems. In many instances, members of this population have not had access to effective health care services. In other cases, they have not seen health as a priority and frequently do not engage in practices that are conducive to good health. In addition, drug and alcohol use, which may result in incarceration, have both physical and psychological consequences for health. Incarceration, in and of itself, may have adverse health consequences.

Correctional facilities provide a relatively new practice setting for population health nursing compared to the settings discussed in previous chapters. Correctional nursing, however, is congruent with the primary focus of population health nursing—the health of groups of people and the general public. Correctional nursing frequently involves challenges not encountered in other population health nursing settings. Practice in a correctional setting requires autonomy and excellent assessment skills. Nurses are often responsible for triaging inmates during entry or sick call and identifying those who need to be seen by physicians, nurse practitioners, or other providers. Nurses may also provide routine treatments, including medication, under agency protocols. Nursing in correctional settings operates within the constraints of the security system, which may contribute to increased job stress and frustration. Another source of stress is the fear of litigation by a population that is prone to threats of litigation. Although there is some risk to the nurse's physical safety, many correctional nurses feel safer than they would in other settings such as emergency departments.

Another source of stress in the correctional setting is the potential for conflict between nursing values and those of corrections personnel. Differences in values frequently give rise to the need for population health nursing advocacy in correctional settings to ensure that health care needs are balanced with custodial and security needs. For example, the primary concerns of the nurse are health care and meeting the health needs of inmates. For custodial personnel, however, the primary concern must be security. The priority placed on security may often make it difficult for the nurse to meet inmates' needs. For instance, giving medications such as insulin in a timely fashion may be impeded by security measures like lockdowns, when nurses are not ordinarily allowed into the areas where inmates are housed. Similarly, nurses may be asked to share information obtained while taking a health history (e.g., past drug use) with custodial or law enforcement personnel, when confidentiality and privacy are primary values of the nursing profession.

Correctional nursing takes place in three general types of facilities: prisons, jails, and juvenile detention facilities. **Prisons** are state and federal facilities that house persons convicted of crimes, usually those sentenced for longer than 1 year. Municipal or county facilities are usually called **jails** and house both convicted inmates and detainees. Convicted inmates in jails are usually serving sentences under a year in length (Lee et al., 2012). **Detainees** are people who have not yet been convicted of a crime. They are being detained pending a trial either because they cannot pay the set bail or because no bail has been set. They may also have violated the terms of probation or parole. **Juvenile detention facilities** house children and adolescents convicted of crimes and those who are awaiting trial but who cannot be released in the custody of a responsible adult. Jails and juvenile detention facilities tend to be smaller and house fewer inmates than prisons.

Whatever the size of the facility or the terminology used, nurses working in correctional facilities must be committed to the belief that inmates retain their individual rights as human beings despite incarceration and that they have the same rights to health care as any other individual. Society does not categorically deprive any other group of individuals of access to adequate health care. In fact, there are carefully monitored standards of health care in such institutions as nursing homes, mental health facilities, and orphanages. It has only been as recently as 1979, however, that a program for accrediting health services in prisons was developed by the American Medical Association. Development of accreditation standards occurred at the request of the U.S. Department of Justice following a landmark court decision that depriving inmates of access to health care violated their civil rights (Rold, 2011). Only since 1985 have published standards for nursing practice in such settings been available (American Nurses Association [ANA], 1985).

The Correctional Population

Crime is a fact of life in modern-day society. In 2009, for example, 10.6 million crimes were committed in the United States for a crime rate of 3,466 for every 100,000 population. Violent crime (murder, rape, robbery, and aggravated assault) accounted for 1.3 million of these incidents and property crimes (burglary, theft, and automobile theft) for another 9.3 million (U.S. Census Bureau, 2013b). Homicide rates decreased by almost half from 10.2 per 100,000 population in 1980 to 5.4 per 100,000 in 2009 (U.S. Census Bureau, 2013d). In 2009, however, murders still claimed the lives of 13,756 people, more than 2,000 of them in the commission of a felony. More than 700 of those murders were the result of juvenile gang killings (U.S. Census Bureau, 2013c).

Globally, 9.8 million people were incarcerated in 2008 with a median incarceration rate of 145 inmates per 100,000 population (Zlodre & Fazel, 2012). The U.S. incarceration rate for 2009 was 250 per 100,000 population, the highest of any country (U.S. Census Bureau, 2013j). On any given day in 2009, more than 2.3 million people were housed in U.S. correctional institutions, but as many as 10 million people may pass through the local, state, and federal correctional systems each year (Lee et al., 2012). More than 11 million people were arrested in the United States in 2009, and more than 2.1 million people were held in U.S. adult correctional facilities (U.S. Census Bureau, 2013a, 2013e). Federal and state prisons held 1.6 million people, 89% of whom were housed in state facilities (U.S. Census Bureau, 2013h). Another 4.2 million persons were on probation, and 819,308 on parole. Overall, 7.12 million people in the United States (3.1% of the population) were under some form of correctional supervision (U.S. Census Bureau, 2013i).

City and county jails account for an even larger number of incarcerated individuals. For example, from June 2010 to June 2011, the average daily census in U.S. jails was 735,000, and the total jail population for the year was 11.8 million people (Smith et al., 2013). The Los Angeles County jail alone houses a population of 20,000 on any given day, with 400 to 600 admissions daily and 180,000 people over the course of a year (Malek et al., 2011). Similarly, the New York City jail reports a daily census of 13,000 people, with approximately 90,000 admissions per year (Ludwig, Cohen, Parsons, & Venters, 2012).

Incarceration rates have increased dramatically in the United States. From 1980 to 2004, for example, the number of people incarcerated in the United States quadrupled. Despite increases in bed capacity, many jails and prisons are operating far over capacity. For example, California prisons had been operating at 200% of capacity for several years when the Supreme Court mandated the release of large numbers of inmates due to the system's inability to effectively meet their needs (Rold, 2011).

There are several reasons for this marked increase in correctional populations. First, there have been significant changes in sentencing guidelines, such as "truth in sentencing" and "three strikes" laws. Truth in sentencing refers to legislation mandating that persons convicted of a crime serve a minimum percentage of their sentence before being eligible for parole (Polk, 2011). Three strikes laws mandate life imprisonment for defendants with two prior convictions for serious or violent crimes. In effect, most such laws are often applied to sentencing for nonviolent crimes as well (Stanford Law School, 2013). As a result, the United States now has the dubious distinction of having the highest rate of incarceration in the developed world (Zlodre & Fazel, 2012).

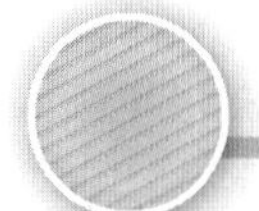

Global Perspectives

Conditions of Incarceration

Although conditions in U.S. jails and prisons are not ideal, for large portions of more than 10 million people incarcerated throughout the world, conditions may be significantly worse. A recent report by the U.S. Department of State (2012) indicated three main areas of concern in international prison conditions: unsafe conditions, mistreatment of prisoners, and inadequate legal protection. Unsafe conditions include overcrowding, unsanitary conditions, barriers to basic hygiene, malnutrition, contaminated water, and poor quality health care. In some parts of the world, correctional facilities are two to five times over capacity, to the extent that inmates in some facilities must sleep in shifts. Elsewhere, irregular facilities such as unventilated shipping containers, basements, or open-air holding facilities are used to house inmates. Much of the overcrowding and other safety issues stem from large numbers of pretrial detainees who in some places may be held for months to years before being tried.

Abuse of prisoners is another common concern. Abuse most commonly occurs among pretrial detainees in attempts to elicit confessions and among political prisoners and prisoners of conscience (persons who voice beliefs contrary to those of people in power). Abuse may also be used to control or punish inmates. Inadequate legal protection may involve incarceration for indefinite periods without conviction, prohibition of access to legal counsel or family members, or secret trials. Other areas of concern include arbitrary or discriminatory criteria for evidence and judicial corruption. Convicted inmates may also be denied their rights during incarceration.

The United Nations Office on Drugs and Crime (UNODC) has developed a set of international standards and norms for prisons that have been used by more than 100 countries in the development of their criminal justice policies (UNODC, 2013). General standards address such issues as nondiscrimination and religious tolerance, inmate registration and valid confinement orders, physical environmental conditions, sanitation and hygiene facilities, suitable clothing and bedding, adequate nutrition and exercise, adequate medical care, family communication, custody of personal property, and notification to family members of an inmate's death, illness, or transfer. The standards also address the need to separate male from female inmates, youth from adults, pretrial detainees from convicted inmates, and those accused of civil or political offenses from those accused of criminal offenses. Finally, the standards address appropriate discipline and use of restraints only to prevent escape during transfer or to protect the inmate or others from harm and never for punishment (UNODC, 2006). For further information about the standards, see the *External Resources* section of the student resources site.

The Need for Correctional Health Services

Health care in correctional facilities is an appropriate endeavor for several reasons. First, the right to adequate health care is a constitutionally recognized right. In 1976, a Supreme Court decision in *Estelle vs Gamble* ruled that neglect of serious medical needs constitutes "cruel and unusual punishment" and violates the Eighth Amendment to the U.S. Constitution (Smith et al., 2013). Similarly, failure to provide needed health services constitutes deliberate indifference under the Fifth Amendment and violates civil rights protected by the Fourteenth Amendment (Muse, 2011).

In addition to the constitutional right to health care, correctional care is good common sense for a variety of other reasons. Because of poverty, lower education levels, and unhealthy lifestyles that frequently involve substance abuse, inmates may enter a correctional facility with significant health problems (Spaulding et al., 2010). Because many of these individuals cannot afford to pay for care on the outside, the cost of care will be borne by society. Societal costs for this care will be lower if interventions occur in a timely fashion, before health problems become severe. Provision of care within the correctional facility also saves taxpayers the cost of personnel and vehicles to transport inmates to other health care facilities. Health promotion and illness and injury prevention in correctional settings are also cost-effective.

Another possible societal cost of failure to provide adequate health care to inmates lies in the potential for the spread of communicable disease from correctional facilities to the community (Malek et al., 2011). Environmental conditions and behaviors within correctional facilities lend themselves to the transmission of communicable diseases such as tuberculosis, HIV, and hepatitis. When inmates are released back into society, they may constitute a source of infection for the rest of the population.

Finally, correctional settings have been described as unhealthy environments in and of themselves and may give rise to a variety of health problems. Correctional environments limit inmate autonomy; promote social isolation and communicable diseases; limit exercise; and foster boredom, stress, hostility, and depression. Services are needed to deal with these effects of incarceration as well as the myriad health problems inmates bring with them to correctional settings.

Population Health Nursing and Correctional Health

Population health nurses working in correctional settings employ the nursing process to design interventions to meet identified health needs. Care begins with an assessment of needs that informs the planning and implementation of interventions to address those needs. Finally, population health nurses evaluate the effectiveness of care in meeting the identified needs.

Assessing the Health Status of Correctional Populations

Factors related to each of the six categories of determinants of health influence the health status of inmates and staff in correctional settings. The nurse assesses biological, psychological, environmental, sociocultural, behavioral, and health system determinants of health to identify health problems and the factors contributing to them and to direct interventions to resolve those problems.

BIOLOGICAL DETERMINANTS. Biological determinants affecting health in correctional populations include age, gender, and race; mortality; infectious and chronic conditions, injury, and other conditions. The nurse in the correctional setting assesses individual clients for existing physical health problems as well as identifying problems that have a high incidence and prevalence in the overall institutional population.

Age, gender, and race/ethnicity. Correctional populations vary greatly in their composition. There are growing numbers of youth and the elderly in U.S. correctional facilities. In 2009, for example, 1.5 million arrests were made among people under 18 years of age and more than 7,000 juveniles were housed in jails throughout the country; a threefold increase from 1990 (U.S. Census Bureau, 2013e, 2013j). In fact, there are now more youth involved in the juvenile justice system than in foster care (Smith et al., 2013). In 2009, 0.5% of the population in correctional settings was 15 to 17 years of age (U.S. Census Bureau, 2013a).

Juvenile inmates tend to have higher prevalence rates of a variety of physical and mental health conditions than their counterparts in the general population and usually have less access to care prior to incarceration. Based on data from the Northwest Juvenile Project, a long-term follow-up study of juveniles in Cook County, Illinois, 80% of the adolescents arrested were undocumented or unaddressed victims of abuse (Teplin et al., 2013). According to a National Academies report, adolescent involvement in criminal activity stems from developmental factors that make juveniles very different from adult perpetrators of crime. These factors relate to biological immaturity in the brain stem, with more rapid development in brain stem functions supporting pleasure seeking behaviors than those that foster self-control. This immaturity leads to an inability to engage in self-regulation, heightened sensitivity to external influences on behavior, and a present orientation that results in the inability to consider future consequences of one's actions. The report also notes that the majority of juvenile offenders are not engaged in serious crimes (Bonnie, Chemers, & Schuck, 2012). In addition, juveniles are often arrested for **status offenses**, conduct that would not be considered criminal if committed by an adult, such as truancy, running away, curfew violation, and alcohol or tobacco possession (Coalition for Juvenile Justice, n.d.).

Incarcerated youth also display significant levels of mental illness and substance abuse. In 2009, for example, more than 130,000 youth were arrested for drug abuse offenses, 86% of which dealt with possession of illegal drugs (U.S. Census Bureau, 2013g). Approximately two thirds of male juvenile offenders and nearly three fourths of females have at least one psychiatric disorder, and 51% of males and 47% of females have a substance abuse disorder. Post-traumatic stress disorder (PTSD) was also found in 11% of juveniles in one study (Teplin et al., 2013).

Because of the move to try more juveniles as adults, particularly for violent crimes, the number of youth incarcerated in adult correctional facilities is growing. Because of the potential for victimization by older and stronger inmates, younger inmates should be in areas segregated by sight and sound. Removing juveniles from adult facilities and sight and sound segregation are two core provisions of the Juvenile Justice and Delinquency Prevention Act (Coalition for Juvenile Justice, n.d.).

Incarcerated youth have different needs than adult inmates. For example, they have greater nutritional needs than adults (Robbins, 2009a). In addition, correctional protocols are often based on the needs of adult inmates. For example, juvenile suicide prevention plans and staff training are often modeled on information from adult prisoners or from youth in the community and may not be effective with incarcerated youth. For instance, factors associated with youth suicide in correctional settings are considerably different than those for adults, including time and location of suicides and the role of intoxicants (Robbins, 2008). Because of these differences, the National Commission on Correctional Health Care (NCCHC) (2014b) has developed standards for juvenile detention facilities separate from those for adult facilities. For further information on the standards for juvenile detention facilities, see the *External Resources* section of the student resources site.

The American Academy of Pediatrics (Braverman & Murray, 2011) revised its policy statement on care of juvenile offenders to include the following recommendations:

- Provision of care on a par with that provided to non incarcerated youth
- Housing of children and adolescents in facilities appropriate to their level of development
- Coordination of care between justice system providers and community providers
- Provision of evidence-based mental health and substance abuse services for youth
- Coordination of efforts to address funding for adequate health services for incarcerated youth (Braverman & Murray, 2011).

Population health nurses may need to advocate for the application of these sets of standards and recommendations in the care of the juvenile correctional population.

The fastest-growing segment of corrections populations is the elderly, primarily because of extended sentences, with a large proportion of the population growing old in the correctional setting. From 1990 to 2012, the proportion of people over 55 years of age in the general population increased by 50%, but the population in this age group in state and federal prisons increased by 550% (Smith et al., 2013). People over 50 years of age are considered "old" in correctional systems due to the accelerated aging that occurs in correctional populations. This accelerated aging process is due to life histories that often include substance abuse and withdrawal, poor health care, and high-risk behaviors as well as the stress of incarceration.

According to U.S. Census Bureau data (2013a), 1.2% of the total population in adult correctional facilities in 2009 were 65 years of age or older. Older inmates have more chronic diseases and disabilities and more cognitive impairments than younger prisoners. For example, the presence of people with dementias is increasing in correctional facilities as well as in the general population, and it is estimated that the prevalence of these conditions in correctional settings may be two to three times that in the general population (Wilson & Barboza, 2010). In addition, older inmates may have more difficulties conforming to prison life, experiencing difficulties climbing into upper bunks or dropping to the floor in an alarm situation (Smith et al., 2013).

Correctional facilities are often unprepared to address the health care needs of older inmates, nor are budgets designed to accommodate these needs. In addition, the shift of older inmates from state and federal prisons to county jails to address overcrowding places them in facilities that are least able to address their needs. Population health nurses may need to be actively involved in assuring that facilities and services are available to meet the needs of elderly inmates as well as to protect them from victimization by younger inmates.

Correctional populations are significantly unbalanced with respect to gender and racial/ethnic composition. In 2009, men constituted 92% of the U.S. adult correctional population (U.S. Census Bureau, 2013a). Unfortunately, correctional facilities are often not well equipped to address the special needs of female inmates and their needs are often overlooked (Matheson, Doherty, & Grant, 2011).

Similar, but not as pronounced, differences in population composition are noted among incarcerated youth, with boys accounting for 75% and girls for 25% of juvenile arrests (U.S. Census Bureau, 2013e), but arrest rates are increasing faster for female juveniles than males (Coalition for Juvenile Justice, 2013). Women tend to be arrested more often for minor property crimes and drug offenses than violent crimes.

Women inmates often have high rates of physical and mental health problems such as histories of physical and sexual abuse and early initiation of sexual intercourse and drug and alcohol use. Incarcerated women also have more unplanned and frequent pregnancies than women in the community and 5% to 6% of female prisoners are pregnant during incarceration. One positive side to these pregnancies is that they often have better outcomes due to improved health care and access to antepartum services in the correctional setting. Female prisoners have higher rates of mental illness than men, and experience a 10- to 20-fold greater rate of sexually transmitted infections (STIs) (Smith et al., 2013). The prevalence of recent or current mental disorders ranges from 48% to 71% of women compared to only 31% of men (Shelton, Ehret, Wakai, Kapetanovic, & Moran, 2010).

Women inmates have special needs not experienced by men. For example, they require both routine and nonroutine gynecologic care and tend to have more difficulty with sleep disturbances due to anxiety and apprehension than men. In addition, their nutritional needs differ. Incarcerated women are more likely than men to gain weight, with an average weight gain of one pound per week, leading to obesity and a variety of adverse health consequences (Smith et al., 2013). Similarly, pain management needs may be influenced by higher levels of depression. Women's substance abuse treatment needs also differ from men's and treatment often must address their histories of trauma and abuse. Women are more likely to request health care and mental health services than men, so staff levels in these areas may need to be higher than in facilities for men. Unfortunately, because they are fewer in number, incarcerated women are less visible than men and services may be less available. Because of gender socialization, women inmates may also be less able to articulate and advocate for themselves, leading to a need for population health nursing advocacy to assure that their health and social service needs are met.

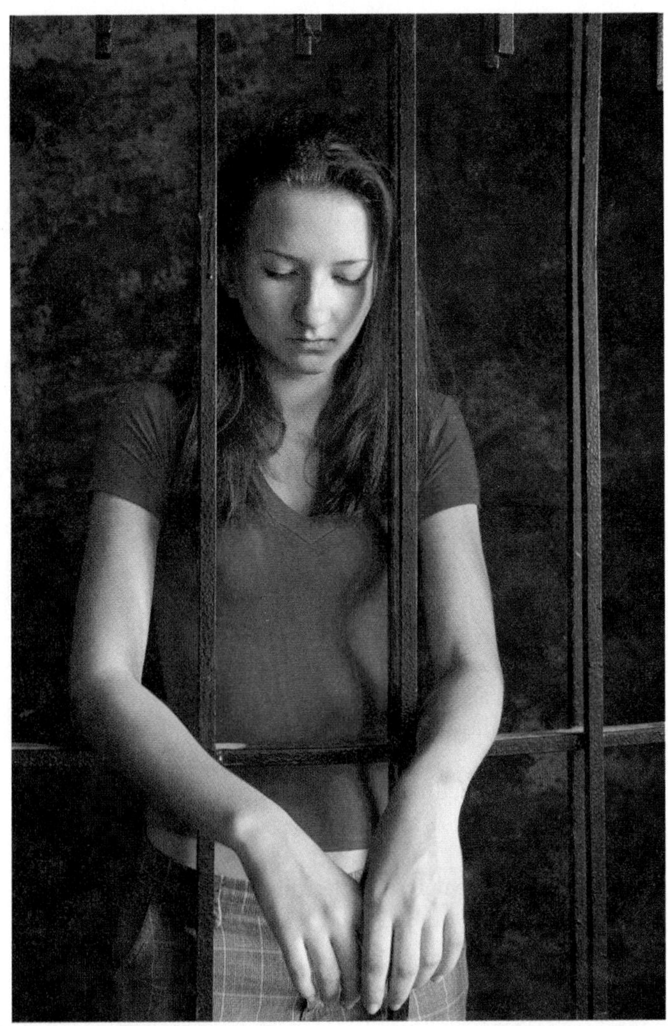

Because of their lower numbers, the health needs of women in correctional settings are often overlooked. *(Andreykr/Fotolia)*

Men and women also respond differently to the experience of being incarcerated. Men have been found to be most distressed by the loss of freedom, social rejection and loss of social status, autonomy, and self-control. Women, on the other hand, have similar concerns, but consider separation from family to be the most difficult aspect of incarceration. Other areas of concern for women include the constant stress of living in close proximity to others and lack of privacy with respect to personal property, modesty, and invasion of personal space. Women, in particular, need support in dealing with family separation and in maintaining family relationships. Unfortunately, because of fewer numbers, women's correctional facilities are less likely to be located close to their place of residence than men's facilities.

Another issue related to gender in correctional settings is the presence of transgendered individuals in the population. Concerns around transgendered individuals include housing decisions, safety, mental health issues, and maintenance of hormone therapy (NCCHC, 2009b). Decisions need to be made whether to place these inmates in male or female housing. It is recommended that they be housed in the general correctional population if possible, with attention given to privacy for hygiene, appropriate clothing, and protection from assault by other inmates. These decisions will best be made in light of where the inmate is in the process of transition. Mental health services may also be needed to address issues of gender dysphoria or stigma. Because of the growth in this population, the NCCHC (2009b) has issued a policy statement on the care of transgendered individuals in correctional settings.

Members of racial and ethnic minority groups are disproportionately represented in correctional settings. In 2009, for example, although the actual number of White inmates was more than twice that of Black inmates, rates of incarceration are higher among Blacks. The U.S. adult correctional population was 49% White, 41% Black or African American, and 1.9% American Indian or Alaskan Native. Nearly 20% of the incarcerated population was Hispanic (U.S. Census Bureau, 2013a, 2013f). A similar disproportionate rate of incarceration exists among racial and ethnic minority youth (Coalition for Juvenile Justice, n.d.).These and other similar figures have prompted concerns for inequities and prejudice within the justice system. In addition, the ethnic and racial diversity of correctional populations may result in racial tensions and violence within facilities as well as the need for culturally sensitive health care. Population health nurses may need to actively advocate for correctional health care services that meet the needs of a culturally and linguistically diverse population as well as advocate for fair treatment for all inmates regardless of race or ethnicity.

Physiologic health status. Assessment considerations related to physical health status in correctional populations include mortality, infectious and chronic illnesses, injury, and other conditions.

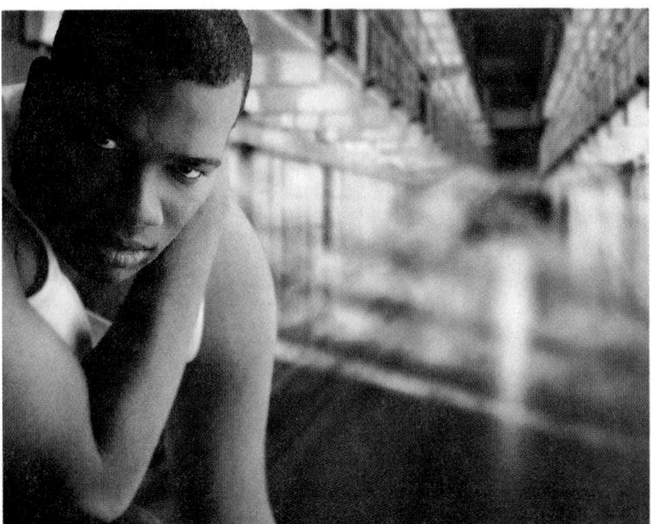

Members of ethnic and racial minority groups may be overrepresented in correctional populations due to discriminatory judicial processes. *(CURAphotography/Fotolia)*

Mortality. Risk of mortality is higher among correctional populations than in the general population, in large part because of poor access to health care and health-risk behaviors prior to incarceration. In a study of New York City jails from 2001 to 2009, an average of 27 deaths occurred each year mostly due to chronic diseases or infections. Suicide and cardiovascular disease were the leading causes of death, and inmates experienced higher mortality than the general population for heart disease, HIV/AIDs, chronic liver disease, homicide, and suicide. On the other hand, lower rates were noted for cancer, influenza and pneumonia, and accidents. During that time period, annual mortality declined despite increases in the age of the population, primarily due to a decrease in HIV mortality with the advent of highly active antiretroviral therapy (HAART) (Brittain, Axelrod, & Venters, 2013).

Members of the correctional population are at increased risk for mortality even after release. For example, a National Academies report noted that released prisoners were 13 times more likely to die in the 2 weeks after their release than members of the general population. In addition, they were 129 times more likely to die of substance overdoses due to decreased opioid tolerance developed during incarceration (Smith et al., 2013). Another study found that this increased rate of mortality continued for the first few years after release (Zlodre & Fazel, 2012).

Infectious diseases. Environmental conditions and behavioral patterns in correctional settings foster the spread of communicable diseases. Although many communicable diseases are found in this population, four are of particular concern: tuberculosis (TB), HIV infection and AIDS, hepatitis, and other sexually transmitted infections (STIs). Overcrowding and generally poor health status are two of the factors that promote the spread of TB in inmate populations. Moreover, co-infection with both TB and HIV is occurring in large segments of some correctional populations. Additional complicating factors in the problem of TB in correctional facilities are the prevalence of multi-drug-resistant (MDR) TB and the tendency of inmates not to complete a full course of treatment.

The large portion of inmates with TB in correctional facilities makes them ideal settings for minimizing the spread of TB in the general population. Population health nurses working in correctional settings should assess inmates for signs of TB as well as provide routine screenings for TB according to agency policy. Tuberculin skin test screening in jails may be inappropriate for many inmates who stay only one or two days, so the nurse should ask about TB symptomatology and history of exposure during the intake assessment to isolate potentially infectious inmates.

HIV infection and confirmed cases of AIDS are another growing problem in correctional facilities. Many inmates are at increased risk of infection because of injection drug use, and the potential for exposure during incarceration via continued drug use and homosexual activity is high. Confirmed AIDS prevalence in U.S. correctional facilities is approximately 2.4 times that in the general population, and an estimated one in seven persons with HIV infection will pass through correctional facilities (Division of HIV/AIDS Prevention, 2014).

Rates of HIV infection and AIDS diagnoses vary from one area of the country to another, and nurses should be aware of the overall prevalence of infection in their jurisdictions. Correctional nurses should assess all inmates for a history of HIV infection, high-risk behaviors, and a history or symptoms of possible opportunistic infections. In addition, population health nurses should advocate for effective treatment for HIV-infected inmates during incarceration and following their release into the community.

Drug use behaviors contribute to the increased incidence of TB and HIV infection in inmates. Such behaviors also place inmates at risk for other STIs and hepatitis B (HBV) and C (HCV). In addition to drug use, sexual activity and tattooing are other risk factors for HBV and HCV common in correctional populations. In assessing individual inmates for health problems, the nurse should ask about a history of STIs and hepatitis B and C and should be alert to the presence of physical signs and symptoms of these diseases.

Other communicable diseases are also prevalent in correctional populations. For example, methicillin-resistant *Staphylococcus aureus* (MRSA) is a common occurrence in institutional settings, including jails and prisons. For example, MRSA was colonized in 16% of Los Angeles County jail inmates (Malek et al., 2011). Similarly, *Chlamydia trachomatis* infection has been found in roughly 15% of girls and 7% of boys admitted to juvenile detention facilities, and gonococcal infection was found in 4% of girls and 10% of boys. Similarly, 7% of adult women and 7% of men screened positive for *Chlamydia*, while gonorrhea was found in slightly less than 2% of women and just over 1% of men (Miller, 2011).

Outbreaks of other infectious diseases, such as influenza and mumps, also occur in correctional facilities (Ringsdorf, Heerema, Ruiz, & Sanchez, 2010). During the 2009 H1N1 influenza pandemic, for example, high rates of infection occurred in correctional settings. Unfortunately, 55% of U.S. jails did not receive supplies of influenza vaccine, and only 11% of state prisons and 14% of federal facilities had vaccine available (Lee et al., 2012).

The problem of infectious diseases in correctional settings is one of international, as well as national, concern. Prevalence rates for HIV infection in the correctional populations throughout the world range from 6 to 50 times those of the non-incarcerated population. These high rates are accounted for primarily by drug use, commercial sex work, tattooing, and men who have sex with men (United Nations Office on Drugs and Crime [UNODC], n.d.).

Chronic conditions. The prevalence of chronic illness in correctional populations is approximately four times that of the general population. Chronic illnesses of particular concern in correctional settings include diabetes, hypertension, heart disease, and chronic lung conditions such as asthma. Other common physical health problems include incontinence, sensory impairments, arthritis, limited mobility, and cancer. Seizure disorders are also common, and inmates may also exhibit seizure activity during withdrawal from drugs and alcohol. Diabetes may be particularly difficult to control given the rigid structure of the correctional routine and the need to time hypoglycemic medications, meals, and exercise periods appropriately. The availability of vending machines and the use of commissary privileges as a reward may also complicate dietary control for inmates with diabetes.

Many inmates with chronic conditions, particularly those with substance abuse problems, enter the correctional facility after prolonged periods without medications or may not know what medications they have been taking. In many instances, the nurse has to exert considerable ingenuity to obtain an accurate health history from clients, family members, and health care providers in the community. Because of poor overall health status, inmates may also be especially susceptible to exacerbations of chronic conditions. The nurse should assess individual inmates for existing chronic conditions and should also identify problems with high incidence and prevalence in the correctional population with whom he or she works.

Incontinence may also be a problem in the correctional population, and population health nurses should assess for problems with incontinence during intake assessments. In one study, for example, 43% of women prisoners reported urinary symptoms that may be difficult to address in a correctional setting (Drennan, Goodman, Norton, & Wells, 2010). Other problems that complicate life for prisoners include sensory impairments and functional incapacity. All of these are issues that population health nurses working in correctional settings can help to address.

Members of the correctional population may also experience terminal illness. A workshop sponsored by the Institute of Medicine identified the need for long-term treatment facilities and palliative care for inmates with serious illnesses, as well as policies for compassionate release for nonviolent offenders with terminal illnesses (Smith, et al., 2013). In addition, the growing prevalence of terminal illness in this population has led to a growing trend toward hospice care within correctional facilities (Hufft, 2013).

Injury. Injury is another area of physiologic function that should be assessed by the nurse. Injury may result from activities preceding arrest, from actions taken by arresting officers, or from accidents or assaults occurring during incarceration. The nurse should be aware of the potential for internal as well as visible injuries and should assess inmates for signs of trauma. In a survey of inmates of state correctional facilities, 31% reported an injury since admission. Accidental injuries were more common than those resulting from violence. The incidence rate for injuries related to violence was 50% higher than that for the general public, and the accidental injury rate was more than twice as high as in the general population (Sung, 2010). Slightly different results were noted in a study of injuries occurring in New York City jails over a 4-month period in 2010. Two thirds of those injuries were the result of violence and only one third were unintentional. Nearly two thirds of the incidents resulted in detectable injuries that required medical attention, and 39% required outside referral for treatment (Ludwig et al., 2012).

Violence resulting in injuries in correctional settings may be associated with traumatic brain injury in the perpetrators. In a meta-analysis, for example, 60% of prisoners were found to have traumatic brain injury, decreasing impulse control and making management of their behavior more difficult (Shiroma, Ferguson, & Pickelsimer, 2010).

Self-injury may also be a problem in correctional settings and accounted for 8% of injuries reported in New York City jails (Ludwig et al., 2012). Self-injury may also be referred to as self-harm or deliberate self-harm, parasuicide, or self-mutilation. **Self-injurious behavior** may be defined as purposeful behavior resulting in mild to moderate injury to self that is not intended to result in death and does not arise from psychosis or intellectual impairment (Fagan, Cox, Helfand, & Aufderheide, 2010). Self-injury may occur in the context of other mental disorders such as depression or among transgender individuals who are prevented from engaging in desired sexual transitions (National Commission on Correctional Health Care, 2009b).

Other conditions. Dental health problems are also common among inmates. One particular problem that nurses in correction settings may encounter is a condition called "meth mouth." Meth mouth is characterized by severe erosion and decay of teeth and usually requires emergency dental services. Meth mouth results from several factors associated with methamphetamine use, including gnashing of the teeth, poor oral hygiene, and dry mouth, which increases the acidic effects of methamphetamine. Methamphetamine use also leads to cravings for high-calorie, high-sugar soft drinks that further contribute to tooth decay (American Dental Association, 2013).

Pregnancy is the final biophysical consideration in assessing the health of correctional populations. As noted earlier, the number of female inmates increases annually. Because of prior drug use and poor health care, pregnant women in correctional settings may be at higher risk for poor pregnancy outcomes than women in the general population. Conversely, incarceration may improve pregnancy outcomes because it interrupts drug use and provides access to prenatal care that the women might not otherwise receive. Care of pregnant women in correctional settings, however, is often hampered by lack of special diets to support pregnancy, lack of exercise, and inappropriate work assignments. Fetal health may also be compromised by problems encountered in drug and alcohol withdrawal in the correctional setting. Finally, the timely transfer of women in labor to obstetrical facilities is often hampered by the security constraints of the correctional facility.

In assessing female inmates, the nurse should ask about the last menstrual period and solicit any symptoms of possible pregnancy. Because drug use can interfere with menses, menstrual history is not always reliable for indicating pregnancy or for suggesting length of gestation when pregnancy is confirmed. The nurse should also ask about high-risk behavior that may affect the fetus, such as smoking, drug and alcohol use, and so on. The pregnant inmate's nutritional status should also be assessed. Other physical problems common in this population that may affect pregnancy outcomes include urinary tract infections and STIs, and the nurse should assess for symptoms of these conditions. Depression and anxiety are also common phenomena among these women. Advocacy may be required to assure adequate prenatal and perinatal care for pregnant inmates. For example, population health nurses may need to convince correctional personnel of the necessity of keeping outside appointments for high-risk pregnancy care, even when these require pulling security personnel away from the correctional facility.

PSYCHOLOGICAL DETERMINANTS. Psychological factors can have a profound influence on health in correctional settings. The presence of mental illness in the correctional population is one of the major psychological factors influencing the health of this population. The level of mental illness in correctional facilities has tripled in the last 30 years, with a current estimate of 16% of the population affected. In addition, an estimated 40% of mentally ill persons will be incarcerated at some time in their lives (Torrey, Kennard, Eslinger, Lamb, & Pavle, 2010). A 2010 study by the Treatment Advocacy Center found three times more severely mentally ill persons in jails and prisons than under treatment in hospitals (Stettin, Frese, & Lamb, 2013). The authors of the study concluded that U.S. correctional facilities have replaced hospitals as a place of containment for the mentally ill and described the increasing trend toward incarceration as a return to the conditions of the 1840s (Torrey et al., 2010). Mental illness is also frequently criminalized in the rest of the world.

Mentally ill inmates are often significantly disabled by their conditions and have a more difficult time adjusting to prison life than other inmates. Overcrowding and isolation units in correctional facilities may contribute to poor mental health even among those without psychiatric diagnoses (Smith et al., 2013). Incarceration itself is stressful and can lead to psychological effects, including depression and suicide. Incarceration also exacerbates existing mental illness. Correctional nurses should be alert to signs of depression and other mental or emotional distress in inmates, and assessment of suicide potential is a critical part of every intake interview. Suicide is the leading cause of death in jails and "lockups," and is the cause of nearly 100% of deaths among incarcerated juveniles. A **lockup** is a temporary holding facility in which inmates are placed prior to transportation to a jail or other facility or to being freed on bail. Detention in a lockup is generally for less than 48 hours (Hufft, 2013).

Attempted suicide is a particularly prevalent problem among incarcerated individuals. In the United States, suicide rates in correctional populations are eight times those of the general population, and are five times higher in England and Wales (Zlodre & Fazel, 2012). Jails tend to have higher rates of

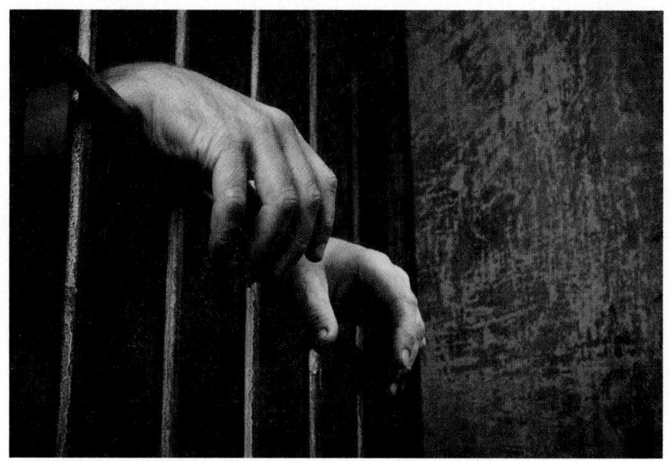

Isolation increases the risk for depression and suicide in correctional populations. *(BortN66/Fotolia)*

successful suicides than prisons (43 per 100,000 inmates versus 16 per 100,000 in prisons), with smaller jails having higher rates yet.

Most adult suicides occur within the first 24 to 48 hours of incarceration, while juvenile suicides are more evenly spaced over 12 months, with a large number still occurring within the first 72 hours. Adolescent suicides shortly after incarceration are often related to intoxication. Adult inmate suicides tend to occur at night when there is less intensive supervision, but juvenile suicides occur primarily in the daytime, particularly in the early evening and are often associated with room confinement (Robbins, 2008). General risk factors for suicide include a prior attempt, mental illness (particularly depression or bipolar disorder), dual diagnosis of mental illness and substance abuse disorders, a family history of suicide, hopelessness, impulsiveness or aggressiveness, and experiencing barriers to mental health treatment. Additional risk factors include recent loss, physical illness, easy access to lethal methods, unwillingness to seek help due to stigma, the influence of significant others who have committed suicide, cultural or religious beliefs, and feelings of isolation (Fagan et al., 2010). Population health nurses should identify inmates at risk for suicide and initiate immediate interventions as well as referral for long-term treatment of underlying factors.

Another group of young offenders may be developmentally disabled, and an additional segment of this population may experience learning disabilities and other developmental disorders. Developmentally disabled individuals, particularly youth, may be persuaded to participate in group crimes in order to be accepted by their peers without fully realizing the consequences of their actions. They may display deficits in both cognitive/intellectual function and adaptive capabilities, leading to greater difficulty adjusting to life in a correctional facility. Because of their diminished mental capabilities, this group of inmates may have difficulty understanding instructions and display impulsivity and low frustration tolerance, earning them frequent punishment for infractions in the correctional setting. This group of individuals may require particular advocacy on the part of population health nurses to assist them in their adjustment, help correctional personnel recognize their limitations, and prevent their victimization by other inmates.

Another mental health issue that correctional health nurses may encounter is acute psychotic delirium, which may result from many causes. Drug overdose, traumatic head injuries, poisoning, and a variety of medical conditions, such as acidosis, insulin reaction, or infection, may all contribute to delirium. The typical reaction to a delirious inmate is to restrain him or her, but that may result in oxygen deprivation worsening delirium or resulting in sudden death (Mathis, 2010). Correctional nurses should be alert to the signs of delirium and take appropriate actions to determine and deal with the cause. They may also need to educate correctional staff on this condition and on appropriate interventions for controlling dangerous behaviors to protect both the inmate and others.

By law, inmates are entitled to mental health services as well as medical treatment. Mental health services, however, may be lacking in some correctional systems, or the need for these services may go unrecognized. This is particularly true among women inmates, the elderly, and youth.

Another subgroup within the inmate population with significant mental health needs includes persons under a sentence of death. In the United States in 2009, more than 3,000 prisoners had been sentenced to be executed. This figure was 4.6 times higher than in 1980 (U.S. Census Bureau, 2013k). Being given a sentence of death does not always result in execution. The number of actual executions was at its highest in the United States in the 1930s, and declined precipitously due to a moratorium on executions during the 1970s. Since that time, some states have reinstituted the death penalty, but from 1973 to 2009, less than 15% of death sentences issued resulted in execution (Nagin & Pepper, 2012). Despite these figures, however, persons under a sentence of death live with constant uncertainty and may develop a variety of mental health problems. Correctional nurses working in systems with "death-row" inmates should assess them for evidence of psychological problems and refer them for counseling as appropriate.

Mental health challenges in dealing with correctional populations are many and varied. Some of these challenges include determining who has mental health problems and how they should be treated, managing behavior and symptoms associated with psychiatric illness, and recognizing and dealing with the negative mental health effects of incarceration. Other challenges include understanding the difficulty in adjusting to incarceration that might be experienced by inmates with mental illness and determining the need for and providing specialized services. For example, few correctional settings deal effectively with the mental health needs of older inmates. Similarly, women and youth exposed to psychological trauma need therapy to deal with issues of abuse as well as co-occurring substance abuse. Population health nurses in correctional settings can engage in advocacy to assure that appropriate services are provided to these vulnerable population groups.

ENVIRONMENTAL DETERMINANTS. Factors in the physical environment also influence the health of correctional populations. The physical environment of the correctional setting is constrained by the need for security. Inmates may be relegated to specific spaces at specific times of the day. Because of the tremendous growth in the incarcerated population, jails and prisons are extremely overcrowded and few jurisdictions are not in violation of space standards for inmates. Overcrowding is often due to delayed court processes and the large numbers of people awaiting trial.

Other physical environmental problems common in correctional settings include poor ventilation, lack of temperature control, and unsanitary conditions. Lack of funds for maintenance may lead to buildings in poor repair, creating safety hazards for both inmates and staff. In New York City jails, for example, 17% of inmate injuries resulted from slips and falls (Ludwig et al., 2012). Other areas that should be assessed by the nurse include the safety of recreational areas, fire protection, lighting, plumbing, solid waste disposal, and safety of the water supply. Additional environmental considerations that may affect health in correctional populations include vermin control, noise control, and lack of privacy (Smith et al., 2013).

Because correctional facilities are often situated in areas away from the general population, they may be located in sites with disaster potential such as flooding, earthquake, and so on. The nurse should assess the potential for such disasters as well as the adequacy of the facility's disaster response plan. Disaster potential may also arise from prison industries. For example, prisoners in work programs may be employed in production industries using processes or materials that create the potential for fires or explosions. Inmate occupations may also present other physical hazards for individual clients that need to be assessed.

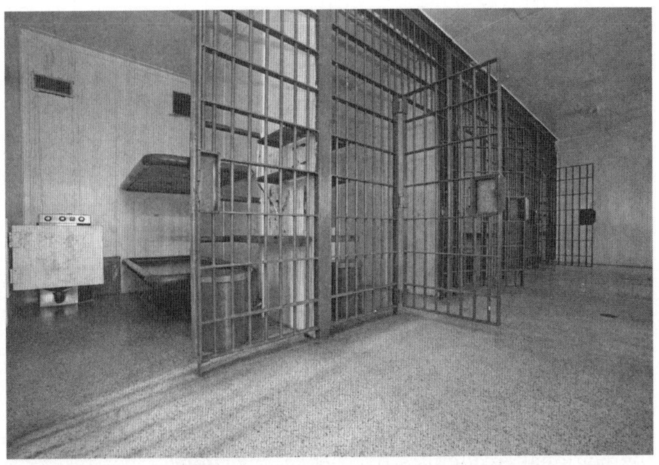

Overcrowding and lack of privacy contribute to the stress of incarceration. *(Intoit/Shutterstock)*

SOCIOCULTURAL DETERMINANTS. A wide variety of sociocultural factors influence the health status of correctional populations. An estimated 80% of law enforcement activity addresses social problems, yet police personnel are often ill-equipped to deal with them because of lack of understanding of the underlying dynamics of social problems. Like health care providers in correctional settings, law enforcement personnel may experience conflict between their law enforcement role and a role in resolving social problems. In addition, social problems that lead to criminal activity are given low priority at the societal level. Particular elements of the sociocultural dimension that influence health in correctional settings include socioeconomic and cultural influences, political and legal influences, the potential for violence in the setting, the needs of special populations, and the social consequences of incarceration. The subculture of the correctional setting itself is another sociocultural factor that may influence the health of inmates and staff.

Socioeconomic and cultural influences. To a large extent, correctional populations tend to be at the low end of economic and educational spectrums. Women offenders, in particular, often come from poverty-stricken neighborhoods with low levels of social capital. Lower socioeconomic status is also associated with worse health status among inmates.

Housing is another socioeconomic issue that may contribute to incarceration. As we saw in Chapter 21∞, many activities performed by homeless individuals to ensure their survival have been criminalized, with the result that they are often arrested for activities that would be tolerated in other members of society. The homeless are overrepresented in correctional populations, and recently released prisoners often become homeless due to poor reentry planning. Incarceration may also lead to homelessness due to the disruption of family and community ties and decreased employment and housing opportunities associated with the stigma of incarceration.

As we saw earlier, correctional populations include many ethnic minority group members who are frequently culturally and linguistically, as well as economically and educationally, disadvantaged. In addition, many more inmates are being incarcerated as a result of immigration offenses than in the past.

Political and legal influences. Historically, jails and prisons have served five distinct purposes and the focus of incarceration has shifted back and forth among these purposes since the inception of correctional institutions. The five purposes are (a) retribution or punishment for crimes, (b) deterrence from crime, (c) incapacitation or rendering people incapable of further crime, (d) rehabilitation or correcting deviant behavior, and (e) to render restorative justice or repair social injuries resulting from crime (Hufft, 2013). The ability of incarceration to address any of these purposes effectively is questionable. For example, a study by the National Research Council of the National Academies of Science determined that research on capital punishment does not provide a clear indication of the deterrent effects on violent crime (Nagin & Pepper, 2012). Similarly, recidivism and re-incarceration rates argue against the effectiveness of jail and prison sentences in rehabilitating offenders.

Correctional policy is in flux and the purpose of incarceration is not always clear. For example, as we saw earlier, jails and prisons have reverted to being settings in which the mentally ill or substance abusers can be removed from society. For example, in 2012, ten times more severely mentally ill people were in U.S. jails and prisons than in state psychiatric hospitals (Treatment Advocacy Center & National Sheriff's Association, 2014) The lack of psychiatric beds in public hospitals and closure of public mental hospitals have greatly contributed to this shift of the mentally ill to correctional facilities. For example, from 2005 to 2010 there was a 14% decrease in state psychiatric beds throughout the nation, with the per capita number of beds reduced to 1850 levels. Nationwide, bed availability only met an estimated 28% of the treatment need. These figures result in a significant negative impact on correctional systems and hospital emergency departments. In addition, relationships have been shown between psychiatric bed availability and the incidence of violent crime and arrest-related deaths (Treatment Advocacy Center, 2012). A joint report by the Treatment Advocacy Center and the National Sheriff's Association (2014) recommended the following changes in public policy:

- Prevention of incarceration by eliminating barriers to treatment for mental illness
- Legislation to promote effective treatment for mentally ill inmates
- Development and implementation of jail diversion programs
- Use of court-ordered outpatient treatment programs for mentally ill offenders
- Research on the costs of incarceration to those of treatment for people with serious mentally illnesses
- Careful screening of mentally ill inmates to determine medication, suicide prevention, and other needs
- Mandatory release planning and community support to facilitate recovery (Treatment Advocacy Center & National Sheriff's Association, 2014).

The U.S. response to drug abuse also involves inappropriate criminal sanctions, with drug-related incarcerations increasing from 41,000 in 1980 to half a million in 2010, 40% of which were for possession of illegal substances. This increase has resulted in an annual cost of $22,000 per incarcerated inmate, far above the cost of treatment (Fiscella, 2010).

Recently, however, there has been more of a trend to diverting individuals with mental illness and substance abuse out of the correctional system and into treatment (Stettin et al., 2013). More and more law enforcement agencies are attempting to identify individuals whose crimes arise from mental illness and divert them to psychiatric treatment settings. **Diversion** is a group of practices, including parole and probation, designed to prevent reincarceration by linking mentally ill offenders to mandated community-based treatment services

(Stettin et al., 2013). Diversion is intended to decriminalize mental illness. Diversion relies on intersectoral collaboration between legal and mental health care systems to address factors that contribute to **recidivism** (rearrest, re-incarceration, or frequent rehospitalization) among mentally ill and substance-abusing inmates.

There are two general approaches to diversion: crisis intervention team policing (CIT) and specialized mental health courts. **Crisis intervention teams (CITs)** are specialized units of police officers trained as mental health specialists who are able to determine if diversion, rather than arrest, is an appropriate option. These officers are knowledgeable about local resources and often get to know local mentally ill offenders quite well and can take them to hospitals for evaluation or to outpatient treatment facilities or initiate court proceedings for assisted outpatient treatment. **Assisted outpatient treatment (AOT)** is the application of coercion through threats of hospitalization for noncompliance with mental illness treatment (Stettin et al., 2013).

The second approach to diversion is the establishment of specialized mental illness courts. Mental illness courts are one of several types of specialized courts including domestic violence courts, drug courts, and so on. These specialized courts seek to work with nonviolent offenders to address the underlying causes of criminal behavior, mental illness in the case of mental illness courts. Like assisted outpatient treatment, mental health courts attempt to foster compliance with mental health treatment through threats of incarceration (Stettin et al., 2013). Similar approaches are used to divert substance abusers into treatment programs. Unfortunately, less than half of the U.S. population lives in jurisdictions that have CITs or mental health courts available, and availability varies significantly from state to state from 100% in Washington, DC (which has a single criminal justice agency), to 0% in Rhode Island. In only four states are these diversion options available to more than 60% of the population (Stettin et al., 2013).

A similar approach may be taken to drug-related criminal activity. For example, California's Substance Abuse and Crime Prevention Act of 2002 marked a major shift in criminal justice policy. Under this legislation, nonviolent adult offenders can be sentenced to probation with substance abuse treatment. Similar provisions affect drug offenders on parole or probation, and offenders are allowed up to three chances to re-enter treatment without penalty. In the first 5 years of operation, this approach cost $120 million, mostly for substance abuse treatment services, but resulted in incarceration cost savings of $2,137 per person served (Anglin, Nosyk, Jaffe, Urada, & Evans, 2013).

For young people, zero tolerance policies in schools have led to more school dropouts and greater justice system involvement. Healthy psychological development at this age requires effective and concerned adult role models, opportunities to interact with peers who value and model academic success and prosocial behavior, and involvement in activities that promote critical thinking and autonomous decision making. Unfortunately, the current juvenile justice system focuses on confinement and control, removing youth from positive influences on behavior and promoting further criminal activity (Bonnie et al., 2012).

Some efforts have been made to change these negative policies related to youth and criminal justice. For example, the Juvenile Justice and Delinquency Prevention Act (JJDPA) funds a variety of programs designed to prevent youth criminal justice involvement. Core requirements for program funding include a focus on deinstitutionalization of status offenders, removal of juvenile offenders from adult correctional facilities or sight and sound separation from adult inmates, and efforts to reduce the disproportionate number of minority youth in contact with the juvenile justice system (Coalition for Juvenile Justice, n.d.). The act, originally passed in 1974, was reauthorized in 2002. Unfortunately, reauthorization failed in 2008 and again in 2009, and the legislation was due to expire in 2013 (Coalition for Juvenile Justice, 2013). Reauthorization legislation was reintroduced in 2013 and contains new provisions for evidence-based assessment of at-risk youth, greater community and family support, and funding for mental and behavioral health services. Other provisions address prevention of bullying and gang activity, substance abuse and mental health screening and treatment, and reentry assistance for juvenile offenders. Congress authorized additional funds for programs under JJDPA for fiscal year 2014 (Coalition for Juvenile Justice, 2014), but the act itself had not been reauthorized as of February 2014 (Jenkins, 2014).

The Affordable Care Act (ACA) is another policy initiative that has implications for correctional populations. Incarcerated individuals are not allowed to receive government supported health insurance. According to the ACA, inmates cannot enroll in insurance exchanges if they are incarcerated at the time of enrollment, but because of a lack of clear definition of incarceration, pretrial detainees and persons on parole or probation may be eligible to enroll. In some states, insurance may be terminated during incarceration, but the Centers for Medicare and Medicaid Services (CMS) is recommending suspension of coverage rather than termination. Under the law, persons with mental illness or substance abuse disorders will be eligible for coverage regardless of incarceration status, and correctional facilities have been urged to establish linkages with Medicare, Medicaid, and other health plans to offset the cost of care for these inmates. Such linkages will necessitate the development of billing and accounting systems and electronic medical records in correctional facilities. Meeting constitutional standards of care with independent oversight of services and appropriate "through care," including continuity of care and effective discharge planning to meet health care needs on release, will also be essential (Blair & Greifinger, 2011).

Violence. Violence within correctional settings is another sociocultural factor that influences the health of the incarcerated population. For example, 40% of injuries in New York City jails were found to be related to inmate violence (Ludwig et al., 2012). Similarly, one in ten state prison inmates have been injured in fights (Smith et al., 2013). Transgender individuals and youth, particularly GLBT youth, are at particular risk for physical and emotional victimization and violence (Coalition for Juvenile Justice, 2013; NCCHC, 2009b). Approximately 12% of youth have been sexually abused in correctional facilities by other inmates or by staff (Greifinger, 2010), and nearly 10% of state and federal prison inmates report sexual abuse (Smith et al., 2013). Cross-gender pat down searches can be particularly traumatic for women who have been sexually abused. Correctional staff may also exercise inappropriate levels of physical force in dealing with inmates (Smith et al., 2013).

Special correctional populations. The special needs of youth, the elderly, pregnant women, and transgender individuals in correctional settings have already been addressed. Another population that may have special needs is former members of the military. Approximately 140,000 veterans are in prisons. Veterans tend to be older than the rest of the correctional population (12 years on average) and are more likely to be incarcerated for violent crimes, particularly against women and children. One in four sex offenders is a military veteran. Most veterans who are incarcerated have served in wartime, but combat service has not been linked to mental illness in this segment of the correctional population. Veterans tend to be better educated than other inmates and are less likely to use drugs (National Coalition for Homeless Veterans, n.d.).

Social consequences of incarceration. Incarceration also has a variety of social consequences including its effects on families, societal costs, and effects on suffrage and future socioeconomic status.

Family effects. Incarceration disrupts families significantly. An estimated 2.7 million U.S. children have a parent who has been incarcerated (Osborne Association, n.d.). Children of incarcerated parents often have behavior problems and exhibit poor academic performance and high levels of psychological distress. Incarceration also decreases relationship commitments on the part of the incarcerated individual as well as his or her spouse or partner. Furthermore, incarceration may lead to family stress and inability to cope with the loss of the incarcerated member. Conversely, for some families, incarceration may decrease family stress related to prior illegal behavior, mental illness, or substance abuse (Dyer, Pleck, & McBride, 2012).

Family members may be the only support available to inmates on release, and weakening of family ties makes reentry that much more difficult. Maintenance of family relationships can be achieved by strategies that help families interact positively. This may include visitation by entire families, including children, eating meals with the incarcerated member, and maintaining family rituals (Dyer et al., 2012).

Concerns for children may be a source of stress for some inmates, particularly women. Because of fewer female detention facilities, women may be incarcerated at a distance from families, making it difficult to maintain contact.

Women's facilities may be more likely than men's institutions to provide parenting education, but most such programs are provided without children present, prohibiting inmates from modeling learned skills with their own children. Problems caused by separation of children from their mothers have led some correctional facilities to allow young children, particularly newborns, to remain with their mothers in custody. Areas for concern in these types of programs that need to be addressed by correctional nurses and other correctional personnel include the security of children, liability issues, costs and mechanisms for providing health care and other services for children, and the effects of incarceration on child development.

Societal costs of incarceration. Incarceration is a costly, and largely unsuccessful, approach to containing crime. In 2008, federal, state, and local governments spent $75 billion on correctional activities, most of it for incarceration, and correctional spending is only exceeded by Medicaid expenditures in terms of government costs (Welsh & Farrington, 2011). Incarceration also diverts state and local funds from other needed services and programs. For example, nearly half of the $15.5 million federal budget allocation for substance abuse in 2011 went to law enforcement activities, compared to $1.7 billion for prevention programs and $3.9 billion for substance abuse treatment (Anglin et al., 2013).

Incarceration has other social consequences as well. For example, laws in 48 states prohibit persons convicted of felonies from voting even after serving their sentences. This inability to vote has a disproportionate effect on racial and ethnic minority populations who may already lack a voice in the body politic. Approximately 1 in 45 people (5.3 million Americans) are disenfranchised by this restriction on voting. Some jurisdictions have processes by which released felons can have their voting rights reinstated, but these vary from state to state and are often cumbersome and difficulty to negotiate (Purtie, 2013).

Incarceration also damages opportunities for work, education, and housing. Some former inmates, for example those convicted of sexual crimes, are restricted from living in certain communities. Persons on probation and parole are also restricted from travel outside the area, which may put them at a disadvantage in areas with few employment opportunities.

The correctional subculture. The primary purpose of correctional institutions is custody and punishment, not health care. This custodial culture may pose considerable challenges to health care providers who must balance their health care and advocacy roles against security concerns.

Security concerns may also hamper provision of health care. In some institutions, nurses do not have immediate access to inmates unless security personnel are present. In other instances, transportation of inmates for outside services may be postponed if there are insufficient security personnel available to accompany them. There is also the potential for violence against health care providers and their use as hostages.

The nurse should be alert to the use of excessive force or punitive conditions to which inmates may be subjected. Correctional nurses will also assess the extent of social support available to inmates. Social support may arise from interactions and programs available within the correctional system or from continued interactions with persons or agencies outside the system (e.g., family). Development of social support systems may be particularly important for clients about to be released from the facility.

Some correctional facilities have programs that promote rehabilitation and permit inmates to earn some money. In some states, there are even provisions for inmates to work to repay the victims of their crimes. Such opportunities are less readily available to women inmates than men and are rarely adequate to meet the rehabilitation needs of all inmates. The presence of occupational opportunities, however, may contribute to a variety of occupational risks to health that should be assessed by nurses in correctional facilities. Occupational hazards for correctional facility staff, as well as those for inmates, should be considered. Corrections personnel, for example, are at higher risk for infectious disease exposure. Physical and psychological safety considerations also present the need for constant vigilance among health care and other personnel in correctional settings.

There is also a subculture within the inmate population that members must adhere to. This subculture has its own rules and norms for behavior among inmates. Five common elements in such subcultures include (a) not interfering with the interests of other inmates, particularly not informing on others, (b) maintaining a low profile and not getting involved in others' issues, (c) not exploiting other inmates, stealing from them, or lying to them, (d) not whining, and (e) not trusting correctional personnel (Hufft, 2013). Some of these elements may make it difficult for correctional health care personnel to develop trusting relationships with clients or to obtain accurate health-related information.

BEHAVIORAL DETERMINANTS. Behavioral factors that influence the health of inmates and staff in correctional settings include diet, substance abuse, smoking, opportunities for exercise and recreation, and sexual activity.

Nutrition. Some subpopulations in correctional settings have unique dietary needs that have already been addressed, but all inmates need adequate nutritional intake. Unfortunately, a report of an Institute of Medicine study found that prison diets are often calorie dense and high in fats (Smith et al., 2013), and prisoners worldwide often have inadequate diets. In addition, cuts in food budgets may limit offerings. Conversely, some correctional systems have found that budget cuts have permitted them to eliminate empty calories (e.g., coffee and sugar, margarine), provide healthier alternatives (e.g., fresh fruits in place of baked goods, use of skim or powdered milk), and offer nutrient dense foods. Such changes can also be accompanied by educating inmates on nutritious diets.

Drug, alcohol, and tobacco use. Inmates are three to four times more likely than the general public to smoke. With little to occupy their time, inmates may find themselves smoking more after incarceration than before. In addition, there are often limited options for smoking cessation. Smoking coupled with overcrowding, lack of exercise, and inadequate diet may increase inmates' risk of both communicable and chronic diseases. Access to tobacco is also a traditional reward for compliant behavior in correctional settings. Approximately 70% to 80% of all inmates and 46% of juveniles smoke and only a few correctional facilities have or enforce smoking bans or promote smoke-free environments (Cropsey et al., 2010). In addition, health care providers may see other addictive behaviors as having higher priority than smoking cessation.

Alcohol and other substance abuse are also common among correctional populations. Approximately 80% of correctional populations have a history of illicit drug use or abuse (Spaulding et al., 2010), and half of the correctional population in the United States meet the criteria for abuse or dependence disorders. Of the 1.5 million arrestees with drug abuse disorders, only 55,000 receive treatment (Fiscella, 2010).

Alcohol misuse is also common among correctional populations, even during incarceration. In fact, inmates may make an illicit alcoholic beverage known as "pruno" from fruit, water, and sugar. This concoction may also incorporate other foods, such as root vegetables, left over from meals. In one correctional setting, pruno consumption caused botulism poisoning in several inmates (Thurston et al., 2012).

The correctional nurse should assess substance use and abuse in individual clients as well as in the inmate population as a whole. The nurse should also assess nutritional status and particular dietary needs for individual inmates (e.g., those with diabetes). Nurses may need to advocate for special diets to accommodate medical or religious needs. Types of diets that may be needed include kosher diets, low-salt diets, diabetic diets, consistency-modified diets, allergy diets, bland diets, and diets to address specific renal problems or gastric reflux.

Rest and physical activity. Rigid schedules may constrain inmates' abilities to get adequate rest or exercise. Inmates may complain of difficulty sleeping due to medical conditions, stress, poor sleep hygiene, noise and other environmental factors, or shift work. Other causes of sleep disturbances may include medical conditions, medication side effects, or rebound from use of sleep aids. Nurses need to carefully assess and address root causes of sleep difficulties rather than relying on pharmacologic sleep aids.

Some inmates may engage in vigorous physical activity as a way to pass time, and the nurse needs to be alert to the potential for overuse and muscle injury. Conversely, other inmates may become physically inactive, contributing to risks for cardiovascular disease and other obesity-related conditions.

Physical activity may be particularly important for incarcerated women engaged in smoking cessation which has been linked to significant weight gain (Cropsey et al., 2010). Potential safety hazards posed by exercise and recreation activities should also be assessed.

Sexual risk behaviors. Sexual behaviors prior to and during incarceration can also influence inmate health status. Early initiation of sexual activity is common among inmate populations, and the incidence of sexually transmitted diseases is high in this population. Among incarcerated youth, 90% of juveniles in one study engaged in more than three HIV risk behaviors, and 65% engaged in more than ten risk behaviors, many of them for more than 3 years (Teplin et al., 2013).

Sexual activity also occurs within the correctional setting. Such behavior may be consensual or nonconsensual, and high-risk behaviors such as anal intercourse are common. As many as 45% of state and federal prisoners and 3.2% of local jail inmates may be sexually assaulted while incarcerated (Greifinger, 2010). Lack of access to condoms and the prevalence of STIs in correctional populations promote the spread of disease to others in the setting. The nurse should assess the extent of sexual activity among the correctional population and the availability and use of condoms within correctional systems. Nurses may also need to advocate for provision of condoms to sexually active inmates.

HEALTH SYSTEM DETERMINANTS. Factors related to the correctional health system also influence the health status of correctional populations. Correctional facilities are the only settings in which people have a constitutional right to health care (Muse, 2011). Because many inmates enter the correctional setting with multiple health problems, the adequacy of the correctional health care system has a significant influence on the health status of the population. Depending on several factors, including size and financial capabilities, correctional facilities may take one of two approaches to the provision of health care services for inmates. Services may be provided in-house by staff employed by the facility, or the agency may contract with other provider agencies for needed services. In many institutions, a combination of both approaches is used.

Specific areas to be addressed in the correctional health care system include health promotion and illness prevention services, medical and dental services, mental health services, and emergency response capabilities. Health promotion services will be discussed in more detail later in this chapter. Minimum medical services should include screening, diagnostic, treatment, and follow-up services.

The correctional health care system should also make adequate provision for diagnostic and treatment services with access to health personnel evaluation in a timely fashion. In some situations, this may mean curtailing the discretion of corrections personnel in determining whether an inmate should be brought to the attention of health care providers. If needed diagnostic and treatment services are not available within the facility, arrangements should be in place for securing these services elsewhere. The need for diagnostic and treatment services extends to dental health and mental health needs as well as to physical health problems.

Correctional health services tend to be chronically underfunded, and some correctional systems have instituted copayments for medical and dental services provided. The intent of this practice is to decrease service utilization rates and generate funds. The courts have upheld the initiation of small fees for care. In a 2004 survey, less than 20% of correctional systems surveyed did not require some form of copayment from inmates. In one setting, institution of copayments decreased trips from emergency departments from 65 per month to fewer than 15 (Su, 2009).

Copayments may deter inmates from obtaining needed health care (Smith et al., 2013) and contribute to the spread of communicable diseases as well as increased costs for care of chronic conditions allowed to deteriorate. Correctional nurses may need to be actively involved in evaluating the effect of copayment systems on the health of inmates and the implications for the health of the general public if legitimate needs for services are not being addressed. They may also need to advocate for elimination of copayments if they are found to impede access to care.

The extent of emergency response capabilities (including suicide prevention programs) is another important aspect of the correctional health system. Emergencies may be inmate-specific or general. Examples of inmate-specific emergencies are medical emergencies (e.g., heart attack), psychiatric emergencies (e.g., suicide attempt), or traumatic injury. System-wide emergencies could include inmate-generated emergencies (e.g., riots) or natural or human-caused disasters affecting the correctional setting. Population health nurses should advocate for and be involved in disaster planning for correctional settings. Disaster planning may include plans for evacuation of inmates as well as staff. In addition to plans for safe evacuation and provision for the health and survival needs of inmates and staff, correctional disaster plans must address public safety issues and prevent escape during evacuation. Disaster planning will be dealt with in more detail in Chapter 25∞.

The health care system within a correctional setting should also make adequate provision for efforts to control communicable diseases. This means screening programs, isolation of infectious inmates, and follow-up on contacts both within and outside the correctional system.

For health care services to be adequate to meet clients' needs, health care personnel must be available in adequate numbers and with adequate preparation for practice in correctional settings.

Another consideration related to health system determinants is inmates' use of health care services prior to their incarceration. For example, the nurse might ask the female inmate when she had her last pap smear or mammogram. The nurse would also want to explore prior interactions with health care providers related to existing health problems. For example, was the client being seen for hypertension or other health problems? Or has the client not been taking antihypertensive medications because he or she did not have the prescription renewed?

Correctional health nursing. Nurses are a crucial element of the correctional health care system. Correctional or "forensic" nursing is a specialized area of population health nursing with a special target population. **Correctional nursing** is defined as nursing care designed to promote health and prevent or treat illness or injury in populations involved with the criminal justice system (American Nurses Association [ANA], 2013). **Forensic nursing**, on the other hand, is nursing practice directed toward investigation of injury or death resulting from violence, criminal activity, or accident. Forensic nursing also addresses issues of liability (International Association of Forensic Nurses & ANA, 2009). Advanced practice correctional nursing involves the performance of traditional and advanced practice nursing roles within jails and prisons (Hufft, 2013). Population health nurses working in correctional settings are more often focused on correctional nursing or advanced practice correctional nursing than forensic nursing. Correctional nursing roles include screening and evaluation, specific health screening, direct care, teaching, counseling, and providing linkages to continued care on release (Muse, 2009).

Work in correctional settings requires nurses to function within specific security parameters and to understand both the legal and public health implications of care in this setting. Correctional settings place constraints on how nurses may care for clients, and nurses must often balance custodial and care functions. Correctional nurses are actively involved in advocacy and may need to take professional risks within the setting to meet inmates' needs or initiate changes in the system. Nursing in correctional settings also requires superlative interpersonal skills and skills in collaborating with corrections personnel who often have a philosophical perspective far different from that of the nurse. Certification for correctional nurses is available from NCCHC (2014a) and the American Correctional Association (n.d.). For further information about certification requirements and processes, see the *External Resources* section of the student resources site. Certification provides recognition of the specialized expertise required for nursing practice in correctional settings (Schoenly, 2011).

Standards and guidelines for correctional health care. Standards have been established for both correctional health care systems and for nursing practice within those systems. As noted earlier, NCCHC has developed sets of standards for health care systems in jails, prisons, and juvenile facilities, as well as for mental health services and opioid treatment programs for correctional populations (NCCHC, 2014b). For further information about specific standards, see the *External Resources* section of the student resources site. In addition, NCCHC accredits correctional health systems. Accreditation is based on adherence to the relevant sets of standards.

Standards for nursing practice in correctional settings have been developed by the American Nurses Association and were last revised in 2013. The set of 16 standards address use of the nursing process in correctional settings as well as professional performance of nurses practicing in such settings (ANA, 2013). The revised standards also address a new standard related to the nurse's environmental health capabilities, focusing on knowledge of environmental concepts, and the use of strategies to reduce environmental health risks (Knox, 2013). For more information on correctional nursing standards, see the *External Resources* section of the student resources site.

Ethical concerns in correctional nursing. There are several ethical considerations that are particularly relevant to nursing in a correctional facility. The right to health care is an ethical as well as legal issue that has already been addressed. Other ethical issues include confidentiality and appropriate use of health care personnel, refusal of care, abuse of prisoners, and advocacy. Many of these issues are addressed in the various sets of standards discussed above, and readers should review NCCHC (2014b) documents for information with respect to these issues. Confidentiality issues may be a source of conflict in correctional settings when health care providers have access to information that may be of use in criminal proceedings against inmates. Health professionals in correctional institutions may be pressured to divulge client information or to assist with procedures designed to provide evidence for criminal proceedings (e.g., body cavity searches, blood alcohol levels) (Olsen, 2013). When these procedures need to be performed by trained personnel (e.g., venipuncture), they should be the task of personnel hired specifically for these types of responsibilities to prevent conflict of interest for health care providers and to avoid jeopardizing a relationship of trust between provider and client. Similarly, health care professionals should not be called on to engage in security measures or to participate in disciplinary decisions or in execution by lethal injection. Assuring appropriate use of personnel in the correctional setting may also mean making sure that nonprofessionals (including inmates) are not allowed to perform medical tasks or dispense medications.

Confidentiality, particularly with respect to HIV status, may be more difficult to achieve in a correctional environment. The intensive nature of treatment and the need for multiple doses of medication may serve to label inmates as infected, even when official confirmation of disease is not provided. This potential for lack of confidentiality may act as a deterrent to HIV testing and noncompliance with treatment in infected individuals. Another potential conflict related to confidentiality is the question of whether security personnel should be alerted to inmates' HIV-infection status to ensure their use of universal precautions.

In addition to maintaining confidentiality, nurses may be called on to support an inmate's refusal of care, including forcible administration of psychotherapeutic medications. Inmates have the right to refuse care unless they are determined to be legally incompetent to make that decision. Inmates' right to refuse care, however, must be balanced against community safety (Muse, 2011; Olsen, 2013). Decisions regarding abrogation of the right to refuse treatment should be based on facts in the individual situation, including the inmate's medical condition, prognosis, benefits and burdens of treatment, and the impact of refusal on other inmates. Refusal of care should be carefully documented, including the nature of the care refused, the inmate's stated reason for refusal, the date and time of refusal, provision of education on the possible consequences of refusal, and the inmate's signature or initials.

Aggressive or potentially suicidal inmates may be subjected to physical restraint if they are deemed a danger to themselves or to others. This includes the use of medical isolation when clients suspected of infectious diseases refuse screening procedures or treatment. Medical isolation may also be legitimately employed to protect inmates with symptomatic AIDS from opportunistic infection. Although the U.S. Supreme Court has upheld segregation of HIV-infected inmates, segregation breaches confidentiality and denies segregated inmates access to programs, such as work release and other programs available to other inmates. In addition, segregation may contribute to exacerbation of psychoses or depression.

Because of the imbalance of power inherent in a correctional setting, there is always the potential for abuse of inmates in the name of punishment. Preventing this and other forms of abuse of inmates (e.g., denial of health care services) is another ethical aspect of nursing in correctional settings. Finally, nurse advocacy may be needed in the correctional setting. Advocacy may be required at the level of the individual client to ensure that rights are upheld and that appropriate health care services are received or at the aggregate level to assure adequate health care delivery systems in correctional institutions.

NCCHC (2012) has delineated three guiding ethical principles for health care in correctional settings. These principles include the following:

- Medical autonomy: The health professional acts first in promoting the patient's interest and judgments should be based on patient needs not legal issues.
- Non-maleficence: Health care providers should not engage in any actions that would lead to patient harm.
- Medical neutrality: Providers should provide care to all inmates regardless of background, status, reason for incarceration, and so on.

Furthermore, an NCCHC position statement on health professionals' responsibility in the event of witnessing harm to inmates indicates that they (a) should not participate in any form of interrogation or abuse, including not providing consultation on such activities; (b) should not gather forensic information or share confidential information with authorities for use in abuse; (c) should not authorize or approve any physical punishment; (d) should promote policies that protect correctional employees who report abuse; and (e) should support training for staff to prevent abuse (NCCHC, 2012).

Features of the correctional setting that influence health are assessed by the population health nurse and then used to derive nursing diagnoses. Assessment tips for use with correctional populations are provided on the next page. In addition, a comprehensive tool for assessing the health status of correctional populations is provided on the student resources site.

Diagnostic Reasoning and Care of Correctional Populations

Based on information obtained in assessing the determinants of health, the nurse in the correctional setting formulates nursing diagnoses. Diagnoses should be validated with the client, significant others, or other health care providers when possible. Population health nurses working in correctional settings determine nursing diagnoses for individual clients as well as diagnoses related to the health needs of the total population of inmates and staff. For example, an individual diagnosis might be "uncontrolled diabetes mellitus due to substance abuse." A diagnosis related to the population group might be "increased potential for violence due to racial tensions and unrest." This second diagnosis would affect facility personnel as well as inmates since all might be involved in any violence that occurs.

Planning and Implementing Health Care for Correctional Populations

Planning to meet identified health problems in correctional settings may be accomplished independently by the nurse or in conjunction with other personnel within and outside the institution. Interventions may take place at any of the four levels of health care: health promotion, injury and illness prevention, resolution of existing health problems, and health restoration.

HEALTH PROMOTION. Health promotion in correctional settings involves provision of adequate nutrition, rest and exercise, health education, prenatal care, and contraceptive services. Health promotion in correctional settings differs from that in other settings in a number of ways. First, the general purpose of health promotion in correctional settings is to protect the health of others rather than to enhance the health of the particular inmate. Second, group health promotion efforts may be hampered by the compulsory nature of inmates' presence in the institution. For example, inmates may be resistant to health education because they perceive themselves as a "captive audience" with little option regarding participation. Third, the great majority of offenders are men who tend not to be as highly motivated with respect to health promotion as women. Health promotion in correctional settings often needs to focus less on information transmission than on attitude development or change, and behavioral change may not be as easy within the

FOCUSED ASSESSMENT Assessing Health and Illness in Correctional Settings

Biological Determinants

- What is the age, gender, and ethnic composition of the correctional population (inmates and staff)?
- What communicable and chronic health problems are prevalent among inmates? Among staff?
- What is the extent of injury in the population? What factors contribute to injuries?
- What is the prevalence of pregnancy among inmates?
- What are the immunization levels in the population?

Psychological Determinants

- What procedures are in place for dealing with suicidal ideation or attempts? Are these procedures followed?
- What is the psychological effect of incarceration? Does the individual inmate exhibit signs of depression? Does the inmate express thoughts of suicide?
- What is the extent of sexual assault among inmates? What are the psychological effects of assault?
- Are there inmates in the setting under sentence of death? If so, what psychological effects does this have? Are there terminally ill inmates in the population?
- What is the prevalence of mental illness among inmates?

Environmental Determinants

- Are there health or safety hazards present in the correctional facility?
- Is there potential for disaster in the area? Is there a disaster plan?

Sociocultural Determinants

- What political/legal issues influence the health of the correctional population?
- What is the socioeconomic status of members of the correctional population? What is the general educational level?
- What ethnic/cultural groups are represented in the correctional population? How does this influence the health status or risks of the population?
- What are the attitudes of health and correctional personnel toward inmates?
- What is the attitude of the surrounding community to the correctional facility and to the inmates?
- Are there intergroup conflicts within the population? Do these conflicts result in violence?
- What is the extent of violence in the correctional population? What factors contribute to violence?
- What family concerns influence the health of inmates? What is the effect of incarceration on the families of inmates?
- What is the extent of mobility in the population?
- Are inmates employed in the correctional setting? Are they employed outside? What health hazards, if any, are posed by the type of work done?
- How do security concerns affect the ability of health care personnel to provide services?
- What are the elements of the correctional subculture? How do they affect the health of the correctional population?

Behavioral Determinants

- Are there inmates with special nutritional needs? How well are these needs being met? What is the nutritional quality of food served in the correctional setting?
- What are the health-related behaviors of the correctional population? How do they affect health?
- What is the prevalence of tobacco use in the population?
- What is the prevalence of alcohol or drug abuse in the population?
- Do inmates have access to illegal drugs or alcohol within the correctional setting?
- How are medications dispensed in the correctional setting? Are there procedures in place to prevent inmates from selling medications or accumulating them for use in a suicide attempt?
- Do conditions in the correctional setting support adequate rest?
- Do conditions in the correctional setting promote physical activity?
- What is the extent of sexual activity in the correctional setting? To what extent do inmates engage in unsafe sexual practices? What is the availability of condoms?

Health System Determinants

- What health services are offered in the correctional setting? Are they adequate to meet needs?
- Are there isolation procedures in place for inmates with communicable diseases? Are these procedures followed?
- How are health care services funded? Is funding adequate to meet health needs? Are inmates charged a fee for health care services?
- What is the quality of interaction between internal and external health care services?
- What is the extent of emergency response capability of the correctional facility (e.g., to myocardial infarction, stab wound)?
- What provisions are made for continuity of care after release from the correctional facility?

constraints of the correctional setting as in the outside world. In addition, the correctional emphasis on punishment for crimes may result in political interference with health promotion efforts. Finally, given the extensive health problems encountered in this population, there may be little time or few resources available for health promotion efforts, which may receive lower priority than curative activities.

Nutritional intake in correctional settings may be far from adequate. NCCHC recommendations include the initiation of heart-healthy diets as a routine aspect of correctional settings (Wakeen, 2008). The nurse in this setting may need to monitor the diet of inmates and may need to influence administrative decisions regarding the nutritive value of meals served. There may also be a need to suggest changes in food served to facility personnel if meals are provided for them as well. In addition, the nurse may need to make arrangements to meet the special dietary needs of specific inmates based on their health status. Examples include a diabetic diet or a liquid diet for an inmate recuperating from a broken jaw. Juveniles, in particular, have special dietary needs, including the need for increased calories, calcium, phosphorus, and iron.

Juvenile facilities may participate in the U.S. Department of Agriculture's Child Nutrition National School Lunch Programs or School Breakfast programs, and population health nurses can encourage facility participation in these programs. Such participation involves meeting specific nutritional requirements and limitations on nonnutritive foods. Juveniles in adult facilities may be given adult meals with additional milk, fruits, and snacks (Robbins, 2009a). Women also have special nutritional needs, particularly pregnant women. As noted earlier, women have a tendency to gain weight during incarceration, so attention should be given to lower calorie foods.

Attention should also be given to provisions for adequate rest and physical activity by inmates. Nurses may need to advocate for adequate space and facilities for sleeping in inmate housing units. In addition, the nurse should work to assure that time and facilities are provided for inmates to engage in physical activity. In some instances, this may mean curtailing certain activities that place inmates at risk because of existing health problems. Nurses can also educate both inmates and staff on the benefits of activity and suggest forms of physical activity congruent with health status and available opportunities. Physical activity is particularly important for women who are engaged in smoking cessation programs as they have been shown to experience significant weight gain (Cropsey et al., 2010).

Both inmates and facility staff may be in need of a variety of health education efforts. Areas of importance include the elimination of risk factors for disease. Education programs that may be planned and implemented by nurses may include smoking cessation campaigns or stress management classes. Nurses can also advocate for access to smoking cessation assistance and aids such as nicotine patches. Education regarding problem solving and positive coping strategies may also benefit both staff and inmates.

Prenatal care is a significant health promotion activity for pregnant female inmates. NCCHC recommendations include provision of pregnancy screening for all women inmates and further screening of pregnant women for HIV and other STIs. Areas to be addressed in prenatal care include adequate nutrition, the effects of smoking and other substances on the fetus, parenting skills, discomforts of pregnancy, and planning for childcare if the child is delivered while the client is still in custody. Contraceptive education may benefit both pregnant and nonpregnant inmates. Health promotion strategies for correctional populations are summarized in Table 24-1●.

PREVENTION. Three aspects of prevention are pertinent to correctional health care. These include preventing incarceration as well as injury and illness prevention.

Preventing incarceration. As we saw earlier, CITs and special drug and mental illness courts are aimed at preventing incarceration of persons whose crimes are the result of substance abuse or mental illness. Similarly, programs funded by the Juvenile Justice and Delinquency Prevention Act are designed to prevent gang activity and other avenues of contact with the juvenile justice system. Other social programs may also serve to prevent youth involvement in criminal activity. For example, the Perry Preschool Project was credited with decreasing arrests, preventing school dropouts, and promoting education and employment among at-risk children. The program involved a daily preschool program with weekly home visits to address family problems over a 2-year period. Cost estimates indicate that $17 were saved for every dollar invested in the program, primarily in reduced criminal activity and better educational attainment (Welsh & Farrington, 2011). Population health nurses can advocate for and help initiate similar programs in low-income, high-risk communities.

Preventing illness. Preventing the spread of communicable diseases in correctional settings is an important primary prevention activity.

Possible approaches to infectious disease prevention include the use of universal precautions in the handling of blood and body fluids (National Institute for Occupational Safety and Health [NIOSH], 2011), isolation of infected persons when appropriate, immunization, and education on hygiene and

TABLE 24-1 Health Promotion Strategies for Correctional Populations

- Provision of adequate nutrition
- Provision of opportunities for adequate rest and exercise
- Health education for self-care, risk factor elimination, stress reduction, etc.
- Prenatal care for pregnant inmates
- Contraceptive education
- Advocacy for available health promotion services in correctional settings

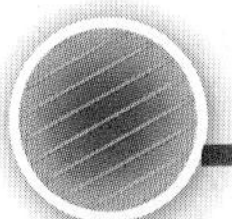

Evidence-Based Practice

Preventing Incarceration

A significant body of research suggests that prevention of delinquency and later criminal activity is much more effective than incarceration of offenders. In 2007, for example, Washington State allocated $48 million to evidence-based crime prevention and intervention programs. Although this was a political decision, unlike many such decisions, it was based on research findings related to effective interventions. A series of research studies conducted by the Washington State Institute for Public Policy explored the effects and cost-effectiveness of several adult and juvenile intervention programs. Based on their analysis of 571 evaluations of crime prevention and criminal justice programs, the institute was able to project the potential benefits and costs of certain intervention approaches. The evidence suggests that alternatives to prison can achieve cost savings to the public as well as some reduction in crime rates (Welsh & Farrington, 2011).

condom use during sexual encounters. Isolation is appropriate for diseases spread by airborne transmission such as measles and influenza. Isolation of HIV-infected individuals is not generally recommended. During community- or facility-based influenza outbreaks, isolation of infected inmates, removal of infected staff from duty, and prohibiting visitors with recent symptoms also help to prevent the spread of disease (NCCHC, 2009a).

Immunization is particularly recommended for HBV (Malek et al., 2011), but other immunizing agents may be needed as well, depending on the incidence of specific diseases in the general community. For example, measles immunizations may be warranted for all inmates and staff during a measles outbreak in the community, and hepatitis A vaccine is recommended for inmates at risk for hepatitis A (e.g., inmates who engage in oral–anal intercourse). Corrections staff, particularly health care personnel, should also receive HBV immunization. Condom use and substance abuse education on harm reduction strategies (e.g., use of clean needles and syringes for injection drug use) can also help to prevent the spread of hepatitis B and C in correctional populations.

Because correctional settings house a large proportion of inmates who are infected with or at risk for hepatitis, provision of HBV vaccine is a good way to minimize disease prevalence within correctional settings and in the larger community. Similarly, seasonal influenza immunization is recommended for correctional populations (Malek et al., 2011). As noted earlier, many correctional facilities do not receive adequate supplies of influenza vaccine, and states and local jurisdictions may need to re-evaluate vaccine allocation policies to address the needs of this vulnerable population (Lee et al., 2012). Population health nurses in correctional settings may be actively involved in providing immunizations and advocating vaccine availability to inmates.

Periodic outbreaks of other infectious diseases may also necessitate immunization programs to prevent the spread of disease. For example, several recent mumps outbreaks have been reported in correctional facilities. In addition to immunization, isolation of infected inmates and quarantine of exposed inmates or staff are warranted. If infected inmates are scheduled for release, immunization of household members may also be indicated (Ringsdorf et al., 2010).

Recommended TB control measures in correctional settings include screening of all inmates for infection, isolation of suspected and confirmed cases, and treatment of persons with active or latent TB infection. Preventing the spread of TB may also employ engineering controls related to adequate ventilation systems, air filtration, and irradiation of areas where infected persons are housed. **TB prophylaxis** is the treatment of persons with reactive tuberculin skin tests but without evidence of active TB (in other words, those with latent infection), to prevent their development of disease. TB prophylaxis is also recommended for persons with HIV infection even in the absence of evidence of latent TB. Corrections personnel with positive skin tests should also receive prophylaxis. In addition, all inmates and personnel should be educated on infection control procedures and universal precautions, and health care providers should use appropriate protective barriers to prevent infection (e.g., gloves, aprons, face shields, goggles, and gowns, as needed) (NIOSH, 2011). Population health nurses are often responsible for providing directly observed TB therapy and in monitoring its effectiveness. They also monitor clients receiving therapy for potential adverse reactions to medication.

HIV prevention education is another area of importance among incarcerated women (and men) who are often at high risk for infection. Population health nurses may need to advocate for the availability of condoms for use by inmates who are sexually active. There is considerable debate on providing condoms for incarcerated inmates, but a recent study in California's state prison system indicated that condom availability in prisons would minimize the spread of HIV infection and other STIs and significantly reduce treatment costs (California HIV/AIDS Policy Research Centers, 2013).

Other more mundane avenues for preventing communicable diseases include routine skin screening for infectious lesions and effective wound infection control procedures. Promotion of inmate hygiene, use of alcohol-based hand rubs for hand washing, and effective laundry procedures can also prevent the spread of infections, particularly methicillin-resistant *staphylococcus aureus* (MRSA) infections. Pregnancy prevention using emergency contraception may also be warranted, particularly for young girls in juvenile detention facilities (Robbins, 2009b).

Illness prevention efforts may also be required for chronic conditions. For example smoking cessation, obesity reduction, and promotion of physical activity may serve to prevent a variety of chronic illnesses. Specific prevention strategies for chronic illness are similar to those discussed in Chapter 27∞.

Preventing injury. Injury prevention is also needed in correctional settings. For example, population health nurses may identify environmental hazards or occupational hazards in the correctional setting that present injury risks and can advocate for their removal or modification. Nurses may also provide safety education for inmates and staff. Specific injury prevention strategies may also be warranted for certain at-risk populations in the setting. For instance, the nurse may need to advocate for a lower bunk for an inmate with limited mobility or ensure the availability of assistive devices such as walkers or canes. Nurses may also identify chemical hazards or rodent infestations that need to be addressed.

Other avenues for injury prevention include suicide prevention and prevention of violence. The primary mode of suicide prevention is identification of inmates at risk for suicide. Those at risk for suicide should be closely monitored and receive timely referrals for psychiatric services. Suicide assessment involves obtaining information regarding past personal or family history of suicide attempts, the extent of life stress and social support, presence of suicidal ideation, and presence of mental illness.

Components of an effective suicide prevention plan include initial screening and ongoing identification of inmates at risk, staff training, inmate assessment by qualified mental health professionals, appropriate housing, and referral to needed mental health services. Other elements of effective plans include adequate communication between corrections and health care staff, immediate intervention for a suicide attempt or suicide in progress, and availability of needed equipment and supplies (e.g., resuscitation breathing masks, gloves, defibrillators, and tools for opening jammed cell doors and cutting down a hanging inmate). Suicide prevention may also involve judicious and carefully supervised use of suicide prevention cells (Suicide Prevention Resource Center, 2014). Additional guidelines and resources for suicide prevention in correctional settings have been compiled by the Jail Suicide Task Force of the American Association of Suicidology (Kennedy & McKeon, n.d.). For more information about the guidelines, see the *External Resources* section of the student resources site.

Violence prevention activities may need to be directed to both inmates and corrections staff. The purpose of such activities is to teach alternative behavioral responses to violence (Sung, 2010). Recommended components of violence prevention programs in correctional settings include incorporation of violence assessment (including prior exposure to violence) as part of intake screening, referral of inmates with a history of personal violence or violence exposure for counseling, education on alternative responses to potentially violent situations for both inmates and corrections staff, and referral of inmates for continued counseling on release. Prevention emphases in correctional health care are summarized in Table 24-2●.

RESOLVING EXISTING HEALTH PROBLEMS. Strategies for addressing existing health problems in correctional settings focus on screening and diagnostic and treatment activities.

Screening. Standards related to screening have been described as some of the more important standards for correctional health care. Screening has a threefold purpose: identifying and addressing the health needs of inmates, promoting early identification of key problems prior to more comprehensive assessments, and identifying and isolating potentially communicable inmates.

Screening begins with medical clearance or a determination that a specific inmate is well enough to be admitted to the facility. Medical clearance is intended to ensure that emergent health needs are met. Based on NCCHC standards, medical clearance screening is followed within 2 to 4 hours of admission by receiving screening. *Receiving screening* is the collection of health-related information to identify newly arrived inmates who pose a health threat to themselves or the general facility population. The goal of receiving screening is to identify needs for care and continued treatment of existing conditions. Receiving screening includes a comprehensive health history; observation of appearance, behavior, ease of movement, breathing, and skin integrity; and presence of suicidal ideation (Kistler & Chavez, 2011a). Receiving screening also includes an initial assessment for mental health issues that may be conducted by correctional staff, but mental health screening, required within 14 days of admission, must be conducted by qualified mental health professionals (Kistler & Chavez, 2011b). Receiving screening should also include assessment for substance abuse and signs of intoxication or withdrawal (NCCHC, 2010b).

Screening may also include specific tests for infectious diseases. For example, tuberculin skin testing is recommended for inmates who will be incarcerated long enough for the results to be read. The Centers for Disease Control and Prevention (CDC) has also recommended routine screening for sexually transmitted diseases in correctional populations, particularly among adolescent and young females (Miller, 2011). Recommendations have also been made for routine screening for sexual abuse or for risk of being abusive (Greifinger, 2010) and for evidence of dementia (Wilson & Barboza, 2010).

Routine screening for infectious diseases may be conducted on either an opt-in or opt-out basis. In opt-in screening, screening is conducted for inmates who agree to it. In opt-out screening, the screening test is performed unless the inmate specifically refuses it. CDC specifically recommends opt-out

TABLE 24-2 Prevention Foci and Related Strategies for Correctional Populations

Focus	Strategies
Preventing incarceration	• Community support programs for high-risk families • Delinquency prevention programs for youth • Advocacy for CITs, mental health courts, and substance abuse courts
Preventing infectious diseases	• Immunization • Isolation of persons with infectious diseases • Quarantine of exposed persons • Restriction of infected staff from work • Restriction of visitors with symptoms of disease • Use of universal precautions for blood and body fluids • TB prophylaxis • Education for safe sex • Advocacy for condom availability • Hygiene education
Pregnancy prevention	• Provision of emergency contraception
Preventing chronic conditions	• Risk factor modification • Smoking cessation • Obesity reduction
Preventing injury	• Modification of environmental safety hazards • Safety education
Preventing suicide	• Identification of high-risk inmates • Referral for mental health services • Staff education for recognition of risk and response to attempted suicide • Effective communication with correctional personnel regarding inmate risk status • Advocacy for emergency response equipment and supplies • Judicious use and careful supervision of isolated inmates • Immediate response and first aid for suicide attempt
Preventing violence	• Violence risk assessment • Referral for mental health services • Anger management counseling • Education on conflict management strategies

screening for HIV infection. Opt-out screening tends to be more effective, achieving a 90% screening rate, compared to a 72% rate for opt-in screening, and only 5% when screening is provided on the basis of inmate request (Strick, MacGowan, & Belcher, 2011). Opt-out screening has the potential for identifying inmates with hepatitis B and C, TB, syphilis, gonorrhea, and chlamydia, in addition to HIV infection, thereby promoting early treatment and preventing the spread of disease in the facility (Malek et al., 2011). Offering routine HIV screening at intake resulted in the diagnosis of 52 new cases in one correctional setting (Spaulding et al., 2013). In large volume settings in which universal screening of all inmates is impractical, screening targeted to specific arrest charges (e.g., drug charges, sex charges, parole violation) has been suggested, but evidence for the effectiveness of this approach is limited (Harawa et al., 2009).

Subsequent assessments may take one of two approaches: full population assessment or individual assessment. In the full population approach, every inmate receives a comprehensive assessment after intake screening. The individual approach provides comprehensive assessment when clinically indicated for an individual inmate. Both approaches include a review of screening information, a comprehensive health history, further inquiry into problem areas, a physical examination, and routine diagnostic and laboratory tests. Assessments result in treatment plans tailored to the needs of particular inmates (Kistler, 2008).

Screening for mental health problems is another important element in resolving existing health problems. Mental health screening is needed to identify inmates at risk for harm to themselves or others, determine inmates' functional capabilities, identify the need to transfer inmates to a specific mental health unit, and determine the inmate's potential to benefit from treatment. There is also a need for ongoing assessment for suicide risk, particularly among inmates that may engage in self-injury (Fagan et al., 2010).

Suggested elements of mental health assessment in correctional settings include an inmate's psychiatric history, current use of psychotropic medications, presence of suicidal ideation, and a history of suicide attempt. Other relevant screening information includes drug and alcohol use, history of violence or victimization, history of special education placement, and history of traumatic brain injury. Assessment also includes evaluation of the inmate's response to incarceration and evidence of developmental disability. Population health nurses may also assess inmates' readiness and motivation for treatment.

Population health nurses may also be involved in other screening activities with inmates. For example, they may be involved in screenings for work clearance or periodic screening for work-related conditions or prior to transfer to another facility or court. In addition, they may be called upon to screen for harm following a use-of-force incident or when an inmate is restrained (Knox, 2013). In addition, they may screen for infectious diseases or chronic conditions based on risk factors or inmate health histories.

Nurses in correctional settings are also involved in triage during sick call activities. Inmates with health complaints can ask to be seen during sick call. At this time, the nurse determines the need for treatment of specific conditions under specific protocols, advice for self-care, or referral for a higher level of care (Knox, 2013). Protocols would cover, at a minimum, a problem definition and etiology, subjective and objective information to be collected, relevant nursing diagnoses with possible differential diagnoses, interventions to be considered, patient education, and disposition and follow-up care (Smith, 2009).

Diagnosis and treatment. Diagnosis and treatment may be required for medical conditions, mental illness, or substance abuse. Correctional nurses may be actively involved in the diagnosis and treatment of existing medical conditions. Many minor illnesses are handled exclusively by nurses working under medical protocols as noted earlier. In other instances, nurses are responsible for implementing medical treatment plans initiated by physicians or nurse practitioners. This may involve giving medications or carrying out treatment procedures. Treatment procedures would be handled in much the same way as in any health care facility. Dispensing medications in a correctional setting, however, requires that the nurse directly observe the client taking the medication, and often only a single dose is dispensed at a time rather than giving the client several doses of medication to be taken at prescribed times. This precaution is necessary because of the potential for inmates to sell medications to other inmates or to stockpile certain medications for use in a suicide attempt. In some instances (e.g., epidemics of communicable diseases), mass treatment of the entire correctional population or subpopulation in a given setting may be warranted.

Treatment for TB and HIV infection in correctional settings is complicated by the long-term nature of the therapies. Inmates with TB (except those also infected with HIV) should be placed in respiratory isolation in negative-pressure rooms until they are no longer contagious. If negative-pressure rooms are not available in the correctional facility, arrangements should be made to transport the inmate to a local hospital with such facilities. Respiratory isolation should also be instituted for all inmates with respiratory symptoms suspicious of TB disease. Treatment should involve a multi-drug regimen, particularly when exposure to MDR infection is suspected. Drug susceptibility testing should be carried out on all inmates with active TB, and treatment should rely on directly observed therapy (DOT).

HIV/AIDS therapy is also difficult in correctional settings because of the number of factors that promote noncompliance. As noted earlier, having to receive multiple doses of medication each day may "tag" inmates as infected and leave them open to discrimination and assault. Security practices such as lockdowns and search and seizure may interfere with dispensing of medications or attendance at support group or education programs. A **lockdown** occurs when inmates are locked in their cells at times when they would ordinarily have greater freedom to come and go throughout the facility, usually in response to a security incident or to permit a search for contraband items (drugs, alcohol, weapons) or a **search and seizure** procedure. During search and seizure, all medications are taken away, so clients in some facilities where self-medication is permitted may have their medications removed and be unable to take doses as directed.

Strategies that can increase compliance with TB treatment regimens include simplifying the regimen to include fewer doses or combining medications into a single pill, protecting confidentiality, using medications with fewer side effects, and dealing with those side effects that occur. DOT has also been found to be effective in promoting compliance with highly active antiretroviral therapy (HAART) for inmates with HIV/AIDS. Treatment is also more effective if provided by health care professionals who have expertise with HIV/AIDS. In larger systems, inmates with HIV infection may be moved to facilities with this expertise or where this expertise is available in the community.

Treatment may also be needed for a variety of chronic health problems experienced by correctional populations. Again, population health nurses working in correctional settings may provide treatment and monitor treatment effectiveness under approved protocols. They may also be responsible for making referrals for specialty services to outside health care agencies. This may require particular advocacy on the part of population health nurses to assure that outside appointments are kept when they are jeopardized by security concerns or lack of security personnel to escort inmates to community facilities.

Treatment should also be available for substance abuse and mental health problems. There are a number of sound reasons for mental health care in correctional settings. These include the need to reduce the disabling effects of mental illness and to maximize the ability of inmates to participate in rehabilitation programs. A second reason is to minimize the suffering of the inmates themselves. Finally, treatment of inmates with mental illness and substance abuse problems promotes the safety of all, both within the correctional setting and in the community when the inmate is released. Unfortunately, many inmates with mental illness or substance abuse disorders do not receive treatment, or medications being prescribed for treatment are discontinued on incarceration despite evidence that medication-assisted treatment and cognitive behavioral therapy have been shown to be effective in addressing these problems (NCCHC, 2010b). In one large longitudinal study of incarcerated youth, for example, only 15% of juvenile offenders with major psychiatric disorders were treated when incarcerated and only 8% received treatment on release (Teplin et al., 2013). Population health nurses may need to advocate for the availability of treatment for mental illness and substance abuse disorders in correctional settings. They may also need to campaign at state legislative levels for authorization and funding of diversion programs to promote treatment options rather than incarceration (Stettin et al., 2013).

Methadone maintenance is a special area of consideration in treatment for substance abuse. For many opiate abusers, methadone may be an important step in treatment for addiction. Although a significant proportion of persons in methadone treatment programs get arrested during their enrollment, few correctional settings make provision for continuing methadone treatment except for pregnant inmates. Involuntary cessation of methadone leads to painful withdrawal symptoms and risk of death, as well as relapse to opiate use and subsequent rearrest. NCCHC standards require mental health services for all inmates in need of them that include both individual and group counseling (Kistler & Chavez, 2010). Provision of mental health services in correctional settings is often hampered by variables related to correctional systems, personnel, and inmates. System-level variables include limited fiscal allocations for services and privatization of correctional facilities, the institutional climate, and limitations in access to care posed by inmate classification systems. Privatization of correctional settings (government contracting with private corporations for operation of correctional facilities) often leads to cost cutting to remain competitive, and cost cutting may eliminate services, such as mental health services, that are considered "nonessential." In addition to entire correctional systems run by private for-profit companies under contract to government agencies, health care services in correctional settings may also be privatized. For example, a county sheriff's department may contract with a private firm for health care personnel and services within the correctional setting rather than hiring health care personnel as county employees. Government service contracts are usually given to the lowest bidder, providing an incentive to decrease the quality or frequency of services in the interests of cost containment. In addition, privatization may lead to less official oversight of correctional facilities and the quality of care provided. On the other hand, privatization has the advantage of services provided by people who have a health care perspective rather than a custodial focus.

The institutional climate is frequently one of punishment rather than treatment, so inmates may not receive needed mental health services. Finally, classification of inmates as security risks may put them at risk for isolation, exacerbation of mental health problems, and lack of access to many services available to other inmates.

Personnel variables that affect mental health treatment services in correctional settings include staff attitudes to mentally ill inmates and training of correctional and health care personnel relative to mental health needs. Cultural diversity and differences between correctional personnel and inmates may also make identification of mental health problems more difficult. Cultural factors related to mental health and illness are discussed in more detail in Chapters 5∞ and 28∞.

Inmate-related variables include mental health treatment history, a slower response to medication among inmates than in the general population due to the prevalence of substance abuse, and peer pressure within the setting to not appear weak or vulnerable. In addition, the nuisance side effects associated with psychotropic medications may lead many inmates to be noncompliant with treatment plans.

Issues that need to be addressed, in addition to mental health or substance abuse treatment needs, include continuity of public assistance, housing support, and the need for social service referrals and treatment of other medical conditions.

Research has indicated that treatment of substance abuse while an inmate is in prison reduces the likelihood of rearrest and reduces the return to previous drug use patterns. For example, treatment mandated by drug courts has successfully reduced crime rates and rearrests by 11% to 14% (Anglin et al., 2013). Promoting self-care for mental illness and using educational, behavioral, and motivational strategies have also been effective in minimizing the effects of mental illness (Shelton et al., 2010).

Treatment may also be needed for a variety of chronic conditions. Treatment would be similar to that provided to the general population, but may need to be modified to fit the correctional setting. For example, self-medication may be constrained by facility regulation, as in the case of inmates giving themselves insulin. Foci for chronic disease management in correctional settings are similar to those in community settings and include self-care when possible, development of inmate support groups, patient education, assistance in dealing with medication side effects, and reinforcing compliance to achieve treatment goals.

There may also be a need to arrange for physical and psychological treatment of sexual abuse (Greifinger, 2010) and treatment of acute psychosis as mentioned earlier (Mathis, 2010). Other areas of concern in treating existing problems are sleep disorders, dealing with violent and agitated inmates, and addressing dementia in the correctional population. Treatment for sleep disturbances usually focuses on promoting sleep hygiene (e.g., regular sleep–wake patterns, avoidance of stimulants, environmental modifications to minimize noise and light, etc.) and life changes, such as a healthier diet, stress management, and daily exercise (Anderson, 2010). Pharmacologic sleep aids, medical conditions, and medications that affect sleep may also need to be addressed.

Four basic approaches can be used to deal with aggressive and agitated inmates: de-escalation, seclusion, physical restraint, and pharmacologic restraint (Savage, 2010). De-escalation involves talking to the inmate to calm him or her, and involves listening with empathy, giving a context to the agitation, providing options, confirming non-cooperation, and more definitive action. Seclusion should be used only for immediate protection of the inmate or others, not for punishment, and the inmate should be carefully observed. Physical restraint may be necessary, but may have serious health consequences and should be minimized, and pharmacologic restraint has the potential for drug side effects. Nurses need to keep in mind that agitation may be the result of physical illness. They may also need to advocate for judicious use of restraints and monitor the health status of inmates under physical or pharmacologic restraint (Savage, 2010). Restraint of pregnant women poses particular risks for both the women and the fetus, and should be accomplished in the least restrictive manner possible with consultation from medical staff. Wrist restraints, in particular, should be applied, if necessary, in such a way as to allow the women to protect herself in the event of a fall (NCCHC, 2010a).

Treatment for inmates with dementia involves planning ahead for a possible influx of patients as time goes by. Management includes informing inmates of their diagnosis, structuring the environment to minimize confusion, and developing and using nonpharmacologic interventions such as praise for positive behaviors, relaxation training, support of remaining skills and abilities, and promoting exercise and group interaction. Effective management also involves training staff to communicate effectively with inmates with dementia, promoting client choices, repeating introductions, using strategies for getting clients' attention, using gestures, giving simple instructions, and giving clients time to process their thoughts and responses (Wilson & Barboza, 2010).

When physical or mental health services needed by inmates are not available within the correctional health care setting, correctional health nurses are often responsible for arranging appointments with outside consultants or providers. In addition to arranging for appointments, correctional nurses usually have to arrange transportation and security supervision. This often means that scheduling of appointments can be extremely complicated. Once inmates have been seen by outside providers, correctional nurses also need to follow through on recommendations for treatment. Because many outside providers do not understand the constraints of correctional systems, nurses may need to be creative in promoting treatment compliance. For example, in some small rural jails, there are no facilities for warm soaks to injuries, and special diets may also be difficult to arrange. Other recommendations that pose security hazards may not be able to be fulfilled (e.g., metal braces that can be converted to weapons). Population health nurses may need to advocate for treatments that are not typically used in the setting, or may need to explain to outside providers why a particular treatment option is not feasible in a correctional setting.

Nurses will also be involved in emergency response to life-threatening situations. Emergency situations likely to be encountered include seizures, cardiac arrest, diabetic coma or insulin reaction, attempted suicide, and traumatic injury due to inmate violence. The nurse would respond to these situations with actions designed to relieve the threat to life and stabilize the client's condition prior to transportation to a hospital facility either within or outside the correctional system. Correctional nurses may also find themselves involved in emergency care of large numbers of persons injured in human-caused or natural disasters involving the correctional facility (Kistler, 2009). Major foci in resolving existing health problems in correctional settings are summarized in Table 24-3●.

HEALTH RESTORATION AND END-OF-LIFE CARE. Health restoration in correctional settings focuses on areas similar to that in any setting, preventing or dealing with complications of disease and preventing problem recurrence when possible. Intervention directed toward preventing complications of existing health problems depends on the conditions experienced by inmates. For example, health restoration for the inmate with diabetes will be directed toward preventing circulatory changes, diabetic ketoacidosis, and hypoglycemia. For the client with arthritis, restoration will focus on pain management and prevention of mobility limitations.

Population health nurses may also help inmates deal with the long-term consequences of chronic conditions. An example might be providing a walker to an inmate with mobility limitations. Health restoration activities may also be directed toward preventing the recurrence of problems once they have been resolved. For example, the nurse may educate an inmate who has been treated for gonorrhea on the use of condoms to prevent reinfection.

In addition, there are three special considerations in health restoration in correctional settings: long-term care planning, reentry planning, and end-of-life care. Each of these major foci will be addressed briefly.

Long-term care planning. With the aging of the correctional population and longer sentences without option for parole, there is a need to engage in long-term care planning for elderly inmates and those with chronic conditions. Correctional systems have taken a variety of approaches to long-term care planning for these subpopulations. Older inmates or those with disabilities related to chronic illness may be transferred to appropriate facilities or housing conditions separate from the general inmate population. Usually such facilities have an infirmary where exacerbations of chronic conditions requiring hospitalization can be addressed in-house. In other instances, inmates may be transferred to assisted living facilities that provide assistance with the activities of daily living. Terminally ill inmates may be transferred to specialized hospice units or to community hospices (Hufft, 2013). Alternatively, hospice services can be provided to inmates housed in the general population, at least until inmates become severely debilitated.

When inmates with chronic illnesses or disability are housed in the general population, correctional systems may provide "home care" services and case management to address their long-term care needs. In such systems, nurses might go to inmate housing units to provide care in the same way that they would provide home care in community settings. Another alternative is to have other inmates function as "personal care attendants" for disabled inmates, assisting them with certain activities of daily living (e.g., bathing).

TABLE 24-3 Foci and Related Strategies for Resolving Existing Health Problems in Correctional Populations

Focus	Related Strategies

Screening	• Screening for communicable diseases
	  • Tuberculosis
	  • HIV infection
	  • Hepatitis B
	  • Sexually transmitted diseases
	• Routine screening for chronic conditions
	  • Asthma, hypertension, obesity, seizure disorder
	  • Mammography
	  • Papanicolaou smear
	  • Colorectal cancer
	• Provision of specialized screening services for inmates at risk (e.g., diabetes)
	• Screening for suicide risk
	• Screening for pregnancy
	• Screening for mental illness and substance abuse
	• Screening for treatment motivation
	• Advocacy for availability of routine and specialized screening services

Diagnosis and treatment	• Provision of diagnostic services relevant to inmate needs • Treatment of existing acute and chronic conditions • Education for self-management of chronic conditions • Treatment of mental illness and substance abuse • Methadone maintenance for opiate users • Emergency care for accidental and intentional injuries • Treatment of sleep disorders • Treatment of violent and agitated inmates • Treatment of inmates with dementia • Care for psychiatric emergencies • Emergency care in the event of a disaster • Advocacy for effective and available diagnostic and treatment services in correctional settings

Other health restoration activities related to long-term care include providing assistive devices, monitoring the status of chronic conditions and treatment compliance, monitoring for adverse effects of treatment, and providing support in dealing with the emotional and physical consequences of long-term physical or mental illness. Population health nurses may be involved in providing these interventions or in advocating their availability in the correctional setting. They may also need to advocate for access to these kinds of services for specific inmates.

Reentry planning. Approximately 95% of the 2 million state and federal and 10–12 million jail inmates will eventually be released back into the community (Bureau of Justice Assistance, 2013). In 2009, for example, 729,295 state and federal prisoners were released back into the community, and many more were released from local jails. Many of these inmates re-enter the larger society as probationers or parolees. A **probationer** is an adult offender who has been remanded to community-based supervision, often as an alternative to incarceration. Probationers usually are held in correctional facilities for only a short time until their case has been tried in court. A **parolee** is an adult released from a correctional facility to community supervision after serving all or part of his or her sentence. Both probationers and parolees are subject to re-incarceration if they violate the terms of probation or parole. In 2009, there were 4.2 million U.S. men and women under federal, state, or local probation and 819,308 on parole (U.S. Census Bureau, 2013i).

The dual process of incarceration and reentry has been cited as a public health opportunity. Reentry provides opportunities for addressing health care and other issues and preventing re-incarceration. Unfortunately, little planning may be initiated toward meeting inmates' reentry needs. The Second Chance Act, enacted in 2008, was designed to assist released inmates in the transition from jail or prison into the community and to prevent rearrest and incarceration. The act provides funding at federal, state, and local levels for a variety of reentry programs as well as research on reentry needs and strategies that support successful reentry (Bureau of Justice Assistance, 2013). Unfortunately, organized reentry programs are few and may not be available to the majority of inmates released from jails or prisons. A National Academies report found that less than 10% of released prisoners receive reentry planning services (Smith et al., 2013).

Reentry, in the correctional context, is the process of leaving jail or prison and being reintegrated into the larger society. Two challenges inherent in reentry are protecting the public and promoting effective reintegration into the community.

Reentry also poses risks for the spread of communicable diseases within the general population if infected inmates have not been effectively treated.

Released inmates often have limited job skills and social support networks, so many of them have difficulty reintegrating into the larger community. For example, half of released inmates lack a high school diploma, and more than half have been fired from a prior job. Prior to incarceration, many supported themselves with income from illegal activities (Urban Institute, 2014). For these reasons, released inmates may have difficulty finding employment and housing due to the stigma attached to incarceration (Bonnie et al., 2012). At the same time, the social capital or infrastructure of communities that reabsorb large numbers of released inmates are often stretched beyond their capacity (Underwood, 2011). Given the lack of support services, resources, and opportunities for legitimate employment, many released inmates return to criminal activities. An estimated two thirds of inmates released in any given year will be rearrested within 3 years of release (Bureau of Justice Assistance, 2013). Effective reentry planning and support following release can help to prevent rearrest and incarceration.

Reentry planning begins with the development of systematic discharge protocols to be used with all inmates to be released from a correctional setting. Such protocols should be developed with input from the communities to which inmates will be released. Population health nurses can be active advocates for reentry planning for all inmates. They can also advocate community involvement in the development of reentry planning protocols and in designing community infrastructures to support reentry.

Planning considerations related to individual inmates are based on an individualized needs assessment and include issues related to health care and social and financial needs. As many as 80% of persons released from correctional facilities have ongoing physical or mental health conditions that require long-term management (Wang et al., 2012). These clients need copies of their medical records, a sufficient supply of medications, referrals (and possibly actual appointments) for physical and mental health services in the community, and assistance with health insurance coverage. This may mean advocacy on the part of population health nurses to get Medicaid, Medicare, or Veteran's Administration benefits reinstated, or assisting inmates to find low-cost health care services. Advocacy may also be required to ensure that inmates have a sufficient supply of necessary medications until they can find employment and purchase medications on their own. This is particularly important for inmates who are receiving long-term therapy for HIV/AIDS or TB. Population health nurses may also need to advocate for continuing therapy for mental illness or substance abuse or for hormonal therapy for transgender individuals (NCCHC, 2009b). Released women prisoners may also need contraceptive assistance, particularly former narcotics abusers for whom cessation of use may result in increased fertility (Smith et al., 2013).

There is a particular need for effective communication between the correctional system and community health agencies. Too often, inmates are discharged with ongoing health needs (e.g., HIV/AIDS or TB treatment) without local health authorities being notified. In addition to making referrals and links to community services, population health nurses in correctional settings should also develop systems for monitoring service continuation and its effects on inmate health status.

Reentry planning should also address a variety of social and financial needs of released inmates. For example, many inmates have alienated family members and may not be able to find shelter with their families. In this case, population health nurses may need to assist in arranging housing for former inmates. Referrals may also be needed for employment assistance or job training. Unfortunately, federal spending on employment training in correctional settings has been drastically reduced in recent years, and a third of inmates in one large study would have liked to receive programs that were not available to them in correctional facilities. However, in-prison job training, holding a job while incarcerated, and earning a GED while incarcerated have been linked with successful employment on release (Urban Institute, 2014). Population health nurses may need to advocate at the societal level for job training programs for inmates and others with low levels of employability. They may also need to advocate for relaxation of restrictions on financial and other assistance benefits for people who have been incarcerated.

For some inmates, reentry planning may entail assistance with family reintegration. Population health nurses may assist families to deal with concerns about bringing a released inmate back into the family constellation, particularly if the inmate was incarcerated for a crime involving family violence. There are also some instances in which inmates should not return to families if their presence may put family members at risk of harm.

Specific programs have been found to promote effective reentry and prevent recidivism. For example, reentry housing units help ease the transition to the community for juvenile offenders. They have also been found to forestall attempts by other inmates to prevent early release by involving soon-to-be released adolescents in fights or other infractions. Such programs, which involve moving to special housing units 4 to 6 weeks prior to release, allow adolescents to develop healthy relationships with adult staff, address anxiety about release, and engage in prerelease employment activities (Maynard & Alston, 2011). Similarly, a holistic aftercare program for women drug abusers has been successful in preventing relapse, with participants being significantly less likely to return to jail within a year after release (Matheson et al., 2011).

End-of-life care. End-of-life care for inmates with terminal illnesses may be similar to that on the outside. For example, population health nurses may need to discuss advance directives with inmates and help those who wish to execute advance directives. Nurses may also need to advocate adherence to advance directives when they have been executed by an inmate. In addition to discussing advance directives with inmates, correctional health care personnel need to develop policies regarding the timing of advance directives, communicating information about advance directives when inmates are transferred to outside hospitals or hospice settings, and addressing effective pain control for seriously ill inmates.

Just as in the general population, referral for hospice care may be appropriate for terminally ill inmates. Some correctional facilities have in-house hospice units, and others may transfer inmates to community hospices when there is no security risk to the public. Whether in a hospice setting, in an infirmary, or in the general correctional population, terminally ill inmates are likely to need assistance in setting their affairs in order. For some inmates, there may also be a need to reconcile with family members. Population health nurses can be instrumental in facilitating these end-of-life activities. For example, they may advocate with family members for reconciliation or assist inmates to obtain legal assistance in settling any assets the inmates may have on their heirs. Symptom control and palliative care are also important aspects of end-of-life care in correctional settings.

There are also two unique aspects to end-of-life care that need to be addressed in correctional settings. The first is the concept of "compassionate release" or "medical parole." **Compassionate release** is the release of a seriously ill or disabled inmate back into the community to receive needed health care services from community agencies and, often, to permit time with family members. Compassionate release is most often used for terminally ill inmates; however, the Federal Bureau of Prisons also makes provisions for compassionate release for elderly inmates, death or incapacitation of a family caregiver of an inmate's child, or incapacitation of a spouse or registered partner of an inmate. In all instances, inmates granted compassionate release should be judged as not posing a threat to the safety of the community (U.S. Department of Justice, 2013). Similar provisions may exist in state and local jurisdictions as well. As noted in Table 24-4●, population health nursing advocacy may be required to initiate or support a compassionate release decision. In addition to advocating for compassionate release when appropriate, community health nurses will assist with arranging for follow-up care after release.

The second unique aspect of end-of-life care in correctional settings relates to inmates who have been sentenced to death. These inmates have the same needs for psychological end-of-life care as those with terminal illnesses, but their care is often complicated by feelings of hopelessness and attendant security measures (e.g., the use of handcuffs and shackles and constant supervision). Aspects of health restoration and end-of-life care in correctional settings are summarized in Table 24-4.

TABLE 24-4 Health Restoration and End-of-life Strategies for Correctional Populations

Focus	Related Activities
Long-term care planning	• Transfer to appropriate facility as needed • Provision of "home care" in general population • Use of assistive devices as needed • Continued monitoring of the status of chronic conditions • Monitoring treatment compliance • Monitoring for adverse effects of treatment • Provision of support in dealing with long-term consequences of chronic illness • Advocacy for effective long-term care service availability
Reentry	• Development of systematic discharge protocols • Development of individual discharge plans • Provision for continuity of health care • Arrangement for a supply of necessary medications on discharge • Arrangement for health insurance coverage • Provision for housing and financial assistance needs • Assistance with job training and employment as needed • Assistance with family reintegration as needed • Coordination of community health care and correctional activities • Advocacy for effective prerelease planning for all inmates • Advocacy for development of community infrastructure to support reentry • Advocacy for civil rights of released inmates
End-of-life care	• Development of advance directives as desired by inmates • Symptom control and palliative care • Advocacy for compassionate release and arrangement for follow-up care • Advocacy for adherence to advance directives by personnel • Provision of emotional and spiritual support to inmates and significant others • Referral to hospice care • Assistance with setting life in order • Assistance with family reconciliation as needed

Evaluating Health Care for Correctional Populations

The principles that guide the evaluation of health care in correctional settings are the same as those applied in other settings. The nurse evaluates the outcomes of care for individual clients in light of identified goals. Correctional nurses may also be involved in evaluating health outcomes for groups of inmates or for the entire facility population, including staff. In addition, the nurse examines processes of care and makes recommendations for improvements in terms of quality, efficiency, and cost-effectiveness.

CHAPTER RECAP

Correctional facilities present a useful setting in which population health nurses can engage in health-promotive and illness-preventive activities with clients who may have little knowledge of these activities. Clients in correctional settings may be less motivated than those in other settings, but can realize substantial health benefits through the efforts of population health nurses during incarceration and in promoting follow-up on release. Population health nursing efforts in correctional settings also help to prevent the flow of health problems back into the larger population, thereby benefiting society as a whole.

CASE STUDY Nursing in the Correctional Setting

You are the correctional nurse responsible for sick call. So far today you have seen eight inmates with fever and severe upper respiratory symptoms; your diagnosis is influenza infection which has been prevalent in the surrounding community for the last several weeks. Several of the inmates seen describe other inmates housed in their cell block with similar symptoms. Further checking reveals that three guards from the affected cell blocks came to work earlier in the week with symptoms of influenza, but all three went home sick when their symptoms worsened.

The affected inmates are from two cell blocks that house 30 inmates each. The inmates from these two cell blocks share a communal dining facility not used by other cell blocks. Inmates at high risk for complications of influenza received influenza vaccine, but other inmates in the facility did not due to a lack of available vaccine. One of the infected inmates was recently transferred from another facility and is severely immunocompromised due to HIV infection. He did not receive immunization at a prior facility despite his health status. The facility infirmary is staffed round the clock, but only has a capacity of four beds.

1. What are the biological, psychological, environmental, sociocultural, behavioral, and health system factors operating in this situation?
2. What actions would you take related to illness prevention, resolution of health problems, and health restoration in this situation? Why?

REFERENCES

American Correctional Association. (n.d.). *Professional certification: Corrections certification program*. Retrieved from https://www.aca.org/certification/

American Dental Association. (2013). *Meth mouth*. Retrieved from http://www.mouthhealthy.org/en/az-topics/m/meth-mouth

American Nurses Association. (1985). *Standards of nursing practice in correctional facilities*. Kansas City, MO: Author.

American Nurses Association. (2013). *Correctional nursing: Scope and standards of practice* (2nd ed.). Silver Spring, MD: Author.

Anderson, J. R. (2010). "I can't sleep": Treating complaints of sleep disturbances in corrections. *Correct Care, 24*(1), 14–15.

Anglin, M. D., Nosyk, B., Jaffe, A., Urada, D., & Evans, E. (2013). Offender diversion into substance use disorder treatment: The economic impact of California's Proposition 39. *American Journal of Public Health, 103*, 1106–1102. doi:10.2105/AJPH.2012.301168

Blair, P., & Greifinger, R. B. (2011). The health care reform law: What does it mean for jails? *Correct Care, 25*(1), 10–12.

Bonnie, R. J., Chemers, B. M., & Schuck, J. (Eds.). (2012). *Reforming juvenile justice: A developmental approach*. Washington, DC: National Academies Press.

Braverman, P. K., & Murray, P. J. (2011). American Academy of Pediatrics policy statement: Health care for youth in the juvenile justice system. *Pediatrics, 128*, 1219–1235. doi:10.1542/peds.2011-1757

Brittain, J., Axelrod, G., & Venters, H. (2013). Deaths in New York City jails, 2001-2009. *American Journal of Public Health, 103*, 638–640. doi:10.2105/AJPH.2012.301042

Bureau of Justice Assistance. (2013). *Second Chance Act (SCA)*. Retrieved from https://www.bja.gov/ProgramDetails.aspx?Program_ID=90

California HIV/AIDS Policy Research Centers. (2013). *Proposal to mandate condom distribution in prisons would reduce correctional facility costs for inmate health care in California*. Retrieved from http://www.californiaaidsresearch.org/initiatives_programs/_files/condom%20distribution%20in%20prisons%20bill.pdf

Coalition for Juvenile Justice. (n.d.). *Juvenile Justice and Delinquency Prevention Act: Core requirements*. Retrieved from http://www.juvjustice.org/juvenile-justice-and-delinquency-prevention-act/core-requirements

Coalition for Juvenile Justice. (2013). *Reauthorize the Juvenile Justice and Delinquency Prevention Act (JJDPA): Invest in what works*. Retrieved from http://www.juvjustice.org/sites/default/files/resource-files/resource_903_0.pdf

Coalition for Juvenile Justice. (2014). *Overview of FY14 appropriations for juvenile justice*. Retrieved from http://www.juvjustice.org/sites/default/files/resource-files/Act4jj%20OVerview%20of%20FY14%20Appropriations%20Bill%20FINAL.PDF

Cropsey, K. L., McClure, L. A., Jackson, D. D., Villalobos, G., Weaver, M. F., & Stitzer, M. L. (2010). The impact of quitting smoking on weight among women prisoners participating in a smoking cessation intervention. *American Journal of Public Health, 100,* 1142–1148. doi:10.2105/AJPH.2009.172783

Division of HIV/AIDS Prevention. (2014). *HIV in correctional settings*. Retrieved from http://www.cdc.gov/hiv/risk/other/correctional.html

Drennan, V., Goodman, C., Norton, C., & Wells, A. (2010). Incontinence in women prisoners: An exploration of the issues. *Journal of Advanced Nursing, 66,* 1953–1967. doi:10.1111/j.1365-2648.2010.05377.x

Dyer, W. J., Pleck, J. H., & McBride, B. A. (2012). Imprisoned fathers and their family relationships: A 40 year review from a multi-theory view. *Journal of Family Theory & Review, 4*(1), 20–47. doi:10.1111/j.1756-2589.2011.00111.x

Fagan, T. J. (2003). Mental health in corrections: A model for service delivery. In T. J. Fagan & R. K. Ax (Eds.), *Correctional mental health handbook* (pp. 1–19). Thousand Oaks, CA: Sage.

Fagan, T. J., Cox, J., Helfand, S. J., & Aufderheide, D. (2010). Self-injurious behavior in correctional settings. *Journal of Correctional Health Care, 16,* 48–66. doi:10.1177/1078345809348212

Fiscella, K. (2010). Drug treatment policy: Time for Reform. *Correct Care, 24*(1), 3.

Greifinger, R. B. (2010). Sexual abuse: What is the health professional's role in prevention and response? *Correct Care, 24*(1), 12–13.

Harawa, N. T., Bingham, T. A., Butler, Q. R., Dalton, K. S., Cunningham, W. E., Behel, S., & MacKellar, D. A. (2009). Using arrest charge to screen for undiagnosed HIV infection among new arrestees: A study in Los Angeles County. *Journal of Correctional Health Care, 15,* 105–117. doi:10.1177/1078345809331466

Hufft, A. G. (2013). Correctional nursing. In R. M. Hammer, B. Moynihan, & E. M. Pagliaro (Eds.), *Forensic nursing: A handbook for practice* (2nd ed., pp. 375–399). Burlington, MA: Jones & Bartlett Learning.

International Association of Forensic Nurses & American Nurses Association. (2009). *Forensic nursing: Scope and standards of practice*. Silver Spring, MD: American Nurses Association.

Jenkins, R. (2014). *My 2014 wishlist for a reauthorized but improved JJDPA*. Retrieved from http://www.juvjustice.org/blog/760

Johnston, N. (n.d.). *Prison reform in Pennsylvania*. Retrieved from http://media.wix.com/ugd//4c2da0_41bed342ea390827839e1ffa4b3dca97.pdf

Kennedy, D., B., & McKeon, R. (n.d.). *Jail/custody suicide: A compendium of suicide prevention standards and resources*. Retrieved from http://www.suicidology.org/c/document_library/get_file?folderId=231&name=DLFE-107.pdf

Kistler, J. E. (2008). Spotlight on the standards. *Correct Care, 22*(2, 18), 6–7

Kistler, J. E. (2009). Spotlight on the standards. *Correct Care, 23*(4), 7.

Kistler, J. E., & Chavez, S. (2010). Spotlight on the standards. *Correct Care, 24*(3), 6.

Kistler, J. E., & Chavez, S. (2011a). Spotlight on the standards. *Correct Care, 25*(1), 7–8.

Kistler, J. E., & Chavez, S. (2011b). Standards Q&A: Expert advice on NCCHC standards. *Correct Care, 25*(1), 28.

Knox, C. (2013). *Essentials of correctional nursing*. Retrieved from http://essentialsofcorrectionalnursing.com/2013/06/14/the-new-scope-and-standards-of-practice-for-correctional-nursing/

Lee, A. S., Brendes, D. M., Seib, K. G., Whitney, E. A. S., Berkelman, R. L., Omer, S. B., ..., Meyer, P. L. (2012). Receipt of a(H1N1)pdm09 vaccine by prisons and jails—United States, 2009–10 influenza season. *Morbidity and Mortality Report, 60,* 1737–1740.

Ludwig, A., Cohen, L., Parsons, A., & Venters, H. (2012). Injury surveillance in New York City Jails. *American Journal of Public Health, 102,* 1108–1111. doi:10.2105/AJPH.2011.300306

Malek, M., Bazazi, A. R., Cox, G., Rival, G., Baillargeon, J., Miranda, A., & Rich, J. (2011). Implementing opt-out programs at Los Angeles County Jail: A gateway to novel research and interventions. *Journal of Correctional Health Care, 17,* 69–76. doi:10.1177/1078345810385916

Matheson, F. I., Doherty, S., & Grant, B. (2011). Community-based aftercare and return to custody in a national sample of substance-abusing women offenders. *American Journal of Public Health, 101,* 1126–1132. doi:10.2105/AJPH.20102.300094

Mathis, H. (2010). Acute psychotic delirium and sudden death in custody: Tips for prevention. *Correct Care, 24*(4), 14–15.

Maynard, M., & Alston, V. (2011). Juvenile voice: Special housing unit smooths reentry. *Correct Care, 25*(1), 23.

Miller, J. L. (2011). New STD screening guidelines for corrections. *Correct Care, 25*(1), 3.

Morse, R. (2007). *The relationship between crime and poverty in black antebellum Boston*. Retrieved from http://www.primaryresearch.org/bh/research/morse/index.php.

Muse, M. V. (2009). Correctional nursing: The evolution of a specialty. *Correct Care, 23*(1), 3–4.

Muse, M. V. (2011). Correctional nursing practice: What you need to know (part 5). *Correct Care, 25*(1), 16–17.

Nagin, D. S., & Pepper, J. V. (Eds.). (2012). *Deterrence and the death penalty*. Washington, DC: National Academies Press.

National Coalition for Homeless Veterans. (n.d.). *Background and statistics*. Retrieved from http://nchv.org/index.php/news/media/background_and_statistics/

National Commission on Correctional Health Care. (2009a). CDC issues H1N1 influenza guidance for corrections and detention facilities. *Correct Care, 23*(2), 3.

National Commission on Correctional Health Care. (2009b). *Transgender health care*. Retrieved from http://www.ncchc.org/transgender-health-care-in-correctional-settings

National Commission on Correctional Health Care. (2010a). *Restraint of pregnant inmates*. Retrieved from http://www.ncchc.org/restraint-of-pregnant-inmates

National Commission on Correctional Health Care. (2010b). *Substance use disorder treatment for adults and adolescents*. Retrieved from http://www.ncchc.org/substance-use-disorder-treatment-for-adults-and-adolescents

National Commission on Correctional Health Care. (2012). *Correctional health care professionals' response to inmate abuse*. Retrieved from http://www.ncchc.org/correctional-health-care-professionals'-response-to-inmate-abuse

National Commission on Correctional Health Care. (2014a). *CCHP-RN certification*. Retrieved from http://www.ncchc.org/CCHP-RN

National Commission on Correctional Health Care. (2014b). *Standards: A framework for quality*. Retrieved from http://www.ncchc.org/standards

National Institute for Occupational Safety and Health. (2011). *Correctional health care workers: Information for workers—Simple and safe work practices*. Retrieved from http://www.cdc.gov/niosh/topics/correctionalhcw/workers.html

Olsen, D. (2013). Ethical considerations in forensic nursing. In R. M. Hammer, B. Moynihan, & E. M. Pagliaro (Eds.), *Forensic nursing: A handbook for practice* (2nd ed., pp. 45–71). Burlington, MA: Jones & Bartlett Learning.

Osborne Association. (n.d.). *Children of incarcerated parents fact sheet*. Retrieved from http://www.osborneny.org/images/uploads/printMedia/Initiative%20CIP%20Stats_Fact%20Sheet.pdf

Polk, S. (2011). *Truth in sentencing: A process that works*. Retrieved from http://azsentencing.org/issues/117-truth-in-sentencing

Prison and asylum reform. (n.d.). Retrieved from http://www.ushistory.org/us/26d.asp

Purtie, J. (2013). Felon disenfranchisement in the United States: A health equity perspective. *American Journal of Public Health, 103*, 632–637. doi:10.2105/AJPH.2012.300933

Ringsdorf, L., Heerema, B., Ruiz, J., & Sanchez, R. (2010). Mumps: A jail outbreak and public health response. *Correct Care, 24*(4), 12.

Robbins, J. (2008). Juvenile suicide and prevention: An interview with expert Lindsay Hayes. *Correct Care, 22*(2), 23–27.

Robbins, J. (2009a). Juvenile voice. *Correct Care, 23*(2), 23.

Robbins, J. (2009b). Juvenile voice: Emergency contraception in Maryland. *Correct Care, 23*(4), 23.

Rold, W. J. (2011). Supreme Court Oks overcrowding reduction to protect inmate health rights. *Correct Care, 25*(3), 10–12.

Savage, S. (2010). Violent and agitated inmates: A review of management and a call for research. *Correct Care, 24*(3), 12–13.

Schoenly, L. (2011). Correctional nursing practice: What you need to know (part 7). *Correct Care, 25*(3), 18.

Shelton, D., Ehret, M. J., Wakai, S., Kapetanovic, T., & Moran, M. (2010). Psychotropic medication adherence in correctional facilities: A review of the literature. *Journal of Psychiatric and Mental Health Nursing, 17*, 603–613. doi:10.1111/j.1365-2850.2010.01587.x

Shiroma, E. J., Ferguson, P. L., & Pickelsimer, E. E. (2010). Prevalence of traumatic brain injury in an offender population: A meta-analysis. *Journal of Correctional Health Care, 16*, 147–159. doi:10.1177/1078345809356538

Smith, A. (Rapporteur), Committee on Causes and Consequences of High Rates of Incarceration, Committee on Law and Justice, Division of Behavioral and Social Science and Education, Board on the Health of Select Populations, & Institute of Medicine. (2013). *Health and incarcerations: A workshop summary*. Washington, DC: National Academies Press.

Smith, S. (2009). The nurse is in: Designing effective nursing sick call guidelines. *Correct Care, 23*(3), 14–15.

Spaulding, A. C., Bowden, C. J., Kim, B. I., Mann, M. C., Miller, L., Mustaafaa, G. R., … Belcher, L. (2013). Routine HIV screening during intake medical evaluation at a county jail—Fulton County, Georgia, 2011–2012. *Morbidity and Mortality Weekly Report, 62*, 495.

Spaulding, A. C., Perez, S. D., Seals, R. M., Hallman, M. A., Kavasery, R., & Weiss, P. S. (2010). Diversity of release patterns for jail detainees: Implications for public health interventions. *American Journal of Public Health, 101*, S347–S352. doi:10.2105/AJPH.2010.300004

Stanford Law School. (2013). *Three strikes basics*. Retrieved from http://www.law.stanford.edu/organizations/programs-and-centers/stanford-three-strikes-project/three-strikes-basics

Stettin, B., Frese, F. J., & Lamb, H. R. (2013). *Mental health diversion practices: A survey of the states*. Retrieved from http://tacreports.org/storage/documents/2013-diversion-study.pdf

Strick, L. B., MacGowan, R. J., & Belcher, L. (2011). HIV screening of male inmates during prison intake medical evaluation—Washington, 2006–2010. *Morbidity and Mortality Weekly Report, 60*, 811–813.

Su, I. J. (2009). How our medical co-pay program improved health care delivery. *Correct Care, 23*(3), 18.

Suicide Prevention Resource Center. (2014). *The role of corrections professionals in preventing suicide*. Retrieved from http://www.sprc.org/sites/sprc.org/files/CorrectionOfficers.pdf

Sung, H.-E. (2010). Prevalence and risk factors of violence-related and accident-related injuries among state prisoners. *Journal of Correctional Health Care, 16*, 178–187. doi:10.1177/1078345810366287

Teplin, L. A., Abram, K. M., Washburn, J. J., Welty, L. J., Hershfield, J. A., & Dulcan, M. K. (2013). *The northwestern juvenile project: Overview*. Retrieved from http://www.ojjdp.gov/pubs/234522.pdf

Thurston, D., Risk, I., Hill, M. B., Vitek, D., Bogdanow, L., Robertson, J., et al. (2012). Botulism from drinking prison-made illicit alcohol—Utah, 2011. *Morbidity and Mortality Weekly Report, 61*, 782–784.

Torrey, E. F., Kennard, A. D., Eslinger, D., Lamb, R., & Pavle, J. (2010). *More mentally ill persons are in jails and prisons than hospitals: A survey of the states*. Retrieved from http://tacreports.org/storage/documents/2010-jail-study.pdf

Treatment Advocacy Center. (2012). *No room at the inn: Trends and consequences of closing public psychiatric hospitals*. Retrieved from http://tacreports.org/bed-study

Treatment Advocacy Center & National Sheriff's Association. (2014). *The treatment of persons with mental illness in jails and prisons: A state survey*. Retrieved from http://tacreports.org/storage/documents/treatment-behind-bars/treatment-behind-bars.pdf

Underwood, R. L. (2011). Public health implications of medical care discontinuity for imprisoned black men. *American Journal of Public Health, 101*, 1540–1541.

United Nations Office on Drugs and Crime. (n.d.). *HIV and prisons in Sub-Saharan Africa: Opportunities for action*. Retrieved from http://www.unodc.org/documents/hiv-aids/Africa%20HIV_Prison_Paper_Oct-23-07-en.pdf

United Nations Office on Drugs and Crime. (2006). *Compendium of united nations standards and norms in crime prevention and criminal justice*. Retrieved from http://www.unodc.org/pdf/criminal_justice/Compendium_UN_Standards_and_Norms_CP_and_CJ_English.pdf

United Nations Office on Drugs and Crime. (2013). *United nations prison-related standards and norms*. Retrieved from http://www.unodc.org/newsletter/en/perspectives/no02/page004a.html

Urban Institute. (2014). *Returning home: Understanding the challenges of prisoner reentry*. Retrieved from http://www.urban.org/center/jpc/returning-home/index.cfm#findings

U.S. Census Bureau. (2013a). *Table 73. Group quarters population by type of group quarter and selected characteristics: 2009. In the 2012 statistical abstract: The national data book, population, households, families, group quarters*. Retrieved from http://www.census.gov/compendia/statab/cats/population/households_families_group_quarters.html

U.S. Census Bureau. (2013b). *Table 306. Crimes and crime rates by type of offense: 1980-2009. In the 2012 statistical abstract: The national data book, law enforcement, courts and prisons*. Retrieved from http://www.census.gov/compendia/statab/cats/law_enforcement_courts_prisons.html

U.S. Census Bureau. (2013c). *Table 310. Murder victims—circumstances and weapons used or cause of death: 2000–2009. In the 2012 statistical abstract: The national data book, law enforcement, courts and prisons*. Retrieved from http://www.census.gov/compendia/statab/cats/law_enforcement_courts_prisons.html

U.S. Census Bureau. (2013d). *Table 312. Homicide trends: 1980–2008. In the 2012 statistical abstract: The national data book, law enforcement, courts and prisons.* Retrieved from http://www.census.gov/compendia/statab/cats/law_enforcement_courts_prisons.html

U.S. Census Bureau. (2013e). *Table 324. Arrests by sex and age: 2009. In the 2012 statistical abstract: The national data book, law enforcement, courts and prisons.* Retrieved from http://www.census.gov/compendia/statab/cats/law_enforcement_courts_prisons.html

U.S. Census Bureau. (2013f). *Table 325: Arrests by race: 2009. In the 2012 statistical abstract: The national data book, law enforcement, courts and prisons.* Retrieved from http://www.census.gov/compendia/statab/cats/law_enforcement_courts_prisons.html

U.S. Census Bureau. (2013g). *Table 326: Juvenile arrests for drug abuse offenses: 1980 to 2009. In the 2012 statistical abstract: The national data book, law enforcement, courts and prisons.* Retrieved from http://www.census.gov/compendia/statab/cats/law_enforcement_courts_prisons.html

U.S. Census Bureau. (2013h). *Table 347: Prisoners under jurisdiction of federal or state correctional authorities â€" summary by state: 1990–2009. In the 2012 statistical abstract: The national data book, law enforcement, courts and prisons.* Retrieved from http://www.census.gov/compendia/statab/cats/law_enforcement_courts_prisons.html

U.S. Census Bureau. (2013i). *Table 348. Adults under correctional supervision. In the 2012 statistical abstract: The national data book, law enforcement, courts and prisons.* Retrieved from http://www.census.gov/compendia/statab/cats/law_enforcement_courts_prisons.html

U.S. Census Bureau. (2013j). *Table 349. Jail inmates by sex, race, and Hispanic origin: 1990–2009. In the 2012 statistical abstract: The national data book, law enforcement, courts and prisons.* Retrieved from http://www.census.gov/compendia/statab/cats/law_enforcement_courts_prisons.html

U.S. Census Bureau. (2013k). *Table 351. Prisoners under sentence of death by characteristic: 1980–2009. In the 2012 statistical abstract: The national data book, law enforcement, courts and prisons.* Retrieved from http://www.census.gov/compendia/statab/cats/law_enforcement_courts_prisons.html

U.S. Department of Justice. (2013). *Program statement: Compassionate release /reduction in sentence.* Retrieved from http://www.bop.gov/policy/progstat/5050_049.pdf

U.S. Department of State. (2012). *Report on international prison conditions.* Retrieved from http://www.state.gov/documents/organization/210160.pdf

Venters, H., Lainer-Vos, J., Razvi, A., Crawford, J., Venable, P. S., & Drucker, E. (2008). Bringing health care advocacy to a public defender's office. *American Journal of Public Health, 98,* 1953–1955.

Wakeen, B. (2008). Turning lemons into (sugar-free) lemonade: How food budgets cuts can improve diets. *Correct Care, 22*(3), 18–20.

Wang, E. A., Hong, C. S., Shavit, S., Sanders, R., Kessell, E., & Kushel, M. B. (2012). Engaging individuals recently released from prison into primary care: A randomized trial. *American Journal of Public Health, 102,* 222–229.

Welsh, B. C., & Farrington, D. P. (2011). The benefits and costs of early prevention compared with imprisonment: Toward evidence-based policy. *The Prison Journal, 91,* 120S–137S.

Wilson, J., & Barboza, S. (2010). The looming challenges of dementia in corrections. *Correct Care, 24*(2), 12–14.

Zlodre, J., & Fazel, S. (2012). All cause and external mortality in released prisoners: Systematic review and meta-analysis. *American Journal of Public Health, 102,* 267–275.

CHAPTER

25 Care of Populations Affected by Disaster

Learning Outcomes

After reading this chapter, you should be able to:

1. Describe ways in which disaster events may vary.
2. Describe the elements of a disaster.
3. Describe two aspects of disaster-related assessment.
4. Identify biological, psychological, environmental, sociocultural, behavioral, and health system considerations to be assessed in relation to a disaster.
5. Describe two aspects of health promotion related to disasters.
6. Discuss foci in prevention related to disaster events.
7. Identify the component elements of an effective disaster response plan.
8. Analyze the role of community health nurses with respect to health promotion, prevention, response, and health restoration or recovery related to disaster situations.

Key Terms

bioterrorism
community resilience
community resource maps
community risk maps
complex emergencies
disaster
disaster preparedness
early warning systems
emergency
health care disaster
human-generated disasters
immediate care
internally displaced persons (IDPs)
logistical coordination
natural disasters
pandemics
preimpact mobilization
reconstitution
reconstruction
refugee
rescue chains
syndromic surveillance
synergistic disasters
technological disasters
terrorism
triage
vulnerability analysis

Advocacy Then

Responding to the San Francisco Earthquake

Early on an April morning in 1906, San Francisco experienced an 8.25-magnitude earthquake that caused massive fires. More than 3,000 people died, and 28,000 buildings burned. Half of the city's population was homeless, and more than 225,000 people were injured. Because the Central Emergency Hospital had been destroyed, nurses hastened to tent hospitals, which were being established all over the city including in Golden Gate Park, Ft. Mason, and the grounds of the Presidio. At one point, one of the makeshift hospitals was threatened by uncontrolled fires and more than 350 patients were evacuated to safer locations. Later, one of those locations was threatened by fire, but the fire was diverted before it reached the site.

Physicians who had been attending the California Medical Convention in the city also volunteered their services. Personal accounts described volunteers raiding local pharmacies for needed supplies. Some of the health care volunteers worked 7 days and nights with little rest. Although later accounts by nurses indicated a relatively well-organized response, particularly in the light of the lack of advance planning, they also described the tendency of "charity workers" to "pauperize a self-respecting community" treating displaced citizens as if they were dependent paupers. Chinese survivors were also badly treated by outside volunteers and local citizens. Despite these blots on the record, the nurses engaged in heroic work. As one of them later noted, if "continuity of life is dependent upon adaptability to the environment, we possessed that qualification in a high degree" (Lucy Fisher, as quoted in Wall & Kelly, 2011, p. 51).

Advocacy Now

Promoting Disaster Preparedness

Disaster preparedness can save lives as well as minimize physical damage. Each year, the American Public Health Association (APHA) sponsors a "Get Ready Day" when local chapters engage in advocacy activities to promote emergency preparedness in their own communities. Preparedness initiatives range from development of personal/family readiness kits including the "big six" items identified by the American Red Cross (bottled water, nonperishable food, a battery-operated or hand-cranked radio, flashlights with extra batteries, medications and first aid supplies, and important documents) (Kukaswadia, 2013) to holding preparedness fairs in schools or other community sites to working with grocers to promote stockpiling of nonperishable foods among their customers. Less labor-intensive initiatives include sharing "Get Ready Day" information with others on your Facebook or Twitter page or with people at school or work (APHA, 2014). For information on planning "Get Ready" activities for your community, see the *External Resources* section of the student resources site.

Every day, a disaster occurs somewhere in the world (Baack & Alfred, 2013). In the last two decades, worldwide disasters cost $629 billion (Bosher & Dainty, 2011), and from 2000 to 2012, disasters affected 2.9 billion people and caused 1.2 million deaths throughout the world. In 2012 alone, disaster damage costs were more $138 billion (United Nations Office for Disaster Risk Reduction [UNODRR], 2013). In the United States, an average of 50 federally declared disasters occurred each year from 1980 to 2011 with a peak of 99 disasters in 1999 alone (Veenema & Woolsey, 2013).

Defining and Categorizing Disasters

A **disaster** is a destructive event that interferes with normal everyday function, the consequences of which cannot be effectively managed by the population experiencing it (Veenema & Woolsey, 2013). This definition highlights the difference between an emergency and a disaster. An **emergency** is a sudden event with serious adverse consequences that requires an immediate response but lies within the capabilities of those affected. A house fire, for example, is an emergency. A disaster, on the other hand, cannot be addressed with usual procedures and requires assistance beyond the ordinary. The wildfire that destroyed more than 300 homes and caused 16 deaths in San Diego in 2003 is an example of a fire-related disaster.

The Center for Research on the Epidemiology of Disasters (CRED) maintains a database of disasters that occur throughout the world. Four criteria are used to define disasters for inclusion in the database. These criteria include: (a) more than 10 deaths, (b) more than 100 people affected, (c) declaration of a state of emergency, and (d) a call for international assistance (CRED, 2009b). Based on the final criteria, the majority of U.S. disasters would not meet the definition since the bulk of them are handled without assistance from abroad.

Disasters are classified into two broad categories: natural and man-made or human-generated. **Natural disasters** are destructive events arising from natural forces, such as severe weather patterns; epidemics of human, plant, or animal diseases; or insect infestations (Baack & Alfred, 2013). **Human-generated disasters**, on the other hand, are catastrophic events arising from human actions, either intentional or unintentional, that cause significant damage to people, the environment, or property (Baack & Alfred, 2013). Both categories can result in a **health care disaster**, which is an event that overwhelms health care resources (Veenema & Woolsey, 2013).

These general categories can be further classified into several subcategories. For example, human-generated disasters may be complex emergencies, technological disasters, or synergistic disasters. **Complex emergencies** are situations that cause numerous casualties and numerous other adverse events (e.g., starvation, displacement) and populations exposed to war, political conflict or civil unrest (Veenema & Woolsey, 2013). **Technological disasters** are events caused by major transportation accidents, industrial accidents, unplanned nuclear energy release, fires, explosions, or releases of hazardous substances that have direct or indirect adverse effects on large numbers of people (Veenema & Woolsey, 2013). **Synergistic disasters**, also called NA-TECH disasters, are a combination of natural and technological disasters.

The Centers for Disease Control and Prevention (CDC, 2014c) categorizes disasters as (a) natural disasters and severe weather, (b) bioterrorism, (c) chemical emergencies, (d) mass casualties, and (e) radiation emergencies. Natural disasters and severe weather are definitely not human-generated, whereas bioterrorism results from intentional human actions. Chemical and radiation emergencies and mass casualty events (e.g., the collapse of a building or an explosion) may be either intentionally caused or unintentional.

Natural disasters can be further broken down into geophysical, meteorological, hydrological, climatological, and biological disasters (CRED, 2009a). Geophysical disasters are those resulting from movements within the earth and include earthquakes and resultant tsunamis, volcanic eruptions, rock falls, avalanches, landslides, and subsidence. Meteorological disasters include severe winter weather, severe thunderstorms, hurricanes, tornadoes, cyclones, severe sandstorms, and tropical storms. Hydrological disasters include floods and wet land mass movements, such as mud slides. Climatologic disasters include extreme temperatures due to heat or cold waves, drought, and wildfires. Finally, biological disasters result from epidemics of disease in people, plants, or animals (CDC, 2014d, CRED, 2009a). Epidemics that affect major segments of the world are called **pandemics**.

CDC distinguishes among a number of different types of chemical emergencies including biotoxins, blister agents, blood agents, caustics, choking/lung/pulmonary agents, incapacitating agents, long-acting anticoagulants, and metals. Additional chemical agents include nerve agents, organic solvents, riot control agents, toxic alcohols, and vomiting agents (CDC, 2014b). Table 25-1 • summarizes the various types of natural and chemical disasters.

War and civil conflict and terrorism are specific forms of human-generated disasters that occur with increasing frequency throughout the world. War and civil conflict are usually long-term events that have a singular capacity to destroy societal infrastructures leading to significant suffering among those affected (Burkle, 2013). War is defined as widespread conflict between groups of people, often motivated by religious or political differences or socioeconomic factors.

War and civil conflict result in a number of adverse effects for populations in addition to the numbers of people killed and injured. Some of these effects include destruction of a population's economic structure, food and water systems, electrical power sources, and transportation and communication systems. Other effects include famine, poor health, and violation of human rights. In large part, these effects are due to the diversion of resources from meeting population needs to supporting a war effort (Klare, Levy, & Sidel, 2011). A further significant effect lies in the displacement of large numbers of people. Displaced persons may include those who move from one area of

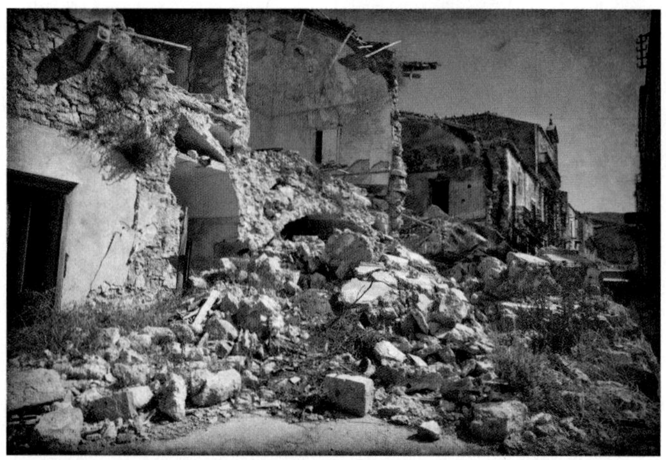

Some parts of the world experience frequent earthquakes that result in widespread devastation. *(lapas77/Fotolia)*

TABLE 25-1 Types and Examples of Natural Disasters and Chemical Emergencies

Types of Natural Disasters	Examples
Biological: Disasters caused by exposure of living organisms to pathogenic microorganisms	Epidemics of human, animal, or plant diseases
Climatological: Disasters resulting from extreme changes in climate	Heat wave, cold wave, drought, wildfire
Geophysical: Disaster events originating from solid earth movements	Earthquake, tsunami, volcanic eruption, rock fall, avalanche, landslide, subsidence
Hydrological: Disasters related to deviations in the normal water cycle or overflow of bodies of water	Floods, mudslides
Meteorological: Disasters due to severe weather conditions	Severe winter storms, blizzards, severe thunderstorms, sandstorms, hurricanes, tornados, cyclones, tropical storms

Types of Chemical Emergencies	Examples
Biotoxins	Digitalis, nicotine, ricin
Blister agents/vesicants	Mustards, chlorasine
Blood agents	Arsine, carbon monoxide, cyanide
Caustics (acids)	Hydrofluoric acid, hydrogen chloride
Choking/lung/pulmonary agents	Ammonia, bromine, chlorine, phosphine
Incapacitating agents	Fentanyls and other opioids
Long-acting anticoagulants	Super warfarin
Metals	Arsenic, mercury, thallium
Nerve agents	Sarin
Organic solvents	Benzene
Riot control agents	Tear gas
Toxic alcohols	Ethylene glycol
Vomiting agents	Adamsite

Data from: Centers for Disease Control and Prevention. (2014b). *Chemical categories.* Retrieved from http://emergency.cdc.gov/agent/agentlistchem-category.asp; Centers for Disease Control and Prevention. (2014d). *Natural disasters and severe weather.* Retrieved from http://emergency.cdc.gov/disasters/

a country to another to avoid the effects of civil unrest. These people are known as **internally displaced persons (IDPs)**. Refugees are another category of displaced persons. A **refugee** was defined by the 1951 United Nations Convention Relating to the Status of Refugees as a person who "owing to a well-founded fear of being persecuted for reasons of race, religion, nationality, membership of a particular social group, or political opinion, is outside the country of his nationality and is unable to, or owing to such fear, is unwilling to avail himself of the protection of that country" (quoted in United Nations High Commissioner for Refugees [UNHCR], 2012, p. 4).

Other categories of displaced persons include asylum seekers and stateless people. Asylum seekers consider themselves refugees fleeing persecution, but their claim has not yet been accepted by the country in which they are seeking asylum. Stateless people are those who are not considered to be nationals of any country or who may be outside the protection of their country of residence (UNHCR, 2012). In 2012, 14 million refugees, 15.4 million IDPs, more than 850,000 asylum seekers, and 3.4 million stateless people were of concern to the UNHCR with respect to protection of human safety and rights. An additional 3.7 million people who had returned to their homelands were also of concern. The plight of these displaced populations is more challenging than ever because of restricted access to countries of relocation following the September 11, 2001, bombing of the World Trade Center and the U.S. Pentagon (UNHCR, 2012).

War and civil conflict can have devastating consequences for those affected. For example, Iraq, which has experienced almost continuous periods of war from 1980 to the present has suffered worker shortages and skill-set imbalances, unreliable supply distribution, unstable leadership, and land degradation. Other effects have included destruction of much of the water supply system and industrial contamination of the Tigres and Euphrates rivers with consequent increases in waterborne diseases and toxic chemical exposures. Sanctions resulting from the Gulf war have led to decreased food importation and availability (Zolnikov, 2013). A March 2013 news report estimated that the war in Iraq resulted in an estimated 116,900 civilian fatalities as well the deaths of 4,487 U.S. and 197 British troops (Blair, 2013). Similarly, Somali refugees fleeing to Kenya experienced high mortality rates prior to departure (primarily due to malnutrition), during their journey to safety, and after arrival in Kenyan refugee camps (Spiegel et al.,

2011). In addition, repeated civil wars in Sudan have resulted in hundreds of deaths. Even after South Sudan declared its independence from Sudan, hundreds of thousands have fled the country or become internally displaced due to continued fighting (*South Sudan Profile*, 2014). Among Sudanese refugees in one camp, crowded living conditions and lack of sanitation resulted in more than 5,000 cases of hepatitis E with high case fatality rates, particularly among pregnant women (Thomson et al., 2012).

Terrorism is a growing concern and source of disasters throughout the world. Although there is no commonly accepted definition of terrorism, most definitions include the targeting of civilian populations and the intention of creating fear and social disruption. Some definitions also include a purpose of achieving change in policies or practices. The People's Health Movement, Medact, and Global Equity Gauge Alliance (2008) indicated a need for a comprehensive definition of terrorism that encompasses four elements:

- Actual or threatened violence, particularly targeted at civilians, to create fear
- Perpetration by state or non-state individuals or organizations
- Occurrence within or across national boundaries
- Perpetration during war, peace, and periods of internal or civil conflict

The following definition has been recommended: "politically motivated violence or the threat of violence particularly against civilians, with the intent to instil (sic) fear, whether conducted by nation-states, individuals, or sub-national groups" (People's Health Movement et al., 2008, p. 114).

Terrorism is defined in the U.S. Code of Federal Regulations as "the unlawful use of force and violence against persons or property to intimidate or coerce a government, the civilian population, or any segment thereof, in the furtherance of political or social objectives" (Federal Bureau of Investigation, 2005). **Bioterrorism** is "the intentional release of viruses, bacteria, or other germs that can sicken or kill people, livestock, or crops" (CDC, 2014a). Potential agents for bioterrorism are classified as category A, B, or C on the basis of the ease of spread of disease and the anticipated severity of effects. Category A includes organisms or toxins that pose the greatest risk to public health and national security based on their ease of transmission, high death rates and potential for major public health impact, ability to cause panic and social disruption, and requirements for specific public health preparedness activity. Examples of category A agents include anthrax, botulism, plague, smallpox, tularemia, viral hemorrhagic fevers (e.g., Ebola and Marburg viruses), and arenaviruses (CDC, n.d.).

Category B agents are moderately easily spread, result in moderate illness and low death rates, and may require specific enhancement of laboratory and disease surveillance and monitoring systems. Examples include brucellosis; food safety threats, such as *salmonella*, *E. coli*, and *shigella* species; psittacosis; Q fever; ricin toxin; staphylococcal enterotoxin B; typhus fever; viral encephalitis; and water safety threats, such as cholera and cryptosporidium. Category C agents include emerging pathogens that could be engineered for mass dissemination in the future due to their easy availability, ease of production and transmission, and the potential for high morbidity and mortality and severe health impact. Examples might include nipah virus and hantavirus (CDC, n.d.).

Disaster Trends

Disasters seem to be occurring with greater frequency than ever before. In part, this may be due to more extensive news coverage of catastrophic events around the world. It is clear, however, that disasters are having more horrendous effects than in the past. For example, between 2000 and 2012, disasters affected 2.9 billion people, caused 1.2 million deaths, and resulted in $1.7 trillion in damage (UNODRR, 2013). In 2012 alone, natural disasters resulted in $1 trillion in damage in Asia, $800 billion in the Americas, more than $200 billion in Europe, and significantly less in Africa. Most damage in the Americas was due to storms, with earthquakes causing the most damage in Asia. The 2011 earthquake in Honshu, Japan, for example, was the most expensive disaster in terms of damages since 1975 followed by hurricane Katrina in 2005, the Wenchuan earthquake in China in 2008, and the 1995 Kobe earthquake in Japan (CRED, 2014a). Africa suffered minimal physical damage because the built environment is considerably less well developed than in other parts of the world.

Mortality due to disasters decreased significantly for biological disasters from 1900 to 2012, primarily due to the advent of antimicrobial therapies. Deaths from other types of natural disasters have generally declined in the same period, with periodic peaks. The exception is geophysical disasters for which mortality has increased due to increased population density in areas subject to such events. Conversely, the numbers of people affected by disasters from 1900 to 2012 has increased

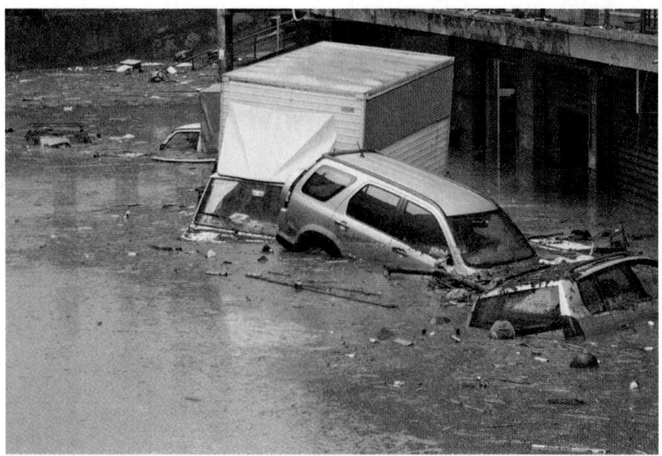

Hydrological disasters may result in severe flooding and population displacement. *(Fotonazario/Fotolia)*

for all types of natural disasters except for biological disasters, with the greatest number affected by hydrological disasters, again because of increased population density in areas prone to flooding (CRED, 2014a).

With respect to technological disasters from 1900 to 2012, the number of disasters peaked at more than 350 events in 2000 and then again in 2006, with approximately 160 technological disasters occurring in 2012. The greatest extent of damages occurred in the Americas ($25 billion), primarily due to fires, with the second-highest damages seen in Europe ($13.5 billion), mostly related to flooding. Two major oil spills caused significant damage in 2010 and 2012. Transportation incidents comprised a significant portion of technological disasters and their frequency has been increasing over the last two decades. Overall deaths due to technological disasters, on the other hand, have declined from more than 12,000 in 2002 to about 6,000 in 2012. Unlike other parts of the world, however, deaths related to technological disasters show increasing trends in Africa and Asia, possibly due to lack of effective building codes and other regulatory measures. Similarly, the number of people affected by disasters has declined from a peak of more than 1 million in 1981 to somewhat over 3,000 in 2012 (CRED, 2014b).

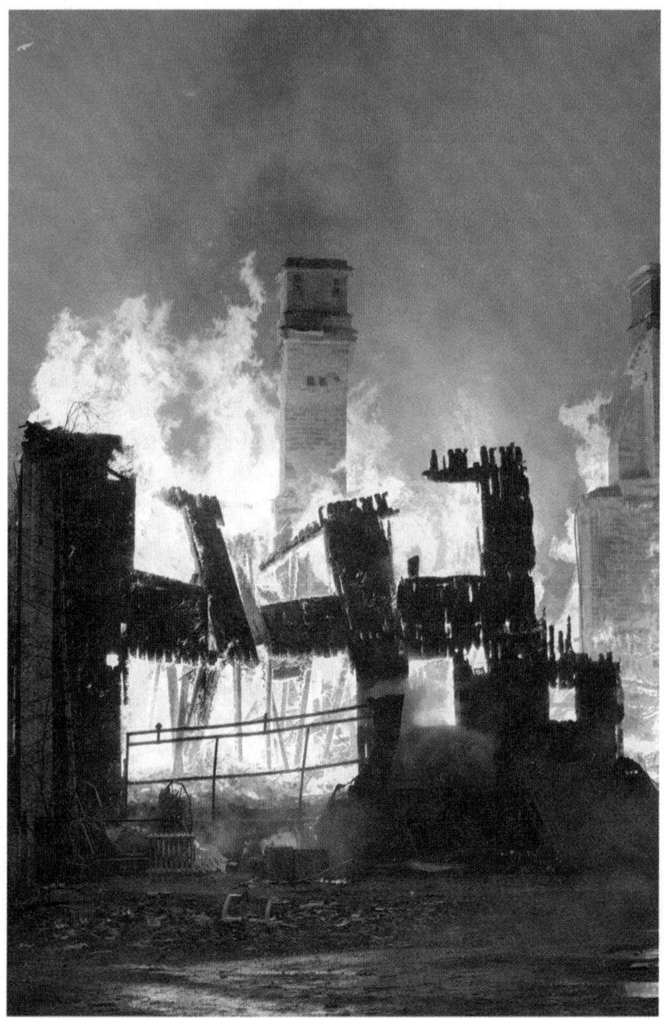

Wildfires can spread rapidly resulting in extensive property damage and loss of life. *(Gemenacom/Fotolia)*

In the United States, from 2003 to 2013, CDC's Emergency Operations Center (EOC) implemented a full Emergency Management Plan 55 times in response to disease outbreaks, natural disasters, national security events, and man-made disasters. Another 109 events required CDC support but did not necessitate full EOC activation (Leidel, Groseclose, Burney, Navin, & Wooster, 2013).

Worldwide, terrorist activities have declined somewhat in the last few years. U.S. Department of State statistics include 10,283 incidents of terrorism in 2011, down slightly from 14,415 in 2007. Declines in attacks resulting in at least one death, injury, or kidnapping have decreased even further dropping from 11,085 incidents in 2007 to 7,453 in 2011, and the number of attacks resulting in the death of 10 or more people declined from 353 to 193 in the same time period. Overall, the number of people killed as a result of terrorist activity has decreased by almost half from 22,720 to 12,533 (National Counterterrorism Center, 2012).

Although terrorist attacks occurred in more than 70 countries, approximately three fourths of them took place in the Near East and South Asia. Approximately two thirds (64%) of all attacks occurred in three countries, Afghanistan, Iraq, and Pakistan. Terrorist attacks increased by nearly 40% from 2010 to 2011, mostly related to the activities of the Revolutionary Armed Forces of Columbia. The majority of attacks (80%) in 2011 involved armed attacks and bombings, with suicide bombings accounting for 21% of terrorism-related deaths. Half of those deaths occurred among civilians (National Counterterrorism Center, 2012). Table 25-2● provides information on some recent disaster events.

The increasing severity of disaster effects is due to a number of societal changes. Human populations are more densely concentrated and increasingly found in areas with high disaster potential (Landesman, 2011). Global climate changes are also altering weather patterns, creating more severe storms with resulting damage. In addition, technological advances increase the potential for human-generated disasters such as toxic leaks, transportation disasters, and massive electrical power outages. Finally, recent events have demonstrated the willingness of some radical groups to engineer massive disasters to achieve their political goals through terrorism.

Characteristics of Disasters

Disasters vary with respect to a number of characteristics, including their frequency, predictability, preventability, imminence, and duration. Disasters also vary in terms of the extent of their effects. Some disasters occur relatively frequently in certain parts of the world. Consequently, people in those areas have some knowledge of what to expect and what can be done to minimize the effects of the event. For example, earthquakes

TABLE 25-2 Recent Disaster Events

Date	Event/Locale	Category	Effects
January, 2010	Earthquake in Haiti	Natural: Geophysical	222,570 deaths 300,000 injuries
July–August, 2010	Flooding in Pakistan	Natural: Hydrological	18 million people affected, 1,700 deaths, 1.9 million homes damaged or destroyed, 10 million people without shelter
October, 2010	Cholera epidemic in Haiti and the Dominican Republic	Natural: Biological	121,518 cases, 63,711 hospitalizations, 2,491 deaths
April, 2011	351 tornadoes in Alabama, Arkansas, Georgia, Mississippi, and Tennessee	Natural: Meteorological	338 deaths
May, 2011	Tornado in Joplin, Missouri	Natural: Meteorological	159 deaths, 1,000 injuries, fatal fungal infections due to soft tissue injuries
October, 2012	Hurricane Sandy, eastern United States	Natural: Meteorological	117 deaths, 7 to 8 million people without power, 20,000 people in shelters
April, 2013	Boston marathon bombing	Terrorism	3 deaths, 260 injured

Data from: Benedict, K., Adebanjo, T., Harris, J., Lockhart, S., Peterson, J., McClinton, S., . . . Lo, Y.-C. (2011). Fatal fungal soft-tissue infections after a tornado—Joplin, Missouri, 2011. *Morbidity and Mortality Weekly Report, 60,* 992; Casey-Lockyer, M., Donald, C. M., Moulder, J., Aderhold, D. Harris, D., Woodall, G., . . . Chin, C. (2013). Tornado-related fatalities—Five states, southeastern United States, April 25–28, 2011. *Morbidity and Mortality Weekly Report, 62,* 529–533; Casey-Lockyer, M., Heick., R. J., Mertzlufft, C. E., Yard, E. E., Wolkin, A. F., Noe, R. S., . . . Murti, M. (2013). Deaths associated with hurricane Sandy—October–November 2012. *Morbidity and Mortality Weekly Report, 62,* 393–397; Hotz, G., Ginzburg, E., Wurm, G., DeGennaro, V., Andrews, D., Basaravaju, S., . . . Selent, M. (2011). Post-earthquake injuries treated at a field hospital—Haiti, 2010. *Morbidity and Mortality Weekly Report, 59,* 1673–1677; Jenkins, P. H., Montejano, H. J., Broward, M.S., Abbassi, M. J., Crowley, M. S., O'Brien, M. G., . . . Merlo, E. (2010). Update on cholera—Haiti, Dominican Republic, and Florida, 2010. *Morbidity and Mortality Weekly Report, 59,* 1637–1641; Ray, M. (2013). *Boston Marathon bombing of 2013.* Retrieved from http://www.britannica.com/EBchecked/topic/1924021/Boston-Marathon-bombing-of-2013; Sabatinelli, G., Kakar, S. R., Malik, M., Kazi, B. M., Khan, M. R., Aurakzai, J. K., . . . Shapar, C. (2012). Early warning disease surveillance after a flood emergency—Pakistan, 2010. *Morbidity and Mortality Weekly Report, 61,* 1002–1007.

occur periodically in California, and residents in earthquake-prone areas are encouraged to be prepared in the event of a large quake. Similarly, hurricanes and other severe storms are frequently experienced during certain seasons in other parts of the country.

Some disaster events are predictable. In general, the probability of destructive tornadoes increases from April through June in the United States. Similarly, many rivers are known to flood periodically with heavy spring rains. Severe blizzards can also be predicted, allowing people to stockpile food supplies, medications, or fuel for heating in case they are isolated by the storm. Other events, such as a plane crash, a fire in a chemical plant, or a terrorist attack are not predictable.

Some types of disasters are more easily prevented than others. For example, periodic flooding can be prevented by rerouting waterways or by building dams. Others, such as earthquakes and severe winter storms, cannot be controlled or prevented. Increased security measures are one attempt to prevent disasters resulting from terrorist activities, but their effectiveness remains to be seen.

Disasters also vary with respect to their imminence in terms of their speed of onset and may have a period of forewarning before striking. Some disasters provide evidence of their imminent occurrence and allow time for preparation prior to impact. For example, blizzards, hurricanes, and other severe storms can be tracked and their probable path determined. People along that path usually have sufficient warning to take preventive actions that minimize the potential for death and destruction. Other disasters such as fires and explosions occur instantaneously, with no prior warning. Catastrophic disasters tend to have a rapid onset, whereas pervasive disasters, such as drought or famine have a more gradual onset (Institute of Medicine, 2013). In some cases, the disaster event itself is of

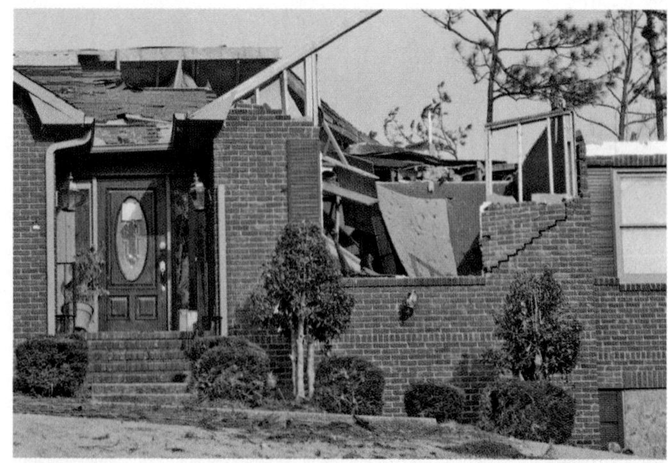

Tornadoes are somewhat more predictable than other types of disasters allowing more time for preparation or evacuation.
(Michael Ballard/Fotolia)

short duration (Veenema & Woolsey, 2013), as in the case of an earthquake or a transportation disaster. At other times, the disaster event lasts some time. Examples of prolonged disasters are epidemics, famine, and war. Disasters such as hurricanes and blizzards have an intermediate duration.

Finally, disasters vary in terms of their impact and their destructive potential. Some disasters are fairly limited in scope, affecting a small geographic area or a relatively small number of people. For example, the effects of a mine cave-in are generally restricted to the area where the mine is located. The effects of war or famine, on the other hand, may be more far-reaching. For a particular organization, the extent of a disaster may be conceptualized as internal or external. External disasters do not affect the organization directly but tax its resources. For example, an explosion at an industrial plant probably does not affect a local hospital directly, but caring for the injured will tax the hospitals resources. Internal disasters, on the other hand, result in disruption of organizational function due to loss of personnel or damage to the facility (Veenema & Woolsey, 2013). The extent of disaster effects will be discussed in more detail later in this chapter.

The Disaster Role of the Public Health System

Disasters are events that have significant effects on the health of the public. It is not surprising, then, that the public health system should play a major role in planning for and responding to a wide variety of disaster occurrences. Disaster-related public health responsibilities include the following:

- Preventing and responding to epidemics and the spread of disease
- Protecting the public from environmental hazards
- Preventing injury
- Promoting healthy behavior and mental health
- Responding to actual disaster events and assisting in community recovery
- Ensuring access to quality health services in the event of a disaster (Reed, Veenema, & Rains, 2013)

These responsibilities might be executed in activities before, during, and after a disaster event. Before a disaster, members of the public health care system should be involved in identifying disaster risks and particularly vulnerable populations. They should then educate those populations regarding disaster prevention and preparedness. In addition, they should cooperate with other agencies to develop plans to prevent disasters when possible and to limit effects of disasters that cannot be prevented. They can also assist in the identification of resources available for disaster response. This may include the recruitment and training of volunteer health professionals to deal with the potential health effects of a disaster. Finally, public health professionals, including population health nurses, can advocate for and help develop public policies that reduce the potential for and effects of disasters (Landesman, 2011). For example, they might advocate for building codes that create structures that will withstand major earthquakes, or brush removal ordinances in fire-prone areas.

During a disaster event, public health professionals will assess and communicate information regarding health-related effects to relevant government agencies. They will also coordinate the provision of needed emergency and routine health care immediately after the disaster. Other activities include advising and assisting in the prevention of injury and promotion of food and water safety, vector control, and control of communicable diseases. They may also be involved in inspecting shelter sites for health risks (Landesman, 2011).

Following a disaster, public health professionals would be involved in assuring that follow-up care is available to disaster victims with continuing needs. They would also participate in a collaborative evaluation of the disaster response and subsequent redrafting of response plans for future disasters (Landesman, 2011).

The public health system also has a similar role in responding to the health consequences of terrorist activities. Public health activities to prevent terrorism may include reducing access to biological agents. In addition, public health professionals should assure that a balance is maintained between terrorism preparedness and addressing other public health issues and between preventing terrorism and protecting individual civil rights. Both of these latter responsibilities may require concerted advocacy initiatives on the part of public health professionals, particularly population health nurses. Preparedness and prevention should not lead to inappropriate responses that infringe on civil rights or that draw resources from other important public health initiatives.

Elements of a Disaster Event

Disaster literature typically addresses three main elements of a disaster occurrence: the temporal element, the spatial element, and the role element. In this chapter, we will also address a fourth element, the effects element.

The Temporal Element: Stages of Disaster Response

Disaster experts characterize disasters as cyclic phenomena unfolding in five stages: (a) the nondisaster or interdisaster stage, (b) the predisaster stage, (c) the impact stage, (d) the emergency stage, and (e) the recovery stage. Other classifications of the stages of a disaster focus on the preimpact, impact, and postimpact stages (Veenema & Woolsey, 2013).

THE NONDISASTER STAGE. The nondisaster stage, also referred to as the interdisaster phase, is the period of time before the threat of a disaster materializes. This period should be a time of planning and preparation. During this stage, communities should engage in such activities as identifying potential disaster risks and mapping their locations in the community.

Vulnerability assessment and capability inventory are other features of this stage in which the community assesses the potential consequences of disasters likely to occur within the community and its ability to cope with these consequences. **Vulnerability analysis** involves predisaster determination of groups most likely to be adversely affected, property most likely to be damaged, and community capacity to deal with the effects of a disaster (CRED, 2009c; Veenema & Woolsey, 2013). Loss may be conceptualized in terms of death or injury, damage to or destruction of homes, or economic losses. Elderly persons, those with disabilities, and members of ethnic minority groups are examples of highly vulnerable populations. The extent and location of vulnerable populations should be determined and plans made for meeting their unique needs in the event of a disaster. Capability inventory involves determination of the adaptive capacity of the community through inventory of resources that are likely to be needed in the event of specific types of disasters and their availability in the community.

During the nondisaster stage, the community should also engage in prevention, preparedness, and mitigation activities. As we saw in Chapter 22∞, mitigation is action taken to prevent or reduce the harmful effects of a disaster on human health or property (Federal Emergency Management Agency [FEMA], 2013c). Mitigation may be either structural or nonstructural. Structural mitigation involves construction or alteration of the built environment to withstand the effects of disasters. Nonstructural mitigation is reflected in measures to protect critical supplies, systems, and functions (Davis, Hansen, Kushma, Peek, & Phillips, 2013). Retrofitting or reinforcing major highway overpasses is an example of hard mitigation being used in California to prevent the collapse of highways and bridges in the event of an earthquake. Examples of nonstructural mitigation include stockpiling vaccines in the event of an epidemic, and creating backup communication systems and early warning systems. Other examples related to mitigation include enforcing strict building codes for new construction and repair of existing structures; adapting zoning ordinances to minimize building in disaster-prone areas; relocating structures in danger areas; and building community shelters and safe rooms in schools, homes, and other locations (FEMA, 2013a).

Some of the major foci in mitigation activities include developing cost-effective strategies agreed upon by major stakeholders and the public for reducing risks, focusing resources on the greatest risks and vulnerabilities, and building partnerships and collaborations. Additional mitigation foci include increasing public risk awareness, communicating priorities to state and federal officials, and aligning risk reduction with other community goals (FEMA, 2013b).

The final area of activity in the nondisaster planning period is the education of both professionals and the public regarding disaster prevention and preparation. Unfortunately, many communities deny the need for disaster planning when they are not faced with the direct threat of a disaster. Even when disaster planning occurs, if the plan is not widely disseminated, disaster response can be impeded.

THE PREDISASTER STAGE. The predisaster stage occurs when a disaster event is imminent but has not yet occurred. This stage may also be referred to as the warning or threat stage. Major activities during this stage are warning, preimpact mobilization, and, in some cases, evacuation. Warning involves apprising members of the community of the imminence of a disaster event and of the actions that should be taken to minimize its consequences. For example, storm warnings are broadcast in many areas when there is potential for a severe storm, but people do not immediately go to a storm cellar or leave the area because the possibility remains that the storm will bypass the area.

The U.S. federal government has developed the Integrated Public Alert and Warning System (IPAWS) to "enable rapid dissemination of authenticated alert information over as many communication pathways as possible" (FEMA, 2012b, para 1). The system allows authenticated local, state, tribal, territorial, or federal authorities to create location-specific messages regarding emergency situations for specific populations at risk. The resulting messages are broadcast by existing communication systems including the Emergency Alert System through radio and television stations, National Oceanic and Atmospheric Administration Weather Radio, and other national weather service systems. In addition, the Commercial Mobile Alert System sends alerts to cell phones and other mobile devices in specified locales. Alerts may also be sent to giant voice sirens or digital road signs increasing the warning capacity of the system (FEMA, 2012b).

Just as communities may accept or deny the need for disaster planning, members of the community may respond positively or negatively to warnings of possible disasters. Several factors can influence a person's response, including the source, content, and mechanism for warning, and individual perceptions and beliefs. Warning messages that are clear, practical, and relevant or that originate from credible sources are more likely to be acted on than vague or impractical warnings. Warnings need to specify the exact nature of the threat and provide specific recommendations for action. For example, vague warnings of the potential for additional terrorist activities following the September 11, 2001, attacks provided little direction for action. Specific guidelines on how to handle mail potentially contaminated with anthrax spores, on the other hand, were more effective in promoting action. Warnings should also contain sufficient information to allow people to decide on an appropriate course of action. It is sometimes erroneously believed that detailed information about a disaster will cause panic. In effect, failure to provide information usually leads to failure to act on warnings; providing information does not seem to contribute to panic among individual citizens.

Response to a warning is also affected by each individual's perceptions about the possibility of disaster. These perceptions arise from past experiences with disaster, psychological traits, and sociocultural factors. For example, if people have previously been only on the fringes of a hurricane path, they may not perceive a hurricane as a very frightening event, and they

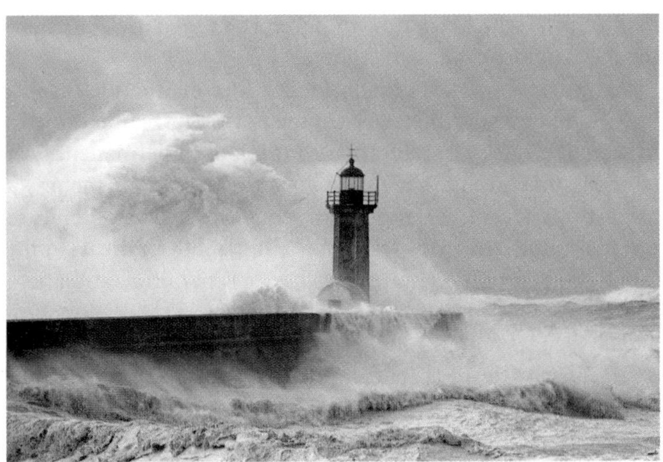

Because of the lack of imminence, tsunami warnings following distant earthquakes may be ignored. *(Zacarias da Mata/Fotolia)*

may ignore storm warnings. Similarly, if the individual has a fatalistic attitude that one's own actions will not make much difference in the outcome of an event, he or she might not act in response to warnings. Such an attitude may be the result of an individual personality trait or a sociocultural norm in the group.

Warning confirmation also influences the way people respond. Warnings tend to be believed if the source of the warning is official, if the probability of the event is increasing, and if one is in close geographic proximity to the area where the disaster is likely to occur. For example, people who live on a recognized geological fault line are more likely to take warnings about potential earthquakes seriously than those who do not live on a fault line.

Belief also influences action with respect to warnings. Again, belief in the potential for disaster is enhanced if the source of the warning is an official agency and if that agency has credibility. For example, if there have been numerous false alarms in the past, people are less likely to pay attention to warnings. Belief is also enhanced if the medium of the warning is personal rather than impersonal. People are more likely to evacuate their homes if they receive a targeted telephone message than if they hear a warning on the radio. Previous experience also influences the likelihood of belief. If one has experienced the full force of a hurricane before, one is more likely to believe and act on a hurricane warning than would otherwise be the case.

The frequency with which the warning is received also influences belief, as do observable changes in the situation. For example, if people see evidence of flames on a nearby hill, they are more likely to believe in the imminence of danger posed by a wildfire. Perceived behavior of others can influence belief either positively or negatively. When others act in response to the warning, belief is enhanced. If others appear to be ignoring the warning, however, belief is less likely. Factors influencing responses to disaster warnings are summarized in Table 25-3●.

Preimpact mobilization involves initiation of activities designed to avert an imminent disaster or minimize its effects. Activities involved in this stage might include efforts to prevent the disaster or its effects, seeking shelter from the effects of the disaster, evacuating people from areas threatened by the disaster, and implementing plans to deal with the effects of a disaster. For example, in the threat of a flood, people may sandbag riverbanks to divert floodwaters from a town, or board up windows and tie down equipment when a hurricane is forecast. People may seek shelter from tornadoes or other storms by moving to a basement, a storm cellar, or an interior room of a house. Preimpact mobilization might also involve evacuating people from an area threatened by fire, radiation, or chemical leakage. Finally, the initial phases of a disaster response plan may be implemented. For example, off-duty health care

TABLE 25-3 Factors Influencing Response to Disaster Warnings

Warning Feature	Influencing Factors
Warning message	• Clarity • Practicality • Relevance • Informativeness
Individual perceptions	• Past experience with disasters • Psychological traits • Sociocultural attitudes
Warning confirmation	• Official source • Increasing evidence and probability of disaster • Geographic proximity to the expected disaster location
Beliefs	• Credibility of warning sources • Personal rather than impersonal contact • Previous experience of disaster • Observable changes in the situation • Frequency of warning • Belief and action by others

personnel may be recalled to health facilities in preparation for treating anticipated casualties.

THE IMPACT STAGE. In the impact stage of a disaster, the disaster event has occurred and its immediate effects are experienced by the community. One major activity in this stage is the assessment of the impact of the disaster with an inventory of the immediate needs of the community. Inventory is a rapid assessment of the damage to buildings and the type and extent of injuries suffered. This information is used to determine actions needed in carrying out the efforts of the emergency stage.

THE EMERGENCY STAGE. The focus of the emergency stage of a disaster is on saving lives through rescue efforts, first aid, and emergency treatment (Landesman, 2011). The emergency response to a disaster usually begins with community members because there has not been time for assistance to arrive from outside sources. If the community is geographically isolated or access to the community is impeded by the disaster, this isolation period will be prolonged. Later, relief assistance is provided from sources outside of the area affected by the disaster. The activities performed are essentially the same, although performed by different agents in the two phases, and include search and rescue operations, first aid, emergency medical assistance, establishment or restoration of modes of communication and transportation, surveillance for public health effects of the disaster (e.g., infectious diseases, mental health problems), and, in some cases, evacuation of community members from affected areas.

THE RECOVERY STAGE. In the recovery stage, the focus is on returning the community to equilibrium. This stage can be divided into substages of restoration and actual reconstruction and ends in reconstitution. Mitigation may also occur in the recovery stage with efforts to prevent a recurrence of a disaster or to enhance preparedness and response capabilities.

Restoration is the reestablishment of a basic way of life following a disaster, usually occurring within the first 6 months. Activities of this stage include returning to homes or seeking alternative shelter, removing debris, and replacing lost or damaged property. At the community level, restoration involves reestablishing community services that may have been disrupted by the disaster (Landesman, 2011). After a flood, for example, people may return to their homes, clean up the mud, and replace water-damaged furniture. Schools reopen and residents return to work. If a prominent community official was killed in the flood, someone is appointed to fill that post until an election can be held.

Reconstruction involves the rebuilding and reordering of the physical and social environments following a disaster (Landesman, 2011). Homes, schools, businesses, and other structures may need to be rebuilt. Dams or levees may be constructed to prevent future flooding. Reconstruction may also entail alterations in the social environment. For example, terrorist activity has led to enhanced security provisions in airports, at international borders, and even in educational institutions, which are now required to more closely account for the activities of foreign students.

Reunification is a special instance of reconstruction for refugee families who may have been separated during their travels in search of safety. Immigration restrictions in permanent host countries may result in lengthy separations of family members as portions of families migrate in sequence. Refugee literature has identified three stages of separation and reunification for families—before the separation, during separation, and afterwards—each of which creates an imbalance in family function and challenges families' abilities to function effectively.

Reconstitution is a state of affairs that occurs when the life of the community has returned, as far as possible, to normal after a disaster. This return to normal may take several months to several years, depending on the degree of damage sustained in the disaster. It may take several years after a flood, for example, to restore the landscape of the community to its former state or to replenish the city treasury after disaster costs have depleted it. It may also take some time for individuals to adjust to the loss of loved ones or for the community government to be reconstituted. In extreme disasters, full reconstitution may never occur. For example, many people believe that life in the United States was completely changed by the terrorist attacks on September 11, 2001, and the full effects of that disaster are not yet known.

The final stage of recovery after a disaster is mitigation, which involves future-oriented activities to prevent subsequent disasters or to minimize their effects. For example, a community that has experienced a flood may take engineering action to prevent the likelihood of subsequent floods, or a community that was unprepared for disaster may develop a disaster response plan. Increased security measures are another example of efforts aimed at preventing subsequent terrorist activities and their effects. These activities cycle the community back into the nondisaster stage. Stages and related activities in the development of and response to a disaster are summarized in Table 25-4●.

The Spatial Element

The spatial elements of a disaster refer to the extent of its effects on specific geographic regions. These regions include the area of total impact, the area of partial impact, and outside areas (Figure 25-1●).

The area of total impact is the zone where the most severe effects of the disaster are found. In an earthquake, for example, this would include the area where the greatest damage to buildings has occurred and where the greatest number of injuries was sustained.

In the area of partial impact, evidence of the disaster can be seen but the effects are not of the magnitude of those in the total impact area. Using the earthquake example, windows may be broken or objects shaken from shelves in the partial impact area, but buildings are intact. Injuries, if any, are infrequent and relatively minor, or only telephone and electrical services might be disrupted in the partial impact area.

TABLE 25-4 Stages and Activities in Disaster Occurrence and Response

Disaster Stage	Related Activities
Nondisaster/interdisaster stage	• Identification of potential disaster risks • Vulnerability analysis • Capability inventory • Prevention and mitigation • Response planning and plan dissemination • Stockpiling necessary supplies • Public and professional education
Predisaster stage	• Warning • Preimpact mobilization • Evacuation
Impact stage	• Damage inventory • Injury assessment
Emergency stage	• Search and rescue • First aid • Emergency medical assistance • Restoration of communication and transportation • Public health surveillance • Further evacuation, as needed
Recovery stage	• Restoration of functional capabilities • Reconstruction of physical and social environments • Reunification of families • Reconstitution • Mitigation of future disaster events

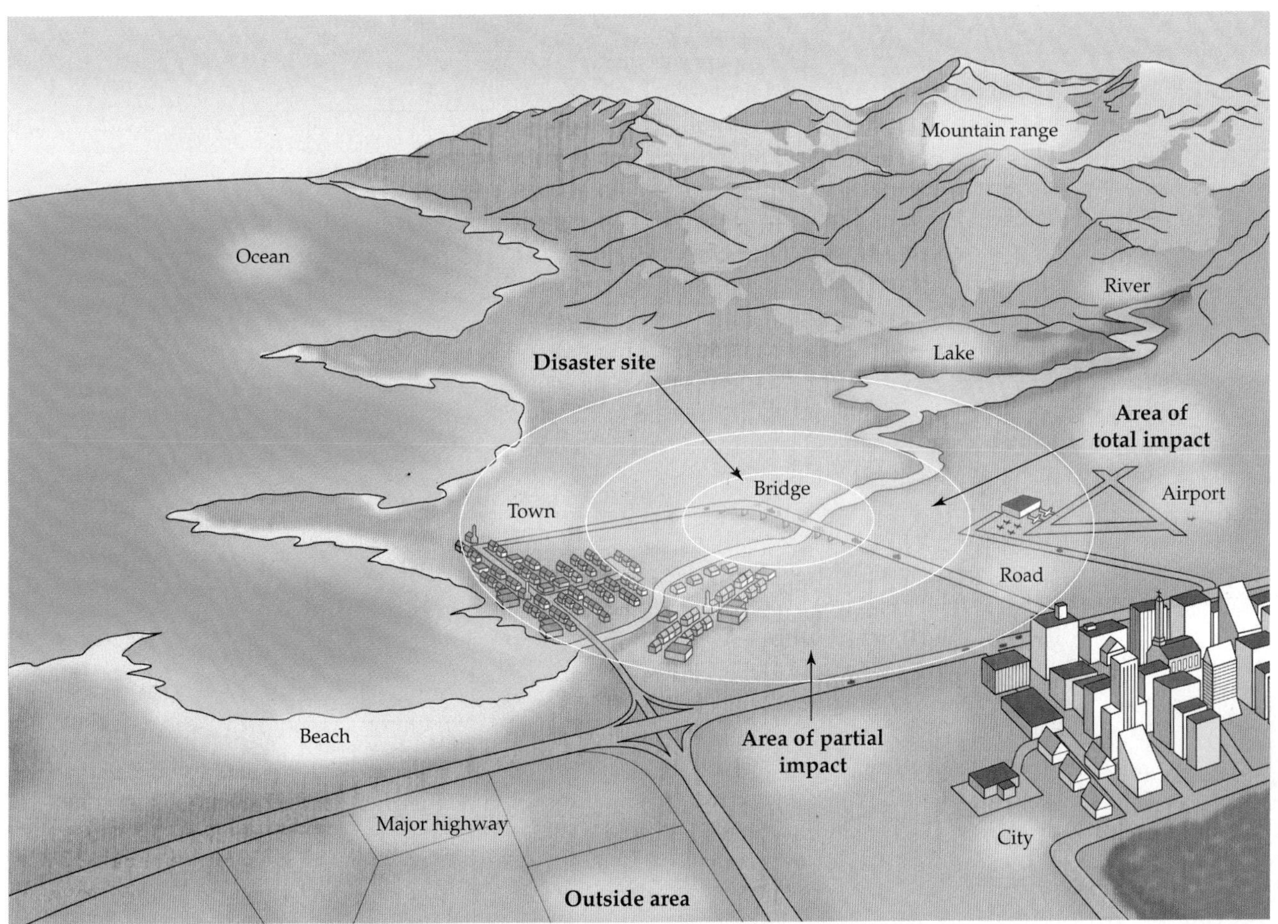

FIGURE 25-1 Areas of Disaster Impact

The outside area is not directly affected but may be a source of assistance in response to the disaster. Areas immediately adjacent to the disaster area are called on first to provide assistance, with further outlying areas being involved later as needed. In a major disaster, the federal government may be called on to provide assistance. This occurs once the area affected has been declared an official disaster area. Figure 25-2● depicts the process by which a presidential declaration of a major disaster or emergency is initiated and federal assistance is provided. As indicated in the figure, when a disaster occurs, local emergency personnel respond and assess the magnitude of the disaster. They inform local government officials of the extent of the problem and the need for outside assistance. Local officials request assistance from the state governor. The governor executes the state emergency plan. If it is determined that dealing with the disaster and its effects is beyond available state and local resources, the governor may initiate a request for federal assistance through the regional FEMA office. In initiating such a request, the governor certifies that the magnitude of the disaster falls outside the ability of state resources and that federal assistance is needed. The governor must also certify adherence to cost sharing requirements for assistance. A preliminary damage assessment (PDA) is conducted by FEMA and state officials. Regional and national FEMA offices review the PDA and the governor's request and make a recommendation for a presidential emergency disaster declaration. Once the President of the United States has made the official declaration, elements of the federal response plan are implemented and federal disaster assistance is provided to the local jurisdiction (FEMA, 2012a, 2012c).

Spatial elements of a disaster vary greatly from event to event. For example, the total and partial impact areas affected

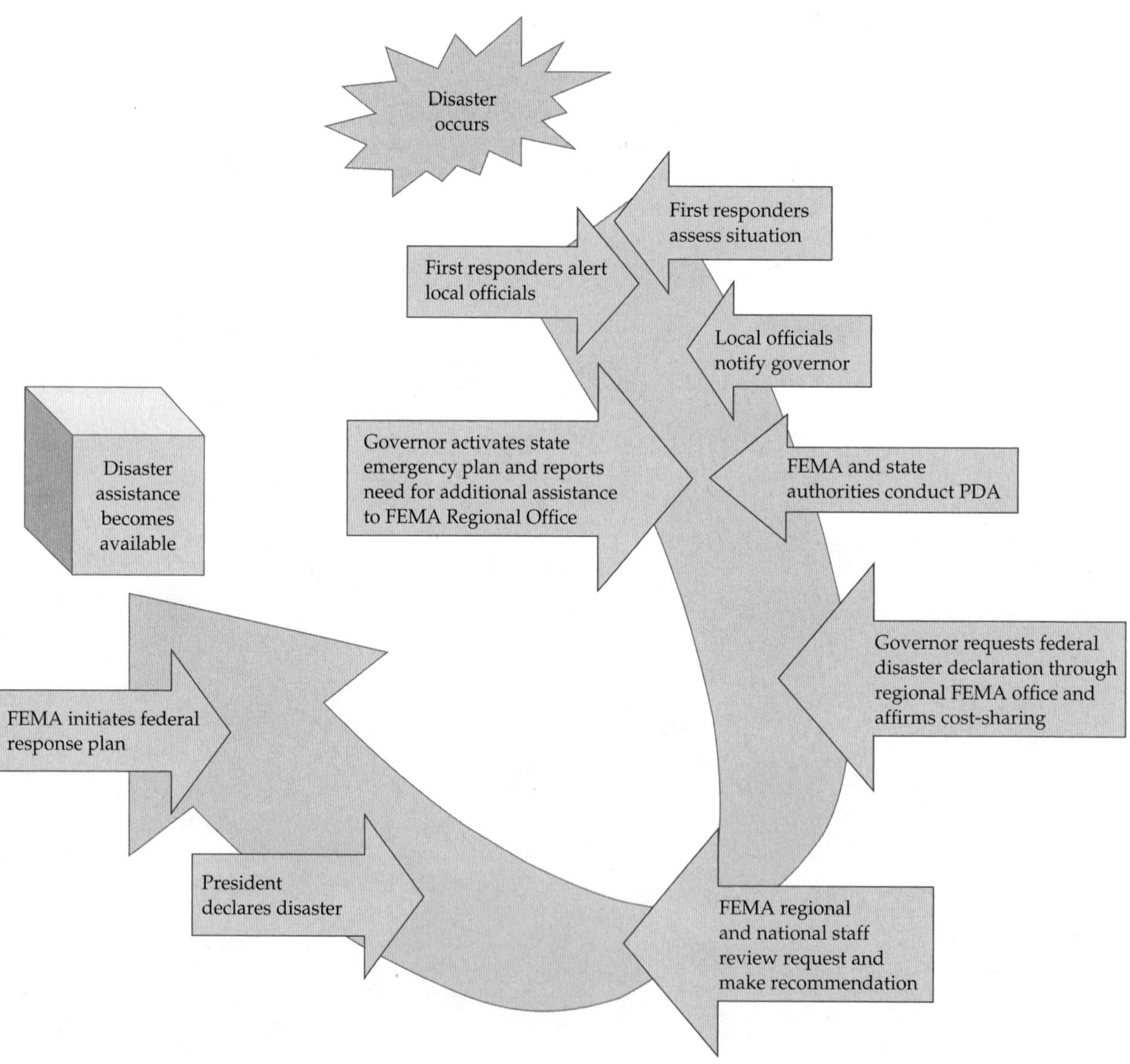

FIGURE 25-2 The Federal Process of Disaster Declaration

by a nuclear accident would be far larger than those affected by a fire at an industrial chemicals plant. The area from which assistance might be requested would also be larger given the greater magnitude of the problem, the number of victims involved, and the damage sustained.

Spatial elements of a potential disaster can also be explored prior to a disaster event. Creation of hazard maps to identify and locate potential disaster hazards in a country, state, or local area has been suggested. At the community level, community risk maps and community resource maps are used to help delineate spatial dimensions in disaster planning. **Community risk maps** are geographic representations pinpointing the locations of disaster risks within a community. Risk maps also delineate probable areas of effect for different types of disasters. Figure 25-3● is an example of a community risk map. Two primary disaster risks are identified in the community risk map in the figure: a dam and reservoir that could result in flooding and a chemical manufacturing plant on the south side of the river. In addition, this community is in an area that experiences periodic tornadoes. The community risk map delineates the areas of the community likely to be affected by a flood (along the river) and a fire or explosion at the chemical plant. The area affected

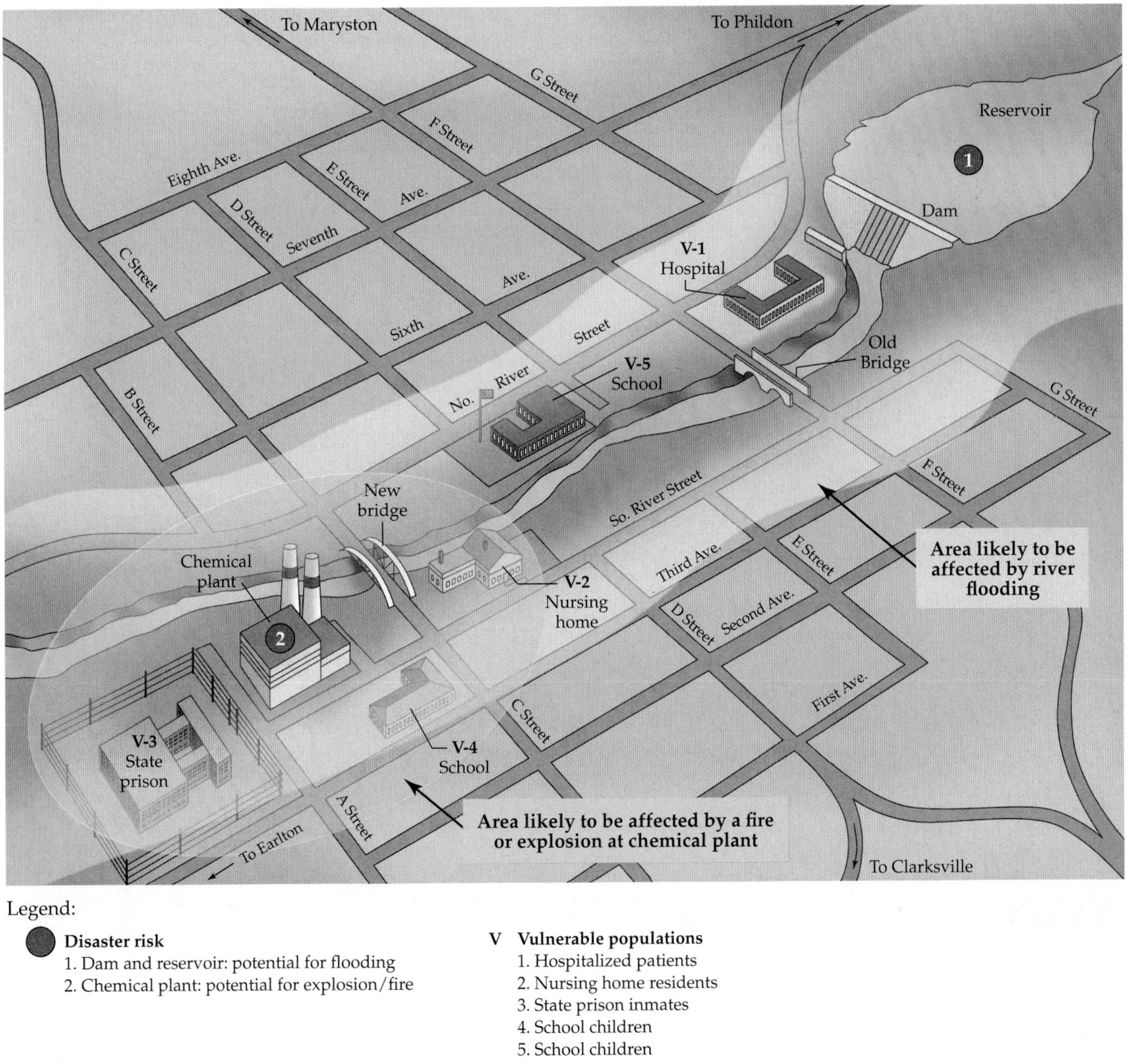

Legend:

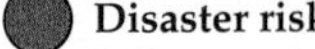

Disaster risk
1. Dam and reservoir: potential for flooding
2. Chemical plant: potential for explosion/fire

V **Vulnerable populations**
1. Hospitalized patients
2. Nursing home residents
3. State prison inmates
4. School children
5. School children

FIGURE 25-3 Sample Community Risk Map

by a tornado would depend on where the tornado touched down. The map also indicates several pockets of particularly vulnerable populations in areas likely to be affected by disasters. These include residents of a nursing home, prison inmates, and schoolchildren in the vicinity of the chemical plant. These same groups, along with patients at the hospital at F and North River Streets and children in the school just north of the river, would be at risk in the event of a flood on the river.

Community resource maps are maps indicating the locations of resources likely to be needed in the event of each of the types of disasters for which a particular community is at risk. Notations on a community resource map include, for example, potential shelter locations, designated command headquarters (and alternates if advisable), storage places for supplies, areas where heavy equipment is available, health care facilities, and proposed emergency morgue areas for the dead. Resource maps also indicate primary and alternate evacuation and transportation routes. Figure 25-4● is a sample resource map related to the community risks identified in Figure 25-3. Looking at Figure 25-4, we see that city hall is adjacent to the river and likely to be affected by a flood. Therefore, the command headquarters has been situated at the television station in the northern part of town. It was believed that placement at the station would facilitate communication because of the equipment available there. A southern command post has also been established in the event that both bridges are impassable and

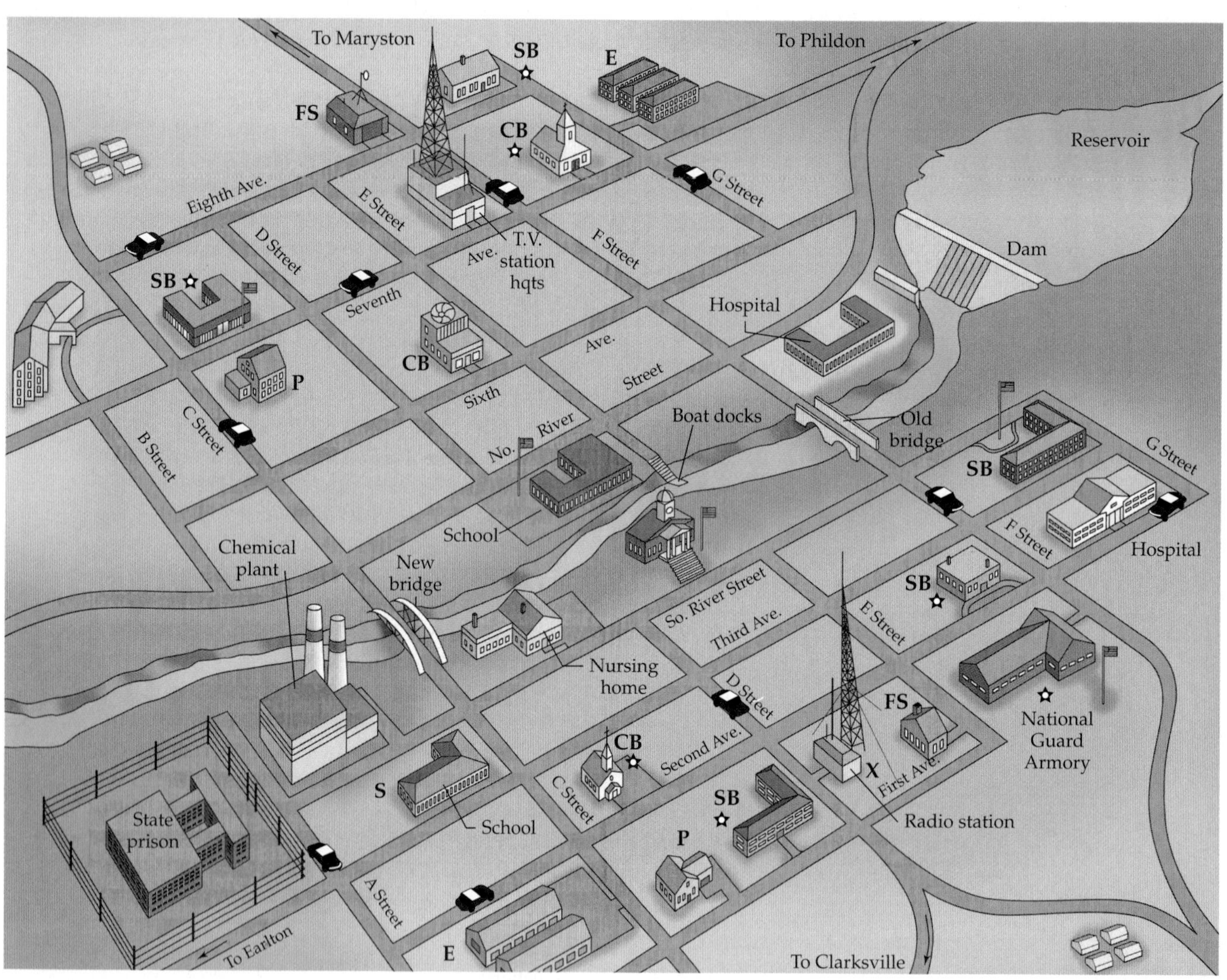

Legend:

✩	Stored supplies	SB	School with basement, shelter site	FS	Fire station
E	Heavy equipment	CB	Church with basement, shelter site	P	Police station
hqts	Command headquarters				Evacuation route
X	Southern command post		Tent shelter site		

FIGURE 25-4 Sample Community Resource Map

response operations on the two sides of the river cannot be coordinated. Because of the potential for splitting the community and lack of access across the river, potential shelter sites have been established and supplies have been stored on both sides of the river. Health services are also available on both sides even if the hospital at F and North River Streets has to be evacuated due to flooding. Rescue operations for people stranded along the river would have to be handled from the north side of the river because that is where the boat docks are located. Personnel and supplies can be brought in from other towns in several different directions and could be brought directly to tent shelter sites if necessary. Only the road from Phildon is likely to be impassable if flooding reaches that far from the reservoir. Both the community risk and resource maps allow disaster planners to visualize what is likely to occur in a disaster event and to plan the most effective response to a disaster.

The Role Element

The third element of a disaster is its role element. Two basic roles for people involved in a disaster are *victim* and *helper roles.*

One of the ways in which the role aspect of a disaster influences disaster response lies in the actions taken by those affected. As we will see later, disaster planning needs to take into consideration the likely response of people to the occurrence of a disaster. Disaster planning can be completely ineffective if it fails to account for public response. People affected by a disaster are likely to take whatever actions seem best to them at the moment. When people are not educated regarding appropriate disaster response, those actions may not actually be in their own best interests or those of the community at large.

The second aspect of the role element of a disaster involves persons that play helper roles. Helpers include designated rescue and recovery personnel as well as community members who help provide care or who assist in the provision of necessities such as food, shelter, and clothing. Victim and helper roles may overlap, and rescue and recovery personnel or other community helpers may themselves have suffered injury or loss as a result of the disaster.

Both victims and helpers are under stress as a result of the disaster. Stressors for victims may be quite obvious and include injury and the loss of loved ones or property. Additional stressors for helpers during the rescue and recovery periods include encounters with multiple deaths that are frequently of a shocking nature, experiencing the suffering of others, and role stress. Frequently, the overwhelming nature of role demands or needs for assistance by victims leads to feelings of helplessness and depression. Other sources of role stress include communication difficulties, inadequacies in terms of resources or staff, lack of access to people needing assistance or resources to help them, bureaucratic difficulties, exhaustion, uncertainties regarding role or authority, and intragroup or intergroup conflicts. Stress may also arise from conflicts between the demands of the helper's family members and the needs of victims, and between the demands of one's regular job and one's disaster role.

The Effects Element

The final element of a disaster is the effects element. We have already discussed the geographic distribution of disaster effects in the spatial element of a disaster, but there are also various categories of effects that may result from disasters.

Many experts distinguish between direct or primary and indirect or secondary and tertiary effects of disasters (Nelson, 2013). Primary disaster effects are the immediate effects of the disaster event itself, such as the extent of death, injury, and destruction of property. Rapid-onset natural disasters, such as earthquakes, often have severe primary effects. Secondary disaster effects are those that occur indirectly as a result of the disaster. Examples include homelessness resulting from damage to residences or flooding due to the collapse of a dam as a result of an earthquake. Tertiary effects are long-term effects of the disaster, such as increased rates of post-traumatic stress disorder (PTSD), malnutrition due to disruption of food supplies, or the disruption of the local economy. Disaster effects may also be tangible or intangible. Tangible effects are usually those that can be measured in economic costs. Intangible effects are those that cannot be measured in terms of monetary losses, such as death and suffering.

Disasters also vary in terms of the severity of their effects. Some disasters cause moderate loss of life or property and result in only temporary inability to function, whereas others are devastating. The destructive potential of a nuclear explosion, for example, is far greater than that of a single plane crash.

Another way of categorizing the effects of disasters is into physical and mental health effects, economic effects, structural effects, and social effects. Physical health effects may arise as a direct result of the disaster itself (e.g., deaths or injuries) or as secondary effects (e.g., an epidemic of diarrheal disease among shelter residents). Mental health effects may be seen immediately after a disaster or surface days, weeks, or months later. Structural effects include homes, roads, and other structures destroyed by the disaster, and economic effects include the cost of rebuilding these structures as well as the economic costs of lost productivity, lost income, and care for disaster victims. Finally, social effects may occur that are either positive or negative. An example of a positive social effect might be an increased sense of community cohesion, whereas distrust and scapegoating of persons believed responsible for a disaster would be a negative effect. Change in the health care delivery system is another example of a social effect of a disaster. Each of these categories of disaster effects will be addressed in more detail in the discussion of disaster assessment later in this chapter.

Population Health Nursing and Disaster Care

As public health professionals, population health nurses have a significant role to play in both disaster preparedness and response. Effective disaster response by population health nurses and other health professionals rests on development of certain competencies. The Columbia University School of Nursing has developed a set of competencies for health care professionals involved in disaster response. These competencies include an understanding of their role in a disaster; abilities to recognize possible disaster-related health effects, use effective infection control and decontamination practices, and accurately report cases of disease; expertise in referral; use of reliable information sources, abilities to communicate effectively with others and to educate the public on risks and appropriate actions; and abilities to assist others with stress management and dealing with psychological effects of a disaster (American Nurses Association, 2008).

In addition, the Association of Community Health Nurse Educators has identified competencies in disaster assessment, planning, intervention, and process and outcome evaluation as core components of population health nursing education (Kuntz, Frable, Qureshi, & Strong, 2008). For more information about the competencies, see the *External Resources* section of the student resources site.

Further responsibilities of population health nurses in disaster preparedness and response include assessing community needs and disaster risk, surveillance for adverse effects, communication to promote accurate dissemination of information, management of points of supply distribution or mass countermeasure centers (e.g., mass immunization campaigns for disease outbreaks), on-site triage, and education of families and community groups to foster disaster preparedness (Spencer & Spellman, 2013). Finally, the International Council of Nursing has identified several disaster-related roles for nurses in two categories: (a) prevention, mitigation, and preparedness and (b) relief response. Responsibilities related to prevention, mitigation, and preparedness include developing awareness of disaster potential and human behavior, lobbying for disaster preparedness at multiple levels, participating in disaster planning and implementation, development of chain of command policies, training nurses for disaster response, and networking with other health care professionals. Response-related responsibilities include mobilizing resources, helping with emergency care, advocating for and addressing the needs of vulnerable groups, assisting with recovery, and caring for responders (Speraw & Persell, 2013). Execution of these responsibilities occurs in the context of the nursing process.

Disaster-related Assessment

The assessment activities of population health nurses with respect to disaster care have two major aspects: the types of assessment conducted and specific assessment considerations.

TYPES OF ASSESSMENT. Assessment with respect to disaster preparation and response occurs in two stages: before and after a disaster occurs. Population health nursing involvement in predisaster assessment involves assessing the potential for disaster and response capabilities within a specific community. Assessment during a disaster focuses on identification of disaster effects and related health needs.

Assessing disaster risk and capacity. Earlier we discussed the need to create community risk and resource maps. Because of familiarity with communities and their physical and social features, population health nurses are often in a prime position to identify potential disaster risks in a community. Not only are they aware of the types of industries in a community that may pose disaster hazards, but they may also recognize early signs of pending civil unrest among segments of the population that they serve. Identifying the potential for disaster in a particular community involves forecasting the types of disasters possible and the likelihood of their occurrence (Gebbie & Qureshi, 2013). The possible types of disasters, of course, vary from community to community. Disaster potential and the probable effects can be systematically assessed by examining factors related to each of the six categories of determinants of health. The determinants-of-health perspective can also be used to assess the effects of an actual disaster. Both of these aspects of disaster assessment are discussed in the section on assessment considerations.

Assessment of response capability is another aspect of predisaster assessment. This is closely tied to an assessment of the degree of disaster preparedness in the community and community attitudes to disaster planning. The population health nurse should assess the attitudes of community members toward disaster preparedness. Some of the questions to be addressed might include the following:

- To what extent are individuals and families in the area prepared for potential disasters?
- Have families in an earthquake-prone region, for example, gathered supplies that will be needed in the event of an earthquake and placed them in an accessible location?
- Have emergency escape routes from homes, schools, and other buildings been identified?
- Have families discussed an emergency contact person who can relay messages for and about family members separated in a disaster?
- Or are these types of preparation largely ignored?

Population health nurses also have knowledge of resources that might be brought to bear in a disaster situation. For example, they may be aware of community residents who should be involved in disaster response planning, or they may have a better grasp of potential public response to proposed disaster response initiatives than others involved in disaster planning. Again, specific categories of response capability are addressed in the discussion of the determinants of health later in this chapter.

Postdisaster assessment. Postdisaster assessment includes both rapid assessment and surveillance. Following the occurrence of an actual disaster event, population health nurses will be actively involved in rapid assessment of disaster effects. Rapid assessment involves determination of the extent of damage caused by the disaster as well as the number of deaths, injuries, and/or illnesses resulting from the disaster. Population health nurses may be involved in identifying and reporting the extent of health-related disaster effects.

Surveillance is intended to provide early warning of severe consequences of a disaster. Most disaster plans make provision for early warning systems based on surveillance data. Disease early warning systems (DEWS), for instance, are intended to foster early identification of and response to epidemic-prone diseases. As an example, DEWS in Afghanistan were intended to provide early warning of disease outbreaks. Due to reporting problems, however, only 130 outbreaks were reported after flooding in 2010. Following improvements in the system, more than 5,000 outbreaks were captured by the system after similar flooding in 2011 (Sabatinelli et al., 2012).

The World Health Organization (WHO) has developed guidelines for what it terms Early Warning and Response Network or EWARN systems (early warning systems for epidemic diseases). These include focusing data collection on information that would trigger a major response rather than normal surveillance data, monitoring suspicious symptom syndromes (e.g., fever and diarrhea) rather than confirmed disease diagnoses, which may take time, providing for immediate alerts as well as weekly reporting, and focusing on clusters of deaths rather than overall mortality. Additional recommendations include collecting data from all available sources using standardized reporting forms, aggregation and analysis of data at local levels to promote immediate action, inclusion of threshold indicators for action, and inclusion of information on outbreak preparedness and response (WHO, 2011). Population health nurses will be actively involved in recognition of symptom clusters and may have major responsibility for the collection and reporting of surveillance data.

ASSESSMENT CONSIDERATIONS. Both risk and capacity assessment and assessment of the health-related effects of an actual disaster can be framed in terms of the determinants of health as they influence a disaster situation.

Biological determinants. One determinant in forecasting potential disasters is that of human biology. Certain groups of people are more likely than others to be affected by a disaster. For example, if the anticipated disaster is an epidemic of influenza, those most likely to be severely affected are the very young and the elderly; however, there also will be illness among the health care workforce that may impede efforts to halt the spread of disease. On the other hand, if there is potential for an explosion in a local chemical plant, those affected are likely to be company employees and persons in surrounding buildings. Again, this might include children if there is a school nearby. In disasters requiring evacuation, the elderly and disabled are at particular risk because of potential mobility limitations (Davis et al., 2013). The elderly and disabled are also the most likely groups to have necessary health care services disrupted and quality of life diminished by a disaster.

Human biology is also a factor in predicting the types of effects expected as a result of the disaster. In the case of an influenza epidemic, illness potentially accompanied by dehydration and electrolyte imbalance may be expected. In an earthquake, many deaths result from injuries due to falling debris. After the earthquake in Haiti, for example, 42% of hospitalizations were due to injuries including fractures, dislocations, wound infections, and head, face, and neck injuries, and 28% were earthquake-related (Hotz et al., 2011). In the classic 1906 San Francisco earthquake, on the other hand, the majority of damage was caused by the ensuing fires and rupture of city water mains. Similarly, soft tissue injuries incurred during tornados in Joplin, Missouri resulted in 13 cases of a rare fungal infection causing five deaths (Benedict et al., 2011). Floods result primarily in drownings, but the floodwaters in New Orleans after hurricane Katrina also led to clusters of diarrheal disease, wound infections, and skin infestations from working in contaminated water. Terrorist dissemination of anthrax spores, on the other hand, may result in cutaneous, inhalation, or intestinal forms of disease with related symptoms and complications (CDC, 2014a). War and other civil unrest can contribute to a variety of biological effects. For example, large numbers of Bhutanese refugees admitted to the United States suffer from hematologic and neurological disorders stemming from vitamin B12 deficiencies after two decades of poor nutrition (Walker et al., 2011).

The overall health status of the community also influences disaster planning requirements. For example, if hypertension is prevalent in the community, provisions need to be made in a disaster plan for ongoing treatment of hypertension or other prevalent diseases, particularly communicable diseases such as tuberculosis (TB) and HIV infection. For example, nearly 1,900 people in the areas most affected by hurricane Sandy were being treated for TB at the time of the disaster and special initiatives were needed to maintain treatment continuity (Burzynski et al., 2013).

It has been suggested that people with disabilities and other complex chronic conditions establish "go packs" that can be ready in case of the need for evacuation. Go packs should contain essential medication for at least 7 days, easily accessible assistive devices (e.g., canes), food and water for guide animals, and emergency health information. People with chronic conditions should also know where to evacuate so their own particular needs can be met (Landesman, 2011).

In the event of a disaster, the population health nurse assesses the physiologic effects of the event on human biology. The most catastrophic effect of disasters is, of course, death. Disaster-related deaths may be of three types: direct deaths, indirect deaths, and disaster-related natural deaths. Direct deaths are those caused by the disaster itself. For example, fires directly cause death through burns and smoke inhalation. Indirect deaths are due to circumstances caused by the disaster.

For example, starvation is indirectly attributable to drought and famine. Disaster-related natural deaths are the result of existing conditions that are exacerbated by the disaster. For example, a death due to myocardial infarction during a hurricane would most likely be a disaster-related naturally caused death. The terrorist attacks of September 11, 2001, actually led to development of a new category of mortality and morbidity in both the WHO *International Classification of Diseases, Tenth Revision* (ICD-10) and clinical modification to classify deaths and injuries related to terrorist activities in the U.S. ICD-10 (Centers for Medicare and Medicaid Services [CMS], 2010).

The nurse appraises the extent of injuries incurred by victims and relief workers and may also assess other needs for health care. For example, the nurse might need to assess the health status of a disaster relief worker with diabetes or of a child with a fever. The nurse assists in assessing the health status of groups of people including both victims and rescue workers. Other people not immediately affected by the disaster may also develop disaster-related illnesses. For example, worsening asthma is frequently noted by many people following wildfires and volcanic eruptions. Possible biological effects of several types of disasters are presented in Table 25-5●.

Psychological determinants. Psychological determinants can profoundly influence the effects of a disaster on health.

Many people who experience disasters, either as victims or helpers or both, will experience some level of psychological distress as a result. An estimated 54% to 60% of those affected will develop immediate psychiatric symptoms. The proportion of those affected drops to about 41% within 10 weeks or so, but approximately 22% will have continuing psychological problems after a year. Depression is the most common long-term result, affecting about 41% of people, PTSD may be experienced by 22% to 59% of people, generalized anxiety disorder by 10%, and substance abuse disorder by 14% to 22% (Plum & Meeker, 2013).

Suicide is another relative common psychological effect. For example, the suicide rate among Bhutanese refugees settled in the United States (21.5 per 100,000 people) is far higher than the rate for the general U.S. population (12.4/100,000) or the international rate of 16 per 100,000. In addition, nearly one third of the refugees knew someone who had committed suicide. Other psychological problems noted in this group were anxiety, depression, and PTSD. Contributing factors included lack of nationality, sudden flight, lack of freedom of movement, language difficulties, and concerns about family members left

TABLE 25-5 Potential Biological Effects of Selected Disasters

Type of Disaster	Potential Biological Effects
All disasters	Greater loss of life and injury among the elderly, young children, and chronically ill and disabled persons
Avalanches	Asphyxiation; frostbite and other exposures to cold; fractures or other forms of trauma
Bioterrorism	Widespread communicable disease, death, and disability
Chemical spills or chemical terrorism	Chemical burns of the skin, respiratory irritation and illness; poisoning with a variety of symptoms depending on the chemical involved; eye irritation
Earthquakes	Crushing injuries and fractures from falling bricks, masonry, and other objects; may also cause crushing syndrome Burns suffered in fires and explosions due to ruptured natural gas mains Waterborne diseases because of ruptured water mains and lack of safe drinking water Electrocutions from fallen power lines
Epidemics	Communicable diseases with a variety of symptoms depending on the diseases involved
Explosions	Burns due to associated fires; fractures or crushing injuries die to explosion impact or falling bricks, masonry, and other debris
Famine	Developmental delay in young children; failure to thrive in nursing infants due to inadequate lactation by mothers; protein-energy malnutrition and other nutritional deficiencies
Fire	Minor to severe burns; secondary infections; respiratory problems due to inhalation of smoke and hazardous fumes from burning objects
Floods	Waterborne and insect-borne diseases from contaminated water supplies and insect breeding grounds; drownings
Nuclear attacks or radiation leakage	Radiation burns or radiation sickness; later cancer; later infertility, spontaneous abortion, or fetal defects
Storms	Crushing injuries due to windblown objects and debris; minor to severe lacerations due to flying glass from broken windows
Transportation disasters	Crushing injuries and other trauma; burns from associated vehicle fires; drowning or asphyxiation if disaster occurs over water or in a tunnel; exposure to the elements if disaster occurs in a remote area
Volcanic eruptions	Toxic gas or radiation exposure; respiratory or eye irritations

in Bhutan. In addition, 36% reported experiencing four to seven presettlement trauma events (Cochran et al., 2013).

A number of factors have been identified that influence the psychological response of individuals to disaster. These include traumatic bereavement or loss of loved ones, being injured or hospitalized as a result of the disaster, loss of one's home or employment, and disruption of one's life. People with existing mental illness and disaster workers who handle severely injured victims or the dead are also at greater risk for long-term psychological effects of disasters. Psychological effects may manifest as emotional, behavioral, cognitive, or somatic symptoms of psychological distress (Plum & Meeker, 2013).

Similar factors influence the prevalence of psychological distress in communities recovering from a disaster. These factors include a high incidence of deaths and traumatic injuries, severe widespread property damage in the area affected, and ongoing economic problems in the community. Generally speaking, communities and individuals with good coping skills usually respond more effectively in a disaster situation than those who have poor coping skills.

As noted earlier, both victims and relief workers may experience stress related to a disaster, and the nurse should be alert to signs of emotional distress in both groups.

Types of immediate psychological responses to disasters range along a continuum from calm, collected action to confusion and hysteria. Plans should be made for services to address each level of response. Health care providers should also keep in mind that psychological responses may change with time and with the progression of the disaster event. Psychological recovery occurs for most people within 6 to 12 months of the disaster, but a small segment of the population may exhibit ongoing problems and require therapy.

Population health nurses working in disaster situations can assess the extent and severity of psychological reaction in individual clients (victims, rescue personnel, and others) and population groups. They can use this information to make appropriate referrals for individual assistance and to help in the development of services to address identified mental health needs in the population.

Environmental determinants. Many disasters arise out of features of the physical environment. For example, the presence of a river near the community and the likelihood of heavy rainfall both contribute to the potential for flooding, as does the construction of homes and businesses on floodplains. In fact, the number of people in the United States at risk for flooding is expected to double from 1 to 2 million before 2050 (Bosher & Dainty, 2011). A geological fault, a nuclear reactor, and a chemical plant are other examples of factors in the physical environment that may increase the potential for a disaster. Similarly, the potential effects of climate change may give rise to increased frequency, duration, and intensity of tropical storms as well as emergence and reemergence of tropical diseases (Yumul, Cruz, Servando, & Dimalanta, 2011).

Elements of the physical environment can either help or hinder efforts to control the effects of a disaster. For example, limited traffic access to the part of town where an explosives plant is located could hinder movement of emergency vehicles in the event of a fire or explosion. Similarly, the physical isolation of a mountain community may impede rescue efforts in the event of a forest fire or flood. On the other hand, such isolation might spare the community from the effects of an epidemic in the surrounding area.

In conducting a community assessment, the population health nurse identifies physical environmental factors that might contribute to the occurrence of a disaster. The nurse also determines whether the community is prepared for potential disasters. When the community is not prepared, the nurse would advocate the planning activities described later in this chapter.

The nurse also identifies factors that might impede the community's response in the event of a disaster. The nurse can then share these observations with others involved in disaster planning, and interventions to modify or circumvent these factors can be incorporated into the community's disaster response plan.

Disasters may also contribute to a wide variety of environmental health hazards. For example, hurricane Katrina gave rise to many wound infections with methicillin-resistant *Staphylococcus aureus* and other pathogens due to exposure to floodwaters. Flooding may also contaminate drinking water supplies, whereas fires and explosions result in exposure to smoke and other air pollutants. Mosquito infestations are another potential result of extensive flooding. Population health nurses can be actively involved in educating the public to prevent health effects of environmental hazards arising from disasters.

Crowding and congregate living in shelters, as well as lack of access to adequate sanitary facilities and facilities for bathing, washing clothes and bedding, and washing dishes, may also contribute to health problems for disaster survivors. Population health nurses can identify poor shelter conditions and assist in planning to improve environmental conditions in shelters and refugee camps.

Finally, community responses to disaster conditions may give rise to environmental conditions that imperil health. For example, hurricane Sandy, for instance, resulted in 263 reports of carbon monoxide poisoning mostly due to improper placement of generators and indoor use of charcoal grills after power failures (Clower et al., 2012). Population health nurses can advocate for safe use of such equipment and help educate residents on the hazards of portable generators and their safe use based on the client education tips provided on the next page.

Environmental factors may also promote effective response and disaster recovery. For example, public parks may serve as settings for congregate shelters. In addition, they may foster physical activity and stress reduction among affected populations as well as serving as a social outlet (Rung, Broyles, Mowen, Gustat, & Sothern, 2011).

CLIENT EDUCATION

Preventing Carbon Monoxide (CO) Poisoning

- Do not use portable generators or other gasoline-powered tools indoors.
- Place gasoline-powered equipment away from doors, windows, and air intakes.
- Do not use gasoline-powered equipment in enclosed spaces (e.g., garage, basement, carport).
- Do not heat homes with gas oven or charcoal.
- Properly vent space heaters and use in well-ventilated spaces.
- Install carbon monoxide detectors in home.
- Open windows and fans are not enough to prevent CO buildup.
- Leave the area and seek medical help if CO alarm sounds or if symptoms of CO poisoning are noted (headache, fatigue, dizziness, nausea, vomiting, loss of consciousness).

Data from: Clower, J., Henretig, R., Trella, J., Hoffman, R., Wheeler, K., Maxted, A., . . . Schier, J. G. (2012). Carbon monoxide exposures reported to poison control centers and related to hurricane Sandy—Northeastern United States, 2012. *Morbidity and Mortality Weekly Report, 61,* 905.

Sociocultural determinants. In assessing disaster potential, the population health nurse identifies social factors that might influence the way people respond to a disaster or even give rise to one. For example, the presence of racial tensions could trigger outbreaks of violence in some communities. War is another disaster arising out of social environmental conditions.

Terrorism, like war, arises out of sociocultural factors. Terrorist activity is fueled by perceptions of the United States as being arrogant, decadent, and indifferent to the plight of others. Similarly, terrorism is often a strategy used by those who lack political or military power to address what they perceive as social wrongs. Poverty is another sociocultural factor that motivates terrorist activity, particularly in the face of affluence in other segments of society. Environmental justice issues, such as loss of biodiversity or perceived highjacking of natural resources without consideration for others who depend on them for their livelihood, also fuel terrorist initiatives. Many politically motivated terrorists are generally motivated by a single issue, which if effectively addressed may defuse terrorist activity.

Terrorism also has roots in religious beliefs and may surface in conflicts between religious groups at the national or international level. Concepts of national honor and shame may also motivate terrorist activity—for example, in response to perceptions that adoption of Western values is corrupting women or youth. Ethnic/nationalist conflicts may have a religious component to them, but there is often a long history of intolerance of social and cultural differences outside of religious beliefs.

Sociocultural factors may also contribute to the ability of terrorists to achieve their goals. Media attention to terrorist attacks, for example, provides perpetrators with the public attention to their position that they need. Some authors have described terrorism as a Western phenomenon dependent on a free press. Media coverage can be controlled in countries without a free press, thereby denying terrorists the showcase for their political ideology that is one of the major intents of terrorism. The same may be true of media coverage of other disasters designed to promote giving or to highlight specific political perspectives. For example, media coverage of hurricane Katrina tended to portray minority victims as passive individuals with little expertise, overreported crime, and underreported acts of kindness and heroism. It has also been suggested that media treatment of the disaster may have delayed outside responses due to fear for personal safety of volunteers (People's Health Movement et al., 2008). Treating disaster victims as individuals with dignity rather than as hopeless objects is one of the tenets of the *Code of Conduct* for the International Federation of Red Cross and Red Crescent Societies (n.d.).

Other aspects of society may lend themselves to terrorism. For example, dependence on mass-produced foods makes the United States more vulnerable to agroterrorism. Widespread destruction of food crops or animals would have significant effects on the health of the population as well as on national economics. Similarly, disruptions in electrical power or telecommunications could bring much of everyday life to a halt. Access to the Internet and other technological advances also make information on weapons that can be used for terrorist activity readily available to the general public. For example, from 2003 to 2011, 134 reports of homemade chemical bombs were received in the United States, more than four times the number reported between 1996 and 2003 (Strain et al., 2013).

Elements of the sociocultural dimension also may increase or limit the effects of a disaster on a community. For example, the economic status of community members and of the community at large may limit the ability of people to prepare for potential disasters or to recover after a disaster event. Language barriers may hamper evacuation or rescue efforts. Strong social networks in the community that can be tied into disaster planning aid in effective disaster response; intragroup friction hampers response effectiveness. The nurse identifies social and cultural factors present within the community that may decrease the effectiveness of the community's response to a disaster and participates in planning efforts to modify these factors.

Community resilience is an important factor that assists communities to recover from disasters. **Community resilience** is the ability of a community to recover from an adverse event or situation (Chandra et al., 2011). Components of community resilience include social and economic well-being;

the physical and psychological health of the population; effective risk communication; integration and involvement of government and nongovernmental organizations in planning, response and recovery; social connectedness; community engagement; and development of community self-sufficiency (Chandra et al., 2013). Community resilience includes preparedness at the individual-citizen level as well as a supportive social context (Plough et al., 2013). Population health nurses can assist communities to develop the components of resilience.

Community engagement is a related sociocultural determinant that influences community disaster preparation. There is a need for community engagement in disaster planning and preparedness. Unfortunately, although most people recognize the need for preparation, few actually are prepared for a disaster. In one study, for example, less than 31% of people responded that they were prepared for disasters, 26% indicated that they did not have time to engage in preparation, and 22% reported that they did not know what to do to be prepared (Miller, Adame, & Moore, 2013). Behavioral Risk Factor Surveillance System (BRFSS) data for 14 states from 2006 to 2010 also indicated differing levels of household preparedness. For example, although 94% of households had working battery-operated flashlights and 90% of people had at least a 3-day supply of necessary medications, only 83% had stored a 3-day food supply, 78% had a working-battery-operated radio, and 54% had a 3-day supply of water for family members. In addition, only 21% had developed a written evacuation plan (DeBastiani & Strine, 2012).

This lack of engagement in disaster preparedness extends beyond the individual or family household level. In a study by the Trust for America's Health (2012), most states were not adequately prepared for disaster events, epidemics, or bioterrorism. For example, only two states had met the target for 90% immunization rates of children. Similarly, 35 states and the District of Columbia did not have plans to address extreme weather events, and 20 states did not mandate all-hazard response evacuation plans for child care facilities. In addition, 29 states had cut public health funding that supports disaster preparedness, 16 of them for the second year in a row, and 13 state public health laboratories did not have the capacity to address infectious disease outbreaks. The study scored states for their level of preparedness on a scale of 1 to 10; no state received a score greater than 8, and only 6 states received a score that high. Two states received scores of 2 (Trust for America's Health, 2012).

Based on study findings, the organization recommended reauthorization of the Pandemic and All-hazards Preparedness Act and assurance of sufficient funds for public health preparedness. Other recommendations included providing ongoing support for community-level preparedness; modernization of biosurveillance systems; efforts to address continually developing antimicrobial resistance; increased readiness for extreme weather conditions; updating the nation's food safety system; and facilitating research, development, and manufacture of medical countermeasures for disease (Trust for America's Health, 2012).

The Institute of Medicine (2013) has recommended actively involving community members in disaster planning. Five tenets for community engagement were put forth in the Institute's report, "Engaging the Public in Critical Disaster Planning and Decision Making." These included (a) acknowledging that engagement may be sought for a variety of reasons (e.g., fostering public awareness of the need for preparedness, incorporation of community values and priorities, and promoting adherence to plan elements), (b) recognizing that engagement requires resources that promote community input, (c) the need for inclusion of widespread participation in planning, (d) the need for meaningful support of opportunities for input, and (e) the need for transparency regarding how community input will be used in disaster planning. An earlier IOM publication, "Crisis Standards of Care" (Hanfling, Altevogt, Viswanathan, & Gastin, 2012), identified essential principles of public engagement. These principles include the following:

- Policy makers are committed to considering public input.
- Participants represent community diversity.
- Participants receive information and meaningful opportunities to engage in discussion.
- Deliberation is a goal in and of itself.
- Public input is considered in decision making processes.
- Top-down support and sufficient resources are available to promote meaningful input. (Hanfling et al., 2012)

Economic capacity is another sociocultural factor that influences community response to a disaster. Economic capacity includes local resources as well as the availability of outside assistance. Obviously, a more affluent community would be able to better withstand the effects of a major disaster than a poverty-stricken one. However, the nurse would need to assess the extent to which the economic foundation of the community is affected by the disaster. For example, if a disaster event damages a large portion of local industry, jobs are lost, tax revenues decrease, and even affluent communities may have diminished recovery capabilities. Even more simple economic effects may be felt by a community following a disaster. For example, access to supermarkets declined by 42% in New Orleans following hurricane Katrina and still had not returned to predisaster levels by 2009, making access to healthy foods difficult in the areas most affected (Rose, Bodor, Rice, Swalm, & Hutchinson, 2011).

External economic assistance is also a factor in community recovery from disasters. Humanitarian aid may be available from a variety of sources, but it is usually short-term funding and may not assist in rebuilding of community infrastructures damaged by a disaster. In addition, aid resources may not effectively prioritize recovery needs, misallocating resources. Provision of aid may be restricted by perceptions of responsibility for a disaster or other political considerations. For example, foreign policy considerations may weigh more heavily in aid decisions than humanitarian needs. In addition, with the exception of assistance by the International Red Cross, foreign aid requires a request for assistance from the host country that, again, may not be forthcoming for political reasons (People's Health Movement et al., 2008). Funding streams for global disaster response identified by the People's Health Movement include government funding; private foundations (e.g., the Gates, Ford, and Rockefeller foundations, Wellcome Trust); other private organizations (e.g., individuals and corporate social responsibility programs); multilateral funding agencies, such as the World Bank; bilateral programs, such as PEPFAR and USAID; global health funding agencies, such as the Global Fund and GAVI; and United Nations agencies like WHO, UNICEF, and UNAIDS. In the United States, disaster relief and recovery assistance is often provided by a variety of governmental and humanitarian organizations, making coordination of efforts difficult and resulting in gaps and overlaps in services.

Economic endeavors may also contribute to disaster occurrence. For example, there is some concern that human-induced seismic activity may contribute to earthquakes. Such activities usually involve either extraction of substances from the earth or injection of wastewater into the earth. A recent IOM report by the Committee on Induced Seismicity Potential in Energy Technologies and others (2013) found that fracturing or fracking, a process of injecting water and sand into the earth under high pressure to create fractures allowing release of oil and gas, is not a major contributor to seismic activity, and that injection of wastewater from oil and gas production poses minimal risk. Carbon capture and storage, another process that involves injection of large volumes of fluid into the earth, may have considerable potential for seismic activity although the risk is less if a balance is maintained between extraction and injection of substances. The report concluded that further research is needed to determine the risk posed by these newer energy technologies.

The population health nurse assists in identifying social factors that enhance or impede the community's ability to respond effectively in the event of a disaster. Planning groups could then capitalize on positive factors in designing an effective disaster plan. For example, well-established cooperative relationships between groups and agencies in the community are an asset in designing and implementing a disaster plan, whereas the presence of relatively isolated cultural groups may impede planning and response efforts.

Occupational factors are another element of the sociocultural dimension that contribute to the potential for disaster in a community and should be assessed by the nurse. Occupational disasters are events related to a particular business or industry in which more than five deaths occur. The population health nurse should be aware of industries in the area that pose hazards related to fire or explosion. The potential for radiation exposure or leakage of toxic chemicals in the community should also be determined. The nurse may also want to appraise the extent to which local industries adhere to safety regulations related to hazardous conditions. Population health nurses working in industrial settings would be particularly likely to have access to this type of information. Other population health nurses may need to advocate for regular inspection of industrial conditions by the appropriate authorities.

The population health nurse also identifies occupational factors that may enhance a community's abilities to respond effectively in the event of a disaster. The nurse and others involved in disaster planning would explore the adequacy of rescue services and personnel for dealing with potential disasters. Is the number of firefighters in the community, for example, adequate to deal with an explosion and fire in a local chemical plant? Do firefighting units possess the equipment needed to deal with such an event? Planners also assess the existence of other occupational groups that may assist with disaster response. For example, are there construction companies in the community that could supply heavy equipment that might be needed for rescue operations?

In the event of an actual disaster, the nurse might also assess sociocultural factors influencing the community's disaster response. For example, the nurse might identify growing intergroup tensions in shelters for disaster victims or disorganization in efforts to reunite families separated by the disaster. Other areas for consideration include the degree of cooperation among groups providing disaster relief and, following the disaster, the availability of recovery assistance to individuals and families. Failure of government agencies and other organizations to interact effectively may be a sociocultural factor that hampers adequate disaster response. For example, lack of coordination between local, state, and federal agencies delayed control of the San Diego wildfires in 2003, resulting in increased loss of life and extensive property damage. Steps have been taken since to improve coordination and collaboration.

Another social response to disasters, particularly those caused by terrorist activities, may include anger and hostility toward groups deemed responsible for the disaster. These emotions may be demonstrated in prejudice, discrimination, and attacks on innocent parties believed to be related to the perpetrators. Population health nurses may need to be involved in advocacy to prevent discrimination and violence against such groups. Anger may also be directed at public officials. Other related social responses may include loss of faith in social institutions, demoralization, and social isolation (Plum & Meeker, 2013). Even well-intentioned social responses to disaster may have adverse effects. For example, food aid provided to countries experiencing famine may do as much harm as good. Potential negative effects of food aid include undermining the local economy and promoting black market sales of food goods. Other effects may include promoting rural to urban migration of people seeking relief assistance. Foreign aid may also create national dependency rather than promoting self-sufficiency. Misuse of supplies is also a problem. In addition, the costs and problems of shipping, storage, and dissemination of food supplies exhaust funds that could be used more effectively to promote local economies and infrastructures that prevent disaster. A balance of food and economic aid is recommended to promote the ability of developing countries to address their own needs while meeting the current survival needs.

One particular social group that needs to be considered in disaster response planning is jail and prison inmates. Evacuation of these populations poses special considerations related to public safety and security. Correctional officials may need to be able to safely relocate major inmate populations to multiple locations.

Finally, assessment of sociocultural determinants in a disaster setting includes exploration of the availability and adequacy of basic social services. Areas to be addressed include the availability of shelter, transportation, financial assistance, communication networks, and other goods and services. Population health nurses can help in the rapid assessment of postdisaster conditions, making referrals for assistance, and planning to assure that assistance is available to those in need.

Behavioral determinants. Behavioral factors related to consumption patterns and even leisure pursuits can influence the occurrence of disasters and their effects on the health of community members. Consumption patterns such as smoking, drinking, and drug use can contribute to disasters. Smoking, for example, is often the cause of residential fires and wildfires that result in loss of life as well as extensive property damage. Drinking and drug abuse have both been known to contribute to transportation disasters, and they may also contribute to industrial disasters when the abuser is working in a setting with disaster potential. For example, if a person responsible for monitoring the safety of a nuclear reactor is intoxicated, he or she is unlikely to recognize or respond appropriately to signs of danger. The population health nurse assesses the extent of smoking and substance abuse in the community in relation to the potential for disaster. The nurse may also want to assess (or encourage others to assess) the effectiveness of substance abuse policies in transportation services and industries where there is potential for disaster. Another area for assessment is the extent of safety education with regard to smoking (e.g., not smoking in bed) that occurs in the community. Population health nursing advocacy may be needed to assure attention to these concerns.

Consumption patterns may also intensify the effects of a disaster on the health of a population. A community whose members are poorly nourished, for example, is at greater risk for consequences of disaster such as communicable diseases. Substance abuse may limit one's potential for appropriate behavior in an emergency and lead to injury and even death due to failure to respond appropriately. For example, intoxication may prevent someone from fleeing a burning building.

Consumption patterns and their effects are particularly relevant in disasters involving famine and large displaced or refugee populations. Famine is a population-wide condition involving substantial mortality from malnutrition. Common nutritional effects of famine among refugee populations include *protein-energy malnutrition (PEM)*, a severe state of undernutrition that may be either acute or chronic, and deficiencies of specific micronutrients such as vitamin A, iron, vitamin C, niacin, and thiamine. In some cases, famine is less a function of lack of food than of the inability of some segments of the population to afford what food is available.

Lack of exercise in the population can limit the ability to engage in strenuous labor that might be demanded in a disaster situation. Unaccustomed activity may result in exhaustion or heart attack. The nurse assesses the levels of exercise engaged in by the general population. Population health nurses in occupational settings may also be responsible for determining the physical fitness of personnel who would be involved in rescue operations in the event of a disaster (e.g., firefighters).

The leisure pursuits of community members may, on occasion, contribute to the occurrence of a disaster event. Careless campers, for example, could ignite a forest fire, or skiers might trigger an avalanche. Fires can be started by sparks from recreational vehicles. The population health nurse and others involved in disaster planning assess the extent of such leisure pursuits in the community, the existence of safety regulations related to these pursuits, and the degree of adherence to safety regulations. Advocacy may also be required for the development or enforcement of such regulations.

Leisure pursuits can also enhance the community's response to a disaster event, and the nurse assesses the presence of leisure pursuits that may have this effect. For example, the existence of a group with an interest in wilderness survival may be an advantage in the event of an avalanche or a plane crash in a remote area. Social groups within the community may also serve as a vehicle for preparedness education.

Finally, disasters may affect consumption patterns other than dietary intake. For example, smoking, alcohol consumption, and drug use may increase as means of coping with the negative psychological effects of a disaster.

Health system determinants. The adequacy of the health care system's response capability in the event of a disaster influences the extent to which a disaster affects a community and the health of its members. Assessing the ability of the health care system to respond to a disaster includes examining facilities and personnel as well as the organizational framework in which they operate. A community that has a variety of health care facilities joined in a cooperative network can respond more effectively to the health care demands of a disaster situation than can a community with limited facilities or no existing system for coordinating efforts.

The nurse and other disaster response planners identify the types of health care facilities available in the community and the number and type of health care personnel that could be called on in the event of a disaster. Planners might also determine the existence and adequacy of disaster plans developed by health care facilities. For example, has a local hospital developed a plan for evacuating patients if the hospital is affected by the disaster? Is there a plan for handling mass casualties of various types in the event of a disaster?

Large populations affected by a disaster increase the demand for services by health systems and hospitals. These effects can be mitigated by widespread preparedness in the population. Health care systems need to assess the likelihood of specific disasters in the area and prepare accordingly. The IOM has recommended that health care and other organizations identify indicators and triggers for initiating specific actions in response to disaster events. Indicators are measures, events, or other data that predict a change in demand for services or the availability of resources. Indicators may be either actionable or predictive. Actionable indicators are those that can be influenced by action taken within the organization or as an element of the emergency response system. An example of an actionable indicator might be an increasing number of cases of a particular communicable disease in the dormitories of your school. A predictive indicator is one that cannot be influenced by action, such as notification of isolation of H1N1 cases in the local community (Hanfling, Hick, & Stroud, 2013).

Triggers are decision points that require a change in activity based on information about available resources. For example, a specific number of disaster-related traumatic injuries needing surgical intervention might trigger a hospital decision to cancel all elective surgeries, reserving surgical resources for disaster victims. Crisis care triggers mark the point at which the scarcity of resources requires movement from routine care to crisis care. Cancellation of elective surgeries is an action taken in response to a crisis care trigger; a decision to call in additional personnel to address increased needs would be an example of a noncrisis care trigger. Triggers may be either scripted or nonscripted (Hanfling et al., 2013). Scripted triggers are predetermined points at which action is to be taken. For example, when the number of cases of disease in the dormitories reaches a certain predetermined level, classes may be canceled. Nonscripted triggers are not predetermined. For example, a countywide power outage in San Diego resulted in cancellation of all university classes for several days.

Indicators and triggers lead to tactics or actions to be taken to address the issue of concern. Tactics may also be scripted or unscripted. Scripted tactics are predetermined actions to be taken in the event of the occurrence of certain specified indicators or triggers (e.g., establishing mass immunization sites when the incidence of a particular disease reaches a predetermined level). Nonscripted tactics vary based on the situation and what seems to be the most effective approach to solving an identified problem (Hanfling et al., 2013). The IOM has developed a toolkit to assist organizations, agencies, and jurisdictions in identifying indicators, triggers, and tactics for disaster response. For further information about the toolkit, see the *External Resources* section of the student resources site.

Specific public health preparation for disasters should also be assessed. Preparation includes:

- Establishing close working relationships and mutual-aid agreements with other health and emergency agencies
- Participating in vulnerability and risk assessment
- Conducting system capacity assessments
- Acquiring resources and surge capacity needed to continue basic services
- Developing plans, procedures, and guidelines congruent with those of other response agencies
- Developing operational objectives for public health emergency response
- Developing basic surveillance systems for morbidity, mortality, syndromic, and mental health issues
- Developing guidelines and procedures for risk communication
- Engaging in resource typing and credentialing of personnel, resources, and assets
- Ensuring training and certification of agency personnel regarding safety and health practices and use of personal protective equipment
- Providing orientation and training to response personnel, including volunteers
- Participating in planning and implementing preparedness exercises
- Participating in after-action performance reviews (CDC, 2011)

Population health nurses and others assessing disaster preparedness should determine the extent to which state and large local public health agencies (e.g., those in large metropolitan areas) are capable of carrying out these responsibilities.

In the event of an actual disaster, there is also a need to assess the effects of the disaster on the health care system and its ability to respond effectively. For example, are facilities badly damaged or unusable for other reasons? In some instances, health care facilities have collapsed in earthquakes or become inaccessible due to floodwaters or highway damage. Damage to the health system, as well as other elements of the community infrastructure that permit access to health care services (e.g., roads, electricity, communication networks), can have negative consequences for the population's health.

Questions for assessing disaster potential and the health-related effects of a disaster are included in the *Focused Assessment* on pages 723–724. Two assessment tools are included on the student resources site. One is the "Community Disaster Preparedness Checklist" a tool for rapid assessment of the level of community disaster preparedness. The other tool is the more detailed "Disaster Assessment and Planning Guide" designed to assist with assessment of disaster potential and planning to deal with disaster occurrences.

Diagnostic Reasoning and Care of Populations in Disaster Settings

Based on the assessment of biological, psychological, environmental, sociocultural, behavioral, and health system determinants of health, the nurse derives nursing diagnoses related to disaster care. These diagnoses may reflect the potential for disaster occurrence, the adequacy of disaster preparation, or the extent of effects in an actual disaster. A diagnosis related to disaster forecasting is "potential for major earthquake

FOCUSED ASSESSMENT Disaster-related Assessment Considerations

Biological Determinants

- What is the age, gender, and ethnic composition of the population involved in the disaster? Are the effects of the disaster likely to be worse for some subgroups than others (e.g., the disabled, elderly)?
- What is the extent of injury or disease resulting from the disaster?
- What existing health problems are prevalent among those involved in the disaster?
- Are there pregnant women involved in the disaster?

Psychological Determinants

- How does the population respond to disaster warnings? What is the public's attitude to disaster preparedness?
- What is the extent of community/individual ability to cope with the disaster?
- What is the extent of existing mental illness among those involved in the disaster?
- What is the extent of damage or loss of life involved in the disaster?
- Does the disaster present the potential for continuing damage or loss of life?
- What is the effect of the disaster on rescue workers? On victims? What are the long-term psychological effects of the disaster on the community?

Environmental Determinants

- What physical features of the community create the potential for disaster? What types of disasters are likely to occur?
- What structures are likely to be threatened by a disaster? To what extent are vital structures likely to withstand a disaster?
- What structures could be used as emergency shelters?
- Will weather conditions influence the effects of the disaster?
- Are there elements of the physical environment that will hinder response to the disaster (e.g., blockage of roads)?
- Have buildings been structurally damaged? Is there potential for additional structural damage? Does structural damage pose further risk to victims? To rescuers?
- Is there a need for sources of shelter for persons displaced by the disaster?
- Is there a safe water source available to victims of the disaster?
- To what extent are animals involved in the disaster? What health effects might this have?

Sociocultural Determinants

- Do relationships in the community have the potential to create a disaster (e.g., civil strife, war)?
- What is the level of community resilience? What factors contribute to or impede resilience?
- How cohesive is the community? Are community members able to work together for disaster planning? What level of priority is given to disaster planning by official agencies? By private organizations and individuals?
- What provisions have been made for reuniting families separated by disaster?
- What is the extent of social support available to disaster victims?
- What is the extent of collaborative interaction among relief agencies involved in the disaster?
- Has the community disaster plan been communicated to residents? How are disaster warnings communicated to residents? Are there language barriers that impede communication in the disaster setting? What is the effect of disaster on normal channels of communication?
- What community groups are responsible for disaster planning? Who is available to provide leadership in responding to the disaster? What is the level of credibility of leaders among those affected by the disaster?
- What community industries pose disaster hazards? What types of hazards are present? To what extent do local industries adhere to safety procedures that would prevent a disaster? Is adherence monitored by regulatory bodies?
- What occupational groups in the community are available to respond to the disaster?
- What is the extent of property damage and loss resulting from the disaster?
- What is the economic status of those affected by disaster? Do they have economic resources available to them? What is the effect of the disaster on the local economy?
- What external sources of economic assistance are available?
- What is the effect of the disaster on transportation?
- What is the effect of the disaster on community services? What community services are available to assist with recovery?
- Is equipment needed to deal with the disaster available and in good repair?

Behavioral Determinants

- To what extent do consumption patterns (e.g., drugs or alcohol) create the potential for disaster in the community?
- Do community members engage in leisure pursuits that pose a disaster hazard? To what extent do community members engage in recreational safety practices that can prevent disasters? What leisure pursuits by community members could enhance the community's disaster response?

(Continued)

FOCUSED ASSESSMENT (Continued)

- What is the availability of food and water to disaster victims? To rescuers? Are there special dietary needs among those affected by the disaster? What provisions have been made to meet these needs?
- To what extent have psychological effects of the disaster increased the incidence or prevalence of substance abuse?

Health System Determinants

- How well prepared are health service agencies to respond to a disaster?
- What health care facilities are available to care for disaster victims? What are their capabilities? What health care personnel are available to meet health needs in a disaster? How can they best be mobilized?
- What is the extent of basic first aid and other health-related knowledge in the community?
- What is the effect of a disaster on health care facilities? On health care services?
- What physical and mental health care services are needed as a result of disaster? Are available services adequate to meet the need?

damage and injury due to community location on a geological fault." A diagnosis of "inadequate disaster planning due to fragmentation of planning efforts among community agencies" is a possible nursing diagnosis related to disaster preparedness. A diagnosis derived from information about the effects of an actual disaster is "need for additional shelter sites due to destruction of planned shelters by fire."

In the event of an actual disaster, nursing diagnoses might relate to individual clients as well as to the status of the overall community. Examples of individual level diagnoses include "grief due to loss of husband" and "pain due to leg fracture suffered in building collapse." Nurses may derive diagnoses related to disaster helpers as well as victims, such as "role overload due to need to rescue disaster victims and care for own family" and "stress related to constant exposure to death."

Planning: Disaster Preparedness

Activities related to disaster preparedness and response occur at all four levels of health care, but the terminology used is somewhat different.

HEALTH PROMOTION. General health promotion activities such as good nutrition, physical activity, and development of effective coping skills assist individuals and communities in withstanding the effects of disasters. In addition, specific activities designed to enhance community resilience are an element of health promotion related to disaster care. The Committee on Increasing National Resilience to Hazards and Disasters, Committee on Science, Engineering, and Public Policy, and The National Academies (2012) have identified several universal steps in fostering community resilience. These include engaging the whole community in policy making and planning, linking public and private performance and interests to resilience goals, improving public and private infrastructure and essential services, and promoting a culture of resilience by communicating risks and connecting community networks. Other steps include organizing communities, neighborhoods, and communities to prepare for disasters.

In the event of a disaster, actions that promote overall physical and mental health within the population will assist in disaster recovery. Goals of health promotion in a disaster include meeting basic survival needs for food, water, shelter, and security, ensuring access to goods and services, empowering survivors to advocate for themselves and promoting the highest achievable level of health in the population affected (Reed et al., 2013). Table 25-6● presents health promotion foci and population health nursing strategies related to disasters.

PREVENTION. Prevention, in the context of disaster, has two main foci: preventing disasters from occurring and minimizing their effects. Disaster prevention relies on risk analysis and hazard identification with subsequent activities to reduce risks.

Preventing disasters. Population health nurses may be involved in identifying and eliminating factors that may contribute to disasters to the extent that they identify these factors and report their existence to the appropriate authorities. For example, the population health nurse working in an occupational setting may note that an employee who is responsible for monitoring pressure levels in a boiler may be drinking heavily. This employee's drinking problem may lead to lack of attention to rising pressures and an explosion and fire in the plant. In such a case, the nurse would call the employee's drinking behavior to the attention of a supervisor.

Population health nurses may also become politically active to ensure that risk factors for potential disasters present in the community are eliminated or modified. For example, the nurse might campaign for stricter building codes or serve as a mediator in an attempt to defuse social unrest in the community.

TABLE 25-6 Health Promotion Foci and Strategies Related to Disasters

Focus	Strategies
General community health promotion	• Educate community members for good nutrition • Advocate for availability of nutritious foods • Educate community members for physical activity • Promote effective individual coping
Promotion of community resilience	• Engage the whole community in policy making and planning • Link public and private performance and interests to resilience goals • Improve public and private infrastructure and essential services • Promote a culture of resilience by communicating risks and connecting community networks • Organize communities, neighborhoods, and communities to prepare for disasters
Promotion following a disaster event	• Meet basic survival needs for food, water, shelter, and security • Ensure access to goods and services • Empower survivors to advocate for themselves • Promote the highest achievable level of health in the population affected

Population health nurses can also advocate for maintenance and repairs of structures to promote disaster resistance or the creation of surveillance systems to identify covert biological or chemical terrorism. There may also be a need for advocacy regarding identification of potential terrorist targets or for strategies to minimize terrorist resources. For example, there may need to be stricter controls on access to agents that can be used for biological or chemical terrorism. Safeguards should be developed related to production, storage, transport, and use of such substances. International treaties and national regulation of the sale of weapons and the production, distribution, storage, and use of biological, chemical, and nuclear agents may also be of some help in preventing international terrorist activities.

Prevention of resource wars may also reduce the risk of complex emergencies. Such preventive efforts might include promoting and conserving renewable energy, documenting the impact of such wars and advocating for peaceful resolution of disputes, and protecting the rights of noncombatants (Klare et al., 2011).

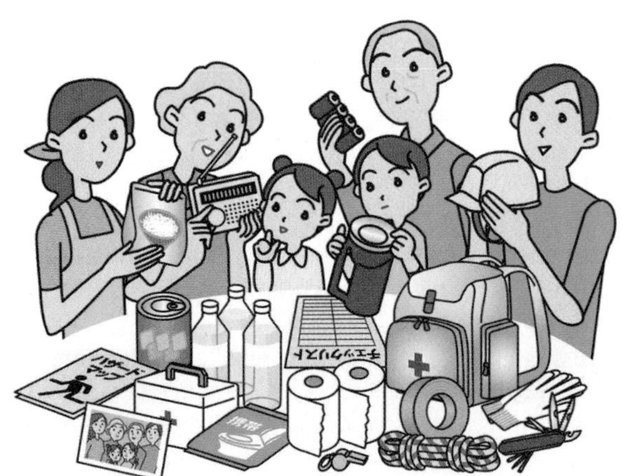

Disaster planning by families contributes to more effective community disaster response. *(alphabetMN/Fotolia)*

Immunization is another preventive measure for epidemics of communicable disease that might occur naturally or result from biological terrorism. Population health nurses can educate the public regarding routine immunization as well as immunization for selected bioterrorism agents.

Population health nurses are often involved in educating the public about major disaster risks, how to prevent disasters, and minimize their consequences. This may involve planning education for individuals, families, or groups of clients on home safety practices to prevent fires and explosions, how to prepare for a possible community disaster, and what to do in the event of a disaster situation.

The nurse would plan to acquaint clients with whom he or she works with the types of disasters possible in their community and actions they can take to minimize the consequences should an emergency arise. The nurse can also guide clients to resources that help them prepare for the possibility of a disaster. A variety of government agencies publish literature containing guidelines for emergency preparation by individual citizens. For example, the San Diego County Office of Emergency Services (n.d.) has developed a *Family Disaster Plan and Personal Survival Guide*. Similarly, the American Red Cross has prepared a series of toolkits to promote home and family, school, and workplace preparedness. For further information about the toolkits, see the *External Resources* section of the student resources site. Potential topics for family disaster education are presented on the next page.

Minimizing disaster effects. As we saw earlier, mitigation efforts may be undertaken prior to a disaster with the intent of minimizing the adverse effects on a population. In addition, population health nurses can be involved in activities to minimize effects after occurrence of a disaster event. For example, they can educate clients on immediate safety measures, such

CLIENT EDUCATION Family Disaster Planning

Important Information

- Provide each family member with emergency contact information (name, phone number, location) for someone out of the immediate area
- Develop and inform family members of the family disaster plan, including:
  - Where and how to safely shut off utilities (electrical circuit breaker, main water valve, gas valve, location of a wrench, manual garage door override, other utilities)
  - Floor plan with marked window and door exits, utility shutoffs, first aid and emergency supplies (also inform babysitters and guests of this information)
  - Avenues of escape from the home or other buildings
  - Two possible reunion locations: immediately outside the home and away from home if family members cannot get home.
  - Alternative evacuation routes out of the neighborhood
- Obtain information on school and employment disaster policies (keeping children to be picked up, etc.)
- Record medication information for each family member
- Obtain and post utility phone numbers, police, medical, contact information
- Obtain information on local emergency plans, shelter locations, and evacuation plans
- Obtain information on community disaster warning signals and their meaning
- Assign activities related to evacuation (e.g., designate the person responsible for taking the baby or family pets)
- Know the general plan and designated routes for evacuating the community
- Know what actions should be taken when warning is given
- Know where to seek additional information

Important Papers

- Medical consents for children
- Insurance papers, bank account numbers
- Identification papers
- Emergency release permissions provided to children's schools
- Pet immunization records
- Significant medical information
- Cash

Important Skills

- Utility shut off
- First aid/CPR as age appropriate
- Personal protection in case of storms, fire, earthquake, toxic fumes

Home Inspection and Risk Reduction

- Install and maintain smoke detectors in homes
- Identify potential risks and evacuation routes
- Secure water heater and heavy furniture to wall studs
- Move heavy items to lower shelves
- Remove or isolate and secure flammable materials
- Install locking devices on cabinet doors
- Install and support flexible connections on gas appliances
- Install fire escape ladders as needed at upper windows
- Keep stairways and doors free of obstacles to permit an easy way out

Disaster Supplies

- Medications, glasses, and first aid supplies
- Flashlights, radio, and extra batteries and bulbs
- Food and water sufficient for 72 hours
  - Water (one gallon per person per day)
  - Nonelectric can opener
  - Canned, dehydrated, or precooked food requiring minimum heat or water
  - Special dietary needs (baby formula, pets)
- Blankets and extra clothing (at least one complete change of clothes per person), outer wear
- Other: fire extinguisher, first aid kit and book, watch or nonelectric clock
- Sanitation supplies: powdered chlorinated lime (to add to sewage), large plastic bags, pre-moistened towelettes, sealable bags, newspapers, hand soap/liquid detergent, shampoo, toothpaste and toothbrushes, dentures, feminine supplies, infant supplies, toilet paper, paper towels, deodorant
- Safety items: heavy shoes, gloves, candles and waterproof matches, garden hose, knife or razor blades, tools, household bleach
- Cooking items: sealable plastic bags, paper plates, utensils, paper towels, cooking pots, barbecue or gas grill, charcoal and lighter or propane
- Tent or other type of shelter

Immediate Response

- Get to a safe location
- Seek shelter from hurricanes or tornadoes in basements or inner rooms without windows
- Seek high ground in the event of a flood
- Assist family members with mobility limitations and functional needs
- Check for injuries and provide first aid as needed
- Check for fires and hazards
- Turn off utilities (only turn off gas in the event of a suspected leak)
- Check on neighbors

CLIENT EDUCATION *(Continued)*

- Stay apprised of events with a battery-powered radio
- Do not touch downed power lines
- Clean up or avoid potentially harmful materials
- Check for damage if safe to do so
- Do not use the telephone except in emergency
- For updated information and shelter information call the Red Cross
- Open doors carefully
- Cooperate with safety officials
- Be prepared to evacuate if necessary
- Purify water if needed by boiling, adding ¼ tsp household bleach/gallon of clear water (2½ tsp/gallon for cloudy water) or water purification tablets
- Engage in safe use of electric generators
- Do not use charcoal grills or other carbon monoxide–producing fuels indoors

Other

- Practice implementing the plan
- Replace stored food, water, and medications periodically

as seeking shelter from severe storms, moving to safer parts of the house in the event of an earthquake, or turning off utilities and safe use of portable generators, and can encourage the placement of CO monitors in all homes. Public education with respect to response to nuclear or radiological attacks would include staying indoors, limiting consumption of milk and locally produced food, and use of potassium iodide prophylaxis following exposure. Population health nurses may need to advocate for the availability of prophylactic antidotes for a variety of potentially hazardous substances depending on the disaster potential in the community.

Postdisaster prevention may also involve use of personal protective equipment (PPE) for those working in disaster-affected areas. For example, those working in floodwaters should wear heavy boots and other protective gear to avoid wound exposure to contaminated water. PPE (e.g., respirators) should also be used in disasters such as fires and the collapse of buildings in which smoke and lingering particulate matter pose health hazards for rescue and clean-up workers. PPE should be standardized across agencies when possible, and all responders, including volunteers, should be adequately trained in its use. Similarly, work to identify the dead poses risks for morgue personnel, who should use PPE during examinations and arrange for appropriate disposal of bodies and autopsy fluids and samples.

Postdisaster immunization campaigns (e.g., for hepatitis A, influenza, varicella) may be warranted in shelter settings depending on conditions such as crowding, poor sanitation, or contamination of food and water. Vaccination may also be needed for autopsy workers and mortuary personnel and their families in the event of disease outbreaks with multiple deaths. Population health nurses may be involved in the design and implementation of immunization campaigns and in educating the public about the need for immunization.

Prevention of mental health problems resulting from disaster may involve preventing group panic by providing reliable risk communication focusing on specific actions that can be taken to promote safety. Health officials should also avoid "knee-jerk" responses to circumstances (e.g., imposing mass quarantine regulations for disease outbreaks). Prevention of mental health effects can also be fostered by assisting people to manage fear and anger and restoring them to a useful social role. Provision of respite may also be warranted for rescue and other personnel and other people with significant care burdens (e.g., single women with children, caretakers of persons with disabling conditions) (Plum & Meeker, 2013). Table 25-7• presents some of the specific activities of population health nurses related to prevention in disaster settings.

RESOLVING PROBLEMS: RESPONSE PLANNING. Resolving problems arising from a disaster involves implementing the disaster response plan. Prior to implementation, however, the plan needs to be developed. Disaster response is based on disaster planning that occurs in the nondisaster stage. In discussing disaster response, we will address purposes and principles and challenges in disaster planning, general considerations in planning, and specific elements of a disaster response plan.

Disaster response planning should be a collaborative effort that incorporates members of the community in plan development, dissemination, and implementation. Planning activities should encourage personal and community responsibility for preparedness rather than relying on the actions of governmental bodies (Chandra et al., 2011).

Purposes of disaster planning. Emergency or **disaster preparedness** involves the development of knowledge, skills, and plans for action needed to prepare for or respond to a disaster (Baack & Alfred, 2013). The general intent of disaster preparedness is to limit the morbidity and mortality resulting from a disaster and to decrease the population's vulnerability to the effects of a disaster. A second general purpose of disaster planning is to ensure that resources are available for effective response in the event of a disaster. This aspect of planning involves determining procedures that will be employed in response to a disaster event

TABLE 25-7 Prevention Foci and Strategies Related to Disasters

Focus	Strategies
Disaster prevention	• Assist in the identification of disaster risks • Advocate for the elimination or modification of disaster risks • Advocate for appropriate controls on the production, transport, storage, and use of hazardous materials • Advocate for measures to promote human dignity and prevent civil unrest • Advocate for effective building codes, maintenance, and security • Advocate for adoption of sound land use planning practices • Provide immunization services and educate the public on the needs for immunization • Educate the public regarding disaster preparedness
Minimizing disaster effects	• Assist in communicating community disaster response plans to the public • Educate the public about major disaster risks, how to prevent disasters, and how to minimize their consequences • Advocate for the availability and use of PPE by disaster responders • Educate responders on the use of PPE • Initiate postdisaster immunization campaigns and educate the public regarding the need for immunization
Preventing psychological effects	• Prevent group panic through timely and honest risk information and direction for action to foster safety • Provide reassurance and assistance in dealing with anxiety • Advocate avoidance of knee-jerk responses • Assist with the management of fear and anger • Provide people with useful social roles • Provide respite as needed

and obtaining material and personnel that will be required to implement the disaster plan.

Principles and challenges of disaster planning. Effective disaster planning is based on several principles that include the following:

- Planning must be based on a scientific understanding of human behavior.
- Planning should incorporate findings from current research.
- Preparedness must go beyond routine response to everyday emergencies.
- Planning should be based on regularly updated community assessment information.
- Planning needs to incorporate establishment of a chain of command prior to a disaster event.
- Disaster response plans should incorporate measures to mobilize local resources during the first 24 to 48 hours after a disaster.
- Planning needs to be based on identification of the needs of vulnerable populations and address those needs.
- Planning should incorporate development of mutual aid agreements with state and federal organizations and include knowledge of what assistance can be expected.
- Plans also need to be flexible.
- Plans need to consider the training and resource needs of response personnel.
- Plans need to incorporate mechanisms for early damage assessment of the overall magnitude of the disaster, health effects, integrity of health system function, specific health care needs of survivors, disruption of public services needed for survival, and the extent of local response (Veenema & Woolsey, 2013).

Disaster preparedness, particularly as it relates to responses to bioterrorist threats, poses several challenges. These include preventing disaster (e.g., the spread of disease) without unduly infringing on individual freedom, supporting economic stability in the face of security controls that may disrupt commerce, supporting and restoring social bonds in the face of suspicion and uncertainty, and alerting the public to the occurrence of a crisis without creating fear and panic. Additional challenges include earning public confidence and support regarding the use of resources in responding to the disaster, maintaining credibility in situations in which information on which to base sound decisions is lacking, and promoting collaboration among multiple social sectors to promote effective response.

Population health nurses should be actively involved in disaster response planning and can help to assure that principles of effective planning are incorporated and that the challenges are met. For example, population health nurses might advocate for collection of community perspectives prior to developing a response plan or might help to assure that civil liberties are protected as much as possible. Similarly, population health nurses might advocate for a response plan that meets the needs of diverse segments of the community (e.g., non-English-speaking residents or those who cannot afford recommended disaster preparation activities).

General considerations in disaster response planning. General considerations in planning the response to a disaster event include designating authority, developing communication mechanisms, providing transportation, and developing a record-keeping system.

Authority. An effective disaster response plan designates a central authority and delineates the responsibilities that are delegated to specific persons and organizations. For example, if it is clear that evacuation decisions are made by the mayor and implemented by members of a local military installation, while police have the responsibility for keeping roads open, there will be less confusion, and evacuation efforts will be carried out more smoothly. Central authority may be assigned to several people in a hierarchical order so that in the absence of the first person designated, the second person has authority to implement the plan. In this individual's absence, a third person would assume that authority, and so on.

Authority for on-the-spot decisions should be delegated, whenever possible, to persons at the scene of a disaster to avoid time-consuming delays in response to an emergency situation. At the same time, there needs to be a balance between immediate response and overall coordination of activities. Areas in which authority will be needed should be identified and responsibility designated. Gaps in authority should be prevented since this results in inability to engage in timely response. For example, one of the policies that prevented effective response to the San Diego wildfires in 2003 was the routine grounding of U.S. Forest Service helicopters half an hour before sundown. There was no one with local authority to invalidate this policy and allow at least one flight with fire retardant chemicals that could have helped contain the fires. Pilots of one helicopter that was already en route had to return to base even though they believed they could safely drop their load of chemicals before flight conditions became too dangerous.

Communication. Communication is critical to the effective implementation of a disaster response plan. Effective communication serves a number of purposes. First, it increases the likelihood of appropriate action by responders and the general public. Second, it reduces anxiety and unnecessary action by segments of the population that are not threatened by the disaster. Third, and most important, effective communication facilitates relief efforts.

Modes of communication should be established and disaster personnel and the general public should be familiarized with them. Specific considerations in this area include how warnings of an imminent disaster will be communicated, how communication between various emergency teams and facilities will be handled, and how communication with the outside world will be facilitated. It is important to remember that normal means of communication may be disrupted during an emergency, and that there is a need for "redundant communication systems" using multiple modes of communication from and to multiple locations (Davis et al., 2013).

Some consideration should also be given to facilitating communication among members of the community. For example, there may be a central bulletin board where messages can be left or a specific agency that is responsible for handling personal communications that permit family members separated by a disaster to locate each other. There should also be two-way communication between authorities and the public so disaster response best meets community needs. This may be facilitated by emergency information systems that collect data about disaster effects during impact, response, and recovery phases (Landesman, 2011).

Disaster-related communication should be factual, positive, and reassuring whenever possible. CDC has adopted the acronym STARCC to reflect the characteristics of effective disaster communication: **S**imple, **T**imely, **A**ccurate, **R**elevant, **C**redible, and **C**onsistent. Trust and credibility may be fostered by expressing empathy and caring, competence and expertise, honesty and openness, and commitment and dedication. Additional communication tips include avoiding over reassurance, acknowledging uncertainty, explaining the processes to be used to find answers, acknowledging peoples' fears, providing direction for specific action, and asking people to share risk. In addition, risk communication messages and information "hot lines" should be updated regularly and coordinated with other responding organizations (CDC, 2011).

Communication mechanisms and messages may need to be targeted to specific audiences, which may necessitate developing ongoing relationships with public media prior to a disaster. Media representatives may need to be educated regarding their potential role in disaster communications (Chandra et al., 2011). Ethnic radio and television stations can broadcast warnings and instructions in a variety of languages, but specific contacts should be established before a disaster event occurs. Development of media dissemination plans will support disaster-related communication with the public. Specific messages should be developed based on communication and behavioral theory to promote positive responses, and messages should be accurate, clear, consistent, and timely in their delivery. Another consideration is the need for interoperable communication systems between response agencies that interface well. In addition, plans should be made to accommodate communication between and among fixed and mobile locations. There is also a need for emergency alert systems that will be easily understood by the general public (e.g., the air raid sirens designed to warn of enemy attack in the 1940s and 1950s). Other aspects of communication include designating reporting sites for rescue and health care personnel and mechanisms for identifying who these people are. For example, color-coded vests might be used to distinguish health care providers from rescue workers. Several prepared public service announcements (PSAs) and podcasts are available from CDC to inform residents of emergency preparedness and appropriate actions. For further information about these media messages, see the *External Resources* section of the student resources site.

Communication-related components of a disaster response plan should consider three possible scenarios and develop contingency plans for each. In the first scenario, normal communication channels remain intact and can be used for disaster response purposes. In the second scenario, some normal channels are intact, but others have been incapacitated. In the third scenario, there is little intact communications technology and other means of communication need to be employed.

Communication considerations in disaster response planning must also include dissemination of the plan to the general public, the scientific and professional community, and other stakeholders to permit them to take appropriate action regarding their own preparation for and response to a disaster. Again, these communications should be targeted to specific audiences and be delivered by trusted spokespersons. Population health nurses can help identify appropriate mechanisms for communicating with particular segments of the community and draft meaningful messages.

A final, highly specialized consideration with respect to disaster communication is how notification regarding the death of a family member will be handled. Protocols should be developed regarding how significant others will be notified of deaths and may necessitate coordination with mental health personnel (Landesman, 2011).

Transportation. General plans for the provision of necessary transportation must also be considered in disaster response planning. There will be a need to transport personnel and equipment to the disaster site as well as to transport victims away from the site. There will also be a need to move personnel to areas where they are most needed. Another consideration with respect to transportation is keeping access roads open so that emergency vehicles can pass. There is also a need to provide alternate transportation routes, especially for evacuating people from a high-risk area, in case first-choice routes are blocked.

Records. Records are needed prior to a disaster regarding the availability of supplies and equipment and areas where they are stored. This information should be updated on a regular basis, and a systematic process for its updating should be established. Local institutions such as schools and businesses should be encouraged to keep records of all those present at any given time so that everyone can be accounted for and those missing can be identified as early as possible. Institutional records may also include emergency contact and health-related information that will facilitate reunification of families or meeting ongoing health needs. One of the disaster plan elements that facilitated continued TB treatment for infected individuals following hurricane Sandy was the maintenance of duplicate records and emergency contact information for patients. All of the 1,899 people under treatment for TB in the most affected areas were located and their care continued without interruption (Burzynski et al., 2013).

During the disaster itself, a variety of other types of records are needed. Victims must be identified and their condition and treatment documented. Deaths should also be recorded. Records are also needed of the use of supplies and equipment so that additional materials can be obtained if required. Records of the deployment of rescue personnel are needed to ensure the most effective use of personnel. It would be difficult to develop systematic record-keeping systems during an actual disaster, so it is important that such systems be in place before a disaster occurs.

Elements of a disaster response plan. A comprehensive disaster plan should address notification, warning, control, coordination, evacuation, and rescue. Additional elements of the plan should specify protocols for immediate care, supportive care, recovery, and evaluation. These last two elements will be discussed under health restoration or recovery, and the others will be briefly examined here.

Notification. An effective disaster response plan specifies in a systematic fashion the means of notifying the person or persons who can set the plan in motion. Persons who might be in a position to have advance warning of a disaster (e.g., local weather service personnel) should have a clear understanding of who should be apprised of the potential for disaster. There must also be specific plans for notifying personnel and organizations involved in the disaster response. Notification should always include the fact of occurrence of a disaster, the type of disaster involved, and the extent of damage as far as it is known at the time. Notification should also convey any other relevant information that is known about the situation.

Warning. The disaster plan should also spell out the procedures for disseminating disaster warnings to the general public. Procedures should specify the content of warnings, who will issue the warnings, and the manner in which warnings will be communicated. For example, the plan might specify that warnings include the type of disaster involved, the area affected, and specific directions on actions to be taken by community members. Warnings may be issued by local radio and TV stations and by police vehicles with loudspeakers. Sirens may be used to alert people if they have been informed beforehand of the meaning of the siren and where to turn for more information. If warnings are to be communicated by media personnel, the plan should specify contact persons at radio and TV stations. Recent technological developments have allowed information to be disseminated in a variety of other ways, for example, through social media or by means of mobile telephones (FEMA, 2012b).

There is also a need to consider mechanisms to provide warning for certain particularly vulnerable segments of the population. For example, sign language or closed caption messages may accompany audio messages on television stations or vibrating alarms may be used. Use of other high-tech mechanisms for warning messages may miss low-income households, and the tendency to provide media messages in English does not meet the needs of non-English-speaking segments of the population (DeBastiani & Strine, 2012).

Control. A disaster plan also specifies how the effects of a disaster are to be controlled. Different control efforts are required for different types of disasters, and a community should be prepared to implement a variety of control activities. In the case of an earthquake, for example, control measures are directed at preventing and extinguishing fires before further damage is caused. Again, the procedures, materials, and personnel needed to carry out control measures must be specified in the plan. Disaster response plans frequently include measures to prevent looting of evacuated homes; however, research has indicated that looting is not generally a widespread problem and such measures may siphon off protective services personnel who could be better used in other capacities.

Logistical coordination. Another element of a community disaster plan deals with logistical coordination. **Logistical coordination** is the coordination of attempts to procure, maintain, transport, and disburse needed materials in a disaster. The disaster plan specifies where and how supplies and equipment will be obtained, where these will be stored, and how they will be transported to the disaster site.

Traffic control is another aspect of logistical coordination. The disaster plan should specify personnel and procedures for controlling access to the disaster site. Traffic control procedures should also specify means by which access to the disaster site is ensured for rescue vehicles and vehicles carrying personnel, supplies, and equipment.

Evacuation. An effective disaster plan also specifies evacuation procedures. The plan should indicate how those to be evacuated will be notified, what they can take with them, and how the evacuation will be accomplished. The plan may need to specify several contingency evacuation procedures, depending on the type of disaster.

The disaster response plan also provides for the logistics of evacuation, including the personnel needed to carry out the evacuation, how they are to be recruited and assigned, and how they will be notified. The plan also specifies the forms of transportation to be used during evacuation, where appropriate vehicles can be obtained, and how they will be refueled.

Rescue. The response plan should specify the process to be used to assess rescue needs and who is responsible for carrying out the assessment. Once the assessment is made, procedures should be in place for obtaining the appropriate personnel and equipment. For example, in the event of an earthquake, heavy construction equipment and operators are needed, whereas fire department personnel are needed in a fire-related disaster.

The rescue operation should focus on removing victims from hazardous conditions and providing first aid as needed. **Rescue chains** are the logistical component of emergency health services including plans for moving injured persons to appropriate health care facilities. Rescue personnel should refrain from providing other forms of care as much as possible. This care can be provided by others, thus freeing rescue personnel to carry out the rescue operation.

Immediate care. Provision of immediate care is another consideration detailed in a disaster response plan. **Immediate care** is health care required on the spot to ensure a disaster victim's survival or a disaster worker's continued ability to function. Plans for providing immediate care in four areas in the vicinity of the disaster site should be detailed in the disaster response plan (Figure 25-5•). Immediate care begins at the actual site of the disaster, with a rapid initial assessment of all victims by the first health care provider on the scene. This phase of immediate care is geared to correcting any life-threatening problems.

The second area of immediate care is the triage area. **Triage** is the process of sorting disaster casualties on the basis of urgency and their potential for survival to determine priorities for treatment, evacuation, and transportation. Triage decisions are intended to maximize the number of survivors of a disaster event without consuming excessive resources (Romig, 2013). When victims are easily accessible, triage can take place at the site of the disaster. Victims are then removed to treatment areas based on their triage priority. In a disaster occurring in an enclosed environment (e.g., in a mine or in a building), victims may not be easily accessible and will probably need to be removed to a more distant triage area as they are found. Triage in the event of exposure to hazardous materials may occur in hot, warm, and cold zones. Hot zones are those immediately adjacent to the exposure area and triage and treatment in this area are minimal. Warm zones are located at least 300 feet from the exposure area; triage here addresses essential stabilization prior to transportation to other area. In the cold zone, victims who have undergone decontamination are retriaged and directed to appropriate treatment areas based on their conditions and prognosis (Romig, 2013).

The triage process usually involves placing color-coded tags on victims. Typically, black tags are attached to victims who are already dead and those for whom death is imminent without heroic measures or extensive resource utilization. Red tags indicate top priority and are attached to victims who have life-threatening injuries but who can be stabilized without undue resource utilization and who have a high probability of survival (Romig, 2013). Priority is automatically given to injured rescue workers, their family members, hysterical persons, and children. Yellow tags, indicating second priority, are assigned to victims who have injuries with systemic complications that are not yet life threatening and who are able to withstand a wait of 45 to 60 minutes for medical attention, but whose condition could deteriorate with significant delay. Green tags indicate victims with local injuries without immediate systemic complications who can wait several hours for treatment without risk of deterioration in their conditions (Romig, 2013).

Triage in an epidemic setting is designed to prevent secondary spread of disease. Those at least risk are persons who have been immunized or are receiving prophylactic medication. Persons who are "removed" are those who are no

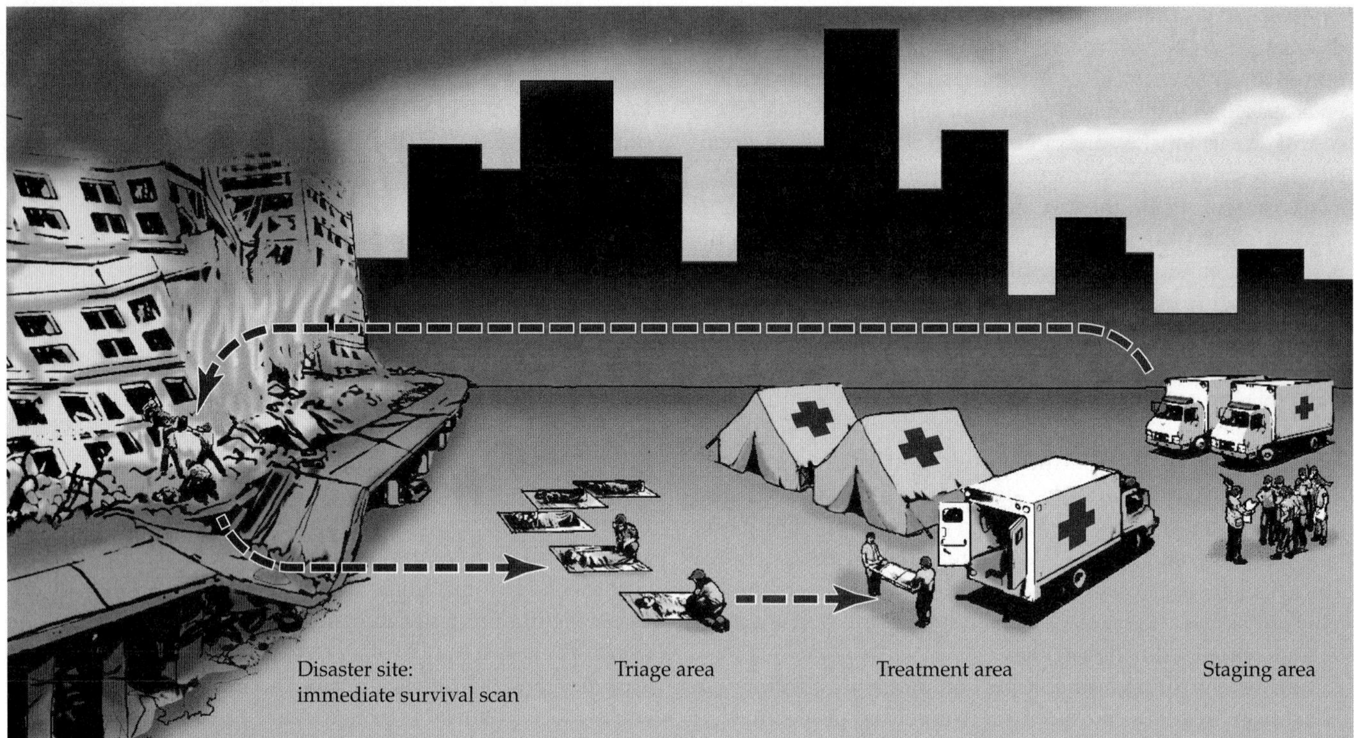

FIGURE 25-5 Areas of Operation in Immediate Care

longer considered infectious or who have died. The next level is persons who are infectious, followed by those who have been exposed, but do not yet exhibit symptoms, and finally by persons who are susceptible, but unexposed (Romig, 2013).

The third area of immediate care at the disaster site is the treatment area to which victims are removed after triage. In this area, medical stabilization, temporary care, and emergency surgical stabilization are provided as needed. There may also be a need for psychological first aid at this point. The final area at the site of the disaster is the staging area. It is here that immediate care operations are coordinated and vehicles and personnel are directed to areas of greatest need. The disaster plan should specify the procedures for setting up and operating each of the four areas of immediate care. The plan should also address the supplies, equipment, and personnel needed in each area, how they will be obtained, and how they will be transported to the area.

Another aspect of immediate care that should be addressed in the disaster plan is care of the dead. Plans should be included for procedures to identify bodies and transport them to a morgue of some sort. Records of deaths should be kept, and procedures for rapid disposal of bodies should be specified should contagion be a problem. Plans should also include where and how body bags and identification tags will be obtained.

Plans should be made for casualty distribution and transport of persons with specific types of health problems to specific facilities (Veenema & Woolsey, 2013). Casualty distribution plans prevent overloading health care facilities closest to the disaster, and may be based on the specific capabilities of certain health care facilities. For example, victims with severe burns may be sent directly to a facility with a burn unit, whereas physical trauma patients may be taken to other facilities.

Supportive care. Supportive care is another component of an effective disaster response plan. Supportive care includes providing food, water, and shelter for victims and disaster relief workers. Other considerations in this area are sanitation and waste disposal, providing medications and routine health care, and reuniting families separated by the disaster.

Shelter is required for those who are evacuated from their homes or whose homes are damaged in the disaster. The disaster response plan should specify which community buildings can be used to shelter victims and how victims are to be transported to shelters. There may also be a need to use the homes of private citizens to shelter victims if public shelters are insufficient. When such is the case, the plan should specify how to notify concerned citizens of the need to place victims in their homes and how placement is to be handled. It is helpful to have a list of people willing to provide shelter to others should a disaster occur. In the case of large groups of displaced persons, refugee camps may be set up. Potential camp sites should be carefully selected in relation to possible physical hazards or water runoff.

Within the shelter, there is a need for supplies to sustain daily living (Chandra et al., 2011). Shelters should have adequate sanitation and sleeping facilities. There should be plans for heating shelters and cooking food if area gas and electrical power systems are disrupted. Shelters should also meet accessibility standards for disabled individuals and provide separate space, if possible, for families with children or persons with dementia. Additional considerations include privacy for breastfeeding women, durable medical equipment (e.g., wheelchairs, walkers) for those in need, auxiliary power supplies for persons on oxygen or respirators, and private examination and counseling areas (Davis et al., 2013). Mechanisms should also be specified for governance and security within the shelter, particularly if the shelter will be in use for some time. Shelter leaders can be appointed or elected, and persons within the shelter should have a means of providing input into governance in long-term shelter situations.

Food supplies should be planned and obtained prior to a disaster. There should also be a mechanism for obtaining more food and other supplies from outside the community in the event of damage to stores and stockpiled supplies. A source of clean water is needed, and the disaster plan should identify how and where water will be supplied. Equipment and supplies for water purification should be stored in case of need. Considerations that need to be addressed in planning to feed large groups, in addition to the availability of food supplies, include toilet and hand- and dishwashing facilities, waste storage and removal (both liquid and solid), cooking and refrigeration facilities, serving dishes and utensils, and food preparation personnel and equipment. Rodent control and food safety information for preparers are other elements of this part of the disaster response plan (Landesman, 2011).

Victims may have other health care needs unrelated to the disaster that need to be met, so plans for providing basic health care in shelters should also be specified. These plans should include stores of medications most likely to be needed by the general public and critical to survival. For example, diabetics will continue to need insulin or oral hypoglycemics, whereas individuals with heart conditions may need a variety of medications. Priority should be given to medications required for serious illnesses rather than for minor conditions. Because communicable diseases spread more rapidly in a debilitated population following a disaster, antibiotics and vaccines should be stored in case of need.

Actions to meet population health needs after a disaster are dependent on identification of those needs. Such identification can occur through early warning systems or syndromic surveillance. **Early warning systems** are planned surveillance systems designed to alert health care personnel of potential large-scale health problems resulting from a disaster. For example, an effective early warning system would identify early cases of communicable disease in a refugee camp, permitting immunization or other control measures to prevent an epidemic. Local surveillance for cases of anthrax or smallpox is another example of an early warning system. The success of early warning systems is dependent on timely reporting and investigation of case reports of specific conditions, pattern recognition, and monitoring of new types of data that can suggest disease outbreaks (Sabatinelli et al., 2012). As we saw earlier, WHO (2011) has developed guidelines for effective early warning systems.

Syndromic surveillance is a special form of early warning system in which data are collected regarding specific clusters of symptoms or syndromes from a variety of sources (WHO, 2011). Surveillance activities in the case of chemical releases or nuclear attacks may include environmental sampling as well as evidence of disease.

Specific screening activities may also be needed in a postdisaster situation. For example, TB screening may be warranted in extended shelter situations such as refugee camps. Similarly, screening for scabies or other infestations might be needed when outbreaks occur in sheltered populations. Screening may also be undertaken to identify people with mental health problems arising from the disaster.

Health care providers may need to be educated to recognize covert releases of biological or chemical agents. Covert releases are often difficult to recognize because initial symptoms of exposure might be mild or nonexistent or might be similar to those of other conditions. In addition, health care providers may not be familiar with symptoms of diseases or chemical exposures that are not often seen in their practice. Finally, cases of diseases may occur over a long period of time in various locations, making it difficult to identify any particular patterns. Epidemiologic cues that suggest covert chemical releases include an increase in the number of people presenting specific symptoms, unexplained deaths in healthy young people, clients emitting unusual odors, and clusters of illness in people that display common characteristics. Other potential signs of covert release include rapid onset of symptoms following exposure to potentially contaminated media (e.g., food or water supplies), unexplained wildlife deaths, and symptoms suggestive of syndromes associated with chemical exposures.

Resolving existing health problems in a disaster situation will also include treatment for conditions identified. As noted earlier, antidotes for potential chemical and radiological agents should be readily available and providers should know how to administer them. Treatments for chemical exposures should be based on syndrome categories (e.g., respiratory effects) rather than on specific agents to minimize time spent in identifying specific agents. Appropriate treatment should also be provided for diseases caused by biological agents as well as for existing illness in the population affected by the disaster (e.g., hypertension, diabetes, HIV/AIDS, TB).

Supportive care also includes psychological counseling for those who are not coping adequately with the situation. Counseling may be required by both victims and disaster workers, and plans should be made to provide crisis intervention services during the response stage of the disaster. General principles of psychological disaster response include the following:

- Interventions generally need to be taken to survivors who will often not seek help on their own.
- Survivors and bereaved members of the affected population are sensitive to perceived voyeurism so assessment for mental health problems should not be intrusive.

- Children should not be separated from family members unless unavoidable.
- Exposure of survivors and helpers to dead and mutilated bodies should be minimized as much as possible.
- Those affected should be given accurate and truthful information.
- Victims' privacy should be protected and exposure to the media limited.
- Use naturally occurring support systems whenever possible.
- Avoid medicalizing reactions and assure victims of the normalcy of their responses.
- Minimize retraumatization of victims (e.g., through interviews with police) and do not force them to recount details of their experiences.
- Do not mandate psychological debriefing of rescue workers, but provide assistance as needed. (Meeker, Plum, & Veenema, 2013)

Interventions for psychological effects include reducing distress and providing for immediate needs, promoting adaptive functioning, crisis intervention as needed, social support, psychological triage, referral for mental health services if needed, and attention to the needs of disaster workers as well as victims and survivors (Meeker et al., 2013).

Elements of psychological intervention that should be incorporated into disaster response planning include mental health triage, emergency psychological first aid and crisis intervention, provisions for meeting physical health needs, and establishment of a calm, stable environment that provides a sense of safety and protection. Disaster victims may require goal orientation and guidance, and they can be directed to perform specific tasks that help them achieve a sense of control. Support is needed for those who must identify loved ones among the dead. Expression of feelings should be fostered, and victims should be encouraged to make use of available support networks. Immediate referral to mental health personnel may be required in some instances. Structuring the environment and regularizing schedules, particularly in shelters, can also help to reestablish a sense of security.

Some relief from psychological stress can frequently be obtained if victims can be assured that family members are safe. Disaster plans should therefore include mechanisms for locating people and reuniting families. Names of persons admitted to shelters or health care facilities should be recorded and communicated to a central location where others can check for word of loved ones. Deaths should also be reported if the dead can be identified, and information should be kept on the assignment of disaster workers to specific areas. It is helpful if institutions, such as schools and businesses, compile the names of those who were present prior to a disaster so that they can be accounted for afterward.

Aside from advocacy for and participation in the development of disaster response plans, population health nursing involvement in resolution of existing problems in disaster response lies primarily in the areas of immediate care and supportive care. Population health nurses may be involved in triage activities and immediate first aid for disaster victims or rescue workers. Population health nurses may also be responsible for shelter supervision and action to meet the supportive care needs of the population after a disaster. They will most likely be involved in assessing health care needs in shelters and addressing those needs directly or making referrals to needed physical and psychological health services. Population health nurses can also advocate for participation in shelter governance by those housed there and help to address areas of conflict among shelter residents.

Population health nurses will also be involved in surveillance activities, and, because of their interactions with disaster victims, may be among the first to recognize signs of disease outbreaks. They may also identify symptoms in the general population suggestive of covert biological or chemical terrorism. If specific screening activities are warranted in shelter situations, population health nurses will probably be involved in developing and implementing screening programs. Finally, population health nurses may be involved in educating the public and other health care providers regarding recognition and treatment of health conditions related to the disaster. Areas of emphasis and related population health nursing strategies to resolve health problems in disaster situations are presented in Table 25-8•.

HEALTH RESTORATION: RECOVERY. Health restoration is referred to as recovery in a disaster context. Recovery has two major goals. The first is recovery of the community and its members from the effects of the disaster and return to normal. The second aspect of recovery is preventing a recurrence of the disaster. Recovery issues include physical rebuilding, restoration of livelihoods, provision of permanent shelter, and coordination of humanitarian aid. One other issue has been referred to as "disaster diplomacy" or sensitivity to the needs of victims and efforts to empower them and reduce dependence on external sources of assistance (Veenema, 2013). During the recovery period, there may be a need to reestablish medical care and other services in the community.

Population health nurses have responsibilities in both community recovery and prevention of subsequent disasters. Nurses may be called on to provide sustained care to both victims and disaster workers following the disaster. They may also be involved in identifying health and psychosocial problems that require further assistance. Population health nurses should plan to provide counseling or referral for persons with psychological problems stemming from their experiences during the disaster. There may also be a need to refer disaster victims to continuing sources of medical care. Population health nurses may also need to plan referrals for clients in need of social and financial assistance. For example, disaster victims may require help in finding housing or in getting financial aid to rebuild homes or businesses.

Population health nurses may also provide input into interventions designed to prevent future disasters or to minimize

TABLE 25-8 Foci and Strategies for Resolving Health Problems in Disaster Settings

Focus	Strategies
Immediate care	**Triage** • Assess disaster victims for extent of injuries/illness • Determine priority for treatment, evacuation, and transportation • Place appropriate colored tag on victim depending on priority **Treatment of injuries** • Render first aid for injuries • Provide additional treatment
Supportive care	**Shelter supervision** • Coordinate activities of shelter workers • Oversee records of those admitted and discharged from shelters • Promote effective interpersonal and group interactions among shelter residents • Promote independence and involvement of those housed in the shelter **Surveillance and screening** • Participate in specific surveillance activities • Recognize evidence of disaster-related health effects • Recognize other health needs in the disaster population • Implement screening activities as needed • Educate health care providers and others regarding recognition and treatment of disaster-related health effects **Treatment** • Provide treatment as needed for disease and injury under medically approved protocols • Refer for additional medical or psychological treatment as needed

their effects. For example, if the disaster involved rioting by members of oppressed groups, the population health nurse might advocate measures to meet the needs of minority group members to prevent further rioting; or the nurse might campaign for stronger building codes to prevent the collapse of buildings in subsequent earthquakes. Population health nurses can also help to educate the public on disaster preparedness to minimize the effects of subsequent disasters. A particular challenge following disasters resulting from terrorist activities involves protection of civil liberties while promoting national security. Health restoration/recovery foci in disaster settings and related population health nursing strategies are summarized in Table 25-9●.

Implementing Disaster Care

Prior to the occurrence of a disaster, the population health nurse may be involved in activities preliminary to implementing a disaster plan, particularly in disseminating the plan to others. Dissemination needs to occur among persons and agencies that will have designated responsibilities

TABLE 25-9 Restoration/Recovery Foci and Related Strategies in Disaster Care

Focus	Strategies
Follow-up care for injuries and illnesses	• Monitor response to treatment • Provide continued care for people injured as a result of the disaster or during rescue operations • Provide rehabilitative care for injury or illness or make referrals for care as needed • Monitor disaster effects on existing chronic health problems and refer for assistance as needed
Follow-up care for psychological problems resulting from the disaster	• Provide counseling for those with psychological problems resulting from the disaster • Refer clients for counseling as needed • Monitor progress in resolving psychological problems
Recovery assistance	• Refer clients for financial assistance • Provide assistance in finding housing, employment, etc.
Prevention of future disasters and their consequences	• Advocate measures to prevent future disasters • Educate the public about disaster preparation to minimize the effects of subsequent disasters • Advocate for protection of civil liberties while promoting national security

during a disaster. Population health nurses participating in disaster planning are responsible for communicating elements of the plan to members of their employing agency. They may also ensure that the plan is disseminated to nursing organizations in the area (e.g., to members of a district nurses' association). The nurse who assumes this responsibility should be sure that the general plan, as well as the specific part to be played by members of the agency or organization, is understood.

The essential features of the community's disaster response plan should also be communicated to the general public so residents will be prepared to follow the plan in the event of a disaster. The population health nurse may be involved in helping to communicate the plan to the public by apprising clients with whom he or she works of relevant aspects of the plan. Population health nurses may also involve community advocacy groups in disseminating information to particularly vulnerable populations, such as members of ethnic minority groups, or recipients of home health care (Chandra et al., 2011). The public should be alerted to mechanisms that will be used to inform them of a disaster and where to go for additional information. Community members should also know the general procedures to be followed in terms of caring for disaster victims and setting up shelters. They should also be informed of the locations of proposed shelters. Finally, community members should be told of specific disaster preparations that should be undertaken by individuals and families.

When a disaster occurs, population health nurses will be actively involved in implementing the disaster plan. Some of the activities involved in implementation were discussed earlier in the section on resolving health problems in a disaster setting or in promoting recovery.

Evaluating Disaster Preparedness and Response

The final responsibility of population health nurses with respect to disaster care is evaluating that care. Nurses and others involved in the disaster participate in evaluative activities outlined in the disaster plan. Evaluation focuses on the adequacy of the plan for curtailing the disaster and meeting the needs of those affected by it.

In this effort, it may be helpful to examine the disaster response in light of the six determinants of health. Did the plan adequately provide for the needs of the people affected and the kinds of health problems that resulted? Did environmental, psychological, or sociocultural determinants impede implementation of the plan or limit its effectiveness? What influence did behavioral factors have on plan implementation, if any? Were health care services adequate to meet the health needs posed by the disaster itself as well as those encountered in the period after the disaster? Data obtained in the evaluative process are used to assess the adequacy of the community disaster plan and to guide revisions of the plan to better deal with future disasters.

The effectiveness of care provided to individual disaster victims should also be assessed. Evaluation in this area focuses on the degree to which individual needs were met and the extent to which problems resulting from the disaster were resolved.

The Sphere Project's (2011) *Humanitarian Charter and Minimum Standards in Disaster Response* provides a set of guidelines that may be used to evaluate the effectiveness of disaster response planning. The Sphere Project (2011), a group of humanitarian non-governmental agencies and Red Cross and Red Crescent Societies, has developed a handbook to address international disaster response. The handbook incorporates basic principles of protection, six core standards, and related actions and key indicators that can be used to evaluate the effectiveness of disaster response. Guidance notes and points to consider in applying the standards are also included. A description of the Sphere Project standards and related considerations are included in the *Global Perspectives* feature on the next page. For further information about the standards, see the *External Resources* section of the student resources site. Population health nurses would participate in using the standards to evaluate the response to a particular disaster. In addition,

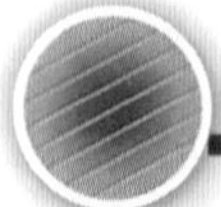

Evidence-Based Practice

Community Involvement in Generating Evidence

Svendsen et al. (2010) have noted that epidemiologic research following disasters has often been imposed from outside researchers and government agencies. This often leads to resentment among community members who are trying to rebuild lives shattered by disaster and its short- and long-term effects. The authors proposed that a community-based participatory research (CBPR) strategy be used to address questions of particular interest to those affected by the disaster to enable them to better prepare for future disaster events. They noted that some of the earliest CBPR research, although not given that label, occurred many years after the bombings of Hiroshima and Nagasaki, after health and reconstruction needs of the population had been addressed and trust in U.S. officials, including researchers, had been established. They emphasized the vulnerable status of those affected by disasters and stressed the need for special care to "address the immediate health needs of the community first, rather than the pressing needs to answer important scientific questions" (p. 77).

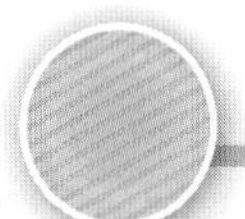

Global Perspectives

The Sphere Project

The Sphere Project was established in 1997 by several non-governmental disaster relief organizations as a way to monitor and improve their performance in disaster response throughout the world. The result was the development of a handbook incorporating a set of minimum standards for humanitarian response to disaster based on three core beliefs: (a) that people affected by disasters have a right to lives with dignity, (b) that they have a right to humanitarian assistance, and (c) that they have a right to protection and security. In keeping with these principles, actions taken by humanitarian organizations should incorporate consultation with and accountability to those affected.

These beliefs are reflected in four protection principles that include:

- Avoid causing further harm in the course of providing assistance
- Ensure access to impartial assistance
- Protect people from physical or psychological harm due to violence or coercion
- Assist people with rights claims, access to remedies, and recovery from abuse

The handbook includes core standards in six key areas, as well as key actions to achieve the standard, indicators of accomplishment, and guidance notes on addressing practical difficulties. The key areas addressed include the following:

- *People-centered humanitarian response*: Focuses on widespread inclusion of those affected in decision making and evaluation related to assistance activities, support for local capacity, use of local labor and self-help initiatives when possible, cultural sensitivity, and provision of avenues for airing grievances.
- *Coordination and collaboration*: Addresses collaboration and coordination with governmental and other non-governmental organizations in the provision of assistance, intersectoral collaboration of activities (e.g., health-related and development activities), sharing of knowledge and progress information, strengthening overall advocacy among organizations to deal with shared concerns, and development of policies for interaction with non-humanitarian organizations (e.g., business or industrial concerns).
- *Assessment*: Addresses participation in interorganizational assessment, use of predisaster capacity data, rapid assessment of needs, consideration of a wide variety of perspectives in assessment (particularly vulnerable populations), systematic collection of data, assessment of capacity of in-country systems and those affected, assessment of psychosocial as well as other aspects of well-being, and sharing of assessment information.
- *Design and response*: Focuses on development of programs based on needs and capacity of those affected, filling gaps between local capacity and need; prioritization of urgent needs; addressing the needs of vulnerable populations; providing equitable access to assistance; minimizing negative effects of assistance (e.g., undermining local economies); promoting risk reduction and resilience to future disasters; modifying programs to maintain relevance and appropriateness; and planning exit strategies.
- *Performance, transparency, and learning*: Focuses on continual monitoring of agency performance and effectiveness, adapting programs based on monitoring data, conducting final effectiveness evaluation and sharing results, and participating in collaborative learning to inform future disaster responses.
- *Aid worker performance*: Addresses the adequacy of leadership and management training of supervisors, appropriate worker recruitment and orientation, providing for the physical and psychological needs of workers, promoting respectful interactions between workers and recipients of services, monitoring worker performance, developing worker safety, health, security, and evacuation guidelines, investigating and addressing complaints about worker performance.

population health nurses would advocate for the evaluation of disaster services from the perspective of service recipients. One further consideration in disaster evaluation is the cost of the disaster response and mechanisms to decrease the cost of future responses while maintaining quality of services to those affected (Landesman, 2011).

Healthy People 2020 also addresses four national objectives that can be used to evaluate some aspects of disaster preparation. Some of these objectives are developmental in nature, so there are as yet no data related to the achievement of most of them. Data are available for objectives PREP-3.2 dealing with the ability of Laboratory Response Network (LRN) chemical laboratories to meet professional competencies. Unfortunately, the objective is moving away from the 95% target, declining from 92% of laboratories in 2008 to 91% in 2011 (U.S. Department of Health and Human Services [USDHHS], 2014). The preparedness objectives may be viewed on the *Healthy People 2020* website.

CHAPTER RECAP

Although disasters occur infrequently in population health practice, population health nurses should be prepared to respond effectively when they do occur. They should also be instrumental in assuring that individual clients and families, as well as communities, are prepared to respond effectively in the event of a disaster. Preparation for a disaster event includes assessment of disaster potential as well as the effects of a disaster from the perspective of the six categories of determinants of health. Activities at each level of health care are relevant to disaster nursing. For example, basic health promotion and promotion of community resilience can help to mitigate the effects of disasters and promote recovery after a disaster. Prevention focuses on prevention of disaster events and prevention or mitigation of their effects. Resolution of health problems resulting from a disaster are based on the type of disaster involved, but should be addressed by the basic elements of a community disaster plan. Finally, population health nurses also have a role in health restoration or recovery after a disaster.

CASE STUDY Nursing in a Disaster Setting

Two commuter trains have collided in a tunnel at rush hour. Both trains derailed and one of them struck the side of the tunnel, causing it to collapse on two of the derailed cars. There were approximately 300 passengers on the two trains, and 50 or more people are trapped in the two buried cars. The accident occurred approximately one quarter mile from the west end of the tunnel and two miles from the east end. The largest portions of both trains lie on the west side of the collapsed portion of the tunnel.

One of the passengers is a population health nurse. The nurse was not injured in the accident and was able to get out of the wreckage to the west end of the tunnel, where most of the survivors are gathered.

1. What are the biological, psychological, environmental, sociocultural, behavioral, and health system determinants that may influence this disaster situation?
2. What role functions might the population health nurse carry out in this situation?
3. What health promotion, prevention, resolution, and restoration activities might be appropriate in this situation? Why?

REFERENCES

American Nurses Association. (2008). *Adapting standards of care under extreme conditions: Guidance for professionals during disasters, pandemics, and other extreme emergencies.* Retrieved from http://nursingworld.org/MainMenuCategories/WorkplaceSafety/Healthy-Work-Environment/DPR/TheLawEthicsofDisasterResponse/AdaptingStandardsofCare.pdf

American Public Health Association. (2014). *Get ready day planning tips for your event.* Retrieved from http://www.getreadyforflu.org/GetReadyDayPlanning.htm

Baack, S., & Alfred, D. (2013). Nurses' preparedness and perceived competence in managing disasters. *Journal of Nursing Scholarship, 45,* 281–287.

Benedict, K., Adebanjo, T., Harris, J., Lockhart, S., Peterson, J., & McClinton, S. (2011). Fatal fungal soft-tissue infections after a Tornado—Joplin, Missouri, 2011. *Morbidity and Mortality Weekly Report, 60,* 992.

Blair, D. (2013). *Iraq war 10 years on: At least 116,000 civilians killed.* Retrieved from http://www.telegraph.co.uk/news/worldnews/middleeast/Iraq/9932214/Iraq-war-10-years-on-at-least-116000-civilians-killed.html

Bosher, L., & Dainty, A. (2011). Disaster risk reduction and "built in" resilience: Towards overarching principles for construction practice. *Disasters, 35,* 1–18.

Burkle, F. M. (2013). Complex humanitarian emergencies. In T. G. Veenema (Ed.), *Disaster nursing and emergency preparedness for chemical, biological, and radiological terrorism and other hazards* (3rd ed., pp. 333–343). New York, NY: Springer.

Burzynski, J., Varma, J. K., Rodriquez, E., Oxtoby, M. J., Privett, T., Forbes, A., et al. (2013). Tuberculosis control activities before and after hurricane Sandy—Northeast and Mid-Atlantic states. *Morbidity and Mortality Weekly Report, 62,* 206–208.

Casey-Lockyer, M., Donald, C. M., Moulder, J., Aderhold, D., Harris, D., Woodall, G., et al. (2013). Tornado-related fatalities—five states, Southeastern United States, April 25–28, 2011. *Morbidity and Mortality Weekly Report, 62,* 529–533.

Casey-Lockyer, M., Heick, R. J., Mertzlufft, C. E., Yard, E. E., Wolkin, A. F., Noe, R. S., et al. (2013). Deaths associated with hurricane Sandy—October–November 2012. *Morbidity and Mortality Weekly Report, 62,* 393–397.

Center for Research on the Epidemiology of Disasters. (2009a). *Classification.* Retrieved from http://www.emdat.be/classification

Center for Research on the Epidemiology of Disasters. (2009b). *Criteria and definition.* Retrieved from http://www.emdat.be/criteria-and-definition

Center for Research on the Epidemiology of Disasters. (2009c). *The EM-DAT glossary.* Retrieved from http://www.emdat.be/glossary/9

Center for Research on the Epidemiology of Disasters. (2014a). *Disaster trends: Natural disasters.* Retrieved from http://imgur.com/a/KdyTV" \l "16

Center for Research on the Epidemiology of Disasters. (2014b). *Disaster trends: Technological disasters*. Retrieved from http://imgur.com/a/gxkrh#0

Center for Research on the Epidemiology of Disasters. (2014c). *Disaster trends: Natural disasters*. Retrieved from http://imgur.com/a/KdyTV#16

Centers for Disease Control and Prevention. (n.d.). *Bioterrorism agents/diseases, by category*. Retrieved from http://emergency.cdc.gov/agent/agentlist-category.asp

Centers for Disease Control and Prevention. (2011). *Public health emergency response guide for state, local, and tribal public health directors*. Retrieved from http://emergency.cdc.gov/planning/pdf/cdcresponseguide.pdf

Centers for Disease Control and Prevention. (2014a). *Anthrax: Bioterrorism*. Retrieved from http://www.cdc.gov/anthrax/bioterrorism/index.html

Centers for Disease Control and Prevention. (2014b). *Chemical categories*. Retrieved from http://emergency.cdc.gov/agent/agentlistchem-category.asp

Centers for Disease Control and Prevention. (2014c). *Emergency preparedness and response: Specific hazards*. Retrieved from http://emergency.cdc.gov/

Centers for Disease Control and Prevention. (2014d). *Natural disasters and severe weather*. Retrieved from http://emergency.cdc.gov/disasters/

Centers for Medicare and Medicaid Services. (2010). *ICD-10CM: Official guidelines for coding and reporting*. Retrieved from http://www.cms.gov/Medicare/Coding/ICD10/downloads/7_Guidelines10cm2010.pdf

Chandra, A., Acosta, J., Stern, S., Uscher-Pines, L., Williams, M. V., Yeung, D., et al. (2011). *Building community resilience to disasters: A way forward to enhance national health security*. Santa Monica, CA: Rand Corporation.

Chandra, A., Williams, M., Plough, A., Stayton, A., Wells, K. B., Horta, M., et al. (2013,). Getting actionable about community resilience: The Los Angeles county community disaster resilience project. *American Journal of Public Health, 103,* 1181–1189.

Clower, J., Henretig, R., Trella, J., Hoffman, R., Wheeler, K., Maxted, A., et al. (2012). Carbon monoxide exposures reported to poison control centers and related to hurricane Sandy—Northeastern United States, 2012. *Morbidity and Mortality Weekly Report, 61,* 905.

Cochran, J., Gelman, P. L., Ellis, H., Brown, C., Anderton, S., Montour, J., et al. (2013). Suicide and suicidal ideation among Bhutanese refugees—United States, 2009–12. *Morbidity and Mortality Weekly Report, 62,* 533–536.

Committee on Increasing National Resilience to Hazards and Disasters; Committee on Science, Engineering, and Public Policy; The National Academies. (2012). *Disaster resilience: A national imperative*. Retrieved from http://www.nap.edu/download.php?ecord_id=13457#

Committee on Induced Seismicity Potential in Energy Technologies, Committee on Earth Resources, Committee on Geological and Geotechnical Engineering, Board on Earth Science and Resources, Division on Earth and Life Studies, and National Research Council of the National Academies. (2013). *Induced seismicity potential in energy technologies*. Retrieved from http://www.nap.edu/download.php?record_id=13355

Davis, E. A., Hansen, R., Kushma, J., Peek, L., & Phillips, B. (2013). Identifying and accommodating high-risk, high-vulnerability populations in disasters. In T. G. Veenema (Ed.), *Disaster nursing and emergency preparedness for chemical, biological, and radiological terrorism and other hazards* (3rd ed., pp. 519–537). New York, NY: Springer.

DeBastiani, S. D., & Strine, T. W. (2012). Household preparedness for public health emergencies—14 states, 2006–2010. *Morbidity and Mortality Weekly Report, 61,* 713–719.

Degutis, L. C. (2013). Epidemiology of violence. In R. M. Hammer, B. Moynihan, & E. M. Pagliaro (Eds.), *Forensic nursing: A handbook for practice* (2nd ed., pp. 31–44). Burlington, MA: Jones & Bartlett Learning.

Federal Bureau of Investigation. (2005). *Terrorism 2000-2005*. Retrieved from http://www.fbi.gov/stats-services/publications/terrorism-2002-2005

Federal Emergency Management Agency. (2012a). *Declaration process fact sheet: The emergency response process*. Retrieved from http://www.fema.gov/declaration-process-fact-sheet

Federal Emergency Management Agency. (2012b). *Integrated public alert and warning system overview*. Retrieved from http://www.fema.gov/integrated-public-alert-and-warning-system-overview

Federal Emergency Management Agency. (2012c). *The declaration process*. Retrieved from http://www.fema.gov/declaration-process

Federal Emergency Management Agency. (2013a). *Federal insurance mitigation administration*. Retrieved from http://www.fema.gov/what-mitigation/federal-insurance-mitigation-administration

Federal Emergency Management Agency. (2013b). *Multi-hazard mitigation planning*. Retrieved from http://www.fema.gov/multi-hazard-mitigation-planning

Federal Emergency Management Agency. (2013c). *What is mitigation?* Retrieved from http://www.fema.gov/what-mitigation

Gebbie, K. M., & Qureshi, K. (2013). Disaster management. In T. G. Veenema (Ed.), *Disaster nursing and emergency preparedness for chemical, biological, and radiological terrorism and other hazards* (3rd ed., pp. 181–199). New York, NY: Springer.

Hanfling, D., Altevogt, B. M., Viswanathan, K., & Gastin, L. O. (2012). *Crisis standards of care: A systems framework for catastrophic disaster response*. Retrieved from http://www.nap.edu/download.php?record_id=13351

Hanfling, D., Hick, J. L., & Stroud, C. (2013). *Crisis standards of care: A toolkit for indicators and triggers*. Retrieved from http://www.nap.edu/download.php?record_id=18338

Hotz, G., Ginzburg, E., Wurm, G., DeGennaro, V., Andrews, D., Basaravaju, S., et al. (2011). Post-earthquake injuries treated at a field hospital—Haiti, 2010. *Morbidity and Mortality Weekly Report, 59,* 1673–1677.

Institute of Medicine. (2013). *Engaging the public in critical disaster planning and decision making: Workshop summary*. Retrieved from http://www.nap.edu/download.php?ecord_id=18396

International Federation of Red Cross and Red Crescent Societies. (n.d.). *Code of conduct*. Retrieved from http://www.ifrc.org/en/publications-and-reports/code-of-conduct

Jenkins, P. H., Montejano, H. J., Broward, M. S., Abbassi, M. J., Crowley, M. S., O'Brien, M. G., et al. (2010). Update on cholera—Haiti, Dominican Republic, and Florida, 2010. *Morbidity and Mortality Weekly Report, 59,* 1637–1641.

Klare, M. T., Levy, B. S., & Sidel, V. W. (2011,). The public health implications of resource wars. *American Journal of Public Health, 101,* 1615–1619.

Kukaswadia, A. (2013). *APHA get ready day planning: How preparation can save lives (including your own)*. Retrieved from http://blogs.plos.org/publichealth/2013/09/17/apha-get-ready-day-how-preparation-can-save-lives-including-your-own/

Kuntz, S., Frable, P., Qureshi, K., & Strong, L. (2008). *Disaster preparedness white paper for community/public health nursing educators*. Retrieved from http://www.achne.org/files/public/DisasterPreparednessWhitePaper.pdf.

Landesman, L. Y. (2011). *Public health management of disasters: The practice guide* (3rd ed.). Washington, DC: American Public Health Association.

Leidel, L., Groseclose, S. L., Burney, B., Navin, P., & Wooster, M. (2013). CDC's emergency management program activities—Worldwide, 2003–2012. *Morbidity and Mortality Weekly Report, 62,* 498–500, 709–713.

Meeker, E. C., Plum, K. C., & Veenema, T. G. (2013). Management of the psychosocial effects of disasters. In T. G. Veenema (Ed.), *Disaster nursing and emergency preparedness for chemical, biological, and radiological terrorism and other hazards* (3rd ed., pp. 111–130). New York, NY: Springer.

Miller, C. H., Adame, B., J., & Moore, S. D. (2013). Vested interest theory and disaster preparedness. *Disasters, 37,* 1–27.

National Counterterrorism Center. (2012). *Developing statistical information*. Retrieved from http://www.state.gov/j/ct/rls/crt/2011/195555.htm

Nelson, S. A. (2013). *Natural hazards and natural disasters*. Retrieved from http://www.tulane.edu/~sanelson/Natural_Disasters/introduction.htm

People's Health Movement, Medact, & Global Equity Gauge Alliance. (2008). *Global health watch 2: An alternative world health report*. London, UK: Zed.

Plough, A., Fielding, J., E., Chandra, A., Williams, M., Eisenman, E., Wells, K. B., et al. (2013). Building community disaster resilience: Perspectives from a large urban county department of health. *American Journal of Public Health, 103,* 1190–1197.

Plum, K. C., & Meeker, E. C. (2013). Understanding the psychosocial impact of disasters. In T. G. Veenema (Ed.), *Disaster nursing and emergency preparedness for chemical, biological, and radiological terrorism and other hazards* (3rd ed., pp. 93–110). New York, NY: Springer.

Ray, M. (2013). *Boston marathon bombing of 2013.* Retrieved from http://www.britannica.com/EBchecked/topic/1924021/Boston-Marathon-bombing-of-2013

Reed, J., Veenema, T. G., & Rains, A. B. (2013). Restoring public health under disaster conditions: Basic sanitation, water, food supply, and shelter. In T. G. Veenema (Ed.), *Disaster nursing and emergency preparedness for chemical, biological, and radiological terrorism and other hazards* (3rd ed., pp. 287–304). New York, NY: Springer.

Romig, L. (2013). Disaster triage. In T. G. Veenema (Ed.), *Disaster nursing and emergency preparedness for chemical, biological, and radiological terrorism and other hazards* (3rd ed., pp. 201–222). New York, NY: Springer.

Rose, D., Bodor, J. N., Rice, J., Swalm, C. M., & Hutchinson, P. L. (2011,). The effects of hurricane Katrina on food access disparities in New Orleans. *American Journal of Public Health, 101,* 1181–1189.

Rung, A. L., Broyles, S. T., Mowen, A. J., Gustat, J., & Sothern,, M. S. (2011,). Escaping to and being active in neighborhood parks: Park use in a post disaster setting. *Disasters, 35,* 383–403.

Sabatinelli, G., Kakar, S. R., Malik, M., Kazi, B. M., Khan, M. R., Aurakzai, J. K., et al. (2012). Early warning disease surveillance after a flood emergency—Pakistan, 2010. *Morbidity and Mortality Weekly Report, 61,* 1002–1007.

San Diego County Office of Emergency Services. (n.d.). *Family disaster plan and personal survival guide.* San Diego, CA: Author.

South Sudan profile: A chronology of key events. (2013). Retrieved from http://www.bbc.com/news/world-Africa-14019202

Spencer, L., & Spellman, J. (2013). The role of the public health nurse in disaster response. In T. G. Veenema (Ed.), *Disaster nursing and emergency preparedness for chemical, biological, and radiological terrorism and other hazards* (3rd ed., pp. 687–698). New York, NY: Springer.

Speraw, S., & Persell, D. J. (2013). National nurse preparedness: Achieving competency-based practice. In T. G. Veenem (Ed.), *Disaster nursing and emergency preparedness for chemical, biological, and radiological terrorism and other hazards* (3rd ed., pp. 669–685). New York, NY: Springer.

Sphere Project. (2011). *Humanitarian charter and minimum standards in humanitarian response.* Retrieved from http://www.sphereproject.org/resources/download-publications/?search=1&keywords=&language=English&category=22

Spiegel, P. B., Burton, A., Tepo, S., Jacobson, L. M., Anderson, M. A., Cookson, S. T., et al. (2011). Mortality among refugees fleeing Somalia—Dadaab Refugee Camps, Kenya, July–August 2011. *Morbidity and Mortality Weekly Report, 60,* 1133.

Strain, S. L., Welles, W. L., Larson, T. C., Orr, M. F., Wu, J., & Horton, K. (2013). Homemade chemical bomb incidents—15 states, 2003–2011. *Morbidity and Mortality Weekly Report, 62,* 498–500.

Svendsen, E. R., Whittle, N. C., Sanders, L., McKeown, R. E., Sprayberry, K., Heim, M., et al. (2010). GRACE: Public health recovery methods following an environmental disaster. *Archives of Environmental and Occupational Health, 65*(2), 77–85. doi:10.1080/19338240903390222

Thomson, K., Dvorzak, J. L., Lagu, J., Laku, R., Dineen, B., Schilperoord, M., et al. (2012). Investigation of hepatitis E outbreak among refugees—Upper Nile, South Sudan, 2012–2013. *Morbidity and Mortality Weekly Report, 61,* 581–586.

Trust for America's Health. (2012). *Ready or not? Protecting the public from diseases, disasters, and bioterrorism.* Retrieved from http://healthyamericans.org/report/101/

United Nations High Commissioner for Refugees. (2012). *Protecting refugees & the role of UNHCR.* Retrieved from http://www.unhcr.org/509a836e9.html

United Nations Office for Disaster Risk Reduction. (2013). *Disaster impacts/2000-2012.* Retrieved from http://www.preventionweb.net/files/31737_20130312disaster20002012copy.pdf

U.S. Department of Health and Human Services. (2014). *Preparedness.* Retrieved from http://www.healthypeople.gov/2020/topicsobjectives2020/objectiveslist.aspx?topicId=34

Veenema, T. G. (2013). Disaster recovery: Creating sustainable disaster-resistant communities. In T. G. Veenema (Ed.), *Disaster nursing and emergency preparedness for chemical, biological, and radiological terrorism and other hazards* (3rd ed., pp. 719–722). New York, NY: Springer.

Veenema, T. G., & Woolsey, C. (2013). Essentials of disaster planning. In T. G. Veenema (Ed.), *Disaster nursing and emergency preparedness for chemical, biological, and radiological terrorism and other hazards* (3rd ed., pp. 1–20). New York, NY: Springer.

Walker, P. F., O'Fallon, A., Nelson, K., Mano, B., Dicker, S., Chute, S., et al. (2011). Vitamin b deficiency in resettled Bhutanese refugees—United States, 2008–2011. *Morbidity and Mortality Weekly Report, 60,* 343–346.

Wall, B. M., & Kelly, M. E. (2011). The San Francisco earth quake and fire, 1906: "Lifetime of experience." In B. M. Wall & A. W. Keeling (Eds.), *Nurses on the front line: When disaster strikes—1878 to 2010* (pp. 45–67). New York, NY: Springer.

World Health Organization. (2011). *Early warning surveillance and response in emergencies: Report of the second WHO technical workshop.* Retrieved from http://whqlibdoc.who.int/hq/2011/WHO_HSE_GAR_DCE_2011.2_eng.pdf

Yumul, G. P., Jr., Cruz, N. A., Servando, N. T., & Dimalanta, C. B. (2011). Extreme weather events and related disasters of the Philippines, 2004–08: A sign of what climate change will mean? *Disasters, 35,* 262–282.

Zolnikov, T. R. (2013). The maladies of water and war: Addressing poor water quality in Iraq. *American Journal of Public Health, 103,* 980–987.

UNIT

5

Population Health Issues

Chapters

CHAPTER

26 Communicable Diseases

Learning Outcomes

After reading this chapter, you should be able to:

1. Analyze major trends in the incidence of communicable diseases.
2. Identify the modes of transmission for common communicable diseases.
3. Describe the influence of biological, psychological, environmental, sociocultural, behavioral, and health system determinants on communicable disease incidence and prevalence.
4. Analyze the role of population health nurses in controlling communicable diseases as it interfaces with those of other health professionals.
5. Provide examples of health promotion strategies that minimize communicable disease incidence.
6. Describe major considerations in prevention of communicable diseases.
7. Discuss population health nursing strategies for resolving health problems related to communicable diseases.
8. Identify health restoration strategies related to communicable diseases and possible population health nursing roles in each.

Key Terms

anergy
chain of infection
co-infection
communicable diseases
contact investigation and notification
control
cross-immunity
directly observed therapy (DOT)
endemic disease
epidemic
expedited partner therapy (EPT)
extinction
immunity
incubation period
induration
infectious diseases
isolation
mass screening
nosocomial infection
opportunistic infections (OIs)
outbreak
preexposure prophylaxis (PrEP)
prodromal period
quarantine
reservoir
selective screening
social distancing
superinfection
vector
vehicle

Advocacy Then

Sled Dogs and Communicable Disease

In the winter of 1925, Nome, Alaska, experienced a diphtheria epidemic that threatened the entire population of the region. Lacking a supply of diphtheria antitoxin, the local physician sent dozens of telegrams requesting help. The closest large supply of antitoxin was more than 600 miles away in Anchorage. Sea ice around Nome prevented sea delivery of the antitoxin; there were no roads or rail lines and air service was unavailable. Mail delivery was by sled dogs and "mushers" (sled dog drivers). Traveling day and night over rugged terrain, through blizzards and in temperatures of 50 degrees below zero, 20 teams of mushers and 150 dogs made the trip over the Iditarod Trail in 5 days and 7 hours to deliver the needed supplies in a third to a quarter of the usual time (Centers for Disease Control and Prevention [CDC], 2013b).

This heroic feat required the cooperation of hundreds of people from across the nation. It captured the attention of the media and the general public and became a significant motivator for the use of diphtheria vaccine. The event is commemorated each year by the Iditarod Trail Sled Dog Race (CDC, 2013b).

Advocacy Now

One Little Candle

In 1952, Perry Como sang "One Little Candle" extolling the virtues of bearing light rather than stumbling in the dark. Sometimes when we reflect on the chapters of our lives, a song heard from the distant past makes more sense than when it was a pop tune on the radio.

In 1997, my son Jeremy worked at an internationally staffed YMCA Camp in the mountains of southern California, with counselors from all over the world—Holland, Germany, even Tanzania, East Africa. Those from far flung regions weren't able to go home for weekends, so Jeremy invited Frank Manase, a counselor from Tanzania, to our house for the weekend.

Frankie nearly fell over when I called out a Swahili greeting: "Jambo, habari!" I only know a few Swahili words, learned when I spent part of a summer in a Seventh-Day Adventist mission compound in Kenya, Kendu Bay, at age 15. Frank's musical laughter, gratitude, and loving heart made him an easy addition to our family. His skills in tracking animals, illustrating the mysteries of nature to the children at the camp, made him such a valued counselor that the YMCA extended his visa for a year. In that role, he continued to inspire children, not only with the beauties of nature, but with the goodness of getting along, working as a team, and enjoying the outdoors. At the end of the year, he had made so many friends and learned to love America so much that he wondered about the possibilities of staying and studying in the United States.

However, he had a place in medical school back in Tanzania, a rare privilege and a secure opportunity. After thinking it through I said, "Frankie, some people are tempted by drugs, some are tempted by alcohol, and some are tempted to stay in America. Your people need you." So Frank went back to Tanzania. On a 2001 visit to meet our Tanzanian family and lecture at the university there, he laughingly introduced me as "my American mom, who made me come back to Africa!"

Five years later, as a new physician, Dr. Frank Manase was given the opportunity to study hospice and palliative care through the international scholars program at San Diego Hospice. He then received a scholarship from the International Hospice & Palliative Care Association to study for his Master's degree in Hospice and Palliative Care in South Africa. His work at Pastoral Activities and Services for people with AIDS Dar es Salaam Archdiocese (PASADA) enabled him, as medical director, to implement radical models of care that were family-centered and included the use of volunteers to facilitate care of patients. PASADA serves approximately 40,000 patients, 11,000 of whom are children. Some of the highest risk children who have lost everything—family, property, their health—are also given the opportunity to participate in a year-long art or music/drama therapy program where they are able to express their grief as well as their resilience and joy through art and song. In a country where the typical antiretroviral (ARV) drug adherence rate is 30–40%, PASADA's personal approach to caring for patients and families has dramatically increased adherence to ARVs to 89%, thereby promoting both length and quality of life for their patients.

Recently, 14 years after our relationship began, 10 years after my last visit to Tanzania, I was able to visit and witness Frank's accomplishments. I asked him if, in 1998, I had given the right advice to go home, become a doctor, and help his people. His answer: "so much, Mom, so much." As we stood with a gathering of HIV-infected children served through PASADA, the family-centered care staff lighting candles and remembering those affected by HIV/AIDS around the world, the power of light through God working in his people who are everywhere in this world burned brightly in my heart.

The following is a song written by the PASADA children's choir that symbolizes their need for care and understanding.

WE ARE FULL ORPHANED, WE ARE LEFT ALONE

Due to loss of both of our parents as a result of HIV and AIDS, we are left depressed with many of life's uncertainties. We do feel lonely. Some of us are living with relatives, good Samaritans, or family friends. As orphans, we have encountered a lot of practical life difficulties. These include: stigma and discrimination, lack of education, inadequate availability of food and shelter, lack of involvement in issues that touch our lives and legal limitations. It was not our choice to be orphaned, please listen to our cry.

Our message to the Tanzanians and the whole world is as follows:

There are so many orphaned children who live in the most risky environment here in Tanzania and over the world. Being a Tanzanian community member, you have valuable contribution to offer to this vulnerable group of people.

Many children wish to get a reasonable education and medical care but it has not been possible for them. Dear uncle, father, mother, brother and sisters, government and non-government sector and all citizens, it is your turn to participate and provide support to these children so that they get education and quality medical care. By doing so, you will enable children to celebrate their childhood just like many other children.

Many children have experienced relatives taking their family belongings by force encountering many legal barriers when they try to recover. Many children are considered young and therefore less responsible. Our message to the community is, despite our young age, we strongly believe we have legal rights of owning our late parents' belongings. Will you please listen and attend to our expressed needs.

It was not our choice to be orphaned.

(Written by the PASADA children's choir—Simba wa Afrika Group—used with permission). Gail Reiner, DNP, RN

Human beings have been subject to illnesses caused by pathogenic microorganisms throughout history. For example, testing of mummies has provided evidence of tuberculosis (TB) in a mother and child who lived 9,000 years ago, and the earliest evidence of disease caused by the malaria parasite dates from 3,500 years ago. Similarly, smallpox DNA has been recovered from a 300-year-old frozen mummy from Siberia, and similar findings indicate that up to 80% of the population of medieval Britain may have suffered from sinusitis exacerbated by air pollution from local industries such as brewing, tanning, and lime burning (Williams, 2013).

Although these and other illnesses can be considered infectious illnesses, not all of them are communicable diseases. **Infectious diseases** are those illnesses that result from the growth of pathogenic microorganisms in the body. **Communicable diseases**, on the other hand, are diseases caused by pathogens that are transmitted directly or indirectly from one person to another. Bacterial otitis media and wound infections are infectious diseases. Measles, hepatitis A, and HIV infection are examples of diseases that can be transmitted from one person to another and are communicable diseases.

Historical events and human migrations have led to the spread of communicable diseases. For example, smallpox is thought to have originated in Africa and was possibly brought to Europe by Arab invaders. Similarly, there is no evidence that diseases such as measles and smallpox existed in the Western Hemisphere until after the advent of Europeans. Both Aztec and Incan rulers died of smallpox in the 1500s after the arrival of

Spanish conquistadors (Smallpox History, 2011). Conversely, travel from the new world may have been responsible for the introduction of syphilis in Europe (Syphilis, 1494–1923, n.d.). Changes characteristic of syphilis have been identified in bones found in the area of the Dominican Republic where Columbus first landed. No similar changes have been identified in pre-Columbian Europe, supporting the theory of transfer from the New World to the Old (Rothschild, 2005). Similarly, it is believed that tuberculosis originated in East Africa and spread to Europe and Asia, and from Asia to the Americas prior to the arrival of the first European explorers (McDaniel, 2006).

In the last century-and-a-half, immunization has enabled control of a number of communicable diseases. Incidence of vaccine-preventable diseases has decreased significantly from peak incidence rates prior to vaccine availability. However, periodic outbreaks continue to occur, and new diseases continue to emerge to challenge human ingenuity. In spite of the remarkable decline in mortality due to communicable diseases in the United States and other developed nations, these conditions continue to exact a toll in worldwide suffering, death, and economic costs.

General Concepts Related to Communicable Diseases

Several communicable disease concepts must be understood before control efforts can be undertaken. These include concepts related to the "chain of infection," such as modes of transmission and portals of entry and exit, and the concepts of incubation and prodromal periods.

Chain of Infection

In communicable diseases, epidemiologic factors related to biological, psychological, environmental, sociocultural, behavioral, and health system determinants create what is often called a chain of infection. A **chain of infection** is a series of events or conditions that lead to the development of a particular communicable disease. The "links" in the chain are the infected person or source of the infectious agent, the reservoir, the agent itself, the mode of transmission of the disease, the agent's portals of entry and exit, and a susceptible new host. The concepts of agent and host were introduced in Chapter 3∞. This discussion focuses on the remaining links in the chain: reservoirs, modes of transmission, and portals of entry and exit.

Modes of Transmission

The mode of transmission of a particular disease is the means by which the infectious agent that causes the disease is transferred from an infected person or animal to an uninfected one. Infected people or animals are one type of reservoir, but there are other reservoirs that do not have the infection or disease. A **reservoir** is an animal, person, plant, soil, or substance where an infectious microorganism lives and from which it is transmitted to a susceptible host (CDC, 2012b). People are the reservoir for illnesses like measles or varicella (chickenpox) that can be spread directly from one person to another. Animals may also serve as reservoirs or sources of infection for human beings. For example, infected animals, like dogs, bats, raccoons, and so on, are reservoirs for rabies. In some instances, inanimate objects serve as reservoirs. For instance, soil is a reservoir for tetanus bacilli.

Communicable diseases may be spread to a susceptible new host by any of several modes of transmission: airborne transmission, fecal–oral (gastrointestinal) transmission, direct contact, sexual contact, direct inoculation, insect or animal bite, or via inanimate objects or soil. Two general mechanisms for transmission of infectious agents are direct and indirect transmission. In direct transmission, the microorganism passes directly from one person to another. In indirect transmission, the microorganism is transmitted by a living or nonliving entity. Contaminated food would be a nonliving means of indirect transmission of a disease-causing microorganism, also called a **vehicle**. A living means of indirect transmission of diseases, or **vector**, might be a mosquito that transmits West Nile virus (CDC, 2012b). The mosquito does not have the disease, but merely transmits it from one person that it bites to another.

AIRBORNE TRANSMISSION. Airborne transmission occurs when the infectious organism is present in the air and is inspired (inhaled) by a susceptible host during respiration. Diseases transmitted by the airborne route include the exanthems (diseases characterized by a rash, such as measles and chickenpox), infections of the mouth and throat (such as streptococcal infections), and infections of the upper and lower respiratory system (such as tuberculosis, pneumonia, influenza, and the common cold). Ccrtain systemic infections are also products of airborne transmission. Examples of these are meningococcal meningitis and pneumococcal pneumonias, hantavirus pulmonary infections, coccidioidomycosis, anthrax, and smallpox. In the case of anthrax and smallpox, disease may also be transmitted by aerosolized dissemination of microorganisms.

FECAL–ORAL TRANSMISSION. Fecal–oral transmission of an infectious agent may be either direct or indirect. Direct transmission occurs when the hands or other objects (fomites) are contaminated with organisms from human feces and then put into the mouth. Indirect transmission occurs via contaminated food or water. For example, a person with hepatitis A may defecate, fail to wash his or her hands properly, and then prepare a sandwich for someone else. The second person would ingest the virus with the sandwich and, if susceptible, might develop hepatitis A. Additional examples include *Salmonella*- or *Shigella*-caused diarrheas. Botulism is another disease in which the causative organism is ingested with contaminated food or water. Contamination usually occurs by accident through inadequate canning and preserving processes, but could potentially occur as a result of bioterrorist activity. Ingestion of anthrax may also result from the intentional introduction of spores into food supplies.

DIRECT CONTACT. Direct contact transmission involves skin-to-skin contact or direct contact with mucous membrane discharges between the infected person and another person.

Diseases typically spread by this route include infectious mononucleosis, impetigo, scabies, and lice. Smallpox may also be transmitted by contact with the lesions of infected persons. Scabies, lice, and other parasitic diseases also may be transmitted through contact with clothing and other items containing the eggs of the parasites. Similarly, the cutaneous form of anthrax is transmitted by handling contaminated objects (CDC, 2013a).

SEXUAL TRANSMISSION. Transmission of diseases via sexual contact is a special instance of direct contact transmission. Diseases spread by this mode of transmission are usually referred to as sexually transmitted infections (STIs) or sexually transmitted diseases (STDs). Diseases spread during sexual intercourse include (but are not limited to) HIV/AIDS, gonorrhea, syphilis, genital herpes, and hepatitis B, C, and D. These diseases may also be spread by other modes of transmission. For example, hepatitis B, C, and D and AIDS may be spread by direct inoculation.

TRANSMISSION BY DIRECT INOCULATION. Direct inoculation occurs when the infectious agent (a bloodborne pathogen) is introduced directly into the bloodstream of the new host. Direct inoculation can occur transplacentally from an infected mother to a fetus, via transfusion with infected blood or blood products, through the use of contaminated hypodermic equipment, or through a splash of contaminated body fluid to mucous membrane or nonintact skin. With the advent of several screening tests for blood donors, transmission via transfusion has been significantly decreased. Health care workers are particularly at risk for several communicable diseases caused by bloodborne pathogens. Diseases commonly spread by direct inoculation include HIV/AIDS and hepatitis B, C, and D.

TRANSMISSION BY INSECT OR ANIMAL BITE. Insect and animal bites can also transmit infectious agents. For example, the bite of the *Anopheles* mosquito is the mode of transmission for malaria, a disease that is widespread in much of the world. West Nile virus infection is another disease that is primarily transmitted by mosquitoes (Kelly et al., 2013). Rabies frequently is transmitted via a bite from infected, warm-blooded animals such as dogs, skunks, and raccoons. Incidence of diseases such as rabies is low in the United States, due to widespread immunization of pets. Approximately 90% of rabies cases occur as a result of the bite of a wild animal (Kellogg et al., 2013). Rabies can also be transmitted from one person to another, however, placing family contacts and health care personnel caring for someone with rabies at risk for infection. Lyme disease and Rocky Mountain spotted fever are transmitted by the bite of infected ticks, and plague can be transmitted by fleas on infected rodents. Human encroachment into wildlife areas is increasing the potential for exposure to diseases caused by insect and animal bites.

TRANSMISSION BY OTHER MEANS. Some communicable diseases are transmitted through contact with spores present in the soil or with inanimate objects. For example, exposure to the bacillus that causes tetanus frequently occurs through a dirty puncture wound. Modes of transmission and typical diseases most often transmitted by each mode are summarized in Table 26-1 •.

Portals of Entry and Exit

Communicable diseases also differ in terms of the portals through which the infectious agent that causes the disease enters and leaves an infected host. Portals of entry include the respiratory system, the gastrointestinal tract, and the skin and mucous membranes.

Portals of exit also differ among communicable diseases. Infectious agents may leave an infected host through the respiratory system or through feces passed from the gastrointestinal tract. Blood and other body fluids such as semen, vaginal secretions, and saliva are the portals of exit for infectious agents causing diseases such as HIV/AIDS, gonorrhea, and hepatitis B. The skin acts as a portal of exit as well as a portal of entry for conditions such as impetigo, cutaneous anthrax, and syphilis. Portals of entry and exit and related modes of disease transmission are summarized in Table 26-2 •.

TABLE 26-1 Modes of Disease Transmission and Typical Diseases

Mode of Transmission	Diseases Transmitted
Airborne	Measles, mumps, rubella, poliomyelitis, *Haemophilus influenzae* type B (HiB) infection, tuberculosis, influenza, scarlet fever, diphtheria, pertussis, hantavirus, respiratory anthrax, coccidioidomycosis, smallpox, plague (pneumonic form)
Fecal–oral/ingestion	Hepatitis A and E, salmonellosis, shigellosis, typhoid, polio (in poor sanitary conditions), botulism, ingestion anthrax
Direct contact	Impetigo, scabies, lice, smallpox, cutaneous anthrax
Sexual contact	Chlamydia, gonorrhea, hepatitis B, C, and D, HIV infection, herpes simplex virus (HSV) infection, human papilloma virus (HPV), syphilis
Direct inoculation	Syphilis, hepatitis A, B, C, and D, HIV infection
Insect or animal bite	Malaria, rabies, Lyme disease, plague (bubonic form)
Other means of transmission	Tetanus, hookworm

TABLE 26-2 Portals of Entry and Exit for Each Mode of Disease Transmission

Mode of Transmission	Portal of Entry	Portal of Exit
Airborne	Respiratory system	Respiratory system
Fecal–oral/ingestion	Mouth	Feces
Direct contact	Skin, mucous membrane	Skin, mucous membrane
Sexual contact	Skin, mouth, urethra, rectum, vagina	Skin lesions, vaginal or urethral secretions
Direct inoculation	Across placenta, bloodstream	Blood
Animal or insect bite	Wound in skin	Blood, saliva
Other means of transmission	Wound in skin, intact skin	Animal feces, soil

Incubation and Prodromal Periods

The **incubation period** of a communicable disease is the interval from exposure to an infectious organism to development of the symptoms of the disease (Gerstman, 2013). The length of the incubation period for a particular disease may influence the success of efforts to halt the spread of the disease. Some diseases, such as influenza and scarlet fever, have incubation periods of less than a week. Others typically require incubation periods of one to two weeks (gonorrhea, measles, pertussis, and polio), two to three weeks (rubella, chickenpox, and mumps), or months (viral hepatitis, syphilis). In some diseases, such as AIDS, the incubation period can be years.

The **prodromal period** of a communicable disease is the period between the first symptoms and the appearance of the symptoms that typify the disease. For example, prior to the appearance of the jaundice that is characteristic of viral hepatitis, the client may experience prodromal symptoms of nausea, fatigue, and malaise. Similarly, a cough, runny nose, and watery eyes are prodromal symptoms for measles. In many diseases, the prodromal period is the time of greatest ability to infect others.

Immunity

Immunity is another concept of great importance in the control of communicable diseases. **Immunity** is a state of nonsusceptibility to a disease or condition. Physiologic immunity is based on the presence of specific antibodies to disease and is described as passive or active depending on the role of the host in developing those antibodies. In *active immunity*, the host is exposed to antigens, substances related to the disease-causing microorganism, which prompt the host's immune system to create antibodies that render the antigen harmless. Exposure to the antigen may occur as a result of having the disease or through immunization with active antigens (e.g., bacterial toxins such as tetanus or diphtheria toxoid or portions of live viruses that cause diseases such as measles and mumps). Active immunity is relatively long lasting, waning over several years if at all. In *passive immunity*, externally produced antibodies are provided to the host by way of immunization (e.g., immune serum globulin from someone who has had a specific disease and developed active immunity) or transfer (e.g., from a mother with active immunity to her fetus across the placenta).

Cross-immunity occurs when immunity to one microorganism or disease also confers immunity to a related disease-causing agent. Cross-immunity was the basis for the smallpox vaccine developed by Edward Jenner. Jenner inoculated people with material from cowpox lesions to prevent smallpox after noticing that milkmaids who developed cowpox from exposure to infected cows did not develop smallpox.

Herd immunity is another concept related to physiologic immunity that has particular relevance for population groups. Herd immunity is generalized resistance to a particular disease within the population that arises because the majority of people have developed specific immunity to the condition. Herd immunity decreases the potential for exposure to the disease among those few people who do not have immunity.

Other Communicable Disease Concepts

Additional concepts related to communicable diseases reflect the extent of a particular disease within a specific population. An **endemic disease** is one that is constantly present in a particular geographic area (Gerstman, 2013). Prior to the advent of adequate sanitation, a wide variety of diarrheal diseases were endemic in the United States and remain endemic in many developing nations. Endemic diseases contrast with those that occur with epidemic frequency. An **epidemic** involves the occurrence of a great number of cases of a disease, beyond what would ordinarily be expected in a given population (Gerstman, 2013). Earlier in U.S. history, for example, periodic epidemics of cholera swept the country. At that time, cholera was generally an endemic disease, with low incidence rates most of the time. Influenza epidemics continue to occur with some frequency in the United States, and there have also been periodic epidemics of pertussis when incidence rates far exceed those normally seen in a given year. A disease **outbreak** is an increased number of cases in the population that does not approach epidemic proportions. Disease outbreaks may be defined differently for different diseases depending on the usual number of cases of a disease typically encountered in the population. For example, a particular city might experience an outbreak of diarrheal disease when drinking water has been accidentally contaminated by sewage. As we saw in Chapter 25∞, a pandemic is the simultaneous experience of extensive disease outbreaks or epidemics in several parts of the world.

Four other related concepts are important in the consideration of communicable diseases: control, elimination, eradication, and extinction. **Control** refers to a reduction in disease incidence or prevalence or a decrease in its associated morbidity and mortality to an acceptable level in a given locale as a result of deliberate intervention. Elimination, as noted in Chapter 8∞, is the reduction of the incidence of a specific disease to zero in a defined geographic area, again as a result of deliberate efforts, while eradication involves worldwide reduction in disease incidence to zero. In **extinction**, on the other hand, the infectious agent that causes a specific disease no longer exists, either in nature or in the laboratory (CDC, 2014). To date, only one disease has been eradicated worldwide (smallpox); measles and some other diseases have been eliminated in some areas; and no currently known microorganism is extinct.

Trends in Communicable Diseases

As noted above, overall mortality from communicable diseases has declined significantly in some parts of the world, but these trends are not universal. Because of the potential for rapid spread of disease throughout the world, population health nurses need to be aware of trends in communicable disease incidence, prevalence, and mortality in their local areas as well as nationally and internationally. Communicable disease incidence also varies among geographic areas within the United States and among ethnic groups. Generally speaking, most communicable diseases have higher incidence rates among ethnic minority groups than among Caucasians, due to a number of social conditions such as poverty and lack of access to care.

As noted above, one communicable disease, smallpox, has been completely eradicated from the world, although there is potential for its reintroduction through bioterrorism. The goal of the World Health Organization (WHO) is the elimination of several diseases, with their eventual eradication throughout the world. Information about elimination and eradication efforts for several communicable diseases is presented in the *Global Perspectives* feature on the next page. Trends related to common vaccine-preventable diseases, STIs, foodborne and waterborne diseases, bloodborne diseases, tuberculosis, hepatitis, arthropod-borne diseases, and selected emerging diseases will be discussed.

Vaccine-preventable Diseases

A number of communicable diseases are preventable using vaccines. Such diseases include measles, mumps, rubella, pertussis, tetanus, diphtheria, varicella (chickenpox), influenza and pneumonia, poliomyelitis, *Haemophilus influenzae* type b, meningococcal disease, and rotavirus infection. Human papilloma virus (HPV) infection is also vaccine preventable, but will be discussed with other STIs. Hepatitis A and B are also discussed separately with other forms of hepatitis. Vaccines are also available for other diseases, such as cholera, typhoid, and tuberculosis, but are not routinely used in the United States, except for certain populations (e.g., persons traveling to endemic areas).

Measles has been eliminated in the United States since 2000 (defined as interruption of continuous transmission for at least 12 months). Unfortunately, cases of measles continue to be imported from other parts of the world. Approximately 20 million cases of measles still occur worldwide each year, and from 2001 to 2012 a median of 60 imported cases occurred each year in the United States (Wallace et al. 2013).

Decline in immunization rates and failure to be vaccinated led to a resurgence of measles as well as other diseases (McLean, Fiebelkorn, Temte, & Wallace, 2013). For example, the number of measles cases reported in 2011 was the highest since 1996. The vast majority of cases (87%) occurred in persons who were not vaccinated or whose vaccination status was unknown, and 36% of cases were known to have claimed a vaccine exemption (a waiver of the requirement for immunization for school enrollment) based on personal, religious, or philosophical beliefs. The WHO European region, which experienced more than 30,000 cases of measles in 2011, was the source of 41% of imported U.S. cases (Adams et al., 2013). During that year, measles outbreaks occurred in 36 of the 53 nations in the European region, accounting for 26,074 cases, mostly in unvaccinated older children and adults (Martin et al., 2011).

From January 1 to August 24, 2013, a total of eight outbreaks and 159 cases of measles were reported in the United States, 82% in unvaccinated individuals. Details of one outbreak highlight the potential for spread of the disease when cases are imported from endemic regions. In 2013, a measles outbreak occurred in a religious community in New York. The source of the outbreak was an intentionally unvaccinated adolescent exposed during a trip to London. The outbreak consisted of six generations of cases in 58 individuals in two neighborhoods. More than three fourths (79%) of the cases occurred in three extended families who declined immunization. The outbreak necessitated 3,500 contact investigations in health care, home, and school settings, school immunization audits, a mass immunization campaign using measles, mumps, and rubella (MMR) vaccine or immune globulin, and testing and vaccinating of several pregnant women (Arciuolo et al., 2013), which heavily burdened the local health jurisdiction.

U.S. mumps incidence in 2011 was 0.13 cases per 100,000 population (National Center for Health Statistics [NCHS], 2014). MMR vaccine effectiveness in preventing mumps is 78% for one dose and 88% for two doses of vaccine. Although required as part of the routine immunization program in the United States, only 62% of countries worldwide include mumps in their national immunization programs, and vaccination rates in Europe have declined in response to vaccine safety concerns. These conditions have led to periodic outbreaks and importation of cases into the United States. For example, one mumps outbreak on a university campus resulted in 29 cases, mostly in unvaccinated students. Again, the source case was an unvaccinated student who had traveled to Europe prior to the start of the school year. Public colleges and universities

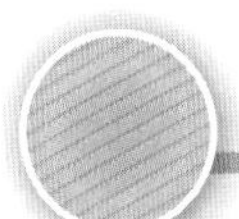

Global Perspectives

Eliminating Communicable Diseases Worldwide

Complete eradication of a communicable disease has only, thus far, been achieved for smallpox. However, the World Health Assembly has established targets for the elimination of several communicable diseases moving eventually to complete eradication. For example, measles has been eliminated in the WHO Region of the Americas since 2002. In 2010, the World Health Assembly established three milestones for measles eradication to be achieved by 2015: (a) increasing to at least 90% the number of children who have had at least one dose of measles vaccine in all countries, (b) reducing annual measles incidence to less than five cases per million population, and (c) reducing measles mortality by 95% from 2000 figures. Elimination of measles from four WHO regions is targeted for 2015 and five regions by 2020. By 2011, global vaccine coverage had increased to 84% of the world's children; measles incidence had decreased to 52 cases per million population, and mortality decreased by 71%. During 2010–2011, however, measles activity increased with several outbreaks reported (Perry et al., 2013). Work remains to be done to increase vaccine coverage and eradicate measles.

Malaria is another communicable disease that is being addressed worldwide as a significant source of morbidity and mortality. In 2000, leaders of 44 African nations committed their countries to decreasing malaria deaths. The estimated costs of global malaria control are $5.1 billion per year. A combination of domestic and international funding provided less than half of the required amount in 2012 (WHO, 2013c).

Recommendations for malaria control include insecticide-treated bed nets (ITNs), and by 2012, a total of 110 countries had adopted this recommendation, 88 of which provide the nets free of charge. Overall requirements to meet the need for protection in sub-Saharan Africa amounts to 150 million nets per year; an estimated 136 million nets were expected to be delivered in 2013. The proportion of individuals with access to nets varies across countries from 7% to 84%, but 89% of persons with nets use them (WHO, 2013c).

Another recommendation is the use of indoor residual spraying for mosquitoes in 88 high-malaria-risk countries. In 2012, only 4% of the population at risk lived in homes that were protected. In addition, a number of countries reported mosquito resistance to at least one commonly used insecticide (WHO, 2012).

Intermittent preventive therapy (IPT) for malaria is also recommended for pregnant women and infants. In 2012, 37 countries had national policies related to IPT for pregnant women, and a mean of 44% of pregnant women in high-burden countries received two doses of IPT. Only one country had adopted IPT for infants and two had adopted a 2012 recommendation for seasonal IPT for children aged 3 to 59 months (WHO, 2013c).

Overall, these interventions have prevented 274 million cases of malaria and more than 1.1 million deaths. Despite these achievements, malaria resulted in 219 million cases and an estimated 660,000 deaths in 2010 indicating the need for additional concerted prevention and treatment initiatives (WHO, 2013c).

Polio is a third disease with catastrophic global impact that has been slated for eradication. In 2012, the World Health Assembly designated completion of polio eradication activities to be a public health emergency. To date, polio has been eliminated from much of the world, but wild polio virus transmission remains endemic in three countries: Afghanistan, Nigeria, and Pakistan. Efforts to eliminate transmission have focused on increasing immunization levels among children. During 2012 and 2013, for example, Nigeria engaged in an N-STOP program (National Stop Transmission of Polio), one focus of which was locating and vaccinating susceptible children. As part of this initiative, public health workers engaged in outreach activities to enumerate children in more than 40,000 remote settlements. Enumeration resulted in identification of 53,738 children who had never been immunized as well as detection of 211 cases of unreported polio. N-STOP is operated entirely by Nigerian citizens, expanding public health capacity to deal with polio as well as other public health problems (Gidado et al., 2013). Outbreaks of imported wild poliovirus transmission have occurred in 21 previously polio-free countries due to importation from endemic countries. Until WPV transmission is eliminated from all parts of the world there is a continued risk for importation in other countries (WHO, Regional Office for Africa, 2013).

Overall, significant strides have been made, however, in the effort to eradicate polio. For example, annual global polio incidence decreased 99% from the launch of the Global Polio Eradication Initiative (GPEI) in 1988 to 2012, and the number of new cases decreased by 66% from 2011 to 2012. Similarly, the number of imported cases in polio-free countries decreased from 309 in 12 countries to 6 in 2 countries. From January to March 2013, only 22 wild poliovirus cases had been reported worldwide, less than half of the number in the same time period in 2012 (Polio Eradication Department, WHO, 2013b).

Vaccination rates have also increased. By the end of 2011, approximately 84% of the world's children had received the routine three doses of vaccine. In 2012, 2.05 billion doses of OPV were administered to 448 million people, most children under 5 years of age. Supplemental immunization activities (SIAs), including national and subnational immunization days, child health days, and mop-up rounds, were conducted in 46 countries, and no new wild poliovirus outbreaks had been reported in polio-free countries as of April 2013 (Polio Eradication Department, WHO, 2013b).

in 22 states and the District of Columbia require two doses of mumps vaccine prior to enrollment to prevent such outbreaks, but many more campuses have no such requirement (Zipprich et al., 2012).

U.S. 2011 rubella incidence was zero cases per 100,000 population (NCHS, 2014), with similar rates for 2009 and 2010, exceeding the *Healthy People 2020* target of 10 or fewer cases per year (U.S. Department of Health and Human Services [USDHHS], 2014). Rubella has been targeted for elimination in the WHO region of the Americas by 2010 and in the European region by 2015. In addition, accelerated control targets have been identified for the Western Pacific region, in part in response to a 2013 epidemic in Japan that resulted in 5,442 cases and 10 infants with congenital rubella syndrome. More than three fourths (77%) of the Japanese cases occurred in adult men who typically not targeted by vaccination programs, which focus on children and childbearing women (Tanaka-Taya et al., 2013).

Like many other vaccine-preventable diseases, the incidence of pertussis declined sharply with the advent of an effective vaccine, dropping from 265,269 cases in 1934 to 1,010 cases in 1976. Unfortunately, the number of cases increased to 25,827 in 2004 and averaged slightly more than 18,000 cases per year from 2004 to 2008 (Pour et al., 2011). The 2009 incidence in the United States was 5.54 cases per 100,000 population, but climbed again to 8.9 per 100,000 in 2010 and dropped to 6.1 in 2011 (Adams et al., 2013).

Periodic outbreaks of pertussis continue to occur. For example, there was a 1,300% increase in the number of pertussis cases in Washington State between 2011 and 2012, primarily in infants and 10-year-old to adolescent children, suggesting early waning of immunity (Tondella et al., 2012). In 2012, 41,880 cases and 14 deaths in infants under a year of age were reported in the United States (Sawyer, Liang, Messonnier, & Clark, 2013).

The availability of vaccine has resulted in a 95% decrease in tetanus cases and a 99% reduction in mortality since 1947. From 2001 to 2008, only 233 cases occurred in the United States. Unfortunately, when cases do occur, fatality rates are relatively high at 13.2% of those affected. The average incidence across all age groups is 0.1 per million persons, but increases to 0.23 per million for people over 65 years of age, primarily due to lack of immunization among older persons. Approximately 40% of older people in the United States have not been immunized. In addition, persons seen for wounds for whom treatment status was known did not receive adequate tetanus prophylaxis, putting them at risk for developing tetanus (Tiwari, Clark, Messonnier, & Thomas, 2011).

No cases of diphtheria were reported in the United States in 2011. Globally, however, an estimated 25,000 deaths occurred in the same year. During 2012, 4,489 cases were reported worldwide. Varicella or chickenpox, on the other hand, continues to occur in the United States, with an incidence of 8.3 per 100,000 population in 2011. This figure represents a decrease of roughly 74% from 2006 and is the result of increasing vaccine coverage (Adams et al., 2013).

Poliomyelitis due to wild poliovirus (WPV) has been eliminated in the United States, and the incidence in 2011 was zero cases per 100,000 population (NCHS, 2014). In 1988, the Global Polio Eradication Initiative (GPEI) established a partnership between WHO, Rotary International, CDC, and the United Nations Children's Fund (UNICEF) to promote polio immunization throughout the world. By 2012, the annual incidence of polio had decreased by 99% worldwide (Polio Eradication Department, 2013a). The number of new cases decreased by 66% from 2011 to 2012 and only three countries (Afghanistan, Nigeria, and Pakistan) continued to experience endemic WPV transmission in 2013. From January to March, 2013, only 22 cases of WPV were reported compared to 48 cases in the same time period in 2012 (Polio Eradication Department, 2013b). Imported cases of polio continue to occur in countries that have eliminated WPV, but only 223 cases were reported globally in 2012. In 2013, WPV was reintroduced in Somalia and Kenya and 50 cases had been reported by June of that year (WHO, Division of Global Migration and Quarantine, 2013a).

Two other diseases of young children that can be prevented by vaccines are *Haemophilus influenzae* type b (Hib) and rotavirus. Since the advent of Hib vaccine in 1987, incidence of invasive disease in children under 5 years of age decreased by 99% to less than one case per 100,000 children (Adams et al., 2013). Rotavirus is the leading cause of diarrheal death in children under 5 years of age resulting in an estimated 8,000 deaths per year in this age group. In 2007, WHO recommended the inclusion of rotavirus vaccine as part of routine national immunization programs in the Americas and Europe. This recommendation was expanded to all children under 32 months of age in 2009 (de Oliviera et al., 2011).

Meningococcal disease also affects young infants, but is also found among adolescents and young adults. Although cases are at a historic low since vaccine availability, cases continue to occur. In 2011, for example, a total of 257 vaccine preventable invasive meningococcal infections occurred in the United States, with the highest rate among children under 1 year of age (0.34/100,000 population) and a second peak in the 15 to 24 age group (0.10/100,000). Overall vaccine-preventable invasive meningococcal disease incidence decreased from 0.10 per 100,000 people in 2001 to 0.08 per 100,000 in 2011 (Adams et al., 2013).

Influenza and pneumococcal pneumonia are two other vaccine-preventable diseases. Influenza virus infection exhibits different seasonal patterns in different areas of the world. For example, the disease tends to appear in early August in Australia and New Zealand. In 2013, peak disease incidence in South Africa occurred in June and then again in August, while incidence in temperate areas of South America peaked in June and declined through September (WHO Collaborating Center for Surveillance, Epidemiology and Control of Influenza, 2013). The typical influenza season in the United States is from late fall to early spring (Grohskopf et al., 2013).

Both influenza and pneumonia contribute to considerable morbidity and mortality. For example, influenza and pneumonia are the eighth leading cause of death in the United States (American Lung Association, 2014). Similarly, influenza accounted for anywhere from 55,000 to 431,000 hospitalizations each year from the 1976–1977 season to the 2002–2006 seasons. The highest influenza complication rates occur among young children and those over 65 years of age (Grohskopf et al., 2013). In 2001, 115 influenza deaths occurred among U.S. children, 46% of them under 5 years of age (WHO Collaborating Center, 2011).

U.S. pneumonia hospitalizations decreased by 20% overall from 2000 to 2010 with slightly larger decreases in older age groups (NCHS, 2012). Among children, introduction of the seven-valent pneumococcal conjugate vaccine resulted in a 77% decrease in invasive pneumococcal disease from 1998 to 2005, and 2008 rates had exceeded the *Healthy People 2010* target (National Center for Immunization and Respiratory Diseases, 2008). Unfortunately, pneumonia continues to account for 20% of child deaths throughout the world (CDC, 2012d).

Sexually Transmitted Infections

A variety of diseases are transmitted by means of sexual contact and result in more than 20 million cases per year at a cost of $16 billion per year in direct medical costs alone (CDC, 2013g). Sexually transmitted diseases to be addressed here include *Chlamydia trachomatis* infection, gonorrhea, HIV infection and AIDS, syphilis, and HPV infection. Some forms of viral hepatitis can be transmitted sexually as well, but they will be discussed in the section on viral hepatitis.

Chlamydia and gonorrhea are the two most frequently reported infectious diseases in the United States (Rotblatt, Montoya, Plant, Guerry, & Kerndt, 2013). Because many cases of both diseases are asymptomatic, their actual frequency is probably far underreported. Both diseases can result in significant reproductive problems, including pelvic inflammatory disease, infertility, and chronic pelvic pain in women. An estimated 4 to 5 million cases of *Chlamydia trachomatis* occur each year in the United States (Singh, Fine, & Marrazzo, 2011). In 2011, 1.4 million cases were reported for an incidence rate of 457.6 cases per 100,000 population. This figure represents an 8% increase over the 2010 incidence rate (Adams et al., 2013).

Reported incidence of gonorrhea declined by 79% from 1975 to 2009, but increased by 6% from 2009 to 2011 for an incidence rate of 104 cases per 100,000 population (Adams et al., 2013). This translates to more than 300,000 cases reported with many more that are undetected because of the frequently asymptomatic nature of the disease. In addition to the female reproductive consequences noted above, gonorrhea may result in disseminated disease and neonatal conjunctivitis and blindness. Gonorrhea also facilitates HIV transmission (Hook, Shafer, Deal, Kirkcaldy, & Iskander, 2013).

Approximately 1.1 million people were living with HIV infection/AIDS in 2013 and 50,000 new infections occur each year (McCree et al., 2013). Worldwide more than 3.3 million people are affected and 2 million deaths occur each year (Talman, Bolton, & Walson, 2013). With the advent of antiretroviral therapy (ART), mortality rates due to AIDS have declined significantly in areas where ART is available. For example, age-adjusted AIDS mortality among men in the United States declined from 16.2 per 100,000 population in 1995 to 2.6 per 100,000 in 2010 (NCHS, 2014).

The incidence of primary and secondary syphilis, the two most infectious and treatable stages of the disease, decreased by 90% from 1990 to 2000, but has recently begun to increase. In 2011, the incidence of primary and secondary syphilis was 4.52 per 100,000 population. Congenital syphilis, acquired through transplacental transmission from mother to fetus, declined from a high of 368.3 per 100,000 live births in 1950 to a low of 7.7 in 1980, but rose again to 92.95 cases per 100,000 live births in 1990. In 2011, congenital syphilis incidence had decreased to 8.48 (NCHS, 2014), but remained above the *Healthy People 2010* target of one case per 100,000 births (U.S. Department of Health and Human Services [USDHHS], 2013).

Unlike many STIs, HPV not only contributes to immediate conditions, such as genital warts, but is also a significant risk factor for several types of cancer. Several HPV serotypes have different effects. For example, types 16 and 18 cause approximately 70% of cervical cancers and most other HPV-related cancers (e.g., vulvar, vaginal, penile, or oropharyngeal cancers). Types 6 and 11, on the other hand, contribute to 90% of cases of genital warts. An estimated 26,200 new HPV-related cancers occur each year in the United States, with women accounting for nearly twice as many cases as men (Stokley et al., 2013). In 2008, more than 529,000 cases of cervical cancer and 275,000 deaths occurred worldwide. In the United States, more than 12,000 new cervical cancer diagnoses and 4,000 deaths were anticipated in 2013 (Henry J. Kaiser Family Foundation, 2014).

Globally, 44% of the world's population is infected by one or more types of HPV, most commonly young men and women under 25 years of age (Mah, Deber, Guttmann, McGeer, & Krahn, 2011). An estimated 79 million people in the United States are HPV infected, and approximately 14 million new cases occur each year (Stokley et al., 2013).

Viral Hepatitis

Viral hepatitis occurs in several different forms based on the causative organism: hepatitis A virus (HAV), hepatitis B virus (HBV), hepatitis C virus (HCV), hepatitis D virus (HDV), and hepatitis E virus (HEV). Hepatitis A and E are transmitted primarily by the fecal oral route and usually produce acute infection, although sexual transmission of hepatitis A has occurred among men who have sex with men (MSM). Hepatitis B, C, and D are transmitted via infected blood (e.g., transfusions, injecting drug use, paraoccupational exposure, or perinatal transmission) and can cause both acute and chronic disease. Chronic hepatitis B and C are the leading causes of cirrhosis and liver cancer (Kirkey et al., 2013).

In 2011, U.S. HAV incidence was 0.45 cases per 100,000 people, while HBV incidence was more than twice as high at

0.94 per 100,000 (NCHS, 2014). Hepatitis B occurs frequently throughout the world and has an estimated prevalence of more than 8% in the Western Pacific region of WHO, resulting in approximately 325,000 deaths per year due to cirrhosis and liver cancer (Xeuatvongsa et al., 2013).

HCV infection is the most common bloodborne infection in the United States. Approximately 70% of cases are mild or asymptomatic leading to under diagnosis and reporting. An estimated 75% to 85% of those affected develop chronic HCV infection, and of those 60% to 70% will develop active liver disease (Division of Viral Hepatitis, 2014). In the United States, an estimated 4.1 million people have ever been infected with HCV (Getchell et al., 2013), and approximately 3.2 million people are living with chronic HCV infection, 45% to 85% of whom are unaware of the infection (Mahajan, Liu, Klevens, & Holmberg, 2013). In 2008, for example, 144,015 cases were reported in the United States, but it is believed that figure represents only approximately half of the actual cases that occurred due to the largely asymptomatic nature of the disease, reporting failures, and insufficient follow-up to establish infection status (Hart-Malloy et al., 2013). HCV appears to be more common in persons born from 1945 to 1965, and this population has been specifically targeted for routine screening for the disease (Bornschlegel, Holtzman, Klevens, & Ward, 2013). WHO estimates that 130 to 170 million people are infected with HCV worldwide, with 10% of the population of countries like Egypt affected (El-Sayed et al., 2012).

HCV creates a significant societal burden. For example, HCV mortality now exceeds that of HIV infection in the United States (Iverson, Wand, Topp, Kaldor, & Maher, 2013). In addition, the estimated direct medical costs of HCV infection in the United States are expected to be $10.7 billion from 2010 to 2019, with additional costs of $54.2 billion related to premature mortality and lost productivity, and $21.3 billion in disability costs (Klevens & Tohme, 2010).

HDV and HEV virus infections occur far less frequently in the United States than hepatitis A, B, or C. Hepatitis D occurs only in conjunction with hepatitis B as a co-infection or as a superinfection (CDC, 2013d). **Co-infection** means that the two diseases occur simultaneously, in the case of hepatitis B and D, usually as a result of injection drug use (IDU). **Superinfection** occurs when one disease is superimposed on an existing disease; hepatitis D is superimposed on an existing HBV infection. HDV infection is uncommon in the United States and occurs primarily through percutaneous (e.g., IDU or needlestick) or mucous membrane exposure (CDC, 2013d).

Hepatitis E occurs primarily in areas of poor sanitation and, in the United States, is usually diagnosed in travelers returning from endemic areas such as South Asia and North Africa. HEV infection is unusual in the United States, but approximately 20 million people become infected annually worldwide, resulting in 3.4 million cases of disease and 70,000 deaths. Case fatality rates are relatively high at 0.2% to 4% in the general population and as high as 25% among pregnant women (Thomson et al., 2012).

Given the disease burden caused by viral hepatitis, particularly hepatitis B and C, the USDHHS has developed a comprehensive viral hepatitis action plan for control of these diseases. Major foci of the plan include preventing health-care-associated viral hepatitis, reducing hepatitis incidence and prevalence among injecting drug users, and strengthening disease surveillance systems (CDC, 2012c). Strategies related to these foci will be addressed later in this chapter.

Tuberculosis

TB is another communicable disease of interest to population health nurses. TB occurs in two forms: active infection or TB disease, and a quiescent form, latent TB infection (LTBI). Persons with active TB disease and positive sputum are capable of transmitting the disease by coughing, singing, or talking. Cases tend to be clustered based on their molecular characteristics, suggesting a common source of infection (Feske, Teeter, Musser, & Graviss, 2013).

TB is spread by the airborne route, particularly in congregate settings, such as long-term care facilities, homeless shelters, or correctional institutions (Bargman et al., 2013). Roughly one third of the earth's population or 2 billion people are infected with tuberculosis, and 1.8 million deaths occur each year worldwide (Otrompke, 2009). In the United States, age-adjusted TB mortality declined 57% from 1999 to 2010, with a 2010 mortality rate of 0.3 per 100,000 population. CDC's goal is to reduce TB incidence to less than one case per million people. In 2012, 9,951 new cases of TB were reported for an incidence rate of 3.2 per 100,000, a decrease of 6.1% from 2011. The TB incidence rate for foreign-born persons in the United States remains high, however, approximately 11.5 times the rate for U.S.-born persons (Miramontes, Pratt, Price, Navin, & Lo, 2013).

Food and Waterborne Diseases

A number of infectious diseases are transmitted through contaminated food and water. For example, approximately 170 million cases of acute gastroenteritis (AGE) per year are transmitted by food or water. These diseases can also occur via person-to-person contact, and from 2009 to 2010, 2,259 person-to-person outbreaks of AGE occurred resulting in 81,491 cases of illness, 1,339 hospitalizations, and 136 deaths (Wikswo & Hall, 2012).

The most common microorganisms implicated in food and waterborne disease outbreaks are norovirus, *Salmonella, Shigella, Escherichia coli*, and rotavirus. Different organisms tend to occur more commonly in some seasons than others. For example, norovirus infections tend to occur primarily in winter in the United States, and *Shigella* and other AGE infections are more common in spring and summer months (Wikswo & Hall, 2012). Many of these microorganisms include multiple disease-causing strains. For example, there are five genotypes of norovirus, more than 34 genotypes, and new strains emerging every 2 to 3 years, often resulting in disease outbreaks (Barclay et al., 2013).

The Foodborne Diseases Active Surveillance Network (FoodNet) identified 19,351 laboratory confirmed cases of foodborne infection in 2012 (Gilliss et al., 2013), and foodborne outbreaks in 2009 and 2010 resulted in 29,444 cases of disease, 1,184 hospitalizations, and 23 deaths. Forty percent of the reported outbreaks were associated with norovirus and 30% with *Salmonella*. Foods most often implicated included beef, dairy, fish, and poultry sources (Gould, Mundai, et al., 2013). A number of other foods, however, can cause disease outbreaks, including crustaceans, mollusks, pork, grains and beans, oils and sugars, fruits and nuts, leafy vegetables, sprouts, and vine or stalk vegetables (Gould, Walsh, et al., 2013). For example, an outbreak of norovirus infection was associated with frozen raw oysters that were distributed internationally (Brucker et al., 2012). Similarly, raw milk produced from one dairy resulted in recurrent outbreaks of *Campylobacter jejuni* (Weltman et al., 2013). In another outbreak, 91 cases of *Salmonella* infection were attributed to mobile lunch trucks selling products from one catering company that was using illegally sourced eggs (Honish et al., 2013). *Salmonella* outbreaks have also been associated with peanut butter and almond butter, as well as raw and roasted shelled and in-shell peanuts, produced by one company (MacDonald et al., 2013) and poultry from another producer (Grinnell et al., 2013).

Waterborne disease outbreaks may be associated with drinking water or water used for recreational or nondrinking purposes. From 2009 to 2010, 33 drinking water outbreaks were reported in the United States resulting in 1,040 cases of illness, 85 hospitalizations, and 9 deaths. Most of these outbreaks were attributed to *Legionella* in plumbing systems, untreated ground water, and distribution system deficiencies (Hillborn et al., 2013). Similarly, from 2007 to 2008, 134 disease outbreaks in the United States were attributed to recreational water (Hlavsa et al., 2011). A significant portion of recreational water-related outbreaks is related to *Cryptosporidium*, which is chlorine tolerant and may not be destroyed by common water treatment approaches (Adams et al., 2013).

Dracunculiasis, or guinea worm disease, is another waterborne infection present in the developing world. The disease is spread by ingestion of the eggs of a parasitic worm in contaminated water. The worms hatch in the new host and burrow to the skin where they cause secondary infection, pain, and disability. The World Health Assembly has called for worldwide dracunculiasis elimination. As of 2013, the disease remained endemic in four countries (south Sudan, Chad, Mali, and Ethiopia), with a total of 542 cases reported in 2012, 83% of which occurred in south Sudan (Hopkins, Ruiz-Tiben, Eberhard, & Roy, 2013).

Bloodborne Diseases

Bloodborne diseases are transmitted through infected blood. Transmission may occur via transfusion, injecting drug use, or cross-placental transmission from mother to fetus. Bloodborne infections may also occur in health care personnel as a result of needlesticks or other exposure to contaminated blood. In the United States, transmission of bloodborne diseases through transfusion is rare, due to screening of donors for major risk factors and testing of donated blood. For example, the risk of HIV transmission via transfusion is approximately one case in 1.5 million transfusions (Laffoon et al., 2010). Transfusion remains a major source of HIV infection in sub-Saharan Africa, however. One of the major foci of the President's Emergency Plan for AIDS Relief (PEPFAR) is the provision of support for improved blood transfusion services in 14 countries in the African region (Holmberg, Basavaraju, Reed, Drammeh, & Qualls, 2011). Another example of bloodborne transmission is transfusion-acquired West Nile Virus (WNV) infection. However, only 12 cases of transfusion-related WNV have been identified in the United States since the implementation of screening of blood supplies for WNV.

Arthropodborne (Arboviral) Diseases

Another group of infectious diseases are spread by the bite of arthropods, primarily mosquitoes and ticks. Common U.S. arboviral diseases include WNV infection, La Crosse virus infection (LACV), Powassan virus infection (POWV), St. Louis encephalitis virus infection (SLEV), Eastern equine encephalitis virus infection (EEEV), and Jamestown Canyon virus (JCV). These diseases are commonly spread from infected vertebrate hosts, such as birds or small mammals, to people via mosquito or tick bites. In 2012, these viruses caused 5,780 cases of illness, 51% of which were neuroinvasive conditions (Lindsey, Lehman, Staples, & Fischer, 2013). Rocky Mountain spotted fever is also spread by ticks.

Two other arthropodborne diseases seen in other parts of the world include lymphatic filariasis (elephantiasis) and malaria, both transmitted by mosquito bites (Mace et al., 2011; Streit et al., 2013). Filariasis affects more than 120 million people worldwide, and WHO has called for the elimination of this disease by 2010 (Streit et al., 2013). Malaria has been targeted by WHO for eradication, and by 2010, 11 countries and the WHO African region had achieved a greater than 50%

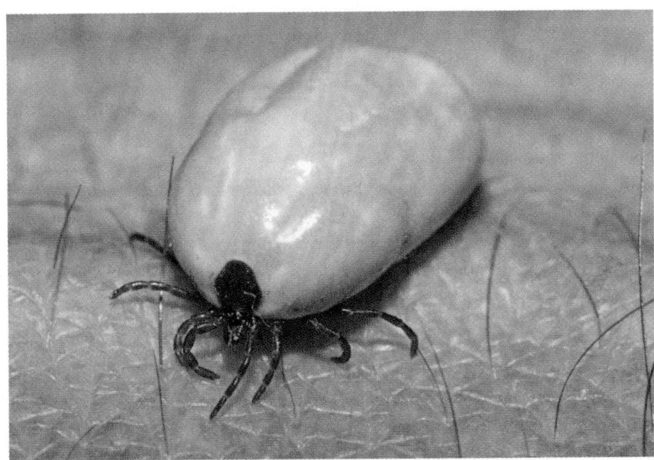

Ticks transmit a number of diseases from animals to humans.
(Bildagentur Zoonar GmbH/Shutterstock)

reduction in malaria cases and deaths (CDC, 2011). Malaria in the United States occurs primarily due to travel to endemic areas of the world, with occasional cases related to infected blood products, congenital transmission, laboratory exposure, and, rarely, local mosquitoes. In 2011, 1,925 cases were reported in the United States, all but four of which were imported. This figure represented an increase of 14% from 2010 and the highest number of cases since 1971 (Cullen & Arguin, 2013).

Globally, half of the world's population lives in malaria transmission areas, and 219 million cases and 660,000 deaths occurred in 2011. Pregnant women and young children are at risk for more severe disease than other groups. More than 40% of children under 10 years of age in central and western Africa are infected. One strain of the causative organism, *Plasmodium falciparum*, has a 15% to 20% fatality rate due to severe anemia, seizures, acute respiratory distress syndrome, and other organ failure (Mace et al., 2011). Two strains of plasmodium have a dormant stage in the human liver that can reactivate months or years later (Cullen & Arguin, 2013).

Emerging Diseases

The diseases discussed here are not the only communicable diseases to affect the health of populations. Each year, new emerging and reemerging diseases occur due to a variety of circumstances. One example of an emerging disease is Middle East Respiratory Syndrome Coronavirus (MERS-CoV) infection. This disease was first reported in humans in September of 2012 and has been designated as a "condition of serious concern." Cases identified thus far have been linked to travel in or near the Arabian peninsula (WHO, Division of Global Migration and Quarantine, 2013c). Reports of MERS-CoV cases in France, Italy, Tunisia, and the United Kingdom and instances of nosocomial transmission to health care personnel in some countries have raised concern about the potential for importation of the disease to other regions of the world (WHO, Division of Global Migration and Quarantine, 2013b).

New pathogens are being identified each year, many of which contribute to significant disease burden. In addition, diseases once thought controlled are becoming more frequent and harder to treat due to development of antimicrobial-resistant strains of microorganisms. Resistance is discussed in more detail in the section of this chapter devoted to treatment of communicable diseases.

Population Health Nursing and Communicable Disease Control

Control of communicable diseases in individuals and population groups entails use of the nursing process. The population health nurse involved in communicable disease control assesses determinants of health contributing to communicable disease, develops related population nursing diagnoses, and plans, implements, and evaluates strategies to prevent or control disease occurrence.

Assessing Determinants of Health in Communicable Disease

The development and effects of any communicable disease are influenced by factors related to each of the categories of determinants of health in the population health nursing model. Population health nurses concerned with control of communicable diseases should be familiar with factors in each category that influence disease development and control. Such knowledge provides guidance for interventions to prevent the disease, deal with it when it occurs, and prevent further spread in the population.

BIOLOGICAL DETERMINANTS. Biological considerations such as age, gender, race/ethnicity, and physiologic health status influence the development of many communicable diseases. In the case of some diseases, age may influence susceptibility to a disease or its effects. For example, the U.S. incidence of cryptosporidiosis for 1- to 4-year-old children in 2011 was more than twice that of any other age group. Similarly, measles incidence was twice as high for infants under a year of age as any other group. On the other hand, adolescents and young adults are at greater risk than other age groups for STIs due to sexual risk behaviors. For instance, the 2011 incidence rate for Chlamydia in 15- to 24-year-olds was four times higher than for any other age group at 2,313.29 cases per 100,000

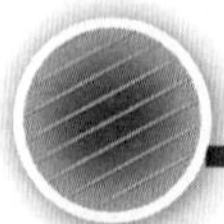

Evidence-Based Practice

Preexposure Prophylaxis (PrEP) for HIV Infection

In PrEP, persons who are uninfected take medication to prevent infection. This is not a new concept and has actually been used for years to prevent malaria in travelers to malaria-endemic regions. It is a relatively new approach to HIV prevention, however, designed to add another preventive strategy to existing behavioral strategies such as safe sexual behaviors and harm-reduction strategies in drug use. Several clinical trials have indicated the efficacy of PrEP for HIV prevention in men who have sex with men as well as heterosexual men and women and injecting drug users (AIDS.gov, 2014). In 2013, CDC updated guidelines on the use of PrEP for these groups at high risk for HIV infection (Smith et al., 2013). Some authors, however, caution that use of PrEP should be considered in light of its costs, the related costs of compliance counseling, potential for development of resistant viral strains, and lost opportunity costs in draining funding from other initiatives (Leibowitz et al., 2011).

population compared to 559.93 per 100,000 for those aged 25 to 39 years, the next highest group. Similarly, invasive disease due to *Haemophilus influenzae* occurred at a higher rate in adolescents and young adults due to lack of immunity. Invasive vaccine preventable meningococcal disease incidence, on the other hand, was highest in infants (0.34/100,000) followed by those over 65 years of age (0.19/100,000), and pertussis incidence was more than three times higher in infants than in any other age group (Adams et al., 2013).

In 2011, TB incidence was higher in persons over 65 years of age than in other age groups. The elderly are also at the greatest risk for tetanus in the United States because they are the least likely to have been immunized. For example, the 2011 incidence rate for tetanus in persons over 65 years of age was three times higher than that of any other age group (Adams et al., 2013). In developing countries with unsafe delivery conditions, neonates are at high risk for tetanus fatality. Neonates are also at risk for diseases that can be passed from mother to child perinatally. Such diseases include congenital rubella syndrome (CRS), HIV infection, syphilis, and hepatitis B and C. As we will see later, treatment of infected women during pregnancy can generally prevent transmission of these diseases to their infants.

Age may also affect the symptoms with which some communicable diseases present. For example, children with hepatitis A are often asymptomatic. Similarly, elderly persons with pneumococcal pneumonia may not present with classic symptoms of cough and fever, but may instead exhibit gastrointestinal symptoms.

Age also influences one's chances of exposure to some communicable diseases. For example, STIs and hepatitis B, C, and D occur more frequently in younger than older people because of their propensity to engage in high-risk sexual behaviors and injecting drug use. As we saw earlier, pertussis and mumps incidence have increased in adolescents and young adults, largely because of waning immunity from initial immunizations.

Communicable disease incidence and prevalence also vary by gender and by race/ethnicity. In 2011, incidence rates for most communicable diseases were higher for males than for females. Exceptions included *Chlamydia trachomatis* infection with a rate of 651.51 cases per 100,000 women compared to 255.36 cases per 100,000 men, some diarrheal diseases, and invasive *Haemophilus influenzae* infection. The incidence of HIV infections was more than four times higher in men than women, and primary and secondary syphilis incidence was more than eight times higher for men than for women (Adams et al., 2013). In addition, transgender females who engage in sex work to pay for hormone therapy or gender recognition surgery are at high risk for HIV-infection, contributing to a 26% infection rate in this population in San Francisco (Rapues, Wilson, Packer, Colfax, & Raymond, 2013).

Racial and ethnic differences in communicable disease incidence are more likely to be the result of differential levels of exposure and other behavioral and sociocultural factors than of differences in inherent susceptibility. For example, disparities in TB incidence, which is more than three times higher among Asians and Pacific Islanders (APIs) than among other racial groups, may reflect crowded living conditions. Similarly, increased incidence of other diseases in some ethnic minority populations (e.g., pertussis, which is highest among American Indians and Alaska Natives [AIAN]) may be a result of lack of access to health-promotive and illness-preventive knowledge and resources. Although disparities do not arise because of gender or ethnic minority group membership per se, population health nurses should be aware of gender and racial/ethnic differences in communicable disease incidence in order to be able to target intervention strategies to those most in need of them.

Racial disparities in STIs are particularly pronounced. In 2011, for example, Blacks had gonorrhea incidence rates 14 times higher than Whites and nearly 5 times higher than AIANs. Similarly, incidence rates for HIV infection were six times higher among Blacks than for any other group, and rates for both primary and secondary and congenital syphilis were approximately five times higher. Conversely, *Chlamydia trachomatis* infection rates were highest in Whites; invasive *Haemophilus influenzae* infection rates were highest among AIANs; and TB incidence rates were more than three times higher in APIs than in other groups. Persons of Hispanic origin tended to have higher incidence rates for some diseases (e.g., *Chlamydia trachomatis*, hepatitis A, HIV infection, mumps, pertussis, salmonellosis and shigellosis, primary and secondary syphilis, and TB) and lower rates for other diseases (e.g., congenital syphilis, hepatitis B and C, measles, and invasive *Haemophilus influenza* infection) than non-Hispanics (Adams et al., 2013).

The presence of other physical health conditions may also influence one's propensity to develop certain communicable diseases. For example, pregnant women are at higher risk for complications and death due to influenza (Newsome et al., 2011) as well as mortality related to HEV infection (Thomson et al., 2012). Similarly, HIV infection increases one's risk of a variety of opportunistic infections. **Opportunistic infections (OIs)** are diseases caused by organisms that either do not usually cause illness in humans or that usually cause only mild disease. For example, HIV infection increases the incidence of TB as well as the rate of progression to active disease. HIV infection and TB form a syndemic in which both diseases act "synergistically" to cause morbidity and mortality beyond what would be expected of either disease alone. For example, the lifetime risk of developing TB disease is 5% to 10% in the general population, but is much higher in those with HIV infection. HIV infection also makes it more difficult to diagnose TB because sputum smears and chest X-rays are less reliable indicators of disease. In addition, individuals with HIV infection are more likely than the general population to have extrapulmonary TB (Getahun et al., 2012).

Conversely, the presence of other STIs increases the potential for HIV infection. This is particularly true for STIs that cause lesions, such as secondary syphilis and herpes simplex virus (HSV) infection, but also occurs with inflammatory STIs such as gonorrhea and *Chlamydia* infections. Syphilis infection may also speed progression from HIV infection to AIDS. The presence of several of these diseases also increases the infectiousness of HIV due to the increased virus present in genital fluids, more so than in peripheral blood (Kalichman et al., 2011). Diseases, such as hemophilia, or other conditions that require transfusions or organ transplantation (e.g., chronic kidney disease) may contribute to exposure to a variety of bloodborne infections, including HIV, hepatitis B, C, and D, WNV, and other communicable diseases.

Another biological consideration with respect to communicable diseases relates to the effects of the diseases themselves. Most childhood diseases are relatively mild and self-limiting. On occasion, diseases such as measles, varicella, and mumps result in death. The overall case fatality rate for untreated tetanus in unimmunized individuals, however, is high as is mortality for HEV infection, particularly in pregnant women (Thomson et al., 2012). As noted in Chapter 3, the case fatality rate is the number of persons who have a disease who will die as a result of it. Hepatitis B, C, and D often result in chronic liver disease with increased risk of death. As noted earlier, persons with hepatitis B and C are also at high risk of cirrhosis and liver cancer, and those with HDV superinfection have a greater risk of developing chronic liver disease than those with HBV alone.

Immunization levels within the population constitute a final biological consideration influencing communicable diseases and their control. Routine immunization recommendations for children and adults were addressed in Chapters 16 through 19. Population health nurses would determine the extent of vaccine coverage for specific diseases for individuals as well as within the overall population.

Worldwide, vaccination coverage for children under 12 months of age in 2012 ranged from a low of 11% for rotavirus infection to highs of 84% for polio and meningococcal vaccines, and 83% for diphtheria, pertussis, and tetanus immunization. Approximately 79% of the world's infants had received three doses of HBV vaccine, and 45% received three doses of Hib vaccine, but immunization rates for pneumococcal conjugate vaccine (PCV) were only 19% (Department of Immunization, Vaccines, and Biologicals, 2013). As of 2012, 68% of WHO member nations had achieved greater than or equal to 90% coverage for three doses of DTP vaccine, and only six countries had DTP immunization levels below 50% (WHO, 2013b). In Latin America and the Caribbean, rotavirus vaccination, the most recently recommended vaccine, had been added to 44% of national immunization programs, and a median of 89% of children under 1 year of age had been immunized across the region as of June 2011 (de Oliviera et al., 2011). Similarly, in Laos, where hepatitis B is endemic, 74% of babies born in health care facilities and 41% of those born at home had received the birth dose of HBV vaccine. Overall, HBV vaccine coverage increased from 3% in 2006 to 34% in 2011 (Xeuatvongsa et al., 2013). As these figures indicate, however, much remains to be done to increase international immunization levels.

Immunization levels also vary among populations and across vaccines in the United States. For example, in 2012, based on National Immunization Survey data, 68% of U.S. children 19 to 36 months of age had received all of the recommended immunizations, and only 1% had received no immunizations. Immunization levels were highest for the completed polio series (92.8%) and lowest for rotavirus (68.6%) (Black, Yankey, & Kolasa, 2013). Similarly, during the 2012–2013 school year, most federally funded immunization programs were at or near the national goal of 95% coverage for all recommended vaccines.

The mean exemption rate (children who have been exempted from immunization requirements for health, religious, or philosophical reasons) across jurisdictions was 1.8% (Seither, Shaw, Knighton, Greby, & Stokley, 2013). Unfortunately, exemptions can cluster within communities, decreasing overall herd immunity and increasing the risk for the spread of disease outbreaks as we saw earlier.

Among adolescents 13 to 17 years of age, nearly 85% had received at least one dose of Tdap, 74% had received at least one dose of meningococcal conjugate vaccine, and nearly 95% had received at least one dose of varicella vaccine. In addition, nearly 21% of males and 54% of females had received at least one dose of HPV vaccine (Curtis et al., 2013). Although the percentage of girls receiving HPV vaccine increased from 25% to 54% from 2007 to 2012, only a third of adolescent girls had received all three recommended doses, and one fourth of parents surveyed did not intend to have their daughters vaccinated against HPV (Stokley et al., 2013).

Annual influenza immunization rates also vary among groups. For example, the immunization rate among children 6 months to 17 years of age during the 2011–2012 influenza season was roughly 57%; among adults over 18 years of age only 38% were immunized (Lu et al., 2013). As we saw in Chapter 19, the influenza immunization rate among people over 65 years of age in the 2009–2010 season was 72% (Serse et al., 2011). Influenza immunization also varies by economic status. For example, only 37.5% of the poor received influenza vaccine in 2010, compared to nearly 48% of the near poor, 51% of middle-income individuals, and 54% of high-income individuals. Despite universal recommendations for annual influenza vaccination for health care personnel (HCPs), only 72% of HCPs were immunized during the 2012–2013 season, with only 58% of those working in long-term care facilities covered (Ball et al., 2013). Immunization levels among HCPs increase in organizations where it is required. For example, during the 2011–2012 influenza season, immunization rates were above 95% in hospitals where it was required, but only 68% if immunization was not required (Ball et al., 2012).

The overall pneumococcal vaccination level in 2012 was 19.8%, but ranged from 8.7% for people aged 18 to 64 years to nearly 60% for those over age 65. Less than 20% of people 18 to 64 years of age at high risk for serious pneumococcal disease, however, had received the vaccine (NCHS, 2014). Slight increases in coverage rates had been achieved by 2011 when 62%

of those over 65 years of age and 20% of younger adults at high risk were immunized (Williams et al., 2013).

Immunization levels for other diseases among adults also vary considerably. For example, in 2008, less than 6% of adults 18 to 64 years of age had received Tdap (Miller, Ahmed, Lu, Euler, & Kretsinger, 2010). Similarly in 2011, the tetanus immunization rate was 64.5% for persons 19 to 49 years of age, and 63.9% for those over 65. Hepatitis B coverage was 12.5% among those 19 to 49 years of age, HPV coverage was 29.5% for those 19 to 26 years of age, and herpes zoster vaccine (HZV) coverage was roughly 16% in people over 60 years of age (Williams et al., 2013). Possible questions for assessing biological determinants contributing to communicable disease incidence in the population are included in the *Focused Assessment* provided below.

PSYCHOLOGICAL DETERMINANTS. Psychological considerations may play a part in the development of some communicable diseases. For example, stress has been shown to contribute to the development of active TB disease in persons with latent infection. Psychological factors may lead to risk-taking behaviors such as unprotected sexual activity or injecting drug use that increase the risk of STIs, HIV infection, and hepatitis B, C, and D. For example, the presence of post-traumatic stress disorder (PTSD) has been associated with high-risk sexual behaviors in low-income inner-city women. Women with PTSD in one study had more sexual partners, were more likely to have sex with a partner at high-risk for STI, and were more likely to experience partner violence related to condom use than women without PTSD (El-Bassel, Gilbert, Vinocur, Chang, & Wu, 2011).

Communicable diseases may also have psychological consequences for those infected. This is particularly true for conditions that have long-term consequences (e.g., HSV infection, HIV infection, or chronic hepatitis C) or require changes in lifestyle and behavior. In addition, clients with HIV/AIDS may develop dementia, which alters behavior and makes them difficult to care for. Depression may also be a significant consequence of stigmatizing diseases such as HIV infection or TB in some cultural groups. Failure to disclose one's HIV-positive status, for example, has been linked to a threefold increased risk for depression (Li et al., 2010). The *Focused Assessment* questions provided on the next page can assist the population health nurse to identify psychological factors related to communicable disease incidence in the population as well as in an individual client.

ENVIRONMENTAL DETERMINANTS. Environmental factors play a part in the development of diseases spread by airborne transmission and those transmitted by fecal–oral means. Overcrowding contributes to the incidence of such diseases as measles, mumps, rubella, polio, diphtheria, pertussis, and varicella. Crowded living conditions also enhance the spread of TB and influenza. For example, an outbreak of 28 cases of TB was associated with a homeless shelter and two neighboring bars frequented by shelter residents (Dobbins et al., 2012). Wind factors are an element of the physical environment that would influence the spread of aerosolized pathogens in the event of a terrorist attack.

Sanitation and disposal of both human and animal feces are other factors in the physical environmental dimension that affect the development of communicable diseases, particularly hepatitis A, tetanus, and polio. The organism causing tetanus is found on a variety of surfaces and is more common in areas where there is animal excrement. In addition, home delivery and poor hygiene on the part of untrained midwives in developing countries contribute to the development of tetanus in neonates and, occasionally, in postpartum women.

In developing countries, poor environmental sanitation contributes to the incidence of diseases such as hepatitis A and E and poliomyelitis. Sanitation is a less likely factor in the development of these diseases in the United States; however, as we saw earlier, contaminated food and water supplies have been implicated in several disease outbreaks related to *Escherichia coli*, hepatitis A, botulism, and other enteric pathogens.

FOCUSED ASSESSMENT
Assessing Biological Determinants Influencing Communicable Diseases

- What age groups are most likely to develop the disease? Are there differences in disease effects among age groups?
- Are there racial/ethnic or gender differences in disease incidence?
- What physiologic conditions, if any, increase the risk of disease?
- Does treatment for existing physiologic conditions increase the risk of disease?
- What are the signs and symptoms of the disease?
- What are the physiologic effects of the disease? What is the effect of the disease in pregnancy?
- What is the mode of disease transmission? What are the physiologic portals of entry and exit?
- Is there a vaccine available for the disease? If so, what are the immunization levels within the population?

FOCUSED ASSESSMENT Assessing Psychological Determinants Influencing Communicable Diseases

- Does exposure to stress increase the risk of disease?
- Do psychological factors increase the risk of exposure to disease?
- What effect, if any, do psychological factors have on high-risk behaviors that contribute to disease?
- Is past trauma or PTSD associated with the risk of disease?
- Does the presence of mental illness (e.g., depression) increase the risk of disease?
- Does the disease have potential psychological consequences (e.g., suicide risk)?

Exposure to tick-bearing animals such as white-tailed deer, elk, and wild rodents in recreational areas or during outdoor work increases the risk of tickborne diseases such as Rocky Mountain spotted fever. Household pets may also be infested by ticks and pose a risk of exposure to humans. Lyme disease is another neurological disease transmitted by ticks. Approximately 30,000 cases of Lyme disease occur each year in the United States in areas where the black-legged tick are common including the northeastern and mid-Atlantic states and in the west (CDC, 2013e). In 2012, the U.S. incidence rate for Lyme disease was 7 cases per 100,000 population (CDC, 2013f). Other species of ticks may also transmit a variety of diseases to humans.

Animals serve as a source of human infection for many diseases. As we saw in Chapter 4∞, zoonoses are diseases that can be transmitted from animals to human beings. Rabies and bubonic plague are two examples of zoonoses. Human rabies is relatively rare in the United States, but can be transmitted by the bite of an infected wild or domestic animal. In one case, for example, a woman was infected with rabies from bats roosting in her home. Prior to becoming ill, the woman had sought help for bat removal, but was not referred to the local health department or warned of the potential for rabies (Rupprecht et al., 2013). In other instances, *E. coli* and *Cryptosporidium* outbreaks have occurred as a result of contact with infected animals in petting zoos, state fairs, and at summer camps that include care of livestock (Collier et al., 2011; Griffin et al., 2012). Similarly, MERS antibodies have been found in camels and bats in the Arabian peninsula suggesting possible transmission to human beings (MERS Antibodies Detected in Camels, 2013). Schistosomiasis or snail fever is another disease with environmental links. Humans are infected after skin contact with water contaminated by parasitic worms that emerge from snails. The worms lay eggs throughout the body that cause extensive damage, particularly to the liver. Global climate changes and construction of dams have led to increases in infected snail populations in some areas resulting in increased disease incidence (Fan, 2012).

Recreational pursuits may increase the risk for exposure to pathogens. For example, walking in brushy or heavily wooded areas may result in exposure to disease-bearing ticks.

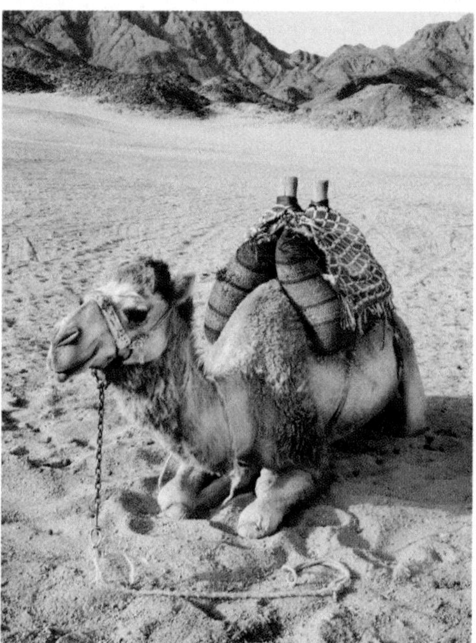

Many animals transmit diseases to humans.

(Hitdelight/Fotolia)

In California, an outbreak of hantavirus pulmonary syndrome occurred as a result of exposure to mouse droppings in cabins at Yosemite National Park (California Department of Public Health, 2012).

Prevention of infection in human beings often depends on disease control in animals. Population health nurses can help educate the public regarding zoonoses and actions that will prevent their spread to people. For example, routine vaccination of pets against rabies has led to marked decreases in the incidence of human rabies. Population health nurses can educate people on the need to immunize their pets and to avoid wild animals that may have rabies. Similarly, nurses can educate the public about the danger of eating raw eggs, which are often contaminated by pathogens such as *Salmonella*.

Because of differences in physical environmental conditions by region and by season, there are geographic and seasonal differences in the incidence of some communicable diseases. As we saw earlier, there are seasonal differences in influenza incidence in different areas of the world. Similarly, urban and rural differences are noted in disease incidence. For example, the incidence of HCV is increasing in some rural communities that are less likely than urban areas to mount prevention initiatives (Stanley et al., 2012). Conversely, TB incidence is higher in urban than rural areas, with 48 large U.S. cities accounting for 36% of all cases from 2000 to 2007. Contributing factors include the extent of homelessness, population density, and declining public health infrastructures for TB control. Another factor is the fact that most immigrants from highly TB-endemic countries tend to settle in urban, rather than rural areas (Oren, Winston, Pratt, Robinson, & Narita, 2011).

Elements of the built environment beyond crowding may influence the development of communicable diseases. For example, the only two cholera epidemics to occur in the Americas in recent memory (Peru in 1991 and Haiti in 2010) both resulted from deteriorating water supply infrastructure. In Peru, a water main collapsed creating a sink hole and allowing sewage to contaminate the local drinking water supply. Similar conditions occurred in Haiti after the 2010 earthquake. Both events reinforce the need for clean water and sanitation and the risks of neglecting upkeep to essential infrastructures (Cerdia & Lee, 2013).

Another example of built environment factors contributing to disease incidence is found in the underlying cause of outbreaks of *Legionellosis* in Alcoi, Spain. After repeated outbreaks over a period of 4 years, an epidemiologic investigation determined that the source of infection was the water tank of a street paving machine. Whenever streets were repaved, microorganisms were propelled into the air to result in increased disease in people living in the area (Coscollá, Fenollar, Escribano, & González-Candelas, 2010).

The relationship between environmental factors and communicable diseases can be extremely complex. For example, the relationship between the environment and HIV infection has been described as a syndemic one in which physical and social environmental factors interact with disease to worsen effects in all areas. Climate change increases migration among "climate refugees" (those leaving poor land conditions) and "conservation refugees" (those displaced from efforts to conserve protected environments). Migration tends to weaken the economy and diminish personal and societal resources to deal with illness and nutritional deficits, which, in turn, make the population more susceptible to HIV infection. Increased susceptibility may be the result of poor overall health or increased high-risk behavior (e.g., sex work) to support life. Conversely, HIV and AIDS decrease productivity among those affected and may lead to abandonment of the land, inability to grow crops due to reduced manpower, and use of natural resources to replace livelihoods (e.g., scavenging for edible foodstuffs or fuel), which depletes resources and leads to food shortages (Talman et al., 2013).

Multiple environmental determinants may contribute to the incidence and prevalence of communicable diseases in individuals and populations. The *Focused Assessment* questions below can assist population health nurses to identify environmental factors influencing communicable disease incidence in a particular population.

SOCIOCULTURAL DETERMINANTS. A variety of social and cultural factors influence the development and course of communicable diseases. For example, congregating with large groups of people indoors during the winter facilitates the spread of airborne diseases, and poverty and poor nutrition increase susceptibility to a variety of diseases, particularly TB. Congregate living in institutional settings also contributes to the spread of disease. For example, TB outbreaks frequently occur in correctional settings, as we saw in Chapter 24∞. College campuses and military installations experience frequent outbreaks of measles, mumps, pertussis, and meningococcal

FOCUSED ASSESSMENT Assessing Environmental Determinants Influencing Communicable Diseases

- What effect, if any, do crowded living conditions have on the incidence of the disease?
- Do elements of the built environment serve as sources of contamination and exposure to disease (e.g., contaminated ventilation systems, aging sewer or water supply systems)?
- Can the disease be transmitted to humans by animals or insects?
- What environmental factors increase the risk of human exposure to animal or insect sources of disease (e.g., standing water where mosquitoes breed)?
- Is the disease spread by contaminated food or water?
- Does poor sanitation affect disease incidence?
- Are there seasonal variations in disease incidence? If so, when is the disease most likely to occur? What environmental factors are present at that time that contribute to disease incidence?
- Do environmental factors impede access to diagnostic or treatment services?
- Are there rural/urban differences in disease incidence? If so, what environmental factors contribute to those differences?
- What effects, if any, does the disease have on physical or social environments?

meningitis among young adults in close quarters who are not immunized or whose levels of immunity have declined over time. Outbreaks of communicable diseases are also common in conditions of civil unrest. For example, more than 5,000 people were affected in a Sudanese refugee camp due to poor sanitation and personal hygiene and drinking water contamination (Thomson et al., 2012). Similarly, a cholera epidemic broke out in Haiti and the Dominican Republic after an earthquake disrupted safe water supplies (Jenkins et al., 2010).

Poverty and unemployment, with consequent loss of health insurance, are social factors that may limit the ability of parents to have their children immunized or to provide prompt medical care when illness does occur, resulting in more serious consequences of disease. Pregnant women with low incomes might not receive prenatal care and are thus denied the opportunity to obtain screening and counseling for syphilis, HIV, HBV, and HCV infection or susceptibility to rubella. HIV infection among heterosexual populations in high prevalence areas has been associated with low socioeconomic status, lower education levels, unemployment, and poverty (Denning, DiNenno, & Wiegand, 2011). In one study, census tracts with high poverty levels and high population density accounted for three times more pediatric hospitalizations for influenza than low poverty/low density areas (Yousely-Hindes & Hadler, 2011). Likewise, the racial disparities in STIs noted earlier have been associated with income disparities (Owusu-Edusei, Chesson, Leichliter, Kent, & Aral, 2013). Population health nurses will need to function as political advocates to assure the availability of communicable disease prevention and treatment services for all segments of the population, particularly those of low socioeconomic status.

Policy and legal issues also influence communicable disease incidence and control. For example, in 2013, 63 countries criminalized HIV transmission (UNAIDS, 2013), and in the United States most states have laws criminalizing intentional failure to disclose HIV infection to prospective sexual partners, but such laws have little effect. For example, in one study in New Jersey, 51% of HIV-positive respondents were aware of the law, but awareness was not associated with abstinence, condom use, or disclosure. The study found that, while such laws do not seem to increase stigma associated with HIV infection, neither do they reduce disease transmission (Galletly, Glasman, Pinkerton, & Di Franceisco, 2012).

Most states also have laws related to control of TB. CDC has suggested a set of standard provisions for state TB control laws that address general areas of case identification, case management, protection of individual rights, and interjurisdictional collaboration. Case identification provisions include mandated reporting of cases, screening, and investigation of both suspected cases and contacts. Case management provisions focus on state authority to implement control measures related to investigation, treatment, isolation of infectious cases, emergency detention, social distancing measures, penalties, and costs of services as well as "grants of authority to take any necessary action to protect public health" (Thombley & Stier, 2010, p. 53). Isolation or detention features of such laws permit state or local health jurisdictions to isolate infectious patients who refuse treatment under home isolation orders or through incarceration. Provisions related to individual rights address provision of due process, religious exemptions, and confidentiality of information (Thombley & Stier). Social distancing accomplishes the same goals, prevention of the spread of disease, but involves voluntarily staying away from others to avoid exposing them (Kumar, Grefenstette, Galloway, Albert, & Burke, 2013). For further information about the model law provisions, see the *External Resources* section of the student resources site.

Other examples of legal and policy issues that influence communicable disease incidence include mandatory immunizations, police interference with needle exchange programs for IDUs, and school policies on the availability of condoms for use by adolescents. All states mandate specific immunizations for school enrollment, although the specific requirements may vary slightly from state to state. As noted earlier, there are provisions for exemptions for medical, religious, or philosophical reasons. Population health nurses should be knowledgeable regarding immunization requirements in their areas. They should also be aware of the extent of exemption requests and reasons for them and help to educate parents regarding the need for mandated immunizations.

Mandatory HPV vaccination of children has been instituted in some jurisdictions, but has been resisted by some stakeholders on the grounds that immunity to HPV does not protect the general public, but protects the individual from a potential future condition (cancer) and should, therefore, be an individual decision rather than a legal mandate (Mah et al., 2011). During the 2009 H1N1 influenza epidemic, New York State mandated influenza vaccination for all HCPs. At the time, the mandate was resisted on grounds of violating civil liberties, but a significant case can be made for a moral and ethical imperative for immunization of HCPs to protect vulnerable patients (Ottenberg et al., 2011). Immunization of HCPs also helps to maintain the structural integrity of the health care system and its ability to respond to an epidemic.

Many jurisdictions have begun to authorize needle exchange programs and deregulation of syringe sales as a means of preventing the spread of HIV infection and other bloodborne diseases, such as hepatitis B and C and syphilis among IDUs. Unfortunately, local police may interfere with such programs even when they are legal due to lack of legal knowledge, fear of needlestick injuries, and overestimation of occupational risk to themselves (Beletsky et al., 2011).

Finally policies that promote or impede condom access by sexually active adolescents can influence rates of STIs as well as unintended pregnancy rates. Unfortunately, only 5% of U.S. school districts make condoms available to sexually active adolescents (Guttmacher Institute, 2014). Policies that promote STI education in the school setting also influence STI incidence, and population health nurses can advocate for both sexuality education and condom availability in schools.

As noted earlier, travel may be a significant sociocultural factor in the spread of communicable diseases. For example, more than 950,000 travelers enter the United States every day, anyone of whom might have a communicable disease. Legal immigrants and refugees are screened for TB and other diseases prior to entry, but approximately 125 people enter the country each year with active TB disease. Incidence rates for TB are 12 times higher in foreign-born persons than among U.S.-born residents (Kim et al., 2012). Each year, approximately 450,000 legal immigrants and 75,000 refugees enter the United States. In addition to the preentry screening, a medical assessment is recommended for refugees within 30 days after arrival. In 2009, the Electronic Disease Notification System notified state and local health departments of 21,319 refugees with a medical condition, 93% either had evidence of LTBI or X-ray evidence of suspected TB diseases. Approximately one third of the notifications were sent to three states: California, Texas, and New York. Nearly three fourths of notifications resulted in TB follow-up within 30 days of arrival (Lee et al., 2013).

When a report of communicable disease such as TB is received for persons arriving in the United States, an investigation is initiated. Federal isolation orders are issued until the person can be shown to be noncommunicable and travel is restricted. If the person arrived by air on a flight of 8 or more hours, contact investigation is initiated for passengers seated in the same row and two rows ahead and behind the source case (Kim et al., 2012). In an investigation of measles infection acquired during air travel, however, many of those who developed measles were seated more than two rows away from the source case, suggesting that exposure potential may extend beyond those limits. In addition, travelers may be exposed in jetways, departure terminals, or transit lounges (Hoskins et al., 2011). Some countries have instituted border screening based on self-report of symptoms and temperature for international arrivals, but these measures have not been shown to be effective in decreasing disease transmission (Priest, Jennings, Duncan, Brunton, & Baker, 2013).

Persons traveling from the United States to other countries may also become ill after exposures abroad. Approximately 8% of those traveling from developed to developing countries become ill. Diseases related to international travel are monitored by the GeoSentinel Surveillance System. The most commonly acquired diseases include acute unspecified diarrheas, bacterial diarrhea, febrile or systemic illness (approximately 19% of which is due to malaria), giardiasis, and dermatologic conditions (Harvey et al., 2013).

The magnitude of the potential for disease spread through international travel is reflected in many such events. In one case, a traveler returning from India with measles resulted in an outbreak with an additional 22 cases, most of which occurred in a large unvaccinated religious community. The outbreak resulted in over 1,000 persons exposed in various settings and required 2,200 hours of control efforts including written quarantine orders for 81% of susceptible contacts who did not receive vaccine within 72 hours of exposure and oral quarantine orders of the remaining 18% at tremendous cost to the local health jurisdiction (Sullivan, Moore, & Fleischauer, 2013).

Language barriers, cultural beliefs and values, and lower education levels among some ethnic and socioeconomic groups may impede awareness of the need for immunization or other preventive measures for communicable diseases. In addition, the beliefs of some religious groups prohibit immunizations, thus increasing the size of the susceptible population among their members and in the community at large. Other factors related to religion may impede or promote communicable disease control. For example, a strong religious foundation among African Americans has been shown to be associated with an increase in the stigma attached to HIV infection for Black MSM and to impede disclosure of HIV status to prospective partners (Bird & Voisin, 2013). Conversely, a faith-based HIV prevention intervention for African American women has been associated with increased abstinence and safer sexual practices (Wingood et al., 2013).

In some cases, religious practices may actually contribute to the development of communicable diseases. For example, cases of amebic meningoencephalitis have been attributed to ritual nasal rinsing as part of ablution prior to prayer in some Islamic groups (Hunte et al., 2013).

Gender socialization may also play a part in risk factors that promote STIs, particularly among women. In one study of condom negotiation among sexually active women, participants were found to rely on their male partners to initiate condom use. They cited unequal gender dynamics and beliefs that they were in a monogamous relationship. Even when faced with an STI diagnosis, the women did not feel able to engage in condom negotiation, highlighting the need to consider gender factors in programs to promote condom use (East, Jackson, O'Brien, & Peters, 2010). Socialization and peer group position have also been found to influence high-risk behaviors among runaway homeless youth. In one study, for example, the extent of risk behavior was associated with the strength of a particular youth's

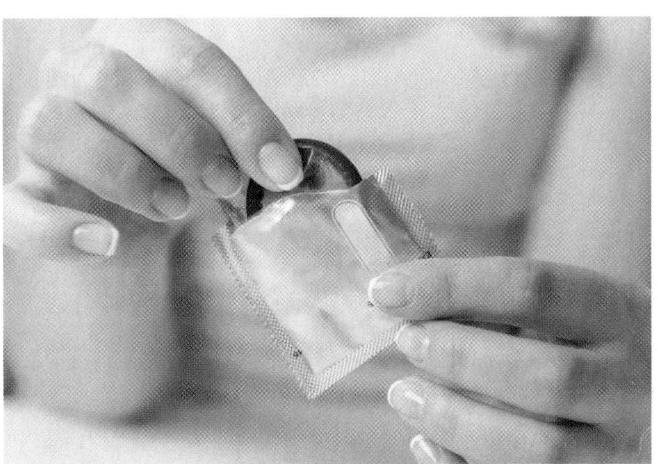

Women can be assisted to develop skills for negotiating condom use with their partners. *(Petro Feketa/Fotolia)*

connections to other youth engaged in high-risk behaviors (Rice, Barman-Adhukari, Milburn, & Monro, 2012).

Occupational factors are another part of the sociocultural dimension that may contribute to communicable diseases. Work with animals or animal products, for example, may contribute to transmission of zoonoses (Anderson et al., 2013) and sex work increases the potential for HIV infection and other STIs, as well as hepatitis B. Health care personnel and "first responders" (e.g., emergency personnel) are at increased risk for bloodborne diseases, and health care workers are frequently exposed to a variety of other communicable diseases. HCPs have the potential for both exposure to and transmission of diseases such as influenza, yet as noted earlier, vaccine coverage among health care personnel is relative low. As another example, hepatitis B and hepatitis C infections occur in HCPs after occupational exposures. Both employees and children are at risk for hepatitis A when outbreaks occur in child care settings. Certain occupations may contribute to the spread of disease as well as increased potential for exposure. For example, food service personnel may spread hepatitis A, and health care workers may expose clients to a number of communicable diseases.

Social stigma is another aspect of the sociocultural dimension that influences exposure to communicable diseases and attitudes to people who have them. Stigma may derive from fear of people who are different or from fear of exposure to disease, and affects people with communicable diseases in several ways. For example, stigma may increase the personal burden experienced by those with the disease or prevent them from seeking health care when stigmatized diseases are suspected. Stigma may also attach to professionals and community volunteers who provide services to those with certain communicable diseases.

Social norms that contribute to high-risk behaviors also foster the spread of some communicable diseases. For example, relaxed sexual mores have led to greater sexual promiscuity and increased risk of exposure to HIV infection, STIs, and some forms of hepatitis. Similarly, a social environment in which it is relatively easy to obtain drugs for injecting drug use promotes infection with HIV, syphilis, and hepatitis B, C, and D.

In addition to social factors that contribute to disease, communicable diseases may have social effects. For example, congenital rubella syndrome and congenital syphilis lead to long-term consequences in newborns that have extensive costs for society. Similarly, treatment of persons with chronic hepatitis or HIV infection imposes a costly burden on society, and care of children orphaned by parental death due to AIDS poses another social dilemma. On the other hand, social conditions may have positive effects on the incidence and prevalence of communicable diseases. For instance, raising the taxes on alcohol and increasing the age for legal consumption have been associated with lower incidence of gonorrhea. Alcohol lowers inhibitions to risky sexual behaviors, so control of alcohol use can minimize such behaviors. Sociocultural factors influencing communicable disease incidence in the community can be identified using the *Focused Assessment* questions provided below.

FOCUSED ASSESSMENT Assessing Sociocultural Determinants Influencing Communicable Diseases

- Does society condone behaviors that increase the risk of disease (e.g., sexual activity)?
- How does socioeconomic status influence disease incidence?
- Does social interaction increase the risk of the spread of disease?
- Is the disease spread easily in congregate living situations? What factors in congregate living situations contribute to the spread of disease?
- What are societal attitudes to the disease? Do they hamper control efforts? Is there social stigma attached to having the disease?
- Does gender or other socialization influence disease incidence?
- Does travel increase the potential for exposure to the disease?
- What influence do policy or legal issues have on incidence of the disease or its control?
- What effect do media messages have on attitudes to the disease? On behaviors that contribute to disease? On willingness to seek care for the disease?
- Do occupational factors influence the incidence of the disease?
- Does socioeconomic status affect risk for the disease? Consequences of the disease?
- Is the disease more common in the homeless population?
- What effect, if any, do language and cultural beliefs and behaviors have on the incidence of the disease?
- How, if at all, do religious beliefs and practices influence the disease?
- What effect does education level have on disease incidence?
- To what extent does gender socialization contribute to disease incidence?
- Is the disease more common in immigrant populations?
- What effects do war and social unrest have on disease incidence, if any?
- What are the social effects of having the disease for the individual or of increased incidence of the disease for the population?
- Does the disease have potential for use as a biological weapon?

BEHAVIORAL DETERMINANTS. Major behavioral determinants that influence the development of communicable disease are related to diet, sexual activity, and injecting drug use. Malnutrition makes people more susceptible to a number of diseases, particularly TB and childhood diseases in unimmunized populations. Malnutrition may also contribute to more severe disease and a greater chance of complications.

Sexual activity obviously increases the risk of STIs, but hepatitis B and D are also spread by sexual activity. Hepatitis C is usually transmitted via percutaneous exposure, but MSM who engage in high-risk sexual behaviors (e.g., anogenital and orogenital sex, use of sex toys, and group sex) are at risk for HCV (Fierer et al., 2011). Similarly, hepatitis A may be transmitted through orogenital sexual activity, particularly among MSM. Sexual transmission of *Shigella* has also been reported among MSM (Adams et al., 2013).

Roughly 27% of new HIV infections in 2009 were acquired by heterosexual activity (Miles et al., 2013), but the bulk of new infections occur in MSM. In 2011, for example, MSM accounted for 78% of all new HIV infections among men in 2011 (Harris et al., 2013). Young Black MSM are at particular risk for infection, and from 2001 to 2006, there was a 93% increase in new HIV infections in this group (Biedrzycki et al., 2011). Youth in general are also at higher risk for HIV infection through sexual activity than other groups. Risk factors for sexual acquisition of HIV infection among youth include early initiation of sexual activity, unprotected intercourse, older partners, sexual abuse, and the presence of other STIs (Division of HIV/AIDS Prevention, 2011).

MSM also account for most new cases of syphilis. For example, 70% to 80% of cases of syphilis in California occurred among MSM, and 57% of MSM with syphilis were also infected with HIV. In addition, California Syphilis Surveillance System data indicated that nearly 6% of MSM in California had repeated primary or secondary syphilis infections within 2 years (Cohen et al., 2012). MSM who seek sexual partners online are more likely than other MSM to be exposed to syphilis due to higher numbers of partners and more anonymous partners (Ng et al., 2013).

Globally, female sex workers are 13.5 times more likely than other women to develop HIV infection (UNAIDS, 2013). Factors contributing to risk for HIV and other STIs among female sex workers include large numbers of partners, unsafe working conditions, inability to negotiate condom use, and criminalization of sex work, which impedes STI screening and treatment (HIV/AIDS Programme, 2012). Transgender women who engage in sex work are also at high risk for HIV infection. In San Francisco, for example, HIV prevalence among transgender females who also engage in injecting drug use is 51% (Rapues et al., 2013).

Women who have sex with women (WSW) are also at greater risk for some STIs. For example, *Chlamydia trachomatis* infection is more prevalent among WSW and those who have sex with both men and women than among strictly heterosexual women. In the National Survey of Family Growth, 11% of U.S. women between the ages of 15 and 44 reported same sex behavior at some point in their lives, and more than 90% of self-identified lesbians have had sex with men as well as women increasing their risk for STIs. WSW are at higher risk for HPV, HIV, herpes, trichomoniasis, and bacterial vaginitis than heterosexual women (Singh et al., 2011).

Combining sexual activity with drug and alcohol use (other than IDU) also increases the risk for STIs. For example, 40% of HIV-infected adults reported illicit drug use other than marijuana in the prior 12 months. In addition, 40% reported heavy alcohol or crack cocaine use, 14% used stimulants, and 38% used marijuana. Drug use is associated with increased numbers of sexual partners and unprotected sexual activity increasing the risk for STIs (Mimiaga et al., 2013).

Concurrent sexual partnerships also increase one's risk for STIs. Concurrent partnerships are those that overlap in time, and are a significant factor in the spread of sexually transmitted infections. Based on data for the National Survey of Family Growth, 5.7% to 8.3% of U.S. women engaged in concurrent relationships (Adimora, Schoenbach, Taylor, Kahn, & Schwartz, 2011). Studies among men who have sex with men in China (Ha, Liu, Liu, Cai, & Feng, 2010) and New York City (Tieu et al., 2014) reported concurrent sexual partners, and 38% of the men in the Chinese study had concurrent partnerships with both men and women. Concurrent partnerships among women have been associated with younger age and younger age at first intercourse; being formerly married, rather than single or currently married; having a nonmonogamous partner, having sex while under the influence of drugs or alcohol; binge drinking; and cocaine use (Adimora et al., 2011). Men with concurrent partnerships were considerably more likely to report inconsistent condom use (Ha et al., 2010; Tieu et al., 2014), but did not perceive themselves as being at any higher risk for HIV than those with single partners (Ha et al., 2010).

Another behavior that increases the potential for HIV exposure and other STIs (e.g., chronic HBV) is the failure of infected persons to disclose their status to sexual partners. Conversely, use of condoms is a behavioral factor that can protect against exposure to STIs. Unfortunately, the prevalence of condom use by sexually active persons waxes and wanes. Among adolescents, access to condoms may influence their use, but many people are reluctant to provide condoms to sexually active young people out of a fear of promoting sexual activity. Population health nurses may educate sexually active clients, particularly adolescents, about the use of condoms. They may also need to advocate for condom availability to those who are sexually active.

Injecting drug use is another behavioral determinant that influences the incidence of several communicable diseases. For example, globally, IDUs are 22 times more likely to develop HIV infection than the general population in reporting countries (UNAIDS, 2013). In fact, because of easy access to the bloodstream, IDU is more efficient than sexual contact in spreading HIV; however, harm reduction strategies, such as needle exchange programs among IDUs can decrease percutaneous transmission, making sexual transmission more significant. In addition, use of certain drugs increases the potential for unsafe sexual activity (Des Jarlais et al., 2011). In 2010, 8% of new HIV infections occurred in IDUs, and only 19% of IDUs reported participating in risk reduction interventions (Smith, Martin, Lansky, Mermin, & Choopanya, 2013).

HCV prevalence among IDUs is estimated at 50% (Iverson et al., 2013), and IDUs engaged in sex work are more likely than non-sex workers to develop syphilis. IDUs are also at higher risk than nonusers for several bacterial infections, particularly wound infections such as anthrax, botulism, and *Clostridium* (Hope et al., 2012). In addition, the self-neglect and poor nutrition that frequently accompany injection drug use increases the risk for a variety of other diseases such as tuberculosis, influenza, and pneumonias.

Drug abuse, particularly opiate use, may also result in anergy, reducing the validity of tuberculin tests as a screening tool in these high-risk populations. **Anergy** is an inability to react to antigens commonly used in TB skin testing due to a weakened immune system (Division of Tuberculosis Elimination, 2011). Anergy also occurs in the presence of HIV infection, making it more difficult to diagnose TB in HIV-infected individuals.

Smoking, breast-feeding, and tattooing are other examples of behavioral determinants that may increase one's risk for communicable diseases. Smoking may result in respiratory irritation, increasing the potential for respiratory diseases. Breast-feeding can promote vertical transmission of HIV infection from mother to infant, but transmission is prevented when mothers receive ART. Tattoos may contribute to a variety of skin infections. For example, an outbreak of nontuberculous mycobacterial skin infections was attributed to contamination of tattoo ink (Bedard et al., 2012). The *Focused Assessment* below includes questions that can assist population health nurses to identify behavioral factors influencing communicable disease incidence in population groups or individuals.

HEALTH SYSTEM DETERMINANTS. Factors related to the health care system may also influence the development and course of communicable diseases. For example, charging fees for immunizations may limit the ability of people in lower socioeconomic groups to become adequately immunized. Similarly, missed opportunities for immunizations and provider failure to give immunizations because of mythical contraindications (e.g., presence of mild fever) also increase the risk of communicable diseases.

Health care providers may also fail to provide screening or health education related to communicable diseases. For example, providers often fail to elicit a sexual history thereby missing clients who are at risk for STIs (Satterwhite et al., 2011). Even among providers caring for clients with communicable diseases, the frequency of preventive counseling may be low. The lack of national guidelines for routine health promotion and wellness activities for young men has been cited as a cause of missed opportunities for health promotion, preventive interventions, and screening (Lanier & Sutton, 2013).

Health care providers may also fail to recognize atypical forms of illnesses or emerging or reemerging diseases and treat them effectively. For example, because of its relative infrequency in modern society, providers may lack clinical experience with pertussis or fail to consider it as a possible diagnosis. Similarly, they may fail to consider a diagnosis of HIV in a client with no known risk factors. Health care providers who are unfamiliar with the symptoms of anthrax or other rarely seen conditions may misdiagnose them, leading to inappropriate treatment and greater spread of disease. Providers may also be unfamiliar with recommended treatment guidelines for certain communicable diseases. For example, gonorrhea treatment guidelines were modified in 2006, but a study conducted in 2008 found that the revised guidelines were followed approximately 20% of the time in primary care settings and only slightly more often in STI clinics (28%) (Dowell et al., 2012).

FOCUSED ASSESSMENT — Assessing Behavioral Determinants Influencing Communicable Diseases

- Does diet play a part in the incidence of the disease (e.g., malnutrition as a risk factor for TB)? Does nutritional status influence the consequences of the disease?
- Does alcohol or drug use contribute to the incidence of the disease?
- Does sexual activity increase the risk of the disease? Do specific sexual behaviors increase or decrease the risk of the disease?
- Are people with the disease likely to disclose their infection to others? What barriers to disclosure exist? What effect does willingness to disclose have on controlling spread of the disease?
- Does breast-feeding increase the risk of infection in young children?
- Does smoking increase the risk of disease?
- What other behaviors contribute to the development of disease (e.g., tattooing)?

In addition, inappropriate use of antibiotics by providers may contribute to the development of resistant strains of microorganisms. For example, approximately 258 million courses of antibiotics are prescribed in the United States each year, many of them inappropriate for the conditions being treated. Half of all hospitalized patients receive some form of antibiotic, and nearly half of those are unnecessary or inappropriate (CDC, 2013c).

Health system factors may also contribute more actively to communicable diseases and their effects. For example, **nosocomial infection** (disease spread as a result of exposure in a health care setting) is a significant factor in the spread of communicable diseases. For example, an outbreak of hepatitis B occurred in an assisted living facility due to assisted monitoring of residents' blood glucose levels using inappropriate lancets (Rossheim et al., 2013). An outbreak of *Streptococcus pneumonia* in another assisted living facility highlighted the need for effective infection control processes in assisted living facilities (Bamberg et al., 2013). In other instances, methylprednisolone injections have resulted in outbreaks of spinal and paraspinal fungal infections and meningitis due to contaminated medication received from compounding pharmacies (Finks et al., 2013; Peterson et al., 2013). As we saw earlier, transfusion and organ transplantation are other health care procedures that may contribute to the development of bloodborne diseases in recipients.

Measles exposure in a hospital emergency department (ED) led to an outbreak that necessitated 4,000 contact investigations and resulted in cases of measles in four other patients and one ED physician. In this particular outbreak, 43% of potentially exposed employees had no documented measles immunity putting them and their patients at risk for disease (Green et al., 2012).

As noted earlier, HCPs are at particular risk for developing and spreading communicable diseases. This is particularly true of HCPs with chronic HBV infection. HBV infection, however, does not preclude health care practice by infected individuals if adequate precautions are taken. U.S. recommendations for preventing HBV exposure of patients by HCPs include screening all providers who engage in exposure prone procedures, vaccinating those who do exposure prone procedures, using safer devices to minimize risk of exposure, and implementing safe work practice controls (e.g., not recapping needles) (Holmberg, Suryaprasad, & Ward, 2012). Similarly, recommended procedures for investigating possible infections associated with health care, such as HBV or HCV, have also been developed (Bornschlegel, Dentinger, Layton, Balter, & France, 2012).

Even routine health care interventions such as immunization may result in unintended illness. For example, rare cases of vaccine-associated paralytic poliomyelitis may occur in persons who receive oral polio vaccine or their close contacts. Such vaccine-associated cases may contribute to outbreaks in populations with low oral polio vaccine (OPV) coverage. Once worldwide polio eradication has been achieved, OPV use can be discontinued and inactivated polio vaccine (IPV) used to maintain vaccination coverage (Polio Eradication Department, WHO, 2012). Although the risk of vaccine-induced disease occurs, it is lower than the risk of exposure through travel to endemic areas, and immunization prior to travel is recommended.

Other medical treatment interventions have also been associated with communicable diseases in their recipients. For example, medical treatment for conditions such as asthma and autoimmune diseases that require immunosuppressive therapy places individuals at greater risk for complications of influenza. In addition, inappropriate prescription of antimicrobials by health care providers has led to the development of antibiotic-resistant strains of several microorganisms, which will be discussed in more detail later in this chapter.

Provider attitudes to persons with stigmatizing diseases may also influence care. Such attitudes may be reflected in refusal of care, blaming and humiliation, poor quality of care, or violation of confidentiality (Li et al., 2013). Lack of infrastructure support and drug shortages are other health system factors that may influence communicable disease control. For example, a 2010 survey of state health departments indicated that many states lacked sufficient capacity to effectively investigate foodborne disease outbreaks due to delays in notification, lack of personnel, and lack of epidemiologic expertise (Boulton & Rosenberg, 2011). With respect to drug shortages, 178 impending shortages were reported to the Food and Drug Administration (FDA) in 2010. Shortages are most often due to recall of medications due to poor quality or to difficulty procuring raw materials for manufacture. Early FDA notification of anticipated shortages can often help to circumvent them (e.g., through authorization of purchase of foreign-made drugs or other strategies) (Seaworth et al., 2013). Currently, drug shortages are being experienced for both first-line and second-line antituberculosis drugs.

Potential questions for exploring health system determinants in the development of communicable diseases are presented in the *Focused Assessment* on the next page. A communicable disease risk inventory for assessing the risk of communicable diseases in population groups is included on the student resources site.

Diagnostic Reasoning and Control of Communicable Diseases

The population health nurse may derive a variety of nursing diagnoses related to communicable diseases. These diagnoses may reflect the health needs of individuals, families, or population groups. Diagnoses may also reflect the potential for infection or the presence of active disease. For example, the nurse working with a family may diagnose "inadequate immunization status due to poor knowledge of children's immunization needs." Possible nursing diagnoses related to individual

FOCUSED ASSESSMENT Assessing Health System Determinants Influencing Communicable Diseases

- What preventive measures are available for the disease? Are they widely used?
- To what extent do health care providers educate the public on prevention of the disease?
- Is there a vaccine available for the disease? Do vaccine-associated cases of the disease occur? If so, what is the incidence of vaccine-associated disease?
- To what extent are health care personnel immunized against the disease?
- Is there a screening test for the disease? If so, are persons at risk for the disease screened?
- How is the disease diagnosed?
- To what extent are health care providers conversant with the signs and symptoms of the disease?
- To what extent are health care providers conversant with recommended treatments for the disease?
- To what extent do health care providers report cases of the disease? Do they engage in contact notification?
- To what extent do health care settings or provider behaviors contribute to the development of disease? What is the extent of nosocomial infection in the community?
- To what extent do routine medical interventions contribute to the incidence of communicable disease?
- Is there an effective treatment for the disease? Are diagnostic and treatment services for the disease available and accessible to infected persons?
- Are the drugs needed to treat the disease available?
- Do health care systems have the capacity needed to investigate outbreaks of disease?
- To what extent do health care providers engage in practices that might lead to the development of drug-resistant microorganisms?
- Do health care personnel with the disease engage in effective infection control practices?
- Do health care facilities engage in effective infection control practices?
- What are the attitudes of health care providers to persons with the disease? How do these attitudes affect willingness to seek diagnostic and treatment services? To what extent do they affect the quality of care provided?

clients might include "potential for infection with tetanus due to increased risk of occupational injury and lack of recent immunization," or "failure to obtain routine immunizations due to lack of transportation." A diagnosis related to the presence of active disease might be "probable tuberculosis as evidenced by symptoms of cough, weight loss, and night sweats and a history of recent travel to an endemic area."

Nursing diagnoses related to communicable diseases may also be derived for population groups. Diagnoses at the community level may reflect the current incidence of disease or the potential for spread of infection. Examples of such diagnoses are "increased incidence of HCV due to injection drug use" and "potential for increased transmission of HIV infection due to widespread use of unsafe sexual practices among MSM."

Nursing diagnoses may also reflect the presence of risk factors that affect the development of communicable diseases in individuals or population groups. For example, the nurse may diagnose an "increased risk of hepatitis A due to shellfish contamination in local waters" or "increased risk of tuberculosis transmission from refugees emigrating from endemic areas."

Planning and Implementing Control Strategies for Communicable Diseases

Many previously known as well as emerging communicable diseases contribute to a significant worldwide burden of disease, death, and suffering. Control of communicable diseases rests on an understanding of the factors that lead to their development and knowledge of interventions to prevent or treat them. Such understandings allow population health nurses and others to engage in effective control strategies related to health promotion, illness prevention, resolution of existing communicable diseases, and health restoration.

HEALTH PROMOTION. Basic health promotion strategies can reduce susceptibility to communicable diseases in individuals or in population groups. Adequate nutrition is an essential facet of health promotion with respect to communicable diseases. As we saw earlier, malnutrition is a significant contributor to communicable disease morbidity, and particularly mortality, throughout the world. Similarly, maintaining one's health through adequate rest and physical activity can also reduce one's susceptibility to illness. Finally, promotion of good coping skills can reduce the contribution of stress to the development of chronic diseases. Population health nurses can educate individuals, families, and population groups regarding good nutrition, rest and exercise, and coping. In addition, they can advocate for the availability of adequate resources to promote overall health.

ILLNESS PREVENTION. Major emphases in preventing communicable diseases include immunization, contact tracing and notification, pre- and postexposure prophylaxis, and other preventive measures specific to particular communicable diseases.

Immunization. Immunization is the most effective method of preventing the occurrence of communicable diseases for which vaccines are available. The modern concept of immunization originated with William Jenner, and the first smallpox vaccine was developed in 1796, but its use did not become widespread for more than 100 years. Similarly, four other vaccines (rabies, cholera, typhoid, and plague) were developed between 1885 and 1897 but were not widely used (Immunization Action Coalition, 2013). Based on U.S. immunization recommendations, discussed in Chapter 16∞, children should receive a recommended set of vaccines before the age of 2 years. These immunizations are intended to protect them from multiple diseases. Immunization with selected vaccines is also recommended for adults, as noted in Chapters 17∞, 18∞, and 19∞, and for members of specific groups at high risk for infection. For example, people in certain occupational categories (e.g., health care providers) are at high risk for exposure to a variety of pathogens, and inmates in correctional settings are at increased risk for diseases such as HIV/AIDS, TB, and hepatitis (see Chapters 23∞ and 24∞ for more in-depth discussion of immunization needs in these populations). Other immunizations are recommended for people traveling to areas with a high incidence of specific diseases. For example, a booster dose of polio vaccine is recommended for travel to countries with high polio risk (World Health Organization, Division of Global Migration and Quarantine, 2013a). Similarly, the Advisory Committee on Immunization Practices has recommended use of the Japanese Encephalitis vaccine (JE-VC) for persons (including young children) traveling to JE-endemic areas (e.g., rural areas in Asia and the western Pacific), whose planned activities promote exposure to mosquito bites (Bocchini, Rubin, Fischer, Hills, & Staples, 2013). As another example, meningococcal vaccine is recommended for all adolescents, but also for military recruits and travelers to or residents of hyperendemic or epidemic areas (Cohn et al., 2013).

Influenza vaccine is recommended for people over 6 months of age in the United States (Grohskopf et al., 2013) and worldwide (WHO, Collaborating Center for Surveillance, Epidemiology, and Control of Influenza, 2013), but is particularly important for young children, the elderly, and persons with chronic illnesses who are at high risk for complications of influenza. Unfortunately, vaccine efficacy is reduced in the elderly due to suboptimal immune responses (Sagawa, Kojimahara, Otsuka, Kimura, & Yamaguchi, 2011), so immunization of health care workers in long-term care facilities is even more critical than in other health care settings. Health care worker immunization is fostered when employers provide onsite availability at no cost to employees (Ball et al., 2013).

Overall, influenza vaccine effectiveness during the 2012–2013 season was estimated at 56% (Jackson et al., 2013). Despite variability in preventing disease, vaccination has been found to be effective in preventing death and hospitalizations among those at risk of complications. In one cost-benefit analysis, influenza immunization for the general population resulted in cost savings of $6 per vaccination to employers, rising to $83 per person vaccinated among those with high-risk comorbidities and $107 per person among older adults (Duncan, Taitel, Zhang, & Kirkham, 2012). Similarly, the New York Department of Health (2013) estimated a cost savings of $13 per vaccination among health care providers.

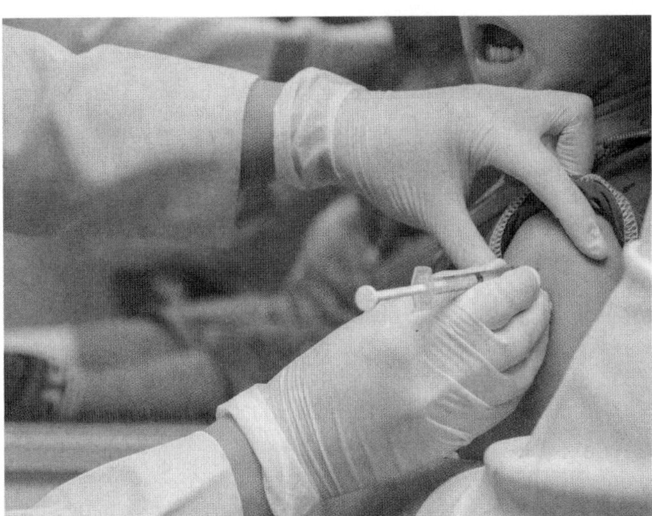

Immunization is a highly effective preventive measure for many communicable diseases. *(casanowe/Fotolia)*

HBV vaccine is recommended for all U.S. children under 19 years of age, and WHO has recommended that all countries incorporate HBV vaccine into their routine childhood immunization. Immunization of pregnant women prevents approximately 90% of mother-to-child transmission of HBV. Some countries, however, target vaccine delivery to high-risk women and children born to HBV-positive mothers leaving other children at risk for later development of HBV (Børresen et al., 2012).

Updated tetanus vaccination is particularly recommended for persons with diabetes, IDUs, and those over 65 years of age, who may never have been immunized (Tiwari et al., 2011). Similarly, TDaP is recommended for pregnant women, health care providers, and others who will be caring for young infants to protect them from exposure. Reimmunization may occur as soon as 2 years after a prior dose in this situation (Miller et al., 2010; Sawyer et al., 2013).

Persons who have immune deficiencies can and should receive many of the recommended vaccines. For example, MMR can be given to HIV-positive individuals without severe immunosuppression, and HIV-exposed infants should be revaccinated after initiation of ART (McLean et al., 2013).

HPV vaccine is now recommended for both boys and girls after age 11 (Guttmacher Institute, 2014). The vaccine is relatively expensive, costing approximately $390 for the three-dose series. Fortunately, vaccine coverage will be required of private insurers under ACA, and the Vaccines for Children Program covers vaccine costs for Medicaid enrollees. State Children's Health Insurance Programs (SCHIP) separate from Medicaid are also required to provide coverage. Internationally, the Global Alliance for Vaccines and Immunization (GAVI) is expected to support HPV vaccine in 28 countries by 2017 (Henry J. Kaiser Family Foundation, 2014).

Bacille Calmette–Guerin (BCG) vaccine is used for TB prevention in some parts of the world, but has been found to be only partially effective. In addition, use of BCG vaccine causes tuberculin skin tests to become reactive and invalidates skin tests as a screening measure for tuberculosis. New vaccines for TB are being developed, and several are currently being tested in animals, so a more effective vaccine may be available in the future. An effective vaccine for malaria may also be available soon. International trials have been promising and the vaccine has been shown to be safe (Ogwang et al., 2013). At present, there are no vaccines for most STDs, for hepatitis C or D, or for HIV infection. There is a vaccine available for HEV, but it is not used in the United States due to the relatively low incidence of the disease, and is not widely used elsewhere in the world (Thomson et al., 2012).

Widespread use of vaccines is a 20th-century phenomenon, but barriers still exist to the use of immunization services. Some of these barriers include lack of access to services (e.g., due to cost), lack of knowledge regarding the need for immunization, parental concerns regarding the discomfort associated with administration of some vaccines (e.g., localized swelling with DTP), and health system limitations such as differences in school entry requirements across jurisdictions, poor enforcement of immunization requirements, and poor data management. Other system barriers are the failure of providers to encourage immunizations other than those required for school entry and missed opportunities for immunization in the course of providing other services. Population health nurses can advocate for the availability of immunization services to all segments of the population and can educate the public and providers on the need for immunization as well as possible adverse reactions. In fact, in some studies, information provided by nurses was the most significant factor in parental decisions to immunize their children (Austvoll-Dahlgren & Helseth, 2010).

Several of the 2020 national health objectives are related to increasing immunization coverage for a variety of communicable diseases (U.S. Department of Health and Human Services, 2014). Some of these objectives with baseline data, current status, and 2020 targets are presented later in this chapter. Additional objectives may be viewed on the *Healthy People 2020* website. For updates on immunization recommendations, see the *External Resources* section of the student resources site.

The problem of data management has also been addressed in the *Healthy People 2020* objectives with the recommendation to develop population-based immunization information systems (IISs) to consolidate records and generate reminders of subsequent immunization needs. IISs record and consolidate confidential information regarding immunizations given by multiple providers. In 2011, 84% of U.S. children under 6 years of age were included in an IIS (Cardemil, Pabst, & Gerlach, 2013). Immunization levels in the community are fostered by systems that can generate reminder messages. For example, text messages reminding parents of their children's need for immunizations have improved immunization rates, particularly in low-income populations (Stockwell et al., 2012). Similarly, population-based recall systems generated by state IISs have been even more effective in promoting up-to-date immunizations than reminders generated by individual provider offices (Kempe et al., 2013). Population health nurses can advocate for the development of local IISs where they do not already exist and for health care provider participation in existing IISs.

The extent of vaccine coverage in a population is affected by a number of variables, including perceptions of vaccine effectiveness and fear of possible adverse consequences of immunization. Vaccination coverage is also influenced by vaccine availability and distribution. Some authors have questioned the advisability of adding new vaccines into routine immunization schedules in developing countries for fear of overwhelming vaccine storage and delivery infrastructures and causing problems with access to previously required immunizations (Lee et al., 2012). Population health nurses in these countries can help to ascertain the potential effects of the addition of new vaccines to immunization schedules and collaborate in addressing infrastructure constraints. Population health nurses educate the public regarding the need for immunizations. They are also frequently involved in planning, implementing, and evaluating immunization campaigns and in giving immunizations to susceptible individuals. When nurses actually provide immunizations, they are also involved in educating clients regarding normal reactions to vaccines and comfort measures that may be taken to address them (e.g., nonaspirin antipyretics for fever or pain following DTP immunization) as well as signs of potential adverse reactions.

Population health nurses may also advocate for access to immunization services for all segments of the population and may be involved in the enactment and enforcement of immunization policies designed to protect the general public. For example, population health nurses might advocate requirements that college entrants provide evidence of measles immunity or that rotavirus immunization be required for preschool or elementary school entry.

Contact investigation and notification. Contact investigation and notification is a prevention strategy used for some communicable diseases with a relatively long incubation period. **Contact investigation and notification** involves identifying people who might have been exposed to someone with a case of a particular disease, making them aware of the exposure and offering prophylactic treatment and/or screening for the disease. Typically, the source case is interviewed and names of persons who might have been exposed to the disease are elicited. Who constitutes a contact depends on the mode of transmission of the disease. For example, sexual contacts would be elicited in the case of a sexually transmitted disease, while persons who might share needles and other drug paraphernalia would be obtained from an IDU with syphilis or HIV, HBV, or HCV infection. For airborne diseases, such as TB or measles, family members, coworkers, or school classmates would be considered contacts. People identified are then located and informed of their exposure status. In many instances, they may be required to submit to testing for the disease or be shown to be noncommunicable. For example, health care providers whose children develop streptococcal infection are frequently required to have negative cultures or be placed on antibiotic therapy before they will be allowed to return to work.

Contact notification can be an expensive undertaking, so contacts should be prioritized in terms of the likelihood of developing the disease. For example, TB contacts would be prioritized on the basis of the infectiousness of the source case, the age and immune status of the contacts, and the intensity and duration of exposure. The World Health Organization has suggested that each person with infectious TB will have at least three close contacts and that approximately 2.5% of those contacts will also have active TB. Routine contact investigation could promote early identification of 300,000 cases of TB per year permitting early treatment and minimizing the spread of disease (WHO, 2012). Many more people may have latent TB and, with treatment, can be prevented from progressing to active disease. As we saw earlier, some people with communicable disease may have significantly more contacts who may have already spread the disease to others leading to widespread and costly contact investigations.

Contact investigation may be more effective when those exposed can be screened on the spot rather than having to go to a health care setting for screening and treatment. For example, the use of rapid HIV screening kits in the field when contacting sex and needle-sharing partners of HIV-positive individuals in New York City increased the percentage of partners screened from 52% to 76% (Renaud et al., 2011).

Population health nurses are frequently involved in contact investigation and notification. They may interview clients with communicable diseases to elicit the names of relevant contacts. In addition, they are often the ones to notify contacts of their status and offer them needed screening and treatment services. Nurses involved in contact investigations may make home visits or approach contacts at work or any other place where they can be located. When they approach contacts, nurses should speak to them in a setting that ensures privacy and inform them that they have been exposed to a communicable disease. Nurses frequently need to exercise creativity to protect both the confidentiality of the source case and the contact and prevent others from knowing why the person is being contacted by a nurse.

Pre- and postexposure prophylaxis. One of the advantages of contact identification and notification is the ability to offer treatment to people prior to exposure to or development of a particular disease. **Preexposure prophylaxis (PrEP)** involves provision of treatment to people who have not yet been exposed to a disease, but who are at high risk for exposure. For example, IDUs and MSM in areas of high HIV infection prevalence might be offered prophylactic ART to prevent them from becoming infected. CDC recommends daily ART preexposure prophylaxis to prevent HIV infection in MSM, IDUs, and heterosexual men and women in high prevalence areas (Leibowitz, Parker, & Rotherham-Bonus, 2011; Smith et al., 2013).

Postexposure prophylaxis (PEP) was defined in Chapter 23∞ and involves the use of medications or vaccines to prevent the onset of disease in exposed individuals. When individuals are prevented from developing symptomatic disease, they are usually also prevented from spreading the disease to others. PEP has been used for a variety of diseases. For example, people at high risk for complications, pregnant women, and infants exposed to measles should be given MMR vaccine or measles immune globulin to prevent disease (McLean et al., 2013). Similarly, varicella immune globulin is recommended for persons exposed to varicella who have no evidence of immunity and are at high risk for severe disease (CDC, 2012a; Marin, Bialek, & Seward, 2013). PEP is also used for rabies and meningococcal disease exposures (Cohn et al., 2013; Rupprecht et al., 2013).

Postexposure prophylaxis has been used extensively to prevent contacts to cases of tuberculosis and persons with latent TB infection from developing active disease (Miramontes et al., 2013). Traditional contact notification for STIs may be replaced by a newer strategy of **expedited partner therapy (EPT)**, which involves providing an individual with a STI with medication to be given to his or her sexual partners without an examination or screening test. CDC recommends EPT for treatment of partners of persons infected with gonorrhea and *Chlamydia trachomatis* (Division of STD Prevention, 2014). Other recommendations are to advocate for legal support of EPT through exceptions to prescription laws, promoting professional support of EPT, and advocating for third-party reimbursement for EPT.

Health care workers are often the recipients of PEP after occupational exposures to a variety of organisms. PEP is highly recommended for health care workers with LTBI and for those with HIV exposures, as well as for HBV and HCV exposure. Population health nurses may need to advocate for effective PrEP and PEP policies for specific vulnerable populations (e.g., homeless persons or inmates in correctional settings). They may also need to advocate for funding for and development of easily accessible services for the general public.

Other prevention measures. Other prevention strategies for communicable diseases may be directed toward the mode of transmission of specific diseases. Prevention for tetanus due to puncture wounds, for example, involves educating clients on the use of protective clothing (e.g., gloves, boots) to prevent injuries and the need for adequate cleansing of wounds with soap and water when injuries do occur. Effective wound care is also critical in preventing rabies after animal bites. Vaccine-laden bait can also be used to immunize wildlife against rabies in high prevalence areas (Kellogg et al., 2013). Disinfection of equipment in health care settings also helps to prevent the spread of communicable diseases.

For STIs, refraining from sexual activity is the most effective means of preventing diseases. For those who are sexually active, however, use of condoms and refraining from unsafe sexual practices may limit exposure to disease. MSM and others who engage in high-risk sexual behaviors (e.g., with multiple partners, anal receptive intercourse) should also be encouraged to use condoms. Population health nurses can advocate for condom use with sexually active clients who engage in high-risk behaviors. They may also educate clients on the correct use of condoms or may advocate for condom availability to special groups like adolescents or correctional inmates. Population health nurses can also inform clients who engage in oral–genital intercourse as a mode of contraception that they continue to be at risk for STI transmission.

Serosorting is another effective strategy for preventing the spread of HIV infection among MSM. As we saw in Chapter 20∞, serosorting involves limiting one's sexual partners to people who are of the same HIV status as oneself (Eaton, Cherry, Cain, & Pope, 2011). Population health nurses can encourage serosorting among MSM without steady partners. Another approach to STI prevention involves focusing on the ABCs of abstinence, being faithful, and condom use promulgated by the United States President's Emergency Plan for AIDS Relief (PEPFAR, n.d.), although such strategies may be difficult for women in unequal power relationships.

WHO has identified several additional strategies to prevent STIs in sex workers, thereby preventing the spread of disease in the general public. Recommendations include decriminalizing sex work, providing health service access for sex workers, preventing violence against sex workers, empowering this segment of the population to advocate for themselves, and providing periodic screening for STIs and HIV infection. Additional prevention strategies include providing presumptive STI treatment for asymptomatic sex workers in high prevalence settings, providing ART for HIV-infected sex workers, engaging in harm-reduction strategies for sex workers who inject drugs, and providing HBV vaccinations (HIV/AIDS Programme, 2012).

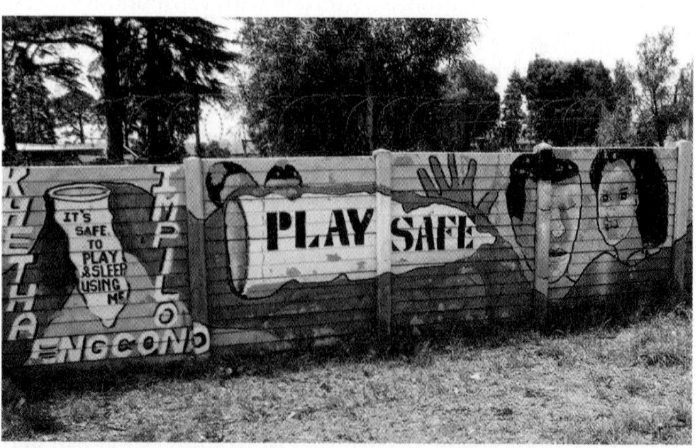

Sexually transmitted infections, as well as unwanted pregnancies, can be prevented with condom use. *(Urbanhearts/Fotolia)*

Preventing bloodborne diseases such as HIV/AIDS and hepatitis B, C, and D involves prevention of drug use or promotion of harm-reduction strategies such as needle exchanges and education on safer drug use procedures. Because these strategies are often not acceptable to the general public or to health policy makers, population health nurses may be involved in advocacy to establish needle exchange programs and other harm-reduction strategies. Infection through occupational exposure to bloodborne diseases can be prevented by means of universal precautions for the handling of blood and other bodily secretions and excretions. Unfortunately, many persons in these occupations fail to use universal precautions, increasing their risk of disease. Screening of blood and tissue donors for HIV and for hepatitis B, C, and D has virtually eliminated transmission of these diseases by means of transfusion.

For foodborne and waterborne diseases, control measures are aimed at improving sanitation, protecting food and water from contamination, and promoting adequate hand washing. Washing fruits and vegetables before eating, boiling contaminated water, and discouraging use of human waste as fertilizer may also serve to prevent diseases in developing countries. Population health nurses can educate people regarding adequate hygiene and the need to wash fruits and vegetables before eating them, particularly those imported from other countries. They can also discourage consumption of shellfish retrieved from contaminated waters and promote environmental policies that prevent contamination of shellfish beds. In addition, nurses can advocate for safe water supplies, effective sanitation and enforcement of food processing techniques that minimize the potential for bacterial contamination (Honish et al., 2013). Promotion of good hygiene and sanitation in areas where animals are kept can also help to prevent the spread of zoonoses (Collier et al., 2011).

Population health nurses may also collaborate with environmental specialists to address issues of food or water contamination with pathogens. For example, the nurse might alert water authorities regarding a sudden increase in diarrheal diseases in a particular neighborhood, suggesting that water sources may be contaminated. Or the nurse might identify unsanitary conditions in a restaurant and notify the appropriate inspectors.

Prevention of crowding is a control measure for conditions such as TB and influenza. Other primary prevention measures include the use of adequate ventilation and ultraviolet light in areas that increase the risk of TB transmission. For example, areas in which aerosol sputum specimens are collected provide an environment conducive to the spread of disease that can be modified using these measures. Providing appropriate facilities for isolating infectious clients in hospitals and other institutions also minimizes the risk of transmission to health care personnel. Population health nurses can work with environmental engineers to address such problems or collaborate with housing authority personnel to address housing conditions conducive to diseases. Grouping patients with drug-resistant strains of microorganisms and personnel caring for them can also help prevent the spread of drug-resistant infections (Jacob et al., 2013).

Prevention of tickborne diseases involves use of tick repellents, avoidance of tall grass and other vegetation, and use of protective clothing. Daily inspection of people and pets for ticks is also recommended. Wearing light-colored clothing may make ticks more visible. Environmental measures for preventing exposure to tickborne diseases include use of pesticides on lawns, removal of brush and leaf litter from around homes, and creating buffer zones of wood chips or gravel between wooded or brushy areas and human habitations. Similarly, removal of standing water and other breeding grounds for mosquitoes can help prevent mosquitoborne diseases such as WNV infection. Pregnant women, in particular, should avoid mosquito exposure, use insect repellent, wear long sleeves and long pants, and avoid being outdoors at dawn and dusk to minimize the risk of WNV infection for themselves and their infants. Use of long-lasting insecticide treated bed nets and indoor spraying can minimize the spread of malaria (Cullen & Arguin, 2013; Mace et al., 2011). Population health nurses often work with environmental specialists and veterinarians to address diseases transmitted from animals to humans.

Other measures that aid in the control of communicable diseases include legislation requiring screening for specific diseases in high-risk groups, mandatory reporting of cases of communicable disease with contact notification and follow-up, and regulation of potential vehicles of transmission such as insects. Population health nursing involvement in other control measures for communicable diseases generally lies in educating the public and individual clients regarding prevention and in identifying and helping to eliminate risk factors for exposure and disease.

Pandemic and bioterrorism preparedness. One further aspect of prevention related to communicable disease addresses preparation for a possible pandemic or bioterrorist event. As we saw in Chapter 25∞, population health nurses are actively involved in identifying the potential for and probable community effects of such disasters. For example, they would identify risk factors for infection in the population in the event of a pandemic (e.g., segments of the population with poor nutritional status that puts them at particular risk for serious disease). They would also be involved in planning for community response to a pandemic or bioterrorist attack. In addition, population health nurses would be actively involved in informing the public regarding preventive measures or other appropriate responses to the threat of a pandemic or bioterrorist event.

Bioterrorism and pandemic preparedness are important not only because of the potential for significant morbidity and mortality resulting from either event, but also because of other population effects that might occur. For example, either a pandemic or a bioterrorist-caused epidemic might cause severe economic effects as a result of business closures to prevent spread of the disease. Availability of food and other essential goods might also be impaired if production and transportation systems are severely affected. Short-term educational effects might also be noted if schools are closed for extended periods of time. One of the most serious effects might be the burden placed on an already overburdened health care system if significant numbers of health care personnel become ill. There is also the problem of inadequate facilities and supplies (including drugs and vaccines) needed to address widespread communicable disease incidence. Preparedness will help to mitigate these potential effects, although it is unlikely that they can be prevented altogether. Health promotion and disease prevention strategies for communicable diseases, including pandemic and bioterrorism preparedness, are summarized in Table 26-3●.

RESOLVING EXISTING PROBLEMS OF COMMUNICABLE DISEASE. Resolution activities in relation to communicable diseases include case finding and surveillance, screening, diagnosis and reporting, and treatment.

Case finding and surveillance. Because they serve large segments of the population who may not receive care from other health care providers, population health nurses are in a unique position to identify possible cases of communicable diseases. Once a person with a potential communicable disease has been identified, the population health nurse may make a referral for further diagnosis and treatment. In some cases, the nurse may be involved in diagnosing and treating communicable diseases on the basis of medically approved protocols. The case finding function of the population health nurse was discussed in general in Chapter 1∞.

To identify a possible case of a communicable disease, population health nurses need to be familiar with the signs and symptoms of communicable diseases commonly seen in their area. They should also be familiar with the signs and symptoms of diseases that may result from bioterrorist activities.

Case finding related to outbreaks of communicable diseases within populations may require some creative strategies. For example, electronic messaging and other media were used to find cases of *Cyclospora* during an outbreak in Iowa. Alerts were also sent to all hospitals, emergency departments, public health agencies, and providers to alert them to the possibility of a *Cyclospora* diagnosis in patients with symptoms of watery diarrhea, nausea, anorexia, abdominal cramping, fatigue, and weight loss. Similarly, e-mail press releases were sent to news media to alert the public (Kalas & Quinlisk, 2013). Contact tracing may also be used to find cases of disease.

Case finding at the population level contributes to surveillance. As we saw in Chapter 1∞, surveillance involves the gathering and analysis of data that reflect trends in disease incidence and prevalence as well as information on the effects of disease within the population. Population health nurses may collect surveillance data or identify cases of disease that are reported to local epidemiologists for inclusion in surveillance

TABLE 26-3 Health Promotion and Prevention in Communicable Disease Control

Health Promotion Foci	Population Health Nursing Interventions
Nutrition	• Educate clients and the public on good nutrition • Advocate for access to adequate nutrition sources
Rest and physical activity	• Promote adequate rest and physical activity to maintain health
Coping	• Model and teach effective coping strategies to minimize stress • Advocate for living conditions than minimize stress
Disease Prevention Foci	**Population Health Nursing Interventions**
Immunization	• Educate clients and the public regarding the need for immunizations • Refer clients for immunization services • Provide immunization services • Advocate for access to immunization services for all segments of the population • Ascertain the potential effects of introducing new vaccines in constrained environments and collaborate to address infrastructure issues
Contact investigation and notification	• Educate providers regarding the legal requirements for reporting communicable diseases • Interview clients with communicable diseases for names and locating information for close contacts • Inform contacts of their exposure to a communicable disease • Refer contacts for testing and PrEP or PEP as needed • Educate clients regarding preventive measures and the need to prevent the spread of disease to others • Advocate for and plan effective contact notification services • Promote contact notification by other health care providers and educate them regarding contact notification • Advocate for/provide field screening services for contacts
Pre- and postexposure prophylaxis	• Refer clients for services as needed • Provide PrEP/PEP under established protocols • Monitor and promote compliance with PEP among contacts • Monitor for adverse effects and side effects of PEP and refer for medical evaluation if needed • Advocate for the availability of PEP for clients in need • Provide expedited partner therapy (EPT) • Advocate changes in prescribing laws and for insurance coverage of EPT
Other primary prevention measures	• Educate clients and the public regarding effective wound care • Educate clients and the public on safe sexual practices, use of condoms, etc. • Prevent drug abuse or refer clients for drug abuse treatment • Promote harm-reduction strategies to prevent infection among IDUs • Promote use of universal precautions for bloodborne diseases • Promote adequate hand washing, washing of produce, etc. • Advocate for adequate sanitation and safe water supplies • Advocate for policies and processes that prevent contamination of food and water supplies • Promote adequate housing to prevent crowding and allow for adequate ventilation • Promote use of ultraviolet light in settings where exposure to pathogens is common • Advocate for preventive education and services • Advocate for STI prevention strategies among commercial sex workers and for decriminalization of sex work
Pandemic and bioterrorism preparedness	• Assist in identifying the potential for a pandemic or bioterrorist event • Assist in identifying particularly vulnerable populations and factors influencing their vulnerability • Participate in planning community response to a pandemic or bioterrorist event • Educate the public and other health care providers regarding prevention of illness or self-care during a pandemic or bioterrorist event • Educate the public regarding the signs and symptoms of disease resulting from a pandemic or bioterrorist event and sources of treatment

systems. Analysis of surveillance data is usually undertaken by epidemiologists or health information system specialists and the results of the analysis conveyed to public health officials and other health policy makers.

Screening. Screening is presumptive identification of asymptomatic persons with disease. Screening may involve either selective or mass screening. **Selective screening** is screening directed toward persons exhibiting risk factors for a particular disease. **Mass**

screening involves screening an entire population regardless of the level of risk among individuals. For example, prior screening recommendations for HCV infection were risk-based, focusing screening activities on persons at risk for HCV (e.g., IDUs; hemodialysis, transfusion, and transplant recipients; exposed health care workers, and children born to HCV-positive mothers). More recent recommendations have added a one time mass screening of persons born between 1945 and 1965 (Mahajan et al., 2013; U.S. Preventive Services Task Force [USPSTF], 2013a).

Screening is not generally done for communicable diseases that have a short incubation period such as measles, rubella, influenza, and so on. Screening tests are available, however, for diseases such as HIV/AIDS, hepatitis A, B, and C, TB, and STIs such as gonorrhea, syphilis, *Chlamydia*, and HSV infection.

Screening for HIV infection is recommended for all pregnant women at entry into prenatal care or during labor if HIV status is unknown. In addition, screening is routinely recommended for all people aged 15 to 65 years in the United States and persons over age 65 if at risk (e.g., sexually active or IDUs) (USPSTF, 2013b). Overall, in 2010, 9% of U.S. adults had been screened for HIV in the prior year (Cohen et al., 2011). Based on National HIV Behavioral Surveillance (NHBS) system data, 25% of heterosexual participants in high HIV prevalence areas had never been tested for HIV until they participated in the survey. Slightly over 2% of participants were found to be HIV-positive, and increased screening outreach was particularly recommended for low-income, low-education groups in high prevalence areas (Miles et al., 2013).

HIV screening is least effective during the period between the appearance of HIV RNA and detection of HIV-specific antibodies in the blood. For this reason, a new diagnostic algorithm has been suggested, in which those with negative immunoassay screening results receive RNA testing. The availability of rapid screening tests makes provision of same-day screening results possible, increasing the number of HIV-positive individuals who are referred for treatment services (Geren et al., 2013).

One strategy that has been suggested to improve identification of those with undiagnosed HIV infection is social networking. A social network strategy involves using HIV-infected clients and those at high risk for infection to recruit people from their social, sexual, and drug-use networks for HIV screening, counseling, and referral for treatment, if needed. This strategy has been particularly effective in promoting HIV screening among MSM, but because of its resource-intensive nature, research is needed to determine its cost-effectiveness in this and other populations (McCree et al., 2013).

Opt-out testing is another strategy that is recommended for certain populations (e.g., correctional inmates). In opt-out testing, screening for HIV is performed at entry unless the inmate specifically refuses testing as opposed to opt-in testing in which inmates are offered the test and must choose to receive it, or testing on request initiated by the inmate. CDC recommends opt-out testing in correctional settings (Strick, McGowan, & Belcher, 2011).

Screening of all sexually active women 24 years of age and under and pregnant women of all ages for *Chlamydia trachomatis* infection is also recommended (Singh et al, 2011). In fact, *Chlamydia* screening has been identified by the USPSTF as "one of the 10 most beneficial and cost-effective preventive services" (Satterwhite et al., 2011, p. 370), but is greatly underutilized. In 2009 for example, less than 60% of women under 25 years of age were screened. The Los Angeles County Health Department initiated the use of free home screening kits for *Chlamydia* and gonorrhea as a means of fostering screening for these STIs among sexually active women. In the first year of the program, nearly 3,000 kits were dispensed and more than half were returned with testable specimens. Among those with positive screening results, 88% retrieved their results and confirmed treatment (Rotblatt et al., 2013). Population health nurses can advocate for screening of sexually active women for a variety of STIs during routine health promotion visits. They may also be involved in educating other health care providers regarding the need for screening or in promoting self-screening programs like that initiated in Los Angeles.

There are two approaches to identification of tuberculosis—a tuberculin skin test (TST) or use of interferon γ release assay (IGRA). A positive or significant reaction to TST is based on the degree of induration that results. **Induration** is a palpable, hard, raised area around the injection site with clearly defined margins. *Induration* does not refer to redness around the injection site. In a person without known risk factors, an area of induration of 15 mm or greater is considered a significant reaction. For recent immigrants, IDUs, residents or employees of

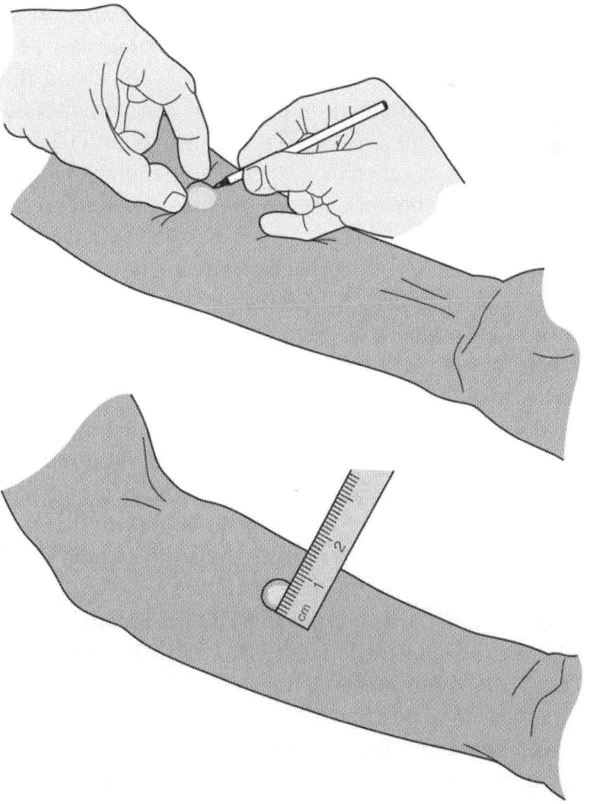

A positive TB skin test showing induration (National Medical Slide).

congregate settings, mycobacteriology lab personnel, those at high risk for disease, children under 4 years of age, and children and adolescents exposed to adults at high risk, 10 mm or more induration is considered positive, and 5 mm is considered a positive reaction for persons with HIV infection or other cause of immunosuppression, transplant recipients, close contacts to an infectious case of TB, or persons with chest X-ray results consistent with prior untreated TB (Division of Tuberculosis Elimination, 2011). A positive tuberculin skin test is shown in the picture on the previous page. The area of induration in the picture is demarcated with ink on all four sides.

There is a shortage of TST antigens in some areas, so IGRA, a more expensive test, can be used instead if available. IGRA has the advantage of being of use with people who have received BCG vaccine as BCG invalidates TST results. In areas with limited supplies of TST antigens or IGRA capacity, screening should be prioritized to those at greatest risk for developing TB (Jereb, Mase, Chorba, & Castro, 2013).

Reaching people at greatest need for TB screening can sometimes be difficult. One suggestion to reach immigrant populations is to offer screening in adult education centers that provide services to immigrants. One such project, for example, found 18.5% of program participants to have positive TSTs (Wieland et al., 2011). Another approach was used by a Texas county health department. Incidence data were used to identify the two neighborhoods with the highest incidence and density of TB cases and persons with LTBI. Outreach workers then went door to door offering TSTs. Results were read in the homes in the appropriate timeframe, and positive reactors were escorted by outreach workers to a mobile clinic for X-ray, clinical evaluation, and treatment services. Using this approach 57% of the population of the two areas was tested, with nearly 18% testing positive. Treatment was initiated for 147 people who might otherwise not have been found. Over the subsequent 10 years, no new cases of TB disease were reported from either neighborhood (Cegielski et al., 2013). Congregate living settings, such as correctional facilities and homeless shelters, are other places in which TB screening is warranted.

Because of the complex interaction between TB and HIV infection, persons with HIV infection should be screened for TB. Conversely, people with TB disease or latent TB infection at risk for HIV infection, should be screened. Population health nurses should keep in mind, however, that people with HIV infection or AIDS may have negative sputum smears for TB and up to a third of them may have normal chest X-rays. In addition, persons with HIV infection are more likely to develop extrapulmonary TB (Getahun et al., 2012).

In resource-constrained settings, WHO has recommended screening all individuals with HIV/AIDS for three symptoms: cough, fever, and night sweats. If none of the three are present, the individual should be offered a 6-month course of isoniazid prophylactic treatment (IPT) for TB. If a tuberculin skin test is positive, but none of the three symptoms is present, IPT should also be considered for 6 months. IPT may be continued for life if feasible. Finally, if any of the three symptoms is present, a TB diagnostic workup should be conducted (Getahun et al., 2012).

HBV screening is recommended for all pregnant women at the first prenatal visit (USPSTF, 2009) and for those at risk of disease (e.g., exposed health care workers, IDUs, sexual or drug contacts to infected persons). As noted earlier, HCV screening is recommended for persons at high risk of exposure as well as those born between 1945 and 1965. This age cohort accounts for approximately 75% of HCV infections in the United States and 73% of HCV-related mortality. One time screening is recommended for this group followed by a brief screening for alcohol abuse and referral for care if needed (Smith et al., 2013). It is anticipated that cohort-based screening of this age group could prevent 120,000 deaths with subsequent treatment with antiviral therapy (Mahajan et al., 2013).

Because of the link between HCV and injecting drug use, drug treatment programs have been suggested as an ideal setting in which to conduct HCV screening. Unfortunately, only 34% of drug treatment programs responding to a national survey offered HCV screening (Frimpong, 2013).

Population health nurses may need to actively advocate for screening as a regular practice in correctional and drug treatment settings. They may refer individuals at risk for disease to appropriate screening resources. Many population health nurses may also be involved in conducting screening examinations and tests and in counseling clients regarding test results and their implications. Population health nurses may also need to advocate for the availability of screening services and for follow-up and treatment (therapeutic or prophylactic) of persons with positive screening tests.

Diagnosis and reporting. Diagnosis of many communicable diseases relies on serologic evidence of disease markers or the actual presence of causative organisms. For example, diagnostic tests for syphilis and hepatitis A, B, C, and D rely on the presence of specific antibodies in the blood of infected persons. More sophisticated tests for syphilis, on the other hand, are based on demonstration of the presence of the actual causative organism in the bloodstream and are used when antibody-based tests are inconclusive. Similarly, tests for gonorrhea involve cultures of urine or urethral, vaginal, anal, or pharyngeal specimens for growth of *Neisseria gonorrhoeae*, and diagnostic tests for *Chlamydia* infection include culture of specimens for *Chlamydia trachomatis*. Diagnosis of many childhood diseases is based on physical signs and symptoms, with laboratory confirmation for some diseases (e.g., measles, pertussis, diphtheria, tetanus, etc.).

Population health nurses may refer suspected cases of communicable diseases for diagnostic confirmation. In addition, nurses may educate clients regarding the types of diagnostic procedures likely to be used. Population health nurses may also be involved in conducting some diagnostic tests for communicable diseases. For example, population health nurses in some agencies routinely draw blood for diagnostic tests for syphilis and collect urine samples for gonorrhea testing.

Diagnosis of TB is of particular concern worldwide, and the Tuberculosis Coalition for Technical Assistance (2014), a group composed of several national and international agencies, has developed *International Standards for Tuberculosis Care*, which address diagnostic and treatment standards, standards for addressing comorbid conditions, and standards for public health and prevention. Elements of the standards are summarized in Table 26-4●.

In the United States, diagnosis of TB is most often based on X-ray findings. However, given the lack of reliability of X-rays in diagnosing TB in persons with HIV infection, newer diagnostic tests have been developed. For example, the Xpert MTB/RIF assay of unprocessed sputum or concentrated sediments can provide a diagnosis of TB within 2 hours. The assay can also detect rifampin-resistant strains of *Mycobacterium tuberculosis*. Because of its relatively high cost, it is not used routinely for people for whom X-rays provide definitive results (Division of Tuberculosis Elimination, 2013; Getahun et al., 2012).

Diagnosis of viral hepatitis is frequently based on the presence of viral antibodies and rapid testing is available for HCV using the OraQuick® HCV Rapid Antibody Test (Getchell et al., 2013). In order to determine if positive results are due to past or current HCV infection, HCV RNA testing is required. In one large study of newly reported cases, just over half of them were current infections (Bornschlegel et al., 2013).

Effective control of communicable diseases requires that diagnoses of many communicable diseases, including TB, be reported to local public health authorities. These reports are then forwarded to state and federal agencies. In the case of some

TABLE 26-4 Summary of International Standards for Tuberculosis Care

Focus	Related Standards
Diagnosis	• Clinician awareness of risk factors and prompt testing of persons with symptoms • TB evaluation for all persons with unexplained cough two weeks or longer or radiographic findings suggestive of TB • Submission of two sputum specimens for smear microscopy by all patients capable of producing sputum, including children. Performance of Xpert MTB/RIF tests performed as the initial diagnostic test for those with HIV risk, risk of resistance, or who are seriously ill • Diagnostic specimens collected from relevant sites for persons suspected of extrapulmonary TB, including children. Use of Xpert MTB/RIF testing for suspected tuberculous meningitis • Use of sputum culture for all those suspected of TB who have negative sputum smears. Initiation of antituberculin treatment in persons with negative smears with strong clinical evidence for TB disease after cultures are collected • Use of smear microscopy and/or culture of respiratory secretions (via expectorated or induced sputum or gastric lavage) for all children with suspected intrathoracic TB
Treatment	• Prescription and monitoring of appropriate treatment for all diagnosed cases of TB • Use of first-line WHO-approved quality assured drugs for all patients who have not been previously treated and do not have risk factors for drug resistance • Use of a patient-centered approach to promote treatment adherence, improve quality of life, and relieve suffering • Monitoring of treatment effects with follow-up sputum smears after 2–3 months with sensivity testing for continued positive smears • Assessment of the likelihood of drug resistance with sensitivity testing and changes in therapeutic regimens as indicated • Use of specialized treatment regimens with quality drugs for persons likely to have drug-resistant TB • Maintenance of systematic records of treatment, incuding medications given, response, and adverse reactions for all clients
Addressing comorbidities	• HIV testing and counseling for all clients with suspected TB in the absence of HIV testing in the last 2 months. Use of integrated TB and HIV treatment approaches in high HIV prevalence areas • Initiation of ART within 2 weeks of TB treatment initiation in those with HIV and TB with profound immunosuppression, unless TB meningitis is present and within 8 weeks for all others with HIV and TB infection • Treatment of persons with HIV infection for presumed latent TB for at least 6 months • Thorough assessment for other comorbid conditions that could affect TB treatment response or outcomes and provision of additional services as needed
Public health and prevention	• Evaluation and appropriate management of all persons in close contact with persons with infectious TB, with special emphasis on children, immunocompromised persons, persons with symptoms suggestive of TB, and contacts to patients with MDR/XDR TB • Treatment for latent TB for all children and persons with HIV infection who do not currently have active TB • Development of infection control plans to prevent the spread of disease to others, including health care workers • Reporting of new and re-treatment of cases of TB and treatment to local health authorities

Data from: Tuberculosis Coalition for Technical Assistance. (2014). *International standards for tuberculosis care: Diagnosis, treatment, public health* (3rd ed.). Retrieved from http://www.thoracic.org/assemblies/mtpi/resources/istc-report.pdf

diseases, national agencies report diagnosed cases to WHO. The list of reportable diseases varies somewhat from one jurisdiction to another (usually at the state level), and population health nurses should inform themselves regarding the reportable diseases in their own locale. Laboratories are required to report positive test results for reportable diseases to official public health agencies, and health care providers who make the actual diagnosis are also required to submit a disease notification report. Reports are usually completed by the physician, nurse practitioner, or other health care provider who makes the diagnosis, but in some settings, reports may be made by population health nurses or other nurses.

In the United States, three categories of diseases are reportable at the national level. The first category includes diseases that are extremely urgent and should be reported to CDC within 4 hours by telephone, followed by electronic submission of a report the next business day. Extremely urgent diseases include anthrax, botulism, plague, paralytic polio, SARS-associated coronavirus, smallpox, tularemia, and viral hemorrhagic fevers. Urgent diseases are to be reported by telephone within 24 hours, with an electronic report with the next regularly scheduled electronic data submission. The final category encompasses diseases to be reported in the next regular reporting cycle. An information resource for diseases in each category from the Council of State and Territorial Epidemiologists (2012) is provided on the student resources site.

There are also two categories of communicable disease reports: case reports and outbreak reports. Case reports are those related to the diagnosis of individual cases of a particular disease (e.g., measles or HIV infection). Outbreak reports address an increased incidence in the number of cases of a particular disease above that normally expected in the population. Outbreak reports may include diseases that are not normally officially reportable in a given jurisdiction or diseases of unknown etiology in the case of emerging infectious diseases. For example, outbreak reports of an unusual respiratory disease among people attending a Legionnaires' convention in Philadelphia led to the identification of Legionnaires' disease.

Some diseases are also reportable to WHO under the *International Health Regulations* (IHR). Mandatory reporting under IHR includes any single case of smallpox, poliomyelitis due to wild poliovirus, a new subtype of influenza, and severe acute respiratory syndrome (SARS). In 2005, however, the IHR were revised to include mandatory investigation of "events involving epidemic-prone diseases of special national or regional concern which 'have demonstrated the ability to cause serious public health impact and to spread rapidly internationally.'" Notification occurs based on a decision algorithm contained in the IHR document (WHO, n.d., p. 2). The revised IHR also require nations to respond to requests for information regarding such events and to designate an IHR focal point and contact person to interface with WHO. Additional requirements include development of basic public health capacities to detect, report, and respond to potential public health emergencies and to implement control measures at airports and other international border points (WHO, 2008). Unfortunately, several WHO member states have not yet fully developed their surveillance, reporting, and control capacities and have requested an extension of capacity development deadlines until 2014 or beyond (WHO, 2013a).

Treatment. Many communicable diseases are treated with antibiotics or antiviral medications, but some diseases such as varicella and uncomplicated measles are treated symptomatically. Antimicrobial treatment is recommended for tickborne diseases as well as for TB, HIV, hepatitis, sexually transmitted diseases, and influenza. Pertussis is another disease for which treatment is available. Treatment guidelines for selected communicable diseases commonly encountered by population health nurses are available from CDC.

In many instances, treatment for communicable diseases is highly effective, both for the infected individual and in terms of preventing the spread of the disease to others. For example, treatment of all HIV-infected pregnant women can reduce transmission of HIV infection to their infants to less than 5%. Unfortunately, in 2011, only 57% of HIV-infected pregnant women received treatment in low- and middle-income countries (Chimbwandira et al., 2013). HIV treatment is often dependent on CD4 cell counts, but many developing countries do not have the laboratory capacity to monitor eligibility for treatment. To address this issue, the recommendation is to provide all pregnant and breast-feeding women in these countries with lifelong ART. This new approach, which is supported by PEPFAR, has increased the number of pregnant and breastfeeding women on treatment by nearly 75%, with 77% of those continuing treatment beyond 1 year.

In the United States, approximately 77% of HIV-infected persons who were aware of their status were linked to care and just over half of them remained in care. In addition, 45% of those in care received counseling on transmission prevention, 89% received ART, and 77% achieved viral suppression (Cohen et al., 2011). ART reduces infectiousness and improves health for those with HIV infection; however, these outcomes require at least 85% adherence to suppress viral replication and avoid drug resistance (Kalichman et al., 2011). Because drug abuse is associated with ART adherence, concurrent drug abuse treatment services are particularly important for those IDUs with HIV infection (Mimiaga et al., 2013). Integrated behavioral interventions focusing on adherence support, sexual risk reduction, and amelioration of risk compensation resulted in increased ART adherence, less unprotected sexual activity, and fewer new STIs in one study (Kalichman et al., 2011).

Treatment for tuberculosis disease and LTBI relies primarily on the strategy of directly observed therapy. **Directly observed therapy (DOT)** is a medication administration strategy in which a client takes his or her medication in the presence of a nurse or other health care provider. Recommended treatment for LTBI consists of weekly DOT with isoniazid (INH) and rifapentine for 12 weeks. This is a considerably shortened time frame and is more likely to promote compliance than the prior recommended 9 months of therapy (Jereb et al., 2011). Standard treatment for active infection incorporates a combination of four first-line drugs: INH, rifampin, pyrazinamide, and ethambutol for 6 months (Burzynski et al., 2013). Treatment of multi-drug-resistant TB requires an 18- to 24-month course of five to six drugs that are less effective, more toxic, and more expensive, with less effective outcomes (Seaworth et al., 2013). DOT is credited with saving 7 million lives globally since 1990 (Getahun et al., 2012).

Population health nurses are often involved in providing DOT as well as monitoring clients for adherence and for adverse drug effects. Population health nurses are actively involved in supervising DOT and in motivating clients to continue compliance with therapy. In addition, population health nurses are often involved in locating clients who are noncompliant and encouraging them to continue therapy. Promoting continued compliance often requires that population health nurses assist clients to deal with factors that interfere with compliance. For example, they may assist a homeless client in his or her search for shelter or employment to eliminate life circumstances that impede DOT compliance. They may also need to be actively involved in promoting access to DOT or to other needed services that support DOT compliance.

Antiviral agents are recommended for treatment of persons with severe influenza, those at high risk for complications, and children under 1 year of age. Antivirals may also be provided to those without risk factors if available and provided within 48 hours of symptom onset (Fiori et al., 2011). Treatment of HCV with antiviral medications can also achieve a sustained response in 40% to 70% of cases (Drobnik et al., 2011). Unfortunately, there has been little use of HCV treatment among IDUs who are at greatest risk for long-term consequences of the disease (Iverson et al., 2013).

Other approaches have been taken in treating other communicable diseases. For example, treatment of malaria with artemisinin-based combination therapy has been shown to cure the disease as well as limit transmission to others (Mace et al., 2011). In addition, WHO has developed a strategy to address all of the major causes of child mortality that integrates services for malaria, pneumonia, and diarrheal disease through case management, strengthened health care systems, and promoting family and community health practices. In combination with insecticide-treated nets, this integrated approach has decreased malaria mortality in intervention areas where it has been implemented (Rowe, Onikpo, Lama, Osterholt, & Deming, 2012). Annual mass medication administration to entire populations has been recommended by WHO for treatment of lymphatic filariasis in endemic areas. This strategy has been implemented in Port-au-Prince in Haiti, one of only four countries in the Americas with endemic filariasis. It is estimated that annual coverage of 65% of the population for 5 years will interrupt disease transmission (Streit et al., 2013). Finally, voluntary isolation of infected persons, first aid for lesions, manual extraction of worms, and use of occlusive bandages have been used to treat dracunculiasis (Hopkins et al., 2013).

Some disease-causing agents are becoming resistant to some of the antimicrobials used in treatment. CDC and WHO recommend that a specific drug no longer be used to treat communicable diseases when 5% of cases in a given population are drug resistant. For example, fluoroquinolone was no longer recommended for treatment of gonorrhea in Hawaii as of 2000. By 2002, the recommendation of nonuse of the drug had extended to California and to MSM by 2004. As of 2007, fluoroquinolone is no longer recommended for treatment of gonorrhea at all (Dowell et al., 2012). Gonorrhea has a long history of developing resistance to successive antimicrobials beginning with sulfonamides, and progressing to penicillin, tetracycline, and fluoroquinolone. Current treatment recommendations are for the use of increased doses and combination therapy with ceftriaxone and either azithromycin or doxycycline (Adams et al., 2013). There is some suggestion, however, that resistance to this regimen has surfaced in Asia and may be occurring in the United States as well (Hook et al., 2013).

Similarly, a growing proportion of TB is caused by multi-drug-resistant (MDR) strains. MDR TB is resistant to at least INH and rifampin. Extensively drug-resistant TB (XDR TB) is also resistant to fluoroquinolone and at least one of three injectable antituberculin drugs. In 2011, there were an estimated 630,000 cases of MDR TB worldwide, with nearly 4% of those occurring as new cases and 20% in persons previously treated for TB. XDR TB has been found in 84 countries and affects an estimated 9% of persons with TB. The mortality rate for drug-resistant TB is about 15% (Mase, Chorba, Lobue, & Castro, 2013).

Antibiotic resistance is fostered by inappropriate use of antibiotics, and population health nurses can be actively involved in educating the general public and health care providers to minimize inappropriate use. They can also advocate for completion of recommended antibiotic therapies (e.g., for TB) to prevent development of resistant microorganisms.

Population health nurses can be active in advocating national policies that support international treatment initiatives for a variety of diseases. For example, U.S. nurses can advocate for federal assistance to international AIDS endeavors. In addition, nurses may be involved in the efforts of non-governmental organizations to support HIV, malaria, or other therapies through their churches or other social organizations. Nurses involved at the international level can assist in the development of policies and procedures that address concerns related to access to care. In the United States, population health nurses can be involved in research that tests various approaches to treatment for communicable diseases that may have implications for international implementation.

In addition to referring clients and assisting with treatment of communicable diseases with antimicrobial agents, population health nurses may provide supportive care for clients with self-limiting diseases that have no specific treatment. Supportive care may include educating clients and families about measures to reduce fever or enhance comfort until the disease has run its course. For example, parents should be informed of the dangers in giving aspirin for fever in children. Other supportive measures may include encouraging a low-fat diet for clients with hepatitis A to deal with nausea.

Population health nurses may provide treatment for some communicable diseases under medical protocols, but are more likely to be involved in educating clients about treatment and promoting compliance. The role of population health nurses in treating communicable diseases may also involve political activity and advocacy. For example, the nurse might be actively engaged in efforts to assure access to health care for persons with AIDS or to change policies for providing treatment to drug users with chronic HCV infection. Strategies for resolving problems of communicable disease are summarized in Table 26-5•.

HEALTH RESTORATION. Health restoration with respect to communicable diseases may occur with individual clients or with population groups. At the individual level, emphasis is on preventing complications and long-term sequelae, monitoring treatment compliance and effects, monitoring treatment side effects and assisting clients to deal with them, and providing assistance in dealing with long-term consequences of some communicable diseases.

Population health nurses can educate clients to prevent complications of communicable diseases with their attendant long-term sequelae. For example, clients with influenza can be encouraged to rest and to refrain from resuming normal activities until they are recovered. Similarly, parents can discourage scratching in children with varicella to prevent secondary infection in lesions and encourage clients with hepatitis to refrain from alcohol use to prevent further liver damage.

Population health nurses also monitor clients with HIV infection for signs and symptoms of opportunistic infections and refer them for treatment when OIs are suspected. Nurses may also be involved in assisting clients with prophylactic regimens to prevent opportunistic infections. The Panel on Opportunistic Infections in HIV-exposed and HIV-infected Children (2014) has developed guidelines for the prevention and treatment of opportunistic infections in HIV-exposed and infected children. Similar guidelines for adults and adolescents have been developed by the Panel on Opportunistic Infections in HIV-infected Adults and Adolescents (2014). For further information about the guidelines, see the *External Resources* section of the student resources site.

Clients with HIV infection may also experience a number of nutritional difficulties that may require nursing intervention. For example, weight loss and wasting may occur as a result of reduced food or calorie intake due to anorexia, nausea and vomiting, changes in taste or smell, fatigue, or painful oral or esophageal lesions. Weight loss, loss of muscle mass, and vitamin deficiencies may also result from malabsorption due to lactose or fat intolerance, gastrointestinal infection, malignancies,

TABLE 26-5 Strategies for Resolving Problems of Communicable Disease

Focus	Population Health Nursing Strategies
Case finding and surveillance	• Recognize symptoms of communicable diseases in clients and refer them for diagnostic and treatment services as needed • Educate the public regarding signs and symptoms of specific communicable diseases • Recognize signs of disease outbreaks in the population • Collect surveillance data regarding communicable disease incidence, prevalence, contributing factors, and effects
Screening	• Recognize and refer possible cases of communicable diseases • Educate clients and the public regarding the need for screening for communicable diseases • Provide selective screening services • Plan and implement mass screening programs • Advocate for screening availability for populations at risk for communicable diseases
Diagnosis and reporting	• Refer clients for diagnostic procedures as needed • Educate clients regarding diagnostic procedures • Provide diagnostic services • Interpret diagnostic test results and counsel clients accordingly • Advocate for the availability of needed diagnostic services • Report cases of communicable diseases in accord with local, state, or national regulations • Educate other health care providers regarding reporting requirements • Follow up on reports of communicable diseases to obtain relevant epidemiologic information
Treatment	• Provide antimicrobial therapies • Educate clients regarding antimicrobial therapy • Supervise DOT • Educate clients and their families for supportive care • Educate health care providers, clients, and the public to prevent inappropriate use of antimicrobials and development of drug-resistant organisms • Advocate for the availability of needed treatment services for all segments of the population

and so on. Finally, HIV-infected clients may experience metabolic alterations due to HIV, medications, and other circumstances. Population health nurses engaged in health restoration activities would assist clients to overcome these nutritional deficiencies through nutritional counseling, promoting food and water safety, dealing with medication side effects, and suggesting complementary and alternative nutritional therapies such as the use of nutritional supplements. Population health nurses may also work closely with public health social workers and mental health counselors to address the health restoration needs of clients with HIV/AIDS and other conditions (e.g., hepatitis C). Although ART has increased health and quality of life and workforce participation among people with HIV/AIDS tremendously, unemployment continues to be a significant problem in this group. Population health nurses may need to engage in political advocacy to assure the availability of health restoration services for clients with these diseases. This may include services needed to address psychosocial as well as physical consequences of disease (e.g., unemployment, housing, discrimination).

Another issue related to HIV infection that requires intervention involves resumption of high-risk sexual or drug use behaviors. Because many people perceive ART to be a "cure" for HIV infection, treatment may lead to continuation or reinitiation of behaviors that may transmit the disease to others. Resumption of unsafe sexual practices may be the result of several factors. Treatment may lead to improved health and functional status, increasing sexual activity as well. In addition, treatment may give rise to unrealistic expectations regarding the potential for disease transmission, leading those with HIV infection to be less cautious in their sexual practices. Prevention case management, however, has led to a decrease in transmission risk behaviors. Prevention case management involves providing follow-up counseling and educational services to clients as well as assistance in dealing with other psychosocial effects of HIV infection.

Population health nurses also monitor communicable disease treatment compliance and treatment effects, particularly in diseases such as tuberculosis and HIV infection that require long-term therapy. Treatment of chronic hepatitis B, C, or D may also involve prolonged use of medications. In addition, population health nurses monitor the occurrence of adverse effects of treatment. For example, antituberculin drugs may result in hepatitis or visual disturbances, and the nurse should be alert to signs and symptoms of adverse effects. Treatment for other diseases may result in medication side effects as well, and population health nurses should educate clients regarding these effects and what clients should do about them.

Promoting treatment adherence in the face of multiple side effects can be difficult. Some strategies that may be effective in promoting compliance include reducing side effects where possible, simplifying the regimen to include fewer doses and fewer pills, establishing client trust in the efficacy of treatment, and tailoring therapy to fit the client's lifestyle whenever possible. Additional approaches may include clarifying treatment instructions and making sure that clients understand them, simplifying distribution systems (e.g., providing easy access to medication refills), and providing frequent follow-up.

Rehabilitation may be required following some communicable diseases. For example, rehabilitation may be needed to strengthen affected muscles or to promote individual and family adjustment to permanent disabilities from paralytic poliomyelitis. Active and passive range of motion may help restore muscle strength and prevent contractures. Maintaining skin integrity for clients with braces or those confined to a bed or wheelchair is also important. Observation for recurrent disease (even many years later) is also needed. Families may also require assistance in financing rehabilitative care and procuring needed equipment and appliances, and population health nurses may collaborate with public health social workers in efforts to address these needs. In addition, population health nurses may need to be involved in political advocacy to assure that needed services are available to clients and their families.

Population health nurses may also need to help clients deal with the long-term consequences of communicable diseases. For example, children with anomalies or developmental disabilities due to congenital rubella syndrome or congenital syphilis will need ongoing care, and their families will need emotional support and assistance in finding resources to deal with their children's disabilities. Support may also be needed for long-term behavior changes required to prevent infecting others with HIV or hepatitis. Population health nurses may also need to function as advocates to prevent stigmatization and discrimination and to foster clients' integration into the community to the extent permitted by their health status. For example, nurses may need to educate those who interact with HIV-infected clients about how HIV infection is and is not transmitted. Similarly, when working with children with AIDS, advocacy by the population health nurse may necessitate planning activities that foster normal growth and development in each child.

Assistance may also be needed in dealing with the financial impact of HIV infection and other diseases that have long-term treatment needs. The population health nurse can help in this respect by referring clients and their families to sources of financial assistance. Advocacy by population health nurses may be required to ensure client eligibility for financial assistance programs. This may involve political advocacy for health policy changes at state or national levels.

For a few communicable diseases, health restoration with individual clients entails preventing reinfection. This does not apply to the majority of the diseases discussed in this chapter because they result in immunity. For example, hepatitis A confers immunity against reinfection with hepatitis A, but does not provide immunity to other forms of hepatitis. Similarly, varicella, measles, and mumps usually confer immunity, and clients do not become reinfected. Some diseases, however, do not produce immunity, and reinfection is possible and even likely if clients do not change risk behaviors. For example, clients may be reinfected with gonorrhea or *Chlamydia* as a result of continued unprotected sexual activity. Similarly, reinfection with syphilis is possible unless the disease has progressed to the point of immunity, by which time the risk for long-term complications is quite high. Population health nurses need to educate clients about the potential for reinfection and the need for behavior changes to reduce the risk of reinfection. For example, nurses might educate clients about the need for condoms during sexual intercourse or educate IDUs on harm-reduction strategies such as not sharing needles or other drug paraphernalia.

Health systems must also be in place to meet the health restoration needs of clients with communicable diseases. At the level of public policy, population health nurses may need to engage in political advocacy to assure necessary funding for assistance programs for clients experiencing long-term needs related to the effects of communicable diseases.

Health restoration at the community level is directed toward preventing the spread of disease and providing access to long-term care services. Measures to prevent the spread of disease in the population include many primary prevention measures for individuals such as immunization and identification, notification, and prophylactic treatment of contacts. Changes in risk behaviors among persons who are chronic carriers of infection can also serve to prevent dissemination of disease.

Isolation or quarantine of infected or exposed persons may also prevent further spread of some communicable diseases within the community. **Isolation** is the process of limiting the movement and interactions of people who have a communicable disease to prevent the spread of the disease to others. **Quarantine**, on the other hand, is a restriction on the movements of healthy people who have been exposed to a particular disease. In both strategies, people who have the disease or have been exposed to it are kept separated from the well population.

Both isolation and quarantine may be voluntary procedures in which people who are infected or exposed self-limit their activities to prevent the spread of the disease to others. Staying home from work or school when one is ill is a simple example of voluntary isolation. Isolation or quarantine may also be mandated by legal authority at local, state, or national levels. As we saw in Chapter 2∞, quarantine was initiated as a strategy for containing the spread of epidemics from one population to another. The length of the period of quarantine varies from disease to disease, but generally is for a period of time equal to the farthest limits of the incubation period for the disease. For example, the incubation period for diphtheria is 2 to 5 days. Adults who work with unimmunized children or handle food are restricted from work for 7 days or until treated and found not to be carriers by means of nose and throat cultures. In other instances, quarantine may only be imposed until people exposed to a microorganism such as aerosolized anthrax spores can be *decontaminated* through a shower and a change of clothes. Quarantine and isolation may also be imposed on a long-term basis for certain diseases. For example, people with communicable TB who refuse treatment may be forcibly isolated from others.

Population health nurses may need to be advocates for long-term isolation of people who pose a risk of communicable disease to the public and initiate isolation procedures when absolutely necessary. At the same time, they need to be advocates for those with communicable diseases to be sure that mandatory isolation and quarantine procedures are warranted, that designated legal processes are followed, and that neither process is used to discriminate against vulnerable population groups. For example, population health nurses have been actively involved, with other civil rights activists, in resisting proposed efforts to quarantine or isolate people with HIV/AIDS.

Outbreak response is another strategy for controlling the spread of communicable diseases in the population. Outbreak response is the corollary to epidemic or bioterrorism preparedness discussed in relation to primary prevention and is initiated once an outbreak has occurred. The two facets of a response to an outbreak of communicable disease are the management of those with the disease and interrupting disease transmission in the population. Steps in an outbreak response include verifying the diagnosis, confirming the existence of an outbreak, identifying those affected and factors contributing to their illness, defining the population at risk, identifying the source and factors contributing to the spread of the disease, and containing the outbreak. Verification of diagnosis may involve the collection of specific specimens from those believed to have a particular disease. For example, population health nurses may collect stool specimens from neighborhood residents who exhibit diarrhea. The existence of an outbreak is confirmed by examining incidence figures in light of past trends in disease incidence. This step in the response to an outbreak is most often carried out by public health officials or epidemiologists rather than population health nurses.

Population health nurses are often involved, however, in obtaining case histories of those affected to determine factors contributing to disease. They may also be actively involved in identifying additional cases of disease. For example, nurses may go door to door asking about family members who have recently experienced diarrhea in an outbreak of diarrheal disease. The data gathered from these disease investigations can then be used by epidemiologists and others to identify persons at risk for the disease and to assist in the determination of the source of infection and factors influencing its spread. Population health nurses may be involved in identifying the source of the infection by collecting samples of suspected food or water sources and conveying them for laboratory testing.

Population health nurses are also actively involved in strategies to control the disease. Control may include managing cases of illness in those affected, and population health nurses are involved in educating people regarding disease management and referring them for medical care as needed. They are also involved in educating the public on measures to prevent the spread of disease or on the need for mass immunization or PEP if available. Population health nurses may also be involved in surveillance for evidence of disease among people at risk, with follow-up care for those who become symptomatic.

Social distancing is a third approach to preventing the spread of communicable diseases within the population. **Social distancing** involves voluntarily limiting one's interactions with others in order to prevent potential exposure to pathogenic microorganisms (Thombley & Steir, 2010). Social distancing measures taken by individuals (e.g., avoiding crowded places during an epidemic or disease outbreak, not sharing food or beverages or personal items with others, wearing a mask in public places, washing hands) would be a form of illness prevention. Some people may also choose to engage in *reverse* quarantine, in which well persons may choose to avoid contact with others as much as possible.

Social distancing measures taken at the population level would be interventions aimed at preventing the spread of existing disease in the community. Population-based examples of social distancing include closing schools and businesses or restricting access to certain places. For example, hospitals might be closed to all but essential personnel in the event of an avian influenza epidemic, minimizing the exposure of well people to those who are ill. Canceling public events that would promote interaction among groups of people is another example of social distancing at the population level.

Population health nurses can educate individuals regarding relevant social distancing strategies to prevent exposure to disease. They may also participate in policy decisions related to population-level social distancing activities when these are warranted by the mode of transmission of a particular disease. They can also help to avoid excessive response to the threat of communicable diseases by educating the public and policy makers regarding factors influencing disease transmission. For example, participation in the gay bar scene has been associated with increased risk of HIV infection, but closing gay bars would not be an appropriate social distancing strategy for preventing the spread of HIV infection in the gay population. Strategies for health restoration related to communicable diseases, including social distancing, are summarized in Table 26-6●.

Evaluating Communicable Disease Control Strategies

Evaluating prevention related to communicable diseases with individual clients is based on the prevention of occurrence of disease. If drug users educated for harm reduction do not develop HBV or HIV infection, intervention has been successful. At the population level, the effectiveness of prevention of communicable diseases is reflected in declining incidence and prevalence rates.

The effectiveness of resolution strategies is reflected in communicable disease mortality and continued morbidity. For example, ART for HIV infection has decreased HIV/AIDS-related mortality and prolonged survival time for infected persons. Similarly, the effectiveness of TB therapy is reflected in the number of clients whose TB has been cured.

Evaluation of health restoration measures focuses on the extent to which complications of communicable diseases have been prevented, the extent to which reinfection occurs for those diseases where reinfection is possible, and the extent of

TABLE 26-6 Health Restoration Strategies for Communicable Disease

Focus	Population Health Nursing Strategies
Monitoring compliance	• Monitor client compliance with therapy • Promote compliance with treatment regimens • Locate noncompliant clients and promote reinitiation of therapy
Monitoring treatment effects	• Monitor side effects and adverse effects of therapy and refer for medical evaluation as needed • Monitor treatment effects by referring clients for follow-up testing as needed
Dealing with consequences	• Prevent complications of communicable diseases • Refer clients with complications to rehabilitation services as needed • Promote adjustment to long-term consequences • Advocate for the availability of long-term services as needed
Preventing reinfection	• Educate clients and the public regarding safe sexual practices • Refer clients for drug abuse treatment, as needed • Promote/advocate for harm-reduction strategies for IDUs
Preventing the spread of disease	• Plan and conduct mass immunization campaigns • Engage in contact notification • Promote screening of blood and tissue donors • Advocate for and provide screening and treatment for infected pregnant women • Promote behavior change to decrease subsequent exposure risks • Promote isolation/quarantine of infected persons when required and educate them regarding the need for quarantine • Prevent the use of isolation and quarantine as discriminatory procedures against vulnerable populations • Advocate for and participate in effective response to disease outbreaks, including case identification and investigation, specimen collection, source identification, disease management, and control strategies • Educate the public regarding social distancing strategies to prevent exposure to disease • Participate in decisions regarding population-based social distancing strategies and educate policy makers regarding their advisability and utility in specific diseases

disability and adverse consequences resulting from communicable diseases. Evaluation at each of the levels of health care is also reflected in the national objectives related to communicable diseases discussed earlier in this chapter. The current status of some of these objectives is presented in the *Healthy People 2020* feature below.

In addition, the Joint United Nations Program on HIV/AIDS (UNAIDS) has developed reporting indicators that can be used to evaluate country-level progress in meeting targets for HIV/AIDS control established in a 2011 "Political Declaration on HIV/AIDS" by the United Nations General Assembly High Level Meeting on AIDS. These targets, intended to be achieved by 2015, include the following:

- Reducing sexual transmission of HIV by 50%
- Reducing HIV transmission via injecting drug use by 50%
- Eliminating new HIV infection among newborns and reducing AIDS-related maternal deaths
- Providing ART to 15 million people
- Reducing tuberculosis mortality in people with HIV/AIDS by 50%
- Increasing annual global funding for HIV/AIDS control to $22 billion to $24 billion in low- and middle-income countries
- Eliminating gender-based abuse and increasing women's abilities to protect themselves from HIV
- Eliminating stigma and discrimination among people living with HIV through legislative provisions
- Eliminating HIV-related restrictions on entry, stay, and residence in other countries, and
- Strengthening integration of AIDS response into global health and development efforts (UNAIDS, 2014)

Healthy People 2020

Selected Objectives Related to Communicable Diseases

OBJECTIVE	BASELINE (YEAR)	TARGET	CURRENT DATA (YEAR)	DATA SOURCES
HIV-4. Reduce new AIDS cases among adolescents and adults (per 100,000 population over age 13)	13.8 (2007)	12.4	13 (2010)	National HIV Surveillance System (NHSS), CDC/NCHHSTP
HIV-6. Reduce new AIDS cases among adolescent and adult men who have sex with men	15,966 cases (2007)	14,369	16,796 (2010)	NHSS, CDC/NCHHSTP
HIV-7. Reduce new AIDS cases among adolescents and adults who inject drugs	5,638 cases (2007)	5,074	4,497*	NHSS, CDC/NCHHSTP
HIV-8.2. Reduce new cases of perinatally acquired AIDS	34 (2007)	31	18* (2010)	NHSS, CDC/NCHHSTP
HIV-11. Increase the proportion of persons surviving more than 3 years after a diagnosis with AIDS	84% (2006)	92.4%	NDA	NHSS, CDC/NCHHSTP
HIV-12. Reduce deaths from HIV infection (per 100,000 population)	3.7 (2007)	3.3	2.6* (2010)	National Vital Statistics System—Mortality (NVSS-M), CDC/NCHS
HIV-14.1. Increased the proportion of adolescents and adults tested for HIV in the past 12 months	17.2% (2006–2010)	18.9%	NDA	National Survey of Family Growth, CDC/NCHS
HIV-14.3. Increase the proportion of pregnant women tested for HIV in the past 12 months	72% (2006–2010)	79.2%	NDA	National Survey of Family Growth, CDC/NCHS
HIV-15. Increase the proportion of adults with TB tested for HIV	73.3% (2008)	80.6%	NDA	National TB Surveillance System (NTSS), CDC/NCHHSTP
HIV-17.1. Increase the proportion of unmarried sexually active females aged 15–44 years who use condoms	35.1% (2006–2010)	38.6%	NDA	National Survey of Family Growth, CDC/NCHS

Healthy People 2020 (Continued)

OBJECTIVE	BASELINE (YEAR)	TARGET	CURRENT DATA (YEAR)	DATA SOURCES
HIV-17.2. Increase the proportion of unmarried sexually active males aged 15–44 years who use condoms	45.8% (2006–2010)	50.4%	NDA	National Survey of Family Growth, CDC/NCHS
IID-1. Reduce, eliminate, or maintain elimination of cases:				National Notifiable Disease Surveillance System (NNDSS). CDC/PHSPO National Health Interview Survey (NHIS), CDC/NCHS
1.1. Congenital rubella syndrome	0/100,000 (2008)	0.0	0.0 (2011)	
1.2. *Haemophilus influenzae type b* (Hib)	0.3/100,000 (2008)	0.27	0.18* (2010)	
1.3. Hepatitis B (2–18 years)	0.1/100,000 (2007)	0.0	NDA	
1.4. Measles (U.S. acquired)	115 cases (2008)	30	142 (2011)	
1.5. Mumps	421 cases (2008)	500	376* (2011)	
1.6. Pertussis (children <1 year of age)	2,777 cases (2004–2008)	2,500	2,744 (2006–2010)	
1.8. Wild poliovirus	0/100,000 (2008)	0.0	0.0 (2011)	
1.9. Rubella	10 cases (2008)	10	2 (2011)	
1.10. Varicella (<18 years)	586,000 cases (2008)	100,000	266,000 (2011)	
IID-2. Reduce early onset group B *Streptococcal* disease	0.28/1,000 newborns (2008)	0.25	0.27 (2010)	National Vital Statistics System- Natality (NVSS-N). CDC/NCHHSTP
IID-3. Reduce meningococcal disease	1,215 cases (2004–2008)	1,094	1,051* (2006–2010)	NNDSS, CDC/PHSPO
IID-8. Increase the proportion of vaccination coverage among children 19–35 months for DTaP, polio, MMR, Hib, hepatitis B, varicella, & PCV	44.3% (2009)	80%	68.5% (2011)	National Immunization Survey (NIS), CDC/NCHS
IID-12.12. Increase the percentage of persons 18 years of age and older vaccinated against influenza annually	38.1 (2010–2011)	70%	39.2% (2011–2012)	NIS, CDC/NCHS
IIID-12.13. Increase the percentage of health care personnel vaccinated against influenza	55.8% (2010–2011)	90%	61.5% (2011–2012)	NIS, CDC/NCHS
IIID-12.14. Increase the percentage of pregnant women vaccinated against influenza	DEV	DEV	NDA	Pregnancy Risk Assessment Monitoring System (PRAMS), CDC/NCCDPHP
IID-15.3. Increase hepatitis B vaccine coverage in health care personnel	64.3%	90%	NDA	National Health Interview Survey (NHIS), CDC/
IID-23. Reduce new cases of hepatitis A	1/100,000 (2007)	0.3	NDA	NNDSS, CDC/PHSPO
IID-25. Reduce new cases of hepatitis B in persons 19 years of age and older	2.0/100,000 (2007)	1.5	NDA	NNDSS, CDC/PHSPO
IID-26. Reduce new cases of hepatitis C	0.28/100,000 (2007)	0.25	NDA	NNDSS, CDC/PHSPO
IID-29. Reduce new cases of tuberculosis	4.8/100,000 (2005)	1.0	3.4 (2011)	NTSS, CDC/NCHHSTP

* Objective has achieved target. NDA = No data available

Data from: U.S. Department of Health and Human Services. (2014). *Healthy people 2020: Topics and objectives.* Retrieved from http://healthypeople.gov/2020/topicsobjectives2020/default.aspx

For further information on achievement of these goals in specific countries, see the *External Resources* section of the student resources site.

As of 2013, 172 countries had reported their progress on meeting the HIV/AIDS control targets. Overall, 35.3 million people were infected with HIV in 2012, but new infections had declined 33% from 2001. HIV/AIDS mortality had also decreased from 2.3 million deaths in 2005 to 1.6 million in 2012. Increases were seen in the use of safer sexual practices, but little progress had been made among sex workers and MSM. From 2009 to 2012, a 35% decrease in the number of newly infected children was achieved. ART coverage among 62% of pregnant women with HIV infection contributed to the reduction in new HIV infections in children. Similarly, some progress has been made in the provision of ART to HIV-infected individuals, with 9.7 million infected people receiving therapy in 2012, but more work in this area is needed. TB mortality among HIV-infected individuals declined by 36% from 2004 to 2012, but only two countries with large populations of people with comorbid TB and HIV infection provided treatment to more than 50% of those affected. Finally, the global funding available for HIV/AIDS control in 2012 was $18.9 billion, with increased domestic spending in many countries (UNAIDS, 2014).

Population health nurses may be involved in collecting evaluative data regarding communicable disease control, including HIV/AIDS control measures. They may also contribute to the interpretation of those data and their use in developing and implementing new control strategies.

CHAPTER RECAP

Communicable diseases occur through a process that involves a "chain of infection" in which the causative organism is transmitted from an infected host through a specific mode of transmission that involves defined portals of entry and exit. Communicable disease control can involve interruption of this chain of events anywhere along the way.

Disease transmission occurs through airborne, fecal–oral, direct contact (including sexual contact), direct inoculation, insect or animal bite, or other mechanisms. Each mode of transmission involves specific portals by which the disease causing organism enters and leaves a host. Communicable diseases also vary in terms of their incubation periods and the presence or absence of a prodromal period.

Population health nurses assist in determining factors related to each of the six categories of determinants of health that contribute to the development and extent of a particular communicable disease in the population. They are also actively involved in general health promotion strategies and illness prevention strategies to prevent communicable diseases in individuals and populations. When communicable diseases do occur, population health nurses may be involved in their identification and treatment. They are also involved in strategies to restore health following a communicable disease or to prevent reinfection. Finally, population health nurses are actively involved in evaluating the effects of communicable disease control measures.

Although remarkable progress has been made in controlling communicable diseases, they remain significant contributors to morbidity and mortality in the United States and throughout the world. Population health nurses can be actively involved in preventing communicable diseases and in identifying and treating them when they do occur.

CASE STUDY A Communicable Disease Outbreak

Jane is an 18-year-old college student. She lives in the dorm with her roommate, Sally. Shortly after Jane returned from Christmas vacation, she developed a fever and severe cough. Sally persuaded her to see a doctor. Because it was Saturday, Jane went to the emergency department (ED) of the local hospital. The physician there made a diagnosis of pertussis. Later that night, he and the nurses in the ED became very busy with victims of a multivehicle accident. As a result, no one completed the health department form reporting Jane's pertussis until 2 days later.

By the time a population health nurse contacted Jane to complete a pertussis case report, Sally and several other girls in Jane's dorm had also developed pertussis. Sally gave it to her boyfriend, who exposed those in his classes. One of the women in his English class just had a baby a month ago.

The university has a policy that all students provide verification of immunizations on admission before enrolling in classes. The student health center reviews student immunization records and notifies students of any deficiencies. They do not, however, follow up on whether the deficient immunizations were obtained. There is also no mechanism for creating a registration "hold" for students with deficient immunizations. A review of cases in this outbreak indicated that approximately three quarters of those affected, including the woman with the new baby, had not received a pertussis booster as adolescents and the remaining quarter had never been immunized for pertussis.

1. Based on the information presented in the case description, what biological, psychological, environmental, sociocultural, behavioral, and health system factors are operating in this situation? What additional determinants might influence the situation? How might you assess for the presence or absence of these determinants?
2. What preventive measures could have been employed to prevent this situation? What prevention measures are appropriate at this point?
3. What problem resolution and health restoration interventions by the population health nurse are appropriate at this time?
4. What roles might the population health nurse perform in dealing with this situation? What other public health personnel might the population health nurse collaborate with in addressing the situation?
5. How would you evaluate the effectiveness of interventions in this situation?

REFERENCES

Adams, D. A., Gallagher, K. M., Jajosky, R. A., Kriseman, J., Sharp, P., Anderson, W. J., . . . Onweh, D. H. (2013). Summary of notifiable diseases—United States, 2011. *Morbidity and Mortality Weekly Report, 103*(53), 1–117.

Adimora, A. A., Schoenbach, V. J., Taylor, E. M., Kahn, M. R., & Schwartz, R. J. (2011). Concurrent partnerships, nonmonogamous partners, and substance use among women in the United States. *American Journal of Public Health, 101*, 839–848. doi:10.2105/AJPH.2009.174292

AIDS.gov. (2014). *Pre-exposure prophylaxis (PrEP)*. Retrieved from http://www.aids.gov/hiv-aids-basics/prevention/reduce-your-risk/pre-exposure-prophylaxis/

American Lung Association. (2014). *Pneumonia fact sheet*. Retrieved from http://www.lung.org/lung-disease/influenza/in-depth-resources/pneumonia-fact-sheet.html

Anderson, A., Bijlmer, H., Fournier, P.-E., Graves, S., Hartzell, J., Kersh, G. J., . . . Sexton, D. J. (2013). Diagnosis and management of Q fever—United States, 2013: Recommendations from CDC and the Q fever working group. *Morbidity and Mortality Weekly Report, 62*(RR-3), 1–28.

Arciuolo, R. J., Brantley, T. R., Asfaw, M. M., Jablonski, R. R., Fu, J., Giancotti, F. R., . . . Zucker, J. R. (2013). Measles outbreak among members of a religious community—Brooklyn, New York, March–June 2013. *Morbidity and Mortality Weekly Report, 62*, 752.

Austvoll-Dahlgren, A., & Helseth, S. (2010). What informs parents' decision making about childhood vaccinations? *Journal of Advanced Nursing, 66*, 2421–2430. doi:10.1111/j.1365-2648.2010.05403.x

Ball, S. W., Donahue, S. M. A., Izrael, D., Walker, D. K., DiSogra, C., Martonik, R., . . . Laney, A. S. (2013). Influenza vaccination coverage among health-care personnel—United States, 2012–2013 influenza season. *Morbidity and Mortality Weekly Report, 62*, 781–786.

Ball, S. W., Walker, D. K., Donahue, S. M. A., Izrael, D., Zhang, J., Euler, G. L., . . . MacCannell, T. F. (2012). Influenza vaccination coverage among health-care personnel—2011–2012 influenza season, United States. *Morbidity and Mortality Weekly Report, 61*, 753–757.

Bamberg, W., Moore, M., Stone, N., Perz, J., Dantes, R., & Wendt, J. (2013). Outbreak of severe respiratory illness in an assisted-living facility—Colorado, 2012. *Morbidity and Mortality Weekly Report, 62*, 230.

Barclay, L., Wikswo, M., Gregoricus, N., Vinjé, J., Lopman, B., Prashar, U., . . . Leshem, E. (2013). Emergence of new norovirus strain GII.4 Sydney—United States, 2012. *Morbidity and Mortality Weekly Report, 62*, 55.

Bargman, G., Reves, R., Parker, M., Belknap, R., Bettridge, J., Bedell, D. T., . . . Jereb, J. A. (2013). Transmission of Mycobacterium tuberculosis in a high school and school-based supervision of an isoniazid and rifapentine regimen for preventing tuberculosis—Colorado, 2011–2012. *Morbidity and Mortality Weekly Report, 62*, 805–809.

Bedard, B., Kennedy, B., Escuyer, V., Mitchell, K., Duchin, J. S., Pottinger, P., . . . Kinzer, M. (2012). Tattoo-associated nontuberculous mycobacterial skin infections—multiple states, 2011-2012. *Morbidity and Mortality Weekly Report, 61*, 653–656.

Beletsky, L., Agrawal, A., Moreau, B., Kumar, P., Weiss-Laxer, N., & Helmer, R. (2011). Police training to align law enforcement and HIV prevention: Preliminary evidence from the field. *American Journal of Public Health, 101*, 2012–2015. doi:10.2105/AJPH.2011.300254

Biedrzycki, P., Vergeront, J., Gasiorowicz, M., Bertolli, J., Oster, A., Spikes, P. S., . . . Nielsen, C. F. (2011). Increase in newly diagnosed HIV infections among young black men who have sex with men—Milwaukee County, Wisconsin, 1999–2008. *Morbidity and Mortality Weekly Report, 60*, 99–102.

Bird, J. D. P., & Voisin, D. R. (2013). "You're an open target to be abused": A qualitative study of stigma and HIV self-disclosure among black men who have sex with men. *American Journal of Public Health, 103*, 2193–2199. doi:10.2105/AJPH.2013.301437

Black, C. L., Yankey, D., & Kolasa, M. (2013). National, state, and local area vaccination coverage among children aged 19–35 months—United States, 2012. *Morbidity and Mortality Weekly Report, 62*, 733–740.

Bocchini, J. A., Rubin, L., Fischer, M., Hills, S. L., & Staples, J. E. (2013). Use of Japanese encephalitis vaccine in children: Recommendations of the Advisory Committee on Immunization Practices, 2013. *Morbidity and Mortality Weekly Report, 62*, 898–900.

Bornschlegel, K., Dentinger, C., Layton, M., Balter, S., & France, A. M. (2012). Investigation of viral hepatitis infections possibly associated with health care delivery—New York City, 2008–2011. *Morbidity and Mortality Weekly Report, 61*, 333–338.

Bornschlegel, K., Holtzman, D., Klevens, M., & Ward, J. W. (2013). Vital signs: Evaluation of hepatitis C virus infection testing and reporting—Eight U.S. Sites, 2005–2011. *Morbidity and Mortality Weekly Report, 62,* 357–361.

Børresen, M. L., Koch, A., Biggar, R. J., Ladefoged, K., Melbye, M., Wohlfahrt, J., et al. (2012). Effectiveness of the targeted hepatitis B vaccination program in Greenland. *American Journal of Public Health, 102,* 277–284. doi:10.2105/AJPH.2011.300239

Boulton, M. L., & Rosenberg, L. D. (2011). Food safety epidemiology capacity in state health departments—United States, 2010. *Morbidity and Mortality Weekly Report, 60,* 1701–1704.

Brucker, R., Bui, T., Kwan-Gett, T., Stewart, L., Hall, A. J., & Kinzer, M. H. (2012). Norovirus infection associated with frozen raw oysters—Washington, 2011. *Morbidity and Mortality Weekly Report, 61,* 110.

Burzynski, J., Varma, J. K., Rodriquez, E., Oxtoby, M. J., Privett, T., & Forbes, A. (2013). Tuberculosis control activities before and after hurricane Sandy—Northeast and Mid-Atlantic states. *Morbidity and Mortality Weekly Report, 62,* 206–208.

California Department of Public Health. (2012). Hantavirus pulmonary syndrome in visitors to a National Park—Yosemite Valley, California, 2012. *Morbidity and Mortality Weekly Report, 61,* 952.

Cardemil, G., Pabst, L., & Gerlach, K. (2013). Progress in immunization information systems—United States, 2011. *Morbidity and Mortality Weekly Report, 62,* 48–51.

Cegielski, J. P., Griffith, D. E., McGaha, P. K., Wolfgang, M., Robinson, C. B., Clark, P. A., . . . Wallace, C. (2013). Eliminating tuberculosis one neighborhood at a time. *American Journal of Public Health, 103,* 1292–1300. doi:10.2105/AJPH.2012.300781

Centers for Disease Control and Prevention. (2011). World malaria day—April 25, 2011. *Morbidity and Mortality Weekly Report, 60,* 481.

Centers for Disease Control and Prevention. (2012a). FDA approval of an extended period for administering VariZIG for postexposure prophylaxis of varicella. *Morbidity and Mortality Weekly Report, 61,* 212.

Centers for Disease Control and Prevention. (2012b). *Glossary of terms.* Retrieved from http://www.cdc.gov/hantavirus/resources/glossary.html

Centers for Disease Control and Prevention. (2012c). Hepatitis awareness month and national hepatitis testing day—May 2012. *Morbidity and Mortality Weekly Report, 61,* 333.

Centers for Disease Control and Prevention. (2012d). World Pneumonia day—November 12, 2012. *Morbidity and Mortality Weekly Report, 61,* 906.

Centers for Disease Control and Prevention. (2013a). *Anthrax: Bioterrorism.* Retrieved from http://www.cdc.gov/anthrax/bioterrorism/index.html

Centers for Disease Control and Prevention. (2013b). *Diphtheria and the Alaskan Iditarod.* Retrieved from http://www.cdc.gov/Features/Diphtheria/

Centers for Disease Control and Prevention. (2013c). Get smart about antibiotics week—November 18–24, 2013. *Morbidity and Mortality Weekly Report, 62,* 905.

Centers for Disease Control and Prevention. (2013d). *Hepatitis D.* Retrieved from http://www.cdc.gov/hepatitis/HDV/index.htm

Centers for Disease Control and Prevention. (2013e). *Lyme disease frequently asked questions (FAQ).* Retrieved from http://www.cdc.gov/lyme/faq/index.html

Centers for Disease Control and Prevention. (2013f). *Lyme disease incidence rates by state, 2003-2012.* Retrieved from http://www.cdc.gov/lyme/stats/chartstables/incidencebystate.html

Centers for Disease Control and Prevention. (2013g). STD awareness month—April 2013. *Morbidity and Mortality Weekly Report, 62,* 256.

Centers for Disease Control and Prevention. (2014). *Preferred usage.* Retrieved from http://wwwnc.cdc.gov/eid/pages/preferred-usage.htm

Cerdia, R., & Lee, P. T. (2013). Modern cholera in the Americas: An opportunistic societal infection. *American Journal of Public Health, 103,* 1934–1937. doi:10.2105/AJPH.2013.301567

Chimbwandira, F., Mhango, E., Makombe, S., Midiani, D., Mwansambo, C., Njala, J., . . . Houston, J. (2013). Impact of an innovative approach to prevent mother-to-child transmission of HIV—Malawi, July 2011–September 2012. *Morbidity and Mortality Weekly Report, 62,* 148–151.

Cohen, S. E., Chew, R. A., Katz, K. A., Bernstein, K. T., Samuel, M. C., Kerndt, P. R., . . . Valleroy, L. A. (2012). Repeat syphilis among men who have sex with men in California, 2002–2006: Implications for syphilis elimination efforts. *American Journal of Public Health, 101,* e1–e8. doi:10.2105/AJPH.2011.300383

Cohen, S. M., Van Handel, M. M., Branson, B. M., Blair, J. M., Hall, H. I., Hu, X., et al. (2011). Vital signs: HIV prevention through care and treatment—United States. *Morbidity and Mortality Weekly Report, 60,* 1618–1623.

Cohn, A. C., MacNeil, J. R., Clark, T. A., Ortega-Sanchez, I. R., Briere, E. Z., Meissner, H. C., . . . Messonnier, N. E. (2013). Prevention and control of meningococcal disease: Recommendations of the Advisory Committee on Immunization Practices (ACIP). *Morbidity and Mortality Weekly Report, 62*(2), 1–28.

Collier, S. A., Smith, S., Lowe, A., Hawkins, P., McFarland, P., Salyers, M., . . . Meites, E. M. (2011). Cryptosporidiosis outbreak in a summer camp—North Carolina, 2009. *Morbidity and Mortality Weekly Report, 60,* 918–922.

Coscollá, M., Fenollar, J., Escribano, I., & González-Candelas, F. (2010). Legionellosis outbreak associated with asphalt paving machine, Spain, 2009. *Emerging Infectious Diseases, 16,* 1381–1387. doi:10.3201/eid1609.100248

Council of State and Territorial Epidemiologists. (2012). *CSTE list of nationally notifiable conditions.* Retrieved from http://c.ymcdn.com/sites/www.cste.org/resource/resmgr/PDFs/CSTENotifiableConditionListA.pdf

Cullen, K. A., & Arguin, P. M. (2013). Malaria surveillance—United States, 2011. *Morbidity and Mortality Weekly Report, 62*(SS-5), 1–17.

Curtis, C. R., Yankey, D., Jeyarajah, J., Dorell, C., Stokley, S., MacNeil, J., . . . Hariri, S. (2013). National and state vaccination coverage among adolescents aged 13–17 years—United States, 2012. *Morbidity and Mortality Weekly Report, 62,* 685–693.

Denning, P. H., DiNenno, E. A., & Wiegand, R. E. (2011). Characteristics associated with HIV infection among heterosexuals in urban areas with high AIDS prevalence—24 cities, United States, 2006–2007. *Morbidity and Mortality Weekly Report, 60,* 1045–1049.

de Oliviera, L. H., Sanwogou, J., Ruiz-Matus, C., Tambini, G., Wang, S. A., Agocs, M., . . . Desai, R. (2011). Progress in the introduction of rotavirus vaccine—Latin America and the Caribbean, 2006–2010. *Morbidity and Mortality Weekly Report, 60,* 1611–1614.

Department of Immunization, Vaccines, and Biologicals, World Health Organization. (2013). Global routine immunization coverage, 2012. *Morbidity and Mortality Weekly Report, 62,* 858–861.

Des Jarlais, D. C., Arasten, K., McKnight, C., Hagan, H., Perlman, D. C., & Semaam, S. (2011). Associations between herpes simplex virus type 2 and HCV with HIV infection among injecting drug users in New York City: The current importance of sexual transmission of HIV. *American Journal of Public Health, 101,* 1277–1283. doi:10.2105/AJPH.2011.300130

Division of HIV/AIDS prevention. (2011). *HIV among youth.* Retrieved from http://www.cdc.gov/hiv/youth/pdf/youth.pdf

Division of STD Prevention. (2014). *Expedited partner therapy.* Retrieved from http://www.cdc.gov/STD/ept/default.htm

Division of Tuberculosis Elimination. (2011). *Targeted tuberculosis (TB) testing and treatment of latent TB infection.* Retrieved from www.cdc.gov/tb/publications/slidesets/LTBI/images/LTBI.pptx

Division of Tuberculosis Elimination. (2013). Availability of an assay for detecting Mycobacterium tuberculosis, including rifampin-resistant strains, and considerations for its use—United States, 2013. *Morbidity and Mortality Weekly Report, 62,* 821–824.

Division of Viral Hepatitis. (2014). *Hepatitis C: FAQs for the Public.* Retrieved from http://www.cdc.gov/hepatitis/c/cfaq.htm

Dobbins, C., Marishta, K., Kuehnert, P., Arbisi, M., Darnall, E., Conover, C., . . . Haddad, M. (2012). Tuberculosis outbreak associated with a homeless shelter—Kane County, Illinois, 2007–2011. *Morbidity and Mortality Weekly Report, 61,* 186–189.

Dowell, D., Tian, L. H., Stover, J. A., Donnelly, J. A., Martins, S., Erbelding, E. J., . . . Newman, L. M. (2012). Changes in fluoroquinolone use for gonorrhea following publication of revised treatment guidelines. *American Journal of Public Health, 102,* 148–155. doi:10.2105/AJPH.2011.300283

Drobnik, A., Judd, C., Banach, D., Egger, J., Konty, K., & Rude, E. (2011). Public health implications of rapid hepatitis C screening with an oral swab for community-based organizations serving high risk populations. *American Journal of Public Health, 101,* 2012–2015. doi:10.2105/AJPH.2011.300251

Duncan, I. G., Taitel, M. S., Zhang, J., & Kirkham, H. S. (2012). Planning influenza vaccination programs: A cost benefit model. *Cost Effectiveness and Resource Allocation, 10*(10). Retrieved from http://www.resource-allocation.com/content/pdf/1478-7547-10-10.pdf

East, L., Jackson, D., O'Brien, L., & Peters, K. (2010). Condom negotiation: Experiences of sexually active young women. *Journal of Advanced Nursing, 67,* 77–85. doi:10.1111/j.1365-2648.2010.05451.x

Eaton, L. A., Cherry, C., Cain, D., & Pope, H. (2011). A novel approach to prevention for at-risk HIV-negative men who have sex with men: Creating a teachable moment to promote informed sexual decision-making. *American Journal of Public Health, 101,* 539–545. doi:10.2105/AJPH.2010.191791

El-Bassel, N., Gilbert, L., Vinocur, D., Chang, M., & Wu. (2011). Posttraumatic stress disorder and HIV risk among poor inner-city women receiving care in an emergency department. *American Journal of Public Health, 101,* 839–848. doi:10.2105/AJPH.2009.181842

El-Sayed, N., Kandeel, A., Genedy, M., Esmat, G., El-Sayed, M., Bernier, A., . . . Averhoff, F. (2012). Progress toward prevention and control of hepatitis C virus infection—Egypt, 2001–2012. *Morbidity and Mortality Weekly Report, 61,* 545–549.

Fan, K.-W. (2012). Schistosomiasis control and snail elimination in China. *American Journal of Public Health, 102,* 2231–2231. doi:10.2105/AJPH.2012.300809

Feske, M. L., Teeter, L. D., Musser, J. M., & Graviss, E. A. (2013). Counting the homeless: A previously incalculable tuberculosis risk and its social determinants. *American Journal of Public Health, 103,* 839–848. doi:10.2105/AJPH.2012.300973

Fierer, D. S., Factor, S. H., Uriel, A. J., Carriero, D. C., Dieterich, D. T., Mullen, M. P., . . . Holmberg, S. D. (2011). Sexual transmission of hepatitis C virus among HIV-infected men who have sex with men—New York City, 2005–2010. *Morbidity and Mortality Weekly Report, 60,* 945–950.

Finks, J., Collins, J., Miller, C., Fiedler, H., Johnson, S., Coyle, J. R., . . . Nyaku, M. K. (2013). Spinal and paraspinal infections associated with contaminated methylprednisolone acetate injections—Michigan, 2012–2013. *Morbidity and Mortality Weekly Report, 62,* 377–381.

Fiori, A. E., Fry, A., Shay, D., Gubareva, L., Bresee, J. S., & Uyeki, T. M. (2011). Antiviral agents for the treatment and chemoprophylaxis of influenza: Recommendations of the Advisory Committee on Immunization Practices (ACIP). *Morbidity and Mortality Weekly Report, 60*(1), 1–25.

Frimpong, J. A. (2013). Missed opportunities for HCV testing in opioid treatment programs. *American Journal of Public Health, 103,* 1028–1030. doi:10.2105/AJPH.2012.301129

Galletly, C. L., Glasman, L. R., Pinkerton, S. D., & Di Franceisco, W. (2012). New Jersey's HIV exposure law and the HIV-related attitudes, beliefs, and sexual and seropositive status disclosure behaviors of persons living with HIV. *American Journal of Public Health, 102,* 2135–2140. doi:10.2105/AJPH.2012.300664

Geren, K., Moore, E., Tomlinson, C., Hobohm, D., Gardner, A., Reardon-Maynard, D., . . . Peters, P. J. (2013). Detection of acute HIV infection in two evaluations of a new HIV diagnostic testing algorithm—United States, 2011–2013. *Morbidity and Mortality Weekly Report, 62,* 489–494.

Gerstman, B. B. (2013). *Epidemiology kept simple.* Hoboken, NJ: Wiley-Blackwell.

Getahun, H., Raviglione, M., Varma, J. K., Cain, K., Samandari, T., Popovic, T., et al. (2012). CDC grand rounds: The TB/HIV syndemic. *Morbidity and Mortality Weekly Report, 61,* 484–489.

Getchell, J. P., Wroblewski, K. E., DeMaria, A., Bean, C. L., Parker, M. M., Pandori, M., . . . Ward, J. W. (2013). Testing for HCV infection: An update of guidance for clinicians and laboratorians. *Morbidity and Mortality Weekly Report, 62,* 362–365.

Gidado, S., Nguku, P. M., Ohuabunwo, C. J., Waziri, N. E., Etsano, A., Mahmud, M. Z., . . . Wiesen, E. S. (2013). Polio field census and vaccination of underserved populations—Northern Nigeria, 2012–2013. *Morbidity and Mortality Weekly Report, 62,* 663–666.

Gilliss, D., Cronquist, A. B., Carter, M., Tobin-D'Angelo, M., Blythe, D., Smith, K., . . . Hall, A. J. (2013). Incidence and trends of infection with pathogens transmitted commonly through food—Foodborne Diseases Active Surveillance Network, 10 U.S. sites, 1996–2012. *Morbidity and Mortality Weekly Report, 62,* 283–287.

Gould, L. H., Mundai, E. A., Johnson, S. D., Richardson, L. C., Williams, I. T., Griffin, P. M., et al. (2013). Surveillance for foodborne disease outbreaks—United States, 2011. *Morbidity and Mortality Weekly Report, 62,* 41–47.

Gould, L. H., Walsh, K. A., Vieira, A. R., Herman, K., Williams, I. T., Hall, A. J., et al. (2013). Surveillance for foodborne disease outbreaks—United States, 1998–2008. *Morbidity and Mortality Weekly Report, 62*(SS-2), 1–34

Green, M., Levin, J., Michaels, M., Vosbinder, S., Vorhees, R., Lute, J., . . . Han, G. (2012). Hospital-associated measles outbreak—Pennsylvania, March–April 2009. *Morbidity and Mortality Weekly Report, 61,* 30–32.

Griffin, D., Springer, D., Moore, Z., Njord, L., Njord, R., Sweat, D., . . . Griese, S. (2012). Escherichia coli O157:H7 gastroenteritis associated with a state fair—North Carolina, 2011. *Morbidity and Mortality Weekly Report, 61,* 1745–1746.

Grinnell, M., Provo, G., Marsden-Haug, N., Stigi, K. A., DeBess, E., Kissler, B., . . . Laufer, A. (2013). Outbreak of Salmonella Heidelberg infections linked to a single poultry producer—13 states, 2012–2013. *Morbidity and Mortality Weekly Report, 62,* 553–557.

Grohskopf, L. A., Shay, D. K., Shimabukuro, T. T., Sokolow, L. Z., Keitel, W. A., Bresee, J. A., & Cox, N. J. (2013). Prevention and control of seasonal influenza with vaccines: Recommendations of the Advisory Committee on Immunization Practices—United States, 2013–2014. *Morbidity and Mortality Weekly Report, 62*(7), 1–43.

Guttmacher Institute. (2014). *American teens' sexual and reproductive health.* Retrieved from http://www.guttmacher.org/pubs/FB-ATSRH.pdf

Ha, T. H., Liu, H., Liu, H. Cai. Y., & Feng, T. (2010). Concurrent sexual partnerships among men who have sex with men in Shenzhen, China. *Sexually Transmitted Diseases, 37,* 506–511. doi: 10.1097/OLQ.0b013e3181d707c9

Harris, N., Johnson, C., Siomean, K., Ivy, W., Singh, A., Wei, S., . . . Lansky, A. (2013). Estimated percentages and characteristics of men who have sex with men and use injection drugs—United States, 1999–2011. *Morbidity and Mortality Weekly Report, 62,* 757–762.

Hart-Malloy, R., Carrascal, A., DiRienzo, G., Flanigan, C., McClamroch, K., & Smith, L. (2013). Estimating HCV prevalence at the state level: A call to increase and strengthen current surveillance systems. *American Journal of Public Health, 103,* 1402–1405. doi:10.2105/AJPH.2013.301231

Harvey, K., Esposito, D. H., Han, P., Kozarsky, P., Freedman, D. O., Plier, D. A., et al. (2013). Surveillance for travel-related disease—Geosentinel Surveillance System, United States, 1997–2011. *Morbidity and Mortality Weekly Report, 62*(3), 1–23

Henry J. Kaiser Family Foundation. (2014). *The HPV vaccine: Access and use in the U.S.* Retrieved from http://kff.org/womens-health-policy/fact-sheet/the-hpv-vaccine-access-and-use-in/

Hillborn, E. D., Wade, T. J., Hicks, L., Garrison, L., Adam, E., Mull, B., . . . Gargano, J. W. (2013). Surveillance for waterborne disease outbreaks associated with drinking water and other nonrecreational water—United States, 2009–2010. *Morbidity and Mortality Weekly Report, 62,* 714–721.

HIV/AIDS Programme, World Health Organization. (2012). *Prevention and treatment of HIV and other sexually transmitted infections for sex workers in low- and middle-income countries.* Retrieved from http://apps.who.int/iris/bitstream/10665/77745/1/9789241504744_eng.pdf

Hlavsa, M. C., Roberts, V. A., Anderson, A., R., Hill, V. R., Kahler, A. M., Orr, L. E., . . . Yoder, J. S. (2011). Surveillance for Waterborne disease outbreaks and other health events associated with recreational water—United States, 2007–2008. *Morbidity and Mortality Weekly Report, 60*(SS-12), 1–37.

Holmberg, J. A., Basavaraju, S., Reed, C., Drammeh, B., & Qualls, M. (2011). Progress toward strengthening national blood transfusion services—14 countries, 2008–2010. *Morbidity and Mortality Weekly Report, 60,* 1577–1582.

Holmberg, S. D., Suryaprasad, A., & Ward, J. W. (2012). Updated CDC recommendations for the management of hepatitis B virus-infected health-care providers and students. *Morbidity and Mortality Weekly Report, 61*(RR-3), 1–12.

Honish, L., Greenwald, D., McIntyre, K., Lau, W., Nunn, S., Nelson, D., . . . Wilkinson, K. (2013). Salmonella enteritidis infections associated with foods purchased from mobile lunch trucks—Alberta Canada, October 2010–February 2011. *Morbidity and Mortality Weekly Report, 62,* 567–569.

Hook, E. W., Shafer, W., Deal, C., Kirkcaldy, R. D., & Iskander, J. (2013). CDC grand rounds: The growing threat of multidrug-resistant gonorrhea. *Morbidity and Mortality Weekly Report, 62,* 103–106.

Hope, V., Palmeteer, N., Weissing, L., Marongiu, A., White, J., Nicune, F., . . . Goldberg, D. (2012). A decade of spore forming bacterial infections among European injecting drug users: Pronounced regional variation. *American Journal of Public Health, 102,* 122–125. doi:10.2105/AJPH.2011.300314

Hopkins, D. R., Ruiz-Tiben, E., Eberhard, M. L., & Roy, S. L. (2013). Progress toward global eradication of dracunculiasis—January 2012–June 2013. *Morbidity and Mortality Weekly Report, 62,* 829–833.

Hoskins, R., Volma, R., Vlack, S., Young, M., Humphrey, K., Selvey, C., . . . Lyon, M. (2011). Multiple cases of measles after exposure during air travel—Australia and New Zealand, January 2011. *Morbidity and Mortality Weekly Report, 60,* 851.

Hunte, T., Morris, T., da Silva, A., Nuriddin, A., Visvesvara, G., Hill, V., . . . Morris, J. (2013). Primary amebic meningoencephalitis associated with ritual nasal rinsing—St. Thomas, U. S. Virgin Islands, 2012. *Morbidity and Mortality Weekly Report, 62,* 903.

Immunization Action Coalition. (2013). *Vaccine timeline: Historic dates and events related to vaccines and immunization.* Retrieved from http://www.immunize.org/timeline/

Iverson, J., Wand, H., Topp, L., Kaldor, J., & Maher, L. (2013). Reduction in HCV incidence among injection drug users attending needle and syringe programs in Australia: A linkage study. *American Journal of Public Health, 103,* 1436–1444. doi:10.2105/AJPH.2012.301206

Jackson, L., Jackson, M. L., Phillips, C. H., Benoit, J., Belongia, E. A., Cole, D., . . . Cox, N. (2013). Interim adjusted estimates of influenza vaccine effectiveness—United States, February, 2013. *Morbidity and Mortality Weekly Report, 62,* 119–123.

Jacob, J. T., Klein, E., Laxminarayan, R., Beldavs, S., Lynfield, R., Kallen, A. J., . . . Cardo, D. (2013). Vital signs: Carbapenem-resistant enterobarteriaceae. *Morbidity and Mortality Weekly Report, 62,* 165–170.

Jenkins, P. H., Montejano, H. J., Broward, M. S., Abbassi, M. J., Crowley, M. S., O'Brien, M. G., . . . Merlo, E. (2010). Update on cholera—Haiti, Dominican Republic, and Florida, 2010. *Morbidity and Mortality Weekly Report, 59,* 1637–1641.

Jereb, J., Mase, S., Chorba, T., & Castro, K. (2013). National shortage of purified protein derivative tuberculin products. *Morbidity and Mortality Weekly Report, 62,* 312.

Kalas, N., & Quinlisk, P. (2013). Use of electronic messaging and the news media to increase case finding during a cyclospora outbreak—Iowa, July, 2013. *Morbidity and Mortality Weekly Report, 62,* 613–614.

Kalichman, S. C., Cherry, C., Kalichman, M. O., Amaral, C. M., White, D., Pope, H., . . . Cain, D. (2011). Integrated behavioral intervention to improve HIV/AIDS treatment adherence and reduce HIV transmission. *American Journal of Public Health, 101,* 531–538. doi:10.2105/AJPH.2010.197608

Kellogg, F., Niehus, N., DiOrio, M., Smith, K., Chipman, R., Kirby, J., . . . Vora, N. M. (2013). Human contacts with oral rabies vaccine baits distributed for wildlife rabies management—Ohio, 2012. *Morbidity and Mortality Weekly Report, 62,* 267–269.

Kelly, S., Le, T. N., Brown, J. A., Lawaczek, E. W., Kuehnert, M., Rabe, I. B., . . . Fischer, M. (2013). Fatal West Nile virus infection after probable transfusion-associated transmission—Colorado, 2012. *Morbidity and Mortality Weekly Report, 62,* 622–624.

Kempe, A., Saville, A., Dickinson, L. M., Eisert, S., Reynolds, J., Herrero, D., . . . Calonge, N. (2013). Population-based versus practice-based recall for childhood immunizations: A randomized controlled comparative effectiveness trial. *American Journal of Public Health, 103,* 1116–1123. doi:10.2105/AJPH.2012.301035

Kim, C., Buckley, K., Marienau, K. J., Jackson, W. L., Escobedo, M., Bell, T. R., . . . Marano, N. (2012). Public health interventions involving travelers with tuberculosis—U.S. ports of entry, 2007–2012. *Morbidity and Mortality Weekly Report, 61,* 570–573.

Kirkey, K., MacMaster, K., Xu, F., Klevens, M., Roberts, H., Moorman, A., . . . Webeck, J. (2013). Completeness of reporting of chronic hepatitis B and C virus infections—Michigan, 1995–2008. *Morbidity and Mortality Weekly Report, 62,* 99–102.

Klevens, R. M., & Tohme, R. A. (2010). Evaluation of acute hepatitis C infection surveillance—United States, 2008. *Morbidity and Mortality Weekly Report, 59,* 1407–1410.

Kumar, S., Grefenstette, J. L., Galloway, D., Albert, S. M., & Burke, D. S. (2013). Policies to reduce influenza in the workplace: Impact assessments using an agent-based model. *American Journal of Public Health, 103,* 1406–1411. doi:10.2105/AJPH.2013.301269

Laffoon, B., Crutchfield, A., Levi, M., Bower, W. A., Kuehnert, M., Brooks, J. T., . . . Juliano, A. D. (2010). HIV transmission through transfusion—Missouri and Colorado, 2008. *Morbidity and Mortality Weekly Report, 59,* 1335–1339.

Lanier, Y., & Sutton, M. Y. (2013). Reframing the context of preventive health care services and prevention of HIV and other sexually transmitted infections for young men: New opportunities to reduce racial/ethnic sexual health disparities. *American Journal of Public Health, 103,* 262–269. doi:10.2105/AJPH.2012.300921

Lee, B. Y., Assi, T.-M., Rajgopal, J., Norman, B., Chen, S.-I., Brown, S. T., . . . Burke, D. S. (2012). Impact of introducing the pneumococcal and rotavirus vaccines into the routine immunization program in Niger. *American Journal of Public Health, 102,* 269–276. doi:10.2105/AJPH.2011.300218

Lee, D., Philen, R., Wang, Z., McSpadden, P., Posey, D. L., Ortega, L. S., . . . Painter, J. A. (2013). Disease surveillance among newly arriving refugees and immigrants—Electronic Disease Notification System, United States, 2009. *Morbidity and Mortality Weekly Report, 62*(7), 1–20.

Leibowitz, A. A., Parker, K. B., & Rotherham-Bonus, M. J. (2011). A U.S. policy perspective on oral preexposure prophylaxis. *American Journal of Public Health, 101,* 982–985. doi:10.2105/AJPH.2010.300066

Li, L., Lee, S.-J., Jiraphongsa, C., Khumtong, S., Iamsirithawom, S., Thammawijaya, P., & Rotherham-Borus, M. J. (2010). Improving the health and mental health of people living with HIV/AIDS: 12-month assessment of a behavioral intervention in Thailand. *American Journal of Public Health, 100,* 2418–2425. doi:10.2105/AJPH.2009.18546

Li, L., Wu, Z., Liang, L.-J., Lin, C., Guan, J., Jia, M., . . . Yan, Z. (2013). Reducing HIV-related stigma in health care settings: A randomized controlled study in China. *American Journal of Public Health, 103,* 286–292. doi:10.2105/AJPH.2012.300854

Lindsey, N. P., Lehman, J. A., Staples, J. E., & Fischer, M. (2013). West Nile virus and other arboviral diseases—United States, 2012. *Morbidity and Mortality Weekly Report, 62,* 513–517.

Lu, P.-J., Santibanez, T. A., Williams, W. W., Zhang, J., Ding, H., Bryan, L., . . . Singleton, J. A. (2013). Surveillance of influenza vaccine coverage—United States, 2007–2008 through 2011–2012 influenza seasons. *Morbidity and Mortality Weekly Report, 62*(SS-4), 1–28.

MacDonald, J. K., Julian, E., Chu, A., Dion, J., Boden, W., Viazis, S., . . . Hancock, W. T. (2013). *Salmonella Bredeney* infections linked to a brand of peanut butter—United States, 2012. *Morbidity and Mortality Weekly Report, 62,* 107.

Mace, K. E., Lynch, M. F., MacArthur, J. R., Kachur, S. P., Stutsker, L., Steketee, R. W., . . . Popovic, T. (2011). Grand rounds: The opportunity for and challenges to malaria eradication. *Morbidity and Mortality Weekly Report, 60,* 476–480.

Mah, C. L., Deber, R. B., Guttmann, A., McGeer, A., & Krahn, M. (2011). Another look at the human papillomavirus vaccine experience in Canada. *American Journal of Public Health, 101,* 1850–1857. doi:10.2105/AJPH.2011.300205

Mahajan, R., Liu, S. J., Klevens, M., & Holmberg, S. D. (2013). Indications for testing among reported cases of HCV infection from enhanced hepatitis C surveillance sites in the United States, 2004–2010. *American Journal of Public Health, 103,* 1445–1449. doi:10.2105/AJPH.2013.301211

Marin, M., Bialek, S. R., & Seward, J. F. (2013). Updated recommendations for use of variZIG—United States, 2013. *Morbidity and Mortality Weekly Report, 62,* 574–576.

Martin, R., Jankovic, D., Goel, A., Mulders, M., Dabbagh, A., Khetsuriani, N., et al. (2011). Increased transmission and outbreaks of measles—European region, 2011. *Morbidity and Mortality Weekly Report, 60,* 1605–1610.

Mase, S., Chorba, T., Lobue, P., & Castro, K. (2013). Provisional CDC guidelines for the use and safety monitoring of bedaquiline fumarate (Sirturo) for the treatment of multidrug-resistant tuberculosis. *Morbidity and Mortality Weekly Report, 62*(RR-9), 1–12.

McCree, D. H., Millett, G., Baytop, C., Royal, S., Ellen, J., Halkitis, P. N., . . . Gillen, S. (2013). Lessons learned from use of social network strategy in HIV testing programs targeting African American men who have sex with men. *American Journal of Public Health, 103,* 1851–1856. doi:10.2105/AJPH.2013.301260

McDaniel, T. M. (2006). The history of tuberculosis. *Respiratory Medicine, 100,* 1862–1870.

McLean, H. Q., Fiebelkorn, A. P., Temte, J. L., & Wallace, G. S. (2013). Prevention of measles, rubella, congenital rubella syndrome, and mumps, 2013: Summary recommendations of the Advisory Committee on Immunization Practices (ACIP). *Morbidity and Mortality Weekly Report, 62*(4), 1–34.

MERS antibodies detected in camels. (2013). *The Nation's Health,* 11.

Miles, I. J., Le, B. C., Wejnert, C., Oster, A., DiNenno, E., & Paz-Bailey, G. (2013). HIV infection among heterosexuals at increased risk—United States, 2010. *Morbidity and Mortality Weekly Report, 62,* 183–185.

Miller, B. L., Ahmed, F., Lu, P. J., Euler, G. L., & Kretsinger, K. (2010). Tetanus and pertussis vaccination coverage among adults aged > 18 years—United States, 1999 and 2008. *Morbidity and Mortality Weekly Report, 59,* 1302–1306.

Mimiaga, M., J., Resiner, S. L., Grasso, C., Crane, H., Safren, St., Kitahata, M. M., . . . Mayer, K. H. (2013). Substance use among HIV-infected patients engaged in primary care in the United States: Findings from the Centers for AIDS Research Network of integrated clinical systems cohort. *American Journal of Public Health, 103,* 1457–1467. doi:10.2105/AJPH.2012.301162

Miramontes, R., Pratt, R., Price, S. F., Navin, T. R., & Lo, T. Q. (2013). Trends in tuberculosis—United States, 2012. *Morbidity and Mortality Weekly Report, 62,* 201–205.

National Center for Health Statistics. (2012). Rates of hospitalization for pneumonia by age group—National Hospital Discharge Survey, United States, 2000–2010. *Morbidity and Mortality Weekly Report, 61,* 657.

National Center for Health Statistics. (2014). *Health, United States, 2013: With special feature on prescription drugs.* Retrieved from http://www.cdc.gov/nchs/data/hus/hus13.pdf

National Center for Immunization and Respiratory Diseases. (2008). Invasive pneumococcal disease in children 5 years after conjugate vaccine introduction—Eight states, 1998–2005. *Morbidity and Mortality Weekly Report, 57,* 144–148.

Newsome, K., Williams, J., Way, S., Honein, M., Hill, H., Rasmussen, S., . . . Zoti, S. (2011). Maternal and infant outcomes among severely ill pregnant and postpartum women with 2009 pandemic influenza A (H1N1)—United States, April 2009–August 2010. *Morbidity and Mortality Weekly Report, 60,* 1193–1196.

New York State Department of Health. (2013). *Health care facility influenza immunization toolkit.* Retrieved from http://www.health.ny.gov/prevention/immunization/toolkits/hc_personnel_hospital/

Ng, R. A. C., Samuel, M. C., Lo, T., Bernstein, K. T., Aynalem, G., Klausner, J. D., et al. (2013). Sex, drugs (methamphetamines), and the Internet: Increasing syphilis among men who have sex with men in California, 2004–2008. *American Journal of Public Health, 103,* 1450–1456. doi:10.2105/AJPH.2012.300808

Ogwang, C., Afolabi, M., Kimani, D., Jagne, Y. J., Sheehy, S. H., Bliss, C. M., . . . Bojang, K. (2013). Safety and immunogenicity of heterologous prime-boost immunization with Plasmodium falciparum malaria candidate vaccines, chAd63 ME-TRAP and MVA ME-TRAP, in healthy Gambian and Kenyan adults. *PLOS One, 8*(3), e57726. doi:10.1371/journal.pone.0057726

Oren, E., Winston, C. A., Pratt, R., Robison, V. A., & Narita, M. (2011). Epidemiology of urban tuberculosis in the United States, 2000–2007. *American Journal of Public Health, 101,* 1256–1263. doi:10.2105/AJPH.2011.300030

Otrompke, J. (2009). *Case studies for global health: Building relationships. Sharing knowledge.* Retrieved from http://www.lilly.com/SiteCollectionDocuments/Media%20Kits/MDR-TB/Case%20Studies%20for%20Global%20Health.pdf.

Ottenberg, A., Wu, J. T., Poland, G., A., Jacobsen, R. M., Koenig, B. A., & Tilburt, J. C. (2011). Vaccinating health care workers against influenza: The ethical and legal rationale for a mandate. *American Journal of Public Health, 101,* 212–216. doi:10.2105/AJPH.2009.190751

Owusu-Edusei, K., Chesson, H. W., Leichliter, J. S., Kent, C. K., & Aral, S. O. (2013). Association between racial disparity in income and reported sexually transmitted infections. *American Journal of Public Health, 103,* 910–916. doi:10.2105/AJPH.2012.301015

Panel on Opportunistic Infections in HIV-exposed and HIV-infected Children. (2014). *Guidelines for the prevention and treatment of opportunistic infections in HIV-exposed and HIV-infected children.* Retrieved from http://aidsinfo.nih.gov/contentfiles/lvguidelines/oi_guidelines_pediatrics.pdf

Panel on Opportunistic Infections in HIV-infected Adults and Adolescents. (2014). *Guidelines for the prevention and treatment of opportunistic infections in HIV-infected adults and adolescents.* Retrieved from http://aidsinfo.nih.gov/contentfiles/lvguidelines/adult_oi.pdf

Perry, R. T., Gacic-Dobo, M., Dabbagh, A., Strebel, P. M., Okwo-Bele, J.-M., & Goodson, J. (2013). Global control and regional elimination of measles, 2000–2011. *Morbidity and Mortality Weekly Report, 62,* 27–31.

Peterson, A., Clark, L., Oh, T., Pavlin, J., Russell, K. L., & Chitale, R. A. (2013). Department of Defense response to a multistate outbreak of fungal meningitis—United States, October 2012. *Morbidity and Mortality Weekly Report, 62,* 800.

Polio Eradication Department, World Health Organization. (2012). Update on vaccine-derived polioviruses—Worldwide, April 2011–June 2012. *Morbidity and Mortality Weekly Report, 61,* 741–746.

Polio Eradication Department, World Health Organization. (2013a). The global polio eradication initiative Stop Transmission of Polio (STOP) program, 1999–2013. *Morbidity and Mortality Weekly Report, 62,* 501–503.

Polio Eradication Department, World Health Organization. (2013b). Progress toward eradication of polio—Worldwide, January 2011–March 2013. *Morbidity and Mortality Weekly Report, 62,* 335–338.

Pour, A. M., Allensworth, C. D., Clark, T. A., Liang, J. I., Bonner, C., Messonnier, M. I., et al. (2011). *Morbidity and Mortality Weekly Report, 60,* 5–9.

Priest, P. C., Jennings, L. C., Duncan, A. R., Brunton, C. R., & Baker, M. G. (2013). Effectiveness of border screening for detecting influenza in arriving airline travelers. *American Journal of Public Health, 103,* 1412–1418. doi:10.2105/AJPH.2012.300761

Rapues, J., Wilson, E. C., Packer, T., Colfax, G., & Raymond, H. F. (2013). Correlates of HIV infection among transfemales, San Francisco, 2010: Results from a respondent-driven sampling study. *American Journal of Public Health, 103,* 1485–1492. doi:10.2105/AJPH.2012.301109

Renaud, T. C., Wong, M. R., Boccur, A., Udeagu, C. N., Pickett, L., Alt, E. N., . . . & Bergier, E. (2011). The effect of HIV field-based testing on the proportion of notified partners who test for HIV in New York City. *American Journal of Public Health, 101,* 1168–1171. doi:10.2105/AJPH.2011.300129

Rice, E., Barman-Adhukari, A., Milburn, N. G., & Monro, W. (2012). Position-specific risk in a large network of homeless youths. *American Journal of Public Health, 102,* 141–147. doi:10.2105/AJPH.2011.300295

Rossheim, B., Goodman, S., Bryant, N., Winters-Callender, M., Kurkjian, K., White-Comstock, M. B., . . . Collier, M. (2013). Transmission of HBV among assisted living facility residents—Virginia, 2012. *Morbidity and Mortality Weekly Report, 62,* 389.

Rotblatt, H., Montoya, J. A., Plant, A., Guerry, S., & Kerndt, P. R. (2013). There's no place like home: First year use of the "I know" home testing program for chlamydia and gonorrhea. *American Journal of Public Health, 103,* 1376–1380. doi:10.2105/AJPH.2012.301010

Rothschild, B. M. (2005). History of syphilis. *Clinical Infectious Diseases, 40,* 1454–1463.

Rowe, A., Onikpo, F., Lama, M., Osterholt, D., & Deming, M. S. (2012). Impact of a malaria-control project in Benin that includes the integrated management of childhood illness strategy. *American Journal of Public Health, 102,* 2333–2341. doi:10.2105/AJPH.2010.300068

Rupprecht, C. E., Brenner, E., Cox, S., Giurgiutiu, D., Drociuk, D., Blanton, J. D., . . . Tack, D. (2013). Human rabies—South Carolina, 2011. *Morbidity and Mortality Weekly Report, 62,* 642–644.

Sagawa, M., Kojimahara, N., Otsuka, N., Kimura, M., & Yamaguchi, N. (2011). Immune response to influenza vaccine in the elderly: Association with nutritional and physical status. *Geriatrics & Gerontology International, 11,* 63–68. doi: 10.1111/j.1447-0594.2010.00641.x

Satterwhite, C. L., Gottlieb, S. L., Romaguera, R., Bolan, G., Burstein, G., Schuler, C., et al. (2011). CDC grand rounds: Chlamydia prevention: Challenges and strategies for reducing disease burden and sequelae. *Morbidity and Mortality Weekly Report, 60,* 370–373.

Sawyer, M., Liang, J. L., Messonnier, N., & Clark, T. (2013). Updated recommendations for use of tetanus toxoid, reduced diphtheria toxoid, and acellular pertussis vaccine (Tdap) in pregnant women—Advisory Committee on Immunization Practices (ACIP), 2012. *Morbidity and Mortality Weekly Report, 62,* 131–135.

Seaworth, B. J., Field, K., Flood, J., Saliba, J., Mase, S. R., Cronin, A., . . . Chorba, T. (2013). Interruptions in supplies of second-line antituberculosis drugs—United States, 2005–2012. *Morbidity and Mortality Weekly Report, 62,* 23–26.

Seither, R., Shaw, L., Knighton, C. L., Greby, S. M., & Stokley, S. (2013). Vaccination coverage among children in kindergarten—United States, 2012–2013 school year. *Morbidity and Mortality Weekly Report, 62,* 607–612.

Serse, R., Euler, G. L., Gonzalez-Feliciano, A. G., Bryan, L. N., Furlow, C., Weinbaum, W., & Singleton, J. A. (2011). Influenza vaccination coverage—United States, 2000–2010. *Morbidity and Mortality Weekly Report, 60*(Suppl.), 38–41.

Singh, D., Fine, D. N., & Marrazzo, J., M. (2011). Chlamydia trachomatis infection among women reporting sexual activity with women screened in family planning clinics in the Pacific northwest, 1997–2005. *American Journal of Public Health, 101,* 1284–1290. doi:10.2105/AJPH.2009.169631

Smallpox history. (2011). Retrieved from http://www.news-medical.net/health/Smallpox-History.aspx

Smith, D. K., Martin, M., Lansky, A., Mermin, J., & Choopanya, K. (2013). Update to interim guidance for preexposure prophylaxis (PrEP) for the prevention of HIV infection: PrEP for injecting drug users. *Morbidity and Mortality Weekly Report, 62,* 463–465.

Stanley, M. M., Guilfoyle, S., Vergeront, J. M., Davis, J. P., Hu, D. J., & Khudyakov, Y. (2012). Hepatitis C infection among young adults—Rural Wisconsin, 2010. *Morbidity and Mortality Weekly Report, 61,* 358.

Stockwell, M. S., Kharbanda, E. O., Martinez, R. A., Lara, M., Vawdrey, D., Natarajan, K., et al. (2012). Text4Health: Impact of a text message reminder-recalls for pediatric and adolescent immunizations. *American Journal of Public Health, 102,* e15–21. doi:10.2105/AJPH.2011.300331

Stokley, S., Curtis, R., Jeyrajah, J., Harrington, T., Gee, J., & Markowitz, L. (2013). Human papillomavirus vaccination coverage among adolescent girls, 2007–2012, and postlicensure vaccine safety monitoring 2006–2013—United States. *Morbidity and Mortality Weekly Report, 62,* 591–595.

Streit, T., Desir, L., Oscar, R., Lemoine, J. F., Purcell, N. C., Keller, A., . . . De Rochars, M. B. (2013). Mass drug administration for the elimination of lymphatic filariasis—Port-au-Prince, Haiti, 2011–2012. *Morbidity and Mortality Weekly Report, 62,* 466–468.

Strick, L. B., MacGowan, R. J., & Belcher, L. (2011). HIV screening of male inmates during prison intake medical evaluation—Washington, 2006–2010. *Morbidity and Mortality Weekly Report, 60,* 811–813.

Sullivan, K., Moore, S. S., & Fleischauer, A. T. (2013). Measles outbreak associated with a traveler returning from India—North Carolina, April–May 2013. *Morbidity and Mortality Weekly Report, 62,* 753.

Syphilis, 1494–1923. (n.d.). Retrieved from http://ocp.hul.harvard.edu/contagion/syphilis.html

Talman, A., Bolton, S., & Walson, J. L. (2013). Interaction between HIV/AIDS and the environment: Toward a syndemic framework. *American Journal of Public Health, 103*, 253–261. doi:10.2105/AJPH.2012.300924

Tanaka-Taya, K., Satoh, H., Arai, S., Yamagishi, T., Yahata, Y., Nakashima, K., . . . Martin, R. (2013). Nationwide rubella epidemic—Japan, 2013. *Morbidity and Mortality Weekly Report, 62*, 457–462.

Thombley, M. L., & Stier, D. D. (2010). *Menu of suggested provisions for state tuberculosis prevention and control laws*. Retrieved from http://www.cdc.gov/tb/programs/laws/menu/TBLawMenu.pdf.

Thomson, K., Dvorzak, J. L., Lagu, J., Laku, R., Dineen, B., Schilperoord, M., . . . Clarke, K. (2012). Investigation of hepatitis E outbreak among refugees—Upper Nile, South Sudan, 2012–2013. *Morbidity and Mortality Weekly Report, 61*, 581–586.

Tieu, H. V., Nandi, V., Frye, V., Stewart, K., Oquendo, H., Bush, B., . . . NYC M2M Study Team. (2014). Concurrent partnerships and HIV risk among men who have sex with men in New York City. *Sexually Transmitted Diseases, 41*, 200–208. doi: 10.1097/OLQ.0000000000000090

Tiwari, T., Clark, T. A., Messonnier, N. E., & Thomas, C. G. (2011). Tetanus surveillance—United States, 2001–2008. *Morbidity and Mortality Weekly Report, 60*, 365–369.

Tondella, M. L., Cassiday, P., Faulkner, A., Messonnier, N. E., Clark, T. A., & Meyer, S. (2012). Pertussis epidemic—Washington, 2012. *Morbidity and Mortality Weekly Report, 61*, 518–521.

Tuberculosis Coalition for Technical Assistance. (2014). *International standards for tuberculosis care: Diagnosis, treatment, public health* (3rd ed.). Retrieved from http://www.thoracic.org/assemblies/mtpi/resources/istc-report.pdf

UNAIDS. (2013). *Global report: UNAIDS report on the global AIDS epidemic, 2013*. Retrieved from http://www.unaids.org/en/media/unaids/contentassets/documents/epidemiology/2013/gr2013/UNAIDS_Global_Report_2013_en.pdf

UNAIDS. (2014). *Global AIDS response progress reporting 2014: Construction of core indicators for monitoring the 2011 Political Declaration on HIV/AIDS*. Retrieved from http://www.unaids.org/en/media/unaids/contentassets/documents/document/2014/GARPR_2014_guidelines_en.pdf

United States President's Emergency Program for AIDS Relief. (n.d.). *ABC guidance #1 (Abstinence, be faithful, and correct and consistent condom use)*. Retrieved from http://www.pepfar.gov/reports/guidance/c19545.htm

U.S. Department of Health and Human Services. (2013). *Healthy people 2010 final review*. Retrieved from http://www.cdc.gov/nchs/data/hpdata2010/hp2010_final_review.pdf

U.S. Department of Health and Human Services. (2014). *Healthy people 2020: Topics and objectives*. Retrieved from http://healthypeople.gov/2020/topicsobjectives2020/default.aspx

U.S. Preventive Services Task Force. (2009). *Screening for hepatitis B virus infection in pregnancy*. Retrieved from http://www.uspreventiveservicestaskforce.org/uspstf/uspshepbpg.htm

U.S. Preventive Services Task Force. (2013a). *Screening for hepatitis C virus infection in adults*. Retrieved from http://www.uspreventiveservicestaskforce.org/uspstf/uspshepc.htm

U.S. Preventive Services Task Force. (2013b). *Screening for human immunodeficiency virus (HIV)*. Retrieved from http://www.uspreventiveservicestaskforce.org/uspstf13/hiv/hivfact.pdf

Wallace, G., Redd, A., Rota, J., Rota, P., Bellini, W., & Lebo, E. (2013). Measles—United States, January 1—August 24, 2013. *Morbidity and Mortality Weekly Report, 62*, 741–743.

Weltman, A., Longenberger, A. H., Moll, M., Johnson, L., Martin, J., & Beaudoin, A. (2013). Recurrent outbreak of Campylobacter jejuni infections associated with a raw milk dairy—Pennsylvania, April–May 2013. *Morbidity and Mortality Weekly Report, 62*, 702.

Wieland, M. L., Weiss, J. A., Olney, M. W., Alemán, M., Sullivan, S., Millington, K., . . . Sia, M. G. (2011). Screening for tuberculosis at an adult education center: Results of a community-based participatory process. *American Journal of Public Health, 101*, 1264–1267. doi:10.2105/AJPH.2010.300024

Wikswo, M. E., & Hall, A. J. (2012). Outbreaks of acute gastroenteritis transmitted by person-to-person contact—United States, 2009–2010. *Morbidity and Mortality Weekly Report, 61*(SS-9), 1–12.

Williams, A. R. (2013, March 13). Mummy finds revealing ancient disease. *National Geographic News*. Retrieved from http://news.nationalgeographic.com/news/2013/03/130321-mummies-diseases-ancient-archaeology-science/

Williams, W. W., Lu, P. J., Greby, S., Bridges, C. B., Ahmed, F., Liang, J. L., . . . Hales, C. (2013). Noninfluenza vaccination coverage among adults—United States, 2011. *Morbidity and Mortality Weekly Report, 62*, 66–72.

Wingood, G. M., Robinson, L. R., Braxton, N. D., Er, D. L., Conner, A. C., Renfro, T. L., . . . DiClemente, R. J. (2013). Comparative effectiveness of a faith-based HIV intervention for African American women: Importance of enhanced religious social capital. *American Journal of Public Health, 103*, 2226–2233. doi:10.2105/AJPH.2013.301386

World Health Organization. (n.d.). *Notification and other reporting requirements under the IHR (2005): IHR brief no.2*. Retrieved from http://www.who.int/ihr/publications/ihr_brief_no_2_en.pdf

World Health Organization. (2008). *International health regulations (2005)* (2nd ed.). Retrieved from http://whqlibdoc.who.int/publications/2008/9789241580410_eng.pdf

World Health Organization. (2012). *Recommendations of investigation of contacts of people with infectious tuberculosis in low- and middle-income countries*. Retrieved from http://apps.who.int/iris/bitstream/10665/77741/1/9789241504492_eng.pdf

World Health Organization. (2013a). *Alert, response, and capacity building under the International Health Regulations (IHR): Alert and response*. Retrieved from http://www.who.int/ihr/alert_and_response/en/

World Health Organization. (2013b). *Diphtheria*. Retrieved from http://www.who.int/immunization_monitoring/diseases/diphteria/en/

World Health Organization. (2013c). *World malaria report 2013*. Retrieved from http://apps.who.int/iris/bitstream/10665/97008/1/9789241564694_eng.pdf?ua=1

World Health Organization, Collaborating Center for Surveillance, Epidemiology, and Control of Influenza. (2011). Influenza-associated pediatric deaths—United States, September 2010–August 2011. *Morbidity and Mortality Weekly Report, 60*, 1233–1238.

World Health Organization, Collaborating Center for Surveillance, Epidemiology, and Control of Influenza. (2013). Update: Influenza activity—United States and worldwide, May 19–September 28, 2013. *Morbidity and Mortality Weekly Report, 62*, 838–842.

World Health Organization, Division of Global Migration and Quarantine. (2013a). Outbreak of poliomyelitis—Somalia and Kenya, May 2013. *Morbidity and Mortality Weekly Report, 62*, 484.

World Health Organization, Division of Global Migration and Quarantine. (2013b). Update: Severe respiratory illness associated with Middle East respiratory syndrome Coronavirus (MERS-Cov)—Worldwide, 2012–2013. *Morbidity and Mortality Weekly Report, 62*, 480–483.

World Health Organization, Division of Global Migration and Quarantine. (2013c). Updated information on the epidemiology of Middle East

Respiratory Syndrome Coronavirus (MERS-Cov) infection and guidance for the public, clinicians, and public health authorities, 2012–2013. *Morbidity and Mortality Weekly Report, 62,* 793–796.

World Health Organization, Regional Office for Africa. (2013). Assessing the risks for poliovirus outbreaks in polio-free countries—Africa, 2012–2013. *Morbidity and Mortality Weekly Report, 62,* 768–772.

Xeuatvongsa, A., Pathammavong, C., Phounphenback, K., Rayburn, R., Feldon, K., Thompson, M. J., . . . Averhoff, F. (2013). Hepatitis B vaccine birthdose practices in a country where hepatitis B is endemic—Laos, December 2011–February 2012. *Morbidity and Mortality Weekly Report, 62,* 587–590.

Yousely-Hindes, K., M., & Hadler, J. L. (2011). Neighborhood socioeconomic status and influenza hospitalizations among children: New Haven County, Connecticut, 2003–2010. *American Journal of Public Health, 101,* 1785–1789. doi:10.2105/AJPH.2011.300224

Zipprich, K., Murray, E. L., Winter, K., Kong, D., Harriman, K., Preas, C., et al. (2012). Mumps outbreak on a university campus. *Morbidity and Mortality Weekly Report, 61,* 986–989.

CHAPTER

27 Chronic Physical Health Problems

Learning Outcomes

After reading this chapter, you should be able to:

1. Describe personal and population effects of chronic physical health problems.
2. Identify biological, psychological, environmental, sociocultural, behavioral, and health system factors that influence the development of chronic physical health problems.
3. Describe strategies for health promotion related to chronic physical health problems and analyze the role of the population health nurse related to each.
4. Discuss major foci in prevention of chronic physical health problems and identify related population health nursing roles.
5. Identify the major aspects of resolving existing chronic physical health problems and analyze population health nursing roles with respect to each.
6. Analyze population health nursing roles related to health restoration in relation to chronic physical health problems.

Key Terms

activity limitation
cancer navigation
cancer survivors
caregiver burden
chronic disease
disability
disabled persons
impairment
participation restriction
prediabetes
racism-related vigilance
risk markers
self-management
social resistance
stigmatization

Advocacy Then

Fostering Research on Kidney Disease

In 1950, Ada and Harry DeBold's young son developed nephrosis, a condition for which there was no known cure. In an attempt to help their son, they initiated the Committee for Nephrosis Research, which became the National Nephrosis Foundation and in 1964 became the National Kidney Foundation (NKF). Despite her child's death at age four, Ada DeBold continued to raise funds for research and patient services. In 1956, the foundation undertook the first major national fund-raising campaign and raised $400,000. Research led to the development of a Teflon shunt in 1960 that permitted dialysis treatment; converting kidney disease to a chronic condition, rather than a terminal illness. NKF continues to provide public- and patient-focused education, support for research, and advocacy for people with kidney disease. NKF has also been instrumental in the development of clinical practice guidelines for nephrology care and helped create an international program "Kidney Disease: Improving Global Outcomes," which published guidelines related to hepatitis C in the context of kidney disease. That effort was followed by publication of seven additional sets of guidelines. Education of health care providers regarding kidney disease is another significant focus for the foundation (National Kidney Foundation, n.d.).

Advocacy Now

Supplying Health Needs

Afya means "good health" in Swahili. Afya is also the name of a charitable organization that works to meet health resource needs in Africa and the Caribbean. Founded by physical therapist Danielle Butin, Afya focuses on supplying needed supplies, equipment, and humanitarian provisions to developing countries in these regions. Rather than just sending truckloads of supplies that may or may not meet local needs, Afya conducts in-county needs assessments to determine specific equipment and supplies needed. Needs are met through donations of surplus equipment and supplies from U.S. health care institutions, corporations, and private individuals. Individuals and families can donate home care equipment, such as walkers and wheelchairs, when it is no longer needed. Available goods are entered in a computer-based inventory from which health organizations and professionals can select items to meet specific needs (Afya Foundation, n.d.).

In addition, Afya supports other projects to meet identified needs. For example, in Haiti, plastic bottles gleaned from trash piles are used to create lightweight and portable beds and stools to help people keep themselves and their possessions out of the periodic flooding following heavy storms. Another project involved training "Rehab Techs" to deliver home care rehabilitation services and products in tent cities housing survivors of the 2010 earthquake in Haiti (Afya Foundation, n.d.).

Because of the effectiveness of control measures developed for many previously fatal communicable diseases, chronic health problems have largely replaced communicable diseases as the leading causes of death and disability in the United States and elsewhere in the world. Each year, millions of people worldwide experience the suffering and the economic costs associated with chronic health problems, and many die as a result. An estimated 145 million people in the United States, half of the total population, experience at least one chronic condition. This figure is expected to increase by 1% per year to 171 million people by 2030 (Improving Chronic Illness Care, n.d.). Globally, noncommunicable conditions account for 63% of all deaths and outstrip communicable disease mortality in all World Health Organization (WHO) regions except Africa (WHO, 2011).

A **chronic disease** is a condition that persists over a significant period of time that is not amenable to cure, but can be controlled (University of Michigan, Center for Managing Chronic Disease, 2011). Chronic conditions are characterized by uncertain or complex etiologies, multiple risk factors, typically long periods of latency prior to symptom development, a prolonged course of illness, noncommunicability, functional impairment or disability, and an absence of a cure. The standard definition and characteristic features, however, are somewhat blurred by the advent of long-term communicable diseases such as tuberculosis, HIV/AIDS, and chronic forms of hepatitis. A more useful definition has been proposed by an organization called Improving Chronic Illness Care, which notes that a chronic condition is any condition that requires a protracted period of interaction with the health care system and ongoing lifestyle changes for those affected (Improving Chronic Illness Care, n.d.). Based on this definition, chronic conditions include diseases, injuries with lasting consequences, and other enduring abnormalities.

Chronic health problems may be either physical or emotional, and both types of chronic conditions are addressed in the national health objectives developed for the year 2020. These objectives and current levels of achievement may be viewed at the *Healthy People 2020* website. In this chapter, we address chronic physical health problems. Chronic emotional conditions are addressed in Chapter 28∞. Information on selected objectives and their achievement is included at the end of this chapter.

From a population health perspective, the goals of chronic disease prevention and control include reducing their incidence in the population or delaying their onset or the development of resulting functional disability. Additional goals include alleviation of suffering and improving the quality and length of life for those experiencing chronic physical health problems. Unfortunately, a number of deficiencies have been identified in chronic disease control efforts nationally and internationally. These deficiencies include failure to use established practice guidelines for the prevention and treatment of chronic conditions, lack of coordination of care, lack of active follow-up to determine the effects of care, and inadequate education of the public and those affected relative to prevention and self-management of chronic health problems (Improving Chronic Illness Care, n.d.). Population health nurses can be actively involved in resolving these deficiencies and in changing health care delivery from a reactive stance once problems develop to a proactive focus on prevention and effective management that minimizes consequences of chronic conditions.

Individual, Family, and Societal Effects of Chronic Physical Health Problems

Chronic health problems can arise from a variety of sources. For example, some people are born with chronic health problems. Conversely, a person might develop a chronic disability as a result of a serious accident or because of a disease such as arthritis, cardiovascular disease (CVD), chronic respiratory diseases, or cancer. Some chronic conditions, such as some cancers, may result in death. Others, such as arthritis, although not fatal, cause persistent pain and disability.

The effects of chronic health conditions are not only experienced by individuals. Families, population groups, and society at large are also affected by the consequences of chronic health problems.

Individual Effects

The advent of a chronic condition has many personal effects for individual clients. Possible long-term consequences of disease and injury include pain and suffering, hospitalization, disability, and diminished quality of life.

Pain and suffering are frequent accompaniments to chronic health problems, and chronic pain is itself considered an illness. According to the National Research Council (2011), approximately 100 million Americans experience chronic pain at an annual cost to U.S. society of $560 to $635 million. These costs are the result of medical care for pain and lost productivity among those affected. Pain has physical and physiologic effects as well as psychological and cognitive ones, and is a significant contributor to poor quality of life in people with chronic health problems. The constant battle with chronic pain can be disheartening and can lead to depression and possible suicide. Population health nurses can advocate for effective management of chronic pain and promote the use of appropriate pharmacologic and nonpharmacologic management strategies. Pain management with respect to chronic health problems is addressed in more detail later in this chapter.

Pain and other consequences of chronic health problems often lead to diminished functional capability and disability. The United Nations Convention on the Rights of Persons with Disabilities noted that disability is a fluid concept that reflects societal attitudes and environmental circumstances (Rutkow, Vernick, Tung, & Cohen, 2013). Conditions that result in disability for one person may not be disabling for another individual. WHO has delineated three dimensions of disability: the impairment of bodily structure or function, activity limitations, and consequent restrictions in participation in normal daily activities (Benjamin et al., 2013). The U.S. Census Bureau (2010) defined disability in the context of difficulty with any of six categories of function addressed in the American Community Survey (vision, hearing, ambulation, cognition, self-care, and independent living) within three domains of disability: communication, activities of daily living (ADLs), and instrumental activities of daily living (IADLs). WHO described **disability** as a complex phenomenon arising from interactions between one's physical health and functional status and the society in which one lives (2014). Disability results from impairments, activity limitations, and participation restrictions. **Impairment** involves an alteration in bodily structure or function, whereas an **activity limitation** is difficulty in performing a given task. **Participation restriction** is an inability to take part in ordinary social interactions (WHO, 2014). According to the U.N. Convention on the Rights of Persons with Disabilities, **disabled persons** are people with long-term physical, mental, intellectual, or sensory impairments that may interfere with their ability to participate equally in the society in which they live (Rutkow et al., 2013). Disability results when health conditions and their interaction with contextual factors interfere with one's ability to function in ways that are expected or desired. For example, a person in a wheelchair whose workplace accommodates his or her mobility limitations is not disabled. The same person, however, might be considered disabled in another country where buildings have not been designed to facilitate wheelchair access.

An estimated 16% of U.S. adults (37.5 million people) have some form of disability, and 43% of them experience more than one functional limitation. Although the prevalence of disability tends to increase with age, more than a third of people with disabilities in the United States are between 45 and 64 years of age (Benjamin et al., 2013). According to the National Center for Health Statistics (NCHS, 2014b), in 2012, 45.6 million people 18 to 64 years of age in the United States had at least one limitation in basic activities of daily living, and 23.8 million had at least one complex activity limitation related to self-care, work, or social interaction. Among older adults (over age 65), 22.5 million experienced basic activity limitations and 12.8 million had complex activity limitations. For example, nearly 15% of women and 10% of men needed help with personal care activities (NCHS, 2011d). Based on 2012 National Health Interview Survey data, 16% of the U.S. population experienced hearing problems, 8.8% had vision problems, and more than 7% were unable to walk a quarter of a mile without difficulty (Centers for Disease Control and Prevention [CDC], 2014).

Some chronic health conditions may make a greater contribution to disability than others. For example, nearly 17% of people with diabetes experienced visual impairment in 2010 (Burrows, Hora, Li, & Saaddine, 2011), and stroke and arthritis are significant contributors to overall disability figures (CDC, 2012d, 2013e). In July 2005, the U.S. Surgeon General issued a *Call to Action to Improve the Health and Wellness of Persons with Disabilities*. The four goals of this initiative are to (a) promote public understanding of disability and the capabilities of persons with disability, (b) increase the capability of health care providers to provide holistic care to persons with disabilities, (c) assist persons with disabilities to promote their own health, and (d) enhance access to the care and services required to promote independence among those with disabilities (Office of the Surgeon General, 2005). Population health nursing intervention and advocacy will be required to accomplish these goals. For example, population health nurses may need to advocate for holistic care for people with disabilities that meets more than physical health needs. Political advocacy may also be needed to assure access to needed services or to promote environmental changes that limit the disabling effects of chronic conditions.

In addition to a diminished quality of life, the presence of disability may impede other health-related behaviors. For example, women with disabilities may be less likely than those without disabilities to receive Papanicolau smears or mammograms due to mobility difficulties. People with disabilities are also more likely than those without to report poor health, 39% versus 9% in one report (Benjamin et al., 2013). This leads to increased health care utilization, with people with disabilities accounting for almost 40% of emergency departments visits each year (Rasch, Gulley, & Chan, 2012).

Activity limitations engendered by disability often require a change in lifestyle. Individuals with arthritis, for example, may need to adjust to their inability to do some things that they have done in the past or may need to learn to use special implements to accomplish everyday tasks like closing a zipper or buttoning a shirt. Similarly, clients with chronic respiratory conditions may find that they are less able to engage in vigorous activity than in the past and may require more frequent rest periods. The client seriously injured in an automobile accident may need to adjust to using a wheelchair. Frequently, such physical limitations make it necessary to rely on others to perform routine tasks of daily living. This enforced dependence on others may, in turn, adversely affect an individual's self-image.

Even when activities are not restricted, the presence of a chronic health problem usually requires lifestyle adjustments. For the person with diabetes or a heart condition, for example, changes in diet are required. The person with diabetes may also need to make changes in eating patterns. This might mean not skipping meals or not eating on the run.

The pain, lifestyle changes, decreased activity levels, and impaired mobility associated with chronic conditions can contribute to social isolation. The chronically ill individual may be less able to interact with others in familiar patterns or be unable to engage in activities that friends and family enjoy. Consequently, this person may feel left out unless concerted efforts are made to incorporate him or her into family and community life. Advocacy may also be required to address integration of those with disabilities into the everyday life of society. The David L. Bazelon Center for Mental Health Law has developed a set of principles for societal integration of people with disabilities that include rights to the following:

- Opportunities to live like others with respect to residence, employment, and social interactions
- Control over their own lives and daily schedules
- Control over where and how they live
- Employment in nonsegregated workplaces with access to supports necessary to promote productivity
- Independent housing other than group homes
- Opportunities to make informed choices
- Government funding to support implementation of the principles. (David L. Bazelon Center for Mental Health Law, 2013)

Family Effects

Chronic health problems have effects on families as well as on the individual affected. Family members with chronic conditions may no longer be able to fulfill their normal family roles, necessitating role reallocation and possibly role overload for other family members. Restructuring of family roles may also affect relationships among family members, changes in self-image and anger for the member with a chronic disease, and increased stress for other family members. Family members may also have to give up work to care for a disabled member, limiting both the opportunity for respite and family income.

Finally, chronic health problems often entail considerable financial burden for both individuals and families. Most chronic conditions require the individual to take prescribed medications for the rest of his or her life, and the cost can escalate rapidly. Add to this the cost of frequent visits to health care providers to monitor the condition and the effects of therapy. Moreover, many individuals with chronic conditions require expensive special equipment or services. Disabled individuals are more likely than those who are not disabled to put off needed health care because of costs and are more likely to live in poverty (Beckles & Truman, 2011). Population health nurses may need to advocate for services and financial assistance for families affected by chronic health conditions.

Societal Effects

Chronic conditions also affect the general population. These effects are reflected in financial costs to society, morbidity, and mortality.

FINANCIAL COSTS. Chronic health problems cost society millions of dollars each year, and the annual costs of disability related to chronic health conditions amount to approximately $400 billion in health care costs alone (Benjamin et al., 2013). Societal costs of chronic health conditions include the direct medical costs of care, the indirect medical costs (e.g., home modification, special education), and other indirect costs such as productivity losses due to the inability to work, limitations on work ability, or premature death. Societal costs due to lost productivity may also apply to family caretakers who cannot be employed because of their caretaking responsibilities.

U.S. medical care related to stroke resulted in costs of $18.8 billion in 2008, with half of this amount spent on hospitalization (Hall, Levant, & De Frances, 2012). Cancer costs in the United States amount to 1.7% of the total gross domestic product (GDP), but are higher in other countries. For example, in Hungary an estimated 3.05% of the GDP is spent on cancer care. Worldwide, an estimated $180 billion is spent each year on cancers of the lung, bronchus, and trachea alone. In 2008, the total global cost of cancer in terms of premature death and disability and excluding direct treatment costs was an estimated $895 million or 1.5% of the global GDP. Other chronic conditions account for significant costs as well. For example, the global costs of heart disease (excluding treatment costs) in 2008 was $753 billion, with cerebrovascular disease costing $298.2 billion, diabetes $204.4 billion, and chronic obstructive pulmonary disease (COPD) $203.1 billion (American Cancer Society, 2010).

In the United States, 2010 expenditures for cardiovascular diseases, including heart disease and stroke, amounted to $444 billion (Farley et al., 2012), and direct medical care costs related to hypertension amount to $47.5 billion per year (CDC, 2013a). In 2007, the direct medical costs for diabetes care were $116 billion, with another $58 billion related to disability, lost productivity, and premature mortality, for a total cost of $174 billion (CDC, 2011a). Arthritis, the most common cause of disability, accounts for $128 billion in expenditures per year (Cheng, Hootman, Murphy, Langmaid, & Helmick, 2010), and the medical costs for obesity amount to $147 billion annually (Hootman, Helmick, Hannan, & Pan, 2011). Similarly, secondhand smoke exposure related to mortality and years of productive life lost amounted to $6.6 billion in 2006 (Max, Sung, & Shi, 2012).

Accidental injuries also contribute a major portion of societal costs related to chronic conditions. In 2009, for example, productivity and lost wages costs for all unintentional injuries amounted to $357.4 million, with another $147.3 for medical costs (National Safety Council, 2011). According to a report prepared for the Institute of Medicine (IOM), the annual direct and indirect costs of epilepsy are estimated at $15.5 billion (National Center for Chronic Disease Prevention and Health Promotion [NCCDPHP], 2011b), with direct medical costs amounting to $9.6 billion per year. Indirect costs of epilepsy due to lost productivity and quality of life are believed to be far higher (England, Liverman, Schultz, & Strawbridge, 2012). It would seem clear from these cost figures alone that the United States can no longer bear the burden of chronic disease and must take steps to control these and other chronic conditions.

MORBIDITY AND MORTALITY. Societal costs of chronic health conditions are measured not only in dollars but also in terms of the extent of morbidity resulting from these conditions. Although some progress has been made in preventing mortality due to chronic conditions, their prevalence has been increasing over the years. Because the reporting of chronic health conditions is not mandatory, however, prevalence figures probably

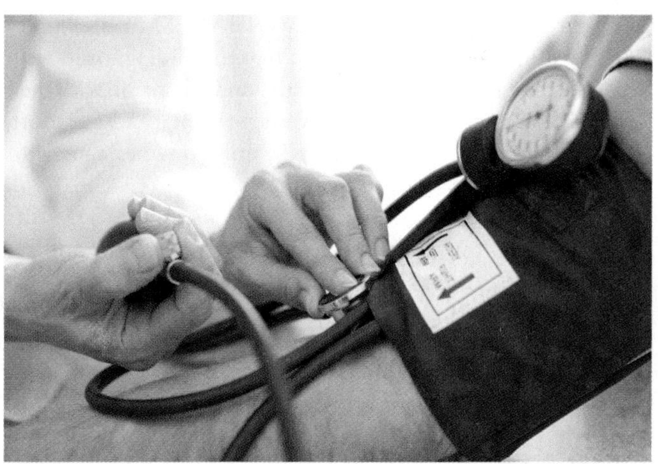

Hypertension is one of the most prevalent chronic health problems. *(Kurhan/Fotolia)*

grossly underrepresent the extent of these conditions in the population.

Approximately half of all Americans are dealing with some form of chronic condition in themselves or in family members. Twelve percent of U.S. children have special care needs, and 23% of those children experience significant effects of their conditions. Among adults, 7% of those 45 to 54 years of age and 37% of those over age 75 are managing three or more chronic conditions (Ryan & Sawin, 2009). Chronic disease mortality also poses a significant burden in the United States and worldwide. In 2008, for example, noncommunicable diseases accounted for 63% of all deaths worldwide or 36 million deaths (WHO, 2011). U.S. age-adjusted heart disease mortality in 2010 was 179.1 per 100,000 population, while cerebrovascular mortality was 39.1 per 100,000, and mortality due to malignant neoplasms was 172.8 per 100,000. Mortality rates per 100,000 population for chronic lower respiratory diseases, unintentional injury, diabetes, and cirrhosis were 42.7, 38.0, 20.8, and 9.4 per 100,000 people, respectively (NCHS, 2014b). In 2010, an estimated 200,070 avoidable deaths occurred in the United States as a result of heart disease, stroke, and hypertension, a decline of 29% from 2001 (Schieb, Greer, Ritchey, George, & Casper, 2013). Similarly, declines in mortality for other conditions have been achieved. For example, in-hospital stroke mortality increased from 21% in 2005 to 23.7% in 2009, but ischemic stroke mortality declined from 6.2% to 5.1% (George, Tong, & Yoon, 2011). Age-adjusted cardiovascular mortality decreased by more than 30% from 1999 to 2009, and cancer mortality declined by almost 12% in the same time period (NCHS, 2011a).

In spite of these gains, however, the incidence and prevalence of chronic conditions continue to rise. Approximately one third of Americans have hypertension, and the self-reported prevalence of hypertension increased from nearly 26% to more than 28% from 2005 to 2009, with nearly 60% of people over 65 years of age affected (Fang, Ayala, Loustalot, & Dai, 2013). By 2009–2012, this figure had increased to 30% of the U.S. population (NCHS, 2014b). Based on data from the National Health and Nutrition Examination Survey (NHANES) from 2005 to 2008, less than 44% of people who have been diagnosed with hypertension have their blood pressure under control, with men less likely to achieve control than women (Keenan & Rosendorf, 2011). In addition, approximately 14 million Americans with hypertension are unaware of their disease status (CDC, 2013a). Hypertension accounted for 38.9 million medical office visits and 3.6 million outpatient department visits in 2010 and resulted in 26,634 deaths (NCHS, 2014c).

Hypertension is a major risk factor for heart disease and stroke (Fang et al., 2013). According to the 2009 Behavioral Risk Factor Surveillance Survey (BRFSS), a median of 5.9% of the population across the states had coronary heart disease (Li et al., 2011). Coronary heart disease prevalence decreased from 6.7% of the population to 6% between 2006 and 2010 (Fang, Shaw, & Keenan, 2011). Despite this decline, approximately 300,000 people experience an out-of-hospital cardiac arrest each year, and 92% of them die. Part of the reason for this level of mortality is the failure of bystanders to provide CPR (only a third of cases from 2005 to 2010 received bystander CPR) or treat the arrest with an automated external defibrillator (AED) (3.7%) (McNally et al., 2011).

Over 6.2 million people in the United States have experienced a stroke, and stroke is the fourth leading cause of death. In 2010, the stroke mortality rate was 41.9 deaths per 100,000 population (NCHS, 2012). From 1999 to 2009 the rate of hospitalization for stroke declined by 20% for persons 65 to 74 years of age, 24% for those in the next decade, and 20% for those 85 years of age and older. Despite these gains, more than a million stroke hospitalizations occurred in 2009 (Hall et al., 2012).

Diabetes is another significant contributor to both heart disease and stroke. In 2010, 26 million people in the United States had diabetes, and another 79 million were prediabetics (CDC, 2012b). **Prediabetes** is a condition in which blood glucose and HgA1c levels are higher than normal, but not yet high enough for a diagnosis of diabetes. Only approximately 11% of those with prediabetes are aware of the condition and, without intervention and changes in lifestyle, are at risk for progression to diabetes (Li, Geiss, Burrows, Rolka, & Albright, 2013). Diabetes prevalence increased by more than 82% from 4.5% in 1995 to 8.2% in 2010 among people 18 years of age and older (Geiss et al., 2012). Diabetes incidence and prevalence data are available by state from the web-based atlas created by the Division of Diabetes Translation (2014). For further information about the atlas, see the *External Resources* section of the student resources site.

Cancer incidence across all types of cancers was 443.1 per 100,000 population in 2010 (NCHS, 2014b). In the 2009 BRFSS, a median of 9.9% of U.S. adults reported having had a diagnosis of cancer (Li et al., 2011), and 1.4 million invasive cancers were diagnosed that year (Singh, Henley, Wilson, King, & Eheman, 2013). Survival rates have improved for most cancers. Survival rates reflect the number of people with a diagnosed condition who are still alive after a given period of time (usually 5 or 10 years for most cancers). From 1971, the number of U.S. cancer survivors increased from 3 million to 11.7 million from 1971 to 2007 (Rowland et al., 2011). One of the *Healthy People 2020* objectives is to increase overall 5-year cancer survival rates to 72.8% of those diagnosed. In 2009, 65.5% of those with a cancer diagnosis had survived for at least 5 years (U.S. Department of Health and Human Services [USDHHS], 2014a), and 39% of people with cancer responding to the 2009 BRFSS had survived for more than 10 years (Underwood et al., 2012). Reasons for increased survival rates include earlier diagnosis as a result of cancer screening programs, the availability of more effective therapies, prevention of secondary disease among persons with cancer, and a decrease in mortality from other causes, leading to longer survival with cancer. Care of cancer survivors will assume greater importance as this objective is achieved and will be addressed in more detail later in this chapter.

Asthma affects about 25.7 million adults and children in the United States, and the number of those affected increased by nearly 3% per year from 2001 to 2010 (Moorman et al., 2012). In the 2006–2008 National Health Interview Survey, current asthma prevalence was 9% among children and 7.3% among adults (Moorman, Zahran, Truman, & Molla, 2011). As noted in Chapter 16∞, asthma accounts for more school absences than any other condition, and in 2008 children with asthma missed 10.5 million school days. Asthma is also a significant problem in the workplace, and one in six people with asthma experience a worsening of their condition due to occupational exposures. In addition, approximately 11 million U.S. workers are exposed to at least one asthmagen in the workplace (American Lung Association, 2014a). Typical asthma triggers at work include mold; dust; gases, fumes, and vapors; secondhand smoke; cleaning and personal care products; animal dander; and stress. Outdoor workers may also encounter air pollutants and vehicle exhaust (American Lung Association, 2014b). In 2008, 34% of workers with asthma missed at least 1 day of work for a total of 14.2 million work days lost (Akinbami, Moorman, & Liu, 2011).

Chronic lower respiratory disease, mostly due to chronic obstructive pulmonary disease or COPD, is the third leading cause of death in the United States and affects 5.1% of the adult population (Herrick et al., 2012). Nearly 30% of those with COPD have a history of asthma (Kosácz et al., 2012), but less than half (48%) report daily use of medications to improve respiratory function and only 82% have ever had a diagnostic breathing test (Herrick et al., 2012).

Arthritis is one of more than a hundred conditions affecting joints and connective tissue. Arthritis contributes to nearly a quarter of disability in older people (Hootman, Helmick, & Brady, 2012). Based on NCHS data for 2012, 22% of the noninstitutionalized population in the United States (51.8 million people) had arthritis, and an additional 303,000 nursing home residents (20%) were affected (NCHS, 2014a). In addition, a third of those with arthritis experience severe pain, and 11% are restricted in social interactions because of the disease (Benjamin et al., 2013). Arthritis also affects 300,000 children. By 2030, an estimated 67 million people will suffer from arthritis, and 25 million will experience activity limitations (CDC, 2012d).

Epilepsy is another chronic condition that contributes to morbidity and mortality in the United States and elsewhere. An estimated 2.2 million persons in the United States have epilepsy, and approximately 150,000 new cases are diagnosed each year. An estimated 1 in 26 people will develop epilepsy at some point in their lives (England et al., 2012). More than a third of people with epilepsy continue to experience seizures despite medications. Epilepsy has been linked to social stigma, lost productivity, and decreased quality of life for those affected (NCCDPHP, 2011b). In addition, people with epilepsy are at increased risk for premature mortality due to cardiovascular disease, stroke, hypertension, and respiratory diseases (Kadima, Kobau, Zack, & Helmers, 2013).

Chronic kidney disease (CKD) is the ninth leading cause of death in the United States (CDC, 2013b). An estimated 26 million people have chronic kidney disease, and millions more are at risk. Diabetes and hypertension are major risk factors for CKD (National Kidney Foundation, 2013).

Accidental injuries are another source of chronic disability, and their long-term consequences constitute chronic health conditions of concern to population health nurses. In 2010, for example, 21,000 deaths and 2.6 million nonfatal injuries occurred as a result of motor vehicle accidents (CDC, 2013c). Worldwide motor vehicle accidents kill 3,500 people each day and injure or disable 50 million more each year (CDC, 2012e), but traffic accidents are not the only cause of unintentional injuries. In 2010, in the United States, 120,589 unintentional injury deaths occurred for an age-adjusted mortality rate of 37.89 deaths per 100,000 population (National Center for Injury Prevention and Control [NCIPC], 2013a). In 2012, the age-adjusted rate for nonfatal unintentional injuries was 9,480.61 per 100,000 people, amounting to 29.4 million injuries (NCIPC, 2013c). NCIPC (2013b) has developed a reporting system for injury statistics that includes injury deaths, violent deaths, and nonfatal injuries that permits population health nurses to determine unintentional injury rates in their own areas and assist in designing appropriate control measures. For further information about the web-based Injury Statistics Query and Reporting System (WISQARS), see the *External Resources* section of the student resources site.

Some of the increase in incidence and prevalence figures for chronic health problems is attributable to better diagnosis as well as to the ability to prevent deaths due to these conditions. These and similar figures for other chronic conditions, however, indicate that Americans are making little progress in the prevention of chronic health problems.

Population Health Nursing and Chronic Physical Health Problems

Factors related to biological, psychological, environmental, sociocultural, behavioral, and health system determinants can increase the risk of an individual or a population group with respect to a particular chronic condition. Conversely, determinants may help protect against chronic health problems. In addition, the presence of a chronic health problem might affect factors in each of these areas.

Assessing Risks for and Effects of Chronic Physical Health Problems

Population health nurses assess both individual clients and populations for risk factors that contribute to the development of chronic physical health problems. They would also assess for the presence of chronic conditions and their effects at both individual and population levels. The assessment would be framed in the context of the six categories of determinants of health.

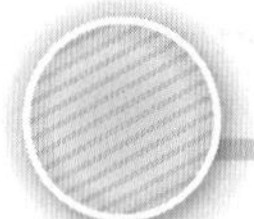

Global Perspectives

The Global Rise of Noncommunicable Diseases

In 2010, the World Health Organization (WHO) published its *Global Status Report on Noncommunicable Diseases* (WHO, 2011). Based on the report, nearly two thirds (63%) of all deaths worldwide in 2008 resulted from noncommunicable conditions, particularly cardiovascular disease, diabetes, cancer, and chronic respiratory diseases. In all regions of the world except Africa, noncommunicable conditions outstripped communicable diseases as a cause of death. Four-fifths of these deaths occurred in low- and middle-income countries, including more than 80% of deaths due to cardiovascular disease and diabetes, nearly 90% of COPD deaths, and two thirds of cancer deaths. In addition, deaths due to these conditions occur at younger ages in lower-income countries, with 29% of deaths occurring before age 60 in low- and middle-income countries compared to only 13% in high-income countries (WHO, 2011).

Four main behavioral risk factors contribute to the global burden of noncommunicable conditions: tobacco use, insufficient physical activity, harmful alcohol use, and unhealthy diet. Worldwide, 6 million deaths are attributed to tobacco use each year. By 2020, this number is expected to increase to 7.5 million, accounting for 10% of all deaths. Among men, smoking is more frequent in lower-middle-income countries, but prevalence is higher for the total population in higher-income countries due to greater participation by women. Physical inactivity causes approximately 3.2 million deaths per year, with those who are inactive having a 20% to 30% increase in their risk of all-cause mortality compared to those who engage in sufficient activity (WHO, 2011).

Harmful alcohol use results in 2.3 million deaths each year, more than half due to chronic conditions such as cancer, cardiovascular disease, and cirrhosis. High-income and upper-middle-income countries have higher per capita alcohol consumption rates than lower-income countries. Increased consumption of salt and saturated fats and trans-fatty acids has been linked to increased prevalence of noncommunicable diseases throughout the world (WHO, 2011).

Biological risk factors, such as elevated blood pressure, overweight and obesity, elevated cholesterol levels, and cancer-related infections also contribute to the global burden of noncommunicable diseases. Hypertension, for example, is estimated to cause 7.5 million deaths per year. Similarly, overweight and obesity result in more than 2.8 million deaths annually, and raised cholesterol is implicated in 2.6 million deaths. Finally, about 18% of cancer deaths are the result of chronic infections with human papillomavirus (HPV), hepatitis B and C, and *Helicobacter pylori*, with a large portion of these deaths occurring in low-income countries (WHO, 2011).

A subsequent report addressed the national capacity of the world's nations to address the growing incidence and prevalence of noncommunicable diseases (WHO, 2012). The report noted that while some countries have some aspects of capacity for addressing noncommunicable conditions, many are woefully lacking in this respect. For example, only 80% of countries had funding available for treatment of these conditions; only 81% had funding for prevention activities. Similarly, although 92% of countries reported at least one policy, plan, or strategy to address noncommunicable conditions, only 79% had at least one operational policy and in only 71% of those countries was policy implementation funded (WHO, 2012).

Surveillance was also an area of concern, with only 48% of countries collecting population-based mortality data, and 23% collecting morbidity data. Similarly, only 59% of countries reported collecting population-based data on chronic disease risk factors. With respect to clinical care activities, only 85% of countries provided prevention and 77% provided risk factor detection services within primary care systems. Even fewer provided self-management support (58%) or home-based care (50%). Although most countries reported having evidence-based practice guidelines for diabetes or hypertension care or nutrition counseling, less than a third had fully implemented any guidelines (WHO, 2012).

WHO (2012) recommended the use of several low-cost "best buys" or strategies that can rapidly contribute to better chronic disease control. Some of these strategies included tobacco and alcohol control, reduced sodium and trans-fat intake, hypertension control, early detection and treatment for cancer, and blood pressure and glycemic control and foot care for persons with diabetes. Recommendations for action also included a comprehensive approach that addresses prevention and treatment interventions; multisectoral action among government, civil society, and the private sector; and improved surveillance and monitoring (WHO, 2011).

BIOLOGICAL DETERMINANTS. Human biological factors related to age, gender, race and ethnicity, specific genetic inheritance, and physiologic function can increase one's risk of developing several chronic health problems. Factors in each of these areas will be addressed here.

Age, Gender, and Race/Ethnicity. Many people think of chronic health problems as occurring primarily among the elderly, despite the fact that approximately 8% of U.S. children experience some form of limitation related to a variety of chronic conditions, many of which were discussed in Chapter 16∞.

More than 50 million Americans under 65 years of age have one or more chronic health conditions (National Health Council, 2013), and both the incidence and prevalence of chronic conditions rise with increasing age. For example, in 2012, 26% of people 18 to 64 years of age had at least one complex activity limitation due to chronic conditions compared to nearly 59% of those over age 65 (NCHS, 2014b).

Both the young and the elderly are at higher risk than other age groups for accidental injuries and resulting disabilities. In part, this increased risk is due to maturational events of childhood and aging. The inability of a young infant to roll over or support his or her head contributes to suffocation as the leading cause of accidental death and disability in this age group. Similarly, normal toddler development involves a great deal of experimentation that may lead to accidental injury and disability if close supervision and safety precautions are not employed. The risk taking and feelings of invulnerability characteristic of preadolescent and adolescent development place young people at risk for motor vehicle accidents. Among the elderly, death and disabilities due to falls are of the greatest concern. In 2010, for example, falls among older adults resulted in 662,000 hospitalizations and 2.3 million nonfatal injuries treated in emergency departments at a cost of $30 billion for direct medical care. In addition, unintentional fall injuries caused 21,700 deaths among the elderly in the United States (Division of Unintentional Injury Prevention, 2013). Leading causes of fatal and nonfatal unintentional injuries by age are presented in Table 27-1●. As can be seen in the table, falls are the leading cause of unintentional injury for all age groups. Population health nurses can help to educate families and the general public regarding age-appropriate safety measures to prevent injuries. They can also engage in political advocacy to promote safe living and working conditions (e.g., legislation mandating functioning smoke alarms in all residences).

Young children and the elderly are also at higher risk for epilepsy than other age groups. By age 80, for instance, 3% of the U.S. population will have a diagnosis of epilepsy (NCCDPHP, 2011b).

Some chronic conditions and their effects are more prevalent in adults. For example, despite the popular belief that people with arthritis are elderly, most cases of arthritis have their onset in the fourth decade of life. For women over age 45, for example, arthritis is the major cause of activity limitation. Older persons do, however, tend to experience greater disability as a result of this condition. The prevalence of COPD tends to increase dramatically in the fifth through the seventh decades of life, and approximately 12% of people 65 to 74 years of age in the United States experience COPD (Kosacz et al., 2012). The incidence of cancer also increases with increasing age. According to the National Cancer Institute's Surveillance, Epidemiology, and End Results (SEER) data, cancer incidence rates from 2005 to 2010 for people over 65 years of age were

TABLE 27-1 Leading Causes of Fatal and Nonfatal Unintentional Injuries in Order of Frequency, by Age Group

Age Group	Fatal Injuries	Nonfatal Injuries
Infants (birth–1 year)	Suffocation, motor vehicle accidents (MVA), drowning, fire/smoke, falls, poisoning, struck by/against an object	Falls, struck by/against an object, bite/sting, foreign body, fire/smoke, cut/pierced, inhalation/suffocation, MVA
1–4 years	Drowning, MVA, fire/smoke, suffocation, pedestrian, struck by or against an object, falls, poisoning, firearms	Falls, struck by/against an object, bite/sting, foreign body. cut/pierced, overexertion, fire/smoke, dog bite
5–9 years	MVA, fire/smoke, drowning, suffocation, other land transport, pedestrian, firearms, struck by or against an object	Fall, struck by/against an object, cut/pierced, bite/sting, pedalcyclist, overexertion, MVA, foreign body, other transports
10–14 years	MVA, drowning, other land transport, fire/smoke, poisoning, suffocation, firearms, falls, pedestrian, other transport	Falls, struck by/against an object, overexertion, cut/pierced, pedalcyclist, MVA, other transport, bite/sting, dog bite
15–24 years	MVA, poisoning, drowning, other land transport, falls, fire/smoke, firearms, pedestrian, other transport	Being struck by or against an object, falls, MVA, overexertion cut/pierced, bite sting, other transport, poisoning
25–34 years	MVA, poisoning, drowning, falls, other land transport, fire/smoke, suffocation, other transport, pedestrian	Falls, overexertion, struck by/against an object, MVA, cut/pierced, bite/sting, poisoning, other transport
35–44 years	Poisoning, MVA, falls, drowning, fire/smoke, suffocation, other land transport, other transport	Falls, overexertion, struck by/against an object, MVA, cut/pierced, poisoning, bite/sting, other transport
45–54 years	Poisoning, MVA, falls, fire/smoke, drowning, suffocation, other land transport	Falls, overexertion, struck by/against an object, MVA, cut/pierced, poisoning, bite/sting, other transport
55–64 years	MVA, poisoning, falls, fire/smoke, suffocation, drowning, other transport	Falls, struck by/against an object, overexertion, MVA, cut/pierced, poisoning, bite/sting, other transport
Over 65 years	Falls, MVA, suffocation, fire/smoke, poisoning, drowning, other land transport	Falls, struck by/against an object, overexertion, MVA, cut/pierced, poisoning, bite/sting, other transport

Data from: National Safety Council. (2011). *Injury facts 2011 edition.* Retrieved from http://www.nsc.org/Documents/Injury_Facts/Injury_Facts_2011_w.pdf

more than nine times higher than those for younger people (2,113.7 per100,000 population and 224.2/100,000, respectively). Cancer mortality was almost twice as high for older people than for those under 65 years of age (104.1 and 56.1 per 100,000 population, respectively) (Howlader et al., 2013).

In 2010, an estimated 215,000 people under 20 years of age had type 1 or type 2 diabetes (Saydah, Geiss, & Gregg, 2012), less than 1% of this segment of the U.S. population (National Diabetes Information Clearinghouse, 2013). Among people over 18 years of age, the 2011 diabetes incidence rate was almost three times higher among persons 65 to 79 years of age than among those aged 18 to 44 years, and 63% of new cases were diagnosed between the ages of 40 and 64 years (Division of Diabetes Translation, 2013a, 2013b). Similarly, although a stroke can occur at any age, two thirds of strokes in the United States occur over 65 years of age, and the rate of hospitalization for stroke is two-and-a-half times higher in people over 85 years of age than in the 65 to 74 age group (Hall et al., 2012). Asthma affects all age groups with 7 million U.S. children and 18.7 million adults affected in 2010. Approximately 3.1 million Americans over 65 years of age also suffer from asthma (Moorman et al., 2012).

Gender can also influence the risk of developing a variety of chronic health conditions. Boys have a higher incidence of asthma than girls, but among adults, women are more likely to be affected than men (Moorman et al., 2012). Men have a higher incidence of coronary heart disease than women (7.8% vs. 4.8%), and invasive cancer incidence is higher in men than women (Singh et al., 2013). Similarly, diabetes prevalence is higher in men, 8.1 per 100,000 population compared to 7.7 per 100,000 for women (Beckles, Zhu, & Moonsinghe, 2011). Men also have higher incidence rates for cancers than women (502.6 per 100,000 men compared to 401 per 100,000 women in 2010) (NCHS, 2014b). With respect to hypertension, White men and women have similar mortality rates (15/100,000 population), but Black women have higher rates than Black men (50/100,000 compared to 40/100,000) (Hicken et al., 2012). Women, in general, experience more arthritis than men. According to the 2007–2009 National Health Interview Survey, 26% of women reported doctor-diagnosed arthritis compared to only 18% of men. Women were also more likely to report arthritis-related activity limitations than men (44% and 40%, respectively) (Cheng et al., 2010).

For many chronic conditions, race and ethnicity are associated with disparities in chronic disease morbidity and mortality. Race and ethnicity are probably markers for differences in health behaviors, access to health care, and other factors that contribute to the development of disease. **Risk markers** are factors that help to identify persons who may have an elevated risk of developing a specific condition but that do not themselves contribute to its development. For example, Black women have lower incidence rates for breast cancer, but have a 41% higher risk for mortality than White women. In part, this disparity is due to more advanced stage at diagnosis than among White women (Cronin et al., 2012). Overall invasive cancer incidence rates are highest in Blacks and lowest in the American Indian/Alaska Native population (AI/AN) (Singh et al., 2013). Conversely, the AI/AN population is far more likely than other racial and ethnic groups to experience diabetes, with prevalence rates two times higher than those for non-Hispanic Whites (CDC, 2011b). In addition, diabetes mortality is three to four times higher in this population than in the overall U.S. population. Because diabetes is a significant factor in cardiovascular disease, increased diabetes prevalence in the AI/AN population also contributes to a cardiovascular mortality rate two-and-a-half times that of the White population.

Furthermore, cardiovascular deaths tend to occur at younger ages in this population (O'Connell, Wilson, Manson, & Acton, 2012). Both hypertension prevalence and mortality are higher among Blacks than Whites (Hicken et al., 2012). In large part, these differences are due to the degree of blood pressure control achieved in the two groups, with 33% of Whites having controlled their blood pressure compared to only 28% of African Americans (Cuffee et al., 2013).

Arthritis occurs with greater frequency among non-Hispanic Whites and AI/ANs than other groups in the United States. For example, arthritis prevalence is roughly 25% for AI/ANs and 24% for non-Hispanic Whites, followed by non-Hispanic Blacks at 19%. The lowest incidence is found among Hispanics (11%) and Asians/Pacific Islanders (8%). Racial and ethnic minority groups, however, are more likely than non-Hispanic Whites to experience arthritis-related activity limitations, work limitations, and severe pain (NCCDPHP, 2011a). For the most part, the disparities noted in the incidence, prevalence, and effects of chronic physical health problems among racial/ethnic groups are associated with differences in socioeconomic status, access to care, and health-related behaviors. Population health nurses can be actively involved in advocating and providing health promotion education and access to health care services to minimize racial and ethnic disparities in the incidence of chronic health problems.

Genetic Inheritance. Some chronic diseases seem to be associated with genetic predisposition. The Center for Surveillance, Epidemiology, and Laboratory Services (CSELS) has noted that genetic factors play a part in nine of the ten leading causes of death in the United States (CSELS, 2014a). Genetic contributions to chronic disease occur in one of three forms: single gene disorders, such as hemophilia, chromosomal abnormalities such as Down syndrome, and multifactorial disease (e.g., cancer or heart disease) in which genetic factors are one of several contributors to disease (Australian Institute of Health and Welfare, 2013).

Genetic factors primarily interact with environmental and behavioral risk factors to promote disease (CSELS, 2014a). Four mechanisms have been proposed for these gene–environment interactions. In the first mechanism, genetic make-up influences one's response to environmental stressors. Second, genetic factors may enhance one's sensitivity to favorable or adverse environmental conditions. In the third mechanism, some inherited characteristics may fit better with some environments than others. Finally, inherited characteristics may only become manifest in certain challenging or favorable environments (Reiss, Leve, & Neiderhiser, 2013).

Genetic factors have been implicated in a variety of cancers. For example, 2% to 7% of women who develop breast cancer have evidence of hereditary BRCA1 or BRCA2 gene mutations, and 10% to 15% of women who develop ovarian cancer have such genetic mutations. Occasionally, other inherited genetic mutations will contribute to breast or ovarian cancer, but these mutations are not common. The majority of breast and ovarian cancer incidence, however, is not related to genetic mutations (CSELS, 2013c). Similarly, colorectal cancer also has a genetic component in which genes interact with behavioral factors such as obesity and physical activity to cause disease. In some rare cases, colorectal cancer is due to hereditary genetic mutations (CSELS, 2013b).

Genetic disorders may also contribute to heart disease. For example, familial hypercholesterolemia, a relatively common condition, increases levels of low density lipoprotein cholesterol (LDL), leading to greater risk of cardiovascular disease. An estimated 1 in 500 people are affected by this inherited condition (CSELS, 2014c). Genetic factors also play a part in stroke risk through contributions to related factors such as hypertension, heart disease, diabetes, and vascular conditions. For example, in one study, 86% of all early strokes occurred in 11% of families in Utah. Stroke may also occur as a complication of other genetic disorders, such as sickle cell disease (CSELS, 2013d).

In addition, genetic factors have been implicated in being overweight and obese, primarily as a result of responses to environmental factors. Genetic variations may affect hunger and food intake contributing to obesity. Genetic–environmental interaction theories of obesity suggest a mismatch between development of "energy-thrifty" genes in periods of restricted food supplies and today's overabundance of food (CSELS, 2013a). Genetic testing has been suggested for several conditions with known genetic contributions. The Office of Public Health Genomics (CSELS, 2014b) has developed guidelines for genetic testing for specific conditions. For further information about the guidelines, see the *External Resources* section of the student resources site.

Population health nurses can obtain a family history of chronic diseases to help determine an individual client's risk for these conditions. Clients may not be knowledgeable regarding family history of disease, and population health nurses can educate the public regarding the need for family health history information and guide them in its collection.

Physiologic Function. Assessment of physiologic factors related to chronic conditions focuses on three areas: presence of physiologic risk factors, physiologic evidence of existing chronic health problems, and evidence of physiologic consequences of chronic conditions.

Physiologic traits over which one has little control may predispose one to certain chronic illnesses. For example, having fair skin, red or blonde hair, or a tendency to sunburn easily increases one's risk for skin cancers. Preventive interventions (e.g., staying out of the sun, use of sunscreen) can, however, mitigate the effects of these risks.

Certain physiologic conditions may predispose one to develop some chronic health problems. Activity limitations and impaired balance and mobility, for example, may contribute to injuries with long-term consequences. Biomedical risk factors, such as overweight and obesity, hypertension, elevated cholesterol levels, and impaired glucose tolerance also contribute to several chronic health problems (Australian Institute of Health and Welfare, 2013).

Obesity, in particular, contributes to a variety of chronic health problems. Approximately 68% of the U.S. population are obese, and obesity affects one third of White women, 43% of Mexican American women, and more than half of Black women. Figures are slightly lower for men, but encompass about a third of U.S. men (Deputy & Boehmer, 2014; Reitzel et al., 2014). Obesity contributes to and worsens conditions such as heart disease, stroke, and diabetes. Obesity also contributes to asthma, worsens symptoms, and impedes asthma control. For example, in 2010, nearly 39% of people with asthma were obese compared to 27% of those without asthma (National Center for Environmental Health, 2013a). Obesity, in the presence of arthritis, has been linked to disease progression, activity limitations, disability, and diminished quality of life (Hootman et al., 2011). Obese adults with arthritis are 44% more likely to be physically inactive than those with obesity alone, increasing their risk for cardiovascular disease and other health problems (Hootman, Murphy, Helmick, & Barbour, 2011). Obesity has also been shown to decrease functional status in persons with COPD (Ade-Oshifogun, 2012), and childhood obesity is 38% higher in the presence of disability than among children without disability (Benjamin et al., 2013). Obesity also increases the risk for occupational injury. Hypertension, a chronic disease in and of itself, is also a major risk factor for heart disease and stroke (Fang et al., 2013). Hypertension is also one of the two main contributors (with diabetes) to CKD, and, in fact, blood pressure elevation is one of the key indicators of CKD, along with urine albumin and serum creatinine. CKD also causes hypertension (National Kidney Foundation, 2013). Arthritis risk and arthritis-related functional limitations are also increased in the presence of diabetes, and heart disease (Barbour et al., 2013).

Epilepsy also increases one's risk of other chronic conditions. For example, persons who experience active seizures are at increased risk of injury. In addition, people with epilepsy have higher prevalence rates of cardiovascular and respiratory diseases, hypertension, asthma, arthritis, cancer, and peptic ulcer disease. Stroke risk for persons with active epilepsy is eight times that for persons without epilepsy; emphysema risk is more than three times higher, and chronic bronchitis rates are twice as high (Kadima et al., 2013).

Past infection may also be implicated in the development of some chronic conditions. For example, viral infection is suspected as a contributing factor in both cancer and diabetes.

A history of recurrent respiratory infections, particularly a history of severe viral pneumonias early in life, has been found to be associated with COPD. Respiratory allergy and asthma may also be predisposing physiologic factors in COPD, whereas viral infection may be a predisposing factor in childhood asthma. Human papillomavirus (HPV) infection in the form of genital warts has been linked to cervical cancer (Stanley et al., 2012). Hepatitis B and C are major factors in the development of liver cancer and cirrhosis, and there is evidence that HIV infection increases one's risk for myocardial infarction by 50% even when CD4 cell counts are controlled and other factors are accounted for (Freiberg et al., 2013).

Other physiologic conditions may be complicated by the existence of chronic illnesses. For example, diabetes places both the pregnant woman and her child at increased risk of adverse outcomes. Conversely, pregnancy complicates diabetes control. In addition, gestational diabetes mellitus (GDM) is an important contributor to later development of type 2 diabetes (Osgood, Dyck, & Grassman, 2011). GDM occurs in 2% to 20% of U.S. pregnancies and 35% to 60% of women with GDM will develop type 2 diabetes in the ensuing 10 to 20 years (CDC, 2011a).

People with chronic health problems may also develop secondary conditions as a result of their illnesses, and population health nurses caring for these clients should be alert to the development of signs of secondary conditions. For example, a client in a wheelchair may develop pressure ulcers, or a client with diabetes might develop diabetic retinopathy. Diabetes also increases the risk of lower extremity disease, often leading to amputation.

Other examples of secondary conditions include pain, sleep disturbances, fatigue, weight gain or loss, respiratory infections, and falls or injuries. When the nurse identifies the presence of secondary conditions, he or she will refer the client for appropriate medical therapy. Population health nurses can advocate for effective care for health problems to prevent the development of these and other secondary conditions. Tips for assessing the influence of biological factors on chronic health problems in the population are included in the *Focused Assessment* questions provided below.

PSYCHOLOGICAL DETERMINANTS. The major psychological factor contributing to chronic health problems is stress. Stress can result in carelessness and contribute to accidents that lead to chronic disability. Similarly, stress has been implicated as a contributing factor in the development of cancer and cardiovascular disease. Stress may also lead to poor compliance with control measures in persons with diabetes, resulting in diabetic complications. Depression and anxiety have also been associated with the onset of cardiovascular disease and with coronary heart disease survival. Conversely, myocardial infarction increases one's risk for major depressive disorder.

People with disability resulting from chronic conditions are more likely than those without disability to report poor mental health. For example, approximately one quarter of people with disabilities report poor mental health compared to only 6% of the general population (Benjamin et al., 2013).

Mental health status also affects treatment and control of chronic health problems. Conversely positive mental health is linked to better health outcome, such as lower cardiovascular disease risk and greater longevity (Perry, Presley-Cantrell, & Dhingra, 2010). Psychological factors may also influence engagement in risk behaviors for chronic conditions or adherence with treatment regimens for chronic health problems. For example, the concept of social resistance has been advanced as a possible contributing factor to the prevalence of high-risk behaviors among nondominant minority populations. **Social resistance** is a propensity to respond to perceived discrimination and alienation by engaging in everyday resistance behaviors, such as high-risk behaviors, in conscious or unconscious opposition to the majority group (Factor, Williams, & Kawachi, 2013). This perspective has received some preliminary research support, but further work is needed to determine its salience in explaining high-risk behaviors in some populations.

Psychological distress has also been found to play a part in exacerbation of symptoms among people who have asthma. Similarly, people with epilepsy have been shown to have higher rates of psychiatric comorbidity than the general population, particularly for depression and anxiety, often as a result of the social stigma attached to having epilepsy (Kadima et al., 2013).

FOCUSED ASSESSMENT — Assessing Biological Determinants Influencing Chronic Physical Health Problems

- What age groups within the population are most likely to develop specific chronic health problems? What age groups will be most seriously affected?
- Are there racial/ethnic or gender differences in disease incidence? What factors influence these differences?
- Is there a genetic predisposition to common chronic health problems in the population?
- Are there other physiologic conditions present in the population that increase the risk of developing chronic health problems?
- What are the signs and symptoms of the problem?
- What are the physiologic effects of specific chronic health problems? Do problems limit functional abilities or contribute to the development of other health problems?

Some chronic conditions have also been found to have effects on mental and emotional function. Alzheimer's disease comes most easily to mind, but traumatic brain injury may also contribute to personality changes and increased aggressiveness. Similarly, insufficient blood circulation to the brain in congestive heart failure has been suggested as an explanation for mental effects such as memory deficit, diminished learning ability, poor executive function, and decreased psychomotor speed.

Population health nurses can assist individual clients to identify personal psychological resources or refer them to support groups and other similar interventions. They can also advocate for access to psychological counseling, as needed, to help with adjustment to a chronic health problem. The *Focused Assessment* provided below can assist population health nurses in exploring factors related to chronic health conditions in individual clients and in population groups.

ENVIRONMENTAL DETERMINANTS. The effects of physical environmental conditions in terms of chronic illness were first observed in terms of scrotal cancer, the first identified occupational illness. Sir Percival Pott noted that English chimney sweeps had a high risk for cancer of the scrotum due to soot exposures while cleaning chimneys. More recently, chimney sweeps in Sweden have been found to have increased risk for ischemic heart disease, nonmalignant respiratory conditions, alcoholism and liver disease, and increased incidence of esophageal, liver, lung, bladder, hematopoietic, and colon cancers as a result of occupational soot and asbestos exposures (Hogstedt, Jansson, Hugosson, Tinnerberg, & Gustavsson, 2013).

Another obvious link to environmental exposures exists between chronic outdoor work and squamous cell carcinoma. Intermittent exposure, on the other hand, increases the risk of melanoma and basal cell carcinoma. In 2008, nearly 60,000 cases of melanoma were diagnosed, resulting in more than 8,000 deaths (CDC, 2012c). The risk of melanoma increases with the number of sunburns experienced in one's lifetime, and in the 2010 National Health Interview Survey, half of all U.S. adults and nearly two thirds of Whites 18 to 29 years of age reported at least one sunburn in the prior year (Holman, Berkowitz, Guy, Saraiya, & Plescia, 2012). In addition, roughly 58% of White women and 20% of White men aged 18 to 25 years reported use of an indoor tanning device more than 10 times in the prior year (Hartman, Guy, Holman, Saraiya, & Plescia, 2012).

Differential exposure to environmental factors may explain some of the health inequalities among population groups (Degeling & Rock, 2012). For example, elevated blood lead levels have been associated with increased systolic blood pressure, among Blacks but not Whites. This difference has been associated with lower socioeconomic status and greater risk of lead exposures among Blacks (Hicken et al., 2012).

Urban and rural differences in disease incidence have also been noted. For example, cardiovascular disease prevalence is higher in rural than urban areas, primarily due to differences in risk behaviors such as smoking, obesity, and physical inactivity (Melvin et al., 2013). Urban density has been associated with lower body mass index (BMI) and more hours per week of physical activity (James et al., 2013). Conversely, the density of fast food restaurants has been associated with higher BMIs for low-income African Americans. Similarly, household proximity to a fast food restaurant was associated with higher BMI for all income groups, but particularly low-income households (Reitzel et al., 2014).

Physical environmental factors also contribute to chronic health problems such as long-term sequelae of accidents, cancer, and COPD. Road conditions, weather, dangerous conditions for swimming, and other physical safety hazards can contribute to accidents that result in permanent physical disability, and the nurse assesses the existence of these types of hazardous conditions in the community.

The population health nurse also assesses the environment for pollutants that may be carcinogenic. Air pollution, in particular, contributes to COPD and asthma. Other environmental factors that may influence chronic respiratory conditions, particularly those with an allergic basis, include house dust, mites, molds, tobacco smoke, and occupational exposures

FOCUSED ASSESSMENT — Assessing Psychological Determinants Influencing Chronic Physical Health Problems

- Does exposure to stress increase the risk of chronic health problems in the population?
- Do existing psychological problems increase the risk for chronic health problems in the population? If so, in what way does this influence occur?
- Does social resistance play a part in high-risk behaviors related to chronic health problems in the population?
- Do existing psychological problems complicate control of physical health problems? If so, how?
- What are the typical psychological effects of chronic health problems common in the population? Are there psychological effects for family members as well as for the person affected by the problem?
- What is the extent of adaptation to chronic health problems? What factors or conditions facilitate or impede adjustment?

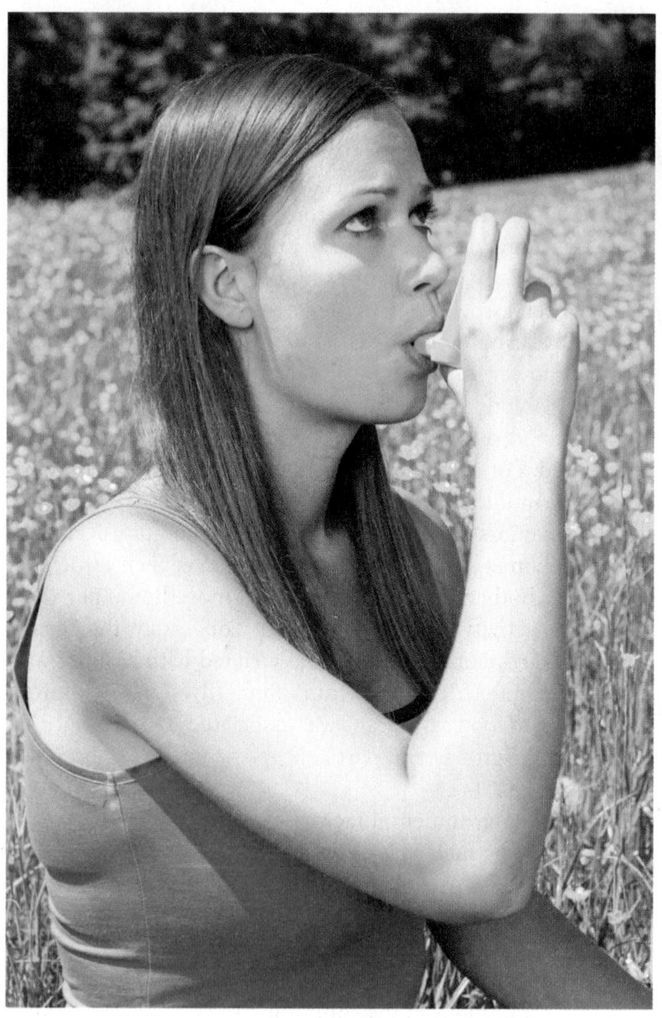

Morbidity and mortality due to asthma are increasing each year.
(Spflaum/Fotolia)

to respiratory irritants. The effects of environmental pollution on health were addressed in more detail in Chapter 4∞.

Global climate changes also affect chronic health problems such as asthma. It is anticipated, for example, that global warming will increase the growth of plant allergens and may prolong periods of seasonal asthma related to pollens.

Population health nurses should also be concerned with the concept of environmental justice. Many environmental hazards are located in low-income neighborhoods, further increasing the effects of poverty and other social factors on health. Advocacy is required to prevent the location of hazardous industries in low-income residential areas and to promote elimination of existing hazards.

The other aspect of the physical environment related to chronic health problems is its effect on the functional abilities of persons with existing chronic conditions. The *disablement process* is influenced by a variety of factors, including the pathology of disease and the environmental conditions that lead to disability in someone with a chronic health problem. For example, substandard housing conditions can lead to fear of falling in older persons with mobility limitations, resulting in social isolation and disability. Similarly, lack of adequate heat increases the growth of molds, exacerbating respiratory problems for people with asthma and other chronic conditions. Population health nurses examine personal and community environmental factors that promote disability in persons with chronic health problems. They may also need to educate clients on dealing with these environmental conditions or advocate for modification of conditions that contribute to chronic disease and/or disability in the population.

The *Focused Assessment* below provides tips for exploring physical environmental considerations as they affect the incidence, prevalence, and effects of chronic health problems in the population.

SOCIOCULTURAL DETERMINANTS. Sociocultural factors contribute to the development of chronic health problems primarily in terms of social conditions, policies, or mores that promote unhealthy behaviors or limit access to care. As some authors have noted, social factors incongruent with health may make it difficult for people to engage in healthy behaviors (Ryan & Sawin, 2009). Major sociocultural determinants to be

FOCUSED ASSESSMENT: Assessing Environmental Determinants Influencing Chronic Physical Health Problems

- Do environmental pollutants contribute to chronic health problems in the population?
- What effect, if any, do weather conditions have on the development or consequences of chronic health problems?
- Do features of rural or urban environments contribute to the development of chronic health problems in the population?
- What influence, if any, do elements of the built environment have on the development of chronic physical health problems in the population?
- Do environmental factors interact with genetic influences to contribute to chronic health problems?
- How do environmental conditions interact with other determinants of health to influence chronic health problems?
- Do chronic health problems in the population or among individuals necessitate environmental changes (e.g., installation of ramps for a wheelchair)?

addressed here include policy issues, employment and income factors, issues of discrimination and isolation, social marketing, and other social factors.

Policy issues. The main policy issue affecting chronic physical health problems is that of tobacco control; 2014 marked the 50th anniversary of the first U.S. Surgeon General's report on smoking and health (Warner, 2014). It is estimated that without the tobacco control efforts during that period, per capita cigarette consumption would be five times what it is today (Warner, Sexton, Gillespie, Levy, & Chaloupka, 2014). In addition, tobacco control policies have been credited with preventing 800,000 deaths from lung cancer alone. States, such as California and Massachusetts, that have most aggressively pursued tobacco control have reduced smoking levels well below averages (roughly 13% for California and 16% for Massachusetts compared to 19% for the nation in 2011 (CDC, 2012a). More recently, the Family Smoking Prevention and Tobacco Control Act of 2009 gave the federal Food and Drug Administration sweeping authority under the Center for Tobacco Products that could be used to control currently unregulated tobacco products such as snuff and little cigars and to mandate reduction of nicotine in cigarettes to nonaddictive levels (Warner, 2014).

Internationally, the World Health Organization's Framework Convention on Tobacco Control requires signatory countries to provide public information on the harm related to tobacco use. Under the convention, warnings on cigarette packages are expected to meet specific criteria related to the size of the message (30% to 50% of the package's principal display area), visibility, and legibility. Warnings are also expected to employ multiple rotating messages and be in the country's main language(s). The 2008–2010 Global Adult Tobacco Survey, conducted in 14 convention countries, indicated that 90% of smokers reported noticing the warnings. In addition more than 50% of those who noticed warnings in six countries considered quitting smoking as a result, and more than 25% considered quitting in all but one of the other countries. Based on these and similar results, WHO has identified package warnings as a "best buy" intervention to promote smoking cessation (Caixeta et al., 2011; 2013a). Warnings have been implemented in 209 countries and have been suggested as a means of reducing disparities related to knowledge of tobacco harm in low literacy groups (Sanders-Jackson, Song, Hiilamo, & Glantz, 2013). The convention has been signed by 177 countries representing 88% of the world's population. Unfortunately, the United States is a notable exception, due to pressure from the tobacco industry (Warner, 2014).

Policies controlling the sale and promotion of tobacco use to minors are also effective in limiting smoking initiation and extent of smoking. In 1992, the Symar amendment to the federal Alcohol, Drug Abuse, and Mental Health Administration Reorganization Act mandated withholding federal funds from states that did not prohibit sales of tobacco to minors. Youth access policies vary from state to state, but generally include warning signs in businesses about youth tobacco purchases and penalties for failure to post such signs, vending machine restrictions, identification requirements, repackaging and free distribution restrictions, and statewide enforcement authority. Most state regulations also include clerk intervention requirements that store clerks retrieve tobacco products from areas other than public-access shelving. Studies have indicated that restricted access during youth results in less smoking in adulthood, but only for women. No single policy has proven to have a significant effect, but it has been suggested that having the full array of policies in effect might reduce lifetime smoking among women by 14%, with a 29% reduction in heavy smoking among those who smoke (Gruzka, Plunk, Hipp, Cavazos-Rehg, & Krauss, 2013). Bans on tobacco product and signage displays have also been effective in reducing tobacco use (Cohen et al., 2011).

Community smoke-free policies and promotion of smoke-free homes are other policy initiatives that can significantly reduce smoking as well as exposure to second-hand smoke (Vijayaraghavan, Messer, White, & Pierce, 2013). In 2000, only one of the 50 largest cities in the United States was covered by comprehensive smoke-free laws. By 2012, this figure had increased to 60%. In 2012 only 20 cities were not covered by either local or state laws, mostly in the South and often in states with laws that preempted local restrictions on smoking (Hopkins et al., 2012). Such laws are not only effective in reducing smoking behavior but also in reducing tobacco-related illnesses. For example, implementation of a statewide smoking ban in Arizona resulted in a significant decrease in hospitalizations for stroke, acute myocardial infarction, angina, and asthma (Herman & Walsh, 2011).

Increased cigarette prices, often through increased taxes, also decrease smoking behaviors. For example, in one study, high cigarette prices (more than $4.50 per pack) were associated with less consumption at all income levels (Vijayaraghavan et al., 2013). From 2010 to 2011, eight states increased their cigarette taxes for a mean state tax of $1.46 per pack. Per pack taxes ranged from a low of 17 cents in Missouri to $4.35 in New York (Tynan, Promoff, & MacNeil, 2012). Some authors caution, however, that increased cigarette taxes may lead to "tax avoidant" behaviors with smokers purchasing untaxed cigarettes "on the street" rather than from authorized dealers. They note a need to pair tax increases with efforts to limit the entry of untaxed cigarettes into the jurisdiction (Coady, Chan, Sacks, Mbamalu, & Kansangra, 2013).

Another policy issue that influences tobacco use includes the current failure to regulate prices and sales of new smokeless tobacco products such as snus (spitless moist snuff), dissolvable oral forms of tobacco in lozenges or breath strips, and electronic cigarettes that vaporize nicotine (Choi, Fabian, Mottey, Corbett, & Forster, 2012). Similarly, the amount of funding available for tobacco control efforts limits the effectiveness of interventions. In 2014, CDC established a minimum nationwide per capita expenditure of $7.41 for tobacco control efforts, with a recommended per capita expenditure of $10.53.Specific expenditure targets have also been established for each state based on the state's socioeconomic outlook. By 2011, however, only two states had met the recommended expenditure targets proposed in 2007 (Office on Smoking and Health, 2014), so concerted effort will be required to meet the new higher recommendations to address tobacco control.

Access to tobacco cessation services is another policy issue that affects smoking prevalence. The Community Preventive Services Task Force (CPSTF, 2014d) has recommended policy changes to limit out-of-pocket expenses for smoking cessation, including medication and counseling. Systematic reviews have indicated that evidence-based cessation strategies increase quit rates and attempts, decrease the prevalence of tobacco use, and can achieve an estimated savings of $2,349 per quality-adjusted life year (QALY) saved. Additional savings related to disability life years averted range from $7,695 to $16,559.

Policy issues influence other factors that contribute to chronic physical health problems. For example, physical activity is known to reduce the risk of multiple chronic problems, yet access to spaces and facilities for physical activity may be limited. One limitation stems from the inability of community members to use school grounds for physical activities due to liability concerns. These concerns can be addressed through careful planning related to community access. For example, school districts can enter into joint use agreements with community organizations that limit school liability. Schools should also address any safety issues in play equipment and facilities through inspection and maintenance (Zimmerman, Kramer, & Trowbridge, 2013).

Income and employment. Economic factors influence both the development of chronic disease and disability and the ability to seek care for existing problems. WHO estimates there are more than 1 billion people with disabilities throughout the world, 200 million of whom have significant functional limitations. Based on World Health Survey data, mean disability levels are higher in low- and lower-middle-income countries than in high-income countries. Even within specific countries disability levels are significantly higher for the poorest segments of the population than the richest (Hosseinpoor et al., 2013).

In the United States, links between socioeconomic status and chronic disease have been established for many illnesses. For example, diabetes prevalence is highest in people living below poverty level (11.7 per 100,000 population) and lowest in those with incomes 400% above poverty (5.5 per 100,000) (Beckles et al., 2011). Similarly, current asthma prevalence among the poor is 11.2% compared to 6.7% for those 450% above the poverty level (Moorman et al., 2012).

Higher income levels are associated with better access to care and better outcomes. For example, the probability of receiving colorectal cancer screening for people at 600% of poverty level is twice as high as for those with incomes below poverty (Huang & Kandi, 2012). Similarly, 21.5% of working adults below poverty level did not get a needed prescription filled due to cost compared to less than 4% of those at 400% of poverty level and above in 2010 (NCHS, 2011b). The effects of poverty are not only experienced at the individual level, but also at the community level. For example, low-income areas are associated with increased risk of asthma rehospitalization and caregiver psychological distress (Beck, Simmons, Huang, & Kahn, 2012). Population health nurses can assess the effects of socioeconomic status on chronic disease incidence and prevalence in the community as well as on access to care.

Occupation, of course, is closely related to income and socioeconomic status, but as we saw in Chapter 23∞, work can also contribute directly to the development of chronic health problems. As one example, nearly 7% of people with asthma, 6% of those with skin conditions, and 69% of those with carpal tunnel syndrome have been told that their condition is work-related (NCHS, 2011c). Safety hazards in the work environment can result in accidents that lead to chronic disability. Clients' occupations may also increase their potential for exposure to various carcinogens found in the workplace. Repetitive movements involved in some jobs can lead to joint injuries and subsequent arthritis. Occupations involving exposure to organic and inorganic dusts or noxious gases increase the probability of COPD. Work-related stress has also been shown to increase the risk of some chronic health problems. Population heath nurses can assess for occupations and working conditions that contribute to chronic health problems in the population or that exacerbate existing problems.

Discrimination, Stigma, and Social Isolation. Perceptions of everyday discrimination have been associated with increased incidence of chronic health problems. Similarly, **racism-related vigilance**, or the expectation that one will be discriminated against as a result of one's race or ethnicity, has been associated with an increase in hypertension risk among African Americans and Hispanics, but not Whites. It is believed that the stress of anticipating discrimination is a contributing factor in hypertension in nondominant groups (Hicken, Lee, Morenoff, House, & Williams, 2014). Perceived racial discrimination may also affect adherence to hypertension medications leading to poor control (Cuffee et al., 2013).

Discrimination may stem from stigmatization of easily recognizable disabilities and other chronic conditions. **Stigmatization** is a social process of attaching unfavorable meaning to behavior and individuals on the basis of certain traits or characteristics. Some chronic health conditions create visible physical evidence, such as the malformed joints often seen in arthritis or the need to use a wheelchair or other assistive devices. The presence of other conditions, such as seizure disorder or developmental disability, may be perceived as evidence of inferiority.

People with disabilities routinely experience social justice issues related to stigma and discrimination. They may be denied the right to make decisions or to marry, and may be subjected to involuntary institutionalization. They also experience lower educational and literacy and higher poverty and unemployment levels than the general population. Stigma is particularly common with respect to epilepsy, which is poorly understood by the general public, and epilepsy is frequently stigmatized in both work and educational settings (NCCDPHP, 2011b).

Stigma and discrimination, as well as functional limitations may contribute to social isolation. Social isolation, in and of itself, has been identified as a significant predictor of illnesses, such as hypertension, and unhealthy behaviors, such as smoking, as well as overall mortality (Pantell et al., 2013). Recent research has shown genetic interactions with social isolation that lead to up-regulation of inflammatory responses and down-regulation of antiviral responses and antibody formation. Ultimately this increases one's risk of inflammatory-type diseases, such as heart disease, neurodegenerative diseases, and some cancers, and decreased immune response to vaccines and viral infections (Cole, 2013).

Conversely, there is convincing evidence that strong social ties may be as influential in preventing mortality as hypertension, smoking, and sedentary lifestyle are in contributing to it. This association is often perceived as one of social support, in which social support from others improves one's health and well-being. Some research, however, suggests that being on the giving, rather than receiving, end of support is beneficial and that actively helping others provides a buffer for the effects of stress in one's own life (Poulin, Brown, Dillard, & Smith, 2013). Further evidence for the effects of social ties lies in findings that increased ethnic density (and potentially increased support networks) is associated with lower cardiovascular disease rates among older African Americans and Mexican Americans (Alvarez & Levy, 2012).

Social marketing. Social marketing strategies have been used extensively to promote unhealthy behaviors such as smoking. For example, tobacco companies have attempted to counteract smoke-free environments policies with the introduction of smokeless tobacco products targeted toward young people. These products are often flavored to attract a younger consumer group and may be gateways to cigarette smoking or substitute for smoking in smoke-free environments (Choi et al., 2012). In 2011, tobacco companies spent 90% of a $8.4 billion budget on advertising and promotion. Point of sale displays have been found to be highly effective in promoting initiation of smoking among youth and in increasing smoking levels in adults. Much of this social marketing has targeted minority and young adult neighborhoods producing environmental triggers to smoking initiation and continuation in these populations (Cantrell et al., 2013). As we saw in Chapter 11∞, however, social marketing strategies can be equally effective in promoting healthy behaviors. Population health nurses can advocate with local and national media for support of health-promoting rather than illness-promoting messages. They may also engage in political advocacy regarding media messages. For example, population health nurses in one community were actively involved in the development of a local ordinance to prohibit billboards advertising tobacco products within a specified distance of elementary and secondary schools.

Cultural factors. Cultural factors may also influence the incidence and consequences of chronic physical health problems. For example, culture may play a role in the extent of support for healthy or unhealthy behaviors that influence the development of chronic health conditions. In many cultures, for instance, use of alcohol is discouraged, so the risk of chronic liver disease due to alcohol intake is reduced. Conversely, nondrinkers would not benefit from the potential positive effects of moderate alcohol intake on cardiovascular disease risk. Cultural factors such as language may influence knowledge of risk factors and health-promoting activities. For example, reading and speaking a language other than English or more fluently than English has been linked to decreased use of screening and preventive services.

Cultural factors may also influence compliance with treatment regimens for chronic conditions. For example, in some cultural groups, health care providers are expected to provide remedies that resolve a problem immediately and group members have difficulty conceiving of conditions that require lifelong use of medications. Similarly, as discussed in Chapter 5∞, traditional cultural remedies may counteract or potentiate the effects of medications prescribed for chronic health conditions.

Tips for assessing the relationship of sociocultural factors to chronic health problems in the community are included in the *Focused Assessment* on the next page.

BEHAVIORAL DETERMINANTS. Behavioral factors are the major contributors to the development of most chronic health problems. Behavioral considerations to be assessed by the nurse include tobacco and alcohol use, physical activity, nutrition, and other health-related behaviors. Usually we think of behavioral factors as negative risk factors that contribute to disease. Research, however, has indicated a positive effect for healthful behaviors. For example, people with four low-risk health behaviors (never smoking, healthy diet, adequate physical activity, and moderate alcohol use) have been found to have significantly lower all-cause mortality risk and mortality risk due to cancers and cardiovascular disease than people who exhibited none of these behaviors (Ford, Zhao, Tsai, & Li, 2011). Whether we focus on health-promoting behaviors or high-risk behaviors, the discussion below highlights the need to modify behaviors related to chronic physical health problems.

Tobacco use. Despite advances in tobacco control, smoking has contributed to 20 million U.S. deaths since 1964 (Warner, 2014). In 2006, 42,000 deaths occurred as a result of secondhand smoke exposure. Nine hundred of those deaths occurred in infants due to in utero exposure to maternal smoking (Max et al., 2012). Although the prevalence of smoking had decreased, the risk of death for smokers compared to nonsmokers increased by more than 25% from 1987 to 2006 (Mehta & Preston, 2012). Worldwide smoking accounts for 6 million deaths per year with

FOCUSED ASSESSMENT Assessing Sociocultural Determinants Influencing Chronic Physical Health Problems

- Do social norms support behaviors that increase the risk of developing chronic health problems (e.g., smoking)?
- How do policy issues affect the development of chronic health problems in the population? What policies are in place for tobacco control? For addressing other risk factors for chronic health problems?
- What effect does socioeconomic status have on the development or effects of chronic health problems?
- Do occupational factors influence the incidence or consequences of chronic physical health problems?
- What are societal attitudes to specific chronic health problems? Do they hamper control efforts? Is there social stigma attached to having the problem? What social support systems are available to people with the problem?
- What is the extent of stigma, discrimination, and social isolation related to chronic health problems? What effects do these conditions have on people with chronic health conditions?
- What effect, if any, do social marketing strategies have on behaviors related to chronic health problems?
- What effect, if any, do cultural beliefs and behaviors have on the incidence of the problem? On treatment of the problem?
- What effect, if any, does legislation have on risk factors for the problem?

600,000 due to second-hand smoke exposure. By 2030, smoking is expected to cause 8 million deaths per year (CDC, 2013d).

Tobacco use is costly to society. For example, U.S. smoking-related costs are approximately $96 billion per year for direct medical care and another $97 billion in lost productivity costs (Agaku, King, & Dube, 2012). Smoking is also costly in terms of property damage. In one study, for example, mean smoking-related costs in California multiunit housing complexes were $4,935 per year in 2008–2009. At that time, slightly more than a third of multiunit housing complexes had completely smoke-free policies, and it was estimated that statewide implementation of such policies would save more than $18 million per year (Ong, Diamant, Zhou, Park, & Kaplan, 2012).

Some headway has been made in controlling tobacco use. For example, the percentage of the U.S. population 18 to 24 years of age who had never smoked increased from 65% in 1999–2001 to 76% in 2011–2012 (NCHS, 2013). Smoking prevalence is highest among persons 26 to 34 years of age and lowest among those over age 65 (Garrett, Dube, Trosclair, Caraballo, & Pechacek, 2011). In spite of laws controlling minors' access to cigarettes, nearly 7% of middle school students and 23% of high school students reported current tobacco use in 2012, and use of cigars, electronic cigarettes, and hookahs increased in these age groups (Arrazola, Dube, & King, 2013).

Use of smokeless forms of tobacco, in general, has been increasing, while cigarette consumption has declined. For example, little cigar sales increased by 221% from 2000 to 2011. Cigar smoking is particularly common among young adults, with first cigar smoking occurring at a mean age of 20.5 years and 11% of people aged 18 to 25 years in the United States reporting smoking little cigars (Cantrell et al., 2013). Similarly, based on the California Tobacco Survey, hookah or bubble pipe use increased more than 40% from 2005 to 2008 and close to 25% of young men in the survey reported ever using a hookah. Hookah smoking is often part of social gatherings. Although there is no research data yet, hookah smoking may be even more harmful than cigarette smoking, but may be perceived as less harmful (Smith et al., 2011). Although advertised as smoking cessation aids, electronic cigarettes or e-cigarettes (battery powered devices that deliver doses of nicotine and other addictive substances by means of an aerosol) are not regulated by the FDA and there are no restrictions on sales to minors. As a result, current use of e-cigarettes increased from 1.1% to 2.1% of 6th- to 12th-grade students from 2011 to 2012 (Corey et al., 2013).

Tobacco use is associated with education level, with college graduates less likely to use tobacco than people with 9 to 11 years of education (7.5% and 36.7%, respectively). Smoking prevalence is highest among the AI/AN population (31.5%), followed by Whites (21%), Blacks (19%), and Hispanics (13%). Lower prevalence among Hispanics is attributed to fewer women smokers in this group (Warner, 2014). Drug use and mental illness are also associated with tobacco use. In fact, people with mental illness (including drug abusers) account for 40% of all tobacco sales in the United States (Hunt, Gajewski, Jiang, Cupertino, & Richter, 2013).

Smoking cessation prior to age 35, results in mortality risks similar to those of nonsmokers. In 2010, nearly 69% of smokers reported wanting to quit and 52% had actually attempted to quit (Malarcher, Dube, Shaw, Babb, & Kaufmann, 2011). Among people with particular needs to stop smoking, fewer than desired have done so. For example, 21% of people with asthma smoke (National Center for Environmental Health, 2013c). Similarly, people with disabilities are more likely to smoke than those without disabilities in some studies (Benjamin et al., 2013), and little change in smoking rates before, during, and after pregnancy occurred from 2000 to 2010 (Tong et al., 2013). Population health nurses can assess the level of tobacco use in the population and its effects on chronic health problems. They can also advocate for and provide education on the harm related to tobacco and provide assistance with smoking cessation. In addition, they can advocate for effective tobacco control policies.

Alcohol use. Alcohol use also contributes to the development of certain chronic health problems and their consequences. For example, alcohol is implicated in motor vehicle accidents, bicycling accidents, fires, falls, and boating accidents, many of which result in chronic disability. Alcohol abuse also contributes to mortality due to chronic liver disease, but moderate alcohol use may have a protective effect for coronary heart disease.

Binge drinking, in particular, has been associated with adverse health outcomes. According to the 2009 BRFSS, more than 20% of men and 10% of women engaged in binge drinking. Men also reported greater frequency of binge drinking and a larger number of drinks per episode than women. Overall prevalence of binge drinking in the U.S. population was 15%. Prevalence was higher among the nondisabled, but frequency and intensity (number of drinks) were higher among disabled individuals (Kanny, Liu, & Brewer, 2011). Population health nurses can assess the extent of alcohol use in the population and its effects in terms of chronic physical health conditions.

Physical activity. Physical activity may enhance the control of diabetes or contribute to hypoglycemic reactions. Physical activity also improves control of arthritis and limits its disabling effects. Both aerobic and strengthening exercises have been linked to improved physical function and decreased disability. Physical activity has also been shown to be directly related to the incidence of heart disease. Several studies have documented that adults with active lifestyles have significantly lower risk of developing heart disease than their less active contemporaries. A sedentary lifestyle, on the other hand, is closely associated with obesity, a risk factor for cardiovascular disease, diabetes, stroke, and arthritis.

An estimated 3.2 million people die each year from the effects of physical inactivity, and inactivity contributes to a 20% to 30% increased risk of all-cause mortality (WHO, 2011). In the United States, a median of just over half of adults engaged in moderate to vigorous physical activity across all states in 2009 (Li et al., 2011). Men were more likely than women to meet aerobic activity and muscle strengthening guidelines, but less than 25% of either gender or any racial/ethnic group did so (Howie, 2013).

Physical activity is beneficial in preventing a number of chronic health problems and in mitigating their effects. Among young adults 25 to 30 years of age, for example, greater levels of physical activity were associated with decreased incidence of hypertension (Parker, Schmitz, Jacobs, Dengel, & Schreiner, 2007). Despite the beneficial effects of physical activity for people with arthritis, however, a 2011 survey indicated that 53% of people with arthritis did no walking, and a median of 66% across states walked less than 90 minutes per week (Hootman, Barbour, Watson, & Fulton, 2013).

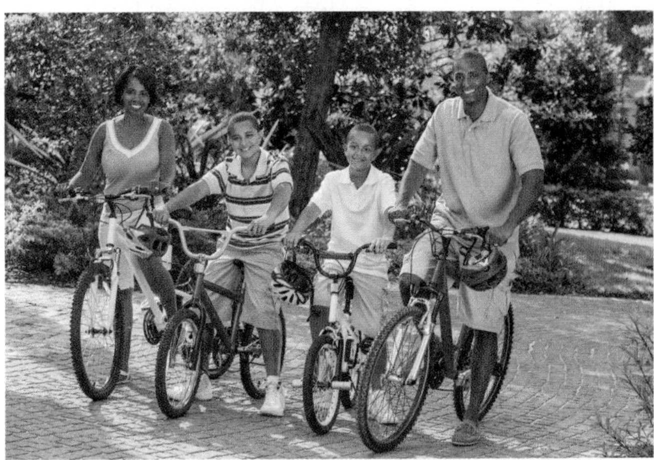

Physical activity helps prevent multiple chronic health problems.
(Spotmatikphoto/Fotolia)

As we saw in Chapter 4∞, elements of the built environment may foster or impede physical activity for the general public. The same is true for individuals with existing chronic illness. For example, some walking trails have exercise stations that promote movement of other muscles than those used in walking. Fewer such trails, however, have activities or facilities designed to promote exercise for someone in a wheelchair or with other limitations. Population health nurses may need to actively advocate for opportunities for physical activity for all segments of the population, including those with disabilities.

Nutrition. Poor dietary patterns contribute to chronic diseases such as diabetes and cardiovascular disease and to obesity, which is a risk factor for these and other chronic conditions. In addition, elevated sodium intake increases the risk for hypertension, heart disease, and stroke. The 2010 Dietary Guidelines for Americans recommended sodium intake less than 2,300 mg per day for the general public, and less than 1,500 grams per day for people over age 50, Blacks, and people with hypertension, diabetes, or CKD. According to the 2005–2008 National Health Assessment and Nutrition Examination Survey (NHANES), 98% of those who should restrict their sodium intake to the lower level failed to do so, and more than 88% of the general population had intake levels above the 2,300 mg recommendation (Loria et al., 2011).

Diet has also been implicated in the development of some forms of cancer. Baseline data for the national health objectives for 2020 indicate that few people meet the targets for 1.1 cup of vegetables per 1,000 calories of dietary intake or 0.6 ounces of whole grains per 1,000 calories. Similarly few people meet the objectives to reduce solid fat and sugar consumption to 16.7% and 10% of daily calories, respectively. Finally, few people achieve the goal of 1,300 mg of calcium per day (USDHHS, 2014b).

Other behavioral factors. Use of complementary and alternative therapies (CAT) is another consumption pattern that should be considered in chronic disease risk and management.

Use of CAT was discussed in Chapter 5. Population health nurses should assess the use of these therapies in terms of their interaction with medications prescribed for chronic diseases and educate clients and the public regarding their safe use. They can also advocate for and conduct research regarding the effectiveness of CAT in controlling chronic health problems, particularly for pain relief.

Another lifestyle behavior that might influence the development and course of chronic conditions includes the use of safety devices and precautions. The use of safety devices and safety precautions can prevent accidents that may result in chronic disability. For example, seat belt use is an important behavioral factor in preventing motor vehicle fatalities. Other safety factors to be considered include the use of bicycle or motorcycle helmets, occupational safety equipment, and so on. Population health nurses would also explore the presence or absence of legislation mandating their use and the extent to which such legislation is enforced.

Other behaviors can contribute to or prevent skin cancer. For example, reducing direct exposure to sunlight (particularly from 10 A.M. to 4 P.M.), using sunscreen protection, and wearing a broad-brimmed hat and other protective clothing can minimize the risk of malignant melanoma.

Another aspect of the behavioral dimension of chronic physical health problems is their effect on client behaviors. Earlier we explored the relationships among chronic illness and functional limitations and disability. The presence of chronic disease may prevent or make it more difficult for people to engage in specific activities. One area that is often neglected is the effect of chronic disease on sexual function. People with asthma and other respiratory conditions may be particularly likely to report sexual limitations. Other conditions that result in fatigue, such as cardiovascular disease and cancer, may also affect sexual function. Finally, as noted in Chapter 17, many medications used to treat chronic conditions may cause sexual dysfunction, particularly among men.

Questions to guide the examination of behavioral influences on the incidence and prevalence of chronic health problems in the population are included in the *Focused Assessment* below.

HEALTH SYSTEM DETERMINANTS. Health system factors may contribute to the development of chronic health problems or influence their course and consequences. Major health system determinants include capacity to address chronic health problems, lack of access to care, lack of a preventive focus, failure to engage in evidence-based practice, and client–provider relationships.

Health system capacity. The World Health Organization (WHO, 2012) has reported limited worldwide capacity to address the problems of noncommunicable diseases, particularly in low- and middle-income countries. It has identified several priorities for improving capacity. These include more effective use of existing health care infrastructures, better surveillance related to morbidity, mortality, and risk factor occurrence, funded policy changes to better support chronic disease control and development of innovative funding strategies, and the development and use of evidence-based guidelines for chronic disease management (WHO, 2012). In the United States, the Council of State and Territorial Epidemiologists (2009) has noted a similar, but less extensive, lack of capacity to monitor chronic disease epidemiology, with less than two thirds of states reporting substantial to full capacity in this area.

Access to care. Access to care is another health system determinant influencing the development and outcomes of chronic physical health problems. This includes lack of access to health care in general and lack of access to disease-specific specialty care. In 2012, for example, nearly 28% of people under 65 years of age with a basic or complex activity delayed or did not receive needed medical care due to cost, and 20.5% did not get a needed prescription filled (NCHS, 2014b). Similarly, in the

FOCUSED ASSESSMENT Assessing Behavioral Determinants Influencing Chronic Physical Health Problems

- Does smoking contribute to the incidence of chronic physical health problem in the population?
- Does alcohol or drug use contribute to chronic physical health problems? What effect does alcohol or drug use have on the development and course of problems?
- What effect does physical activity have on the incidence of chronic physical health problems in the population?
- Do dietary factors influence the incidence of chronic health problems in the population? Does having specific health problems necessitate dietary changes?
- Do chronic physical health problems common in the population necessitate regular medication use or other disease management behaviors (e.g., glucose monitoring)? What is the availability of these treatment modalities? What is the level of compliance with them?
- What effects do self-care behaviors have on the course of chronic physical health problems?
- What effect do safety precautions have on the incidence of chronic physical health problems in the population? To what extent does a common problem necessitate special safety precautions?

2009 National Health Interview Survey, more than half of adults with epilepsy were not seen by a neurological specialist in the prior year (Kobatu, Luo, Zack, Helmers, & Thurman, 2012). Furthermore, people with disabilities are more likely than those without to report not having seen a provider due to cost (Benjamin et al., 2013). People with asthma have also been found to experience cost barriers to adequate care, particularly medications, even when they are insured (National Center for Environmental Health, 2013b). Lack of disability-specific services is another issue with access to care. Some authors have suggested that dental care visits are a good opportunity for oral evaluation for systemic diseases (Strauss, Alfano, Shelley, & Fulmer, 2012), but that presupposes that people obtain dental care, which may not be the case.

Lack of preventive focus. The failure of health care professionals to educate their clients and the general public on the effects of diet, exercise, smoking, alcohol, and other factors in the development of chronic health problems contributes to the increased incidence of these conditions. To some extent this failure may be attributed to time constraints in today's health care system. Some studies have indicated that brief interventions in primary care settings accompanied by telephone counseling and medication assistance have been effective in promoting smoking cessation (Malarcher et al., 2011). A study of screening for tobacco use and cessation advice in 17 countries found wide variation in the extent of provider involvement in these activities (Caixeta, 2013b). Population health nurses and others may need to advocate for changes to reimbursement policies to promote better education for self-management of chronic illnesses.

The extent of screening services for existing chronic conditions may influence their course and effects. The extent to which low-cost screening procedures for various forms of cancer are available varies considerably throughout the country. Although screening services may be obtained from private health care providers, they are often costly, and many low-income people are prevented from taking advantage of them.

Evidence-based practice. Health care system factors influence the availability and quality of treatment obtainable for persons with chronic conditions. For example, provider knowledge and expertise may affect the recognition and treatment of chronic health conditions. Similarly failure to engage in evidence-based practice may also influence the quality of care provided. For example, in the 2009 National Health Interview Survey, only about a third of people with asthma had received a written asthma action plan and just over two thirds had been taught about appropriate responses to symptoms. Likewise, only one third of adults and children with asthma had been given long-acting corticosteroids (Zahran, Bailey, & Garbe, 2011).

Clinical practice guidelines vary in terms of the strength of their underlying evidence base. In one study, the majority of state diabetes programs disseminated a variety of practice guidelines from subspecialty organizations, but had not prioritized them or adapted them for use in specific populations. In addition, 71% of the states indicated that they did not have the capacity to provide guideline-concordant care (Sarkar, Lopez, Black, & Schillinger, 2011). Similarly, in 2009, data from seven states with federally funded stroke registries reported on data related to quality care indicators. According to the report, only 73% of hospitals engaged in dysphagia screening, 70% provided stroke education, and 93% engaged in deep vein thrombosis prophylaxis. In addition, only 57% of hospitals provided intravenous TPA in the event of stroke. Overall, only 69% of the institutions provided "defect-free" in-patient care for ischemic stroke, 57% for hemorrhagic stroke, and 57% for response to transient ischemic attacks (TIAs). In addition, only 72% provided defect-free discharge care for ischemic stroke (George et al., 2011).

Poor quality care occurs in other areas of chronic disease care, as well. For example, methadone is commonly used for chronic noncancer pain relief, yet methadone is responsible for nearly 40% of single opioid deaths, suggesting that providers are not as knowledgeable as they should be in its use for pain relief (Paulozzi, Mack, & Jones, 2012). In other instances, providers may engage in poor care practices even when they know they are inappropriate. For example, two outbreaks of *Staphylococcus aureus* were reported in 2012, both due to multiple injections of pain medications from single dose vials. Reasons given for the inappropriate practice were the inability to obtain single dose vials in the correct dosage amounts and unwillingness to waste medication after first use (Anderson et al., 2012).

Provider failure to provide appropriate screening and preventive services also influences the incidence and course of many chronic physical health problems. The aggressiveness of treatment received also affects the outcome of chronic health conditions. Some studies, for example, suggest that poorer cancer survival rates among low-income populations may be related to reduced access to care. The quality of treatment received for diabetes may also vary widely and affect the consequences of this disease. Medical care, on the other hand, has greatly reduced mortality from cardiovascular and cerebrovascular diseases. This is largely due to a concerted effort to control hypertension, smoking, and diet.

Client–provider relationships. Client–provider relationships are another health system determinant that affects chronic health problems, particularly with respect to adherence to treatment recommendations. Studies have indicated that trust in the medical system in general have been associated with hypertension medication adherence (Cuffee et al., 2013; Elder et al., 2012). Conversely, distrust has been associated with low breast and cervical cancer screening participation (Yang, Matthews, & Hillemeier, 2011) and other health-related behaviors. The *Focused Assessment* on the next page provides questions to guide the examination of health system factors influencing chronic health problems in the population.

Risk factors related to biological, psychological, environmental, sociocultural, behavioral, and health system determinants all influence the development and outcomes of chronic

FOCUSED ASSESSMENT **Assessing Health System Determinants Influencing Chronic Physical Health Problems**

- Do health system factors contribute to the development of chronic physical health problems in the population?
- What health promotion and illness and injury prevention services are available to prevent chronic health problems in the population? Are they widely used? To what extent do health care providers educate the public regarding prevention of chronic health problems?
- Are screening services available for chronic health problems? If so, are persons at risk for the problem adequately screened?
- Are diagnostic and treatment services for chronic health problems available and accessible to those who need them?
- To what extent is evidence-based practice used in the control of chronic physical health problems? Are there alternative therapies that may contribute to the control of problems? Do alternative therapies pose health risks themselves?
- What is the attitude of health care providers to persons with chronic health problems? What is the level of trust accorded to the health care system and health care providers in the population? What effect does trust have on the effectiveness of measures to control chronic physical health problems in individuals and in the population?

physical health problems. Population health nurses use their assessment skills to assess for determinants that contribute to chronic health problems and for existing chronic conditions and their effects. In addition to assessing individual clients for the presence of risk factors for chronic health problems, the population health nurse examines the incidence and prevalence of these risk factors in the general population to determine the potential for chronic health problems in the community. Nurses can also obtain family histories and construct genograms for specific families as described in Chapter 14∞. A *Chronic Disease Risk Factor Inventory* is available on the student resources site to assist the population health nurse in assessing individual and population risk for chronic physical health problems.

Population health nurses are actively involved in efforts to control chronic physical health problems and their effects in individuals and population groups.

Diagnostic Reasoning and Control of Chronic Physical Health Problems

Nursing diagnoses are derived from information collected relative to the incidence and prevalence of chronic health problems in the population and the factors contributing to these conditions. These diagnoses may relate to individual clients or to the general population. Examples of nursing diagnoses related to an individual client are "potential for cardiovascular disease due to smoking and sedentary lifestyle" and "uncontrolled diabetes due to inability to adhere to diabetic diet." At the group level, the nurse might derive diagnoses such as "increased prevalence of lung cancer due to smoking and occupational exposure to carcinogens." In each case, the nursing diagnosis contains a statement of the probable cause or etiology of the problem that directs interventions designed to resolve it.

Planning and Implementing Control Strategies for Chronic Physical Health Problems

Planning interventions related to chronic health problems for individual clients or population groups is based on the understanding of contributing factors derived from the assessment. It is particularly important to involve the client and his or her family or the community in planning solutions to chronic health problems because they will be responsible for implementing the plan or for using services designed. By involving the client/family or community, the nurse can tailor the plan of care to the specific circumstances influencing chronic disease. It is important to remember that the presence of a chronic health problem affects many facets of life. Effective planning accounts for these effects and minimizes the consequences of chronic illness for those affected.

CDC's *Healthy Communities Program* (formerly *Steps to a Healthier US*) is designed to assist local communities to reduce risk factors for chronic diseases and attain health equity within the population. The initiatives are aimed at reducing the incidence and prevalence of heart disease, stroke, diabetes, cancer, obesity, and arthritis. In addition, initiatives focus on reduction of risk factors such as tobacco use and exposure, insufficient physical activity, and poor nutrition (Division of Community Health, 2013). The initiative has produced a series of tools to promote community action related to these chronic conditions. For further information about the tools, see the *External Resources* section of the student resources site.

THE CHRONIC CARE MODEL. The chronic care model was developed to delineate the elements of high-quality chronic disease care and to foster effective interaction between informed clients and providers with the needed expertise to address chronic health issues. Elements of the model include the following:

- A community that mobilizes resources to meet population health needs and fosters partnerships between health care systems and community organizations to enact policies and provide resources needed for effective chronic disease control.
- A health system that embraces change and care improvement, provides incentives for change, and fosters communication and data sharing, evaluation, and correction of errors.
- Self-management support that empowers and prepares patients to manage their health care and engage in assessment, goal-setting, action planning, problem solving, and follow-up. Such support includes information, emotional support, and skill development, and fosters client–provider collaboration in problem definition, priority setting, goal setting, treatment planning, and problem solving.
- A delivery system design with a proactive focus on keeping people healthy that incorporates elements of case management, health literacy, cultural competency, and care coordination and makes routine follow-up part of the standard of care.
- Decision support for health care providers that promotes evidence-based care and use of evidence-based practice guidelines through provider education regarding evidence-based practice and coordination of primary and specialty care.
- Clinical information systems that assure access to key data at individual and population levels to facilitate performance monitoring and quality improvement (Improving Chronic Illness Care, n.d.).

A health system designed around this model will engage in effective care for chronic illness control at all four levels of health care delivery, health promotion, illness and injury prevention, resolution, and health restoration.

HEALTH PROMOTION. General health promotion is aimed at making people healthier and reducing their chances of developing a variety of health problems, including chronic conditions. Health promotion at both the individual and group levels involves promoting a healthier lifestyle and political activity to create conditions that promote health.

Promoting healthy lifestyles. Strategies to promote healthy lifestyles as a means of preventing chronic health problems focus on diet, exercise, and coping skills. The nurse employs the principles of health education discussed in Chapter 11∞ to educate both individual clients and the general public on basic nutrition and specific nutritional requirements based on age and activity level. For example, to prevent obesity the nurse would teach parents about the nutritional needs of infants and young children and encourage a well-balanced diet with minimal amounts of junk food. Similarly, the nurse would teach a pregnant woman, a nursing mother, or a physically active person about their specific nutritional needs. The nurse would also try to inform the general public about proper nutrition.

Access to healthy foods has also been associated with healthier diets. Access to foods such as fruits and vegetables is often related to socioeconomic level. Healthy foods, such as fruits and vegetables, tend to be more expensive when purchased at small neighborhood stores than at supermarkets, thus lessening the ability of low-income families to afford them. Population health nurses may advocate for access to healthy foods in neighborhood stores and may assist local families in cooperative buying to decrease prices. In some areas, nurses may help communities to establish community gardens to improve consumption of fresh produce.

Physical activity is another area in which health education may be required, and nurses would plan to inform both individual clients and the general public about the need for regular physical activity. The nurse might also assist clients to plan ways to incorporate physical activity into their daily routine or develop plans for exercise programs in the community or for employees of local businesses. For example, a simple means of motivating people to climb stairs is to display posters at stairwell entries encouraging use of stairs rather than elevators.

Exercise is also beneficial for people with existing chronic illnesses, and there is a growing emphasis on including people with disabilities in health promotion activities. This includes incorporating them into mainstream programs whenever possible, using approaches common across multiple disabilities (e.g., reduction of physical barriers), and a condition-specific health promotion focus when needed (Benjamin et al., 2013). People with arthritis can be assisted to engage in pain control strategies prior to physical activity and those with COPD can be helped to develop a progressive activity regimen that strengthens their functional capabilities. Population health nurses can help people with these and other chronic conditions to identify avenues for physical activity that are within their capabilities. For certain conditions, such as cardiovascular disease, nurses may suggest a thorough medical evaluation prior to undertaking a rigorous exercise regimen.

Teaching general coping skills is another way for population health nurses to promote health and prevent chronic health problems that are influenced by stress. In this respect, the nurse might assist a harried mother of several small children to develop ways of coping with stress, or the nurse might assist school personnel to develop a program to teach basic coping skills as part of elementary and secondary school curricula. Another approach might be to plan a program to foster adequate coping among employees of local businesses.

Technology provides new avenues for promoting healthy lifestyles among the general public and in clients with chronic diseases. Experts have identified several points at which clients may turn to the Internet for information related to their health. Many people seek information on basic health promotion and health maintenance activities. When symptoms arise, people may seek information on the possible meaning of symptoms, or they may seek to validate a treatment regimen as the appropriate option after diagnosis. Clients may also use the Internet to search for information about their conditions or about specific treatment regimens or options, to identify possible side effects, or to participate in support groups. Population health nurses can make active use of Internet technology to educate clients for health-promoting lifestyles and for self-care when illness occurs. Nurses can also refer clients to credible sources of information and educate them regarding mechanisms for evaluating the credibility of information retrieved from Internet sources.

Political advocacy. Sometimes educational interventions are aimed at informing health policy makers and promoting legislative and regulatory strategies to control chronic illness in the population. Political activity related to health promotion focuses on measures to foster access to health promotion services and to create a healthful environment. Nursing involvement in efforts at this level includes the planning of strategies to influence health policy making discussed in Chapter 9∞. For example, population health nurses might campaign for better access to prenatal care for pregnant women or legislation to prevent or reduce pollution so as to prevent its contribution to chronic respiratory conditions and other chronic health problems.

Political activity by population health nurses might also be required to establish and enforce policies and legislation that foster healthful behaviors. For example, failure to enforce laws related to the sale of tobacco products to minors has enabled youngsters to purchase tobacco. Conversely, enforcement of seat belt legislation has significantly reduced motor vehicle accident fatalities.

ILLNESS AND INJURY PREVENTION. WHO has identified several "best buy" prevention strategies for noncommunicable diseases. These strategies include the following:

- Protection from second-hand smoke and development of smoking bans
- Education on the dangers of tobacco use
- Banning tobacco advertising, promotion, and sponsorship
- Increasing tobacco taxes
- Restricting access to retail alcohol
- Instituting bans on alcohol advertising
- Increasing alcohol taxes
- Reducing salt intake and sodium content in foods
- Replacing trans fats with polyunsaturated fats
- Immunization for hepatitis and HPV (WHO, 2011)

Additional prevention strategies for chronic physical health problems include preventing obesity, promoting tobacco use cessation, and injury prevention.

In the United States, the National Prevention Council developed the *National Prevention Strategy* in 2011. The overall goal of the strategy is to increase the number of people who are healthy at every stage of their lives. The strategy encompasses four strategic directions and seven priorities. The strategic directions include healthy and safe community environments, provision of clinical and community preventive services, empowerment of people for healthful living, and elimination of health disparities among segments of the population. The seven priorities for action are promoting tobacco-free living, preventing drug abuse and excessive alcohol use, promoting healthy eating and active living, and promoting injury and violence-free living, reproductive and sexual health, and mental and emotional well-being (National Prevention Council, 2011). Several of the strategic directions and priorities are relevant to chronic disease prevention and are discussed below.

Preventing obesity. Dietary changes, weight loss, and moderate physical activity can prevent diabetes, obesity, and other related health problems. Increasing food taxes may be a helpful strategy in preventing obesity. Two types of taxes have been suggested: nutrient taxes and category taxes (Franck, Grandi, & Eisenberg, 2013). Nutrient taxes focus on foods that have higher than recommended percentages of fats or sugars (e.g., sugar sweetened fruit juices). Category taxes are taxes assessed on specific categories of foods or beverages. Examples would be a tax on sodas, candy, or snack foods.

Development of modified food products also assists in controlling fat intake. Population health nurses can encourage the food industry to pursue research on food modification. They can also campaign for legislation to require accurate labeling of food packages and disclosure of food contents.

Specific programs for reducing or preventing obesity might focus on increasing physical activity levels. For example, safe walking routes to school and walking school bus programs have been initiated to promote physical activity among children before and after school. In these programs, students walk together to and from school under adult supervision. After-school recreation programs or activity programs in business are other ways of promoting physical activity and preventing obesity.

Smoking cessation assistance. Another approach to preventing multiple chronic health problems is to promote smoking cessation among smokers or prevent smoking initiation among nonsmokers, particularly youth. Efforts to decrease tobacco use constitute one of the most intensive public health initiatives in the last 50 years (Warner, 2014). As effective as these initiatives have been, they are not enough, and even decreasing smoking to 10% of the U.S. population (the *Healthy People 2020* target) will result in more than 100,000 smoking-related deaths per year over the next few decades (Warner, 2014).

Rockland County, New York, has framed its tobacco control efforts in the context of the essential public health services discussed in Chapter 1∞. Application of the essential services model is depicted in Table 27-2•. Application of the model has resulted in a decline in adult smoking prevalence from 16% in 2003 to 9.7% in 2009. In the same time frame smoking prevalence declined to less than 10% among high school students and less than 4% among 8th grade students (Lieberman et al., 2013).

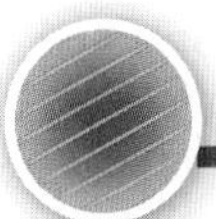

Evidence-Based Practice

Misplaced Evidence

In 2002, the Women's Health Initiative terminated its study of estrogen and progestin due to adverse effects noted in women receiving the study drug Prempro. Because the treatment was often referred to as "hormone therapy" or "estrogen therapy," the study's findings were inappropriately generalized to all forms of hormone replacement, including for women without a uterus who were excluded from the original study. Over a period of 18 months, use of hormone replacement therapy (HRT) for postmenopausal women decreased by about 50%. Both women and providers were anxious to avoid use of HRT despite subsequent findings that estrogen alone provided a protective effect against coronary heart disease for women who had had a hysterectomy. As a result, anywhere from 18,601 to 91,610 women died prematurely as a result of estrogen therapy avoidance (Sarrel, Njike, Vinante, & Katz, 2013).

A similar response was engendered by the results of ethically questionable testing of homeless alcoholic men on New York's Skid Row for prostate cancer in the 1950s and 1960s. A physician recruited members of this vulnerable population in a study to determine the prevalence of prostate cancer using open perineal biopsies. When cancerous cells were found, the surgeons performed radical prostatectomies and orchiectomies with minimal consent, followed by diethylstilbestrol treatment. This practice contributed to the current screen-and-treat paradigm for prostate cancer still in vogue today, despite current evidence that routine screening and radical treatment of prostate cancer are not warranted (Aronowitz, 2014).

These two stories highlight the dangers of relying on the results of one or a few studies and on inappropriate generalization of study findings as a foundation for practice. Population health nurses need to not only keep current with research findings, but also need to examine the strength of the evidence for or against a particular intervention or treatment approach before advocating specific strategies. One strategy to promote the use of evidence-based interventions is to critically evaluate clinical practice guidelines using evaluation guidelines such as SELECT. SELECT is a mnemonic that stands for a six-step process for evaluating and implementing clinical practice guidelines. The six steps are as follows:

- Search: Examination of the practice setting to identify care issues and concerns that suggest a need for a practice change
- Explore the evidence: Identify evidence validating the identified concerns and potential solutions
- Locate existing clinical practice guidelines for best practice interventions relevant to the issue
- Evaluate: Evaluate the process used to develop the practice guidelines and the strength of the evidence base supporting them
- Choose and customize: Select the best guideline recommendations and tailor them to your practice setting
- Translate the guidelines into practice and evaluate their effects (American Professional Wound Care Association, 2010)

TABLE 27-2 Application of the Essential Public Health Services Model to Tobacco Control, Rockland County, New York

Essential Public Health Services	Application
Diagnose and evaluate	Monitored state and local data to set realistic goals
Inform, educate, and empower	Developed student advocacy programs against tobacco industries, created local media campaigns and a smoke-free home campaign
Mobilize community partnerships	Developed a four-county consortium and partnered with multiple local organizations
Develop policies	Created smoke-free school campuses, parks, playgrounds, housing units
Enforce laws	Conducted compliance checks at retail tobacco facilities, bars, and restaurants
Link to/provide care	Provided counseling in multiple languages and links to quitlines
Ensure competent workforce	Trained providers in brief cessation counseling techniques
Evaluate	Conducted an annual tobacco use telephone survey
Monitor	Monitored attitudes and behaviors using an expanded BRFSS survey and a 5-year community assessment

Data from: Lieberman, L., Diffley, U., King, S., Chanler, S., Ferrara, M., Alleyne, O., & Facelle, J. (2013). Local tobacco control: Application of the essential public health services model in a county health departments to Put It Out Rockland. *American Journal of Public Health, 102*, 1942–1948. doi: 10.2105/AJPH.2013.301284

As can be seen in the table, the initiative employed a number of different strategies that have been found to be effective in deterring smoking initiation and promoting smoking cessation among those who smoke. Such strategies include increasing tobacco prices, graphic media campaigns, smoke-free laws, and barrier-free access to cessation assistance (Agaku et al., 2012). CPSTF (2014b) also recommends mass-reach health communications, which have been shown to be effective in decreasing the prevalence of tobacco use, increasing cessation and the use of cessation resources, and decreasing tobacco use initiation. A systematic review of related literature found that mass-reach campaigns resulted in a median increase in quitline calls, decreased median state per capita tobacco consumption to 15 cigarettes per person per year, and increased successful cessation by 2.2% (CPSTF, 2014b). Similarly, CDC's annual national tobacco education campaign resulted in a 75% increase in weekly quitline calls and a 38-fold increase in visitors to its tobacco cessation website (Bright et al., 2013).

Quitlines are effective strategy for promoting smoking cessation, providing information, advice on quitting, and referrals for cessation assistance as well as counseling and support. California was the first state to implement a statewide tobacco quitline, but similar resources are now available in each state and each Canadian province. There have also been calls for the mandatory inclusion of national toll-free quitline numbers on cigarette packages (Leischow et al., 2012). Quitlines are easy to access, cost-free, and can be tailored to individual needs. In addition, they are cost effective, resulting in savings of $2,012 per QALY saved. Even when free cessation assistance medications are included (e.g., nicotine patches), there is a net savings of $795 per QALY (CPSTF, 2014c).

Medications are an important adjunct to smoking cessation that is often neglected in primary care. Studies indicate that people with hypertension are nearly 33 times more likely to receive appropriate medications for their hypertension than smokers are to receive smoking cessation medications. Similarly, diabetes, hyperlipidemia, asthma, and depression are more likely to be treated with medication than smoking. Provider counseling is also more likely for hypertension, diabetes, and hyperlipidemia than for smoking (Bernstein, Yu, Post, Dziura, & Rigotti, 2013).

Tailored interventions may be needed to promote tobacco use cessation in specific target groups. For example, mass media campaigns, insurance coverage of smoking cessation treatment, 100% smoke-free policies, and increased tobacco excise taxes have been particularly recommended for preventing smoking uptake among youth and promoting cessation among pregnant women (Tong et al., 2013). Drug users are another group that needs tailored interventions. As many as 77% to 90% of drug users smoke cigarettes and more than 1 million enter treatment programs each year, but few drug treatment centers provide tobacco cessation treatment. In one study of 405 drug treatment facilities, only 14% provided nicotine replacement therapy, and only two thirds reported their capacity to deal with tobacco addiction as adequate to very good. Similarly, only half had staff with training in tobacco cessation and only one third had protocols, procedures, or curricula in place for addressing smoking. Finally, only 20% reported having the financial resources needed to provide tobacco counseling for their clientele (Hunt et al., 2013).

Population health nurses can be actively involved in providing tobacco cessation counseling or in referring clients for cessation services. They can also advocate for insurance coverage of cessation services and for inclusion of free medication in conjunction with existing tobacco quitlines. Finally, they can be involved in the development of mass media campaigns for the general public or for specific targeted populations such as pregnant women and youth.

Population health nurses may also be involved in political activity to limit smoking. Legislative and regulatory activities to control smoking can be of two types: legislation controlling smoking in public places and taxation of tobacco sales. Public smoking bans and smoke-free workplace policies not only affect smoking behaviors but also limit exposure to *second-hand* or *involuntary* smoking (also called environmental tobacco smoke).

Preventing cardiovascular disease. Prevention of cardiovascular disease has also become a priority in the United States. For example, the *Million Hearts Initiative* was established to prevent 1 million heart attacks by 2017. The initiative is a public–private partnership to decrease cardiovascular disease using evidence-based practice. Two goals of the initiative are to reduce the need for treatment for cardiovascular disease by empowering people to make healthy lifestyle choices and to improve preventive care employing the ABCS (aspirin use for those at risk, blood pressure control, cholesterol management, and smoking cessation). Foci include decreasing tobacco use and second-hand smoke exposure, reducing sodium intake, eliminating artificial trans fats, and providing workplace wellness and media campaigns. Other areas of emphasis are increasing the use of evidence-based practices among health care providers and increasing use of health information technology (Farley et al., 2012).

A similar program, *Healthy Heart, Healthy Family,* has been created to address cardiovascular disease in African Americans, AI/ANs, Filipinos, and Latinos (USDHHS, 2012). The program includes a series of educational materials, heart healthy recipes, and community health worker manuals to minimize cardiovascular disease risk factors in these populations (National Heart, Lung, and Blood Institute [NHLBI], n.d.). For further information about these materials, see the *External Resources* section of the student resources site.

In addition, the CPSTF (2013b) has recommended reducing out-of-pocket costs for treatment for hypertension and hypercholesterolemia to include low- or no-cost medication, behavioral counseling (particularly for weight loss), and behavioral support for gym memberships and weight management programs. In its systematic reviews, the task force found that reducing out-of-pocket costs increased medication adherence and decreased blood pressure and cholesterol levels.

Population health nurses can be involved in educating the public and health care providers regarding interventions to lower cardiovascular disease risk. They can also advocate for better insurance coverage of the cost of preventive strategies.

Injury prevention and other prevention strategies. Other strategies may also help to prevent chronic physical health problems. Injury prevention at home and in occupational settings is one effective approach to the prevention of long-term consequences of unintentional injuries. In addition the "Click It or Ticket" campaign, a national police crackdown on unbelted drivers and passengers conducted every Memorial Day weekend has been shown to be one of the most effective seat belt use strategies.

The use of safety devices and other safety precautions can modify risk factors for accidents that may lead to chronic disability. Population health nurses can encourage clients to install smoke detectors in residences, provide adequate supervision for small children, store hazardous items appropriately, and remove hazards that contribute to falls in the elderly. They can also promote the use of seat belts in vehicles and campaign for legislation that makes seat belt use mandatory in all vehicles (e.g., school buses). Population health nurses can promote use of safety devices and safety precautions in the work setting to prevent accidental injury. Programs to prevent sports and occupational injuries will also help to prevent arthritis. Fall prevention through balance training, correcting visual impairment, limiting medication side effects, and environmental changes can also help to prevent injury, particularly in older populations. Finally, population health nurses can motivate clients to use sunscreen, sunglasses, and protective clothing to prevent melanoma and cataracts. In 2012, the USPSTF recommended counseling for children and young adults to age 24 years on skin cancer prevention (USPSTF, 2012). In addition, CPSTF has developed several recommendations related to parent and caregiver education, policy approaches, and community wide initiatives to promote skin cancer prevention (CPSTF, 2013a).

Modifications of environmental conditions that contribute to chronic health problems may also help to control them. For example, population health nurses can advocate for enforcement of clean-air legislation and promote measures that prevent contamination of drinking water by heavy metals and other agents that cause chronic health problems. Control of environmental conditions, such as radon emissions and air pollution, are particularly important in preventing some forms of cancer. Similarly, nurses and others can campaign for traffic control measures that minimize motor vehicle accidents and subsequent disability. Nurses can also advocate for environmental designs that promote physical activity.

Although usually considered a preventive strategy for communicable diseases, selected immunizations may also prevent chronic diseases. For example, the Advisory Committee on Immunization Practices (ACIP) has recommended hepatitis B vaccine for all adults 19 to 59 years of age with diabetes, and at the discretion of providers for those over age 60 (Sawyer et al., 2011). Similarly, people with chronic diseases are at particular risk for disease and complications due to influenza and pneumococcal pneumonia and should receive the relevant vaccines. In addition, HPV vaccine can prevent genital warts and subsequent cervical cancer and varicella zoster vaccine (VZV) can prevent shingles, particularly in the elderly.

Innovative strategies may need to be employed to inform the public about prevention strategies for chronic health problems. One such strategy is the development of a radio novella series in Spanish "Promesas y Traiciones," produced in Alabama, that focused on chronic disease risk factor reduction. In this project, community members helped develop, implement, and evaluate a series of 48 episodes to address salient chronic disease issues (Frazier, Massingale, Bowen, & Kohler, 2012).

Population health nurses may be involved in educating individual clients and the general public about the need for and availability of vaccines or in designing and providing immunization services. They may also need to advocate for accessible immunization services and coverage of routine immunization under health insurance plans. Health promotion and illness and injury prevention goals in the control of chronic physical health problems and related population health nursing activities are summarized in Table 27-3•.

RESOLVING EXISTING CHRONIC PHYSICAL HEALTH PROBLEMS. Population health nurses are also involved in activities aimed at dealing with chronic health problems once they have occurred. Three major foci in resolving existing chronic conditions are screening and surveillance, early diagnosis, and prompt treatment.

Screening and surveillance. Screening involves identifying individuals who are either at high risk for chronic health problems or who may already have them. Surveillance, on the other hand is a process of monitoring the incidence and prevalence of chronic health problems in the population in order to establish priorities for control efforts. WHO identified three essential components of noncommunicable disease surveillance. These include monitoring exposures and risk factor prevalence, monitoring disease outcomes (e.g., morbidity and mortality), and monitoring health system response. A WHO report on noncommunicable disease capacity indicated that these three components are lacking in most national health information systems and should be integrated into existing systems to promote more effective control of chronic physical health problems (WHO, 2011).

Although the prevalence of many chronic conditions in the population has been increasing, there is less evidence of both upper and lower body limitations that may lead to disability. In all likelihood, this improvement in health status despite increased incidence of disease is due to earlier diagnosis and more effective disease management. Screening is the first step in early diagnosis of many chronic health problems.

Screening tests are available for several chronic health problems but the extent of screening varies across population

TABLE 27-3 Goals for Health Promotion and Injury and Illness Prevention and Related Population Health Nursing Interventions in the Control of Chronic Physical Health Problems

Health Promotion Goal	Nursing Interventions
1. Provide prenatal care.	1. Educate clients and public about the need for prenatal care. Refer to or provide prenatal care.
2. Maintain appropriate body weight through adequate nutrition. • Breast-feed infants. • Delay introduction of solid foods. • Avoid use of food as pacifier or reward. • Establish healthy food habits from childhood.	2. Educate clients and public about adequate nutrition. • Obtain diet history and identify poor food habits. • Assist with breast feeding. • Assist with menu planning and budgeting. • Refer for food-supplement plans as needed. • Encourage use of nonfood reward systems.
3. Engage in graduated program of exercise.	3. Educate public about need for exercise. Assist clients to plan appropriate exercise programs.
4. Develop coping skills.	4. Teach coping skills.
Illness and Injury Prevention Goals	**Nursing Interventions**
1. Decrease obesity prevalence. a. Decrease dietary intake of saturated fats, cholesterol, sodium, and alcohol. b. Provide access to healthy food. c. Modify foods to decrease unhealthy constituents.	1. Educate clients and the public regarding the contribution of obesity to chronic health problems. a. Educate and help clients plan adequate nutritional intake. Foster self-help groups for overeaters. b. Advocate for access to low-cost healthy foods (e.g., fruits and vegetables). c. Advocate for control of fat, sugar, salt content of foods. Promote modification of foods to decrease unhealthy constituents.
2. Decrease tobacco use. a. Prevent initiation of smoking and increase smoking cessation.	2. Educate clients and the public regarding the harm from tobacco a. Foster self-help groups for smokers. • Educate nonsmokers about the hazards of smoking. • Promote no-smoking policies in public places and in the workplace. • Promote smoke-free homes.
3. Decrease cardiovascular disease incidence. a. Identify and treat existing health problems that are risk factors for chronic illness (hypertension, obesity). b. Increase use of evidence-based practices. c. Increase compliance with treatment for diseases contributing to CVD.	3. Educate clients, the public, and providers on strategies to prevent cardiovascular disease. a. Screen for and refer clients with existing conditions. • Educate clients regarding therapy for existing disease. • Educate clients and providers regarding the ABCS of CVD prevention. • Adjust therapy to client's situation when possible. • Monitor for compliance, therapeutic effects, and side effects.
4. Prevent long-term consequences of unintentional injury.	4. Eliminate risk factors for unintentional injury. • Educate client and the public regarding safety hazards and safety precautions. • Advocate for safety legislation and its enforcement. • Prevent occupational and sports injuries through use of safety equipment and practices. • Identify caretaker injury risk factors and plan appropriate interventions. Educate caretakers for injury prevention. Refer for help in obtaining client management equipment and assistive devices. Advocate for funding to provide needed caretaker assistance to prevent injuries.
5. Eliminate environmental pollutants contributing to chronic conditions. a. Decrease exposure to sources of radiation (X-ray, sunlight). b. Eliminate occupational exposure to hazardous substances.	5. Educate public about pollution. Become politically active on environmental legislation. a. Educate public about risks of radiation. • Discourage sunbathing. • Encourage use of sunscreen and protective clothing. b. Monitor occupational safety conditions.
6. Eliminate or modify effects of emotional stress. Avoid stressful situations when possible.	6. Assist clients to identify stressful situations. Explore with clients ways of decreasing stress.
7. Increase immunization to prevent chronic health problems.	7. Educate clients and the public on the need for immunizations that prevent or minimize effects of chronic health problems. Refer for or provide immunization services. Advocate for the availability of immunization services.

groups and conditions. The U.S. Preventive Services Task Force (USPSTF) has recommended several screening tests for chronic health problems many of which have been addressed in other chapters for specific populations (see Chapters 16∞, 17∞, 18∞, and 19∞). Recently, the USPSTF also recommended annual lung cancer screening using computerized tomography for current smokers 55 to 85 years of age or those who quit smoking within the last 15 years who have a 30-pack-year history of smoking (USPSTF, 2013).

Creative strategies may be needed to promote screening in some populations. For example, the emergency department has been suggested as an effective setting to educate clients regarding mammography screening. In one study, for instance, three fourths of respondents indicated their willingness to listen to mammography promotion materials while waiting to be seen (Hatcher, Rayens, & Schoenberg, 2010). Expansion of Medicaid-funded family planning services also served to increase receipt of breast and cervical cancer screening services in low-income populations (Wherry, 2013). Similarly, interventions using tailored motivational messages and peer support by trained volunteers increased mammography screening rates among African American women (Fouad et al., 2010).

Most people with prediabetes are unaware of their status, yet awareness can lead to lifestyle changes that may prevent progression to type 2 diabetes (Li et al., 2013). The latest USPSTF recommendation is for diabetes screening for individuals with treated or untreated blood pressures over 135/80 (USPSTF, 2008), but some authors have recommended routine screening of high-risk populations in emergency departments.

Population health nurses play an important role in screening for chronic illness. They are conversant with the prevalence of various risk factors in the community and can plan screening programs to detect conditions related to the most prevalent risk factors. They may also plan to motivate client participation in screening by educating the public regarding the need for screening. Knowledge of risk factors alone does not motivate the general public to seek screening opportunities, so motivational activities must go beyond educational campaigns. For example, population health nurses may be actively involved in referring clients for screening services and linking disease prevention to other goals valued by clients (e.g., the ability to continue working).

Interpretation of test results and referrals for further diagnosis and treatment of suspected conditions are also functions of population health nurses in relation to chronic health problems. Screening is only effective if clients understand the results of the screening test and the need for further diagnostic evaluation when screening tests are positive. Misunderstanding of screening reports may lead to increased anxiety or failure to act. Population health nurses can be instrumental in helping clients understand the results of screening tests and in educating them regarding next steps when tests are positive.

At the population level, population health nurses may need to advocate for available and accessible screening services for underserved segments of the population. For example, people lacking health insurance were twice as likely as those with insurance not to be screened for colorectal cancer (Klabunde, Joseph, King, White, & Plescia, 2013). Similarly, only 38% of women without health insurance had received a mammogram in the past 2 years in the 2010 National Health Interview Survey, compared to 80% of those with private insurance and 67% with public insurance coverage (Khajuria, 2013). Population health nurses may also need to educate and motivate providers to recommend screening procedures to their clients since provider recommendation has been shown to be a strong predictor of screening for many health conditions.

Early diagnosis. The effects of many chronic health conditions can be minimized when they are diagnosed and treated early in the course of the disease. Positive screening test results are always an indication of a need for further diagnostic testing. Persons with obvious symptoms associated with chronic diseases should also be referred for diagnostic evaluation.

Population health nurses frequently engage in case finding with respect to chronic diseases, identifying community members with possible symptoms of disease and referring them for diagnosis and treatment as appropriate. Population health nurses are also active in educating clients and the general public regarding signs and symptoms of chronic diseases and the need for medical intervention. Population health nurses who are nurse practitioners may also be involved in making medical diagnoses of chronic illnesses.

At the population level, early diagnosis may also involve surveillance for increasing incidence of specific chronic diseases and detection of "outbreaks" in particular populations. For example, a four-step process had been suggested by CDC and the Council of State and Territorial Epidemiologists for investigating reports of cancer clusters. This process includes the following:

- Initial response: Data collection to determine the credibility of the concern and referral to the appropriate agency unit for investigation. Includes exploration of the nature of the concern, demographics of those affected, and any history of prior reporting and response.
- Assessment: Determining if incidence or prevalence figures represent a statistically significant excess of cases, developing a case definition, identifying the population involved and local environmental concerns.
- Major feasibility study: An epidemiologic study of cancer cases and environmental factors of concern, and
- Etiologic investigation of contributing factors (Abrams et al., 2013).

Population health nurses may need to advocate for available and accessible low-cost diagnostic services for chronic health problems. They may also refer individual clients for those services. In addition, they may need to assist clients to deal with the anxiety and uncertainty that accompany the diagnostic process. A systematic review of available research has indicated that increased distress during the diagnostic phase for breast cancer can affect treatment outcomes particularly for women with low education levels and high levels of trait anxiety. It has been suggested that providers may need to engage in interventions to reduce distress from the first mention of a possible cancer diagnosis (Montgomery & McCrone, 2010).

Prompt treatment. The third aspect of resolving chronic health problems is the treatment of existing conditions. The primary public health role in this area lies in promoting and monitoring treatment standards for chronic disease in the personal health care sector. Treatment considerations in chronic conditions include engaging in evidence-based disease management, pay for performance, and promoting and supporting client self-management.

Evidence-based disease management. Unfortunately, many people with chronic illnesses do not receive effective evidence-based clinical services. For example, the percentage of people with self-reported hypertension who reported being treated only increased from 61% in 2005 to 62% in 2009 (Fang et al., 2013) and from 2003 to 2010, only 60% of people with stage 2 hypertension were treated with medication (Valderama, Gillespie, & Mercado, 2013). Similarly, from 2009 to 2010, 17.2% of U.S. adults with diabetes had HgA1c levels indicative of good glycemic control (USDHHS, 2012).

A 2013 report for the Institution of Medicine identified elements of quality cancer care that can be adapted to other chronic health problems as well. The first element is engaged patients who are adequately informed and included in decision making regarding their health and health care. The second element is an adequate health professional workforce that includes coordinated services from generalist and specialist providers who possess core competencies. Use of evidence-based care strategies is the third element of quality care. A fourth element is a "learning" information technology system that supports care decision making, while the fifth element is the translation of evidence into quality care that is supported by quality measurement and performance improvement strategies. The final, and most critical, element is access to affordable care for all who need it. This last element will need to be achieved through reimbursement system reforms and elimination of waste as well as through elimination of disparities in care quality (Levit, Balogh, Nass, & Ganz, 2013). Population health nurses may be involved in evaluating the extent to which chronic care systems address these elements of quality care. They can also be active in advocating changes in care delivery system to promote quality care.

Effective treatment of chronic illness can be facilitated with disease management and decision support systems. The CPSTF defined disease management as "an organized, proactive, multicomponent approach to health care delivery for people with a specific disease, such as diabetes. Care is focused on and integrated across the spectrum of the disease and its complications, the prevention of comorbid conditions, and the relevant aspects of the delivery system" (2014a, para 1). Disease management emphasizes prevention and client–provider collaboration and includes the following components: identification of affected populations; use of evidence-based practice guidelines; collaborative practice including the primary provider, client, and other health care professionals; education of clients for self-management; process and outcomes evaluation; and routine feedback to providers and clients. Disease management has been shown to result in better client health outcomes for several chronic health problems.

Disease management has been shown to be particularly effective in the control of asthma. In 2007, the National Heart, Lung, and Blood Institute (NHLBI) developed expert guidelines for the management of asthma that addressed four essential elements of asthma management: assessment and monitoring, education for a partnership of client and provider in asthma control, control of environmental factors and comorbid conditions, and pharmacologic therapy. The guidelines were subsequently expanded as practice implementation recommendations (NHLBI, 2008). For example, the education guideline was amplified to incorporate collaborative development of an individualized asthma action plan, and pharmacologic recommendations included the use of both rescue medications for acute exacerbations and long-term use of inhaled corticosteroids for better control. Similarly, the assessment and monitoring guideline was operationalized in recommendations for measures of asthma severity, degree of control, and scheduled follow-up visits. Environmental control measures included recommendations for elimination of asthma triggers as well as prevention of comorbidities through influenza immunization. Similar disease management guidelines have been developed for other chronic diseases such as diabetes, cardiovascular disease, and COPD.

Pay for performance. One approach to promoting effective care for chronic physical health problems is to provide incentives for quality care and achievement of specific health outcomes. The Health Care Incentives Improvement Institute has created an innovative reimbursement model called Prometheus that is similar to the Medicare system of diagnosis-related groups (DRGs), but that rewards health systems and providers for prevention of avoidable complications of disease. Approximately one in five Medicare hospitalizations is for potentially avoidable complications of chronic diseases that could be prevented with more effective evidence-based care (de Brantes, Rastogi, & Painter, 2010). An estimated 40 cents of each dollar spent on chronic disease care and 20 cents spent on each hospitalization is the result of potentially avoidable complications (Health Care Incentives Improvement Institute, n.d.b).

Prometheus stands for Provider Payment Reform for Outcomes, Margins, Evidence, Transparency Hassle Reduction, Excellence, Understandability and Sustainability. The Prometheus payment model creates a reimbursement system based on a budget for an entire care episode for a particular disease tailored to a specific patient based on the severity and complexity of their disease. Reimbursement is based on an evidence-informed case rate (ECR), which is a reimbursement rate for a specific package of covered services based on clinical guidelines or expert opinion in the treatment of a particular condition. Whereas Medicare's current practice is to not reimburse providers and health care systems for "never events" or potentially avoidable complications, Prometheus factors in an allowance for these events based on their typical rates of occurrence. Providers would be paid the lump sum based on the ECR including that allowance. If no complications occur, however, the provider retains the allowance as a net gain, thereby rewarding effective care (Health Care Incentives Improvement Institute, n.d.a). It has been estimated that use of such a reimbursement system for six major chronic diseases (congestive heart failure, coronary artery disease, diabetes, hypertension, COPD, and asthma), could reduce the costs of care by approximately 4% (de Brantes et al., 2010), but actual results remain to be seen.

Other approaches to pay for performance are based on the extent to which providers adhere to best practices in disease management. For example, providers would be reimbursed based on whether or not they provide nutrition counseling to diabetic clients or the percentage of patients with asthma who receive a written asthma action plan. Such mechanisms, however, address provider activities, but do not consider actual patient care outcomes.

Promoting and supporting self-management. Another approach to the treatment of chronic physical health problems lies in client self-management. **Self-management** of chronic health problems involves the ability the ability to manage risk factors and deal effectively with symptoms and treatment regimens and to adjust to the physical and psychological effects of a chronic condition. Self-management also requires knowledge of when to seek medical assistance. The impetus for the current emphasis on self-management by clients with chronic health problems lies in the economic burden posed for society by these conditions. Self-management encompasses three phenomena: a process, a program, and outcomes. Self-management programs are intended to prepare clients to assume responsibility for managing their illness or engage in health promotion behaviors. From an outcomes perspective, self-management should result in better control of the chronic condition and better quality of life for the person affected (Ryan & Sawin, 2009).

Self-management differs from self-care, which is the performance of activities of daily living independent of the health care system (Ryan & Sawin, 2009). Rather, self-management involves self-monitoring, decision making, and action. Monitoring includes both awareness and measurement of one's health status and condition, while symptom management includes awareness of and response to physiologic, cognitive, or functional changes (Richard & Shea, 2011). Self-management skills include problem solving, decision making, resource utilization, formation of effective relationships with providers, development of an action plan, and tailoring the plan to address personal needs and conditions. Common self-management foci across multiple chronic conditions include symptom management, medication adherence, recognition of acute episodes, promoting good nutrition and physical activity, smoking cessation, stress reduction, interaction with health care providers, obtaining information, adapting to work, managing relations with others, and managing emotions (Ryan & Sawin, 2009).

Some authors have cautioned against an overemphasis on self-management, suggesting that a focus on client responsibility for managing their own conditions may lead to a greater emphasis on cost-containment than quality of services (Baumann, 2012). Others have noted that health care providers are often ill-equipped to assist clients in the acquisition of self-management knowledge and skills (Ryan & Sawin, 2009).

Effective control of chronic health problems should incorporate both evidence-based disease management by health care providers and appropriate self-management by clients. Population health nurses and other health professionals can support clients in the development of needed self-management skills. The Agency for Health Care Research and Quality (AHRQ, 2014) has collected a number of resources to assist health care providers to promote clients' self-management of chronic conditions. For further information about the AHRQ materials, see the *External Resources* section of the student resources site.

Monitoring treatment effects. Another important aspect of resolving chronic physical health problems for individual clients involves monitoring treatment effects. This includes monitoring both therapeutic effects and side effects of treatment. For instance, the nurse may obtain or review periodic blood pressure measurements for the client with hypertension. If the nurse determines that antihypertensive therapy has not noticeably affected the client's blood pressure, the nurse would make sure that the client is taking the medication appropriately and refer the client to his or her primary provider for further follow-up. The nurse also monitors clients for the presence of side effects related to treatment. For example, the nurse may note that a client is experiencing postural hypotension due to antihypertensive medications and will then educate the client about the need to change position gradually and will continue to monitor blood pressure levels to be sure that they do not drop too low.

At the population level, population health nurses will monitor the effects of health care delivery programs in reducing the incidence of chronic health problems or in promoting their control in the population. The goal of monitoring the therapeutic effectiveness of interventions may also require population health nurses to advocate for routine treatment-monitoring services. For example, although effective diabetes management includes annual dilated eye examinations, foot examinations, and glycosylated hemoglobin (HbA1c) determinations, clients with diabetes may not receive these services. Goals for resolving chronic physical health problems and related population health nursing interventions are summarized in Table 27-4●.

TABLE 27-4 Goals for Resolving Existing Chronic Physical Health Problems and Related Population Health Nursing Interventions

Goal	Nursing Interventions
1. Screening a. Perform periodic health examinations. b. Periodically screen for chronic disease.	1. Screen for existing chronic diseases. a. Educate public about need for health examinations. Provide periodic examinations. b. Educate public about need for periodic screening. Plan and implement screening programs for high-risk groups.
2. Early diagnosis	2. Educate public about warning signs and symptoms of chronic disease. a. Engage in case finding and refer for diagnosis as appropriate. b. Prepare client for diagnostic procedures (physically and emotionally). c. Conduct diagnostic tests as appropriate.
3. Prompt treatment a. Stabilize condition as soon as possible. b. Establish treatment regimen. • Medication • Radiation • Chemotherapy • Surgery c. Provide evidence-based disease management. d. Promote and support self-management. e. Prevent disease progression.	3. Assist with management of chronic disease. a. Provide emergency care as needed. • Educate public to provide emergency care (CPR). • Refer for further treatment. b. Prepare client for treatment procedures (physically and emotionally). • Carry out treatment regimen. • Provide supportive measures during treatment (relief of pain). • Educate clients about medications: dosage, side effects, etc. • Encourage client compliance with treatment. c. Educate providers for evidence-based disease management. • Disseminate evidence-based clinical guidelines. • Advocate for pay-for-performance reimbursement mechanisms. d. Educate and motivate clients for self-management. e. Monitor therapeutic effects of treatment. • Monitor side effects. • Refer for follow-up as needed.

HEALTH RESTORATION. The aim of health restoration with respect to chronic physical health problems in individual clients is to promote the client's optimal level of function despite the presence of a chronic health problem. This entails preventing further loss of function in affected and unaffected systems, restoring function, monitoring health status, assisting the client to adjust to the presence of a chronic condition, and providing palliative and end-of-life care as needed.

Preventing loss of function in affected systems. Chronic health problems frequently result in some loss of function in organ systems affected by the condition, and health restoration activities should be planned to restore function or prevent further loss of function in these systems. Activities may be planned to minimize losses or to eliminate risk factors that might lead to adverse consequences of the condition. Such activities on the part of the population health nurse might include motivating client adherence to treatment recommendations and assisting clients to identify and change risk factors that may lead to further loss of function. For example, the client who has had a myocardial infarction may be assisted to plan a regimen of diet and exercise that will prevent future infarcts. Population health nurses can advocate for the development of and access to restoration services for those in need of them. In addition, nurses can promote clients' active participation in rehabilitation activities for myocardial infarction as well as for stroke, COPD, and other chronic health problems.

Clients with arthritis may be assisted to identify safety factors in the home that might contribute to falls, leading to further mobility limitation. Other interventions aimed at preventing further loss of function in people with arthritis include weight and physical activity counseling and education to address pain management and other problems leading to disability. Population health nurses can provide counseling and education in these areas or refer clients for these services. They may also advocate for access to these services by promoting coverage under health insurance plans or fostering the development of such services for the uninsured.

Pain management may be another intervention that helps to limit loss of function in both affected and unaffected body systems. Pain management will be discussed in more detail in the section on promoting adjustment to chronic health problems.

Preventing loss of function in unaffected systems. Chronic health problems may also result in loss of function in other physical and nonphysical systems not directly affected by the condition. For example, the client with arthritis may develop skin lesions due to limited mobility, or the client with COPD may become malnourished because meal preparation is too exhausting.

Nursing interventions will be directed toward preventing both physical and social disability. Physical complications of chronic conditions may be prevented by activities such as teaching breathing exercises to clients with COPD and providing good skin care and teaching foot care for clients with diabetes. Clients may also need help in managing fatigue, a frequent effect of chronic health problems, particularly COPD and asthma. Prevention of additional physical effects may also entail immunization. Clients with diabetes and COPD, for example, are in particular need of influenza and pneumonia immunizations. The use of statewide immunization information systems to send reminders regarding influenza vaccine for children with chronic diseases has helped to limit comorbidity in this population (Dombkowski et al., 2014).

Other measures to prevent loss of function in people with diabetes include tight glycemic control, control of hypertension, and lipid management as well as screening for diabetic retinopathy (CPSTF, 2014a). Laser therapy for early diabetic eye disease can minimize the risk of severe vision loss, and foot care can reduce the risk of amputation by 50% to 60% (CDC, 2011a). Population health nurses will be actively involved in educating clients with diabetes regarding strategies to control hyperglycemia (e.g., medication use, diet, exercise, glucose monitoring) and prevention of hypoglycemic reactions. They will also assist in monitoring clients' blood pressure and referring them for treatment if needed. In addition, they will educate clients regarding dietary fat intake and treatment measures for hyperlipidemia if prescribed. Population health nurses also educate clients with diabetes regarding skin and foot care and appropriate footwear. In addition, advocacy may be required to assure the availability of these and other services to all segments of the population. Population health nurses can also refer clients to sources of services to prevent deterioration in other body systems.

Nurses can also help prevent social disability by encouraging clients to interact with others, assisting clients to maintain their independence as much as possible, assisting with necessary role changes within the family, and referring the client to appropriate self-help groups. At the group level, population health nurses can work to prevent social isolation of those with chronic illnesses by advocacy and political activities to assure access to services. They can also work to educate the public and to develop positive attitudes to persons with chronic or disabling conditions. Nurse-led clinics have been found to be an effective approach to preventing further loss of function in clients with many chronic health problems (Melville, 2011). Use of community outreach workers is another effective strategy for controlling chronic health problems such as asthma (Hootman et al., 2012) and diabetes (McEwen, Pasvogel, Gallegos, & Barrera, 2010; Spencer et al., 2011). For clients with cancer, navigation services have resulted in improved patient outcomes. The addition of weatherization interventions to community health worker home visits has also improved asthma outcomes. Examples of weatherization interventions included promoting air tightness, heating system cleaning and maintenance, dealing with moisture-related problems, replacing carpets, and installing stove and dryer hoods (Breysse et al., 2014). For some clients and populations, telemedicine case management can improve function and chronic disease outcomes (Shea et al., 2013).

Cancer navigation involves assisting people to obtain timely access to necessary cancer-related screening, treatment, and survivorship services (Nguyen, Tran, Kagawa-Singer, & Foo, 2011). Nurse navigators, in particular, have been shown to result in better emotional support and feeling better informed and better able to manage care (Brooks, 2013). Navigators can also promote influenza and pneumonia vaccine for cancer survivors (Underwood et al., 2012).

Restoring function. Specific rehabilitation services are needed to offset the consequences of many chronic health conditions, including accidental injury, stroke, and myocardial infarction. Unfortunately, many clients in need of rehabilitation services do not receive them. Population health nurses can refer clients to rehabilitation programs or advocate for their accessibility to those in need. They can also help design programs that meet the perceived needs of the client population.

Particular areas to be addressed in rehabilitation programs include functional status related to activities such as positioning, range of motion, transfer abilities, dressing, bowel and bladder control, hygiene, locomotion, and eating. Other functional considerations include vision, hearing, speech, mental ability, and capacity for social interaction. The nurse, together with the client and his or her significant others, can foster renewed abilities to perform these functions. For example, the nurse may develop a plan and teach the client and family how to reestablish bowel control following a stroke, or the nurse might assist the client with passive and active range-of-motion exercises to restore function after a broken arm has healed. Other considerations include teaching stress management, dealing with the limitations imposed by a chronic condition, and addressing the financial burden of disease that may limit clients' abilities to regain function.

Other interventions may necessitate referral to other health care providers. For example, clients may need physical therapy to regain lost function after a stroke. Clients may also need rehabilitation services following myocardial infarction or to minimize the effects of arthritis or stroke. Population health nurses may assist individual clients to obtain these services or advocate for their availability and accessibility in the community.

Promoting adjustment. Movement to an optimal level of health entails adjustment to the constraints of a chronic physical health problem. Areas for special consideration in promoting adjustment to chronic health problems include functional and psychological adjustment, pain management, and survivorship care.

Adjustments to the presence of a chronic disease occur in both functional and psychological realms. Functional adjustments reflect changes in lifestyle necessitated by the illness. Such changes may involve diet, activity patterns, restrictions (e.g., limiting alcohol use or caloric intake), and the need to take medications. Some diseases necessitate learning special skills. For example, insulin-dependent diabetic clients need to learn to give themselves insulin injections, and hypertensive clients may need to learn how to take their blood pressure. In other chronic conditions, such as arthritis, there may be a need for special apparatus to assist in performing routine activities. The need for medication may also necessitate budgetary changes that the client must adjust to.

Adjustment in the work setting is a special consideration for many people with chronic conditions. Promoting adjustment in the work setting usually combines a variety of approaches. First, population health nurses in occupational settings can enhance the employee's personal ability to cope with illness. This might be accomplished through education regarding medication management or self-monitoring skills or other interventions. Second, the nurse can advocate for the support of management or colleagues for self-care activities (e.g., scheduling flexible breaks or meals) and advocate for working conditions that accommodate any limitations or special needs (e.g., redesign of work stations to prevent exacerbation of carpal tunnel syndrome, assuring wheelchair access to all areas of the work setting). Third, nurses can connect employees to support groups and services outside the work setting, and finally, the nurse can assure adequate access to care and advocate for insurance benefits to cover the costs of care. Case management is also an effective approach to keeping employees with chronic health problems on the job. Disease management programs may also be helpful for groups of employees with similar conditions.

Psychological adjustments are also necessary. Psychological adjustment to a chronic condition may be required in a number of areas. Self-esteem is one of these areas. A chronic disease may make a client more dependent on others and less able to engage in activities that promote a positive self-image. For example, the client may need to stop working or begin to rely on others for assistance with basic functions such as eating and toileting. This dependence may be demeaning to one who has been self-reliant. The nurse should encourage the client to maintain as many functions as possible and help families to see the client's need for independence.

Loss of independence also necessitates adjustments in one's sense of control. Clients may feel they are not in control of events when the food they eat or the activities they perform are dictated in part by the chronic health problem. For some clients, noncompliance with recommendations might be an attempt to regain control over their own lives. Nurses can help prevent noncompliance by providing the client with other avenues for exercising control. Ways of doing this include involving the client in planning interventions and providing, whenever possible, choices in which the client can exercise control over actions and outcomes. Population health nurses may also help clients obtain assistive technology devices (e.g., braces, chairlifts, railings, shower seat, grab bars) that can decrease their dependence on the assistance of other.

Another area that may require adjustment for clients with chronic conditions is that of intimacy. Among men, for example, some chronic conditions or their treatments may result in impotence. In other cases, pain or changes in self-image may limit a client's ability to maintain intimate relationships with others. Another potential problem may be the withdrawal of significant others. Clients and their families can be encouraged to discuss intimacy issues openly, and significant others can be assisted to find ways of fulfilling intimacy needs that are congruent with the presence of a chronic health problem.

Stigma is another psychological issue in adjustment to a chronic health problem. Many chronic health conditions are stigmatized by the general population. Clients with visible evidence of disease may attempt to deal with stigma by minimizing the perceived consequences of the disease or covering them up as much as possible while still acknowledging their existence. Those whose condition is invisible are faced with decisions of whether to disclose their chronic illness, how much to disclose, and to whom. Clients who fear rejection on the basis of stigma attached to the disease may attempt to pass themselves off as healthy, but then endure the stress of possible discovery and loss of credibility as well as rejection. Population health nurses can assist clients to deal with perceptions of stigma and to make decisions regarding disclosure. For clients suffering from the psychological effects of stigmatization, referrals for counseling services may be warranted. Nurses may also engage in public education campaigns to diminish the stigma attached to certain chronic conditions.

Population health nurses may also need to help clients and their families deal with caregiver burden. **Caregiver burden** is the effect of the stress of caring for a family member with a physical or mental illness on those providing the care. Caregiver burden can stem from the extent of care required or from behaviors exhibited by the family member receiving care. For example, caregiver burden may be increased when the person to whom care is given exhibits behavioral disturbances.

Population health nurses can refer clients and caregivers to self-help groups or other community agencies that provide assistance in dealing with problems arising from chronic health conditions. When self-help groups are not available in the local area, population health nurses may be involved in their development. Nurses may also advocate for the provision of services to promote functional and psychological adjustment to chronic health problems. For example, they may advocate for funding for homemaker assistance to permit people with disabilities to remain in their homes. Or they may advocate for insurance coverage for psychological counseling for clients with chronic physical health problems or for respite for caregivers.

Pain management. Pain management is an important component of management of chronic physical health problems. Effective pain management is important not only for improving the quality of life of individual clients, but also for decreasing the economic costs of chronic health problems for society in general. According to an Institute of Medicine report, an estimated 37% of the adult population in 10 countries experience chronic pain. In the United States, this figure rises to 43%. The prevalence of pain is increasing and is anticipated to continue to increase, primarily due to diabetic neuropathies and orthopedic problems. The overall cost of pain in the United States is conservatively estimated to be between $560 and $635 billion each year when medical care costs and lost productivity costs are considered (National Research Council, 2011).

Goals of pain management in chronic illness include preventing pain whenever possible, reducing the severity or frequency of pain, improving physical function, reducing psychological distress, and improving the overall quality of life. Health care providers often prescribe pharmacologic agents for pain management, but population health nurses may be able to assist clients to find other means of dealing with pain. For example, they can refer clients for acupuncture services, which have been shown to be effective in decreasing some types of chronic pain. Population health nurses can refer clients for these services. They may also advocate for reimbursement for nonpharmacologic pain management strategies under insurance coverage.

Population health nurses can work to educate health policy makers, providers, legislators, clients and their families, and the general public regarding the need for effective pain control and appropriate pain management strategies. They can also advocate for changes in laws or insurance coverage to promote effective pain management. In addition, population health nurses can assess the pain management needs of individual clients with chronic illnesses. *Partners Against Pain* (n.d.) provides a number of pain assessment tools and pain management tools. An information resource regarding the tools is provided in the student resources site for this book.

Survivorship care. Survivorship is another aspect of health restoration care for people with some chronic health problems. **Cancer survivors** include persons with cancer from the time of diagnosis through the balance of their lives as well as their families, friends, and caregivers (Levit et al., 2013). The vast majority of cancer survivors will need some level of continuing care for the rest of their lives because of their increased risk for recurrent cancers. Survivors may also need assistance in dealing with the psychosocial effects of their diagnosis. The concept of survivorship care was developed to address these ongoing needs. Although the concept was developed in relation to cancer survivors, elements of survivorship care are relevant to other health conditions that threaten life and have long-term consequences for survivors (e.g., HIV/AIDS and severe traumatic injuries).

Survivorship care encompasses care provided not only to clients who survive life-threatening conditions, but also to families, friends, and caregivers who are affected by the condition. Life for all of these people is irrevocably changed. Survivors and those around them who are affected by their condition are subjected to physical, emotional, social, spiritual, and financial issues that require long-term care. Additional needs may include dealing with pain or side effects of treatment, many of which may occur well after treatment is completed. Psychological issues of anxiety and depression may also need to be addressed. Cancer survivors may also have special nutritional needs or increased susceptibility to infection. Survivors also need information about health promotion activities such as exercise and weight control as well as ongoing surveillance and periodic screening for recurrent cancer, although the type and frequency of screening recommendations will vary with the type of cancer involved.

Survivorship care includes:

- Prevention of recurrent and new cancers and late treatment effects
- Surveillance for recurrent or new cancer and medical or psychological effects of the cancer and its treatment
- Interventions to address the consequences of disease and treatment
- Coordination of care between oncology specialists and primary care providers to assure that all the health needs of survivors are met (Levit et al., 2013)

Survivorship care should be grounded in a *survivorship care plan* that includes information about the cancer diagnosis, treatment received, and possible consequences; recommended follow-up interventions (e.g., screening for cancer recurrence, reconstructive surgeries, dietary recommendations); recommendations for health promotion; information on legal protections related to employment and health insurance; and referral for psychosocial services (e.g., financial assistance, job training) as needed.

Population health nurses can be instrumental in developing cancer survivorship plans for clients or for assuring that assistance in developing such plans is available. They may also need to advocate for insurance coverage for plan development services and services needed to implement the survivorship plan. There is also a need to develop clinical practice guidelines for survivorship care for specific types of cancer, and population health nurses can advocate for or conduct research in this area. Nurses may also need to engage in political advocacy to promote insurance reforms that prohibit denial of health insurance based on a past history of cancer and to include coverage of survivorship care as an integral part of cancer care.

Palliative and end-of-life care. A few chronic physical health problems are terminal in nature, and population health nurses may be involved in providing care to clients who are facing death, and to their families. In other instances, care is directed primarily toward palliation of symptoms, with no real expectation of improvement in the condition. Palliative and hospice care were addressed in Chapter 13∞ in the context of home health care and home visiting.

The National Consensus Project for Quality Palliative Care (2013) has developed clinical practice guidelines for quality palliative care. The guidelines address seven domains of practice that encompass structure and processes of care with an emphasis on an interdisciplinary approach; physical aspects of care, including multidimensional symptom management; psychological and psychiatric aspects of care, including bereavement services for families; and social, spiritual, and cultural aspects of care. Additional domains include end-of-life care, including communication and documentation of signs and symptoms of the dying process, and ethical and legal aspects of palliative care. For further information about the palliative care practice guidelines, see the *External Resources* section of the student resources site.

Another consideration in end-of-life care is attending to clients' care wishes. In one study, 60% of people surveyed indicated that they wanted their end-of-life wishes respected, yet only one third of them had completed an advance directive. Many people were not knowledgeable regarding advance directives and others indicated that they were not yet ready to execute one. It is estimated that greater use of advance directives could reduce health care costs considerably, since approximately a quarter of costs are related to unnecessary care provided in the last few months of life (Morhaim & Pollack, 2013). Population health nurses can educate clients and the general public regarding advance directives and can assist clients in their completion. They can also advocate for making provider discussion of advance directives a reimbursable health care activity and promote such discussions with clients.

Health restoration goals for end-of-life care and other aspects of chronic disease care and related nursing interventions are summarized in Table 27-5●.

Evaluating Control Strategies for Chronic Physical Health Problems

Evaluating control strategies for chronic health problems is done in terms of care outcomes. Care may be evaluated in relation to the individual client or to a population group. In the case of the individual client, the nurse evaluates the status of the chronic condition as well as the client's adjustment to having a chronic health problem. If medical, nursing, or self-management interventions have been effective, the condition will be controlled or may even be improving. Failing improvement, the condition will provide the least disruption possible to the life of the client and his or her significant others. Evaluative criteria reflect both the client's physiologic status and his or her quality of life.

Evidence of success in controlling chronic health problems at the community or population level lies primarily in changes in morbidity and mortality figures. Are there fewer cases of hypertension or cardiovascular disease in the population now than before the initiation of control efforts? Are there fewer disabilities due to accidental injuries? Do those individuals with diabetes live longer or have fewer hospitalizations for diabetic complications? Based on the evaluative data, decisions can be made regarding the need to attempt other control strategies or to continue with current measures.

Evaluation of population-based control strategies may focus on the status of national objectives for 2020 for selected chronic diseases. Baseline and target information and the current status of several of these objectives are presented on the next page.

TABLE 27-5 Goals for Health Restoration and Related Community Health Nursing Interventions in the Control of Chronic Physical Health Problems

Goal	Nursing Interventions
1. Prevent further loss of function in affected systems. Decrease risk factors for recurrence, exacerbation, or development of crises.	1. Motivate client to comply with treatment regimen. Assist client to identify risk factors amenable to change. Assist client to identify ways of decreasing risk factors.
2. Prevent loss of function in unaffected systems.	2. Assist client to maintain function in unaffected systems.
a. Prevent physical disability.	a. Prevent physical complications of illness through: • Breathing exercises • Skin care • Range-of-motion exercises and physical activity • Adequate nutrition and fluids Provide physical care as required. Refer for assistance with physical care as needed.
b. Prevent social disability.	b. Accept client as a unique person. Encourage interaction with others. Assist significant others to deal with feelings about client's illness. Assist client to maintain independence as much as possible. Assist with identification of need for changes in family roles. Work to change public attitudes toward the disabled. Promote legislation to aid chronically ill to maintain their independence.
3. Restore function.	3. Assist with planning and implementation of programs to regain function (bowel training, physical therapy). Teach client and others to carry out program and evaluate effects.

TABLE 27-5 *(Continued)*

Goal	Nursing Interventions
4. Promote adjustment.	4. Assist client to adjust to presence of chronic disease.
a. Deal with feelings about disease.	a. Accept client at his or her level of development and acceptance of disease. Encourage client to discuss fears and apprehensions. Refer to self-help groups as appropriate.
b. Adjust lifestyle to accommodate chronic disease and its effects.	b. Assist client to identify needed changes in lifestyle. Assist client to plan and carry out lifestyle changes.
c. Adjust environment to meet changed needs.	c. Identify need for self-help devices and help client obtain them. Identify environmental changes needed to foster independence. Assist client to make necessary environmental changes.
d. Adjust self-image.	d. Assist client to adjust to change in self-image. Refer for counseling as needed.
e. Adjust to expense of chronic care.	e. Refer for financial aid as needed.
f. Deal with stigma.	f. Assist with decisions regarding disclosure. Assist client to cope with effects of stigma. Educate public to minimize stigma.
g. Effectively manage pain.	g. Accurately assess client pain levels. Assist in identifying appropriate pharmacologic and nonpharmacologic approaches to pain control. Refer for pain management services, as needed. Educate clients, family, providers, and the public regarding effective pain control. Advocate for available and accessible pain management services and insurance coverage for services. Monitor the effectiveness of pain control strategies.
5. Meet survivorship care needs.	5. Identify survivorship care needs and participate in developing a survivorship care plan. Refer clients and families for survivorship care services as needed. Advocate for insurance coverage of survivorship care planning and needed survivorship care. Conduct research to identify care needs and best practices in survivorship care.
6. Adjust to impending death.	6. Provide end-of-life care. a. Provide pain management. b. Provide comfort care. c. Provide palliative care. d. Encourage advance directives. e. Refer to hospice services as needed.

Healthy People 2020

Selected Health Objectives Related to Chronic Physical Health Problems

OBJECTIVE	BASELINE (YEAR)	TARGET	CURRENT DATA (YEAR)	DATA SOURCES
AOCBC-1. Reduce the mean level of joint pain in adults with doctor-diagnosed arthritis	5.6 (on a 10-point scale) (2006)	5	5.7 (2009)	National Health Interview Survey (NHIS), CDC/ NCHS
AOCBC-2. Reduce the proportion of adults with doctor-diagnosed arthritis with limitation in activity	39.4% (2008)	35.5%	40.5% (2011)	NHIS, CDC/ NCHS
AOCBC-10. Reduce the proportion of adults with osteoporosis	5.9% (2005–2008)	5.38%	NDA	National Health and Nutrition Examination Survey (NHANES), CDC/ NCHS
CKD-1. Reduce the proportion of the population with chronic kidney disease	15.1% (1994–2004)	13.6%	NDA	US Renal Disease System (USRDS), NIH/NIDDK
CKD-8. Reduce the rate of new cases of end-stage renal disease (per million population)	358.9 (2007)	323	349.7 (2010)	USRDS, NIH/NIDDK

Healthy People 2020 (Continued)

OBJECTIVE	BASELINE (YEAR)	TARGET	CURRENT DATA (YEAR)	DATA SOURCES
CKD-9.1. Reduce kidney failure due to diabetes (per million population)	154.6 (2007)	139.1	150.6 (2010)	USRDS, NIH/NIDDK
D-1. Reduce the annual number of new cases of diabetes in people aged 18–64 (per 1,000 population)	8 2006–2008	7.2	7.3 (2010–2012)	NHIS, CDC/ NCHS
D-3. Reduce the diabetes death rate (per 100,000 population)	74 (2007)	66.6	70.7 (2010)	National Vital Statistics System—Mortality (NVSS-M), CDC/NCHS
D-14. Increase the proportion of persons with diagnosed diabetes who receive formal diabetes education	56.8% (2008)	62.5%	58% (2010)	Behavioral Risk Factor Surveillance System (BRFSS), DCD/PHSPO
HDS-2. Reduce coronary heart disease deaths (per 100,000 population)	129.2 (2007)	103.4	113.6 (2010)	NVSS-M, CDC/NCHS
HDS-3. Reduce stroke deaths (per 100,000 population)	43.5 (2007)	34.8	39.1 (2010)	NVSS-M, CDC/NCHS
HDS-5.1. Reduce the proportion of adults with high blood pressure	29.9% (2005–2008)	26.9%	NDA	NHANES, CDC/ NCHS
HDS-7. Reduce the proportion of adults with high total blood cholesterol levels	15% (2005–2008)	13.5%	NDA	NHANES, CDC/ NCHS
HDS-12. Increase the proportion of adults with high blood pressure whose blood pressure is under control	43.7% (2005–2008)	61.2%	45.9% (2009–2010)	NHANES, CDC/ NCHS
NWS-8. Increase the proportion of adults who are at healthy weight	30.8% (2005–2008)	33.9%	NDA	NHANES, CDC/ NCHS
PA-1. Reduce the proportion of adults who engage in no leisure-time physical activity	36.2% (2008)	32.6%	31.6% (2011)	NHANES, CDC/ NCHS
RD-4. Reduce activity limitations among persons with asthma	12.7% (2008)	10.2%	10%* (2012)	NHIS, CDC/ NCHS
RD-7.1. Increase the proportion of persons with asthma who receive written asthma management plans	33.4% (2008)	36.8%	NDA	NHIS, CDC/NCHS
TU-1.1. Reduce cigarette smoking by adults	20.6% (2008)	12%	19% (2011)	NHIS, CDC/NCHS
TU-2.1. Reduce use of tobacco products by adolescents (grades 9–12) (last month)	26% (2009)	21%	23.4% (2011)	Youth Risk Behavior Surveillance System (YRBSS), NCHHSTP

NDA = No data available

*Objective has met target.

Data from: U.S. Department of Health and Human Services. (2014a). *Healthy People 2020 - Topics and objectives.* Retrieved from http://healthypeople.gov/2020/topicsobjectives2020/default.aspx

CHAPTER RECAP

Chronic physical health problems have largely replaced communicable diseases as the major contributors to death and disability, and significant morbidity and mortality due to chronic physical conditions are seen throughout the world. Factors related to each of the six categories of determinants of health contribute to the development and/or control of chronic physical health problems. Population health nurses are actively involved in efforts to educate the public to prevent these diseases as well as in the design, implementation, and evaluation of programs to provide diagnostic, treatment, and support services for persons with existing disease.

CASE STUDY Reducing Hypertension Incidence

You have just started working as a population health nurse for the Wachita County Health Department in Mississippi. During your employment interview, the nursing supervisor mentioned that one of your responsibilities would be to participate in developing plans for dealing with the high rate of hypertension in the county. The incidence rate for hypertension here is three times that of the state and twice that of the nation. The population of the county is largely African American, with high unemployment rates and little health insurance. Folk health practices are quite common, one of them being drinking pickle brine for a condition called "high blood." Although this condition is not related to high blood pressure, the two terms are frequently confused by lay members of the community and professionals alike. Dietary intake is typical of the rural South, consisting of a variety of fried foods, beans and other boiled vegetables, and corn bread.

Most of the adult members of the community work in service industry jobs that involve little vigorous physical activity. In addition, few community members engage in leisure time physical activity. The local Baptist and Methodist churches are interested in initiating health ministries, but have not made much headway in organizing related activities yet. Few health services are available in the county itself, although there is a major hospital 50 miles away. There are two general practitioners in the area and one pediatrician. Both of the general practitioners are older physicians, and you doubt that they are incorporating current practice guidelines for hypertension control. The health department holds well-child, immunization, tuberculosis, and family planning clinics regularly, and all are well attended. Transportation is a problem for many community residents.

1. What are the biological, psychological, environmental, sociocultural, behavioral, and health system factors influencing the incidence and prevalence of hypertension in this county?
2. Write two objectives for your efforts to resolve the county's problem with hypertension.
3. What health promotion, illness prevention, problem resolution, and health restoration activities might be appropriate in dealing with the problem of hypertension? Which of these activities might you carry out yourself? Which would require collaboration with other community members? Who might these other people be?
4. How would you evaluate the outcome of your interventions?

REFERENCES

Abrams, B., Anderson, H., Blackmore, C., Bove, F. J., Condon, S. K., Eheman, C. T., . . . Wartenberg, D. (2013). Investigating suspected cancer clusters and responding to community concerns: Guidelines from CDC and the Council of State and Territorial Epidemiologists. *Morbidity and Mortality Weekly Report, 62*(RR-8), 1–24.

Ade-Oshifogun, J. B. (2012). Model of functional performance in obese elderly people with chronic obstructive pulmonary disease. *Journal of Nursing Scholarship, 44*, 232–241. doi:10.1111/j.1547-5069.2012.01457.x

Afya Foundation. (n.d.). *International in-country assessments and sourcing.* Retrieved from http://www.afyafoundation.org/assessment.html

Agaku, I., King, B., & Dube, S. R. (2012). Current cigarette smoking among adults—United States, 2011. *Morbidity and Mortality Weekly Report, 61*, 889–894.

Agency for Healthcare Research and Quality. (2014). *Self-management support.* Retrieved from http://www.ahrq.gov/professionals/prevention-chronic-care/improve/self-mgmt/self/index.html

Akinbami, L. J., Moorman, J. E., & Liu, X. (2011). Asthma prevalence, health care use, and mortality: United States, 2005–2009. *National Health Statistics Reports, 32.* Retrieved from http://www.cdc.gov/nchs/data/nhsr/nhsr032.pdf

Alvarez, K. J., & Levy, R. R. (2012). Health advantages of ethnic density for African American and Mexican American elderly individuals. *American Journal of Public Health, 102*, 2240–2242. doi:10.2105/AJPH.2012.300787

American Cancer Society. (2010). *The global economic cost of cancer.* Retrieved from http://www.cancer.org/acs/groups/content/@internationalaffairs/documents/document/acspc-026203.pdf

American Lung Association. (2014a). *Asthma in the workplace.* Retrieved from http://www.lung.org/lung-disease/asthma/creating-asthma-friendly-environments/asthma-in-the-workplace/

American Lung Association. (2014b). *Guide to controlling asthma at work.* Retrieved from http://www.lung.org/lung-disease/asthma/creating-asthma-friendly-environments/asthma-in-the-workplace/guide-to-controlling-asthma-at-work.html

American Professional Wound Care Association. (2010). SELECT: Evaluation and implementation of clinical practice guidelines: A guidance document from the American Professional Wound Care Association. *Advances in Skin and Wound Care, 23,* 161–168. doi:10.1097/01.ASW.0000363529.93253.dd

Anderson, S., Rigler, J., Oberoi, V., Christ, C., Eggers, P., Lempp, J., . . . Perz, J. (2012). Invasive staphylococcus aureus infections associated with pain injections and reuse of single-dose vials—Arizona and Delaware. *Morbidity and Mortality Weekly Report, 61,* 501–504.

Aronowitz, R. (2014). "Screening" for prostate cancer in New York's skid row: History and implications. *American Journal of Public Health, 104,* 70–76. doi:10.2105/AJPH.2013.301446

Arrazola, R. A., Dube, S. R., & King, B. A. (2013). Tobacco product use among middle and high school students—United States, 2011 and 2012. *Morbidity and Mortality Weekly Report, 62,* 893–897.

Australian Institute of Health and Welfare. (2013). *Risk factors to health.* Retrieved from http://www.aihw.gov.au/risk-factors/

Barbour, K. E., Helmick, C. G., Theis, K. A., Murphy, L. B., Hootman, J. M., Brady, T. J., & Cheng, Y. J (2013). Prevalence of doctor-diagnosed arthritis and arthritis-attributable activity limitation—United States, 2010–2012. *Morbidity and Mortality Weekly Report, 62,* 869–872.

Baumann, S. L. (2012). What's wrong with the concept of self-management? *Nursing Science Quarterly, 25,* 362–363.

Beck, A. F., Simmons, J. M., Huang, B., & Kahn, R. S. (2012). Geomedicine: Area-based socioeconomic measures for assessing risk of hospital reutilization among children admitted for asthma. *American Journal of Public Health, 102,* 2308–2314. doi:10.2105/AJPH.2012.300806

Beckles, G. L., & Truman, B. I. (2011). Education and income—United States, 2005 and 2009. *Morbidity and Mortality Weekly Report, 60*(Suppl. 1), 13–17.

Beckles, G. L., Zhu, J., & Moonsinghe, R. (2011, January 14). Diabetes—United States, 2004 and 2008. *Morbidity and Mortality Weekly Report, 60*(Suppl.), 90–93.

Benjamin, G., Mitra, M., Graham, C., Krahn, G., Luce, S., Fox, M., . . . Popovic, T. (2013). CDC grand rounds: Public health practices to include persons with disabilities. *Morbidity and Mortality Weekly Report, 62,* 697–701.

Bernstein, S. L., Yu, S., Post, L. A., Dziura, J., & Rigotti, N. A. (2013). Undertreatment of tobacco use relative to other chronic conditions. *American Journal of Public Health, 103,* e59–e65. doi:10.2105/AJPH.2012.301112

Breysse, J., Dixon, S., Gregory, J., Philby, M., Jacobs, D. E., & Krieger, J. (2014). Effect of weatherization combined with health worker in-home education on asthma control. *American Journal of Public Health, 104,* e57–e64. doi:10.2105/AJPH.2013.301402

Bright, M. A., Davis, K., Bann, S., Bunnell, R., Rodes, R., Alexander, R., . . . McAfee, T. (2013). Impact of a national tobacco education campaign on weekly numbers of quitline calls and website visitors—United States, March 4–June 23, 2013. *Morbidity and Mortality Weekly Report, 62,* 763–767.

Brooks, M. (2013). *Nurse navigator helpful after cancer diagnosis.* Retrieved from http://www.medscape.com/viewarticle/815466?nlid=41743_785&src=wnl_edit_medp_nurs&uac=3108CT&spon=24

Burrows, N. R., Hora, I. A., Li, Y., & Saaddine, J. B. (2011). Self-reported visual impairment among persons with diagnosed diabetes—United States, 1997–2010. *Morbidity and Mortality Weekly Report, 60,* 1549–1553.

Caixeta, R. B., Blanco, A., Fouad, H., Khoury, R. N., Sinha, D. N., Rarick, J., . . . Pechacek, R. (2011). Cigarette package health warnings and interest in quitting smoking—14 countries, 2008–2010. *Morbidity and Mortality Weekly Report, 60,* 645–651.

Caixeta, R. B., Sinha, D. N., Khoury, R. N., Rarick, J., Fouad, H., d'Espaignet, E. T., . . . Asma, S. (2013a). Antismoking messages and intention to quit—17 countries, 2008–2011. *Morbidity and Mortality Weekly Report, 62,* 417–422.

Caixeta, R. B., Sinha, D. N., Khoury, R. N., Rarick, J., Fouad, H., d'Espaignet, E. T., . . . Asma, S. (2013b). Health care provider screening for tobacco smoking and advice to quit—17 countries, 2008–2011. *Morbidity and Mortality Weekly Report, 62,* 920–927.

Cantrell, J., Kreslake, J. M., Pearson, J. L., Vallone, D., Anesetti-Rothermel, A., Xiao, H., & Kirchner, T. R. (2013). Marketing little cigars and cigarillos: Advertising, price, and associations with neighborhood demographics. *American Journal of Public Health, 103,* 1902–1909. doi:10.2105/AJPH.2013.301362

Center for Surveillance, Epidemiology, and Laboratory Services. (2013a). *Behavior, environment, and genetic factors all have a role in causing people to be overweight and obese.* Retrieved from http://www.cdc.gov/genomics/resources/diseases/obesity/index.htm

Center for Surveillance, Epidemiology, and Laboratory Services. (2013b). *Colorectal cancer awareness.* Retrieved from http://www.cdc.gov/genomics/resources/diseases/colorectal.htm

Center for Surveillance, Epidemiology, and Laboratory Services. (2013c). *Quick facts about family health history and genetic testing for breast and ovarian cancer.* Retrieved from http://www.cdc.gov/genomics/resources/diseases/breast_ovarian_cancer/quick_facts.htm#1

Center for Surveillance, Epidemiology, and Laboratory Services. (2013d). *Stroke awareness.* Retrieved from http://www.cdc.gov/genomics/resources/diseases/stroke.htm

Center for Surveillance, Epidemiology, and Laboratory Services. (2014a). *Genomics and health.* Retrieved from http://www.cdc.gov/genomics/public/index.htm

Center for Surveillance, Epidemiology, and Laboratory Services. (2014b). *Genomic tests and family history by levels of evidence.* Retrieved from http://www.cdc.gov/genomics/gtesting/tier.htm

Center for Surveillance, Epidemiology, and Laboratory Services. (2014c). *Heart disease and family history.* Retrieved from http://www.cdc.gov/genomics/resources/diseases/heart.htm

Centers for Disease Control and Prevention. (2011a). *National diabetes fact sheet: National estimates and general information on diabetes and prediabetes in the United States, 2011.* Retrieved from http://www.cdc.gov/diabetes/pubs/pdf/ndfs_2011.pdf

Centers for Disease Control and Prevention. (2011b). Native Diabetes Wellness Programs commemorates Native American heritage month—November, 2011. *Morbidity and Mortality Weekly Report, 60,* 1587.

Centers for Disease Control and Prevention. (2012a). Great American smoke out—November 15, 2012. *Morbidity and Mortality Weekly Report, 61,* 889.

Centers for Disease Control and Prevention. (2012b). National diabetes month—November, 2012. *Morbidity and Mortality Weekly Report, 61,* 869.

Centers for Disease Control and Prevention. (2012c). Skin cancer awareness month—May 2012. *Morbidity and Mortality Weekly Report, 61,* 328.

Centers for Disease Control and Prevention. (2012d). World arthritis day 2012. *Morbidity and Mortality Weekly Report, 61,* 821.

Centers for Disease Control and Prevention. (2012e). World day of remembrance for road traffic victims—November 18, 2012. *Morbidity and Mortality Weekly Report, 61,* 928.

Centers for Disease Control and Prevention. (2013a). National blood pressure education month—May 2013. *Morbidity and Mortality Weekly Report, 62,* 372.

Centers for Disease Control and Prevention. (2013b). National kidney month—March 2013. *Morbidity and Mortality Weekly Report, 62,* 152.

Centers for Disease Control and Prevention. (2013c). Click it or ticket campaign—May 20–June 2, 2013. *Morbidity and Mortality Weekly Report, 62,* 390.

Centers for Disease Control and Prevention. (2013d). World no tobacco day. *Morbidity and Mortality Weekly Report, 62,* 417.

Centers for Disease Control and Prevention. (2013e). World stroke day—October 29, 2013. *Morbidity and Mortality Weekly Report, 62,* 845.

Centers for Disease Control and Prevention. (2014). *Disability and functioning (adults).* Retrieved from http://www.cdc.gov/nchs/fastats/disability.htm

Cheng, Y. J., Hootman, J. M., Murphy, L. B., Langmaid, G. A., & Helmick, C. G. (2010). Prevalence of doctor-diagnosed arthritis and arthritis-attributable activity limitation—United States, 2007–2009. *Morbidity and Mortality Weekly Report, 59,* 1261–1265.

Choi, K., Fabian, L., Mottey, N., Corbett, A., & Forster, J. (2012). Young adults' favorable perceptions of snus, dissolvable tobacco products, and electronic cigarettes: Findings of a focus group study. *American Journal of Public Health, 102,* 2088–2093. doi:10.2105/AJPH.2011.300525

Coady, M., H., Chan, C. A., Sacks, R., Mbamalu, I. G., & Kansagra, S. M. (2013). The impact of cigarette excise tax increases on purchasing behaviors among New York City smokers. *American Journal of Public Health, 103,* e54–e60. doi:10.2105/AJPH.2013.301213

Cohen, J. E., Planinac, L., Lavack, A., Robinson, D., O'Connor, S., & Di Nardi, J. (2011). Changes in retail tobacco promotions in a cohort of stores before, during, and after a tobacco product display ban. *American Journal of Public Health, 101,* 1879–1881. doi:10.2105/AJPH.2011.300172

Cole, S. W. (2013). Social regulation of human gene expression: Mechanisms and implications for public health. *American Journal of Public Health, 103,* S84–S92. doi:10.2105/AJPH.2012.301183

Community Preventive Services Task Force. (2013a). *Cancer prevention and control.* Retrieved from http://www.thecommunityguide.org/cancer/index.html

Community Preventive Services Task Force. (2013b). *Cardiovascular disease prevention and control: Reducing out-of-pocket costs for cardiovascular disease preventive services for patients with high blood pressure and high cholesterol.* Retrieved from http://thecommunityguide.org/cvd/ropc.html

Community Preventive Services Task Force. (2014a). *Diabetes prevention and control: Disease management programs.* Retrieved from http://www.thecommunityguide.org/diabetes/diseasemgmt.html

Community Preventive Services Task Force. (2014b). *Reducing tobacco use and secondhand smoke exposure: Mass-reach health communication interventions.* Retrieved from http://thecommunityguide.org/tobacco/massreach.html

Community Preventive Services Task Force. (2014c). *Reducing tobacco use and secondhand smoke exposure: Quitline interventions.* Retrieved from http://www.thecommunityguide.org/tobacco/quitlines.html

Community Preventive Services Task Force. (2014d). *Reducing tobacco use and secondhand smoke exposure: Reducing out-of-pocket costs for evidence-based tobacco cessation treatments.* Retrieved from http://www.thecommunityguide.org/tobacco/outofpocketcosts.html

Corey, C., Wang, B., Johnson, S. E., Apelberg, B., Husten, C., King, B. A., . . . Dube, S. (2013). Electronic cigarette use among middle and high school students—United States, 2011–2012. *Morbidity and Mortality Weekly Report, 62,* 729–730.

Cronin, K. A., Richardson, L. C., Henley, J., Miller, J. W., Thomas, C. C., White, A., & Plescia, M. (2012). Vital signs: Racial disparities in breast cancer severity—United States, 2005–2009. *Morbidity and Mortality Weekly Report, 61,* 922–926.

Council of State and Territorial Epidemiologists. (2009). *2009 Assessment of epidemiology capacity: Findings and recommendations.* Retrieved from http://c.ymcdn.com/sites/www.cste.org/resource/resmgr/Workforce/2009ECA.pdf?hhSearchTerms=%22Chronic+and+disease+and+epidemiology+and+capacity%22

Cuffee, Y. L., Hargraves, L., Rosai, M., Briesacher, B. A., Schoenthaler, A., Person, S., . . . Adison, J. (2013). Reported racial discrimination, trust in physicians, and medication adherence among inner-city African Americans with hypertension. *American Journal of Public Health, 103,* e55–e62. doi:10.2105/AJPH.2013.301554

David L. Bazelon Center for Mental Health Law. (2013). *Community integration for people with disabilities: Key principles.* Retrieved from http://www.bazelon.org/portals/0/ADA/7.30.13%20Key%20Principles%20-%20Community%20Integration%20for%20People%20with%20Disabilities.pdf

de Brantes, F., Rastogi, A., & Painter, M. (2010). Reducing potentially avoidable complications in patients with chronic diseases: The Prometheus payment approach. *Health Services Research, 45,* 1854–1868. doi:10.1111/j1475-6773.2010.01136.x

Degeling, C., & Rock, M. (2012). Hemoglobin A1c as a diagnostic tool: Public health implications from an actor-network perspective. *American Journal of Public Health, 102,* 99–106. doi:10.2105/AJPH.2011.300329

Deputy, N. P., & Boehmer, U. (2014). Weight status and sexual orientation: Differences by age and within racial and ethnic groups. *American Journal of Public Health, 104,* 103–109. doi:10.2105/AJPH.2013.301391

Division of Community Health. (2013). *CDC's healthy communities program: Program overview US.* Retrieved from http://www.cdc.gov/nccdphp/dch/programs/healthycommunitiesprogram/overview/index.htm

Division of Diabetes Translation. (2013a). *Distribution of age at diagnosis of diabetes among adult incident cases aged 18–79 years, United States, 2011.* Retrieved from http://www.cdc.gov/diabetes/statistics/age/fig1.htm

Division of Diabetes Translation. (2013b). *Incidence of diagnosed diabetes per 1,000 population aged 18–79 years, 1980–2011.* Retrieved from http://www.cdc.gov/diabetes/statistics/incidence/fig3.htm

Division of Diabetes Translation. (2014). *Diabetes interactive atlas.* Retrieved from http://www.cdc.gov/diabetes/atlas/

Division of Unintentional Injury Prevention. (2013). *Falls among older adults: An overview.* Retrieved from http://www.cdc.gov/homeandrecreationalsafety/falls/adultfalls.html

Dombkowski, K. J., Cowan, A. E., Potter, R. C., Dong, S., Kolasa, M., & Clark, S. J. (2014). Statewide pandemic influenza vaccination reminders for children with chronic conditions. *American Journal of Public Health, 104,* e39–e44. doi:10.2105/AJPH.2013.301662

Elder, K., Ramamonjianrivelo, Z., Wiltshire, J., Piper, C., Horn, W. S., Gilbert, K. L., . . . Allison, J. (2012). Trust, medication adherence, and hypertension control in South African American men. *American Journal of Public Health, 102,* 2242–2245. doi:10.2105/AJPH.2012.300777

England, M. J., Liverman, C. T., Schultz, A. M., & Strawbridge, L. M. (Eds.). (2012). *Epilepsy across the spectrum: Promoting health and understanding.* Washington, DC: National Academies Press.

Factor, R., Williams, D. R., & Kawachi, I. (2013). Social resistance framework for understanding high-risk behavior among nondominant minorities: Preliminary evidence. *American Journal of Public Health, 103,* 2245–2251. doi:10.2105/AJPH.2013.301212

Fang, J., Ayala, C., Loustalot, F., & Dai, S. (2013). Self-reported hypertension and use of antihypertensive medication among adults—United States, 2005–2009. *Morbidity and Mortality Weekly Report, 62,* 237–244.

Fang, J., Shaw, K. M., & Keenan, N. L. (2011). Prevalence of coronary heart disease. *Morbidity and Mortality Weekly Report, 60,* 1377–1381.

Farley, T., DeMaria, A. N., Wright, J., Conway, P. H., Valderama, A. L., Blair, N. A., . . . Popovic, T. (2012). CDC grand rounds: The Million Hearts Initiative. *Morbidity and Mortality Weekly Report, 61,* 1017–1021.

Ford, E. S., Zhao, G., Tsai, J., & Li, C. (2011). Low-risk lifestyle behaviors and all-cause mortality: Findings from the National Health and Nutrition Examination Survey III Mortality Study. *American Journal of Public Health, 101,* 1922–1929. doi:10.2105/AJPH.2011.300167

Fouad, M. N., Partridge, E., Dignan, M., Holt, C., Johnson, R., Nagy, C., . . . Scarinci, I. (2010). Targeted intervention strategies to increase and maintain mammography utilization among African American women. *American Journal of Public Health, 101,* 2526–2531. doi:10.2105/AJPH.2009.167312

Franck, C., Grandi, S., & Eisenberg, M. J. (2013). Taxing junk food to counter obesity. *American Journal of Public Health, 103,* 1949–1953. doi:10.2105/AJPH.2013.301279

Frazier, M., Massingale, S., Bowen, M., & Kohler, C. (2012). Engaging a community in developing an entertainment—education Spanish-language radio novella aimed at reducing chronic disease risk factors, Alabama, 2010–2011. *Preventing Chronic Disease, 9,* 110344. doi:10.5888/pcd9.110344

Freiberg, M. S., Chang, C.-C. H., Kuller, L. H., Skanderson, M., Lowy, E., Kraemer, K. L., . . . Justice, A. C. (2013). HIV infection and the risk of acute myocardial infarction. *JAMA Internal Medicine, 173,* 614–622. doi:10.1001.jamainternmed.2013.3728

Garrett, B. E., Dube, S. R., Trosclair, A., Caraballo, R. S., & Pechacek, T. E. (2011, January 14). Cigarette smoking—United States, 2003–2007. *Morbidity and Mortality Weekly Report, 60,* 109–113.

Geiss, L. S., Li, Y., Kirtland, K., Barker, L., Burrows, N. R., & Gregg, E. W. (2012). Increasing prevalence of diagnosed diabetes—United States and Puerto Rico, 1995–2010. *Morbidity and Mortality Weekly Report, 61,* 918–921.

George, M. G., Tong, X., & Yoon, P. W. (2011). Use of a registry to improve acute stroke care—Seven states, 2005–2009. *Morbidity and Mortality Weekly Report, 60,* 206–210.

Gruzka, R. A., Plunk, A. D., Hipp, P. R., Cavazos-Rehg, P., & Krauss, M. J. (2013). Long-term effects of laws governing youth access to tobacco. *American Journal of Public Health, 103,* 1493–1499. doi:10.2105/AJPH.2012.301123

Hall, M. J., Levant, S., & DeFrances, C. J. (2012). *Hospitalization for stroke in U. S. hospitals, 1989–2009* (NCHS data Brief, No. 95). Retrieved from http://www.cdc.gov/nchs/data/databriefs/db95.htm

Hartman, A. M., Guy, G. P., Holman, D. M., Saraiya, M., & Plescia, M. (2012). Use of indoor tanning devices by adults, United States, 2010. *Morbidity and Mortality Weekly Report, 61,* 323–326.

Hatcher, J., Rayens, M. K., & Schoenberg, N. E. (2010). Mammography promotion in the emergency department: A pilot study. *Public Health Nursing, 27,* 520–527. doi:10.1111/j-1525-1446.2010.00894.x

Health Care Incentives Improvement Institute. (n.d.a). *Evidence-informed case rates.* Retrieved from http://www.hci3.org/what_is_prometheus/framework/evidence_informed_case_rates

Health Care Incentives Improvement Institute. (n.d.b). *The framework of Prometheus payment.* Retrieved from http://www.hci3.org/what_is_prometheus/framework

Herman, P. M., & Walsh, M. E. (2011). Hospital admissions for acute myocardial infarction. Angina, stroke, and asthma after implementation of Arizona's comprehensive statewide smoking ban. *American Journal of Public Health, 101,* 491–496. doi:10.2105/AJPH.2009.179572

Herrick, H., Pleasants, R., Wheaton, A. G., Liu, Y., Ford, E. S., Presley-Cantrell, L. R., & Croft, J. B. (2012). Chronic obstructive pulmonary disease and associated health care resource use—North Carolina, 2007 and 2009. *Morbidity and Mortality Weekly Report, 61,* 143–146.

Hicken, M. T., Gee, G. C., Morenoff, J., Connell, C. M., Snow, R. C., & Hu, H. (2012). A novel look at racial health disparities: The interaction between social disadvantage and environmental health. *American Journal of Public Health, 102,* 2344–2351. doi:10.2105/AJPH.2012.300774

Hicken, M. T., Lee, H., Morenoff, J., House, J. S., & Williams, D. R. (2014). Racial/ethnic disparities in hypertension prevalence: Reconsidering the role of chronic stress. *American Journal of Public Health, 104,* 117–123. doi:10.2105/AJPH.2013.301395

Hogstedt, C., Jansson, C., Hugosson, M., Tinnerberg, H., & Gustavsson, P. (2013). Cancer incidence in a cohort of Swedish chimney sweeps, 1958–2006. *American Journal of Public Health, 103,* 1708–1714. doi:10.2105/AJPH.2012.300860

Holman, D. M., Berkowitz, Z., Guy, G. P., Saraiya, M., & Plescia, M. (2012). Sunburn and sun protective behaviors among adults aged 18–29 years—United States, 2000–2010. *Morbidity and Mortality Weekly Report, 61,* 317–320.

Hootman, J. M., Barbour, K. E., Watson, K. B., & Fulton, J. E. (2013). State-specific walking among adults with arthritis—United States, 2011. *Morbidity and Mortality Weekly Report, 62,* 331–334.

Hootman, J. M., Helmick, C. G., & Brady, T. J. (2012). A public health approach to addressing arthritis in older adults: The most common cause of disability. *American Journal of Public Health, 102,* 426–433. doi:10.2105/AJPH.2011.300423

Hootman, J. M., Helmick, C. G., Hannan, C. J., & Pan, L. (2011). Prevalence of obesity among adults with arthritis—United States, 2003–2009. *Morbidity and Mortality Weekly Report, 60,* 509–513.

Hootman, J. M., Murphy, L. B., Helmick, C. G., & Barbour, K. E. (2011). Arthritis as a potential barrier to physical activity among adults with obesity—United States, 2007 and 2009. *Morbidity and Mortality Weekly Report, 60,* 614–618.

Hopkins, M., Hallett, C., Babb, S., King, B., Tyman, M., & MacNeil, A. (2012). Comprehensive smoke-free laws—50 largest U.S. cities, 2000 and 2012. *Morbidity and Mortality Weekly Report, 61,* 914–917.

Hosseinpoor, A. R., Williams, J. A. S., Gautam, J., Posarac, A., Officer, A., Verdes, E., . . . Chatterji, S. (2013). Socioeconomic inequality in disability among adults: A multicountry study using the World Health Survey. *American Journal of Public Health, 103,* 1278–1286. doi:10.2105/AJPH.2012.301115

Howie, L. D. (2013). Percentage of adults aged >18 years who met the aerobic activity and muscle strengthening guidelines by sex and selected race/ethnicity—National Health Interview Survey, United States, 2009–2011. *Morbidity and Mortality Weekly Report, 62,* 635.

Howlader, N., Noone, A. M., Krapcho, M., Garshell, J., Neyman, N., Altekruse, S. F., . . . Cronin, K. A. (Eds.). (2013). *SEER cancer statistics review, 1975–2010.* Retrieved from http://seer.cancer.gov/csr/1975_2010/browse_csr.php?sectionSEL=2&pageSEL=sect_02_table.07.html

Huang, D. T., & Kandi, D. (2012). Percentage of adults aged 50–75 years who received colorectal cancer screening, by family income level—National Health Interview Survey, United States, 2010. *Morbidity and Mortality Weekly Report, 61,* 955.

Hunt, J. J., Gajewski, B. J., Jiang, Y., Cupertino, P., & Richter, K. P. (2013). Capacity of U.S. drug treatment facilities to provide evidence-based tobacco treatment. *American Journal of Public Health, 103,* 1799–1801. doi:10.2105/AJPH.2013.301427

Improving Chronic Illness Care. (n.d.). *The chronic care model.* Retrieved from http://www.improvingchroniccare.org/index.php?=The_Chronic_Care_Model&s=2

James, P. J., Troped, P. J., Hart, J. E., Joshu, C. E., Colditz, G. A., Brownson, R. C., . . . Laden, F. (2013). Urban sprawl, physical activity, and body mass index: Nurses' health study and nurses' health study II. *American Journal of Public Health, 103,* 369–375. doi:10.2105/AJPH.2011.300449

Kadima, N. T., Kobau, R., Zack, M. M., & Helmers, S. (2013). Comorbidity in adults with epilepsy—United States, 2010. *Morbidity and Mortality Weekly Report, 62,* 849–853.

Kanny, D., Liu, Y., & Brewer, R. D. (2011, January 14). Binge drinking—United States, 2009. *Morbidity and Mortality Weekly Report, 60*(Suppl.), 101–104.

Keenan, N. L., & Rosendorf, K. A. (2011, January 14). Prevalence of hypertension and controlled hypertension—United States, 2005–2008. *Morbidity and Mortality Weekly Report, 60,* 94–97.

Khajuria, H. (2013). Percentage of women aged 50–64 years who reported receiving a mammogram in the past 2 years, by health insurance status—National Health Interview Survey, United States, 1993–2010. *Morbidity and Mortality Weekly Report, 62,* 651.

Klabunde, C. N., Joseph, D. A., King, J. B., White, A., & Plescia, M. (2013). Vital signs: Colorectal cancer screening test use—United States, 2012. *Morbidity and Mortality Weekly Report, 62,* 881–888.

Kobatu, R., Luo, Y.-H., Zack, M. M., Helmers, S., & Thurman, D. J. (2102). Epilepsy in adults and access to care—United States, 2010. *Morbidity and Mortality Weekly Report, 61,* 909–913.

Kosacz, N. M., Punturieri, A., Croxton, T. L., Ndenecho, M. N., Kiley, J. P., Weinmann, G. G., . . . Giles, W. H. (2012). Chronic obstructive pulmonary disease among adults—United States, 2011. *Morbidity and Mortality Weekly Report, 61,* 938–943.

Leischow, S. J., Provan, K., Beagles, K., Bonito, J., Ruppel, E., Moor, G., et al. (2012). Mapping tobacco quitlines in North America: Signaling pathways to improve treatment. *American Journal of Public Health, 102,* 2123–2128. doi:10.2105/AJPH.2011.300529

Levit, L., Balogh, E., Nass, S., & Ganz, P. (Eds.). (2013). *Delivering high-quality cancer care: Charting a new course for a system in crisis.* Retrieved from http://www.nap.edu/download.php?record_id=18359

Li, C., Balluz, L. S., Okoro, C. A., Strine, T. W., Lin, J.-M. S., Town, M., . . . Valluru, B. (2011). Surveillance of certain health behaviors and conditions among states and selected local areas—Behavioral Risk Factor Surveillance System, United States, 2009. *Morbidity and Mortality Weekly Report, 60*(9), 1–248.

Li, Y., Geiss, L. S., Burrows, N. R., Rolka, D. B., & Albright, A. (2013). Awareness of prediabetes—United States, 2005–2010. *Morbidity and Mortality Weekly Report, 62,* 209–212.

Lieberman, L., Diffley, U., King, S., Chanler, S., Ferrara, M., Alleyne, O., et al. (2013). Local tobacco control: Application of the essential public health services model in a county health department's efforts to put it out Rockland. *American Journal of Public Health, 102,* 1942–1948. doi:10.2105/AJPH.2013.301284

Loria, C. M., Mussolino, M. E., Cogswell, H. E., Gillespie, C., Gunn, J. P., Labarthe, D. R., . . . Pavkov, M. E. (2011). Usual sodium intakes compared with current dietary guidelines—United States, 2005–2008. *Morbidity and Mortality Weekly Report, 60,* 1413–1417.

Malarcher, A., Dube, S., Shaw, L., Babb, S., & Kaufmann, R. (2011). Quitting smoking among adults—United States, 2001–2010. *Morbidity and Mortality Weekly Report, 60,* 1513–1519.

Max, W., Sung, H.-Y., & Shi, Y. (2012). Deaths from secondhand smoke exposure in the United States: Economic implications. *American Journal of Public Health, 102,* 2173–2180. doi:10.2105/AJPH.2012.300805

McEwen, M. M., Pasvogel, A., Gallegos, G., & Barrera, L. (2010). Type 2 diabetes self-management social support intervention at the U.S. Mexico border. *Public Health Nursing, 27,* 310–319. doi:10.1111/j.1525.1446.2010.00860x

McNally, B., Robb, R., Mehta, M., Vellano, K., Valderama, A. L., Yoon, P. W., & Kellerman, A. (2011). Out-of-hospital cardiac arrest surveillance—Cardiac Arrest Registry to Enhance Survival (CARES), United States, October 1, 2005 to December 31, 2010. *Morbidity and Mortality Weekly Report, 60*(8), 1–19.

Mehta, N., & Preston, S. (2012). Continued increase in the relative risk of death from smoking. *American Journal of Public Health, 102,* 2181–2186. doi:10.2105/AJPH.2011.300489

Melville, N. A. (2011). *Nurse-led clinics show success for chronic disease management.* Retrieved from http://www.medscape.com/viewarticle/753418?src=mp&spon=24

Melvin, C. L., Corbie-Smith, G., Kumanyika, S. K., Pratt, C. A., Nelson, C., Walker, E. R., . . . Workshop Working Group on CVD Prevention in High-risk Rural Communities. (2013). Developing a research agenda for cardiovascular disease prevention in high-risk rural communities. *American Journal of Public Health, 103,* 1011–1021. doi:10.2105/AJPH.2012.300984

Montgomery, M., & McCrone, S. H. (2010). Psychological distress associated with the diagnostic phase for suspected breast cancer. *Journal of Advanced Nursing, 66,* 2372–2390. doi:10.1111/j.1365-2648.2010.05439x

Moorman, J. E., Akinbami, L. J., Bailey, C. M., Zahran, H. S., King, M. E., Johnson, C. A., & Liu, X. (2012). *National surveillance of asthma—United States, 2001–2010.* Retrieved from http://www.cdc.gov/nchs/data/series/sr_03/sr03_035.pdf

Moorman, J. E., Zahran, H., Truman, B. I., & Molla, M. T. (2011, January 14). Current asthma prevalence—United States, 2006–2008. *Morbidity and Mortality Weekly Report, 60*(Suppl.), 84–86.

Morhaim, D. K., & Pollack, K. M. (2013). End-of-life care issues: A personal, economic, public policy, and public health crisis. *American Journal of Public Health, 103,* e8–e10. doi:10.2105/AJPH.2013.301316

National Center for Chronic Disease Prevention and Health Promotion. (2011a). *Differences in the prevalence and impact of arthritis among racial/ethnic groups in the United States.* Retrieved from http://www.cdc.gov/arthritis/data_statistics/race.htm

National Center for Chronic Disease Prevention and Health Promotion. (2011b). *Targeting epilepsy: Improving the lives of people with one of the nation's most common neurological conditions: At a glance 2011.* Retrieved from http://www.cdc.gov/chronicdisease/resources/publications/aag/epilepsy.htm

National Center for Environmental Health. (2013a). *Asthma and obesity.* Retrieved from http://www.cdc.gov/asthma/asthma_stats/percentage_people_asthma_obese.pdf

National Center for Environmental Health. (2013b). *Insurance coverage and barriers to care for people with asthma.* Retrieved from http://www.cdc.gov/asthma/asthma_stats/Insurance_Asthmasta.pdf

National Center for Environmental Health. (2013c). *Percentage of people with asthma who smoke.* Retrieved from http://www.cdc.gov/asthma/asthma_stats/asthma_stats_factsheet.pdf

National Center for Health Statistics. (2011a). Age-adjusted death rates for heart disease and cancer—United States, 1999–2009. *Morbidity and Mortality Weekly Report, 60,* 713.

National Center for Health Statistics. (2011b). Percentage of adults aged 18–64 years who did not get a needed prescription drug because of cost, by poverty status—National Health Interview Survey, United States, 1999–2010. *Morbidity and Mortality Weekly Report, 60,* 1495.

National Center for Health Statistics. (2011c). Percentage of employed adults aged 18-64 years with current asthma, skin condition, or carpal tunnel syndrome who were told their condition was work-related, by sex—National Health Interview Survey, 2010. *Morbidity and Mortality Weekly Report, 60,* 1712.

National Center for Health Statistics. (2011d). Percentage of noninstitutionalized adults aged >80 years who need help with personal care, by sex—United States, 2008–2009. *Morbidity and Mortality Weekly Report, 60,* 819.

National Center for Health Statistics. (2012a). *Cerebrovascular disease or stroke.* Retrieved from http://www.cdc.gov/nchs/fastats/stroke.htm

National Center for Health Statistics. (2013). Percentage of adults aged 18–24 years who had never smoked cigarettes, by sex – National Health Interview Survey, United States, 1999-2001 through 2011–2012. *Morbidity and Mortality Weekly Report, 62,* 814.

National Center for Health Statistics. (2014a). *Arthritis.* Retrieved from http://www.cdc.gov/nchs/fastats/arthrits.htm

National Center for Health Statistics. (2014b). *Health, United States, 2013: With special feature on prescription drugs.* Retrieved from http://www.cdc.gov/nchs/data/hus/hus13.pdf

National Center for Health Statistics. (2014c). *Hypertension.* Retrieved from http://www.cdc.gov/nchs/fastats/hyprtens.htm

National Center for Injury Prevention and Control. (2013a). *2010, United States, unintentional injury deaths and rates per 100,000*. Retrieved from http://webappa.cdc.gov/sasweb/ncipc/mortrate10_us.htm

National Center for Injury Prevention and Control. (2013b). *Injury prevention and control: Data and statistics (WISQARS)*. Retrieved from http://www.cdc.gov/injury/wisqars/

National Center for Injury Prevention and Control. (2013c). *Unintentional all injury causes nonfatal injuries and rates per 100,000*. Retrieved from http://webappa.cdc.gov/sasweb/ncipc/nfirates2001.html

National Consensus Project for Quality Palliative Care. (2013). *Clinical practice guidelines for quality palliative care* (3rd ed.). Retrieved from http://www.nationalconsensusproject.org/NCP_Clinical_Practice_Guidelines_3rd_Edition.pdf

National Diabetes Information Clearinghouse. (2013). *National diabetes statistics*. Retrieved from http://diabetes.niddk.nih.gov/dm/pubs/statistics/#ddY20

National Health Council. (2013). *About chronic diseases*. Retrieved from http://www.nationalhealthcouncil.org/NHC_Files/Pdf_Files/AboutChronicDisease.pdf

National Heart, Lung, and Blood Institute. (n.d.). *Materials for African American audiences*. Retrieved from http://www.nhlbi.nih.gov/health/healthdisp/aa.htm

National Heart, Lung, and Blood Institute. (2007). *Expert panel report 3: Guidelines for the diagnosis and management of asthma*. Retrieved from http://www.nhlbi.nih.gov/guidelines/asthma/asthgdln.pdf

National Heart, Lung, and Blood Institute. (2008). *Guidelines implementation panel report for: Expert panel report 3: Guidelines for the diagnosis and management of asthma: Partners putting guidelines into action*. Retrieved from https://www.nhlbi.nih.gov/guidelines/asthma/gip_rpt.pdf

National Kidney Foundation. (n.d.). *History: The early years*. Retrieved from http://www.kidney.org/about/history.cfm

National Kidney Foundation. (2013). *About chronic kidney disease*. Retrieved from http://www.kidney.org/kidneydisease/aboutckd.cfm

National Prevention Council. (2011). *National prevention strategy: America's plan for better health and wellness*. Retrieved from http://www.surgeongeneral.gov/initiatives/prevention/strategy/report.pdf

National Research Council. (2011). *Relieving pain in America: A blueprint for transforming prevention, care, education, and research*. Washington, DC: The National Academies Press.

National Safety Council. (2011). *Injury facts 2011 edition*. Retrieved from http://www.nsc.org/Documents/Injury_Facts/Injury_Facts_2011_w.pdf

Nguyen, T.-U. N., Tran, J. H., Kagawa-Singer, M., & Foo, M. A. (2011). A qualitative assessment of community-based breast health navigation services for Southeast Asian women in Southern California: Recommendations for developing a navigator training curriculum. *American Journal of Public Health, 101*, 87–93. doi:10.2105/AJPH.2009.176743

O'Connell, J. M., Wilson, C., Manson, S. M., & Acton, K. J. (2012). The costs of treating American Indian adults with diabetes within the Indian health service. *American Journal of Public Health, 102*, 301–308. doi:10.2105/AJPH.2011.300332

Office of the Surgeon General. (2005). *The Surgeon General's call to action to improve the health and wellness of persons with disabilities, 2005*. Retrieved from http://www.ncbi.nlm.nih.gov/books/NBK44667/

Office on Smoking and Health. (2014). *Best practices for comprehensive tobacco control programs 2014*. Retrieved from http://www.cdc.gov/tobacco/stateandcommunity/best_practices/pdfs/2014/comprehensive.pdf

Ong, M. K., Diamant, A. L., Zhou, Q., Park, H.-Y., & Kaplan, R. M. (2012). Estimates of smoking-related property costs in California multiunit housing. *American Journal of Public Health, 102*, 490–493. doi:10.2105/AJPH.2011.300170

Osgood, N. D., Dyck, R. F., & Grassman, W. K. (2011). The inter- and intragenerational impact of gestational diabetes on the epidemic of type 2 diabetes. *American Journal of Public Health, 101*, 173–179. doi:10.2105/AJPH.2009.186890

Pantell, M., Rehkopf, D., Jutte, D., Syme, L., Balmes, J., & Adler, N. (2013). Social isolation: A predictor of mortality comparable to traditional clinical factors. *American Journal of Public Health, 103*, 2056–2062. doi:10.2105/AJPH.2013.301261

Parker, E. D., Schmitz, K. H., Jacobs, D. R., Dengel, D. R., & Schreiner, P. J. (2007). Physical activity in young adults and incident hypertension over 15 years of follow-up: The CARDIA study. *American Journal of Public Health, 97*, 703–709. doi:10.2105/AJPH.2004.055889

Partners Against Pain. (n.d.). *Pain management tools*. Retrieved from http://www.partnersagainstpain.com/hcp/pain-assessment/tools.aspx

Paulozzi, L. J., Mack, K. A., & Jones, C. M. (2012). Vital signs: Risk for overdose from methadone used for pain relief —United States, 1999–2010. *Morbidity and Mortality Weekly Report, 61*, 493–496.

Perry, G. S., Presley-Cantrell, L. R., & Dhingra, S. (2010). Addressing mental health promotion in chronic disease prevention and health promotion. *American Journal of Public Health, 100*, 2337–2339. doi:10.2105/AJPH.2010.205146

Poulin, M. J., Brown, S. L., Dillard, A. J., & Smith, D. M. (2013). Giving to others and the association between stress and mortality. *American Journal of Public Health, 103*, 1649–1655. doi:10.2105/AJPH.2012.300876

Rasch, E. K., Gulley, S. P., & Chan, L. (2012). Use of emergency departments among working age adults with disabilities: A problem of access and service needs. *Health Services Research* (online version). Retrieved from http://onlinelibrary.wiley.com/doi/10.1111/1475-6773.12025/full

Reiss, D., Leve, L. D., & Neiderhiser, J. M. (2013). How genes and the social environment moderate each other. *American Journal of Public Health, 103*, S111–S121. doi:10.2105/AJPH.2013.301408

Reitzel, L. R., Regan, S. D., Nguyen, N., Cromley, E. K., Strong, L. L., Wetter, D. W., et al. (2014). Density and proximity of fast food restaurants and body mass index among African Americans. *American Journal of Public Health, 104*, 110–116. doi:10.2105/AJPH.2012.301140

Richard, A. A., & Shea, K. (2011). Delineation of self-care and associated concepts. *Journal of Nursing Scholarship, 43*, 555–564. doi:10.1111/j.1547-5069.2011.01404.x

Rowland, J. H., Mariotto, A., Alfana, C. M., Pollack, L. A., Weir, H. K., & White, A. (2011). Cancer survivors—United States, 2007. *Morbidity and Mortality Weekly Report, 60*, 269–272.

Rutkow, L., Vernick, J. S., Tung, G. J., & Cohen, J. E. (2013). Creating smoke-free places through the UN convention on the rights of persons with disabilities. *American Journal of Public Health, 103*, 1748–1753. doi:10.2105/AJPH.2012.301174

Ryan, P., & Sawin, K. J. (2009). The individual and family self-management theory: Background and perspectives on context, process, outcomes. *Nursing Outlook, 57*, 217–225. doi:10.1016/j.outlook.2008,10.004

Sanders-Jackson, A. N., Song, A. V., Hiilamo, H., & Glantz, S. A. (2013). Effect of the Framework Convention on Tobacco Control and voluntary industry health warning labels on passage of mandated cigarette warning labels from 1965 to 2012: Transition probability and event history analysis. *American Journal of Public Health, 103*, 1748–1753. doi:10.2105/AJPH.2013.301324

Sarkar, U., Lopez, A., Black, K., & Schillinger, D. (2011). The wrong tool for the job: Diabetes public health programs and practice guidelines. *American Journal of Public Health, 101*, 1871–1873. doi:10.2105/AJPH.2011.300148

Sarrel, P. M., Njike, V. Y., Vinante, V., & Katz, D. L. (2013). The mortality toll of estrogen avoidance: An analysis of excess deaths among hysterectomized women aged 50 to 59 years. *American Journal of Public Health, 103*, 1583–1588. doi:10.2105/AJPH.2013.301295

Sawyer, M. H., Hoerger, T. J., Murphy, T. V., Schillie, S. F., Hu, D., Spradling, P. R., . . . Zhou, F. (2011). Use of Hepatitis B vaccination for adults with diabetes mellitus: Recommendations of the Advisory Committee on Immunization Practices (ACIP). *Morbidity and Mortality Weekly Report, 60,* 1709–1711.

Saydah, S., Geiss, L., & Gregg, E. (2012). Diabetes death rates among youths aged < 19 years—United States, 1968–2009. *Morbidity and Mortality Weekly Report, 61,* 869–872.

Schieb, L. J., Greer, S. A., Ritchey, M. D., George, M. G., & Casper, M. L. (2013). Vital signs: Avoidable deaths from heart disease, stroke, and hypertensive disease—United States, 2001–2010. *Morbidity and Mortality Weekly Report, 62,* 721–727.

Shea, S., Kothari, D., Teresi, J. A., Kong, J., Eimike, J. P., Lantigua, R. A., . . . Weinstock, R. S. (2013). Social impact analysis of the effects of a telemedicine intervention to improve diabetes outcomes in an ethnically diverse, medically underserved population: Findings from the IDEATel study. *American Journal of Public Health, 103,* 188801894. doi:10.2105/AJPH.2012.300909

Singh, S., Henley, J., Wilson, R., King, J., & Eheman, C. (2013). Invasive cancer incidence—United States, 2009. *Morbidity and Mortality Weekly Report, 62,* 113–118.

Smith, J. R., Edland, S. D., Novotny, T. E., Hofstetter, R., White, M. M., Lindsay, S. P., & Al-Delaimy, W. K. (2011). Increasing hookah use in California. *American Journal of Public Health, 101,* 1876–1879. doi:10.2105/AJPH.2011.300196

Spencer, M. S., Rosland, A.-M., Kieffer, E. C., Sinco, B. R., Valerio, M., Palmisano, G., . . . Heisler, M. (2011). Effectiveness of a community health worker intervention among African American and latino adults with type 2 diabetes: A randomized controlled trial. *American Journal of Public Health, 101,* 2253–2260. doi:10.2105/AJPH.2010.300106

Stanley, M. M., Guilfoyle, S., Vergeront, J. M., Davis, J. P., Hu, D. J., & Khudyakov, Y. (2012). Hepatitis c infection among young adults—Rural Wisconsin, 2010. *Morbidity and Mortality Weekly Report, 61,* 358.

Strauss, S. M., Alfano, M. C., Shelley, D., & Fulmer, T. (2012). Identifying unaddressed systemic health conditions at dental visits: Patients who visited dental practices but not general health care providers in 2008. *American Journal of Public Health, 102,* 253–255. doi:10.2105/AJPH.2011.300420

Tong, V. T., Dietz, P. M., Morrow, B., D'Angelo, D. V., Farr, S. L., Rockhill, K. M., & England, L. J. (2013). Trends in smoking before, during, and after pregnancy—Pregnancy Risk Assessment Monitoring System, United States, 40 sites, 2000–2010. *Morbidity and Mortality Weekly Report, 62*(SS-6), 1–19.

Tynan, M. A., Promoff, M. A., & MacNeil, A. (2012). State cigarette excise taxes. *Morbidity and Mortality Weekly Report, 61,* 201–204.

Underwood, J. M., Townsend, J. S., Stewart, S. L., Buchannan, N., Ekwueme, D. U., Hawkins, N. A., . . . Fairley, T. L. (2012). Surveillance of demographic characteristics and health behaviors among adult cancer survivors—Behavioral Risk Factor Surveillance System, United States, 2009. *Morbidity and Mortality Weekly Report, 61*(SS-1), 1–23.

University of Michigan, Center for Managing Chronic Disease. (2011). *What is chronic disease?* Retrieved from http://cmcd.sph.umich.edu/what-is-chronic-disease.html

U.S. Census Bureau. (2010). *Disability among the working age population: 2008 and 2009.* Retrieved from http://www.census.gov/prod/2010pubs/acsbr09-12.pdf

U.S. Department of Health and Human Services. (2012, July). *Leading health indicators.* Retrieved from http://content.govdelivery.com/bulletins/gd/USOPHSODPHPHF-4b54cc

U.S. Department of Health and Human Services. (2014a). *Healthy people 2020 – Topics and objectives.* Retrieved from http://healthypeople.gov/2020/topicsobjectives2020/default.aspx

U.S. Department of Health and Human Services. (2014b). *Nutrition and weight status.* Retrieved from http://healthypeople.gov/2020/topicsobjectives2020/objectiveslist.aspx?topicId=29

U.S. Preventive Services Task Force. (2008). *Screening for type 2 diabetes mellitus in adults.* Retrieved from http://www.uspreventiveservicestaskforce.org/uspstf/uspsdiab.htm

U.S. Preventive Services Task Force. (2012). *Behavioral counseling to prevent skin cancer.* Retrieved from http://www.uspreventiveservicestaskforce.org/uspstf/uspsskco.htm

U.S. Preventive Services Task Force. (2013). *Screening for lung cancer.* Retrieved from http://www.uspreventiveservicestaskforce.org/uspstf/uspslung.htm

Valderama, A. L., Gillespie, C., & Mercado, C. (2013). Racial/ethnic disparities in the awareness, treatment, and control of hypertension—United States, 2003–2010. *Morbidity and Mortality Weekly Report, 62,* 351–355.

Vijayaraghavan, M., Messer, K., White, M. M., & Pierce, J. P. (2013). The effectiveness of cigarette price and smoke-free home on low-income smokers in the United States. *American Journal of Public Health, 103,* 2276–2283. doi:10.2105/AJPH.2013.301300

Warner, K. E. (2014). 50 years since the first Surgeon General's report on smoking and health: A happy anniversary? *American Journal of Public Health, 104,* 5–7.

Warner, K. E., Sexton, D. W., Gillespie, B. W., Levy, D. T., & Chaloupka, F. J. (2014). Impact of tobacco control on adult per capita cigarette consumption in the United States. *American Journal of Public Health, 104,* 83–89. doi:10.2105/AJPH.2013.301591

Wherry, L. R. (2013). Medicaid family planning expansions and related preventive care. *American Journal of Public Health, 103,* 1577–1578. doi:10.2105/AJPH.2013.301266

World Health Organization. (2011). *Global status report on noncommunicable diseases.* Retrieved from http://whqlibdoc.who.int/publications/2011/9789240686458_eng.pdf

World Health Organization. (2012). *Assessing national capacity for the prevention and control of noncommunicable diseases.* Retrieved from http://www.who.int/cancer/publications/national_capacity_prevention_ncds.pdf

World Health Organization. (2014). *Disabilities.* Retrieved from http://www.who.int/topics/disabilities/en/

Yang, T.-C., Matthews, S. A., & Hillemeier, M. M. (2011). Effect of health care system distrust on breast and cervical cancer screening in Philadelphia, Pennsylvania. *American Journal of Public Health, 101,* 1297–1305. doi:10.2105/AJPH.2010.300061

Zahran, H. S., Bailey, C., & Garbe, P. (2011). Vital signs: Asthma prevalence, disease characteristics, and self-management education—United States, 2001–2009. *Morbidity and Mortality Weekly Report, 60,* 547–552.

Zimmerman, S., Kramer, K., & Trowbridge, M. J. (2013). Overcoming legal liability concerns for school-based physical activity promotion. *American Journal of Public Health, 103,* 1962–1968. doi:10.2105/AJPH.2013.301319

CHAPTER

28 Mental Health and Mental Illness

Learning Outcomes

After reading this chapter, you should be able to:

1. Define mental health and mental illness.
2. Analyze the personal, family, and societal impact of mental illness and mental health problems.
3. Analyze factors influencing the development of mental health problems.
4. Identify symptoms characteristic of common mental health problems.
5. Describe strategies for promoting mental health and analyze the population health nurse's role in each.
6. Analyze the role of the population health nurse in strategies to prevent mental health problems.
7. Discuss approaches to resolving mental health problems and analyze the population health nurse's role in each.
8. Describe areas of emphasis in health restoration related to mental health problems and analyze the role of the population health nurse in maintenance.

Key Terms

community mental health problems
dual diagnosis
dysthymia
ethnopsychopharmacology
label avoidance
mental health
mental health problems
mental health promotion
mental illness
psychological flexibility
recovery
resilience
seasonal affective disorder (SAD)
serious mental illness
somatization
transinstitutionalization
treatment gap

Advocacy Then

Dorothea Dix and Asylum Reform

Dorothea Lynde Dix was born to parents who had mental health problems, although the exact nature of those problems is debated in various sources and includes alcoholism, depression, or mental retardation (Bumb, n.d.; Casarez, 2000; Dorothea Lynde Dix, 2014). At a young age, she began teaching young girls in schools supported by her grandmother. She was first exposed to the inhumane conditions in which both prisoners and the mentally ill were kept when she volunteered to teach a Sunday school class to inmates at the jail in East Cambridge, Massachusetts. Appalled by what she saw, she went to court and was successful in securing heat for the inmates (Dorothea Dix, 2014). She then embarked on a fact-finding tour that took her to most of the jails, almshouses, and houses of correction within the state. She compiled her findings in a report presented to the Massachusetts legislature that led to funding for an institution specifically for the mentally ill (National Women's Hall of Fame, 2011). She extended her efforts throughout the United States and in Europe and was responsible for multiple changes in how the mentally ill were perceived and treated, including the establishment of several hospitals for the mentally ill (Dorothea Dix, 2014).

When she volunteered at the beginning of the U.S. Civil War, Dix was made Superintendent of Nurses for the Union Army (Prison and Asylum Reform, n.d.). In that capacity, although she had no nursing background, she was responsible for the administration of military hospitals and supplies as well as for recruiting nurses. She was the first women to serve in a high-level federally appointed role (Dorothea Lynde Dix, 2014). After the war, she continued to be politically active in advocating for humane care of the mentally ill.

Advocacy Now

Advocating for Mental Illness Treatment

The Treatment Advocacy Center is a national nonprofit organization that advocates for access to timely treatment for persons with mental illness. The organization works to influence legislation and policy related to mental health treatment and supports research on innovative treatments for mental disorders. Organizational activities have resulted in changes in commitment and treatment laws in 22 states. Foci for activities include educating policy makers abut mental illnesses and their treatment, assisting grassroots activism for effective legislation, promoting innovative strategies for preventing diversion of mentally ill people to correctional facilities, and promoting strategies to enhance treatment adherence after hospital discharge (Treatment Advocacy Center, 2011).

Mental health and mental illness are not mutually exclusive and have been conceptualized as dual continua: one reflecting mental health and the other reflecting mental illness. Mental health is a state of flourishing, characterized by positive emotions and high levels of psychological and social function. Mental illness, on the other hand, is a state of languishing, characterized by feelings of emptiness and stagnation accompanied by specific symptoms. Some level of mental illness may be present even in the context of general mental health and vice versa (Perry, Presley-Cantrell, & Dhingra, 2010).

A 1999 U.S. Surgeon General's report defined **mental health** as "a state of successful performance of mental function, resulting in productive activities, fulfilling relationships with people, and the ability to adapt to change and to cope with adversity" (quoted in Keyes, Myers, & Kendler, 2010, p. 2379). The World Health Organization's (WHO) definition of mental health encompasses achievement of one's potential and abilities to cope with life's stresses, work productively, and contribute to society (2014a). The Surgeon General's definition incorporates two aspects: feeling good and functioning well (Keyes et al., 2010), whereas the WHO definition addresses emotional (feelings of happiness and satisfaction), psychological (effective individual function), and social well-being (effective social function) (Fledderus, Bohlmeijer, Smit, & Westerhof, 2010). The absence of positive mental health has been linked to increased risk of all-cause mortality (Keyes & Simoes, 2012).

Mental illness or mental disorder is defined as "health conditions that are characterized by alterations in thinking, mood, or behavior (or some combination thereof) associated with distress and/or impaired functioning" (National Institute of Mental Health [NIMH], 1999, p. 5). **Serious mental illness** is defined by the U.S. federal government as "a diagnosable mental, behavioral, or emotional disorder of sufficient duration to meet diagnostic criteria specified within the *Diagnostic and Statistical Manual of Mental Disorders (DSM)-III-R*, (4) that has resulted in functional impairment which substantially interferes with or limits one or more major life activities" (Insel, 2013, para 3). **Mental health problems** involve signs and symptoms of mental distress that are of insufficient duration or intensity to qualify as mental disorders diagnosed on the basis of accepted criteria. **Community mental health problems** are those that occur with sufficient frequency in the community or population group to be of serious concern in the overall health status of the population. In this chapter we use the term *mental health problems* to refer to the composite of mental and emotional conditions that result in impaired function.

Individual, Family, and Societal Effects of Chronic Mental Health Problems

Mental health problems have burdensome effects for individuals and their families as well as for society as a whole. Some of these effects will be presented here.

Personal Effects

Suffering and disability are the two most prominent effects of mental health problems for the individuals they affect. There is no objective measure of the suffering endured, but measures of disability are discouraging. Depression is one of the top three disabling conditions in high-income countries throughout the world (Smith & Bielecky, 2012). Although disability related to chronic health problems has decreased in recent years, mental illness-related disability has increased. For example, mental health disability increased from 2% of the U.S. non-elderly adult population in 1997–1999 to 2.7% in 2007–2009, affecting approximately 2 million people (Mojtabai, 2011).

Mental health problems not only result in mental disability but also cause physical and social impairments. Mental illness may result in worsening of physical health problems due to inability or lack of motivation for effective self-care. On average, people with serious mental health problems die 25 years earlier than those without mental health problems (Shim & Rust, 2013).

Family Effects

Mental health problems also exact a toll on the families of people that experience them. The family costs of mental disorders are both economic and emotional. In Chapter 19∞, we reviewed the effects of caregiving on family members with Alzheimer's disease. Other chronic mental health problems also have family effects. For example, families in which one member has schizophrenia may not progress through the normal stages of family development described in Chapter 14∞ due to the difficulty people with schizophrenia have with separating from home and becoming independent. Parents of a child with schizophrenia may find themselves extending the parental role indefinitely.

The increasing move to treat mental health problems in community settings has increased the burden of care for families. The presence of a family member with a mental illness creates demands and stress for families that can affect family interactions and the physical, emotional, and social health of family members (Lowenstein, Butler, & Ashcroft, 2010). The effects of mental illness in a family member include denial and feelings of anxiety and hopelessness. Family members may also suffer the burden of caring for someone who is not fully capable of caring for him or herself. In addition, families may experience the stigma associated with mental illness or suffer with stigmatized family members.

Clients with mental illness may have difficulty holding a job because of the impairments resulting from their conditions. Unemployment and underemployment may lead to poverty for the individual and the family. In addition, family caretakers may be forced to take time from work or even stop working, further diminishing family income. Major mental disorders may also prevent family members from carrying out their expected family roles. Mental illness in a family member often increases stress for the entire family and may contribute to family communication problems and perceptions of social stigma for both client and family.

Strategies that have been suggested for dealing with the burden of caring for family members with mental illness include educating themselves about the disease and becoming involved in the treatment process, seeking out resources, having realistic expectations, reaching out for support, and working closely with the treatment team (Tartakovsky, n.d.). The National Alliance on Mental Illness (NAMI) has developed a family education course, *Family-to-family*, designed to provide support to families with loved ones with mental illness (NAMI, n.d.c). Research on program effectiveness has indicated that it improves knowledge about the illness and fosters empowerment, problem-focused coping, and increased acceptance of the illness, as well as reducing stress (Dixon et al., 2011). For further information about the *Family-to-family* program, see the *External Resources* section of the student resources site.

Societal Effects

Mental illness and less severe mental health problems also pose a burden for society in general. Mental disorders are the leading cause of disability worldwide and account for a substantial portion of the global disease burden. For example, in 2004, depression was the third leading cause of disease burden worldwide and is expected to rise to the second leading cause by 2020. Much of this burden is related to decreased productivity as well as the direct treatment costs for mental health problems (Centers for Disease Control and Prevention [CDC], 2010). Overall, mental health conditions account for 37% of healthy life years lost due to noncommunicable diseases. Unipolar depression alone accounts for nearly a third of mental health disability-adjusted life years lost, and bipolar disorder and schizophrenia account for another 15% (Bloom et al., 2011).

In addition to the burden of disability posed by mental disorders, society experiences considerable economic burden as well. For example, overall costs of mental health care in 2006 amounted to $57.5 billion, equal to the amount spent on cancer care (Insel, 2011). A 2011 World Economic Forum report estimated global costs for mental health in 2010 at $2.5 trillion. These costs are expected to rise to $6 trillion by 2030, about two thirds of which are due to indirect costs, such as lost economic productivity (Bloom et al., 2011).

The importance of chronic mental health problems in the United States is highlighted by the number of objectives related to these disorders in the national health objectives for the year 2020 (U.S. Department of Health and Human Services [USDHHS], 2014). Some of these objectives are presented at the end of this chapter. The complete set of objectives for mental health and mental disorders can be viewed on the *Healthy People 2020* web page.

Trends in Mental Health Problems

WHO estimates that one quarter of all the people in the world who utilize health services have at least one mental health problem (Bloom et al., 2011). Together mental health and substance abuse disorders constitute the second leading cause of worldwide disease burden and disability (Shim & Rust, 2013). In addition, the Organisation for Economic Cooperation and Development (OECD) estimates that 20% of the working age population in OECD countries has a clinical mental disorder, and the lifetime prevalence is estimated at 50% of the world's population. By conservative estimates, mental illness costs account for 3% to 4% of the gross domestic product (GDP) of the European Union, and one third to one half of all disability claims result from mental health problems (OECD, 2011).

The majority of mental illnesses, or common mental disorders (CMDs), are mild or moderate in their effects, but all can evolve to severe mental disorders (SMDs). In addition, most mental illness is recurrent. For example, recurrence occurs in 40% to 80% of people with depression even with medication. An individual may also experience a variety of co-occurring mental disorders as well as comorbidity with chronic physical health problems, with comorbid conditions being more disabling than a single condition (OECD, 2011).

In the United States an estimated quarter of adults experience a diagnosable mental illness in any given year, and approximately two thirds of them do not seek care (Center for Surveillance, Epidemiology, and Laboratory Services [CSELS], 2012). In 2011–2012, 3.1% of the U.S. population reported serious psychological distress within the prior 40 days (National Center for Health Statistics [NCHS], 2014), and in the 2009–2011 National Survey on Drug Use and Health, nearly 20% of U.S. adults over 18 years of age had a mental illness (Gfroerer et al., 2013). According to the 2007–2008 National Ambulatory Medical Care Survey, 5% of all ambulatory care visits in the United States were related to mental health disorders, primarily depression, psychoses, and anxiety disorders. The rate of hospitalization with a primary diagnosis of mental illness was 97.9 per 10,000 population but this rate decreased with increasing age (Reeves et al., 2011).

Prevalence figures for specific mental disorders are equally alarming. Periodic depression, "feeling down" or "having the blues," is a common occurrence in all people, but major depression is not a normal phenomenon. A milder, chronic, ongoing form of depressed mood that prevents one from functioning well or feeling good is called **dysthymia** (Mayo Clinic Staff, 2012). Bipolar disorder is another form of depression. In bipolar disorder, also known as manic-depressive disorder, people experience unusual shifts in mood, energy, and functional ability. Most people with bipolar disorder cycle through periods of depression alternating with periods of energy, excitability, and irritability called *mania*. Symptoms gradually flow through a continuum from severe mania and hyperactivity through hypomania, characterized by mild to moderate manic symptoms, followed by a normal mood state. Normal mood eventually shifts into mild depression and then into severe depression. Some people exhibit symptoms of both mania and depression simultaneously in a mixed state (NIMH, n.d.b). Both major depression and bipolar disorder are risk factors for suicide. Symptoms of depression and mania are presented in Table 28-1●.

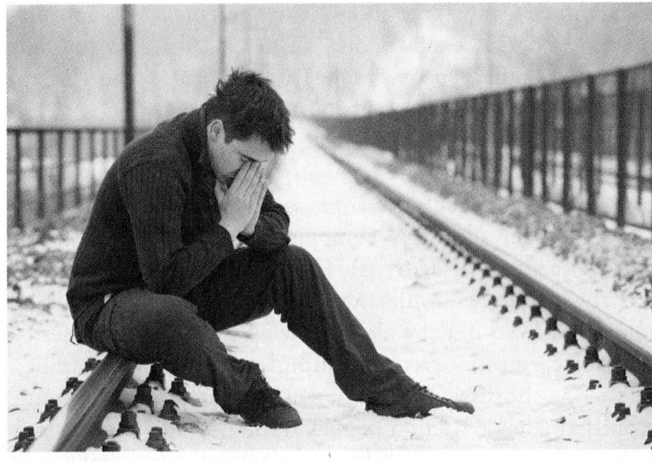

Depression may lead to suicide attempts. *(Chalabala/Fotolia)*

TABLE 28-1 Mood and Behavior Changes Characteristic of Depression and Mania

Depression	Mania
Mood Changes: • Persistent sadness or despair • Loss of interest in formerly pleasurable activities (including sex)	**Mood Changes:** • Persistent feelings of euphoria, overly happy, or outgoing • Irritability
Behavior Changes: • Feeling fatigued or "slowed down" • Problems concentrating, remembering, or making decisions • Restlessness, irritability • Changes in eating, sleeping, or other habits • Thinking of death or suicide, attempting suicide	**Behavior Changes:** • Talking fast, jumping from one topic to another • Psychomotor agitation • Decreased sleep • Racing thoughts and distractibility • Poor judgment and impaired impulse control, engaging in high-risk behaviors • Increasing activities or projects • Unrealistic perceptions of one's abilities

Data from: National Institute of Mental Health. (n.d.b). *Bipolar disorder.* Retrieved from http://www.nimh.nih.gov/health/topics/bipolar-disorder/index.shtml

The lifetime risk of major depression in the United States is 16.5% and approximately 3.5% of the population will experience bipolar disorder (NIMH, n.d.c, n.d.e). In the 2008 Behavioral Risk Factor Surveillance System (BRFSS), more than 8% of the population reported current depression, and similar figures were reported in the National Health and Nutrition Examination Survey (NHANES) from 2007 to 2010 (NCHS, 2012a). In 2009, people responding to the BRFSS reported an average of 3.5 mentally unhealthy days in the last month. Postpartum depression occurs in 14.5% of women after delivery and ranges from 10% in women aged 30 to 39 years to 23% in those less than 19 years of age (Reeves et al., 2011).

Schizophrenia is generally conceived of as a disease of abnormality in the brain. Schizophrenia is characterized by three types of symptoms: positive symptoms, negative symptoms, and cognitive symptoms. Positive symptoms are unusual thoughts or perceptions that are not present in "normal" people. Negative symptoms are an absence of normal behaviors and emotional states, and cognitive symptoms reflect deficits in attention, memory, and executive functions that permit planning and organizing thoughts and behaviors (NIMH, 2013). Positive, negative, and cognitive symptoms of schizophrenia are summarized in Table 28-2●. Schizophrenia affects approximately 1% of the general public (NIMH, 2009b). This amounts to about 2.4 million people in the United States (Wexner Medical Center, Ohio State University, n.d.).

Anxiety disorders are a group of illnesses that result in chronic and overwhelming fear and anxiety that tend to grow progressively worse with time. Anxiety disorders include panic disorder, obsessive-compulsive disorder (OCD), posttraumatic stress disorder (PTSD), phobias, and generalized anxiety disorder. Panic disorder is characterized by episodes of intense fear without any identifiable basis. Panic is manifested in cardiac, respiratory, and gastrointestinal symptoms of distress (e.g., shortness of breath, palpitations) or fear of dying. Approximately 6 million people in the United States experience panic disorders. Full-blown recurrent panic attacks can be extremely disabling, particularly when those affected begin to avoid places or situations in which attacks have occurred (NIMH, 2009a).

OCD manifests as persistent upsetting thoughts (obsessions) and the use of rituals (compulsions) to control the resulting anxiety. For example, an obsession with dirt may lead to constant hand washing. Performance of these rituals is distressing and interferes with daily life, but those affected cannot desist. OCD may be accompanied by other mental health problems such as eating disorders, depression, and other anxiety disorders (NIMH, 2009a).

PTSD, another form of anxiety disorder, arises in response to experiencing or witnessing a traumatic event and is characterized by nightmares, flashbacks, irritability, depression, and poor concentration. About 70% of the U.S. population has experienced at least one major traumatic event in their lives. Approximately 20% of these people develop PTSD. PTSD affects approximately 5% of the U.S. population or 1.5 million people at any given time and will affect about 8% of adults over their lifetimes (PTSD Alliance, n.d.). PTSD is characterized by the presence of three clusters of symptoms present for at least

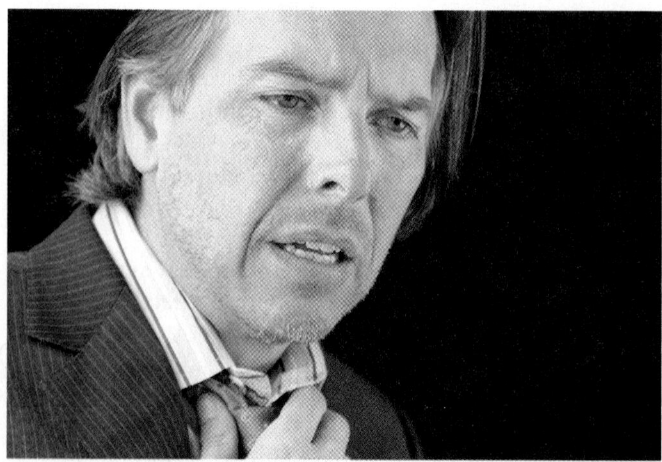

Panic attacks can strike without warning and usually get worse over time. *(David Stuart/Fotolia)*

TABLE 28-2 Positive, Negative, and Cognitive Symptoms of Schizophrenia

Positive symptoms: Symptoms present in people with schizophrenia that are not present in the general population • Hallucinations: Seeing, hearing, smelling, or feeling things that no one else does • Delusions: Unchanging false beliefs that are not part of one's culture • Thought disorders: Unusual or dysfunctional ways of thinking, difficulty organizing thoughts or presenting them coherently, loss of thoughts, creation of meaningless words (neologism) • Movement disorders: Agitated or repetitive body movements or lack of movements and response (catatonia)
Negative symptoms: Disruptions of normal emotions and behaviors • "Flat affect": Lack of facial expression or monotonous voice • Lack of pleasure in everyday life • Lack of ability to begin and sustain planned activities • Speaking little, even when forced to interact
Cognitive symptoms: Inappropriate thought processes • Poor executive function: Inability to understand information and use it to make decisions • Trouble focusing or paying attention • Problems with working memory: Inability to use information immediately after learning it

Data from: National Institute of Mental Health. (2013). *Schizophrenia.* Retrieved from http://www.nimh.nih.gov/health/topics/schizophrenia/index.shtml

6 months. Symptom clusters include reliving the traumatic event through flashbacks or nightmares; avoiding thoughts, people, places, and things that recall memories of the event; and hypervigilance (PTSD Alliance, n.d.). Hypervigilance may manifest as irritability, aggression, or being easily startled (NIMH, 2009a). According to the National Institute for Mental Health (NIMH, 2009a), an estimated 7.7 million U.S. adults experience PTSD.

Phobias are the most common anxiety disorders and include social phobia and specific phobias. People with social phobia, or social anxiety disorder, feel overwhelming anxiety, embarrassment, or self-consciousness that make them incapable of interacting comfortably with others in everyday social situations. Social phobias may be related to one specific type of social interaction (e.g., speaking in public) or to broad categories of interaction. Specific phobias are extreme and unreasonable fears of something that pose little real danger (e.g., heights, being closed in). Approximately 15 million U.S. adults are affected by social phobias, and 19.2 million experience specific phobias (NIMH, 2009a).

Finally, general anxiety disorder is characterized by constant and excessive worry about everyday events. General anxiety disorder affects about 6.8 million U.S. adults (NIMH, 2009a). A given person may experience more than one type of anxiety disorder, and anxiety disorders frequently co-occur with other mental health problems such as depression, eating disorders, and substance abuse.

Eating disorders result in serious disturbances of one's everyday diet. Three types of eating disorders are common: anorexia nervosa, bulimia nervosa, and binge eating disorder. Anorexia nervosa is characterized by a strong resistance to maintaining a minimal weight for one's height and body type, by intense fear of gaining weight, and by a distorted body image that leads one to perceive oneself as fat even when significantly underweight (NIMH, 2011b). An estimated 1% to 4.2% of U.S. women experiences anorexia nervosa in their lifetimes, with prevalence three times higher among women than men (Ekern, 2014).

Bulimia nervosa is characterized by frequent episodes of eating unusually large amounts of food followed by compensatory purging or other behaviors to prevent weight gain that usually occur at least twice a week. Because of the compensatory behaviors, many people with bulimia are able to maintain a normal weight (NIMH, 2011b). Approximately 1.5% of U.S. women and 0.5% of men have bulimia at some point in their lives (Ekern, 2014). Excessive overeating without compensatory purging and other behaviors is referred to as binge eating disorder. Binge eating contributes to obesity and the resulting increased risk for cardiovascular disease, hypertension, and other chronic physical health problems (NIMH, 2011b). An estimated 2.8% of the U.S. adult population engages in binge eating in their lifetimes, including 3.5% of women and 2% of men (Ekern, 2014).

Borderline personality disorder (BPD) is characterized by rapidly changing moods and resulting difficulty with interpersonal relationships and an inability to function effectively in society. BPD affects 1% to 2% of the U.S. population (NAMI, n.d.a). The characteristic mood changes of people with BPD occur rapidly, over a period of hours rather than days as is the case with depression or mania. The impulsivity that accompanies these mood changes may lead to self-injury or suicide, impulsive spending, or sudden shifts in attitudes toward others (e.g., from idealization to anger and dislike). People with BPD may see routine absences of significant others as evidence of rejection and abandonment and may resort to threats of self-harm or suicide in response (NIMH, n.d.d).

Autism spectrum disorders (ASDs), also called pervasive developmental disorders, tend to occur in young children and may be diagnosed as early as 18 months of age. Autism is characterized by persistent difficulties with social interaction and communication and restricted repetitive patterns of behavior or activity. Children with ASD have difficulty learning to

TABLE 28-3 Characteristic Symptoms of Selected Mental Disorders

Disorder	Characteristic Symptoms
Anxiety disorders • Panic disorder • Obsessive compulsive disorder • Post-traumatic stress disorder (PTSD) • Phobias • General anxiety disorder	Symptoms: Feelings of fear/dread, trembling, restlessness, muscle tension, rapid heart rate, dizziness, lightheadedness, increased perspiration, cold hands and feet, shortness of breath
Autism spectrum disorders • Asperger syndrome • Rett syndrome • Childhood disintegrative disorder	Symptoms: Deficits in social interaction and verbal and nonverbal communication, repetitive behaviors or interests, unusual response to sensory stimulation, delayed development
Borderline personality disorder	Symptoms: Chronic instability of moods with intense anger, depression, and anxiety lasting only hours, may be accompanied by periodic aggression, self-injury, or substance abuse, frequent changes in life goals and plans, impulsivity
Eating disorders • Anorexia nervosa • Binge eating • Bulimia nervosa	Symptoms: Intense fear of gaining weight, altered body image, infrequent menses, recurrent and uncontrolled eating followed by purging, misuse of laxative, diuretics, enemas

Data from: National Institute of Mental Health, n.d.a, n.d.c, 2009a, 2011b. (See references at the end of this chapter for full citations.)

interpret social cues from others, which makes communication difficult. They may also under- or overreact to stimuli. Approximately one in 88 children is affected by ASD (NIMH, n.d.a).

In all likelihood, the figures presented here underrepresent the actual prevalence of mental illness in the United States and the world. Due to stigma, lack of knowledge, and lack of access to care, many people with mental health problems do not seek care and remain undiagnosed. This gap between the true prevalence of mental health disorders and those treated, or treatment prevalence, is referred to as the **treatment gap** (Henderson, Evans-Lacko, & Thornicroft, 2013). Symptoms characteristic of autism and other mental illnesses are presented in Table 28-3●.

Population Health Nursing and Mental Health and Illness

Population health nurses may play a significant part in the control of mental health problems with individuals and with population groups. Effective control includes assessment of risks for and factors influencing mental health problems, as well as the planning, implementation, and evaluation of health care programs directed toward mental health.

Assessing Mental Health Status

Factors related to each of the six categories of determinants of health influence the risk for and course of mental health problems for individuals and populations. Population health nurses will be actively involved in assessing for these risks as well as for the presence of mental illness in individual clients and in the population as a whole. Knowledge of factors in each of the categories will enable population health nurses to better promote mental health and contribute to control strategies for community mental health problems.

BIOLOGICAL DETERMINANTS. Biological factors influencing mental health problems include age, gender, and race or ethnicity; genetic inheritance; and physiologic function.

Age, gender, and race/ethnicity. Age influences mental health problems primarily in terms of the typical age at first onset of symptoms. Both children and adults develop mental health problems. One in three or four children has a mental disorder, and one in ten experiences serious mental disturbances. Over the course of their lifetimes one in four to five children can expect to meet criteria for a mental disorder with severe impairment. *The National Comorbidity Survey Replication—Adolescent Supplement* indicated a lifetime prevalence of 32% for anxiety disorder in adolescents and 19% for behavioral disorders. In addition, 40% of those who develop a mental disorder will experience more than one disorder, and 22% will experience severe distress or impairment (Merikangas et al., 2010).

Different mental disorders have their typical age of onset at different ages. For example, the median age for onset of anxiety among children and adolescents is 6 years of age, compared to 11 years for behavior disorders, 13 years for mood disorders, and 15 years for substance use disorders. The median age for all mental disorders is 14 years of age, and 75% of disorders develop before the age of 24. Only mood disorders typically start at older ages with onset typically in the 30s and 40s. There is an estimated 12-year gap between symptom onset and initiation of treatment for most people with mental disorders (OECD, 2011). Given the relatively young age of onset of these disorders, some authors have called for a greater focus on mental health promotion and prevention of mental illness rather than on treatment (Merikangas et al., 2010).

Depression is more common in older age groups than in children and adolescents. As much as 6.6% of U.S. elderly experience a major episode of depression in any given year. In

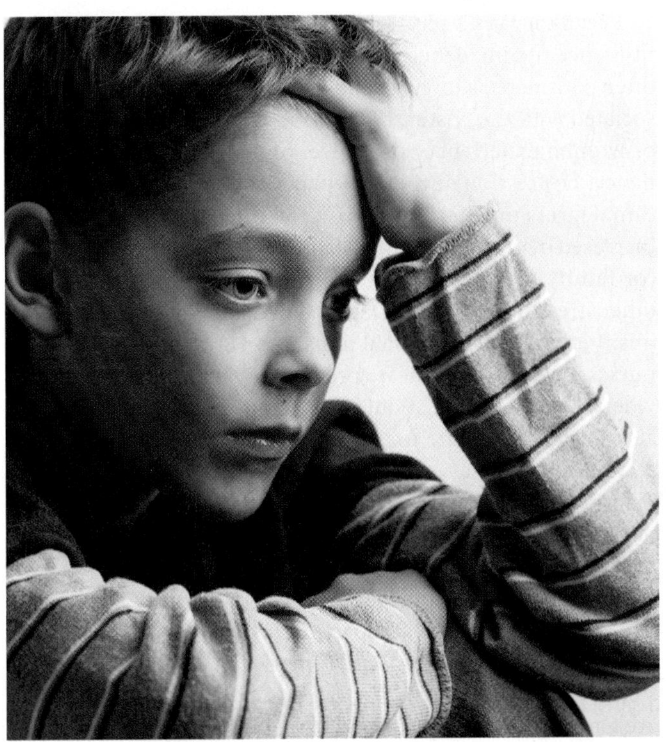

Children also experience mental health problems. *(Tatyana Gladskih/Fotolia)*

this age group, in particular, depression may complicate treatment for other chronic physical health problems (Akincigil et al., 2012).

Generally speaking, women are more likely than men to develop most mental disorders. One exception is ASDs, which occur five times more often in boys than girls (CSELS, 2013). Similarly, while equally prevalent in men and women, men develop symptoms of schizophrenia at earlier ages than women (late teens to early 20s vs. 20s and 30s for women) (NIMH, 2009b; Wexner Medical Center, n.d.). Schizophrenia rarely has its onset in childhood or over age 45, but there may be a prodromal period during adolescence characterized by withdrawal and increases in unusual thoughts and suspicions. This prodromal period is more apt to occur in adolescents with a family history of psychosis (NIMH, 2009b). Both social phobias and OCD may manifest in childhood, and approximately a third of people with OCD first developed symptoms as children (NIMH, 2009a). Eating disorders can manifest throughout life, but often begin in adolescence or young adulthood (NIMH, 2011b).

Women are less likely than men to be exposed to traumatic events at some point in their lives (51% vs. 61%) (Vogt, 2014), but are more than twice as likely as men to develop PTSD (PTSD Alliance, n.d.). The estimated prevalence for PTSD in women is 9.7% compared to 3.6% for men. Women are more vulnerable to sexual assaults and molestation, more likely to have experienced childhood neglect or abuse, and more likely to be affected by domestic violence or the sudden death of a loved one. It has been proposed that women's increased vulnerability to the effects of these traumas is because women's sense of well-being is closely tied to the character of their relationships with others (Vogt, 2014).

In the 2007–2010 NHANES, women were more likely to report current depression at every age than men (NCHS, 2012b), and in the 2010–2011 National Health Interview Survey, 22% of women and 17% of men reported often feeling worried or anxious (NCHS, 2012a).

Although Blacks generally have a lower risk of substance abuse and mental disorders, such as depression and anxiety than Whites, this is not true among some subgroups of the population. For example, the prevalence of mental illness is higher in Caribbean-born Black men than U.S.-born Black men, but the reverse was found to be true for women. Similarly, mental illness rates were found to be lower among Somali-born Blacks than either U.S.-born Blacks or Whites. Among the elderly, however, African Americans were less likely than White elders to receive a diagnosis of depression even in the face of symptoms and were less likely to receive treatment (Akincigil et al., 2012). This finding suggests that there may be less difference in actual occurrence of disease than in its recognition.

Genetic inheritance. Genetics also appear to influence the incidence of some mental health problems. Various studies of families, twins, and adopted children provide strong evidence that some people have a genetic predisposition to develop schizophrenia. Apparently an inherited chemical imbalance in the brain is necessary for schizophrenia to develop, but its development is influenced by the probable interaction of multiple genetic and environmental factors. Siblings of persons with schizophrenia have a 7% to 8% risk of developing the disease, and the risk increases to 10% to 15% of children whose parents have schizophrenia. Risk of disease also increases with the number of family members affected (NIMH, 2009b; Wexner Medical Center, n.d.).

Genetic contributions to vulnerability are implicated in other mental health problems as well. For example, ASDs are believed to be influenced by multiple gene–environment interactions (Johnson, Giarelli, Lewis, & Rice, 2013). The effects of genetic influence, however, are apparent in findings that the chance of an identical twin whose sibling has ASD developing the condition is 35% to 90%. Risk decreases to 0% to 31% of non-identical twins. In addition, parents who have one child with ASD have a 2% to 28% chance of having a second child that is affected (CSELS, 2013).

The heritability of major depressive disorder is estimated at 31% to 42%, but no specific genes influencing transmission have yet been identified (Schutte, Davies, & Goris, 2013). Risk of depression may be as much as three to five times higher for people with a first-degree relative affected than for the general population, and risk seems to increase if the affected relative became symptomatic before 25 to 30 years of age. Similarly, a child of a parent with depression has a 5% to 30% risk of developing the disease. If both siblings and parents have depression, the estimated risk of developing the disease in other children is 50% for bipolar disorder and 30% to 40% for major depression.

Families with a history of depression may also have a history of other comorbid conditions, such as alcohol abuse and eating disorders. There is some evidence, however, that the genetic risk of major depression is mitigated by higher education and upward social mobility (Mezuk, Myers, & Kendler, 2013).

Genetic inheritance may also play a part in Alzheimer's disease and other irreversible dementias. For example, to date, three specific gene mutations have been associated with some forms of Alzheimer's disease (Schutte et al., 2013). Similarly, there is some evidence that genes may play a role in creating fear memories that lead to PTSD. There is also a suggestion that changes in the prefrontal cortex may modify responses designed to control stress when stress is perceived to be controllable. It is hypothesized that these changes may be activated by trauma, head injury, or mental illness, or modified by personality factors such as optimism or negativity or the availability of social support (NIMH, 2012a).

On the positive side, there is also some evidence that factors related to psychological well-being may also be heritable. Genetic influences have been noted with respect to emotional and social well-being (Keyes et al., 2010).

Physiologic Function. The interaction between mental health and physiologic factors is complex. The presence of physiologic conditions may increase one's risk for mental health problems. Conversely, mental health problems may pose risks for physiologic effects. Finally, the presence of either mental or physical conditions may complicate control of problems in the other realm.

There is considerable evidence that some mental health problems have a physiologic basis in brain chemistry and that the resulting neurophysiologic deficits are a major contributor to mental illness. For example, deficits in sensory processing result in the sensory-based behaviors typical of ASDs (Marco, Hinkley, Hill, & Nagarajan, 2011). Similarly, the presence of chronic physical illness, infection, malnutrition, and the effects of hormones and physical trauma have all been shown to play a part in the development of mental health problems. Infectious agents such as human immunodeficiency virus (HIV) and syphilis, for example, are implicated in the development of some forms of dementia. In addition, depression has been associated with declining CD4-T cell counts in people with HIV infection, speeding progression to AIDS and increasing mortality risk (Tsai et al., 2013). Physiologic differences also account for differential effects of psychotropic drugs in different racial and ethnic groups.

Mental health problems may also increase one's risk for physical illness. For example, anxiety and depression have been shown to increase the risk for the onset of coronary heart disease (CHD) and to affect survival in persons with existing CHD. Conversely, people recovering from myocardial infarction are at increased risk for major depressive disorders. Depression may also be implicated in falls among the elderly. Treatment for depression may also increase fall risk and fallers may be prone to anxiety and depression.

Pregnancy, as a physiologic condition, has been found to influence the incidence of depression. Although pregnancy is often considered a joyful event and depression is more often associated with the postpartum period, an estimated 10% to 20% of women experience some level of depression during pregnancy. Depression during pregnancy is also known as antepartum depression. A woman's risk for antepartum depression is increased by relationship problems, a past history of depression (or family history of depression), prior pregnancy loss, and other stressful life events. Depression during pregnancy may be misinterpreted as hormonal imbalance, and population health nurses may need to educate pregnant women, health care providers, and the public about antepartum depression. They may also need to advocate for access to counseling and treatment services for those affected. For example, although many health insurance plans cover care for the pregnancy itself, they may not provide coverage for counseling services related to antepartum depression.

Depression in the postpartum period is more common and better recognized than antepartum depression and may occur in one of three forms: postpartum blues, postpartum depression, or puerperal or postpartum psychosis. Postpartum blues are a mild form of depression characterized by tearfulness and anxiety. They are time-limited, and usually do not require treatment beyond emotional support. Postpartum depression and psychosis are more serious conditions that require treatment. Miscarriage, menstrual cycle difficulties, and menopause may also trigger depression, particularly in the context of a family history of depression.

Receiving a diagnosis of a chronic illness may also lead to depression or anxiety (Al-Modallal, Abuidhail, Sowan, & Al-Rawashdeh, 2010). Conversely, mental health problems of all kinds may interfere with treatment adherence for physical health conditions (Perry et al., 2010). The presence of some chronic physical health problems may also impede recognition of mental health problems. For example, people who are culturally Deaf (meaning they have been deaf from a young age, use American Sign Language [ASL], and perceive themselves to be members of a unique cultural group) may not be recognized as having depression. Many words for depression have no equivalent in ASL, and depression screening tools have not been normed on this population. In addition, some signs used to connote depression are unrecognizable even to people who use ASL. In focus groups with culturally Deaf people, use of signing interpreters was considered intrusive in mental health encounters, and most participants reported never having been asked about depression even in the face of obvious symptoms (Sheppard & Badger, 2010). Similarly, other people who have difficulty with communication (e.g., those with aphasia or dementia) may have unrecognized depression or other mental health problems. The *Focused Assessment* below provides some questions for evaluating the contribution of biological determinants to community mental health problems.

FOCUSED ASSESSMENT Assessing Biological Determinants Influencing Mental Health and Illness

- Is there a family history of mental health problems?
- Is there evidence of heritable personality traits that promote mental health (e.g., optimism)?
- Are there any existing physical health conditions that may contribute to mental health problems? What effects do personal physical health conditions or those of family members have on mental health? Do physical health problems or their treatment cause signs and symptoms suggestive of mental health problems?
- Does the presence of a mental health problem complicate treatment of physical health conditions?
- Does the present of physical health problems impede recognition of mental health concerns?

PSYCHOLOGICAL DETERMINANTS. Psychological considerations to be addressed relative to community mental health problems include psychological risk factors, psychiatric comorbidity, coping skills, and suicide potential.

Psychological risk factors for mental health problems. Personality traits, difficult temperament, experience of stressful life events, and below-average intelligence are some of the psychological factors that have been associated with the development of mental health problems. Some people's personalities appear to place them at increased risk for mental health problems. For example, people who are excessively critical or who have difficult temperaments may alienate others, receiving less social support for dealing with everyday sources of stress that we all encounter.

Psychological stress appears to play an important part in the development of mental disorders (CSELS, 2012). Stress and an emotionally charged environment are also implicated in symptomatic relapses in clients with schizophrenia. Conversely, decreasing stress and increasing personal and interpersonal competencies appear to contribute to mental health and to control of existing mental health problems. Stressful life events may contribute to situational depression or exacerbate major depressive disorders.

Psychiatric comorbidity. Clients with one mental disorder may concurrently experience other disorders. This co-occurrence of two mental disorders is referred to as psychiatric comorbidity. **Dual diagnosis** is the term commonly used to indicate the co-occurrence of a substance abuse disorder with one or more other psychiatric diagnoses. Several forms of comorbidity may occur. For example, preexisting depression and anxiety disorders increase one's risk for PTSD following a traumatic event (Vogt, 2014). Similarly, PTSD, depression, and anxiety disorders frequently co-occur with substance abuse disorders (NIMH, 2009a). Co-occurring PTSD and depression may also be linked to increased suicide risk in some populations. People with borderline personality disorder also have high rates of co-occurring depression, anxiety disorders, substance abuse, and eating disorders, and are at high risk for suicide (NIMH, n.d.d). Similarly, people with panic disorder often experience depression and/or substance abuse as well (NIMH, 2009a).

The presence of comorbidity complicates treatment for any given mental illness, and population health nurses working with clients with comorbid conditions or dual diagnosis may need to assure that clients receive treatment for all the disorders that they experience. Similarly, the combination of HIV infection, depression, and homelessness increases the difficulty of treating depression as well as HIV infection (Tsai et al., 2013).

Coping skills. The extent of an individual's coping abilities mediates the effect of stress on both physical and mental health. Coping strategies are culturally determined, and different cultural groups may display different approaches to coping with life's stress. Specific types of coping strategies have been linked to various mental disorders. For example, adolescents with schizophrenia frequently use emotion-focused coping, particularly in the face of anxiety and fear (Lee & Schepp, 2011). Development of problem-focused coping, however, contributes to mental health and may help in dealing with symptoms associated with mental illness. Negative thinking, excessive worry, and a sense of lack of control of one's life are personal traits that have been associated with depression.

Some clients with mental health problems may turn to substance use or abuse as a coping strategy, which may contribute to the potential for dual diagnosis. Other clients may engage in other, more or less adaptive coping strategies for dealing with stress or with symptoms. Research has indicated, for example, that clients with schizophrenia have fairly well developed coping skills for controlling their symptoms. Some of these coping strategies are healthier than others and can be encouraged by population health nurses working with clients with schizophrenia and their families. One category of coping skills displayed by schizophrenic clients dealt with behavior control by means of distraction (e.g., listening to music, reading, playing an instrument or writing), physical activity (e.g., running), asking for help or interacting with sympathetic others, prayer, and meditation. Other coping strategies include avoiding thinking about or ignoring misperceptions, shifting one's attention to other thoughts, engaging in future planning or problem solving. An innovative suggestion is to engage selectively with voices, informing them that they are not welcome unless they have useful information and requesting that they make an appointment and treat the patient with respect. Other strategies, such as telling voices to "shut up" or doing as told by voices are less healthy approaches to dealing with symptoms of schizophrenia. Similarly, passive acceptance of hallucinations may result in hallucinations consuming one's life. Mindfulness, on the other hand, is a healthier approach in which the client acknowledges voices, but does not agree to be guided by them, relying on his or her own decision-making abilities (Brichford & Jones, 2009).

Suicide potential. Both the stress that contributes to the development of mental disorders and the hopelessness often associated with having a mental disorder place clients at increased risk for suicide, and population health nurses must be particularly alert to evidence of suicidal ideation in clients with mental health problems. Depression, in particular, whether due to major depressive, unipolar, or bipolar disorder or to situational factors, increases the potential for suicide (NIMH, n.d.b). Suicide risk is also increased among people with schizophrenia with about 10% of those affected attempting suicide (NIMH, 2009b). Those with PTSD and borderline personality disorder are also at increased risk for suicide (NIMH, n.d.c, 2009a). The nurse should explore with the client any suicidal tendencies or thoughts of suicide. Suicide tends to occur most frequently when clients are recovering from an episode of depression; this is because the severely depressed client probably does not have the energy to commit suicide. Suicide is addressed in more depth in Chapter 30∞. Possible questions to assist population health nurses in identifying psychological factors contributing to mental health and illness are included in the *Focused Assessment* below.

ENVIRONMENTAL DETERMINANTS. Physical environmental factors influence the development and course of some mental health problems. Chronic exposure to lead and other toxins may cause mental retardation and other forms of mental illness. Cataclysmic environmental events may also contribute to PTSD and depression. For example, many survivors of hurricane Katrina evacuated from New Orleans experienced PTSD for several years after the event. PTSD was also associated with depression, particularly in people with debilitating physical illnesses. For instance, 24% of people with end-stage renal diseases affected by the hurricane developed PTSD and depression (Edmondson et al., 2013). Disasters may also interrupt treatment for many forms of mental illness.

Seasonal changes may also contribute to mental health problems, as in the case of seasonal affective disorder. **Seasonal affective disorder (SAD)** is a form of depression that varies with the seasons, resulting in depression in the fall and winter when exposure to natural light is diminished. For some people, experience of symptoms is reversed, with depression occurring in the spring and summer. The incidence of SAD increases at greater distances from the equator, and some people with bipolar disorder may experience a degree of mania in spring or summer (Mayo Clinic Staff, 2011). Environmental considerations in mental health problems are addressed in the *Focused Assessment* provided on the next page.

SOCIOCULTURAL DETERMINANTS. A number of sociocultural determinants influence risk for and treatment of mental health problems. These factors include societal disorganization, economic factors, family relationships and social support, culture, and societal attitudes, stigma, and societal policies related to mental health and illness.

Societal disorganization and immigration. As noted in Chapter 25∞, social upheaval such as war and disaster increases the incidence of mental health problems in the populations affected, particularly when the effects are long-lasting. Immigration, which may result from social upheaval, has also been linked with a high incidence of mental disorders. Research has suggested that the circumstances of immigration, for instance, if it was planned or unplanned, influence its effects on mental health and illness. In one study of Latinos, for example, being forced to immigrate was associated with increased distress, particularly among women, Cubans, and Puerto Ricans (Torres & Wallace, 2013). Immigration from Mexico to the United States has been associated with increased risk of mental illness, particularly in

FOCUSED ASSESSMENT Assessing Psychological Determinants Influencing Mental Health and Illness

- What life stresses is the client experiencing? Does stress contribute to or exacerbate mental health problems? How does the client cope with stress?
- What signs and symptoms does the client exhibit that suggest the presence of mental health problems?
- What is the extent of adaptation to the mental health problem? How does the client cope with the problem?
- Is there existing psychiatric comorbidity? If so, what form does it take?
- Is the client at risk for suicide as a result of the mental health problem?

FOCUSED ASSESSMENT Assessing Environmental Determinants Influencing Mental Health and Illness

- Have environmental disasters contributed to the incidence and prevalence of mental health problems in the population?
- Have environmental disasters complicated treatment for existing mental health problems?
- Do environmental pollutants contribute to the incidence of mental health problems?
- Are there seasonal fluctuations in the incidence or severity of particular mental health problems? If so, when do these fluctuations occur?

third generation or higher Mexican Americans, who may have twice the risk of mental illness as non-immigrants (Orozco, Borges, Medina-Mora, Aguilar-Gaxiola, & Breslau, 2013). Immigration is associated with multiple stressors, including discrimination, issues related to legal status, and separation from family support systems. Discrimination, in particular, may lead to mental health problem among immigrants.

Mental health problems are also influenced by more contained social events. For example, the risk of depression increases with recent divorce or separation, unemployment, and bereavement. Inability to work and stresses associated with low income have also been associated with mental illness, as have overcrowding and living in an area with a high rate of disorganization.

Socioeconomic Factors. Economic and employment factors may also influence one's mental status. The Center for Surveillance, Epidemiology, and Laboratory Services (2012) has indicated that poverty and other economic circumstances are potential contributors to mental illness. For example, mortgage delinquency was associated with depression as well as less access to care during the height of the mortgage foreclosures in 2009 (Alley et al., 2011).

Employment factors may also influence mental health and mental illness. Job strain and an increase in the psychological demands of one's job have been linked to the incidence of major depression (Smith & Bielecky, 2012). Similarly, jobs that entail exposure to trauma are also associated with mental health problems. For example, health care workers who respond to trauma victims are at risk for PTSD (PTSD Alliance, n.d.). Likewise, military personnel exposed to combat conditions are at risk for a variety of mental disorders (Maguen, Bosch, Marmar, & Seal, 2010). Becoming suddenly unemployed is a risk factor for depression, which may be intense at first due to "unemployment shock," then taper off, and then become worse if the length of unemployment extends and job searches are fruitless (OECD, 2011).

Mental health problems may also interfere with work. Worldwide, 60% to 70% of people with common mental health problems (CMDs) are employed compared to 75% to 85% of those without mental health problems. Employment rates are closer to 45% to 55% among those with severe mental disorders (SMDs). Most people with mental health problems want to work but may have difficulty finding or keeping a job. People with CMDs are two to three times more likely to be unemployed than those without problems, and those with SMDs are six to seven times more likely to be unemployed. They may also be employed in low paying jobs that combine high psychological demands and low decision latitude (OECD, 2011).

Mental health problems may contribute to workplace absences and reduced productivity. For example, 80% of people with SMDs in one international study reported reduced productivity in the prior 4 weeks, compared to 69% of those with CMDs and only 26% of people without mental health problems. There is also a worldwide increase in the rate of disability claims related to mental health issues. In addition, people may move to disability benefits too soon or be on them too long without attempts to find or fit them for successful employment. For example, an estimated half of people with SMDs receive disability benefits and the other half receives some other form of benefits. The Organisation for Economic Cooperation and Development (2011) has indicated a need for sickness monitoring and early intervention for people with mental health problems to minimize the personal and societal effects of mental illness.

Employment is often beneficial for mental health and may aid recovery in the face of mental illness. Key workplace variables that have been identified as preventing worsening of mental health problems among the mentally ill include good management characterized by support, adequate feedback, and recognition of effort. Unfortunately, such conditions are only experienced by about 60% of people with SMDs and 70% of those with CMDs (OECD, 2011). Population health nurses in occupational settings can help to identify employees with mental disorders and advocate for assessment of work capacity and meeting of support needs.

Family relationships and social support. Family interactions may also influence the development and course of mental health problems. For example, women experiencing parenting stress are more likely to report poor mental health than those without such stress. High levels of negative emotional expression have also been associated with anorexia nervosa and depression. Conversely, warmth and positive family relationships may have a protective effect against mental health problems or assist family members to cope more effectively when problems do occur.

Social support may assist clients to cope with the stresses of life and prevent mental health problems. Lack of social support, on the other hand, may increase the risk of mental illness, contributing to the feelings of isolation and poor social skills common among people with mental health problems.

Abuse may also contribute to the development of mental health problems. For example, gender abuse resulting from atypical gender presentation and transgression of gender norms has been linked to high levels of depression in male-to-female transgender individuals. Gender abuse may occur both within and outside of the family constellation (Nuttbrock et al., 2013). Spouse abuse has also been linked to depression, anxiety disorders, and substance abuse (Al-Modallal et al., 2013). Trafficking and sexual exploitation are also associated with PTSD, depression, and anxiety disorders. Abuse and trafficking will be addressed in more detail in Chapter 30∞.

Cultural factors. The effects of culture on mental health are many and pervasive. Culture defines what constitutes mental illness for members of a group, and that definition may not always conform to the diagnostic criteria established in the *DSM-5*. What may be seen as abnormal behavior or feelings in one culture may be perfectly normal in another. Similarly, culture mediates one's experience of distress and how one expresses that distress. Culture, for example, creates what are known as "idioms of distress" or typical ways of expressing mental discomfort. In many cultural groups, for example, mental distress is expressed in terms of somatization. **Somatization** is the expression of mental or emotional distress in terms of physical symptoms. Diagnostic criteria contained in the *DSM-5* are based on Western-Anglo experience, and it is unclear how applicable diagnostic criteria are to members of other cultural groups. Some cultures also have recognized culture-bound syndromes generally reflecting concepts of mental illness that are culture-specific and fall outside Western psychiatric practice. Culture-bound syndromes were discussed in Chapter 5∞.

Cultural differences in diagnostic criteria, expressions of distress, and meanings and value attributed to different symptoms may result in misdiagnosis in cross-cultural encounters. For example, in a qualitative study among African American men, participants described life events that resulted in stressors and led to "the funk" or depression. If not resolved, the funk resulted in a "breakdown," but the men rarely sought assistance for these feelings (Bryant-Bedell & Waite, 2010). In another study, Jordanian women who experienced depression as a result of spousal abuse rarely identified their emotional response as depression and so did not seek care (Al-Modallal et al., 2010). Language barriers between provider and client also increase the potential for misdiagnosis, as do diagnostic measurements that are not linguistically or culturally sensitive.

Culture also influences expectations regarding treatment that may enhance or impede compliance with therapy. Members of many cultural groups engage in the use of herbal remedies. For this reason, they may expect psychotropic medications to act rapidly, as most herbals do. The need to build effective blood levels of medications may be difficult for clients in these cultural groups to understand. Inability to see immediate results may lead to discontinuation of pharmacotherapy. Herbal therapies may also interact with prescription medications to impede or enhance their effects, contributing to therapeutic ineffectiveness or adverse reactions to medications. Increasing use of complementary and alternative medicine (CAM) has been reported among persons with psychotic disorders. In one study, for instance, 88% of people with schizophrenia had used CAM in their lifetimes, and 68% in the prior 12 months (Hazra et al., 2010). In another study, 45% of Asian Americans with probable psychiatric diagnoses had used CAM alone, 26% used CAM in conjunction with conventional mental health services, and 29% had used conventional services alone (Choi & Kim, 2010).

Societal attitudes, stigma, and policy issues. Culture also contributes to the way people view mental illness and to the degree of stigmatization encountered by those who experience mental illness. Stigmatization is characterized by bias, distrust, stereotyping, fear, embarrassment, anger, and avoidance. Stigmatization has the effect of reducing willingness to seek help and thereby reduces access to needed care.

The response to perceived stigma is mediated by culture. For example, members of many ethnic groups may fail to seek care for psychological problems as a result of perceived stigma or because of perceived incongruence between group cultures and the Western mental health care system. Cultural barriers to obtaining mental health services include racial and cultural biases and inappropriate services, philosophical differences regarding disease causation or treatment, cultural attitudes to seeking help , language barriers, a lack of bilingual and culturally sensitive providers, and clients' lack of knowledge about available services. Clients from ethnic cultural groups may also be subjected to *language discrimination*, being treated unfairly because of language differences or accented speech. As we saw earlier, such factors also influence recognition of depression among the culturally Deaf.

Stigmatization of the mentally ill may also decrease their access to needed resources and opportunities, such as those related to employment or housing. For the individual, stigma leads to low self-esteem, hopelessness, and social isolation. Clients with mental illness are faced with the same kinds of decisions regarding disclosure that were discussed in the context of sexual orientation and gender identity in Chapter 20∞. At the population level, stigmatization influences public willingness to pay for services for the mentally ill or to locate treatment facilities in residential neighborhoods.

Stigma and the discrimination that results from belonging to a stigmatized group may also contribute to mental health problems. As we saw in Chapter 20∞, the stigma attached to nonheterosexual orientation has been associated with higher rates of suicide and depression. Discrimination has been reported by 21% of gay, lesbian, and bisexual individuals and is linked to higher incidence rates for mental illness in these populations than in the heterosexual population. Similarly, racism experienced in the general community and homophobia among heterosexual friends have been linked to depression and anxiety disorders in African American, Asian American and Pacific Islander, and Latino men who have sex with men (Choi, Paul, Ayala, Boylan, & Gregorich, 2013).

Stigma encompasses four social-cognitive processes that influence people's perceptions of and behavior toward those who are different, including those with mental illness. These four processes include cues, stereotypes, prejudice, and discriminatory behavior. Cues may be physical symptoms (e.g., tics or repetitive behaviors), social skills deficits, physical appearance (e.g., flat affect), or labels (e.g., a mental illness diagnosis) that trigger cognitive associations with stereotypes. Stereotypes may include some of the core perceptions reported below, such as incompetence, violence, or tendencies to criminal behavior that one believes are typical of people with a particular mental illness or of mental illness in general. These stereotypes then lead to prejudice against people with mental illness that are often acted upon in discriminatory behaviors (Cummings, Lucas, & Druss, 2013).

Stigma occurs at three levels: institutional, community, and individual. Institutional stigma results in discriminatory legislation, funding, and availability of services (Henderson, et al., 2013). Evidence of societal attitudes and the stigma associated with mental illness lies in the number of the mentally ill who are incarcerated in correctional facilities. Mental illness may contribute to unlawful behaviors or to incarceration as an alternative to mental health care. A study by the Treatment Advocacy Center described U.S. corrections institutions as the "new mental hospitals" (Torrey, Kennard, Eslinger, Lamb, & Pavle, 2010). The report further noted "We have now returned to the conditions of the 1840s by putting large numbers of mentally ill persons back into jails and prisons" (Torrey et al., 2010, p. 1). In 2010 in North Dakota, for example, an equal number of mentally ill persons were incarcerated as were hospitalized. In states like Arizona and Nevada, the number of incarcerated mentally ill was 10 times the number hospitalized. Overall, from 1980 to 2009, the U.S. prison population increased fivefold (Nicosia, MacDonald, & Arkes, 2013). In part, these figures are the result of massive closures of psychiatric hospital beds. From 1955 to 2005, for example, the rate of psychiatric beds decreased from one bed per 300 population to one per 3,000 (Torrey et al., 2010). These closures were well intentioned and resulted from a move to treat persons with mental illness in community settings. Unfortunately, community treatment capacity has never been equal to the demand for services (Torrey et al., 2010), and the per capita bed rate has receded to 1850 levels with 14 beds per 100,000 population in 1850 and 14.1 beds per 100,000 in 2010. In 2010, the number of beds available was less than 28% of the estimated need (Treatment Advocacy Center, 2012).

The loss of in-patient psychiatric beds has also resulted in patients with mental illnesses being shunted to other sectors of society. For example, the number of in-patient beds for mental illness in the Veterans Administration (VA) declined from 43,894 in 1999 to 40,928 in 2007 despite increases in veterans from Iraq and Afghanistan who experience myriad mental health problems. In addition, the average length of stay decreased from 33 to 19 days. This decline has been termed the "disaster of the past," and has resulted in a process of **transinstitutionalization**, or movement from one category of institution to another. Increased rates of incarceration are one example of transinstitutionalization. In the VA system, persons with mental illness were relegated to nursing homes that were ill-equipped to deal with mental illness treatment (Bowersox, Szymanski, & McCarthy, 2013). Transinstitutionalization results in a significant negative impact on correctional systems, emergency departments, and other segments of society. There is also an association between bed availability and violent crime, including homicide, further adding to the societal costs of not addressing mental health issues (Treatment Advocacy Center, 2012).

Community stigma, the second level of stigma attached to mental illness, is reflected in public attitudes and behaviors (Henderson et al., 2013). An international study conducted in 16 countries indicated that while large segments of the population believe that mental illness reflects disease processes and that the mentally ill can be helped, the majority of people exhibited several core elements of prejudice against people with schizophrenia. These elements of prejudice centered on not wanting those affected to associate with children (e.g., as teachers or child caretakers), not wanting them to marry into one's family, and perceptions of unpredictability or tendencies to violence against self or others. Less widely held, but still significant prejudices, related to perceptions of unproductivity, unsuitability for leadership positions or public office, and perceptions that the mentally ill were difficult to interact or communicate with (Pescosolido, Medina, Martin, & Long, 2013).

At the individual level, persons with mental illness may experience discrimination or stigma. In addition, people with mental illnesses may internalize stigma, and begin to self-stigmatize. Self-stigma may interfere with help-seeking behaviors, treatment adherence, feelings of self-efficacy, and the ability to achieve personal goals. Some authors have suggested that a process of "coming out" or disclosure of one's mental illness may be liberating and empowering, as suggested by the experience of persons in gender minority groups. Assistance with coming out employs a cognitive behavioral approach in which people are guided to frame self-stigma as irrational self-statements to be challenged and to invalidate through examination of one's personal strengths, acceptance of self, and mindfulness. Research has indicated that, like members of gay, lesbian, bisexual, and transgender groups, persons with mental illness who identify with a mental illness support group are more likely to participate in peer support activities (Corrigan, Kosyluk, & Rüsch, 2013).

As noted by some authors, the primary challenge is to identify and implement interventions to change attitudes and decrease discrimination against those suffering from mental illness (Pescosolido et al., 2013). Legislation has made some strides in overcoming institutional stigma by prohibiting discrimination. Three major pieces of legislation have been enacted in the United States that attempt to prevent discrimination against people with mental illnesses. Each of the three have in common expansion overtime to include persons with mental illness, differential protections for persons with mental illness, implementation challenges related to label avoidance, and an explicit exclusion of substance abuse disorders from protective provisions. **Label avoidance** is the failure to seek the protections afforded by antidiscrimination legislation for fear of being further stigmatized and discriminated against if one admits to membership in a protected group (Cummings et al., 2013).

The first piece of legislation was the Education for All Handicapped Children Act of 1975. Initially drafted to encompass only certain physical handicaps, the Act was later amended to include psychologically handicapping conditions as well. Amendments also expanded coverage to preschool children and to conditions such as attention deficit hyperactivity disorder (ADHD). The second legislative effort to curb discrimination was the Americans with Disabilities Act of 1990, which prohibited workplace discrimination against people with disabilities. Again, the original legislation did not include disabilities due to mental health problems or those that were controlled by medication until amended in 2008. Finally, the Mental Health Parity and Addiction Equity Act of 2008 was expanded by the Affordable Care Act to mandate incorporation of mental health and substance abuse coverage in essential health insurance benefits packages. Unfortunately, the original provisions of the law only applied to large employers and state insurance exchanges (Cummings et al., 2013).

The Community Preventive Services Task Force (CPSTF) conducted a systematic review of research on the effects of legislation to increase parity in mental health services as compared to physical health services. The task force found sufficient evidence to recommend passage of comprehensive mental health parity legislation, noting that such legislation increased access to care, decreased out-of-pocket spending for mental health services, increased service utilization among those in need, increased treatment access, decreased the percentage of people who reported poor mental health, and decreased suicide rates without causing substantial increases in insurance costs for services. At the time of the review, 49 states and the District of Columbia had enacted some form of mandatory parity legislation for mental health services. In 2014, the Affordable Care Act expanded federal parity requirements to new health insurance plans in individual and small group markets (CPSTF, 2014).

Unfortunately, legislation can only address one aspect of stigma—outright discrimination. Legislation may also have a certain symbolic value in that it indicates that those with mental illness should not be discriminated against and may help to change societal values and perceptions. Antidiscrimination laws must be combined with anti-stigma campaigns that are directed to the community and individual levels of stigma (Cummings et al., 2013). One such initiative is the California Mental Health Services Act of 2004, which funds statewide programs designed to reduce the stigma of mental illness (California Department of Mental Health, 2009). The initiative is described in the *Evidence-Based Practice* feature below. The *Focused Assessment*

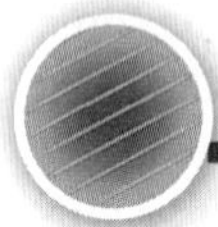

Evidence-Based Practice

Reducing Stigma

The California State Mental Health Services Act, passed in 2004, was designed to fund a series of evidence-based initiatives throughout the state to decrease the stigma of mental illness. Initiatives funded by the Act employ multiple evidence-based strategies related to social marketing, creating public awareness, promoting cultural competence among providers, and capacity building among those affected by mental illness (Clark et al., 2013).

Funded initiatives are supported by a 1% tax on people with annual incomes over $1 million, and 20% of funding is directed toward prevention and early intervention strategies. The intent of the legislation was to improve attitudes toward the mentally ill, decrease stigma, and promote help-seeking behavior. By 2008, more than 100,000 people had participated in planning efforts for programs to reduce stigma. The initiative applies scientific evidence to the development of interventions in one of four strategic directions designed to reduce the stigma attached to mental illness (Clark et al., 2013).

The four strategic directions, as laid out in the *California Strategic Plan on Reducing Mental Health Stigma and Discrimination*, include:

- Creating a supportive environment with social norms that acknowledge that mental health is an integral component of well-being and creating widespread public understanding of mental health and mental illness.
- Promoting changes that encourage respect for and protection of the rights of those with mental illness.
- Upholding and advancing laws that identify and eliminate discriminatory policies and practices.
- Increasing knowledge of programs and practices that effectively decrease discrimination and stigma and incorporate community participation in related activities (California Department of Mental Health, 2009).

FOCUSED ASSESSMENT Assessing Sociocultural Determinants Influencing Mental Health and Illness

- How does the population define mental health and mental illness? Do these definitions hamper recognition of mental health problems or help-seeking behaviors?
- What are the effects of mental health problems on social interactions (with family and others)?
- What are the economic effects of mental health problems on those affected? On the overall population?
- What are societal attitudes to mental health problems? Do they hamper control efforts?
- Is there social stigma attached to having particular mental health problems? What effect does stigma have on clients' willingness to seek care? On public willingness to fund care?
- What effect, if any, do cultural beliefs and behaviors have on mental health problems?
- Do mental health problems contribute to the risk of homelessness for those affected?
- What social support systems are available to persons with mental health illness? What support is available to their families?
- How do social factors (e.g., unemployment) influence mental health problems?
- How do the mental health problems affect community members' ability to work?

above includes questions to assess sociocultural determinants influencing community mental health and illness.

BEHAVIORAL DETERMINANTS. Personal behaviors also influence the development and course of mental health problems, but it is often difficult to determine the direction of influence. In some cases, people engage in drug, alcohol, and tobacco use as a means of coping with symptoms of mental illness. Other times, substance use contributes to mental illness or affects treatment. All that is known for sure is that people with mental illness tend to engage in more substance use than those without illness.

In 2009–2011, 36% of people with mental illness smoked, compared to 21% of those without mental illness. In addition, people with mental illness smoked 31% of all cigarettes consumed in the United States (Gfroerer et al., 2013). In the 2007, National Health Interview Survey, smoking rates increased with the number of comorbid psychiatric conditions, and mental illness was associated with lower quit ratios and less success with smoking cessation (McClave, McKnight-Eily, Davis, & Dube, 2010). Regular smoking has been linked to increased risk of new onset mood or anxiety disorders, particularly among people 18 to 49 years of age. In addition, the level of risk increases with the number of cigarettes smoked (Mojtabai & Crum, 2013). Among people with schizophrenia, 75% to 90% are nicotine addicted, and smoking may reduce the effectiveness of antipsychotic medications (NIMH, 2009b). Alcohol and drug use also have implications for mental illness. For example, veterans who are problem drinkers have been found to have a risk of PTSD 2.7 times that of nondrinkers. Problem drinking has also been linked to depression and chronic fatigue syndrome in this group (Coughlin, Kang, & Mahan, 2011). Conversely, men with PTSD are also at risk for substance abuse disorders although this association has not been demonstrated in women (Vogt, 2014).

Physical activity and sexual activity are two other behavioral considerations in an assessment of mental health problems. For example, clients with mental illness have been shown to be less physically active and have a greater risk for obesity than those without illness. On the other hand, increased physical activity has been associated with improvements in anxiety and depression (NAMI, n.d.b).

Sexual activity is an area that is often ignored in the care of clients with mental illness. Attention should be given to meeting sexual needs as well as to assessing high-risk sexual behaviors that may be exhibited by some mentally ill individuals. Sexuality issues are complicated by possible links with childhood sexual abuse, the sexual content of positive symptoms in clients with schizophrenia, sexual disinhibition in some conditions, and medication side effects such as diminished libido and disabling extrapyramidal effects that promote distancing and social isolation by other people. Use of safe sexual practices and contraception are other sexual behaviors that should be assessed. Sexual orientation and gender identity have also been linked to mental illness, particularly to depression and anxiety disorders. For example, a meta-analysis of relevant research indicated that the lifetime incidence of depression and anxiety disorder was 1.5 times higher in the lesbian, gay, and bisexual population than in the general population, and suicide risk was nearly 2.5 times higher (Choi et al., 2013). Depression related to gender abuse has also been linked to high-risk sexual behaviors (Nuttbrock et al., 2013). The *Focused Assessment* on next page addresses behavioral determinants influencing mental health problems.

HEALTH SYSTEM DETERMINANTS. The health care system is fragmented with respect to mental health promotion and illness prevention. The care provided targets SMDs, and much of the treatment evidence and knowledge addresses this

FOCUSED ASSESSMENT Assessing Behavioral Determinants Influencing Mental Health and Illness

- Does alcohol or drug use influence mental health problems or their effects in the population? Are alcohol or drugs used in an effort to self-manage symptoms?
- What effect, if any, does exercise have on mental health problems in the population?
- Does smoking influence mental health problems?
- What effect do mental health problems have on self-care behaviors among those affected?
- To what extent do mental health problems or their treatment influence sexual activity?

end of the disease spectrum rather than the more commonly encountered, less severe forms of disease. Worldwide, an estimated 80% of people with CMDs receive no treatment, and as much as 50% of those with SMDs do not seek or receive care. Those with CMDs who do receive treatment, primarily receive medications, which are not very effective. Pharmacotherapy for SMDs, on the other hand, is more effective, but frequently does not completely control symptoms (OECD, 2011). Furthermore, there are wide discrepancies in treatment among subgroups in the population, with some groups receiving little to no treatment.

The issue of parity with respect to health insurance coverage of mental health treatment was addressed earlier. Lack of parity, however, is one contributing factor in lack of service access. People with mental health problems tend to use emergency departments (EDs) for acute psychiatric emergencies, injuries, or illness related to their mental illness or when primary care is unavailable. In one study, for example, 10% of all ED visits in North Carolina were related to mental illness diagnoses, with 61% of those visits related to stress, depression, or anxiety. Persons with mental illness seen in EDs are admitted to the hospital twice as often as those without mental illness, and the rate of hospitalization is above 50% for older people with mental illness (Hakenewerth, Tintinallis, Waller, Ising, & DeSlem, 2013).

It has long been noted that people who do seek care for mental health problems most often do so in primary care settings. In part this may relate to greater ease of access, but may also be the result of perceptions of stigma attached to mental illness care. Competing demands in the primary care setting make attention to mental health issues difficult. In addition, managed care carve-outs for mental health services increase institutional level stigma due to unequal funding for services. As a result, some authors have called for better integration of primary care and behavioral health care in one setting. It is often argued that integrated care is too expensive, but fragmented care is actually more costly and results in suboptimal outcomes. Advantages to the integration of primary care and mental health services include primary prevention of mental illness, early risk factor identification and modification, early recognition and treatment of mental illness, and potentially better outcomes (Shim & Rust, 2013). Integrated treatment services could also increase the use of evidence-based treatment approaches by clinicians who are more knowledgeable regarding mental illness treatment.

A report from the Institute of Medicine (2006) indicated that many providers failed to use evidence-based practices in treating mental disorders. Other problems identified in the report included medication errors; excessive use of restraints and seclusion resulting in 150 deaths each year; and failure to provide needed mental health treatment even for people who have access to health care services (IOM, 2006). Additional system flaws include coercion of clients into treatment, a poorly developed structure for assessing treatment outcomes, limited use of information technology to coordinate care, and an educationally diverse workforce (IOM, 2006). Based on the report, the IOM made two overarching recommendations for strengthening the mental health care system in the United States.

These recommendations included treatment services for mental and substance abuse disorders grounded in an understanding of mind—body interactions and tailoring of strategies for health system redesign recommended in *Crossing the Quality Chasm* to the care of mental health problems (Institute of Medicine, 2006).

Other, more specific recommendations include support for client decision making; lack of coercion; dissemination of evidence-based practice information; development of quality assessment instruments and outcome measures; better linkages between health care organizations, providers, and systems; and coordination of health and social services to best meet client needs. In addition, mental health care should be addressed as fully as care for physical health problems, and the Congress and state legislatures should mandate standard health insurance benefits that improve mental health care coverage. Computer technology should be used to standardize billing and information processes, and attention should be given to developing an adequate mental health workforce (IOM, 2006).

Tips for assessing health system factors influencing risk for mental health problems are presented in the *Focused Assessment* on next page. A tool for assessing the broad range of factors contributing to mental health problems is included on the student resources site.

FOCUSED ASSESSMENT Assessing Health System Determinants Influencing Mental Health and Illness

- What are the attitudes of health care providers to persons with mental health problems?
- Are health care providers alert to signs and symptoms of mental health problems?
- What treatment facilities are available to persons with mental health problems? How adequate are they? What types of therapy are available? How effective are they?
- Are diagnostic and treatment services available and accessible to persons with mental health problems?
- To what extent are primary care and mental health care services integrated in the health care system?
- Is there parity in health insurance coverage for mental health services?
- Does the individual client exhibit treatment side effects or adverse effects?
- Does treatment for other health problems cause or exacerbate mental health problem in the population?

At the individual client level, the population health nurse would assess clients for evidence of mental health problems and for individual characteristics and circumstances that may be contributing to mental health difficulties. For example, the nurse might identify poor coping skills, unemployment, or family dysfunction as factors contributing to depression in a particular client. At the population level, the nurse would assess the incidence and prevalence of biological, psychological, environmental, sociocultural, behavioral, or health system determinants influencing mental health and illness.

Diagnostic Reasoning and Mental Health and Illness

Population health nurses may make a variety of nursing diagnoses related to mental health and mental illness. These diagnoses can reflect the mental health status of an individual client, the client's family, or a population group. For example, the nurse might diagnose "high levels of mental health" for an individual client or family or in a population group. Conversely, the nurse might diagnose "impaired reality orientation due to schizophrenic episode" in an individual client or an "exacerbation of depression due to family stress." Another nursing diagnosis at this level might reflect "disruption of family function due to exhibition of symptoms of schizophrenia" on the part of one member.

Nursing diagnoses may also be made that reflect mental health problems affecting population groups. For example, the population health nurse might diagnose an "increased incidence of schizophrenia in the homeless population" or "inadequate treatment facilities for persons with chronic mental health problems due to reduced program funds."

Planning and Implementing Strategies Related to Mental Health and Illness

The Surgeon General's report on mental health (NIMH, 1999) made several recommendations with respect to mental health care in the United States. These recommendations included the need to reduce the stigma attached to mental illness, improve public awareness of the availability of effective treatment for most mental health problems, assure the supply of providers and services for those in need, and ensure the use of state-of-the-art treatments. Additional recommendations addressed the need to tailor treatment to the age, gender, race, and culture of those affected; to facilitate early entry into treatment; and to reduce financial barriers to treatment (NIMH, 1999). Although these recommendations were made a number of years ago, they remain relevant to efforts to control community mental health problems, and population health nurses can be actively involved in efforts to address these recommendations.

MENTAL HEALTH PROMOTION. Prevention of mental illness through risk reduction has not been effective in reducing the incidence or prevalence of mental health problems, so many authors are suggesting a need to focus on active promotion of mental health in addition to specific prevention endeavors. Positive mental health has been linked to less mental illness, decreased ADL limitations, fewer missed work days, better physical health, and less use of health care services and prescription drugs. Gains in mental health over time predict lower risk for future mental illness. Conversely, diminished mental health predicted an increased risk for mental illness (Keyes, Dhingra, & Simoes, 2010).

Promotion of mental health involves moving from a risk reduction model of mental illness control to a competence enhancement model (Fledderus et al., 2010). WHO has defined **mental health promotion** as the creation of conditions that support mental health and adoption of healthy lifestyles (WHO, 2014a). The goal of mental health promotion is to enhance both individual competencies and community assets to prevent mental health problems and improve quality of life (Kobau et al., 2011). General strategies to foster mental health include health-enhancing public policy related to employment and antidiscrimination, creating supportive environments, strengthening community action, developing personal skills, and reorienting health services to address mental health needs (Kobau et al., 2011).

Mental health is also referred to as positive psychology and consists of four aspects. The first aspect is positive emotions which have been shown to reduce autonomic arousal and promote effective engagement with one's environment. Positive emotions have been found to be linked to better immune function, decreased risk of injury and illness, speedier recovery from illness, healthier behaviors, and increased longevity (Kobau et al., 2011).

The second aspect of positive psychology is reflected in individual traits of optimism and resiliency, creativity, bravery, kindness, and perseverance, all of which tend to buffer against psychological disorder. Development of positive relationships with others is the third aspect of positive psychology, and the last is the existence of enabling institutions, such as schools that prohibit bullying, that foster positive psychological outcomes (Kobau et al., 2011).

Psychological flexibility is one specific competency that has been linked to mental health. **Psychological flexibility** involves an attitude of acceptance of negative experiences, rather than attempting to avoid or control them, and engaging in behavior based on personal values. Two approaches can be used to increase psychological flexibility: acceptance and commitment therapy (ACT) and mindfulness. ACT involves learning to detach oneself from negative experiences and focus on behaviors that support personal values. Mindfulness involves awareness of and attention to experiences as they occur in a nonjudgmental and accepting way. Research has indicated that a combination of the two approaches is even more effective in increasing psychological flexibility (Fledderus et al., 2010).

Promotion of coping abilities and resilience also foster mental health. **Resilience** is the ability to withstand chronic stress or to recover from traumatic and stressful events. Population health nurses can assist individual clients to develop coping skills that will increase their resilience in the face of adversity. In addition, nurses can be instrumental in developing programs that promote coping in school, work, or other settings. Population health nurses might also organize stress management education programs as part of a school health curriculum or in a work setting.

Strategies to promote mental health should be employed across the life span. For example, strategies to promote mental health in young children include support for effective parenting and improved parent–child interaction, both of which may require attention to parental stressors such as poverty, unemployment, and so on. Effective strategies include parental education, home visiting and support programs, and child care programs outside the home. During the school years, programs that develop personal coping and social skills and foster inclusion, identity, and connectedness have been shown to enhance mental health. Other successful strategies include improving problem-solving ability and self-control, addressing learning problems, bullying prevention, promotion of self-awareness and self-esteem, and programs to foster social and emotional skills.

For adults, mental health promotion focuses on two primary areas: prevention of unemployment and dealing with work-related stress. Job training programs and assistance with employment can help to promote mental health. Similarly, programs to reduce work stress and burnout, creation of balance between job demands and skills, promoting job control and decision latitude, and creating work climates that are socially and emotionally supportive can also enhance mental health in adults. Noise reduction, relaxation training, and conflict management strategies can also be helpful. For older adults, climates of respect and emotional and material support that help to maintain independence can enhance mental health. Prevention of social isolation and loneliness can also foster mental health. Population health nurses can be actively involved in the development of community programs to promote mental health at all age levels or can refer individuals to existing programs. Table 28-4• summarizes foci and strategies for mental health promotion.

ILLNESS AND INJURY PREVENTION. Prevention of mental health problems and mental disorders involves reduction of risk factors. Population health nurses may be actively involved in risk-reduction efforts. The support provided to clients with mental distress and efforts to ameliorate or eliminate sources of stress may prevent the occurrence of mental health problems. Population health nurses can assist individuals and families to identify sources of stress and plan strategies to eliminate or minimize them. For example, referral for financial assistance may alleviate economic stresses that can contribute to depression. The nurse may also refer clients experiencing situational stressors such as divorce or care of a chronically ill family member to support groups to help them deal with stress. Assisting clients and families to expand social support networks may also prevent mental health problems.

Population health nurses can also assist clients with chronic physical health problems to cope effectively with their illnesses and refer them for counseling when they are experiencing adjustment difficulties. Referral for family counseling may also help to prevent mental health problems arising out of poor family dynamics. Families can also be assisted by population health nurses to develop communication and interaction patterns that promote the mental health of family members.

At the population level, population health nurses can advocate for societal conditions that minimize stress and prevent mental illness. They can assist communities to identify and develop strategies to address existing sources of stress for community members. For example, population health nurses in one community were actively involved with other community members in advocating for a local ordinance mandating a living wage for people working for organizations that received city contracts to minimize the stress of poverty.

TABLE 28-4 Mental Health Promotion Foci and Strategies

Health Promotion Focus	Strategies
Promote positive personal traits	• Advocate for programs that promote creativity and kindness. • Role model perseverance.
Promote positive relationships with others	• Teach and role model effective communication and relationship skills.
Develop institutions that foster positive psychological outcomes	• Assist in the development and implementation of mental health promotion curricula in schools. • Advocate for policies that promote inclusiveness and connectedness. • Advocate for anti-bullying programs and policies.
Promote coping skills and resilience	• Teach and role model coping skills. • Advocate for coping education in schools.
Promote psychological flexibility	• Assist clients to accept negative events and to engage in personal responses consistent with personal values. • Promote mindfulness and attention to experiences and behavioral responses consistent with personal values.
Promote effective parenting	• Teach parenting skills. • Assist with development of parenting programs. • Role model effective parent–child interaction. • Modify parental stressors. • Advocate for parenting support programs.
Prevent unemployment	• Advocate for and refer clients to job training programs and employment services.
Reduce work-related stress	• Advocate for or implement worksite stress-reduction programs. • Advocate for job control and decision latitude in the work setting. • Promote noise reduction in work settings. • Advocate for strategies that improve work–family balance. • Provide relaxation training in workplaces. • Assist with conflict management in the workplace.
Provide emotional and material support for older clients	• Advocate for programs that provide material support for the elderly. • Make referrals to prevent social isolation. • Assist older clients to maintain independence.

Interventions may also be undertaken to prevent postpartum depression (PPD). Population health nurses often work with pregnant women so they are in an ideal position to take steps to prevent PPD. Interventions that may help to prevent PPD include good nutrition, development of social support networks, exercise, discussion of and education about parenting expectations, promoting coping skills, and assisting parents to seek the help of others in dealing with other household tasks. Population health nurses can also engage in campaigns to change public perceptions of "good parents" to incorporate more realistic parenting expectations and to change policies that require women to return to work soon after delivery. Cultural pressures to regain one's figure may also lead to excessive dieting, nutritional imbalance, and increased risk for PPD. Women may also need to have avenues for processing feelings about perceived birth trauma and population health nurses may help to create groups or programs that allow this processing to occur. Supportive home visits by health professionals have also been shown to be helpful in preventing PPD and population health nurses can advocate for and create home visiting programs for all mothers, not just those with high-risk infants, where such services do not exist.

There is also a need to promote health in clients with existing mental health problems. For example, second-generation antipsychotic medications increase the risk of weight gain and metabolic disorder, and people taking these drugs for schizophrenia need preventive interventions to control weight, such as diet instruction and encouraging physical activity. Population health nurses can educate clients regarding the effects of psychotropic drugs and assist them to minimize these effects through counseling and structured physical activity programs. In addition, population health nurses can advocate for smoking cessation assistance for people in mental illness facilities (Gfroerer et al., 2013).

At the population level, clients with mental health problems should have access to routine health promotion services tailored to meet their needs. For example, walk-in services may be needed for clients who, because of cognitive or emotional deficits, have difficulty making or keeping appointments. Conversely, routine health promotion and illness prevention services (e.g., influenza immunization) could be provided in the context of mental health services to promote ease of access. Population health nurses can educate clients with mental health problems about the need for immunization as well as use of safety precautions and avoidance of high-risk behaviors such as substance abuse, mixing psychotropic medications with alcohol, or driving when taking certain medications or under the influence of drugs or alcohol. Population health

TABLE 28-5 Illness and Injury Prevention Foci and Strategies Related to Mental Health

Focus	Strategies
Modifying risk factors for mental illness	• Assist with identification of risks for mental illness. • Assist clients to modify sources of stress. • Refer clients for counseling to deal with situational stressors as needed. • Promote adjustment to chronic physical health problems. • Teach effective family interactions. • Promote employment and social support strategies.
Preventing postpartum depression	• Advocate for and provide support to new mothers. • Promote realistic expectations of parenthood. • Promote physical activity and good nutrition. • Assist in identification or development of social support networks.
Preventing or modifying treatment side effects	• Assist clients to deal with medication side effects.
Preventing other illnesses	• Promote smoking cessation. • Promote immunization.
Preventing injury	• Educate clients about safety issues. • Prevent high-risk behaviors.
Providing accessible health promotion and illness prevention services	• Advocate for and refer clients to mental health promotion and illness prevention services.

nurses can also assist in the development of mental health services that address health promotion and illness prevention as well as therapy for mental illness. Finally, they can advocate for accessible health promotion and illness prevention services for people with mental illness. Table 28-5 summarizes illness and injury prevention strategies related to mental health.

RESOLVING EXISTING MENTAL HEALTH PROBLEMS. Resolution of existing mental health problems involves screening and treatment interventions.

Screening. Early entry into treatment for mental disorders requires identification of those in need of treatment. Although there are no specific screening examinations for most mental illnesses as there are for some communicable diseases or chronic physical health problems, two aspects of screening are important in identifying clients who are in need of and will benefit from mental health services. The first aspect of screening is a mental health evaluation that includes a client's psychiatric history, use of current psychotropic drugs, presence of suicidal ideation or suicide attempt, drug and alcohol use, and a history of sex offenses, victimization, or violence. Additional components of the mental health evaluation for an individual client include a history of special education placement, history of traumatic brain injury, incarceration, and evidence of mental retardation.

The second aspect of screening is assessment of a client's motivation for treatment. Areas to be considered include perceptions of the seriousness of mental health problems, desire for and perceived importance of treatment, and past attempts at treatment and their effects.

There are screening tools for selected mental health problems. For example, the U.S. Preventive Services Task Force has recommended routine depression screening in adults when mechanisms are in place for dealing with positive screening results (CDC, 2010). Tools for screening for depression and other conditions in the elderly were addressed in Chapter 18. The Edinburgh Postnatal Depression Scale (EDPD) is available for screening for postpartum depression, although the American College of Obstetricians and Gynecologists (2010) has found insufficient evidence for its use in routine screening for pregnant and postpartum women. The need for better screening tools for PTSD, as well as means of tracking disease incidence in mass trauma survivors has been identified, and approaches have been suggested for guiding self-evaluation and referral in the general public (NIMH, 2012a). Similarly, researchers are looking for biomarkers that may identify ASDs, but this effort is complicated by the number of gene expressions implicated in recent research (Johnson et al., 2013). Once population health nurses have identified people in need of and desiring assistance with mental health problems, they can help them find appropriate diagnostic and treatment services. Population health nurses should ensure that any screening tools used for mental health conditions are culturally and age appropriate to the populations for which they are being used. Population health nurses should be knowledgeable about and alert to signs and symptoms of mental illness. They can also educate the general public regarding signs and symptoms of conditions such as depression to promote self-screening or recognition of problems in friends or family members.

Treatment. Primary treatment goals for depression include relief of symptoms and return to effective function (Katon & Ciechanowski, 2014). Additional goals include preventing personal and societal effects of mental health problems, improving the client's (and family's) quality of life, and preventing suicide. These goals can be adapted to the treatment of other mental health problems.

Several general approaches may be implemented for the treatment of mental illness. These approaches include pharmacotherapy, individual or group psychotherapy, family intervention, and use of self-help groups. Multimodal therapy involves a combination of approaches. It is beyond the scope of this book to discuss these therapeutic approaches in detail, but each will be addressed briefly.

Pharmacotherapy relies on the use of medications alone or in conjunction with other treatment approaches to mental illness. Most pharmacologic agents used in the treatment of mental disorders alter the action of neurotransmitters in the brain, either increasing or decreasing their activity. Major categories of pharmacotherapeutic agents include antipsychotics (neuroleptics), antidepressants, stimulants (used for ADHD), mood stabilizers, anxiolytics, and cholinesterase inhibitors (used for Alzheimer's disease). The National Alliance on Mental Illness (NAMI) provides information on a wide variety of medications used in the treatment of mental illness. The role of population health nurses with respect to pharmacotherapy for mental disorders lies primarily in monitoring and motivating medication adherence, monitoring therapeutic effects, assisting with side effects, and identifying adverse effects. Population health nurses may also need to advocate for access to therapeutic drugs for clients without health insurance or those whose insurance does not cover prescription medications. For example, one population health nurse was able to convince the County Medical Services (CMS) division to cover psychiatric medications for a low-income client even though CMS services were usually reserved for addressing physical health needs rather than psychiatric illness. At the population level, population health nurses can advocate for changes to assistance programs to achieve parity for mental health conditions in comparison to physical health needs.

Population health nurses, as well as other providers who deal with clients with mental health problems, need an awareness of ethnopsychopharmacology. **Ethnopsychopharmacology** is the study of ethnic and cultural alterations in response to medication. These alterations reflect genetic differences in drug metabolism as well as cultural practices related to medication adherence, placebo effect, diet and its effects on medication absorption and effect, and the concomitant use of traditional therapies. Members of many ethnic groups have slowed drug metabolism compared to Caucasians, which may result in higher blood levels with typical dosages, leading to adverse effects (Wong & Edmond, 2012). Members of ethnic groups and others may also use herbal remedies for a variety of conditions that interfere with prescription medications or have other adverse effects. For example, St. John's Wort is an herb frequently used for depression that has been found to affect metabolic pathways used by medications to treat conditions such as heart disease, cancer, and seizures and may interfere with treatment for these conditions (NIMH, 2011a). Population health nurses can educate clients, other health care providers, and the general public regarding ethnopsychopharmacologic implications and the potential for adverse drug effects. They can also engage in research to evaluate the effectiveness of ethnopsychopharmacologic approaches to mental health therapy.

Monitoring clients on psychotropic medications for side effects is an important role for population health nurses. Population health nurses educate clients about the intended effects and potential side effects and adverse effects of medications used to treat specific mental illnesses. The nurse also monitors the client closely for signs of toxicity. Population health nurses may need to advocate for coverage of psychotropic medications for individual clients. They may also be involved in political advocacy to promote coverage of psychiatric services, including medication, as a mandated health insurance benefit on par with coverage for physical illnesses.

Psychotherapy may be used with individual clients or with groups of people. The intent of psychotherapy is to develop an understanding of one's problems and ways of dealing with them (NIMH, 2012a). Psychotherapy may be used alone or in conjunction with medication. Several different approaches to psychotherapy are used, including cognitive behavioral therapy, dialectical behavior therapy, interpersonal therapy, family-focused therapy, psychodynamic therapy, and light therapy (NIMH, 2012b), which is used primarily for SAD.

Some other newer therapies have been found to be effective in assisting people with schizophrenia to deal with symptoms that are not eliminated by medication. One such therapy is metacognitive training, which is intended to help clients be aware of cognitive biases that lead to symptoms, and to critically analyze them and the problem-solving behaviors used to address them. Metacognitive training improves one's ability to examine one's own mental processes, identify reasoning or memory errors, and modify their behavioral responses (Favrod, Maire, Bardy, Pernier, & Bonsack, 2010). The University Medical Center Hamburg-Eppendorf (2014) has developed a metacognitive training program to assist people in identifying inappropriate thinking and modify their responses. For further information about the training modules, see the *External Resources* section of the student resources site.

Psychotherapy may not be effective with clients from some cultural groups because it is incongruent with cultural norms of not dwelling on or thinking about problems. A description of key features of several psychotherapeutic approaches is presented in Table 28-6●.

One other approach to treatment of bipolar disorder is electroconvulsive therapy (ECT), or the use of low-level electric shock to stimulate the brain. Although previously discounted as a treatment for depression, newer technologies that deliver more focused stimulation that is not even consciously perceived by the client have been shown to be highly effective for severe depressive, manic, or mixed episodes of bipolar disorder. ECT is also useful in conditions, such as pregnancy, when medications may not be safe (NIMH, n.d.b).

Additional types of therapy might be warranted for some population groups. For example, directly observed therapy has been effective in promoting medication adherence in homeless and marginally housed HIV-infected individuals with depression (Tsai et al., 2013). Similarly, people with schizophrenia may benefit from specialized education programs to promote

TABLE 28-6 Characteristic Features of Selected Psychotherapies

Psychotherapeutic Approach	Characteristic Features
Cognitive behavioral therapy (CBT)	A mix of cognitive and behavioral therapy that focuses on changing one's thoughts and beliefs to be more adaptive and promote changes in unhealthy behaviors.
Dialectical behavioral therapy	A form of CBT in which the provider points out unhealthy behaviors and teaches more effective strategies for dealing with underlying needs.
Interpersonal therapy (IPT)	Focuses on improving communication patterns and relationships with others, identifying emotional triggers to behavior and promoting healthy expression of emotions.
Interpersonal and social rhythm therapy	Combines IPT with regular routines.
Family-focused therapy	Addresses family conflict that may be making the mental health problem worse. Helps with family caretaker stress.
Psychodynamic therapy	Focuses on self-awareness, unconscious emotions, and motivations influencing behavior.
Light therapy	Exposure to bring light. Used with low dose melatonin for seasonal affective disorder.
Metacognitive therapy	Focuses on making clients aware of cognitive biases and faulty thinking. Assists them to critique their own thought processes, identify errors, and change behavioral responses.

Data from: Favrod, J., Maire, A., Bardy, S., Pernier, S., & Bonsack, C. (2010). Improving insight into delusions: A pilot study of metacognitive training for patients with schizophrenia. *Journal of Advanced Nursing, 67*, 401–407. doi: 10.1111/j.1365-2648.2010.05470.x; National Institute of Mental Health. (2012b). *Psychotherapies.* Retrieved from http://www.nimh.nih.gov/health/topics/psychotherapies/index.shtml; University Medical Centre Hamburg-Eppendorf. (2014). *Metacognitive training in psychosis.* Retrieved from http://www.uke.de/kliniken/psychiatrie/index_17380.php#Metacognitive_Training_for_Patients_with_Schizophrenia_MCT

social skills, as well as vocational, speech, and language therapies (Wexner Medical Center, n.d.). A horticulture program has also resulted in decreased rumination and increased attention in people with depression (Gonzalez, Hartig, Patil, Martinsen, & Kirkevold, 2010). Integration of a psychiatric liaison into the ED at night has also been shown to improve integration of care (Waghorn, 2010). Other programs have focused on family education and support of people with eating disorders (Gísladóttir & Svavarsdóttir, 2011) and people caring for family members experiencing a first psychotic episode (Lowenstein et al., 2010). Finally, a web-based information center for people with severe mental health problems was found to be acceptable and helpful by patients once nurses had supported them in learning to use the computer and Internet (Kuosmanen, Jakobsson, Hyttinen, Koivunen, & Valimäki, 2010).

Population health nurses also need to be conversant with the kinds of services available to the individual client and within the population. When appropriate services are not available, population health nursing intervention may focus on advocacy and assurance of access to needed services. For example, nurses may campaign for legislation to include mental health treatment as a mandatory health insurance benefit in their state or to eliminate time limits and other constraints on existing coverage. Foci and related population health nursing strategies for resolving existing mental health problems are summarized in Table 28-7●.

TABLE 28-7 Foci and Strategies for Resolving Mental Health Problems

Focus	Strategies
Promoting early identification of mental health problems	• Advocate for availability of screening for mental health problems for populations at risk. • Assist in developing and implementing screening programs. • Assess need and motivation for screening. • Refer for screening as needed. • Assist in interpreting screening results and refer for diagnosis and treatment as needed. • Educate clients and the public on signs and symptoms of mental health problems. • Assure that screening tools are age- and culture-appropriate.
Providing effective evidence-based treatment for mental health problems	• Advocate for the availability of diagnostic and treatment services. • Refer clients for diagnosis and treatment. • Educate clients and the public on treatment options. • Advocate for insurance coverage for mental health services and medications. • Monitor treatment adherence and effects. • Monitor clients for treatment side effects. • Identify ethnopharmacologic influences on treatment. • Educate providers, clients, and the public on aspects of ethnopharmacology.

HEALTH RESTORATION. In the context of mental illness, health restoration is usually thought of in terms of recovery. **Recovery** involves restoration of a meaningful life rather than symptom relief, which is the emphasis in the medical model of care. In many cases, recovery does not imply a return to full function or the ability to discontinue medication use in chronic mental illnesses. Self-help groups usually focus on recovery. Self-help groups will be discussed in more detail in the context of substance abuse disorders in Chapter 29∞, but population health nurses may be actively involved in initiating and supporting self-help groups for clients with mental health conditions.

Health restoration, in the context of mental illness, also includes maintenance. As was the case with the chronic physical health problems discussed in Chapter 27∞, there is a need to focus on disease management rather than crisis-oriented care for chronic mental health problems. Maintenance involves long-term management of chronic mental illness and focuses on rehabilitating the client and preventing relapse. The goal of maintenance in chronic mental illness is to maintain the client's level of function and to prevent recidivism or frequent rehospitalization. Maintenance may include medications and a variety of other interventions. Population health nurses may be asked to follow clients with diagnoses of chronic mental illness to provide support, encourage treatment adherence, and monitor the effects of treatment. Population health nurses can assist clients to plan regular lifestyles and to minimize sources of stress in their lives. For example, the nurse might help clients with bipolar disorder to reduce stress and to maintain regular sleeping and waking cycles to prevent relapses.

Clients using pharmacologic agents should also be cautioned about potential interactions of medications and alcohol. The nurse can also help clients and their families to identify symptoms that signal a symptomatic relapse and to seek professional assistance when these symptoms are noted. Population health nurses can educate clients and family members regarding signs of relapse and assist them to seek help when relapses occur.

Client and family involvement is an important aspect of maintenance in the control of chronic mental health problems. Population health nurses can promote client and family participation in clinical decision making as well as provide them with information on which to base decisions regarding treatment interventions. In addition, they can regularly monitor clients for medication side effects and offer suggestions for ameliorating them. If side effects cannot be effectively managed or threaten to undermine adherence with treatment, population health nurses can advocate with mental health providers for a change in the treatment regimen to minimize side effects.

It is important that population health nurses learn to assess levels of depression and suicide risk and refer clients at risk to a mental health provider immediately if they are not already involved in ongoing therapy. Population health nurses are also using approaches such as diary writing and physical exercise to help individuals deal more effectively with depressive symptoms. For example, journaling may allow the client to identify triggers for depressive episodes or to recognize initial symptoms of depression so that medical assistance can be sought. Journaling may serve a similar function for clients with schizophrenia, allowing clients or family members to identify early signs of relapse and seek assistance. Open lines of communication are imperative among nurse, mental health provider, family, and client, particularly at times when the client is deeply depressed or actively suicidal.

Persons with chronic mental illness often have a high incidence of physical health problems and sometimes lack the capacity to seek health care in today's complex delivery systems. The population health nurse may be in the situation of following a person for a physical health problem who suddenly begins to show signs of mental illness. The nurse's role in this case is to refer the client for further diagnosis and treatment, as well as to assist in addressing the physical health problem. The population health nurse also refers clients who are exhibiting signs of exacerbation of their disorders.

Respite is another aspect of maintenance in the care of chronic mental illness. Respite has been shown to benefit both clients with serious mental illness and family caregivers. Population health nurses can refer clients and family members to existing respite services, which may be provided in the home or in specialized residential facilities. They may also be actively involved in advocating for the availability of respite for these families. Families and clients with mental illness may also benefit from participation in mutual support groups, and population health nurses can either make referrals to existing groups or work with clients and family members to establish such groups. Table 28-8● summarizes foci and strategies for health restoration related to mental health problems.

Evaluating Interventions for Mental Health and Illness

Evaluation of mental health interventions occurs at the individual and family level as well as the population level. Evidence of effective intervention for the individual client may lie in improved mental health, diminished mental distress, or a decrease in symptoms of a specific mental disorder. Similarly, effective family care may result in improved family dynamics or decreased disruption of family life by a mentally ill family member.

At the population level, evidence of effective health promotion and prevention activities would lie in improved mental health in the population and decreased incidence and prevalence of mental disorders as well as decreased reports of mental distress in the population. National health objectives for 2020 may also be used as guidelines for evaluating mental health care, particularly care related to resolution of existing problems and health restoration. Baseline data and 2020 targets for selected objectives are provided on the next page.

TABLE 28-8 Foci and Strategies for Health Restoration Related to Mental Health Problems

Focus	Strategies
Promoting disease self-management	• Educate clients on long-term management of chronic mental health conditions. • Promote development of and refer to mental illness support groups. • Encourage regular schedules and healthy lifestyles. • Promote physical activity. • Assist clients/families to minimize sources of stress. • Advocate for services to support self-management.
Promoting adherence to therapeutic regimens	• Advocate for client involvement in decision making. • Educate clients regarding the need for continued adherence. • Educate clients/families about drug/alcohol interactions. • Monitor treatment adherence and effects. • Assist clients to deal with treatment side effects.
Preventing relapse or recognizing early symptoms of relapse	• Assist clients and families to identify and modify risk factors for relapse. • Educate clients and families regarding early signs and symptoms of relapse. • Encourage seeking mental health care for early signs of relapse. • Assess for depression and signs of suicidal ideation and refer as needed.
Promoting quality of life	• Assist clients with economic issues, job training, and so on. • Educate clients and families for health interpersonal interactions. • Teach or refer for assistance in development of life skills.
Providing caregiver support	• Educate families about mental illness and ways to help affected family members. • Advocate for availability of respite services. • Refer to respite services as needed.
Preventing stigma and discrimination	• Educate the public about mental health and illness. • Advocate for antidiscrimination laws. • Support antidiscrimination policies in social and health care institutions. • Develop and implement programs to decrease stigma associated with mental illness. • Assist client and families to deal with stigma and discrimination.

Healthy People 2020

Selected *Healthy People 2020* Objectives Related to Mental Health and Mental Illness

OBJECTIVE	BASELINE (YEAR)	TARGET	CURRENT DATA (YEAR)	DATA SOURCES
MHMD-3. Reduce the proportion of adolescents engage in eating disordered behavior	14.3% (2009)	12.0%	16.3% (2011)	Youth Risk Behavior Surveillance System (YRBSS), CDC/NCHHSTP
MHMD-4.1. Reduce the proportion of adolescents who experience major depressive episodes	8.3% (2008)	7.4%	8.2% (2011)	National Survey on Drug Use and Health (NSDUH), SAMHSA
MHMD-4.2. Reduce the proportion of adults who experience major depressive episodes	6.4% (2008)	5.8%	6.6% (2011)	NSDUH, SAMHSA
MHMD-5. Increase the proportion of primary care providers that provide mental health care on site or by paid referral	79% (2006)	87%	NDA	Uniform Data System, HRSA/BPHC
MHMD-8. Increase the proportion of persons with serious mental illness who are employed	58.6% (2008)	64.4%	53.4% (2011)	NSDUH, SAMHSA

Healthy People 2020 (Continued)

OBJECTIVE	BASELINE (YEAR)	TARGET	CURRENT DATA (YEAR)	DATA SOURCES
MHMD-9.1. Increase the proportion of adults with serious mental illness who receive treatment	58.7% (2008)	64.6%	59.6% (2011)	NSDUH, SAMHSA
MHMD-9.2. Increase the proportion of adults with major depressive episodes who receive treatment	71.1% (2008)	78.2%	68.1% (2011)	NSDUH, SAMHSA
MHMD-11.1. Increase the proportion of primary care physicians who screen adults for depression	2.2% (2007)	2.4%	2.4%* (2010)	National Ambulatory Medical Care Survey (NAMCS), CDC/NCHS
MHMD-12. Increase the proportion of homeless adults with mental health problems who receive mental health services	37% (2006)	41%	NDA	Projects for Assistance in Transitioning from Homelessness

NDA = No data available

*Objective has met target.

Data from: U.S, Department of Health and Human Services. (2014). *Healthy people 2020 – Topics and objectives.* Retrieved from http://healthypeople.gov/2020/topicsobjectives2020/default.aspx

Internationally, MiNDbank, an international data base of resources launched by WHO in 2013, will assist in evaluating the state of mental health and mental illness throughout the world. The intent of MiNDbank is to allow resource and best practice sharing and promote integration of mental and physical health, substance abuse, disability, and human rights initiatives to promote a holistic approach to health (WHO, 2013).

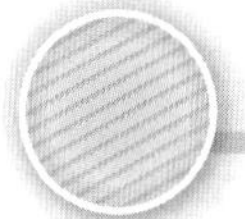

Global Perspectives

WHO QualityRights Project

WHO has established a QualityRights project that is designed to improve the quality and human rights conditions in mental health and social care facilities. The project will also empower organizations to advocate for the rights of people with mental and psychosocial disabilities. Major foci of the project include:

- Improving service quality and human rights conditions in mental health and social care facilities.
- Promoting human rights, recovery, and independent living in the community.
- Developing a movement of people with mental disabilities to provide mutual support, conduct advocacy, and influence policy making.
- Reforming national policies and legislation (WHO, 2014b).

MiNDbank is an international database of resources launched by WHO as part of the QualityRights campaign. The intent of MiNDbank is to allow resource and best practice sharing and promote integration of mental and physical health, substance abuse, disability, and human rights initiatives to promote a holistic approach to health. MiNDbank will also help to reduce the fragmentation and duplication of efforts across sectors of society. Areas of focus within MiNDbank include mental health and substance abuse policies and legislation, disability-related policies and legislation, human rights of persons with mental illness, and mental health services standards. Other resources will include international and regional human rights conventions and treaties, United Nations (UN) special reports, and UN and WHO resolutions (WHO, 2013). For further information about the database, see the *External Resources* section of the student resources site.

CHAPTER RECAP

Population health nurses are actively involved in the development and implementation of programs to promote mental health for clients and populations at all age levels. In addition, because of their presence in the community and familiarity with many community members experiencing adverse life situations, population health nurses are in a position to identify clients at risk for mental health problems. Nurses can engage in activities designed to ameliorate these risks and to promote resilience and coping. Population health nurses are also able to recognize clients with symptomatic mental illness and refer them for mental health services. Assisting clients with chronic mental illness to adjust to their conditions and live as normally as possible is another significant role for population health nurses. Finally, population health nurses may be actively involved in advocacy to assure that culturally appropriate health promotion and illness preventive, diagnostic, and treatment services are available to those in need of them.

CASE STUDY Caring for a Client with Depression

You are the population health nurse assigned to see Donna for a well-baby visit several weeks after she delivered a healthy son. Donna is 39 and has been married to Jack, 48, for a year. Stephen is their first child. When you arrive at Donna's house, you note that she and her family live in a comfortable home in an upper-middle-class neighborhood. Donna answers the door, and you see that her eyes and nose are red as though she has been crying. You explain the purpose of your visit and examine the baby, who is in a freshly painted nursery with a bright mobile over the crib and plenty of stuffed animals and toys around. Stephen is neat, clean, and appears to be well fed, happy, and healthy.

When you finish with the baby, you ask how Donna is doing. Donna bursts into tears. She tells you that she has been feeling desperately unhappy since her pregnancy began. She has been feeling so depressed, she reports that she is not sure she will be able to get out of bed anymore to take care of her son. You say, "Tell me about this past year." Donna tells you that this is a first marriage for her and for Jack, and neither of them has children from previous relationships. In their discussions prior to marriage, she and Jack had never resolved their differences about having children. Donna was ambivalent about having a child; her husband was sure he did not want one. Because they are devout Roman Catholics, they used the rhythm method of birth control. When Donna told Jack she was pregnant after 2 months of marriage, he became very angry and blamed Donna for tricking him into having a baby. Although she had not tricked him, Donna felt guilty and blamed herself for becoming pregnant. Terrified that Jack would leave her if she told him how she felt, she kept all her own feelings of sadness, anger, and depression inside. She did not want to be a single parent. Abortion was never considered because of their religious beliefs.

During the pregnancy, Jack was emotionally withdrawn, depressed, and refused to take part in any activity related to the upcoming birth. Donna's sister attended Lamaze classes with her and coached her during the birth because Jack would not attend. Donna felt jealous of the women whose husbands were so attentive during these classes. Ever since her son's birth, Donna says that she has had "postpartum depression." She has told no one how depressed she feels because she is afraid she will have to be hospitalized as she was several times in her late twenties and early thirties for episodes of clinical depression.

When you do a genogram with her, you discover a family history of depression. Both her grandmother and mother suffered bouts of deep depression, and her grandmother had been hospitalized for a year in a psychiatric institution following menopause. Donna's father is an emotionally withdrawn man whose only sister committed suicide when she was 40. Donna's sister has an eating disorder; she is bulimic.

Now that Donna has been home for 3 weeks with her son, she sees her sister twice a week. Jack is pleased that they have a son, and he is beginning to spend time after he comes home from work playing with Stephen. Donna cannot understand why it makes her angry instead of happy that Jack is becoming involved with their child. Because Jack has refused to support them in a manner that would allow Donna to stay home with Stephen, Donna must return to work after her 6-week maternity leave. She is afraid she will be unable to function at work and has yet to arrange child care for Stephen. Donna worries about these things and has difficulty both falling asleep and getting up during the night to feed her son. She says she cries "at the drop of a hat" and has lost weight. She weighs less now than before she was pregnant. She has little interest in anything, including her baby, and she says that life does not really seem worth living anymore.

1. Does Donna have any typical signs of depression? If so, describe them.
2. How would you assess her potential for suicide?

3. Do you think Donna's depression is "normal" postpartum depression or clinical depression requiring psychiatric assessment and treatment? Why?
4. Based on your assessment, will you follow Donna yourself or refer her to a psychiatrist or mental health worker?
5. How will you involve Donna's husband and sister in the plan of care?
6. What other interventions might be warranted with this family?

REFERENCES

Akincigil, A., Olfson, M., Siegel, M., Zurio, K. A., Walkup, J. T., & Crystal, S. (2012). Racial and ethnic disparities in depression care in community-dwelling elderly in the United States. *American Journal of Public Health, 102,* 319–328. doi:10.2105/AJPH.2011.300349

Alley, D. E., Lloyd, J., Pagân, J., Pollack, C. E., Shardell, M., & Cannuscio, C. (2011). Mortgage delinquency and changes in access to health resources and depressive symptoms in a nationally representative cohort of Americans older than 50 years. *American Journal of Public Health, 101,* 2293–2298. doi:10.2105/AJPH.2011.300245

Al-Modallal, H., Abuidhail, J., Sowan, A., & Al-Rawashdeh, A. (2010). Determinants of depressive symptoms in Jordanian working women. *Journal of Psychiatric and Mental Health Nursing, 17,* 569–576. doi:10.1111/j.1365-2850.2010.01562.x

American College of Obstetricians and Gynecologists. (2010). *Screening for depression during and after pregnancy.* Retrieved from http://www.acog.org/Resources_And_Publications/Committee_Opinions/Committee_on_Obstetric_Practice/Screening_for_Depression_During_and_After_Pregnancy

Bloom, D. E., Cafiero, E. T., Jané-Llopis, E., Abrahams-Gessel, S., Bloom, L. R., Fathima, S., . . . Weinstein, C. (2011). *The global economic burden of noncommunicable diseases.* Retrieved from http://www3.weforum.org/docs/WEF_Harvard_HE_GlobalEconomicBurdenNonCommunicableDiseases_2011.pdf

Bowersox, N. W., Szymanski, B. J., & McCarthy, J. F. (2013). Associations between psychiatric impatient bed supply and the prevalence of serious mental illness in Veterans Affairs nursing homes. *American Journal of Public Health, 103,* 1325–1331. doi:10.2105/AJPH.2012.300783

Brichford, C., & Jones, J. (2009). *Coping with schizophrenic hallucinations and delusions.* Retrieved from http://www.everydayhealth.com/schizophrenia/hallucinations-and-delusions.aspx

Bryant-Bedell, K., & Waite, R. (2010). Understanding major depressive disorder among middle-aged African American men. *Journal of Advanced Nursing, 66,* 2050–2060. doi:10.1111/j.1365-2648.2010.05345.x

Bumb, J. (n.d.). *Dorothea Dix.* Retrieved from http://www2.webster.edu/~woolflm/dorotheadix.html

California Department of Mental Health. (2009). *California strategic plan on reducing mental health stigma and discrimination.* Retrieved from http://www.dhcs.ca.gov/services/medi-cal/Documents/CDMH_MH_Stigma_Plan_09_V5.pdf

Casarez, T. B. (2000). *Dorothea Lynde Dix.* Retrieved from http://www.muskingum.edu/~psych/psycweb/history/dix.htm

Center for Surveillance, Epidemiology and Laboratory Services. (2012). *Mental health awareness.* Retrieved from http://www.cdc.gov/genomics/resources/diseases/mental.htm

Center for Surveillance, Epidemiology and Laboratory Services. (2013). *Autism and family history.* Retrieved from http://www.cdc.gov/genomics/resources/diseases/autism.htm

Centers for Disease Control and Prevention. (2010). National depression screening day—October 7, 2010. *Morbidity and Mortality Weekly Report, 59,* 1229.

Choi, K.-H., Paul, J., Ayala, G., Boylan, R., & Gregorich, S. E. (2013). Experiences of discrimination and their impact on the mental health among African American, Asian and Pacific Islander, and Latino men who have sex with men. *American Journal of Public Health, 103,* 868–874. doi:10.2105/AJPH.2012.301052

Choi, N. G., & Kim, J. (2010). Utilization of complementary and alternative medicines for mental health problems among Asian Americans. *Community Mental Health Journal, 46,* 570–578. doi:10.1007/s10597-010-9322-4

Clark, W., Welch, S., Berry, S. H., Collentine, A. M., Collins, R. M., Lebron, D., & Shearer, A. L. (2013). California's historic effort to reduce the stigma of mental illness: The Mental Health Services Act. *American Journal of Public Health, 103,* 786–794. doi:10.2105/AJPH.2013.301225

Community Preventive Services Task Force. (2014). *Improving mental health and addressing mental illness: Mental health benefits legislation.* Retrieved from http://www.thecommunityguide.org/mentalhealth/benefitslegis.html

Corrigan, P. W., Kosyluk, K. A., & Rüsch, N. (2013). Reducing self-stigma by coming out proud. *American Journal of Public Health, 103,* 794–800. doi:10.2105/AJPH.2012.301037

Coughlin, S. S., Kang, H. K., & Mahan, C. M. (2011). Alcohol use and selected health conditions of 1991 Gulf War veterans: Survey results, 2003–2005. *Preventing Chronic Disease: Public Health Research, Practice, and Policy, 8*(3), 1–11. Retrieved from http://www.cdc.gov/pcd/issues/2011/may/pdf/10_0164.pdf

Cummings, J. R., Lucas, S. M., & Druss, B. G. (2013). Addressing public stigma and disparities among persons with mental illness: The role of federal policy. *American Journal of Public Health, 103,* 781–785. doi:10.2105/AJPH.2013.301224

Dixon, L. B., Lucksted, A., Medoff, D. R., Burland, J., Stewart, B., Lehman, A. F., . . . Murray-Swank A. (2011). Outcomes of a randomized study of a peer-taught family-to-family education program for mental illness. *Psychiatric Services, 62,* 591–597.

Dorothea Dix. (2014). *The Biography Channel website.* Retrieved from http://www.biography.com/people/dorothea-dix-9275710#awesm=~oGQjPfeopiEcKa

Dorothea Lynde Dix. (2014). *The History Channel website.* Retrieved from http://www.history.com/topics/dorothea-lynde-dix

Edmondson, D., Gamboa, C., Cohen, A., Anderson, A., Kutner, N., Kronish, I., . . . Muntner, P. (2013). Association of posttraumatic stress disorder and depression with all-cause and cardiovascular disease mortality and hospitalization among Hurricane Katrina survivors with end-stage renal disease. *American Journal of Public Health, 103,* e130–137. doi:10.2105/10AJPH.2012.301146

Ekern, J. (2014). *Eating disorder statistics and research.* http://www.eatingdisorderhope.com/information/statistics-studies

Favrod, J., Maire, A., Bardy, S., Pernier, S., & Bonsack, C. (2010). Improving insight into delusions: A pilot study of metacognitive training for patients with schizophrenia. *Journal of Advanced Nursing, 67,* 401–407. doi:10.1111/j.1365-2648.2010.05470.x

Fledderus, M., Bohlmeijer, E. T., Smit, F., & Westerhof, G. J. (2010). Mental health promotion as a new goal in public mental health care: A randomized controlled trial of an intervention enhancing psychological flexibility. *American Journal of Public Health, 100*, 2372–2378. doi:10.2105/AJPH.2010.196196

Gfroerer, J., Dube, S. R., King, B. A., Garrett, B. E., Babb, S., & McAfee, T. (2013). Vital signs: Current cigarette smoking among adults aged >18 years with mental illness—United States, 2009–2011. *Morbidity and Mortality Weekly Report, 62*, 81–87.

Gísladóttir, M., & Svavarsdóttir, E. K. (2011). Educational and support intervention to help families assist in the recovery of relatives with eating disorders. *Journal of Psychiatric and Mental Health Nursing, 18*, 122–130. doi:10.1111/j.1365-2850.2010.01637.x

Gonzalez, M. T., Hartig, T., Patil, G. G., Martinsen, E. W., & Kirkevold, M. (2010). Therapeutic horticulture in clinical depression: A prospective study of active components. *Journal of Advanced Nursing, 66*, 2002–2013. doi:10.1111/j.1365-2648.2010.05383.x

Hakenewerth, A. M., Tintinallis, J. E., Waller, A. E., Ising, A., & DeSlem, T. (2013). Emergency department visits by patients with mental health disorders—North Carolina, 2008–2010. *Morbidity and Mortality Weekly Report, 62*, 469–472.

Hazra, M., Noh, S., Boon, H., Taylor, A., Moss, K., & Mamo, D. C. (2010). Complementary and alternative medicine in psychiatric disorders. *Journal of Complementary and Integrative Medicine, 7* (online). doi:10.2202/1553-3840.1239

Henderson, C., Evans-Lacko, S., & Thornicroft, G. (2013). Mental illness stigma, help seeking, and public health programs. *American Journal of Public Health, 103*, 777–780. doi:10.2105/AJPH.2012.301056

Insel, T. (2011). *Director's blog: The global cost of mental illness*. Retrieved from http://www.nimh.nih.gov/about/director/2011/the-global-cost-of-mental-illness.shtml

Insel, T. (2013). *Director's blog: Getting serious about mental illness*. Retrieved from http://www.nimh.nih.gov/about/director/2013/getting-serious-about-mental-illnesses.shtml

Institute of Medicine. (2006). *Improving the quality of health care for mental and substance-use conditions*. Retrieved from http://www.nap.edu/openbook/0309100445/html/2.html

Johnson, N., L., Giarelli, E., Lewis, L., & Rice, C. E. (2013). Genomics and autism spectrum disorder. *Journal of Nursing Scholarship, 45*, 69–78. doi:10.1111/j.1547-5069.2012.01483.x

Katon, W., & Ciechanowski. (2014). *Unipolar major depression in adults: Choosing initial treatment*. Retrieved from http://www.uptodate.com/contents/unipolar-major-depression-in-adults-choosing-initial-treatment#H12

Keyes, C. L. M., Dhingra, S. S., & Simoes, E. J. (2010). Change in level of positive mental health as a predictor of future risk of mental illness. *American Journal of Public Health, 100*, 2366–2371. doi:10.2105/AJPH.2010.192245

Keyes, C. L. M., Myers, J. M., & Kendler, K. S. (2010). The structure of the genetic and environmental influences on mental well-being. *American Journal of Public Health, 100*, 2379–2384. doi:10.2105/AJPH.2010.193615

Keyes, C. L. M., & Simoes, E. J. (2012). To flourish or not: Positive mental health and all-cause mortality. *American Journal of Public Health, 102*, 2164–2172. doi:10.2105/AJPH.2012.300918

Kobau, R., Seligman, M. E. P., Peterson, C., Diener, E., Zack, M. M., Chapman, D., & Thompson, W. (2011). Mental health promotion in public health: Perspectives and strategies from positive psychology. *American Journal of Public Health, 101*, e1–e9. doi:10.2105/AJPH.2010.300083

Kuosmanen, L., Jakobsson, T., Hyttinen, J., Koivunen, M., & Valimäki, M. (2010). Usability evaluation of a web-based patient information system for individuals with severe mental health problems. *Journal of Advanced Nursing, 66*, 2701–2710. doi:10.1111/j.1365-2648.2010.05411.x

Lee, H., & Schepp, K. G. (2011). Ways of coping in adolescents with schizophrenia. *Journal of Psychiatric and Mental Health Nursing, 18*, 158–165. doi:10.1111/j.1365-2850.2010.01643.x

Lowenstein, J. A., Butler, D. W., & Ashcroft, K. (2010). The efficacy of a cognitively orientated carers groups in an early intervention in psychosis service—a pilot study. *Journal of Psychiatric and Mental Health Nursing, 17*, 569–576. doi:10.1111/j.1365-2850.2010.01564.x

Maguen, S., Bosch, J. O., Marmar, C. R., & Seal, K. H. (2010). Gender differences in mental health diagnoses among Iraq and Afghanistan Veterans enrolled in Veterans Affairs health care. *American Journal of Public Health, 100*, 2450–2456. doi:10.2105/AJPH.2009.166165

Marco, E. J., Hinkley, L. B. N., Hill, S. S., & Nagarajan, S. (2011). Sensory processing in autism: A review of neurophysiologic findings. *Pediatric Research, 69*, 48R–54R. doi:10.1203/PDR.0b013e3182130c54

Mayo Clinic Staff. (2011). *Seasonal affective disorder*. Retrieved from http://www.mayoclinic.org/diseases-conditions/seasonal-affective-disorder/basics/definition/CON-20021047?p=1

Mayo Clinic Staff. (2012). *Dysthymia: Definition*. Retrieved from http://www.mayoclinic.org/diseases-conditions/dysthymia/basics/definition/con-20033879

McClave, A. K., McKnight-Eily, L. R., Davis, S. P., & Dube, S. R. (2010). Smoking characteristics of adults with selected lifetime mental illnesses: Results from the 2007 National Health Interview Survey. *American Journal of Public Health, 100*, 2464–2472. doi:10.2105/AJPH.2009.188136

Merikangas, K. R., He, J., Burstein, M., Swanson, S. A., Avenevoli, S., Cui, L., . . . Swendsen, J. (2010). Lifetime prevalence of mental disorders in U.S. adolescents: Results from the National Comorbidity Study-Adolescent Supplement (NCS-A). *Journal of the American Academy of Child and Adolescent Psychiatry, 49*, 980–989. doi:10.1016/j.jaac.2010.05.017

Mezuk, B., Myers, J. M., & Kendler, K. S. (2013). Integrating social science and behavioral genetics: Testing the origin of socioeconomic disparities in depression using a genetically informed design. *American Journal of Public Health, 103*(S1), S145–S151. doi:10.2105/AJPH.2013.301247

Mojtabai, R. (2011). National trends in mental health disability, 1997–2009. *American Journal of Public Health, 101*, 2156–2163. doi:10.2105/AJPH.2011.300258

Mojtabai, R., & Crum, R. M. (2013). Cigarette smoking and onset of mood and anxiety disorders. *American Journal of Public Health, 103*, 1656–1665. doi:10.2105/AJPH.2012.300911

National Alliance on Mental Illness. (n.d.a). *Borderline personality disorder*. Retrieved from http://www.nami.org/Template.cfm?Section=By_Illness&Template=/TaggedPage/TaggedPageDisplay.cfm&TPLID=54&ContentID=44780

National Alliance on Mental Illness. (n.d.b). *Exercise and mental illness*. Retrieved from https://www.nami.org/template.cfm?section=exercise

National Alliance on Mental Illness. (n.d.c). *Family-to-family*. Retrieved from http://www.nami.org/template.cfm?section=Family-to-Family

National Center for Health Statistics. (2012a). Percentage of adults aged > 18 years who often felt worried, nervous, or anxious, by sex and age group—National Health Interview Survey, United States, 2010–2011. *Morbidity and Mortality Weekly Report, 60*, 197.

National Center for Health Statistics. (2012b). Prevalence of current depression among persons aged >12 years, by age group and sex—United States, National Health and Nutrition Examination Survey, 2007–2010. *Morbidity and Mortality Weekly Report, 60*, 1747.

National Center for Health Statistics. (2014). *Health, United States, 2013: With special feature prescription drugs*. Retrieved from http://www.cdc.gov/nchs/data/hus/hus13.pdf

National Institute of Mental Health. (n.d.a). *Autism spectrum disorder*. Retrieved from http://www.nimh.nih.gov/statistics/1AUT_CHILD.shtml

National Institute of Mental Health. (n.d.b). *Bipolar disorder*. Retrieved from http://www.nimh.nih.gov/health/topics/bipolar-disorder/index.shtml

National Institute of Mental Health. (n.d.c). *Bipolar disorder among adults*. Retrieved from http://www.nimh.nih.gov/statistics/1bipolar_adult.shtml

National Institute of Mental Health. (n.d.d). *Borderline personality disorder*. Retrieved from http://www.nimh.nih.gov/health/topics/borderline-personality-disorder/index.shtml

National Institute of Mental Health. (n.d.e). *Major depressive disorder among adults*. Retrieved from http://www.nimh.nih.gov/statistics/1mdd_adult.shtml

National Institute of Mental Health. (1999). *Mental health: A report of the Surgeon General*. Rockville, MD: Author.

National Institute of Mental Health. (2009a). *Anxiety disorders*. Retrieved from http://www.nimh.nih.gov/health/publications/anxiety-disorders/nimhanxiety.pdf

National Institute of Mental Health. (2009b). *Schizophrenia*. Retrieved from http://www.nimh.nih.gov/health/publications/schizophrenia/schizophrenia-booket-2009.pdf

National Institute of Mental Health. (2011a). *Depression*. Retrieved from http://www.nimh.nih.gov/health/publications/depression/index.shtml

National Institute of Mental Health. (2011b). *Eating disorders*. Retrieved from http://www.nimh.nih.gov/health/publications/eating-disorders/eating-disorders.pdf

National Institute of Mental Health. (2012a). *Post traumatic stress disorder research fact sheet*. Retrieved from http://www.nimh.nih.gov/health/publications/post-traumatic-stress-disorder-research-fact-sheet/index.shtml

National Institute of Mental Health. (2012b). *Psychotherapies*. Retrieved from http://www.nimh.nih.gov/health/topics/psychotherapies/index.shtml

National Institute of Mental Health. (2013). *Schizophrenia*. Retrieved from http://www.nimh.nih.gov/health/topics/schizophrenia/index.shtml

National Women's Hall of Fame. (2011). *Dorothea Dix*. Retrieved from http://www.greatwomen.org/component/fabrik/details/2/47

Nicosia, N., MacDonald, J. M., & Arkes, J. (2013). Disparities in criminal court referrals to drug treatment and prison for minority men. *American Journal of Public Health, 103*, e77–84. doi:10.2105/AJPH.2013.301222

Nuttbrock, L., Bockting, W., Rosenblum, A., Hwahng, S., Mason, M., Macri, M., et al. (2013). Gender abuse, depressive symptoms, and HIV and other sexually transmitted infections among male-to-female transgender persons: A three year prospective study. *American Journal of Public Health, 103*, 300–307. doi:10.2105/AJPH.2011.300568

Organisation for Economic Cooperation and Development. (2011). *Sick on the job? Myths and realities about mental health and work*. Retrieved from http://www.oecd.org/els/emp/49227343.pdf

Orozco, R., Borges, G., Medina-Mora, M. E., Aguilar-Gaxiola, S., & Breslau, J. (2013). A cross-national study on prevalence of mental disorders, service use, and adequacy of treatment among Mexican and Mexican American populations. *American Journal of Public Health, 103*, 1610–1618. doi:10.2105/AJPH.2012.301169

Perry, G. S., Presley-Cantrell, L. R., & Dhingra, S. (2010). Addressing mental health promotion in chronic disease prevention and health promotion. *American Journal of Public Health, 100*, 2337–2339. doi:10.2105/AJPH.2010.205146

Pescosolido, B. A., Medina, T. R., Martin, J. K., & Long, J. S. (2013). The 'backbone' of stigma: Identifying the global core of public prejudice associated with mental illness. *American Journal of Public Health, 103*, 853–860. doi:10.2105/AJPH.2012.301147

Prison and asylum reform. (n.d.). Retrieved from http://www.ushistory.org/us/26d.asp

PTSD Alliance. (n.d.). *What is PTSD?* Retrieved from http://www.ptsdalliance.org/about_what.html

Reeves, W. C., Strine, T. W., Pratt, L. A., Thompson, W., Ahluwalia, I., Dhingra, A., . . . Safran, M. A. (2011, September 2). Mental illness surveillance among adults in the United States. *Morbidity and Mortality Weekly Report, 60*(3, Suppl.), 1–29.

Schutte, D. L., Davies, M. A., & Goris, E. D. (2013). The implications of genomics on the nursing care of adults with neuropsychiatric conditions. *Journal of Nursing Scholarship, 45*, 79–88. doi:10.1111/jnu.12006

Sheppard, K., & Badger, T. (2010). The lived experience of depression among culturally Deaf adults. *Journal of Psychiatric and Mental Health Nursing, 17*, 783–789. doi:10.1111/j.1365-2850.2010.01606.x

Shim, R., & Rust, G. (2013). Primary care, behavioral health, and public health: Partners in reducing mental health stigma. *American Journal of Public Health, 103*, 774–776.

Smith, P. M., & Bielecky, A. (2012). The impact of changes in job strain and its components on the risk of depression. *American Journal of Public Health, 102*, 352–358. doi:10.2105/AJPH.2011.300376

Tartakovsky, M. (n.d.). *15 ways to support a loved one with serious mental illness*. Retrieved from http://psychcentral.com/lib/15-ways-to-support-a-loved-one-with-serious-mental-illness/0007039

Torres, J. M., & Wallace, S. P. (2013). Migration circumstances, psychological distress, and self-rated physical health for Latino immigrants in the United States. *American Journal of Public Health, 103*, 1619–1627. doi:10.2105/AJPH.2012.301195

Torrey, E. F., Kennard, A. D., Eslinger, D., Lamb, R., & Pavle, J. (2010). *More mentally ill persons are in jails and prisons than hospitals: A survey of the states*. Retrieved from http://tacreports.org/storage/documents/2010-jail-study.pdf

Treatment Advocacy Center. (2011). *Who we are and what we do*. Retrieved from http://www.treatmentadvocacycenter.org/about-us

Treatment Advocacy Center. (2012). *No room at the inn: Trends and consequences of closing public psychiatric hospitals*. Retrieved from http://tacreports.org/bed-study

Tsai, A. C., Karasic, D. H., Hammer, G. P., Charlebois, E. D., Ragland, K., Moss, A. R., . . . Bangsberg, D. R. (2013). Directly observed antidepressant medication treatment and HIV outcomes among homeless and marginally housed HIV-positive adults: A randomized controlled trial. *American Journal of Public Health, 103*, 308–315. doi:10.2105/AJPH.2011.300422

University Medical Centre Hamburg-Eppendorf. (2014). *Metacognitive training in psychosis*. Retrieved from http://www.uke.de/kliniken/psychiatrie/index_17380.php#Metacognitive_Training_for_Patients_with_Schizophrenia_MCT

U.S, Department of Health and Human Services. (2014). *Healthy people 2020—Topics and objectives*. Retrieved from http://healthypeople.gov/2020/topicsobjectives2020/default.aspx

Vogt, D. (2014). *Research on women, trauma, and PTSD*. Retrieved from http://www.ptsd.va.gov/professional/treatment/women/women-trauma-ptsd.asp

Waghorn, J. (2010). The impact of basing mental health liaison nurses in an emergency department at night. *Journal of Psychiatric and Mental Health Nursing, 17*, 647–650. doi:10.1111/j.1365-2850.2010.01580.x

Wexner Medical Center, Ohio State University. (n.d.). *Schizophrenia*. Retrieved from http://medicalcenter.osu.edu/patientcare/healthcare_services/mental_health/mental_health_about/schizophrenia/Pages/index.aspx

Wong, F. K., & Edmond, H. (2012). Ethnopsychopharmacology considerations for Asians and Asian Americans. *Asian Journal of Psychiatry, 5*, 18–23. doi:10.1016/j.ajp.2012.01.003

World Health Organization. (2013). *WHO MiNDbank*. Retrieved from http://www.who.int/mental_health/mindbank/flyer_EN.pdf?ua=1

World Health Organization. (2014a). *Mental health: Strengthening our response*. Retrieved from http://www.who.int/mediacentre/factsheets/fs220/en/

World Health Organization. (2014b). *WHO QualityRights project—addressing a hidden emergency*. Retrieved from http://www.who.int/mental_health/policy/quality_rights/en/index.html

CHAPTER

29 Substance Abuse

Learning Outcomes

After reading this chapter, you should be able to:

1. Identify signs and symptoms of psychoactive substance dependence.
2. Distinguish between psychoactive substance dependence and abuse.
3. Identify substances that lead to dependence and abuse.
4. Analyze personal, family, and societal effects of substance abuse.
5. Analyze biological, psychological, environmental, sociocultural, behavioral, and health system factors that influence substance abuse.
6. Discuss aspects of population health nursing assessment in relation to substance abuse.
7. Identify major approaches to prevention of substance abuse and analyze the role of the population health nurse with respect to each.
8. Discuss harm reduction as a preventive measure for substance abusers.
9. Describe the components of the intervention process in resolving problems of substance abuse.
10. Identify general principles in the treatment of substance abuse.
11. Describe treatment modalities in substance abuse control and analyze the role of the population health nurse in their implementation.
12. Analyze the role of the population health nurse in health restoration with regard to substance abuse.

Key Terms

addiction
ARV diversion
brief intervention
codependence
corporate social responsibility
crack
designer drugs
drug use
epigenetics
exposome
freebasing
harm reduction
intoxication
market segmentation
physical dependence
polydrug use
psychoactive substance misuse
psychoactive substances
relapse
relapse prevention therapy (RPT)
relapse risk maps
substance-related disorders
supervised injection facilities (SIFs)
teratogenic substances
tolerance
withdrawal

Advocacy Then

Drug Addiction Prevention at the Local Level

Charles E. Terry, MD, became city health officer of Jacksonville, Florida, in 1910. In addition to promoting strict enforcement of sanitary laws and medical examinations for school children, Terry began a concerted campaign against drug addiction while advocating for humane treatment of "drug addicts," the term most often used at the time. He established a system to identify opiate and cocaine users and received legal authority for the health department to provide addicts with drugs if necessary (Fee, 2011).

In 1912, Terry was instrumental in the passage of a city ordinance regulating the sale of drugs containing opium and other addictive drugs, such as cocaine. Sale of these drugs required a written prescription from a physician, prohibited prescription refills, and required that records of sales be kept with copies sent to the health department. The law also provided for the health officer to provide free prescriptions to users if deemed appropriate. These provisions curtailed illegal sales of drugs and brought habitual users into contact with the health officer who obtained histories of use and identified major contributing factors for addiction. The primary contributing factor in more than half of cases was physician prescription or administration of the drugs. Other factors included the encouragement of acquaintances, "dissipation and evil companions," and the presence of chronic and incurable disease. Terry emphasized the need for community level data on the extent of abuse and free publically funded treatment for abusers, noting that merely cutting off the supply of drugs would be "inhumane" (Terry, 1914/2011).

Advocacy Now

Promoting Effective Drug Policies

The Drug Policy Alliance (DPA) is an advocacy organization that contends current U.S. drug policies do more harm than good and seeks to foster more effective policies that recognize individual rights and minimize the personal and societal harm related to drug abuse (DPA, 2014a, para 2). DPA uses legislative avenues to promote sensible drug policy reform.

DPA was formed in 2000 with the merger of the Lindesmith Center, an activist drug policy think-tank and the Drug Policy Foundation, a drug policy reform organization. DPA is a nonprofit organization that advocates for policy reform as it relates to substance use and abuse (DPA, 2014b). DPA's mission is to promote policies that minimize the harm resulting from both drug abuse and prohibition of use and foster individual choice in the matter of drug use (DPA, 2014c). DPA members include a wide array of disciplines, including legislators, health care professionals, members of the legal profession, and others (DPA, 2014a).

The DPA-supported initiatives have led to legalization of marijuana use in Colorado and Washington state, as well as in Uruguay, decriminalization of marijuana use in Rhode Island, and legalization of medical marijuana use in several states. Other initiatives have focused on criminal justice reforms, such as modification of California's "three strikes law" such that life imprisonment is no longer imposed on people convicted of repeated minor nonviolent drug law offenses. DPA has also contributed to the passage of legislation in New Jersey that protects persons who report a drug overdose from prosecution for drug possession and expands access to naloxone to prevent drug overdose deaths. Improving access to clean syringes in New Jersey was another DPA initiative. DPA has also been involved in legislation to promote drug diversion programs and is currently advocating establishment of safe injection facilities in the United States that have been shown to be effective in reducing harm among injection drug users (DPA, 2014d, 2014e, 2014f). Several of these policy initiatives are discussed in more detail later in this chapter.

Most drugs are used appropriately for medicinal purposes. Even when used appropriately, however, drugs may result in substance-related disorders. Substance-related and addictive disorders is one of the diagnostic categories included in the fifth edition of the *Diagnostic and Statistical Manual of Mental Disorders* (*DSM-5*) of the American Psychiatric Association (2013a). This diagnostic category combined the prior separate diagnoses of substance abuse and substance dependence and conceptualizes the occurrence of substance-related disorders on a continuum from mild to severe. Addictive disorders are also included in the diagnostic category and, at present, encompass only gambling disorder (American Psychiatric Association, 2013b). **Substance-related disorders** are defined as maladaptive patterns of substance use resulting in impairment or distress and manifested in specific criteria over a period of time (National Alliance on Mental Illness, n.d.). In this chapter, we are concerned with substance-related disorders resulting from inappropriate use of psychoactive substances. **Psychoactive substances** are drugs or chemicals that alter brain and nervous system function (Hartney, 2011). In the International Classification of Diseases (ICD-10), the World Health Organization (WHO, 2014c) defined psychoactive substance use disorders as mental and behavioral disorders resulting from psychoactive substance abuse and including acute intoxication, harmful use, dependence, and withdrawal.

Substance abuse is a growing world problem. The illegal drug trade is big business, and the fact that many substances with the potential for abuse also have legitimate uses has made control of substance abuse difficult. **Drug use** is the taking of a drug in the correct amount, frequency, and strength for its medically intended purpose. **Psychoactive substance misuse**, or drug abuse, on the other hand, is the deliberate use of a substance for a purpose not consistent with its intended legal or medical purpose. The term misuse is preferred by many experts as being less judgmental than abuse (WHO, 2014b).

Other terms that are important in an understanding of substance abuse include addiction, physical dependence, tolerance, withdrawal, and polydrug abuse. **Addiction** is a "chronic relapsing disease, characterized by compulsive drug seeking and use, despite serious adverse consequences, and by long-lasting changes in the brain" (National Institute on Drug Abuse [NIDA], 2011, p. 1). Dependence or **physical dependence** is "an adaptive physiological state that occurs with regular drug use and results in withdrawal symptoms when the drug is stopped" (NIDA, 2011, p. 1). Dependence can also occur with appropriate use of many medications and does not, by itself, constitute addiction. Signs of psychoactive substance dependence include the following:

- Increasing amounts of substance used, or use extending over a longer period than intended
- Persistent desire for the substance or one or more unsuccessful attempts to control its use
- Increased time spent in obtaining, using, or recovering from the effects of the substance
- Frequent symptoms of intoxication or withdrawal interfering with obligations
- Elimination or reduction of important occupational, social, or recreational activities as a result of substance use
- Continued use of the substance despite recurrent problems caused
- Increased tolerance to the substance
- Experience of characteristic withdrawal symptoms
- Increased substance use to decrease withdrawal symptoms

Tolerance occurs when higher doses of a drug are required to produce the same effect achieved with its initial use; tolerance is often associated with dependence. **Withdrawal** involves the development of a complex set of symptoms that occur when drug use is abruptly stopped or reduced, usually characterized by severe discomfort, pain, nausea, vomiting, and possibly convulsions (NIDA, n.d.). The severity of withdrawal may vary with the abusive substance and the degree of dependence experienced by the client.

In the United States, the abuse of alcohol and other drugs and the use of tobacco products are of particular concern. For example, more than 1.1 million people in the United States sought substance abuse treatment in 2010 (U.S. Census Bureau, 2013a). The magnitude of concern for problems of substance use and abuse is also seen in the development of more than 100 national health promotion and disease prevention objectives and sub-objectives for the year 2020 related to tobacco use and the abuse of alcohol and other drugs (U.S. Department of Health and Human Services [USDHHS], 2014). These objectives can be reviewed on the *Healthy People 2020* website. Baseline data, targets, and current data for selected objectives are provided at the end of this chapter.

In this chapter, effects of and trends in substance use and abuse are examined. Risk factors contributing to all forms of substance abuse, signs and symptoms of specific types of abuse, and population health nursing interventions in the control of substance abuse are addressed.

Individual, Family, and Societal Effects of Substance Abuse

Substance abuse contributes to adverse effects for the abusing individual, for his or her family, and for society at large.

Individual Effects

The effects of substance abuse on the individual are physical, psychological, and social. Physical effects include increased morbidity directly related to the effects of the drug or drugs abused, as well as increased risk of a variety of diseases and conditions. Some physiologic effects may be immediate and some may constitute long-term effects. For example, marijuana users have an estimated risk of heart attack 4.8 times that of nonusers in the first hour after use. *Cannabis* species of plants are the source of marijuana and hashish. The primary psychoactive substance in these drugs is delta-9-tetrahydrocannabinol (THC). THC may be inhaled by smoking marijuana or hashish or ingested and produces relaxation, euphoria, and occasionally altered perceptions of time and space. Marijuana use also results in a productive cough and increased risk for acute respiratory illnesses and infections (NIDA, 2014a). Synthetic cannabinoids, synthetic designer drugs used as a marijuana alternative, have been associated with severe illness resulting from hyperglycemia, hypokalemia, acidosis, and tachycardia. Other effects include nausea and vomiting, seizures, pneumonia, and myocardial infarction. Another serious adverse effect of these drugs is rhabdomyolysis (Drenzek et al., 2013). Rhabdomyolysis is the breakdown of muscle fiber and release of contents into the bloodstream resulting in severe kidney damage (National Center for Biotechnology Information, 2013).

Methamphetamine use is associated with hyperthermia; cardiovascular problems, such as tachycardia, arrhythmias, and increased blood pressure; severe dental problems referred to a "meth mouth," weight loss, and skin lesions from scratching to relieve feelings of "bugs under the skin." Some of these effects are reversible with long-term abstinence, but others are permanent (Gruenewald et al., 2013; NIDA, 2013, 2014b).

Alcohol misuse also contributes to a variety of physical health problems as well, including cirrhosis and liver cancer. Medical emergencies related to drug abuse resulted in 2.5 million emergency department visits in 2011 for an incidence rate of 790 visits for every 100,000 people in the United States. More than half of those visits (51%) involved use of illicit drugs; 51% involved nonmedical use of prescription medications (some in combination with illicit drugs); and 25% involved drugs combined with alcohol (Substance Abuse and Mental Health Services Administration [SAMHSA], 2013a). Methamphetamine use accounted for 103,000 emergency department visits in 2011, the fourth most frequent cause after cocaine, marijuana, and heroin. This figure, however, represents a decrease in methamphetamine-related emergency visits from 132,576 in 2004. Substance abuse treatment admissions were also down from just over 8% of admissions in 2005 to 5.6% in 2011 (NIDA, 2013).

Alcohol use during pregnancy can result in fetal alcohol syndrome, preterm labor, and a variety of fetal abnormalities as indicated in Chapter 16∞. Fetal exposure to nicotine adversely affects brain development, and smoking during pregnancy may result in preterm delivery and stillbirth, and has been associated with attention deficit hyperactivity disorder (ADHD) and disruptive behavioral disorders, although there is insufficient evidence at present to support a causal link between smoking and these neurobehavioral disorders (Office of the Surgeon General, 2014). Other substances of abuse result in equally serious physical health problems.

Substance misuse also increases the potential for exposure to diseases such as HIV/AIDS and hepatitis when abuse involves use of contaminated needles or results in sexual promiscuity as a means of financing a drug habit or because of lowered inhibitions. For example, approximately one in ten new HIV infections worldwide result from injection drug use (IDU), and as much as 80% of all HIV infections in parts of Eastern Europe and Central Asia are due to drug use (WHO, 2014a). In the United States, 6% of new HIV infections in men in 2010 occurred in IDUs, and 4% of HIV infections among men in 2011 were associated with combined IDU and sexual intercourse with other men (Harris et al., 2013). Injection drug users are also at high risk for hepatitis B and C and for resulting liver cancer, cirrhosis, and death (Frimpong, 2013; Masson et al., 2013).

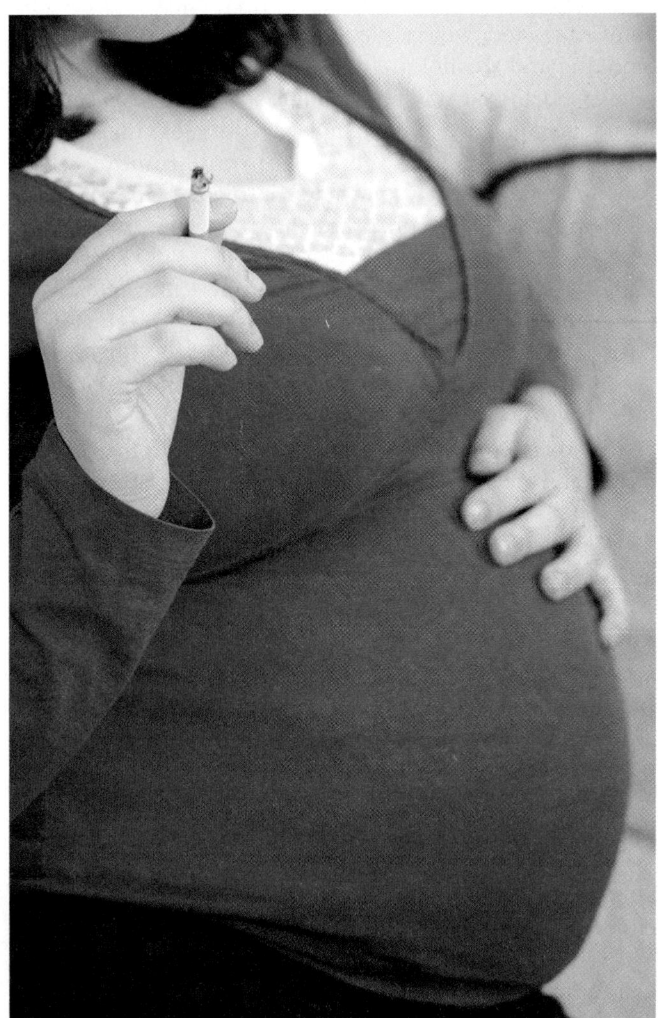

Smoking during pregnancy contributes to a variety of problems for mother and baby. *(Jasmin Merdan/Fotolia)*

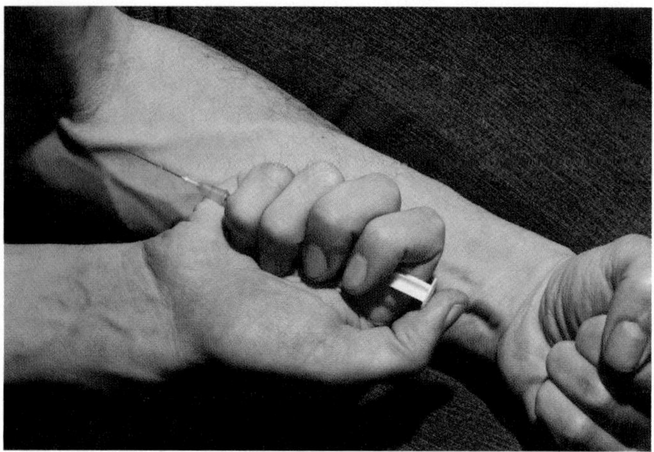

Injection drug users are at high risk for bloodborne diseases.
(terekhov igor/Shutterstock)

Other physical effects of substance abuse include unintentional injury and unintended pregnancy. Substance use also contributes to a wide variety of other unintended injuries. Smoking and alcohol use are often contributing factors in house fires and burn injuries. In one study of persons burned in mobile home fires, for example, 74% of those injured were smokers and 64% reported alcohol abuse (Mullins et al., 2009). Alcohol is widely known to contribute to motor vehicle accidents (MVA), but other substances contribute to MVA injuries as well. For example, in one study cannabis use resulting in blood levels of 2 ng/mL THC (the psychoactive substance in marijuana) increased the risk of accidents four times that of the lowest levels of THC, and stimulants combined with sedatives posed the highest risk for MVAs (Kim, Kuypers, Legrand, Ramaekers, & Verstraete, 2012). Alcohol and drug use also contribute to other forms of injury. For example, in one study of unnatural deaths involving high alcohol concentrations, nearly 15% of the deaths were the result of accidental injury, 11% resulted from suicide, and nearly 7% involved homicide (Darke, Duflou, Torok, & Prolov, 2013).

Some drugs, such as alcohol, nicotine, opiates, and barbiturates, also result in withdrawal symptoms when the drug is removed from the client's system. Some drugs also produce chromosomal changes that cause congenital malformations in children as well as increased potential for spontaneous abortion. Death is the ultimate adverse effect of drug use and may result from a drug overdose, from withdrawal, or from the long-term effects of drug use such as cirrhosis, cancer, cardiovascular disease, and stroke. Assessment for both short-term and long-term physical effects of specific substances is discussed later in this chapter.

In addition to the desired effects that promote drug use and abuse, psychological effects of drug abuse can include personality disturbances, anxiety, and depression. Organic mental disorders characterized by hallucinations, delusions, dementia, delirium, and disorders of mood or perception may also be caused by substance abuse. Aggressive behavior may also result from the use of some drugs (e.g., phencyclidine [PCP], anabolic steroids). In addition, substance abuse may trigger exacerbations of existing mental disorders, such as schizophrenia, depression, and anxiety (NIDA, 2012b).

Preoccupation with the abused substance can lead to a variety of social problems for the substance abuser. Relationships with family and friends may be impaired, or abusers may become incapable of or disinterested in performing their jobs and may be fired. Substance abuse may also lead to poor educational outcomes, limiting the abuser's employability. Initiation of substance use at a young age has been linked to lower income and lower occupational and educational attainment at midlife (Sloan & Grossman, 2011). Unemployment can lead to difficulties in obtaining housing and can contribute to homelessness. Furthermore, the need to obtain money to support a drug habit or to obtain necessities may lead to criminal activity.

Family Effects

The effects of substance abuse on the family of the abuser can be many and severe. These families are characterized by frequent conflict, anger, ambivalence, fear, guilt, confusion, mistrust, and violence as a mode of conflict resolution. The family frequently becomes socially isolated in efforts to cover up the problem of abuse and so may not be able to make use of sources of assistance that might be available to them.

Substance abuse may also be a factor in poor parental role execution, leading to neglect and abuse of children. Children of substance-abusing parents are three to four times more likely to abuse substances themselves than children whose parents do not abuse alcohol or drugs. In addition, they are more likely to exhibit depression, eating disorders, conduct disorders, emotional problems, and poor school performance (American Academy of Experts in Traumatic Stress, 2012).

Direct exposure of children to psychoactive substances within the family and home setting has a variety of adverse physical and psychological effects. Children with perinatal exposure to alcohol, nicotine, or other drugs may be lower in birth weight, be particularly irritable and difficult to comfort, and experience poor school performance later in life. Drug use during pregnancy may also contribute to premature labor. Home exposure to tobacco smoke also affects the health status of children and may contribute to a variety of respiratory conditions as well as childhood cancers. The health effects of drug exposures for infants and children are discussed in more detail later in this chapter.

Other familial effects of substance abuse may include increased illness among nonabusers, poor psychological and interpersonal function, social adjustment difficulties, and lack of family cohesion (American Psychological Association, 2014). These families may also experience interpersonal conflict; divorce is seven times more common among families with substance-abusing members than other families. Family violence is also six times more common in families experiencing substance abuse than in other families (Academy of Experts in Traumatic Stress, 2012). Legal and financial difficulties are also common, and health care utilization rates by family members may be as much as four times higher than those of the average American family (American Psychological Association, 2014)

Family members may exhibit the phenomenon of codependence. **Codependence** is a dysfunctional relationship in which one or more family members attempt to deny the existence of a substance abuse, mental health, or other problem (e.g., compulsive gambling) in a family member and sacrifice their own needs to care for the abuser and try to "fix" his or her problems. Codependence is sometimes referred to as "relationship addition" because the codependent person tends to form relationships that are one-sided and emotionally destructive in order to meet their own need to be needed. Codependents practice maladaptive behaviors to cope with the problem of abuse. Characteristics of codependents center on patterns of denial of feelings, emotional repression, conflict avoidance, and low self-esteem (Mental Health America, n.d.). Codependents may also engage in enabling behaviors in which they ignore the behavior of the substance abuser or make excuses for that behavior, thereby enabling the behavior to continue without challenge (Schimelpfening, 2011).

Co-dependents Anonymous (CoDA), a support group to foster healthy interpersonal relationships, has developed a set of characteristics and behavior patterns that can help people determine if they are codependent (CoDA, 2013). The patterns focus on behaviors demonstrating characteristics of denial, low self-esteem, compliance with the wishes of others, control, and avoidance typical of codependents (CoDA, 2010). In addition, the organization has developed tools for recovery that may assist people in overcoming their codependence (CoDA, 2013). For more information about these behavior patterns, characteristics, and tools, see the *External Resources* section of the student resources site.

Societal Effects

Societal effects of substance abuse include increased morbidity and mortality, economic costs, and increased crime. Physical morbidity related to psychoactive substance abuse was addressed in relation to the personal effects of substance abuse. At the societal level, abuse leads to increased incidence and prevalence of these conditions.

MORTALITY. As noted earlier, substance abuse leads to increased mortality, either directly as a result of drug overdose or withdrawal or indirectly due to other conditions related to abuse. The contribution of smoking to increased mortality was discussed in Chapter 27∞. Alcohol accounts for 2.5 million deaths per year and is the third most common cause of premature mortality worldwide (Pridemore, Chamlin, & Andreev, 2013). Most of these deaths are the result of chronic alcohol-related diseases, such as cirrhosis, liver cancer, and cardiovascular disease (World Health Organization [WHO], 2011). In the region of the Americas, alcohol is the most frequent cause of disease and disability with more than 9% of the total disease burden in the region related to alcohol (Stockwell et al., 2013).

In the United States, excessive alcohol use resulted in approximately 79,000 deaths and 2.3 million years of productive life lost (YPLL) each year from 2001–2005. Half of those deaths and two thirds of YPLL were the result of binge drinking (Kanny, Liu, Brewer, Garvin, & Balluz, 2010). From 2006 to 2010, an average of 88,000 deaths per year occurred as a result of alcohol use (McKnight-Eily et al., 2014). In 2010, alcohol was directly related to 25,692 deaths, excluding deaths resulting from indirect effects related to MVAs, suicide, and homicide. The mortality rate for alcohol-induced deaths was 8.3 per 100,000 population (Murphy, Xu, & Kochanek, 2013a, 2013b). Globally, the World Health Organization considers alcohol use a leading factor for death and disability. Worldwide alcohol consumption contributes to 3.8% of all deaths and 4.6% of disability-adjusted life years (DALYs) (Babor & Robaina, 2013).

Accidental mortality related to alcohol abuse is of particular concern. In spite of decreases in the number of alcohol-related motor vehicle fatalities, 37% of motor vehicle fatalities among people 16 to 20 years of age in 2012 involved alcohol, a decrease from 60% in the mid-1970s (National Institutes of Health [NIH], 2013). Alcohol use is also implicated in other injury fatalities, including falls, drowning, and burns. In addition to accident fatalities, alcohol is a factor in other deaths, including homicide; suicide; deaths due to cancers of the lip, oral cavity, pharynx, esophagus, stomach, liver, and larynx; cardiovascular deaths; and deaths due to respiratory diseases, digestive diseases, and diabetes mellitus. A meta-analysis of

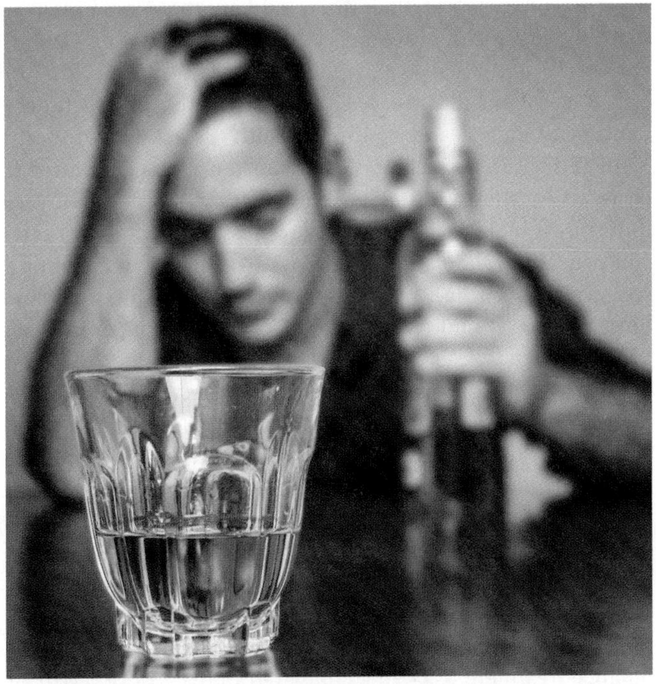

Alcohol misuse is a leading cause of death and disability worldwide. *(kmiragaya/Fotolia)*

relevant studies concluded that alcohol consumption led to an estimated 18,200 to 21,300 cancer deaths in the United States. This amounts to 3.2% to 3.7% of all cancer deaths. People who consumed more than one-and-a-half drinks per day accounted for 26% to 35% of cancer deaths, and each death resulted in 17 to 19.1 years of productive life lost (Nelson et al., 2013).

Other addictive substances also contribute to significant mortality. In 2010, for example, 40,393 drug-induced deaths occurred in the United States, for a mortality rate of 13.1 per 100,000 population. Again, these figures exclude indirect contributions of drug abuse to accidental deaths, suicides, and homicide (Murphy et al., 2013a, 2013b). Drug overdose is the leading cause of accidental death in the United States, outpacing even MVAs. Based on data from the Centers for Disease Control and Prevention (CDC), overdose rates have increased approximately 500% since 1990 (Harm Reduction Coalition, n.d.a), and in 2007, 100 drug overdose deaths occurred daily in the United States (Paulozzi, Jones, Mack, & Rudd, 2011).

Most of these deaths are due to opioid analgesics. From 2002 to 2006, deaths due to prescription opioid pain relievers increased by 98% (Momper, Delva, Tauiliili, Muehller-Williams, & Goral, 2013) exceeding combined mortality rates for heroin and cocaine (Cerdá et al., 2013). In 2010, the U.S. opioid poisoning mortality rate was 5.4 per 100,000 population (National Center for Health Statistics [NCHS], 2014).

COST. Substance abuse also affects society in terms of its economic costs. Estimates of the total economic cost for alcohol and drug abuse in the United States are more than $600 billion per year. Approximately $193 billion is spent each year in relation to abuse of illicit drugs, and another $193 billion is spent in addressing problems caused by tobacco use. Alcohol abuse costs another $235 billion per year (NIDA, 2012b). These costs include health care costs related to substance-related accidents and chronic health problems, property damage related to accidents, and substance abuse treatment costs. In addition, substance abuse poses costs for employers in terms of increased absences, tardiness, accidents, workers' compensation claims, and employee turnover and training costs (NIDA, 2014a). In addition, the estimated lifetime cost of caring for a child with fetal alcohol syndrome (FAS) is $2 million, and the estimated annual cost of FAS in the United States is $4 billion (Division of Birth Defects and Developmental Disabilities, 2012).

Without doubt, drug and alcohol abuse are costly public health problems that the nation can ill afford. Prevention and treatment of substance abuse, on the other hand, are cost-effective. NIDA (2012d) estimated that every dollar invested in substance abuse treatment, for example, saves $4 to $7 in reduced crime, criminal justice, costs, and theft. For example, the average per person cost of 1 year of methadone maintenance treatment is $4,700, compared to the cost of 1 year of incarceration at $24,000 per person. When reduced health care costs are included, savings exceed costs by about 12 to 1. These figures do not even consider the reduction in costs due to lost productivity and drug-related accidents (NIDA, 2012d).

CRIME. One final social effect associated with the abuse of many substances (excluding nicotine) is increased crime. According to data from the Arrestee Drug Abuse Monitoring Program (ADAM-II) across selected major cities, arrests for drug-related crimes ranged from 19% in Denver to 43% in Chicago. Drug use is also implicated in crimes that are not drug-related, and 62% to 86% of all arrestees across sites tested positive for one or more drugs, and 12% to 34% in different jurisdictions were positive for multiple drugs. The most commonly used drug was marijuana (Office of National Drug Control Policy, 2013).

Alcohol use is also implicated in criminal activity. Alcohol use is a factor in 40% of violent crimes, and 36% of people under correctional supervision were drinking at the time of their criminal offense (National Council on Alcoholism and Drug Dependence [NCADD], n.d.b). With the exception of robberies, alcohol use is more common among perpetrators of violent crimes than other drug use (NCADD, n.d.a), and alcohol was a contributing factor in 40% of murder convictions of prisoners in jails or state prisons (NCADD, n.d.b).

Crimes may be committed as a result of the lowering of inhibitions caused by alcohol and other drugs. In other cases, crimes such as theft may be a means of supporting a drug or alcohol habit.

Trends in Substance Use and Abuse

Psychoactive substances are abused because of their desirable initial effects. Some of these effects and the drugs associated with them are presented in Table 29-1●. Rates of psychoactive substance use in general are relatively high in the United States. The most current statistics indicate that the percentage of people over 12 years of age who reported ever using any illicit drug increased from 46.4% in 2003 to 47% in 2008. The percentage of people who reported current illicit drug use declined slightly over the same period from 8.2% to 8% (U.S. Census Bureau, 2013b), but increased to 9.2% in 2012 (NCHS, 2014). Psychoactive substances commonly involved in either dependence or abuse include tobacco, alcohol, prescription drugs, illicit drugs, and other drugs. Each category is briefly discussed below and selected characteristics are summarized in Table 29-1.

Tobacco may be consumed either by smoking or in smokeless forms. As noted in Chapter 27∞, approximately 19% of the U.S. adult population smokes cigarettes. In 2008, nearly 24% of the population 12 years of age and older smoked cigarettes, 5% smoked cigars, and 0.8% smoked pipes. Overall, 3.5% of people reported current use of smokeless forms of tobacco (U.S. Census Bureau, 2013b).

Although the use of smokable forms of tobacco has declined over the last several years, use of smokeless tobacco

TABLE 29-1 Selected Psychoactive Substances, Street Names, Typical Routes of Administration, and Effects Promoting Abuse

Substance	Street Names	Typical Route of Administration	Effects Promoting Abuse
Alcohol	Beer, wine, spirits, booze, various brand names	Orally ingested	Relaxation, decreased inhibitions, increased confidence, euphoria
Sedatives, hypnotics, and anxiolytics		Orally ingested, injected	Calming effect, decreased nervousness and anxiety, improved sleep, relaxation, mild intoxication, loss of inhibition
Barbiturates			
Amytal	Blues, downers		
Nembutal	Yellows, yellow jackets		
Phenobarbital	Phennie, purple hearts		
Seconal	Reds, F-40s, Redbirds		
Tuinal	Rainbows, tooies		
Quaalude	Ludes, 714s, Q's, Quay, Quad, mandrex		
Tranquilizers (minor)	Tranks, downs, downers, goof balls, sleeping pills, candy		
Dalmane			
Equanil/Miltown	Muscle relaxants, sleeping pills		
Librium			
Valium			
Serax			
Opioids			
Codeine	Schoolboy	Orally ingested	Pain relief, euphoria
Demerol	Demies, dolls, dollies, Amidone	Injected	
Dilaudid	Little D, Lords	Injected	
Heroin	Smack, junk, downtown, H, black tar, horse, stuff	Injected, smoked, sniffed	
Methadone	Meth, dollies	Injected	
Morphine	M, Miss Emma, morph, morpho, tab, white stuff, monkey	Injected	
Opium	Blue velvet, black stuff, Dover's powder, paregoric	Orally ingested, smoked, injected	
Percodan	Perkies	Orally ingested	
Cocaine	Coke, snow, uptown, flake, crack, bump, toot, c, candy	Snorted, injected, Smoked	Increased alertness, confidence, euphoria, reduced fatigue
Amphetamines		Orally ingested	Increased alertness, confidence, decreased fatigue, euphoria
Benzedrine	Bennies, pep pills, uppers, truck drivers		
Biphetamine	Black beauties		
Desoxyn	Co-pilots		
Dexedrine	Dex, speed, dexies		
Methedrine	Meth, crank, speed, crystal, go fast		
MDMA	Ecstasy		
Hallucinogens		Orally ingested, smoked, injected	Altered perceptions, mystical experience
Phencyclidine	Angel dust, krystal, DOA, hog, PCP, peace pill	Smoked, orally ingested, injected	Dreamlike state producing hallucinations
LSD	Acid, microdot, cubes		
MDA	The love drug		
Mescaline	Cactus, mesc		
Peyote	Buttons		
Psilocybin	Magic mushrooms, shrooms, sacred mushrooms		
Cannabis		Smoked, orally ingested	Relaxation, euphoria, altered perceptions
Hashish	Kif, herb, hash		
Hashish oil	Honey, hash oil		

(Continued)

TABLE 29-1 (*Continued*)

Substance	Street Names	Typical Route of Administration	Effects Promoting Abuse
Marijuana	Grass, ganja, weed, dope, reefer, Thai sticks, pot, Acapulco gold, roach, loco weed, Maui wowie, joint, Mary Jane		
Inhalants Amyl nitrate Butyl nitrate Nitrous oxide	 Poppers Locker room, rush Laughing gas	Inhaled	Relaxation, euphoria, intoxication
Nicotine	Various brand names of tobacco products	Smoked, chewed	Relaxation, mild stimulation

has increased. Snus (pronounced "snoose") or "Swedish tobacco" is a spit-free moist fermented tobacco product packaged in tea-bag-like pouches that are placed between the upper lip and gums to allow absorption of its psychoactive components (Tobacco Control Legal Consortium, 2013). In 2009, just over 5% of U.S. adults reported use of snus in their lifetimes and nearly 2% reported current use. Electronic cigarettes or e-cigarettes provide aerosolized nicotine, flavoring, and other chemicals via a battery-powered electronic device. The resultant vapors are then inhaled by the user (U.S. Food and Drug Administration [FDA], 2014). Lifetime use of e-cigarettes quadrupled from 0.6% in 2009 to 2.7% in 2010, with current use reported by 1.2% of the U.S. population over age 12. Snus and other dissolvable tobacco products and e-cigarettes provide an alternative in smoke-free environments, promote dual use of smoked and smokeless tobacco, and are considered gateways to smoking initiation by youth (Popova & Ling, 2013). These products are generally free from regulatory control except that e-cigarettes used therapeutically to assist with smoking cessation are regulated (FDA, 2014).

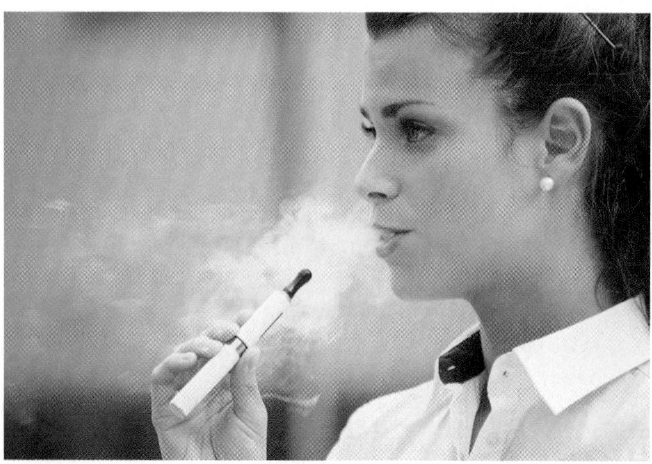

E-cigarettes may be used in the mistaken belief they are less harmful than regular cigarettes. *(Diego cervo/Fotolia)*

Although moderate alcohol intake has been suggested to have possible positive health effects, alcohol abuse remains a serious problem in the United States and elsewhere in the world. The alcohol contained in alcoholic beverages is ethyl alcohol created by the fermentation of grain mixtures or the juice of fruits and berries. After ingestion, alcohol is rapidly absorbed into the bloodstream through the gastrointestinal tract and functions as a central nervous system (CNS) depressant.

In 2012, more than half of the U.S. (52.1%) population over age 12 reported using alcohol. Almost a fourth of the population (23%) reported binge drinking, and 6.5% reported heavy drinking (NCHS, 2014). Binge drinking is defined as five or more alcoholic drinks in one session for men and four or more drinks for women. Heavy drinking is defined as more than two drinks per day for men and more than one drink per day for women (Li et al., 2011). Some authors note that the figures reported here are probably an underrepresentation of binge drinking and heavy drinking because heavy alcohol consumers are likely to underrepresent the extent of their drinking (Heath, 2012).

A variety of prescription drugs are misused, but abuse of opioid pain relievers (OPRs) is the most common occurrence. In terms of overall drug abuse, misuse of OPRs is second only to marijuana abuse (Cerdá et al., 2013). CDC and the Office of National Drug Control Policy have declared prescription drug misuse epidemic (Spoth et al., 2013). OPR sales quadrupled between 1999 and 2010 to a level estimated to be sufficient to medicate every U.S. adult with a standard dose every 4 hours for a month (Paulozzi et al., 2011). In 2010, reported misuse of a prescription drug at least once in a lifetime was reported by 22% of 12- to 18-year-olds and 26% of those 18 to 25 years of age (Spoth et al., 2013). In 2008, 2.5% of the U.S. population over 12 years of age engaged in current use of any psychotropic drug, and pain relievers were routinely used by nearly 20% of the population (U.S. Census Bureau, 2013b).

OPRs and other prescription drugs such as sedatives, hypnotics, and anxiolytics are frequently routinely prescribed in primary care and mental health settings to relieve pain or reduce anxiety and tension and promote sleep. Unfortunately, their prescription for legitimate use often creates dependence. In low doses, these drugs produce a mild state of euphoria, reduce inhibitions, and create feelings of relaxation and decreased tension. Their major pharmacologic action is CNS depression. Because of their widespread use for both legitimate and illegitimate reasons and their easy availability, precise figures on the abuse of these drugs are difficult to obtain. However, in 2008, 0.7% of the population reported current use of tranquilizers and 0.1% reported use of sedatives (U.S. Census Bureau, 2013b).

Illicit drug use involves substances such as marijuana, cocaine, heroin, methamphetamine, hallucinogens such as LSD and ecstasy, inhalants, and steroids. Marijuana is the most commonly used illegal drug in the United States (NIDA, 2014a) even though its possession and use are legal in some jurisdictions and for some purposes. In 2008, more than 6% of the U.S. population over 12 years of age reported current use of marijuana; 0.1% of the population engaged in current heroin use (U.S. Census Bureau, 2013b).

Current cocaine use was reported by 0.7% of the population (U.S. Census Bureau, 2013b). Use of cocaine may be accompanied by the practice of "freebasing." Normally, to maintain its stability, cocaine is combined with a hydrochloride base, creating a substance that is usually only about 25% cocaine. **Freebasing** involves the use of heat and ammonia or sodium bicarbonate and water to free the cocaine from its hydrochloride base, thus creating a purer product that produces a more intense effect. Because of the combination of heat and the highly volatile and explosive ether, freebasing is an extremely dangerous practice. To eliminate the need for freebasing, drug dealers created **crack**, a stable form of cocaine without the hydrochloride base that can be smoked rather than inhaled, for a more rapid and more intense effect (NIDA, 2010).

Methamphetamine use is a growing problem in the United States, particularly in the western states. The 2012 National Survey on Drug Use and Health (NSHUD) indicated that 1.2 million people (0.4% of the U.S. population) had used methamphetamine in the prior year, and 440,000 (0.2%) had used it in the prior month. This latter figure is a decrease from 0.3% in 2006. In 2012, 133,000 people over 12 years of age initiated methamphetamine use for the first time (NIDA, 2013). In California, methamphetamine abuse increased by 17% per year from 1999 through 2008. This growth occurred in three distinct phases, interrupted by laws limiting access to ingredients needed for methamphetamine production and resuming when production processes were modified to incorporate unregulated ingredients (Gruenewald et al., 2013).

Amphetamines in general lend themselves to chemical modifications to create "designer" or "club" drugs. **Designer drugs** are chemical modifications of drugs whose use in their original form is restricted (Bellum, 2011). Club drugs are used at night clubs, bars, concerts, and parties, and include 3,4-methylenedionymethamphetamine (MDMA), better known as "ecstasy"; ketamine; gamma-hydroxybutyrate (GHB); and Rohypnol (a tranquilizer). Reports of club drugs use by 12th graders in 2013 ranged from 0.9% for Rohypnol to 1.4% for ketamine (NIDA, 2012a). Club drugs may cause brain damage and coma as well as long-term effects on memory and learning abilities, seizures, malignant hyperthermia, paranoia, and hostility. Rohypnol is also known as the "date rape" drug because of its strong hypnotic properties.

Hallucinogens distort the distinction between self and the environment, making the user extremely vulnerable to environmental stimuli. Common effects of these drugs include changes in mood (euphoria or terror and despair), heightened sensation or synesthesia (merging of the senses so colors, for example, are experienced as odors or vice versa), changes in perceptions of time and objects, and changes in relationships, leading to depersonalization and feelings of merging with other people and objects.

Inhalants are abused by sniffing products such as airplane model glue, nail polish remover, gasoline, aerosols, and anesthetics such as nitrous oxide. They usually produce a sense of euphoria, loss of inhibition, and excitement. Inhalants are often used by people who do not have the financial resources to support more expensive drug habits. In addition to a variety of adverse physical effects such as kidney and heart damage, there is the potential for suffocation while inhaling these substances from a plastic bag. Because of their volatile nature, explosion is another hazard presented by inhalants. Hallucinogens and inhalants are used by relatively small numbers of people. In 2008, for example, only 0.4% of persons aged 12 years and older reported current use of hallucinogens, and 0.3% reported inhalant use.

Most steroid use occurs under medical direction for treatment of a variety of conditions in which immunosuppression is a desired outcome (e.g., severe arthritis and other inflammatory conditions). Steroids are abused by a small segment of the population, however, particularly adolescents. Anabolic steroids, more properly called anabolic-androgenic steroids due to their dual effects on muscle building and male sex characteristics, are increasing in use, particularly among youth. Anabolic steroids may be used by adolescents and athletes because of their potential to increase strength and weight and to improve body image and athletic performance. In 2013, for example, 2.1% of 12th graders reported lifetime use of steroids, 1.5% reported use in the past year, and 1% reported past month use. Among eighth-grade users, lifetime, past year, and past month use rates were 1.1%, 0.6%, and 0.3%, respectively (NIDA, 2012f).

Prolonged use of anabolic steroids leads to acne, diminished breast size, ovulatory and menstrual difficulties, deepened voice, clitoral enlargement, and male-pattern baldness in women. In men, effects of prolonged use include continuing erections (priapism), difficult urination, gynecomastia, and impotence. Both men and women may experience liver impairment, urinary calculi, anemia, gastrointestinal problems (e.g., anorexia, nausea), and insomnia.

Over-the-counter (OTC) substances are also subject to misuse. Energy drinks, for example, contain caffeine levels equivalent to one to three cups of coffee or cans of caffeinated soda. An estimated 6% of adolescents and young adults consume energy drinks daily. At present their use is unregulated. Extensive use may result in caffeine intoxication or overdose, withdrawal, interactions with alcohol, sleep difficulties, daytime drowsiness, and potential for diminished performance and accidents. As noted in Chapter 23∞, excessive energy drink use is common among military personnel deployed in combat areas (Toblin, Clark-Walper, Kok, Sipos, & Thomas, 2012).

OTC laxatives and diet pills may also be abused for weight control, primarily by youth with eating disorders, particularly bulimia nervosa. An estimated 6% of adolescent girls and 4% of boys use diet products without a health professional's advice. Chronic use of laxatives and diet pills can lead to acute and chronic gastrointestinal and cardiovascular impairments, dehydration, chronic diarrhea or constipation, metabolic acidosis, hypokalemia, and other fluid and electrolyte imbalances. In a meta-analysis of 70 studies, the lifetime prevalence of laxative abuse for weight control was 4% of the general population and 15% to 62% of people with bulimia or other unspecified eating disorders. In 2007, the FDA approved the first OTC diet drug (orlistat or *alli*). Since its OTC designation, approximately 6% of persons with eating disorders have misused the drug (Pomeranz, Taylor, & Austin, 2013).

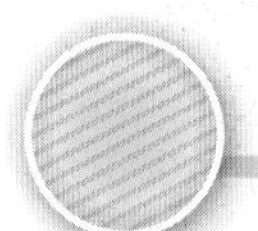

Global Perspectives

Betel Quid Abuse and Oral Cancers

In addition to substances of abuse common in the Western world, much of Asia is faced with an epidemic of betel quid abuse. Betel quid is an addictive combination of areca nut, betel leaf, slaked lime, and regional flavoring ingredients that is widely chewed throughout Asia. Its use is socially accepted in all levels of society for both men and women and for young children. This is true even in societies where tobacco use is considered objectionable. Regular chewers develop tolerance and experience withdrawal symptoms when not using betel quid. Betel quid abuse has been linked to oral premalignant disorders and cancers of the oral cavity, pharynx, esophagus, and larynx. When tobacco is added, abuse rates increase. In one study rates of abuse varied from 0.8% to 46.3% across six Asian populations. Among current chewers abuse rates were over 40%. Factors associated with abuse include lower education level, younger age at initiation, and familial history of use (Lee et al., 2012).

The combination of betel quid with other addictive substances increases the risk of oral cancer. For example, in studies in India and Taiwan, the risk or oral cancer for users of betel quid alone was 7.9 times that of nonusers; more than double the increased risk for those who only smoked tobacco and three times that for people who only drank alcohol. Combining betel quid and smoking increased the risk to 16 times that of nonusers, and the combination of tobacco smoking, betel quid, and alcohol increased the risk of oral cancer to 40 times higher than that for people who used none of the three substances (Petti, Massood, & Scully, 2013).

Population Health Nursing and Substance Abuse

Population health nurses use the nursing process in the context of the population health nursing model to identify problems related to substance use and abuse and to design, implement, and evaluate control strategies for substance abuse.

Assessing Risks for and Effects of Substance Abuse

The epidemiology of substance abuse indicates that there are contributing factors in each of the six categories of determinants of health (biological, psychological, environmental, sociocultural, behavioral, and health system determinants). Population health nurses should keep in mind that the interplay among factors in each of the six areas that leads to substance abuse is unique to each individual and to each population group. For this reason, nurses should assess the factors contributing to abuse in a given situation prior to developing interventions to address substance abuse in an individual or a population group. Assessment in the control of substance abuse problems occurs at two levels: the population or community level and the level of the individual client.

BIOLOGICAL DETERMINANTS. Human biological factors influencing substance abuse and its effects include age, gender, and race/ethnicity, genetic inheritance, and physiologic function.

Age, gender, and race/ethnicity. Age influences one's risk of exposure to tobacco, alcohol, and other drugs through social factors. For example, young people are more likely to be exposed to peer pressure supporting drug use or smoking than are older people. Adolescents and preadolescents are particularly vulnerable to this type of influence because of their developmental need to conform to peer expectations and to be part of a group. Often, being part of the group depends on engaging in behaviors that place the individual at risk, such as sexual activity, smoking, and drug and alcohol use. In addition, youth are at particular risk for substance use and abuse because areas of the brain that deal with decision making, judgment, and self-control are poorly developed in adolescence, leading to engagement in risk-taking behaviors (NIDA, 2012b).

Younger age at onset of substance use has been linked to greater risk of progression to serious abuse (NIDA, 2012b). For example, approximately 9% of marijuana users become addicted, but the rate of addiction prevalence increases to 17% for those who initiate marijuana use at a young age. Similarly, daily marijuana use increases the risk of addiction to 25% to 50% (NIDA, 2014a).

Alcohol is the substance most commonly misused by youth. Data from the Behavioral Risk Factor Surveillance System

(BRFSS) in 2009 indicted that nearly 42% of high school students reported current alcohol use, and 60% of those were binge drinkers (Kanny et al., 2010). From 2001 to 2005, excessive alcohol use accounted for 4,700 deaths and 280,000 years of productive life lost among people less than 20 years of age in the United States (Jernigan, Ross, Ostroff, McKnight-Eily, & Brewer, 2013).

Other drugs are also misused by youth. For example, the 2012 *Monitoring the Future* survey of adolescent drug use indicated that approximately 1% of 8th, 10th, and 12th graders had used methamphetamine in the prior year (NIDA, 2013). Similarly, a 2009 survey of 400 Native American tribes in the Midwest indicated that nonmedical use of OxyContin was highest in people 18 to 25 years of age (Momper et al., 2013). Population health nurses working with young people should assess their level of maturity and their ability to resist pressure to conform.

Perinatal exposures to drugs and alcohol have a variety of adverse effects on the fetus. Some psychoactive substances, such as alcohol, amphetamines, and cocaine, have teratogenic effects when taken during pregnancy. **Teratogenic substances** are those that cause physical defects in the developing embryo. Other drugs do not affect fetal development per se, but have other adverse health effects for the neonate or long-term effects for the child. For example, fetal alcohol exposure may result in prenatal and postnatal growth deficits, CNS abnormality, and delayed psychomotor development. Fetal, neonatal, and developmental effects of selected psychoactive substances are presented in Table 29-2•.

The true incidence of fetal alcohol syndrome (FAS) and fetal alcohol spectrum disorders (FASD) is not known. An estimated 0.2 to 1.5 cases of FAS occur for every 1,000 live births in the United States, and experts speculate that there may be as many as three times as many cases of FASD (Division of Birth Defects and Developmental Disabilities, 2012). From 2006 to 2010, 76% of pregnant women reported some alcohol use during pregnancy, and 1.4% engaged in binge drinking (Marchetta et al., 2012).

Use of other drugs during pregnancy can also harm the fetus. For example, methamphetamine use by pregnant women may result in prematurity, placental abruption, small gestational size, lethargy, and heart and brain abnormalities. Long-term effects may include attention deficits and increased stress (NIDA, 2013).

Population health nurses are often involved in assisting either biological or foster parents to care for infants and children exposed to alcohol in utero. As noted in Chapter 16∞, FAS is a condition resulting from maternal alcohol consumption during pregnancy and is characterized by growth retardation, facial malformations, and CNS dysfunctions that may include mental retardation. Long-term effects of FAS include inability to hold down a job, impulsivity, social withdrawal, poor judgment, and mental retardation. In working with newborns and young children, the population health nurse should be alert to

TABLE 29-2 Fetal, Neonatal, and Developmental Effects of Perinatal Psychoactive Substance Exposure

Substance	Fetal Effects	Neonatal Effects	Developmental Effects
Alcohol	Growth deficiency, microcephaly, stillbirth, low birth weight (LBW), joint and facial anomalies, cardiac and kidney anomalies	Acute withdrawal with sedation, seizures, poor feeding	Developmental delay, low IQ, hyperactivity
Sedatives, hypnotics	Sedation at delivery	Tremors, hypertonicity, poor suck, high-pitched cry	Unknown
Opioids	Intrauterine growth retardation, microcephaly, prematurity, hyperactivity	Withdrawal with tremors, hypertonicity, poor feeding, diarrhea, seizures, irritability	Increased rate of sudden infant death syndrome (SIDS)
Cocaine	Spontaneous abortion	Tremors, hypertonicity, muscle weakness, seizures	Developmental delay, increased rate of SIDS
Amphetamines	Intrauterine growth retardation, biliary atresia, transposition of great vessels	Stillbirth, LBW, cardiac anomalies, withdrawal	Poor school performance
Hallucinogens	Agitation at delivery, microcephaly	Irritability, poor fine-motor coordination, sensory input problems	Unknown
Cannabis	Bleeding problems in delivery	Sedation, tremors, excessive response to light	Unknown
Inhalants	Unknown	Unknown	Unknown
Nicotine	Intrauterine growth retardation, microcephaly	Jitteriness, poor feeding	Poor school performance, increased rate of SIDS

signs of perinatal drug exposure. He or she also assesses for risk factors that would make children and youth particularly vulnerable to substance abuse and its effects.

Lower rates of binge drinking are found among the elderly at only 3.8% of the population over 65 years of age. Binge drinking occurs with greater frequency in this age group but at lower levels of intensity (number of drinks per episode) (Kanny, Liu, & Brewer, 2011). Although generally less likely to abuse alcohol and drugs than their younger counterparts, older people may experience more severe consequences because of their diminished ability to detoxify toxic substances. In addition, substance abuse problems in older clients may not be diagnosed because health care providers are not alert to signs and symptoms of abuse in this age group.

Gender differences in substance use and abuse are also common. For example, 2009 BRFSS data indicated twice as many men as women engaged in binge drinking. Men also engaged in binge drinking more often and consumed a greater number of drinks per episode than women (Kanny et al., 2011). Similarly, men are slightly more likely to be admitted to a hospital for methamphetamine-related problems than women (NIDA, 2013). In addition, age-adjusted alcohol-induced mortality among men was three times that for women in 2010 (11.7 and 3.9 per 100,000 population respectively), and drug induced mortality was 59% higher for men than for women (15.9 vs. 10 per 100,000 population) (Murphy et al., 2013b).

There is also variability among racial and ethnic groups in terms of substance abuse and its effects. For example, in 2010, the age adjusted rate for alcohol-induced deaths for the American Indian/Alaska Native (AI/AN) population was 25.4 per 100,000 population, more than three times that of the next highest group—Whites at 8 per 100,000. The lowest alcohol-induced mortality was experienced by the Asian/Pacific Islander (API) population at 1.6 deaths per 100,000 population (Murphy et al., 2013b).

Drug-induced mortality in 2010 was highest for the White population (14.6/100,000 population), followed by the AI/AN population (11.4/100,000), and lowest in the API population. People of Hispanic origin had higher alcohol-induced mortality than non-Hispanics (9.1 vs. 7.4 per 100, 000 population), but the Hispanic drug-induced mortality rate was less than half of that for non-Hispanics (6.1 and 14.2 per 100,000 population, respectively) (Murphy et al., 2013b). Population health nurses can initiate public education campaigns targeted at and relevant to high-risk groups. For example, prevention campaigns among Native American groups should be culturally relevant and address the myriad social factors that may contribute to abuse as well as the physiologic differences in drug metabolism that influence development of substance-related problems. Programs may also need to be modified for targeted subpopulations within racial or ethnic groups. For example, U.S.-born African Americans have been shown to have higher rates of alcohol dependence and drug abuse than Caribbean Blacks (Gibbs et al., 2013).

Genetic inheritance. A growing body of evidence suggests that substance abuse is associated with some form of genetic predisposition. Studies of adopted children, for example, indicate that alcohol abuse by one or both of the biological parents is associated with alcohol and drug abuse by the child, but no increased risk has been noted when adoptive parents drink. The National Institute on Drug Abuse estimates that genetic factors, in combination with environmental influences, account for about half of population vulnerability to addiction. In addition, gene–environment interactions that occur at particularly critical periods of development add to the risk of substance abuse (NIDA, 2012b).

In assessing individuals and families for the level of risk for substance abuse, the population health nurse prepares a detailed genogram that includes information about the family history of substance abuse as well as the presence of physical and emotional illnesses with a genetic component. Population health nurses can also educate the public about the potential heritability of substance abuse risks and advocate for prevention among people who are at risk due to a family history of abuse.

Physiologic function. The relationship between substance abuse and physiologic function is bidirectional. Persons with chronic physical health problems or disability may abuse drugs or alcohol as an escape from pain, depression, or stress related to the disability. Substance abuse may stem from a desire for gratification when other avenues are denied or as a method of regaining control over one's choices and actions. Data from the 2009 BRFSS indicated that binge drinking prevalence, for example, was slightly lower among disabled individuals than in the nondisabled population (14.3% vs. 16%), but that frequency and intensity of binge drinking were higher in the disabled population (Kanny et al., 2011). In working with disabled clients, population health nurses assess clients' responses to disability and their vulnerability to substance abuse as a means of coping with disability.

Rates of substance abuse are also high among HIV-infected individuals. IDU, of course, is a mode of transmission for HIV infection, but even among non-IDUs, rates of substance use and abuse are high. In one national sample, for example, 40% of HIV-positive individuals reported illicit drug use other than marijuana in the prior year, and 12% screened positive for substance dependence. In another eight-city study, 40% of HIV-infected individuals reported heavy alcohol or crack cocaine use in the prior year; 38% reported marijuana use; 14% used heroin or stimulants; and 25% were polydrug users (Mimiaga et al., 2013). **Polydrug use** is the use of more than one psychoactive substance (NIDA, 2010). HIV-infected substance abusers have also been known to divert their antiretroviral (ARV) medications, selling them on the street to support their drug habits. **ARV diversion** is movement of legal regulated drugs to illegal markets (Surratt, Kurtz, Cicero, O'Grady, & Levi-Minzi, 2013). In one study, diverters were significantly less likely than non-diverters to maintain the 95% adherence to treatment required to suppress viral load and prevent HIV transmission (Surratt et al., 2013).

Substance use and abuse may result in physiologic changes. The trajectory of substance abuse usually begins with occasional use and may progress to regular use. In some people, changes in brain metabolism and activity lead to the compulsive, uncontrollable use that characterizes abuse and dependence. These

TABLE 29-3 Signs of Intoxication with Selected Psychoactive Substances

Substance	Typical Indications of Intoxication
Alcohol	Decreased alertness, impaired judgment, slurred speech, nausea, double vision, vertigo, staggering, unpredictable emotional changes, stupor, unconsciousness, increased reaction time
Sedatives, hypnotics, anxiolytics	Slurred speech; slow, shallow respiration; cold and clammy skin; nystagmus; weak and rapid pulse; drowsiness, blurred vision, unconsciousness; disorientation; depression; poor judgment; motor impairment
Opioids	Sedation, hypertension, respiratory depression, impaired intellectual function, constipation, pupillary constriction, watery eyes, increased pulse and blood pressure
Cocaine	Irritability, anxiety, slow weak pulse, slow shallow breathing, sweating, dilated pupils, increased blood pressure, insomnia, seizures, disinhibition, impulsivity, compulsive actions, hypersexuality, hypervigilance, hyperactivity
Amphetamines	Sweating, dilated pupils, increased blood pressure, agitation, fever, irritability, headache, chills, insomnia, agitation, tremors, seizures, wakefulness, hyperactivity, confusion, paranoia
Hallucinogens	Dilated pupils, mood swings, elevated blood pressure, paranoia, bizarre behavior, nausea and vomiting, tremors, panic, flushing, fever, sweating, agitation, aggression, nystagmus (PCP)
Cannabis	Reddened eyes; increased pulse, respirations, and blood pressure; laughter; confusion; panic; drowsiness
Inhalants	Giddiness, drowsiness, increased vital signs, headache, nausea, fainting, stupor, fatigue, slurred speech, disorientation, delirium
Nicotine	Headache; loss of appetite; nausea; increased pulse, blood pressure, and muscle tone

changes occur through two mechanisms: imitation of the brain's normal neurotransmitters or overstimulating the brain's "reward circuits" (NIDA, 2012b). Unfortunately, many psychoactive drugs with potential for abuse have rebound effects that are usually the opposite of their initial effects and lead to repeated use to eliminate the undesirable symptoms created by the rebound. These adverse effects are discussed later in this chapter. Because of the phenomenon of tolerance defined earlier, the user requires larger and larger doses of many drugs to combat rebound effects and to achieve the desired pleasurable effect.

Population health nurses assess individual clients for signs of intoxication with psychoactive substances, as well as for signs of withdrawal from psychoactive substance use. **Intoxication** is a state of diminished physical or mental control that occurs as a result of the current use of psychoactive drugs. Intoxication with different drugs may be reflected in differing symptoms. For example, cocaine intoxication is characterized by disinhibition, impaired judgment and impulsivity, grandiosity, and compulsively repeated actions. Other common symptoms include hypersexuality, hypervigilance, and hyperactivity. Nicotine intoxication, on the other hand, is characterized by increased blood pressure, heart rate, and muscle tone. Table 29-3● summarizes individual signs of intoxication with selected psychoactive substances, while Table 29-4● provides indicators of withdrawal from specific substances. The nurse also assesses the incidence and prevalence of intoxication and withdrawal in the population.

Substance abuse disorders increase the risks of death and disability due to cirrhosis, heart disease, hepatocellular carcinoma,

TABLE 29-4 Indications of Withdrawal from Selected Psychoactive Substances

Substance	Indications of Withdrawal
Alcohol	Anxiety, insomnia, tremors, delirium, convulsions
Sedatives, hypnotics, anxiolytics	Anxiety, insomnia, tremors, delirium, convulsions (may occur up to 2 weeks after stopping use of anxiolytics)
Opioids	Restlessness, irritability, tremors, loss of appetite, panic, chills, sweating, cramps, watery eyes, runny nose, nausea, vomiting, muscle spasms, impaired coordination, depressed reflexes, dilated pupils, yawning
Cocaine	*Early crash:* agitation, depression, anorexia, high level of craving, suicidal ideation
	Middle crash: fatigue, depression, no craving, insomnia
	Late crash: exhaustion, hypersomnolence, hyperphagia, no craving
	Early withdrawal: normal sleep and mood, low craving, low anxiety
	Middle and late withdrawal: anhedonia, anxiety, anergy, high level of craving exacerbated by conditioned cues
	Extinction: normal hedonic response and mood, episodic craving triggered by conditioned cues
Amphetamines	Fatigue, hunger, long periods of sleep, disorientation, severe depression
Hallucinogens	Slight irritability, restlessness, insomnia, reduced energy level, depression
Cannabis	Insomnia, hyperactivity, decreased appetite
Inhalants	None reported
Nicotine	Nervousness, increased appetite, sleep disturbances, anxiety, irritability

and stroke. IDUs also have a high risk of impairment due to drug impurities and infection. As we saw in Chapter 26∞, injection drug use is associated with high incidence of HIV infection and hepatitis B, C, and D. Drug use is also associated with unprotected sexual activity and an increased number of sexual partners, increasing the risk for sexually transmitted infections (STIs) (Mimiaga et al., 2013). Tetanus and abscesses at the injection site also occur with IDU. Substance abuse also increases the risk for other communicable diseases such as tuberculosis and influenza. In addition, substance abuse acts as a barrier to effective TB treatment, control, and prevention. For example, examination of a cluster of TB patients in one county indicated that 88% were engaged in methamphetamine use, and use was reported by 67% of their contacts, with 25% of contacts screening positive for TB infection (Pevzner et al., 2010). As noted earlier, substance use and abuse may also contribute to long-term physical consequences related to accidental injury.

According to the U.S. Surgeon General's 2014 report on the health consequences of smoking and nicotine, the primary psychoactive substance in tobacco, is acutely toxic in high doses. In addition, tobacco use affects multiple biological pathways contributing to elevated risk for diseases such as lung, liver, colorectal, and breast cancers and chronic obstructive pulmonary disease. In addition, smoking increases the risk of tuberculosis disease and related mortality, and both smoking and second-hand smoke exposure increase the risk of stroke. Other effects of smoking include contributions to age-related macular degeneration, erectile dysfunction, diabetes, immune system compromise, and rheumatoid arthritis. Evidence also suggests causal relationships between smoking and asthma incidence and exacerbation, dental caries, and inflammatory bowel disease (Office of the Surgeon General, 2014).

In addition to assessing clients for signs and symptoms of intoxication and withdrawal, population health nurses also assess individual clients for symptoms of long-term effects of substance abuse. These effects can be physical or psychological and vary with the psychoactive substance. For example, long-term effects of alcohol abuse include malnutrition, cirrhosis, and liver cancer, and typical effects of phencyclidine abuse are psychoses and insomnia. Long-term effects of selected psychoactive substances for individuals are summarized in Table 29-5●. The population health nurse would assess individual clients for long-term effects of substance abuse. He or she would also determine the incidence and prevalence of these effects in the population. Biological factors contributing to or resulting from substance abuse can be identified using the *Focused Assessment* questions provided on the next page.

PSYCHOLOGICAL DETERMINANTS. Both personality traits and the presence of psychopathology may contribute to problems of substance abuse. There seem to be some commonalities in the personalities of substance abusers regardless of the type of substance abused. Personality traits that may place one at risk for substance abuse include rebelliousness and nonconformity that may lead to substance abuse as an expression of defiance or as an escape from the constraints and expectations of the adult world. Other common traits in abusers are a greater tolerance of deviant behavior, a poor self-concept, and passive surrender to belief in their own inevitable failure in life. Abusers of psychoactive substances also tend to be impulsive, be unable to value themselves, and have poor tolerance for frustration and anxiety. They may also have difficulty in acknowledging their feelings and in developing interests and deriving pleasure from them. In addition, people who abuse psychoactive substances frequently feel alienated from those around them and are socially isolated. They may also feel powerless, and they usually have poor coping skills.

Substance abusers also tend to display a common set of defense mechanisms that include denial, projection, rationalization, and conflict minimization and avoidance. Abusers frequently deny that they have a problem with substance abuse and assert that they can change their behavior. They may

TABLE 29-5 Long-Term Effects Associated with Abuse of Selected Psychoactive Substances

Substance	Long-Term Effects of Abuse
Alcohol	Malnutrition; impotence; ulcers; cirrhosis; esophageal, stomach, and liver cancers; organic brain syndrome; deafness
Sedatives, hypnotics, anxiolytics	Potential for death due to overdose from increasing doses due to tolerance, impaired sexual function
Opioids	Lethargy, weight loss, sexual disinterest and dysfunction, increased susceptibility to infection and accidents, constipation
Cocaine	Damage to nasal tissue, high blood pressure, weight loss, muscle twitching, paranoia, hallucinations, disrupted sleeping and eating patterns, irritability, liver damage
Amphetamines	Depression, paranoia, hallucinations, weight loss, impotence
Hallucinogens	Memory loss, inability to concentrate, insomnia, chronic or recurrent psychosis, flashbacks
Cannabis	Chromosome changes, reduced sperm count, impaired concentration, poor memory, reduced alertness, inability to perform complex tasks
Inhalants	Organic brain syndrome, liver and kidney damage, bone marrow damage, anemia, hearing loss, nerve damage
Nicotine	Cardiovascular disease, lung cancer, bladder cancer, chronic disease, diabetic complications

FOCUSED ASSESSMENT Assessing Biological Determinants Influencing Substance Abuse

- Are there existing physical health problems contributing to substance abuse? What effects does substance abuse have on efforts to control existing physical health problems (e.g., diabetes) at individual or population levels?
- Is there a family history of substance abuse?
- Does the individual client exhibit signs of intoxication or withdrawal? Does the client exhibit long-term effects of substance use or abuse? What are the incidence and prevalence of intoxication, withdrawal, and long-term effects of substance abuse in the population?
- What influence, if any, does age have on the development of substance abuse in the individual or population? What is the extent of substance use by among various age groups in the population?
- Is the individual client pregnant? What effects will substance abuse have on the fetus? What is the extent of drug or alcohol use during pregnancy in the population?
- What physiological effects has substance use or abuse had for the individual client?
- What are the incidence and prevalence of substance-related morbidity and mortality in the population?

exhibit inability to accept responsibility for their own behavior in other areas as well, and they frequently project or transfer the blame for their own behavior onto others. They also rationalize their behavior without developing true insights into the reason for that behavior. They tend to try to avoid conflict, and may turn to substance abuse as a means of escaping from the stress generated by conflict rather than engaging in positive modes of conflict resolution.

The relationship between substance abuse and other mental illness is often a reciprocal one. For example, the presence of other mental disorders increases the risk for substance abuse. Psychological stress contributes to substance abuse as well (NIDA, 2012b). Similarly, the presence of ADHD has been linked to increased tobacco use, higher rates of hazardous alcohol use, and greater impairment with the use of drugs such as marijuana and other illicit drugs (Rooney, Chronis-Tuscano, & Yoon, 2014). In addition, ADHD has been associated with younger initiation of use of tobacco and other addictive substances, more severe abuse, and a shorter time period from initiation to dependence or abuse (Kousha, Shahrivar, & Alaghband-rad, 2014).

Conversely, substance use and abuse may contribute to or worsen mental illness. For example, marijuana use has been found to worsen schizophrenia and is associated with depression, anxiety, and other personality disorders (NIDA, 2014a). Similarly, methamphetamine use is associated with affective psychoses, schizophrenia, and depression (Gruenewald et al., 2013). Substance use and abuse is also linked to suicide. For example, alcohol use has been associated with suicide, but somewhat differently depending on age, ethnicity, and the method of suicide chosen. Among young and middle adults, alcohol use frequently accompanies suicide by firearms or hanging. For older people, alcohol use is more often associated with suicide by poisoning. Asian/Pacific Islanders often combine alcohol with poisoning as a method of suicide, whereas Blacks combine alcohol with hanging. Overall, in one study, alcohol was associated with 35% of suicides using firearms, 26.8% of hanging suicides, and 32.7% of suicides by poisoning (Conner et al., 2014). In all probability, the use of alcohol lessens inhibitions against suicide. Questions to help identify psychological determinants influencing substance abuse in the population are included in the *Focused Assessment* below.

FOCUSED ASSESSMENT Assessing Psychological Determinants Influencing Substance Abuse

- Does the individual client have a poor self-image?
- What are the client's life goals? Are they realistic?
- Does the client exhibit poor impulse control? What is the client's level of frustration tolerance?
- What life stresses is the client experiencing? What is the extent of the client's coping abilities? What defense mechanisms does the client display?
- What sources of stress in the population may contribute to substance abuse?
- Is there underlying psychopathology contributing to substance abuse? What is the extent of mental illness in the population and what are the associations with substance abuse?
- To what extent is substance use or abuse associated with suicide or suicide attempts in the population?

ENVIRONMENTAL DETERMINANTS. Recent research is confirming the view of substance abuse or addiction as being a product of gene–environment interactions. The interaction between genetic inheritance and environmental factors to result in disease is referred to as **epigenetics**. The environmental component of this interaction is termed the **exposome**, which is defined as critical environmental factors that interact with genetic and psychological variables to result in addiction (Stahler, Mennis, & Baron, 2013). Based on the findings of relevant research, it is believed that memories of physical, social, and community environmental stimuli and contexts associated with prior drug use are stored in the brain. These memories then act as triggers for subsequent use resulting eventually in addiction (Stahler et al., 2013).

It has been proposed that geospatial technology pinpointing the environments in which drug use occurs can help to understand how place and environment influence behavior. It has even been suggested that tracking movement and activities of abusers over time through GPS technology might lead to real-time interventions via mobile devices to prevent drug use (Stahler et al., 2013). For example, one's phone might locate one in an area with ready access to alcohol. If someone is at risk for alcohol abuse, an immediate automatic text message or telephone call might be generated to help him or her refrain from alcohol use in that environment. Part of the community environment may include local attitudes to drug use and tolerance of the use of specific drugs in that locale. Abuse of specific drugs is known to vary widely by geographic region within the United States. For example, methamphetamine use is more common in western states than elsewhere in the country, with the highest rates of treatment admissions for methamphetamine dependence occurring in Hawaii, followed by San Diego, San Francisco, Denver, and Phoenix (NIDA, 2013). Similarly, adolescent prescription drug misuse has been found to be more common in rural than urban areas (Spoth et al., 2013).

Other elements of the environment that may contribute to substance use and abuse include the ease of access to drugs of choice. For example, the density of alcohol outlets has been found to be associated with rates of binge drinking, with 13% of people in areas with 130 alcohol outlets per square mile engaged in binge drinking compared to 8% in areas with only 20 outlets per square mile. Research has also linked alcohol outlet density to arrests for driving under the influence, MVA, injuries, suicide, violence, mean per person alcohol consumption, and alcohol-related disorders (Ahern, Margerison-Ziko, Hubbard, & Galea, 2013), as well as alcohol-related hospital admissions (Stockwell et al., 2013). Another environmental factor linked to increased rates of substance abuse is the extent of abandoned housing in the area (Stahler et al., 2013). This link may be a product of low socioeconomic status and increased stress in neighborhoods or an easy venue for drug exchanges and use.

Environmental exposure to drug-related advertising is another factor in substance use, particularly among youth. For example, one study in Boston found that public school students in grades 5 through 12 were routinely exposed to advertising in subway stations and the exposure to such advertising was 4.5 times more likely in stations in high poverty areas than in more affluent neighborhoods. The authors concluded that the equivalent of every adult and every 5th to 12th grade public school student in the region received daily exposure to alcohol advertising (Gentry et al., 2011).

The environment in which drugs are used may also contribute to adverse effects on health beyond triggers for subsequent use. For instance, many smoke-free workplace regulations provide exemptions for indoor hookah lounges, where tobacco is smoked through water or "bubble" pipes. A study of air quality in indoor hookah lounges found that air quality ranged from unhealthy to distinctly hazardous (Fiala, Morris, & Pawlak, 2012).

Finally, substance use and abuse may contribute to safety hazards in the environment. Earlier we discussed the effects of drug and alcohol use in terms of MVA, but substance use and abuse also contribute to a variety of accidents in occupational and other settings. In addition, the environment involved in methamphetamine production may result in fires or explosions. Furthermore, methamphetamine production includes a variety of toxic chemicals that may affect people living in the surrounding area (NIDA, 2014b). The *Focused Assessment* below provides questions that can assist the population health nurse in assessing environmental determinants influencing substance use and abuse in the population.

FOCUSED ASSESSMENT: Assessing Environmental Determinants Influencing Substance Abuse

- Do the incidence and prevalence of abuse of specific drugs vary by geographic region or neighborhood?
- What is the density of alcohol outlets in the area?
- How accessible are drugs of abuse in the area?
- What is the extent of abandoned housing in the area?
- Where do drugs tend to be used within the area?
- What environmental factors are associated with drug use and may trigger subsequent use?
- To what extent are members of the population exposed to advertising for alcohol and other substances?
- What are the contributions of substance use and abuse to safety and other health hazards in the environment?

SOCIOCULTURAL DETERMINANTS. Sociocultural factors may also contribute to problems of substance abuse. Sociocultural factors addressed here include cultural influences; interpersonal interactions; factors related to socioeconomic status, employment, and occupation; social policies related to substance use and abuse; and addictive substance marketing.

Cultural influences. Family attitudes derive from cultural perceptions of substance use and abuse. Different cultures may have different perceptions of the acceptability of substance use. For example, there is a growing cultural acceptance of recreational or medical use of marijuana in the United States. These changing perceptions are exemplified by the fact that two states to date have legalized recreational use of marijuana by adults and 20 states have legislation permitting medical marijuana use (NIDA, 2014a).

Different cultural groups also have different norms regarding the use of legitimate substances such as alcohol and tobacco. For example, cultural groups vary with respect to norms regarding who should drink alcohol (e.g., men, women, or both), the appropriate age for initiating alcohol use, and what beverages are appropriate (e.g., beer or hard liquor). Norms may also specify when alcohol should be consumed. For example, alcohol may be used primarily for celebratory reasons or at holidays in some cultures and on any occasion in others. Similarly, there may be restrictions on the time of day one should consume alcohol (e.g., never before noon) or specific forms of alcohol (e.g., champagne at a fancy brunch or mimosas in the morning). Other norms may involve the "etiquette" of drinking; for example, should one drink a beer from the bottle or from a glass? Whether or not to sip one's drink or belt it down may also be dictated by cultural norms (Heath, 2012). Knowledge of cultural norms for the use of alcohol and other legitimate substances, such as tobacco and prescription medications, can assist population health nurses in identifying factors that may contribute to the risk for misuse and abuse in different segments of the population.

Interpersonal interactions. Day-to-day interpersonal interactions also influence initiation of substance use and risk for abuse. Family interactions and relationships with peers are two common elements influencing substance abuse in populations.

Families with low cohesion, high levels of conflict, few shared interests and activities, poor coping strategies, and marital dissatisfaction increase the risk of substance abuse in their members. Families who encounter multiple stressors and have inadequate resources are also at risk. Episodes of violence within the family can also lead family members to abuse substances as a means of escape from family tensions. Good parent–child communication, maternal use of reasoning with children, and adequate supervision of children, on the other hand, may have a protective effect on initiation and use of substances with the potential for abuse. Family attitudes toward and use of alcohol, tobacco, and other substances of abuse also influence substance use by family members. Population health nurses should assess families for conditions that may contribute to substance abuse by family members.

Peer influence is another interaction factor in the social environment that may contribute to substance abuse. In adolescents and preadolescents, in particular, pressure from peers to smoke, drink, or use other psychoactive drugs is a powerful motivator for initiating these behaviors (NIDA, 2012b). In working with young people, in particular, the nurse carefully assesses peer attitudes toward substance use and abuse as well as the degree to which the individual feels a need to conform to peer-dictated norms.

Modes of social interaction may also contribute to access to and misuse of psychoactive substances. For example, the Internet makes it much easier to obtain controlled substances. Similarly, cellular telephones and social networking sites can facilitate drug distribution (Stahler et al., 2013).

Socioeconomic status, employment, and occupation. Social factors related to one's socioeconomic status, employment, and occupation may also contribute to substance use and abuse. For example, *community level income inequality*, or the magnitude of differences between the richest and poorest members of a population, has been associated with both light and heavy drinking, with these associations found to be stronger for Blacks and Hispanics than for Whites (Karriker-Jaffe, Roberts, & Bond, 2013). Binge drinking is more common among people with annual incomes over $75,000 than among those with incomes under $25,000. Persons with cellular telephones also have higher rates of binge drinking at both high and low socioeconomic levels than those with landline telephones only (Kanny et al., 2010), perhaps reflecting the availability of disposable income. Heavy drinking is more prevalent at higher-income levels than among people with lower annual incomes; however, lower-income levels are associated with greater frequency and intensity of heavy drinking (Kanny et al., 2011).

Social factors such as poverty, unemployment, and discrimination may create a sense of hopelessness and powerlessness that leads to substance abuse as an escape or to enhance one's own feelings of competence. In addition, income levels may affect the extent and severity of substance-related health problems. For example, in one study in New York City, analgesic overdose fatalities were less common in higher-income neighborhoods than in lower-income area. Neighborhoods with high rates of analgesic overdose fatalities were characterized by fragmentation, increased levels of divorce, low employment and education levels, lack of health care resources, and neighborhood deprivation (Cerdá et al., 2013).

Substance abuse disorders are prevalent among homeless individuals, but the direction of the relationship may be unclear. In many cases, individuals become homeless as a result of substance abuse disorders and inability to maintain suitable housing. In others, homeless people may turn to alcohol or drug abuse as a means of coping with their homelessness. Substance abuse has been found to be the strongest predictor of returning to homelessness (Zur & Mojtabai, 2013).

Occupation is another sociocultural determinant that may contribute to substance abuse. Some occupational groups may be at increased risk for substance abuse, particularly those who are expected to entertain clients who drink. Similarly, substance abuse may occur among health care providers because of easy access to controlled drugs. An estimated 10% to 15% of nurses, for example, may be impaired by or recovering from substance abuse disorders. The legal obligation of coworkers to report an impaired nurse varies among jurisdictions, but nurses have an ethical obligation to clients, colleagues, the profession, and the public to assure that impaired nurses do not compromise patient safety (Thomas & Siela, 2011).

Employer attitudes toward and sanctions for alcohol, drug, and tobacco use also influence the extent of use among employees. As we saw in Chapters 23∞ and 27∞, smoke-free workplaces lead to reduced smoking among employees as well as decreased exposure to second-hand smoke for nonsmoking employees. Some businesses and industries also perform drug testing at the time of employment or periodically throughout employment. Unemployment and attendant stress and hopelessness may contribute to substance abuse. The effects of unemployment are also seen in the aftermath of substance abuse among recovering substance abusers who experience difficulty obtaining work.

Social policy issues. Societal attitudes and policies related to drug use and abuse also influence the extent of substance abuse in the population. Legal jurisdiction for policies related to substance use and abuse occurs at multiple levels. For example, states and municipalities have jurisdiction over laws that govern tobacco and alcohol use and, increasingly, use of marijuana for recreational or medicinal purposes. The multiplicity of jurisdiction leads to differences in access to addictive substances, substance control spending, smoke-free air laws, advertising regulations, and excise taxes. Increased excise taxes on tobacco and alcohol have been shown to affect per capita consumption. For example, in one study of state tobacco excise taxes, every ten-cent increase in taxes on a pack of cigarettes reduced cigarette consumption by nearly three fourths of a pack per person per month (Sanders & Slade, 2013). Similarly, a 10% increase in the minimum price per unit of alcohol was associated with an almost 9% decrease in acute alcohol-related hospital admissions and a slightly greater decrease in admissions for chronic problems related to alcohol use (Stockwell et al., 2013).

States and municipalities also vary with respect to the extent and strength of tobacco-free legislation. Throughout the nation, coverage under such legislation differentially affects certain groups. For example, one national study indicated better coverage and more comprehensive laws in areas with high Asian and Hispanic populations, and less coverage in primarily White or Black populations, suggesting a need for regionally tailored policy interventions to equalize disparities in coverage (Gonzalez, Sanders-Jackson, Song, Chen, & Glantz, 2013).

Tobacco control in the military falls under federal jurisdiction. Some authors have noted that Congressional opposition has impeded tobacco control in military settings. This opposition may even be abetted by the views of civilian public health leaders. In one study of national public health leaders, several were opposed to banning tobacco use on military installations as a violation of smokers' rights (Smith & Malone, 2013).

In Russia, alcohol control policy is federally mandated and regulates the production and sale of alcohol-containing products. Legislation requires registration of production and distribution facilities at relatively high fees. This has resulted in fewer producers because many producers were forced to close when they could not afford the registration fees. Fewer producers has increased the price of alcohol and decreased consumption. As a result, Russia experienced a drastic decline in alcohol-related transportation fatalities, male alcohol-poisoning deaths, male and female cirrhosis deaths, and suicide rates. The policy change, initiated in 2006, has been credited with saving more than 4,000 lives per year (Pridemore et al., 2013).

In the United States, *internal possession laws* enacted in several states have been associated with decreased probability of past month drinking among youth. Internal possession laws prohibit minors from possessing alcohol within their bodies and permit arrests based on behavioral assessment or blood or urine alcohol levels rather than being caught with alcohol in one's possession (Disney, Lavallee, & Yi, 2013).

Policy initiatives such as internal possession laws can contribute to substance control, but may also have unanticipated consequences. For example, implementation of age-related restrictions on the purchase, possession, and consumption of alcohol among youth have resulted in decreased hospital admissions for alcohol-related conditions among youth under the legal drinking age. Among youth just over the legal age, however, hospitalization rates for alcohol use disorders, self-inflicted injury, and alcohol-related MVA increased. Increased rates were also noted for emergency department visits, assaults, and alcohol-related suicide in the group just over the legal drinking age (Callaghan, Sanches, Gatley, & Cunningham, 2013). These figures suggest that youth who are freed from age-related restrictions on alcohol use may tend to engage in overuse in celebration of that freedom.

Other policies also influence control of substance abuse, some more successfully than others. For example, California has made several attempts to control methamphetamine production, use, and abuse by restricting purchase of chemicals needed for production. Such legislation has resulted in transient decreases in methamphetamine arrests and hospitalizations, but has inevitably been followed by changes in production and distribution processes and subsequent increases in abuse (Gruenewald et al., 2013).

As noted earlier, recent policy changes in some jurisdictions reflect changing societal attitudes to marijuana use and decreased perception of the associated risks. As of early 2014, two states had legalized recreational use of marijuana by adults and 20 states had enacted medical marijuana use laws (NIDA,

2014a). Medical marijuana use laws typically include four main provisions. Users must possess a state issued registry or identification card authorizing marijuana possession and use. The laws also address specific conditions for which marijuana may be used and include provisions prohibiting disciplinary action against physicians who prescribe marijuana for these conditions. Additional provisions regulate access to and possession and cultivation of marijuana. Finally, the legislation provides protection from prosecution for the medical marijuana user. Despite concerns that legalization of marijuana for medical purposes might lead to increased use by adolescents, research has indicated that has not occurred (Lynne-Landsman, Livingston, & Wagenaar, 2013).

Recreational use of marijuana is proving a bit more difficult to control, however. In Colorado, recreational use was approved in 2014 making it legal for persons over 21 years of age to possess up to one ounce of marijuana for any purpose. Unlike medicinal marijuana, recreational marijuana is being sold in a variety of food and beverage items that require child-proof packaging. Like regulation of tobacco sales, prevention of purchase of these items by minors is difficult with retailers not engaging in mandated age verification procedures. In addition, these products contain less than 10 mg of tetrahydrocannabinol (THC), the main psychoactive ingredient in cannabis preparations, resulting in a slower high and temptations to use larger amounts (James, 2014).

Attitudes that promote incarceration rather than treatment are another example of societal policy issues that influence substance abuse and its effects. As noted in Chapter 24∞, many jurisdictions are opting for drug courts and mandatory treatment rather than incarceration for first-time offenders. Goals of drug court programs include reducing substance abuse and criminal justice recidivism among abusers and increasing the likelihood of drug offenders' successful rehabilitation. Drug courts provide access to substance abuse treatment and minimize use of incarceration as a control strategy (Judicial Council of California, 2014). The National Association of Drug Court Professionals (NADCP) has developed a set of key principles for court-directed treatment programs. These principles include the following:

- Integration of substance abuse treatment with justice system case processing
- Use of a non-adversarial approach by prosecution and defense lawyers, focusing on public safety while protecting offenders' right to due process
- Early identification of eligible offenders
- Assured access to substance abuse treatment and other rehabilitative services
- Objective monitoring of continued substance use by testing
- A coordinated response to noncompliance
- Ongoing interaction between offenders and the court
- Evaluation of program outcomes
- Continuing interdisciplinary education of program officials and providers
- Development of partnerships between courts and public and community-based agencies for program support
- Ongoing case management and support for social reintegration
- Appropriate program flexibility to address the needs of special populations (e.g., women, ethnic minorities)
- Provision of post-treatment and aftercare services and support (NADCP, n.d.).

In addition, NADCP (2013) has developed a set of best practice standards for drug courts. For further information about the standards, see the *External Resources* section of the student resources site.

Other jurisdictions are choosing to reduce sentences for nonserious, nonviolent crimes, including possession and use of drugs. For example, California voters passed the Three Strikes Reform Act of 2012 (proposition 36), which shortens the sentences for prisoners convicted of nonserious, nonviolent crimes, including substance abuse–related crimes. As of August, 2013 only 1,000 eligible inmates had been released, and less than 2% of them had been rearrested, a recidivism rate far below state and national averages. Unfortunately, those released are not eligible for state or county employment, housing, or substance abuse treatment assistance putting them at a disadvantage in successfully reorienting their lives. In the first year of implementation, the early release program saved the state $10 to $13 million (Stanford Law School Three Strikes Project & NAACP Legal Defense and Education Fund (n.d.).

Addictive substances marketing. In today's world, cultural attitudes toward specific behaviors may be strongly influenced by media messages. For example, media portrayals of drinking and smoking as desirable behaviors influence use of alcohol and tobacco. Media are also being used to send messages to discourage inappropriate use of drugs and alcohol. Some of these media messages are being generated by firms that produce alcoholic beverages in an attempt to convey an image of corporate social responsibility. **Corporate social responsibility** has been defined as business practices that assist companies to maintain a positive public image and exert favorable influence on policy makers (Babor & Robaina, 2013).

Typical health-related corporate social responsibility activities of the alcohol industry center on research sponsorship, efforts to mold public perceptions of alcohol policy research, sponsorship of scientific documents and conferences, and efforts to influence public health policy. Independent scientific evidence generally supports reducing alcohol consumption through regulatory measures, but industry-supported researchers frequently criticize the methodology and findings of independent research. As a result, the alcohol industry has engaged in research and policy related activities that fall under the guise of corporate social responsibility, but are primarily intended to further the industry's own interests and policy agenda (Babor & Robaina, 2013).

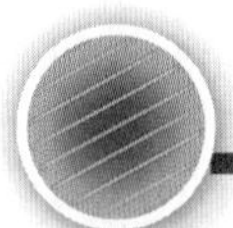

Evidence-Based Practice

Understanding Attempts to Derail Evidence-based Policy

A significant body of research is available that underscores the effects of addictive substances and behaviors, such as alcohol, tobacco, drug use, and uncontrolled gambling, on personal and population health. Unfortunately, this evidence base is rarely used in developing control policies. Adams (2013) contended that another body of evidence is needed regarding what he referred to as "addiction studies research" to understand the influence exerted by addiction product industries (e.g., tobacco and alcohol producers and advertisers, casinos, etc.). Such research could inform strategies to counteract industry attempts to derail or modify legislative policies that might reduce industry profits. Adams described three approaches to addiction industries research, all of which will be needed to develop a sufficient evidence base to counteract addiction industry influence in policy making.

The first area of research involves understanding the pathways by which industry influence occurs. Examples found in recent literature include the expected advertising, targeted marketing, and lobbying strategies, but other forms of influence include research and event sponsorship and charitable giving. The second focus of addiction industries research should be on determining and making public the amount of money spent by addiction industries on influencing policy and public opinion. Finally, research is needed on effective strategies to minimize industry influences (Adams, 2013). Some of this research is already being conducted, but more is needed. Armed with this three-pronged evidence base, public health organizations would be better equipped to promote effective policies for addiction prevention and control.

The value of underage drinking is estimated at $22.5 billion per year, while excessive drinking among adults accounts for another $48.3 billion in revenues the alcohol industry is reluctant to give up. To forestall regulatory initiatives, the alcohol industry tends to support research that emphasizes the positive effects of moderate drinking to offset data on the burden of illness derived from independent studies. Although moderate drinking has been shown to have some positive effects at the individual consumer level, these effects have not held up in aggregate level studies. The alcohol industry provides research support for grant-making organizations that often have industry representatives on boards that award funds and target studies that are likely to be favorable to the industry. For this reason, some scientists have called for a moratorium on accepting alcohol (and tobacco) industry funding for research because of the potential for conflicts of interest.

The alcohol industry has also attempted to sway public perceptions of alcohol-related research. For example, a report on alcohol policies generated for the British government with the assistance of the Portman Group, a major alcohol producer, has been criticized for opposing, minimizing, or ignoring evidence-based alcohol control policies in favor of approaches such as school-based alcohol education, which have proven less effective, but are less detrimental to industry interests. In addition, the industry has also paid academics to write letters to editors of professional journals criticizing and discrediting the findings of independent research. Similarly, industry-sponsored publications and conferences have been criticized for ignoring dissenting findings and being overly enthusiastic about the positive effects of alcohol use. Finally, the industry consistently supports policy initiatives that do not conflict with industry interests, such as drunken driving legislation, responsible drinking initiatives, and industry self-regulation (Babor & Robaina, 2013). The Smirnoff company, for example, has engaged in a campaign to convince policy makers of its commitment to preventing underage drinking and reducing harmful effects of alcohol use. Company efforts have emphasized funding prevention programs focused on education, public awareness, and responsible retail practices, which have been shown to be ineffective, broadcasting "responsibility" ads, establishing partnerships with government and public health agencies, and establishing a self-regulatory structure to regulate advertising (Mosher, 2012).

Industry self-regulation typically focuses on industry pledges not to market addictive substances to youth. For example, the alcohol industry voluntarily agreed not to advertise alcohol on television when more than 30% of the audience is expected to be less than 21 years of age. The National Research Council of the Institute of Medicine proposed lowering the standard to times when more than 15% of viewers would be expected to be youth. A study of advertisements in 25 market areas indicated that nearly 24% of the ads violated the industry standard and 35% would violate the more stringent IOM standard (Jernigan et al., 2013). Similarly, the beer industry has developed a self-imposed advertising code that addresses types of content and exposure markets to be avoided. A study of beer advertising during NCAA basketball tournaments from 1999 to 2008 indicated that 35% to 74% of the ads had code violations, primarily related to the association of beer drinking with social success and use of content that would appeal to people under 21 years of age (Babor, Xuan, Damon, & Noel, 2013).

Media marketing for addictive substances such as tobacco and alcohol often relies on **market segmentation**, which involves the development of tailored marketing plans for specific segments of the population. The intent of segmentation is to identify groups of potential consumers who share certain characteristics and can be anticipated to respond in similar ways to particular marketing strategies. Segmentation requires a substantial population segment that is measurable in terms of its size and purchasing power, is accessible, and is "actionable," meaning that specific marketing strategies can be designed to influence its members (Iglesias-Rios & Parascandola, 2013).

Segmented marketing approaches are typically based on sophisticated analyses of the target population's characteristics. As an example, the R. J. Reynolds Tobacco Company identified young Hispanics as an undersold market and developed a sophisticated surveillance system to track tobacco use in this population. Their research identified five key population segments, those who were concerned with being ruggedly masculine, the "cool" group, those focused on being stylish, those who believed in moderation, and those concerned with savings. Acknowledging the heterogeneity of the Hispanic market, the company then developed marketing strategies to address each of these market segments. They also focused on personality traits characteristic of the population. For example, to address the cultural trait of sociability, ads stressed that tobacco products were "for sharing and savoring." In addition, because certain segments of the market valued attending Hispanic functions, the company sponsored major events (Iglesias-Rios & Parascandola, 2013). Similar tactics were used in marketing tobacco to White and African American men, focusing on the image of the masculine, independent loner (the "Marlboro Man") in marketing to White males and the "Kool" connected and influential man among African Americans (White, Oliffe, & Bottorff, 2013).

Diageo, the company that produces the Smirnoff brand of vodka, used a marketing approach to undo the effects of prohibition on attitudes to distilled spirits or hard liquor. Control policies at the end of the prohibition era in the United States were focused on high alcohol content beverages with prior links to organized crime and bootlegging operations. At the time, beer and wine were viewed as "beverages of moderation" and control strategies promoted a shift to beer and wine through higher taxes on distilled spirits, limitation of outlets where hard liquor could be sold, and allowing beer and wine to be advertised on electronic media. As a result, from 1970 to 1997, hard liquor was associated with older generations, and beer was the beverage of choice for younger consumers. In an effort to increase sales of its Smirnoff vodka brand to a younger market, the company created beverages with vodka that tasted like soft drinks; marketed the products as malt beverages to compete with beer in regard to pricing, availability, and advertising restrictions on hard liquor; and posed their products as a young people's drink using fruit flavors and other marketing strategies. Such strategies were effective in increasing vodka consumption among younger people (Mosher, 2012). Marketing and other sociocultural factors influencing substance abuse in the population can be assessed using the questions provided in the *Focused Assessment* on the next page.

BEHAVIORAL DETERMINANTS. Recreational activities can contribute to the use of psychoactive substances in that alcohol and tobacco use is a frequent adjunct to such activities.

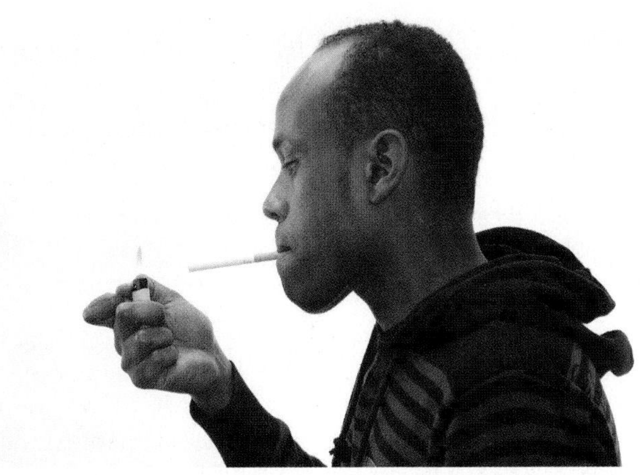

Tobacco companies target their marketing strategies to attract specific segments of the population. *(Dominique VERNIER /Fotolia)*

People tend to drink and smoke when they socialize with others. Friday or Saturday night binges are a relatively common phenomenon, when people can "let go" and drink because they know they will have time to recover before returning to work on Monday. Next to alcohol, marijuana is the most widely used recreational drug, but cocaine is also used recreationally and has the connotation of high status, glamour, and excitement. PCP and the club drugs are also used for recreational purposes.

Alcohol use and frequenting bars are also associated with higher rates of tobacco use and with binge drinking. In addition, alcohol use and bar attendance also make smoking cessation more difficult. Alcohol use has been negatively associated with attempts to quit smoking among light smokers, but has a positive association with successful quitting among heavy smokers (Jiang & Ling, 2013). Smoking in hookah lounges contributes to inhalation of 40 times the volume of smoke as cigarette smoking, exacerbating the negative effects of smoking (Fiala et al., 2012). Drug use is also often combined with smoking (Hunt, Gajewski, Jiang, Cupertino, & Richter, 2013), and early marijuana use has been liked to use of other addictive substances (NIDA, 2014a).

Drug and alcohol use and abuse may also contribute to unsafe sexual activity, particularly among members of sexual minority groups. Substance abuse is more prevalent among sexual minorities, probably as a result of exposure to chronic socially based stressors (Newcomb, Birkett, Corliss, & Mustanski, 2014). Sexual minority youth, in particular, are more likely than their heterosexual counterparts to report lifetime and past month use of alcohol, heavy episodic drinking, and early initiation of alcohol use (Talley, Hughes, Aranda, Birkett, & Marshall, 2014).

Specific behaviors related to actual abuse of drugs also contribute to physical and mental health problems. Injection drug use, for example, increases the risk of HIV infection and related behaviors. For example, in one study of IDUs in 20 cities, 69% engaged in unprotected sexual activity, 34% shared injection equipment, and 23% engaged in unprotected heterosexual

FOCUSED ASSESSMENT Assessing Sociocultural Determinants Influencing Substance Abuse

- To what extent do cultural attitudes and social mores contribute to substance abuse?
- What effect does legislative activity have on substance abuse? What other policy issues influence the incidence and prevalence of substance in the population? How do policies support or impede control of substance misuse and abuse in the population?
- Do peer networks support substance use and abuse? Is substance use a regular part of social interaction in the population?
- Does the individual client's family exhibit characteristics of codependence?
- What cultural or religious values or practices influence substance abuse among individuals and in the population?
- Has the individual client been a victim or perpetrator of family violence? To what extent does victimization contribute to substance abuse in the population?
- What social factors (e.g., unemployment, poverty) contribute to substance abuse?
- How readily available are abused substances?
- What contribution, if any, does occupation make to substance abuse? What is the effect of substance abuse on the individual client's ability to work?
- What is the contribution of substance abuse to criminal activity? To homelessness?
- What is the extent of substance abuse among homeless individuals? How does homelessness influence substance abuse treatment?
- To what extent do alcohol and tobacco producers influence health policy and control of substance abuse? How is this influence exerted?
- Does alcohol and tobacco advertising employ market segmentation approaches?

anal sex. In 2009, 9% of all new HIV infections occurred among men who had sex with men (Wejnert et al., 2012). Methamphetamine use also contributes to sexual transmission of HIV, HBV, and HCV infections due to drug-related short-term increases in libido. Long-term methamphetamine use, however, leads to decreased sexual function (NIDA, 2013, 2014a).

One other surprising behavioral factor that has been linked to substance misuse and abuse is participation in high school athletics. High school sports result in a high incidence of injuries for which Vicodin and OxyContin are increasingly prescribed for pain relief. In fact, the number of prescriptions for controlled pain medications for adolescents nearly doubled from 6.4% in 1994 to 11.2% in 2007. Prescription of these drugs often leads to sharing among friends and teammates (Veliz, Boyd, & McCabe, 2013). Assistance for assessment of behavioral determinants influencing substance abuse is provided in the *Focused Assessment* below.

HEALTH SYSTEM DETERMINANTS. Many of the psychoactive substances with abuse potential originated within the health care system. Opioids were widely used for pain control even during the American Civil War and are still the drug of choice for relief of severe pain. Cocaine and PCP were first used as surgical anesthetics, and marijuana has some legitimate medical use in the treatment of glaucoma and chronic pain. Sedatives and hypnotics are widely used for controlling anxiety, and amphetamines were originally developed as diet aids, although they no longer have any accepted medical use.

FOCUSED ASSESSMENT Assessing Behavioral Determinants Influencing Substance Abuse

- What substances are abused by members of the population?
- What is the extent of substance use and abuse in various segments of the population (e.g., among sexual minority group members, members of particular ethnic groups)?
- Are abused substances used recreationally? Is substance use associated with leisure activities?
- To what extent do substance abusers engage in other high-risk behaviors (e.g., driving while intoxicated, high-risk sexual activity)? What are the health effects of these behaviors in the population?
- What is the extent of injection drug use in the population?
- To what extent do members of the population combine alcohol and other substance use? What is the extent of polydrug use in the population?

Several aspects of the U.S. health care system have contributed to the growing problem of substance abuse. Lack of attention to educating clients and the public about the hazards of substance abuse and failure to identify clients with substance abuse problems have impeded efforts to control abuse. In one study, primary care physicians failed to document conducting screening or intervention in 62% of encounters with patients with risky alcohol use and 59% of encounters with patients engaged in risky drug use even when patients had been screened by health educators prior to the encounter (Kim et al., 2013). Similarly, 2011 BRFSS results from 44 states and the District of Columbia indicated that not quite 16% of U.S. adults had ever discussed alcohol use with a health care provider and only slightly higher percentages of drinkers (17.4%) and binge drinkers (25.4%) had ever had a health care provider discuss the dangers of excessive alcohol intake (McKnight-Eily et al., 2014). At the same time, some health care providers have actively fostered drug abuse by prescribing psychoactive drugs inappropriately or by not monitoring the extent of clients' use of these drugs.

In the past, the health care system has impeded control of substance abuse by failing to provide adequate insurance coverage for substance abuse treatment. In 2009, spending on substance abuse treatment accounted for only 1% of all health care spending in the United States (SAMHSA, 2013a). In a 2008 report, only 65% of substance abuse treatment facilities accepted private insurance reimbursement for services, whereas 96% accepted self-payment (Center for Behavioral Health Statistics and Quality, 2011). In addition, coverage for services may be constrained by a variety of regulations. For example, Medicare Part A only covers inpatient care for substance abuse with out-of-pocket expenditures similar to those for hospitalization for physical illnesses. Coverage in a psychiatric hospital extends to a total of 190 days over an entire lifetime. Some additional care for substance abuse services in general hospitals may also be covered. As of 2014, Medicare Part B covered 80% of outpatient substance abuse services from a clinic or hospital outpatient department. Methadone maintenance, however, is only covered if provided in an inpatient setting. Medicare Part D drug plans can cover medically necessary drugs to treat substance abuse under a formulary list, but do not cover methadone maintenance treatment. Medicare will also reimburse providers for assessment and brief intervention services for drug abuse or dependence and screening and counseling for persons who exhibit substance misuse but are not dependent (Medicare Rights Center, 2011). Medicaid coverage for substance abuse treatment services varies widely from state to state, although all states provide some form of substance abuse treatment under their Medicaid programs.

Under the provisions of the Affordable Care Act (ACA), insurance purchased through state or federal insurance exchanges is required to cover substance abuse services as an essential benefit. In addition, any limitations on services, copayments and out-of-pocket expenditure limits, and requirements for prior authorization of services will have to be comparable to those for medical and surgical services (Centers for Medicare and Medicaid Services, n.d.). These provisions will undoubtedly increase access to treatment services for some substance abusers. As an example, Medicaid eligibility expansion in Massachusetts resulted in a 21% increase in treatment admissions for substance abuse (Zur & Mojtabai, 2013).

Coverage for smoking cessation treatment has also been lacking for some groups. Medicare, for example, covers medications and counseling for a maximum of two treatment attempts per year for people over 65 years of age. Under the provisions of ACA, the Medicare Part D "donut hole" for medication coverage is being reduced, resulting in more affordable medications. Medicaid has covered cessation services for pregnant women since 2010, but will expand coverage to all low-income adults in 2014 under ACA. Coverage of comprehensive tobacco cessation treatment under state health insurance exchanges has not yet been delineated, and all new employer-sponsored insurance plans will need to cover tobacco cessation (American Lung Association, 2014).

In addition, an estimated 77% to 90% of drug abusers also smoke, yet few drug treatment centers provide access to tobacco cessation treatment. In one study of 405 drug treatment facilities, only 14% provided nicotine replacement therapy for smoking cessation, while only one third had protocols, procedures, or curricula for smoking cessation and only 20% reported having the financial resources to support tobacco counseling (Hunt et al., 2013).

Another health system factor that impedes control of substance abuse is failure to refer clients to appropriate sources of treatment. For example, in 2011, approximately 250,000 emergency department visits were made by patients seeking detoxification or substance abuse treatment. Unfortunately, only about 60% of those patients received any follow-up care. About 30% of them were hospitalized, 20% were referred to detoxification or treatment facilities, and 7% were transferred to other facilities (SAMHSA, 2013a).

Provision of adequate treatment of substance abuse may be further impeded by negative feelings on the part of health care providers toward those who abuse psychoactive substances. For example, despite knowledge of the effectiveness of harm-reduction strategies and the prevalence of periodic relapse during substance abuse treatment, many programs expel clients who revert to drug use during treatment. In addition, many clients in need may not have access to supportive services. For example, many shelters for the homeless refuse abusers despite the fact that a large proportion of homeless individuals abuse alcohol and other drugs. It may also be difficult for pregnant abusers or women with children to find appropriate treatment programs.

The health care system may pose additional barriers to care that are particularly burdensome for some population groups. For instance, most treatment programs are geared toward the needs of younger people and may not recognize the unique needs of the elderly substance abuser. In addition, because older people are often considered nonproductive

FOCUSED ASSESSMENT — Assessing Health System Determinants Influencing Substance Abuse

- What are the attitudes of health care providers toward clients with substance abuse problems?
- Are health care providers alert to signs and symptoms of substance abuse? To what extent do health care providers screen for substance misuse and abuse?
- To what extent do health care providers educate clients about substance abuse?
- What health system factors contribute to substance abuse (e.g., inappropriate prescription of psychoactive drugs)?
- What treatment facilities are available to substance abusers? To special populations of substance abusers (e.g., pregnant women, adolescents)?
- How is substance abuse treatment financed?

members of society, priority for placement in overburdened treatment facilities may be given to younger people. Tips for assessing health system factors influencing substance abuse in individuals and in the population are included in the *Focused Assessment* above. A Substance Abuse Risk Factor Inventory is provided on the student resources site.

Diagnostic Reasoning and Control of Substance Abuse

Population health nurses make nursing diagnoses related to substance abuse at two levels. The first level involves diagnoses related to individuals who have problems of substance abuse and their families. For example, the nurse might make a diagnosis for the individual client of "increased risk of substance abuse due to family history of alcohol abuse" or "abuse of sedatives due to increased life stress and poor coping skills." Nursing diagnoses related to the family of a substance abuser might include "codependency due to family feelings of guilt related to daughter's cocaine abuse" and "school behavior problems due to children's anxiety over mother's alcoholism."

At the second level, the population health nurse might make diagnoses of community problems related to substance abuse. For example, the nurse might diagnose an "increased incidence of motor vehicle fatalities due to driving under the influence of psychoactive drugs," or "increased prevalence of drug abuse among minority group members due to discrimination and feelings of powerlessness." Another example of a population-based diagnosis is "increased prevalence of fetal alcohol syndrome due to alcohol use by pregnant women."

Planning and Implementing Control Strategies for Substance Abuse

Strategies for controlling problems of substance abuse can involve health promotion, prevention of substance abuse and its consequences, resolution of existing substance-related problems, and health restoration.

HEALTH PROMOTION AND PREVENTION. Health promotion with respect to substance abuse primarily reflects efforts to improve coping skills and promote sound decision making related to initiation of substance use. Teaching effective coping skills and providing opportunities for their implementation may assist individual clients to decrease stress that might otherwise lead to substance abuse. Similarly, providing people, particularly youth with effective problem-solving and decision-making strategies may lead to healthier decisions regarding initiation of psychoactive substance use and subsequent abuse.

Specific prevention strategies may have one of four foci: preventing initiation of substance use, preventing progression from experimental use to regular use, preventing substance dependence, and preventing adverse consequences of substance use and abuse.

Preventing or delaying initiation of tobacco and alcohol use are major emphases in the *Healthy People 2020* objectives. Specific substance abuse objectives reflect efforts to modify attitudes toward and perceptions of risk involved in substance use and abuse. In addition, tobacco-related objective TU-3 addresses initiation of tobacco use among children, adolescents, and young adults. More information on these and other substance abuse–related objectives is presented at the end of this chapter. Similarly, prevention of drug abuse and excessive alcohol use is one of the priority areas in the National Prevention Strategy put forth by the U.S. Surgeon General's Office (National Prevention Council, 2011).

Universal prevention interventions targeted to overall prevention of risk behaviors among youth have been shown to be effective in preventing prescription opioid and overall prescription drug misuse in adolescents and young adults, particularly among youth at greatest risk for misuse (Spoth et al., 2013). Universal preventive interventions frequently involve school-based programs designed to target multiple risk behaviors including those related to substance abuse. For example, the *All Stars* program addresses substance abuse, fighting, and bullying. Program foci include identifying positive goals and aspirations, establishing positive norms in the school population, developing personal commitments to avoid high-risk behaviors, promoting bonding to the school or peer group, and fostering positive parental attention (Tanglewood Research, 2013). Other similar programs focus on life skills training related to personal self-management skills, social interaction skills, and drug resistance skills (National Health Promotion Associates, n.d.). For further information on three such programs, see the *External Resources* section of the student resources site.

Prevention of substance use initiation and escalation may involve modification of risk factors for use and abuse. Risk factor modification can occur with individuals, families, or society at large. Population health nurses may assist individuals to modify factors that put them at increased risk for substance abuse. For example, the nurse might assist clients experiencing stress to eliminate or modify sources of stress in their lives, or the nurse can assist clients and families to develop more effective coping skills.

In addition, the nurse may make referrals for social services to eliminate financial difficulties and other sources of stress. Or, the nurse might assist a harried single parent to obtain respite care. Nurses can also assist families to enhance family communication and cohesion to minimize the risk of substance abuse among children. Preventing alcohol use and/or promoting contraceptive use among childbearing women can help to reduce the incidence of FAS.

At the societal level, population health nurses can engage in political activity to control access to and limit the availability of psychoactive substances as well as to modify societal factors that contribute to abuse. For example, the nurse might advocate enforcement of laws restricting the sale of alcohol and tobacco to minors, or the nurse might work to reduce discrimination against members of minority groups or to ensure a minimal income for all families. Systematic research reviews have indicated that control of alcohol outlet density is an effective control measure for alcohol abuse (Ahern et al., 2013), and nurses may advocate for legislative control of outlet availability. Similarly, nurses may advocate for legislative and regulatory controls on the availability of laxatives and diet drugs and access by youth. Other control measures for these drugs that have been recommended include specific package labeling with the intended purposes of the medications, appropriate duration of use, warnings regarding possible organ damage and other adverse effects, and age verification for consumers (Pomeranz et al., 2013). Preventing adverse effects of substance use and abuse involves harm reduction. **Harm reduction** involves actions to minimize the harmful effects of drug use rather than preventing drug use *per se* (Harm Reduction Coalition, n.d.b). Harm reduction has also been described as a social justice movement based on respect for the rights of those who use drugs. The following principles underlie a harm reduction philosophy:

- Use of illicit substances is a fact of modern life, so control strategies should focus on addressing the adverse effects of use rather than on its control.
- Drug use is a complex phenomenon and some approaches to use are more harmful than others and should be discouraged in favor of safer approaches.
- The quality of individual and community life should be the focus of intervention, not cessation of use.
- Services provided to drug users should be nonjudgmental and noncoercive.
- Drug users should be involved in harm-reduction program design.
- A harm-reduction approach emphasizes reduction of harm as the primary responsibility of users and promotes mutual sharing of information and support among users.
- Harm reduction recognizes the contribution of societal and personal factors such as poverty, discrimination, social isolation, past trauma, and social inequalities to substance use.
- Harm reduction does not attempt to minimize or ignore the dangers of substance abuse, but seeks to reduce its potential effects (Harm Reduction Coalition, n.d.b).

The initial focus of harm reduction was on preventing infection-related harm from injection drug use, but has since been expanded to encompass other risks of substance abuse. Harm reduction may include prevention of overdose fatalities, a variety of infections, family disruption, social marginalization, and legal risks entailed in substance use (Jauffret-Roustide, 2009). For example, harm-reduction strategies may not only address the provision of clean injection equipment for IDU, but also prohibition of prosecution of people who make use of syringe exchange programs. In fact, the World Health Organization (WHO) supports a wide array of harm-reduction strategies for injection drug users, including needle and syringe exchange programs; drug abuse treatment; HIV testing, counseling, treatment, and care; condom distribution and STI treatment; and tuberculosis and hepatitis management (WHO, 2014a).

The emphasis in harm reduction is on meeting people where they are and reducing the harm of substance use while simultaneously addressing other issues and contributing factors (e.g., homelessness, mental illness, unemployment). Harm reduction focuses on identification of personal goals, not necessarily discontinuation of use, as the criteria for success and may result in a range of outcomes from controlled use, to non-harmful use, to abstinence (Lucas, 2012).

Access to clean needles and syringes is critical to harm reduction from IDU and prevention of HIV, hepatitis, and soft tissue infections. Research has consistently demonstrated the effectiveness of exchange programs in preventing these consequences. Exchange programs also provide opportunities to link drug users with drug treatment and other health services and housing assistance, and to provide overdose prevention education (Harm Reduction Coalition, n.d.c). Exchange programs have also been shown to decrease inappropriate disposal of used syringes and needles, thereby minimizing the potential for needlestick injuries and infection in the general population as well as among IDUs (Wenger et al., 2011).

Other infection prevention strategies include incorporating hepatitis immunization and care coordination into methadone maintenance programs (Masson et al., 2013). Similarly, antiviral prophylactic treatment for IDUs has been suggested as a mechanism for preventing HIV infection, particularly in areas with high HIV prevalence resulting from IDU (Alistar, Owens, & Brandeau, 2014). Another approach to HIV prevention among drug abusers in treatment is a culturally adapted "Real Men are Safe" program, which focuses on safe sexual practices. In one study, 87% of participants completed the program and demonstrated reduced incidence of unprotected sexual encounters (Calsyn et al., 2013).

Overdose prevention is another important aspect of harm reduction. Prevention efforts include education on prevention, recognition, and response to drug overdoses for users, their family members, and service providers (Harm Reduction Coalition, n.d.a). The Substance Abuse and Mental Health Services Administration (SAMHSA) has developed an overdose prevention toolkit that addresses strategies and information for community members; essential steps for first responders; information for prescribers, clients, and family members; and information and resources related to recovery from an overdose (SAMHSA, 2013b). For further information about the toolkit, see the *External Resources* section of the student resources site.

Another approach to harm reduction for persons who abuse alcohol is the installation of ignition interlocks in their cars. Ignition interlocks are connected to a vehicle's ignition system. They are capable of analyzing alcohol on one's breath. If the alcohol level is above the set limit, the lock prevents the vehicle from starting. Some form of ignition interlock legislation exists in all 50 states and the District of Columbia, and several states require all persons convicted of drunken driving offenses to install the locks in their vehicles (Teigen, 2013). Such devices have been estimated to reduce rearrest for driving under the influence of alcohol by a median of 67% across states (National Center for Injury Prevention and Control, 2013).

Supervised injection facilities are another harm-reduction strategy that is gaining acceptance throughout the world, but is not yet approved in the United States. **Supervised injection facilities (SIFs)** are legally sanctioned venues in which IDUs can inject pre-obtained drugs under medical supervision (DPA, 2014e). SIFs may also be referred to as safer injection sites, drug consumption rooms, or supervised injecting centers. In early 2014, 98 SIFs were in operation in 66 cities in ten countries. One of the most widely studied sites is the Canadian *Insite* program in Vancouver. The *Insite* program is funded by the British Columbia Ministry of Health through Vancouver Coastal Health and the Portland Hotel Society. The program is based on a harm-reduction philosophy, focusing on reducing the harm related to IDU without requiring abstinence (Vancouver Coastal Health, n.d.).

Research has consistently demonstrated that SIFs, including *Insite*, increase admissions to drug treatment facilities, reduce public injection and increase public safety, serve a population at high risk for infection and overdose, and reduce HIV and hepatitis risk behaviors related to syringe sharing and unsafe sexual practices. In addition, SIFs have saved hundreds of lives through overdose management and resulted in health care cost savings (DPA, 2014f; Kerr & Montaner, 2013). No evidence has been found that SIFs increase rates of drug use, initiate drug use, or promote drug-related crime (DPA, 2014f). Finally, a ruling by the Supreme Court of Canada in 2011 indicated that "Insite saves lives. Its benefits have been proven. There has been no discernable negative impact on the public safety and health objectives of Canada in its eight years of operation" (quoted in Drug Policy Alliance, 2014f, para 10). The Drug Policy Alliance has developed a toolkit advocating for legislation to promote supervised injection facilities in the United States. For further information about the toolkit, see the *External Resources* section of the student resources site. Table 29-6● summarizes major emphases

TABLE 29-6 Health Promotion and Prevention Strategies in the Control of Substance Abuse

Health Promotion Foci	Related Strategies
Development of effective coping strategies	• Teach coping strategies to individual clients/families. • Advocate for incorporation of coping skills into school curricula. • Develop and implement programs to foster effective coping skills.
Development of effective problem-solving skills	• Teach problem-solving skills to individual clients/families. • Advocate for, develop, and implement programs to foster effective problem solving.
Development of strong self-image	• Foster and reinforce strong self-image in individual clients. • Promote societal attitudes and conditions that foster development of healthy self-images in the public. • Work to change social attitudes to stigmatized groups that might foster substance abuse.
Prevention Foci	**Related Strategies**
Prevention or delayed initiation of substance use	• Educate individual clients regarding substance use risks. • Advocate for, develop, and implement substance risk education programs in schools. • Advocate for, develop, and implement public substance risk-education campaigns.
Control of access to substances of abuse	• Advocate for strong control policies regarding access to alcohol, tobacco, and prescription drugs.
Modification of substance abuse risk factors	• Advocate for social and policy changes to modify or eliminate factors contributing to substance abuse (e.g., poverty, unemployment).
Harm reduction	• Advocate for harm-reduction programs for substance abusers (e.g., syringe exchanges, SIFs, immunizations). • Educate substance abusers and the public regarding harm-reduction strategies. • Educate abusers, family and friends, and service providers for overdose prevention, recognition, and response • Develop and implement harm-reduction programs.

and related population health nursing strategies for health promotion and prevention related to substance abuse.

RESOLVING EXISTING SUBSTANCE ABUSE PROBLEMS. Resolution of existing problems related to substance abuse among individuals and population groups involves screening, brief intervention, and treatment.

Screening. Problem resolution with respect to substance abuse begins with screening for excessive or inappropriate use of psychoactive substances. The U.S. Preventive Services Task Force (USPSTF) has recommended that health care providers ask all adults and pregnant women about tobacco use and provide tobacco cessation interventions for those who use tobacco products, with interventions specially tailored for pregnant women who smoke (USPSTF, 2009). This recommendation is in the process of being updated. USPSTF also recommended universal screening for alcohol misuse for all adults 18 years of age and older, followed by brief behavioral intervention for those engaged in high-risk drinking behaviors (USPSTF, 2013). However, there is insufficient evidence to date to warrant recommending routine screening of adults, adolescents, or pregnant women for illicit drug use (USPSTF, 2008).

In addition, the Community Preventive Services Task Force (CPSTF) has recommended routing electronic screening for excessive alcohol consumption in the general public, with brief intervention for those engaged in high level consumption. This recommendation was based on strong evidence of the effectiveness of electronic screening and intervention in decreasing binge drinking and drinking intensity (CPSTF, 2013). Similarly, the SAMHSA-HRSA Center for Integrated Health Solutions (SAMHSA-HRSA CISH) has recommended screening, brief intervention, and referral to treatment (SBIRT) to identify persons with substance use problems and link them to appropriate services. SBIRT components include screening for risky substance use in any health care setting, brief intervention, and referral to treatment for those needing additional services (SAMHSA-HRSA CISH, n.d.b). Screening for substance misuse usually involves use of a brief initial screening questionnaire such as the National Institute on Alcohol Abuse and Alcoholism's (NIAAA) three-item screening tool or NIDA's quick screen tool. A positive screening result is followed by more in-depth assessment using tools such as WHO's Alcohol, Smoking, and Substance Involvement Screening Test (ASSIST) or Alcohol Use Disorders Identification Test (AUDIT) for those whose initial screening result is positive (SAMHSA-HRSA CISH, n.d.c). For further information about a variety of screening tools, see the *External Resources* section of the student resources site.

Brief intervention. Brief intervention is a 5- to 30-minute interaction between a health care provider who is not a substance abuse expert and substance users who are not drug dependent to motivate changes in high-risk behaviors. Brief intervention is designed to assist people at risk for substance abuse to reduce or eliminate substance use by assisting them to fully understand potential consequences of use and abuse. Brief intervention frequently employs cognitive behavioral therapy (CBT) or motivational interviewing techniques (SAMHSA-HRSA CISH, n.d.a).

Key components of brief interventions for high-risk alcohol use have been identified by the National Institute on Alcohol Abuse and Alcoholism (NIAAA, 2014). These components and their characteristic features are summarized in Table 29-7•. For further information about brief intervention, see the *External Resources* section of the student resources site. Brief interventions have been shown to result in significant reductions in risk scores for cannabis, opioid, cocaine, and amphetamine-type stimulant use and overall illicit drug involvement in several countries (Humeniuk et al., 2012). Population health nurses may provide brief interventions to clients perceived to engage in risky substance use behaviors incorporating the key components included in Table 29-7.

Treatment. Treatment for substance abuse is based on several general principles that have been identified by the National Institute on Drug Abuse (NIDA, 2012c). A similar set of treatment principles has been developed for substance abuse treatment in correctional facilities (NIDA, 2012e). Table 29-8• summarizes these two sets of principles.

Treatment for substance abuse employs many of the same psychotherapeutic modalities used for mental illness and discussed in Chapter 28∞. Evidence-based treatment modalities include medications, behavioral therapies, or some combination of both. The type of treatment modality used is frequently based on client and provider preference and comfort and the type of drug involved. Medications such as methadone, buprenorphine, and naltrexone are often used for opioid addiction, while nicotine patches and other forms of nicotine may assist with tobacco cessation. Disulfiram, acamprosate, and naltrexone may also be used for alcohol dependence (NIDA, 2012a). Currently no medication is available to assist with methamphetamine abuse, although there is some promise for drugs that target glial cell activity or anti-methamphetamine vaccines or antibodies that are currently being studied in human beings (NIDA, 2013). Medications may also be used to help clients deal with the symptoms of withdrawal.

Although smokeless tobacco products have been touted as promoting tobacco use cessation, they are themselves addictive and have not been shown to be of much help in cessation. In some studies, use of such products has been associated with attempts to quit, but not with successful cessation (Popova & Ling, 2013). In fact, in one study of military recruits, initiation of smokeless tobacco use actually led to harm escalation rather than reduction (Klesges, Sherrukk-Mittleman, Ebbert, Talcott, & DeBon, 2010).

Behavioral therapies are often used in conjunction with medication to assist substance abusers to identify and address underlying reasons for their substance misuse and to help develop strategies that will promote abstinence and/or harm reduction. Treatment for dual diagnosis of substance abuse and other psychiatric disorders often requires integrated treatment approaches addressing both conditions at once.

TABLE 29-7 Key Components and Characteristic Features of Brief Interventions

Key Components	Characteristic Features
Feedback related to personal risk	Provision of information on users' personal risks for adverse effects of substance use based on current use patterns, problem indicators (e.g., abnormal lab values), and existing medical problems due to use
Emphasis on client responsibility	Emphasis on personal control and choice to reduce risk behaviors
Advice for changing behaviors	Provision of suggestions on ways to reduce or eliminate risky substance use
Options for reducing use	Provision of several strategies to reduce substance risk (e.g., setting specific limits on use, recognizing and counteracting antecedents to excessive use)
Empathetic counseling style	Use of a concerned and reflective style for delivering the intervention rather than a confrontational or coercive style
Focus on self-efficacy	Emphasis on client strengths and resources, optimistic focus on client ability to change behavior
Goal setting	Development of a specific negotiated goal for behavior change, written as a contract or prescription
Incorporation of follow-up	Periodic follow-up and monitoring of client's success in changing behavior
Timing	Assessment of readiness to change and implementation of strategies to promote readiness

Source: National Institute on Alcohol Abuse and Alcoholism. (2014). *Brief intervention for alcohol problems.* Retrieved from http://alcoholism.about.com/library/blnaa43.htm

TABLE 29-8 General Evidence-Based Principles of Drug Abuse Treatment and Evidence-Based Principles of Drug Abuse Treatment in Correctional Settings

General Evidence-Based Principles of Drug Abuse Treatment	Evidence-Based Principles of Drug Abuse Treatment in Correctional Settings
Addiction is a complex but treatable disease that affects brain function and behavior.	Drug addiction is a brain disease that affects behavior.
No single treatment approach works for everyone.	Recovery from addiction requires effective treatment followed by long-term management.
Treatment services need to be readily available.	Treatment must last long enough to result in stable behavioral changes.
Effective treatment addresses multiple needs of the individual, not just his or her drug abuse.	Assessment is the first step in treatment.
Retention in treatment for sufficient time is critical.	Services need to be tailored to fit the needs of the individual.
Behavioral therapies are the most commonly used forms of drug abuse treatment.	Drugs used in treatment should be carefully monitored.
Medications are an important element of treatment for many abusers, especially in conjunction with behavioral therapies and counseling.	Treatment should target factors associated with criminal activity.
The client's treatment and services plan must be assessed and modified as needed.	Criminal justice supervision should include treatment planning for drug-abusing offenders, and treatment providers should be aware of correctional supervision requirements.
Drug abuse often co-occurs with other mental disorders.	Continuity of care is essential on reentry into the community.
Detoxification is only the first step in substance abuse treatment.	A balance of rewards and sanctions encourages prosocial behavior and treatment participation.
Treatment does not need to be voluntary to be effective.	Persons with co-occurring substance abuse and mental health problems often require integrated treatment.
Drug misuse during treatment must be monitored because lapses frequently occur.	Medications are an important part of treatment.
Treatment programs should incorporate HIV, hepatitis, tuberculosis, and other infection disease testing as well as providing risk-reduction education and treatment for existing health problems as needed.	Treatment planning for community reentry should include treatment of other medical conditions as well.

Data from: National Institute on Drug Abuse. (2012c). *Principles of drug addiction treatment: A research-based guide* (3rd ed.). Retrieved from http://www.drugabuse.gov/sites/default/files/podat_1.pdf; National Institute on Drug Abuse. (2012e). *Principles of drug abuse treatment for criminal justice populations: A research-based guide.* Retrieved from http://atforum.com/addiction-resources/documents/podat_cj_2012.pdf

In today's electronic environment, delivery of treatment modalities might encompass electronic approaches. For example, in one study, face-to-face and telephone treatment strategies were equally effective in treating tobacco addiction. Results varied somewhat based on client characteristics. For example, telephone intervention was more effective among people of higher socioeconomic status than lower status. Whichever modality was used, long-term abstinence was associated with exposure to more content (Sheffer, Stitzer, Landes, Brackman, & Munn, 2013). As we saw earlier, there is increasing potential for delivery of interventions in real time at critical points through geospatial technology.

Some complementary therapies have also been used for treating substance abuse. For example, hypnosis has been used successfully to assist some clients with smoking cessation and alcohol abuse. A novel approach to treatment for families of alcohol abusers using a systemic reflecting intervention has been effective in changing both drinking behavior on the part of the abuser and family behaviors. In this approach, families meet with a therapist and their interaction is watched by a team of observers through one-way mirrors. When the family and therapist agree that they are ready to receive feedback, team members provide reflections and observations on family interactions providing the family with outside perspectives on their behavior and its influence on drinking. Three studies using this technique demonstrated a decrease in drinking behavior, improved family problem-solving abilities, better communication, and retention in treatment (Flynn, 2010).

Population health nurses may be involved in treatment for substance abuse in a number of ways. First, nurses might identify cases of substance abuse and plan to refer clients and their families to treatment resources in the community. Nurses may also educate the general public on the signs and symptoms of substance abuse as well as the availability of treatment facilities. In addition, population health nurses can monitor the use of medications during withdrawal (if this is done on an outpatient basis) or on a long-term basis (e.g., methadone maintenance).

Population health nurses might also be involved in psychosocial therapies by referring clients to sources of group, individual, or family therapy, or the nurse might reinforce contracts made for reducing the use of substances. This is particularly true in measures to help clients stop smoking. In this instance, population health nurses may initiate behavioral contracts with clients to enable them to gradually cut down on tobacco consumption or quit smoking for gradually lengthened periods of time.

At the population level, nursing efforts to control substance abuse might include political activity to support the development of adequate treatment facilities, especially those geared to the needs of currently underserved population groups such as pregnant women, the homeless, and the elderly. Population health nurses might also be involved in political activity and advocacy to encourage insurance coverage of treatment for substance abuse. Major foci and related population health nursing strategies for resolving substance abuse–related health problems are summarized in Table 29-9●.

HEALTH RESTORATION. Health restoration in the context of substance abuse is often referred to as recovery. SAMHSA developed a working definition of substance abuse–related recovery as "a process of change through which individuals improve their health and wellness, live a self-directed life, and strive to reach their full potential" (SAMHSA, 2012, p. 3). The agency has also identified four dimensions that support recovery: health, home, purpose, and community. The health dimension focuses on managing related diseases or symptoms of addiction (e.g., cravings) and making decisions that support physical and mental health. The home dimension reflects the need for a safe and stable residence. The purpose dimension emphasizes the importance of carrying out meaningful daily activities such as work, school, and family responsibilities and having the resources needed to do so effectively. Finally, the community dimension focuses on interpersonal relationships and social networks that provide support and promote abstinence (SAMHSA, 2012).

In addition, SAMHSA has identified ten guiding principles of recovery. These principles include the following:

- Recovery derives from hope and a belief that recovery is possible and will lead to a better future.
- Recovery is person-driven and requires self-determination and self-direction in defining and achieving individually defined goals.

TABLE 29-9 Major Foci and Strategies Related to Resolution of Existing Substance Abuse–Related Problems

Focus	Related Strategies
Early identification of persons with substance use and abuse problems	• Screen individual clients for risk for substance abuse. • Screen individual clients for evidence of excessive substance use, misuse, or dependence. • Educate clients, families, and the public regarding signs of substance use problems. • Promote substance abuse screening in multiple health care venues.
Brief intervention for persons engaged in risky substance use	• Provide brief intervention for clients engaged in high-risk substance use.
Treatment of substance abuse	• Refer substance-abusing clients to treatment services. • Monitor clients during treatment. • Advocate for the availability of substance abuse treatment. • Advocate for insurance coverage of substance abuse treatment.

- There are many pathways to recovery and the recovery needs, goals, and strengths of each individual are unique and dependent on cultural background, life experiences, and other factors.
- Recovery is holistic and addresses all of an individual's needs, not just the substance-abusing behaviors.
- Effective recovery is supported by peers and allies including the support of mutual support and mutual aid groups.
- Recovery is supported through interpersonal relationships and social networks of people who believe in the person's ability to recover.
- Recovery is culturally based and influenced by cultural factors, and recovery services need to be culturally sensitive and congruent with client's cultural values, attitudes, and beliefs.
- Recovery is supported by addressing prior experiences of trauma.
- Recovery involves individual, family, and community strengths and resources; individuals have personal responsibility for their own self-care but may need assistance with self-advocacy. Families have responsibilities in supporting recovering members, and communities have a responsibility to provide resources that support recovery, promote inclusion, and minimize discrimination.
- Recovery is based on respect for the rights of those affected with mental health and substance abuse problems. Self-respect is also essential for successful recovery (SAMHSA, 2012).

Recovery or health restoration is aimed at preventing a relapse into prior substance-abusing behaviors by the individual or into enabling behaviors by family members and significant others. Additional foci in health restoration include dealing with the consequences of substance abuse, and building a foundation for recovery.

Relapse prevention. **Relapse** has been defined as a return to substance use behaviors after a prolonged period of abstinence. Relapse is a common phenomenon among substance abusers, and the emphasis in relapse prevention is elimination of personal triggers for substance use and abuse. Relapse frequently results in response to one of three types of triggers: a small amount of the abused substance, exposure to environmental cues or contexts associated with use and abuse, and stress. Research has indicated that abusers tend to be more susceptible to the action of such cues than nonabusers (Becker, n.d.).

Relapse Prevention Therapy (RPT) is a treatment approach that emphasizes self-control and assists abusers to anticipate and cope with factors that may contribute to relapse (SAMHSA's National Registry of Evidence-based Programs, 2014). Relapse prevention is based on the perspective that drug use behavior is reinforced by external cues that have become linked with rewards (e.g., the positive effects of drugs) and that these cues must be avoided to promote abstinence. Such cues may include people, places, drug use paraphernalia, or sensations previously associated with drug use. Other factors that may contribute to relapse include inadequate skill in dealing with pressures to return to substance use, poor conflict management skills, and a desire to test one's personal control over behavior.

Development of coping skills is central to relapse prevention. RPT focuses on understanding relapse as a process and on identifying and coping with high-risk situations that may precipitate relapse. RPT also emphasizes coping with urges and cravings, minimizing negative consequences of relapse, continued engagement in treatment despite relapse, and creation of a more balanced lifestyle. RPT has been found to be effective in promoting smoking abstinence, treatment for cocaine use and drinking behavior, and in marital adjustment (SAMHSA's National Registry of Evidence-based Programs, 2014).

Relapse prevention may be facilitated by the use of relapse risk maps. **Relapse risk maps** are graphic representations of the factors that contribute to relapse into substance-abusing behaviors drawn by the client with the assistance of a nurse or counselor. For example, the relapse prevention map of a college student with an alcohol problem might include a drawing of the university to represent the stress of making good grades; an endless circle among classrooms, the library, and work representing stressful demands on the student; and the bar where the student stops to relax every night on the way home from class. Other elements of the map might include a demanding employer or girlfriend or friends who encourage drinking. Relapse prevention maps can help clients with substance abuse problems identify factors that contribute to relapse and suggest strategies for dealing with them (e.g., making new friends, cutting back on work, or going to school part-time) (Weegmann, 2008). Similar maps can also be used during the early recovery stage to help identify factors that contribute to substance abuse behaviors.

Mutual-support and self-help groups are another strategy to aid in health restoration and relapse prevention related to substance abuse. Mutual-help groups consist of people who are abusers of the same substance and who provide for each other understanding and support in conquering their substance abuse habit. For example, Alcoholics Anonymous (AA) is a mutual-help group for alcohol abusers, and Potsmokers Anonymous is a mutual-help group for marijuana abusers.

In 2010, AA, the first organized mutual support group, celebrated its 75th anniversary. At that time, the organization included more than 2 million members (1.2 million in the United States alone) in 160 countries. AA originated out of the tenets of the Oxford Group, a Christian sect, but includes no specific religious doctrine. It is better described as a spiritual, rather than a religious program. AA support services are usually used in conjunction with professional care, and there is extensive evidence of its success in helping members maintain sobriety. The emphasis in this and other mutual support groups is voluntary service by recovering substance users helping other users (Gross, 2010). AA, in particular, does not rely on external monetary support, and its funding comes from voluntary contributions of members (AA, 2014).

Self-help therapies usually involve use of publications and educational materials that help people identify underlying reasons and triggers for substance use and suggest specific strategies for curtailing use. *SMART Recovery* is a self-help program that combines self-help education and literature and group interaction to implement its four-point recovery program that includes tools and techniques to help people: (a) build and maintain motivation to stop addictive behaviors, (b) cope with urges to engage in the behavior, (c) manage their thoughts, feelings, and behaviors, and (d) live a balanced life. Unlike AA, which is focused on alcohol addiction, *SMART Recovery* addresses multiple forms of addictive behavior. Group interaction is accompanied by manuals that provide practical tools and strategies for addressing each of the four points (SMART Recovery, n.d.). Recently a tailored manual was developed specifically for use by health care professionals with addictions (SMART Recovery, 2014).

The concepts of self-help or mutual support are predicated on perceptions that "the needs of patients are not adequately taken into account by institutions and professionals" and the concept that substance users are "lay experts" (Jauffret-Roustide, 2009, p. 159). Support groups for substance abusers may be of two types: therapeutic peer support groups, such as AA and SMART Recovery, and interest groups. Interest groups are groups of substance abusers focused on empowerment of group members to advocate for public policies that "change society and make it more tolerant of differences" including drug use (Jauffret-Roustide, 2009, p. 159). The intent of such groups is to advocate for the rights of drug users to choose drug use. These groups are less focused on day-to-day support for abstinence than on advocacy for alternatives based on the concept of harm reduction discussed earlier. The activities of such groups have led to changes in perceptions of users as irresponsible persons with an illness to responsible persons able to adopt behaviors that reduce the personal and societal harm due to substance abuse (Jauffret-Roustide, 2009).

Population health nurses can assist clients with substance abuse problems to identify triggers for relapse and to develop strategies for dealing with them. They can also assist in the development of relapse prevention groups that provide clients with the support of others in dealing with their relapse issues. They may also help to motivate family members and significant others to participate in relapse prevention, educating both clients and significant others about relapse, its causes, and prevention strategies. Population health nurses' involvement with self-help and mutual-help groups usually occurs in the form of referrals for these types of services. In some instances, however, population health nurses are actively involved in initiating support groups. Population health nurses may also be involved in empowerment-focused groups advocating for the rights of substance abusers.

Population health nurses can also contribute to health restoration efforts by providing emotional support to recovering abusers and their families and by linking them with other sources of support. Other health restoration measures might include efforts to eliminate or modify stressors that contribute to relapse. For example, assisting the recovering abuser to find work can alleviate the stress of unemployment and financial worries.

The nurse can also reinforce the individual's motivation to abstain from drug use or engage in harm-reduction strategies by commending and highlighting successes. Development of positive coping skills may also prevent relapse. Other health restoration needs may involve providing information on resources, providing respite from onerous burdens of care, or helping individuals plan time for themselves.

At the population level, population health nurses may be involved in planning and implementing services for people with substance abuse problems (e.g., initiating a mutual-help group or a relapse prevention group). They may also need to participate in political advocacy to assure the availability of health restoration services or to mandate their coverage as a routine health insurance benefit.

Dealing with consequences of abuse. Substance abuse may lead to a variety of physical, psychological, and social consequences with which population health nurses need to assist clients. Population health nurses may provide treatment for physical consequences of substance abuse and assist clients to deal with psychological and social consequences. For example, they may treat abscesses due to injection drug use or refer clients for treatment if necessary. Other examples include assisting clients in recovery to deal with the feelings of guilt engendered by their behavior and its effects on loved ones, or helping them to regain custody of children placed in foster care.

Population health nurses may also need to help family members deal with the consequences of substance abuse in the family. For example, group interventions for schoolchildren whose parents have substance abuse disorders have been shown to reduce feelings of isolation and to improve problem solving, conflict resolution, and social skills as well as enhance academic skills. In addition, such programs provide a sense of personal safety and belonging, and program staff can engage in advocacy for appropriate care of these children. Population health nurses can be actively involved in developing these and similar programs. They can also engage in political activity to assure access to and funding for these types of programs. Political advocacy may also be needed to assure insurance coverage for health services to deal with the physical and emotional consequences of abuse for substance abusers and their family members.

Building a foundation for recovery. Treatment for substance abuse is more than a matter of detoxification and modification of cravings for the drug in question. It is usually a total program of modification that results in changes in modes of thinking and acting. This may be achieved through professional therapy as discussed above, participation in mutual-help groups, changes in environment and lifestyle, self-image enhancement, and development of new coping skills and new patterns of family interaction.

Nurses can also assist clients to plan changes in their environment to minimize stresses that may contribute to substance abuse. For example, the nurse can refer a client for help with financial difficulties or for respite from the care of a handicapped child or elderly parent. Socially isolated older persons who abuse substances can be linked to sources of social support, and unemployed persons can be assisted to find employment or to learn skills that enhance their employability. The provision of housing for homeless substance abusers has been shown to reduce emergency department use, detoxification center use, hospital admission, and jail bookings. One such program cost approximately $18,600 per person, but resulted in per capita savings of $36,579 (Srebnik, Connor, & Sylla, 2013). Similarly, the *Pathways Housing First* program focuses on housing and community-based treatment services for homeless individuals, many of whom have substance abuse disorders. In one study, the program resulted in an 84% rate of retention in treatment after 2 years, reductions in psychiatric symptoms, improvements in alcohol dependence, and declines in community services use (Tsemberis, Kent, & Respress, 2012).

Population health nurses can also help individual clients develop stronger self-images by reinforcing their successes and helping them realistically examine their expectations for themselves. In addition, nurses can help clients who abuse psychoactive substances to develop alternative ways of coping with stress by taking action to modify stressors or changing their perceptions of and responses to stressors.

Treatment efforts are also needed for members of the abuser's family to enable them to recover from codependence. Goals in the care of families of substance abusers include stabilizing the family system, making changes in family interactions, and developing mechanisms for maintaining those changes. Family stabilization may be achieved by linking families to needed support services and engaging in the crisis intervention strategies described in Chapter 14∞. The nurse can also make referrals for marital or family therapy as needed and can assist families to identify their use of defense mechanisms similar to those used by the substance abuser.

The population health nurse might also provide families with anticipatory guidance about the negative effects of life change events and help them deal with these events without resorting to substance abuse. Family members may also need help in working through resentment related to substance abuse and subsequent behaviors by the abuser.

Building positive experiences in the life of the family also fosters cohesion and helps to stabilize the family. The population health nurse can assist the family to plan activities in which all members can participate. It is particularly important to integrate the substance-abusing member into these occasions, if possible, to prevent further alienation.

The population health nurse can also assist families to develop new patterns of interaction. For example, the nurse might help the family realign members into the more usual husband–wife coalition rather than parent–child coalitions by improving family communication and developing joint problem-solving skills. The nurse can also assist family members to identify and express feelings and learn negotiating strategies. The systemic reflecting strategy discussed earlier is one approach to assisting families to develop new patterns of interaction. Even children can be incorporated into such an approach if desired (Flynn, 2010). Areas of focus and strategies for health restoration with respect to substance abuse are summarized in Table 29-10●.

TABLE 29-10 Health Restoration Strategies in the Control of Substance Abuse

Focus	Strategies
Support for abusers	• Provide emotional support and encouragement to individual clients and their families. • Assist with abuser reintegration into the family. • Refer for emotional or material support services as needed. • Advocate for development of and access to support services for abusers and their families.
Relapse prevention	• Educate individual clients and families regarding the process of relapse and relapse prevention. • Assist abusers to identify relapse triggers. • Assist with the development of relapse risk maps and relapse prevention plans. • Assist in minimizing effects when relapse occurs. • Initiate or refer clients to mutual support groups or self-help groups.
Modification or elimination of factors contributing to relapse	• Assist with employment, housing, etc. • Refer for financial assistance as needed. • Refer for respite services to address caregiver burden. • Advocate for societal changes that eliminate stressors that contribute to substance abuse. • Advocate for changes in societal attitudes toward substance abusers.
Dealing with the consequences of abuse	• Provide care to individual clients or refer for services to address physical and psychological consequences of substance abuse. • Advocate for availability of and access to treatment services to address consequences of substance abuse. • Assist family members to deal with the effects of substance abuse on the family or refer for needed services. • Advocate for available services for family members of substance abusers.
Building a foundation for recovery	• Assist substance abusers and family members to develop effective coping strategies. • Promote new family interaction patterns. • Promote family cohesion and reintegration of the substance abuser.

Evaluating Control Strategies for Substance Abuse

Evaluating interventions with individual substance abusers and their families focuses on the extent to which problems of substance abuse have been resolved. Has the abuser been able to abstain from substance use or to engage in harm-reduction strategies? Have stresses contributing to substance abuse been modified? Have personal and family consequences of substance abuse been addressed as far as possible?

At the population level, the nurse could evaluate the effects of intervention programs on the incidence and prevalence of substance abuse as well as indicators of morbidity and mortality related to abuse. The nurse evaluating the effects of programs directed at substance abuse might examine the extent to which national health promotion and disease prevention objectives have been met in the population. The current status of selected *Healthy People 2020* objectives related to substance use and abuse is presented below. As can be seen, very few of the objectives have already reached the targets, but other objectives (e.g., exposure of young people to tobacco marketing on the Internet) are moving away from their targets. For others, the movement toward the target has been slow, suggesting the need for more concerted efforts to control substance use and abuse.

Another source of evaluative information on the overall effectiveness of criminal justice approaches to the control of substance abuse lies in the Office of Management and Budget (OMB) assessment of federal agencies. In its most recent assessment of the Drug Enforcement Administration (DEA) in 2003, the OMB rated the agency's performance as "adequate." In its report, the OMB noted that "the Drug Enforcement Administration is unable to demonstrate its impact on the availability of drugs in the U.S. but has shown sustained progress in disrupting and dismantling high priority drug trafficking organizations" (OMB, 2003, para 2). Based on this assessment and the continued problem of substance abuse, it would seem clear that drug enforcement activities are not having a significant effect on the problem of substance abuse in the United States, and that other strategies are needed.

Healthy People 2020

Selected Objectives Related to Substance Use and Abuse

OBJECTIVE	BASELINE (YEAR)	TARGET	CURRENT DATA (YEAR)	DATA SOURCES
SA-2. Increased the proportion of high school seniors who have never used				
2.3. alcoholic beverages	27.7% (2009)	30.5%	NDA	Monitoring the Future Study (MTF), NIH/NIDA
2.4. illicit drugs	53.3% (2009)	58.6%	NDA	
SA-4. Increase the proportion of adolescents who perceive great risk associated with				
4.1. Binge drinking	40% (2008)	44%	40.7% (2011)	National Survey on Drug Use and Health (NSDUH) SAMHSA
4.2. Marijuana use	33.4% (2008)	36.7%	27.6% (2011)	
4.3. Cocaine use	49.4% (2006)	54.3%	48.1% (2011)	
SA-6. Increase the number of states with mandatory ignition lock laws for first and repeat impaired driving offenders	13 (2009)	50 states and DC	NDA	Mothers Against Drunk Driving
SA-7. Increase the number of admissions to treatment for injection drug use (per year)	254,278 (2006)	279,706	NDA	Treatment Episode Data Set (TEDS), SAMHSA
SA-11 Reduce cirrhosis deaths (per 100,000 population)	9.1 (2007)	8.2	9.4 (2010)	National Vital Statistics System-Mortality (NVSS-M), CDC/NCHS
SA-12. Reduce drug-induced deaths (per 100,000 population)	12.6 (2007)	11.3	12.9 (2010)	NSDUH, SAMHSA

Continued on next page

Healthy People 2020 (Continued)

OBJECTIVE	BASELINE (YEAR)	TARGET	CURRENT DATA (YEAR)	DATA SOURCES
SA-14 Reduce the proportion of people engaged in binge drinking in the last month				
14.3. Adults	21.7% (2008)	24.4%	26.7% (2011)	NSDUH, SAMHSA
14.4 Adolescents 12–17 years of age	9.5% (2008)	8.6%	7.9% (2011	
SA-16. Reduce average annual alcohol consumption (gallons per person)	2.3 gal (2007)	2.1 gal	NDA	Alcohol Epidemiologic Data System (AEDS)
SA-17. Reduce the rate of alcohol impaired driving (per million vehicle miles driven)	0.4 (2008)	0.38	NDA	Fatality Analysis Reporting System (FARS), DOT/NHTSA
SA-18.3 Reduce steroid use by 12th graders (similar objective for 8th and 10th graders)	2.2% (2009)	NT	NDA	MTF, NIH/NIDA
SA-19 Reduce nonmedical use of any psychotherapeutic drug (in past year)	6.1% (2008)	5.5%	5.7% (2011)	NSDUH, SAMHSA
SA-20. Reduce the number of deaths attributable to alcohol	79,646 (Avg 2001–2005)	71,681	NDA	Alcohol Related Disease Impact System (ARDI), CDC
SA-21. Reduce the proportion of adolescents who use inhalants	4% (2008)	NT	3.3% (2011)	NSDUH, SAMHSA
TU-1.1. Reduce cigarette smoking by adults	20.6% (2008)	12%	19% (2011)	National Health Interview Survey (NHIS), CDC/NCHS
TU-2.1. Reduce past month tobacco use by adolescents	26% (2009)	21%	23.4% (2011)	Youth Risk Behavior Surveillance System (YRBSS), CDC/NCHHSTP
TU-3. Reduce initiation of tobacco product use				
3.1 by adolescents (12–17 years)	7.7% (2008)	5.7%	6.9% (2011)	NSDUH, SAMHSA
3.5. by young adults (18–25 years)	10.8% (2008)	8.8%	10.4% (2011)	
TU-5.1. Increase smoking cessation success by adults	6% (2008)	8%	6.7% (2011)	NHIS, CDC/NCHS
TU-6. Increase smoking cessation during pregnancy	11.3% (2005)	30%	18.9% (2010)	NHIS, CDC/NCHS
TU-8. Increase states with Medicaid coverage of treatment for nicotine dependence	6 states (2007)	50 states and DC	5 states (2009)	State Medicaid Coverage for Tobacco Treatment
TU-11. Reduce the proportion of children 3–11 years of age exposed to environmental tobacco smoke (similar objectives for adolescents and adults)	52.2% (2005–2008)	47%	NDA	National Health and Nutrition Examination Survey (NHANES), CDC/NCHS

Healthy People 2020 (Continued)

OBJECTIVE	BASELINE (YEAR)	TARGET	CURRENT DATA (YEAR)	DATA SOURCES
TU-12. Increase the proportion of people covered by indoor worksite polices that prohibit smoking	75.3% (2006–2007)	100%	NDA	Current Population Survey (CPS), Census & DOL,BLS
TU-15.1. Increase tobacco-free environments in junior high schools (similar objectives for middle schools, high schools, and Head Start programs)	65.4% (2006)	100%	NDA	School Health Policies and Practices Study (SHPPS), CDC/ NCHHSTP
TU-18.1 Reduce the proportion of adolescents and young adults exposed to tobacco marketing on the Internet (similar objectives for other media)	36.8% (2009)	33.1%	40.6% (2011)	National Youth Tobacco Survey (NYTS), CDC/ NCCDPHP/OSH

NT = No target set yet, informational data only
NDA = No data available
Data from: U.S. Department of Health and Human Services. (2014). *Healthy people 2020: Topics and objectives.* Retrieved from http://healthypeople.gov/2020/topicsobjectives2020/default.aspx

CHAPTER RECAP

Factors related to each of the six categories of determinants of health influence psychoactive substance use and abuse. Population health nurses engage in a variety of strategies at each level of health to address the problems of substance use and abuse. Health promotion strategies, for example, include development of effective coping and problem-solving strategies and strong individual self-images. Prevention activities focus on preventing substance use initiation, controlling access to drugs and alcohol, modifying substance use and abuse risk factors, and engaging in harm reduction to prevent harmful consequences of substance use and abuse. Strategies designed to resolve existing problems of abuse include screening for excessive use and abuse, brief intervention, and substance abuse treatment. Finally, health restoration involves support for the abuser and his or her family, relapse prevention, modification of factors that promote relapse, dealing with the physical and psychological consequences of abuse, and building a foundation for recovery. Evaluation of control efforts occurs at both the individual client and population levels.

CASE STUDY Alcohol on Campus

Members of the senior class of the baccalaureate nursing program at a state university have noticed that alcohol use is prevalent on their campus. Several friends have been arrested for driving under the influence and one student's boyfriend was killed in a drunk-driving accident. The students have also noted a significant amount of binge drinking at weekend parties when people "let down their hair." The university has a no-drinking-on-campus policy, but enforcement is lax, and alcohol is frequently smuggled into the dorms. The student health center does not really address the problem of excessive alcohol intake and few students use the campus counseling center.

1. What factors related to biological, psychological, environmental, sociocultural, behavioral, and health system determinants of health are operating in this situation?
2. What additional information related to determinants of health might the nursing students need to collect? Where might they obtain that information?
3. What actions by the nursing students might help to address the problem of alcohol use in the campus population? Would these actions primarily reflect health promotion, prevention, resolution of existing problems, or health restoration?
4. How might the students evaluate the effects of their efforts?

REFERENCES

Adams, P. J. (2013). Addiction industry studies: Understanding how proconsumption influences block effective interventions. *American Journal of Public Health, 103,* e35–e38. doi: 10.2105/10AJPH.2012.301151

Ahern, J., Margerison-Ziko, C., Hubbard, A., & Galea, S. (2013). Alcohol outlets and binge drinking in urban neighborhoods: The implications of nonlinearity for intervention and policy. *American Journal of Public Health, 103,* e1–e7. doi:10.2105/AJPH.2012.301203

Alcoholics Anonymous. (2014). *What is A.A.?* Retrieved from http://www.aa.org/lang/en/subpage.cfm?page=1

Alistar, S. S., Owens, D., & Brandeau, M. L. (2014). Effectiveness and cost effectiveness of oral pre-exposure prophylaxis in a portfolio of prevention programs for injection drug users in mixed HIV epidemics. *PLoS ONE, 9*(1), e86584. doi:10.1371/journal.pone.0086584

American Academy of Experts in Traumatic Stress. (2012). *Effects of parental substance abuse on children and families.* Retrieved from http://www.aaets.org/article230.htm

American Lung Association. (2014). *Tobacco cessation treatment: What is covered.* Retrieved from http://www.lung.org/stop-smoking/tobacco-control-advocacy/reports-resources/tobacco-cessation-affordable-care-act/what-is-covered.html

American Psychiatric Association. (2013a). *Diagnostic and statistical manual of mental disorders: DSM-5* (5th ed.). Washington, DC: Author.

American Psychiatric Association. (2013b). *Substance-related and addictive disorders.* Retrieved from http://www.dsm5.org/Documents/Substance%20Use%20Disorder%20Fact%20Sheet.pdf

American Psychological Association. (2014). *Family members of adults with substance abuse problems.* Retrieved from https://www.apa.org/pi/about/publications/caregivers/practice-settings/intervention/substance-abuse.aspx

Babor, T. F., & Robaina, K. (2013). Public health, academic medicine, and the alcohol industry's corporate social responsibility activities. *American Journal of Public Health, 103,* 206–214. doi:10.2105/AJPH.2012.300847

Babor, T. F., Xuan, Z., Damon, D., & Noel, J. (2013). An empirical evaluation of the US Beer institute's self-regulation code governing the content of beer advertising. *American Journal of Public Health, 103,* e45–e51. doi:10.2105/AJPH.2013.301487

Becker, H. C. (n.d.). *Alcohol dependence, withdrawal, and relapse.* Retrieved from http://pubs.niaaa.nih.gov/publications/arh314/348-361.htm

Bellum, S. (2011). *What are designer drugs?* Retrieved from http://teens.drugabuse.gov/blog/post/real-teens-ask-what-are-designer-drugs

Callaghan, R. C., Sanches, M., Gatley, J. M., & Cunningham, J. K. (2013). Effects of the minimum legal drinking age on alcohol-related health service use in hospital settings in Ontario: A regression-discontinuity approach. *American Journal of Public Health, 103,* 2284–2291. doi:10.2105/AJPH.2013.301320

Calsyn, D. A., Burlew, K., Hatch-Maillette, M. A., Beadnell, B., Wright, L., & Wilson, J. (2013). An HIV prevention intervention for ethnically diverse men in substance abuse treatment: Pilot study findings. *American Journal of Public Health, 103,* 896–902. doi:10.2105/AJPH.2012.300970

Center for Behavioral Health Statistics and Quality. (2011). *The N-SSATS report: Acceptance of private health insurance in substance abuse treatment facilities.* Retrieved from http://oas.samhsa.gov/2k11/305/305PrivateIns2k11.htm

Centers for Medicare and Medicaid Services. (n.d.). *Do marketplace insurance plans cover mental health and substance abuse services?* Retrieved from https://www.healthcare.gov/do-marketplace-insurance-plans-cover-mental-health-and-substance-abuse-services/

Cerdá, M., Ransome, Y., Keyes, K. M., Koenen, K. C., Tardiff, K., Vlahov, D., & Galea, S. (2013). Revisiting the role of the urban environment in substance abuse use: The case of analgesic overdose fatalities. *American Journal of Public Health, 103,* 2252–2260. doi:10.2105/AJPH.2013.301347

Co-Dependents Anonymous. (2010). *Patterns and characteristics of codependence.* Retrieved from http://www.coda.org/tools4recovery/patterns-new.htm

Co-Dependents Anonymous. (2013). *What is codependency?* Retrieved from http://www.coda.org/

Community Preventive Services Task Force. (2013). *Preventing excessive alcohol consumption: Electronic screening and brief intervention (e-SBI).* Retrieved from http://www.thecommunityguide.org/alcohol/esbi.html

Conner, K. R., Huguet, N., Caetano, R., Giesbrecht, N., McFarland, B. H., Nolte, K. B., & Kaplan, M. S. (2014). Acute use of alcohol and methods of suicide in a US national sample. *American Journal of Public Health, 104,* 171–178. doi:10.2105/AJPH.2013.301352

Darke, S., Duflou, J., Torok, M., & Prolov, T. (2013). Characteristics, circumstances and toxicology of sudden or unnatural deaths involving very high-range alcohol concentrations. *Addiction, 108,* 1411–1417. doi:10.1111/add.12191

Disney, L. D., Lavallee, R. A., & Yi, H.-Y. (2013). The effect of internal possession laws on underage drinking among high school students: A 12-state analysis. *American Journal of Public Health, 103,* 1090–1095. doi:10.2105/AJPH.2012.301074

Division of Birth Defects and Developmental Disabilities. (2012). *Fetal alcohol spectrum disorders: Data and statistics.* Retrieved from http://www.cdc.gov/ncbddd/fasd/data.html

Drenzek, C., Geller, R. J., Steck, A., Arnold, J., Lopez, G., Gerona, R., & Edison, L. (2013). Severe illness associated with synthetic cannabinoid use—Brunswick, GA, 2013. *Morbidity and Mortality Weekly Report, 62,* 939.

Drug Policy Alliance. (2014a). *About the drug policy alliance.* Retrieved from http://www.drugpolicy.org/about-drug-policy-alliance

Drug Policy Alliance. (2014b). *History.* Retrieved from http://www.drugpolicy.org/mission-and-vision/history

Drug Policy Alliance. (2014c). *Mission and vision.* Retrieved from http://www.drugpolicy.org/mission-and-vision

Drug Policy Alliance. (2014d). *Our victories.* Retrieved from http://www.drugpolicy.org/our-victories

Drug Policy Alliance. (2014e). *Supervised injection facilities.* Retrieved from http://www.drugpolicy.org/supervised-injection-facilities

Drug Policy Alliance. (2014f). *Supervised injection facilities: Overview.* Retrieved from http://www.drugpolicy.org/sites/default/files/DPA_Fact_Sheet_Supervised_Injection_Facilities_Feb2014.pdf

Fee, E. (2011). Charles E. Terry (1978–1945): Early campaigner against drug addiction. *American Journal of Public Health, 101,* 451. doi:10.2105/AJPH.2010.191171

Fiala, S. C., Morris, D. S., & Pawlak, R. L. (2012). Measuring indoor air quality of hookah lounges. *American Journal of Public Health, 102,* 2043–2045. doi:10.2105/AJPH.2012.300751

Flynn, B. (2010). Using systemic reflective practice to treat couples and families with alcohol problems. *Journal of Psychiatric and Mental Health Nursing, 17,* 577–582. doi:10.1111/j.1365-2850.2010.01574.x

Frimpong, J. A. (2013). Missed opportunities for hepatitis C testing in opioid treatment programs. *American Journal of Public Health, 103,* 1028–1030. doi:10.2105/AJPH.2012.301129

Gentry, E., Poirier, K., Wilkinson, T., Nhean, S., Nyborn, J., & Siegel, M. (2011). Alcohol advertising at Boston subway stations: An assessment of exposure by race and socioeconomic status. *American Journal of Public Health, 101,* 1936–1941. doi:10.2105/AJPH.2011.300159

Gibbs, T. A., Okuda, M., Oquendo, M. A., Lawson, W. B., Wang, S., Thomas, Y. F., & Blanco, C. (2013). Mental health of African Americans and Caribbean Blacks in the United States: Results from the National Epidemiological Survey on Alcohol and Related Conditions. *American Journal of Public Health, 103,* 330–338. doi:10.2105/AJPH.2012.300891

Gonzalez, M., Sanders-Jackson, A., Song, A. V., Chen, K. W., & Glantz, S. (2013). Strong smoke-free law coverage in the United States by race/ethnicity: 2000–2009. *American Journal of Public Health, 103,* e62–e66. doi:10.2105/AJPH.2012.301045

Gross, M. (2010). Alcoholics anonymous: Still sober after 75 years. *American Journal of Public Health, 100,* 2361–2363. doi:10.2105/AJPH.2010.199349

Gruenewald, P. J., Ponicki, W. R., Remer, L. G., Waller, L. A., Zhu, L., & Gorman, D. M. (2013). Mapping the spread of amphetamine abuse in California from 1995–2008. *American Journal of Public Health, 103,* 1262–1270. doi:10.2105/AJPH.2012.300779

Harm Reduction Coalition. (n.d.a). *Overdose prevention.* Retrieved from http://harmreduction.org/issues/overdose-prevention/

Harm Reduction Coalition. (n.d.b). *Principles of harm reduction.* Retrieved from http://harmreduction.org/about-us/principles-of-harm-reduction/

Harm Reduction Coalition. (n.d.c). *Syringe access.* Retrieved from http://harmreduction.org/issues/syringe-access/

Harris, N., Johnson, C., Sionean, C., Ivy, W., Singh, S., Wei, S., . . . Lansky, A. (2013). Estimated percentages and characteristics of men who have sex with men and use injection drugs— United States, 1999–2011. *Morbidity and Mortality Weekly Report, 62,* 757–762.

Hartney, E. (2011). *What is psychoactive?* Retrieved from http://addictions.about.com/od/substancedependence/g/psychoactive.htm

Heath, D. B. (2012). *Drinking occasions: Comparative perspectives on alcohol and culture.* New York, NY: Routledge, Taylor & Francis.

Humeniuk, R., Ali, R., Babor, T., Souza-Formigoni, M. L., de Lacerda, R. B., Ling, W., . . . Vendetti, J. (2012). A randomized controlled trial of a brief intervention for illicit drugs linked to the Alcohol, Smoking and Substance Involvement Screening Test (ASSIST) in clients recruited from primary health-care settings in four countries. *Addiction, 107,* 957–966. doi:10.1111/j.1360-0443.2011.03740.x

Hunt, J. J., Gajewski, B. J., Jiang, Y., Cupertino, P., & Richter, K. P. (2013). Capacity of US drug treatment facilities to provide evidence-based tobacco treatment. *American Journal of Public Health, 103,* 1799–1801. doi:10.2105/AJPH.2013.301427

Iglesias-Rios, L., & Parascandola, M. (2013). A historical review of R. J. Reynolds' strategies for marketing tobacco to Hispanics in the United States. *American Journal of Public Health, 103,* e1–e13. doi:10.2105/AJPH.2013.301256

James, S. D. (2014). *Why marijuana edibles are harder to regulate and don't get you as high.* Retrieved from http://abcnews.com/Health/marijuana-edibles-harder-regulate-high/story?id=22350866

Jauffret-Roustide, M. (2009). Self-support for drug users in the context of harm reduction policy: A lay expertise defined by drug users' life skills and citizenship. *Health Sociology Review, 18,* 159–172.

Jernigan, D. H., Ross, C. S., Ostroff, J., McKnight-Eily, L. R., & Brewer, R. D. (2013). Youth exposure to alcohol advertising on television—25 markets, United States, 2010. *Morbidity and Mortality Weekly Report, 62,* 877–880.

Jiang, N., & Ling, P. M. (2013). Impact of alcohol use and bar attendance on smoking and quit attempts among young adult bar patrons. *American Journal of Public Health, 103,* e53–e61. doi:10.2105/AJPH.2013.301014

Judicial Council of California. (2014). *Drug courts.* Retrieved from http://www.courts.ca.gov/5979.htm

Kanny, D., Liu, Y., & Brewer, R. D. (2011, January 14). Binge drinking—United States, 2009. *Morbidity and Mortality Weekly Report, 60*(Suppl.), 101–104.

Kanny, D., Liu, Y., Brewer, R. D., Garvin, W., & Balluz, L. (2010). Vital signs: Binge drinking among high school students and adults—United States, 2009. *Morbidity and Mortality Weekly Report, 59,* 1274–1279.

Karriker-Jaffe, K., Roberts, S. C. M., & Bond, J. (2013). Income inequality, alcohol use, and alcohol-related problems. *American Journal of Public Health, 103,* 649–656. doi:10.2105/AJPH.2012.300882

Kerr, T., & Montaner, J. (2013). *An overview of insite—10 years later.* Retrieved from http://supervisedinjection.vch.ca/media-centre/an-overview-of-insite---10-years-later

Kim, P., Kuypers, C., Legrand, S.-A., Ramaekers, J. G., & Verstraete, A., G. (2012). A case-control study estimating accident risk for alcohol, medicines, and illegal drugs. *PLoS ONE, 7,* e43496. doi:10.1371/journal.pone.0043496

Kim, T. W., Saitz, R., Kretsch, N., Cruz, A., Winter, M. R., Shanahan, W. W., & Alford, D. P. (2013). Screening for unhealthy alcohol and other drug use by health educators: Do primary care clinicians document screening results? *Journal of Addiction Medicine, 7,* 204–209. doi:10.1097/ADM.0b013e31828da017

Klesges, R. C., Sherrukk-Mittleman, D., Ebbert, J. O., Talcott, W., & DeBon, M. (2010). Tobacco use harm reduction, elimination, and escalation in a large military cohort. *American Journal of Public Health, 100,* 2487–2492. doi:10.2105/AJPH.2009.175091

Kousha, M., Shahrivar, Z., & Alaghband-rad, J. (2014). Substance use disorder and ADHD: Is ADHD a particularly "specific" risk factor? *Journal of Attention Disorders, 16,* 325–332. doi:10.1177/1087054710387265

Lee, C.-H., Ko, A. M.-S., Warnakulasuriya, S., Ling, T.-Y., Sunarjo, Rajapakse, O. S., & Ko, Y.-C. (2012). Population burden of betel quid abuse and its relation to oral premalignant disorders in South, Southeast, and East Asia: An Asian Betel Quid Consortium Study. *American Journal of Public Health, 102,* e17–e24. doi:10.2105/AJPH.2011.300521

Li, C., Balluz, L. S., Okoro, C. A., Strine, T. W., Lin, J.-M. S., Town, M., . . . Valluru, B. (2011). Surveillance of certain health behaviors and conditions among states and selected local areas—Behavioral Risk Factor Surveillance System, United States, 2009. *Morbidity and Mortality Weekly Report, 60* (SS-9), 1–248.

Lucas, L. (2012). *Harm reduction and recovery-oriented care.* Retrieved from http://www.samhsa.gov/recoverytoPractice/Resources/wh/2012/2012_04_19/wh_2012_04_19.html

Lynne-Landsman, S. D., Livingston, M. D., & Wagenaar, A. C. (2013). Effects of state medical marijuana laws on adolescent marijuana use. *American Journal of Public Health, 103,* 1500–1506. doi:10.2105/AJPH.2012.301117

Marchetta, C. M., Denny, C. H., Floyd, R. L., Cjeal, N. E., Sniezek, J. E., & McKnight- Eily, L. R. (2012). Alcohol use and binge drinking among women of childbearing age—United States, 2006–2010. *Morbidity and Mortality Weekly Report, 61,* 534–538.

Masson, C., Delucchi, K. L., McKnight, C., Hetterma, J., Khalili, M., Min, A., . . . Perlman, D. (2013). A randomized trial of a hepatitis care coordination model in methadone maintenance treatment. *American Journal of Public Health, 103,* e81–e88. doi:10.2105/AJPH.2013.301458

McKnight-Eily, L. R., Liu, Y., Brewer, R. D., Kanny, D., Lu, H., & Collins, J. (2014). Vital signs: Communication between health professionals and their patients about alcohol use—44 states and the District of Columbia, 2011. *Morbidity and Mortality Weekly Report, 62,* 16–22.

Medicare Rights Center. (2011). *Medicare coverage of treatment for alcoholism and drug abuse.* Retrieved from http://www.medicareinteractive.org/page2.php?opic=counselor&page=script&slide_id=925

Mental Health America. (n.d.). *Codependency*. Retrieved from http://mentalhealthamerica.net/co-dependency

Mimiaga, M. J., Reisner, S. L., Grasso, C., Crane, H. M., Safren, S. A., Kitahata, M. M., . . . Mayer, K. H. (2013). Substance use among HIV-infected patients engaged in primary care in the United States: Findings from the Centers for AIDS Research Network of Integrated Clinical Systems cohort. *American Journal of Public Health, 103,* 1457–1467. doi:10.2105/AJPH.2012.301162

Momper, S. L., Delva, J., Tauiliili, D., Muehller-Williams, A. C., & Goral, P. (2013). OxyContin use on a rural Midwest American Indian reservation: Demographic correlates and reasons for using. *American Journal of Public Health, 103,* 1997–1999. doi:10.2105/AJPH.2012.301372

Mosher, J. F. (2012). Joe Camel in a bottle: Diageo, the Smirnoff brand, and the transformation of the youth alcohol market. *American Journal of Public Health, 102,* 56–63. doi:10.2105/AJPH.2011.300387

Mullins, R. F., Alarm, B., Hug Mian, M. A., Samples, J. M., Friedman, B. C., Brandiqi, C., & Hassan, S. (2009). Burns in mobile home fires—Descriptive study at a regional burn center. *Journal of Burn Care Research, 30,* 694–699. doi:10.1097/BCR.0b013e3181abff34

Murphy, S. L., Xu, J., & Kochanek, K. D. (2013a). Deaths: Final data for 2010. *National Vital Statistic Report, 61*(4), 1–117. Retrieved from http://www.cdc.gov/nchs/data/nvsr/nvsr61/nvsr61_04.pdf

Murphy, S. L., Xu, J., & Kochanek, K. D. (2013b). Deaths: Final data for 2010: Supplemental tables. *National Vital Statistic Report, 61*(4), 1–12. Retrieved from http://www.cdc.gov/nchs/data/nvsr/nvsr61/nvsr61_04_tables.pdf

National Alliance on Mental Illness. (n.d.). *NAMI comments on the APA's draft revision of the DSM-V substance abuse disorders*. Retrieved from http://www.nami.org/Content/ContentGroups/Policy/Issues_Spotlights/DSM5/Substance_Use_Disorder_Paper_4_13_2010.pdf

National Association of Drug Court Professionals. (n.d.). *13 key principles of a drug treatment court*. Retrieved from http://www.nadcp.org/about-us/13-key-principles-drug-treatment-court

National Association of Drug Court Professionals. (2013). *Adult drug court best practice standards* (Vol. 1). Retrieved from http://www.nadcp.org/sites/default/files/nadcp/AdultDrugCourtBestPracticeStandards.pdf

National Center for Biotechnology Information. (2013). *Rhabdomyolysis*. Retrieved from http://www.ncbi.nlm.nih.gov/pubmedhealth/PMH0001505/

National Center for Health Statistics. (2014). *Health, United States, 2013: With special feature on prescription drugs*. Retrieved from http://www.cdc.gov/nchs/data/hus/hus13.pdf

National Center for Injury Prevention and Control. (2013). *Saving lives and protecting people from violence and injuries*. Retrieved from http://www.cdc.gov/injury/overview/index.html

National Council on Alcoholism and Drug Dependence. (n.d.a). *Alcohol and crime*. Retrieved from http://www.ncadd.org/images/stories/PDF/factsheet-alcoholandcrime.pdf

National Council on Alcoholism and Drug Dependence. (n.d.b). *Alcohol and crime*. Retrieved from http://www.ncadd.org/index.php/learn-about-alcohol/alcohol-and-crime/202-alcohol-and-crime

National Health Promotion Associates. (n.d.). *Botvin lifeskills training*. Retrieved from http://www.lifeskillstraining.com/index.php

National Institute on Alcohol Abuse and Alcoholism. (2014). *Brief intervention for alcohol problems*. Retrieved from http://alcoholism.about.com/library/blnaa43.htm

National Institute on Drug Abuse. (n.d.). *Media guide*. Retrieved from http://www.drugabuse.gov/sites/default/files/mediaguide_web_1.pdf

National Institute on Drug Abuse. (2010). *Cocaine abuse and addiction: Glossary*. Retrieved from http://www.drugabuse.gov/publications/research-reports/cocaine-abuse-addiction/glossary

National Institute on Drug Abuse. (2011). *Prescription drugs: Abuse and addiction*. Retrieved from http://www.drugabuse.gov/publications/research-reports/prescription-drugs/glossary

National Institute on Drug Abuse. (2012a). *Club drugs*. Retrieved from http://www.drugabuse.gov/drugs-abuse/club-drugs

National Institute on Drug Abuse. (2012b). *Drug facts: Understanding drug abuse and addiction*. Retrieved from http://www.drugabuse.gov/publications/drugfacts/understanding-drug-abuse-addiction

National Institute on Drug Abuse. (2012c). *Principles of drug addiction treatment: A research-based guide* (3rd ed.), Retrieved from http://www.drugabuse.gov/sites/default/files/podat_1.pdf

National Institute on Drug Abuse. (2012d). *Principles of drug addiction treatment: A research-based guide* (3rd ed.), *Is drug addiction treatment worth its cost?* Retrieved from http://www.drugabuse.gov/publications/principles-drug-addiction-treatment-research-based-guide-third-edition/frequently-asked-questions/drug-addiction-treatment-worth-its-cost

National Institute on Drug Abuse. (2012e). *Principles of drug abuse treatment for criminal justice populations: A research-based guide*. Retrieved from http://atforum.com/addiction-resources/documents/podat_cj_2012.pdf

National Institute on Drug Abuse. (2012f). *Steroids (anabolic)*. Retrieved from http://www.drugabuse.gov/drugs-abuse/steroids-anabolic

National Institute on Drug Abuse. (2013). *Research report series: Methamphetamine abuse and addiction*. Retrieved from http://www.drugabuse.gov/sites/default/files/methrrs_web.pdf

National Institute on Drug Abuse. (2014a). *Drug facts: Marijuana*. Retrieved from http://www.drugabuse.gov/publications/drugfacts/marijuana

National Institute on Drug Abuse. (2014b). *Drug facts: Methamphetamine*. Retrieved from http://www.drugabuse.gov/publications/drugfacts/methamphetamine

National Institutes of Health. (2013). *Alcohol-related traffic deaths*. Retrieved from http://report.nih.gov/nihfactsheets/ViewFactSheet.aspx?csid=24

National Prevention Council. (2011). *National prevention strategy*. Retrieved from http://www.surgeongeneral.gov/initiatives/prevention/strategy/report.pdf

Nelson, D. E., Jarman, D. W., Rehm, J., Greenfield, T. K., Rey, G., Kerr, W. C., . . . Naimi, T. (2013). Alcohol-attributable cancer deaths and years of potential life lost in the United States. *American Journal of Public Health, 103,* 641–648. doi:10.2105/AJPH.2012.301199

Newcomb, M. E., Birkett, M., Corliss, H. L., & Mustanski, B. (2014). Sexual orientation, gender, and racial differences in illicit drug use in a sample of US high school students. *American Journal of Public Health, 104,* 304–310. doi:10.2105/AJPH.2013.301702

Office of Management and Budget. (2003). *Drug Enforcement Administration assessment*. Retrieved from http://www.whitehouse.gov/sites/default/files/omb/assets/omb/expectmore/summary/10000170.2003.html

Office of National Drug Control Policy. (2013). *2012 ADAM II annual report*. Retrieved from http://www.whitehouse.gov/sites/default/files/ondcp/policy-and-research/adam_ii_2012_annual_rpt_web.pdf

Office of the Surgeon General. (2014). *The health consequences of smoking—50 years of progress: A report of the Surgeon General*. Retrieved from http://www.surgeongeneral.gov/library/reports/50-years-of-progress/full-report.pdf

Paulozzi, L. J., Jones, C. M., Mack, K., & Rudd, R. A. (2011). Vital signs: Overdoses of prescription opioid pain relievers—United States, 1999–2008. *Morbidity and Mortality Weekly Report, 60,* 1487–1492.

Petti, S., Masood, M., & Scully, C. (2013). The magnitude of tobacco smoking-betel quid chewing-alcohol drinking interaction effect on oral cancer in South-East Asia. A meta-analysis of observational studies. *PLos ONE, 8*(11), e78999. doi:10.1371/journal.pone.0078999

Pevzner, E. S., Robison, S., Donovan, J., Allis, D., Spitters, C., Friedman, R., . . . Oeltmann, J. E. (2010). Tuberculosis transmission and use of methamphetamines in Snohomish County, WA, 1991–2006. *American Journal of Public Health, 100,* 2481–2486. doi:10.2105/AJPH.2009.162388

Pomeranz, J. L., Taylor, L. M., & Austin, S. B. (2013). Over-the-counter and out-of-control: Legal strategies to protect youths from abusing products for weight control. *American Journal of Public Health, 103,* 220–225. doi:10.2105/AJPH.2012.300962

Popova, L., & Ling, P. M. (2013). Alternative tobacco product use and smoking cessation: A national study. *American Journal of Public Health, 103,* 923–939. doi:10.2105/AJPH.2012.301070

Pridemore, W. A., Chamlin, M. B., & Andreev, E. (2013). Reduction in male suicide mortality following the 2006 Russian alcohol policy: An interrupted time series analysis. *American Journal of Public Health, 103,* 2021–2026. doi:10.2105/AJPH.2012.301405

Rooney, M., Chronis-Tuscano, A., & Yoon, Y. (2014). Substance use in college students with ADHD. *Journal of Attention Disorders, 16,* 221–234. doi:10.1177/1087054710392536

SAMHSA-HRSA Center for Integrated Health Solutions. (n.d.a). *SBIRT: Brief intervention.* Retrieved from http://www.integration.samhsa.gov/clinical-practice/sbirt/brief-interventions

SAMHSA-HRSA Center for Integrated Health Solutions. (n.d.b). *SBIRT: Screening, brief intervention, and referral to treatment.* Retrieved from http://www.integration.samhsa.gov/clinical-practice/sbirt

SAMHSA-HRSA Center for Integrated Health Solutions. (n.d.c). *SBIRT: Screening page.* Retrieved from http://www.integration.samhsa.gov/clinical-practice/sbirt/screening-page

SAMHSA's National Registry of Evidence-based programs. (2014). *Relapse prevention therapy.* Retrieved from http://nrepp.samhsa.gov/ViewIntervention.aspx?id=97

Sanders, A., & Slade, G. (2013). State cigarette excise tax, second hand smoke exposure, and periodontitis in US nonsmokers. *American Journal of Public Health, 103,* 740–746. doi:10.2105/AJPH.2011.300579

Schimelpfening, N. (2011). *Codependence.* Retrieved from http://depression.about.com/od/glossary/g/codependence.htm

Sheffer, C., Stitzer, M., Landes, R., Brackman, L., & Munn, T. (2013). In-person and telephone treatment of tobacco dependence: A comparison of treatment outcomes and participant characteristics. *American Journal of Public Health, 103,* e74–e82. doi:10.2105/AJPH.2012.301144

Sloan, F. A., & Grossman, D. S. (2011). Alcohol consumption in early adulthood and school completed and labor market outcomes at midlife by race and gender. *American Journal of Public Health, 101,* 2093–2101. doi:10.2105/AJPH.2010.194159

Smart Recovery. (n.d.). *SMART recovery: Self-management for addiction recovery.* Retrieved from http://www.smartrecovery.org/

Smart Recovery. (2014). *Motivational guide and workbook for healthcare professionals.* Retrieved from https://smartrecovery.org/SMARTStore/index.php?main_page=product_info&products_id=42&zenid=2d89f9000c39464 1339efb529588971b

Smith, E. A., & Malone, R. E. (2013). Military exceptionalism or tobacco exceptionalism: How civilian health leaders' beliefs may impede military tobacco control efforts. *American Journal of Public Health, 103,* 599–604. doi:10.2105/AJPH.2012.301041

Spoth, R., Trudeau, L., Shin, C., Ralston, E., Redmond, C., Greenberg, M., & Feinberg, M. (2013). Longitudinal effects of universal preventive intervention on prescription drug misuse: Three randomized controls with late adolescents and young adults. *American Journal of Public Health, 103,* 664–672. doi:10.2105/AJPH.2012.301209

Srebnik, D., Connor, T., & Sylla, L. (2013). A pilot study of the impact of housing first-supported housing for intensive users of medical hospitalization and sobering services. *American Journal of Public Health, 103,* 316–321. doi:10.2105/AJPH.2012.300867

Stahler, G., J., Mennis, J., & Baron, D. A. (2013). Geospatial technology and the "exposome": New perspectives on addiction. *American Journal of Public Health, 103,* 1354–1356. doi:10.2105/AJPH.2013.301306

Stanford Law School Three Strikes Project & NAACP Legal Defense and Education Fund. (n.d.). *Progress report: Three strikes reform (Proposition 36), 1,000 prisoners released.* Retrieved from http://www.naacpldf.org/files/publications/ThreeStrikesReport_v6.pdf

Stockwell, T., Zhao, J., Martin, G., Macdonald, S., Vallance, K., Treno, A., . . . Buxton, J. (2013). Minimum alcohol prices and outlet densities in British Columbia, Canada: Estimated impacts on alcohol-attributable hospital admissions. *American Journal of Public Health, 103,* 2014–2020. doi:10.2105/AJPH.2013.301289

Substance Abuse and Mental Health Services Administration. (2012). *SAMHSA's working definition of recovery.* Retrieved from http://store.samhsa.gov/shin/content//PEP12-RECDEF/PEP12-RECDEF.pdf

Substance Abuse and Mental Health Services Administration. (2013a). *National expenditures for mental health services and substance abuse treatment, 1986–2009* (HHS Publication No. SMA-13-4740). Retrieved from http://store.samhsa.gov/shin/content/SMA13-4740/SMA13-4740.pdf

Substance Abuse and Mental Health Services Administration. (2013b). *Opioid overdose prevention toolkit* (HHS publication No. (SMA) 13-4742). Retrieved from http://store.samhsa.gov/shin/content//SMA13-4742/Overdose_Toolkit_2014_Jan.pdf

Surratt, H. L., Kurtz, S. P., Cicero, T. J., O'Grady, C., & Levi-Minzi, M. A. (2013). Antiretroviral medication diversion among HIV-positive substance abusers in South Florida. *American Journal of Public Health, 103,* 1026–1028. doi:10.2105/AJPH.2012.301092

Talley, A. E., Hughes, T. L., Aranda, F., Birkett, M., & Marshal, M. P. (2014). Exploring alcohol-use behaviors among heterosexual and sexual minority adolescents: Intersections with sex, age, and race/ethnicity. *American Journal of Public Health, 104,* 295–303. doi:10.2105/AJPH.2013.301627

Tanglewood Research. (2013). *All stars: Building bright futures.* Retrieved from http://www.allstarsprevention.com/new/about.html

Teigen, A. (2013). Ignition interlocks: Stalling drinkers. *State Legislatures, 39*(5), 8.

Terry, C. E. (1914/2011). Drug addictions: A public health problem. *American Journal of Public Health, 101,* 448–460. (Reprinted from C. E. Terry. (1914). Drug addictions: A public health problem. *American Journal of Public Health, 4*(1), 28–47)

Thomas, C. M., & Siela, D. (2011). The impaired nurse. *American Nurse Today, 6*(8). Retrieved from http://www.medscape.com/viewarticle/748598_print

Tobacco Control Legal Consortium. (2013). *Regulatory options for snus.* Retrieved from http://publichealthlawcenter.org/sites/default/files/pdf/tclc-fs-regulatory-options-snus-2013.pdf

Toblin, R. L., Clark-Walper, K., Kok, B. C., Sipos, M. L., & Thomas, J. L. (2012). Energy drink consumption and its association with sleep problems among U.S. service members on a combat deployment—Afghanistan, 2010. *Morbidity and Mortality Weekly Report, 61,* 895–898.

Tsemberis, S., Kent, D., & Respress, C. (2012). Housing stability and recovery among chronically homeless persons with co-occurring disorders in Washington, DC. *American Journal of Public Health, 102,* 3–15. doi:10.2105/AJPH.2011.300320

U.S. Census Bureau. (2013a). *Statistical abstract of the United States, 2012: Table 206. Substance abuse treatment facilities and clients: 1995 to 2010.* Retrieved from http://www.census.gov/compendia/statab/2012/tables/12s0206.pdf

U.S. Census Bureau. (2013b). *Statistical abstract of the United States, 2012: Table 207. Drug use by type of drug and age group: 2003 and 2008.* Retrieved from http://www.census.gov/compendia/statab/2012/tables/12s0207.pdf

U.S. Department of Health and Human Services. (2014). *Healthy people 2020: Topics and objectives.* Retrieved from http://healthypeople.gov/2020/topicsobjectives2020/default.aspx

U.S. Food and Drug Administration. (2014). *Electronic cigarettes (e-cigarettes).* Retrieved from http://www.fda.gov/newsevents/publichealthfocus/ucm172906.htm

U.S. Preventive Services Task Force. (2008). *Screening for illicit drug use.* Retrieved from http://www.uspreventiveservicestaskforce.org/uspstf/uspsdrug.htm

U.S. Preventive Services Task Force. (2009). *Counseling and interventions to prevent tobacco use and tobacco-caused disease in adults and pregnant women.* Retrieved from http://www.uspreventiveservicestaskforce.org/uspstf/uspstbac2.htm

U.S. Preventive Services Task Force. (2013). *Screening and behavioral counseling interventions in primary care to reduce alcohol misuse.* Retrieved from http://www.uspreventiveservicestaskforce.org/uspstf/uspsdrin.htm

Vancouver Coastal Health. (n.d.). *Insite-supervised injection site.* Retrieved from http://supervisedinjection.vch.ca/

Veliz, P. T., Boyd, C., & McCabe, S. (2013). Playing through pain: Sports participation and nonmedical use of opioid medications among adolescents. *American Journal of Public Health, 103,* e28–e30. doi:10.2105/AJPH.2013.301242

Weegmann, M. (2008). *Recovery maps guide clients.* Retrieved from http://www.addictiontoday.org/addictiontoday/2008/01/recovery-maps-g.html

Wejnert, C., Pham, H., Oster, A. M., DiNenno, E. A., Smith, A., Krishna, N., & Lansky, A. (2012). HIV and HCV-associated behaviors among injecting drug users—20 cities, United States, 2009. *Morbidity and Mortality Weekly Report, 61,* 133–138.

Wenger, L. D., Martinez, A. N., Carpenter, L., Geckeler, D., Golfax, G., & Kral, A. H. (2011). Syringe disposal among injection drug users in San Francisco. *American Journal of Public Health, 101,* 484–486. doi:10.2105/AJPH.209.179531

White, C., Oliffe, J. L., & Bottorff, J. L. (2013). From promotion to cessation: Masculinity, race, and style in the consumption of cigarettes, 1962–1972. *American Journal of Public Health, 103,* e1–e12. doi:10.2105/AJPH.2012.300992

World Health Organization. (2011). *Global status report on alcohol and health.* Retrieved from http://www.who.int/substance_abuse/publications/global_alcohol_report/msbgsruprofiles.pdf?ua=1

World Health Organization. (2014a). *HIV/AIDS: Injecting drug use.* Retrieved from http://www.who.int/hiv/topics/idu/about/en/index.html

World Health Organization. (2014b). *Management of substance abuse: Abuse (drug, alcohol, chemical, substance, or psychoactive substance).* Retrieved from http://www.who.int/substance_abuse/terminology/abuse/en/

World Health Organization. (2014c). *Management of substance abuse: Psychoactive substance use disorders.* Retrieved from http://www.who.int/substance_abuse/terminology/definition4/en/

Zur, J., & Mojtabai, R. (2013). Medicaid expansion initiative in Massachusetts: Enrollment among substance abusing homeless adults. *American Journal of Public Health, 103,* 2007–2013. doi:10.2105/AJPH.2013.301283

CHAPTER

30 Societal Violence

Learning Outcomes

After reading this chapter, you should be able to:

1. Compare types of societal violence.
2. Analyze the influence of biological, psychological, environmental, sociocultural, behavioral, and health system determinants on societal violence.
3. Identify major foci in health promotion and prevention related to societal violence.
4. Describe approaches to resolving existing problems of societal violence.
5. Discuss considerations in health restoration related to societal violence.
6. Analyze the role of population health nurses with respect to control of societal violence.

Key Terms

aggravated assault
alcohol-facilitated sexual abuse
assault
code of the street
collective violence
community violence
dating violence
domestic violence
domestic violence restraining order
family/partner violence
female genital mutilation (FGM)
homicide
interpersonal violence
intimate partner violence (IPV)
psychological violence
self-directed violence
sexual violence
shaken baby syndrome
stalking
street efficacy
suicidal ideation
suicide
suicide attempt
trafficking
violence

Advocacy Then

Protecting Children from Abuse

Until the late 1800s, there was no systematic protection of children from abuse, although isolated instances of criminal prosecution for egregious abuse occurred periodically. Arguments against intervention included parental rights to raise their children as they saw fit. In 1869, however, the Illinois Supreme Court ruled that punitive action could legally be taken against parents who failed to exercise their parental authority "within the bounds of reason and humanity" (Myers, 2008). Similarly, as early as 1642, Massachusetts enacted legislation that enabled magistrates to remove children from parents who did not care for them properly, but such actions were rare.

In 1866, the American Society for the Prevention of Cruelty to Animals (ASPCA) was formed and provided the foundation for similar protective organizations for children. The first such organization in the world was the New York Society for the Prevention of Cruelty to Children (NYSPCC) established in 1875. The impetus for the society's establishment was the case of a young girl named Mary Ellen, who was routinely abused by her guardian. Mary Ellen's plight was reported by a neighbor to a church worker who sought the aid of Henry Berg, founder of the ASPCA. Berg enlisted the aid of the organization's attorney, Elbridge Gerry. Gerry employed an obscure section of the rule of habeas corpus to file a complaint, initiating the child's removal from the home and criminal proceedings against the guardian.

As a result of the case, Berg and Gerry enlisted the aid of philanthropist John D. Wright in establishing the NYSPCC. The organization's purpose was to

> Rescue little children from the cruelty and demoralization which neglect, abandonment and improper treatment engender; to aid by all lawful means in the enforcement of the laws intended for their protection and benefit; to secure by like means the prompt conviction and punishment of all persons violating such laws and especially such persons as cruelly ill-treat and shamefully neglect such little children of whom they claim the care, custody or control. (NYSPCC, 2000, p. 7)

Through links established with local police, the society was notified of all cases of abuse of children, and the New York State Attorney General and the county district attorney authorized the society to act on their behalf in court proceedings. During its first 8 months, the society rescued 72 children and prosecuted 68 criminal cases. In addition, the society was active in promoting legislation to protect children and is credited with being the impetus for most of the body of modern child protective law (NYSPCC, 2000). It was not until 1962 that child protective services were identified as part of public responsibility with amendments to the Social Security Act (Myers, 2008).

Advocacy Now

Establishing a Women's Shelter

Rates of domestic violence against American Indian women are higher than in the general population. In one small town on the Navajo Indian Reservation, community members collaborated to establish a shelter for abused women. For most of the community and residents of surrounding rural homes or sheep camps, domestic violence was not considered a problem, or was not one that outweighed the daily struggle for survival. However, churches and agencies serving abused women were amenable to taking action and provided volunteers to help with establishing the shelter. Other organizations, including members of the tribal police force, also became allies and were kept apprised of progress (Begay, 2011).

Considerable initial resistance to the project was encountered in the community based on denial of a problem or beliefs that domestic violence was a family issue that should be addressed within the confines of the family. Other sources of resistance included beliefs that the problem of domestic violence stemmed from excessive alcohol use, which should be the focus of community efforts (Begay, 2011).

Efforts began with a campaign to educate tribal elders and convince them of the problem within cultural constraints of respect for authority. These efforts were followed by presentations and discussion in multiple community venues, including the weekly flea market, WIC program office, police departments, and schools. The planning group also sponsored an educational float in the high school home coming parade (Begay, 2011).

Barriers to shelter development included difficulties raising funds and finding a site for the shelter. The latter was complicated by community members' reluctance to have the shelter located in their neighborhoods. The initial shelter site was in a mobile home. Due to funding inadequacies, the shelter was forced to close periodically. Development of policies and procedures was another aspect to be considered, and the community group adopted and adapted policies and procedures from another shelter. Assuring the safety of residents from the local community was difficult because the shelter's location was well known, so women from the local area were transferred to another shelter as soon as possible (Begay, 2011).

Lessons learned from the project included the need for clarity in the mission and commitment from the working group and from other supporters, particularly elders and tribal leaders. Developing community awareness of domestic violence was an early issue that needed to be overcome. Continuous outreach to other individuals and groups and flexibility were also essential as was maintaining the enthusiasm and commitment of those involved. Despite the obstacles encountered, the shelter was established and continues to meet the needs of women in the surrounding area (Begay, 2011).

Violence is a pervasive phenomenon in our society. In part, this is a function of the American heritage and the actions required to carve a nation from a wild and uncivilized land. Violence has historically been seen as a mode of resolving conflict and even of ensuring support of law and order. The vigilante approach to justice on the Western frontier is one example of the use of violence to protect society. Excessive attention to "national security" issues may also be used to justify societal violence and is an outcome that population health nurses can help to guard against by advocating the protection of civil liberties. The World Health Organization (WHO) defined **violence** as the purposeful use of actual or threatened force against another individual or a group that results in, or could result in, harm (Violence Prevention Alliance [VPA], 2014).

In societies in which survival is subjected to physical threats that must be countered by physical force, violent behavior may be more or less of a necessity. Some authorities, however, contend that humankind has failed to adapt to changes in survival needs and has continued to exercise proclivities to violence that are not warranted in today's society. Societal violence has become a global as well as national concern.

Violence may occur in one of three forms: self-directed violence, interpersonal violence, and collective violence. **Self-directed violence** is deliberate behavior directed at oneself that results in or has the potential for injury (Haegerich & Dahlberg, 2011). Self-directed violence encompasses self-abuse and neglect and suicide (VPA, 2014). **Interpersonal violence** involves violence between individuals and includes violence within families or intimate partner relationships and community violence. Family/partner violence includes child maltreatment, intimate partner violence (IPV), and elder abuse. **Community violence** occurs outside of family or intimate partner relationships and may involve acquaintances or strangers; examples include youth violence, assault by strangers, violence in the commission of a crime, workplace violence, and so on. **Homicide**, which is the intentional killing of one person by another, overlaps all of the family/partner and community violence categories. **Collective violence** is violence perpetrated by a group of individuals on another group (VPA, 2014). War, genocide, and political or economic repression are examples of collective violence. Figure 30-1● presents on overview of

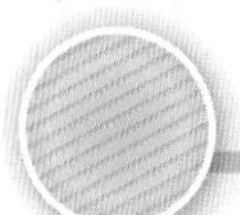

Global Perspectives

Violence Prevention at a Global Level

Violence is a growing global problem. Violence results in 1.4 million deaths per year, or 3,800 deaths per day. More than half (58%) of these deaths are self-inflicted; 36% are caused by others, and 6% resulted from war or other forms of collective violence. Deaths due to violence are particularly prevalent among men aged 15 to 44 years. For every person killed by violence perpetrated by others, another 20 to 40 people receive injuries severe enough to require hospitalization. Similarly for every suicide among people under age 25, another 100 people attempt suicide (World Health Organization [WHO], 2014a).

In 2002, WHO initiated its *Global Campaign for Violence Prevention*. In 2012, the Violence Prevention Alliance established its plan of action for 2012 to 2020. The plan of action is directed toward the achievement of six global goals for violence prevention throughout the world. The first two goals focus on prioritizing violence prevention within the global public health agenda. Goals 3, 4, and 5 address the construction of a foundation for ongoing-violence prevention efforts. The final goal emphasizes the use of evidence-based strategies to prevent multiple forms of violence. The six goals are as follows:

1. Intensify global communication and advocacy for allocation of resources to prevention programs and support for clear violence prevention policy agendas.
2. Enhance integration of violence prevention in global agendas.
3. Strengthen national violence prevention action plans.
4. Increase individual and institutional capacity for violence prevention and provision of services to victims and perpetrators.
5. Promote research and data collection related to violence and its prevention.
6. Implement evidence-based violence prevention strategies, including
    a. Parenting support strategies
    b. Life and social skills training
    c. Initiatives to change social and cultural norms that support violence and to promote nonviolent norms
    d. Reducing access to excessive use of alcohol as a contributing factor in social violence
    e. Programs to reduce firearms-related deaths and injuries
    f. Services to address the consequences of violence and prevent recurrence (Violence Prevention Alliance, 2012)

the types of societal violence. The focus of this chapter is on self-directed and interpersonal violence.

Societal violence seems to be escalating throughout the world and in the United States in particular. In part, the increasing frequency with which violence is reported may be a result of greater recognition of violent behaviors, but the following figures serve to highlight the magnitude of the problem of violence in the United States.

- The U.S. homicide rate is three to five times that of any other Western democracy.
- A violent crime occurs every 23 minutes.
- Someone is murdered every 33 minutes.
- Someone is raped every 6 minutes.
- A child is abused or neglected every 13 to 35 seconds.
- An incident of elder victimization occurs every 3 minutes.
- IPV against a woman occurs every 1.3 minutes and every 6.7 minutes against a man.
- Someone attempts suicide every 39 seconds.
- Someone successfully ends their own life every 16 minutes. (Gellert, 2010)

These factors may actually underrepresent the extent of violence in America. In fact, the Department of Justice estimates that only 37% to half of violent crimes are reported (Gellert, 2010).

Worldwide, violence results in an estimated 1.6 million deaths each year (Centers for Disease Control and Prevention [CDC], 2013). Approximately 55,000 of those deaths occur in the United States (Parks, Johnson, McDaniel, & Gladden, 2014). Violence is one of the top ten causes of death for all age groups from birth to 64 years of age and results in 1.5 million years of productive life lost before age 65 each year (Haegerich & Dahlberg, 2011). In addition, violence results in significant injury as well as fatality. For example, from 2005 to 2010, violence contributed to approximately 388,000 emergency department visits (National Center for Health Statistics [NCHS], 2013b). Dealing with the problem of violence by promoting "injury and violence free living" is one of the national priorities identified in the National Prevention Council's (2011) *National Prevention Strategy*.

Trends in Societal Violence

We will briefly describe features of and trends in the different forms of violence encountered in society. Areas to be addressed include self-directed violence and suicide, family/partner violence, community violence, and homicide.

Self-Directed Violence

Self-directed violence includes both suicidal and nonsuicidal behavior (Haegerich & Dahlberg, 2011). Nonsuicidal self-injury involves deliberately causing physical harm to oneself without the intention to cause death. Self-injurious behavior was discussed in Chapter 24. Cutting and burning are two examples of self-injury that may be employed by young people as a means of coping with emotional pain, anger, or frustration. Self-injury may build to more serious self-aggressive action (Mayo Clinic Staff, 2012). As we saw in Chapter 19, self-injury may also include self-neglect which may be seen among

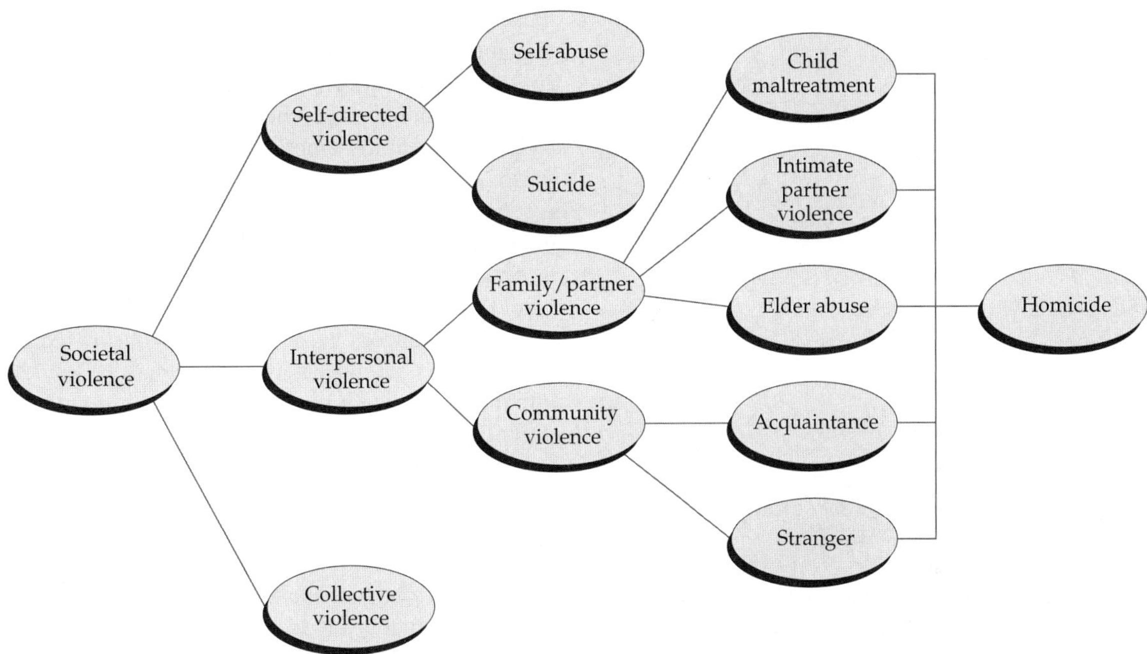

FIGURE 30-1 Categories of Societal Violence

the elderly who fail to address their own physical, emotional, or social needs through inadequate nutrition, shelter, clothing, medication use, or administration of finances (National Center for Injury Prevention and Control [NCIPC], 2014d). Although self-injury is not intended to result in death, those who engage in these behaviors may die as a result of miscalculating the potential effects of their actions.

Suicide, on the other hand, is a "death caused by self-directed injurious behavior with the intent to die as a result" (NCIPC, 2013a, para. 1). A **suicide attempt** is "a nonfatal self-directed potentially injurious behavior with an intent to die as a result" (NCIPC, 2013a, para. 2). **Suicidal ideation** involves thinking about or planning to end one's own life (NCIPC, 2013a).

Suicide rates increased by about 60% in the last 50 years (Demirçin, Akkoyun, Yilmaz, & Gökdoğan, 2011) to the point that suicide has become the tenth leading cause of death in the United States (NCIPC, 2013f). In 2009, suicide surpassed motor vehicle accidents as the leading cause of injury deaths (Rockett et al., 2012). The age-adjusted suicide rate for 2010 was 12.1 per 100,000 population (NCHS, 2014), resulting in 38,000 deaths. Another 1 million people attempted suicide, and 2 million engaged in suicidal ideation (NCIPC, 2013f). On average, 31,000 suicide deaths occur each year in the United States (Degutis, 2013). Suicide is also one of the top ten causes of death throughout the world, with an estimated 10 to 20 suicide attempts for every completed suicide (Demirçin et al., 2011).

U.S. costs for suicide are estimated at $34.6 billion per year. When the costs of lost productivity for lives cut short are calculated, the average cost of suicide is more than $1 million per person. In addition, suicide has long-term psychological costs for survivors of suicide victims. Approximately 7% of the U.S. population knows someone who committed suicide in the last year, and suicide by a family member increases the risk of suicide in survivors (NCIPC, 2013f).

Interpersonal Violence

Forms of interpersonal violence include family or intimate partner violence and community violence. Both will be briefly addressed here.

FAMILY/PARTNER VIOLENCE. Family violence has been defined by Canada's Department of Justice (2013) as "any form of abuse, mistreatment, or neglect that a child or adult experiences from a family member, or from someone with whom they have an intimate relationship" (para. 1). Similarly, Family Law Courts (n.d.) of Australia defined family violence as "violent, threatening or other behavior by a person that coerces or controls a member of the person's family . . . or causes the family member to be fearful" (para. 1). In the United States, the term **domestic violence** is more often used and is defined as a "pattern of abusive behavior in any relationship that is used by one partner to gain or maintain power or control over another intimate partner (U.S. Department of Justice, 2013, para. 1). The definition of **family/partner violence** used here is any form of violence or coercion perpetrated by one family member or partner against another.

Family/partner violence encompasses child maltreatment, elder abuse, and intimate partner violence. In many families, these forms of abuse are intertwined, creating an intergenerational pattern of violence in which children who are subjected

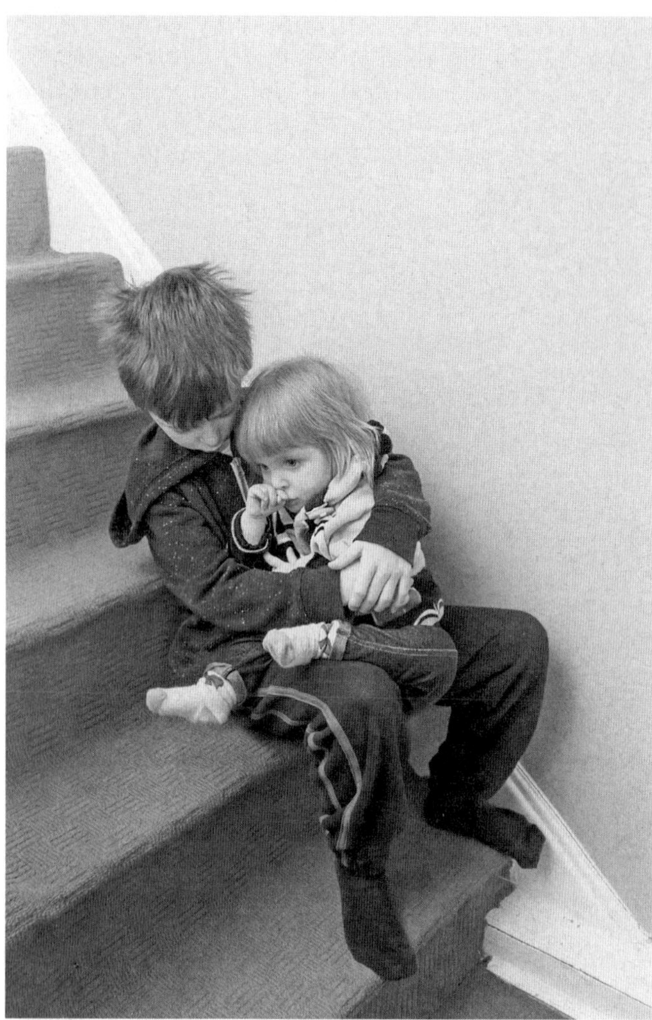

Children exposed to violence in the home experience a wide variety of negative consequences. *(Pixel Memoirs/Fotolia)*

to or witness violence in the family internalize violence as a mode of family interaction. These children may then become abusive or enter abusive relationships in adulthood (Spivak et al., 2014). These abusive relationships may also carry over into care of aging parents, particularly if the parents were abusive themselves.

Child maltreatment. Child maltreatment or abuse was defined in Chapter 16∞ and involves intentional physical or mental harm to a child by someone responsible for the child's welfare including parents, caregivers, or other persons in a custodial role (e.g., a coach, teacher, or clergy person) (NCIPC, 2014b). Child maltreatment includes both acts of commission and omission. Acts of commission are intentional and deliberate actions or words that cause or threaten harm to a child or have the potential to cause harm. Acts of commission include physical, sexual, and psychological abuse (NCIPC, 2014a). Physical violence involves nonaccidental physical injury to a child by a parent or other person responsible for the child's welfare. Sexual abuse encompasses a wide array of sexual activities, such as genital fondling, penetration, incest, rape, sodomy, or exploitation through prostitution or production of pornographic materials. Emotional or psychological abuse involves actions that undermine a child's emotional development or sense of self-worth. These actions may be positive actions, such as engaging in constant criticism, or negative actions, as in withholding love and support (Child Welfare Information Gateway, 2013).

Acts of omission or neglect involve "failure to provide for a child's basic physical, emotional, or educational needs or to protect a child from harm or potential harm" (NCIPC, 2014a, p. 2). In physical neglect, caretakers fail to provide the child with the material requirements for healthy growth. Physical neglect may include failure to feed or clothe a child appropriately. Emotional neglect involves failure to provide a child with the love and affection needed for optimal emotional development. Educational neglect is failure to educate the child or to provide for special education needs. Medical neglect is another aspect of neglect in which caretakers fail to provide needed medical, dental, or mental health treatment (Child Welfare Information Gateway, 2013; NCIPC, 2014a). Abandonment is another form of neglect and occurs when caretakers leave children alone in circumstances that may cause harm or fail to maintain contact with children (Child Welfare Information Gateway, 2013). Finally, failure to provide adequate supervision for children or exposing children to dangerous environments (including drug use) is considered an act of omission constituting child maltreatment (NCIPC, 2014a).

In 2012, more than 3.2 million reports of maltreatment affecting more than 6.3 million children were made to child protective service (CPS) agencies in the United States. Of these, 62% or 2.1 million reports involving 3.2 million children were investigated, and more than 686,000 children were found to be victims of maltreatment. The majority of cases (78%) involved neglect, but more than 18% involved physical abuse, and 9% involved sexual abuse, 7% involved emotional abuse, and 2.2% involved medical neglect. Child maltreatment resulted in 1,649 deaths among children as a result of abuse for a national fatality rate of 2.2 per 100,000 children. Slightly more than 70% of fatalities occurred in children under 3 years of age (Administration for Children and Families, 2012).

Perpetrators of child abuse tend to be family members, typically parents. Other perpetrators include mothers' boyfriends, babysitters, and stepfathers. In 2012, just over 80% of child maltreatment was perpetrated by parents, most of whom were biological parents (Administration for Children and Families, 2012).

Societal costs for child maltreatment are extensive. For example, the lifetime cost for 1 year's worth of confirmed child maltreatment cases was estimated at $124 billion. When lost productivity costs are considered, each death due to child maltreatment costs approximately $1.3 million, and lifetime costs for children who survive are estimated at $210,012 per child, a figure higher than or similar to the lifetime cost of conditions such as stroke and diabetes (Division of Violence Prevention, 2014).

Intimate partner violence. Intimate partner violence (IPV) is defined as violence between two people of the same or opposite sex who are current or past intimate partners (Degutis, 2013). An estimated 1.3 million women and more than 834,000 men experience IPV. In addition 7.7% of women and 0.3% of men report being raped by an intimate partner at some point in their lives (Haegerich & Dahlberg, 2011). Like child maltreatment, there are several forms of IPV: physical violence, sexual violence, threats of physical or sexual violence, and psychological or emotional violence. Physical violence is the intentional use of force with the potential to cause harm and may involve the use of a weapon, restraints, or one's body size or strength to cause damage (NCIPC, 2013c). Physical violence may also be referred to as "battering" (Women against Domestic Violence, n.d.).

Sexual violence involves the use of force to compel sexual activity against one's will. It also includes attempted or completed sex acts against a person who cannot understand the nature of the act (e.g., a cognitively disabled person) or one who cannot communicate their unwillingness. Sexual violence also includes coercion to engage in sexual activity and noncontact sexual acts, such as verbal sexual harassment, being flashed, or being forced to look at sexually graphic materials.

In some parts of the world, sexual violence against women also includes female genital mutilation (Basile & Smith, 2011). **Female genital mutilation (FGM)** includes any procedure involving partial or total removal of external female genitalia or other nonmedical injury to female genital organs. Approaches to FGM may include clitoridectomy (removal of the clitoris), excision (removal of the clitoris and labia minora, with or without removal of the labia majora), or *infibulation* (narrowing of the vaginal opening). FGM may be motivated by social or cultural conventions, efforts to prevent illicit sexual activity, or conceptions of femininity and modesty. FGM is most often performed in African and Middle Eastern countries, but population health nurses may encounter immigrant women who have been subjected to FGM. Although most FGM is performed by unlicensed personnel, WHO has reported that more than 18% of FGM is carried out by health care providers. Consequences of FGM include infection, hemorrhage, urinary retention and infection, cysts, infertility, and increased risk of complications in childbirth. More than 125 million girls and women have been affected in the countries where FGM is most commonly practiced (WHO, 2014b).

Threatening physical or sexual violence also constitutes IPV. **Psychological violence** or "psychological battering" includes

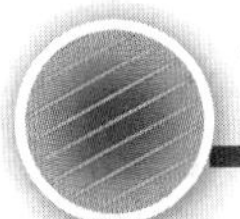

Evidence-Based Practice

Combining Efforts to Address Sexual Violence and HIV/AIDS

International literature suggests that HIV/AIDS and gender violence are twin epidemics resulting from gender inequities in many regions of the world. This underlying cause suggests that approaches to resolving gender inequities can assist in preventing both HIV/AIDS and violence. Two evidence-based approaches have been suggested to address the problem of gender inequity: one focused on empowerment of women and the other focused on changing attitudes and behaviors among men (Dworkin, Dunbar, Krishnan, Hatcher, & Sawires, 2011).

Strategies to empower women focus on changing social and cultural conceptualizations of gender that constrain women in much of the world (Dworkin et al., 2011). Examples of such strategies include the *Intervention for Microfinance and Gender Equity* (IMAGE) program in South Africa and *Shaping the Health of Adolescents in Zimbabwe* (SHAZ). IMAGE combines education for women on gender equity, violence prevention, and HIV prevention with microfinance of women's businesses. The program also includes training on community mobilization for change. The program has been shown to increase participant use of counseling and HIV testing, improved communication with partners and families, and individual and community action related to IPV resulting in a 55% reduction in IPV (Dworkin et al., 2011).

The SHAZ program includes vocational training and microgrants for small businesses, skill development related to HIV prevention and interpersonal communication, development of peer social support networks and counseling, and reproductive health and HIV services. Program results included improved economic status and "relationship power" as well as a 50% reduction in physical and sexual violence (Dworkin et al., 2011).

Because women's ability to even participate in empowerment programs is often constrained by domination by their partners, other programs have focused on masculinity and its effects on the health of men and women. In these programs men are assisted to reflect on conceptualizations of masculinity and their potential to lead to behaviors that put both men and women at risk for poor health outcomes. Viewing current conceptualizations of masculinity as harmful to themselves can lead men to adopt new gender identities that are more conducive to health and may also lead to reduced gender discrimination. For example, the *Men as Partners* program focuses on getting men to question patriarchal attitudes and their effects on family health resulting in more equitable views of gender, particularly with respect to gender-based violence. A similar program, *Stepping Stones*, led to decreases in herpes simplex virus (HSV) infection rates and IPV incidence (Dworkin et al., 2011). Perhaps the most effective response to the problem of gender-based violence would be to combine approaches to address both men and women.

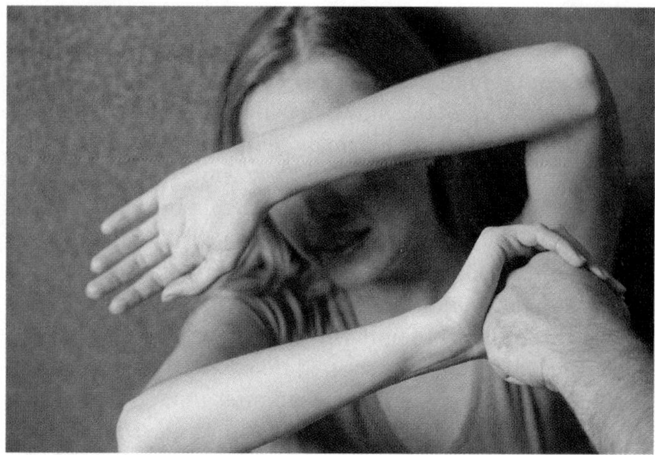

Sexual violence often results from highly traditional gender roles.
(BlueSkyImages/Fotolia)

denigrating the victim, diminishing their sense of self-worth, or socially isolating him or her from others (NCIPC, 2013c; Women against Domestic Violence, n.d.).

IPV is believed to occur in a predictable cycle that includes a period of growing tension in the batterer, culminating in a specific incident of battering followed by a period of remorse and forgiveness (Strengthen Our Sisters, n.d.).

Approximately 24 people per minute experience IPV. This figure is most likely an underrepresentation of the true magnitude of the problem, because many incidents of IPV go unreported. In 2010, IPV accounted for 10% of all homicides in the United States (Spivak et al., 2014). Approximately one in four women will experience some form of domestic violence or IPV in their lifetimes, and IPV is a significant contributor to homelessness among women (National Coalition for the Homeless, 2012).

Stalking is another form of IPV. **Stalking** involves "a pattern of harassing or threatening tactics used by a perpetrator that is both unwanted and causes fear or safety concerns in the victim" (Division of Violence Prevention, 2011, p. 29). Stalking may include following someone, appearing at their home or work place, making harassing telephone calls, leaving threatening messages, or vandalizing their property. Stalking may also employ technological approaches such as text messages, surveillance, and global positioning systems to track victims (Division of Violence Prevention, 2011). An estimated 6.6 million people or 1 in 6 women and 1 in 19 men are subjected to stalking each year. Nearly half (46%) are stalked at least weekly, and 11% have been stalked for 5 years or longer (Stalking Resource Center, 2012).

Stalking may lead to violence, and one in five stalkers uses a weapon to threaten his or her victim. More than three fourths (76%) of women killed by an intimate partner had been stalked beforehand. More than half of these women had reported being stalked prior to being killed (Stalking Resource Center, 2012).

When IPV involves violence that occurs in a dating relationship, it is often referred to as **dating violence**. Nearly one third of high school and college women report dating violence, and dating violence accounts for half of the sexual assaults experienced by women aged 12 to 24 years. Women who have a history of childhood sexual abuse are at higher risk for dating violence than women who were not abused as children (Degutis, 2013). Dating violence may involve physical, sexual, and emotional abuse and stalking (NCIPC, 2012).

The estimated annual direct and indirect cost of IPV is $8.3 billion (NCIPC, 2013b). Mental and physical health care costs may be as high as $4.1 million per year (National Coalition for the Homeless, 2012). Stalking also results in lost worktime and productivity. For example, one in eight stalking victims loses worktime (Stalking Resource Center, 2012). Severe IPV results in the loss of nearly 8 million days of work productivity for employed women and 5.6 million days of lost household productivity (NCIPC, 2013b).

In addition to its economic costs, IPV also has significant health effects for victims as well as for family members who witness the abuse. Health effects are both physical and emotional and include injury, sexually transmitted infections, depression, anxiety, and post-traumatic stress disorder (PTSD). These effects will be discussed in more detail in the section on psychological determinants. Pregnancy is another effect of sexual violence, and pregnancy in the context of IPV may lead to abortion. In a study in one abortion clinic, for example, almost 10% of patients reported a history of physical abuse and 2.5% reported sexual abuse. Most often the violence in these cases was perpetrated by former, rather than current, intimate partners (Saftlis et al., 2010). In another study, IPV was associated with male involvement in a pregnancy ending in abortion and with conflict related to abortion decisions. The authors noted that policies requiring partner consent for an abortion may put women at risk for IPV (Silverman et al., 2010).

IPV occurs throughout the world in all nations and in all social, economic, religious, and cultural groups. IPV is often referred to as *gender-based violence* because in many cultures it arises in part from women's subordinate social status.

Although most people think of IPV as occurring in heterosexual relationships, there is evidence to suggest that IPV also occurs in same-sex relationships (Spivak et al., 2014). IPV in same-sex relationships was discussed in Chapter 20∞.

Elder abuse. As we saw in Chapter 19∞, elder abuse or maltreatment is purposeful physical or psychological harm or exploitation of elderly persons. Elder abuse can occur within families or in institutional settings such as nursing homes and other residential facilities for the elderly. The focus of this chapter, however, is on abuse of older persons within community, rather than institutional, settings.

Excluding financial exploitation, approximately one in ten elderly individuals in the United States experiences maltreatment. This figure probably represents only about a fourth of the actual incidence of elder abuse. In one study in New York State, there are an estimated 24 unknown cases of elder abuse for every known case (National Center on Elder Abuse, n.d.). There are few national studies of the incidence of elder abuse, but in another state study, the average annual rate of elder victimization from 2005 to 2009 was 204.5 per 100,000 population. Half of these incidents involved serious violence against older individuals (National Center for Victims of Crime, 2013).

Several forms of elder abuse occur, many of them similar to the types of abuse found among children and intimate partners. Types of abuse that may be encountered by population health nurses working with elderly clients include physical and sexual abuse, neglect, emotional abuse, abandonment, and financial or material exploitation (NCIPC, 2013h). Physical abuse of the elderly may include injury, inappropriate restraint, or overmedication. Neglect may involve failure to meet physical or emotional needs, failure to attend to medical needs, or self-neglect by the older person himself or herself. Emotional abuse may consist of verbal abuse or disrespect or social isolation. Older clients may also be financially exploited when their funds or material goods are appropriated by others rather than used to meet their needs. Older clients' personal rights may be violated if they are not allowed to participate in decisions regarding their lives when they are capable of making such decisions. Some older clients may be abandoned or deserted by those responsible for their care. In addition, there is an increasing incidence of Internet crime focused on the elderly. For example, people over 60 years of age make 14% of fraud reports to the Federal Trade Commission and as many as 14% may be subjected to identity theft (National Center for Victims of Crime, 2013). Community violence and political violence disproportionately affect the elderly as well as children.

Perpetrators of elder maltreatment are usually family members or acquaintances. In fact, up to 90% of elder abuse is perpetrated by family members, most often spouses (Acierno, Hernandez-Tejeda, Muzzy, & Steve, 2009; National Center on Elder Abuse, n.d.)

In a 2009 national epidemiologic study funded by a National Institute of Justice grant, emotional mistreatment was the form of elder abuse most frequently reported, affecting 4.6% of the respondents. Only 8% of the mistreatment was reported, and more than half was perpetrated by family members—25% by spouses and 19% by children or grandchildren. Physical abuse was reported by 1.6% of the elders in the study. Elders were more likely to report physical abuse to police (31%), and more than three-fourths of the perpetrators were family members. Less than 1% of the elders (0.6%) reported experiencing sexual abuse, but only 16% of those reported it to the authorities. Again, half of sexual abuse against elders was perpetrated by family members, typically a partner or spouse. Slightly more than 5% of the elders were experiencing current potential neglect (defined as at least one essential need not being met, although no one in particular may have been designated responsibility for meeting that need). A total of 11% of the elderly respondents had experienced any of these forms of abuse (Acierno et al., 2009).

In the same study, financial exploitation by family members was reported by 5.2% of the elders. Exploitation was more common among elders who were functionally impaired or those receiving social services whose providers should have been alert to the potential for financial abuse. An additional 6.5% of the elderly reported lifetime experience of financial exploitation by strangers, usually involving fraud (Acierno et al., 2009).

COMMUNITY VIOLENCE. Interpersonal violence also occurs outside of family or partner relationships. Forms of community violence to be addressed here include assault and sexual assault, hate crimes, and trafficking.

Assault and sexual assault. Multiple forms of physical assault take place each day in the United States, with the most extreme form of assault resulting in homicide. **Assault** is defined as "an unlawful physical attack or threat of attack" (Bureau of Justice Statistics, 2013, para. 1). Assault may be classified as either simple or aggravated. An **aggravated assault** is one in which a weapon is used or in which serious injury is inflicted without use of a weapon (e.g., a severe beating). In a simple assault, no weapon is used and no injury or minimal injury results (Bureau of Justice Statistics, 2013). Incidents of rape, attempted rape, and sexual assault are excluded from assault figures. In 2012, more than 1 million aggravated assaults occurred in the United States. These assaults involved more than 1.2 million victims and nearly 1.2 million offenders (Criminal Justice Information Systems Division, 2013b). During the first 6 months of 2013, the number of aggravated assaults decreased by 6.6% from the same period in 2012 (Federal Bureau of Investigation [FBI], 2013).

As we saw earlier, sexual assault not only occurs frequently within family or intimate partner relationships, but also occurs as a form of community violence. In 2012, 73,132 forcible sexual offenses and 6,493 nonforcible offenses were reported to the FBI (Criminal Justice Information Systems Division, 2013b). In the first 6 months of 2013, reports of forcible rape declined by 10.6% (FBI, 2013). Approximately 18.3% of U.S. women and 1.4% of men will be raped at some point in their lives. As we noted earlier, the majority of rape of women in the United States occurs within the context of an intimate partner relationship, but just over 40% of women report being raped by an acquaintance rather than a partner. More than half of men are raped by an acquaintance and 15% by strangers.

Most incidents of sexual violence are perpetrated by single offenders, but sexual violence is often used in civil conflicts, such as war and insurrection, as a systematic tactic to destabilize and demoralize whole populations. For example, over several years of civil war in the Democratic Republic of Congo, an estimated 1 million women and girls have been subjected to sexual violence (Peterman, Palermo, & Bredenkamp, 2011).

Hate crimes. As we saw in Chapter 20∞, hate crimes are motivated by a bias against a particular group of people. In 2012, 1,730 law enforcement agencies reported 5,796 incidents of hate crimes to the Federal Bureau of Investigation. Nearly half of the single-bias incidents (these motivated by a single source of bias) were racially motivated, and nearly 20% were motivated by sexual orientation. Another 17.4% of incidents were based on religious bias, 11.5% on the victim's ethnicity or national origin, and 1.6% on disability bias. Two thirds of racially motivated incidents were directed at Blacks and 22% at Whites. Smaller proportions of incidents were the result of bias against Asians/Pacific Islanders, American Indian/Alaska Native, or people of mixed race (4.1%, 3.3%, and 4.1%, respectively) (Criminal Justice Information Systems Division, 2013a).

Nearly two thirds (59.7%) of religiously motivated hate crimes were directed at Jews, 12.8% toward members of Islam, and 6.8% at Catholics. More than half of hate crimes based on sexual orientation were directed at gay men, and only 12.3% involved lesbian victims. An additional 2% of hate crimes in this category involved anti-heterosexual bias. Nearly 60% of hate crimes based on ethnic bias were directed at Hispanics and the remainder at members of other ethnic groups. Finally, a large majority (82%) of disability bias-motivated incidents involved victims who were mentally ill; only 20% involved bias against physical disability (Criminal Justice Information Systems Division, 2013a).

Trafficking. Trafficking is another form of community violence. **Trafficking** is defined as:

> All acts involved in the recruitment, abduction, transport, harboring, transfer, sale or receipt of persons, within national or across international borders, through force, coercion, fraud or deception, to place persons in situations of slavery or slavery-like conditions, forced labor or services, such as forced prostitution or sexual services, domestic servitude, bonded sweatshop labor, or other debt bondage. (California Department of Justice, n.d., para. 5).

The International Labor Organization has estimated that 12.3 million people, half of them girls and women, are held in situations of forced or bonded labor (Hossain, Zimmerman, Abas, Light, & Watts, 2010). Although there are many forms of trafficking, the most common are forced labor and sex trafficking, and as many as 1.3 million persons may be involved in sexual servitude, 56% of whom are women. Trafficking is a crime in the United States and in many other countries. The Trafficking Victims Protection Act of 2000 makes provision for prosecution of persons engaged in human trafficking and promotes rescue and long-term assistance for trafficking victims (Moynihan & Gaboury, 2013).

Victims of trafficking may be prevented from escape by a number of means, including being illegally confined. Other traffickers use debt bondage, social isolation, confiscation of legal documents, and threats of violence to prevent victims from leaving the situation. Other controlling tactics include threats of shaming, threat of imprisonment or deportation, and control of money (Office of Refugee Resettlement, 2012). Trafficking results in a variety of health and social consequences for victims, including PTSD, depression, anxiety, injury, sexually transmitted infections, pregnancy and abortion, and substance abuse (Hossain et al., 2010; Moynihan & Gaboury, 2013).

A report from the National Academies of Science identified risk factors for trafficking at several levels: individual, relationship, community, and societal. Individual level risk factors include a history of childhood maltreatment, being homeless or a runaway or thrown-away youth, being a member of a sexual minority, and criminal justice or foster care involvement. Relationship factors reflect family conflict or dysfunctional family dynamics. Community level factors include social norms that create a demand for trafficked labor or sexual partners; social isolation; gang involvement; and under-resourced schools, communities, and neighborhoods. Societal level risk factors include lack of awareness of commercial sexual exploitation, sexualization of children, and lack of resources (Clayton, Krugman, & Simon, 2013). For example, in some parts of the world, poverty-stricken families may sell young children into forced labor or prostitution as a means of supporting other family members.

HOMICIDE. As noted earlier, homicide is a form of societal violence that cuts across the family/intimate partner and community categories of violence. For that reason, it is addressed separately. Approximately 37% of intentional injury deaths are the result of homicide (Degutis, 2013). The 2010 age-adjusted homicide rate in the United States was 5.3 deaths per 100,000 population. This figure represents a decline from 5.9 per 100,000 population in 2000 to 5.5 per 100,000 in 2009 (NCHS, 2014). In 2012, 3,943 homicides were reported to the FBI (Criminal Justice Information Systems Division, 2013b). The number of homicides reported from January to June of 2013 decreased by 6.9% from the number of cases reported during the same period in 2012.

Population Health Nursing and Societal Violence

Violence contributes to a variety of physical, psychological, and social problems that can be prevented by population health nursing efforts to modify factors that contribute to violence against self or others. Population health nurses play an active role in responding to societal violence. This role may be enacted in services to individual clients and families or in planning and implementing interventions to control the problem of violence at the community or population level. Control involves use of the nursing process to assess factors contributing to and impeding violence, planning and implementing evidence-based control strategies, and evaluating their effectiveness.

Assessing Risks for and Effects of Societal Violence

The National Academies Panel on the Understanding and Control of Violent Behavior (Gellert, 2010) identified four levels of risk factors for societal violence. These included biological, psychological, microsocial, and macrosocial level factors. Biological factors include hormonal and chemical influences on violence, genetics, and the effects of drug use and traumatic brain injury on cognitive ability and impulse control. Psychological factors include temperament, coping skills, learned responses, and negative emotions. Microsocial factors reflect the influence of encounters and relationships between people. Finally, macrosocial factors include societal characteristics at community or population levels that promote or deter violence. As we will see, these categories of risk factors are encompassed within the discussion of determinants of health as they affect societal violence.

BIOLOGICAL DETERMINANTS. Biological considerations related to violence include both factors that contribute to or protect against violence and those that arise as a consequence of violence. Areas to be addressed include age, gender, race/ethnicity, and physiologic function.

Age. Age influences both one's potential for exposure to violence and the severity of its effects. During 2009–2010, homicide was the 15th leading cause of death for the overall population, but was the 2nd most common cause of death for people 10 to 19 years of age (Kegler & Mercy, 2013). U.S. homicide rates in 2010 were highest among people 20 to 24 years of age at 13.2 per 100,000 population and second highest for those 15 to 19 years old (8.3/100,000). When these two groups are combined, the overall homicide mortality rate was 10.7 per 100,000 people. A shocking 7.9 per 100,000 infants under 1 year of age were victims of homicide, but the rate decreased dramatically to 1.1 for children from 1 to 14 years of age and to 2 per 100,000 for people over 65 years of age (NCHS, 2014).

Infants and toddlers are also at increased risk for injury from abuse. For example, 12% to 20% of fractures in very young children are due to abuse, and premature infants are at greater risk for abuse than infants born at term, possibly due to their greater neediness (Harrison & Vega, 2014). In addition, an estimated 1,300 children experience shaken baby syndrome each year, and death occurs in about 20% of victims (National Center on Shaken Baby Syndrome, n.d.). **Shaken baby syndrome** is a traumatic brain injury that results from violently shaking an infant. Effects include visual, motor, and cognitive impairment (National Institute of Neurological Disorders and Stroke, 2014).

In 2009, 762,940 children were victims of abuse. Three fourths of them (76%) were subjected to neglect, 16.4% experienced physical abuse, 8.8% experienced sexual abuse, and 7% were subjected to emotional abuse. In addition, 2.2% of child maltreatment involved medical neglect. Overall incidence of child maltreatment is highest in 2- to 5-year-olds (25.9% of abuse), followed by 6- to 9-year-olds at 21.5% (U.S. Census Bureau, 2013b). Among the elderly, "younger" elders (those under 70 years of age) are less likely to be subjected to emotional abuse than "older" persons (those over age 70) (Acierno et al., 2009).

The first incident of IPV is also more likely to occur at younger than older ages. For example, 22% of women victims encountered IPV between 11 and 17 years of age, and another 47% before the age of 25 years. The first experience of IPV occurred between the ages of 11 and 17 for 15% of abused men, while 39% experienced IPV for the first time between 18 and 24 years of age. In addition, 21% of women and 31% of men reported their first experience of IPV victimization between 25 and 34 years of age. Overall, 90% of women and 85% of men experience their first episode of IPV before 35 years of age (Spivak et al., 2014). Similarly, most (71%) victims of rape are under 18 years of age and half of those are under age 12 (Basile & Smith, 2011).

The age distribution for suicide mortality shows somewhat different patterns. In one study, people under 30 years of age were significantly more likely than those over age 30 to engage in thoughts of suicide, formulate a plan, and attempt suicide (Crosby, Han, Ortega, Parks, & Gfroerer, 2011). Despite these findings, the highest rate of completed suicide in 2010 was among people 45 to 64 years of age (18.6/100,000 population), then decreased for older ages, to rise again to 17.6 among people 85 years of age and older. In contrast, the 2010 suicide rate for people aged 15 to 24 years was 10.5 (American Foundation for Suicide Prevention, 2014), and for youth 10 to 19 years of age, the rate was 4.5 per 100,000 population (Perou et al., 2013).

Gender. Gender also influences risk of violence. For example, men are approximately three times more likely than women to be victims of homicide (U.S. Census Bureau, 2013a). In 2010, the age-adjusted homicide rate was 8.4 per 100,000 men compared to 2.3 for women (NCHS, 2014). Only among people over 65 years of age are women more likely to be victims of homicide than men (National Center for Victims of Crime, 2013).

With respect to suicide, some research has indicated that women have more suicidal thoughts than men (Crosby et al., 2011), but men have higher rates of completed suicide than women, primarily because men choose more lethal methods for suicide (Haegerich & Dahlberg, 2011). In 2010, the suicide mortality rate for men was 19.8 per 100,000 population, compared to 5 per 100,000 women (NCHS, 2014).

On the other hand, women are more likely than men to experience severe physical and sexual violence related to IPV and are more likely than men to be injured. Women are also twice as likely as men to be killed as a result of IPV. Approximately 24% of women are subjected to physical and/or sexual IPV, whereas only 13.8% of men experience violence from an intimate partner (Spivak et al., 2014). Similarly, women are at higher risk for sexual violence in general (Basile & Smith, 2011), whereas men are nearly always the perpetrators of sexual violence (Black et al., 2011).

Race and ethnicity. Racial and ethnic disparities are also noted in the incidence of particular forms of societal violence. For example, in 2010 suicide rates were highest for non-Hispanic White men at 24.2 per 100,000 men; followed by American Indian/Native Alaskan (AI/AN) men (15.5 per 100,000); and Hispanic, Asian Pacific/Islander, and Black men (at 9.9, 9.5, and 9.1 deaths per 100,000 population, respectively). A similar distribution, but lower rates are noted for suicide among women. Overall, from 1999 to 2010, suicide rates were twice as high for Whites as for Blacks (NCHS, 2013a), with increases of more than 65% in suicide rates among AI/AN populations and 40% among Whites (Sullivan, Annest, Luo, Simon, & Dahlberg, 2013).

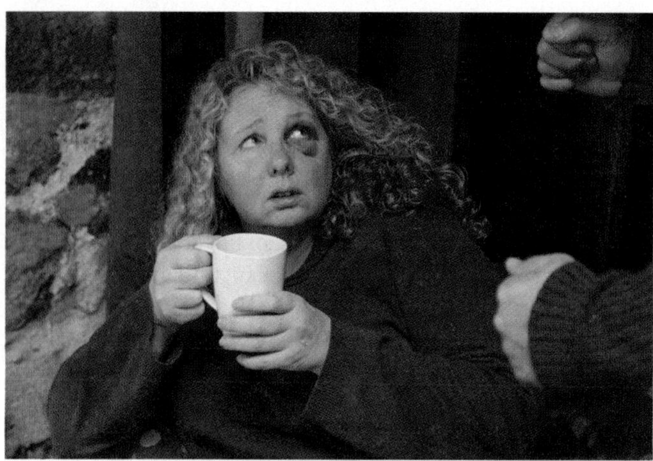

Although both men and women perpetrate intimate partner violence, women are more likely to sustain serious injuries.
(Amyinlondon/Fotolia)

Conversely, homicide rates were highest among Black or African American men (31.5 per 100,000), with rates nearly four times higher than any other racial or ethnic group. The second highest rate was noted for AI/AN men (8.8/100,000), followed by Hispanic men at 8.7, and non-Hispanic Whites at 3.3 per 100,000 population, The lowest homicide rates were noted among API men (2.6/100,000). The distribution of homicide rates by race or ethnicity among women was similar, with the highest rates for Black or African American women, followed by AI/AN women, non-Hispanic White women, Hispanic women, and API women (NCHS, 2014). From 1999 to 2010, age-adjusted homicide rates were four times higher for Blacks than Whites (NCHS, 2013a).

With respect to IPV and sexual violence, Hispanic and AI/AN women have been found in some studies to be at greater risk for rape than other women (Basile & Smith, 2011). IPV has been found to occur in AI/AN women at rates 80% above those of other women, and as many as 65% of urban AI/AN women may be subject to IPV (Begay, 2011). In other studies, approximately 22% of Black women, 27% of AI/AN women, 19% of non-Hispanic White women, and 15% of Hispanic women have been raped at some point in their lives. Among men, 45% of AI/AN men and 40% of Black and multiracial men have been subjected to sexual violence by an intimate partner in their lifetimes (Black et al., 2011). Although racial and ethnic variations in violence occur, studies have found that disparities are explained by a variety of socioeconomic factors, including marital and immigration status and neighborhood social context. These findings suggest that general interventions to improve social and economic factors affecting populations will help to reduce racial and ethnic disparities in the incidence and prevalence of violence. For instance, among immigrant populations, the stresses arising from acculturation and language and economic barriers may contribute to abuse and could also be resolved by improvement in social conditions. Population health nurses can be actively involved in advocacy to improve living conditions for both immigrant and nonimmigrant populations.

Physiologic function. Physiologic status may influence one's risk for violence victimization. Conversely, violence may result in a variety of physiologic effects. Physical illness and disability may increase one's risk of abuse. For example, older persons who need assistance with activities of daily living have been found to be at twice the risk of emotional abuse as those without functional limitations (Acierno et al., 2009). Similarly, poor overall health among the elderly has been associated with greater risk of abuse (National Center for Victims of Crime, 2013) and institutionalized women with disabilities were more likely to report a history of IPV, including sexual and physical abuse, than nondisabled women (National Center on Elder Abuse, n.d.). Physical health problems and disability are also risk factors for suicide (NCIPC, 2013g; Parks et al., 2014).

Violence victimization also leads to a variety of physical health effects. For example, sexual violence may lead to injuries, genital tearing (experienced by 50% to 90% of rape victims), sexually transmitted diseases (4% to 30% of victims), and pregnancy (5%). In addition, IPV may result in a 20% pregnancy rate. Other effects include pelvic inflammatory disease

FOCUSED ASSESSMENT Assessing Biological Determinants Influencing Societal Violence

- What influence does age have on the incidence and prevalence of violence in the population? What is the age distribution among victims of specific types of violence? What is the age distribution among perpetrators of violence?
- Are there gender differences in victimization or perpetration of specific forms of violence in the population?
- What is the racial/ethnic distribution of violence victimization and perpetration in the population?
- Are there physical considerations that place clients at risk for family violence or suicide (e.g., disability, pregnancy)? What is the extent of these conditions in the population?
- Is there physical evidence of abuse?
- What are the physical effects of violence for the individual victim? What is the extent of physical effects of violence in the population?

and other genito-urinary problems (Basile & Smith, 2011). IPV has also been shown to affect endocrine and immune systems as a result of chronic stress, resulting in conditions like fibromyalgia, irritable bowel syndrome, gynecologic disorders, and complications of pregnancy (NCIPC, 2013b). Physical abuse also results in multiple injuries for children and older persons and population health nurses should be alert to signs and symptoms of abuse. *Focused Assessment* questions for assessing biological determinants influencing societal violence are provided on the previous page.

PSYCHOLOGICAL DETERMINANTS. As was the case with biological determinants, psychological factors serve as both contributors to and consequences of violence. For example, caregiver resentment, fatigue, family conflict, and personality traits have been found to contribute to elder abuse. The presence of psychiatric disorders also increases the potential for all forms of violence. For example, major depressive disorder, borderline personality disorder, PTSD, and nicotine dependence have been linked to suicide risk (Bolton & Robinson, 2010). Similarly, other psychological factors such as hopelessness, impulsivity, and aggressiveness may contribute to suicide. Conversely, protective factors include effective coping, problem-solving skills, and conflict resolution skills and knowledge of nonviolent ways of addressing disputes (NCIPC, 2013g). Suicide is often precipitated by mental health problems, intimate partner conflict, or a recent crisis (Parks et al., 2014).

Risk for IPV increases in the presence of low self-esteem on the part of both victims and perpetrators, a history of aggressive or delinquent behavior as a youth, depression, anger and hostility, antisocial or borderline personality disorders, emotional dependence and insecurity, and desires for power and control (NCIPC, 2013d). IPV is also associated with adverse psychological effects, such as depression, suicidal behavior, anxiety, low self-esteem, PTSD, fear of intimacy and inability to trust others, emotional detachment, and difficulties sleeping (NCIPC, 2013b). Sexual assault results in similar psychological consequences. PTSD, in particular, is common, and is more likely to occur in people who experience rape as adults, rather than in childhood, and with forcible rape. Experience of gang rape is also more likely to result in suicide than rape by a single perpetrator (Basile & Smith, 2011). Perpetration of elder abuse is associated with high levels of hostility and poor coping skills, as well as current mental illness in the perpetrator. Exposure to abuse as a child may also contribute to elder abuse (NCIPC, 2014e). Elder abuse may also be the result of caregiver strain or emotional or material dependence on the elder (NCIPC, 2013h). Older persons with dementia may be at higher risk for abuse than those with normal cognitive abilities. An estimated 47% to 50% of people with dementia are abused by their caretakers (National Center on Elder Abuse, n.d.). Psychological effects of elder abuse include fear, anxiety, and distrust (NCIPC, 2013h), as well as lower feelings of self-efficacy and greater psychological distress than in nonabused elders (NCIPC, 2013h; National Center on Elder Abuse, n.d.). Psychological effects of violence experienced by parents may also affect the behavior of their children. For example, the occurrence of a homicide near the home increased caretaker distress and was also associated with decreased attention and impulse control in their children (Sharkey, Tirado-Strayer, Papachristos, & Raver, 2012).

The emotional climate in the family can also contribute to abuse. Families that exhibit increased emotional tension and anxiety, with little display of visible affection or emotional support, are considered emotionally impoverished and are at risk for violence. Similarly, family communication patterns that are non-nurturing, destructive, or ambiguous may also indicate risk for family violence. Couples that experience IPV have been found to have poorer communication skills and less satisfying relationships than other couples. These couples may also be characterized by poor conflict negotiation skills and poor problem-solving skills.

Child abusers may exhibit unrealistic expectations of children, particularly as sources of warmth and love. When they are disappointed in these expectations, abuse may occur. For example, children who are irritable, who cry often, or who do not care to be cuddled may be perceived as rejecting the parent. For parents with low self-esteem, this perceived rejection can set the stage for abuse. Population health nurses can assist parents to develop age-appropriate expectations of their children and engage in strategies that assist parents to recognize and foster normal child development.

Population health nurses can identify risk factors for perpetration of violence or victimization in individuals and families or in population groups. In addition, they can assist individuals and families to deal with the psychological effects of violence. They may also need to advocate for changes in societal perceptions of and attitudes toward victims of abuse to prevent feelings of guilt and diminished self-worth.

Witnessing abuse may also have psychological effects. Consequences of witnessing abuse among children include emotional and behavioral problems, anxiety, poor school performance, low self-esteem, disobedience, nightmares, physical complaints, and aggression. Depression is a particularly common effect of witnessing parental domestic violence, especially among adolescents. Witnessing violence in childhood may also contribute to perpetration of violence as an adult (Haegerich & Dahlberg, 2011). The *Focused Assessment* on the next page includes questions that the population health nurse can use to examine psychological determinants influencing violence in a specific population group or family.

ENVIRONMENTAL DETERMINANTS. Environmental factors may also influence the incidence and prevalence of societal violence. For example, schools have become a source of exposure to violence in today's society. In 2011, for example, 597,500 students 12 to 18 years of age experienced nonfatal violence victimization, with more incidents occurring within than outside of school. During the 2010–2011 school year, 31 violent deaths occurred in schools (25 homicides and 6 suicides) among children 5 to 18 years of age, and 24% of U.S. public

FOCUSED ASSESSMENT Assessing Psychological Determinants Influencing Societal Violence

- What is the level of stress experienced by potential abusers or suicide victims? To what extent are stressors present in the population (e.g., unemployment) that might influence violence or suicide?
- What coping strategies are employed by members of the population? By family members? How effective is coping among members of the population or family?
- Is there evidence of psychiatric disorder in the family? Depression? What is the extent of psychiatric illness in the population and what effect does it have on the incidence of societal violence?
- Are members of the population with mental illnesses subjected to stigma or violence?
- Do potential victims or perpetrators of violence exhibit poor self-esteem? Poor impulse control?
- Is there a negative emotional climate in the setting that might contribute to violence? In the population (e.g., general hostility or feelings of frustration with life circumstances)?

schools reported at least one incident of violence, with 16% reporting incidents involving serious violence (Robers, Kemp, Truman, & Snyder, 2013).

A significant portion of school-related violence is directed at sexual minority youth, but the character of the school environment may have a protective effect for this population group. In one study, for example, gay, lesbian, bisexual, and transgender (GLBT) youth in states and cities with more protective school climates exhibited a decreased prevalence of suicidal ideation. Protective school climates include antibullying policies that address sexual orientation, have active gay-straight student alliances on campus, incorporate information on HIV, STI, and pregnancy prevention relevant to GLBT youth into school curricula, provide safe spaces in which youth can receive support from staff, provide staff training on supportive environments for GLBT youth, and make referrals to offsite providers to meet the needs of this vulnerable population (Hatzenbuehler, Birkett, Van Wagenen, & Meyer, 2014).

The home is another potential environment for violence. Both suicides and homicides occur more frequently in houses or apartments than in any other locale (Parks et al., 2014). Central cities also have higher rates of some forms of homicide than other areas. For example, from 2006 to 2007, two thirds of the 50 largest metropolitan statistical areas (MSAs) in the United States had firearms homicide rates that exceeded national rates, and 86% of center city areas had rates higher than the related MSAs (Kegler, Annest, Kresnow, & Mercy, 2011). Similar distributions were noted for both homicides and suicides employing firearms in 2009–2010, although suicide rates were lower than those for homicides (Kegler & Mercy, 2013). From 2007 to 2009, homicide rates were highest in large central metropolitan counties, and homicide rates for men in these areas were 76% higher than in other locales (NCHS, 2012).

Occupational environment may also contribute to violence. For example, more than 15% of women and 0.7% of men receiving care from the Veteran's Health Administration reported military sexual trauma (Kimerling et al., 2010). Risk for violence also increases in occupational settings associated with the use of alcohol.

One other influence of environment on societal violence lies in the availability of means of suicide or homicide. For example, from 1999 to 2010, there was a more than 81% increase in suicides due to suffocation, a 24% increase in suicides due to poisoning, and a 14% increase in suicides using firearms (Sullivan et al., 2013). Suffocation may result from mixing household chemicals and inhaling the resulting fumes in an enclosed space, or exposure to exhaust fumes in a closed area (McNew et al., 2011).The extent of household gun ownership in a area has been found to be a significant predictor of firearms-related homicide rates. An estimated 1% increase in the number of guns is associated with a 0.9% increase in homicide rates (Siegel, Ross, & King, 2013).

In other locales, jumping from high places may be the preferred form of suicide. For example, falls and firearms were the two most common modes of suicide in 284 incidents in 84 national parks over a period of 7 years (Newman, Akre, Bossarte, Mack, & Crosby, 2010). Similarly, high bridges may be a common venue for suicides. Installation of a bridge barrier on a bridge in Montreal, Canada, effectively reduced suicide rates. Suicides were not found to be displaced to other places because of the iconic value of the bridge as a site for taking one's life (Perron, Burrows, Fournier, Perron, & Ouellet, 2013). Population health nurses should be alert to environmental influences on societal violence and can assess those influences using the *Focused Assessment* questions posed on the next page.

SOCIOCULTURAL DETERMINANTS. Sociocultural factors influence both perpetration of and victimization in societal violence, and risk factors for violence occur at both individual and community levels. Individual level risk factors for perpetration of violence include low educational level, low income, social isolation, association with delinquent peers, gang involvement, family disruption and poor family function, family conflict, unsupportive environments, and poor parent–child relationships

FOCUSED ASSESSMENT Assessing Environmental Determinants Influencing Societal Violence

- Do school environments support or impede violence?
- To what extent do schools incorporate violence prevention strategies into school curricula?
- In what settings does violence typically occur within the population?
- What methods of violence are available within the home or the population (e.g., availability of firearms, iconic suicide locations, such as famous bridges for jumping to one's death)?
- What physical environmental features, if any, deter violence in the population (e.g., bridge barriers, well-lighted streets)? What physical environmental features promote violence (e.g., secluded areas, poor lighting, prevalence of bars and retail alcohol outlets, abandoned building)?

(Haegerich & Dahlberg, 2011). Additional individual risk factors for perpetration of violence include unemployment, marital conflict or instability, and economic stress (NCIPC, 2013d). Elder abuse is associated with caregivers' assumption of responsibility for elder caregiving at a young age, exposure to abuse as a child, lack of formal support, and expectations of caregiving without assistance from others (NCIPC, 2014e).

Risk factors for violence victimization at the individual level include unemployment or retirement among older persons, low household income, and lack of social support (National Center for Victims of Crime, 2013). Having strong relationships with a variety of people and the availability of social support are protective factors against elder abuse (NCIPC, 2014e). IPV risk may be increased by being divorced or separated and by emotional or financial dependence on the abuser (Basile & Smith, 2011).

Family relationships and dynamics may increase the risk for child maltreatment or serve as protective factors. Family risk factors include social isolation, parental lack of understanding of child development, family disorganization, and lack of family cohesion. Negative parent–child interactions and parental stress levels may also contribute to family violence. Protective factors within families include supportive family relationships, nurturing parenting skills, stable family relationships, household rules, and adequate role models outside the family. Population health nurses can work with families to enhance protective factors against violence and to modify those that contribute to violence. For example, the nurse may teach parenting skills or assist with finding employment.

Community or population level sociocultural risk factors for violence include poverty and diminished economic opportunity, residential instability, overcrowding, low levels of social capital, social disorganization, and lack of institutional support. Additional population level factors include a general tolerance for violence and cultural norms that support violence, traditional gender norms and support for male dominance and sexual entitlement, weak laws and policies related to violence, and weak social sanctions against violence (Haegerich & Dahlberg, 2011; NCIPC, 2013d). Other population level factors that influence elder abuse include negative societal beliefs and attitudes toward the elderly, the societal latitude frequently given to their caretakers, and failure to monitor the welfare of elderly community members. Conversely, the availability of support services and respite for caretakers, a strong sense of community cohesion, greater community efficacy, and the presence of effective monitoring systems for older individuals are protective factors against elder abuse (NCIPC, 2014e).

Social networks and attitudes may also contribute to increased incidence and prevalence of violence. For example, membership in social networks of co-offenders (people arrested together for the same crime) that include homicide victims has been shown to increase one's risk of homicide. The closer one's relationship to the homicide victim is within the network, the greater one's own risk of being killed. In another similar study, 85% of gunshot injuries in one community were among members of a single network (Papachristos & Wildeman, 2014).

The social context of violence in some communities reflects a so-called **code of the street**, or informal expectations for interpersonal interaction among various members of the community that both "street" people and "decent" people must adhere to (Richardson, Brown & Van Brakle, 2013). The code relies on the use of violence to acquire, defend, and maintain personal respect within the system. A series of focus groups with violent juvenile offenders in adult prisons indicated that one needed to be willing to engage in violence at any moment to protect and maintain respect leading to desensitization to the threat of violence and belief in the inevitability of violent death (Richardson et al., 2013). Street efficacy is a converse concept to the code of the street. **Street efficacy** is the ability to avoid entanglement in dangerous interpersonal interactions (Gibson, Fagan, & Antle, 2014). While the code of the street necessitates dealing with violence by becoming violent, street efficacy is associated with a decreased likelihood of violent victimization in which youth actively avoid situations where violence is likely to occur. Street efficacious youth are less likely than others to spend time with peers who engage in delinquency and violence (Gibson et al., 2014).

Population level risks for suicide include cultural and religious beliefs that suicide is an "honorable" way out of personal difficulties, easy access to lethal methods of suicide, and unwillingness to seek assistance with mental health problems due to perceived stigma. Conversely, cultural or religious proscriptions against suicide have a protective effect (NCIPC, 2013g). As noted in Chapter 25∞, forced migration is a risk factor for suicide. For example, suicide rates among Bhutanese refugees resettled in the United States were higher than the global suicide rate and were comparable to those of people awaiting resettlement in camps in Nepal, suggesting that resettlement resulted in stressors beyond those that caused migration from their homeland. Some of the stressors identified included language issues, lack of residential and occupational choices, and worry about family members left in Bhutan (Cochran et al., 2013).

The social response to violence also influences its occurrence. Cultural factors, for example, influence the willingness of persons outside the intimate relationship to take action when IPV is suspected. The incidence of abuse tends to be higher in cultures in which family matters are considered "private" and where community sanctions against IPV are weak (NCIPC, 2013d). Being a victim of certain forms of violence may carry with it a level of social stigma that may prevent victims from reporting the violence or taking action to escape it. For example, social stigma attached to rape is often the product of enduring myths such as perceptions that women lead men on, participate willingly in the violation, or make false accusations of rape for their own purposes. Population health nurses can be involved in educating the public to change these perceptions and foster willingness to report and take action to prevent abuse.

Legislation prohibiting violence, protecting victims, and mandating sanctions for abusive behaviors is another social response to violence, particularly family violence. While all U.S. states have legislation related to child abuse, fewer states have adequate legislation and policy addressing IPV and elder abuse. For example, *Futures Without Violence*, a domestic violence advocacy organization, has evaluated state and territorial efforts with respect to six criteria related to domestic violence. The criteria include conducting a state- or territory-wide domestic violence fatality review, mandatory reporting of domestic violence by health care providers, prohibition of insurance discrimination against victims of domestic violence, development of protocols addressing domestic violence, screening for domestic violence by health care professionals, and training of health professionals regarding domestic violence. This evaluation has been conducted three times since 2001. In the most recent edition, only three states, California, New York, and Pennsylvania, and none of the territories or the District of Columbia had effectively addressed all of the criteria. An additional eight states had met five of the six criteria, with the criterion related to screening for domestic violence the one least likely to have been addressed (Durborow, Lizdas, O'Flaherty, & Marjavi, 2013).

Social responses to violence also include the development of support services for victims of violence, particularly family violence. In many U.S. cities, for example, there are safe houses and shelters for abused women, children, and elders. Use of shelters, of course, depends upon the willingness of victims to leave an abusive situation.

Legal alternatives open to victims may also influence response to violence. For example, women may be more likely to seek a domestic violence restraining order or personal protection order (PO) against an abusive partner than to press criminal charges. A **domestic violence restraining order** is a court order that prohibits the restrained person from engaging in abusive activities directed at a family member or intimate partner. Restraining orders and processes for obtaining them vary from state to state, but in many jurisdictions they apply to married or registered domestic partners, divorced or separated individuals, dating or former dating partners, cohabiting partners, or other closely related person (parent, child, sibling, etc.). Depending on the specifications of the order, the restrained person may be prohibited from contacting the person who requested the order or others close to that person, coming to the home or place of work of the person requesting the order, or possessing a gun. The order may also mandate certain behaviors such as support payments, return of property, and so on (California Courts, n.d.).

Research funded by the National Institute of Justice (2011) indicated that restraining orders resulted in decreased abuse and fear of abuse in about 50% of cases, even when the abuser violated the order. POs were also found to save money for justice and social service systems, but ease of obtaining an order and enforcement varied among jurisdictions. Restraining orders may not be as effective among abusers with a history of other criminal activity or juvenile offenders. Similarly, threat of prosecution and the ability to drop charges if warranted provided some protection from further abuse, but mandatory intervention programs for abusers did not seem to be effective in deterring future abuse (National Institute of Justice, 2011).

Restraining orders may also be available to prevent elder abuse and abuse of children. Men subjected to IPV, particularly in same-sex couples, may have more difficulty obtaining restraining orders or other services that are designed primarily to address the needs of abused women. In some jurisdictions, abuse within same-sex couples may not even be acknowledged as IPV (Herek & Sims, 2008). Similarly, although stalking is considered a crime in most jurisdictions, less than a third of states classify stalking as a felony on the first offense, and only half consider it a felony on the second offense or when stalking involves aggravating factors, such as weapons possession or violation of a court order (Stalking Resource Center, 2012).

Another social factor that influences societal violence is media attention. Some authors contend that unbalanced media attention to some types of homicide (e.g., of children or by children) provides the public with an inaccurate view of the problem that hampers their ability to engage in effective problem solving. Others suggest that exposure to media violence is a causal factor in homicide and suicide. The media no longer presents extensive coverage of youth suicides, for example, because of the known effect seen in cluster suicides. The contention is made that similar coverage of adolescent homicide creates inappropriate role models for vulnerable youth. Questions for exploring the sociocultural factors influencing societal violence are included in the *Focused Assessment* below.

BEHAVIORAL DETERMINANTS. Behavioral risk factors contribute to societal violence and may also be a consequence of violence. For example, data from the National Council on Alcoholism and Drug Dependence [NCADD] (n.d.b) indicate that 40% of violent crimes involve alcohol use. In addition, alcohol use is implicated in 3 million crimes each year, including 37% of rapes, 27% of aggravated assaults, and 25% of simple assaults. Approximately two thirds of violent victimizations by a known perpetrator involve alcohol use, as do 1.4 million incidents of violence among strangers. Alcohol use is also a factor in half a million incidents of IPV and 118,000 incidents of other forms of family violence. In addition, use of alcohol is a contributing factor in half of murder convictions among inmates in state prisons (NCADD, n.d.a.). Similarly, IPV and elder abuse have both been linked to heavy alcohol and other drug use and abuse (NCIPC, 2013d, 2013h).

Alcohol use also contributes to suicide, but differentially for different methods of suicide, age groups, and ethnic groups. Alcohol use in general is linked to suicide using firearms, hanging, and poisoning. For young and middle adults, alcohol use is more likely to be associated with use of guns and hanging than among older persons. Among older age groups and members of Asian Pacific Islander groups, alcohol use is more closely associated with suicide by means of poisoning. For Blacks, however, the strongest link between alcohol and suicide method relates to hanging (Conner et al., 2014).

Drugs and alcohol may also be used by perpetrators of sexual violence to facilitate sexual abuse. **Alcohol-facilitated sexual abuse** occurs when someone who is intoxicated or incapacitated due to drugs or alcohol is subjected to sexual behavior to which he or she is unable to consent or refuse (Basile & Smith, 2011). The behavior of the perpetrator in such a situation may be either opportunistic or proactive. An opportunistic perpetrator takes advantage of the fact that a potential victim is intoxicated or incapacitated by drugs or alcohol. In proactive alcohol-facilitated sexual abuse, the perpetrator purposely introduces the drug or alcohol without the victim's knowledge. In either case, the drug or alcohol may either decrease the victim's inhibitions related to sexual activity or may actually incapacitate them rendering them vulnerable to assault. Sexual penetration has been found to be more likely when the victim has been drinking, and perpetrators may be less aggressive when victims are intoxicated. In one emergency department approximately 12% of cases of sexual assault were suspected to be alcohol- or drug-facilitated, and figures have been as high as 18% of cases in other studies. Drug and alcohol use also tend to occur in settings where exposure to sexual predators is more likely (Basile & Smith, 2011).

FOCUSED ASSESSMENT Assessing Sociocultural Determinants Influencing Societal Violence

- Do sociocultural norms support violence?
- Is there evidence of a "street culture" that supports violence as a means of conflict resolution or achieving respect?
- What is the extent of "street efficacy" in neighborhoods with high rates of violence?
- To what extent is the welfare of vulnerable groups within the population monitored (e.g., the elderly)?
- What is the extent of latitude accorded to heads of households or caretakers to control the behavior of others without outside interference?
- What effects do expected gender roles have on violence within families? In the population?
- What is the legal and economic status of women, minors, and the elderly in the population?
- What legislative approaches have been taken to prevent violence? To support victims of violence?
- Is there intergenerational evidence of violence in the family? In the population?
- Are family social interactions positive or negative? What is the quality of social interactions between various segments of the population?
- Do societal conditions contribute to stress (e.g., unemployment, homelessness)?
- Do cultural or religious values influence the risk of violence? Is this influence protective or does it support violence?
- Are there adequate social support networks available to family members? To members of society?
- Are there occupational risks for violence? If so, what occupations are most affected? What features of these occupations increase the risk for violence?
- What is the societal response to violence? What is the media response to violence?
- Is there a perception of social stigma attached to reporting or experiencing violence?
- Is there social unrest in the population that may contribute to increased violence (e.g., war or other social conflict)?

Sexual orientation is another behavioral factor associated with the risk of violence. For example, meta-analyses indicated the lifetime risk of suicide is 2.47 greater for members of sexual minority groups than for the heterosexual population (Choi, Paul, Ayala, Boylan, & Gregorich, 2013). As we saw earlier, sexual orientation and gender identity may put people at risk for hate crime victimization. Experience of physical or sexual abuse by sexual minority youth has also been associated with increased risk of injection drug use and high-risk sexual behavior.

Exposure to violence may also contribute to risky behaviors. For example, sexually abused women have been found to be more likely to use drugs and alcohol than nonabused women (Basile & Smith, 2011). Similarly, sexual abuse of women in childhood has been linked to other negative health-related behaviors such as unprotected sexual activity, multiple sexual partners, early initiation of consensual sexual activity, and participation in sex work. A history of prior sexual abuse has also been associated with smoking, overeating, and failure to use seat belts (Basile & Smith, 2011).

IPV among adult women is also associated with high-risk sexual behaviors, multiple partners, smoking, and unhealthy eating behaviors, such as fasting, purging and vomiting, abuse of diet pills, and overeating (NCIPC, 2013b). A meta-analysis of related research has indicated that victims of IPV, particularly women, are also more likely to smoke than those who are not subjected to violence (Crane, Hawes, & Weinberger, 2013). The *Focused Assessment* below includes questions to identify behavioral determinants influencing societal violence among individuals and in population groups.

HEALTH SYSTEM DETERMINANTS. Health system factors contributing to violence relate primarily to the failure of health care providers to identify clients at risk for or experiencing violence. Providers are generally able to deal with the physical effects of IPV or attempted suicide or homicide but may be less adept at dealing with underlying causes or addressing safety issues. Only a small percentage of health care providers routinely screen clients for risk for violence.

Even when abuse is suspected or confirmed, providers may be hesitant to report findings. Barriers to reporting abuse of older clients also exist. For example, some providers report confidentiality issues, fear regarding the response of the abuser, desires to avoid involvement in court proceedings, distrust of the effectiveness of follow-up, and doubt of their own abilities to accurately recognize abuse as reasons for not reporting abuse. Population health nurses can help to educate providers about the need to identify and report abuse and can help them develop skills in intervening in abusive situations.

Health care providers also often fail to identify clients at risk for suicide. Suicide risk is increased in people with chronic physical illness, particularly illnesses that result in significant long-term pain. This suggests that better disease management for prevalent chronic illnesses could help to reduce suicide. Similarly, better access to care for substance abuse and mental health problems could serve to decrease suicide rates among these populations (NCIPC, 2013g). In addition, victims of IPV and sexual violence have been found to overuse health care services, providing opportunities for alert health care providers to identify problems of violence victimization (Basile & Smith, 2011; NCIPC, 2013b).

In part, the lack of health care provider screening for societal violence may lie in lack of education regarding issues of violence or lack of ability to identify persons at risk for or experiencing violence. For example, health care providers have been found to misdiagnose as much as 20% of fractures related to abuse in children under 3 years of age (Harrison & Vega, 2014). Tables 30-1●, 30-2●, and 30-3● present common physical and psychological indicators of child maltreatment, IPV, and elder abuse, respectively. Even with knowledge, however, providers may be reluctant to address issues of abuse and violence for a variety of reasons (e.g., unwillingness to become involved, lack of comfort in asking about abuse, or lack of knowledge of resources for dealing with abuse).

As we have seen, numerous biological, psychological, environmental, sociocultural, behavioral, and health system factors contribute to the occurrence of violence in individual clients and families and in society at large. Tips for exploring health system factors involved in societal violence are presented in the *Focused Assessment* on p. 927. Tools for assessing individual

FOCUSED ASSESSMENT Assessing Behavioral Determinants Influencing Societal Violence

- Is there evidence of substance abuse in the family situation? What is the extent of substance abuse in the population? How does substance abuse influence societal violence?
- What is the extent of smoking among family members? In the general population?
- Is there evidence of high-risk sexual behavior by family members? In the general population?
- To what extent does sexual orientation or gender identity contribute to risk for violence in the individual or population?
- To what extent do members of the population engage in other behaviors that might lead to violence (e.g., bullying, carrying weapons)?

FOCUSED ASSESSMENT Assessing Health System Determinants Influencing Societal Violence

- Are health care providers alert to risk for or evidence of violence? To what extent do health care providers screen for risk for or evidence of violence perpetration or victimization?
- What is the response of health care providers to evidence of violence or potential for violence?
- To what extent does the health care system provide for support and care of victims of societal violence? For perpetrators of violence?
- To what extent do victims of violence use health care services?

TABLE 30-1 Physical and Psychological Indications of Child Maltreatment

Type of Abuse	Physical Indications	Psychological Indications
Neglect	Persistent hunger Poor hygiene Inappropriate dress for the weather Constant fatigue Unattended physical health problems Poor growth patterns	Delinquency due to lack of supervision School truancy/poor school performance Begging or stealing food Behavior problems
Physical abuse	Bruises or welts in unusual places or in several stages of healing; distinctive shapes Burns (especially cigarette burns; immersion burns of hands, feet, or buttocks; rope burns; or distinctively shaped burns) Fractures (multiple or in various stages of healing, inconsistent with explanations of injury) Joint swelling or limited mobility Long-bone deformities Lacerations and abrasions to the mouth, lip, gums, eye, genitalia Human bite marks Signs of intracranial trauma Deformed or displaced nasal septum Bleeding or fluid drainage from the ears or ruptured eardrums Broken, loose, or missing teeth Difficulty in respirations, tenderness or crepitus over ribs Abdominal pain or tenderness Recurrent urinary tract infection	Wary of physical contact with adults Behavioral extremes of withdrawal or aggression Apprehensive when other children cry Inappropriate response to pain
Emotional abuse	Nothing specific	Overly compliant, passive, and undemanding Extremely aggressive, demanding, or angry Behavior inappropriate for age (either overly adult or overly infantile) Developmental delay Attempted suicide
Sexual abuse	Torn, stained, or bloody underwear Pain or itching in genital areas Bruises or bleeding from external genitalia, vagina, rectum Sexually transmitted diseases Swollen or red cervix, vulva, or perineum Semen around the mouth or genitalia or on clothing Pregnancy	Withdrawn Engages in fantasy behavior or infantile behavior Poor peer relationships Unwilling to participate in physical activities Wears long sleeves and several layers of clothes even in hot weather Delinquency or running away Inappropriate sexual behavior or mannerisms

TABLE 30-2 Physical and Psychological Indications of Intimate Partner Violence

Physical Indications	Psychological Indications
Chronic fatigue Vague complaints, aches, and pains Frequent injuries Recurrent sexually transmitted diseases Muscle tension Facial lacerations Injuries to chest, breasts, back, abdomen, or genitalia Bilateral injuries of arms or legs Symmetric injuries Obvious patterns of belt buckles, bite, fist, or hand marks Burns of hands, feet, buttocks, or with distinctive patterns Headaches Ulcers	Casual response to a serious injury or excessively emotional response to a relatively minor injury Frequent ambulatory or emergency room visits Nightmares Depression Anxiety Anorexia or other eating disorder Drug or alcohol abuse Poor self-esteem Suicide attempts

TABLE 30-3 Physical and Psychological Indications of Elder Maltreatment

Type of Abuse	Physical Indications	Psychological Indications
Neglect	Constant hunger or malnutrition Poor hygiene Inappropriate dress for the weather Chronic fatigue Unattended medical needs Poor skin integrity or decubiti Contractures Urine burns/excoriation Dehydration Fecal impaction	Listlessness Social isolation
Emotional abuse	Hypochondria	Habit disorder (biting, sucking, rocking) Destructive or antisocial conduct Neurotic traits (sleep or speech disorder, inhibition of play) Hysteria Obsessions or compulsions Phobias
Physical abuse	Bruises and welts Burns Fractures Sprains or dislocations Lacerations or abrasions Evidence of oversedation	Withdrawal Confusion Fear of caretaker or other family members Listlessness
Sexual abuse	Difficulty walking Torn, stained, or bloody underwear Pain or itching in genital area Bruises or bleeding on external genitalia or in vaginal or anal areas Sexually transmitted diseases	Withdrawal
Financial abuse	Inappropriate clothing Unmet medical needs	Failure to meet financial obligations Anxiety over expenses
Denial of rights	Nothing specific	Hesitancy in making decisions Listlessness and apathy

risk for family violence and suicide are also provided on the student resources site.

Population health nursing assessment related to societal violence may entail identification of risk factors at individual/family or population levels. For example, nurses working with families would assess them for factors in each of the six dimensions of health that increases their risk for family violence, suicide, or homicide. In addition, nurses would be alert to the signs and symptoms of actual family/partner violence presented in Tables 30-1, 30-2, and 30-3 or signs of impending suicide. At the community or population level, nurses would identify risk factors that lend themselves to high incidence and prevalence of societal violence. For example, they would identify unemployment or other causes of social stress (e.g., homelessness, racial/ethnic tension) as risk factors for social violence. Information on risk factors for and the incidence and prevalence of violence would be used to derive nursing diagnoses and to plan strategies to minimize or control societal violence.

Diagnostic Reasoning and Societal Violence

Nursing diagnoses may be derived from assessment data related to individual clients and families or population groups. An example of a nursing diagnosis for an individual client might be "potential for child abuse due to increased stress of single parenthood and care of a disabled child." A population-based diagnosis might be "increased potential for violence due to prevalence of weapons carrying among high school students."

Planning and Implementing Control Strategies for Societal Violence

Population health nurses are actively involved in planning control strategies for societal violence related to health promotion, prevention, resolution of existing problems, and health restoration. Some interventions at each level are discussed below.

HEALTH PROMOTION. Health promotion related to societal violence involves development of effective coping skills in individuals and adoption of nonviolent conflict resolution strategies by individuals and groups of people. Specific strategies at the population level might include teaching effective coping, conflict resolution, and anger management strategies within school curricula. Similar strategies might be used to develop healthy coping skills and aversion to violence in individuals and families.

Increasing aversion to violence may be accomplished by teaching alternative methods of conflict resolution and by imposing cultural and social sanctions against violent behavior. For example, in societies in which violence is not perceived as an acceptable approach to interpersonal conflict, less violence occurs. Similarly, strong religious convictions may deter attempted suicide. Population health nurses can be actively involved in teaching positive modes of conflict resolution, anger management, and coping strategies and in activities designed to change societal attitudes toward the acceptability of violence.

Population health nurses can also assist clients and families at risk to develop effective parent–child and intimate partner relationships by providing anticipatory guidance, assistance with communication, and so on. For instance, the nurse can educate new parents about child behavioral cues and appropriate parental responses as well as provide reinforcement for positive responses. In addition, the nurse can suggest activities that will enhance the bond between parents and child (e.g., reading to or playing with the child), and educate parents regarding appropriate forms of discipline.

PREVENTION. A public health approach to violence prevention encompasses four major activities: monitoring the incidence and burden of violence over time, identifying contributing and protective factors, developing and testing control strategies to address those factors, and disseminating and promoting adoption and adaptation of effective strategies in families, communities, and populations (Haegerich & Dahlberg, 2011).

Several general evidence-based strategies have been developed to prevent each of the types of violence discussed in this chapter. For example, family support and parenting programs and hospital-based programs to educate new parents on crying and its management have been shown to be effective in reducing child maltreatment, particularly for young children. Similarly, school-based programs to develop social and emotional skills coupled with intensive family and community-based approaches have reduced youth violence. Street-level outreach and conflict mediation strategies among violent youth have also been found to be effective (Haegerich & Dahlberg, 2011).

Effective prevention programs for IPV have included school-based curricula focusing on healthy interpersonal relationships and social norms that inhibit violence as a mode of conflict resolution. Screening for and amelioration of risk factors for violence perpetration or victimization have also been effective in reducing IPV. Similarly, school-based programs focused on healthy relationships and changing social norms have been shown to reduce the incidence of sexual violence (Haegerich & Dahlberg, 2011). Prevention of sexual violence needs to start early with efforts to promote healthy and respectful relationships in families, foster healthy parent–child relationships, and create supportive family environments. Several effective programs have been found to decrease IPV. Examples include the "Start Strong: Building Healthy Teen Relationships Initiative" (Spivak et al., 2014) and "Safe Dates" programs designed to change social norms related to sexual violence and improve problem-solving skills in youth (NCIPC, 2012). These and similar school-based programs have been found to reduce violence among high-school students by as much as 29% and by 15% across all grade levels (NCIPC, 2013e). For further information about the Start Strong and Safe Dates programs, see the *External Resources* section of the student resources site.

Prevention of child maltreatment may employ similar strategies. For example, child–parent centers provide support to economically disadvantaged families focusing on a child-centered approach to services. Such services resulted in a 52% decline in child maltreatment in one study. Similarly, the "Durham Family Initiative" coordinates services to families at high risk for child maltreatment and has resulted in a 57% decline in incidence in the affected county compared to other counties without similar services. Comparable results in decreasing child maltreatment have been noted for other similar programs such as the "Nurse-Family Partnership" program, the "Triple P: Positive Parenting Program," and the "Safe Environment for Every Kid" (SEEK) program (NCIPC, 2014c). For more information about the these programs, see the *External Resources* section of the student resources site. Population health nurses may be involved in providing services through these and other similar programs or may refer families at risk for child maltreatment to appropriate services and programs.

Prevention strategies for elder abuse include listening to elders and their caregivers and addressing their needs. Population health nurses can also encourage both elders and caregivers to seek help and refer them to appropriate services that can minimize the stress of caregiving (NCIPC, 2013h). They may also refer elders to day care centers or assist caregivers to access respite services. Population health nurses may also need to advocate for the availability of such services.

Evidence-based prevention measures for self-directed violence include screening for risk in health care settings, suicide awareness programs in schools, reduced stigma attached to sexual minority membership and mental illness, and restriction of access to lethal means of suicide (Haegerich & Dahlberg, 2011). Programs such as the U.S. Air Force Suicide Prevention Program focus on early recognition and treatment of people at high risk for suicide. Other foci include education and reduction of stigma attached to seeking help. The program is designed to normalize feelings of distress, promote effective coping skills, and eliminate negative career consequences of help seeking and treatment (Knox et al., 2010). The Youth Suicide Prevention Program has developed suicide prevention curricula for elementary, middle, and high school students as well as community programs and initiatives targeted to particularly vulnerable populations such as sexual minority youth (Youth Suicide Prevention Program, n.d.). See the *External Resources* section of the student resources site for sources of information about these programs.

Population health nurses can also help to remove or reduce factors that contribute to stress and the potential for abuse. For example, the nurse might refer caretakers of an elderly client or a child with disabilities for respite services, assist an unemployed parent to find employment, or increase social support networks for socially isolated families. Treatment of substance abuse problems in the individual or family may also decrease the potential for violence. Crisis intervention and hotlines may also prevent suicide.

Decreasing access to weapons has also been suggested as a preventive measure for violence, but the Community Preventive Services Task Force (CPSTF, 2014) has found insufficient evidence that firearms control legislation prevents violence. The task force examined such approaches as bans on specific types of weapons, waiting periods before purchase, purchase restrictions, registration and licensing of firearms, prevention of child access to firearms, and zero tolerance policies in schools and found insufficient evidence to recommend any of them as major foci for violence prevention. Other research has indicated that weapons control is an effective measure against violence in specific circumstances. For example, easy access to firearms has been found to increase the risk of murder by perpetrators of IPV. Federal law prohibits the purchase or possession of firearms by persons convicted of IPV who are under a restraining order. Ten states require and another 20 states authorize courts to order respondents to restraining orders to surrender their firearms for the duration of the order. A California program uses a variety of data sources to identify perpetrators of IPV who own firearms, which are then confiscated under the terms of a restraining order. Such programs have been shown to decrease retaliatory homicides against family members seeking restraining orders (Wintemute, Frattaroli, Claire, Vittes, & Webster, 2014).

Environmental measures to deter suicide include placing barriers at iconic jumping locations (Perron et al., 2013). Recommendations have also been made to erect site-specific suicide barriers in National Parks with a high incidence of suicide (Newman et al., 2010).

Older clients may use several options to safeguard their funds and property from financial abuse. Some of these options include a financial representative trust, durable power of attorney, and joint tenancy. In a *financial representative trust*, the older person transfers to a trustee, selected by himself or herself, responsibility for managing his or her property. A

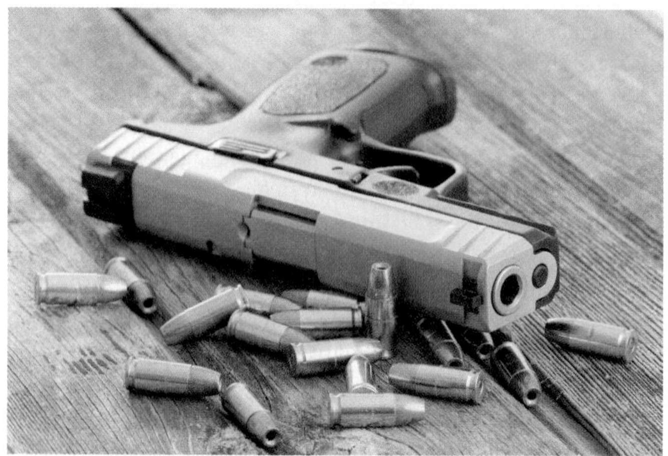

Easy access to lethal weapons contributes to violence-related deaths. *(Oocoskun/Fotolia)*

durable power of attorney is a written document in which the older person grants another person the authority to handle financial matters in his or her stead. In *joint tenancy*, the older person is co-owner of the assets covered with one or more designated others. All parties involved have the use of funds or property covered under joint tenancy. In the event of the death of one party, ownership automatically devolves on other members of the joint tenancy agreement. Each of these options has advantages and disadvantages and population health nurses would be best advised to refer older clients to reputable sources of legal and financial information to assist them in selecting options to protect themselves from financial abuse. Health promotion strategies and prevention strategies related to elder abuse and other forms of societal violence are summarized in Table 30-4●.

RESOLVING EXISTING PROBLEMS OF VIOLENCE. Resolving existing problems related to family/partner violence involves identification of abuse and treatment for its immediate effects. Many victims of abuse choose not to identify themselves or report the abuse for a variety of reasons. Female victims of IPV, for example, may fear additional violence. In other cases, victims may feel stigmatized or wish to protect the abuser.

Identification requires screening for those at risk for or experiencing abuse, and routine screening for abuse has been suggested in emergency departments, women's health clinics, and primary care settings. Workplace screening programs have also been suggested, and population health nurses can be involved in designing and implementing screening programs in the work setting and other venues.

Screening for family/partner violence should be conducted when the client is alone using any of a variety of screening tools. Available tools deal with different issues depending on client characteristics (Sheridan, Nash, Hawkins, Makely, & Campbell, 2013). For example, screening tools for the elderly or disabled individual would include questions about the withholding of needed care or financial abuse in addition to asking about other forms of abuse. Tools for IPV and child maltreatment would address psychological as well as physical and sexual abuse. Child maltreatment screening tools would also explore issues of neglect.

A variety of screening tools have been developed for screening for IPV, most of them directed toward women. NCIPC has published a compendium of assessment tools for IPV screening. For further information about these tools, see the *External Resources* section of the student resources site. Information resources for elder abuse screening tools are also provided.

In 2012, the U.S. Preventive Services Task Force updated its 2004 recommendation related to IPV screening. The previous recommendation had indicated insufficient evidence that screening for IPV was effective in reducing the incidence and prevalence of abuse. The updated recommendation, however, indicates that "screening instruments accurately identify women experiencing IPV" and their use is unlikely to result in adverse effects (Nelson, Bougatsos, & Blazina, 2012, p. 796).

Similarly, the task force found insufficient evidence for the effectiveness of screening for abuse in older clients (Moyer, 2013). Another systematic review by Caldwell, Gilden, and Mueller (2013) found a growing body of evidence that suggests that routine screening for abuse among the elderly is an effective intervention. Once evidence of family/partner violence has been detected, treatment focuses on assessing the client for immediate danger, providing appropriate care for the consequences of violence, documenting the client's condition, developing a safety plan, and making needed referrals to community services. Management of IPV should include assurances that the client is not alone, that he or she is not at fault for the abuse, and that confidentiality of information shared is dependent upon applicable state laws. Injuries must be thoroughly documented, with photographs, if possible. In addition, the victim should be educated regarding available resources and options, including resources, and should be assisted to develop a safety plan for himself or herself or other family members threatened by violence. This may include children who may be harmed by witnessing abuse even if they are not abused themselves. Elements of a safety plan should include hiding money and extra keys, establishing a secret code with friends or family members, asking neighbors to call the police in the event of an altercation, removing weapons from the home, and putting copies of important documents in a handy and secure location. Documents may include Social Security numbers (for the victim and children as well as the abuser), rent and utility receipts, birth certificates and marriage license if relevant, driver's license or other identification (e.g., a passport), bank account and insurance policy numbers, jewelry and other easily transported valuables, names and telephone numbers of important contacts, extra clothing, and essential toiletries. Population health nurses can assist clients at risk for family/partner violence in developing a safety plan and in identifying sources of assistance.

Intervention may include referring an abused family member to a shelter or removing a dependent victim from the abusive situation. Resolution at this point also includes treatment for the perpetrator of violence and for family members who witness violence. Resources may need to be developed to address the needs of male as well as female victims of violence. In addition, criminal justice systems must provide equitable treatment for victims of abuse, whether they are men or women. Population health nurses can advocate for equitable enforcement of laws prohibiting violence as well as for legislation that protects victims from abuse and assures the availability of resources to both victims and perpetrators.

Resolution of violence also involves mandatory reporting of suspected child maltreatment and, in some jurisdictions, reporting of IPV or elder abuse. Reports are generally made initially by telephone to the appropriate agency and are followed,

TABLE 30-4 Individual/Family-Oriented and Population-Oriented Health Promotion and Prevention Strategies Related to Societal Violence

Health Promotion Focus	Individual/Family-Oriented Strategies	Population-Oriented Strategies
Development of effective coping skills	• Teach coping and stress management skills to individuals and families.	• Teach coping and stress management skills to population groups. • Advocate for inclusion of coping and stress management in school curricula.
Development of self-esteem	• Foster self-image.	• Advocate for school programs to foster self-esteem in young people.
Development of realistic expectations of self and others	• Educate parents on child development. • Educate caregivers on the needs of the elderly. • Help clients recognize strengths.	• Educate the public regarding developmental expectations. • Advocate for and implement parenting education programs. • Develop and implement caregiver education programs.
Development of effective parenting and interpersonal skills	• Teach parenting skills. • Teach and role model effective communication skills. • Refer families with communication difficulties for counseling assistance.	• Advocate for communication education in school curricula. • Advocate for and implement parenting education programs. • Advocate for available counseling services to improve family communication.
Promotion of nonviolent conflict resolution	• Teach nonviolent conflict management strategies.	• Advocate for inclusion of conflict management content in school curricula and other education programs.
Prevention Focus	**Individual/Family-Oriented Strategies**	**Population-Oriented Strategies**
Treatment of psychopathology or substance abuse	• Refer for treatment.	• Advocate for available and accessible treatment services.
Provision of emotional and material support	• Refer to sources of assistance as needed. • Assist in development and expansion of social support networks.	• Advocate for supportive services for persons at risk for violence perpetration or victimization. • Advocate for societal changes to minimize sources of stress contributing to violence.
Reduction of risk behaviors	• Encourage clients not to frequent places where violence is likely to occur. • Encourage clients not to use alcohol or drugs in circumstances in which interpersonal conflict is likely.	• Educate the public on the influence of drugs and alcohol on violence. • Advocate for adequate police protection in high crime areas. • Advocate for social mores to promote early intervention to prevent escalation of conflict to violent behaviors.
Decreased availability of weapons, drugs, and alcohol	• Encourage removal of weapons from homes. • Encourage responsible alcohol use.	• Engage in political activity to promote weapons control and limit access to drugs and alcohol.
Change in societal attitudes to violence	• Teach nonviolent modes of conflict resolution. • Teach problem-solving and decision-making skills. • Discuss appropriate approaches to discipline.	• Develop and implement campaigns to change cultural perceptions of violence as a means of conflict resolution.
Development of policies that discourage violence and protect potential victims		• Engage in political activity and advocacy. • Promote positive attitudes toward the elderly and disabled. • Advocate for women's social rights.

usually within 48 hours, by a written report. In making a report, the population health nurse should be careful to focus on objective evidence that suggests violence victimization and to report exactly what he or she has seen or verbatim reports of those involved.

When IPV involves sexual assault or rape, or when such events occur outside intimate relationships, population health nurses should refer victimized clients to a local emergency department for assessment. Most emergency departments have sexual assault response teams (SART) or sexual assault nurse examiners (SANE nurses) that have extensive background in assessment and care of persons who have been sexually assaulted. Members of SART teams and SANE nurses also have expertise in the collection of forensic evidence that may be used in criminal proceedings against the abuser (International Association of Forensic Nurses & American Nurses Association, 2009). SANE nurses also provide emotional support, emergency contraception, STI or injury treatment, education regarding HIV and pregnancy risk, and practical assistance with clothing, transportation, and safety planning (Basile & Smith, 2011). Population health nurses should encourage victims of sexual abuse and other forms of IPV to report the event and to seek help in an emergency department. Clients should be particularly cautioned not to "clean themselves up" following the assault as this destroys physical evidence of the assault.

Programs to prevent violence by chronically delinquent youth have shown some success. Therapeutic foster care is one such program and is recommended by the Community Preventive Services Task Force (2014). Therapeutic foster care is an approach in which young people with emotional, behavioral, physical, or developmental needs unable to be met within their own families are placed with a foster family with special training in providing a structured environment that fosters the development of social and emotional skills (Northern Virginia Family Services, 2014; Oklahoma Department of Health Services, 2014). Foster parents receive intensive training in dealing with youth with special needs and become part of the treatment team to meet those needs. Goals of therapeutic foster care include community integration of services, meeting the health care needs of the child, eliminating inappropriate behaviors, and supporting the child's educational needs (Friends of Youth, n.d.). Based on evaluation of the effectiveness of therapeutic foster care, the Community Preventive Services Task Force has recommended this intervention for use in preventing violence among youth (CPSTF, 2014). Such programs may be used in place of incarceration for juvenile offenders and are more effective. Similarly, research has indicated that programs developed for violent offenders in juvenile justice settings are not appropriate for juveniles held in adult correctional facilities (Richardson et al., 2013). Population health nurses may be involved in the establishment of therapeutic foster care programs or in providing support to foster parents and their young charges.

Much of the nursing research related to IPV and other forms of societal violence is directed toward identifying contributing factors and responses of and effects on victims or witnesses, with few controlled studies of the effectiveness of interventions. Recent research, however, has demonstrated the effectiveness of integrated treatment for substance abuse and IPV among substance-abusing perpetrators (Kraanen, Vedel, Scholing, & Emmelkamp, 2013). Similarly, a telephone intervention providing personalized feedback on factors contributing to IPV among substance-abusing men has demonstrated some effectiveness in reducing IPV perpetration (Mbillinyi et al., 2011).

A systematic review of interventions with victims of domestic violence suggested that brief interventions that included specific foci were effective in addressing the needs of survivors. The recommended foci included provision of information on the dynamics of IPV and safety concerns, development of cognitive reframing and survival skills, culturally competent interventions, promoting social connections, and individualization to specific survivor needs (Warshaw, Sullivan, & Rivera, 2013).

Resolution of problems related to societal violence also involves the early identification of persons who are contemplating suicide or homicide and intervention to prevent the act or limit the consequences. Health care providers, teachers, and counselors may recognize the signs of impending suicide or escalating aggression and should take immediate action. Such action might include counseling, referral, or hospitalization if the danger appears imminent. Population health nurses may also be involved in educating individuals who work with young people, the elderly, and others at risk for suicide to recognize indicators of a potential suicide attempt. Indications of suicide risk are summarized in the *Focused Assessment* on the next page. Foci and strategies for resolving existing problems of violence at individual/family and population levels are summarized in Table 30-5●.

HEALTH RESTORATION IN SOCIETAL VIOLENCE. Health restoration in the context of societal violence involves dealing with the consequences of violence and preventing its recurrence. Interventions intended for the individual or family level include providing treatment for long-term physical or psychological effects of violence. For example, victims of IPV may need a referral for treatment of PTSD, or children who witness or experience abuse can be referred for counseling. Victims of abuse may also need assistance in finding coping strategies as alternatives to subsequent alcohol and drug abuse or high-risk sexual behaviors. Similarly, the loved ones of suicide or homicide victims may need assistance in dealing with their loss. Assistance needed may range from counseling to cope with the loss of a loved one to help with concrete tasks like planning a funeral, filing claims for death benefits, settling the victim's estate, and dealing with the criminal justice sys-

TABLE 30-5 Individual/Family-Oriented and Population-Oriented Strategies to Address Existing Problems of Societal Violence

Focus	Individual/Family-Oriented Strategies	Population-Oriented Strategies
Identification of persons at risk for or experiencing violence	• Engage in case finding. • Teach teachers and counselors to recognize signs of abuse or risk for violence. • Screen for evidence of abuse or potential for violence.	• Educate the public regarding risks and signs of violence victimization. • Develop screening programs for risk or experience of violence.
Provision of counseling for victims and perpetrators of violence	• Refer for counseling. • Provide emotional support to both victims and perpetrators.	• Advocate for available counseling services.
Provision of treatment for victims of violence	• Refer for necessary services.	• Engage in political activity and advocacy to assure availability of adequate treatment facilities.
Identification of episodes of violence	• Report instances of violence.	• Monitor trends in societal violence to identify problem areas.
Provision of safe environments	• Remove victims of abuse to safe environments. • Plan with victims to achieve a safe environment. • Refer to a shelter as needed. • Initiate involuntary commitment proceedings if the person is a clear danger to self or others.	• Advocate for available shelter or other resources for victims of violence.
Education of health care providers for effective response to incidents of violence	• Educate individual providers for sensitive and caring response to victims of violence and family members.	• Advocate for effective training regarding response to violence in health professions curricula.

FOCUSED ASSESSMENT Assessing Suicide Risk

- Is there a family history of suicide? Of other forms of violence?
- Do family or cultural views support suicide? Do cultural beliefs lead to stigma and unwillingness to seek help for depression or other problems?
- Does the client hold religious beliefs that would protect against suicide?
- Is there a history of prior suicide attempt(s) by the client or by significant others?
- Is there a history of mental illness? Is the client exhibiting current symptoms of mental illness? Has the client experienced barriers to obtaining mental health services?
- Is there a history of substance abuse by the client or significant others?
- Does the client exhibit impulsive or aggressive behavior?
- Has the client experienced a recent serious loss (particularly in the last 6 months)?
- Does the client have a chronic illness that is severely affecting his or her quality of life?
- Does the client exhibit signs of depression?
- Does the client express feelings of hopelessness or helplessness?
- Does the client talk about wanting to die or express the wish that he or she were dead?
- Does the client express feelings of being a burden to others?
- Does the client express feelings of isolation?
- Does the client display evidence of anxiety, irritability, or panic?
- Does the client fail to refer to future goals or activities?
- Does the client express frequent or persistent thoughts of suicide?
- Has the client developed a carefully thought-out plan for suicide?
- Has the client chosen a lethal method for suicide with reduced likelihood of rescue?
- Does the client have easy access to lethal methods of suicide?
- Is suicide planned for the near future?
- Does the client exhibit behavior designed to "put one's house in order" (e.g., making a will, giving away prized possessions)?
- Does the client engage in behavior that would be likely to result in death (e.g., provoking fights with others, hazardous driving)?
- Has there been extensive media attention to recent suicides?

tem. Another health restoration measure for suicide and homicide is control of media representations that promote copycat events.

Health restoration for family/partner violence also entails changing circumstances that promote violence. For example, the population health nurse may assist abusive parents to understand the needs and behavioral cues of their children or help caregivers of disabled children or elderly family members to find respite. Other potential health restoration strategies for elder maltreatment include providing alternatives to home care of the elderly and increasing community support services for persons who are caring for older family members.

Population health nurses may also be involved in the development of programs to assist the perpetrators of violence. For example, they may plan and implement anger management programs for people who see violence as a means of dealing with anger. They may also advocate for and assist in initiating treatment programs for abusers. Another approach involves parenting classes for abusive parents and referral to Parents Anonymous, a mutual-help group for parents who have a history of or are at risk for child abuse.

Nurses may also assist family members to improve coping and communication skills as well as to improve self-esteem. This is particularly important for victims of child abuse if the intergenerational cycle of abusive behavior is to be broken. This may involve identifying past family interaction patterns, needed changes in those patterns, and mechanisms to achieve those changes. Table 30-6● summarizes areas of focus and related strategies in the context of societal violence.

Evaluating Control Strategies for Societal Violence

The effectiveness of control strategies for societal violence can be evaluated at the level of the individual client or family or at the population level. For example, the nurse might determine whether or not child abuse has been prevented in a family at high risk for abuse, or whether subsequent instances of abuse have been experienced by an older client or pregnant woman. At the population level, the population health nurse might look for changes in suicide or homicide rates or the frequency of reports to child protective services to evaluate the effectiveness of population-based interventions. As noted earlier, there is a great need for nursing research to examine the effectiveness of interventions to address societal violence. For example, nurses might study the effects of school curricula on culturally prescribed gender roles and their influence on IPV. Or they might contribute to the body of knowledge on the effectiveness of screening for suicide risk in decreasing the incidence of suicide in the elderly.

In assessing the effectiveness of strategies to reduce societal violence, population health nurses and others might evaluate the extent to which national objectives related to violence and suicide have been achieved. Baseline and target information for selected objectives are presented on the next page.

TABLE 30-6 Individual/Family-Oriented and Population-Oriented Foci and Strategies Related to Health Restoration in Societal Violence

Focus	Individual/Family-Oriented Strategies	Population-Oriented Strategies
Prevention of suicide clusters and copycat murders		• Assist in the development of community response plans. • Advocate for control of media exposure to violence.
Provision of care to families of homicide and suicide victims	• Assist families to work through feelings of grief, anger, and guilt. • Assist families to find positive ways to cope with loss. • Refer for assistance with legal and other tasks as needed. • Refer for counseling as needed.	• Advocate for support services for families of victims.
Treatment of consequences of violence	• Refer for physical and psychological treatment services as needed.	• Advocate for available services for victims and perpetrators of violence.
Reduction of sources of stress to prevent recurrence of violence	• Refer to sources of assistance. • Develop or expand social support networks. • Arrange for respite care as needed. • Assist with employment and other social needs.	• Advocate for social changes to minimize sources of stress contributing to violence. • Advocate for development of respite care and other support services.

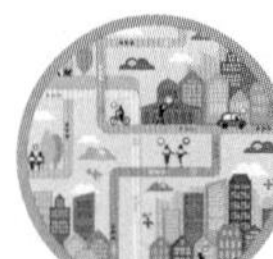

Healthy People 2020

Selected Objectives Related to Societal Violence

OBJECTIVE	BASELINE (YEAR)	TARGET	CURRENT DATA (YEAR)	DATA SOURCES
IVP-29. Reduce homicide deaths (per 100,000 population)	6.1 (2007)	5.5	5.3* (2010)	National Vital Statistics System—Mortality (NVSS-M), CDC/NCHS
IVP-33. Reduce physical assaults (per 1,000 population 12 years and older)	21.3 (2008)	19.2	19.4 (2011)	National Crime Victimization Survey (NCVS), DOJ/BJS
IVP-36. Reduce weapon carrying by adolescents on school property	5.6% (2009)	4.6%	5.4% (2011)	Youth Behavior Risk Surveillance System (YRBSS), CDC/NCHHSTP
IVP-37. Reduce child maltreatment deaths (per 100,000 children)	2.3 (2008)	2.1	2.1* (2011)	National Child Abuse and Neglect Data System (NCANDS), ACF
IVP-38. Reduce nonfatal child maltreatment (per 1,000 children)	9.4 (2008)	8.5	9.1 (2011)	NCANDS, ACF
IVP-41. Reduce nonfatal intentional self-harm requiring medical attention (ED visits per 100,000 population)	125.3 (2008)	112.8	153.0 (2010)	National Electronic Injury Surveillance System—All Injury Program (NEISS-AIP), CDC/NCIPC and CPSC
IVP-42. Reduce children's exposure to violence	58.8% (2008)	52.9%	56.5% (2011)	National Survey on Children's Exposure to Violence (NatSCEV), DOJ/OJJDP
MHMD-1. Reduce the suicide rate (per 100,000 population)	11.3 (2007)	10.2	12.1 (2011)	NVSS-M, CDC/NCHS
MHMD-2. Reduce suicide attempts by adolescents (per 100 population)	1.9 (2009)	1.7	2.4 (2011)	YRBSS, CDC/NCHHSTP

* Objective has met target.

Data from: U.S. Department of Health and Human Services. (2014). *Healthy people 2020: Topics and objectives.* Retrieved from http://healthypeople.gov/2020/topicsobjectives2020/default.aspx

CHAPTER RECAP

Societal violence occurs in many forms including self-directed violence, family/partner violence, and community violence. Collective violence by one social group against another may also occur, but is less amenable to intervention by population health nurses than the forms of violence presented in this chapter.

Factors related to each of the six categories of determinants of health influence the development of problems related to societal violence. In some instances factors related to some determinants of health may be protective against violence (e.g., street efficacy and family or community cohesion). Control strategies related to societal violence may include health promotion and specific prevention strategies as well as strategies for resolving existing problems related to violence and health restoration after violence has occurred.

CASE STUDY Preventing Dating Violence

You are a population health nurse assigned to an adolescent clinic. Part of your responsibility in the clinic is to conduct intake interviews for girls who come to the clinic requesting pregnancy tests. In the last several months, you have identified several girls who indicate that they became pregnant as result of sexual activity in which they were verbally coerced by their boyfriends despite not really wanting to engage in sex. Subsequent focus group interviews with adolescent girls at the local public high school indicated that many girls engage in sex because they are afraid they will lose their boyfriends or because boyfriends have specifically indicated they will end the relationship unless the girls "put out." In addition, several of the girls reported incidents of parties at which girls who had had too much to drink were subjected to unwanted sexual activity. In a few cases, boys had been heard joking about purposely getting their girlfriends drunk to decrease their inhibitions. A small minority of the girls reported being subjected to physical force when their boyfriends wanted to have sex.

None of the girls in the clinic or those in the focus group had reported the sexual coercion to their parents or school officials. In the case of parents, the girls were reluctant to admit to engaging in sexual activity. With respect to school officials, the girls felt they would not be listened to or would be perceived as bringing the problems on themselves by getting into compromising situations with their boyfriends. Most of the girls were also afraid their parents might forbid them to see their boyfriends if they knew about the situation. In addition, they reported not wanting to get their boyfriends in trouble or make them angry.

1. What biological, psychological, environmental, sociocultural, behavioral, and health system factors are contributing to the problem?
2. What interventions might be appropriate for addressing the problem?
3. Who might you collaborate with in resolving the problem?
4. How would you evaluate the effectiveness of your interventions?

REFERENCES

Acierno, R., Hernandez-Tejada, M., Muzzy, W., & Steve, K. (2009). *National elder mistreatment study.* Retrieved from https://www.ncjrs.gov/pdffiles1/nij/grants/226456.pdf

Administration for Children and Families. (2012). *Child maltreatment 2012.* Retrieved from http://www.acf.hhs.gov/sites/default/files/cb/cm2012.pdf

American Foundation for Suicide Prevention. (2014). *Facts and figures.* Retrieved from http://www.afsp.org/understanding-suicide/facts-and-figures

Basile, K. C., & Smith, S. G. (2011). Sexual violence victimization of women: Prevalence, characteristics, and the role of public health and prevention. *American Journal of Lifestyle Medicine, 5,* 407–417. doi:10.1177/1559827611409512

Begay, C. (2011). Women's shelter in a rural American Indian community. *Family & Community Health, 34,* 229–234. doi:10.1097/FCH.0b013e318296039

Black, M. C., Basile, K. C., Breiding, M. J., Smith, S. G., Walters, M. L., M. T. Merrick, . . . Stevens, M. R. (2011). *The National Intimate Partner and Sexual Violence Survey (NISVS): 2010 summary report.* Retrieved from http://www.cdc.gov/ViolencePrevention/pdf/NISVS_Report2010-a.pdf

Bolton, J. M., & Robinson, J. (2010). Population-attributable fractions of axis I and axis II mental disorders for suicide attempts: Findings from a representative sample of the adult, noninstitutionalized US population. *American Journal of Public Health, 100,* 2473–2480. doi:10.2105/AJPH.2010.192262

Bureau of Justice Statistics. (2013). *Assault.* Retrieved from http://www.bjs.gov/index.cfm?ty=tp&tid=316

Caldwell, H. K., Gilden, G., & Mueller, M. (2013). Elder abuse screening instruments in primary care: An integrative review, 2004 to 2011. *Clinical Geriatrics, 21*(1). no page.

California Courts. (n.d.). *Domestic violence.* Retrieved from http://www.courts.ca.gov/selfhelp-domesticviolence.htm

California Department of Justice. (n.d.). *What is human trafficking?* Retrieved from http://oag.ca.gov/human-trafficking/what-is

Centers for Disease Control and Prevention. (2013). *CDC helps prevent global violence.* Retrieved from http://www.cdc.gov/ViolencePrevention/globalviolence/index.html?s_cid=fb_vv445

Child Welfare Information Gateway. (2013). *What is child abuse and neglect? Recognizing the signs and symptoms.* Retrieved from https://www.childwelfare.gov/pubs/factsheets/whatiscan.pdf#page=3&view=What Are the Major Types of Child Abuse and Neglect?

Choi, K.-H., Paul, J., Ayala, G., Boylan, R., & Gregorich, S. E. (2013). Experiences of discrimination and their impact on the mental health among African American,

Asian and Pacific Islander, and Latino men who have sex with men. *American Journal of Public Health, 103,* 868–874. doi:10.2105/AJPH.2012.301052

Clayton, E. W., Krugman, R. D., & Simon, P. (Eds.). (2013). *Confronting commercial sexual exploitation and sex trafficking of minors in the United States.* Retrieved from http://www.nap.edu/download.php?record_id=18358

Cochran, J., Gelman, P. L., Ellis, H., Brown, C., Anderton, S., Montour, J., . . . Ao. (2013). Suicide and suicidal ideation among Bhutanese refugees—United States, 2009–2012. *Morbidity and Mortality Weekly Report, 62,* 533–536.

Community Preventive Services Task Force. (2014). *The community guide.* Retrieved from http://www.thecommunityguide.org/about/conclusionreport.html

Conner, K. R., Huguet, N., Caetano, R., Giesbrecht, N., McFarland, B. H., Nolte, K. B., et al. (2014). Acute use of alcohol and methods of suicide in a US national sample. *American Journal of Public Health, 104,* 171–178. doi:10.2105/AJPH.2013.301352

Crane, C. A., Hawes, S. W., & Weinberger, A. H. (2013). Intimate partner violence victimization and cigarette smoking: A meta-analytic review. *Trauma, Violence, & Abuse, 14,* 305–315. doi: 10.1177/1524838013495962

Criminal Justice Information Systems Division. (2013a). *2012 Hate crime statistics: Incidents and offenses.* Retrieved from http://www.fbi.gov/about-us/cjis/ucr/hate-crime/2012/topic-pages/incidents-and-offenses/incidentsandoffenses_final

Criminal Justice Information Systems Division. (2013b). *Incidents, offenses, victims, and known offenders by offense category, 2012.* Retrieved from http://www.fbi.gov/about-us/cjis/ucr/nibrs/2012

Crosby, A. E., Han, B., Ortega, L. A., Parks, S. E., & Gfroerer, J. (2011). Suicidal thoughts and behaviors among adults aged > 18 years—United States, 2008–2009. *Morbidity and Mortality Weekly Report, 60*(SS-13), 1–22.

Degutis, L. C. (2013). Epidemiology of violence. In R. M. Hammer, B. Moynihan, & E. M. Pagliaro (Eds.), *Forensic nursing: A handbook for practice* (2nd ed., pp. 31–44). Burlington, MA: Jones & Bartlett Learning.

Demirçin, S., Akkoyun, M., Yilmaz, R., & Gökdoğan, M. R. (2011). Suicide of elderly persons: Towards a framework for prevention. *Geriatrics & Gerontology International, 11,* 107–113. doi:10.1111/j.1447-0594.2010.00660.x

Department of Justice. (2013). *Family violence.* Retrieved from http://www.justice.gc.ca/eng/cj-jp/fv-vf

Division of Violence Prevention. (2011). *National Intimate Partner and Sexual Violence Survey, 2010 summary report.* Retrieved from http://www.cdc.gov/violenceprevention/pdf/nisvs_report2010-a.pdf

Division of Violence Prevention. (2014). *Cost of child abuse and neglect rivals other public health problems.* Retrieved from http://www.cdc.gov/violenceprevention/childmaltreatment/economiccost.html

Durborow, N., Lizdas, K. C., O'Flaherty, A., & Marjavi, A. (2013). *Compendium of state and U.S. territory statutes and policies on domestic violence and health care.* Retrieved from http://www.futureswithoutviolence.org/userfiles/file/HealthCare/Compendium%20Final%202013.pdf

Dworkin, S. L., Dunbar, M. S., Krishnan, S., Hatcher, A. M., & Sawires, S. (2011). Uncovering tensions and capitalizing on synergies in HIV/AIDS and antiviolence programs. *American Journal of Public Health, 101,* 995–1003. doi:10.2105/AJPH.2009.191106

Family Law Courts. (n.d.). *What is family violence?* Retrieved from http://www.familylawcourts.gov.au/wps/wcm/connect/FLC/Home/Family+Violence/What+is+family+violence/

Federal Bureau of Investigation. (2013). *January to June, 2012–2013 percent change by population group.* Retrieved from http://www.fbi.gov/about-us/cjis/ucr/crime-in-the-u.s/2013/preliminary-semiannual-uniform-crime-report-january-june-2013/tables/table_1_january_to_june_2012-2013_percent_change_by_population_group.xls

Friends of Youth. (n.d.). *What is therapeutic foster care?* Retrieved from http://www.friendsofyouth.org/whatistfc.aspx

Gellert, G. A. (2010). *Confronting violence: Answers to questions about the epidemic destroying America's homes and communities* (3rd ed.). Washington, DC: APHA Press.

Gibson, C. L., Fagan, A. A., & Antle, K. (2014). Avoiding violent victimization among youths in urban neighborhoods: The importance of street efficacy. *American Journal of Public Health, 104,* e-154–e161. doi:10.2105/AJPH.2013.301571

Haegerich, T. M., & Dahlberg, L. L. (2011). Violence as a public health risk. *American Journal of Lifestyle Medicine, 6,* 392–403. doi:10.1177/1559827611409127

Harrison, L., & Vega, C. P. (2014). *Fractures in children: Identifying abuse.* Retrieved from http://www.medscape.org/viewarticle/818580?src=cmemp.

Hatzenbuehler, M. L., Birkett, M., Van Wagenen, A., & Meyer, L. H. (2014). Protective school climates and reduced risk for suicide ideation in sexual minority youths. *American Journal of Public Health, 104,* 279–286. doi:10.2105/AJPH.2013.301508

Herek, G. M., & Sims, C. (2008). Sexual orientation and violent victimization: Hate crimes and intimate partner violence among gay and bisexual males in the United States. In R. J. Wolitski, R. Stall, & R. O. Valeiserri (Eds.), *Unequal opportunity: Health disparities affecting gay and bisexual men in the United States* (pp. 35–71). New York: Oxford University Press.

Hossain, M., Zimmerman, C., Abas, M., Light, M., & Watts, C. (2010). The relationship of trauma to mental disorders among trafficked and sexually exploited girls and women. *American Journal of Public Health, 100,* 2442–2449. doi:10.2105/AJPH.2009.173229

International Association of Forensic Nurses & American Nurses Association. (2009). *Forensic nursing: Scope and standards of practice.* Silver Spring, MD: American Nurses Association.

Kegler, S. R., Annest, J. L., Kresnow, M.-J., & Mercy, J. A. (2011). Violence-related firearm deaths among residents of metropolitan areas and cities—United States, 2006–2007. *Morbidity and Mortality Weekly Report, 60,* 573–578.

Kegler, S. R., & Mercy, J. A. (2013). Firearms homicides and suicides in major metropolitan areas—United States, 2009–2010. *Morbidity and Mortality Weekly Report, 62,* 597–602.

Kimerling, R., Street, A. E., Pavao, J., Smith, M. W., Cronkite, R. C., Holmes, T. H., & Frayne, S. M. (2010). Military-related sexual trauma among Veterans Health Administration patients returning from Afghanistan and Iraq. *American Journal of Public Health, 100,* 1409–1412. doi:10.2105/AJPH.2009.171793

Knox, K. L., Pflanz, S., Talcott, G. W., Campise, R. L., Lavigne, J. E., Bajorska, A., . . . Caine, E. D. (2010). The US Air Force Suicide Prevention Program: Implications for public health policy. *American Journal of Public Health, 100,* 2457–2463. doi:10.2105/AJPH.2009.159871

Kraanen, F. L., Vedel, E., Scholing, A., & Emmelkamp, P. M. G. (2013). The comparative effectiveness of integrated treatment for substance abuse and partner violence (I-StoP) and substance abuse treatment alone: A randomized controlled trial. *BMJ Psychiatry, 13,* 189. Retrieved, from http://www.biomedicalcentral.com/1471-244X/13/189

Mayo Clinic Staff. (2012). *Self injury/cutting.* Retrieved from http://www.mayoclinic.org/diseases-conditions/self-injury/basics/definition/con-20025897

Mbillinyi, L. F., Neighbors, C., Walker, D. D., Roffman, R. A., Zegree, J., Edelson, J., et al. (2011). A telephone intervention for substance-using adult male perpetrators of intimate partner violence. *Research on Social Work Practice, 21*(1), 41–56. doi:10.1177/1049731509359008

McNew, J. L., Bigouard, S. G., Welles, W. L., Wilburn, R., Anderson, A. R., Orr, M. F., et al. (2011). Chemical suicides in automobiles—Six states, 2006–2010. *Morbidity and Mortality Weekly Report, 60,* 1189–1192.

Moyer, V. A. (2013). Screening for intimate partner violence and abuse of elderly and vulnerable adults: U.S. Preventive Services Task Force recommendation statement. *Annals of Internal Medicine, 158,* 478–486.

Moynihan, B., & Gaboury, M. T. (2013). Hidden in plain sight: Modern-day slavery and the rise of human trafficking. In R. M. Hammer, B. Moynihan, & E. M. Pagliaro (Eds.), *Forensic nursing: A handbook for practice* (2nd ed., pp. 331–348). Burlington, MA: Jones & Bartlett Learning.

Myers, J. E. B. (2008). A short history of child protection in America. *Family Law Quarterly, 42,* 449–463.

National Center for Health Statistics. (2012). Age-adjusted homicide rates, by sex and type of locality—United States, 2007–2009. *Morbidity and Mortality Weekly Report, 61,* 422.

National Center for Health Statistics. (2013a). Annual age-adjusted death rates for suicide and homicide by black or white race—United States, 1999–2010. *Morbidity and Mortality Weekly Report, 62,* 257.

National Center for Health Statistics. (2013b). Average annual rate of emergency department visits for assault among persons aged < 18 years, by age group and race/ethnicity—United States, 2005–2010. *Morbidity and Mortality Weekly Report, 62,* 319.

National Center for Health Statistics. (2014). *Health, United States, 2013: With special feature prescription drugs.* Retrieved from http://www.cdc.gov/nchs/data/hus/hus13.pdf

National Center for Injury Prevention and Control. (2012). *Understanding youth violence: Fact sheet.* Retrieved from http://www.cdc.gov/ViolencePrevention/pdf/YV-FactSheet-a.pdf

National Center for Injury Prevention and Control. (2013a). *Definitions: Self-directed violence.* Retrieved from http://www.cdc.gov/ViolencePrevention/suicide/definitions.html

National Center for Injury Prevention and Control. (2013b). *Intimate partner violence: Consequences.* Retrieved from http://www.cdc.gov/Violence-Prevention/intimatepartnerviolence/consequences.html

National Center for Injury Prevention and Control. (2013c). *Intimate partner violence: Definitions.* Retrieved from http://www.cdc.gov/Violence-Prevention/intimatepartnerviolence/definitions.html

National Center for Injury Prevention and Control. (2013d). *Intimate partner violence: Risk and protection.* Retrieved from http://www.cdc.gov/Violence-Prevention/intimatepartnerviolence/riskprotectivefactors.html

National Center for Injury Prevention and Control. (2013e). *Saving lives and protecting people from violence and injuries.* Retrieved from http://www.cdc.gov/injury/overview/index.html

National Center for Injury Prevention and Control. (2013f). *Suicide: Consequences.* Retrieved from http://www.cdc.gov/ViolencePrevention/suicide/consequences.html

National Center for Injury Prevention and Control. (2013g). *Suicide: Risk and protective factors.* Retrieved from http://www.cdc.gov/ViolencePrevention/suicide/riskprotectivefactors.html

National Center for Injury Prevention and Control. (2013h). *Understanding elder abuse: Fact sheet.* Retrieved from http://www.cdc.gov/violence-prevention/pdf/EM-FactSheet-a.pdf

National Center for Injury Prevention and Control. (2014a). *Child maltreatment: Definitions.* Retrieved from http://www.cdc.gov/ViolencePrevention/childmaltreatment/definitions.html

National Center for Injury Prevention and Control. (2014b). *Child maltreatment prevention.* Retrieved from http://www.cdc.gov/ViolencePrevention/childmaltreatment/index.html

National Center for Injury Prevention and Control. (2014c). *Child maltreatment: Prevention strategies.* Retrieved from http://www.cdc.gov/ViolencePrevention/childmaltreatment/prevention.html

National Center for Injury Prevention and Control. (2014d). *Elder abuse: Definitions.* Retrieved from http://www.cdc.gov/violenceprevention/elderabuse/definitions.html

National Center for Injury Prevention and Control. (2014e). *Elder abuse: Risk and protective factors.* Retrieved from http://www.cdc.gov/violence-prevention/elderabuse/riskprotectivefactors.html

National Center for Victims of Crime. (2013). *Elder victimization.* Retrieved from http://www.victimsofcrime.org/docs/ncvrw2013/2013ncvrw_stats_elder.pdf?sfvrsn=0

National Center on Elder Abuse. (n.d.). *Statistics/data.* Retrieved from http://www.ncea.aoa.gov/Library/Data/index.aspx#problem

National Center on Shaken Baby Syndrome. (n.d.). *General SBS/AHT statistics.* Retrieved from http://dontshake.org/sbs.php?opNavID=3&subNavID=27

National Coalition for the Homeless. (2012). *Domestic violence and homelessness.* Retrieved from http://www.nationalhomeless.org/factsheets/domestic.html

National Council on Alcoholism and Drug Dependence. (n.d.a). *Alcohol and crime.* Retrieved from http://www.ncadd.org/images/stories/PDF/factsheet-alcoholandcrime.pdf

National Council on Alcoholism and Drug Dependence. (n.d.b). *Alcohol and crime.* Retrieved from http://www.ncadd.org/index.php/learn-about-alcohol/alcohol-and-crime/202-alcohol-and-crime

National Institute of Justice. (2011). *Protection orders may reduce intimate partner (domestic) violence.* Retrieved from http://www.nij.gov/topics/crime/intimate-partner-violence/interventions/pages/protection-orders.aspx

National Institute of Neurological Disorders and Stroke. (2014). *NINDS shaken baby syndrome information page.* Retrieved from http://www.ninds.nih.gov/disorders/shakenbaby/shakenbaby.htm

National Prevention Council. (2011). *National prevention strategy.* Retrieved from http://www.surgeongeneral.gov/initiatives/prevention/strategy/report.pdf

Nelson, H. D., Bougatsos, C., & Blazina, I. (2012). Screening of women for intimate partner violence: A systematic review to update the 2004 U.S. Preventive Services Task Force recommendation. *Annals of Internal Medicine, 156,* 796–808.

New York Society for the Prevention of Cruelty to Children. (2000). *History.* Retrieved from http://www.nyspcc.org/nyspcc/history/attachment:en-us.pdf

Newman, S., Akre, E., Bossarte, R., Mack, K., & Crosby, A. (2010). Suicides in National Parks—United States, 2003–2009. *Morbidity and Mortality Weekly Report, 59,* 1546–1549.

Northern Virginia Family Services. (2014). *About therapeutic foster care.* Retrieved from https://www.nvfs.org/fostercare

Office of Refugee Resettlement. (2012). *What is human trafficking?* Retrieved from http://www.acf.hhs.gov/programs/orr/resource/about-human-trafficking

Oklahoma Department of Health Services. (2014). *Therapeutic foster care.* Retrieved from http://www.okdhs.org/programsandservices/tfc

Papachristos, A. V., & Wildeman, C. (2014). Network exposure and homicide victimization in an African American community. *American Journal of Public Health, 104,* 143–150. doi:10.2105/AJPH.2013.301441

Parks, S. E., Johnson, L. L., McDaniel, D. D., & Gladden, M. (2014). Surveillance for violent deaths: National Violent Death Reporting System, 16 states, 2010. *Morbidity and Mortality Weekly Report, 63*(SS-1), 1–33.

Perou, R., Bitsko, R. H., Blumberg, S. J., Pastor, P., Ghandour, R. M., Gfroerer, J. C., . . . Huang, L. N. (2013, May 17). Mental health surveillance among children—United States, 2005–2011. *Morbidity and Mortality Weekly Report, 62*(Suppl.), 1–35.

Perron, S., Burrows, S., Fournier, M., Perron, P. A., & Ouellet, F. (2013). Installation of a bridge barrier as a suicide prevention strategy in Montreal, Quebec, Canada. *American Journal of Public Health, 103,* 1235–1239. doi:10.2105/AJPH.2012.301089

Peterman, A., Palermo, T., & Bredenkamp, C. (2011). Estimates and determinants of sexual violence against women in the Democratic Republic of Congo. *American Journal of Public Health, 101,* 1060–1067. doi:10.2105/AJPH.2010.300070

Richardson, J. B., Brown, J., & Van Brakle, M. (2013). Pathways to early violent death: The voices of serious violent youth offenders. *American Journal of Public Health, 103,* e1–e12. doi:10.2105/AJPH.2012.301160

Robers, S., Kemp, J., Truman, J., & Snyder, T. D. (2013). *Indicators of school crime and safety: 2012.* Retrieved from http://www.bjs.gov/content/pub/pdf/iscs12.pdf

Rockett, I. R. H., Regier, M. D., Kapusta, N. D., Coben, J. H., Miller, T. R., Hanzlick, R. L., . . . Smith, G. S. (2012). Leading causes of unintentional and intentional mortality: United States, 2000–2009. *American Journal of Public Health, 102,* e84–e92. doi:10.2105/AJPH.2012.300960

Saftlis, A. F., Wallis, A. B., Shochet, T., Harland, K., K., Dickey, P., & Peek-Asa, C. (2010). Prevalence of intimate partner violence among an abortion clinic population. *American Journal of Public Health, 100,* 1412–1415. doi:10.2105/AJPH.2009.178947

Sharkey, P. T., Tirado-Strayer, N., Papachristos, A. V., & Raver, C. C. (2012). The effect of local violence on children's attention and impulse control. *American Journal of Public Health, 102,* 2287–2293. doi:10.2105/AJPH.2012.300789

Sheridan, D. J., Nash, C. R., Hawkins, S. L., Makely, J. L., & Campbell, J. C. (2013). Forensic implications of intimate partner violence. In R. M. Hammer, B. Moynihan, & E. M. Pagliaro (Eds.), *Forensic nursing: A handbook for practice* (2nd ed., pp. 129–143). Burlington, MA: Jones & Bartlett Learning.

Siegel, M., Ross, C. S., & King, C., III. (2013). The relationship between gun ownership and firearm homicide rates in the United States, 1981–2010. *American Journal of Public Health, 103,* 2098–2105. doi:10.2105/AJPH.2013.301409

Silverman, J. G., Decker, M. R., McCauley, H. L., Gupta, J., Miller, E., Raj, A., et al. (2010). Male perpetration of intimate partner violence and involvement in abortions and abortion-related conflict. *American Journal of Public Health, 100,* 1415–1417. doi:10.2105/AJPH.2009.17339

Spivak, H. R., Jenkins, E. L., VanAudenhove, K., Lee, D., Kelly, M., & Iskander, J. (2014). CDC grand rounds: A public health approach to prevention of intimate partner violence. *Morbidity and Mortality Weekly Report, 63,* 38–41.

Stalking Resource Center. (2012). *Stalking fact sheet.* Retrieved from http://www.victimsofcrime.org/docs/src/stalking-fact-sheet_english.pdf?sfvrsn=4

Strengthen Our Sisters. (n.d.). *Understanding the cycle of battering.* Retrieved from http://www.strengthenoursisters.org/understanding_abuse_cycle.html

Sullivan, E. M., Annest, J. L., Luo, F., Simon, T. R., & Dahlberg, L. L. (2013). Suicide among adults aged 35–64 years—United States, 1999–2010. *Morbidity and Mortality Weekly Report, 62,* 321–325.

U.S. Census Bureau. (2013a). Table 311. Murder victims by age, sex, and race: 2008. In *The 2012 statistical abstract: The national data book, Law enforcement, courts and prisons.* Retrieved from http://www.census.gov/compendia/statab/cats/law_enforcement_courts_prisons.html

U.S. Census Bureau. (2013b). Table 342. Child abuse and neglect victims by selected characteristics: 2000–2009. In *The 2012 statistical abstract: The national data book, Law enforcement, courts and prisons.* Retrieved from http://www.census.gov/compendia/statab/cats/law_enforcement_courts_prisons.html

U.S. Department of Health and Human Services. (2014). *Healthy people 2020: Topics and objectives.* Retrieved from http://healthypeople.gov/2020/topicsobjectives2020/default.aspx

U.S. Department of Justice. (2013). *Domestic violence.* Retrieved from http://www.ovw.usdoj.gov/domviolence.htm

Violence Prevention Alliance. (2012). *Global campaign for violence prevention: Plan of action for 2012–2020.* Retrieved from http://www.who.int/violence_injury_prevention/violence/global_campaign/gcvp_plan_of_action.pdf?ua=1

Violence Prevention Alliance. (2014). *Definition and typology of violence.* Retrieved from http://www.who.int/violenceprevention/approach/definition/en/

Warshaw, C., Sullivan, C. M., & Rivera, E. A. (2013). *A systematic review of trauma-focused interventions for domestic violence survivors.* Retrieved from http://www.nationalcenterdvtraumamh.org/wp-content/uploads/2013/03/NCDVTMH_EBPLitReview2013.pdf

Wintemute, G. J., Frattaroli, S., Claire, B. E., Vittes, K., & Webster, D. W. (2014). Identifying armed respondents to domestic violence restraining orders and recovering their firearms: Process evaluation of an initiative in California. *American Journal of Public Health, 104,* e113–e118. doi:10.2105/AJPH.2013.301484

Women against Domestic Violence. (n.d.). *What is battering?* Retrieved from http://wadv.org/battering.htm

World Health Organization. (2014a). *10 facts about violence prevention.* Retrieved from http://www.who.int/features/factfiles/violence/en/

World Health Organization. (2014b). *Female genital mutilation.* Retrieved from http://www.who.int/mediacentre/factsheets/fs241/en/

Youth Suicide Prevention Program. (n.d.). *Youth suicide prevention.* Retrieved from http://www.yspp.org/

Index

A

D

H

I

J

K

L

O

S

U

V

W

X

Y

Z